TRADITIONAL CHINESE MEDICINES

Molecular Structures, Natural Sources, and Applications

TRADITIONAL CHINESE MEDICINES

Molecular Structures, Natural Sources, and Applications

Compiled by

X Yan, J Zhou and G Xie

Edited by

G W A Milne

Ashgate

Published by
Ashgate Publishing Limited
Gower House
Croft Road
Aldershot
Hampshire GU11 3HR
England

Ashgate Publishing Company
Old Post Road
Brookfield
Vermont 05036
USA

British Library Cataloguing in Publication Data
Traditional Chinese Medicines : molecular structures,
natural sources, and applications
1. Medicine, Chinese 2. Traditional medicine - China
I. Yan, X. II. Zhou, J. III. Milne, G. W. A. (George William
Anthony), 1937-
610.9'51

ISBN 0 566 08210 1

Library of Congress Cataloging-in-Publication Data
Yan, X. (Xinjian)
Traditional Chinese Medicines : molecular structures, natural
sources, and applications / compiled by X. Yan, J. Zhou, and G. Xie
: edited by G.W.A. Milne.
p. cm.
ISBN 0-566-08210-1 (hbk.)
1. Materia medica, Vegetable. 2. Pharmaceutical chemistry.
3. Medicine, Chinese. I. Zhou, J. (Jiaju). II. Xie, G. (Guirong).
III. Milne, G. W. A. (George William Anthony), 1937- . IV. Title.
RS431.M37Y36 1999
615' .32'0951--dc21 99-39805
CIP

Printed in Great Britain by MPG Books Ltd, Bodmin.

CONTENTS

PREFACE

For many centuries, medical practice has developed in China along a path that is quite distinct from that adopted more recently in the West. Much of the experience gained in China predated twentieth-century chemistry and depended largely upon empirical observation. For medicinal agents the Chinese looked to other living systems, in particular plants and animals, vertebrate and invertebrate. Western medical science, while not neglecting plant sources, has placed a greater reliance upon synthetic chemicals, and the natural materials in the Chinese *materia medica* far outnumber those found in the European and American pharmacopeia.

Transfer to the West of the knowledge of traditional Chinese medicine has been hampered by several factors. The empirical nature of Chinese medicine, which relies more on botany than chemistry, has been a difficulty that is compounded by the language problem. Recent extensive advances in chemistry and biochemistry, both in the West and in China, have facilitated the use of chemistry as a basis for the description of materials used in Chinese medical practice. In the past, parts of specific plants were used in China to treat medical disorders and this is still true, particularly in the rural areas of the country. In thousands of cases, however, research has permitted the identification of the chemical compounds in the plants which are responsible for the medicinal effect. This book, *Traditional Chinese Medicines*, contains a database of all the chemicals that are known to be present in medicinally useful plants (or animals) and which are thought to be responsible for the medical effect of the species or its extracts.

This database will be invaluable to medicinal chemists in the West because it will enable them to bypass the botanical detail and immediately view chemical structures and their related biological activities. This database therefore contains enormously valuable feedstock for the currently fashionable field of structure-activity relationships. It certainly contains many new such relationships which should provide compelling rationale for new drug development efforts. Thus a synthesis of Chinese and Western medicinal chemistry may begin with the information that is presented here.

The compilers of *Traditional Chinese Medicines,* Xinjian Yan, Jiaju Zhou and Guirong Xie, are chemists who work at the Chinese Academy of Sciences in Beijing. Professor Yan, a graduate of Peking University, spent two years working in the National Cancer Institute of the National Institutes of Health in Bethesda, MD and one year at the University of Texas in Austin, TX, where he used techniques of molecular modeling to study the interactions at the molecular level between biologically active materials such as ricin and targets such as ribosomal RNA. He has long been interested in the functions of traditional Chinese drugs and has worked to build a bridge between traditional and modern medicine. Professor Zhou also graduated from Peking University in 1963 and has spent many years developing databases for use in chemistry. He has worked for extended periods at the University of British Columbia, Marseilles University and the US National Institute of Standards and Technology in Gaithersburg, MD where he worked in the design and implementation of chemical data systems. Currently he leads a team working in molecular design in the LCC. Professor Xie graduated from Shandong University in 1965 and has worked as an analytical chemist at the Chinese Academy of Sciences since then. She has worked on the establishment of standard methods at the US National Institute of Standards and Technology in

Gaithersburg, MD and since 1990 has worked in database design. These three scientists have brought their combined skills to the task of extracting and linking the published information on Chinese medicines so as to relate chemicals to their biological activities. The result is this book: *Traditional Chinese Medicines.*

G W A Milne
Brookfield, Vermont

ACKNOWLEDGMENTS

This work has been supported by the Laboratory of Computer Chemistry (LCC) of the Institute of Chemical Metallurgy, Chinese Academy of Sciences, Beijing.

We, the compilers, would like to express our gratitude to George W A Milne, who originally urged us to develop this book in 1996. He not only offered us much encouragement but has also spent much of his time editing the material as it was developed. We would also like to thank Kay Pool, Berry Carroll, Wucheng Tang, Pingan Liu and Li Yan for their editorial help. We are grateful to Professors Zhihong Xu, Zhhangyuan Yang and Hao Wen for their long-term support and guidance. Finally, we would like to give special thanks to our family members; without their total and never-ending support, this book would not have been completed.

Xinjian Yan
Jiaju Zhou
Guirong Xie
Beijing

EXPLANATORY NOTES

Structure and Contents

Traditional Chinese Medicines describes 6,808 chemical compounds that are found in the materials that are used for medicinal purposes in China.

The book is organized in three Parts. Part I presents the structure, molecular formula and molecular weight of 6,808 chemicals which have been identified in plants and animals. All are used in Chinese medical practice. Every entry gives the source of the chemical and the corresponding reference to the Chinese scientific literature where the identification of the chemical was first reported. Part II contains a listing of Chinese medicines, identified by their English name, and gives the source of the medicine, together with a description of its medicinal effects and its indications. Part III contains indexes of traditional Chinese medicines arranged by (1) (transliterated) Chinese Names, (2) English Names and (3) Latin Names. Finally, an index of the chemical names of the compounds in Part I is provided.

Part I

This Part contains the chemical information pertaining to the referenced compounds. Each entry contains the name of the chemical, its molecular formula and molecular weight, the medication containing the chemical and a reference to the appropriate scientific literature. A typical entry from Part I is shown below:

131 Aescigenin
$C_{30}H_{48}O_5$ MW: 488.71 Property: mp 307°C, 317-8°C.
Source: SUO LUO ZI. Ref: 6.

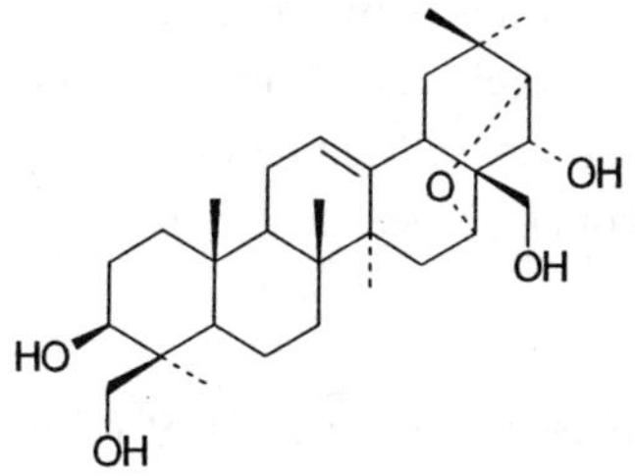

The chemical shown in this entry, Aescigenin, has molecular formula $C_{30}H_{48}O_5$, molecular weight 488.71 and two reported melting points, 307°C and 317-318°C. The origin of the compound is the seed (ZI)* of the plant SUO LUO, whose entry in the Index of Traditional Chinese Medicines by Chinese Name shows it to be the Chinese Buckeye Seed which is further described in Part II of the book. The publication reporting this information is cited as Reference 6, whose full citation will be found in the References section.

---

* See Structure of Traditional Chinese Medicine Names (p. xiii).

Part II

In Part II, all the plant-derived medications are listed alphabetically by their English name. The plant species from which the material is derived, as well as the part of the plant, are given. This Part contains 1,268 medicines, involving 1,548 distinct plant species.

Each entry in Part II describes a single medicinally significant plant, animal, or plant part in cases where different parts of a plant are associated with different medicinal effects. In thc case of materials derived from animal species, each derived medicinal material constitutes an entry. Thus the entry "cow-bezoar (ox-gallstone)" (p. 694) is presented as a single entry even though it originates in at least two species (*Bos taurus domesticus* Gmelin and *Bubalus bubalis* Linnaeus).

Each entry in Part II contains up to six items of information. As an example, the entry for the Chinese Buckeye Seed (SUO LUO ZI) is given below:

> **Chinese Buckeye Seed; SUO LUO ZI** Origin: *Aesculus chinensis* Bge. *(Hippocastanaceae).* Part: ripe fruit without shell. Effects: To rectify *qi*, relieve stuffiness and pain in the epigastrium. Indications: Oppression in the chest, rib-side pain, stomach pain abdominal distention due to liver stomach *qi* stagnation; premenstrual distention and pain of the breasts.

The entry begins with the name of the plant (Chinese Buckeye Seed). This is followed by the Chinese name (SUO LUO ZI) and the Latin name of the species of origin [*Aesculus chinensis* Bge. *(Hippocastanaceae)*]. The part of the plant is identified, and then the effects of the medicine followed by the indications, i.e. the symptoms which suggest its use.

Part III

Four indexes are presented. These are:

- Index of Traditional Chinese Medicines by Chinese Name
- Index of Traditional Chinese Medicines by English Name
- Index of Origin of Traditional Chinese Medicines
- Index of Chemicals in Traditional Chinese Medicines.

Note

Every attempt has been made to ensure the accuracy of the information given in this edition of *Traditional Chinese Medicines*. However, the publishers cannot be held responsible for the accuracy of the information and readers intending to use or suggest the use of of any of the medicines described in this book are encouraged, whenever possible, to consult the original publications that are cited.

Structure of Traditional Chinese Medicine Names

The Traditional Chinese Medicine (TCM) name is the primary identifier of medicines, and this book is organized around these names. The *Index of Traditional Chinese Medicines by Chinese Name* is based on the TCM name and can be used to look up information on any particular TCM.

All TCM names have been defined in the simplified Chinese phonetic alphabet (without the four tone marks) and are written in upper case throughout. The Greenish Lily, for example, can be found in Part II to have the TCM **BAI HE** and recourse with this TCM name to the Chinese Name Index reveals the Latin name of the plant as *Lilium brownii* F. E. Brown var. *colchesteri* Wils, of the family *Liliaceae.*

A TCM name, as expressed here, is organized in a set of upper case letter groups, with each group corresponding to a "square word" in Chinese. For some TCM names, particularly the longer ones, the last letter groups serve to identify the parts of the plant that are important as the source of the TCM. These commonly used letter groups are given below.

Letter Group	Meaning
GEN	root
JING	stem
ZHI	branch
YE	leaf
HUA	flower
GUO (or **ZI**)	fruit or nut
ZI	seed
PI	bark
BAI PI	bast (fiber)

Examples of this construction are given below.

TCM Name	English Name
TAO GEN	Peach root
TAO HUA	Peach flower
TAO JING BAI PI	Peach fiber (bast)
TAO YE	Peach leaf
TAO ZHI	Peach juvenile branch
BAI GUO	Ginkgo nut
BAI GUO GEN	Ginkgo root
BAI GUO SHU PI	Ginkgo bark

(Cont'd)

TCM Name	English Name
BAI GUO YE	Ginkgo leaf
GOU QI YE	Wolfberry leaf
GOU QI ZI	Wolfberry fruit
GOU QI GEN PI	Wolfberry root-bark
HEI DA DOU	Black soyabean
HEI DA DOU YE	Black soyabean leaf
HEI DA DOU PI	Black soyabean spermoderm
BI MA GEN	Castorbean root
BI MA YE	Castorbean leaf
BI MA ZI	Castorbean seed

The first letter groups in TCM names are often modifiers. Thus, as shown below, DA YE means largeleaf, DA HUA, largeflower. YUN NAN (the Chinese province), AN HUI, TIAN SHAN and MENG GU are geographic terms.

TCM Name	English Name
DA YE CHAI HU	Bigleaf Thorowax
DA YE GOU TENG	Largeleaf Gamirplant
DA YE HOU PU	Bigleaf Magnolia
DA YE XIANG CHA CAI	Largeleaf Rabdosia
DA YE ZI ZHU	Bigleaf Beautyberry
YUN NAN BA JIAO	Yunnan Anisetree
YUN NAN GAN CAO	Yunnan licorice
YUN NAN HONG DOU SHAN	Yunnan Yew
AN HUI BEI MU	Anhwei Fritillary
TIAN SHAN DA HUANG	Tianshan Rhubarb
MENG GU LI	Mongolian Oak
DA HUA HONG JING TIAN	Bigflower Rhodiola

Thus, in the TCM name **HEI DA DOU PI** (black soyabean spermoderm), **HEI** is "black" in Chinese, **DA DOU** means soyabean and **PI** identifies the part of the plant (the bark or spermoderm).

Many TCMs have more than one plant source. **HOU PO**, for example, is found in two plant species (*Magnolia officinalis* and *M. biloba*). **DA HUANG** is derived from three species, **BAI HE** from four, **QING YE** from five, and so on. Some details of these examples are given opposite.

TCM Name	English Name	Origin(s)	Family
HOU PO	Officinal Magnolia	*Magnolia officinalis*	*Magnoliaceae* Rehd. *et* Wils
	Two-lobed Officinal Magnolia	*Magnolia biloba*	*Magnoliaceae* (Rehd *et* Wils.)
DA HUANG	Medicinal Rhubarb	*Rheum officinale* Baill.	*Polygonaceae*
	Sorrel Rhubarb	*Rheum palmatum* L.	*Polygonaceae*
	Tangut Rhubarb	*Rheum tanguticum* Maxim. *ex* Balf.	*Polygonaceae*
DA QING YE	Common Baphicacanthus Leaf	*Baphicacanthus cusia* (Nees) Bremek	*Acanthaceae*
	Dyers Woad Leaf	*Isatis tinctoria* L.	*Cruciferae*
	Indigo-colored Woad Leaf	*Isatis indigotica* Fort.	*Cruciferae*
	Indigoplant Leaf	*Polygonum tinctorium* Ait	*Polygonaceae*
	Manyflower Glorybower Leaf	*Clerodendron cyrtophyllum* Turcz	*Verbenaceae*
GUAN ZHONG	Brainea	*Brainea insignis*(Hook.) J. Sm.	*Blechnaceae*
	Japanese Chain Fern	*Woodwardia japonica* (L. F.) Sm.	*Blechnaceae*
	Japanese Osmunda Fern	*Osmunda Japonica* thumb.	*Osmundaceae*
	Lunathyrium Fern	*Lunathyrium acrostichoides* (Sw.) Ching	*Athyriaceae*
	Male Fern Rhizome	*Dryopteris crassirhizoma* Nakai	*Dryopteridaceae*
	Matteuccia Fern	*Matteuccia struthiopteris* (L.) Todaro	*Onocleaceae*
	Oriental Blechnum Frond	*Blechnum orientale* L.	*Blechnaceae*
CHUAN BEI *See*:			
JUAN YE BEI MU		*Fritillaria cirrhosa* D. Don	*Liliaceae*
WU HUA BEI MU		*F. cirrhosa* D. Don var. ecirrhosa Franch.	*Liliaceae*
LENG SHA BEI MU		*Fritillaria delavayi* Franch.	*Liliaceae*
AN ZI BEI MU		*Fritillaria unibracteata* Hsiao et K.C. Hsiao	*Liliaceae*
YI BEI MU		*Fritillaria pallidiflora* Schrenk	*Liliaceae*
PING BEI MU		*Fritillaria ussuriensis* Maxim.	*Liliaceae*

Such examples given in the table above (one TCM to many species) are ubiquitous and can be traced through the indexes of this book. For example, to learn all the origins of **DA HUANG**, the Index of Traditional Chinese Medicines by Chinese Name should be consulted first. This identifies three sources of **DA HUANG** as Medicinal Rhubarb, Sorrel Rhubarb and Tangut Rhubarb. Each of these plants can be found as entries in Part II which list the effects and indications of the medicine.

In some cases, for example, **BEI XIE**, no English name is given; instead, references to other Chinese medicines are provided. Each of these can be found in the Index of Traditional Chinese Medicines by Chinese Name, which leads to specific entries in Part II. Alternatively, the Latin names found in the Index of Origin of Traditional Chinese Medicines lead to the English names which can be used to find the entry in Part II.

The medicine, **BEI XIE,** is found in at least five different plant species and, in each case, a distinct name is applied to it. These names are listed in the Index of Chinese Names, and their entries in the same index lead to English names of the plants involved. Thus, the relationships are:

BEI XIE	**FEN BEI SHU YU**	Hypoglaucous Collett Yam
	CHA RUI SHU YU	Collett Yam
	SHAN BEI XIE	Mountain Yam
	XIAN XI SHU YU	Thinnest Yam
	FU ZHOU SHU YU	Foochow Yam

This subordinate relationship is documented in Part II, where Collett Yam, for example, is identified as "One of the **BEI XIE.**"

Resulting from omission of the Chinese four tone marks, a few pairs of different plants have the same name. Both the Peking Euphorbia and the Japanese Thistle, which are distinct species, are identified here as **DA JI.** For clarity, these are termed **DA JI (a)** and **DA JI (b)**, respectively. Likewise, the Common Butterbush (*Cephalanthus*, family *Rubiaceae*) and the Beautiful Sweetgum (*Liquidambar*, family *Hamamelidaceae*) are both termed **FENG XIANG SHU**. To distinguish between them, the Common Butterbush is identified as **FENG XIANG SHU (a)** and the Beautiful Sweetgum as **FENG XIANG SHU (b)**. Similarly, the Japanese Avens (*Geum*, family *Rosaceae*) is named **SHUI YANG MEI (I)** and the Thinleaf Adina (*Adina*, family *Rubiaceae*) as **SHUI YANG MEI (II)**.

Effects and Indications of Traditional Chinese Medicines

Traditional Chinese medicine uses many words and phrases which defy precise translation into English. The compilers have adopted the Wiseman terminological system* which has the following major rules.

- The English-language terms should be faithful to the original concepts in traditional Chinese medicine. Thus the term "wind-fire eye" is used rather than "acute conjunctivitis," and "flesh goiter" in preference to "exophthalmic goiter." Other phrases common in Chinese medicine are "wind-cold-damp impediment," "wind-heat attacking upward, " and so on.

- The English-language TCM terminology should be susceptible to easy modification so that derivative effects can be described. Thus "quicken the blood" is a general effect meaning "activating blood flow" or "promoting blood circulation." Elaboration produces "quicken the blood and perform stasis," "quicken the blood and free network vessels," or "quicken the blood and move *qi*." Further extensions to "quicken the blood" are:

  - and dissipate stasis
  - and regulate menstruation
  - and resolve toxins
  - and eliminate swelling
  - and stanch bleeding.

This practice will not facilitate the reader's task but it does allow an accurate account of the stated effect of the medicine and as Wiseman has pointed out,* such accuracy is jeopardized by attempts to translate the terminology of Chinese medicine into Western terms.

- Wiseman, N. and Feng, Y. (1998), Practical Dictionary of Chinese Medicine. Second Edition, Paradigm Publications, Brookline, MA.

English Names of Plants and Animals

Plants often have more than one common name or alias and, to avoid confusion, the practice adopted in this book is to use a single common English name for each plant. There is, therefore, a one-to-one correspondence between this English name and the Latin name of the species.

Classification of Plants and Animals

The classification used conforms to that found in Zhang *et al.** The following rules have been used:

- For algae, fungi, lichens and bryophyta, the common classification is used.
- For pteridophyta, the Renchang Qin classification system (1978) is used.
- For gymnospermae, the Wanjun Zheng classification system (1978) is used.
- For angiospermae, the Engler classification system (1964) is used.
- For fauna, the Johnson classification (1977) is used.

---

* Zhang, H. et al. (1994), China Resources - A Brief Flora of Chinese Medicine. Beijing.

Part I

CHEMICAL COMPOUNDS IN TRADITIONAL CHINESE MEDICINES

1 Abamagenin
$C_{28}H_{42}Cl_2O_4$ MW: 513.55 Source: HU WEI LAN. Ref: 6.

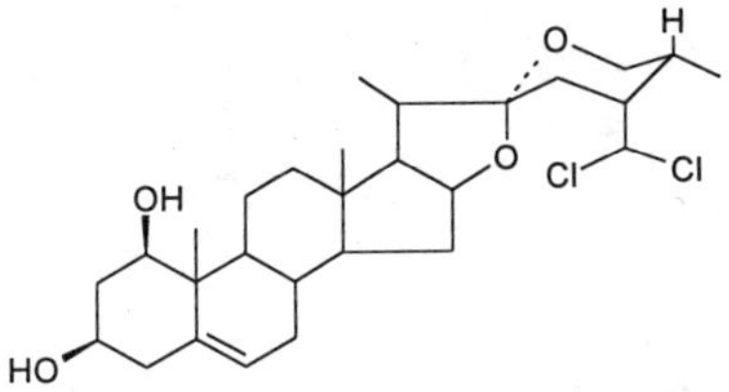

2 Abietic acid
$C_{20}H_{30}O_2$ MW: 302.46 Property: mp (-): 171-3°C, (±): 148-50°C. Source: SONG XIANG. Ref: 6, 631.

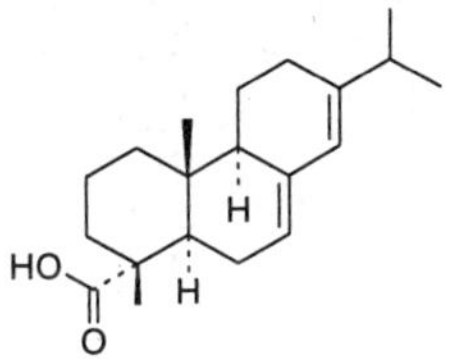

3 Abrine
$C_{12}H_{14}N_2O_2$ MW: 218.26 Property: prismatic crystal (water), mp 295°C (dec). Source: JI GU CAO, XIANG SI ZI. Ref: 1, 5, 6.

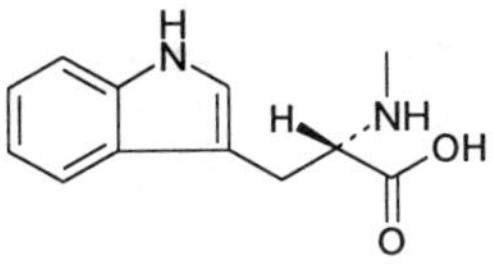

4 Abscisic acid
d-Abscisin II. CAS: 21293-29-8 $C_{15}H_{20}O_4$ MW: 264.32 Property: mp 160-3°C, soluble in diethyl ether. Source: SHAN YAO, XIANG SI ZI. Ref: 2.

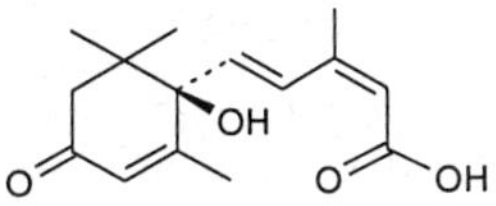

5 Absinthin
$C_{30}H_{40}O_6$ MW: 496.65 Property: orange acicular crystal (anhydrous ether), mp 179-83°C (dec). Source: BAI HAO. Ref: 1, 6.

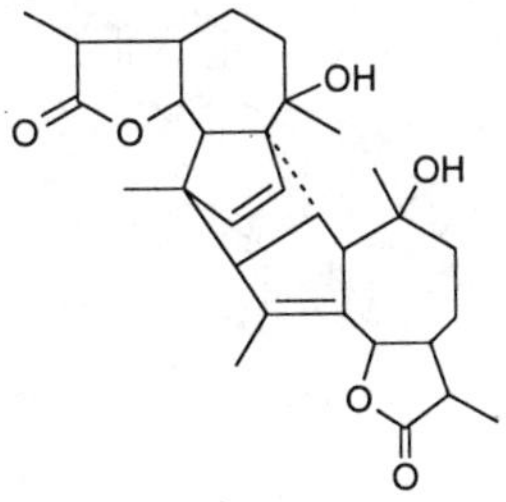

6 Acacetin
5,7-Dihydroxy-4'-methoxyflavone. CAS: 480-44-4 $C_{16}H_{12}O_5$ MW: 284.27 Property: yellow acicular crystals (95% alcohol), mp 263°C, soluble in ethanol. Source: FENG JIAO, HUO XIANG, LI ZHI HAO, MI MENG HUA. Ref: 1, 7, 319, 369, 463.

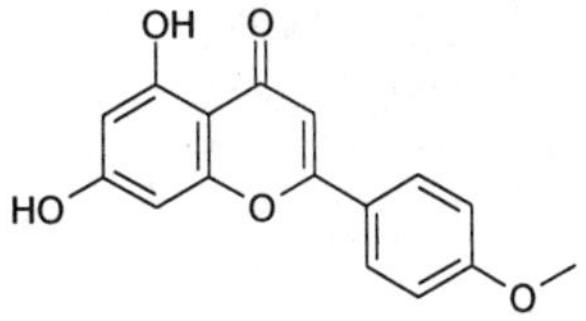

7 Acacetin-7-glucurono-(1→2)-glucuronide
$C_{28}H_{28}O_{17}$ MW: 636.53 Property: mp 191-205°C (dec). Source: CHOU WU TONG. Ref: 6.

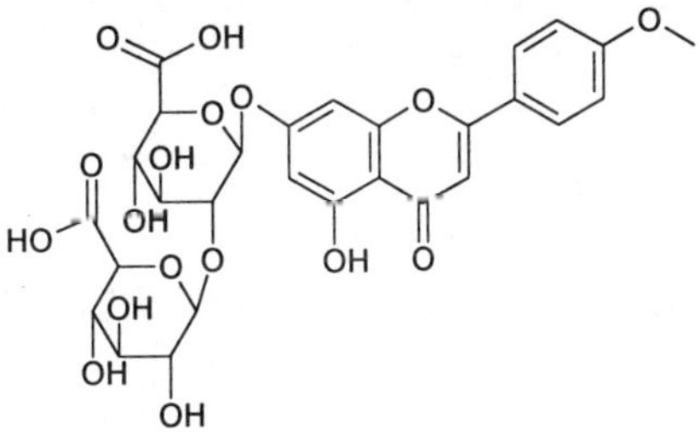

8 Acaciin
Acacetin-7-rhamnosideglucoside. $C_{28}H_{32}O_{14}$ MW: 592.56 Property: mp 263°C. Source: BEI YE JU, CI HUAI HUA, LING MI MENG HUA.Ref: 6, 369, 388.

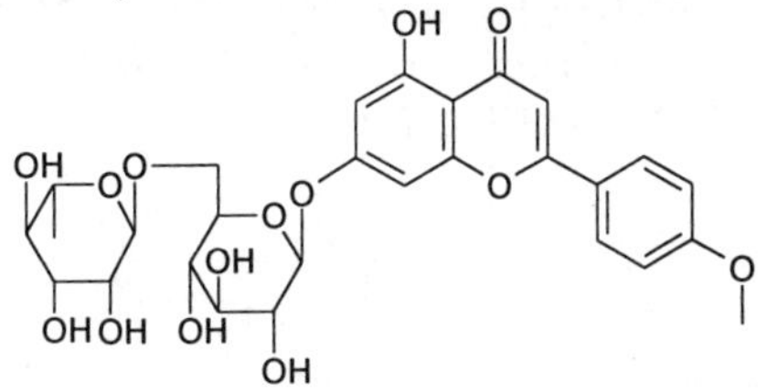

9 Acanthamolide
CAS: 64852-96-6 $C_{19}H_{25}NO_5$ MW: 347.17 Property: colourless prismatic crystal (benzene-methanol), mp 249-51°C. Source: GUANG CI BAO JU. Ref: 1, 5.

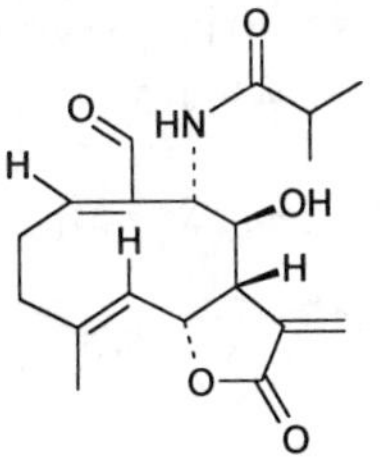

10 Acanthoglabrolide
CAS: 75744-66-0 $C_{23}H_{30}O_7$ MW: 418.49 Source: GUANG CI BAO JU. Ref: 1, 5.

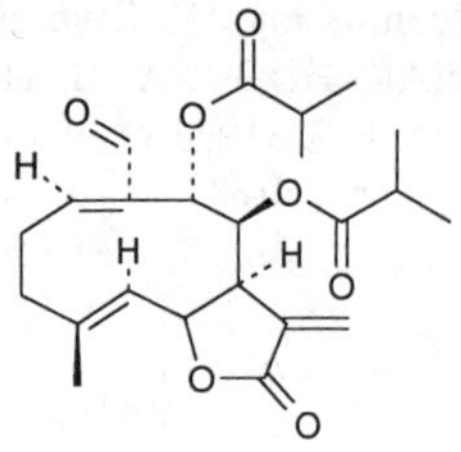

11 Acanthoidine
$C_{16}H_{26}N_4O_2$ MW: 306.41 Source: FEI LIAN. Ref: 6.

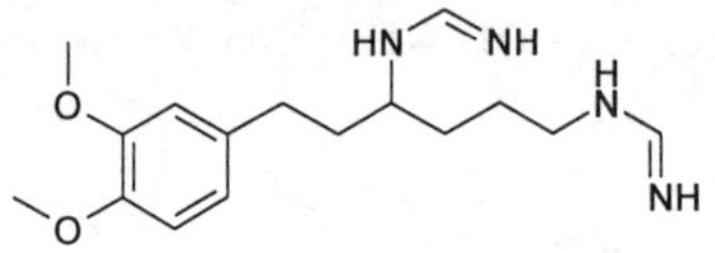

12 Acanthoine
$C_{16}H_{22}N_4O_2$ MW: 302.38 Source: FEI LIAN. Ref: 6.

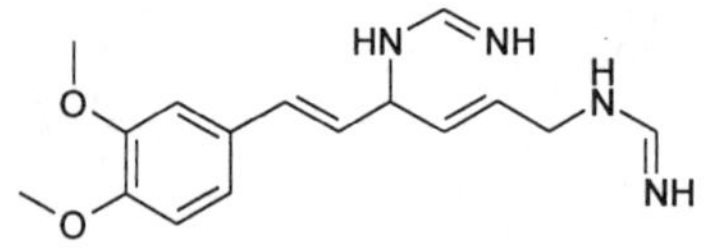

13 Acantholide
CAS: 72548-16-4 $C_{19}H_{24}O_6$ MW: 348.16 Property: colourless acieular crystal, mp 208°C. Source: GUANG CI BAO JU. Ref: 1, 5.

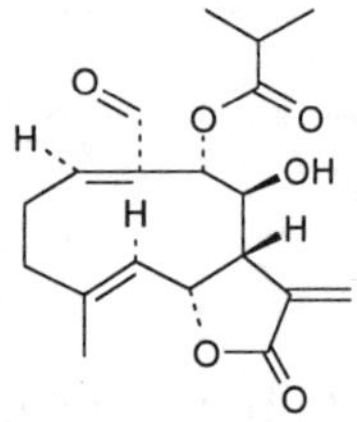

14 Acanthoside B
$C_{28}H_{36}O_{13}$ MW: 580.59 Property: mp 150°C. Source: HUANG HUA REN, WU JIA PI. Ref: 6, 540.

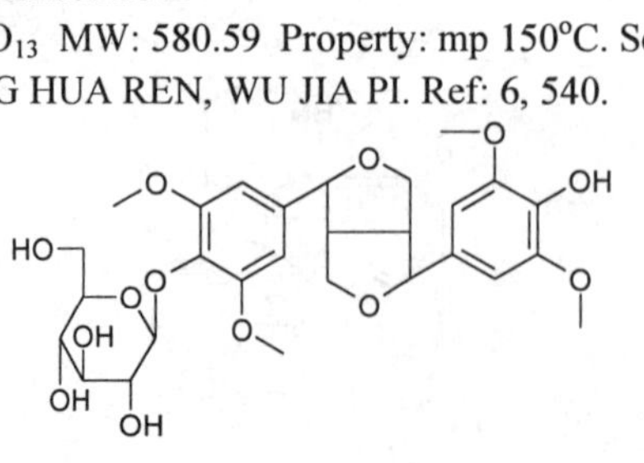

15 Acanthoside D
$C_{34}H_{46}O_{18}$ MW: 742.73 Property: mp 245-7°C. Source: WU JIA PI. Ref: 6, 235.

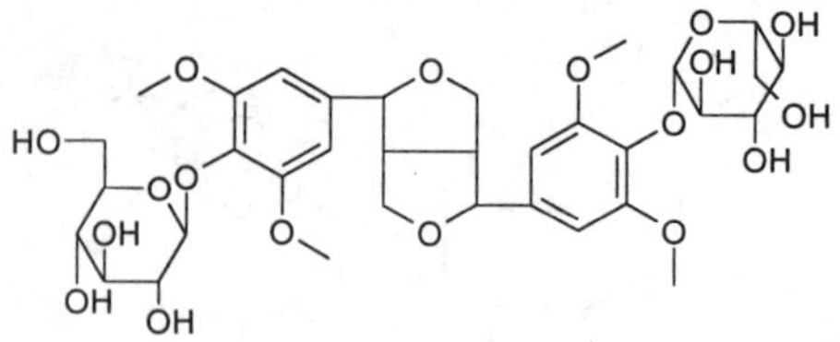

16 Acanthospermal A
CAS: 56689-33-9 $C_{23}H_{30}O_8$ MW: 434.49 Source: GUANG CI BAO JU. Ref: 1, 5.

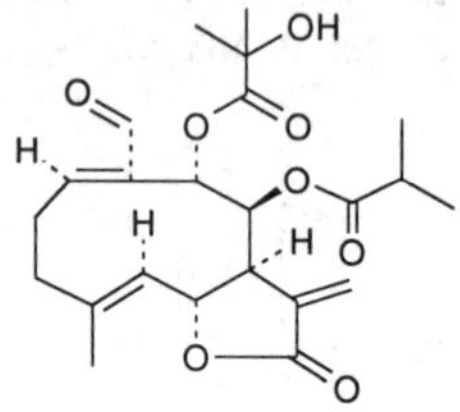

17 Acanthospermolide
CAS: 75744-64-8 $C_{20}H_{26}O_6$ MW: 362.41 Property: mp 154°C. Source: GUANG CI BAO JU. Ref: 1, 5.

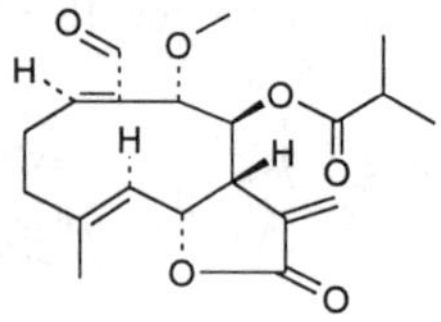

18 Acerinol glycoside
$C_{30}H_{46}O_5$ MW: 486.70 Property: mp 152-3°C. Source: SAN MIAN DAO. Ref: 6.

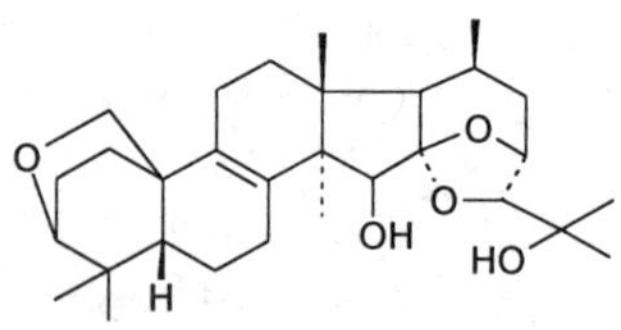

19 Aceritannin
$C_{20}H_{20}O_{13}$ MW: 468.37 Source: Leaves of *Acer ginnala* Maxim. Ref: 1.

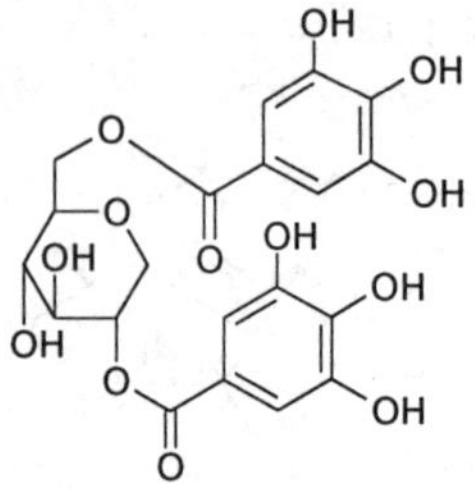

20 Acetal
$C_7H_{16}O_2$ MW: 132.20 Property: bp 103.2°C/761mm. Source: CU. Ref: 6.

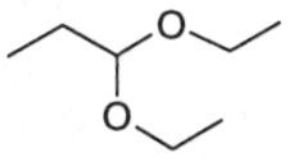

21 Acetamide
C_2H_5NO MW: 59.07 Property: mp 82-3°C. Source: XIANG XUN. Ref: 6.

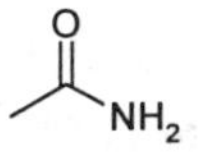

22 Acetic ester of L-βartemisia alcohol
$C_{12}H_{20}O_2$ MW: 196.29 Property: bp 74-6°C/6mm. Source: HUANG HUA HAO. Ref: 6.

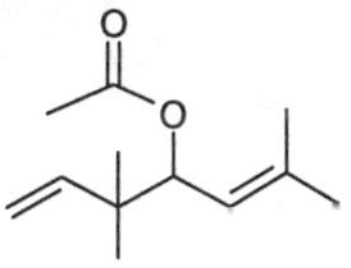

23 Acetoin
$C_4H_8O_2$ MW: 88.11 Property: mp (±): -72°C, bp (+): 142-4°C, (-): 143°C, (±): 148°C. Source: CU. Ref: 6.

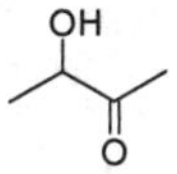

24 Acetovanillone
Apocynin. $C_9H_{10}O_3$ MW: 166.18 Property: mp 115 °C, bp 295-300°C. Source: MIAN HUA GEN. Ref: 6.

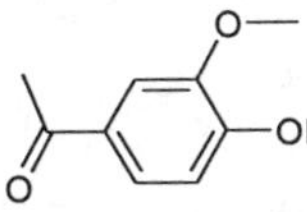

25 3β-Acetoxy-atractylon
$C_{17}H_{22}O_3$ MW: 274.36 Source: CANG ZHU. Ref: 2.

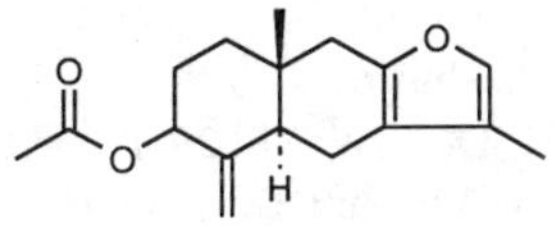

26 d-8-Acetoxycarvotanacetone
$C_{12}H_{18}O_3$ MW: 210.28 Property: mp 45.3-46.2°C, $[\alpha]_D^{20}$ +32.2°(c=10, $CHCl_3$). Source: BO HE. Ref: 1.

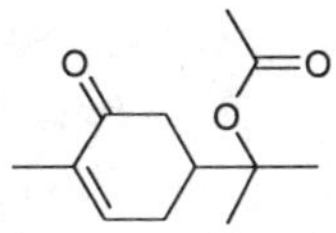

27 1'-Acetoxychavicol acetate
$C_{13}H_{14}O_4$ MW: 234.25 Property: $[\alpha]_D^{20}$ -80° (c=1.0, alcohol). Source: DA LIANG JIANG. Ref: 1.

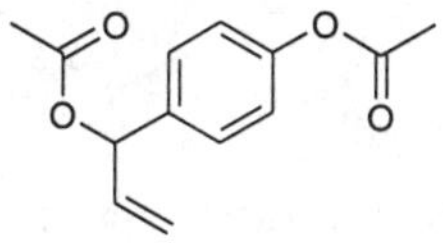

28 1'-Acetoxyeugenol acetate
$C_{14}H_{16}O_5$ MW: 264.28 Source: DA LIANG JIANG. Ref: 1

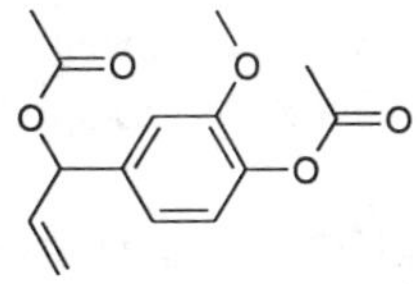

29 9-Acetoxyfukinanolide
$C_{17}H_{24}O_4$ MW: 292.38 Property: mp 96-7°C. Source: FENG DOU CAI. Ref: 6.

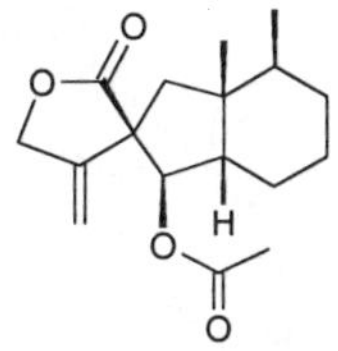

30 16-Acetoxy-7α-methoxyroyleanone
$C_{23}H_{32}O_6$ MW: 404.51 Property: yellow acicular crystal, mp 185-7°C, $[\alpha]_D^{16}$ +12.3° (c=0.3, methanol). Source: CHANG YE XIANG CHA CAI. Ref: 76.

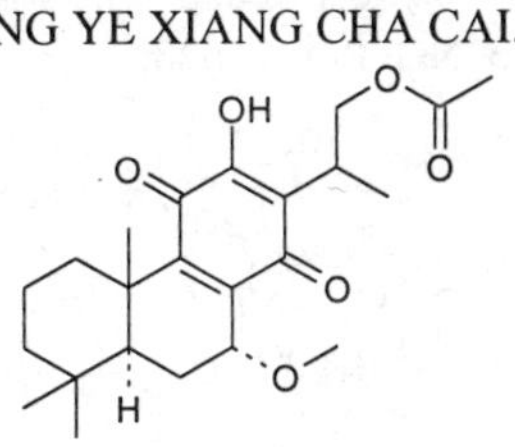

31 7-Acetoxy-2-methylisoflavone
$C_{18}H_{14}O_4$ MW: 294.31 Source: GAN CAO. Ref: 2.

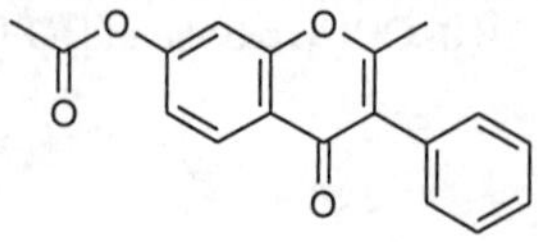

32 3-Acetoxy-1-nonene
$C_9H_{16}O_2$ MW: 156.23 Source: FENG DOU CAI. Ref: 6.

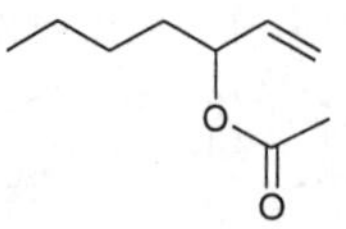

33 3β-Acetoxynorerythrosuamine
CAS: 26523-10-4 Property: mp 173-5°C. Source: *Erythrophleum Chlorostachyus* Baill. Ref: 1, 5.

34 3α-Acetoxy oleanolic acid
$C_{32}H_{50}O_4$ MW: 498 Property: white acicular crystal, mp 265-7°C. Source: CAO CONG RONG. Ref: 471.

35 (5S,6S,7R)-2-[2-(2-Acetoxyphenyl)ethyl]-5a', 6a',7a-triacetoxy-5,6,7,8-tetrahydrochromone (AH9)
$C_{25}H_{26}O_{10}$ MW: 486.48 Property: colourless acicular crystal, mp 147-8°C, $[\alpha]_D$ -11.1°. Source: CHEN XIANG. Ref: 13.

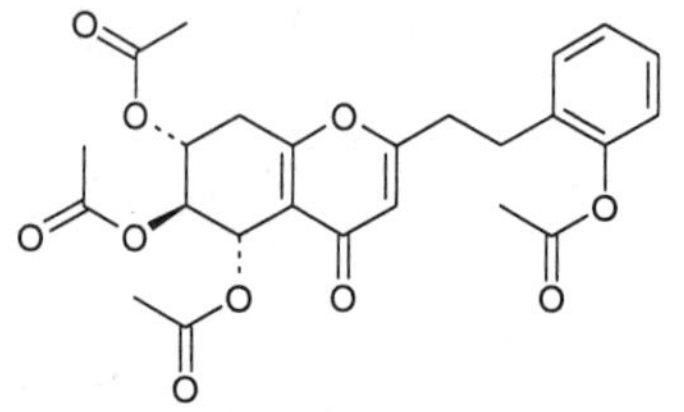

36 2'-Acetylacteoside
$C_{31}H_{38}O_{16}$ MW: 666.64 Source: GAN DI HUANG, ROU CONG RONG. Ref: 2, 628.

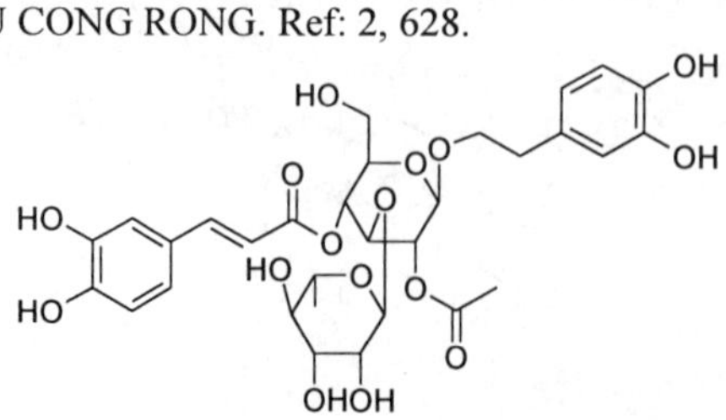

37 Acetylamarolide
$C_{22}H_{30}O_7$ MW: 406.48 Property: mp 264-5°C. Source: CHU BAI PI. Ref: 6.

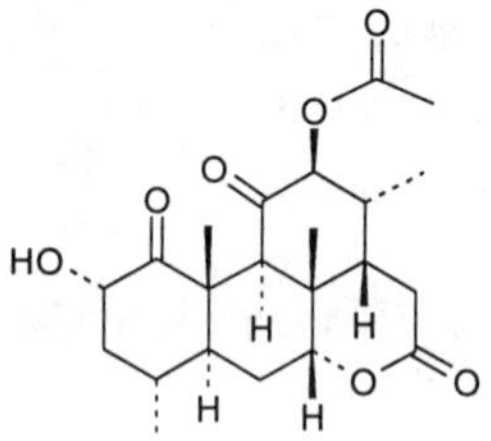

38 2'-Acetylangelicin
$C_{13}H_8O_4$ MW: 228.21 Property: light yellow acicular crystal, mp 200-2°C (ethanol). Source: SHE CHUANG. Ref: 352.

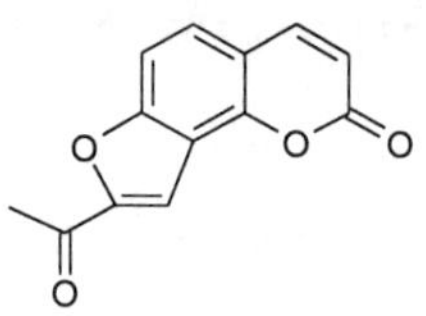

39 3-O-(4-O-Acetyl)-α-L-arabinopyranosyl-hederagenin
28-O-β-D-glucopyranosyl-(1→6)-β-D-gluco-pyranoside. $C_{49}H_{78}O_{19}$ MW: 971.16 Property: white powder, mp 198-201°C, $[\alpha]_D^{19}$ +19.7° (c=0.25, Methanol). Source: CHUAN XU DUAN. Ref: 201.

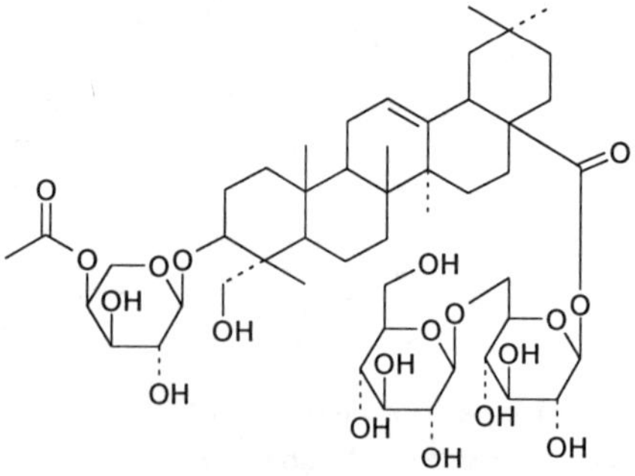

40 6-O-Acetylarbutin
Pyroside. $C_{14}H_{18}O_8$ MW: 314.29 Property: 214-6°C. Source: YUE JU YE. Ref: 6.

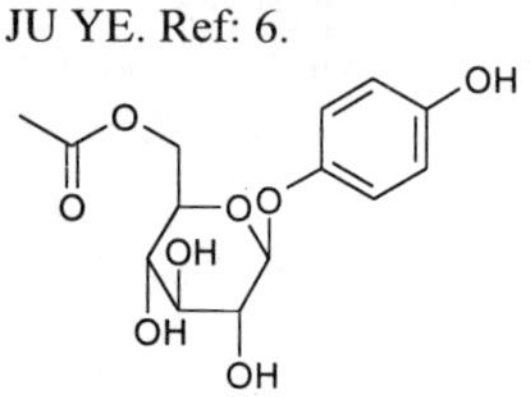

41 6'-Acetyl asperuloside

$C_{20}H_{24}O_{12}$ MW: 456.41 Property: white powder, $[\alpha]_D$ -104.6° (c=0.085, methanol). Source: HUANG MAO ER CAO. Ref: 400.

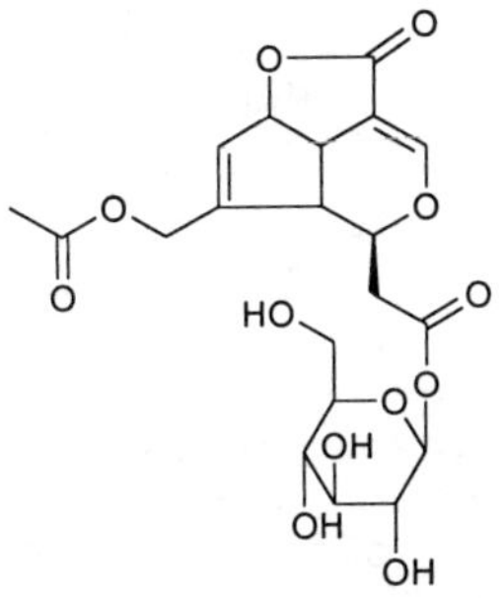

42 Acetyl-atractylodinol

$C_{15}H_{12}O_3$ MW: 240.26 Source: CANG ZHU. Ref: 2.

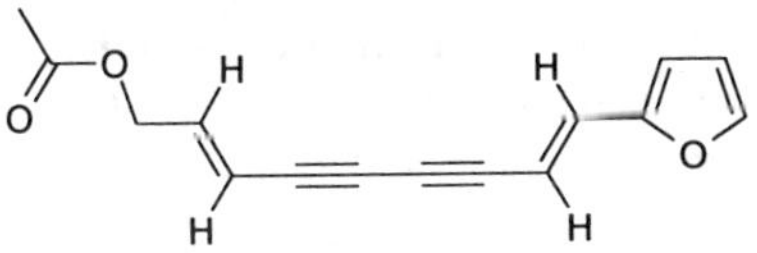

43 8-Acetyl-14-benzoylchasmaninie

$C_{34}H_{47}NO_8$ MW: 597.76 Property: colorless acicular crystal, mp 150-2°C, $[\alpha]_D^{25}$ +9.8° (c=0.08, ethanol). Source: SONG PAN WU TOU. Ref: 107.

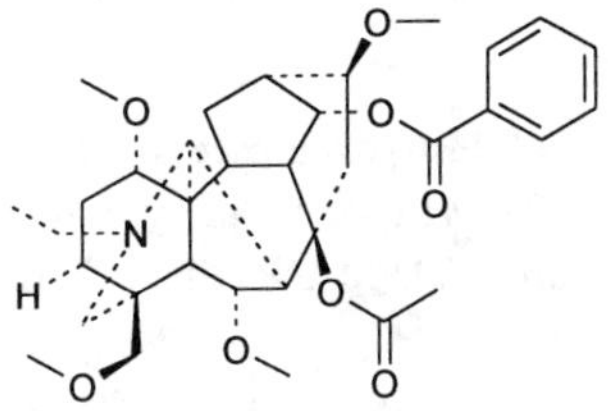

44 Acetylborneol

Bornyl acetate. $C_{12}H_{20}O_2$ MW: 196.29 Property: mp 26.5-29°C, bp 225-6°C. Source: HOU PO, QIANG HUO, QING HAO, SHENG JIANG, WU WEI ZI, XI XIN, YIN CHEN HAO, YU XING CAO, etc. Ref: 1, 2, 6.

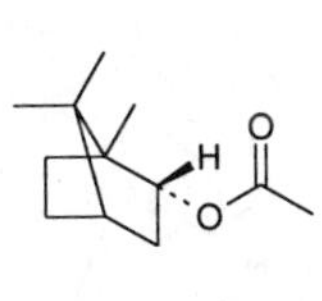

45 Acetyl-bupleurotoxin

$C_{19}H_{24}O_3$ MW: 300.40 Property: colorless lamellar crystal, mp 48°C, $[\alpha]_D^{18}$ -10° (c=0.04, methanol), toxicity. Source: DA YE CHAI HU. Ref: 81.

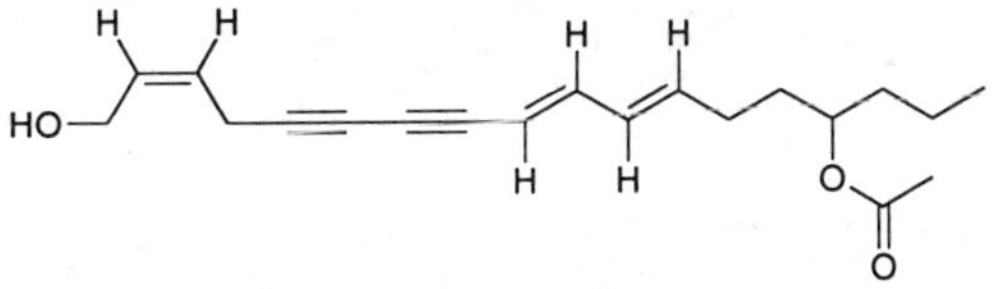

46 1-Acetyl-β-carboline

$C_{13}H_{10}N_2O$ MW: 210.29 Source: KU MU. Ref: 12.

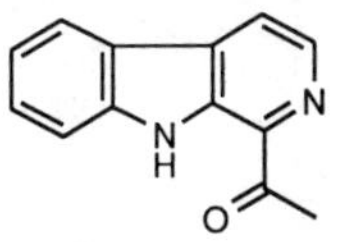

47 Acetylcatalpol

$C_{19}H_{28}O_{10}$ MW: 416.43 Source: GAN DI HUANG. Ref: 2.

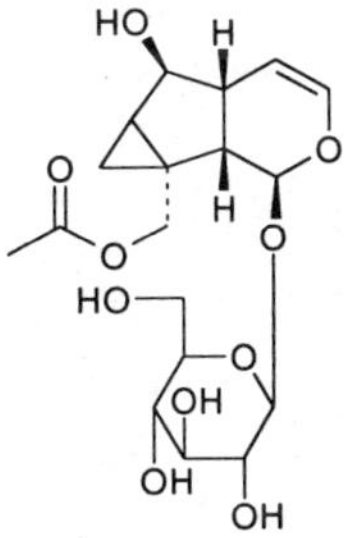

48 Acetylcephalotaxine

$C_{20}H_{23}NO_5$ MW: 357.41 Source: SAN JIAN SHAN. Ref: 2.

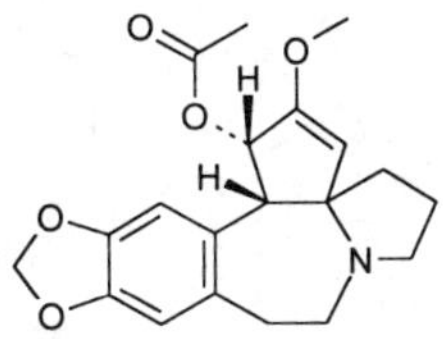

49 Acetylcholic acid

$C_{26}H_{42}O_6$ MW: 450.62 Source: XIANG DAN. Ref: 6.

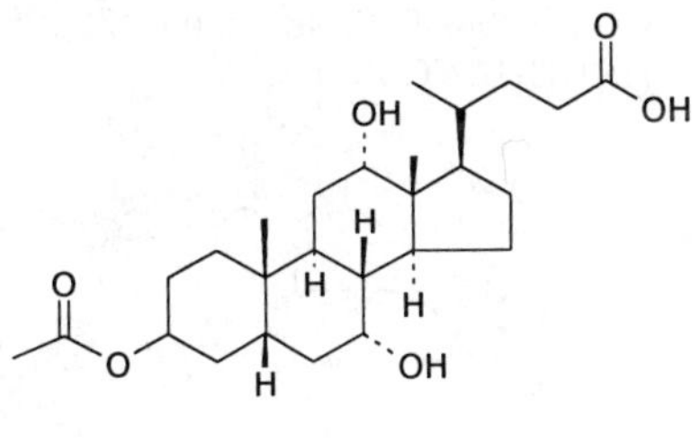

50 Acetyl choline
Source: FENG MI, FENG RU, HE SHI, JI CAI, MAI JIAO, SHAN ZHA, SHAN ZHA YE, SHI QI, XIONG DAN. Ref: 6.

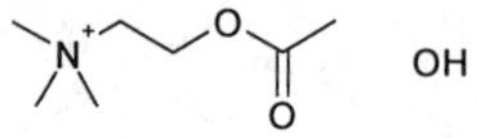

51 Acetylcimifugoside
$C_{36}H_{54}O_{10}$ MW: 646.83 Source: YE SHENG MA. Ref: 6.

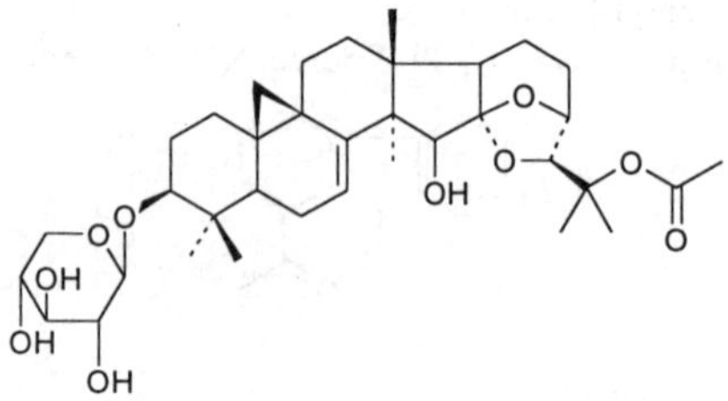

52 25-O-Acetylcimigenol
$C_{32}H_{50}O_6$ MW: 530.75 Property: mp 193-4°C. Source: SAN MIAN DAO. Ref: 6.

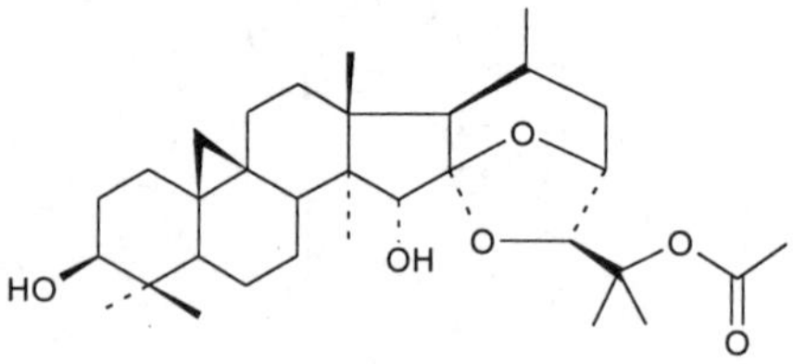

53 25-O-Acetylcimigenoside
$C_{37}H_{58}O_{10}$ MW: 662.87 Property: mp 234-5°C. Source: SAN MIAN DAO, YE SHENG MA. Ref: 6.

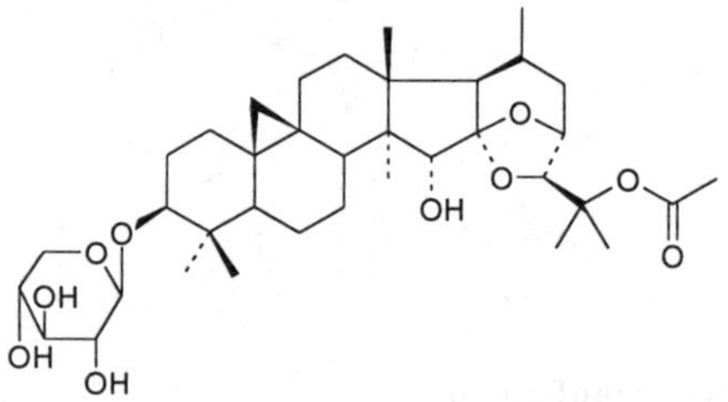

54 O-Acetyl columbianetin
$C_{16}H_{16}O_{10}$ MW: 288.30 Property: mp 127.5-8.5°C. Source: SHE CHUANG ZI. Ref: 6.

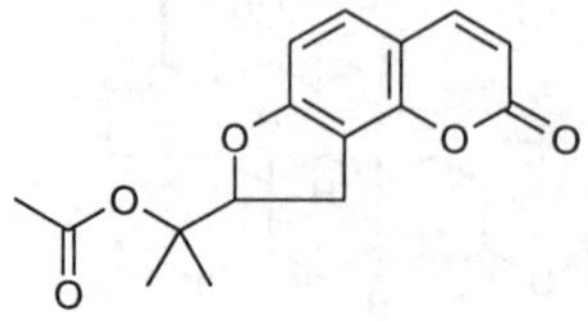

55 Acetylcorynoline
$C_{23}H_{23}NO_6$ MW: 409.44 Property: mp 157-9°C. Source: YUN QIAN HU, ZI HUA YU DENG CAO (LIE BAO ZI JING). Ref: 6, 436.

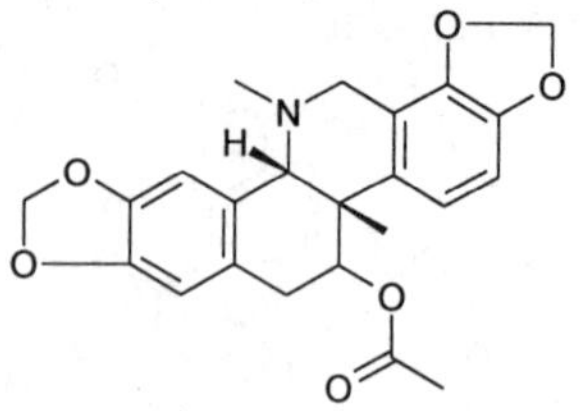

56 2-Acetyl-3-(p-coumaroyl)-meso-tartaric acid
$C_{15}H_{14}O_9$ MW: 338.27 Source: BO CAI. Ref: 6.

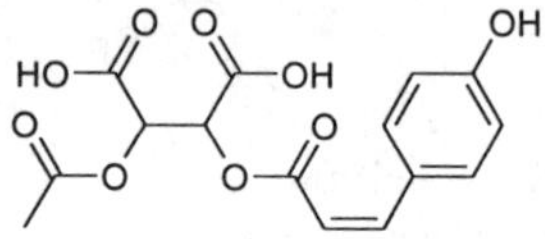

57 22-O-Acetyl-N_b-demethyl-echitamine
$C_{23}H_{28}N_2O_5$ MW: 412.49 Property: white acicular crystals, mp 234°C. Source: DAI YAO XIAO DENG TAI. Ref: 270.

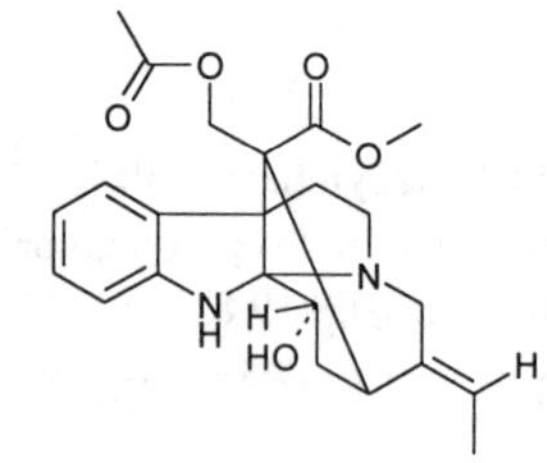

58 19-(R)-Acetyldihydrogelseevirine
$C_{23}H_{28}N_2O_5$ MW: 412.49 Property: mp 186-9°C, $[\alpha]_D$ -6.7°. Source: HU MAN TENG. Ref: 14.

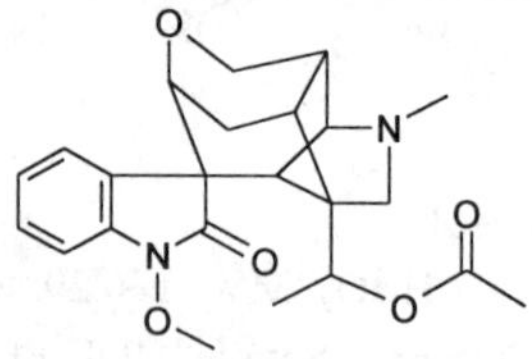

59 8-Acetyldolaconine
$C_{26}H_{39}NO_6$ MW: 461.61 Property: wax solid. Source: WAN ZHUO WU TOU. Ref: 270.

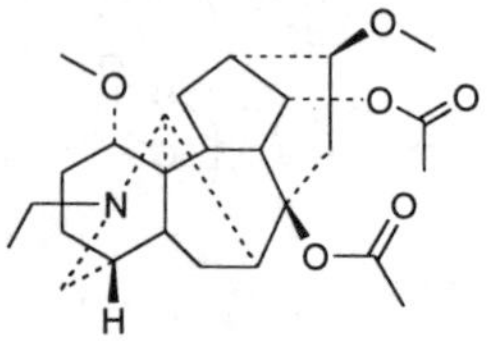

60 Acetyleugenol
$C_{12}H_{14}O_3$ MW: 206.24 Property: mp 30-1°C, bp 281-2°C/752mm. Source: DING XIANG, YUE GUI ZI. Ref: 6.

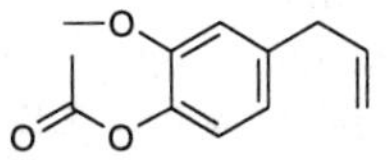

61 6-Acetylfuranofukinol
$C_{17}H_{24}O_4$ MW: 292.38 Source: FENG DOU CAI. Ref: 6.

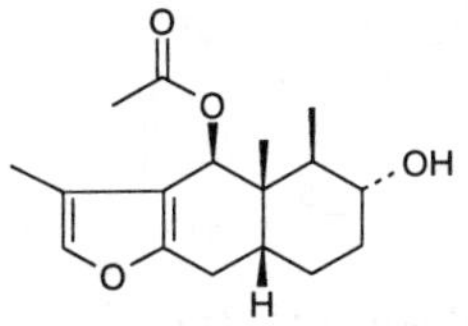

62 10-O-Acetylgeniposide
$C_{19}H_{26}O_{11}$ MW: 430.41 Source: ZHI ZI. Ref: 2, 626.

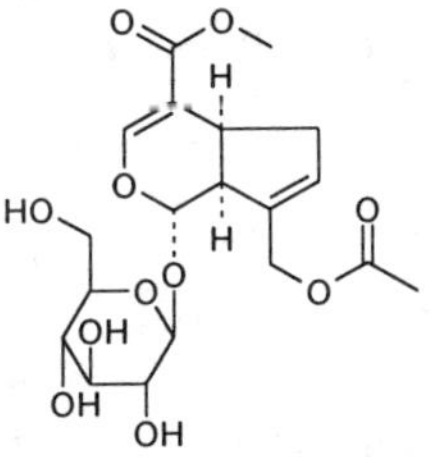

63 16-Acetylgitoxigenin
Oleandrigenin. Source: JIA ZHU TAO. Ref: 6.

64 Acetylglaucarubinone
CAS: 32426-14-0 $C_{27}H_{36}O_{11}$ MW: 536.58 Property: mp 170-172°C. Source: *Pierreodendron kerstingii* Little. Ref: 1, 5

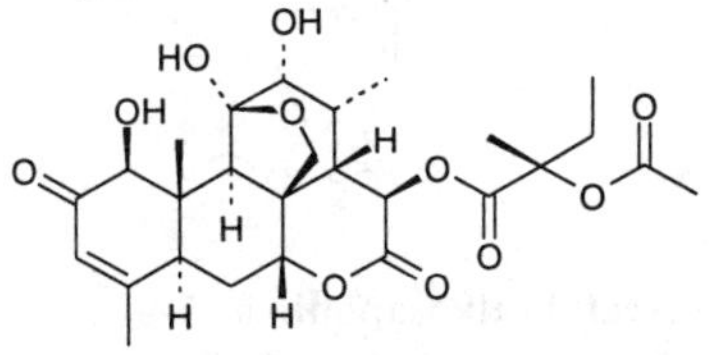

65 N-Acetyl-D-glucosamine
$C_9H_{19}NO_5$ MW: 221.26 Source: XIE KE, YUAN ZHI. Ref: 2, 6.

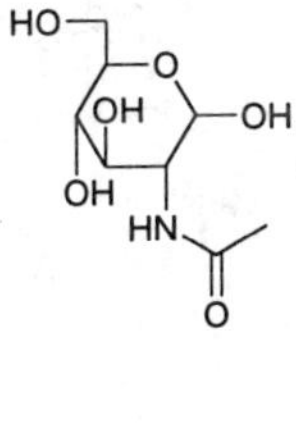

66 3'-O-Acetylhamaudol
$C_{17}H_{18}O_6$ MW: 318.33 Source: FANG FENG. Ref: 2.

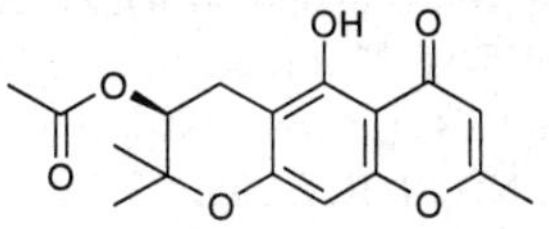

67 5-Acetyl-7-hydroxy-2-methyl-benzopyran-γ-one
$C_{12}H_{10}O_4$ MW: 218.21 Source: DA HUANG. Ref: 2.

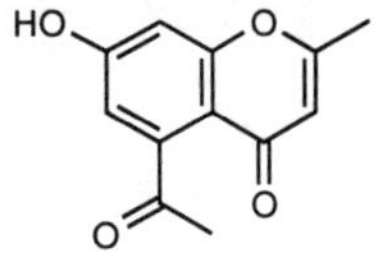

68 Acetylindicine
$C_{18}H_{29}NO_6$ MW: 355.43 Source: DA WEI YAO. Ref: 6.

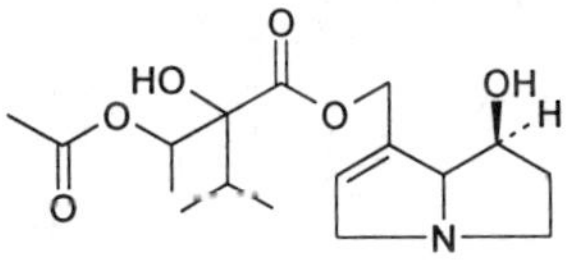

69 Acetylisocorynoline
$C_{23}H_{23}NO_6$ MW: 409.44 Property: mp 205-9°C. Source: YUN QIAN HU, ZI HUA YU DENG CAO (LIE BAO ZI JING). Ref: 6, 436.

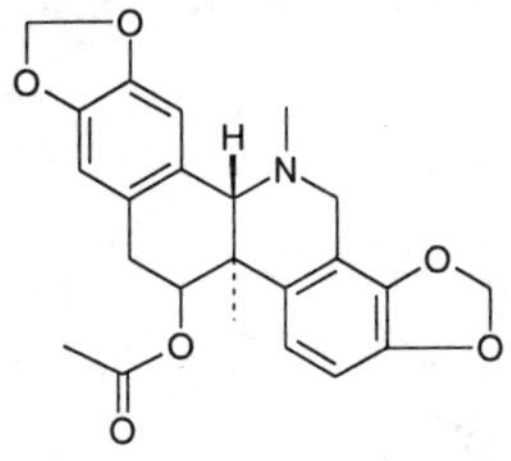

70 1-Acetyl-4-isopropylidene-cyclopentene
$C_{10}H_{14}O$ MW: 150.22 Source: AN YE. Ref: 6.

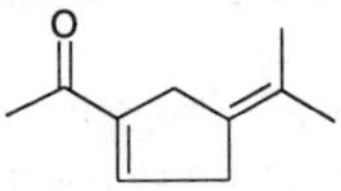

71 16-Acetylkirenol
$C_{22}H_{36}O_5$ MW: 380.53 Source: XI XIAN. Ref: 2.

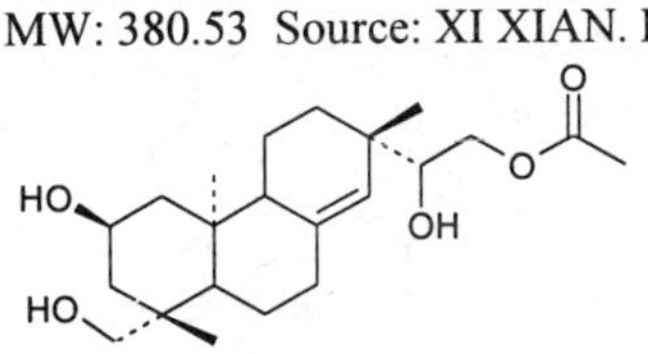

72 3β-O-Acetyl-mangiferolic acid
3β-Acetoxyl-9,19-cyclolanost-24(E)en-26-oic acid. $C_{32}H_{50}O_4$ MW: 498.37 Property: colorless acicular crystal, mp 180-2°C (petroleum spirit-acetic ester). Source: DI FENG PI. Ref: 395.

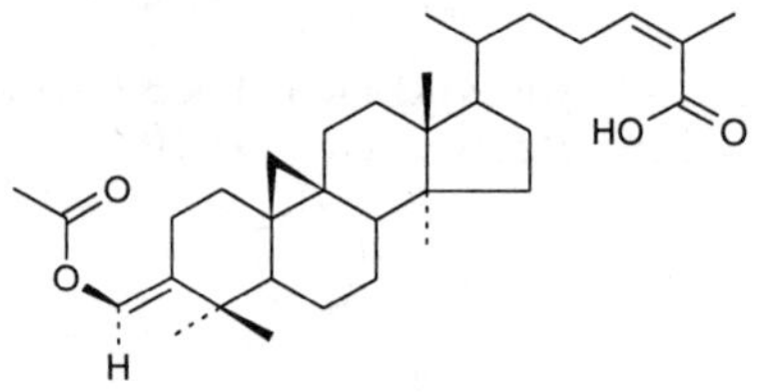

73 Acetyl-*l*-myrtenol
$C_{12}H_{18}O_2$ MW: 194.28 Source: XIE CAO. Ref: 6.

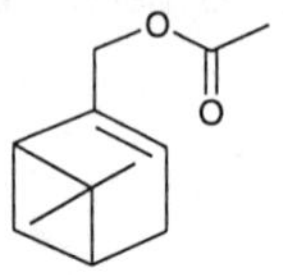

74 Acetyl oleanolic acid
$C_{32}H_{50}O_4$ MW: 498.75 Property: colorless acicular crystal, mp 258-68°C. Source: BAI HUA, BAI TOU WENG, MEI SHANG LU, NU ZHEN ZI, RUAN ZAO MI HOU TAO, YE DONG QING QUO, ZI MEI SHU. Ref: 6

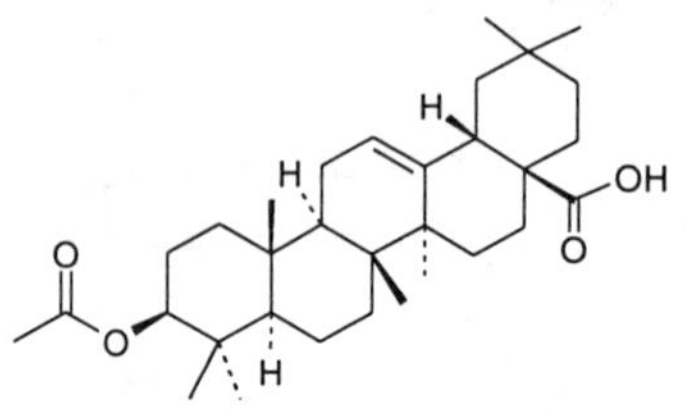

75 (-)-3'-(S)-Acetyloxy-4'-(S)-angeloyloxy-3',4'-dihydroseselin
$C_{21}H_{22}O_7$ MW: 386.41 Property: colorless acicular crystal, mp 172-4°C (petroleum spirit-acetic ester), $[\alpha]_D^{18}$ -27.2° (c=0.25, chloroform). Source: NAN LING QIAN HU. Ref: 373.

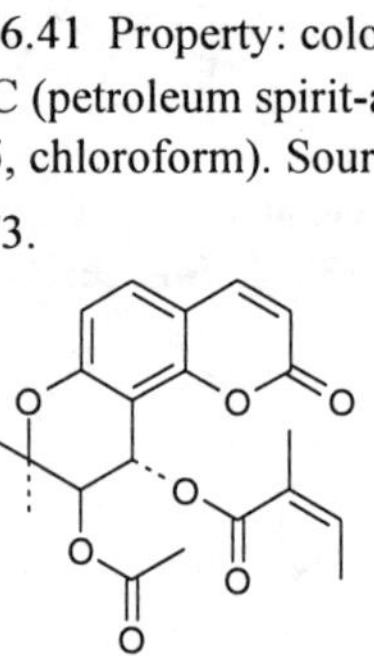

76 O-Acetyl-pachymic acid
Source: FU LING. Ref: 536.

77 Acetylpectolinarin
$C_{31}H_{36}O_{16}$ MW: 664.62 Property: mp 134-8° (ether-petroleum), $[\alpha]_D^{18}$ -68.5°. Source: LIU CHUAN YU. Ref: 1.

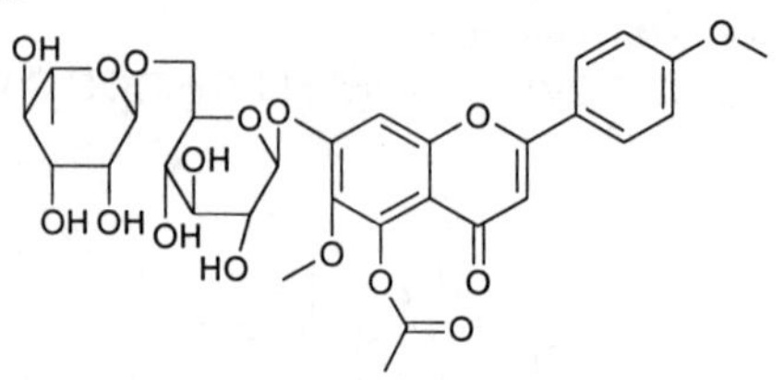

78 3-O-Acetyl pomolic acid
Property: mp 254-6°C. Source: MU GUA. Ref: 610.

79 Acetylpterosin C
$C_{16}H_{20}O_4$ MW: 276.34 Property: mp 115-6°C. Source: JUE. Ref: 6.

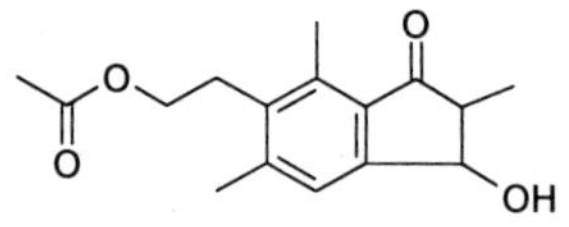

80 2''-O-Acetylquercitrin
$C_{23}H_{22}O_{12}$ MW: 490.42 Source: Flower of *Red wing azalea.* Ref: 1.

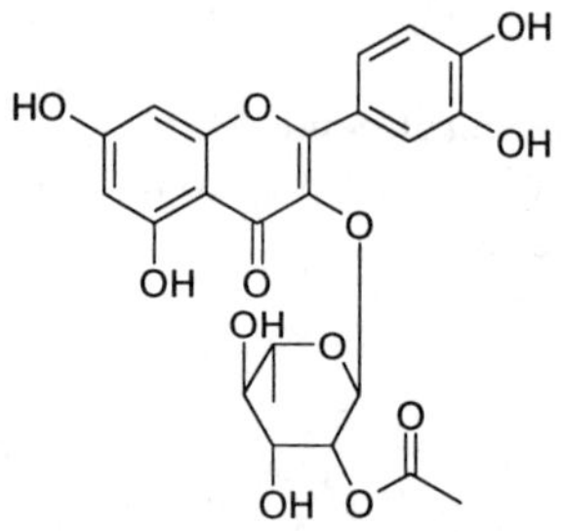

81 3''-O-Acetyl saikosaponin a
Source: CHAI HU. Ref: 7.

82 8-O-Acetyl shanzhiside methyl ester
Source: MENG GU CAO SU. Ref: 381, 560.

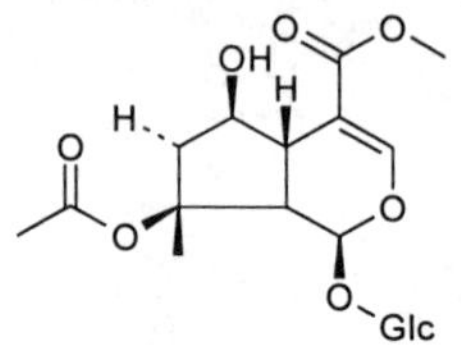

83 Acetylshikonin

$C_{18}H_{18}O_6$ MW: 330.34 Property: Red acicular crystal (petroleum spirit), mp 92-4°C. Source: ZI CAO. Ref: 1, 2.

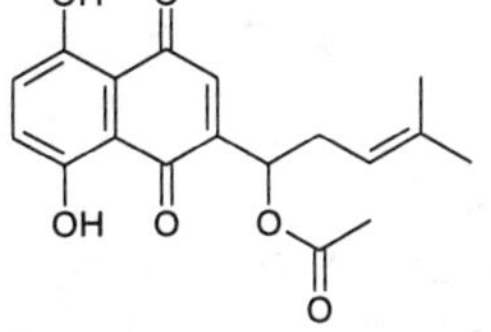

84 3-O-Acetyl ursolic acid

Property: 289-90 °C. Source: MU GUA. Ref: 610.

85 3-O-α-(2''-O-Acetyl)-D-xylopyranosyl-3β-hydroxyolean-12-ene-28,29-dioic acid

$C_{37}H_{56}O_{10}$ MW: 660.85 Property: white powder, mp 267-70°C, $[\alpha]_D^{20}$ +3.55° (c=0.1, methanol). Source: YI YE LIANG WANG CHA. Ref: 216.

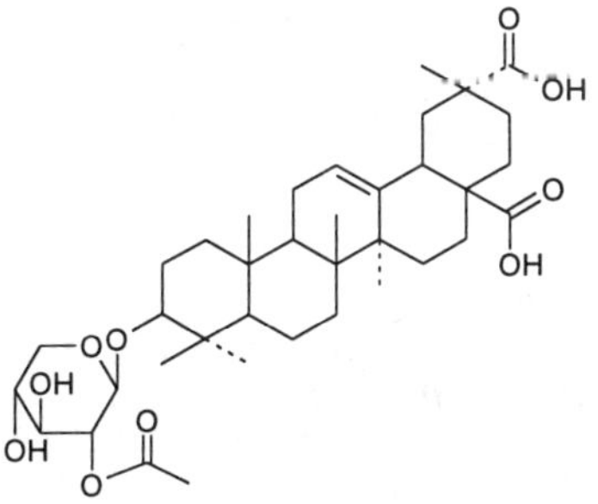

86 Acevaltratum

$C_{24}H_{32}O_{10}$ MW: 480.52 Property: white acicular crystal (ethane), mp 83-4°C, $[\alpha]_D^{24}$ +163.7° (methanol). Source: Root of *valeriana wallichii* DC. Ref: 1.

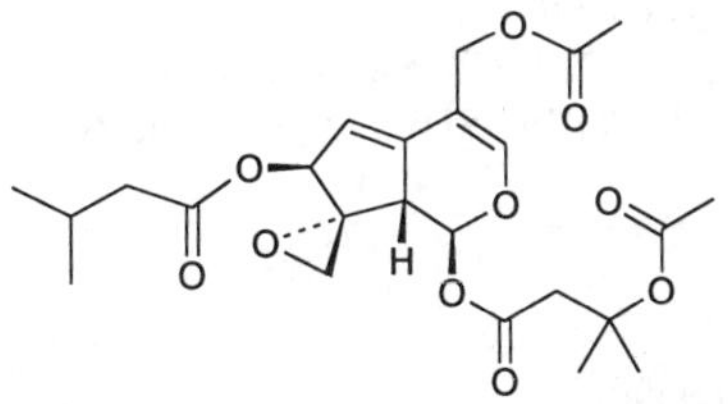

87 Achillin

$C_{15}H_{18}O_3$ MW: 246.31 Property: mp 144-5°C. Source: YANG SHI CAO, YI ZHI HAO. Ref: 6.

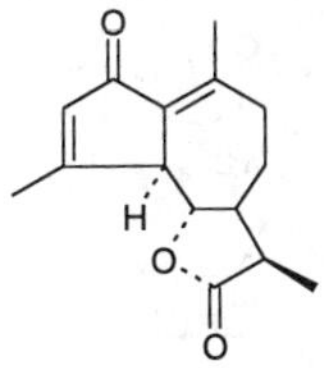

88 Acolamone

$C_{15}H_{24}O$ MW: 220.36 Source: BAI CHANG. Ref: 6.

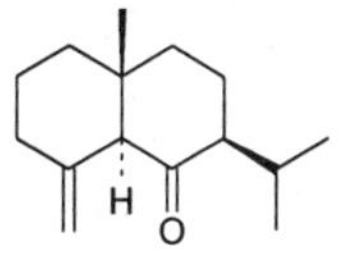

89 Aconifine

$C_{32}H_{43}NO_7$ MW: 553.70 Source: CAO WU TOU. Ref: 6.

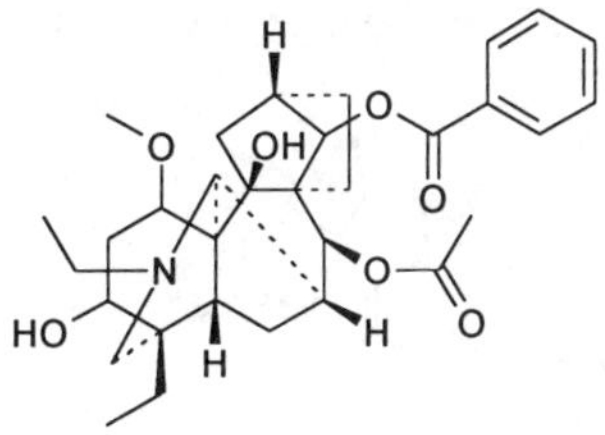

90 Aconitic acid

$C_6H_6O_6$ MW: 174.11 Property: mp cis: 125°C, trans: 194-5°C. Source: GAN ZHE, JIN CAO, GU JIE CAO, HEI DA DOU YE, YI ZHI HAO. Ref: 1, 6.

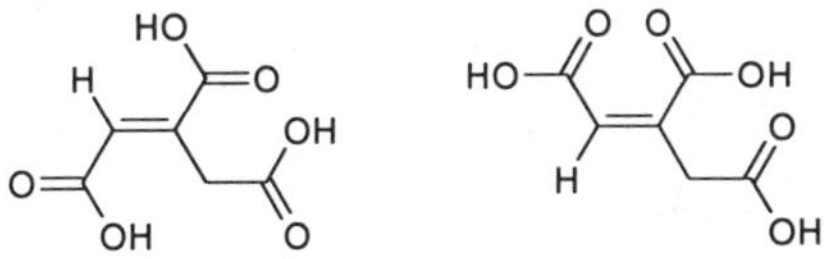

trans- cis-

91 Aconitine

CAS: 302-27-2 $C_{34}H_{47}NO_{11}$ MW: 645.75 Property: mp 204°C, $[\alpha]_D$ +19° (20, Chloroform), soluble in chloroform, benzene, ethanol and ether, insoluble in water. Source: CAO WU TOU, CHUAN WU TOU, FU ZI, XUE SHANG YI ZHI HAO. Ref: 2, 4, 5, 6.

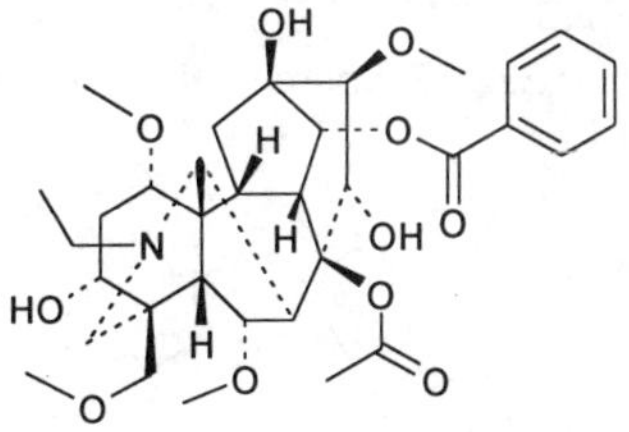

92 α-Acoradiene

$C_{16}H_{24}$ MW: 204.36 Source: DANG GUI, DU SONG SHI. Ref: 2.

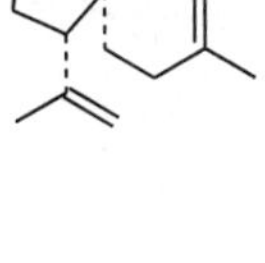

93 β-Acoradiene
$C_{15}H_{24}$ MW: 204.36 Source: DANG GUI, DU SONG SHI. Ref: 2.

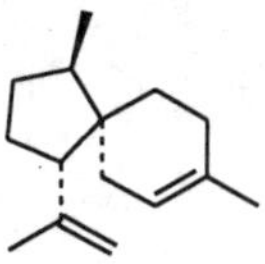

94 γ-Acoradiene
$C_{15}H_{24}$ MW: 204.36 Source: DANG GUI, DU SONG SHI. Ref: 2.

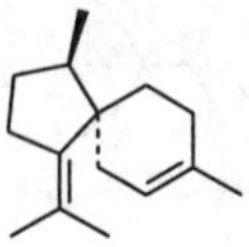

95 δ-Acoradiene
$C_{15}H_{24}$ MW: 204.36 Source: DANG GUI. Ref: 2.

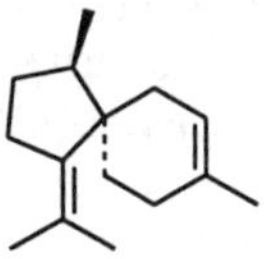

96 α-Acorenol
$C_{15}H_{26}O$ MW: 222.37 Source: DU SONG SHI. Ref: 6.

HO

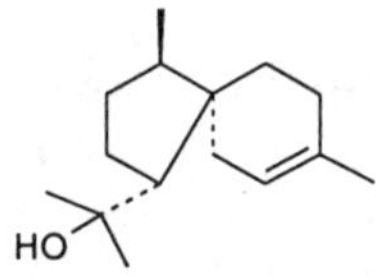

97 β-Acorenol
$C_{15}H_{26}O$ MW: 222.37 Source: DU SONG SHI. Ref: 6.

HO

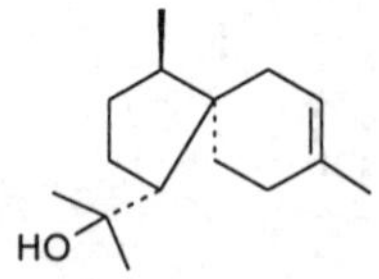

98 Acorenone
$C_{15}H_{24}O$ MW: 220.36 Source: BAI CHANG. Ref: 6.

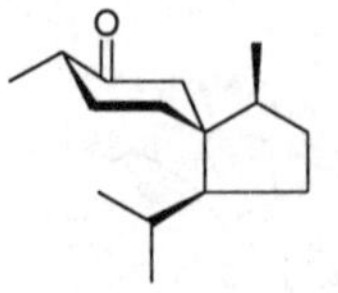

O

99 Acorone
$C_{15}H_{24}O_2$ MW: 236.36 Property: mp 100°C. Source: BAI CHANG. Ref: 6.

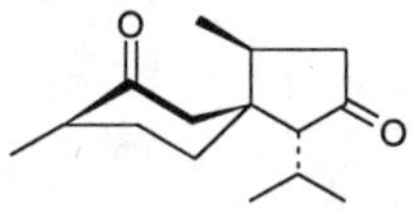

O O

100 Acoronene
$C_{14}H_{19}O_2$ MW: 219.31 Property: mp 69°C. Source: BAI CHANG. Ref: 6.

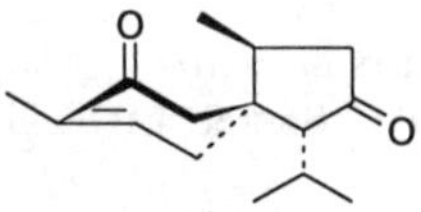

O O

101 Acrifoline
$C_{16}H_{23}NO_2$ MW: 261.37 Property: mp 103-4°C. Source: XIAO JIE JIN CAO. Ref: 6.

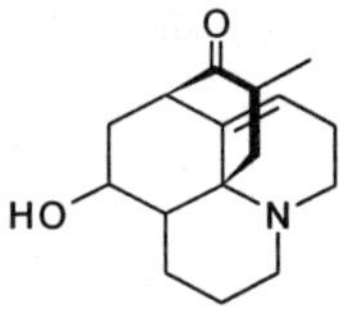

O HO N

102 Acronycine
$C_{20}H_{19}NO_3$ MW: 321.38 Source: JIU LI XIANG, SHA TANG MU. Ref: 1, 6, 11.

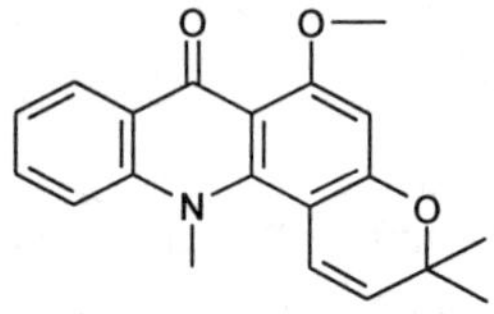

O O N O

103 Acrylic acid
$C_3H_4O_2$ MW: 72.06 Property: mp 13°C, bp 141°C. Source: SHI CHUN, SHUI SONG. Ref: 6.

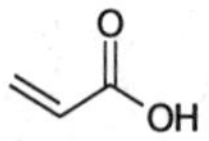

O OH

104 Acteoside
Verbascoside. $C_{29}H_{36}O_{15}$ MW: 624.60 Property: mp 142°C. Source: GAN DI HUANG, ROU CONG RONG. Ref: 2, 529, 628, 629.

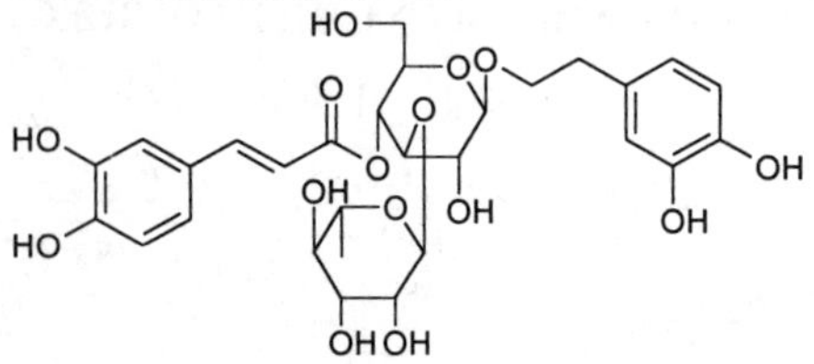

HO O O O O HO HO OH O OH OH OH OH OH

105 Actinidine
CAS: 62624-46-8 $C_{10}H_{13}N$ MW: 147.22 Property: mp (±):142-3°C, bp 100-3°C/9mm, $[\alpha]_D^{22}$ -7.2° (C=17.54, chloroform). Source: MI HOU LI, MI HOU TAO, MU TIAN LIAO, XIE CAO. Ref: 1, 4.

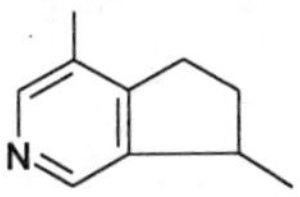

106 Actinodaphnine
$C_{18}H_{17}NO_4$ MW: 311.34 Property: mp (+): 210-1°C. Source: YUE GUI ZI. Ref: 6.

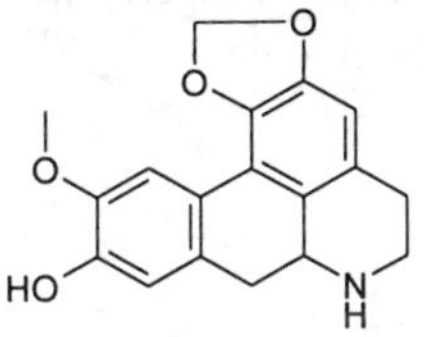

107 Aculcatin
$C_{16}H_{18}O_5$ MW: 290.32 Property: mp 113°C. Source: FEI LONG ZHANG XUE. Ref: 6.

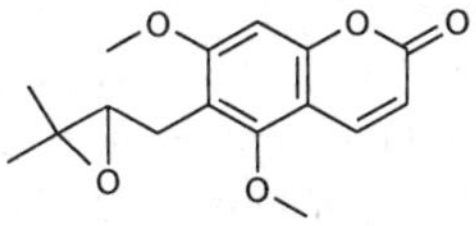

108 Acutifoliside
$C_{88}H_{140}O_{51}$ MW: 2014.07 Source: HUANG JIE GU DAN. Ref: 6.

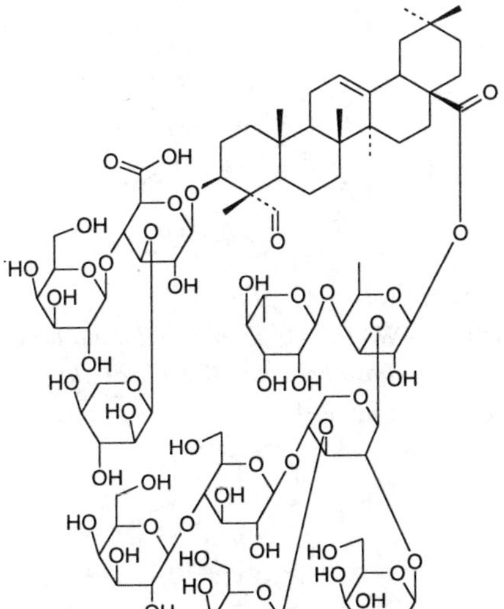

109 Acutumidine
$C_{18}H_{22}ClNO_6$ MW: 383.83 Property: mp 239-41°C (dec). Source: BIAN FU GE GEN, QING FENG TENG. Ref: 6.

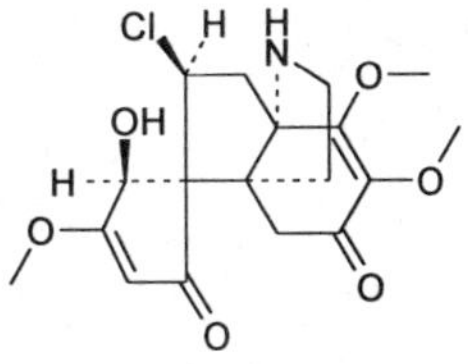

110 Acutumine
$C_{19}H_{24}ClNO_6$ MW: 397.86 Property: mp 238-40°C (dec). Source: BIAN FU GE, BIAN FU GE GEN, QING FENG TENG. Ref: 6.

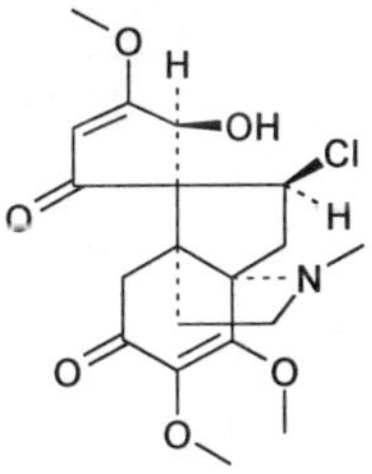

111 Acutuminine
$C_{19}H_{24}ClNO_5$ MW: 381.86 Property: mp 175-7°C. Source: BIAN FU GE, BIAN FU GE GEN. Ref: 6.

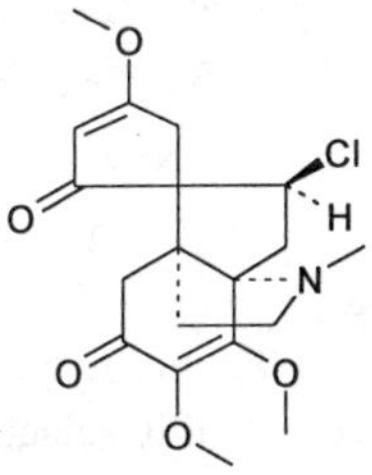

112 Adenosine
9-B-D-ribofuranosyl-9H-purin-6-amine; Adenine riboside. CAS: 58-61-7 $C_{10}H_{13}N_5O_4$ MW: 267.25 Property: mp 235-6°C, soluble in water. Source: (AN HUI) BEU MU, (GAN SU) BEI MU, CHANG CHUN HUA, DA QING YE, MA BIAN CAO, PING BEI MU, REN SHEN, ZHE BEI MU. Ref: 2, 569.

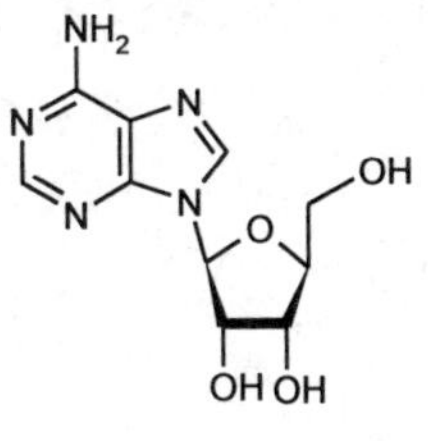

113 5'-Adenosine monophosphate
$C_{10}H_{14}N_5O_7P$ MW: 347.23 Property: mp 195°C. Source: MO GU. Ref: 6.

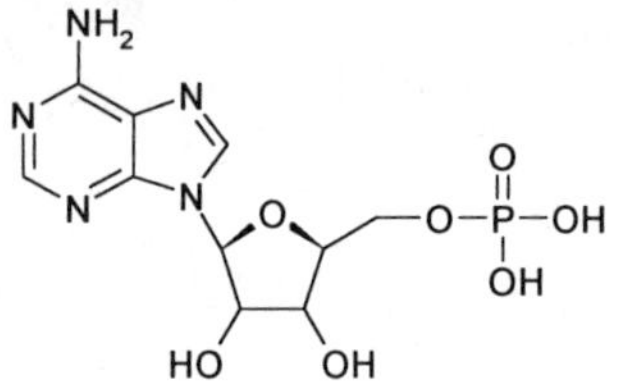

114 Adenosine triphosphate
$C_{10}H_{16}N_5O_{13}P_3$ MW: 507.19 Source: HA SHI MA LU RONG, QING WA, REN SHEN. Ref: 2, 6.

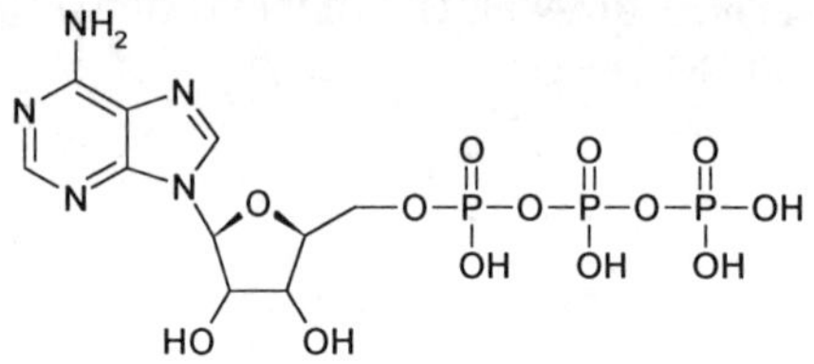

115 Adhatodine
$C_{20}H_{21}N_3O_2$ MW: 335.41 Property: mp 183°C. Source: DA BO GU. Ref: 6.

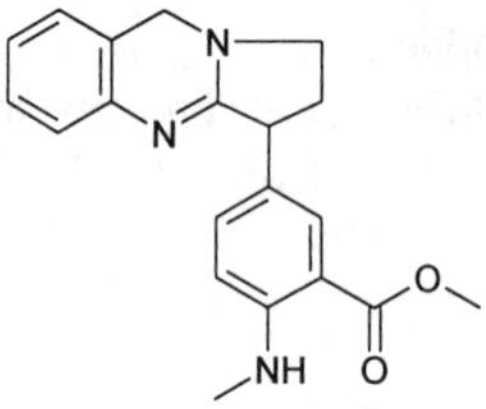

116 Adiantifoline
$C_{42}H_{50}N_2O_9$ MW: 726.87 Property: Dark yellow acicular crystal (alcohol), thin acicular crystal (alcohol-ether), mp 142-3°C, dark yellow needle crystal (anhydrous alcohol), mp 143.5-4°C, $[\alpha]_D^{28}$ +90° (C=0.11, methanol). Source: HE NAN TANG SONG CAO. Ref: 1, 537.

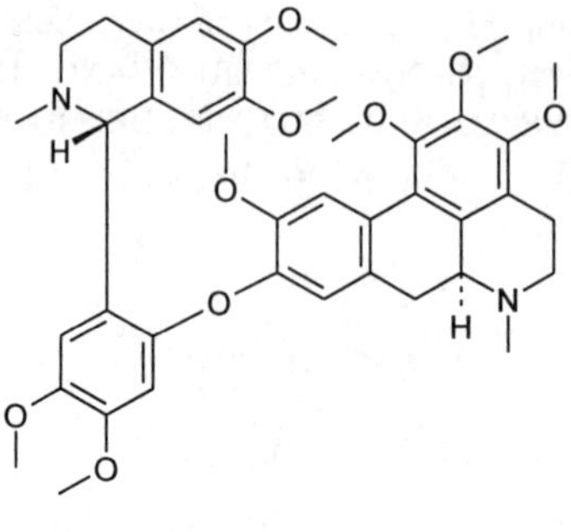

117 Adiantone
$C_{29}H_{48}O$ MW: 412.71 Property: mp 222-4°C. Source: BIAN YE TIE XIAN JUE, GUAN ZHONG, TIE SI QI, ZHU ZONG CAO. Ref: 6.

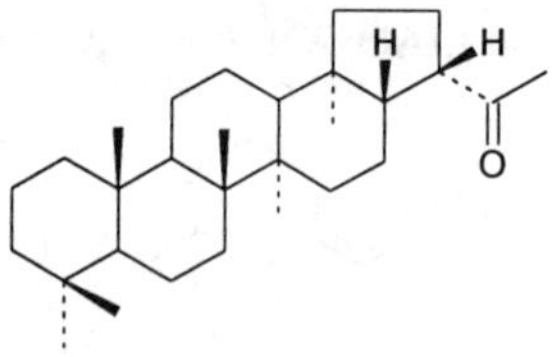

118 Adipedatol
$C_{29}H_{48}O_2$ MW: 428.70 Property: mp 185-8°C. Source: TIE SI QI. Ref: 6.

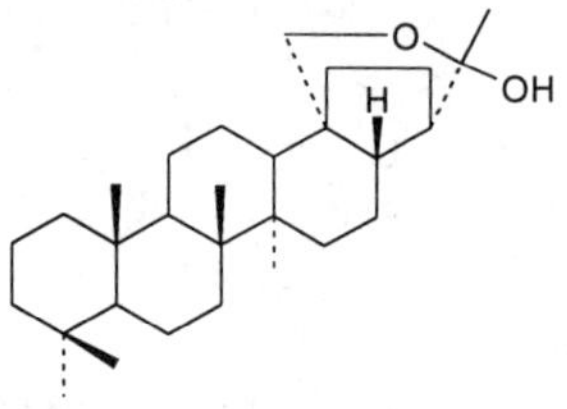

119 Adlumidine
$C_{20}H_{17}NO_6$ MW: 367.36 Property: orthogonal lamellar crystal (chloroform-methanol), mp 236-8°C, $[\alpha]_D^{25}$ + 116.2° (C=22, chloroform), almost insoluble in water, very slightly soluble in alcohol, ether and ethane. Source: XIA TIAN WU, ZI HUA YU DENG CAO (LIE BAO ZI JING). Ref: 1, 6.

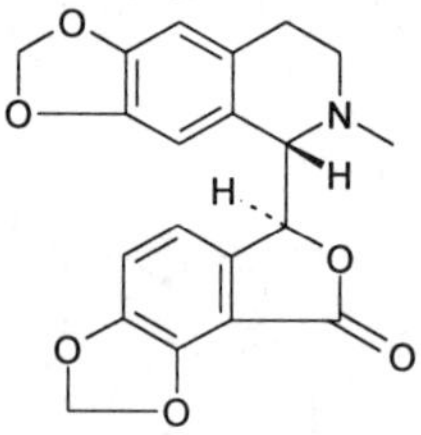

120 Adlumine
$C_{21}H_{21}NO_6$ MW: 383.40 Source: *Adlumia fungoss* Greene (*A. cirrhosa kom. non* Raf.), *Corydalis lineariodes* Maxim. Ref: 1.

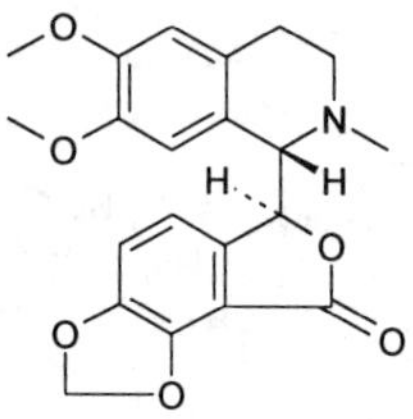

121 Adonilide
$C_{21}H_{28}O_4$ MW: 344.45 Property: mp 268-70°C. Source: FU SHOU CAO. Ref: 6.

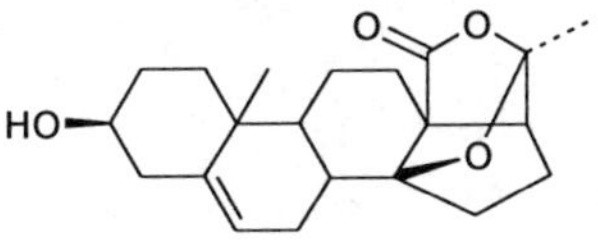

122 Adonitol
CAS: 488-81-3 $C_5H_{12}O_5$ MW: 152.15 Property: mp 104°C, soluble in water and ethanol. Source: CHAI HU, JI CAI. Ref: 2.

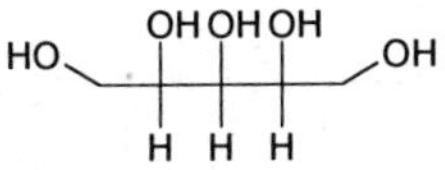

123 Adouetine X
$C_{28}H_{44}N_4O_4$ MW: 500.69 Property: mp 277-9°C. Source: HE TA CAO. Ref: 6.

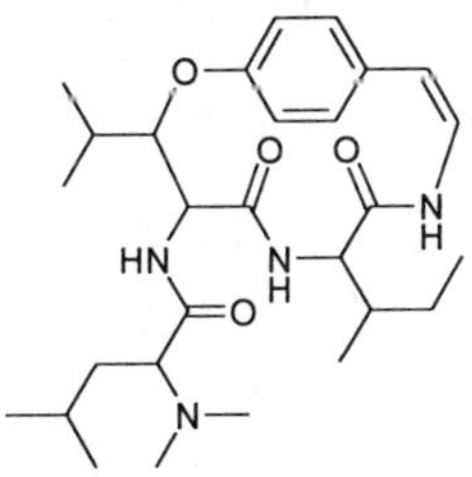

124 Adouetine Y
$C_{34}H_{40}N_4O_4$ MW: 568.72 Property: mp 292°C. Source: HE TA CAO. Ref: 6.

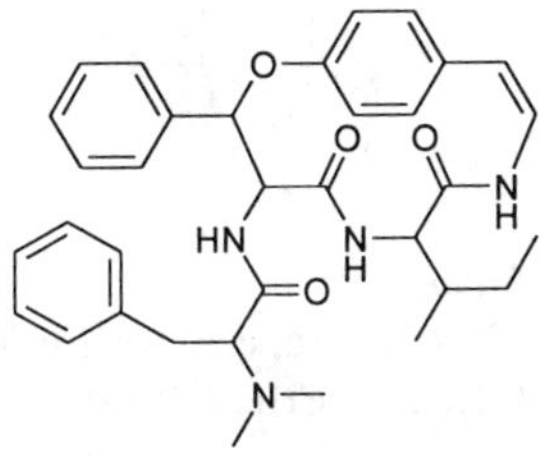

125 Adouetine Y'
$C_{31}H_{42}N_4O_4$ MW: 534.70 Property: mp 289.0-290.5°C. Source: HE TA CAO. Ref: 6.

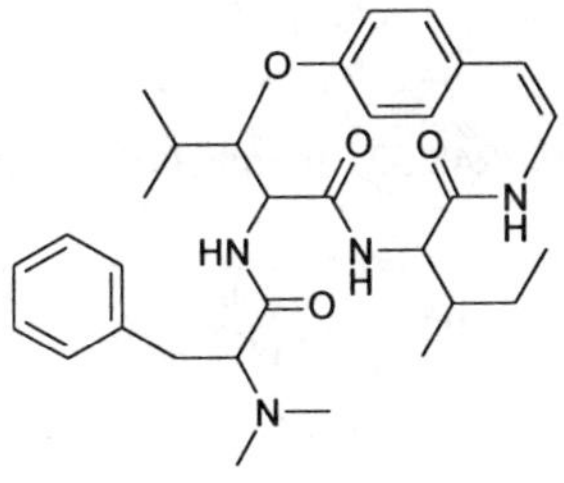

126 Adouetine Z
$C_{42}H_{45}N_5O_5$ MW: 699.86 Property: mp 140-5°C. Source: HE TA CAO. Ref: 1, 6.

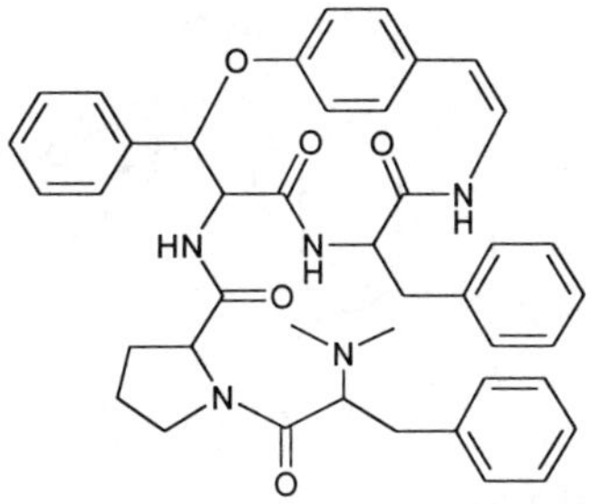

127 Adrenaline(*l*)
l-Epinephrine CAS: 51-43-4 $C_9H_{13}NO_3$ MW: 183.21 Property: mp 211-2°C, soluble in acetic acid. Source: NIU SHEN, JIN YU, WEI NAO, WEI XIN GAN, CHAN SU. Ref: 6.

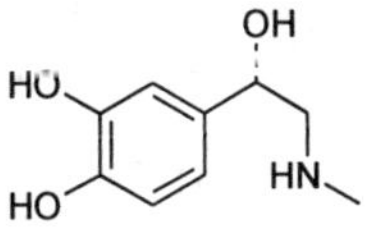

128 Adynerin
$C_{30}H_{44}O_7$ MW: 516.68 Property: mp 234°C. Source: JIA ZHU TAO. Ref: 6.

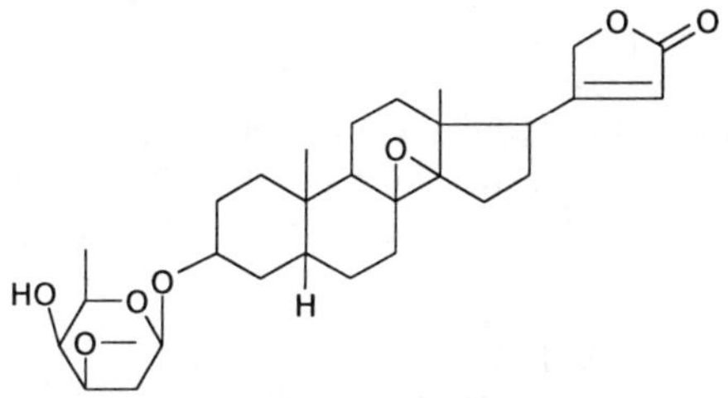

129 Aeginetic acid
$C_{15}H_{24}O_4$ MW: 268.36 Property: mp 205°C. Source: YE GU. Ref: 6.

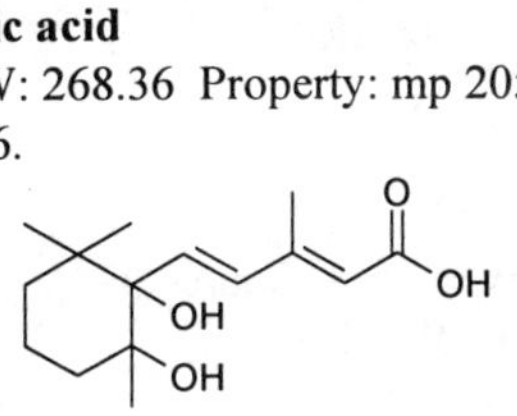

130 Aeginetolide
$C_{11}H_{18}O_3$ MW: 198.26 Property: mp 169-70°C. Source: YE GU. Ref: 6.

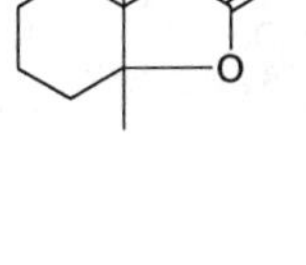

131 Aescigenin
$C_{30}H_{48}O_5$ MW: 488.71 Property: mp 307°C, 317-8°C. Source: SUO LUO ZI. Ref: 6.

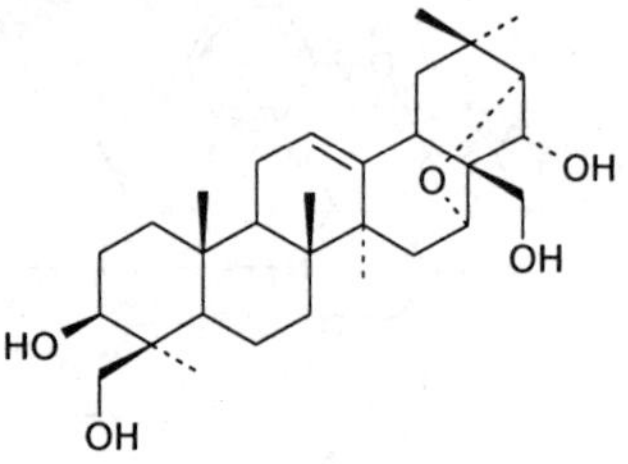

132 Aesculetin
Cichorigenin; Esculetin. CAS: 305-01-1 $C_9H_6O_4$ MW: 178.15 Source: FEI CAI, JU QU, LONG YAN DU HUO, NING MENG YE, PI HAN CAO, QIN PI. Ref: 4, 6, 572.

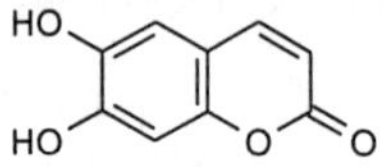

133 Aesculetin dimethylether
Esculetin-6,7-dimethylether. $C_{11}H_{10}O_4$ MW: 206.20 Property: mp 144°C. Source: YE HUA JIAO YE. Ref: 6.

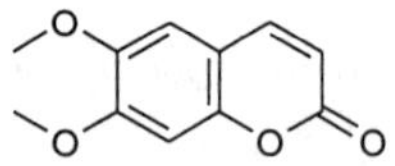

134 Aesculin
Bicoloirin; Enullachromw; Escosyl; Esculin; Esculoside; Polychrome. CAS: 531-75-9 $C_{15}H_{16}O_9$ MW: 340.29 Source: JU QU, QIN PI, PI HAN CAO. Ref: 4, 6.

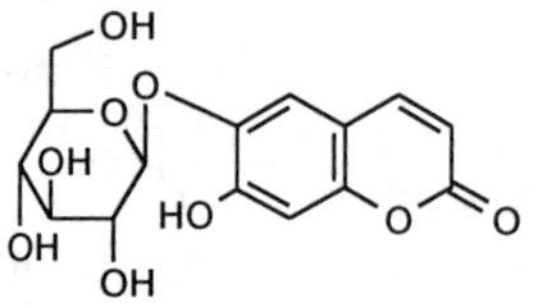

135 Afzelin
$C_{21}H_{20}O_{10}$ MW: 432.39 Source: DA JIN NIU CAO, YU XING CAO. Ref: 2, 6.

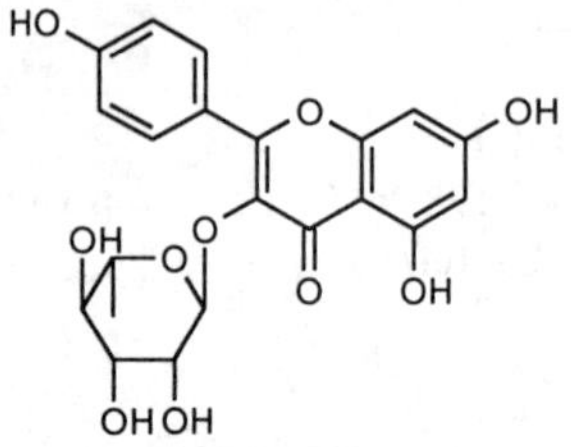

136 Agaricic acid
$C_{22}H_{40}O_7$ MW: 416.56 Property: mp 142°C (dec). Source: SANG HUANG. Ref: 6.

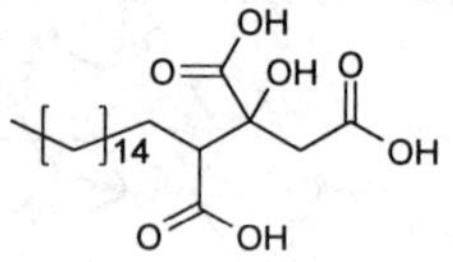

137 Agaritine
β-N-[γ-L-(+)-Glutamoyl]-p-hydroxymethylphenyl hydrazine. $C_{12}H_{17}N_3O_4$ MW: 267.29 Property: mp 205-9°C (dec). Source: MO GU. Ref: 6.

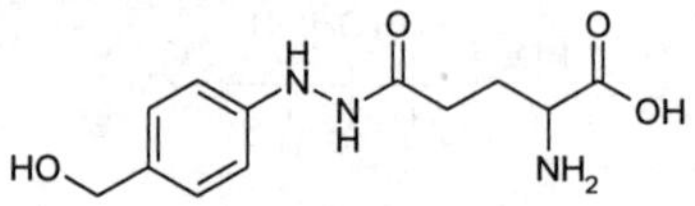

138 Agarobiose dimethylacetal
$C_{14}H_{26}O_{11}$ MW: 370.36 Property: bp 155-6°C/0.052mm. Source: LU JIAO CAI. Ref: 6.

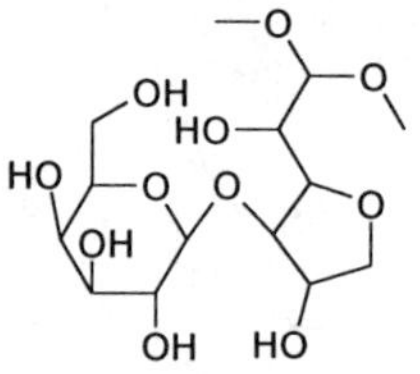

139 α-Agarofuran
$C_{15}H_{24}O$ MW: 220.36 Property: bp 134°C /6mm. Source: CHEN XIANG. Ref: 6, 16.

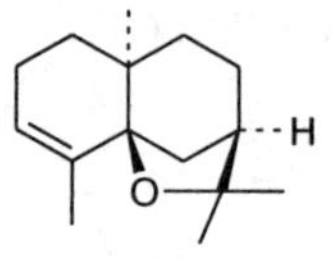

140 β-Agarofuran
$C_{15}H_{24}O$ MW: 220.36 Property: bp 130°C /8mm. Source: BAI MU XIANG, CHEN XIANG. Ref: 6, 13.

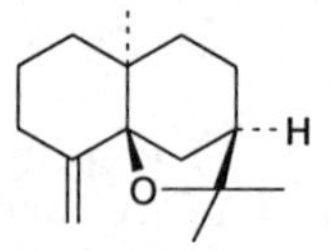

141 Agarol
$C_{15}H_{20}O_3$ MW: 248.32 Source: CHEN XIANG. Ref: 13.

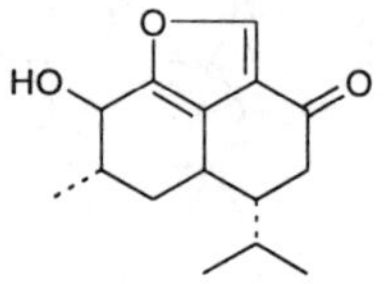

142 Agarospirol

$C_{15}H_{26}O$ MW: 222.37 Property: bp 90-1.0°C/0.1mm. Source: BAI MU XIANG, CHEN XIANG. Ref: 13.

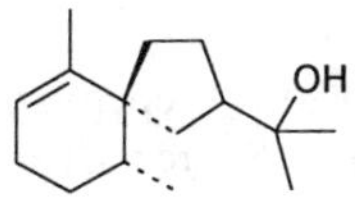

143 Agarotetrol (AH1)

$C_{17}H_{18}O_6$ MW: 318.33 Property: colourless acicular crystal, mp 179-81°C, $[\alpha]_D^{24}$ -21.3C°. Source: CHEN XIANG. Ref: 13.

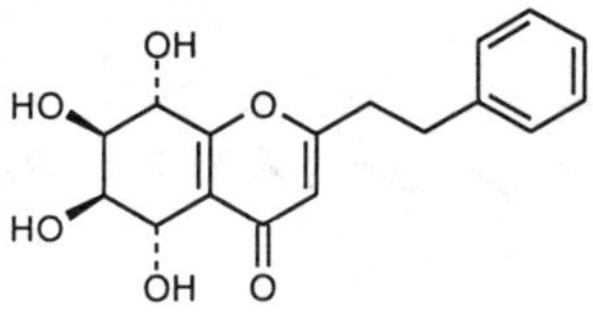

144 Agastachin

$C_{47}H_{48}O_{22}$ MW: 964.89 Source: HUO XIANG. Ref: 2.

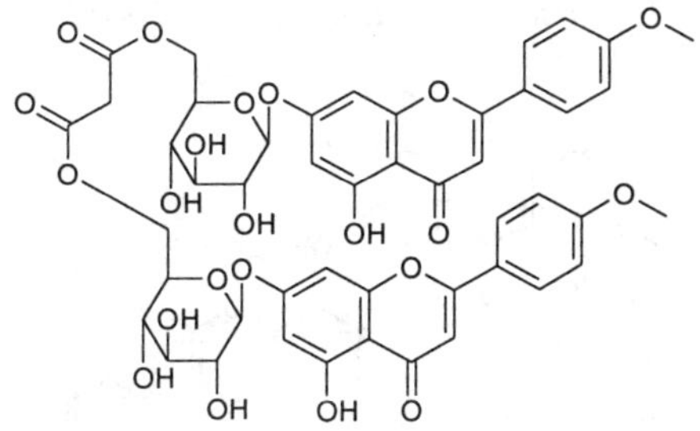

145 Agastachoside

$C_{24}H_{26}O_{11}$ MW: 490.47 Source: HUO XIANG. Ref: 2, 7.

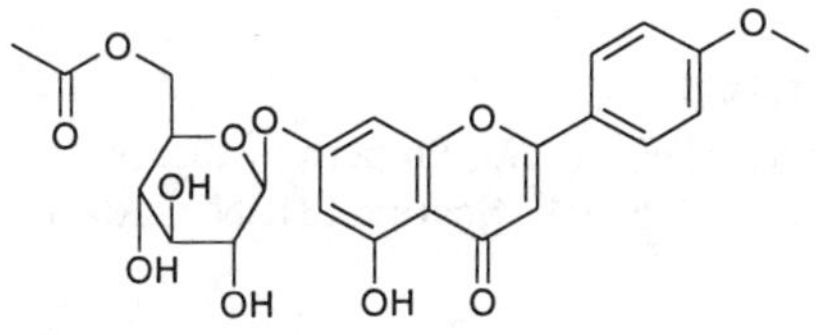

146 Agathodienediol

$C_{20}H_{34}O_2$ MW: 306.49 Property: mp 107-8°C. Source: HAI SONG ZI. Ref: 6

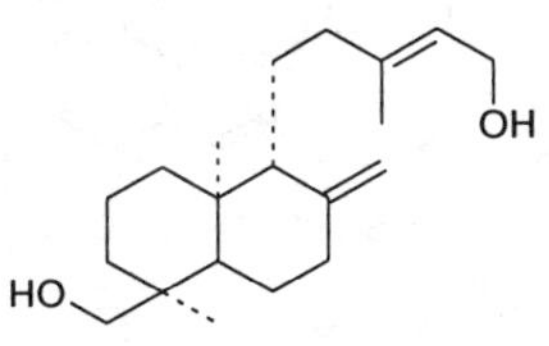

147 Aglaiol

$C_{30}H_{50}O_2$ MW: 442.73 Property: mp 113-4°C. Source: MI ZI LAN. Ref: 6.

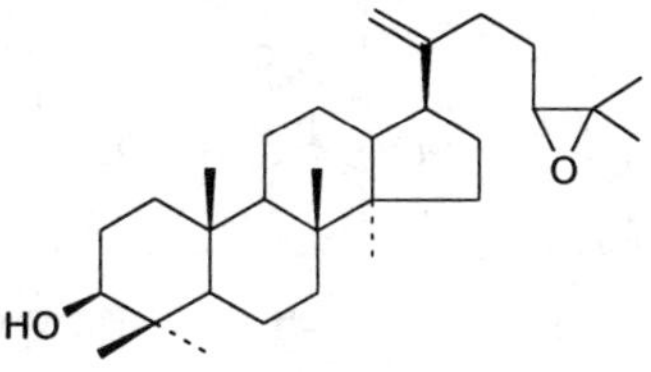

148 Agmatine

$C_5H_{14}N_4$ MW: 130.19 Source: MAI JIAO. Ref: 6.

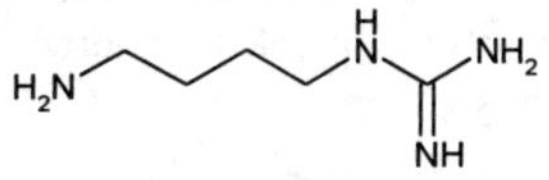

149 (R)-(-)-agrimol B

$C_{37}H_{46}O_{12}$ MW: 682.77 Property: yellow acicular crystal, mp 173-5°C, $[\alpha]_D^{19}$ -3.3° (c=1, $CHCl_3$). Source: XIAN HE CAO. Ref: 129.

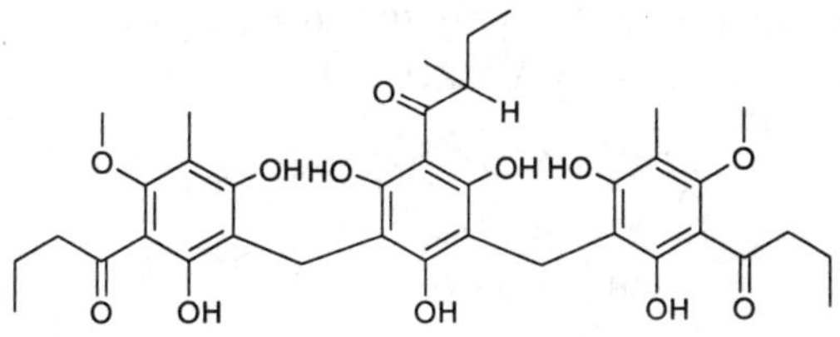

150 Agrimol C

$C_{36}H_{44}O_{12}$ MW: 668.75 Source: XIAN HE CAO. Ref: 2.

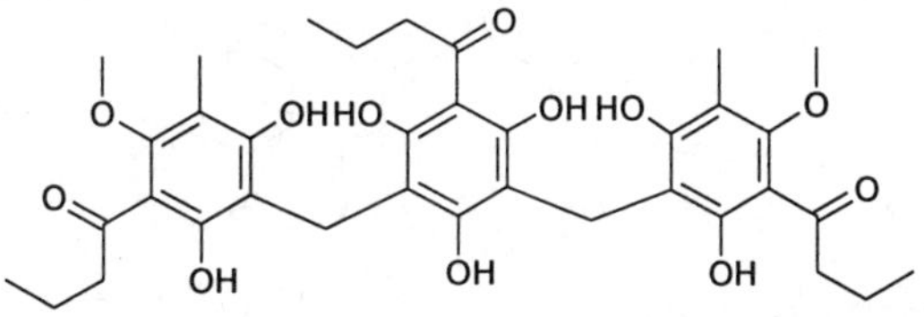

151 Agrimol F

$C_{34}H_{40}O_{12}$ MW: 640.69 Source: XIAN HE CAO. Ref: 2.

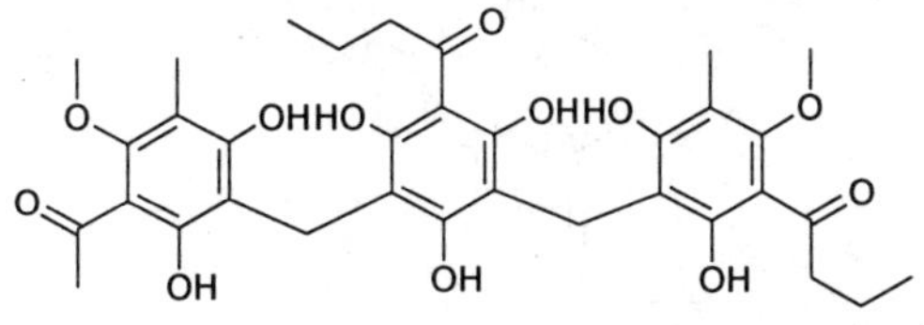

152 Agrimol G
$C_{36}H_{44}O_{12}$ MW: 668.75 Source: XIAN HE CAO. Ref: 2.

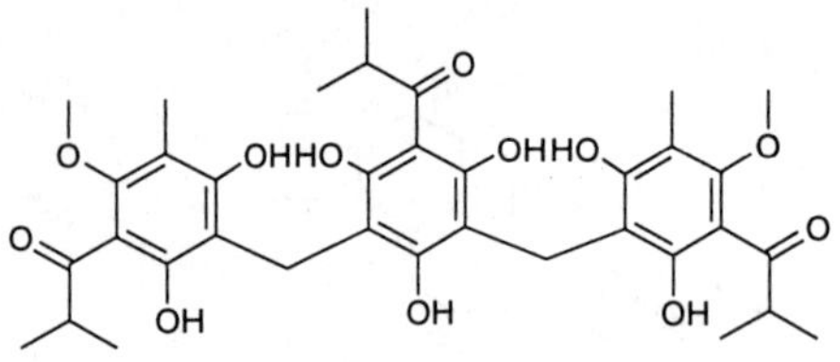

154 Agrimonolide
$C_{18}H_{18}O_5$ MW: 314.34 Property: colorless columnar crystal, mp 173-5°C, $[\alpha]_D^{18}$ +8.1°. Source: XIAN HE CAO. Ref: 1, 2, 5.

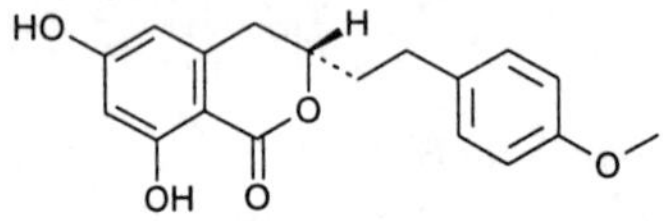

155 Agrimonolide-6-O-β-D-glucopyranoside
$C_{24}H_{28}O_{10}$ MW: 476.48 Property: white acicular crystals, mp 165-7°C, $[\alpha]_D^{14}$ -30.8° (c=1, Me_2CO). Source: XIAN HE CAO. Ref: 144.

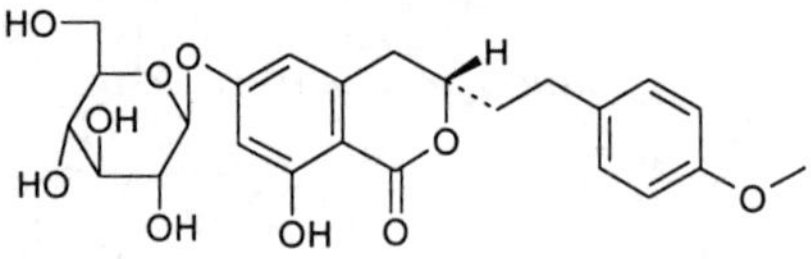

156 Agrimophol(um)
$C_{26}H_{34}O_5$ MW: 474.55 Property: mp 138.4-9.5°C. Source: XIAN HE CAO, XIAN HE CAO GEN YA. Ref: 1, 2, 4, 5, 6.

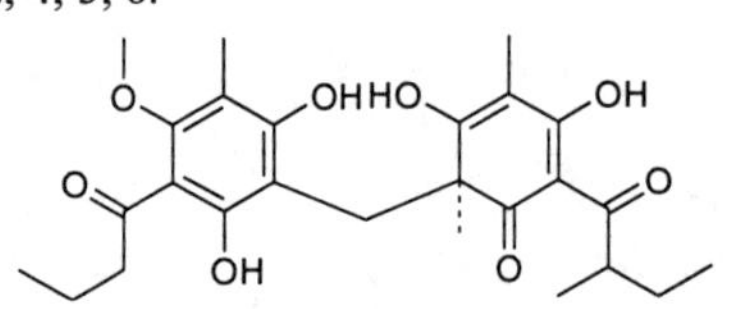

157 Agroclavine
$C_{16}H_{18}N_2$ MW: 238.34 Property: mp 203°C (dec). Source: MAI JIAO. Ref: 1, 6.

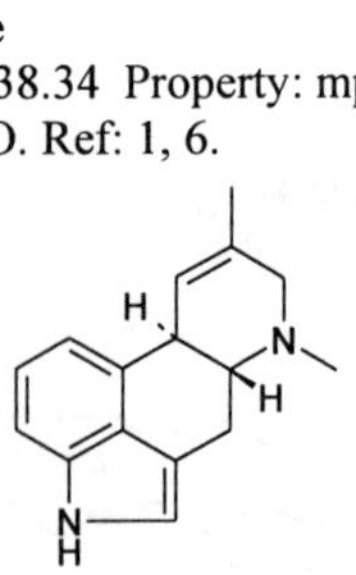

158 Agropyrene
$C_{12}H_{12}$ MW: 156.23 Property: bp 140-3°C/10mm. Source: YIN CHEN HAO. Ref: 6.

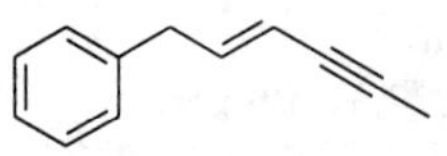

159 AH18
$C_{51}H_{46}O_{14}$ MW: 882.93 Property: white powder, mp 147-8°C, $[\alpha]_D$ -109.1°. Source: CHEN XIANG. Ref: 13.

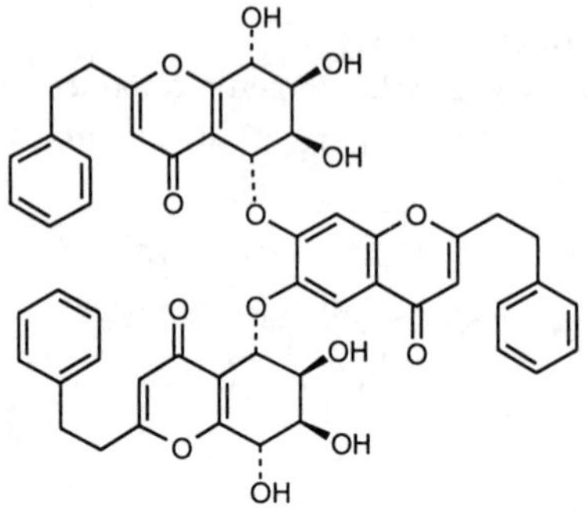

160 AH19a
$C_{51}H_{46}O_{14}$ MW: 882.93 Property: white powder, mp165-7°C, $[\alpha]_D$ -33.89°. Source: CHEN XIANG. Ref: 13.

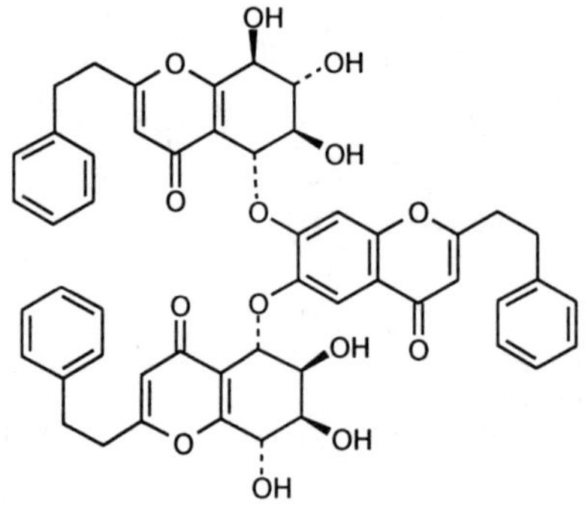

161 AH19 b
$C_{51}H_{46}O_{14}$ MW: 882.93 Property: white powder, mp 130-3°C, $[\alpha]_D$ -64.04°. Source: CHEN XIANG. Ref: 13.

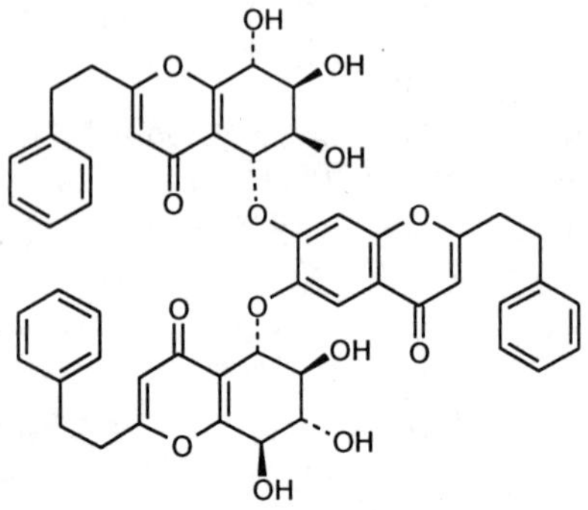

162 AH20

$C_{51}H_{46}O_{14}$ MW: 882.93 Property: white powder, mp 143-5°C, $[\alpha]_D$ -27.83°. Source: CHEN XIANG. Ref: 13.

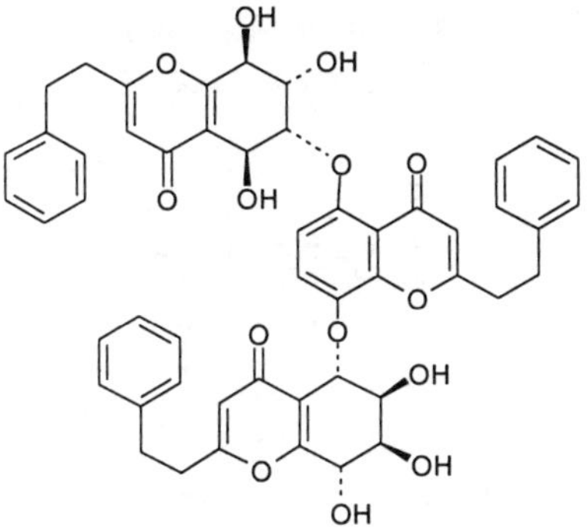

163 AH21

$C_{34}H_{28}O_8$ MW: 564.60 Property: white powder, mp 123-5°C, $[\alpha]_D$ -75.2°. Source: CHEN XIANG. Ref: 13.

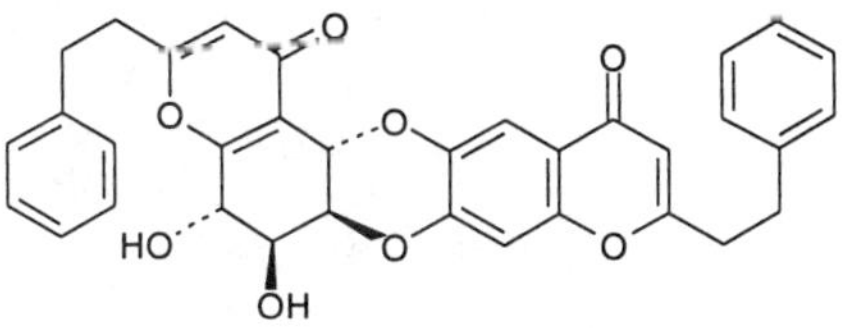

164 Ailanthone

$C_{20}H_{24}O_7$ MW: 376.41 Property: mp 234-8°C. Source: CHU BAI PI. Ref: 6.

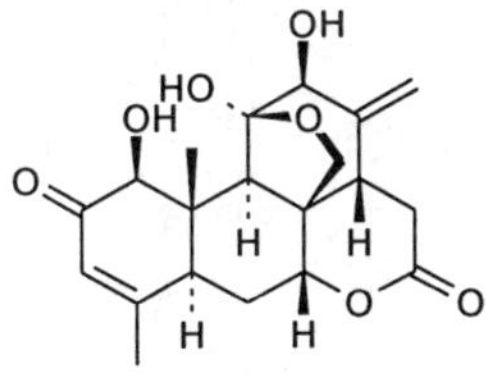

165 Ailanthinone

$C_{25}H_{34}O_9$ MW: 478.51 Property: Acicular crystal (acetone-ethane), mp 227-30°C, $[\alpha]_D^{27}$ +90° (C= 0.10, chloroform). Source: Bark of *Ailanthus altissima* (Mill.) Swingle, *A. excelsa* Roxb., *Pierreodendron kerstingii* Little. Ref: 1,5.

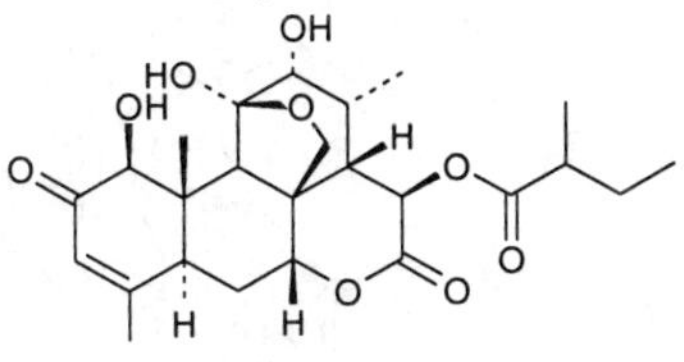

166 Ajacine

$C_{34}H_{48}N_2O_9$ MW: 628.77 Property: acicular crystal (70% alcohol), mp 154°C, $[\alpha]_D^{22}$ +49.5° (C=2, anhydrous alcohol), $[\alpha]_D^{16}$ +53° (C=0.66, chloroform). Source: FEI YAN CAO. Ref: 1, 6.

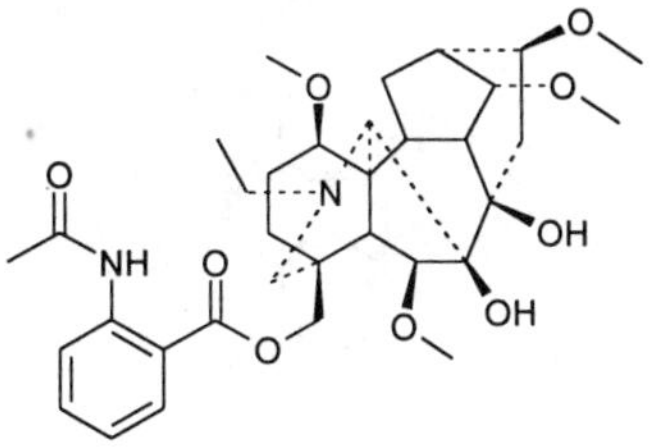

167 Ajaconine

$C_{22}H_{33}NO_3$ MW: 359.51 Property: prismatic crystal (dilute alcohol), mp 172°C, $[\alpha]_D^{18}$ -119° (C=2, anhydrous alcohol)[2], mp 167°C, $[\alpha]_D$ -122° (C= 1.75). Source: FEI YAN CAO. Ref: 1, 6.

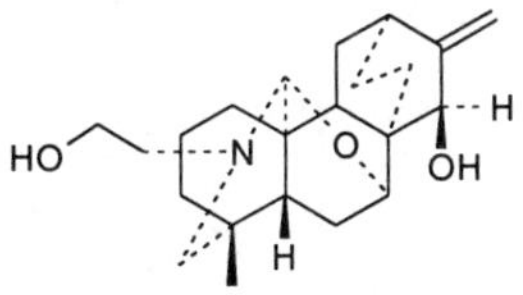

168 Ajmalicine

Tetrahydrosertpentine. $C_{21}H_{24}N_2O_3$ MW: 352.44 Property: prismatic crystal (methanol), mp 257°C (dec), $[\alpha]_D^{20}$ -60° (C=0.5, $CHCl_3$), $[\alpha]_D^{20}$ -45° (C=0.5, pyridine), $[\alpha]_D^{20}$ -39° (C=0.25, methanol). Source: CHANG CHUN HUA, LUO FU MU. Ref: 1, 2, 6.

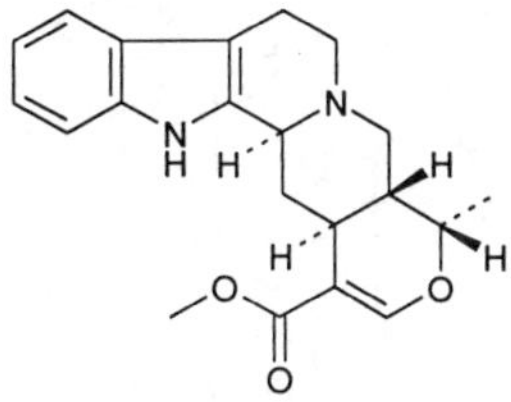

169 Ajmaline

$C_{20}H_{26}N_2O_2$ MW: 326.44 Property: mp 205-7° C. Source: LUO FU MU. Ref: 1, 6.

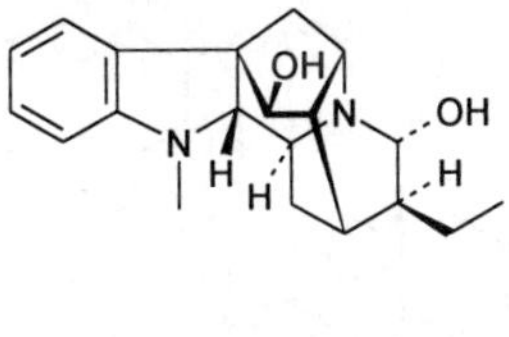

170 Ajuforrestin A
12,16-Epoxy-11,14-dihydroxy-3,5,8,11,13,15-abietahexaene-7-one. $C_{20}H_{20}O_4$ MW: 324.38 Property: red brown crystal, mp 245-8°C, $[\alpha]_D^{28}$ -51.5° (chloroform). Source: LI ZHI HAO. Ref: 319.

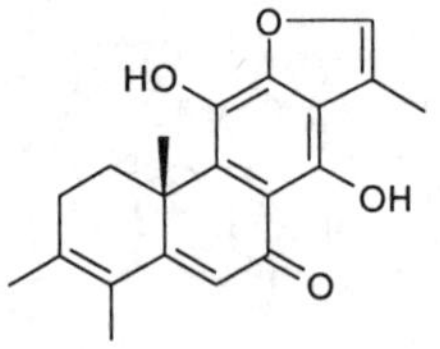

171 Ajuforrestin B
12,16-epoxy-11,14-dihydroxy-3,5,8,11,13-abietapentaene-7-one. $C_{20}H_{22}O_4$ MW: 326.40 Property: yellow crystal, mp 182-5°C, $[\alpha]_D^{28}$ -61.8° (chloroform). Source: LI ZHI HAO. Ref: 319.

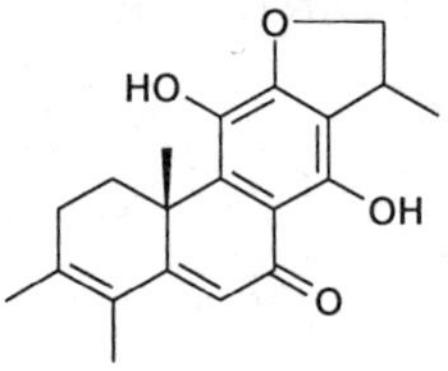

172 Ajugalactone
$C_{29}H_{40}O_8$ MW: 516.64 Property: mp 225-35 °C (dec). Source: BAI MAO XIA KU CAO. Ref: 6.

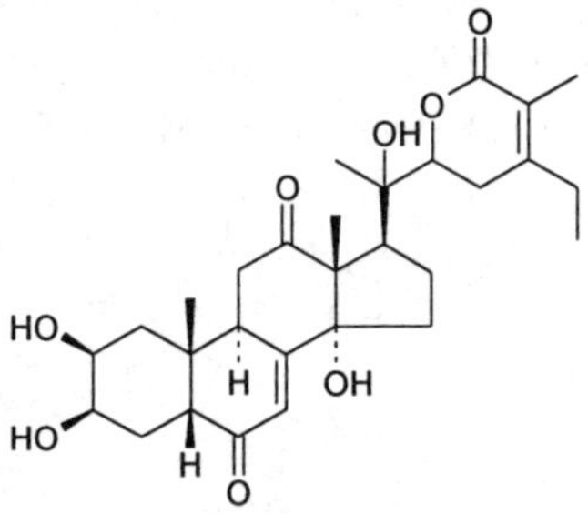

173 Ajugasterone C
$C_{27}H_{44}O_7$ MW: 480.65 Source: BAI MAO XIA KU CAO. Ref: 6.

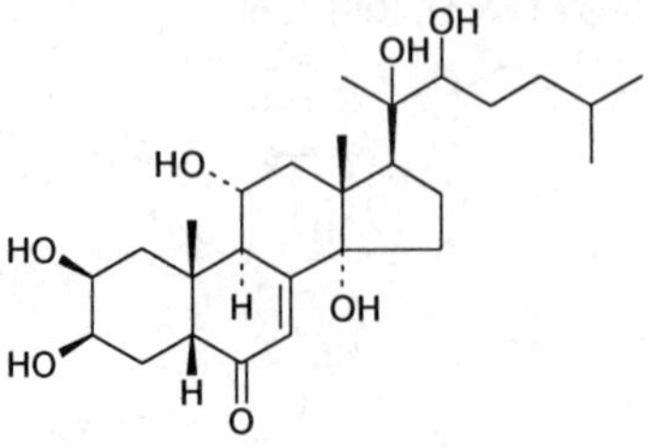

174 Ajugol
Source: GAN DI HUANG. Ref: 7.

175 Ajugoside
$C_{17}H_{26}O_{10}$ MW: 390.39 Source: GAN DI HUANG, DU ZHONG, XIAN DI HUANG. Ref: 2, 7.

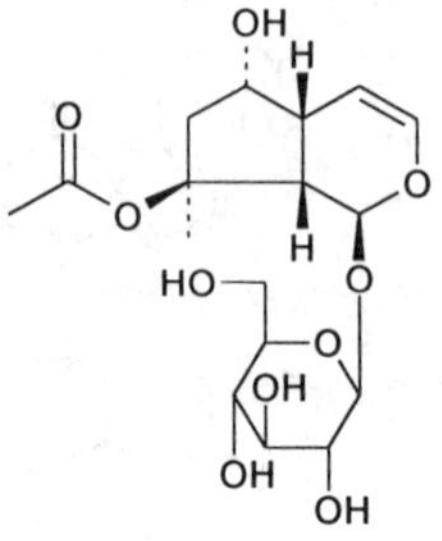

176 Akeboside st$_h$
$C_{59}H_{96}O_{25}$ MW: 1205.41 Property: mp 221-2°C (dec). Source: MU TONG, MU TONG GEN. Ref: 6.

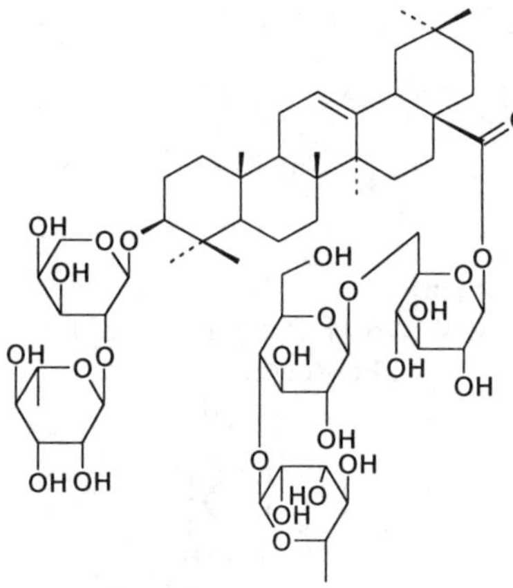

177 Akeboside st$_j$
$C_{65}H_{106}O_{30}$ MW: 1367.55 Property: mp 224-6°C (dec). Source: MU TONG, MU TONG GEN. Ref: 6.

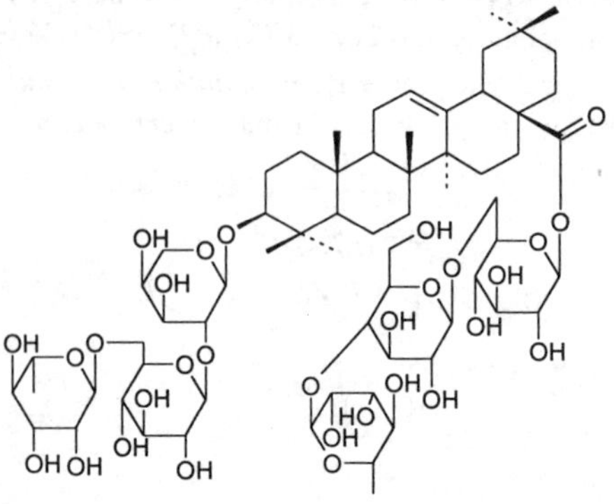

178 Akuammicine
$C_{20}H_{24}N_2O_2$ MW: 324.43 Source: CHANG CHUN HUA, GOU TENG. Ref: 2.

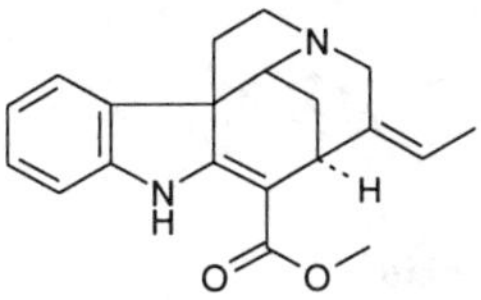

179 19-(Z)-Akuammidine
$C_{21}H_{24}N_2O_3$ MW: 354.24 Property: mp 247-50°C, $[\alpha]_D$ +9°. Source: HU MAN TENG. Ref: 14.

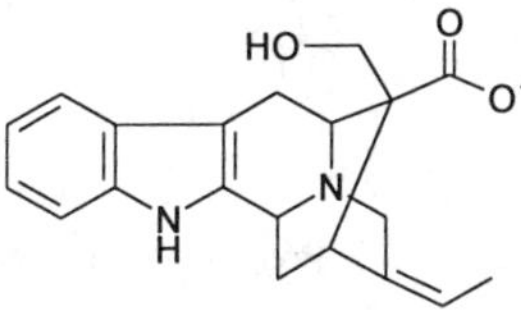

180 Akuammidine N-oxide
$C_{21}H_{24}N_2O_4$ MW: 368.44 Property: mp 250°C (dec) Source: HU MAN TENG. Ref: 14.

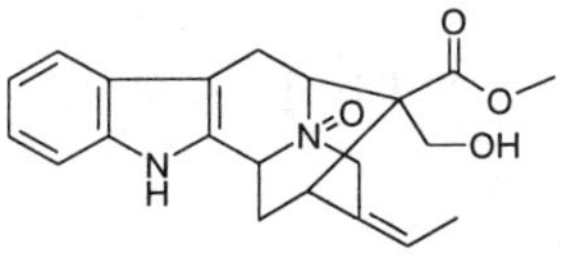

181 Alantolactone
Alant camphor; Elecampane camphor; Helenine; γ-Lactone. $C_{15}H_{20}O_2$ MW: 232.33 Property: mp 76-9°C, bp 275°C, soluble in benzene, diethyl ether, ethanol. Source: DI TANG HUA, KONG QUE CAO, MU XIANG, TU MU XIANG. Ref: 1, 2.

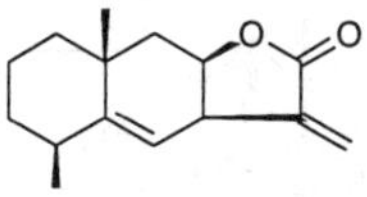

182 Alatolide
$C_{19}H_{26}O_8$ MW: 350.42 Property: mp 59-61°C, $[\alpha]_D^{25}$ +64.4°. Source: *Jurinea alata* Cass. Ref: 1.

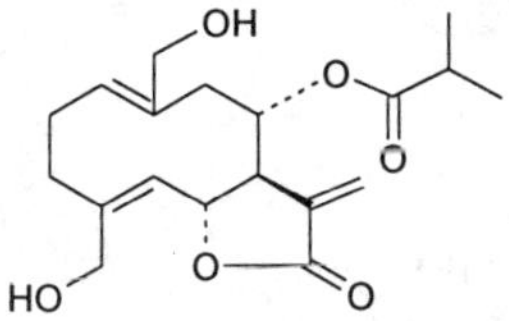

183 Albiflorin
$C_{24}H_{30}O_{11}$ MW: 494.50 Source: BAI SHAO YAO, CHI SHAO YAO. Ref: 2.

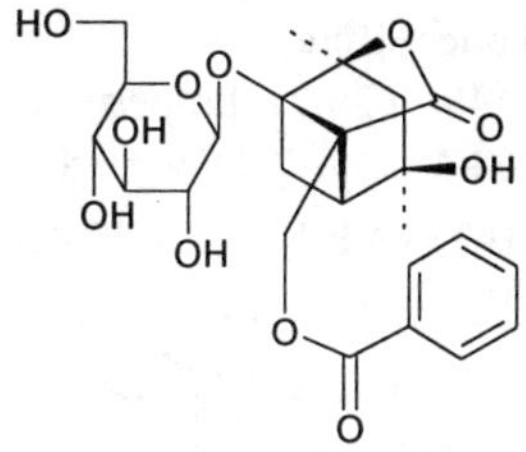

184 Albizzin
$C_4H_9N_3O_3$ MW: 147.13 Property: mp 214-5°C. Source: HE HUAN PI. Ref: 6.

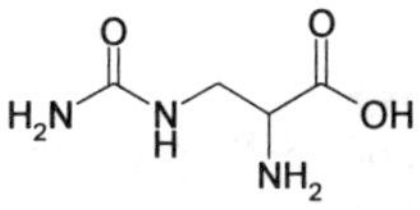

185 Albopetasin
$C_{20}H_{28}O_3$ MW: 316.44 Property: mp 106-7°C. Source: FENG DOU CAI. Ref: 6.

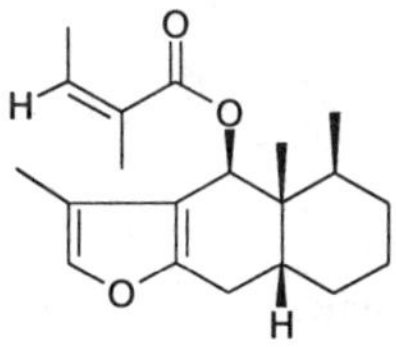

186 6-Aldehydo-isoophipogonone A
6,7-Dihydroxy-8-methyl-6-aldehydo-3-(3',4'-methylene dioxybenzyl) chromone. $C_{19}H_{14}O_7$ MW: 354.32 Property: orange acicular crystal, mp 170-2°C. Source: MAI DONG. Ref: 83.

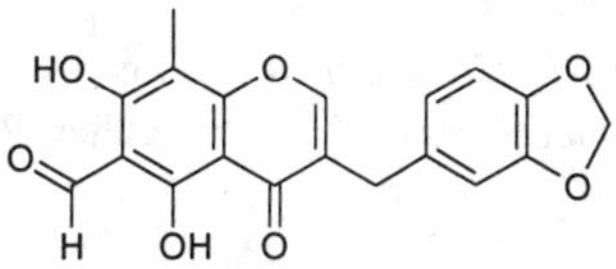

187 6-Aldehydo-isoophipogonone B
5,7-Dihydroxy-8-methyl-6-aldehydo-3-(4'-methoxy-benzyl) chromone. $C_{19}H_{16}O_6$ MW: 340.34 Property: light red acicular crystal, mp 144-5°C. Source: MAI DONG. Ref: 83.

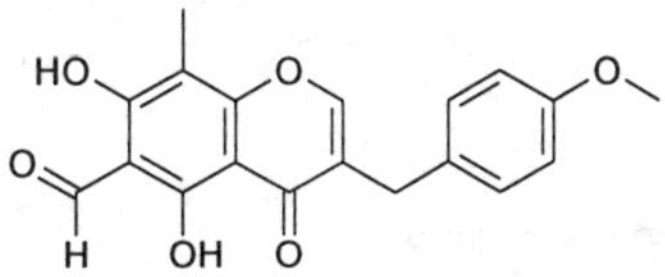

188 Aldohypaconitine
$C_{33}H_{43}NO_{11}$ MW: 629.71 Property: white clustered crystal, mp 262-4°C, $[\alpha]_D^{20}$ -56.9° (c=0.30, $CHCl_3$). Source: E ZHANG YE FU ZI. Ref: 460.

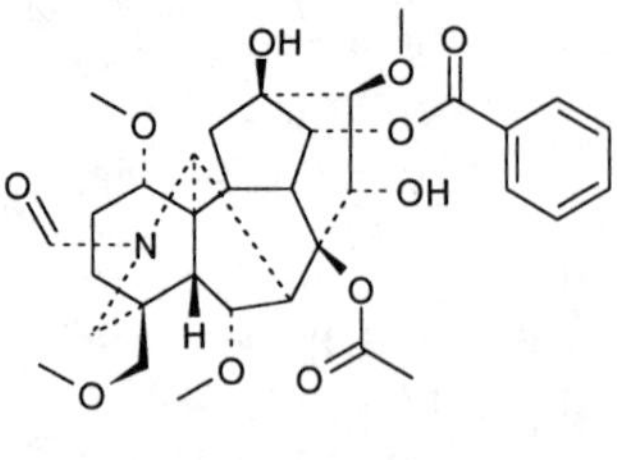

189 Aldosterone
$C_{21}H_{28}O_5$ MW: 360.45 Property: mp 164-9°C. Source: NIU SHEN. Ref: 6.

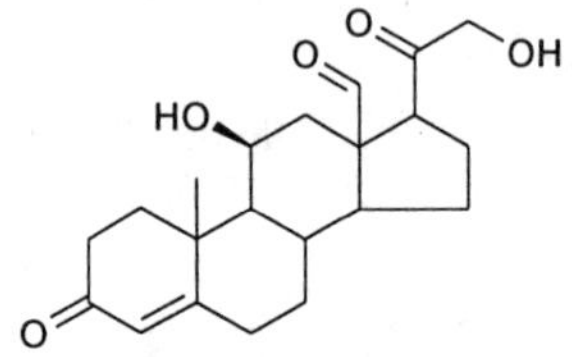

190 Aleprestic acid
$C_{10}H_{16}O_2$ MW: 168.24 Source: Seed of *Hydnocarpus anthelmintica* Pier. Ref: 1.

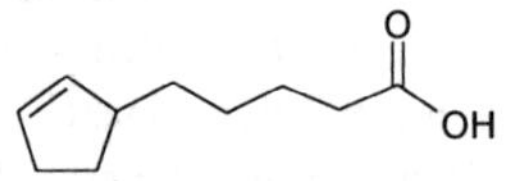

191 Alepric acid
$C_{14}H_{24}O_2$ MW: 224.35 Property: mp 48°C. Source: Seed of *Hydnocarpus anthelmintica* Pier. Ref: 1.

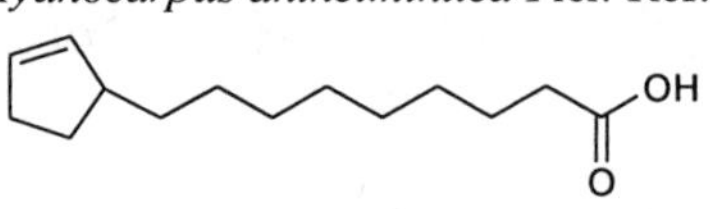

192 Aleprylic acid
$C_{12}H_{20}O_2$ MW: 196.29 Property: mp 32°C. Source: Seed of *Hydnocarpus anthelmintica* Pier. Ref: 1.

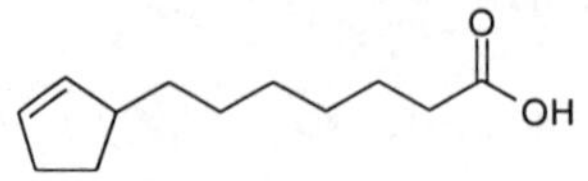

193 Alepterolic acid
$C_{20}H_{32}O_3$ MW: 320.48 Property: mp 162.5-63°C. Source: TONG JING CAO. Ref: 6.

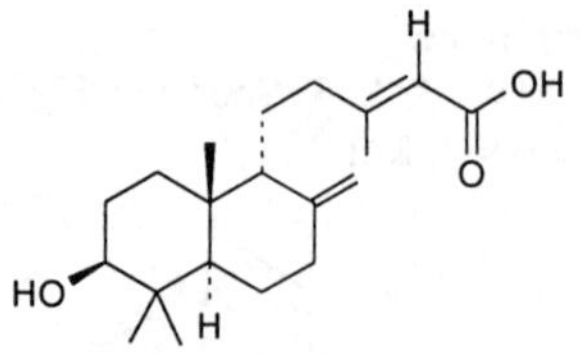

194 Aleuritic acid
$C_{16}H_{32}O_5$ MW: 304.43 Property: mp 102°C. Source: ZI CAO RONG. Ref: 6.

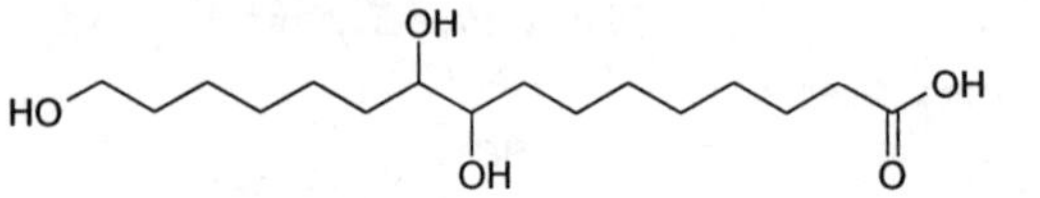

195 Alisol A
$C_{30}H_{50}O_5$ MW: 490.73 Property: mp 90-1°C. Source: ZE XIE. Ref: 1, 6.

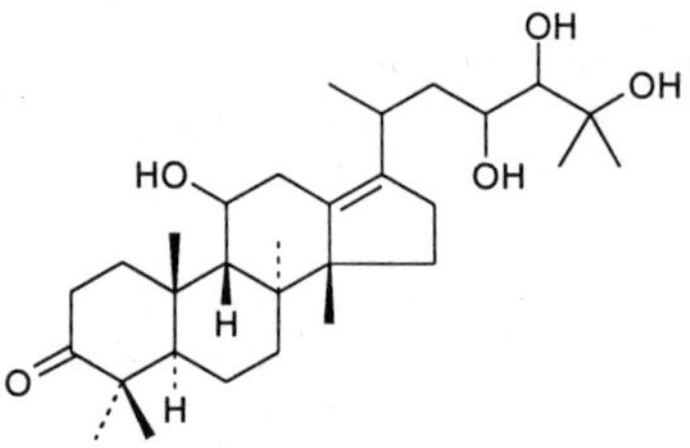

196 Alisol B
$C_{30}H_{48}O_4$ MW: 472.71 Property: mp 166-8°C. Source: ZE XIE. Ref: 6.

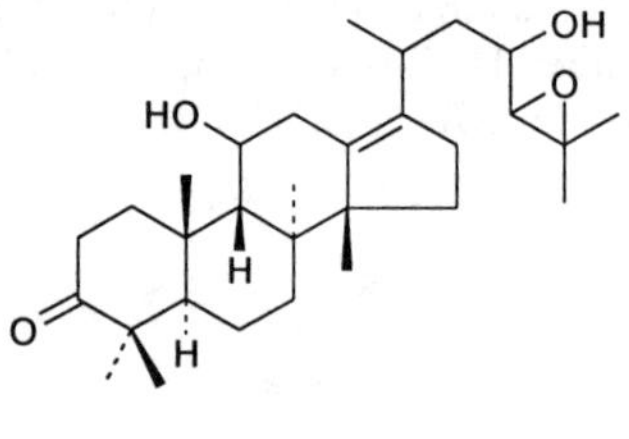

197 Alisol A monoacetate
$C_{32}H_{52}O_5$ MW: 514.75 Property: mp 194-6°C. Source: ZE XIE. Ref: 6.

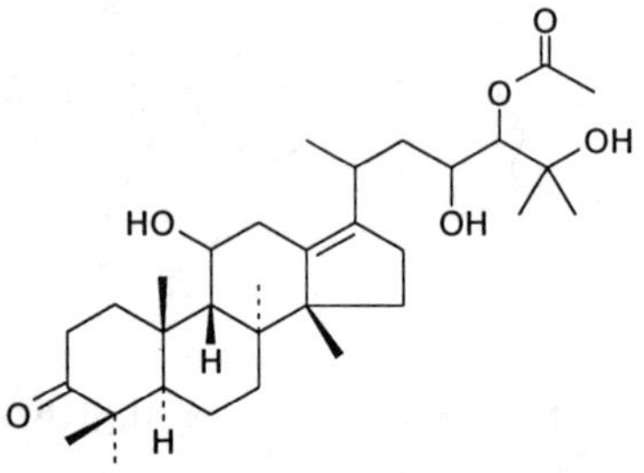

198 Alisol B monoacetate
$C_{32}H_{50}O_5$ MW: 514.75 Property: mp 162-3°C. Source: ZE XIE. Ref: 6.

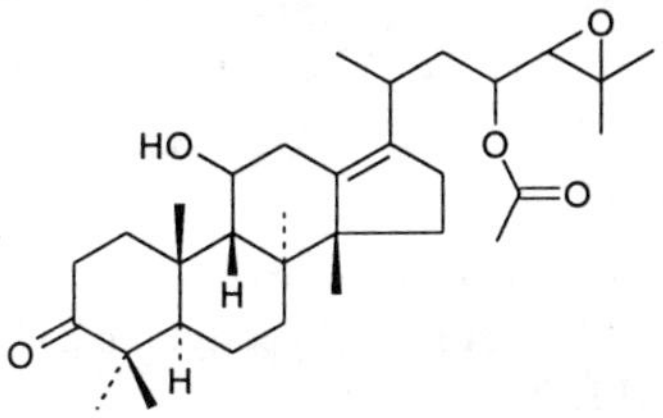

199 Alizarin
1,2-Dihydroxyanthraquinone; Alizarina. $C_{14}H_8O_4$ MW: 240.22 Property: mp 289-290°C, bp 430°C. Source: QIAN CAO, QIAN CAO GEN, YANG JIAO TENG. Ref: 1, 4, 6, 7.

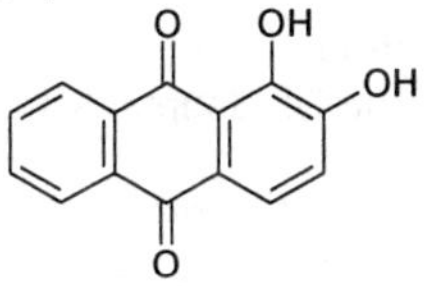

200 Alizarin 1-methylether
$C_{15}H_{10}O_4$ MW: 254.24 Property: mp 179°C. Source: YANG JIAO TENG, HU CI. Ref: 6.

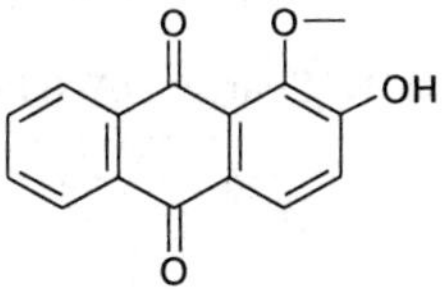

201 Alizarin 2-methylether
$C_{15}H_{10}O_4$ MW: 254.24 Property: mp 232-3°C. Source: YANG JIAO TENG. Ref: 6.

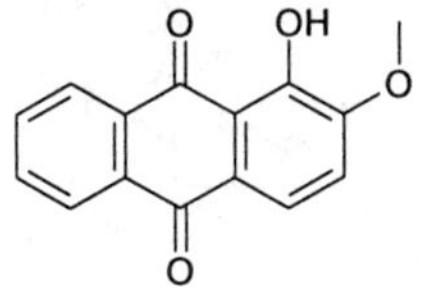

202 Alkannan
$C_{16}H_{18}O_4$ MW: 274.32 Source: ZI CAO. Ref: 2.

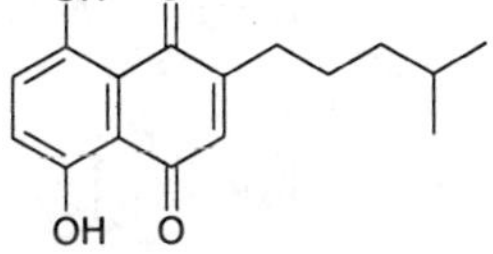

203 Alkannin angelate
$C_{21}H_{22}O_6$ MW: 370.41 Source: ZI CAO. Ref: 2.

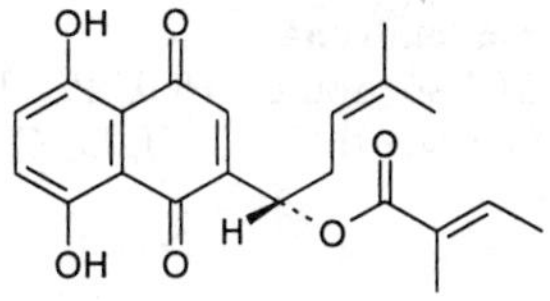

204 Allantoic acid
$C_4H_8N_4O_4$ MW: 176.13 Property: mp 173°C (dec). Source: ZI TENG. Ref: 6.

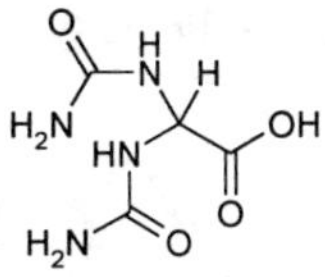

205 Allantoin
Glyoxyldiureide; Ureidohydantoin; 5-Ureido-hydantoin. CAS: 97-59-6 $C_4H_6N_4O_3$ MW: 158.12 Property: mp 238-40°C, soluble in water and ethanol, almost insoluble in diethyl ether. Source: GE GEN, QING MU XIANG, SHE XIANG, XIAO MAI, YAO YONG DAO TI HU, ZI TENG. Ref: 2, 4.

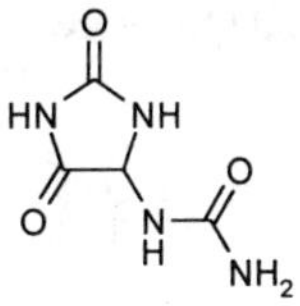

206 Allicin
S-Oxodiallydisulfide. CAS: 539-86-6 $C_6H_{10}OS_2$ MW: 162.27 Property: yellow liquid, soluble in water, ethanol, diethyl ether and benzene. Source: CONG BAI, DA SUAN. Ref: 2, 4.

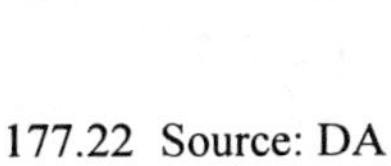

207 Alliin
$C_6H_{11}NO_3S$ MW: 177.22 Source: DA SUAN. Ref: 2.

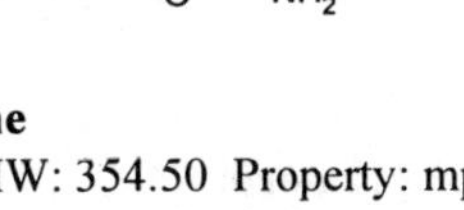

208 Allithiamine
$C_{15}H_{22}N_4O_2S_2$ MW: 354.50 Property: mp 132-3°C (dec). Source: DA SUAN. Ref: 6.

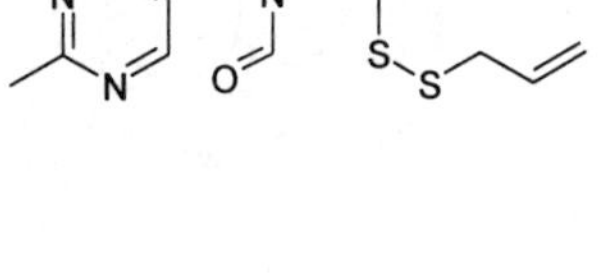

209 Alloaromadendrene
$C_{15}H_{24}$ MW: 204.36 Source: HOU PO, HUO XIANG, REN SHEN, SHENG JIANG, XIE CAO. Ref: 2.

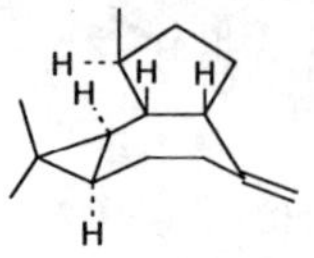

210 Allochenodeoxycholic acid
$C_{24}H_{40}O_4$ MW: 392.58 Property: mp 245-6°C. Source: LI YU DAN. Ref: 6.

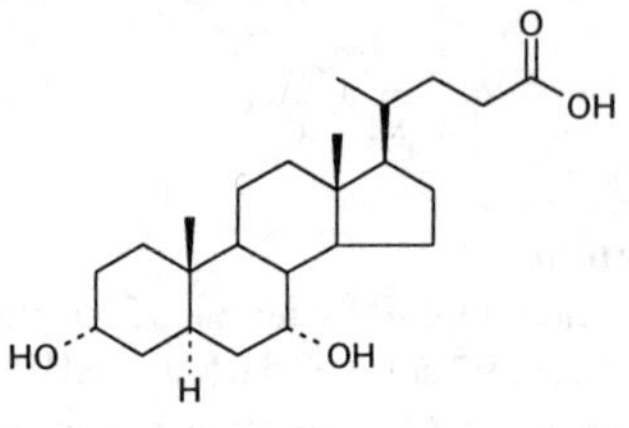

211 Allocryptopine
α-Allocryptopine. $C_{21}H_{23}NO_5$ MW: 369.42 Property: mp 163°C. Source: BAI QU CAI, BO LUO HUI, HE QING HUA, YAN HU SUO. Ref: 6.

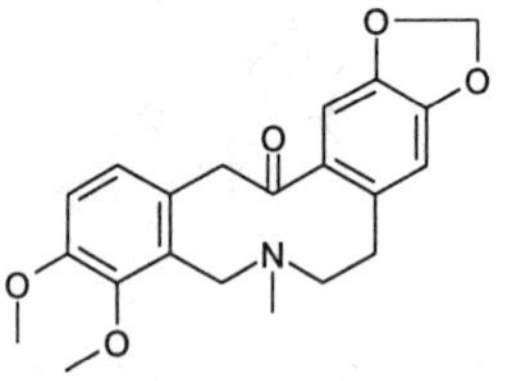

212 β-Allocryptopine
Property: mp 168-71°C. Source: YING SHUI HUANG LIAN. Ref: 6.

213 Alloimperatorine
$C_{16}H_{14}O_4$ MW: 270.29 Source: BAI ZHI, SHE CHUANG ZI. Ref: 2, 6, 7.

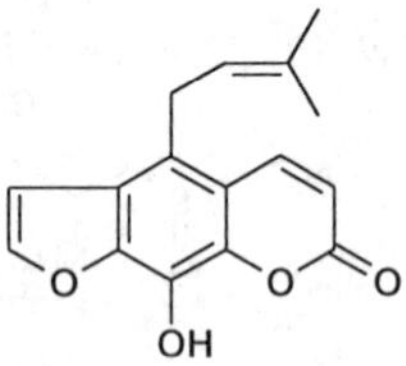

214 Alloisoimperatorin
$C_{16}H_{14}O_4$ MW: 270.29 Source: BAI ZHI. Ref: 2.

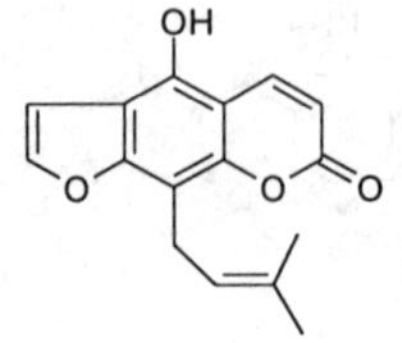

215 Alloisoleucine
$C_6H_{13}NO_2$ MW: 131.18 Property: mp 280-1°C (dec). Source: KUN BU. Ref: 6.

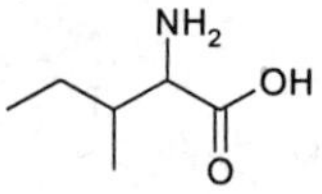

216 α-Allokainic acid
$C_{10}H_{15}NO_4$ MW: 213.24 Property: mp 237-8°C (dec). Source: HAI REN CAO. Ref: 6.

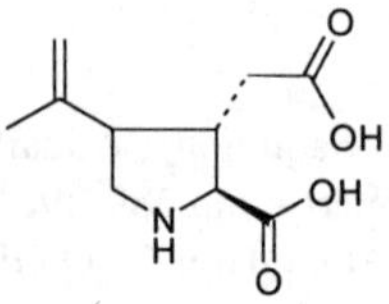

217 Allomatatabiol
$C_{10}H_{16}O_2$ MW: 168.24 Source: MU TIAN LIAO. Ref: 6.

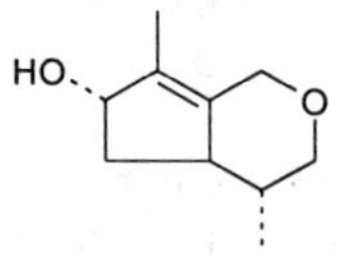

218 Alloocimene
$C_{10}H_{16}$ MW: 136.24 Source: DANG GUI. Ref: 2.

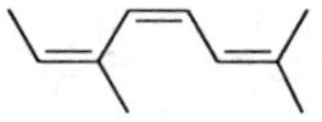

219 Allosecurinine
$C_{13}H_{15}NO_2$ MW: 217.27 Property: mp 136-8°C. Source: YI YE QIU. Ref: 6.

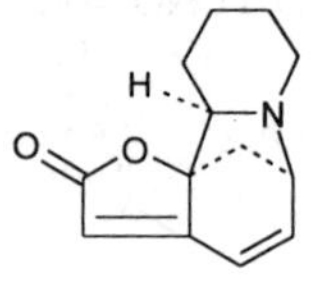

220 Alloyohimbine
$C_{21}H_{26}N_2O_3$ MW: 354.45 Property: white powder, mp 139-40°C, $[\alpha]_D^{24.0}$ -76.7° (c=0.48, pyridine). Source: YANG JIAO MIAN. Ref: 633.

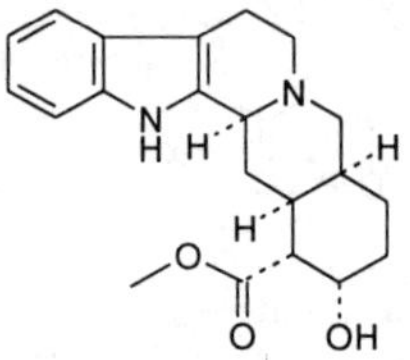

221 1-Allyl-2,4-dimethoxybenzene
$C_{11}H_{14}O_2$ MW: 178.23 Source: XIANG GEN QIN. Ref: 6.

222 Allyl disulfide
Diallyldisulfide. $C_6H_{10}S_2$ MW: 146.27 Property: bp 100°C/48mm. Source: DA SUAN, GE CONG, JIU CAI, TING LI ZI, YANG CONG. Ref: 6.

223 Allyl isothiocyanate
$C_4H_5NS_2$ MW: 99.16 Property: mp -80°C, bp 151 °C. Source: GAN LAN, JIE ZI, TING LI ZI. Ref: 6.

224 Allyl methyl disulfide
$C_4H_8S_2$ MW: 120.24 Source: DA SUAN. Ref: 2.

225 Allyl methyl pentasulfide
$C_4H_8S_5$ MW: 216.43 Source: DA SUAN. Ref: 2.

226 Allyl methyl sulfide
C_4H_8S MW: 88.17 Source: DA SUAN. Ref: 2.

227 Allyl methyl tetrasulfide
$C_4H_8S_4$ MW: 184.36 Source: DA SUAN. Ref: 2.

228 Allyl methyl trisulfide
$C_4H_8S_3$ MW: 152.30 Source: DA SUAN. Ref: 2.

229 Allyl monosulfide
Allyl sulphide; Diallyl sulfide. $C_6H_{10}S$ MW: 114.21 Property: bp 139°C/758mm. Source: CONG BAI, DA SUAN, YANG CONG. Ref: 2, 6.

230 Allyl propyl disulfide
$C_6H_{12}S_2$ MW: 148.29 Source: DA SUAN. Ref: 2.

231 Allylpyrocatechol
$C_9H_{10}O_2$ MW: 150.18 Property: mp 48-9°C. Source: JU JIANG YE. Ref: 6.

232 Allylthiocyanate
C_4H_5NS MW: 99.16 Property: bp 161°C. Source: GUI ZHU TANG JIE. Ref: 6.

233 1-Allyl-2,4,5-trimethoxy-benzene
$C_{12}H_{16}O_3$ MW: 208.26 Property: mp 28°C. Source: CHANG PU YE (SHI CHANG PU YE). Ref: 6.

234 Aloe emodin
$C_{15}H_{10}O_5$ MW: 270.24 Source: DA HUANG, FAN XIE YE, JUE MING ZI, LU HUI, NIU SHE CAO, NIU XI XI, SHU LI, SHAN BIAN DOU ZI, WANG JIANG NAN ZI. Ref: 2, 534, 627.

235 Aloe-emodin diglucoside
$C_{27}H_{30}O_{15}$ MW: 594.53 Source: DA HUANG. Ref: 2.

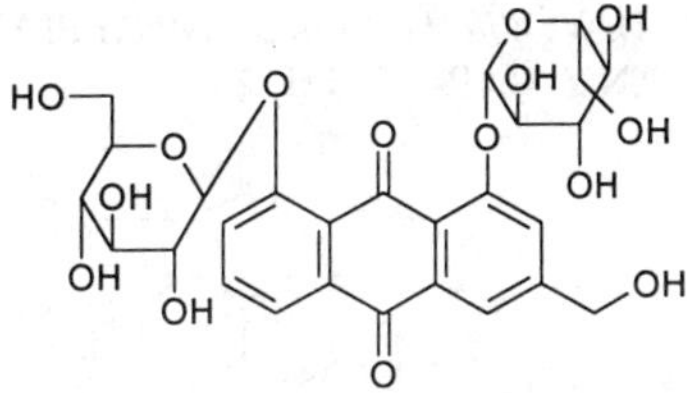

236 Aloe-emodin-ω-O-β-D-glucopyranoside
$C_{21}H_{20}O_{10}$ MW: 432.39 Source: DA HUANG. Ref: 2.

237 Aloenin
$C_{19}H_{22}O_{10}$ MW: 410.38 Source: LU HUI, LU HUI YE. Ref: 2.

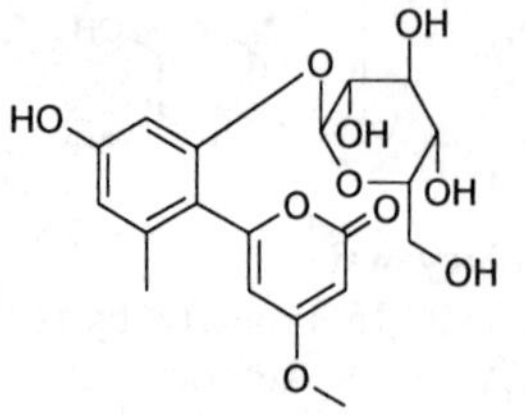

238 Aloesin
$C_{19}H_{22}O_{9}$ MW: 394.38 Source: LU HUI. Ref: 2, 534.

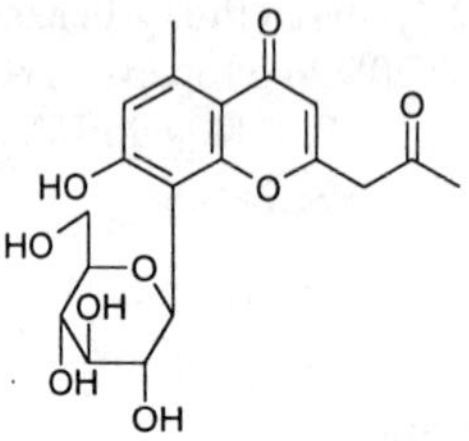

239 Aloin
Barbaloin. $C_{21}H_{22}O_{9}$ MW: 418.40 Source: LU HUI. Ref: 2.

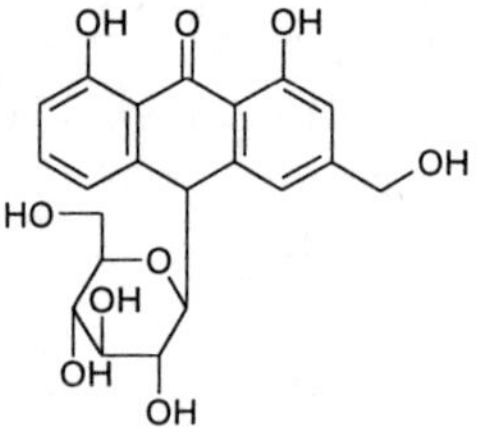

240 Alphitolic acid
$C_{30}H_{48}O_{4}$ MW: 472.71 Source: BING PIAN, DA ZAO, SUAN ZAO REN. Ref: 2.

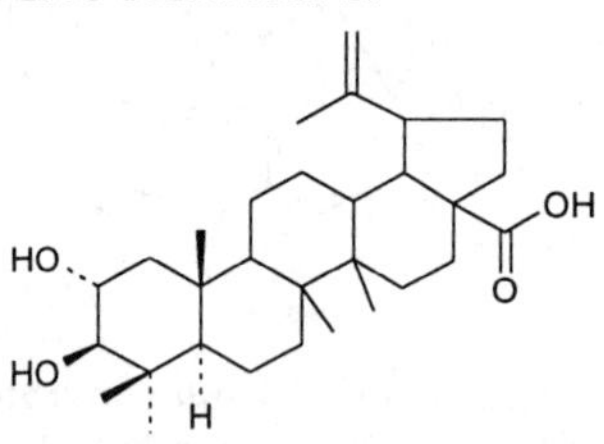

241 Alpinetin
$C_{16}H_{14}O_{4}$ MW: 270.29 Property: mp 225°C. Source: CAO DOU KOU, DA CAO KOU, LIAN JIANG. Ref: 6.

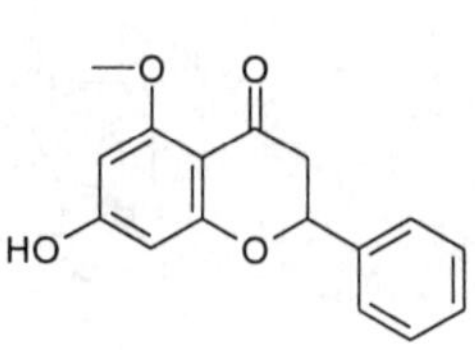

242 Alpinone
$C_{16}H_{14}O_{5}$ MW: 286.29 Property: mp 186-7°C. Source: TU SHA REN. Ref: 6.

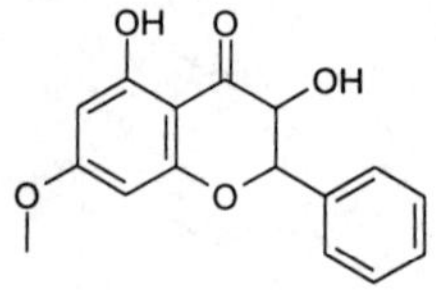

243 Alstonine
$C_{21}H_{22}N_{2}O_{3}$ MW: 350.42 Source: CHANG CHUN HUA. Ref: 2.

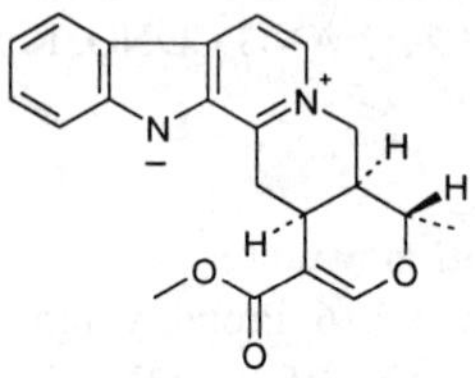

244 3-O-α-L-Alucopyranosyl(1→3)-α-L-rhamnopyranosyl (1→2)-α-L-arabinopyranosyloleanclic acid
$C_{47}H_{76}O_{16}$ MW: 892.12 Source: BAI JIANG. Ref: 2.

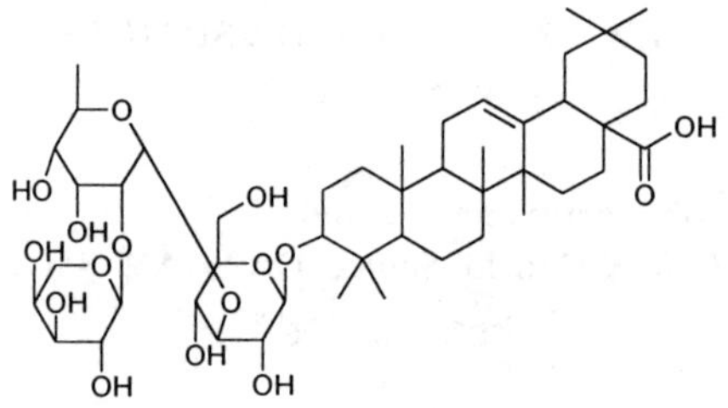

245 Amabiline
$C_{15}H_{25}NO_{4}$ MW: 283.37 Source: GOU SHI HUA. Ref: 6.

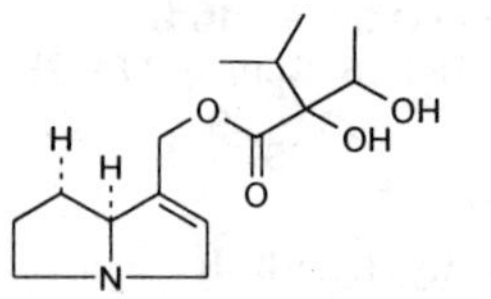

246 Amaranthin
$C_{30}H_{34}N_{2}O_{19}$ MW: 726.61 Source: QIAN RI HONG, YAN LAI HONG. Ref: 5, 15.

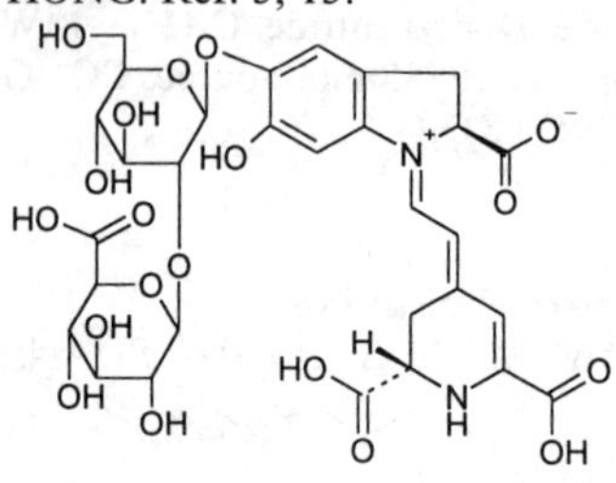

247 Amarasterone A
$C_{30}H_{50}O_7$ MW: 522.73 Property: mp 210-1°C.
Source: CHUAN NIU XI. Ref: 6.

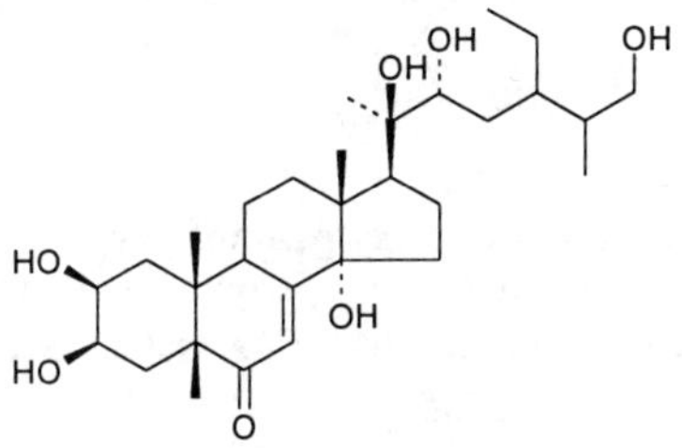

248 Amarasterone B
$C_{30}H_{50}O_7$ MW: 522.73 Property: mp 284-5°C.
Source: CHUAN NIU XI. Ref: 6.

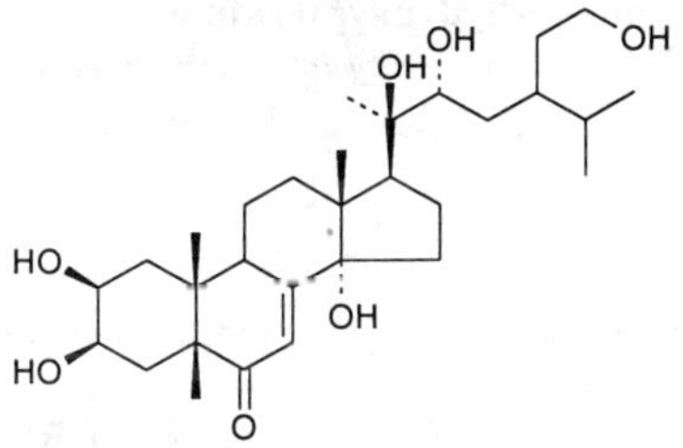

249 Amarogentin
$C_{27}H_{28}O_{14}$ MW: 576.52 Source: LONG DAN. Ref: 2.

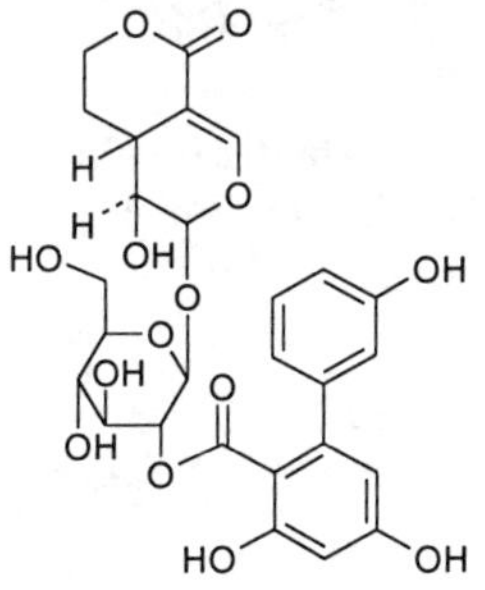

250 Amarolide
$C_{20}H_{28}O_6$ MW: 364.44 Property: mp 253-5°C.
Source: CHU BAI PI. Ref: 6.

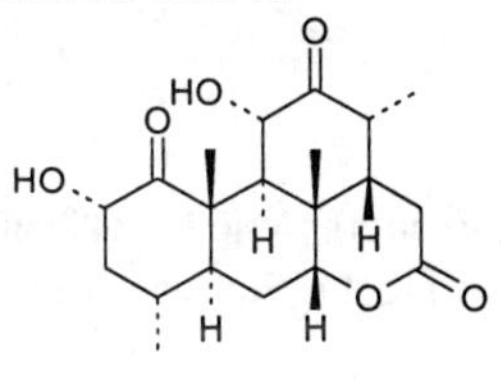

251 Amaroswerin
$C_{29}H_{30}O_{14}$ MW: 602.55 Source: LONG DAN.
Ref: 2, 7.

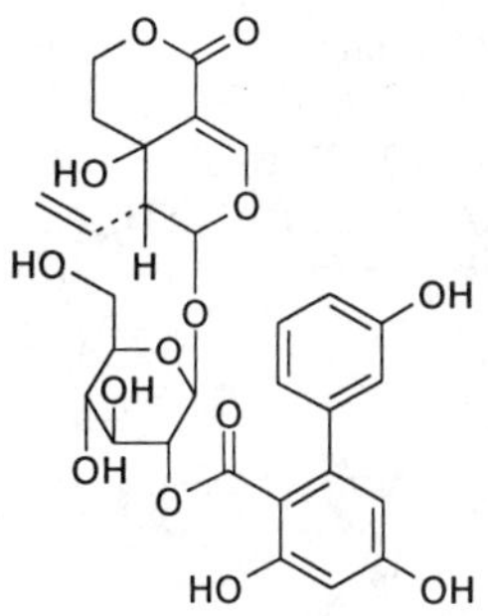

252 Ambolic acid
$C_{31}H_{50}O_3$ MW: 470.74 Property: mp 168-70°C.
Source: MANG GUO. Ref: 6.

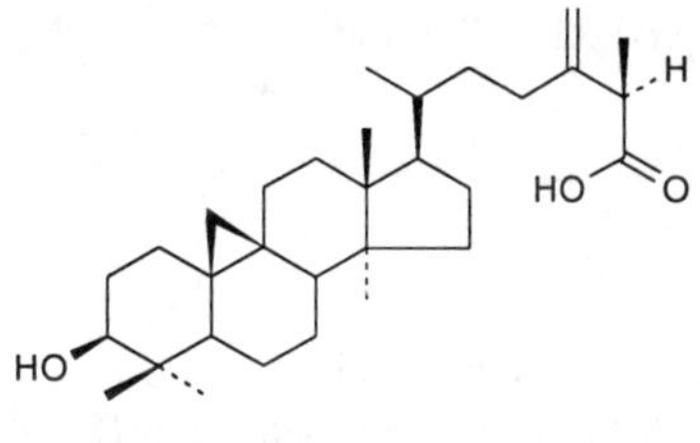

253 Ambonic acid
$C_{31}H_{48}O_3$ MW: 468.73 Property: mp 149-50°C.
Source: MANG GUO, MANG GUO SHU PI. Ref: 6.

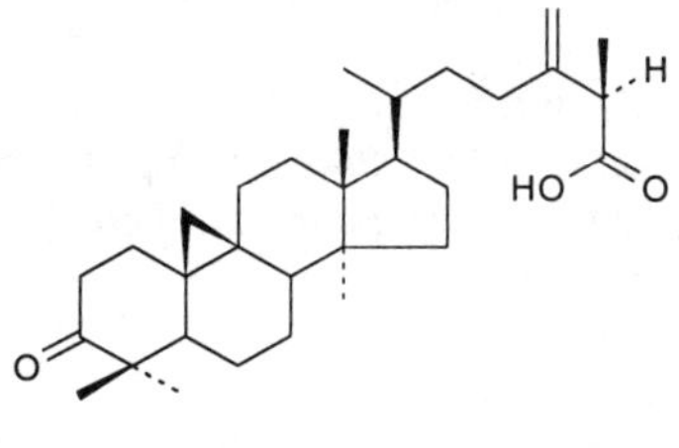

254 Ambrein
$C_{30}H_{52}O$ MW: 428.75 Property: mp 81-3°C. Source:
LONG XIAN XIANG, XIAN CHI SHE PU TAO. Ref: 6.

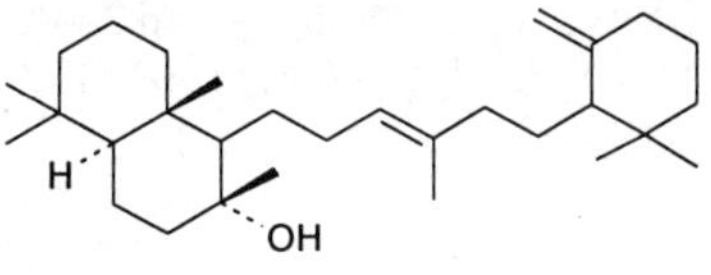

255 Ambrettolid
Property: bp 154-6°C/1mm. Source: HUANG KUI.
Ref: 6.

256 Amellin
Source: YE GAN CAO. Ref: 6.

257 Amentoflavone

$C_{30}H_{18}O_{10}$ MW: 538.47 Property: mp 300°C (dec). Source: BAI GUO, CE BAI YE, DU SONG SHI, GUI YE, JUAN BAI, SAN JIAN SHAN. Ref: 2, 6.

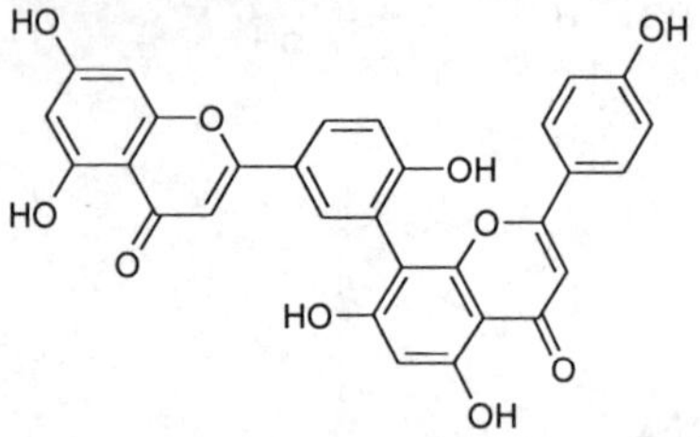

258 α-Aminoadipic acid

$C_6H_{11}NO_4$ MW: 161.16 Property: mp 206°C. Source: MO GU, MU XU GEN. Ref: 6.

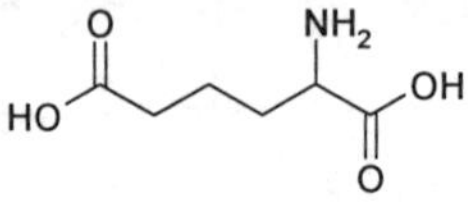

259 p-Aminobenzoic acid

$C_7H_7NO_2$ MW: 137.14 Property: mp 186-7°C. Source: JI ZI BAI, JI ZI HUANG. Ref: 6.

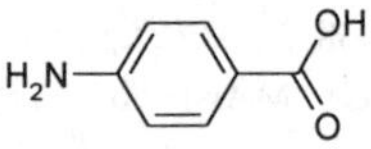

260 α-Aminobutyric acid

$C_4H_9NO_2$ MW: 103.12 Property: mp (+): 292°C (dec), (-): ≈292°C (dec). Source: KU GUA, XI GUA. Ref: 6.

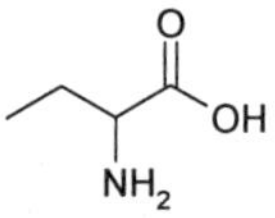

261 β-Aminobutyric acid

$C_4H_9NO_2$ MW: 103.12 Property: mp 220°C (dec). Source: BAN XIA, CAO YUAN LAO GUAN CAO. Ref: 6.

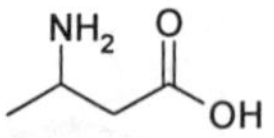

262 γ-Aminobutyric acid

$C_4H_9NO_2$ MW: 103.12 Source: BAN LAN GEN, CHAN SU, GAN DI HUANG, GAN ZHE, JI NAO, LI ZI, MU GU, QIANG HUO, SU MI, TIAN HUA FEN, XI GUA. Ref: Ref: 2, 4, 506.

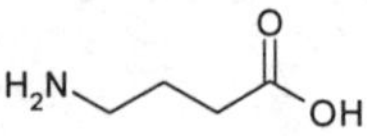

263 4-(2-Aminoethyl)-pyrocatechol

$C_8H_{11}NO_2$ MW: 153.18 Property: mp ≈220°C. Source: WEI XIN GAN. Ref: 6.

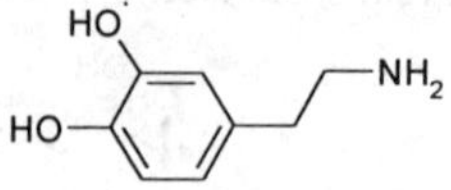

264 3-Amino-2-hydroxy pentandioic acid

$C_5H_9NO_5$ MW: 163.13 Property: white powder, mp 114-6°C, $[\alpha]_D^{25}$ +16.33° (c=0.049, water). Source: PAO PI JUN. Ref: 335.

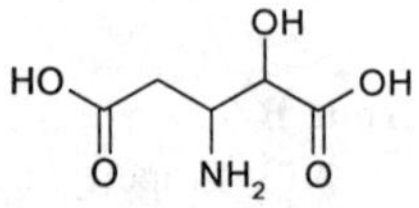

265 2-Amino-6-hydroxypteridine

$C_6H_5N_5O$ MW: 163.14 Source: HEI MA YI. Ref: 6.

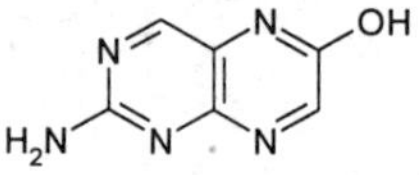

266 2-Amino-4-hydroxy-pteridine-6-carboxylic acid

$C_7H_5NO_3$ MW: 207.15 Source: JIN YU. Ref: 6.

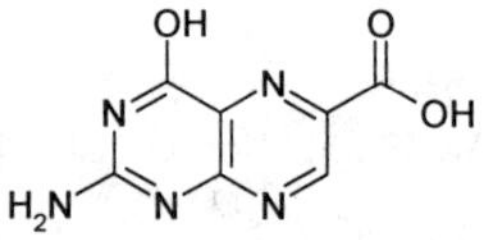

267 L-α-Amino-δ-hydroxyvaleric acid

$C_5H_{11}NO_3$ MW: 133.15 Property: mp 223-4°C. Source: DAO DOU. Ref: 6.

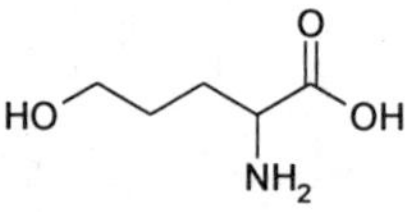

268 Aminoisobutyric acid

$C_4H_9O_2$ MW: 103.12 Property: mp 280°C (sublimation). Source: MO GU. Ref: 6.

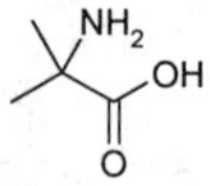

269 γ-Amino-α-methylene butyric acid

$C_5H_9NO_2$ MW: 115.13 Source: LUO HUA SHENG. Ref: 6.

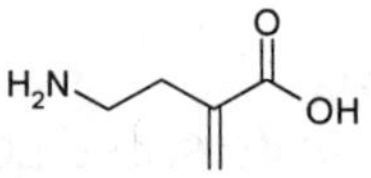

270 Aminophenols
C_6H_7NO MW: 109.13 Source: FU ZI. Ref: 2.

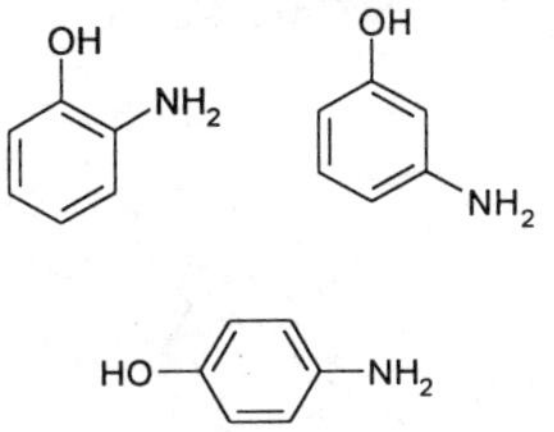

271 α-Amino-β-(pyrazolyl-N)propionic acid
$C_6H_9N_3O_2$ MW: 155.16 Property: mp 236-8°C (dec). Source: XI GUA, XI GUA ZI REN. Ref: 6.

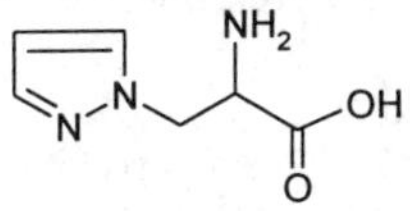

272 Aminozide
$C_6H_{12}NO_3$ MW: 160.17 Source: JU HUA. Ref: 6.

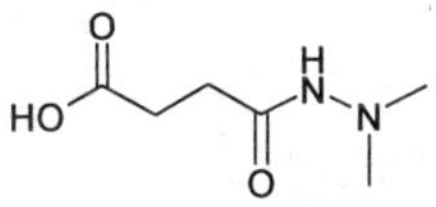

273 Amlaic acid
$C_{27}H_{24}O_{19}$ MW: 652.48 Property: mp 206°C. Source: YOU GAN YE. Ref: 6.

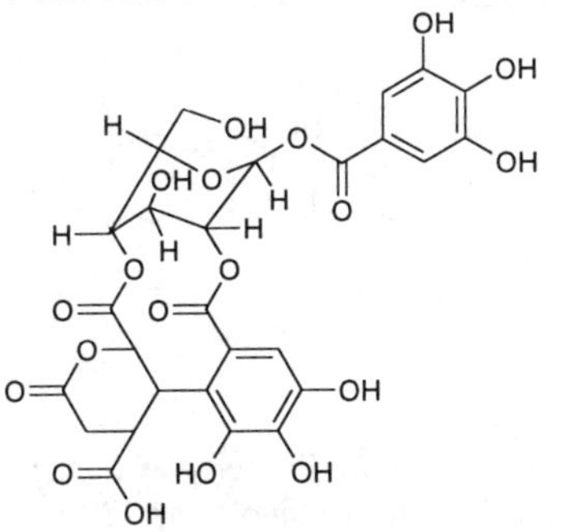

274 Ammiol
$C_{14}H_{12}O_6$ MW: 276.25 Property: mp 211°C. Source: YE SHENG MA. Ref: 6.

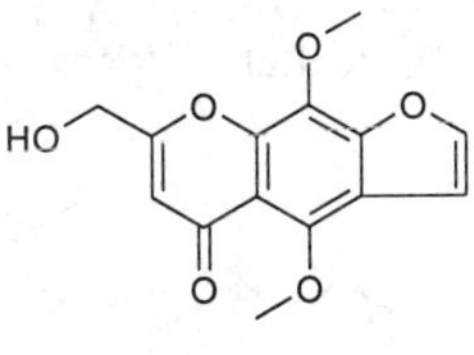

275 Amoenin A$_3$
$C_{21}H_{20}O_{11}$ MW: 448.39 Property: yellow-white acicular crystal, mp 235-6°C. Source: SHAN YE WAN DOU. Ref: 375.

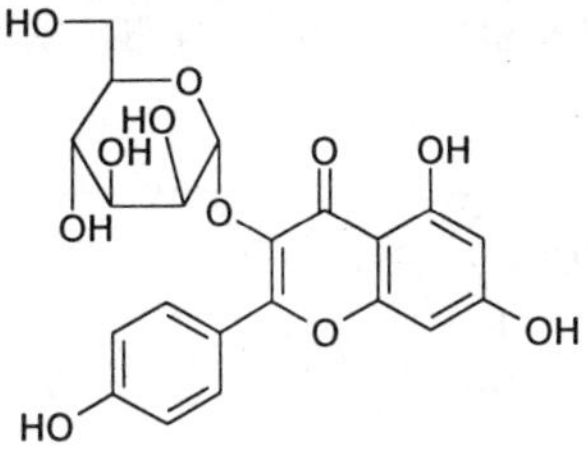

276 Ampelopsin
Property: mp 245-6°C. Source: XIAN CHI SHE PU TAO. Ref: 605.

277 Ampelopsisin
$C_{23}H_{28}O_{12}$ MW: 496.47 Property: white amorphous powder. Source: YU YE SHE PU TAO. Ref: 434.

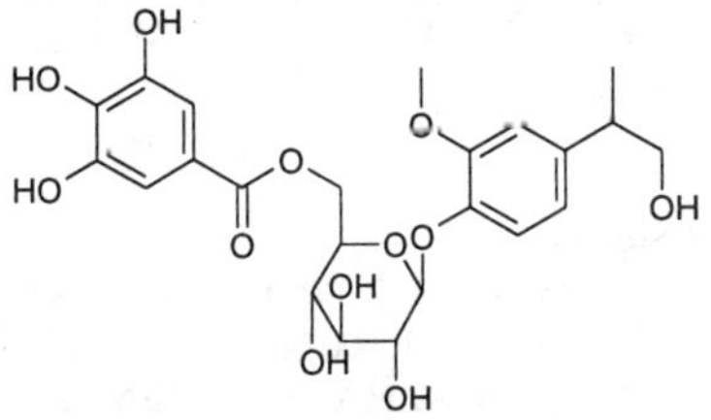

278 Ampeloptin
3,5,7,3',4',5'-Hexahydroxy-flavanone. $C_{15}H_{12}O_8$ MW: 320.26 Property: mp 245-6°C. Source: BAI LIAN. Ref: 6.

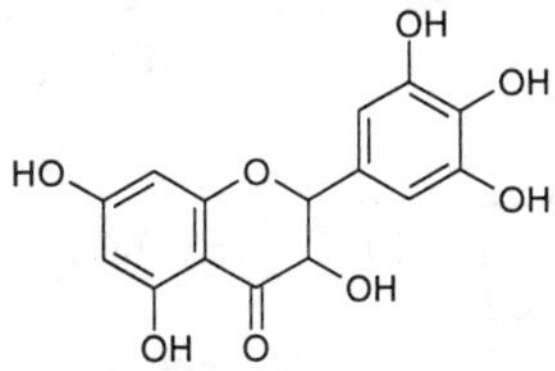

279 Amphibin D
$C_{36}H_{49}NO_5$ MW: 631.82 Source: MIAN ZAO. Ref: 6.

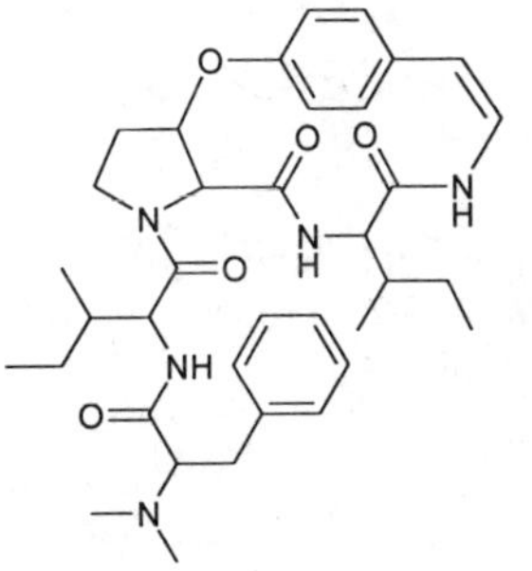

280 Amritoside
$C_{26}H_{26}O_{18}$ MW: 626.49 Property: mp 248-50°C. Source: FAN SHI LIU PI, FAN SHI LIU YE. Ref: 6.

281 Amurensin
$C_{26}H_{30}O_{12}$ MW: 534.52 Property: mp 290°C. Source: HUANG BAI. Ref: 6.

282 Amygdalin
$C_{20}H_{27}NO_{11}$ MW: 457.44 Source: BA DAN XING REN, CI WU JIA, LI HE REN, MEI HE REN, PI PA HE, PI PA YE, SHAN ZHA, TAO REN, TIAN SHAN HUA QIU, WEN PO, XING REN, YU LI REN. Ref: 2, 4, 530.

283 Amyl acetate
$C_7H_{14}O_2$ MW: 130.19 Property: bp 148°C/737mm. Source: JIU. Ref: 6.

284 Amyl butyrate
$C_9H_{18}O_2$ MW: 158.24 Property: bp 185°C. Source: JIU. Ref: 6.

285 n-Amyl ethyl ketone
$C_8H_{16}O$ MW: 128.22 Property: bp 165-6°C. Source: XIANG XUN. Ref: 6.

286 δ-Amyrenol
$C_{30}H_{50}O$ MW: 426.73 Property: mp 212-3.5°C. Source: XIAO JIAN CAO. Ref: 6.

287 α-Amyrenone
$C_{30}H_{48}O$ Property: colorless acicular crystal (chloroform-methanol), mp 119-21°C. Source: QIU HUA NIU NAI CAI. Ref: 464.

288 δ-Amyrenone
$C_{30}H_{48}O$ MW: 424.72 Property: mp 198-201°C. Source: XIAO JIAN CAO. Ref: 6.

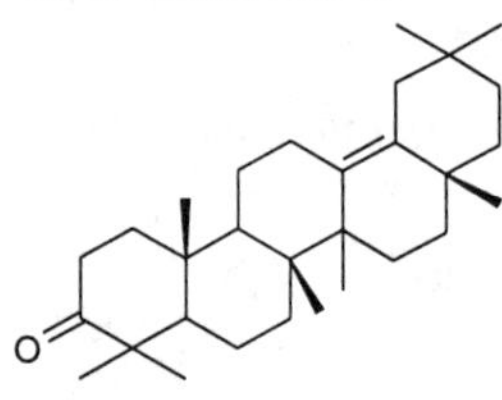

289 β-Amyrenonol
$C_{30}H_{48}O_2$ MW: 440.72 Property: mp 229-30°C. Source: SHAN REN YE. Ref: 6.

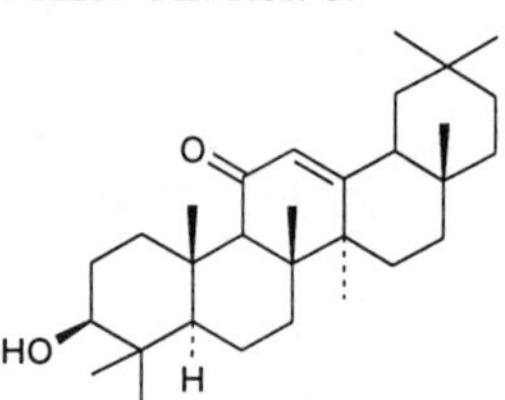

290 α-Amyrin
$C_{30}H_{50}O$ MW: 426.73 Property: white acicular crystal (chloroform-methanol), mp 180-6°C. Source: AI YE, CHI YANG, DA JI (b), GAN LAN, HUI BAO HAO, JU JU, KU DING CHA, LUO DI SHENG GEN, MA QIAN ZI, MAO LIAN HAO, MI DIE XIANG, PAI QIAN CAO GEN, QIU HUA NIU NAI CAI, SAN LI HONG, XIANG JIA PI, XIANG PI MU, YANG MEI, etc. Ref: 6, 464, 474, 503, 620.

291 β-Amyrin

$C_{30}H_{50}O$ MW: 426.73 Property: mp 197.0-197.5°C. Source: CHI YANG, CU LIU GUO (SHA JI), DA FEI YANG CAO, DA JI (b), DUO SUI SHI KE YE, GE XUN, HUO YANG LE, JIU BI YING (BAI MU XIANG), KU DING CHA, LONG XUCAO (II), LUO DI SHENG GEN, MAO YE BA DOU, MI DIE XIANG, PU GONG YING, QIU FENG MU, SANG JI SHENG, SHAN REN YE, SHAN WO JU, SHE PU TAO, WU HUA GUO YE, WU TONG YE, XI YE DA JI, XIANG JIA PI, XIANG SI ZI, YANG MEI. Ref: 2, 6, 408, 552.

292 α-Amyrin acetate

$C_{32}H_{52}O_2$ MW: 468.77 property: white scale crystal (chlorotorm-methanol), mp 220-26°C. Source: AI YE, CHANG CHUN HUA, HUI BAO HAO, LU ZHU GEN, QIU HUA NIU NAI CAI, WU MU XIE, XIANG JIA PI, XIANG PI MU. Ref: 6, 503.

293 β-Amyrin acetate

$C_{32}H_{52}O_2$ MW: 468.77 Property: mp 236°C. Source: BI LI, FU LING, DA JI (b), DI SHAO GUA, HUI BAO HAO, LU ZHU GEN, WU TONG YE, XIANG JIA PI. Ref: 6, 236, 503, 536.

294 α-Amyrin butyrate

$C_{34}H_{56}O_2$ Property: white acicular crystal (chloroform-methanol), mp 186-8°C. Source: QIU HUA NIU NAI CAI. Ref: 464.

295 α-Amyrin caproate

$C_{36}H_{60}O_2$ Property: white acicular crystal(ethanol), mp 127°C. Source: QIU HUA NIU NAI CAI. Ref: 464.

296 α-Amyrin laurate

$C_{43}H_{74}O_2$ MW: 623.07 Source: TIAN WEN CAO. Ref: 6.

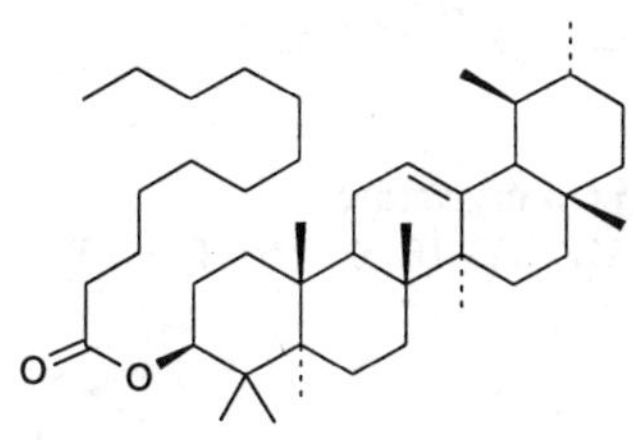

297 β-Amyrin laurate

$C_{42}H_{72}O_2$ MW: 609.04 Source: TIAN WEN CAO. Ref: 6.

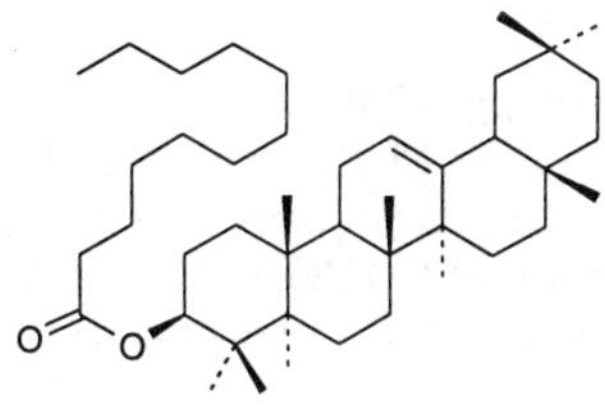

298 α-Amyrin linoleate

$C_{48}H_{80}O_2$ MW: 689.17 Source: TIAN WEN CAO. Ref: 6.

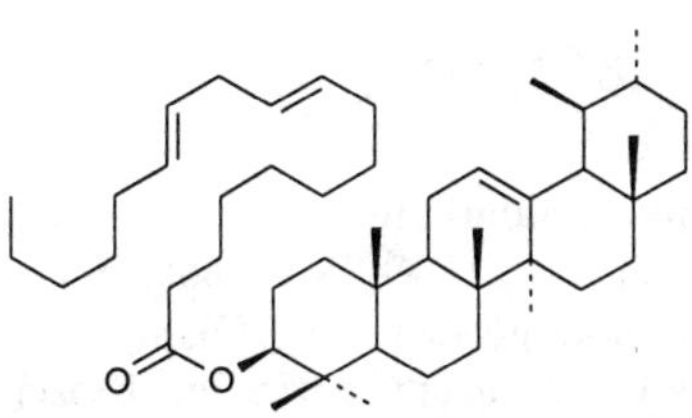

299 β-Amyrin linoleate

$C_{48}H_{80}O_2$ MW: 689.17 Source: TIAN WEN CAO. Ref: 6.

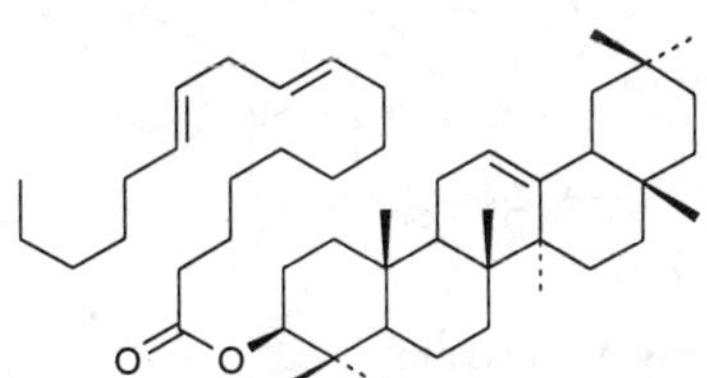

300 α-Amyrin myristate
$C_{44}H_{76}O_2$ MW: 637.10 Source: TIAN WEN CAO. Ref: 6.

301 β-Amyrin myristate
$C_{44}H_{76}O_2$ MW: 637.10 Source: TIAN WEN CAO. Ref: 6.

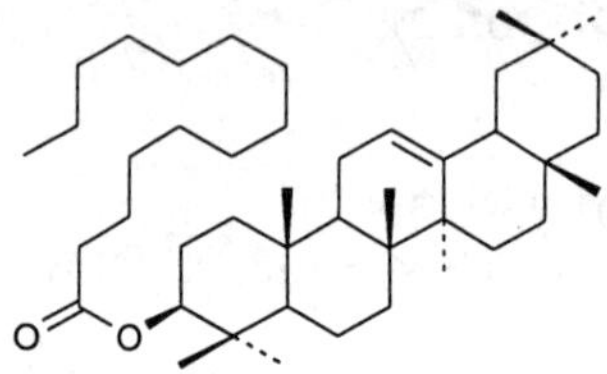

302 α-Amyrin palmitate
$C_{46}H_{80}O_2$ MW: 665.15 Property: white lamellar crystal (acetone-methanol), mp 114-6°C. Source: MENG GU SHAN LUO BO, QIU HUA NIU NAI CAI, TIAN WEN CAO. Ref: 6, 464.

303 β-amyrin palmitate
Balanophorin A. $C_{46}H_{80}O_2$ MW: 665.15 Property: white amorphous powder (Me_2CO), mp 77°C, soluble in chloroform, petroleum benzine and benaene. Source: MU XIANG, TIAN WEN CAO, YIN DU SHE GU. Ref: 2, 6, 423.

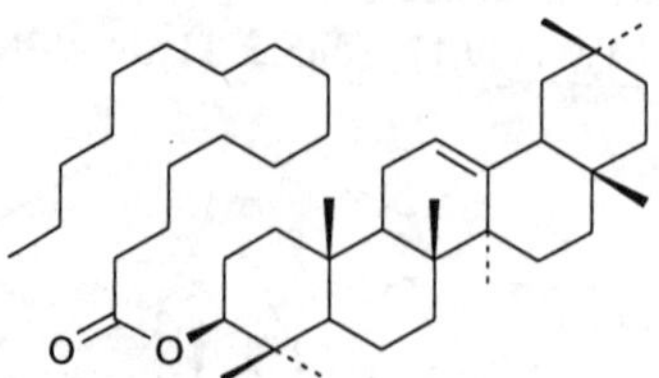

304 α-Amyrin stearate
$C_{48}H_{84}O_2$ MW: 693.20 Source: MU XIANG. Ref: 2.

305 Anabasine
$C_{10}H_{14}N_2$ MW: 162.24 property: bp (-): 276°C. Source: YAN CAO. Ref: 6.

306 Anacardic acid A
$C_{22}H_{36}O_3$ MW: 348.53 Source: BAI GUO. Ref: 2.

307 Anacardic acid B
$C_{22}H_{34}O_3$ MW: 346.51 Source: BAI GUO. Ref: 6.

308 Anacardic acid C
$C_{22}H_{32}O_3$ MW: 344.50 Source: BAI GUO. Ref: 2.

309 Anacardic acid D
$C_{22}H_{30}O_3$ MW: 342.48 Source: BAI GUO. Ref: 2.

310 Anagyrine
$C_{16}H_{22}N_2O$ MW: 258.37 Property: bp (-): 210-5°C /4mm. Source: KU SHEN, MU MA DOU, SHAN DOU GEN. Ref: 6.

311 Anatabine
$C_{10}H_{12}N_2$ MW: 160.22 Property: bp (-): 145-6°C/10mm. Source: YAN CAO. Ref: 6.

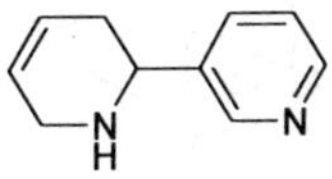

312 Andrographan
$C_{40}H_{82}$ MW: 563.10 Source: CHUAN XIN LIAN. Ref: 2.

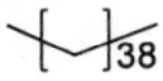

313 Andrographidine A
$C_{23}H_{26}N_{10}$ MW: 462.46 Source: CHUAN XIN LIAN. Ref: 2.

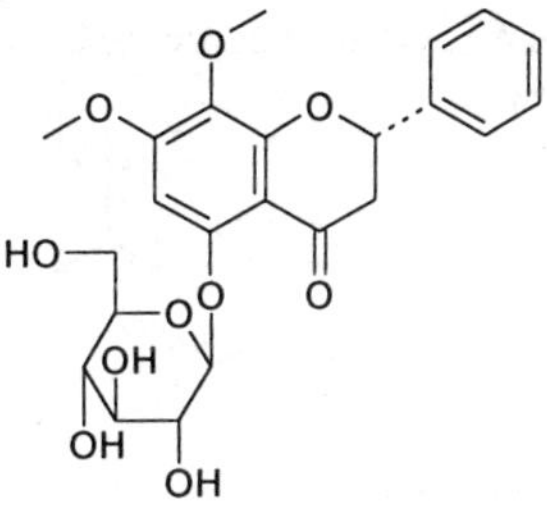

314 Andrographidine B
$C_{23}H_{24}N_{12}$ MW: 492.44 Source: CHUAN XIN LIAN. Ref: 2.

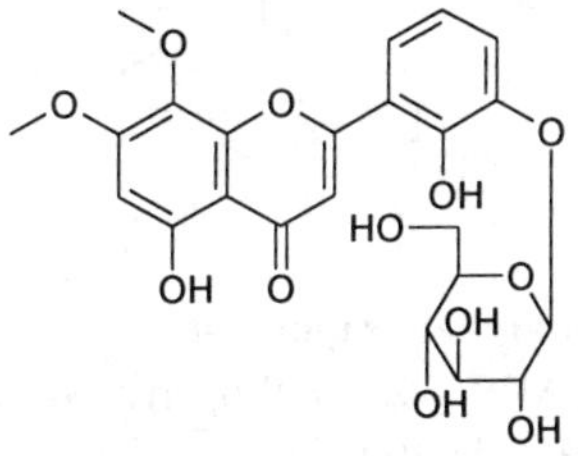

315 Andrographidine C
$C_{23}H_{24}N_{10}$ MW: 460.44 Source: CHUAN XIN LIAN. Ref: 2.

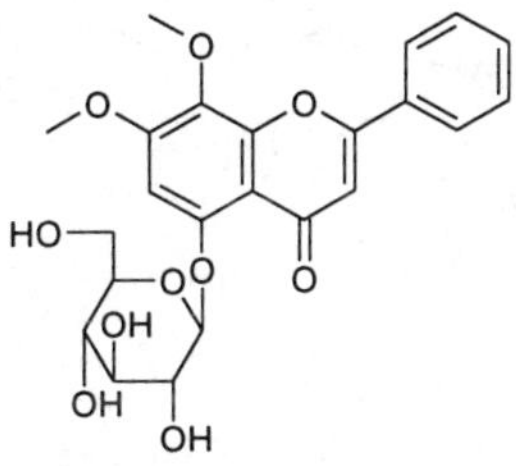

316 Andrographidine D
$C_{25}H_{28}N_{12}$ MW: 520.49 Source: CHUAN XIN LIAN. Ref: 2.

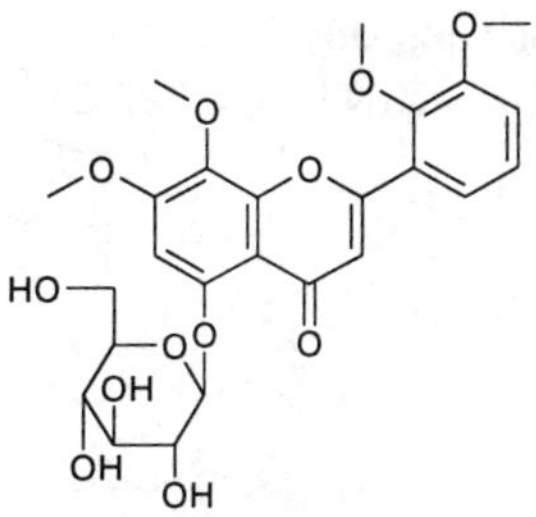

317 Andrographidine E
$C_{24}H_{26}N_{11}$ MW: 490.47 Source: CHUAN XIN LIAN. Ref: 2.

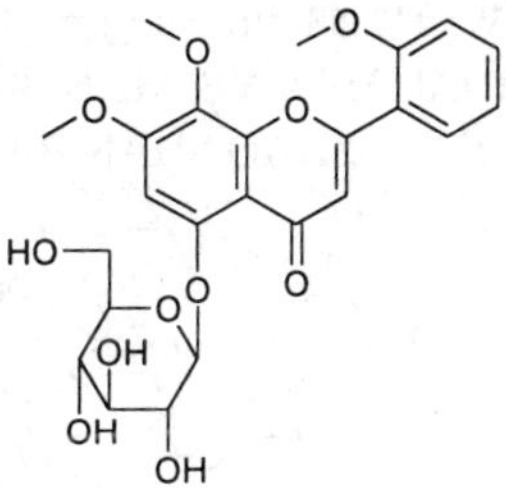

318 Andrographin
$C_{18}H_{16}O_6$ MW: 328.22 Property: mp 190-1°C. Source: CHUAN XIN LIAN. Ref: 2.

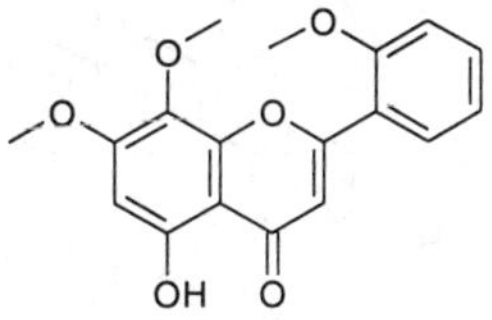

319 Andrographin F
Source: CHUAN XIN LIAN. Ref: 2.

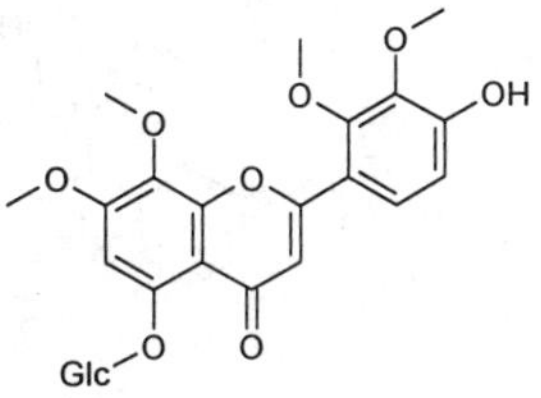

320 Andrographolide
$C_{20}H_{30}O_5$ MW: 350.46 Source: CHUAN XIN LIAN. Ref: 2, 4.

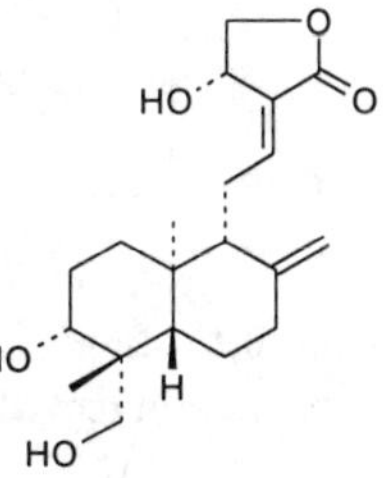

321 Andrographoside
Source: CHUAN XIN LIAN. Ref: 2.

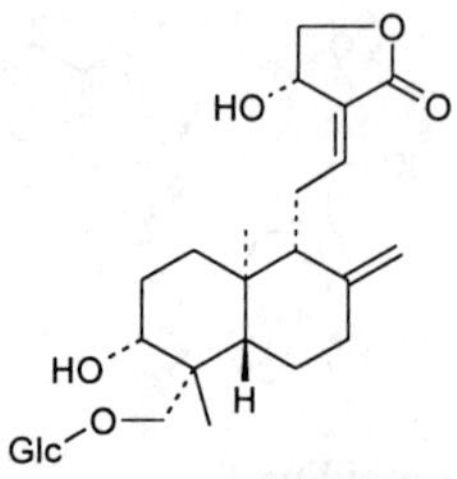

322 Andromedotoxin
$C_{22}H_{36}O_7$ MW: 412.53 Property: mp 267-70°C. Source: DU JUAN HUA YE, MAN SHAN HONG, NAO YANG HUA, ZHAO SHAN BAI. Ref: 4, 6.

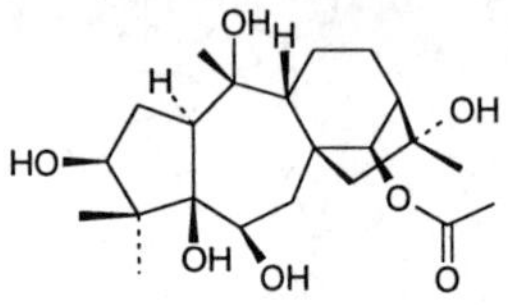

323 5β-Androstan-3α,17α-diol
$C_{20}H_{34}O_2$ MW: 306.49 Source: SHE XIANG. Ref: 2.

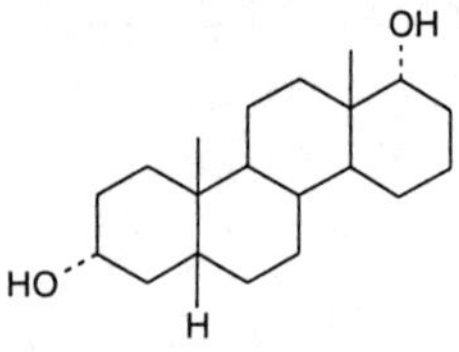

324 5β-Androstan-3α,17β-diol
$C_{20}H_{34}O_2$ MW: 306.49 Source: SHE XIANG. Ref: 2.

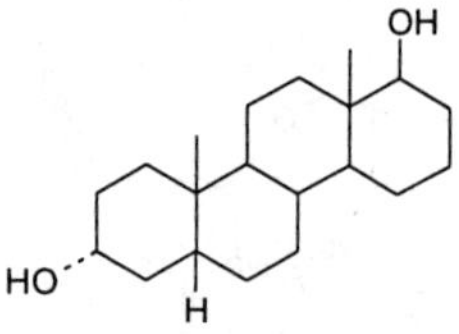

325 5α-Androstan-3,17-dione
$C_{20}H_{30}O_2$ MW: 302.46 Source: SHE XIANG. Ref: 2.

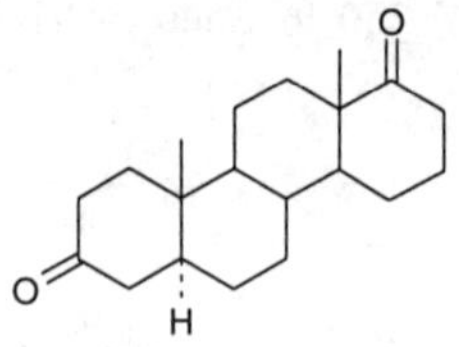

326 5β-Androstan-3,17-dione
$C_{20}H_{30}O_2$ MW: 302.46 Source: SHE XIANG. Ref: 2.

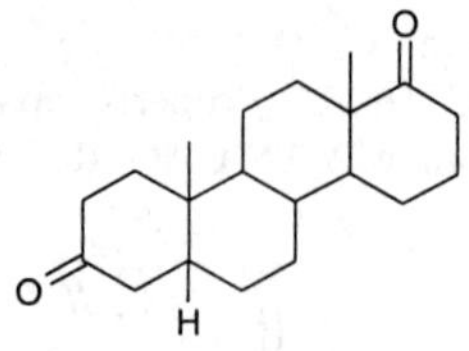

327 Androst-4,6-diene-3,17-dione
$C_{20}H_{26}O_2$ MW: 298.43 Source: SHE XIANG. Ref: 2.

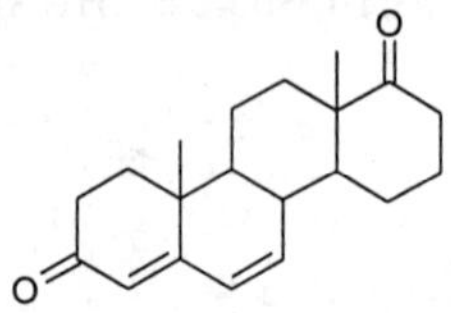

328 Androst-4-ene-3,17-dione
$C_{20}H_{28}O_2$ MW: 300.44 Source: SHE XIANG. Ref: 2.

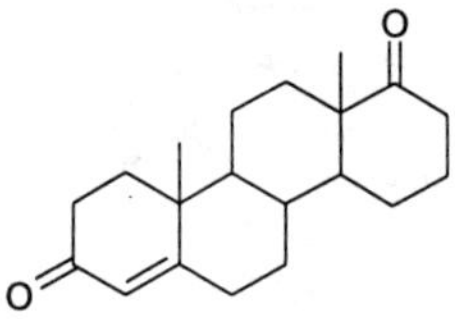

329 Androsterone
$C_{19}H_{30}O_2$ MW: 290.45 Property: mp 178°C. Source: ZI HE CHE. Ref: 6.

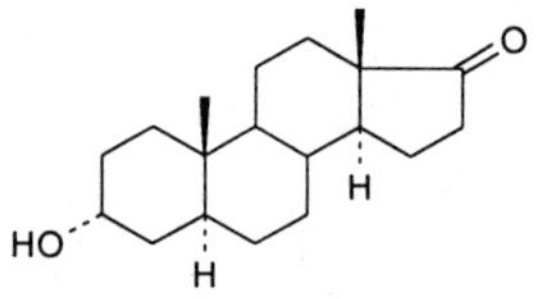

330 Anemarrhenasaponin-I
$C_{31}H_{20}O_{10}$ MW: 552.50 Property: white powder. Source: ZHI MU. Ref: 443.

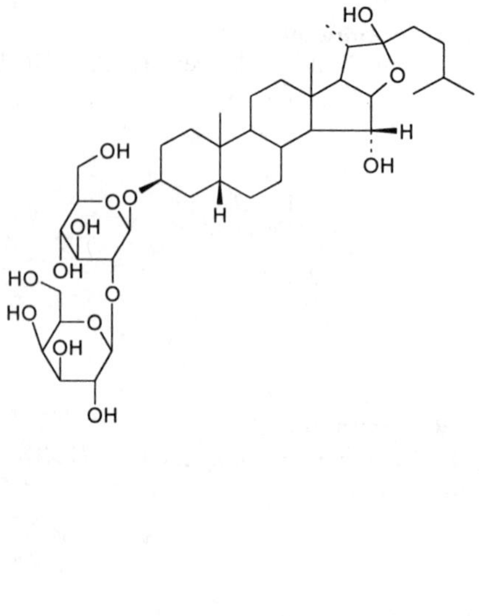

331 Anemarrhenasaponin-Ia
$C_{31}H_{20}O_{10}$ MW: 552.50 Property: white powder. Source: ZHI MU. Ref: 443.

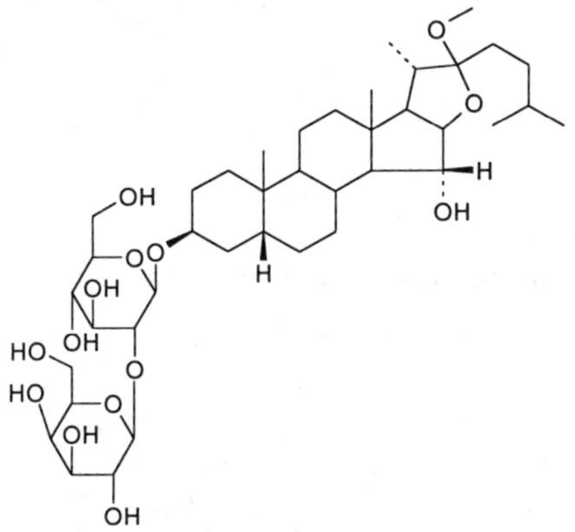

332 Anemarsaponin C
(25S)-O-β-D-glucopyranosyl-5β-furost-20(22)-ene-3β, 26-diol-3-O-β-D-glucopyranosyl-(1→2)-β-D-glucopyranoside. $C_{45}H_{74}O_{18}$ MW: 903.08 Property: white amorphous powder, mp >212°C. Source: ZHI MU. Ref: 353.

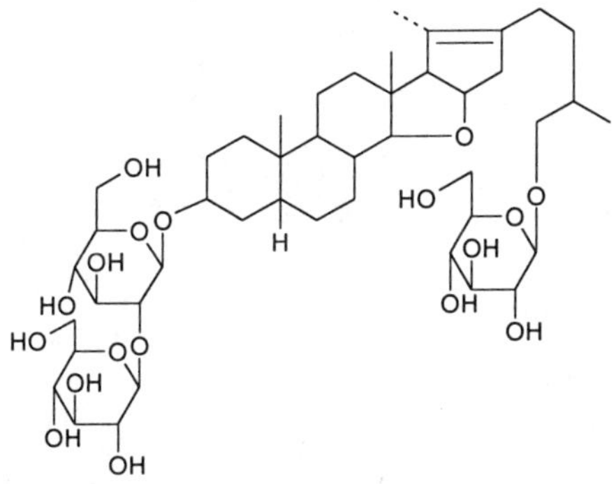

333 Anemonin
$C_{10}H_8O_4$ MW: 192.17 Source: BAI MAO GEN, BAI TOU WENG, DA PO WAN WAN HUA, MA TI YE, MAO GEN, SHI LONG RUI, WEI LING XIAN. Ref: 2, 6.

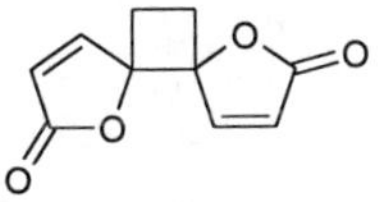

334 Anemonol
$C_5H_4O_2$ MW: 96.09 Source: WEI LING XIAN. Ref: 6.

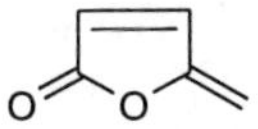

335 Anemosapogenin
$C_{30}H_{48}O_4$ MW: 472.71 Source: BAI TOU WENG. Ref: 2.

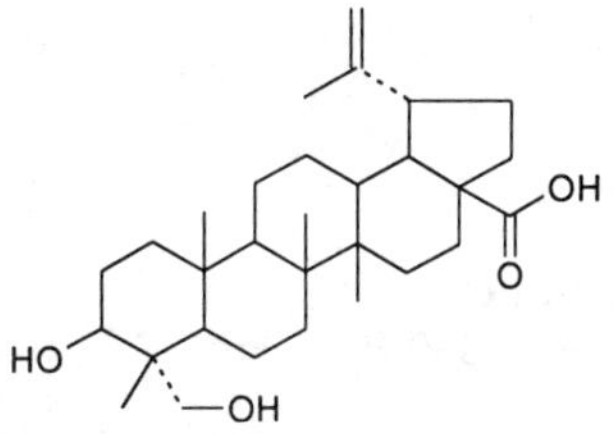

336 Anemoside A3
Source: BAI TOU WENG. Ref: 2.

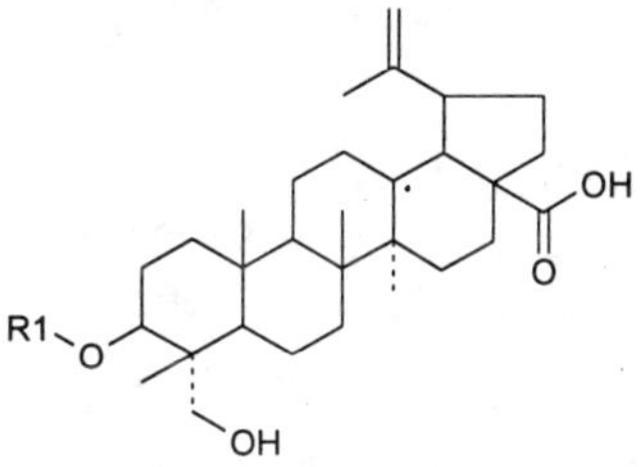

R1 = α-L-rhamnopyranosyl (1→2)-α-L-arabinopyranosyl

337 Anemoside B4
Source: BAI TOU WENG. Ref: 2.

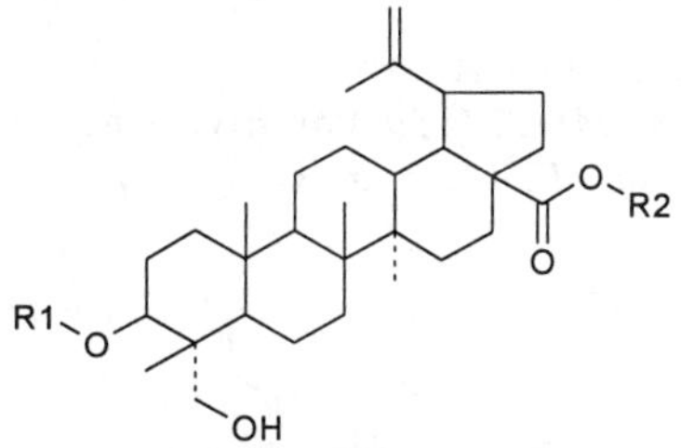

R1 = α-L-rhamnopyranosyl (1→2)-α-L-arabinopyranosyl
R2 = α-L-rhamnopyranosyl(1→4)-β-D-glucopyranosyl (1→6)-β-D-glucopyranosyl

338 Anethole
$C_{10}H_{12}O$ MW: 148.21 Source: BA JIAO HUI XIANG, DU SONG SHI, HUI XIANG, HUO XIANG, LUO LE, SHUI HUI XIANG, XIANG GEN QIN, ZI WAN. Ref: 2, 6, 7.

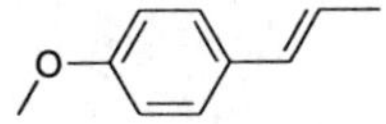

339 cis-Anethole
$C_{10}H_{12}O$ MW: 148.21 Source: HUI XIANG. Ref: 6, 7.

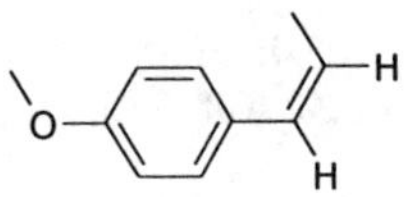

340 Angelic acid
$C_5H_8O_2$ MW: 100.12 Source: DU HUO, FENG DU CAI. Ref: 2.

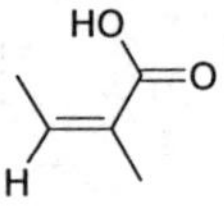

341 Angelicide
$C_{24}H_{28}O_4$ MW: 380.49 Source: DANG GUI. Ref: 2.

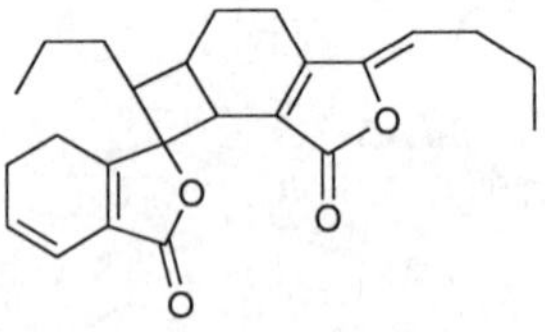

342 Angelicone
Glabralactone. $C_{16}H_{16}O_5$ MW: 288.30 Property: mp 129-30°C. Source: DU HUO. Ref: 2, 6.

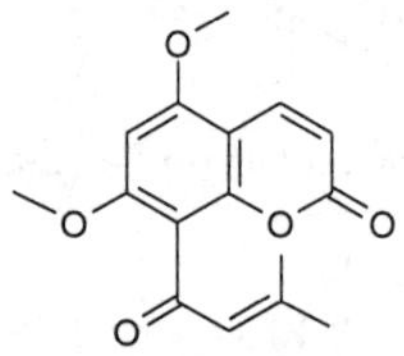

343 Angeliticin A
$C_{20}H_{22}O_7$ MW: 374.39 Property: white granular crystal, mp 177-8°C. Source: GUAI QIN. Ref: 340.

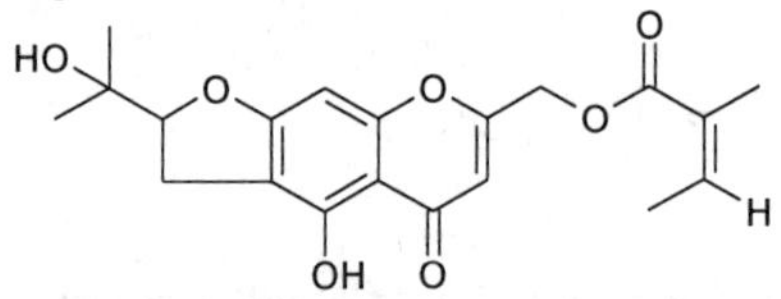

344 Angelol
$C_{20}H_{24}O_7$ MW: 376.41 Property: mp 104-5°C. Source: DU HUO, Ref: 6.

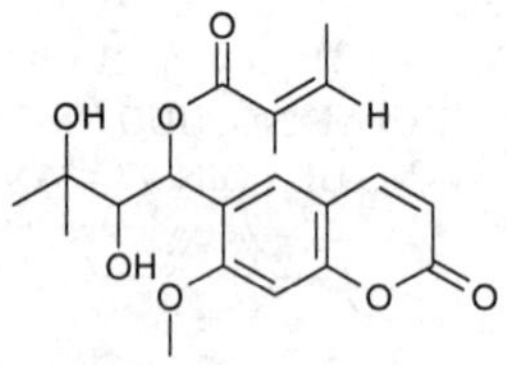

345 Angelol D
Source: DU HUO, Ref: 7.

346 Angeloylgomisin H
Source: WU WEI ZI. Ref: 2.

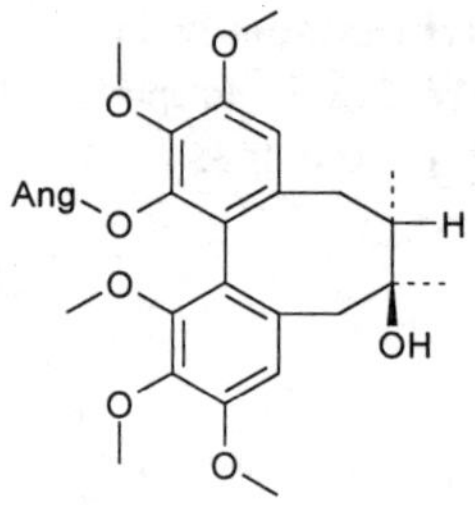

347 Angeloylgomisin O
Source: WU WEI ZI. Ref: 2.

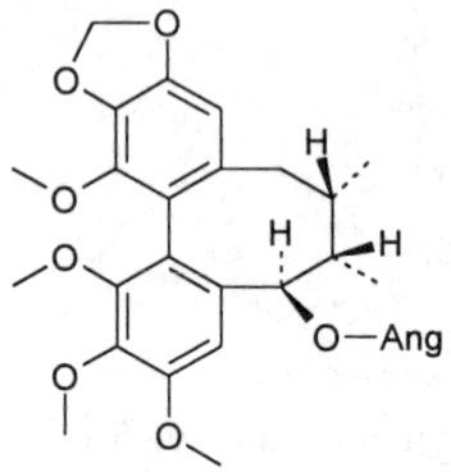

348 Angeloylgomisin P
Source: WU WEI ZI. Ref: 2.

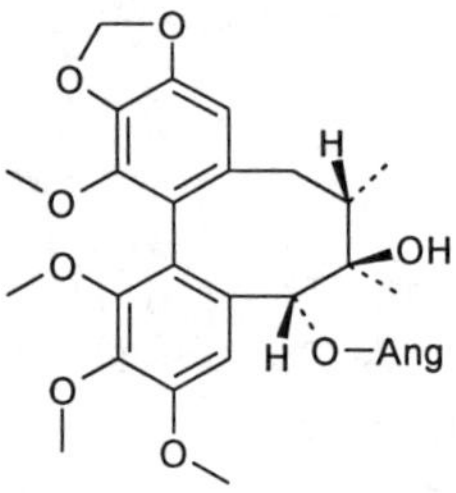

349 Angeloylgomisin Q
Source: WU WEI ZI. Ref: 2.

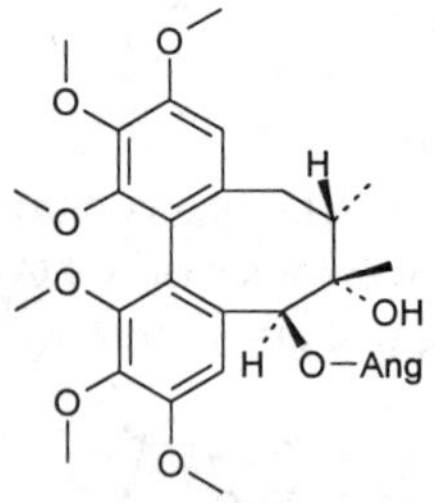

350 3'-O-Angeloylhamaudol
$C_{20}H_{22}O_6$ MW: 358.39 Source: FANG FENG. Ref: 2.

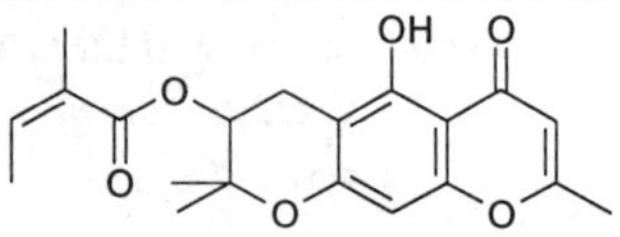

351 Angeloylisogomisin O
Source: WU WEI ZI. Ref: 2.

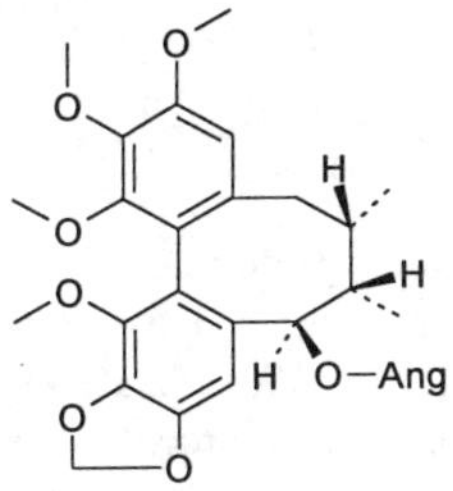

352 6-Angeloylfuranofukinol
$C_{20}H_{28}O_4$ MW: 332.44 Source: FENG DOU CAI. Ref: 6.

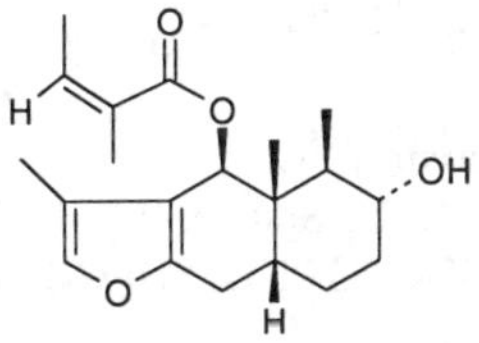

353 22-O-Angeloyl theasapogenol A
Source: PU ER CHA. Ref: 581.

354 22-O-Angeloyl theasapogenol B
Source: PU ER CHA. Ref: 581.

355 22-O-Angeloyl theasapogenol E
Source: PU ER CHA. Ref: 581.

356 Angenomalin
$C_{14}H_{12}O_3$ MW: 228.25 Property: mp 105-126.0°C. Source: BAI ZHI. Ref: 6.

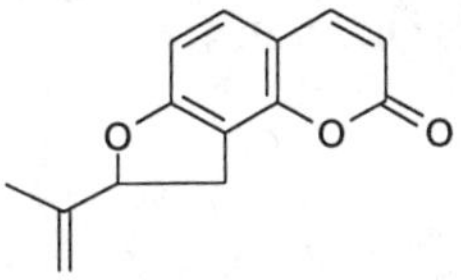

357 Angolensin
$C_{16}H_{18}O_6$ MW: 272.30 Property: mp (-): 120.5-121.0°C. Source: ZI TAN. Ref: 6.

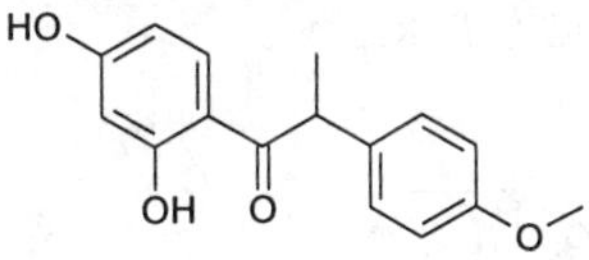

358 Angustiamarin
$C_{26}H_{30}O_{13}$ MW: 550.52 Property: light yellow amorphous powder, mp 115-8°C. Source: XIA YE ZHANG YA CAI. Ref: 340.

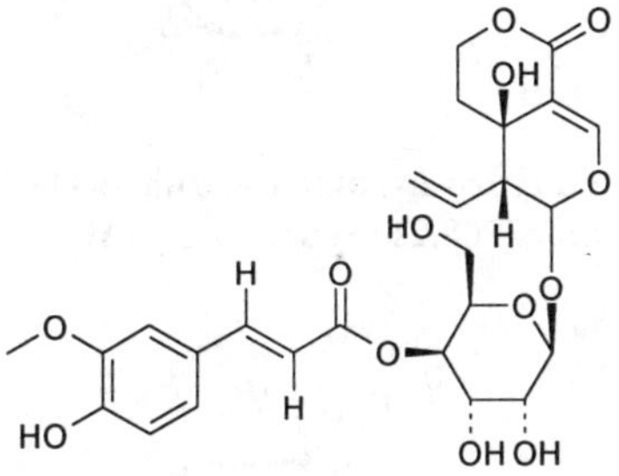

359 Angustidine
$C_{19}H_{15}N_3O$ MW: 301.35 Source: GOU TENG. Ref: 2.

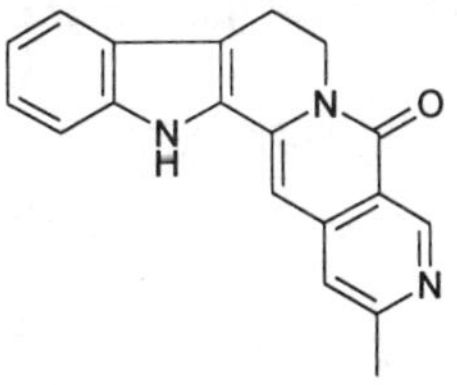

360 Angustioside
$C_{26}H_{30}O_{14}$ MW: 566.52 Property: light yellow amorphous powder, bitter flavour, mp 124-8°C. Source: XIA YE ZHANG YA CAI. Ref: 220.

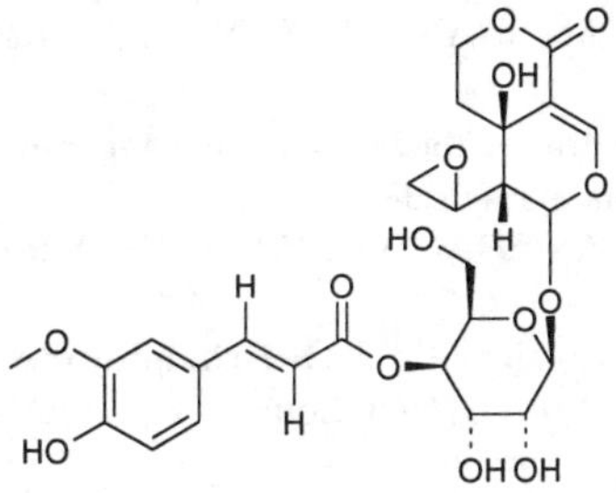

361 Angustoline
$C_{20}H_{17}N_3O_2$ MW: 331.38 Source: GOU TENG. Ref: 2.

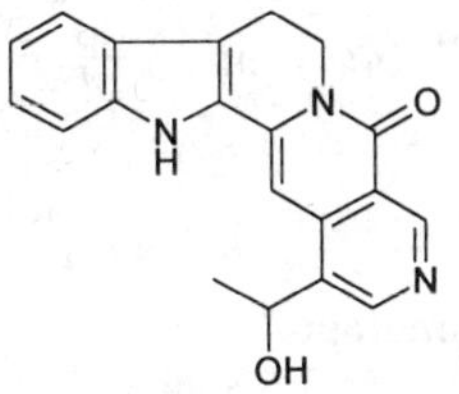

362 3,6-Anhydrogalactose
$C_6H_{10}O_5$ MW: 162.14 Source: QI LIN CAI. Ref: 6.

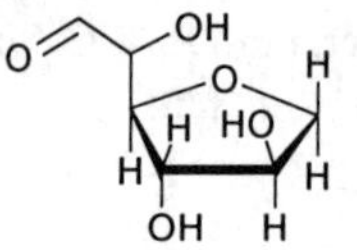

363 3,6-Anhydro-L-galactose dimethyl acetal
$C_8H_{18}O_6$ MW: 208.21 Source: LU JIAO CAI. Ref: 6.

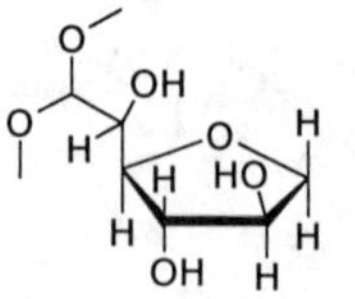

364 Anhydroharringtonine
$C_{29}H_{37}NO_8$ MW: 527.62 Source: SAN JIAN SHAN. Ref: 2.

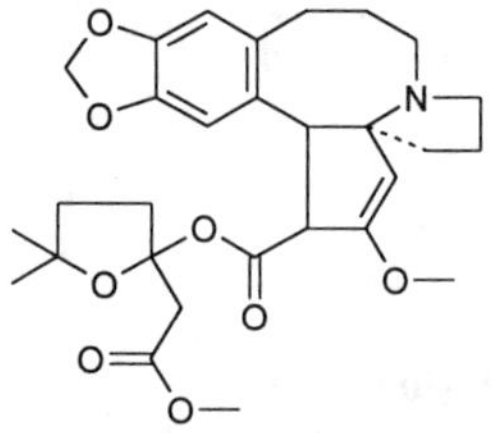

365 Anhydroicaritin
MW: 368 Property: yellow powder, mp 228-9°C. Source: WAN SHAN YIN YANG HUO. Ref: 465.

366 Anhydroicaritin-3-O-α-L-rhamnopyranosyl-(1→2)-α-L-rhamno-pyranoside
Source: WAN SHAN YIN YANG HUO. Ref: 574.

367 Anhydroicaritin-3-O-α-rhamnoside
$C_{33}H_{40}O_{15}$ MW: 676.68 Source: YIN YANG HUO. Ref: 2.

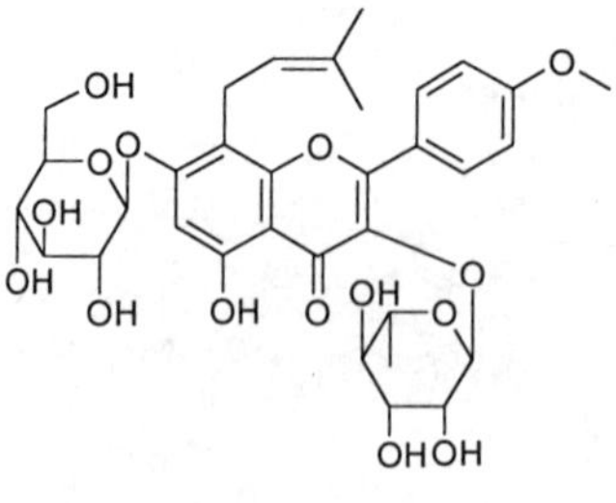

368 Anhydronotoptol
$C_{21}H_{20}O_4$ MW: 336.39 Source: QIANG HUO. Ref: 2, 507.

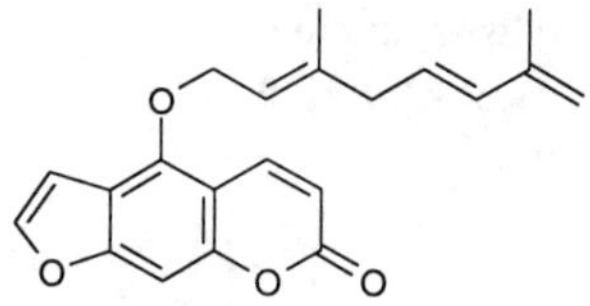

369 Anhydronotoptoloxide
5-[(2E)-3,7-Dimethyl-5,6-epoxy-2,7-octadienyloxy] psoralen. $C_{21}H_{20}O_5$ MW: 352.39 Property: colorless oleaginous substance. Source: QIANG HUO. Ref: 325.

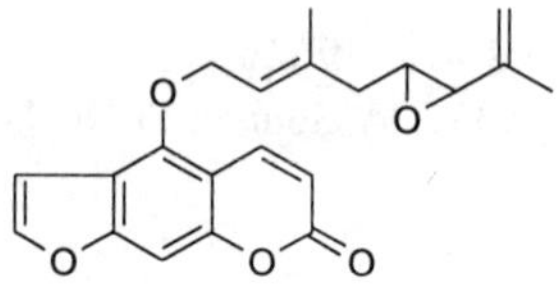

370 Anisaldehyde
$C_8H_8O_2$ MW: 136.15 Source: BA JIAO HUI XIANG, HUI XIANG, HUO XIANG, SHI CHUN, XIANG GEN QIN. Ref: 2, 6.

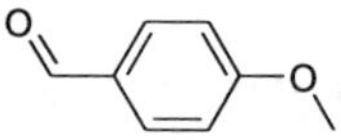

371 Anisic acid
$C_8H_8O_3$ MW: 152.15 Source: BA JIAO HUI XIANG, BAI MU XIANG, DANG GUI, FEI JI CAO, HUI XIANG, HUI XIANG JING YE, SHUI HUI XIANG. Ref: 2, 13.

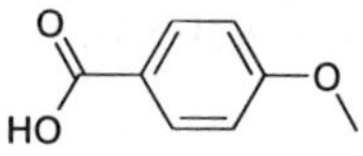

372 Anisodamine
$C_{17}H_{23}NO_4$ MW: 305.38 Property: mp 84.5-85.5°C. Source: ZANG QIE. Ref: 4, 6.

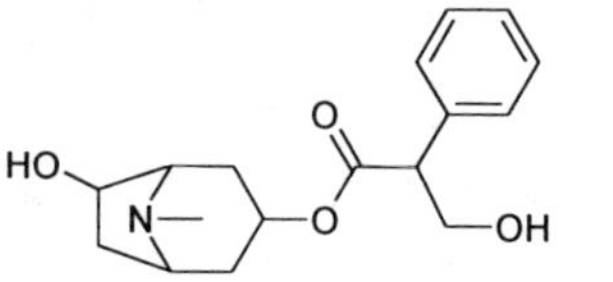

373 Anisodine
$C_{17}H_{21}NO_5$ MW: 319.36 Property: mp 62-4°C. Source: ZANG QIE. Ref: 4, 6.

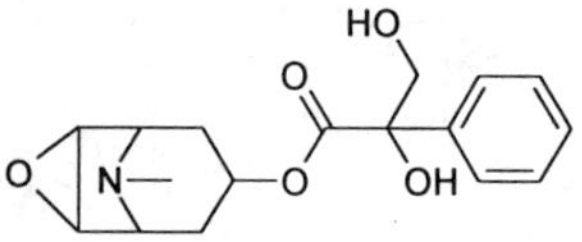

374 Anisotine
$C_{20}H_{19}N_3O_3$ MW: 349.39 Property: mp 189-90°C. Source: DA BO GU. Ref: 6.

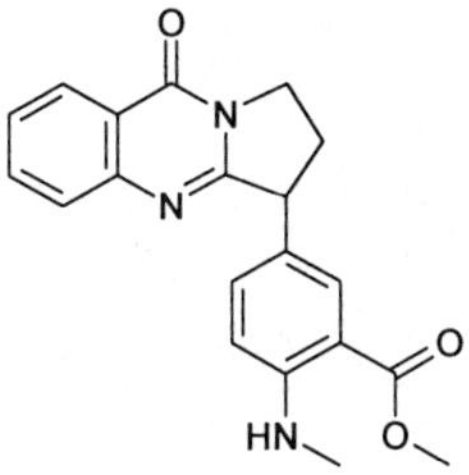

375 Anisylacetone
$C_{10}H_{12}O_2$ MW: 164.21 Property: bp 267-9°C. Source: BA JIAO HUI XIANG, HUI XIANG. Ref: 6.

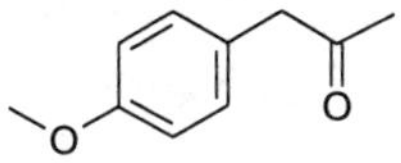

376 Annomonicin
$C_{35}H_{64}O_8$ MW: 612.90 Property: light yellow wax solid, mp 85-7°C. Source: NIU XIN PAN LI ZHI. Ref: 432.

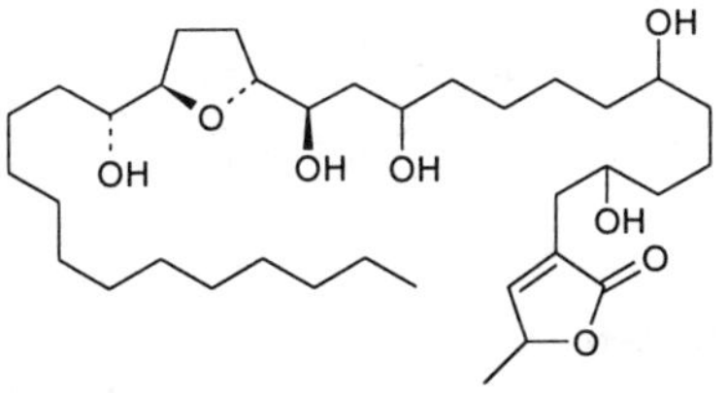

377 Annonacin
$C_{35}H_{64}O_7$ MW: 596.90 Property: white amorphous solid. Source: CI GUO FAN LI ZHI, JIN PING GE NA XIANG. Ref: 385, 420.

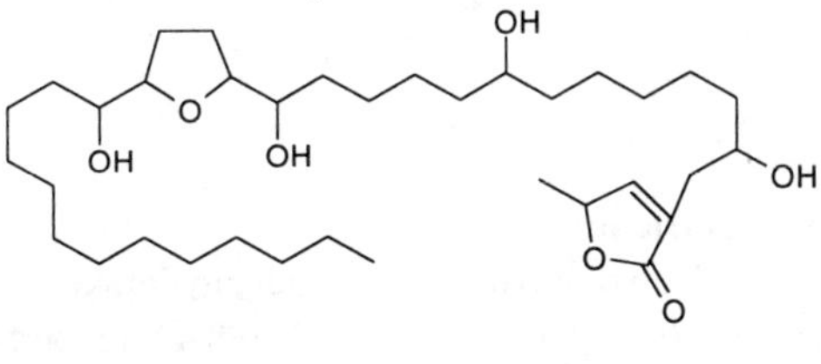

378 Annonareticin
$C_{37}H_{66}O_7$ MW: 622.93 Property: white crystal, mp 72-3°C, $[\alpha]_D^{25}$ +22.3° (c=0.1, MeOH). Source: NIU XIN PAN LI ZHI. Ref: 432.

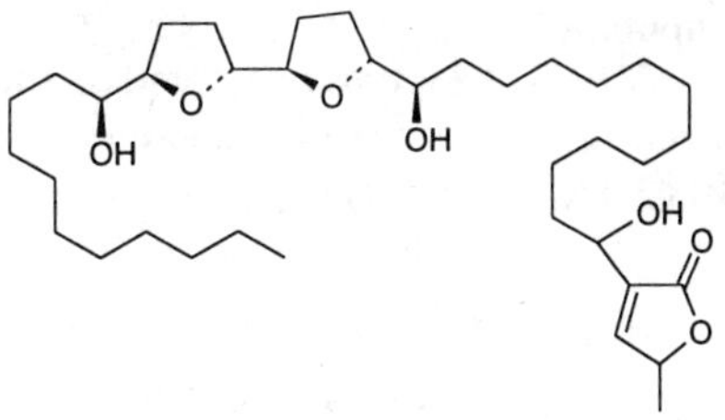

379 Annoreticuin
$C_{35}H_{64}O_7$ MW: 596.90 Property: light yellow wax solid, mp 75-7°C. Source: NIU XIN PAN LI ZHI. Ref: 432.

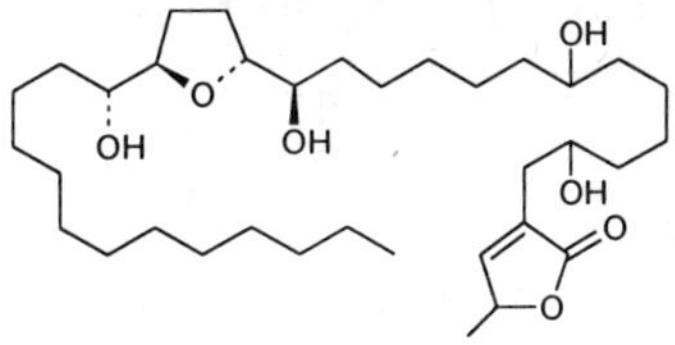

380 Anolobine
$C_{17}H_{15}NO_3$ MW: 281.31 Property: mp 262°C. Source: YE HE HUA. Ref: 6.

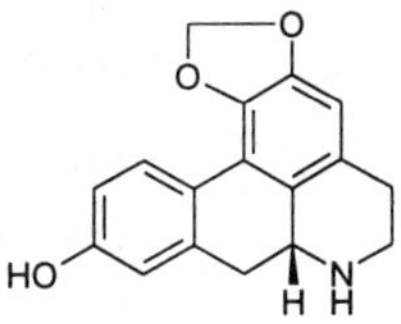

381 Anomalin
$C_{24}H_{26}O_7$ MW: 426.47 Property: mp 173-4°C. Source: BAI ZHI. Ref: 2, 6.

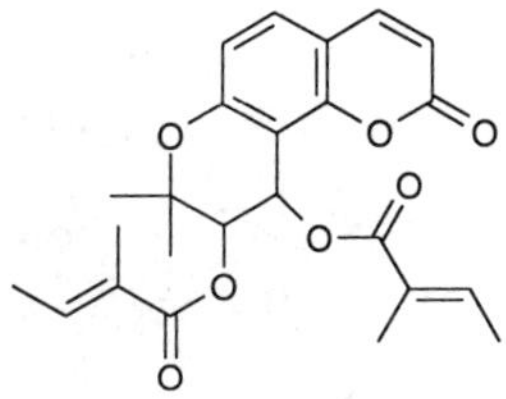

382 (+)-Anomalin
Source: LI JIANG QIAN HU. Ref: 557.

383 Anonaine
$C_{17}H_{15}NO_2$ MW: 265.31 Property: mp 122-3°C. Source: FAN LI ZHI, HE YE, HOU PU. Ref: 6, 221, 625.

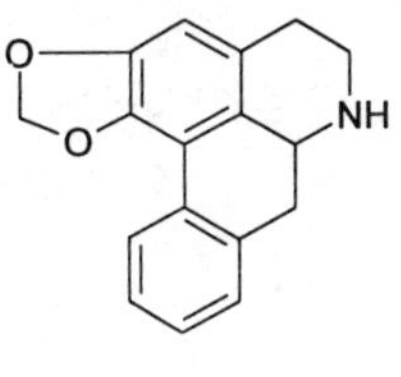

384 Anpubesol

$C_{20}H_{26}O_7$ MW: 378.43 Property: colorless and transparent, $[\alpha]_D^{20}$ -72.5° (c=0.15, chloroform). Source: ZHONG CHI MAO DANG GUI. Ref: 79.

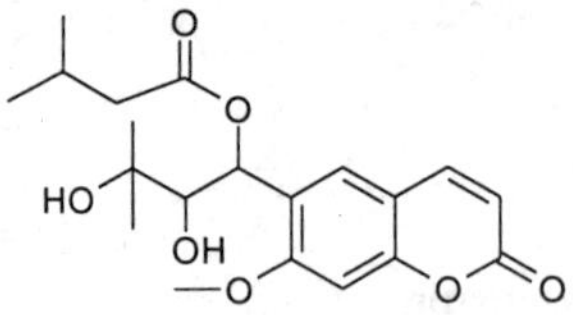

385 Anserine

$C_{10}H_{16}N_4O_3$ MW: 240.26 Property: mp 238-9°C. Source: JI NAO, XIA TIAN GAO, MAN LI YU. Ref: 6.

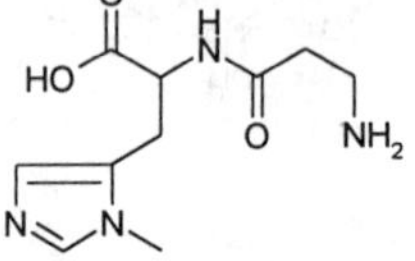

386 Antheraxanthin

$C_{40}H_{56}O_3$ MW: 584.89 Property: mp cis: 110°C, trans: 207°C. Source: BAI HE, DAO CAO. Ref: 6.

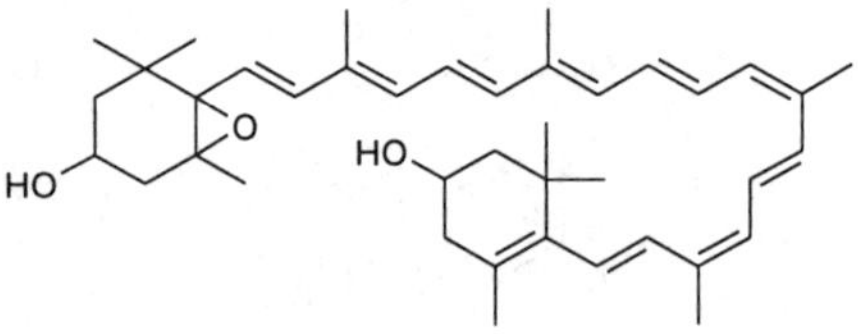

387 Anthragallol

$C_{14}H_8O_5$ MW: 256.22 Property: mp 312-3°C. Source: TU LIAN QIAO. Ref: 6.

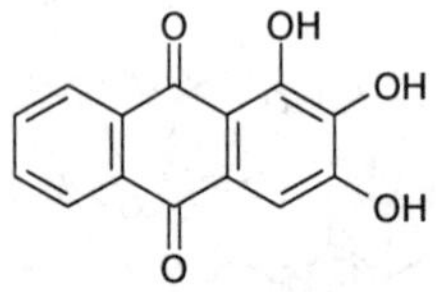

388 Anthraglycoside A

Physcione-8-β-D-glucopyranoside. $C_{22}H_{22}O_{10}$ MW: 446.41 Property: mp 230-2°C. Source: HU ZHANG. Ref: 6.

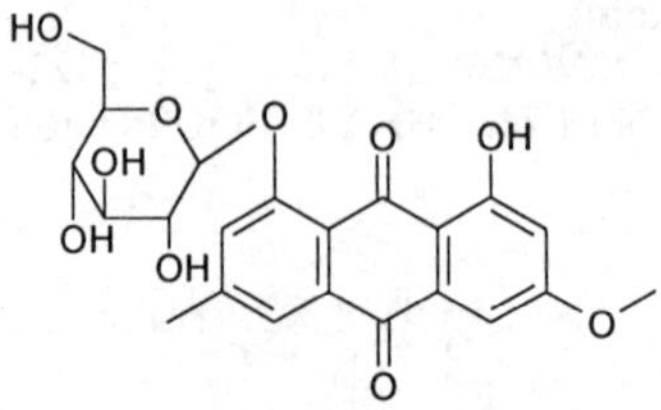

389 Anthraglycoside B

Emodin-8-O-β-D-glucopyranoside. $C_{21}H_{20}O_{10}$ MW: 432.39 Property: mp 190-1°C. Source: DA HUANG, HU ZHANG. Ref: 2, 6.

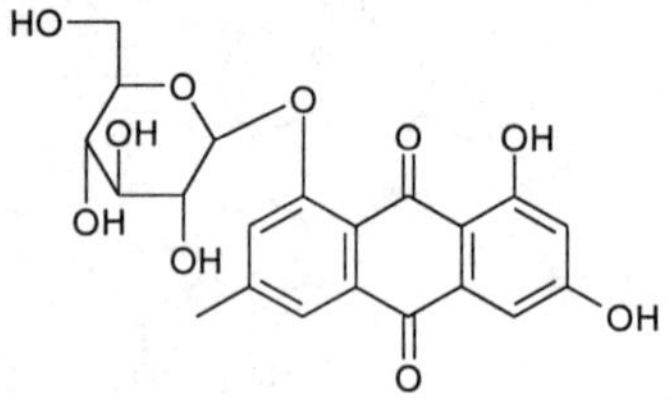

390 Anthranol

$C_{14}H_{10}O$ MW: 194.24 Source: LU HUI. Ref: 2.

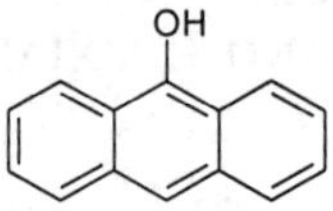

391 Anthraquinone

$C_{14}H_8O_2$ MW: 208.22 Property: mp 286°C, bp 379-81°C (sublimation). Source: HU ZHANG, LUO BU MA. Ref: 6.

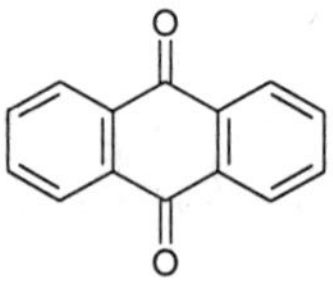

392 Anthraxin

$C_{21}H_{16}O_9$ MW: 412.36 Property: mp 336°C. Source: JIN CAO. Ref: 6.

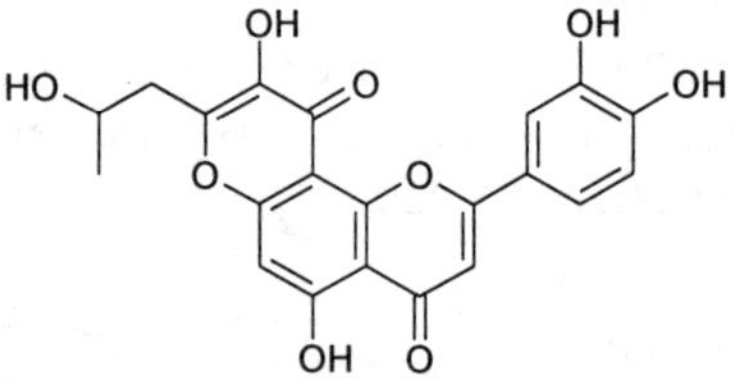

393 Anthricin

Deoxypodophyllotoxin; Desoxypodophyllotoxin. CAS: 24150-39-8 $C_{22}H_{22}O_7$ MW: 398.42 Property: mp 167-8°C. Source: BA JIAO LIAN, E SHEN. Ref: 4, 6.

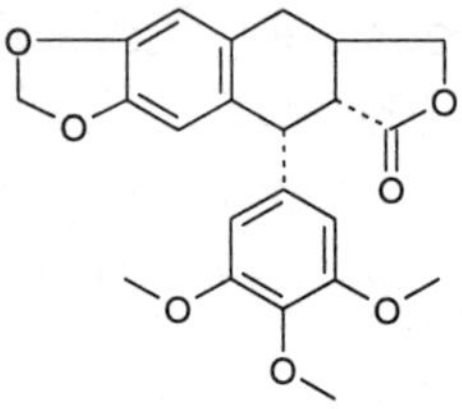

394 Anti-isorhynchophylline N-oxide
$C_{22}H_{28}N_2O_5$ MW: 400.48 Source: FENG XIANG SHU YE (a). Ref: 6.

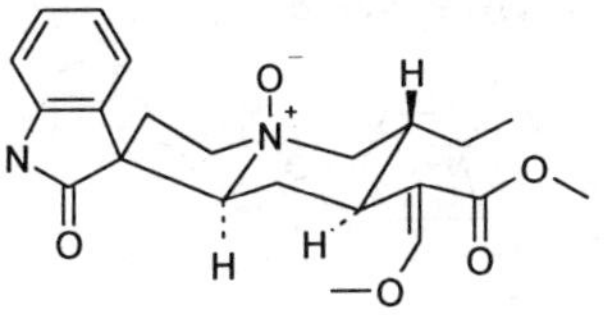

395 Apigenin
4H-1-benzopyran-4-one,5,7-dihydroxy-2-(4-hydroxy-phenyl); 5,7,4'-Trihydroxyflavone. $C_{15}H_{10}O_5$ MW: 270.24 Property: light yellow crystal (methanol), mp 344-7°C. Source: BAI GUO YE, BEI YE JU, FENG JIAO, HU ZHANG, HUO XIANG, LIE YE JU MAI CAI, MA HUANG, MI MENG HUA, PU GONG YING, SAN JIAN SHAN. Ref: 2, 369, 388, 440, 463, 521, 597.

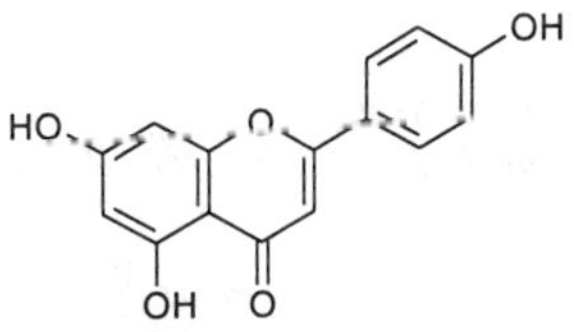

396 Apigenin bioside
$C_{26}H_{28}O_{13}$ MW: 548.51 Property: mp 257-8°C. Source: CI HUAI HUA. Ref: 6.

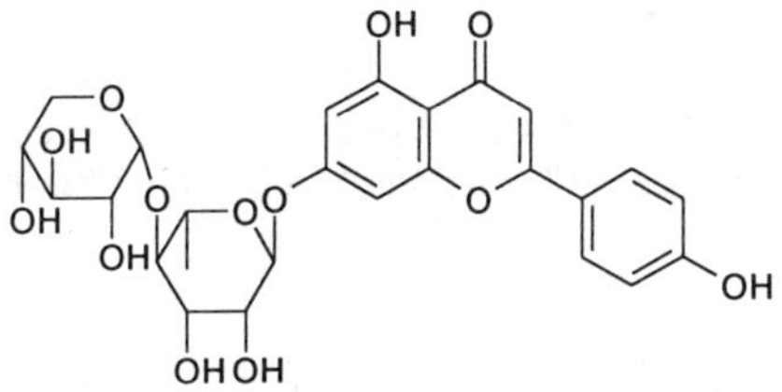

397 Apigenin-7-O-β-D-(6''-p-courmaroyl)-glucoside
$C_{30}H_{26}O_{12}$ MW: 578.53 Property: colourless thin acicular crystal, mp 264-5°C, $[\alpha]_D^{17}$ -143.93° (c=0.06, EtOH). Source: HUO XIANG, MAO BAI YANG. Ref: 2, 269.

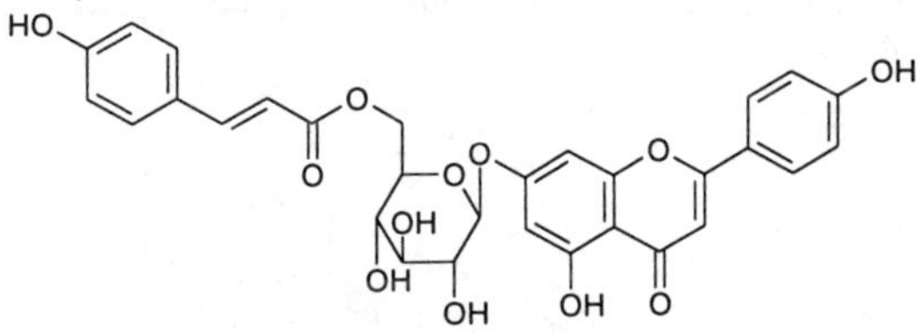

398 Apigenin-7,4'-dimethyl ether
$C_{17}H_{14}O_5$ MW: 298.30 Property: mp 171-2°C.Source: CHUAN XIN LIAN. Ref: 2.

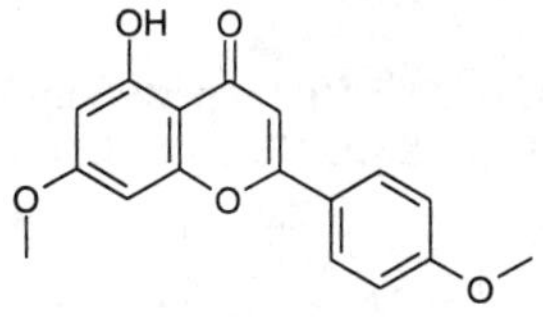

399 Apigenin-7-glucoside
$C_{21}H_{20}O_{10}$ MW: 432.39 Property: mp 226-8°C. Source: JING JIE, XIAN HE CAO. Ref: 2.

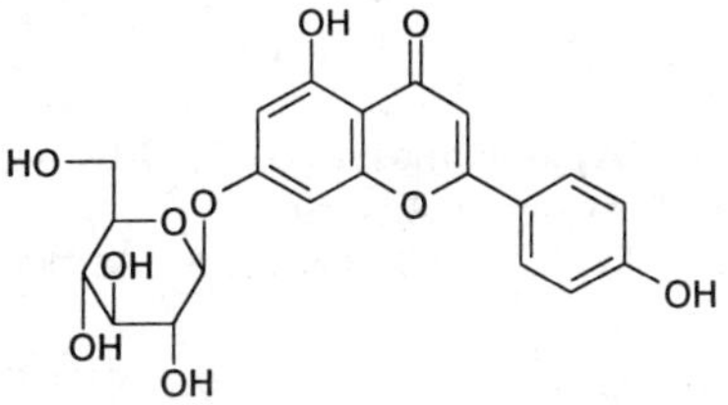

400 Apigenin-7-O-glucoside
Property: yellow powder, mp 178-80°C. Source: PU GONG YING. Ref: 440.

401 Apigenin-7-glucuronide
$C_{21}H_{18}O_{11}$ MW: 446.37 Property: mp 335-42°C. Source: DA YE ZI ZHU, YI NIAN PENG. Ref: 6.

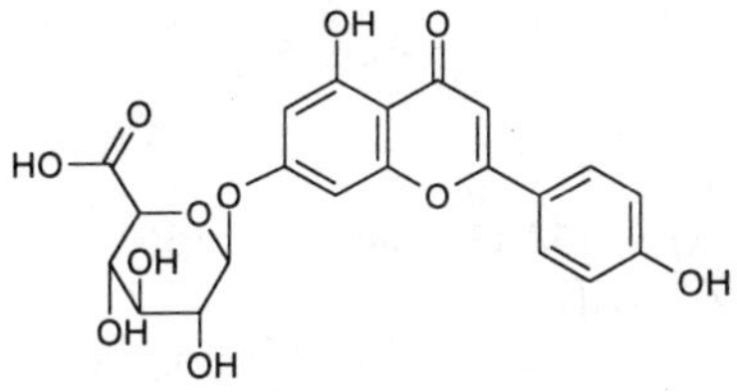

402 Apigenin-5-rhamnoside
Source: MA HUANG. Ref: 2.

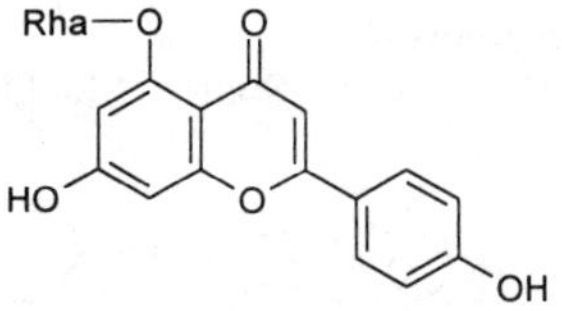

403 Apigetrin
$C_{21}H_{20}O_{10}$ MW: 432.39 Source: HUO XIANG. Ref: 2.

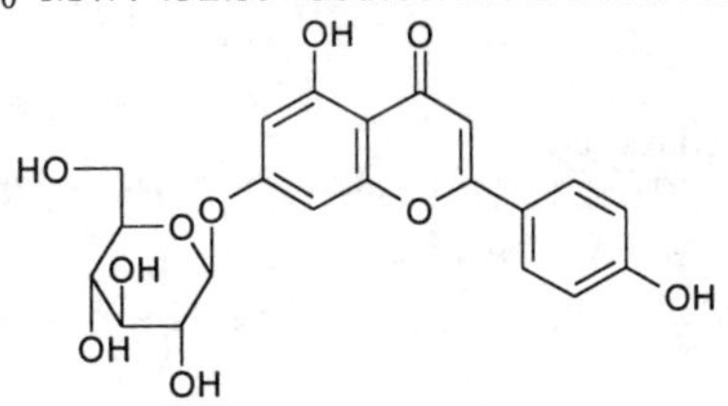

404 Apiin

$C_{26}H_{28}O_{14}$ MW: 564.50 Property: mp 228°C. Source: HAN QIN, MU JU, XIAO CHAO CAI. Ref: 6.

405 6-1(α-Apiofuranosyl-(1→6)-O-β-D-gluco-pyranosyl) oxy-rubrofusarin

$C_{27}H_{30}O_{14}$ MW: 578.53 Source: JUE MING ZI. Ref: 2.

406 Apiol

$C_{12}H_{14}O_4$ MW: 222.24 Source: QIANG HUO. Ref: 2.

407 Apiose

$C_5H_{10}O_5$ MW: 150.13 Source: FU PING, HAI DAI (DA YE ZAO). Ref: 6.

408 Aplopaeonoside

$C_{20}H_{28}O_{12}$ MW: 460.44 Source: MU DAN PI. Ref: 2, 50.

409 Aplotaxene

$C_{17}H_{28}$ MW: 232.41 Property: bp 110-5°C/8mm. Source: MU XIANG. Ref: 6.

410 Apoatropine

Atropamine. $C_{17}H_{21}NO_2$ MW: 271.36 Property: mp 60-2°C. Source: TAI ZI SHEN, TIAN XIAN ZI, LANG DANG GEN. Ref: 6.

411 β-Apopicropodophyllin

$C_{22}H_{20}O_7$ MW: 396.40 Property: mp 220-1°C. Source: WO ER QI. Ref: 6.

412 Aposiopolamine

$C_{16}H_{17}NO_3$ MW: 271.32 Source: HUA SHAN SHEN. Ref: 3.

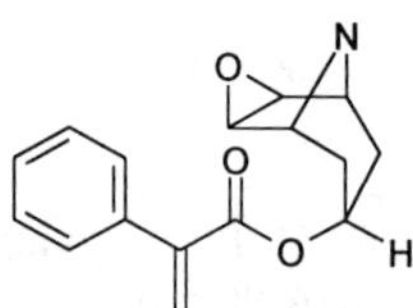

413 Apotutin

$C_{15}H_{18}O_6$ MW: 294.31 Property: white rhomboid crystal, mp 227-9°C. Source: MA SANG. Ref: 413.

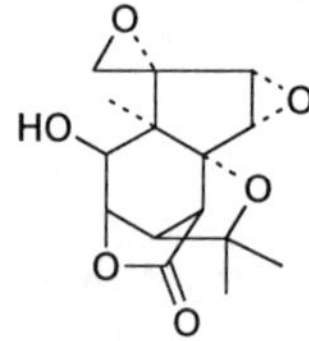

415 3-O-α-L-Arabinopyranosyl-3β,23-dihydroxy-lup-20(29)-en-28-oic acid

$C_{35}H_{56}O_8$ MW: 604.83 Source: BAI TOU WENG. Ref: 2.

416 3-O-α-L-Arabinopyranosyl oleanolic acid 28-O-β-D-glucopyranosyl-(1→6)-β-D-gluco-pyranoside

$C_{47}H_{76}O_{17}$ MW: 913.12 Property: white powder, mp 227-30°C, $[\alpha]_D^{19}$ +6.2° (c=0.25, Methanol). Source: CHUAN XU DUAN. Ref: 201.

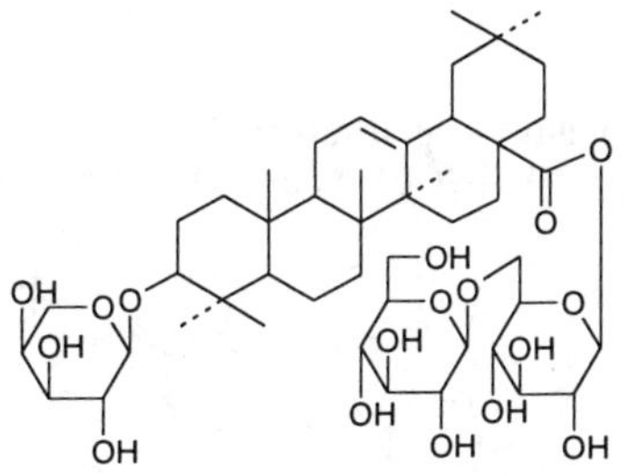

417 D-Arabitol

$C_5H_{12}O_5$ MW: 152.15 Property: mp 103°C. Source: JIN SI DAI, XUE CHA. Ref: 6.

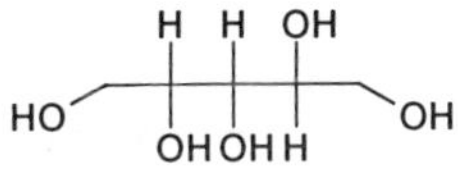

418 Arachidic acid

$C_{20}H_{40}O_2$ MW: 312.54 Property: mp 77°C, Bp 203-5°C. Source: BA DOU, GE GEN, CU LIU GUO (SHA JI), HONG HUA. Ref: 2.

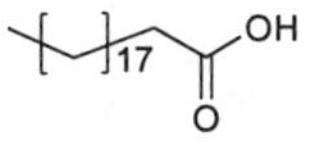

419 Arachidonic acid

$C_{20}H_{32}O_2$ MW: 304.48 Source: PU HUANG. Ref: 2.

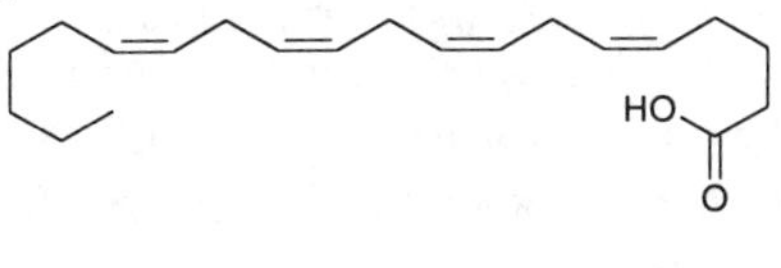

420 Arachidoside

$C_{16}H_{16}O_6$ MW: 304.30 Source: WU ZHU YU. Ref: 2.

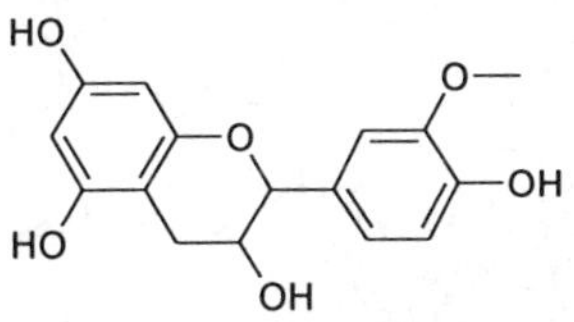

421 Araloside A

Chikusetsu saponin IV. $C_{47}H_{74}O_{18}$ MW: 927.10 Source: CI LAO YA, LIAO DONG SONG MU, REN SHEN, SONG MU, ZHU JIE SAN QI. Ref: 2, 6, 183, 235.

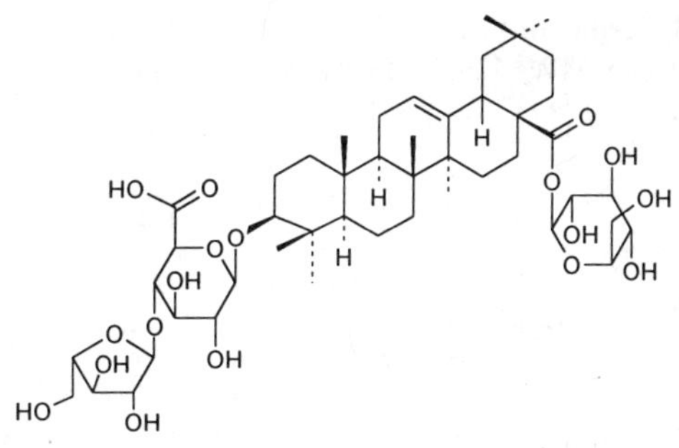

422 Araloside B

$C_{52}H_{82}O_{22}$ MW: 1059.22 Source: CI LAO YA, LIAO DONG SONG MU. Ref: 6, 235.

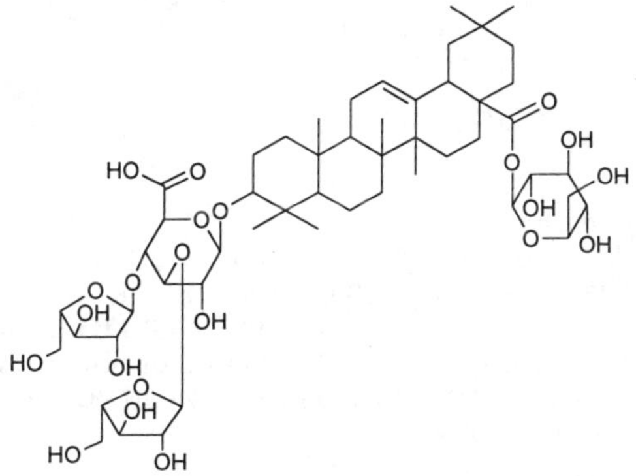

423 Araloside D

3-O-β-D-Glucopyranosyl-(1→2)-β-D-xylopyranosyl-(1→2)-α-L-arabinopyranoside(III). $C_{46}H_{74}O_{16}$ MW: 883.09 Property: white thin acicular powder, mp 157-8°C. Source: CONG MU. Ref: 183.

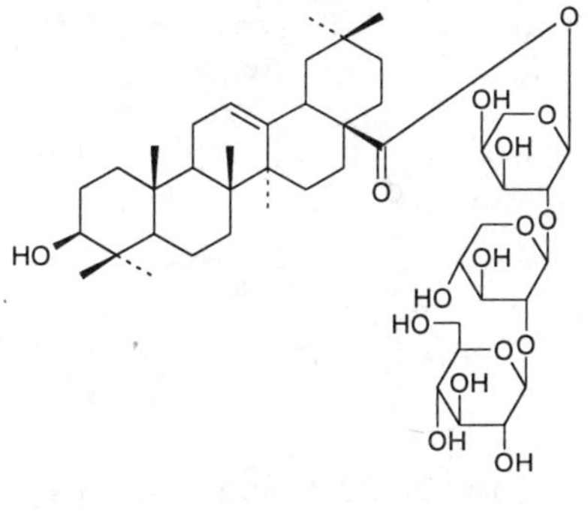

424 Arborinine

$C_{16}H_{15}NO_4$ MW: 285.30 Property: mp 175-6°C. Source: CHOU CAO. Ref: 6.

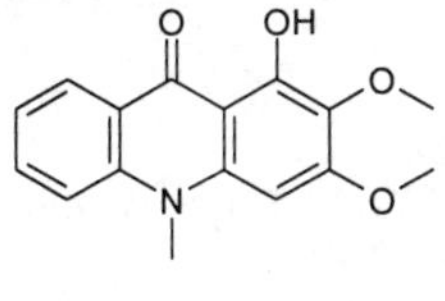

425 Arborinol
$C_{30}H_{50}O$ MW: 426.73 Property: mp 274.0-.5°C. Source: MAO CAO YE. Ref: 6.

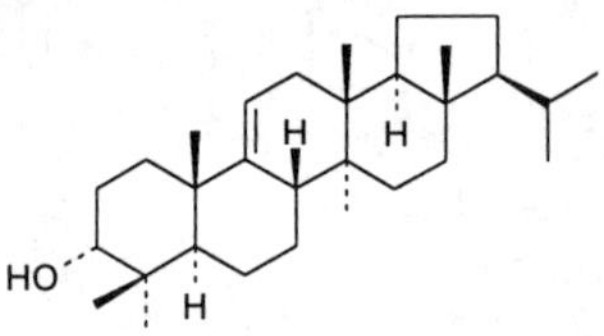

426 Arborinone
$C_{30}H_{48}O$ MW: 424.72 Property: mp 214.0-.5°C. Source: MAO CAO YE. Ref: 6.

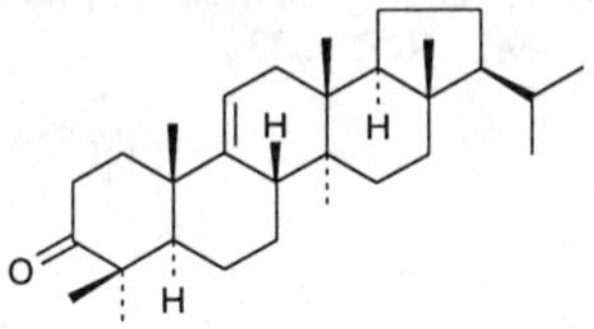

427 Arbutin
Hydroquinone β-D-glucopyranoside. $C_{12}H_{16}O_7$ MW: 272.26 Property: mp 200°C. Source: HU ER CAO, JI SHI TENG, JING TIAN SAN QI GEN, LI YE, LU SHOU CAO, LU XIAN CAO, QING MU XIAN (MA DOU LING GEN), YAN BAI CAI, YE LI ZHI YE, YUE JU YE, ZHEN ZHU MEI. Ref: 4, 6.

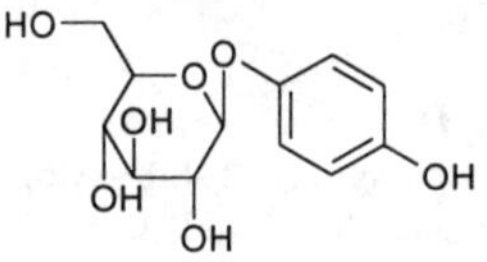

428 Archangelicin
$C_{24}H_{26}O_7$ MW: 426.47 Property: mp 103-5°C. Source: SHE CHUANG ZI. Ref: 6.

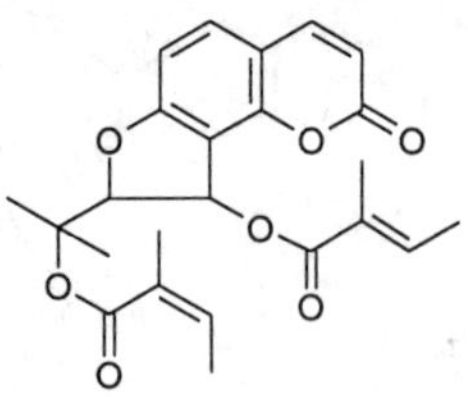

429 Arctic acid
$C_{12}H_8O_2S_2$ MW: 248.32 Source: NIU BANG GEN. Ref: 6.

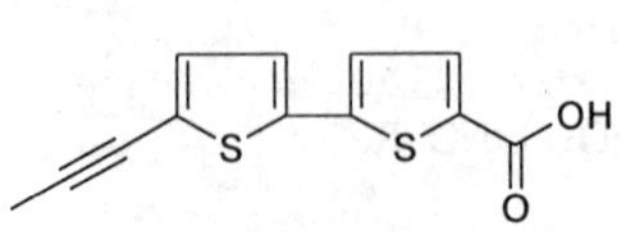

430 *l*-Arctigenin
$C_{21}H_{24}O_6$ MW: 372.42 Property: mp cis(-): 102°C. Source: NIU BANG ZI. Ref: 6.

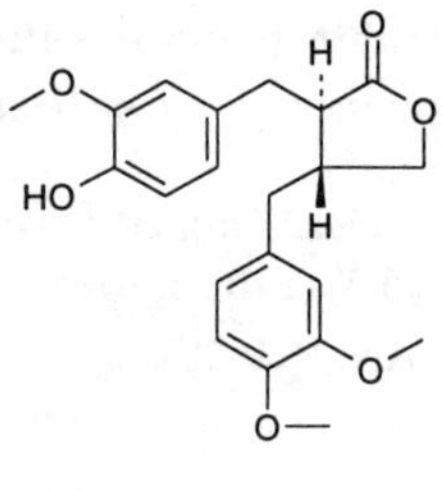

431 Arctigenin 4'-gentiobioside
$C_{33}H_{44}O_{16}$ MW: 696.71 Source: DA JIN NIU CAO. Ref: 6.

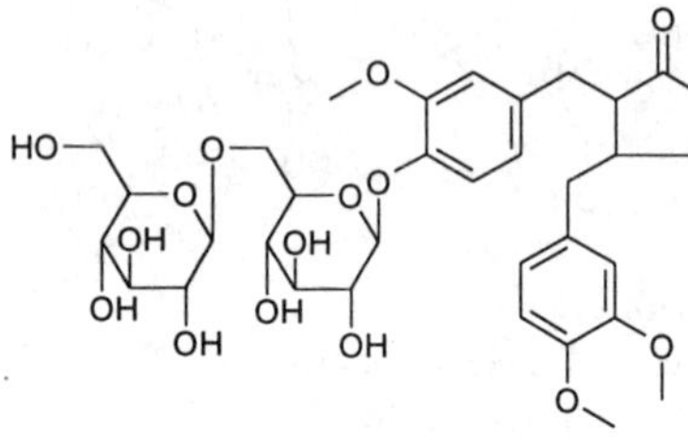

432 Arctiin
$C_{27}H_{34}O_{11}$ MW: 534.57 Property: mp 111-2°C. Source: DA JIN NIU CAO, LUO SHI TENG, NIU BANG ZI. Ref: 6, 7, 288.

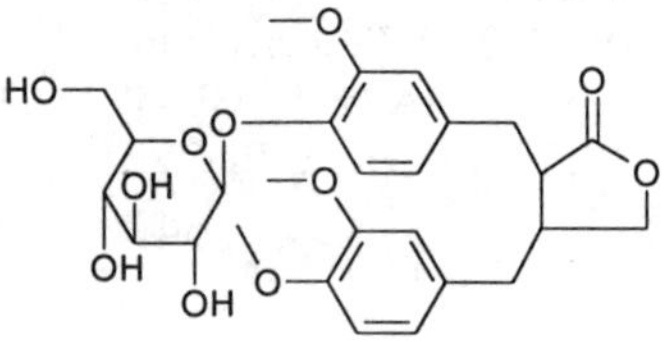

433 Ardipusilloside I
3-O-[α-L-Rhamnopyranosyl-(1→2)-β-D-gluco-pyranosyl-(1→3)][β-D-glucopyranosyl-(1→2)]-α-L-arabinopyranosyl cyclamiretin A. $C_{53}H_{86}O_{22}$ MW: 1075.26 Property: white acicular crystal, mp 239-41°C, $[\alpha]_D^{22.8}$ -26.6° (c=0.93, MeOH). Source: CHUAN CHAN JIU JIE LONG. Ref: 276.

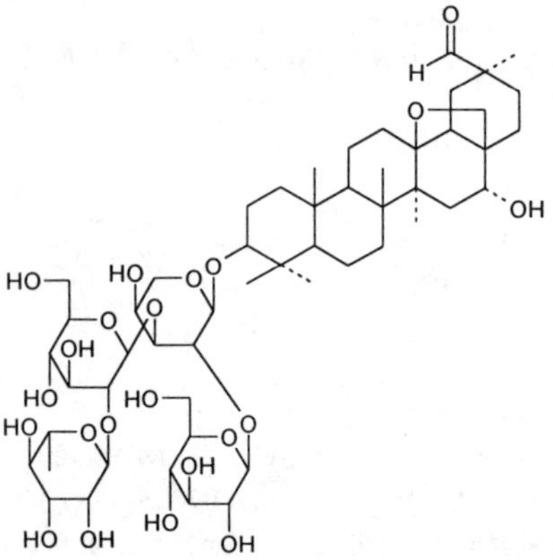

434 Ardipusilloside II

3-O-[α-L-xylopyranosyl-(1→2)-β-D-glucopyranosyl-(1→4)][β-D-glucopyranosyl-(1→2)-β-D-glucopyranosyl-(1→2)]-α-L-rhamnopyranosyl cyclamiretin A. $C_{58}H_{94}O_{27}$ MW: 1223.38 Property: white powder, mp 279-81°C, $[\alpha]_D^{22.5}$ -21.91° (c=0.79, C_5H_5N). Source: JIU JIE LONG. Ref: 276.

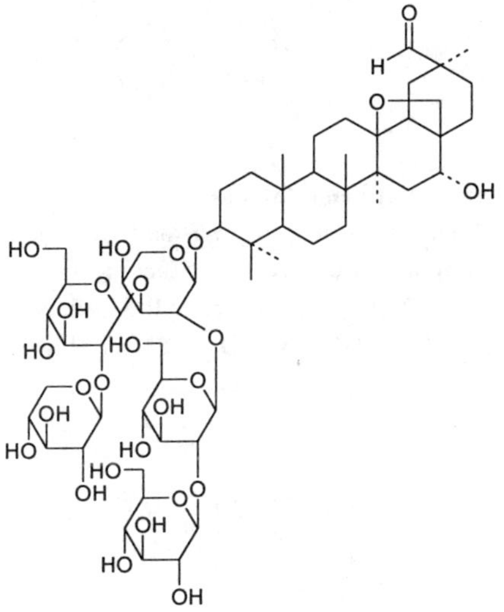

435 Areapillin

$C_{18}H_{16}O_8$ MW: 360.32 Source: YIN CHEN HAO. Ref: 2.

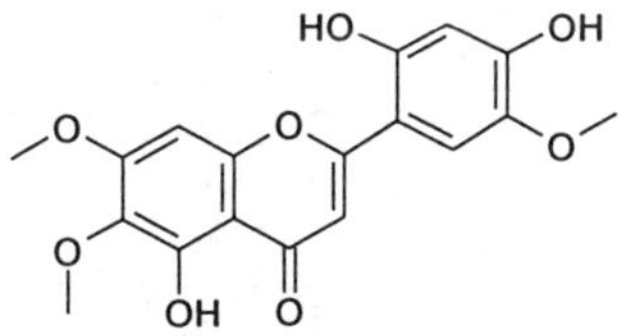

436 Arecaidine

Arecaine. $C_7H_{11}NO_2$ MW: 141.17 Property: mp 223-4°C (dec). Source: BING LANG. Ref: 2.

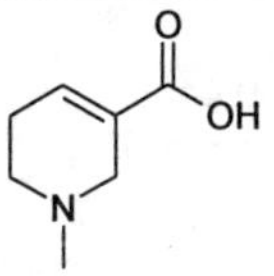

437 Arecolidine

$C_8H_{13}NO_2$ MW: 155.20 Source: BING LANG. Ref: 2.

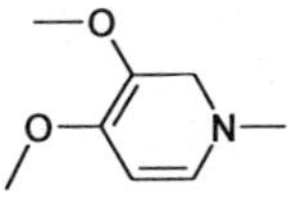

438 Arecoline

$C_8H_{13}NO_5$ MW: 155.20 Property: bp 209°C. Source: BING LANG. Ref: 2, 4.

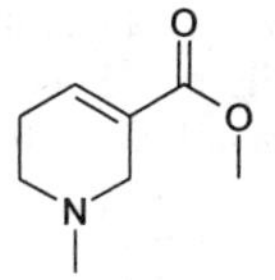

439 Arenobufagin

$C_{24}H_{32}O_6$ MW: 416.52 Source: CHAN SU. Ref: 2.

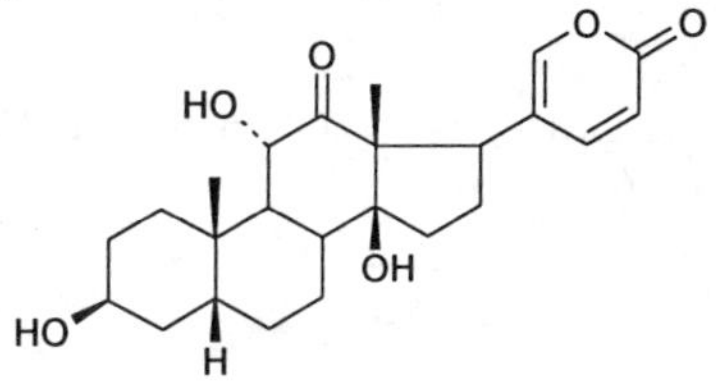

440 Argentine

$C_{23}H_{26}NO_3$ MW: 406.49 Source: MU MA DOU. Ref: 6.

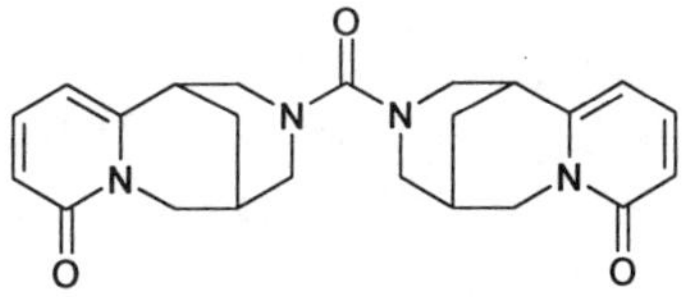

441 Aricine

$C_{21}H_{24}N_2O_4$ MW: 368.44 Property: mp 188-9°C. Source: JIN JI LE, LUO FU MU JING YE. Ref: 6.

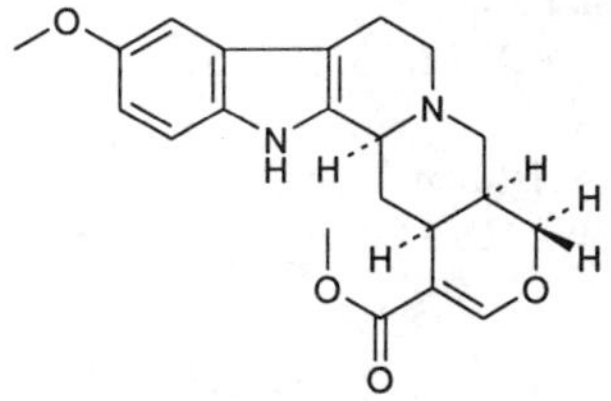

442 Argininyl-fructosyl-glucose

$C_{18}H_{34}N_4O_{12}$ MW: 498.49 Property: white powder, mp 158-60°C. Source: HONG SHEN. Ref: 348.

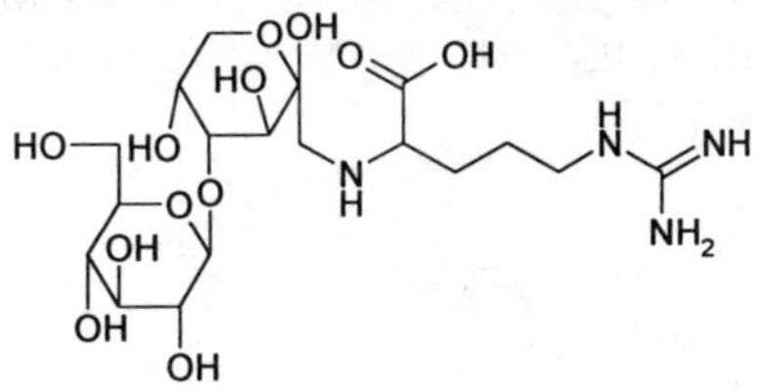

443 Argutone
2-Ethoxymethylene-3,5-dihydroxy-γ-pyrone. $C_8H_{10}O_5$ MW: 186.17 Property: colorless acicular crystal, mp 94°C (sublimate), easy soluble in chloroform, methanol, able to dissolve in benzene, ether, acetone, acetic ester and ethanol, insoluble in water. Source: MA TONG HUA. Ref: 85.

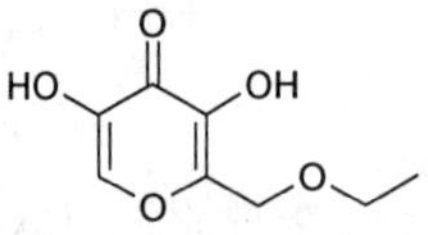

444 Aristolene
9-Aristolene. $C_{15}H_{24}$ MW: 204.36 Source: GAN SONG. Ref: 6.

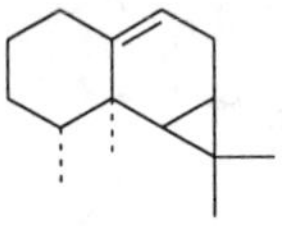

445 Aristolamide-N-hexoside
Source: QING MU XIANG. Ref: 517.

447 9-Aristolen-1-α-ol
$C_{15}H_{24}O$ MW: 220.36 Source: GAN SONG. Ref: 6.

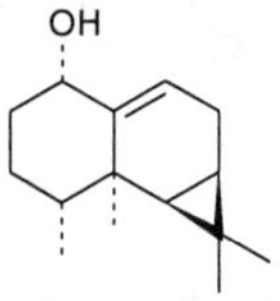

448 Aristolenone
Source: MA DOU LING. Ref: 517.

449 1(10)-Aristolen-2-one
$C_{15}H_{22}O$ MW: 218.34 Source: GAN SONG. Ref: 6.

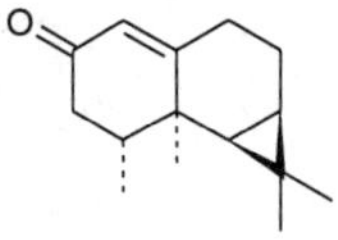

450 Aristolochic acid
$C_{17}H_{11}NO_7$ MW: 341.28 Property: mp 287-92°C (dec). Source: MA DOU LING, GUAN MU TONG, HUAI TONG, MU TONG MA DOU LING, MA DOU LING, QING MU XIANG, ZHU SHA LIAN. Ref: 6, 334, 517.

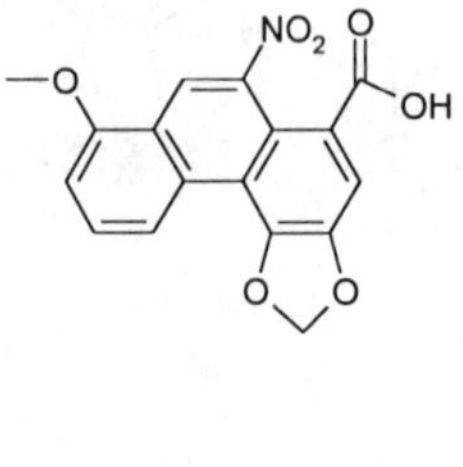

451 Aristolochic acid BII methyl ester
3,4-dimethoxy-10-nitrophenanthrenic-1-acid methyl ester. $C_{18}H_{15}NO_6$ MW: 341.32 Property: yellow acicular crystal, mp 283°C. Source: MU TONG MA DOU LING. Ref: 334.

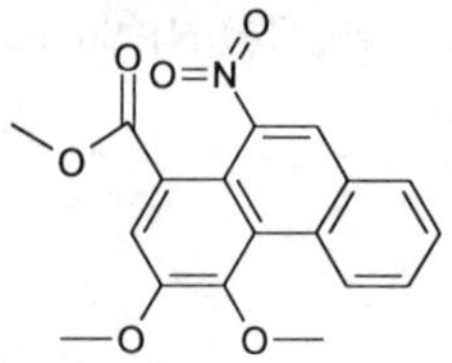

452 Aristolophenanlactone I
9,10-dihydroxy-8-methoxy-3,4-methylenedioxy-phenanthrene-1-carboxylic acid lactone. $C_{17}H_{10}O_6$ MW: 310.27 Property: bright yellow solid, mp 278°C. Source: GUAN HUA MA DOU LING. Ref: 332.

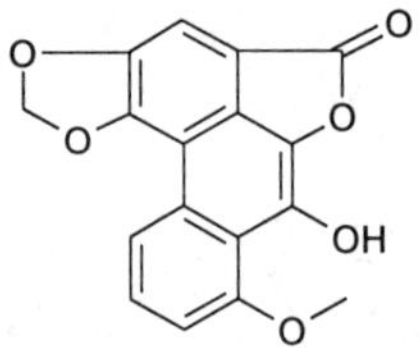

453 Aristoloterpenate
$C_{32}H_{31}NO_8$ MW: 557.61 Property: thin yellow acicular crystal, mp 259°C (chloroform-methanol). Source: MIAN MAO MA DOU LING. Ref: 358.

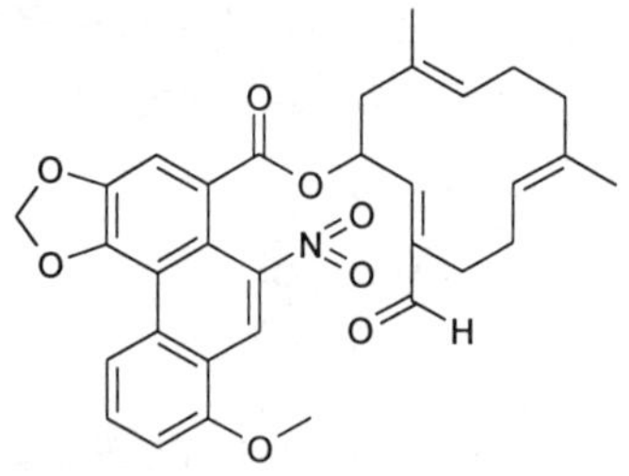

454 Aritasone
$C_{20}H_{28}O_2$ MW: 300.44 Property: mp 105-6°C. Source: TU JING JIE. Ref: 6.

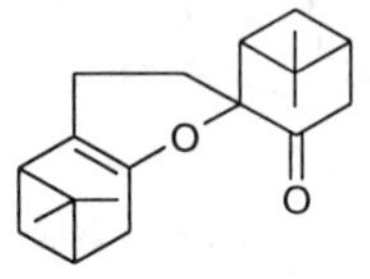

455 Arjunolic acid
$C_{30}H_{48}O_5$ MW: 488.71 Property: mp 337-40°C.
Source: FAN SHI LIU PI, SHAN GAN CAO. Ref: 6.

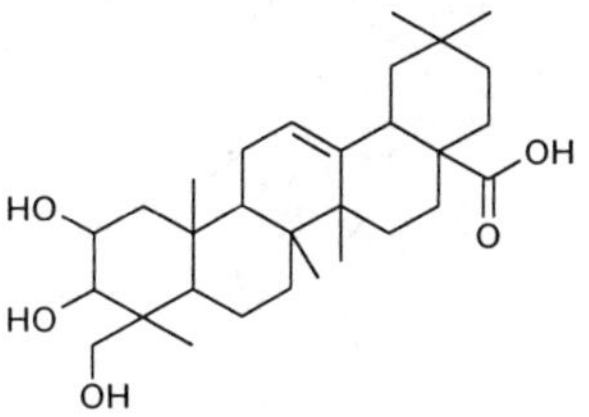

456 Armepavine
$C_{19}H_{23}NO_3$ MW: 313.40 Property: mp 148-9°C.
Source: HE YE. Ref: 6.

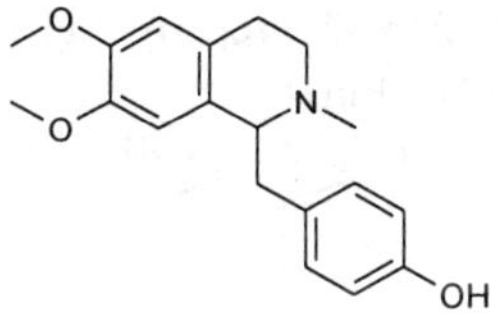

457 Armillarilin
$C_{24}H_{30}O_7$ MW: 430.50 Property: white massive crystal, mp 179-80°C, $[\alpha]_D^{14}$ +162° (chloroform).
Source: MI HUAN JUN. Ref: 147.

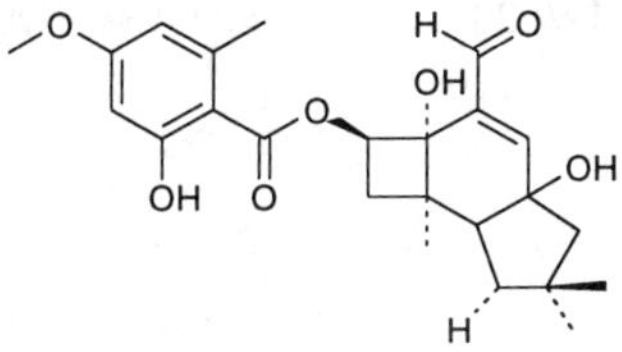

458 Armillarinin
$C_{24}H_{29}ClO_7$ MW: 464.95 Property: white massive crystal, mp 152-5°C, $[\alpha]_D^{17}$ +153.6° (chloroform).
Source: MI HUAN JUN. Ref: 147.

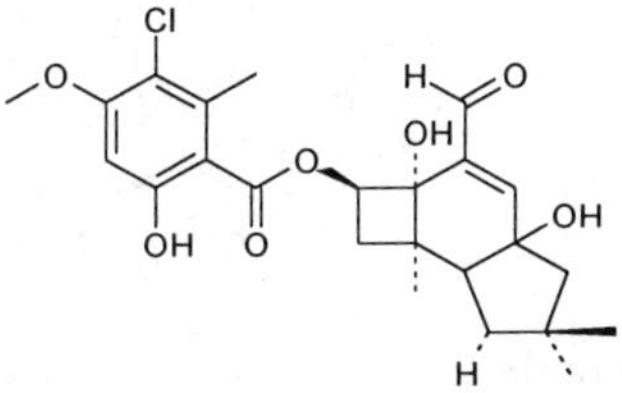

459 Armillaripin
$C_{24}H_{30}O_6$ MW: 414.50 Property: mp 202-4°C.
Source: MI HUAN JUN. Ref: 154.

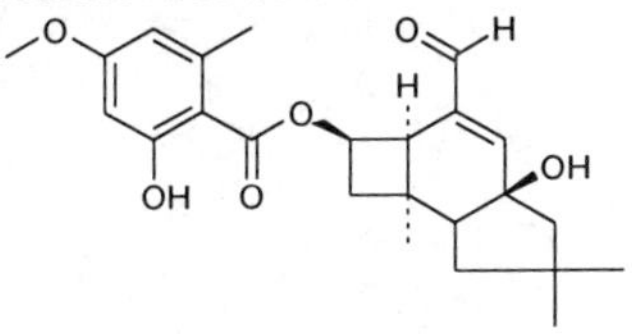

460 Armillarisin A
$C_{12}H_{10}O_5$ MW: 234.21 Property: mp 245-6°C.
Source: LIANG JUN. Ref: 6.

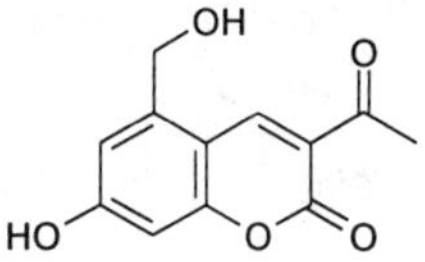

461 Arnidiol
$C_{30}H_{50}O_2$ MW: 442.73 Property: mp 257°C. Source: E BU SHI CAO, JIN ZHAN JU, PU GONG YING. Ref: 6.

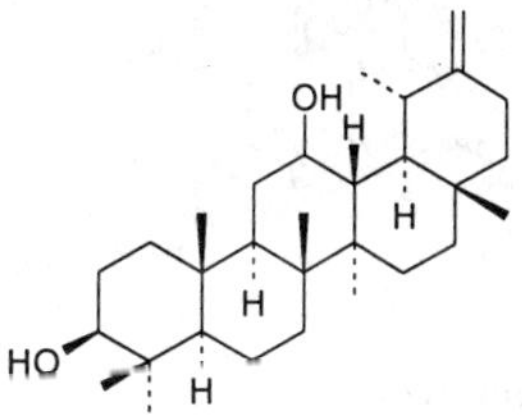

462 Aromadendrene
$C_{15}H_{24}$ MW: 204.36 Source: CHAI HU, HOU PO, JIU LI XIANG. Ref: 2, 11.

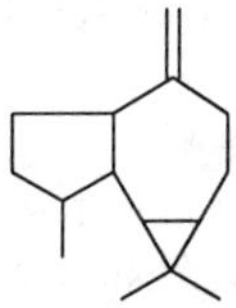

463 Aromadendrin
$C_{15}H_{12}O_6$ MW: 288.26 Property: mp 247-9°C.
Source: BA DAN XING REN, CE BAI YE, TAO JING BAI PI, TAO ZHI. Ref: 6.

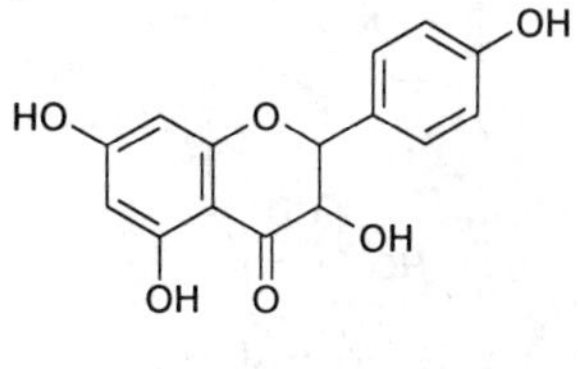

464 Aromadendrin-4',7-dimethyl ether
$C_{15}H_{12}O_5$ MW: 272.26 Property: mp 189-90°C.
Source: NING MENG AN YE. Ref: 6.

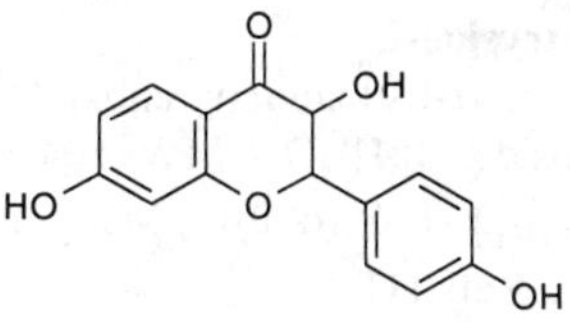

465 Aromadendrin-5,7-dimethyl ether
$C_{15}H_{12}O_5$ MW: 272.26 Property: mp 226-30°C. Source: NING MENG AN YE. Ref: 6.

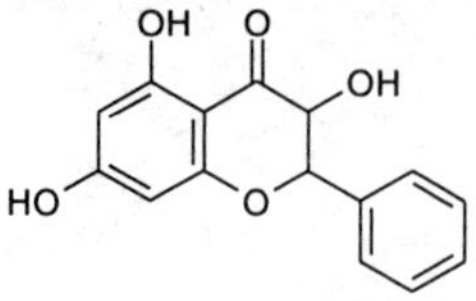

466 Aromadendrin-7-monomethyl ether
$C_{16}H_{14}O_6$ MW: 302.29 Property: mp 193°C. Source: NING MENG AN YE. Ref: 6.

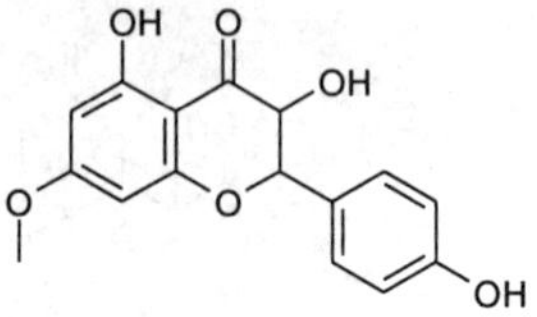

467 Aromadendrol
Source: SHE PU TAO. Ref: 552.

468 Arotopine
Property: colorless rhomboid crystal, mp 208-9°C. Source: YUN QIAN HU. Ref: 436.

469 Artabotryside-A
Quercetin-3-O-α-L-rhamnopyranosyl(1→2)-α-L-rarbinofuranoside. $C_{26}H_{28}O_{15}$ MW: 580.50 Property: white, mp175-7°C, $[\alpha]_D^{30}$ -113°(c=0.1, MeOH). Source: YING ZHUA. Ref: 411.

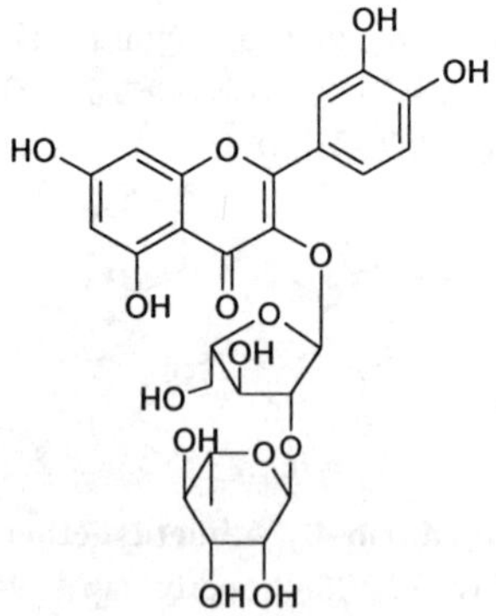

470 Artabotryside-B
Kaempferol-3-O-α-L-rhamnopyranosyl(1→2)-α-L-rarbinofuranoside. $C_{26}H_{28}O_{14}$ MW: 564.50 Property: mp 262-5°C, $[\alpha]_D^{30}$ -146° (c=0.12, MeOH). Source: YING ZHUA. Ref: 411.

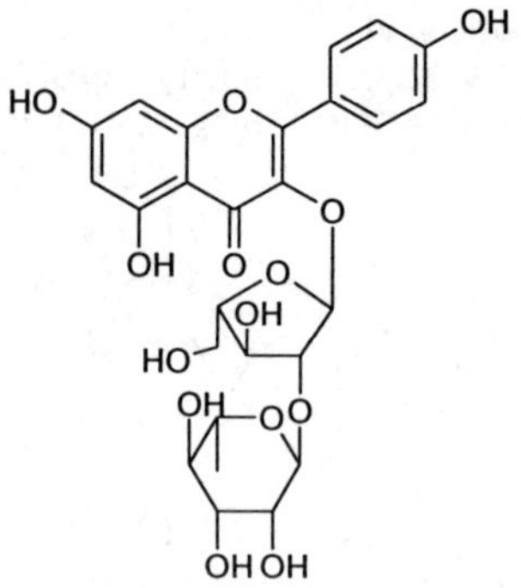

471 Artabsin
$C_{15}H_{20}O_3$ MW: 248.32 Property: mp 133-5°C. Source: BAI HAO. Ref: 6.

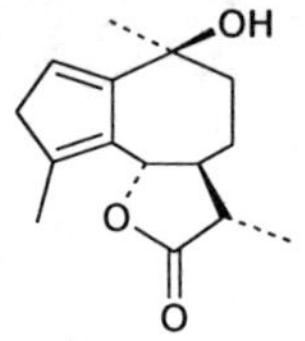

472 Arteamisinine I
$C_{13}H_{18}O_2$ MW: 206.29 Source: QING HAO. Ref: 2.

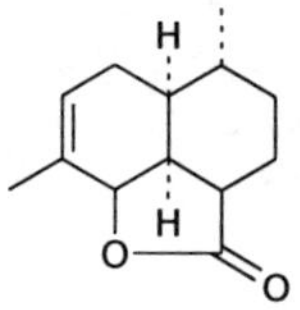

473 Arteamisinine III
$C_{14}H_{22}O_4$ MW: 266.34 Source: QING HAO. Ref: 2.

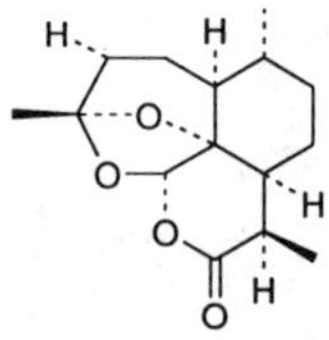

474 Arteannuin B
$C_{15}H_{20}O_3$ MW: 206.29 Source: QING HAO. Ref: 2.

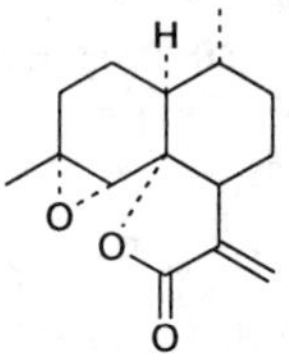

475 Artemisetin

$C_{20}H_{20}O_8$ MW: 388.38 Source: QING HAO. Ref: 2.

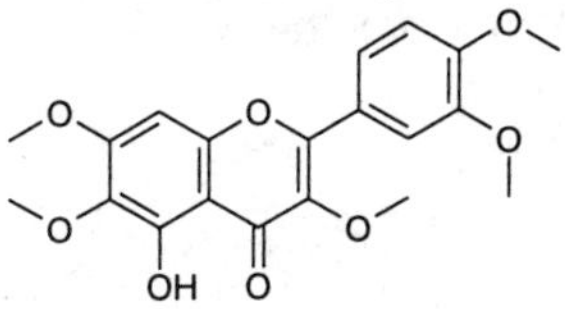

476 Artemisia alcohol

$C_{10}H_{18}O$ MW: 154.25 Property: bp 71°C/6mm. Source: MU HAO. Ref: 6.

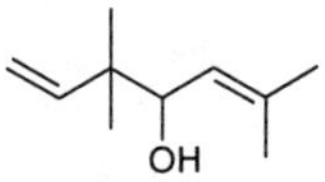

477 Artemisia ketone

$C_{10}H_{16}O$ MW: 152.24 Property: bp 182°C.Source: HUANG HUA HAO, MU XIANG, QING HAO. Ref: 2, 6.

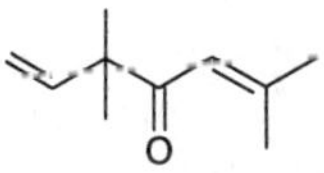

478 Artemisic acid

$C_{15}H_{22}O_2$ MW: 234.34 Source: QING HAO. Ref: 2.

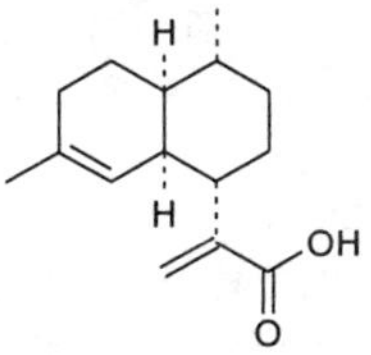

479 Artemisilactone

$C_{15}H_{22}O_3$ MW: 250.34 Source: QING HAO. Ref: 2.

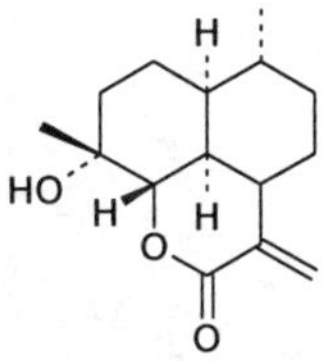

480 Artemisin

$C_{15}H_{18}O_4$ MW: 262.31 Property: mp (-): 203°C, (±): 190-2°C. Source: SHAN DAO NIAN HAO. Ref: 6.

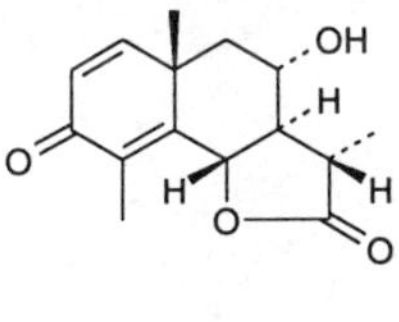

481 Artemisinin

Qinghaosu. $C_{15}H_{22}O_5$ MW: 282.34 Source: QING HAO. Ref: 2.

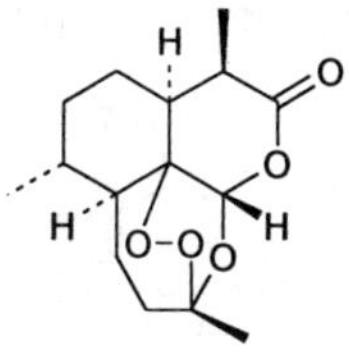

482 Artemisinol

$C_{15}H_{28}O$ MW: 224.39 Source: QING HAO. Ref: 2.

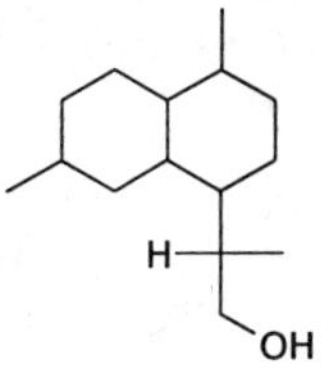

483 Artemisitene

$C_{15}H_{20}O_5$ MW: 280.32 Source: QING HAO. Ref: 2.

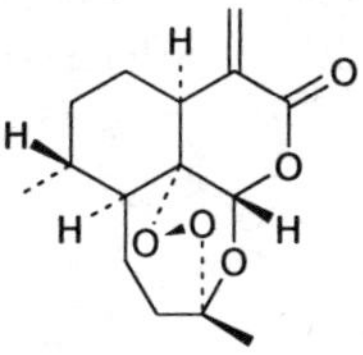

484 Arundoin

$C_{31}H_{52}O$ MW: 440.76 Property: mp 235-7°C, 271-3°C. Source: BAI MAO GEN, DAN ZHU YE, SUI GU ZI, LONG XUCAO (II). Ref: 6.

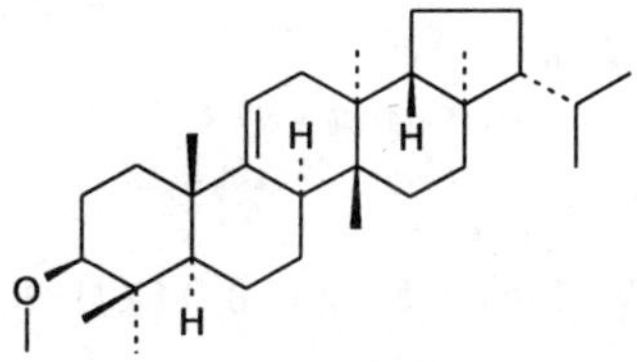

485 Asarinin

$C_{20}H_{18}O_6$ MW: 354.36 Property: mp(+): 121-2°C, (-): 22-4°C. Source: TONG MU, XI XIN. Ref: 6.

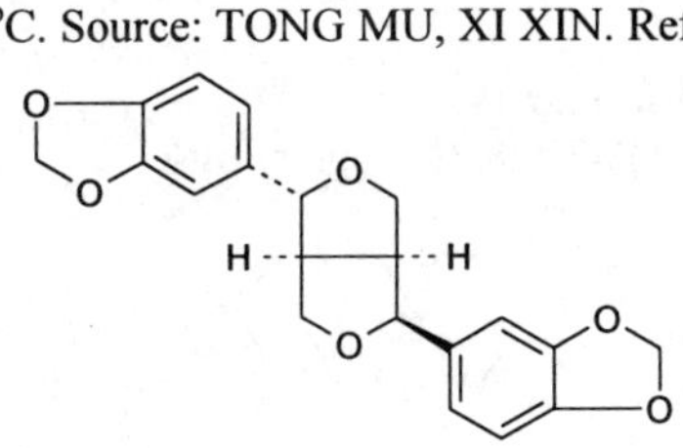

486 Asarone
$C_{12}H_{16}O_3$ MW: 208.26 Property: mp 67°C (62°C), bp 296°C. Source: BAI CHANG, CHANG PU YE, DA YE XIANG, HE SHI, HE SHI FENG, SHICHANG PU, XI XIN. Ref: 2, 4.

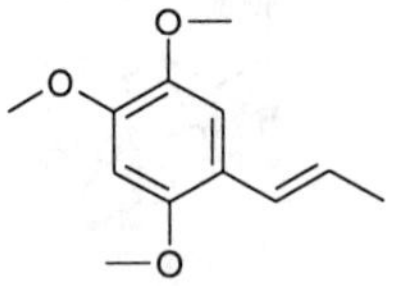

487 β-Asarone
$C_{12}H_{16}O_3$ MW: 208.26 Property: bp 162-3°C/ 12mm. Source: BAI CHANG, CHANG PU YE, SHI CHANG PU. Ref: 6.

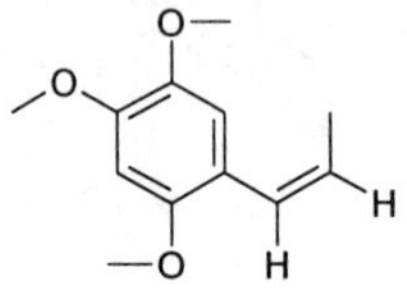

488 Asarylaldehyde
$C_{10}H_{12}O_4$ MW: 196.20 Property: mp 114°C. Source: BAI CHANG, HE SHI, HE SHI FENG. Ref: 6.

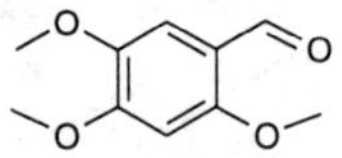

489 Ascaridole
$C_{10}H_{16}O_2$ MW: 168.24 Property: mp 2.5°C, bp 115°C/15mm. Source: TU JING JIE. Ref: 6.

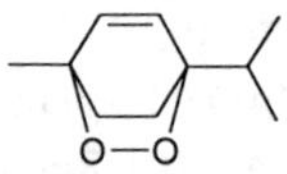

490 Aschantin
Source: WANG CHUN MU LAN. Ref: 543.

491 Ascorbic acid
$C_6H_8O_6$ MW: 176.13 Source: BAI GUO, CU LIU GUO (SHA JI), GOU QI ZI. Ref: 2.

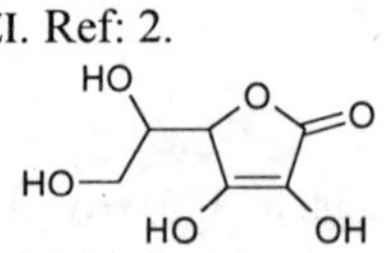

492 Asiatic acid
$C_{30}H_{48}O_5$ MW: 488.71 Source: BING PIAN. Ref: 2.

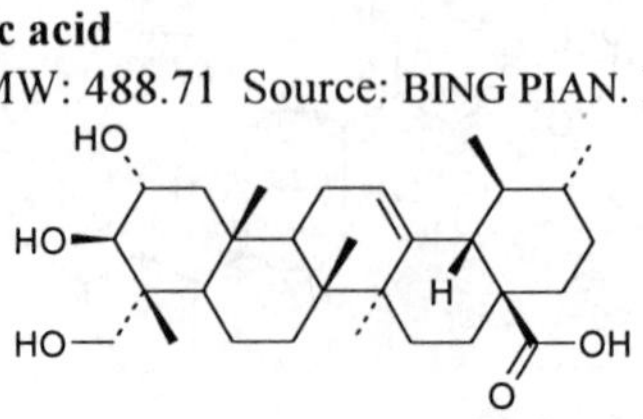

493 Asiaticoside
$C_{48}H_{78}O_{18}$ MW: 943.15 Property: mp 230-3°C. Source: JI XUE CAO. Ref: 6.

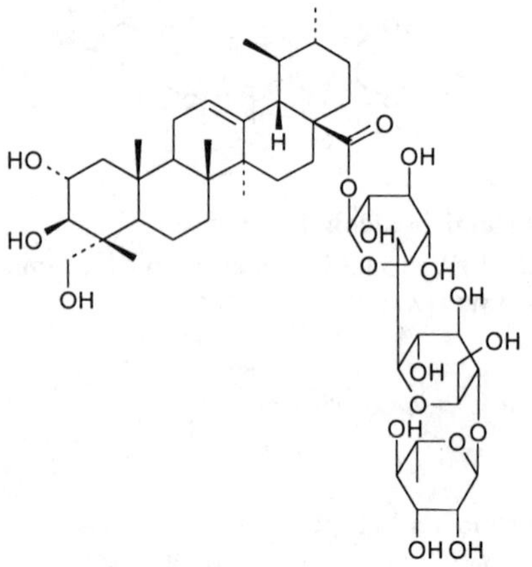

494 Asimilobine
$C_{17}H_{17}NO_2$ MW: 206.29 Property: mp 177-9°C. Source: DA ZAO, HOU PU. Ref: 2, 625.

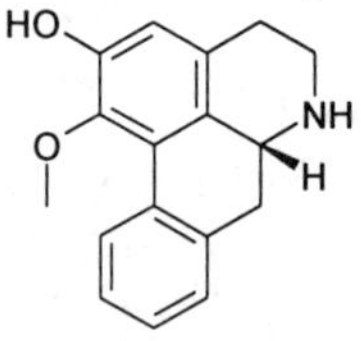

495 Aspafilioside A
$C_{38}H_{62}O_{12}$ MW: 710.91 Property: white acicular crystal (methanol), mp 210-2°C, $[\alpha]_D^{14}$-36.5° (c=0.09, chloroform-methanol). Source: XIAO BAI BU. Ref: 159.

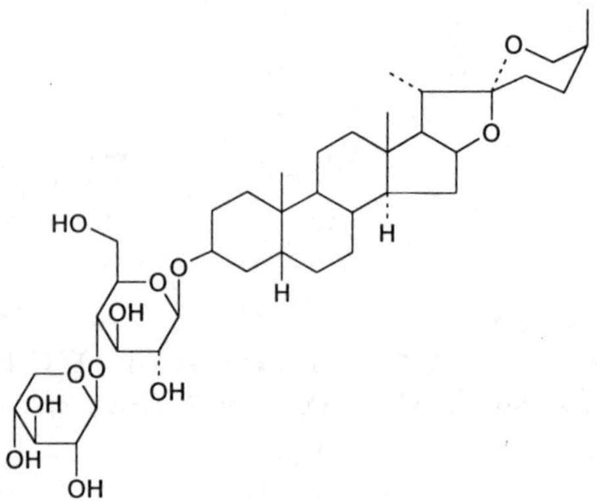

496 Aspafilioside B

$C_{43}H_{70}O_{16}$ MW: 843.03 Property: white acicular crystal, mp 180-2°C (methanol), $[\alpha]_D^{14}$ -47.3° (c = 0.07, chloroform-methanol). Source: XIAO BAI BU. Ref: 159.

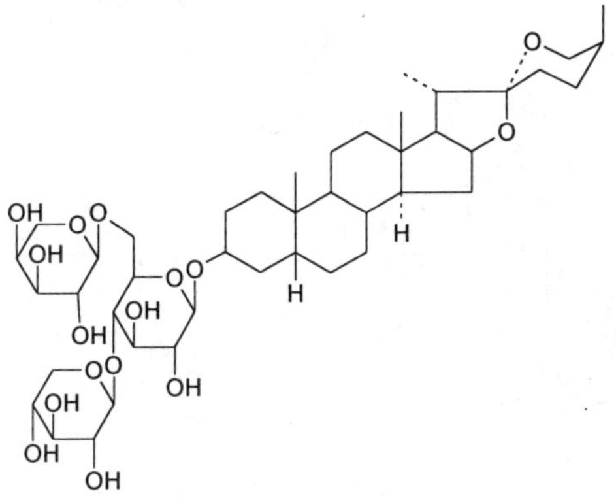

497 Aspafilioside C

$C_{49}H_{82}O_{22}$ MW: 1023.19 Property: white amorphous powder (methanol), mp 178-80°C, $[\alpha]_D^{14}$ -36.5° c=0.09, chloroform-methanol). Source: XIAO BAI BU. Ref: 159.

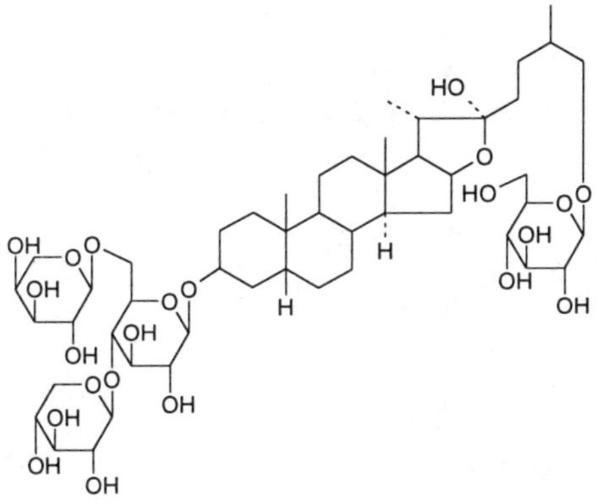

498 Asperosaponins F

3-O-[β-D-xylopyranosyl(1→4)-β-D-(1→4)][α-L-rhamno-pyranosyl(1→3)-β-D-galactopyranosyl (1→3)-α-L-rhamnopyranosyl(1→2)-α-L-arabino-pyranosyl-hederagenin. $C_{64}H_{104}O_{30}$ MW: 1353.52 Property: white powder, mp 244-7°C, soluble in methanol, pyridine and water. Source: CHUAN XU DUAN. Ref: 307.

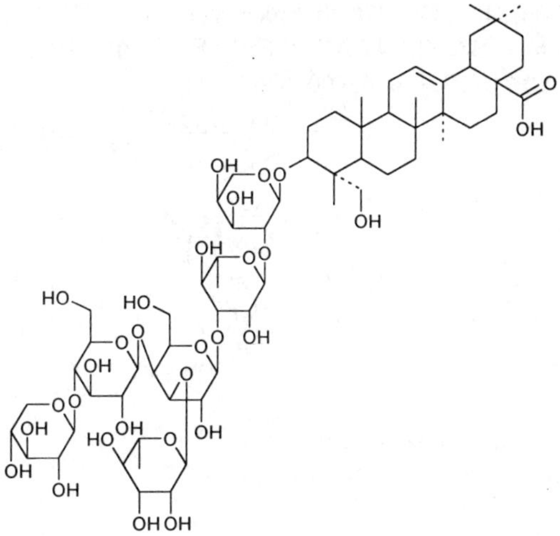

499 Asperosaponins H₁

3-O-[β-D-xylopyranosyl(1→4)-β-D-glucopyranoyl (1→4)][α-L-rhamnopyranosyl(1→3)-β-D-galacto-pyranosyl(1→3)-α-L-rhamnopyranosyl(1→2)-α-L-arabinopyranosyl-hederagenin-28-O-β-D-gluco-pyranosyl(1→6)-β-D-glucopyranoside. $C_{76}H_{124}O_{40}$ MW: 1677.81 Property: white powder, mp 233-6°C, soluble in methanol, pyridine and water. Source: CHUAN XU DUAN. Ref: 307.

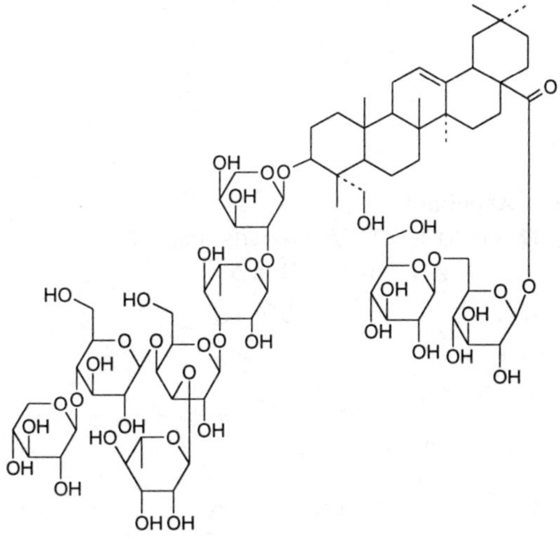

500 Asperuloside
$C_{19}H_{24}O_{11}$ MW: 428.40 Property: mp 125-7°C. Source: BA XIAN CAO, JI SHI TENG, PENG ZI CAI, ZHI ZI. Ref: 6, 400, 626.

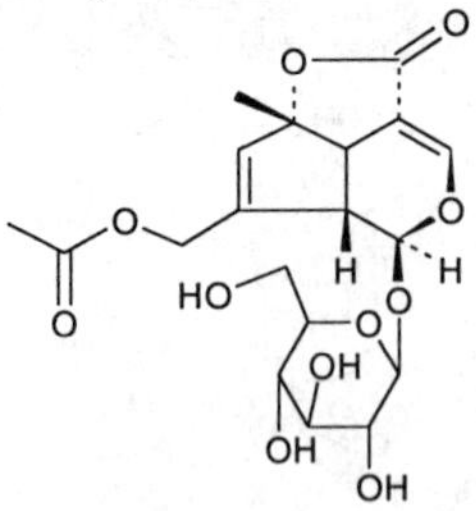

501 Asperulosidic acid
Source: Hedyotis diffusa Willd. Ref: 7.

502 Aspidin
$C_{25}H_{32}O_8$ MW: 460.53 Property: mp 125°C. Source: GUAN ZHONG, MAO GUAN ZHONG. Ref: 6.

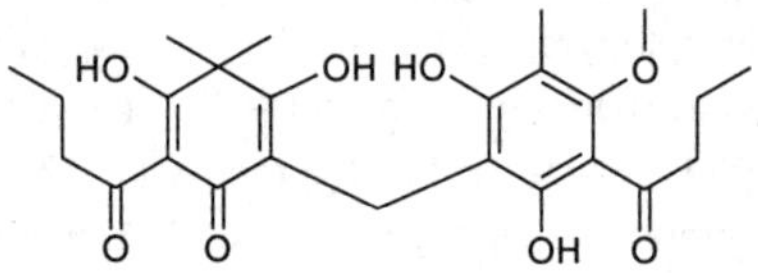

503 Aspidinin
$C_{21}H_{26}O_7$ MW: 390.44 Property: mp 111-2°C. Source: GUAN ZHONG. Ref: 6.

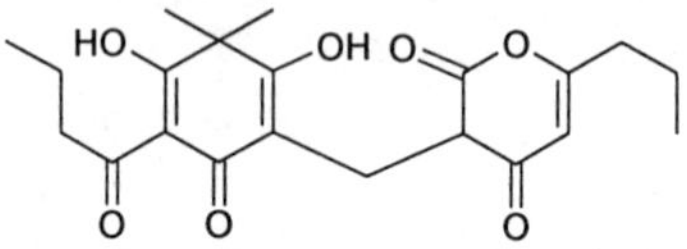

504 Aspidinol
$C_{12}H_{16}O_4$ MW: 224.26 Property: mp 156-61°C. Source: GUAN ZHONG. Ref: 6.

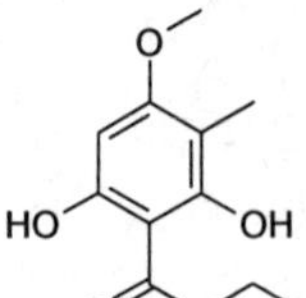

505 Aspidistrin
$C_{51}H_{82}O_{23}$ MW: 1063.21 Property: mp 265-7°C (dec). Source: ZHI ZHU BAO DAN. Ref: 6.

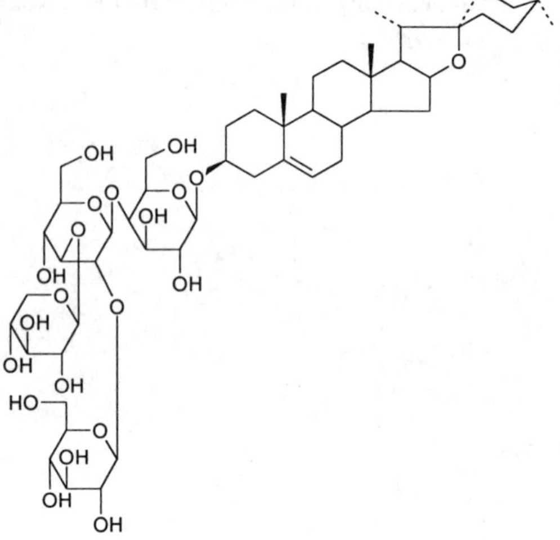

506 Assafoetidin
Source: A WEI. Ref: 7.

507 Astaxanthin
$C_{40}H_{52}O_4$ MW: 596.86 Property: mp 215-6°C (dec). Source: JIN YU, HAI XIA, LI YU PI. Ref: 6.

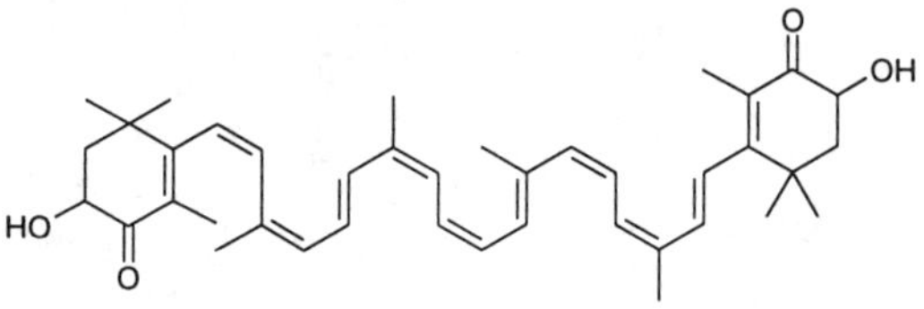

508 Astilbin
$C_{21}H_{22}O_{11}$ MW: 450.40 Property: mp 180°C (dec). Source: LI MU, TU FU LING. Ref: 6, 416, 568.

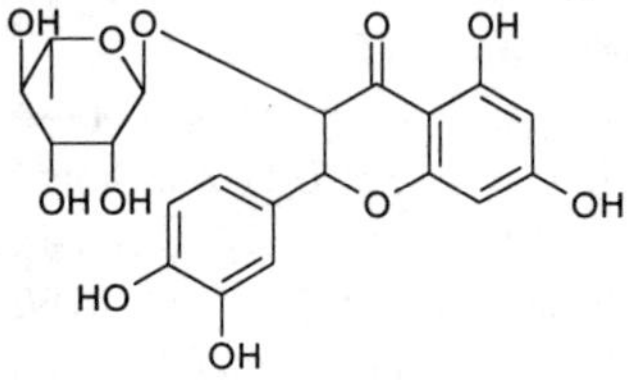

509 Astragaloside I

$C_{45}H_{76}O_{16}$ MW: 869.07 Source: HUANG QI. Ref: 2.

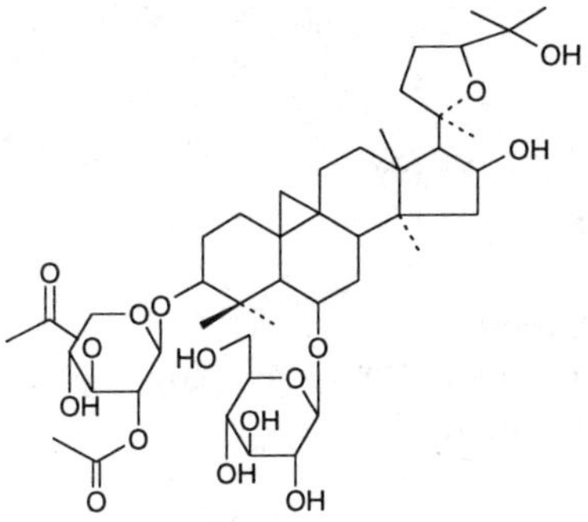

510 Astragaloside II

$C_{43}H_{70}O_{15}$ MW: 827.03 Source: HUANG QI. Ref: 2.

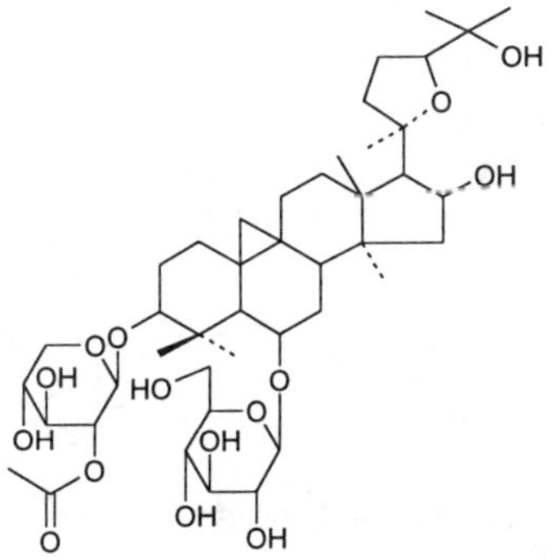

511 Astragaloside IV

$C_{41}H_{68}O_{14}$ MW: 784.99 Source: HUANG QI. Ref: 2.

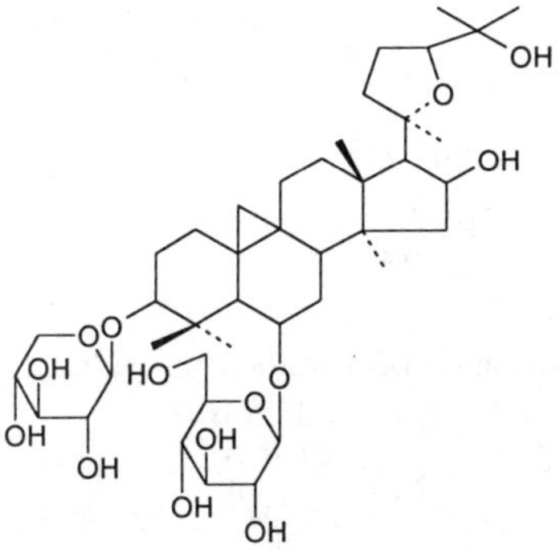

512 Atalafoline B

N-Methyl-1,4,5-trihydroxy-3,6-dimethoxyacridine-9-one. $C_{16}H_{15}NO_6$ MW: 317.30 Property: yellow columnar crystal, mp 192-4°C. Source: DONG FENG JU. Ref: 91.

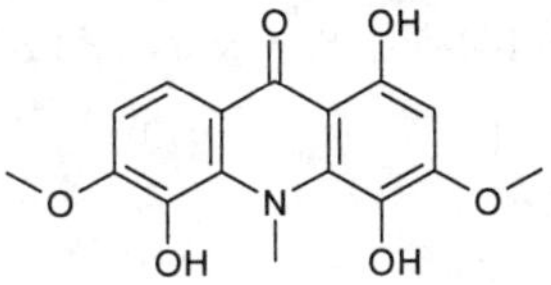

513 Atractylenolide I

$C_{15}H_{18}O_2$ MW: 230.31 Source: BAI ZHU. Ref: 2.

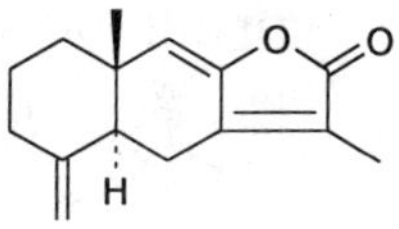

514 Atractylenolide II

$C_{15}H_{20}O_2$ MW: 232.33 Source: DANG SHEN. Ref: 2, 632.

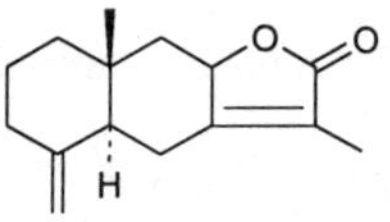

515 Atractylenolide III

$C_{15}H_{20}O_3$ MW: 248.32 Source: DANG SHEN. Ref: 2, 632.

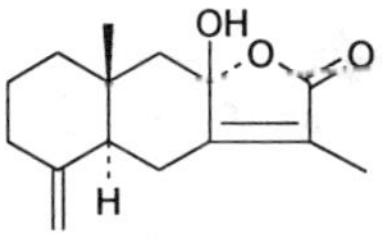

516 Atracty lentrid

$C_{14}H_{16}O_3$ MW: 232.28 Source: BAI ZHU. Ref: 2.

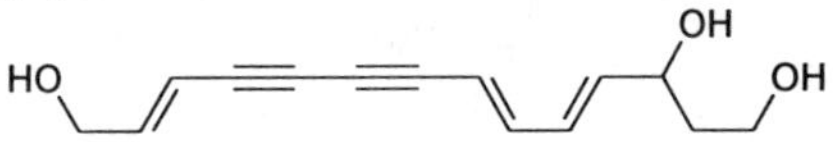

517 Atractylodin

Atractylin. $C_{13}H_{12}O$ MW: 184.24 Property: mp 52°C. Source: CANG ZHU. Ref: 6.

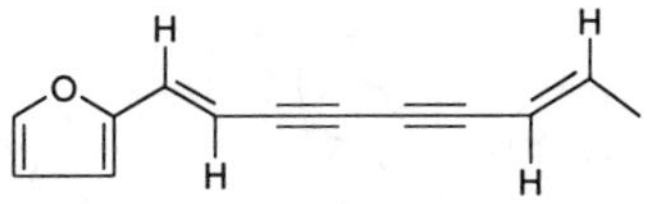

518 Atractylodinol

$C_{13}H_{12}O_2$ MW: 200.24 Source: CANG ZHU. Ref: 2.

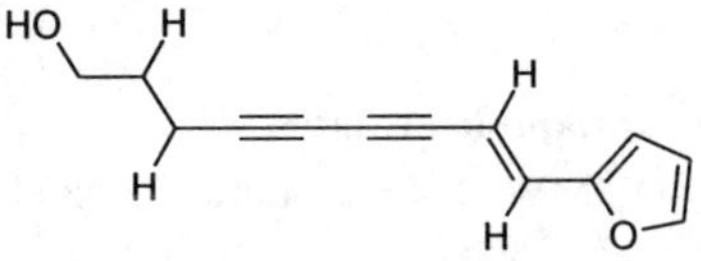

519 Atractylon

$C_{15}H_{20}O$ MW: 216.33 Source: CANG ZHU. Ref: 2.

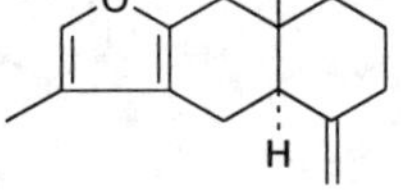

520 Atranorin

$C_{19}H_{18}O_8$ MW: 374.35 Property: mp 196-7°C. Source: SHI HUA, SHI RUI. Ref: 6.

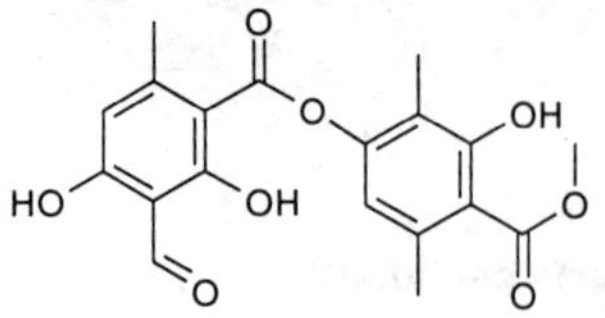

521 Atropine

$C_{17}H_{23}NO_3$ MW: 206.29 Source: GOU QI ZI. Ref: 2.

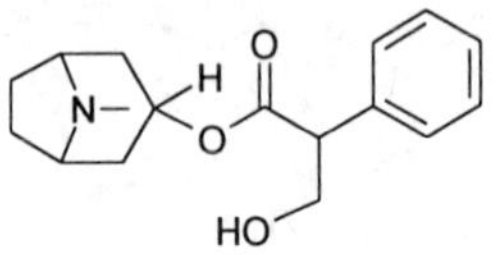

522 Aucubigenin

$C_9H_{12}O_4$ MW: 184.19 Source: TIAN JIAO BAN. Ref: 6.

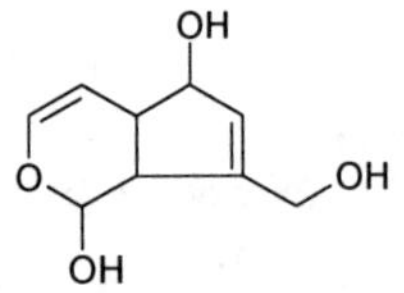

523 Aucubin

$C_{15}H_{22}O_9$ MW: 346.34 Source: GAN DI HUANG, DU ZHONG. Ref: 2.

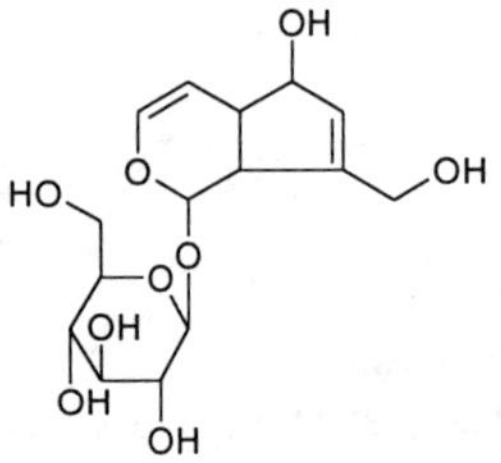

524 Aurantiamide acetate

$C_{29}H_{34}N_2O_4$ MW: 474.60 Source: QING HAO. Ref: 2.

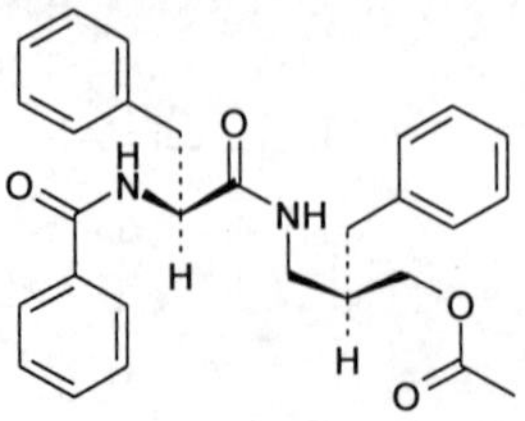

525 Aurantio-obtusin

$C_{17}H_{14}O_7$ MW: 330.30 Source: JUE MING ZI. Ref: 2.

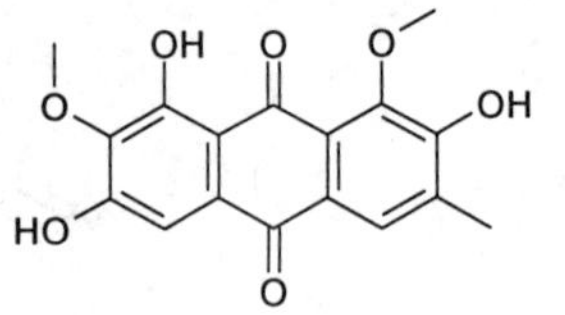

526 Aurapten

$C_{19}H_{22}O_3$ MW: 298.39 Property: mp 68°C. Source: GOU JU HE. Ref: 6.

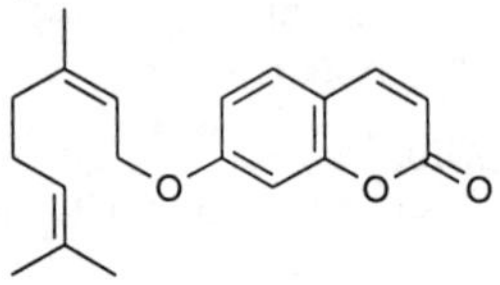

527 Aureusidin

$C_{15}H_{10}O_6$ MW: 286.24 Property: mp 270°C (295°C dec). Source: NING MENG. Ref: 6.

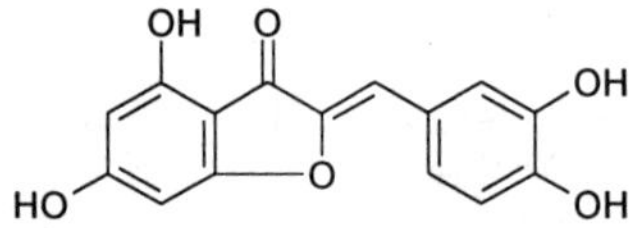

528 Aureusidin-6-glucoside

$C_{21}H_{20}O_{11}$ MW: 448.39 Property: mp 264.5-5.5°C. Source: NING MENG. Ref: 6.

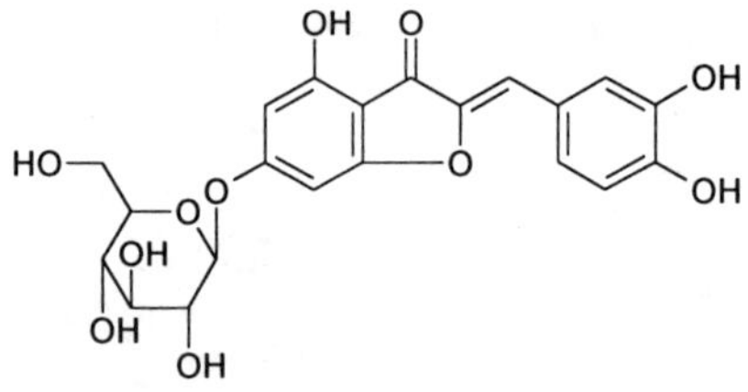

529 Aureusidin-6-rhamnoglucoside

Source: NING MENG. Ref: 6.

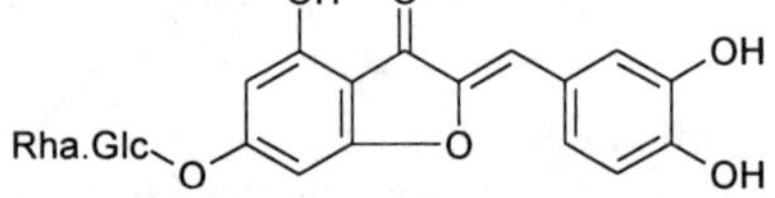

530 Australiside A

4-Oic acid-7-oxokaurene-6α-*O*-β-*D*-glucoside. Property: mp 143-5°C. Source: NAN FANG TU SI ZI. Ref: 589.

531 Avicennin
$C_{20}H_{20}O_4$ MW: 324.38 Property: mp 141-2°C. Source: YING BU BO. Ref: 6.

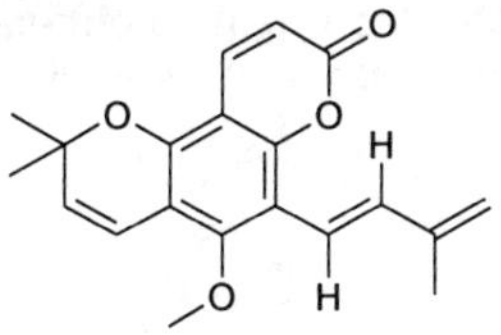

532 Avicine
$C_{20}H_{14}NO_4$ MW: 332.34 Source: YING BU BO. Ref: 6.

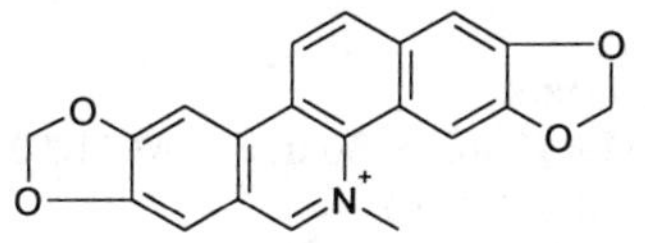

533 Avicularin
$C_{20}H_{18}O_{11}$ MW: 434.36 Property: mp 217°C (hydrate), 222°C (anhydrous). Source: BIAN XU, FAN SHI LIU GAN, FAN SHI LIU YE, LIANG QI LIAO, MAN SHAN HONG, SAN SE JIN, SANG JI SHENG, YUE JU YE. Ref: 6.

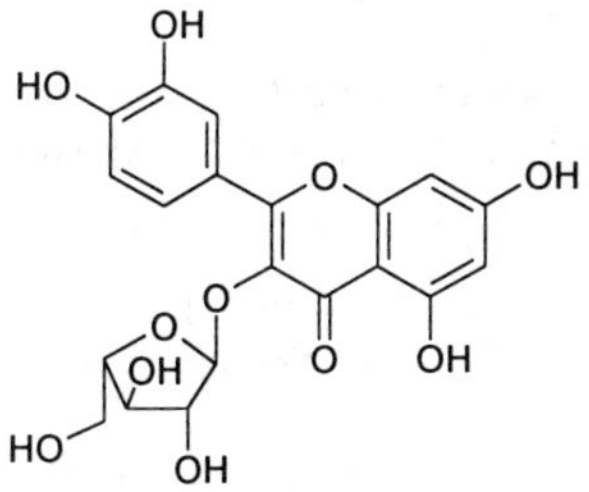

534 Axillarin
$C_{17}H_{14}O_8$ MW: 346.30 Source: QING HAO. Ref: 2.

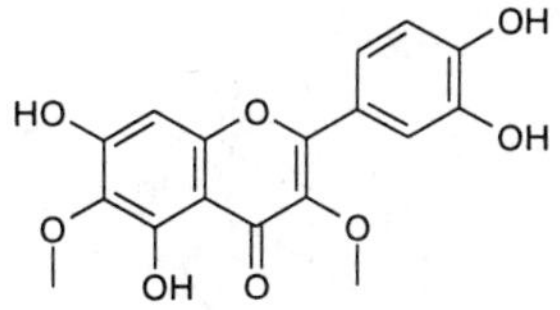

535 Azaleatin
$C_{16}H_{12}O_7$ MW: 316.27 Property: mp 322°C. Source: BAI HUA YING SHAN HONG, MAN SHAN HONG, XI YE TENG, YING SHAN HONG. Ref: 6.

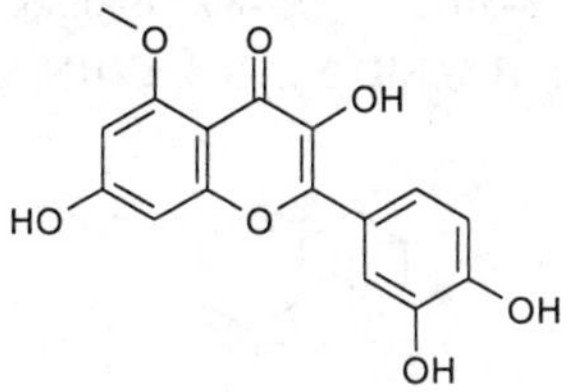

536 Azaleatin 3-rhamnosylglucoside
Source: DU JUAN HUA. Ref: 6.

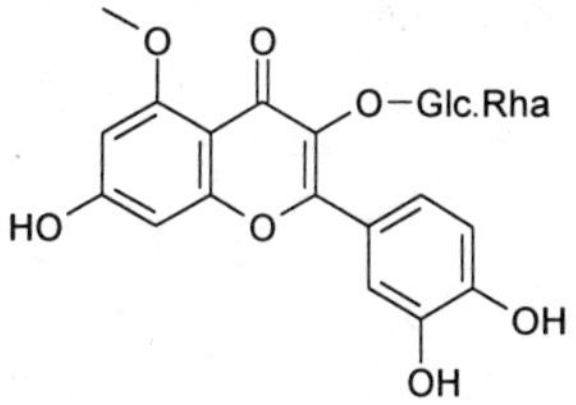

537 Azalein
Property: mp 181-5°C. Source: BAI HUA YING SHAN HONG. Ref: 6.

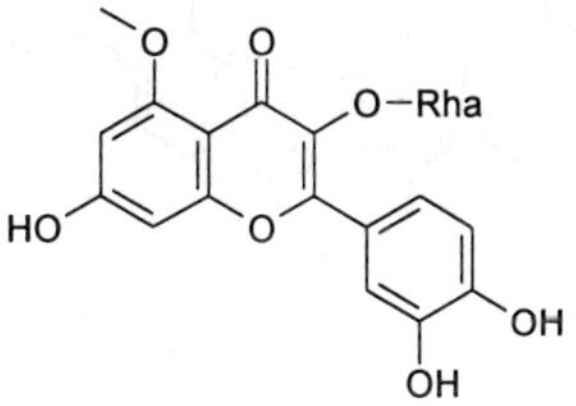

538 Azelaic acid
$C_9H_{16}O_4$ MW: 188.23 Source: DANG GUI, DANG SHEN, YIN CHEN HAO. Ref: 2.

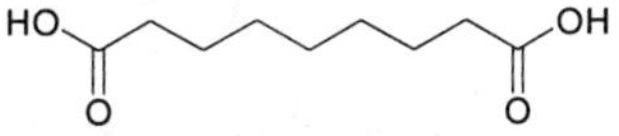

539 Azetidine-2-carboxylic acid
$C_5H_9NO_2$ MW: 115.13 Property: not melt, change to black at 270°C. Source: HUANG JING, YU ZHU. Ref: 6.

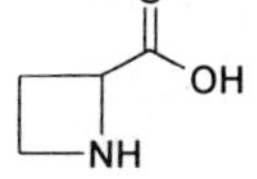

540 Azralidoside
Property: mp 108-10°C. Source: SHEN HUANG DOU. Ref: 6.

541 Azulene
$C_{10}H_8$ MW: 128.18 Property: mp 98.5-9.0°C. Source: MU JU, YANG SHI CAO, ZHANG MU. Ref: 6.

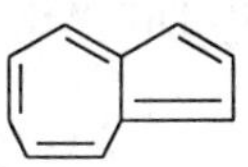

542 Baeckeol
$C_{13}H_{18}O_4$ MW: 238.29 Property: mp 103-4°C. Source: GANG SONG. Ref: 6.

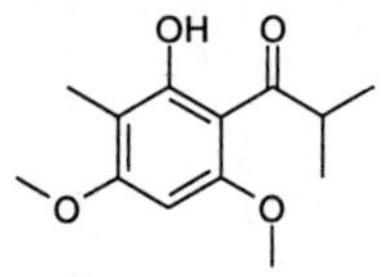

543 Baeomycesic acid
$C_{19}H_{20}O_8$ MW: 376.37 Property: mp 2 33°C. Source: BAN JIU. Ref: 6.

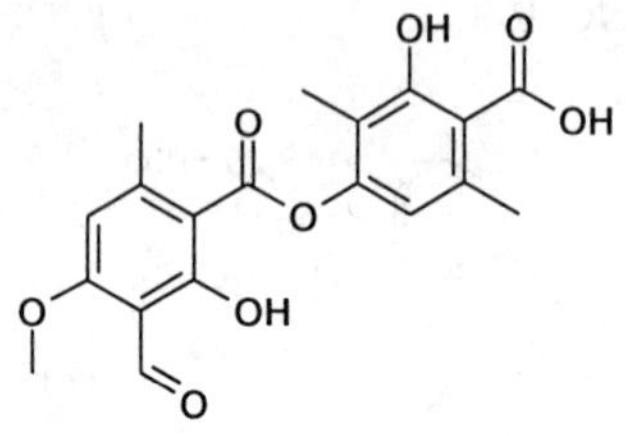

544 Baicalein
Noroxylin. CAS: 491-67-8 $C_{15}H_{10}O_5$ MW: 270.24 Source: HUANG QIN. Ref: 2, 4.

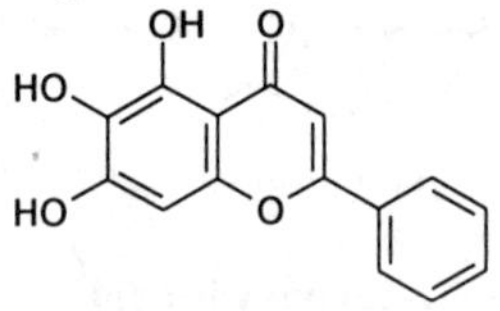

545 Baicalein-6-glucuronide
$C_{21}H_{18}O_{11}$ MW: 446.37 Property: mp 114°C. Source: MU HU DIE. Ref: 6.

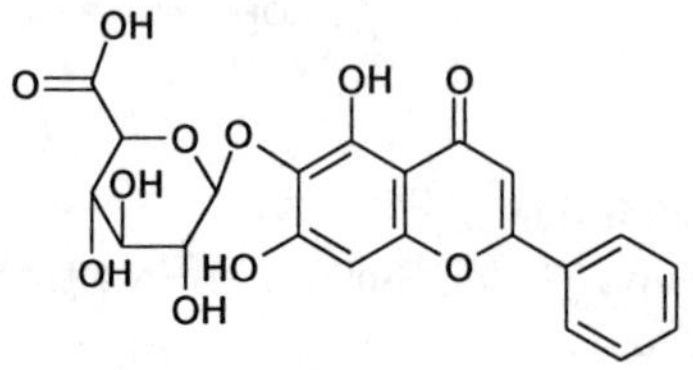

546 Baicalin
Baicalein-7-glucuronide. CAS: 21967-41-9 $C_{21}H_{18}O_{11}$ MW: 446.37Property: mp 223°C. Source: DAN SHEN, HUANG QIN, MU HU DIE, MU HU DIE SHU PI. Ref: 2, 4, 5, 6.

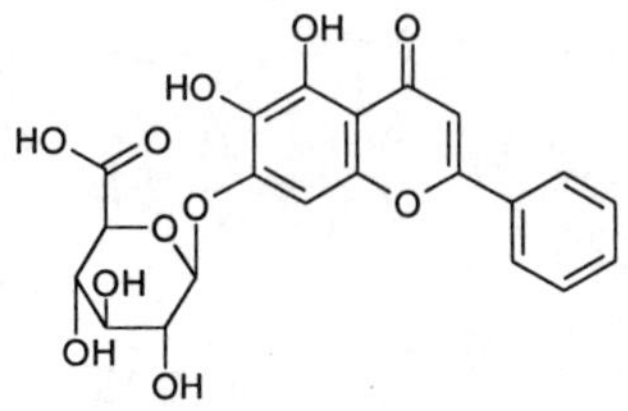

547 Baihuaqianhuoside
3-methoxy-4-O-β-D-glycopyranosylpropiophenone. $C_{16}H_{22}O_8$ MW: 342.35 Property: white crystalline powder, mp 165.5-7.5°C (chloroform-methanol). Source: BAI HUA QIAN HU. Ref: 297.

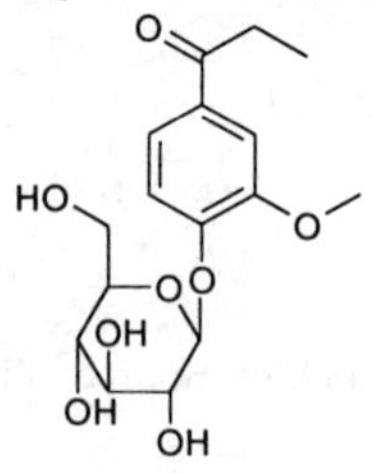

548 Baimuxinal
$C_{15}H_{24}O_2$ MW: 236.36 Source: BAI MU XIANG, CHEN XIANG. Ref: 13.

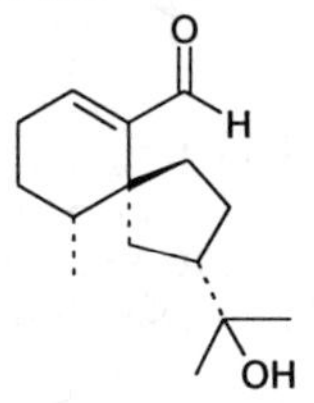

549 Baimuxinfuranic acid
$C_{15}H_{24}O_3$ MW: 252.36 Source: BAI MU XIANG. Ref: 13.

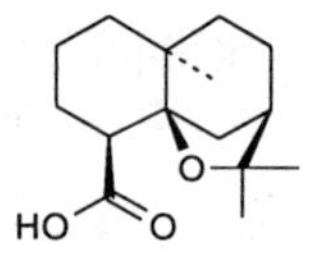

550 Baimuxinic acid
$C_{15}H_{24}O_3$ MW: 252.36 Source: BAI MU XIANG. Ref: 13.

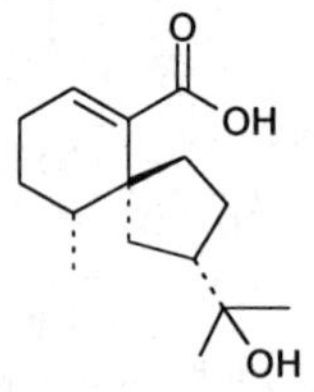

551 Baimuxinol
$C_{15}H_{26}O_2$ MW: 238.37 Property: colorless massive crystal, mp 128-30°C, $[\alpha]_D^{30}$ -83° (c=0.56, chloroform). Source: BAI MU XIANG, CHIN XIANG. Ref: 13, 57.

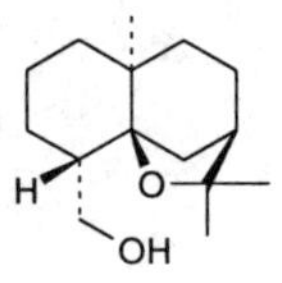

552 Baishouwubenzophenone
$C_{16}H_{14}O_5$ MW: 302.08 Property: light yellow acicular crystal, mp 198-200°C. Source: ER YE NIU PI XIAO. Ref: 103.

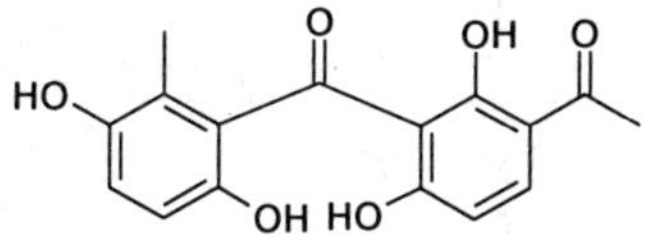

553 Bakuchicin
$C_{11}H_6O_3$ MW: 186.17 Source: BU GU ZHI. Ref: 2, 630.

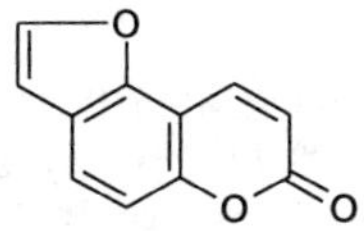

554 Bakuchiol
CAS: 10309-37-2 $C_{18}H_{24}O$ MW: 256.39 Source: BU GU ZHI. Ref: 1, 2, 4.

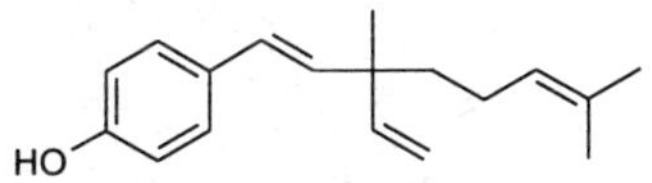

555 Balsaminasterol
$C_{27}H_{40}O$ Property: mp 106.1°C. Source: JI XING ZI. Ref: 6.

556 Balsampear protein
MW: >34,000 Property: white crystal powder, $[\alpha]_D^{25}$ +4° (c= 0.68, water), easily soluble in water, pH of watersolution 7.6, isoelectric point pH 8.4, composed of 17 kinds of aminoacids, N-end amino acid is leucine. Source: KU GUA. Ref: 482.

557 Bannamurpanisin
$C_{21}H_{22}O_8$ MW: 402.40 Source: JIU LI XIANG. Ref: 11.

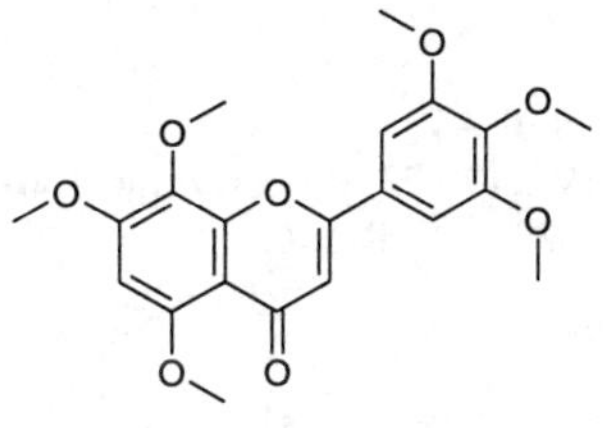

558 Baogongteng C
Source: GUANG YE DING GONG TENG. Ref: 585.

559 Baohuoside I
3,5,7-Trihydroxy-4'-methoxyl-8-prenylflavone-3-O-α-L-rhamnopyranoside. $C_{27}H_{30}O_{10}$ MW: 514.53 Property: yellow crystalline powder, mp 208-10°C, easy soluble in methanol and ethanol, soluble in acetone. Source: CHUAN DIAN YIN YANG HUO, YIN YANG HUO. Ref: 114, 540, 565, 635.

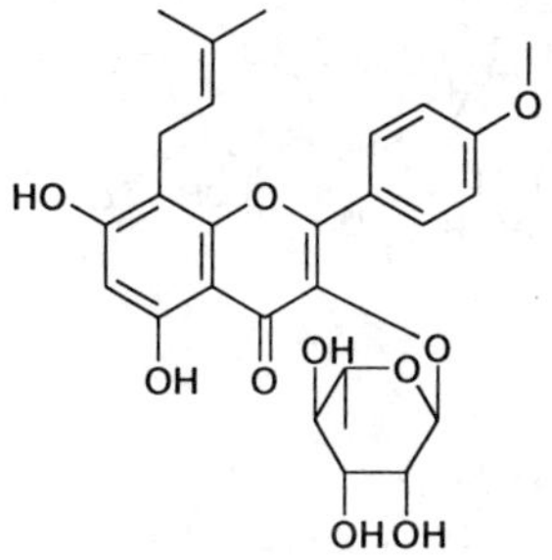

560 Baohuoside-II
3,5,7,4'-Tetrahydroxy-8-prenylflavone-3-O-α-L-rhamnopyranoside. $C_{26}H_{28}O_{10}$ MW: 500.51 Property: yellow crystalline powder, mp 154-6°C, easy soluble in ethanol and methanol. Source: CHUAN DIAN YIN YANG HUO, CU MAO YIN YANG HUO, YIN YANG HUO. Ref: 112, 514, 565.

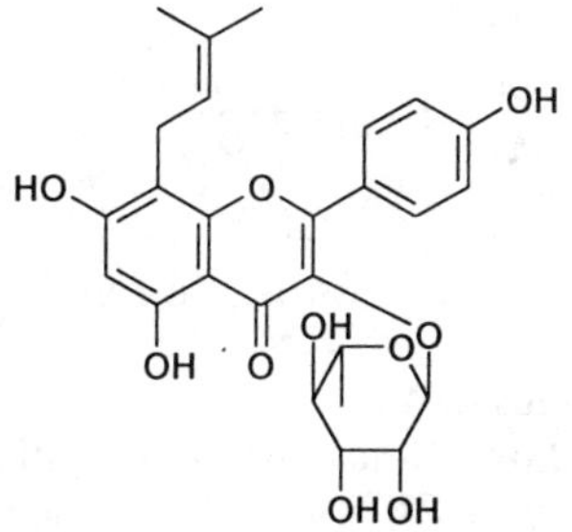

561 Baohuoside-III
3,5,7,4'-Tetrahydroxy-8-prenylflavone-3-O-α-L-rhamnopyranosyl(1→4)-α-L-rhamnopyranoside. $C_{32}H_{38}O_{14}$ MW: 646.65 Property: yellow powder, mp 215-20°C, easy soluble in methanol. Source: CHUAN DIAN YIN YANG HUO. Ref: 112.

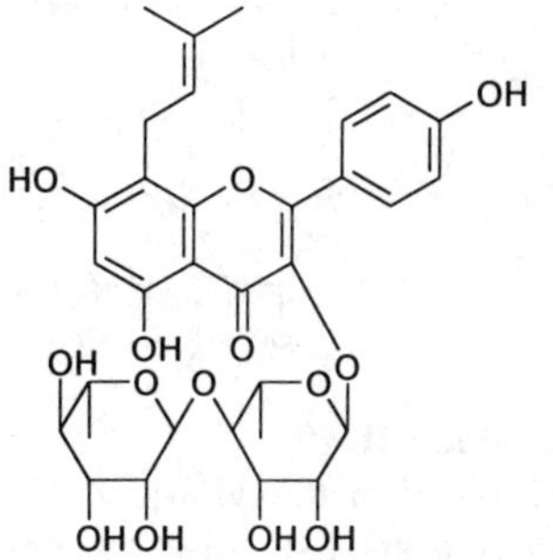

562 Baohuoside-IV
3,5,7,4'-Tetrahydroxy-8-prenylflavone-3,7-O-α-L-dirhamnopyranoside. $C_{32}H_{38}O_{14}$ MW: 646.65 Property: yellow powder, easy soluble in methanol. Source: CHUAN DIAN YIN YANG HUO. Ref: 112.

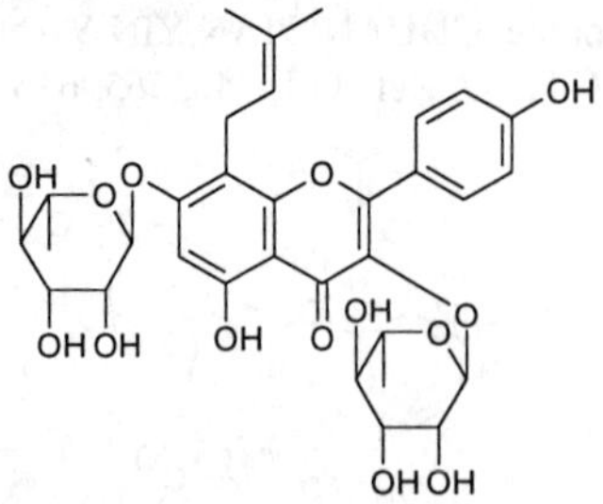

563 Baohuoside-V
3,5,7,4'-Tetrahydroxy-8-prenylflavone-3-O-α-L-rhamnopyranosyl(1→4)-α-L-rhamnopyranosyl-7-O-β-D-glucopyranoside. $C_{38}H_{48}O_{19}$ MW: 808.79 Property: yellow powder, easy soluble in methanol. Source: BAO XING YIN YANG HUO. Ref: 112.

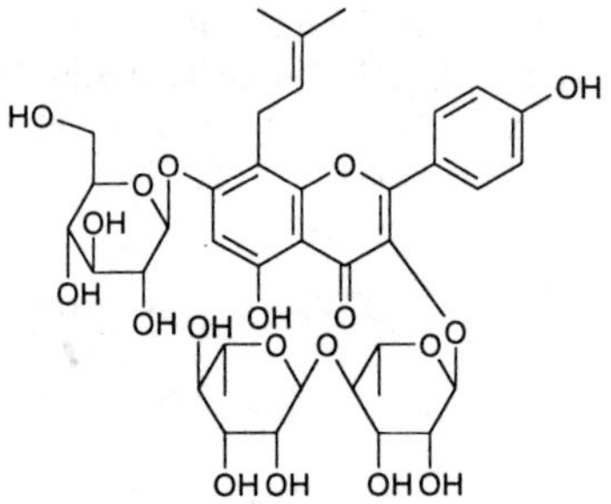

564 Baohuoside VI
3,5,7-trihydroxy-4'-methoxyl-8-prenylflavone-3-O-α-L-rhamnopyranosyl(1→4)-α-L-rhamnopyranosyl-7-O-β-D-glucopyranoside. $C_{39}H_{50}O_{19}$ MW: 822.82 Property: yellow powder, mp 240-5°C, soluble in methanol. Source: BAO XING YIN YANG HUO, XIN YE YIN YANG HUO. Ref: 114, 540, 623.

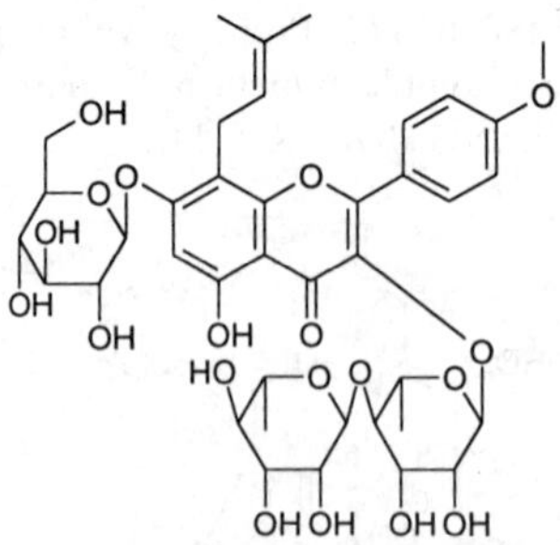

565 Baohuoside VII
3,5,7-Trihydroxy-4'-methoxyl-8-prenylflavone-3-O-α-L-rhamnopyranosyl(1→4)-β-D-glucopyranoside. $C_{33}H_{40}O_{15}$ MW: 676.68 Property: yellow powder, easily soluble in methanol and ethanol. Source: BAO XING YIN YANG HUO. Ref: 114.

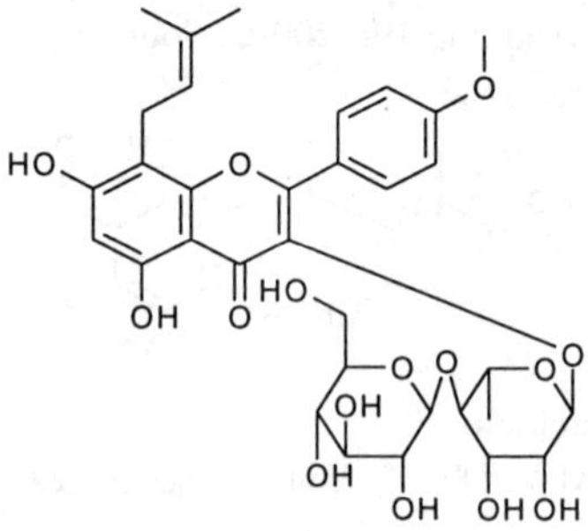

566 Baohuosu
5,7,4'-Trihydroxy-3',5'-dimethoxyl-8-prenylflavone. $C_{22}H_{22}O_7$ MW: 398.42 Property: yellow crystalline powder, mp 254-7°C. Source: BAO XING YIN YANG HUO. Ref: 114.

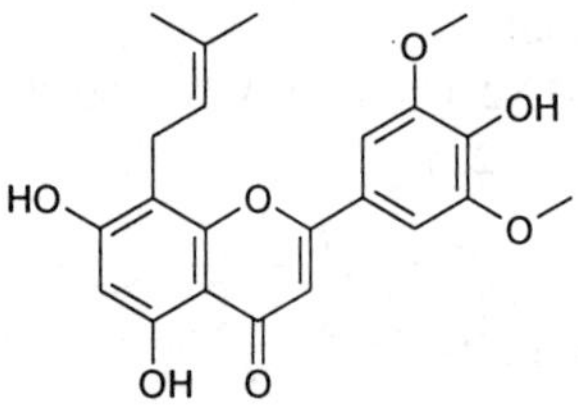

567 Baptifoline
$C_{15}H_{20}N_2O_2$ MW: 260.34 Source: KU SHEN. Ref: 2.

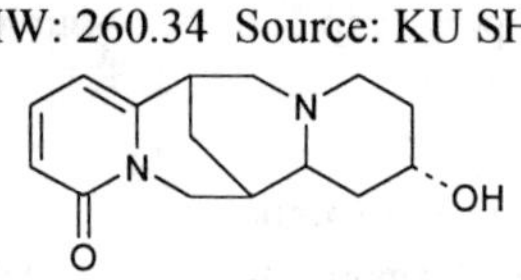

568 Barbatic acid
$C_{19}H_{20}O_7$ MW: 360.37 Property: mp 191°C (186°C). Source: SONG LUO. Ref: 6.

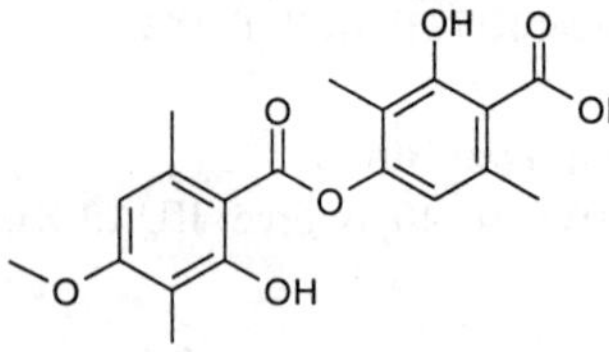

569 Barrigenol-A1
$C_{30}H_{50}O_5$ MW: 490.73 Property: mp 300-2°C. Source: CHA ZI XIN. Ref: 6.

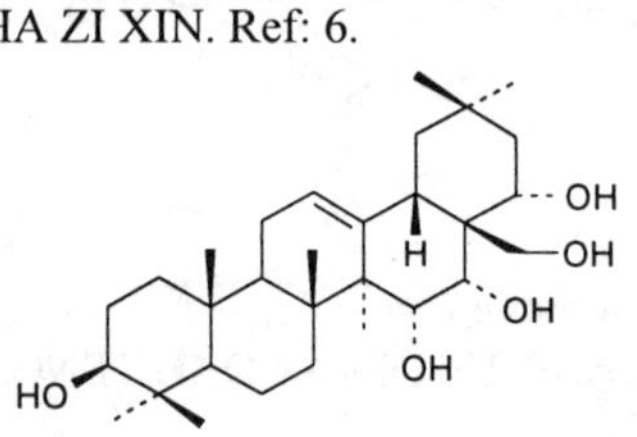

570 Barringtogenol C
Theasapogenol B. $C_{30}H_{50}O_5$ MW: 490.73 Property: mp 326-30°C (dec). Source: SUO LUO ZI. Ref: 6.

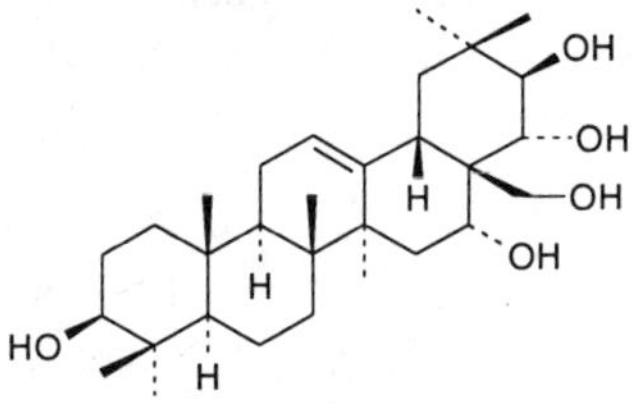

571 Bassianin
$C_{23}H_{29}O_5$ MW: 399.49 Source: BAI JIANG CAN. Ref: 6.

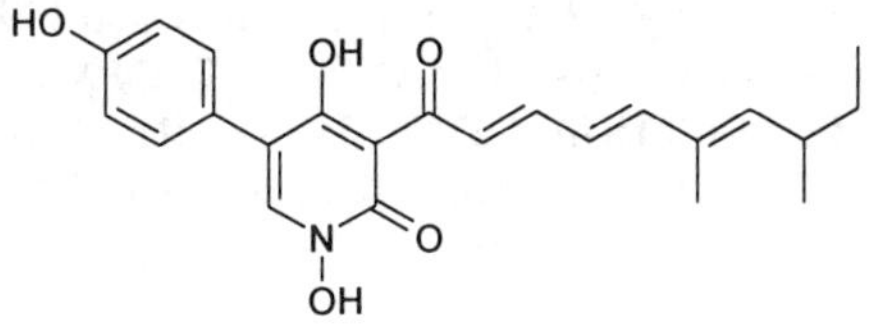

572 Bauerenol
Ilexol. $C_{30}H_{50}O$ MW: 426.73 Property: mp 207-8°C. Source: KUAN DONG HUA, QIAO MU ZI ZHU, SHA TANG MU, WU MU XIE, ZI JIN NIU. Ref: 6.

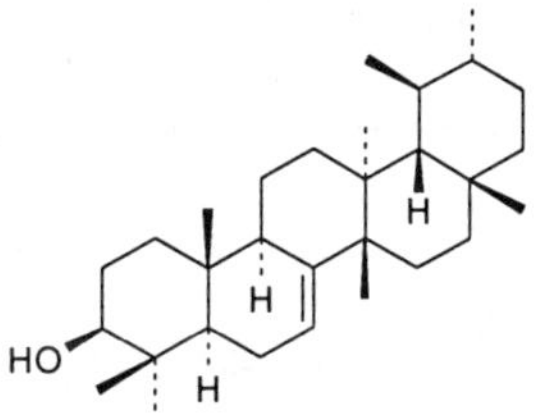

573 Baurenyl acetate
Source: JU JU. Ref: 620.

574 Bavachalcone
$C_{21}H_{22}O_4$ MW: 338.41 Source: BU GU ZHI. Ref: 2, 630.

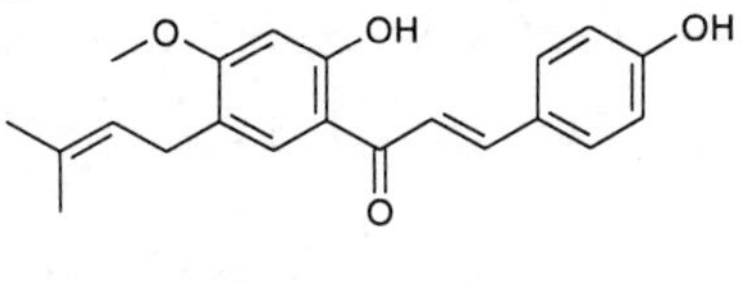

575 Bavachin
$C_{20}H_{20}O_4$ MW: 324.38 Source: BU GU ZHI. Ref: 2, 630.

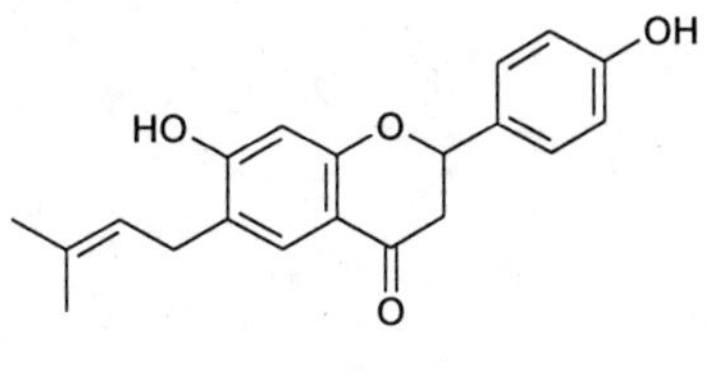

576 Bavachinin
$C_{21}H_{22}O_4$ MW: 338.41 Source: BU GU ZHI. Ref: 2, 630.

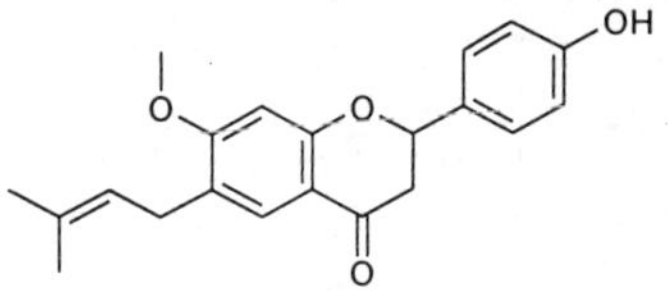

577 Bavachromanol
$C_{20}H_{20}O_5$ MW: 340.38 Source: BU GU ZHI. Ref: 2, 630.

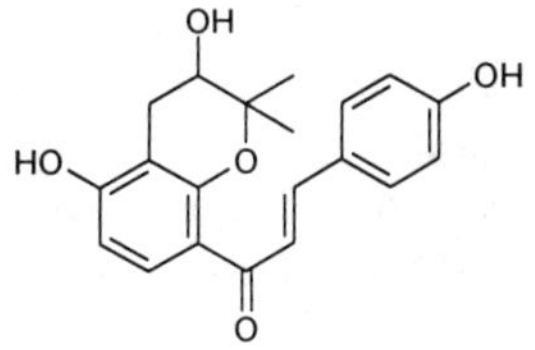

578 Bavachromene
$C_{20}H_{18}O_4$ MW: 322.36 Source: BU GU ZHI. Ref: 2, 630.

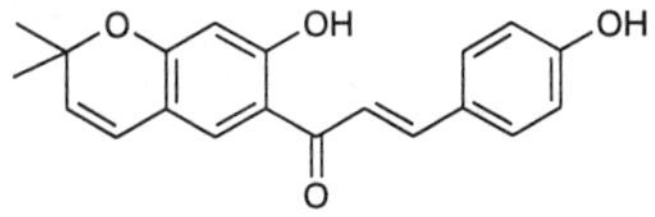

579 Bavacoumestan A
$C_{20}H_{16}O_6$ MW: 352.35 Source: BU GU ZHI. Ref: 2, 630.

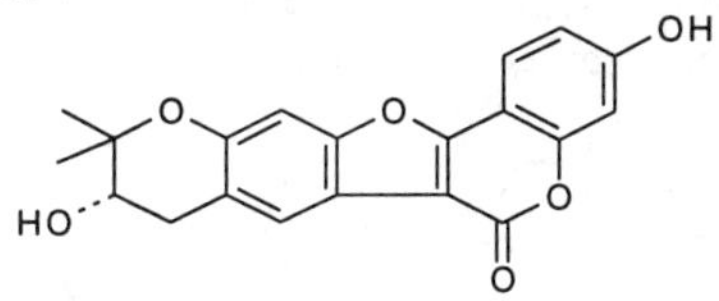

580 Bavacoumestan B
$C_{20}H_{16}O_6$ MW: 352.35 Source: BU GU ZHI. Ref: 2, 630.

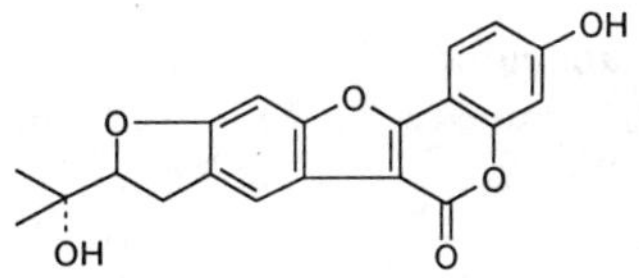

581 Beaumontoside
$C_{30}H_{46}O_7$ MW: 518.70 Property: mp 202-3°C. Source: PAO DAN GUO. Ref: 1, 6.

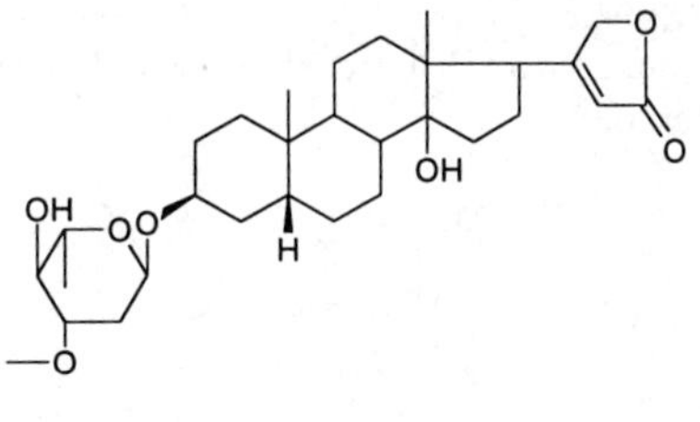

582 Beauverici(a)n
$C_{45}H_{57}O_9$ MW: 783.97 Property: mp 93-4°C. Source: BAI JIANG CAN. Ref: 6.

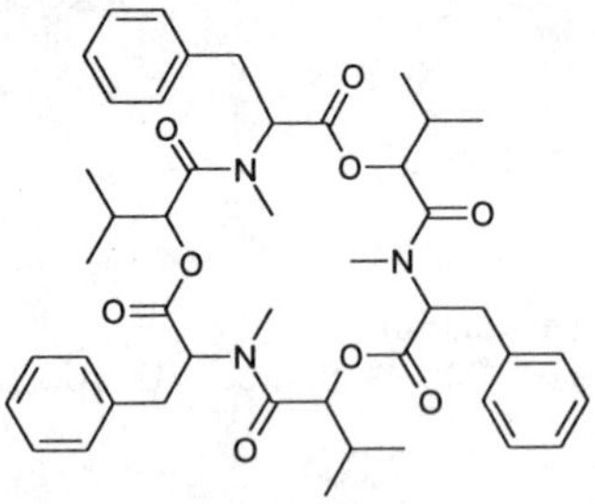

583 Beauwalloside
$C_{32}H_{48}O_9$ MW: 576.73 Property: mp 223-6°C. Source: PAO DAN GUO. Ref: 1, 6.

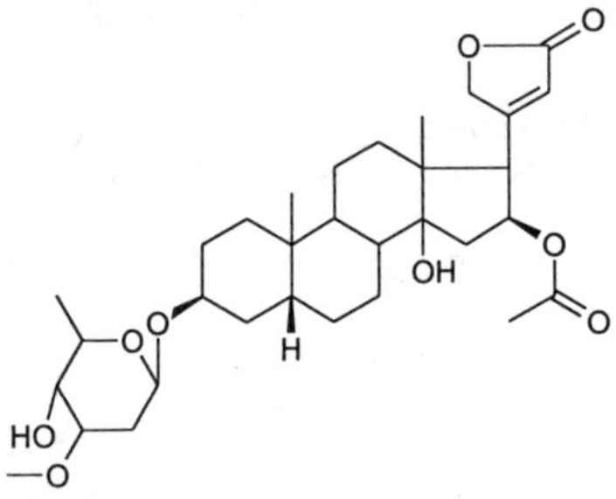

584 *l*-Bebeerine
l-Curine. $C_{36}H_{38}N_2O_6$ MW: 594.71 Property: mp (-) 221°C. Source: XI SHENG TENG. Ref: 6.

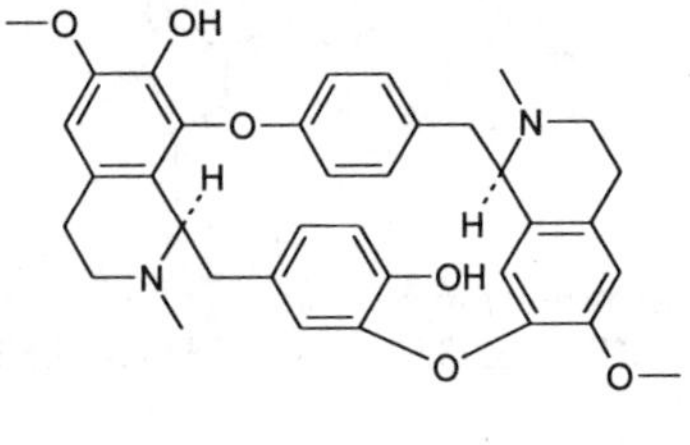

585 Beilupeimine
$C_{27}H_{43}NO_3$ Property: mp 155-7°C. Source: CHUAN BEI MU. Ref: 6.

586 Belamcandin
$C_{24}H_{26}O_2$ Source: SHE GAN. Ref: 6.

587 Bellidifodin
$C_{14}H_{10}O_6$ MW: 274.23 Property: yellow acicular crystal, mp 254-6°C. Source: BAO E ZHANG YA CAI. Ref: 634.

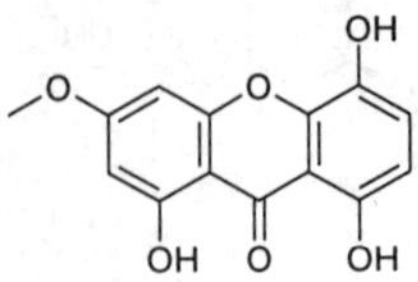

588 Bemeuxin
$C_{34}H_{48}O_5$ MW: 488.71 Property: colorless column crystal (MeOH), mp 295-6°C, $[\alpha]_D^{13}$ +13.8° (c=0.52, pyridine). Source: YAN JIN CAI. Ref: 286.

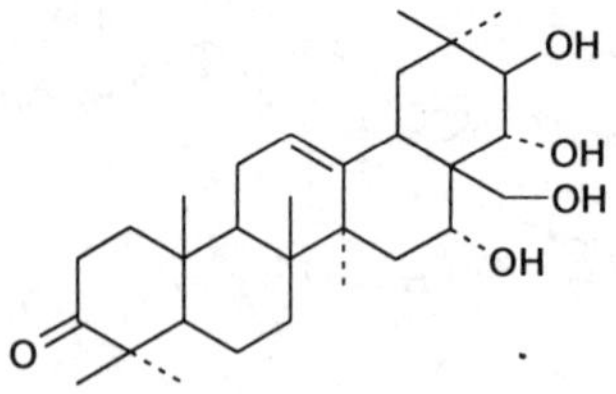

589 Benzaldehyde
C_7H_6O MW: 106.13 Property: mp -26°C, bp 179°C /751mm. Source: AN XI XIANG, BA DAN XING REN, BAI MEI HUA, DING XIANG, HUO XIANG, SHI CHUN, SHUI SONG, SHUI XIAN HUA. Ref: 6.

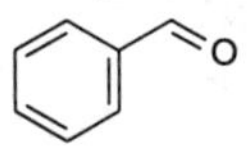

590 Benzoic acid
$C_7H_6O_2$ MW: 122.12 Source: BAI SHAO YAO, CHI SHAO YAO, GAN DI HUANG, JIN QIAO MAI, TIAN NAN XING, WU WEI ZI. Ref: 2, 594.

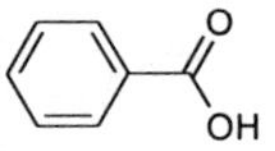

591 3,4-Benzopyrene
$C_{20}H_{12}$ MW: 252.32 Property: mp 176.5-7.5°C, bp 310-2°C/10mm. Source: XIANG RI KUI ZI. Ref: 6.

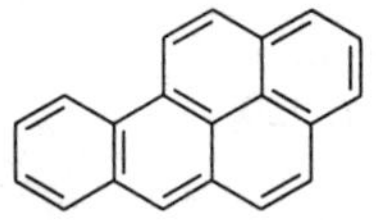

592 Benzoylgomisin H
$C_{29}H_{34}O_7$ MW: 494.59 Source: WU WEI ZI. Ref: 2.

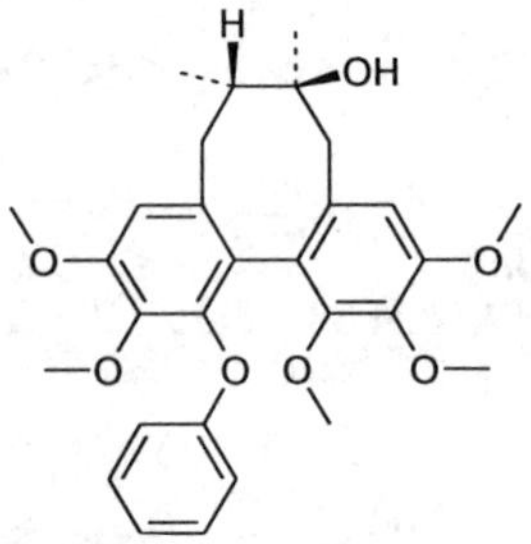

593 Benzoylgomisin O
$C_{29}H_{32}O_7$ MW: 492.57 Source: WU WEI ZI. Ref: 2.

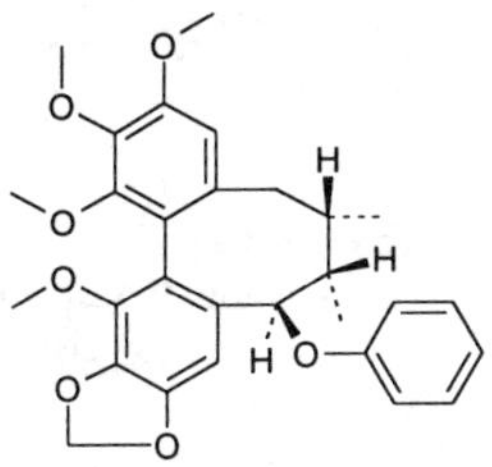

594 Benzoylgomisin P
$C_{29}H_{32}O_8$ MW: 508.57 Source: WU WEI ZI. Ref: 2.

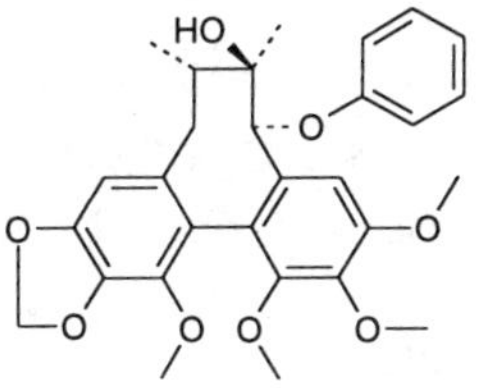

595 Benzoylgomisin Q
$C_{30}H_{36}O_8$ MW: 524.62 Source: WU WEI ZI. Ref: 2.

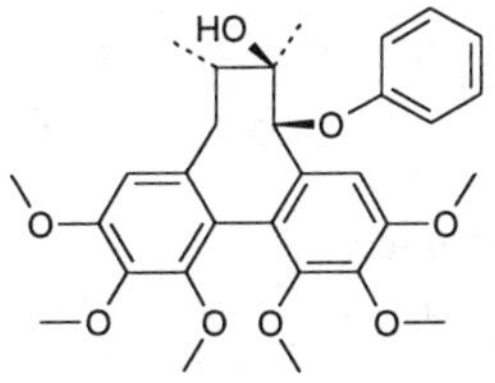

596 12-O-Benzoylisolineolone
$C_{28}H_{36}O_6$ MW: 468.60 Property: mp 245-50°C. Source: FU SHOU CAO. Ref: 6.

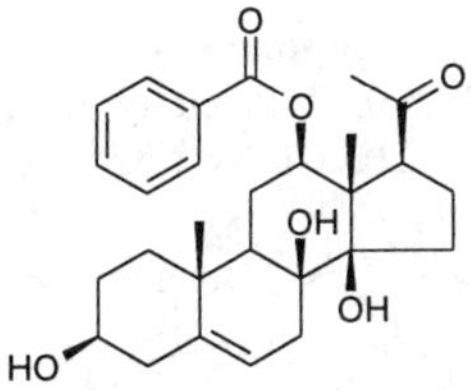

597 14-Benzoyl-8-O-methyl-aconine I
$C_{33}H_{47}O_{10}$ MW: 617.74 Property: amorphous, $[\alpha]_D^{20}$ -2.36° (c=0.721, $CHCl_3$). Source: NI YU LONG WU TOU. Ref: 487.

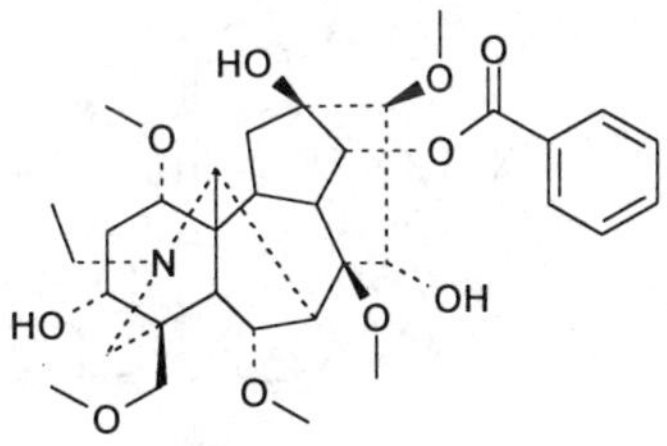

598 Benzoyl-oxypaeoniflorin
$C_{30}H_{32}O_{13}$ MW: 600.58 Source: MU DAN PI. Ref: 1.

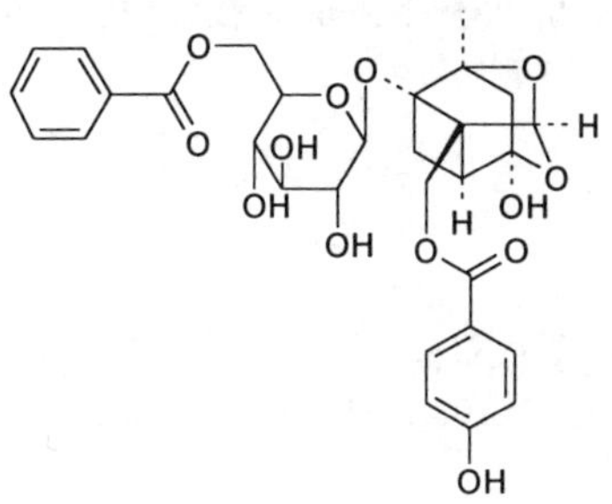

599 Benzoylpaeoniflorin
$C_{29}H_{30}O_{12}$ MW: 584.58 Source: BAI SHAO YAO, CHI SHAO YAO, MU DAN PI. Ref: 1.

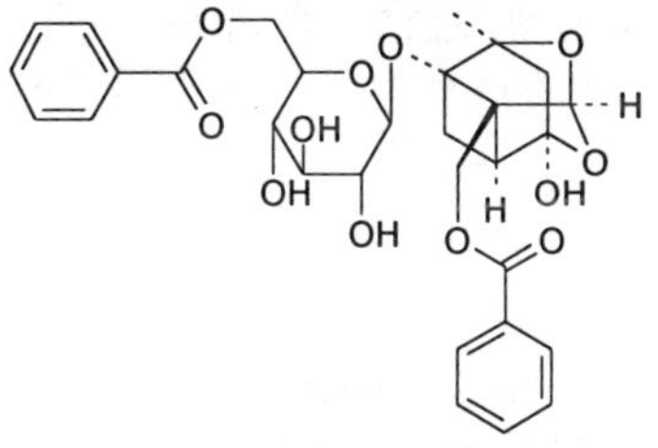

600 Benzoylpterosin B
$C_{21}H_{22}O_3$ MW: 322.41 Property: mp 68-70°C. Source: JUE. Ref: 6.

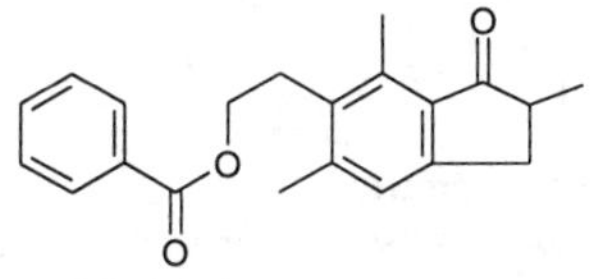

601 Benzoylramanone
$C_{28}H_{36}O_5$ MW: 452.60 Property: mp 222-6°C. Source: LUO MO. Ref: 6.

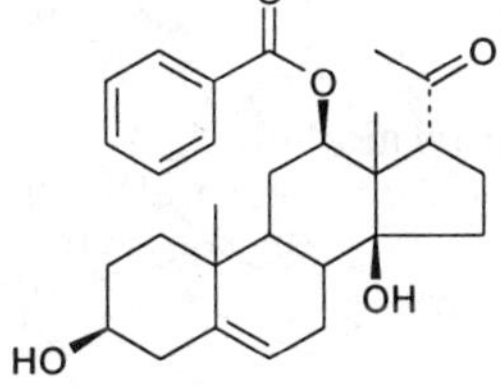

602 Benzyl acetate
$C_9H_{10}O_2$ MW: 150.18 Property: bp 213.5°C /756mm. Source: DING XIANG, HUANG HUA HAO, LA MEI HUA, SHUI XIAN HUA. Ref: 6.

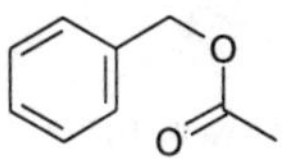

603 Benzyl acetone
4-Phenyl-2-Butanone. $C_{10}H_{12}O$ MW: 148.21 Property: bp 235°C. Source: BAI MU XIANG, CHEN XIANG. Ref: 1, 6, 13.

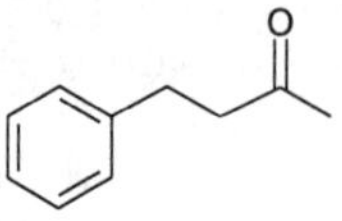

604 Benzyl alcohol
C_7H_8O MW: 108.14 Source: JIN YIN HUA, JU PI. Ref: 2.

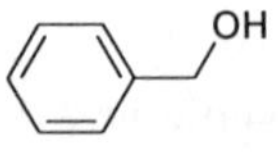

605 Benzyl benzoate
$C_{14}H_{12}O_2$ MW: 212.25 Property: mp 21°C, bp 323-4°C. Source: BI LU XIANG JIAO, QU MAI. Ref: 6.

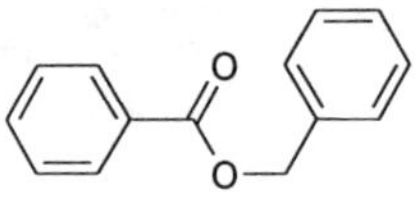

606 Benzyl benzoic acid
$C_{14}H_{12}O_2$ MW: 212.25 Property: mp 117°C. Source: QI ZHOU YI ZHI HAO. Ref: 6.

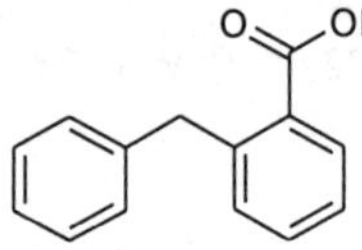

607 Benzyl cinnamate
$C_{16}H_{14}O_2$ MW: 238.29 Property: mp 39°C, bp 195-200°C/5mm. Source: BI LU XIANG JIAO, SHAN ZHU YU. Ref: 2, 6.

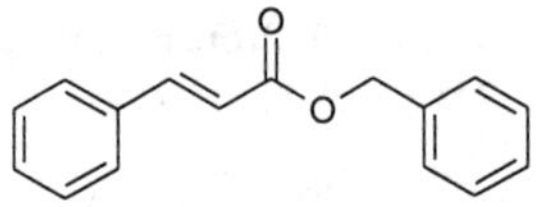

608 Benzyl ethyl alcohol
$C_8H_{10}O$ MW: 122.17 Source: JIN YIN HUA. Ref: 2.

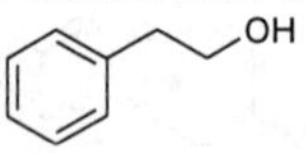

609 Benzyl formate
$C_8H_8O_2$ MW: 136.15 Property: bp 202-3.0°C/747mm. Source: CHA YE. Ref: 6.

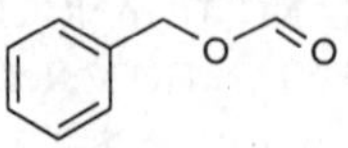

610 Benzyl isothiocyanate
Benzyl mustard oil. C_8H_7NS MW: 149.22 Property: bp 243°C, 124-5.0°C/12mm. Source: FAN MU GUA JIE ZI, HAN LIAN HUA, TING LI ZI. Ref: 1, 6.

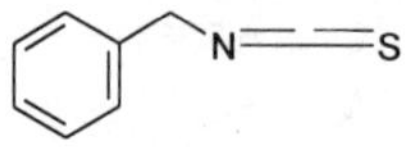

611 Benzyl-methylamine
$C_8H_{11}N$ MW: 121.18 Source: MA HUANG. Ref: 2.

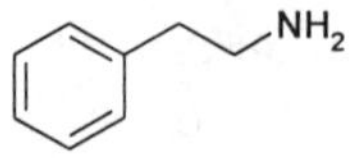

612 Benzyl d-2-methylbutyrate
$C_{12}H_{16}O_2$ MW: 192.26 Source: HUANG HUA HAO. Ref: 6.

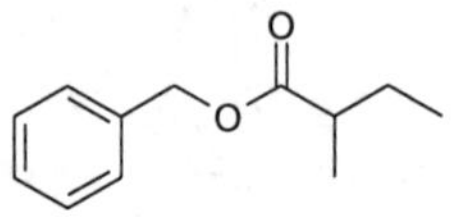

613 Benzyl salicylate
$C_{14}H_{12}O_3$ MW: 228.25 Property: bp 208°C/26mm. Source: QU MA. Ref: 6.

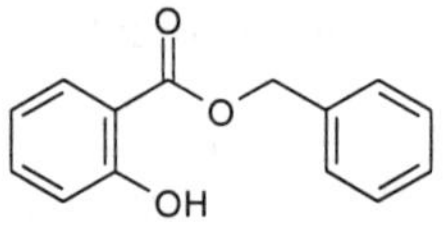

614 Benzyl thiocyanate
C_8H_7NS MW: 149.22 Property: mp 43°C, bp 235°C. Source: HAN LIAN HUA. Ref: 6.

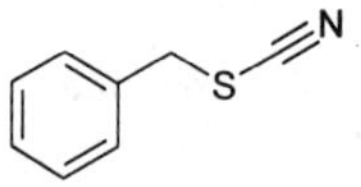

615 2-Benzylxanthopurpurin
$C_{21}H_{14}O_4$ MW: 330.34 Property: mp 300°C. Source: TU LIAN QIAO, HU CI. Ref: 6.

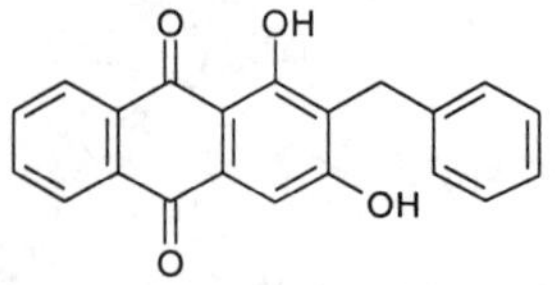

616 Berbamine
CAS: 478-61-5 $C_{37}H_{40}N_2O_6$ MW: 608.74 Source: FANG JI. Ref: 1, 2, 4, 5.

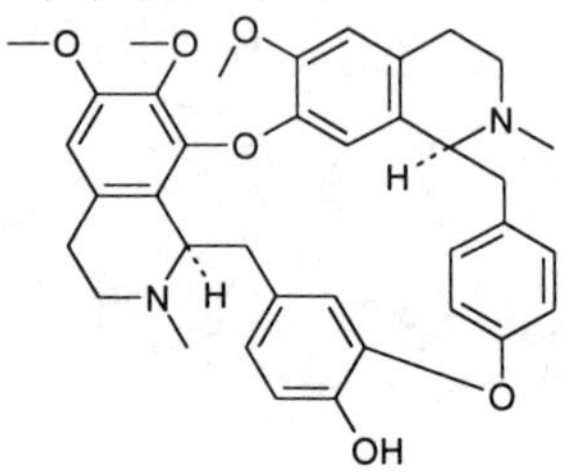

617 Berberine
Umbellatine. CAS: 2086-83-1 $C_{20}H_{18}NO_4$ MW: 336.37 Source: HE NAN TANG SONG CAO, HUANG LIAN, HUANG BAI. Ref: 1, 2, 4, 538.

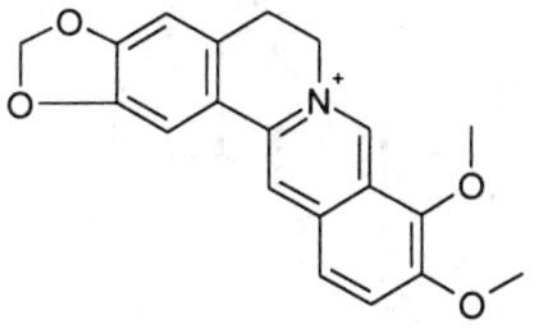

618 Berberrubine
9-Berberoline. $C_{19}H_{15}NO_4$ MW: 321.34 Source: TANG SONG CAO. Ref: 1.

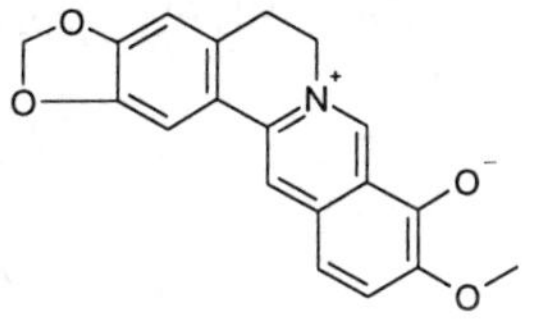

619 α-Bergamotene
$C_{15}H_{24}$ MW: 204.36 Source: DU HUO, SHENG JIANG. Ref: 2

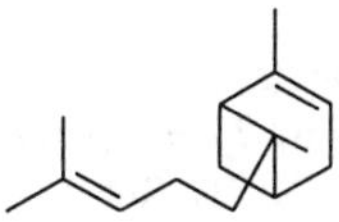

620 9(10)Z,α-trans-Bergamotenol
$C_{15}H_{24}O$ MW: 220.36 Property: colorless oily liquid, $[\alpha]_D$-55.64° (c=0.39, $CHCl_3$). Source: GUO CHAN TAN XIANG MU. Ref: 285.

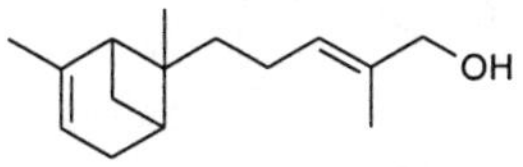

621 Bergapten
CAS: 484-20-8 $C_{12}H_8O_4$ MW: 216.20 Property: mp 188-90°C. Source: BAI ZHI, DANG GUI, DU HUO, FANG FENG, QIANG HUO, SONG YE FANG FENG, YUN NAN QIANG HUO, YONG NING DU HUO, ZHONG CHI MAO DANG GUI. Ref: 2, 5, 344, 507, 542, 549, 551.

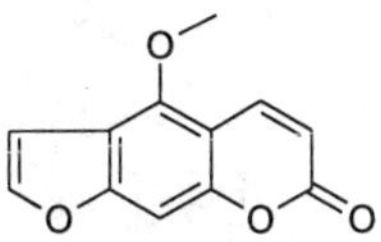

622 Bergaptol
$C_{11}H_6O_4$ MW: 202.17 Source: QIANG HUO. Ref: 2, 507.

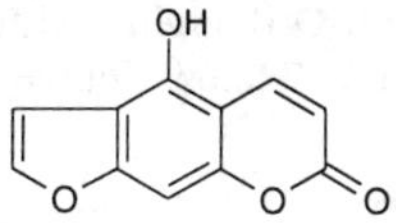

623 Bergenin
Bergenit; Arolisic acid B; Cuscutin; Peltaphorin. $C_{14}H_{16}O_9$ MW: 328.28 Source: BAI LIANG JIN, BAI LIANG JIN YE, LU SONG QIU MAO, LUO XIN FU, LUO XIN FU GEN, MU HE, YAN BAI CAI, YE WU TONG, ZI JIN NIU. Ref: 1, 4, 6.

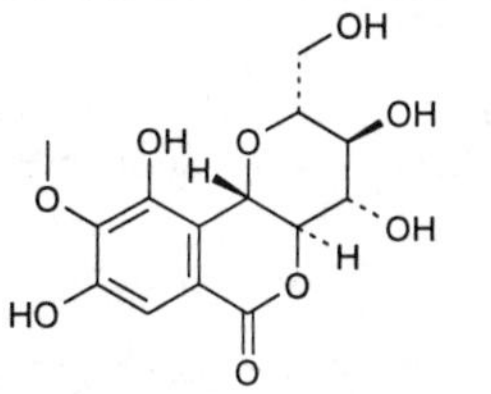

624 Bessisterol
$C_{29}H_{48}O$ MW: 412.71 Property: mp 172-5.0°C. Source: MU ZEI. Ref: 6.

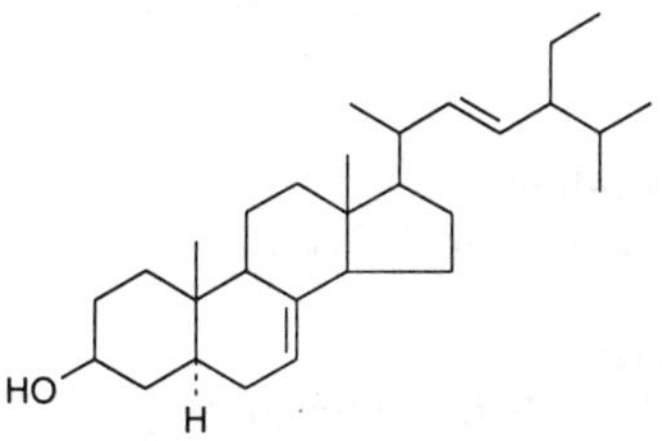

625 Betacyanin
Source: BAN ZHI LIAN. Ref: 6.

626 Betaine
Glycine betaine; Lydine; Oxyneuyine. CAS: 107-43-7 $C_5H_{11}NO_2$ MW: 117.15 Property: mp 293°C. Source: DI GU PI, GOU QI ZI, HUANG QI, LA JIAO, NIU XI, QUAN XIE, ROU CONG RONG. Ref: 1, 2, 4, 15, 530.

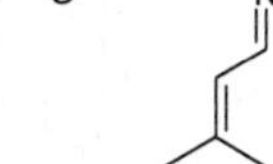

627 Betanidin 6-O-rhamnosylsophoroside
Source: YE ZI HUA. Ref: 6.

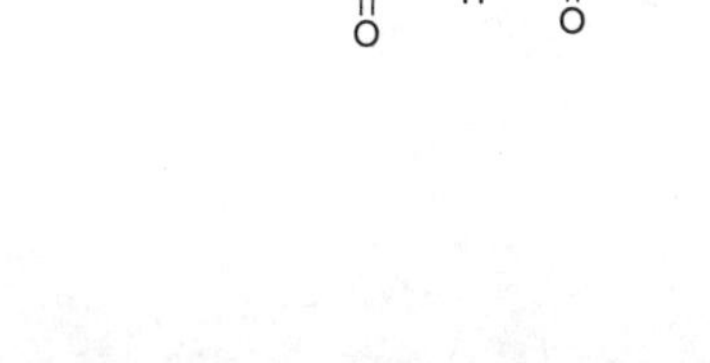

Rha-Sophorose

628 Betanidin 6-O-β-sophoroside
$C_{31}H_{38}N_2O_{18}$ MW: 726.65 Source: YE ZI HUA. Ref: 6.

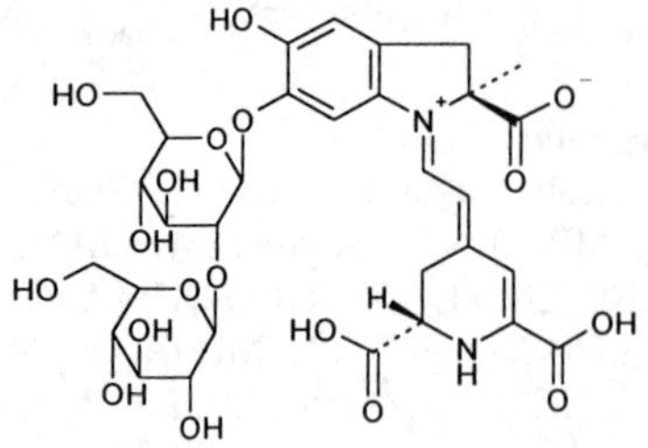

629 Betanin
$C_{25}H_{28}N_2O_{13}$ MW: 564.51 Source: BAN ZHI LIAN. Ref: 6.

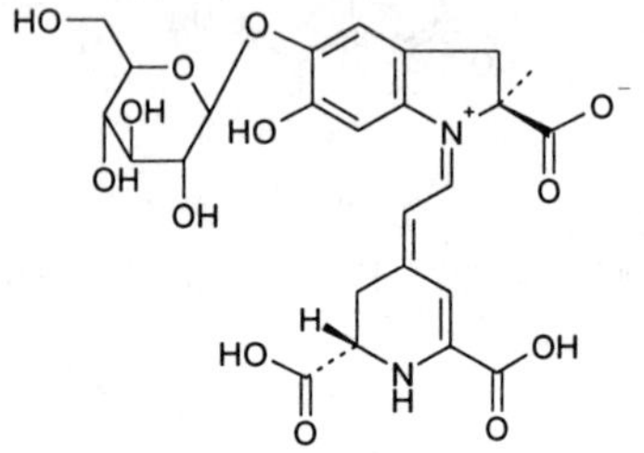

630 Betaxanthins
Source: ZI MO LI GEN. Ref: 6.

631 Bethogenin
$C_{28}H_{44}O_4$ MW: 444.66 Property: mp 193-4.0°C. Source: YU ER QI. Ref: 6.

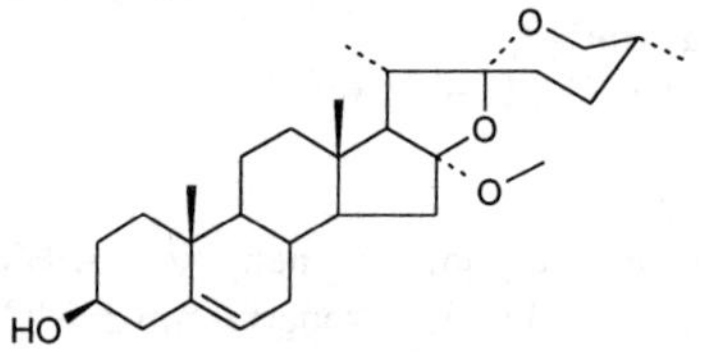

632 Betonicine
$C_7H_{13}NO_3$ MW: 159.19 Property: mp 254-6.0°C. Source: YANG SHI CAO. Ref: 6.

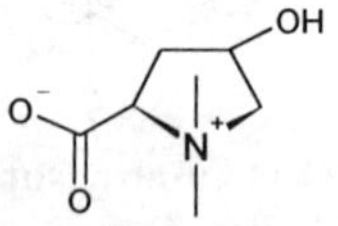

633 Betulafolien(e)tetraol
$C_{30}H_{52}O_4$ MW: 476.75 Property: mp 168-70°C. Source: HUA MU PI. Ref: 6.

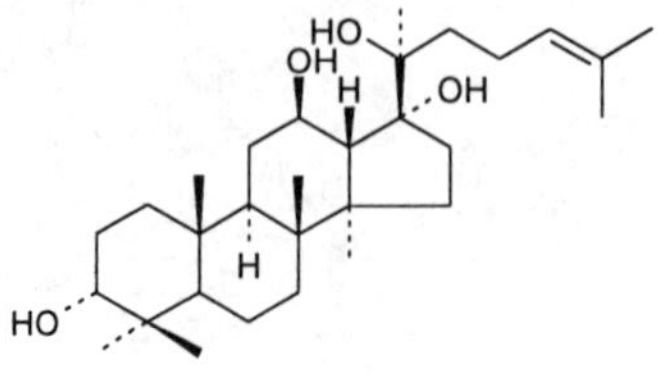

634 Betulafolien(e)triol
$C_{30}H_{52}O_3$ MW: 460.75 Property: mp 127-9.0°C. Source: HUA MU PI. Ref: 6.

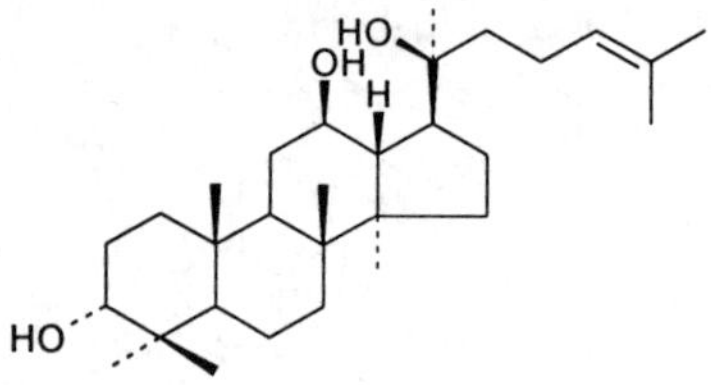

635 Betulin
Betulinol; Trochol. $C_{30}H_{50}O_2$ MW: 442.73 Property: mp 248-54°C Source: BAI HUA, MU JIN PI, DU ZHONG, MU XIANG, SHE PU TAO, SUAN ZAO REN. Ref: 2, 5, 6.

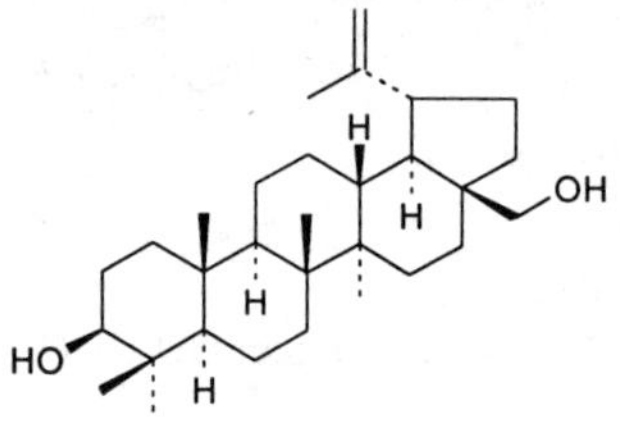

636 Betulin-3-acetate
$C_{31}H_{49}O_3$ MW: 469.73 Property: mp 260°C. Source: LI MU, SHAN REN YE. Ref: 6.

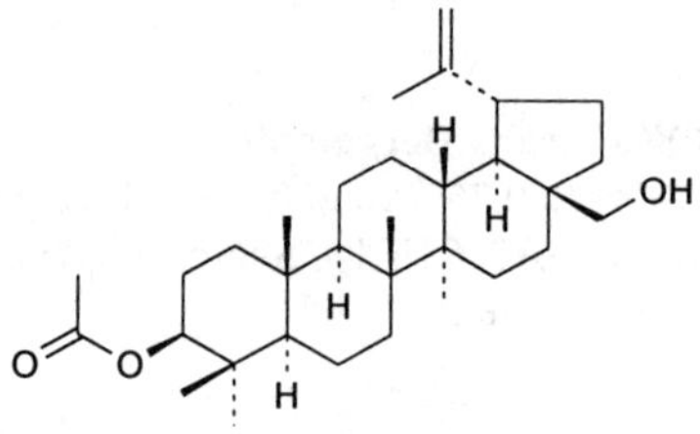

637 Betulinic acid
Betulic acid. $C_{30}H_{48}O_3$ MW: 456.72 Property: white solid, mp 285-7°C, easily soluble in chloroform, acetone, acetic ester, hardly soluble in water. Source: BAI HUA, CI WU JIA, DA ZAO, DU ZHONG, HUANG GAN CAO, LIAN QIAO, SUAN ZAO REN, MU GUA. Ref: 2, 453, 531, 591, 610.

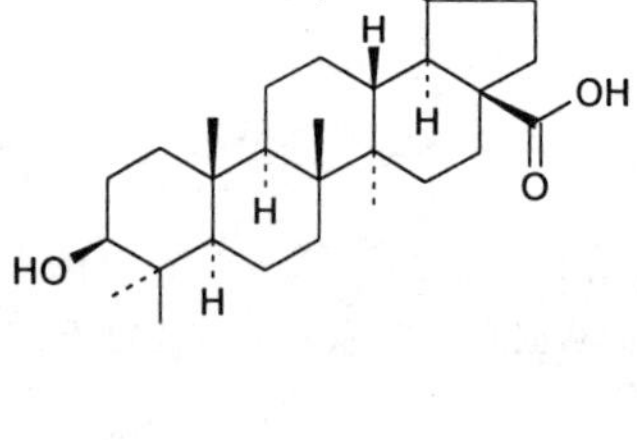

638 Betulol
$C_{15}H_{24}O$ MW: 220.36 Property: bp 157-8.0°C /20mm. Source: LIANG YE HUA PI. Ref: 6.

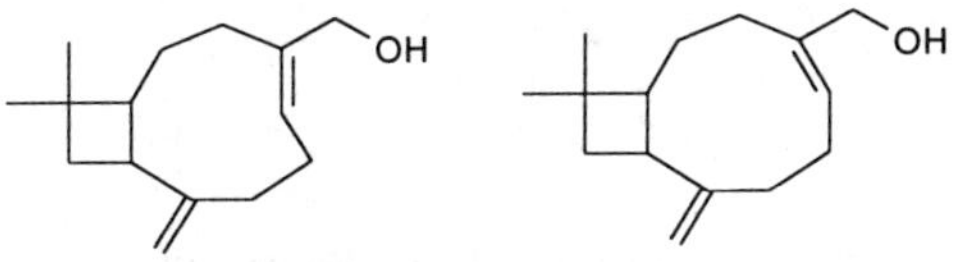

α:- β:-

639 Bianfugecine
5,9-dimethoxy-7H-dibenzo(de,h)quinolin-7-one. $C_{18}H_{13}NO_3$ MW: 291.31 Property: yellow brownish green powder, mp 160°C, sublimating at 160°C and changing into yellow acicular crystal, decomposing at 200-2°C. Source: BIAN FU GE. Ref: 23.

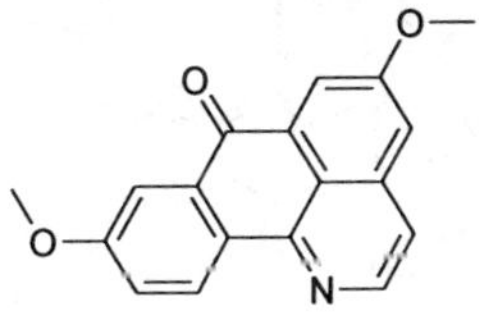

640 Bianfugedine
5,6-methylenedioxy-9-methoxy-7H-dibenzo(de,h) quinoli-7-one. $C_{18}H_{11}NO_4$ MW: 305.29 Property: yellow prismatic crystal, mp 292-6°C (dec). Source: BIAN FU GE. Ref: 23.

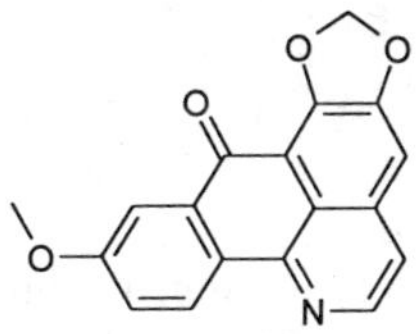

641 Bianfugenine
4,5,6,9-tetramethoxy-7H-dibenzo[de,h]quinoli-7-one. $C_{20}H_{17}NO_5$ MW: 351.36 Property: yellowish green thin acicular crystal, mp 162-164°C, appearing strong yellowish green fluorescence in the solution of chloroform. Source: BIAN FU GE. Ref: 23.

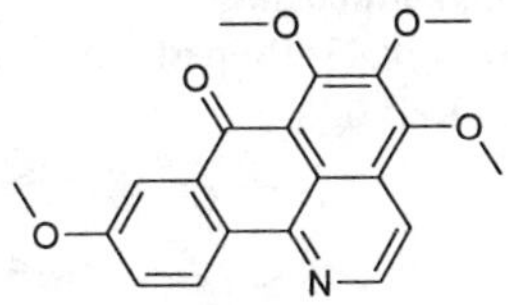

642 Bicuculline
$C_{20}H_{17}NO_6$ MW: 367.36 Property: mp 215°C. Source: YAN HU SUO. Ref: 1, 6.

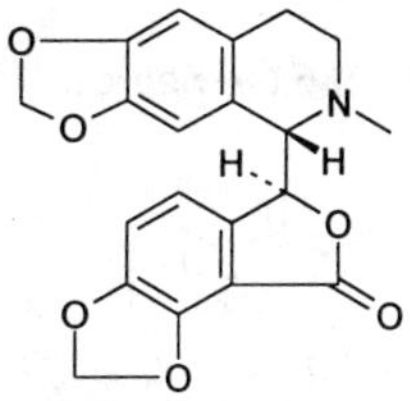

643 Bicyclo[2,2,2]oct-5-en-2-ol
$C_8H_{12}O$ MW: 124.18 Source: ROU CONG RONG. Ref: 2.

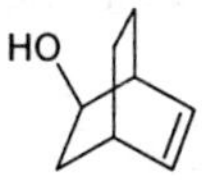

644 Bicyclogermacrene
$C_{15}H_{24}$ MW: 204.36 Source: REN SHEN. Ref: 2.

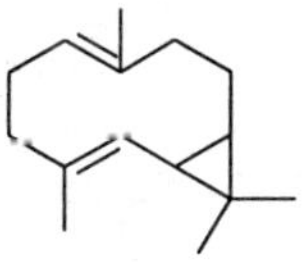

645 Bicyclomahanimbine
$C_{23}H_{25}NO$ MW: 331.46 Source: JIU LI XIANG. Ref: 11.

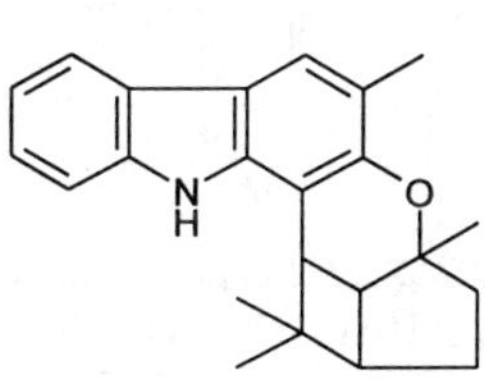

646 Bicyclomahanimbicine
$C_{24}H_{27}NO$ MW: 345.49 Source: JIU LI XIANG. Ref: 11.

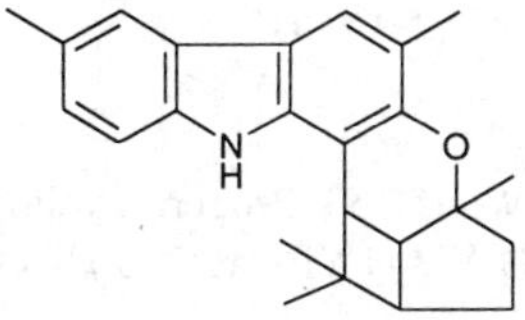

647 Bilatriene
$C_{19}H_{14}N_4$ MW: 298.35 Source: JI NEI JIN. Ref: 6.

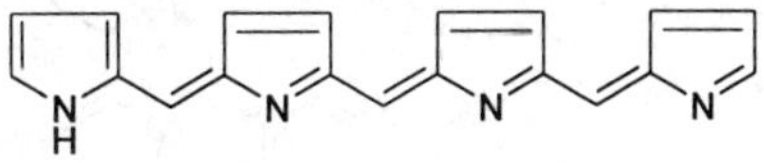

648 Bile acids
Source: LI YU DAN. Ref: 6.

649 Bilirubin
$C_{33}H_{38}N_4O_6$ MW: 586.69 Source: NIU HUANG. Ref: 2.

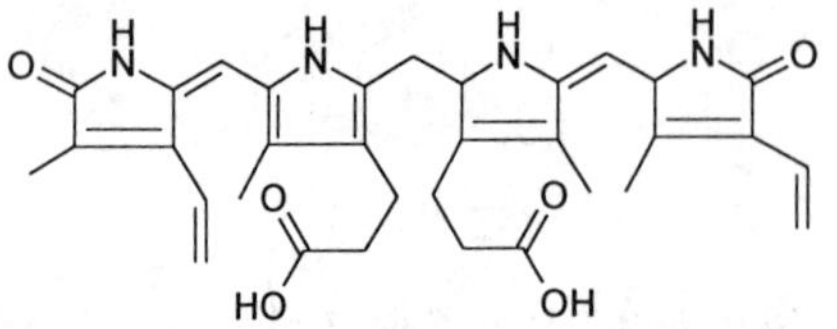

650 Biliverdin
$C_{33}H_{36}N_4O_6$ MW: 584.68 Source: NIU HUANG. Ref: 2.

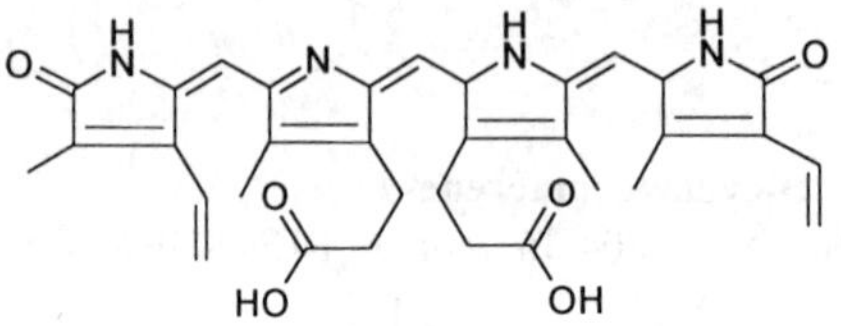

651 Bilobanol
$C_{15}H_{22}O_2$ MW: 234.34 Source: YIN YANG HUO. Ref: 2.

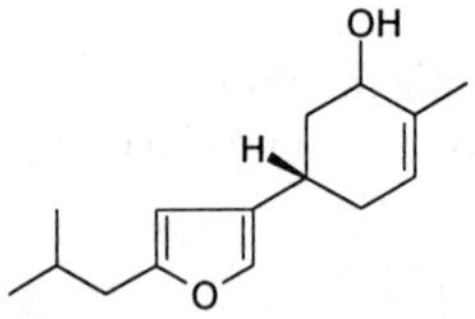

652 Bilobanone
$C_{15}H_{20}O_2$ MW: 232.33 Property: mp 118-22°C /0.09mm. Source: BAI GUO SHU PI. Ref: 6.

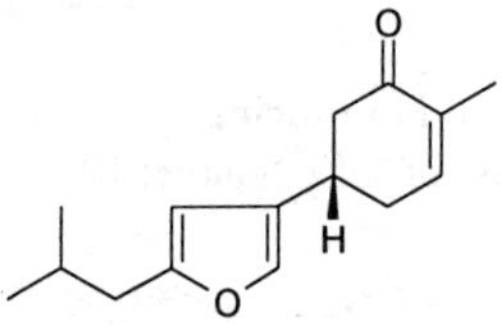

653 Bilobetin
$C_{31}H_{20}O_{10}$ MW: 552.50 Property: yellow powder. Source: CHAO XIAN YIN YANG HUO, BAI GUO. Ref: 1, 2, 442.

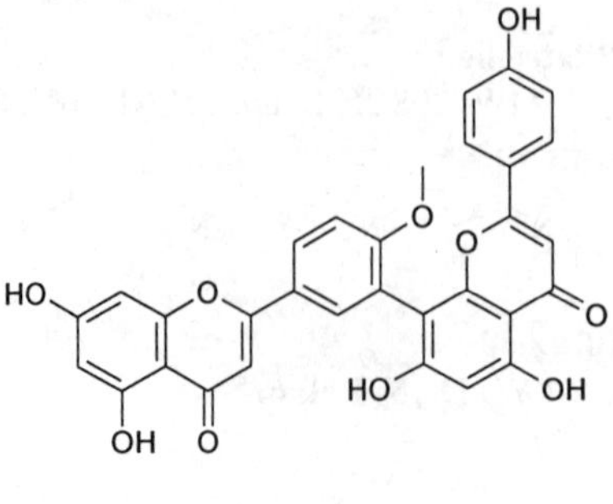

654 Bilobol
$C_{19}H_{30}O_2$ MW: 290.45 Source: BAI GUO. Ref: 2.

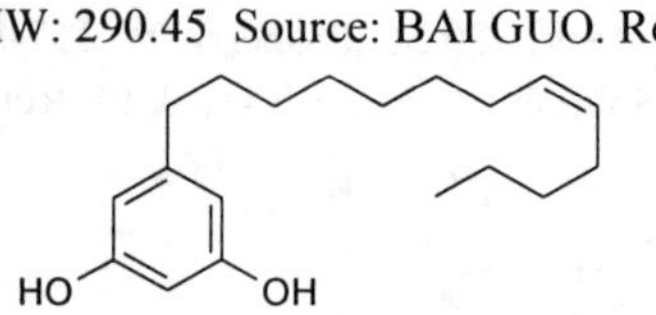

655 3,8''-Binaringenin-7''-O-β-glucoside
$C_{36}H_{32}O_{15}$ MW: 704.65 Source: SHAN ZHU ZI. Ref: 6.

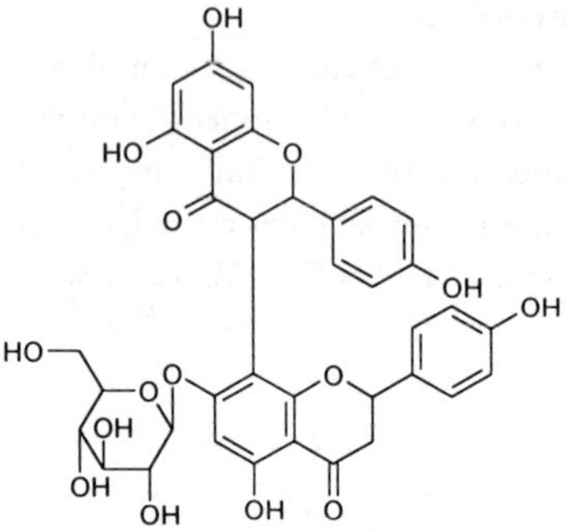

656 Biochanin A
Olmelin. $C_{16}H_{12}O_5$ MW: 284.27 Property: mp 215-6.0°C. Source: HUI HUI DOU, HONG CHE ZHOU CAO. Ref: 1, 6.

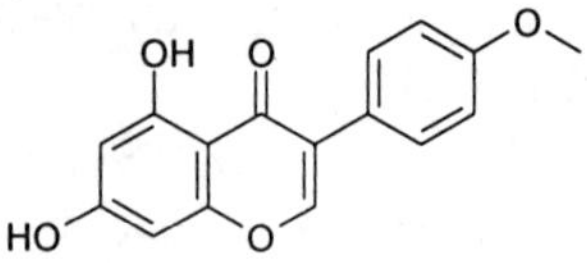

657 Biochanin B
$C_{16}H_{12}O_4$ MW: 268.27 Property: mp 256-7.0°C. Source: HONG CHE ZHOU CAO, HUI HUI DOU. Ref: 6, 2. 6.

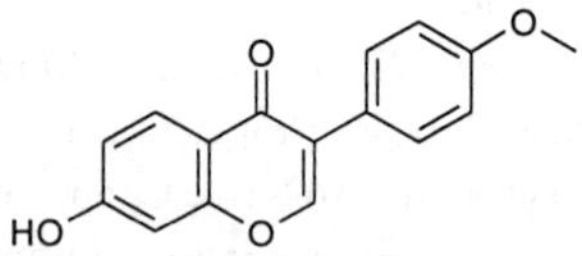

658 Biochanin-7-glucoside
$C_{10}H_{24}O_{10}$ MW: 448.43 Property: mp 220°C. Source: HUI HUI DOU. Ref: 6.

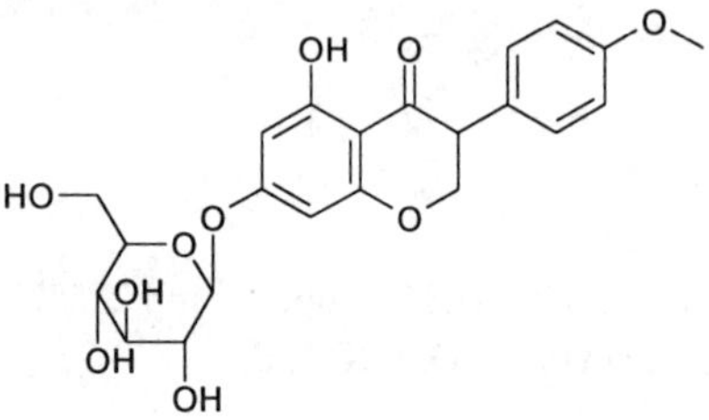

659 Biondnoid I
Kaempferol-7-O-β-D-(6''-O-p-hydrocinnamoyl)-D-glucoside. $C_{30}H_{26}O_{13}$ MW: 594.53 Property: yellow crystal, mp 220-1°C. Source: XIN YI. Ref: 306.

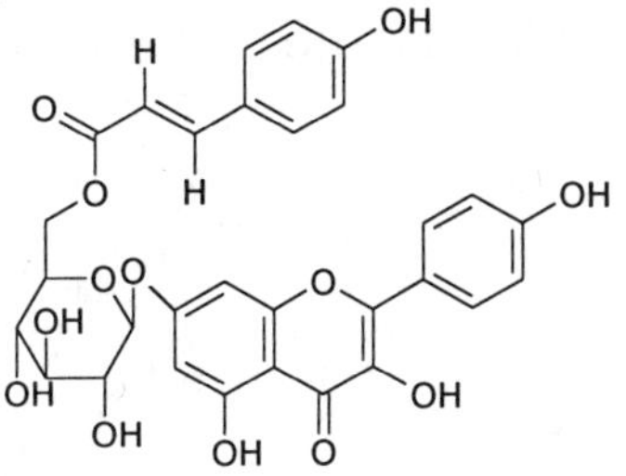

660 Biopterin
$C_9H_{11}NO_3$ MW: 237.22 Source: FENG RU, HEI MA YI, JIN YU. Ref: 6.

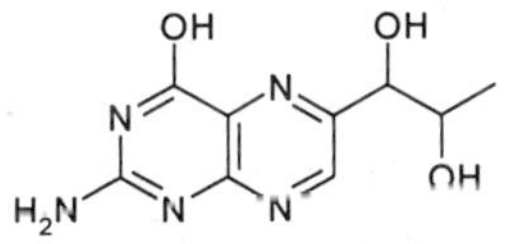

661 Biotin
$C_{10}H_{16}N_2O_3S$ MW: 244.31 Source: REN SHEN. Ref: 2.

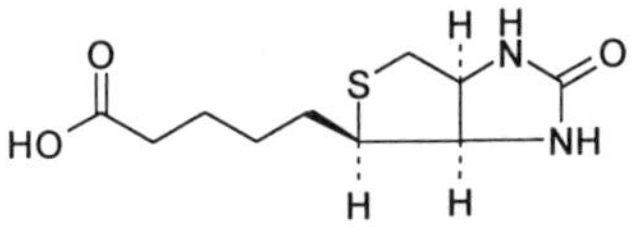

662 α-Biotol
$C_{15}H_{24}O$ MW: 220.36 Property: mp 78°C. Source: BAI ZHI JIE. Ref: 6.

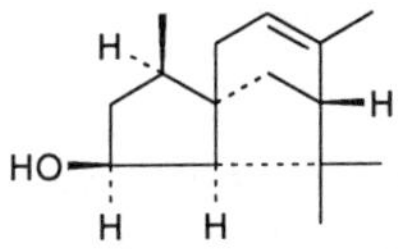

663 β-Biotol
$C_{15}H_{24}O$ MW: 220.36 Property: mp 84°C. Source: BAI ZHI JIE. Ref: 6.

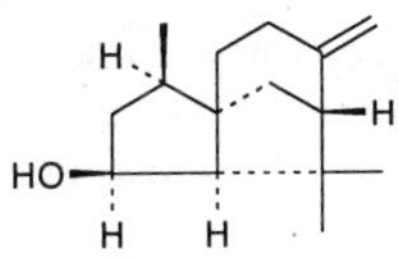

664 3,3'-Biplumbagin
$C_{22}H_{14}O_6$ MW: 374.35 Property: mp 214-6.0°C. Source: BAI HUA DAN. Ref: 6.

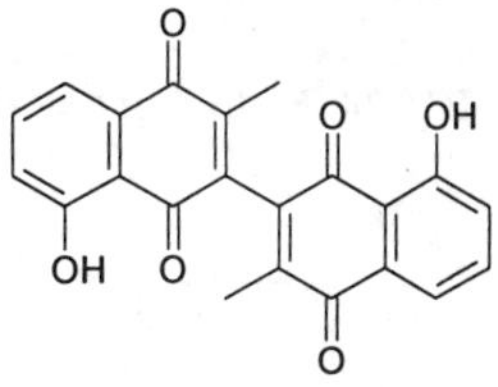

665 α-Bisabolene
$C_{15}H_{24}$ MW: 204.36 Source: DU HUO. Ref: 2.

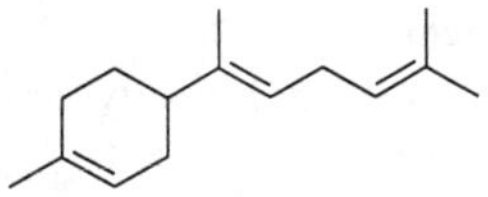

666 β-Bisabolene
l-Bisabolene. $C_{15}H_{24}$ MW: 204.36 Property: bp (-): 129-30°/10.5mm. Source: DA YE XIANG RU, DANG GUI, DU HUO, DU SONG SHI, FANG FENG, FENG DOU CAI, GAN JIANG, HOU PO, JI NING, REN SHEN, SHENG JIANG, WU WEI ZI, XI YANG SHEN, XIE CAO. Ref: 2, 6.

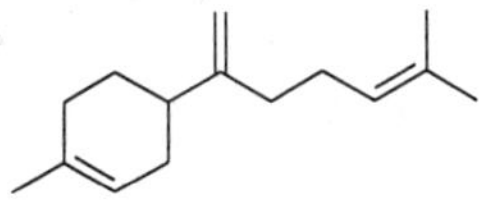

667 β₂-Bisabolene
$C_{15}H_{24}$ MW: 204.36 Source: WU LING ZHI. Ref: 6.

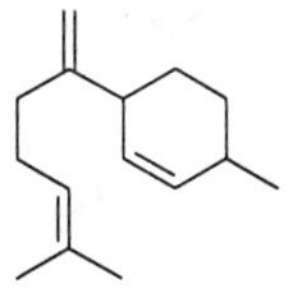

668 Bisabolol
α-Bisabolol. $C_{15}H_{26}O$ MW: 222.37 Property: bp 154-6.0°C/12mm. Source: CANG ZHU, MU JU.
Ref: 1, 2, 6.

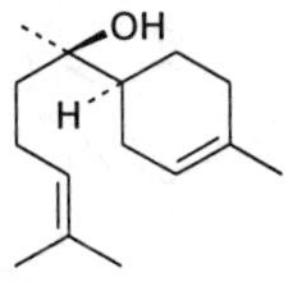

669 Bisabolol oxide-A
$C_{15}H_{26}O_2$ MW: 238.37 Property: bp 156-8.0°C. Source: MU JU. Ref: 6.

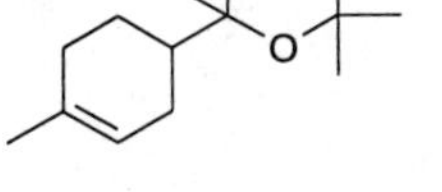

670 Bisacumol
$C_{15}H_{22}O$ MW: 218.34 Source: JIANG HUANG. Ref: 3.

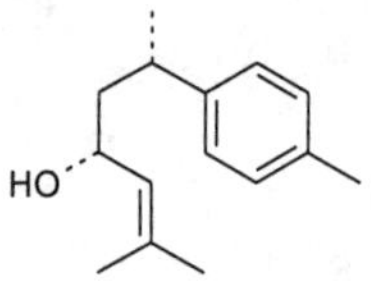

671 Bisasaricin
$C_{24}H_{32}O_6$ MW: 416.52 Property: mp 98.5-100°C. Source: SHI CHANG PU. Ref: 1

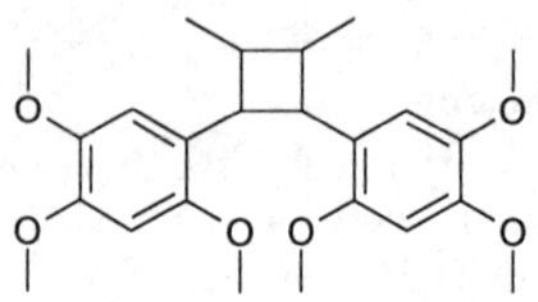

672 Bisdemethoxycurcumin
$C_{18}H_{14}O_4$ MW: 294.31 Source: YU JIN. Ref: 6.

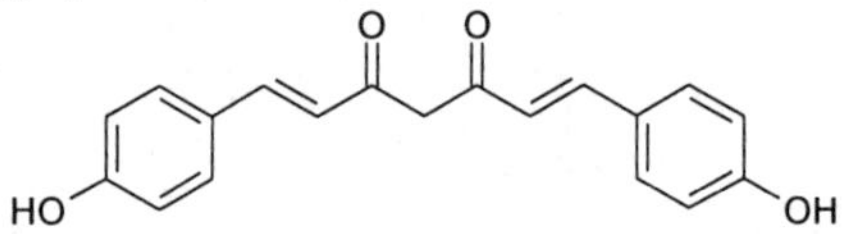

673 2,6-Bis(1,1-dimethylethyl)-4-methyl phenol
$C_{15}H_{24}O$ MW: 220.36 Source: ROU CONG RONG. Ref: 2.

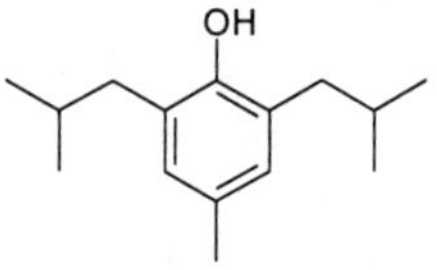

674 Bis(2-ethylbutyl)phthalate
$C_{20}H_{30}O_4$ MW: 334.46 Source: SHUI QIN. Ref: 6.

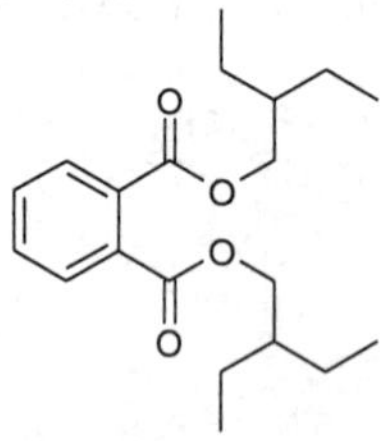

675 Bis-2-ethyl-hexyl-phthalate
$C_{24}H_{38}O_4$ MW: 390.57 Source: ROU CONG RONG. Ref: 2.

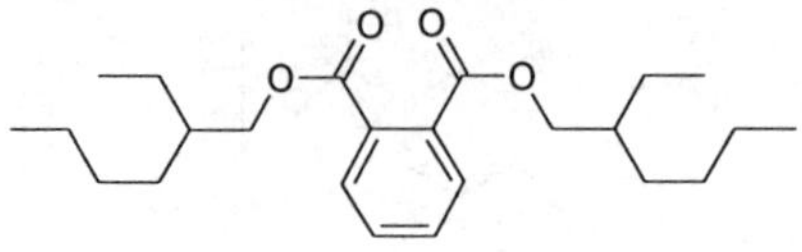

676 Bis[4-(β-D-glucopyranosyloxy) benzyl] (S)-2-butylmalate
$C_{34}H_{46}O_{17}$ MW: 726.74 Property: white amorphous powder, mp 107-110°C, $[\alpha]_D^{20}$ -40.07° (c=2.25, MeOH). Source: SHAN HU LAN. Ref: 280.

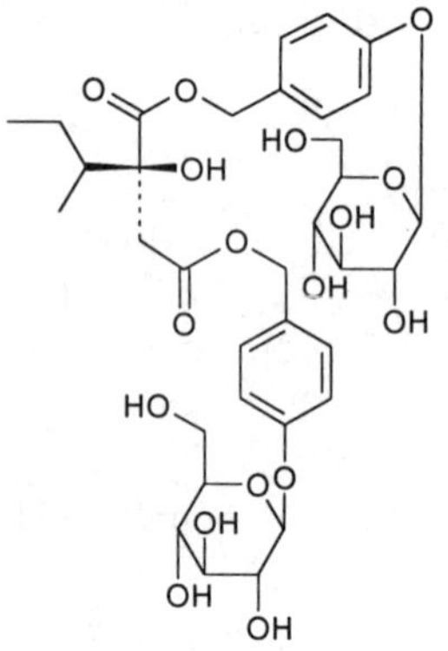

677 6,8-Bis(C-glucosyl)-apigenin
$C_{27}H_{30}O_{15}$ MW: 594.53 Property: mp 220°C (Dec). Source: NING MENG. Ref: 6.

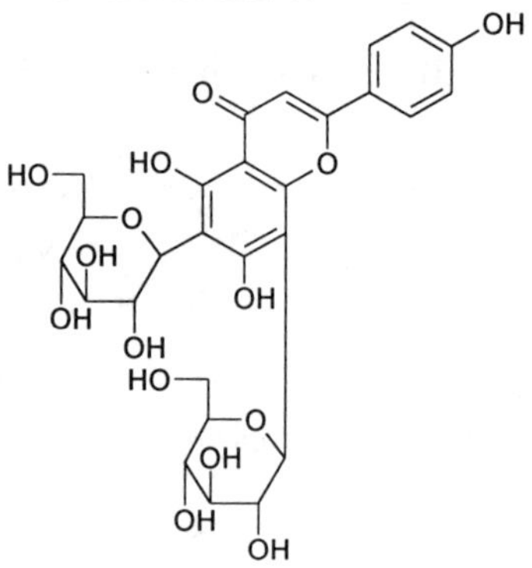

678 Bis(4-hydroxybenzyl) ether
$C_{14}H_{14}O_3$ MW: 230.27 Source: TIAN MA. Ref: 2.

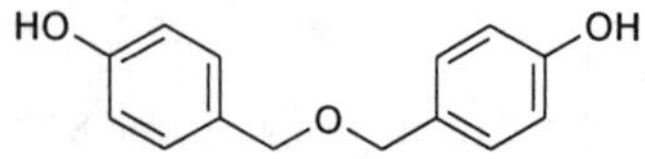

679 Bis(4-hydroxybenzyl) ether mono-β-D-glucopyranoside
$C_{20}H_{24}O_8$ MW: 392.41 Source: TIAN MA. Ref: 2.

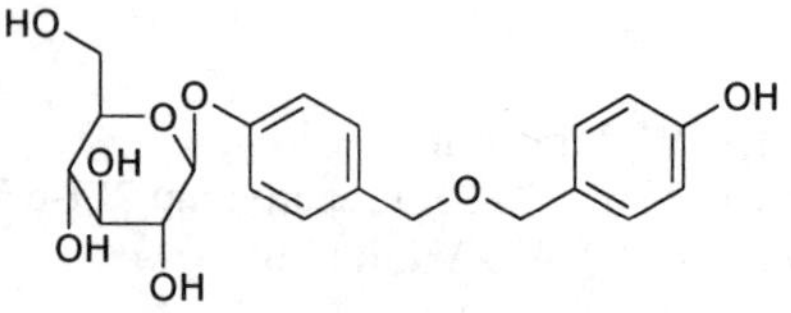

680 3,3'-Bis(indolylmethyl)dimethyl ammonium hydroxide
Source: LU ZHU GEN. Ref: 6.

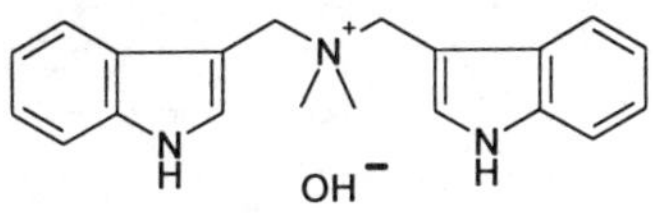

681 Bisisodiospyrin
$C_{48}H_{34}O_{12}$ MW: 802.80 Property: mp >320°C. Source: JUN QIAN ZI. Ref: 6.

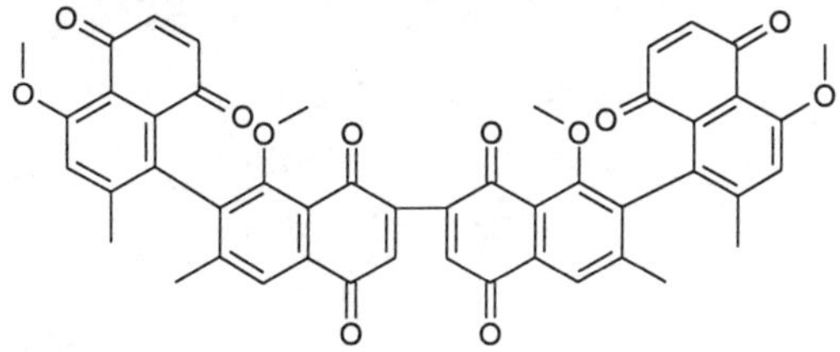

682 Borneol
$C_{10}H_{18}O$ MW: 154.25 Property: mp 208°C, bp 212°C. Source: BING PIAN, GAN JIANG, LIAN QIAO, SHENG JIANG, WU WEI ZI, XI XIN. Ref: 1, 2.

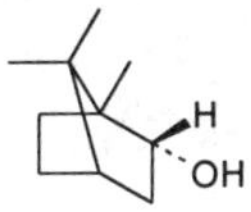

683 d-Borneol
$C_{10}H_{18}O$ MW: 154.25 Source: BING PIAN. Ref: 2.

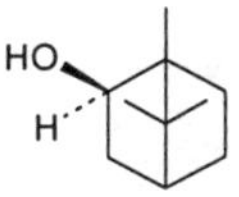

684 *l*-Borneol
$C_{10}H_{18}O$ MW: 154.25 Property: mp 204°C, bp 210°C/779mm. Source: AI NA XIANG, GANG SONG, SHE XIANG CAO, YANG SHI CAO, YE XIANG MAO, ZHI ZHU XIANG. Ref: 6.

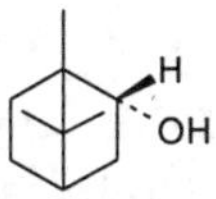

685 L(+)-Bornesitol
$C_7H_{14}O_6$ MW: 194.19 Property: mp 201-3.0°C. Source: HUANG HUA JIA ZHU TAO, JIANG LI MU GEN. Ref: 6.

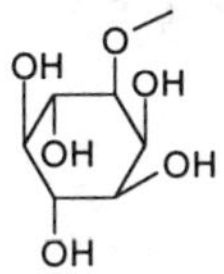

687 Bornyl isovalerianate
$C_{15}H_{26}O_2$ MW: 238.37 Source: QING HAO. Ref: 2.

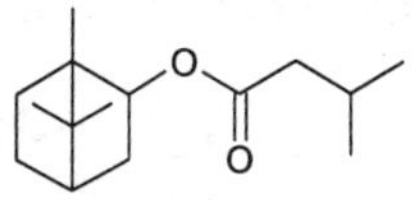

688 Bornyl magnolol
$C_{28}H_{34}O_2$ MW: 402.58 Source: HOU PO. Ref: 2.

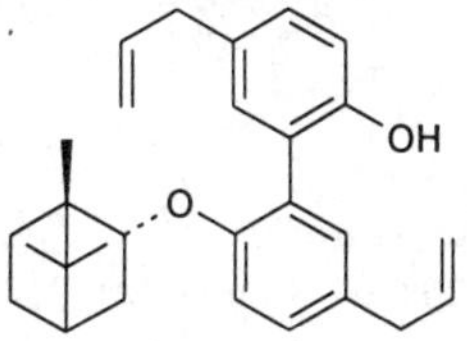

689 Boschnaloside
$C_{16}H_{24}O_8$ MW: 344 Property: white lamellar crystal, mp 102-3°C (acetone). Source: CAO CONG RONG. Ref: 471.

690 Boschniakine
$C_{10}H_{11}NO$ MW: 161.21 Property: bp 80-90°C/3mm. Source: CAO CONG RONG. Ref: 6.

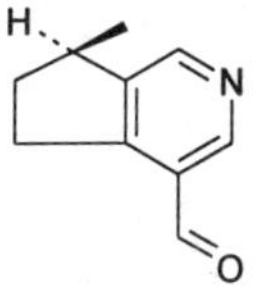

691 Boschnialactone
$C_9H_{14}O_2$ MW: 154.21 Property: bp 105-12°C/6mm. Source: CAO CONG RONG. Ref: 6.

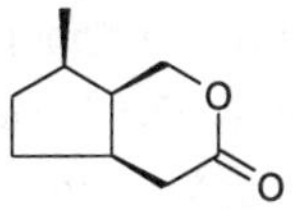

692 α-Boswellic acid
$C_{30}H_{48}O_3$ MW: 456.72 Property: mp 289°C. Source: RU XIANG. Ref: 6.

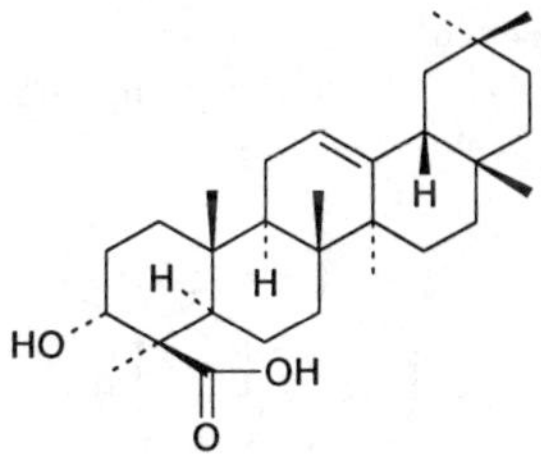

693 β-Boswellic acid
$C_{30}H_{48}O_3$ MW: 456.72 Property: mp 238-40°C. Source: RU XIANG. Ref: 6.

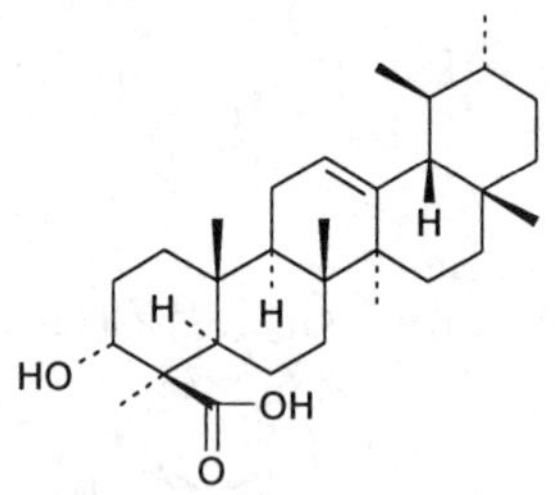

694 β-Bourbonene
$C_{15}H_{24}$ MW: 204.36 Source: MU HAO, QING HAO. Ref: 6.

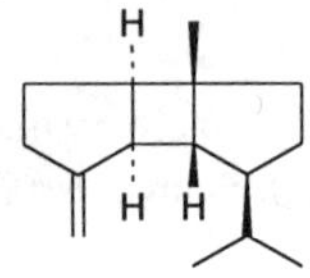

695 Brahmic acid
$C_{30}H_{48}O_6$ MW: 504.71 Property: mp 293°C. Source: JI XUE CAO. Ref: 6.

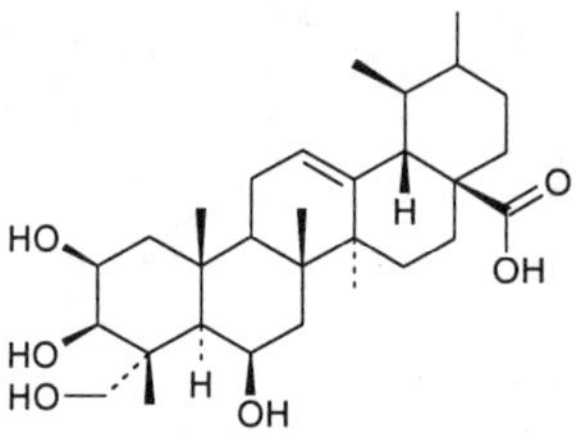

696 Brasilin
Brazilin. $C_{16}H_{14}O_5$ MW: 286.29 Property: mp 250°C. Source: SU MU. Ref: 1, 6.

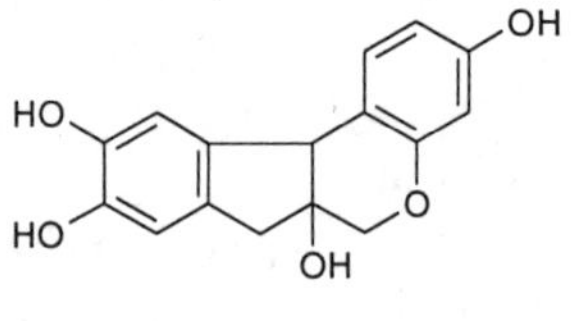

697 Brassicasterol
$C_{29}H_{48}O$ MW: 412.71 Property: mp 148°C. Source: YUN TAI ZI. Ref: 6.

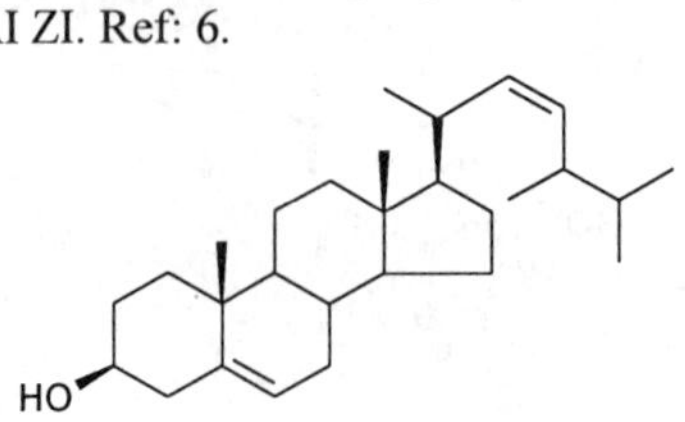

698 Brefeldin A
$C_{16}H_{26}O_4$ MW: 282.38 Source: DANG GUI. Ref: 2.

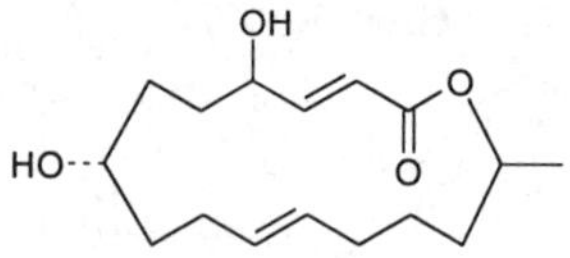

699 Britanin
$C_{19}H_{26}O_7$ MW: 366.41 Property: mp 189-91°C. Source: JIN FO CAO, XUAN FU HUA. Ref: 1, 6.

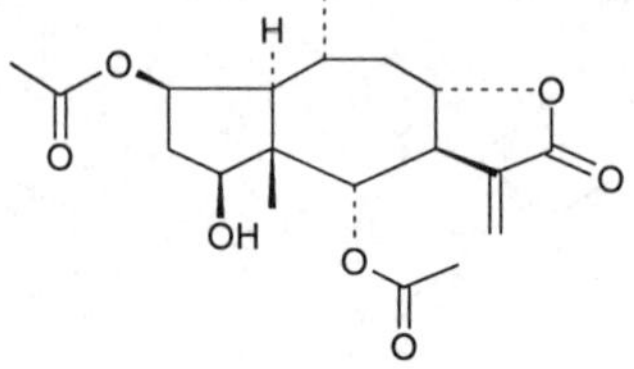

700 Bruceine A
$C_{26}H_{34}O_{11}$ MW: 522.55 Property: mp 267-70°C. Source: YA DAN ZI. Ref: 1, 2, 4, 6.

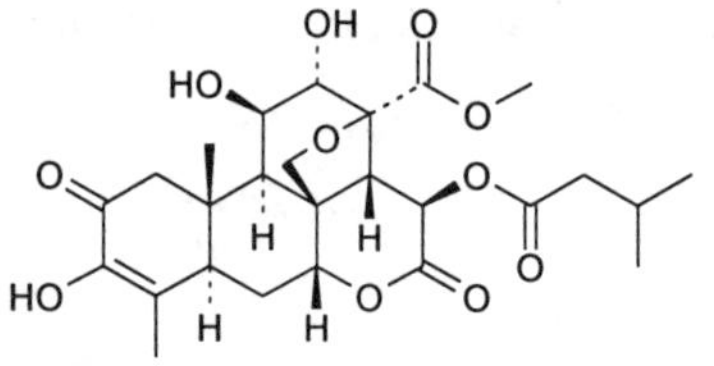

701 Bruceine B
CAS: 25514-29-8 $C_{23}H_{28}O_{11}$ MW: 480.47 Property: mp 262-6°C. Source: YA DAN ZI. Ref: 1, 2, 4, 6.

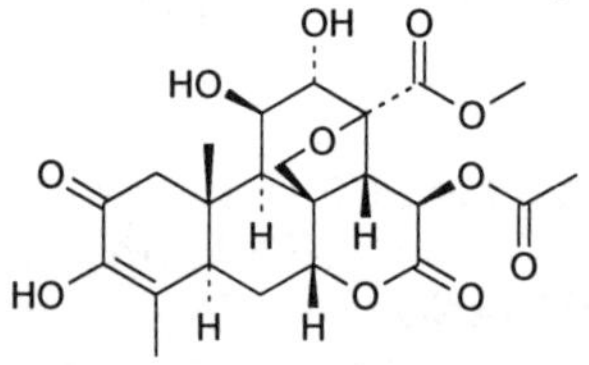

702 Bruceine C
$C_{28}H_{36}O_{12}$ MW: 564.59 Property: mp 175-80°C. Source: YA DAN ZI. Ref: 1, 2, 4, 6.

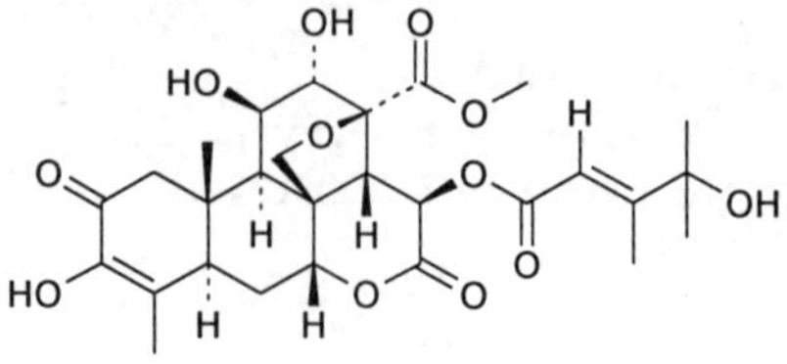

703 Bruceine D

CAS: 21499-66-1 $C_{20}H_{26}O_9$ MW: 410.42 Property: mp 285-90°C. Source: YA DAN ZI. Ref: 1, 2, 4, 6.

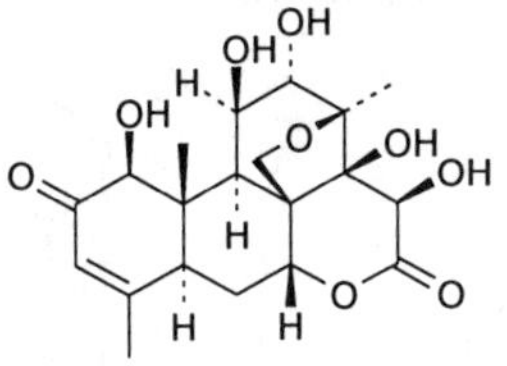

704 Bruceine E

CAS: 21586-90-3 $C_{20}H_{28}O_9$ MW: 412.44 Property: mp 260-4°C. Source: YA DAN ZI. Ref: 1, 2, 4, 6.

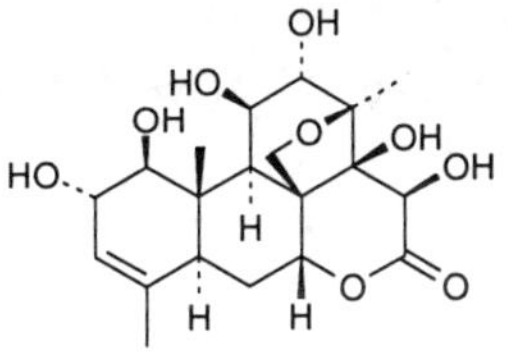

705 Bruceine F

$C_{20}H_{28}O_{10}$ MW: 428.44 Property: mp 224-7°C. Source: YA DAN ZI. Ref: 1, 2, 4, 6.

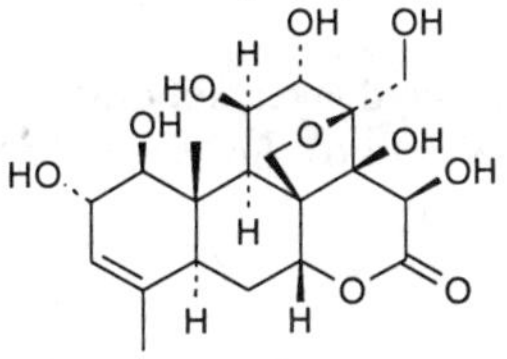

706 Bruceine G

$C_{20}H_{26}O_8$ MW: 394.43 Source: YA DAN ZI. Ref: 1, 2, 4.

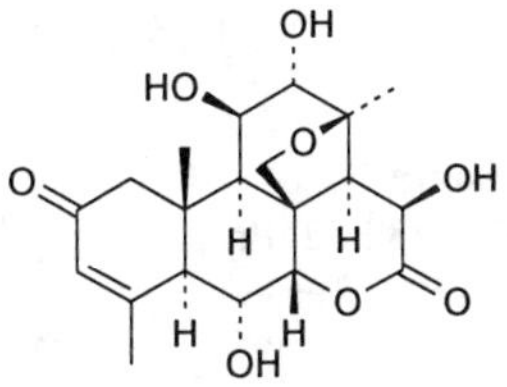

707 Bruceine H

$C_{20}H_{26}O_9$ MW: 410.42 Source: YA DAN ZI. Ref: 2.

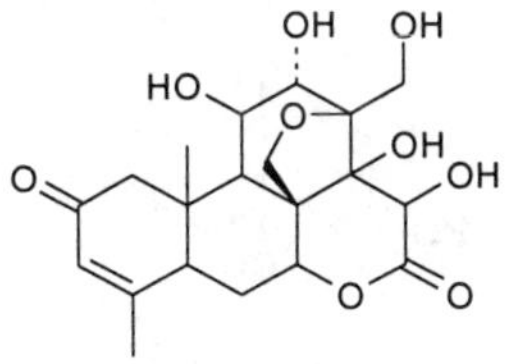

708 Bruceine I

$C_{22}H_{28}O_9$ MW: 436.46 Property: colorless prismatic crystal, mp 293-5°C. Source: YA DAN ZI. Ref: 2, 156.

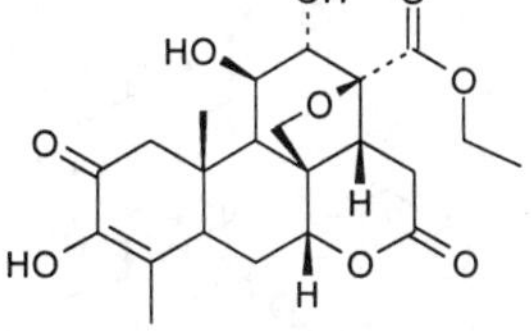

709 Brucenol

$C_{21}H_{25}O_9$ MW: 421.43 Property: mp 260-1.0°C. Source: YA DAN ZI. Ref: 6.

710 Bruceolic acid

$C_{47}H_{94}O_3$ MW: 707.27 Property: mp 88.5°C. Source: YA DAN ZI. Ref: 6.

711 Bruceoside A

$C_{32}H_{42}O_{16}$ MW: 682.66 Source: YA DAN ZI. Ref: 2.

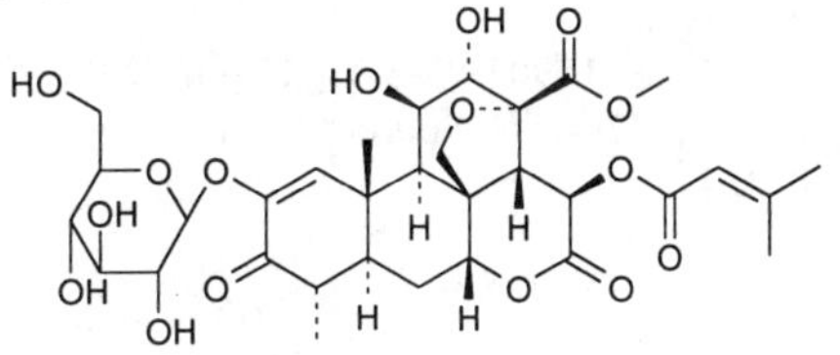

712 Bruceoside B

$C_{32}H_{42}O_{16}$ MW: 682.66 Source: YA DAN ZI. Ref: 2.

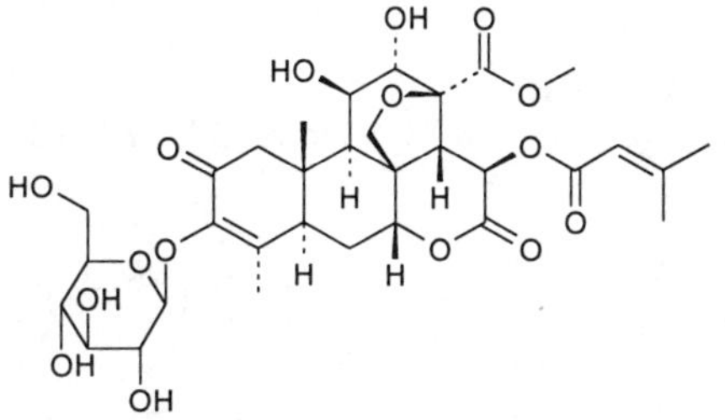

713 Bruceoside C

$C_{32}H_{42}O_{16}$ MW: 682.66 Source: YA DAN ZI. Ref: 2.

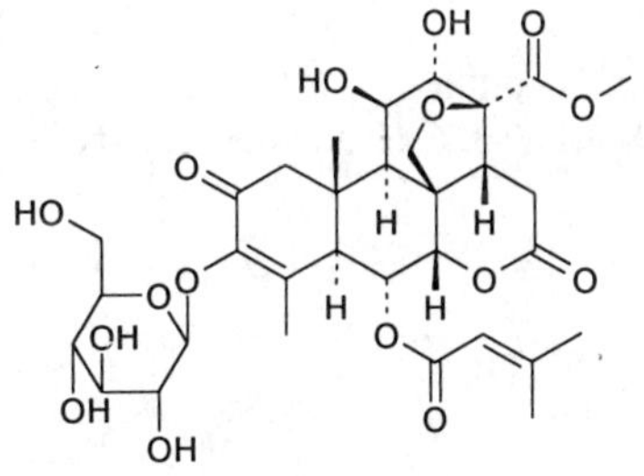

714 Brucine
$C_{23}H_{26}N_2O_4$ MW: 394.47 Property: mp 178°C. Source: MA QIAN ZI, MAO ZHU MA QIAN. Ref: 1, 4, 543, 576.

715 Brucine N-oxide
Brucineoxide. $C_{24}H_{28}N_2O_5$ MW: 424.50 Source: MA QIAN ZI. Ref: 2, 543.

716 Brusatol
Yatansin. CAS: 14907-98-3 $C_{26}H_{32}O_{11}$ MW: 520.54 Property: mp 276-8°C. Source: YA DAN ZI. Ref: 1, 2, 4.

717 Bryonolie
$C_{30}H_{48}O_3$ MW: 456.72 Source: TIAN HUA FEN. Ref: 2.

718 Bufadienolide
$C_{22}H_{30}O_2$ MW: 326.48 Source: CHAN SU. Ref: 2.

719 Bufagin
$C_{24}H_{32}O_5$ MW: 400.52 Property: mp 224-5.0°C. Source: CHAN SU. Ref: 6.

720 Bufalin
$C_{24}H_{34}O_4$ MW: 386.54 Source: CHAN SU. Ref: 2, 618.

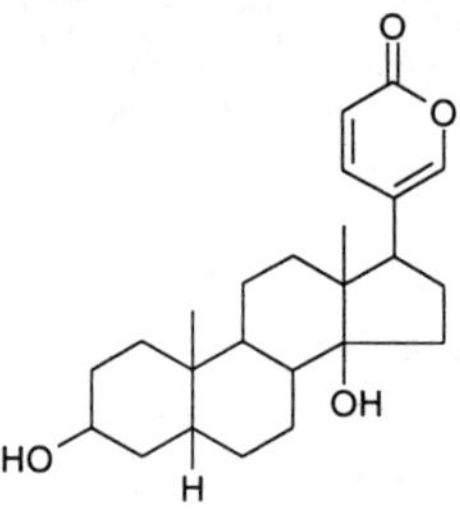

721 Bufalin-3-hydrogen suberate
$C_{30}H_{42}O_7$ MW: 514.67 Source: CHAN SU. Ref: 6.

722 Bufarenogin
$C_{24}H_{32}O_7$ MW: 432.52 Property: mp 230-3.0°C. Source: CHAN SU. Ref: 6.

723 Bufodihydroxycholanic acid
$C_{24}H_{40}O_3$ MW: 376.58 Property: mp 230°C. Source: CHAN CHU DAN. Ref: 6.

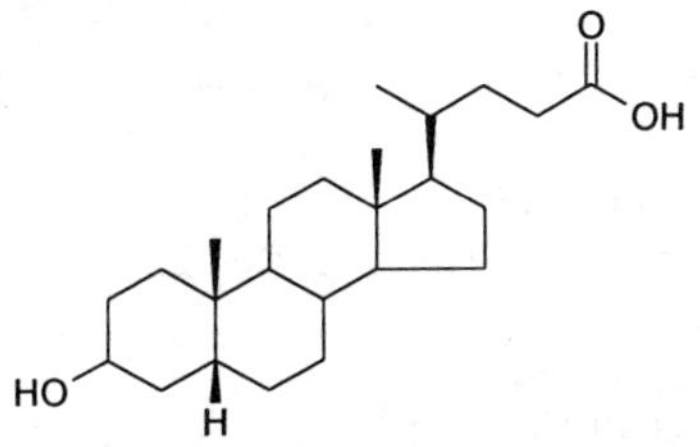

724 5β-Bufol sulfate
$C_{27}H_{48}O_5$ MW: 452.68 Source: XIA MA DAN. Ref: 6.

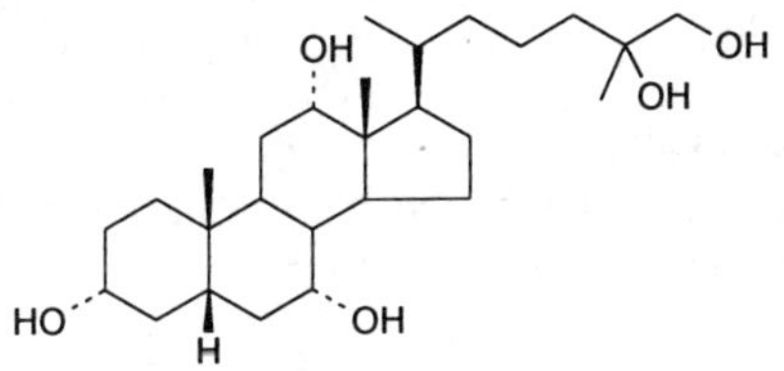

725 Bufotalidin
Hellebrigenin. CAS: 465-90-7 $C_{24}H_{32}O_6$ MW: 416.52 Source: CHAN SU. Ref: 2.

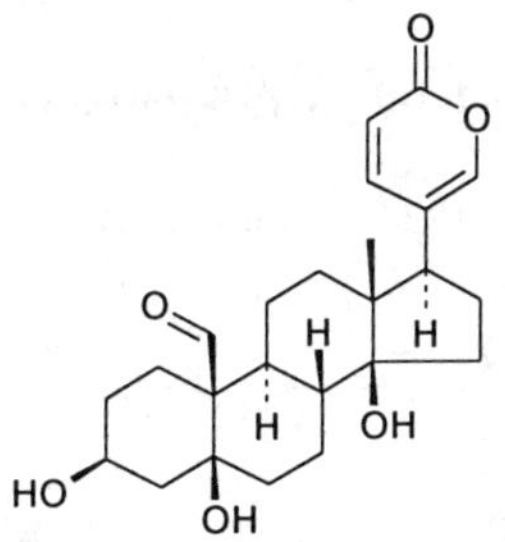

726 Bufotalin
$C_{25}H_{34}O_7$ MW: 446.55 Source: CHAN SU. Ref: 2.

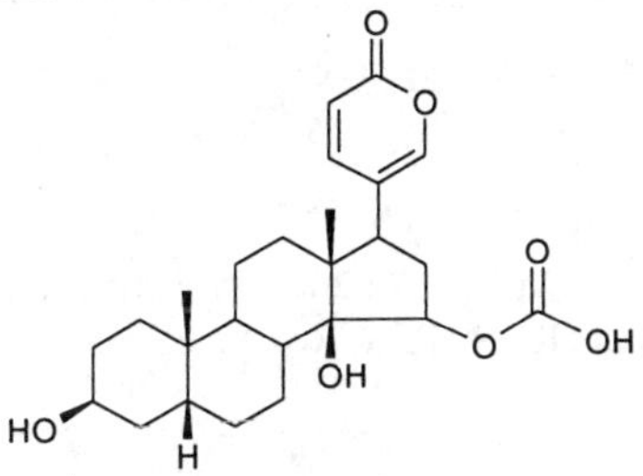

727 Bufotalinin
$C_{24}H_{30}O_6$ MW: 414.50 Source: CHAN SU. Ref: 2.

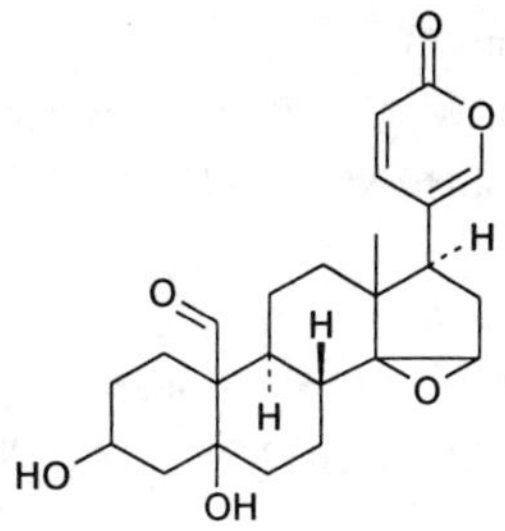

728 Bufotalin 3-succinoylarginine ester(I)
$C_{36}H_{52}N_4O_{10}$ MW: 700.84 Property: colorless amorphous powder, mp 213-5°C. Source: CHAN PI. Ref: 241.

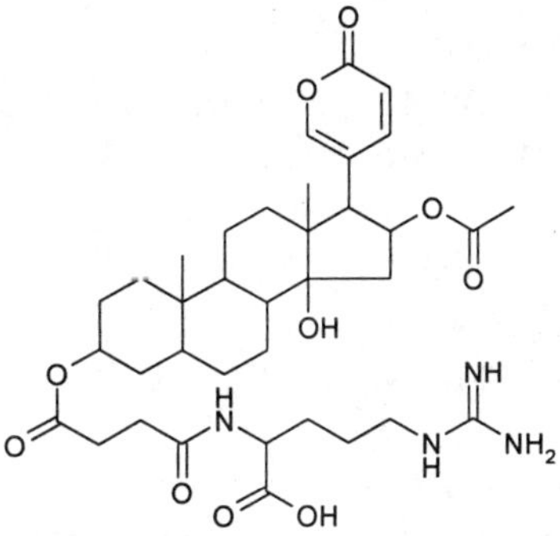

729 Bufotenidine
$C_{13}H_{18}N_2O$ MW: 218.30 Source: CHAN SU. Ref: 1, 2.

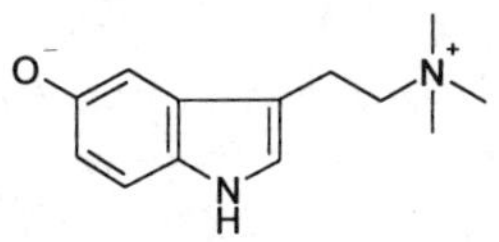

730 Bufothionine
$C_{12}H_{15}N_2O_3S$ MW: 267.33 Source: CHAN SU. Ref: 2.

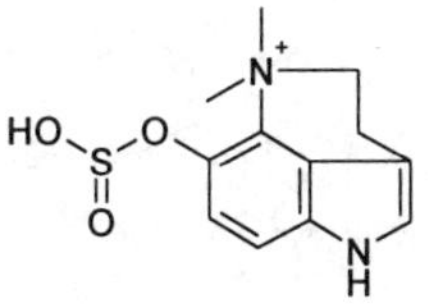

731 Bulbocapnine
$C_{19}H_{19}NO_4$ MW: 325.37 Source: XIA TIAN WU. Ref: 1, 6.

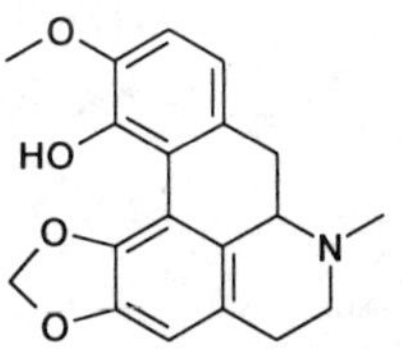

732 Bullatine A
$C_{21}H_{31}NO_2$ MW: 329.49 Property: mp 251-3.0°C. Source: XUE SHANG YI ZHI HAO. Ref: 1, 6.

733 Bullatine B
$C_{24}H_{39}NO_6$ MW: 437.58 Property: mp 158-9.0°C. Source: XUE SHANG YI ZHI HAO. Ref: 1, 6.

734 Bullatine C
$C_{26}H_{41}NO_7$ MW: 479.62 Property: mp 220°C. Source: XUE SHANG YI ZHI HAO. Ref: 1, 6.

735 Bullatine D
$C_{23}H_{37}NO_9$ MW: 471.55 Property: mp 221°C. Source: XUE SHANG YI ZHI HAO. Ref: 1, 6.

736 Bullatine E
$C_{24}H_{39}NO_6$ MW: 437.58 Property: mp 182-3.0°C. Source: XUE SHANG YI ZHI HAO. Ref: 6.

737 Bullatine F
$C_{24}H_{39}NO_7$ MW: 453.58 Property: mp 186°C. Source: XUE SHANG YI ZHI HAO. Ref: 6.

738 Bullatine G
Napellonine; Songorine; Zongorine. CAS: 509-24-0
$C_{22}H_{31}NO_3$ MW: 357.50 Property: mp 210-2°C. Source: CAO WU TOU, E ZHANG YE FU ZI, SI CHUAN JIANG YOU FU ZI, XUE SHANG YI ZHI HAO. Ref: 4, 6, 239, 461.

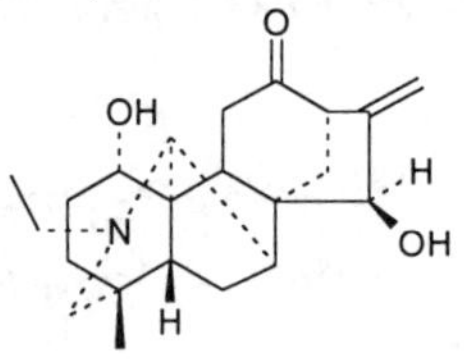

739 Bupleuonol
$C_{18}H_{22}O_2$ MW: 270.37 Property: colorless lamellar crystal, mp 22°C. Source: DA YE CHAI HU. Ref: 81.

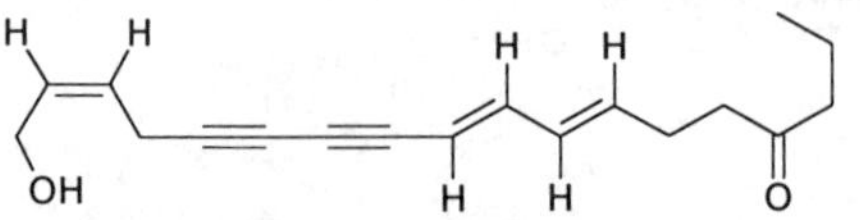

740 Bupleurotoxin
$C_{18}H_{24}O_2$ MW: 272.39 Property: colorless lamellar crystal, mp 54°C (methanol), $[\alpha]_D^{18}$ +20° (c=0.021, methanol). Source: DA YE CHAI HU. Ref: 81.

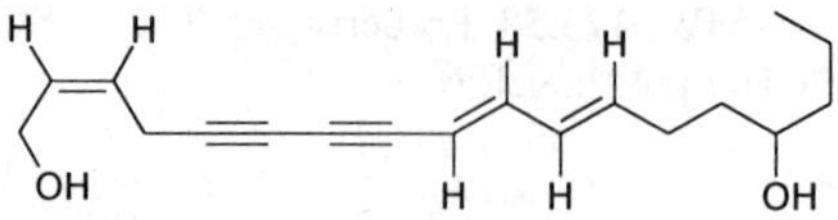

741 Bupleurumol
$C_{37}H_{64}O_2$ Source: CHAI HU. Ref: 2.

742 Bupleurynol
$C_{17}H_{22}O$ MW: 256.39 Property: colorless lamellar crystal, mp 36°C. Source: DA YE CHAI HU. Ref: 81.

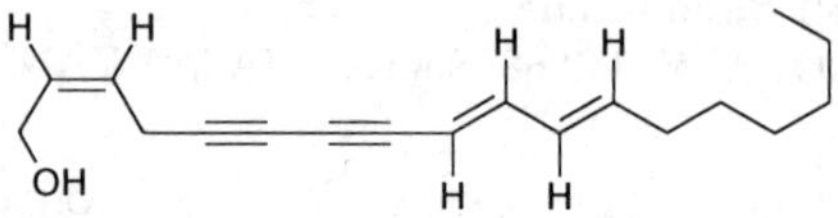

743 Burchellin
$C_{20}H_{20}O_5$ MW: 340.38 Property: white amorphous powder. Source: SHAN JU. Ref: 75.

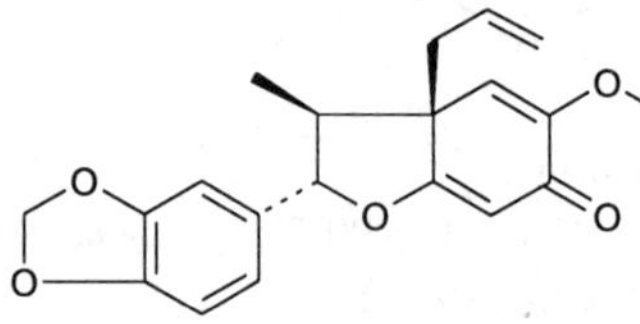

744 2-(Buta-1,3-diynyl)-5-(but-3-en-1-ynyl) thiophene
$C_{12}H_6S$ MW: 182.25 Source: MO HAN LIAN. Ref: 6.

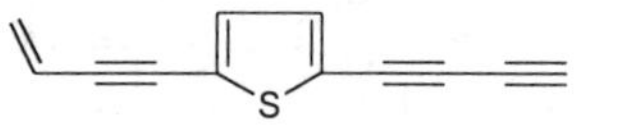

745 2-(Buta-1,3-diynyl)-5-(4-chloro-3-hydroxy-but-1-ynyl) thiophene
$C_{12}H_7ClOS$ MW: 234.71 Source: MO HAN LIAN. Ref: 6.

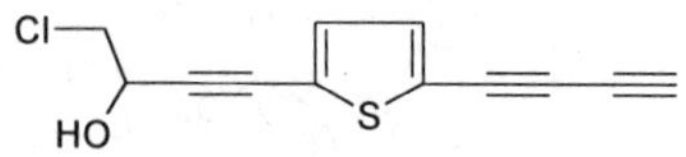

746 Butein
$C_{15}H_{12}O_5$ MW: 272.26 Property: mp 213-5°C. Source: CI HUAI HUA. Ref: 6.

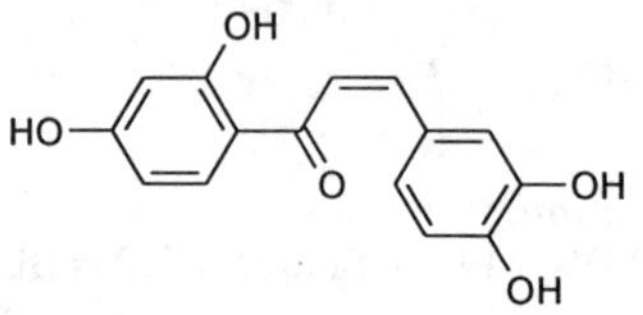

747 3-Butenyl isothiocyanate
C_5H_7NS MW: 113.18 Property: bp 78.5°C/26mm. Source: GAN LAN, JIE ZI. Ref: 6.

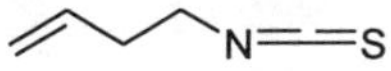

748 5-(3-Buten-1-ynyl)-2,2'-bithienyl
$C_{12}H_8S_2$ MW: 216.33 Source: KONG QUE CAO. Ref: 6.

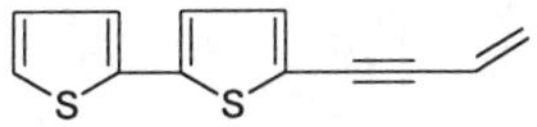

749 5-(3-Buten-1-ynyl)-2,2'-bithienyl-5'-methyl-acetate
$C_{15}H_{12}O_2S_2$ MW: 288.39 Source: MO HAN LIAN. Ref: 6.

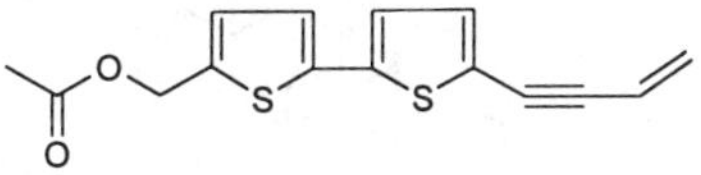

750 Butin
$C_{15}H_{12}O_5$ MW: 272.26 Property: mp 224-6.0°C. Source: CI HUAI HUA. Ref: 6.

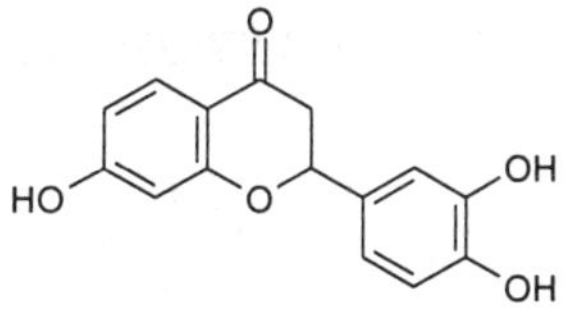

751 Bututic acid
Source: XI YUAN TENG. Ref: 596.

752 n-Butylaldehyde
C_4H_8O MW: 72.11 Source: SHENG JIANG, YIN CHEN HAO. Ref: 2.

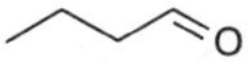

753 n-Butyl allophanate
$C_6H_{12}N_2O_2$ MW: 144.17 Source: DANG SHEN. Ref: 2.

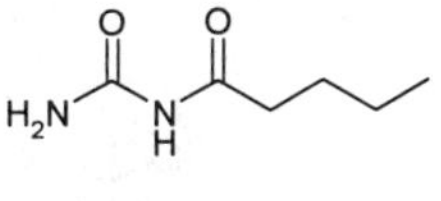

754 Butyl-cyclohexane
$C_{10}H_{20}$ MW: 140.27 Source: SHAN ZHA. Ref: 2.

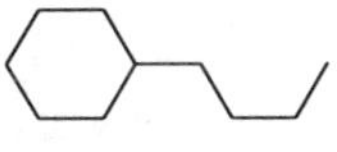

755 3(S)-3-Butyl-4,5-dihydrophthalide
$C_{12}H_{18}O_2$ MW: 194.28 Source: CHUAN XIONG. Ref: 2.

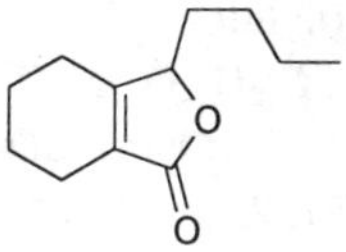

756 n-Butyl-2-ethylbutylphthalate
$C_{18}H_{26}O_4$ MW: 306.41 Source: SHUI QIN. Ref: 6.

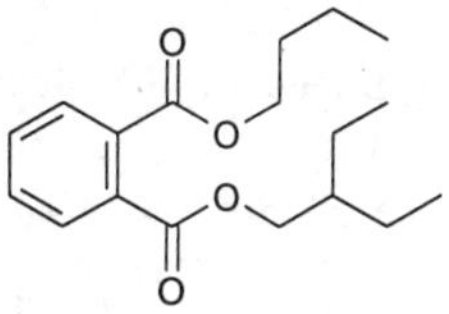

757 3-n-Butyl-3-hydroxy-4,5,6,7-tetrahydro-6,7-dihydroxy phthalide
$C_{12}H_{18}O_5$ MW: 242.27 Source: CHUAN XIONG. Ref: 2.

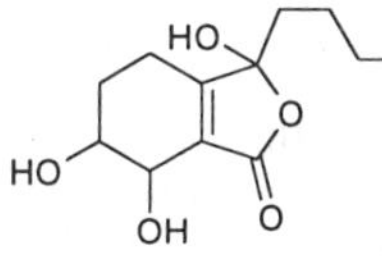

758 Butylidenecyclohexane
$C_{10}H_{18}$ MW: 138.25 Source: HOU PO. Ref: 2.

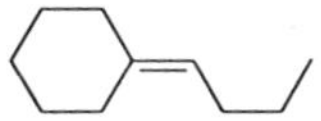

759 3-Butylidene-phthalide
n-Butylidene-phthalide. $C_{12}H_{12}O_2$ MW: 188.23 Source: CHUAN XIONG, DANG GUI. Ref: 1, 2, 601.

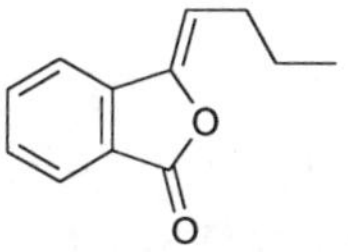

760 Butyl isothiocyanate
C_5H_9NS MW: 115.20 Property: bp 167°C. Source: JIE ZI. Ref: 6.

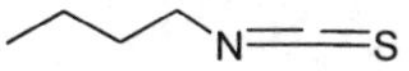

761 sec-Butyl isothiocyanate
C_5H_9NS MW: 115.20 Property: bp 159°C. Source: JIE ZI. Ref: 6.

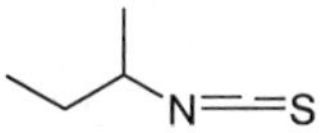

762 3-Butyl-phthalide
n-Butyl-phthalide. $C_{12}H_{14}O_2$ MW: 190.24 Property: bp 140-1°C, 177-8°C /15mm. Source: CHUAN XIONG, DANG GUI. Ref: 1, 2.

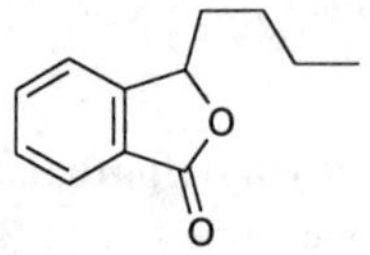

763 2-(Butyn-2-ylidene)-Δ[3]-dihydrofuran[5-spiro-2']tetrahydrofuran
$C_{11}H_{14}O_2$ MW: 178.23 Source: MU JU. Ref: 6.

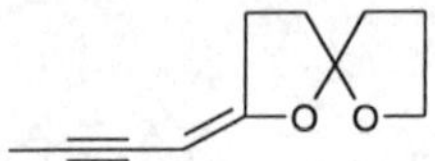

764 Butyric acid
$C_4H_8O_2$ MW: 88.11 Source: BAI GUO, CU LIU GUO (SHA JI). Ref: 2.

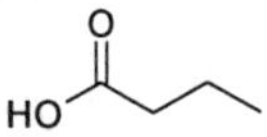

765 Buxamine E
$C_{26}H_{44}N_2$ MW: 384.65 Source: HUANG YANG MU YE. Ref: 6.

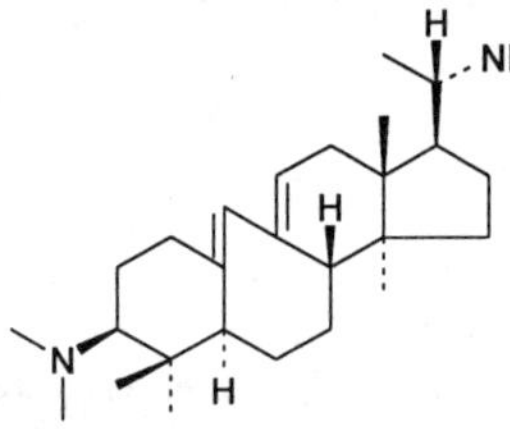

766 Buxaminol E
$C_{26}H_{44}N_2O$ MW: 400.65 Property: mp 199-200°C. Source: HUANG YANG MU YE. Ref: 6.

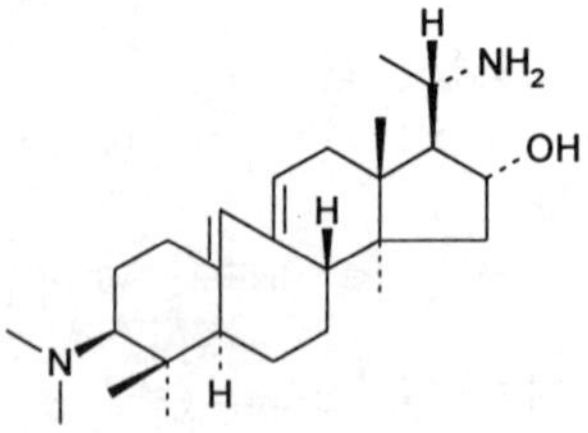

767 Buxpiine
$C_{25}H_{41}NO_2$ MW: 387.61 Property: mp 178-80°C (173°C). Source: HUANG YANG MU YE. Ref: 6.

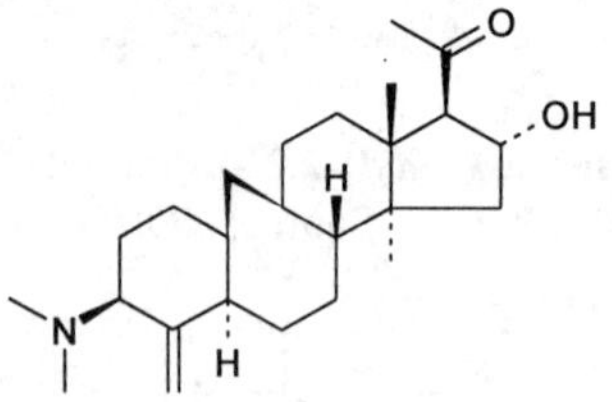

768 Buxtauine
$C_{24}H_{39}NO_2$ MW: 373.58 Property: mp 178-81°C. Source: HUANG YANG MU YE. Ref: 6.

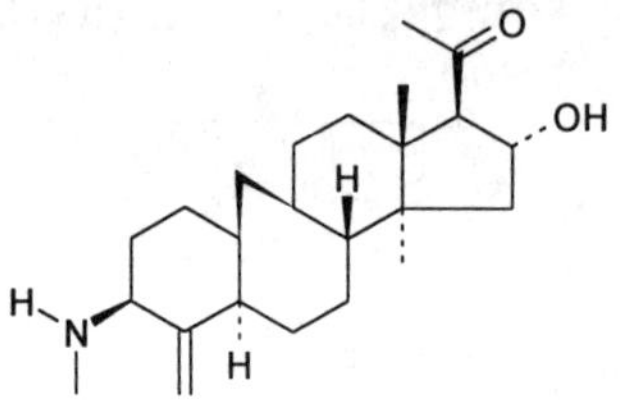

769 Byak-angelicin
CAS: 482-25-7 $C_{17}H_{18}O_7$ MW: 334.33 Source: BAI ZHI. Ref: 2, 5.

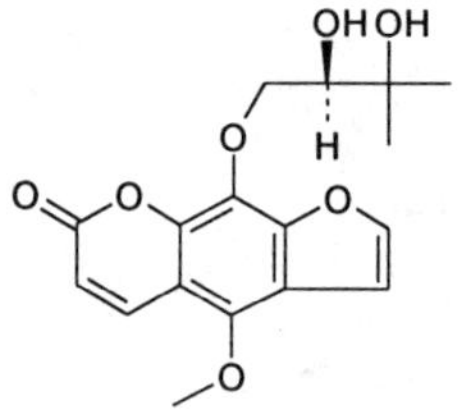

770 Byak-angelicol
$C_{17}H_{16}O_6$ MW: 316.31 Source: BAI ZHI. Ref: 2.

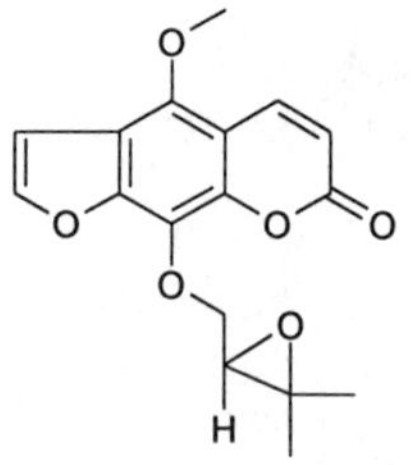

771 Cacticin
$C_{21}H_{20}O_{12}$ MW: 464.39 Source: YIN CHEN HAO. Ref: 2.

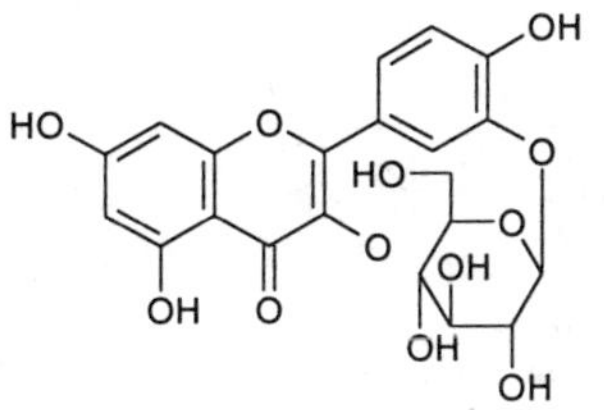

772 Cadambine
$C_{28}H_{34}N_2O_9$ MW: 542.59 Source: GOU TENG. Ref: 2.

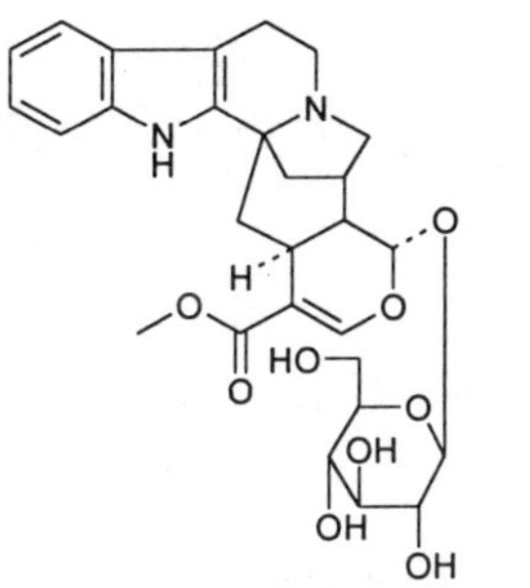

773 Cadaverine
$C_5H_{14}N_2$ MW: 102.18 Property: bp 178-80°C. Source: CHONG CHUN YU, JIANG. Ref: 6.

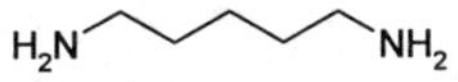

774 Cadina-9,11(12)-diene
$C_{15}H_{25}$ MW: 205.37 Property: bp 94°C/2mm. Source: ZHANG MU. Ref: 6.

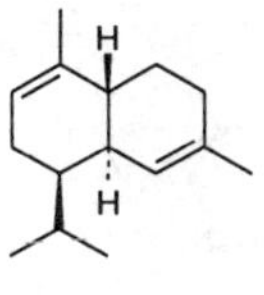

775 α-Cadinene
$C_{15}H_{24}$ MW: 204.36 Source: PI PA YE. Ref: 6.

776 γ-Cadinene
$C_{15}H_{24}$ MW: 204.36 Source: HUO XIANG, QING HAO, REN SHEN. Ref: 2.

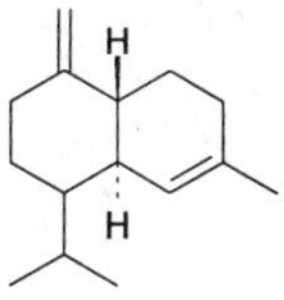

777 δ-Cadinene
$C_{15}H_{24}$ MW: 204.36 property: mp (+): 133-4°C /10mm, (±): 133°C/10mm. Source: QING HAO, REN SHEN, SAN QI, WU WEI ZI, XI XIAN. Ref: 2, 6.

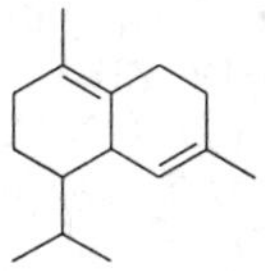

778 Cadinene
$C_{15}H_{24}$ MW: 204.36 Source: YIN CHEN HAO. Ref: 2.

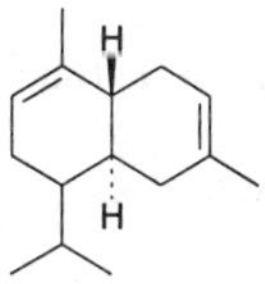

779 L-Cadinene
$C_{15}H_{24}$ MW: 204.36 Property: bp (-): 273-5°C. Source: JIU LI XIANG. Ref: 11.

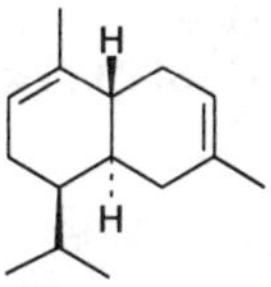

780 ε-Cadinene
$C_{15}H_{24}$ MW: 204.36 Source: MU HAO, QING HAO. Ref: 6.

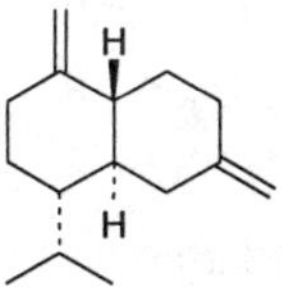

781 α-Cadinol
$C_{15}H_{26}O$ MW: 222.37 Property: mp 74.8-5.4°C. Source: PI PA YE. Ref: 6.

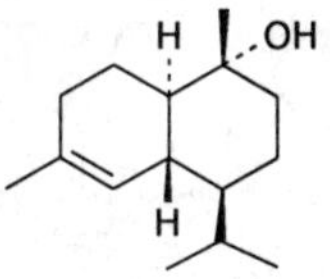

782 δ-Cadinol
$C_{15}H_{26}O$ MW: 222.37 Property: mp (+): 137-8°C, (-): 139-40°C. Source: GOU GU SHU PI. Ref: 6.

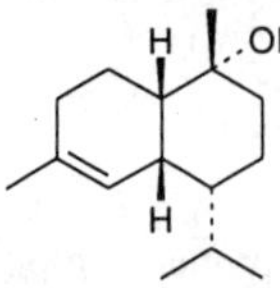

783 Caffeic acid
CAS: 331-39-5 $C_9H_8O_4$ MW: 180.16 Source: BO HE, CHUAN XIONG, DU ZHONG, JIAN DI PU GONG YING, JIN LONG DAN CAO, MU ZEI, NAN FANG TU SI ZI, SI JI QING, XIAN HE CAO. Ref: 1, 2, 4, 589, 602, 604, 527.

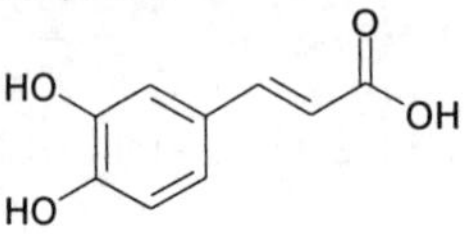

784 Caffeic acid dimethyl ether
$C_{11}H_{12}O_4$ MW: 208.22 Property: mp 179.5-80.5°C. Source: YE SHENG MA. Ref: 6.

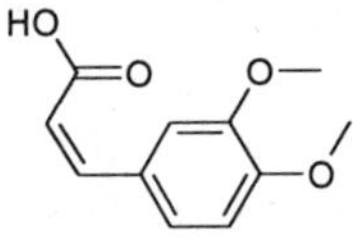

785 Caffeic-β-D-gluside
Source: NAN FANG TU SI ZI. Ref: 589.

786 Caffeine
CAS: 58-08-2 $C_8H_{10}N_4O_2$ MW: 194.19 Property: mp 235-8°C. Source: CHA SHU GEN, CHA YE, GOU GU SHU PI, GOU GU YE, KU DING CHA, WU TONG ZI. Ref: 1, 4, 6.

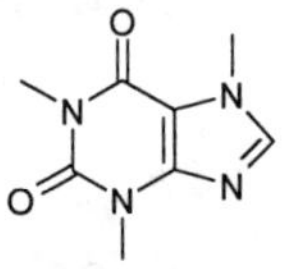

787 2-O-Caffeoyl arbutin
$C_{21}H_{22}O_{10}$ MW: 434.40 Property: mp 165°C. Source: YUE JU YE. Ref: 6.

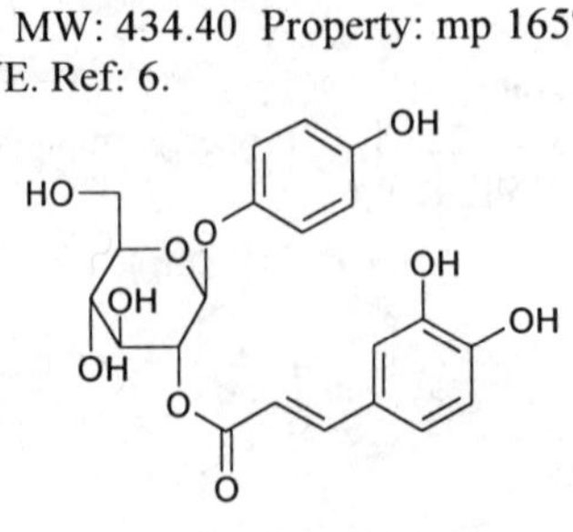

788 Caffeoyl calleryanin
$C_{23}H_{26}O_9$ MW: 446.46 Source: YE LI ZHI YE. Ref: 6.

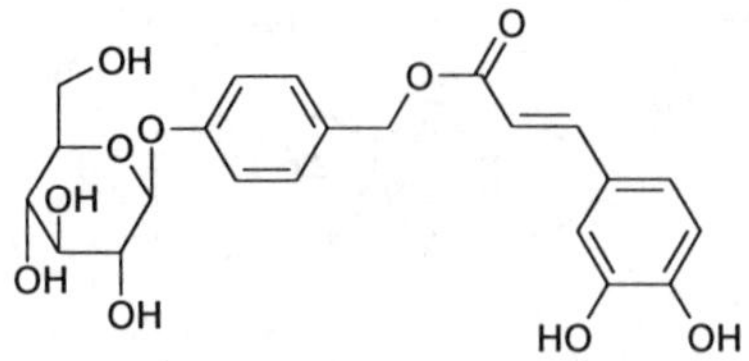

789 4-O-Caffeoylquinic acid
$C_{16}H_{18}O_9$ MW: 354.32 Source: GUANG YE SHUI SU, XIANG RI KUI YE, XIANG RI KUI JING SUI. Ref: 6.

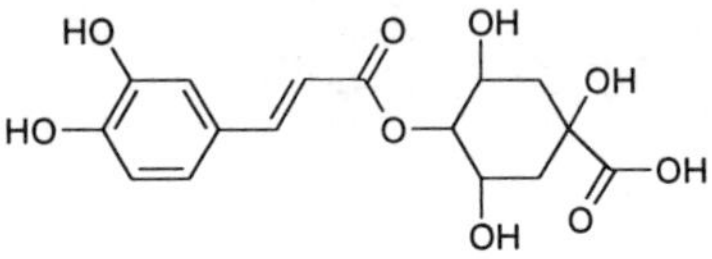

790 4-O-Caffeoyl-D-quinic acid
Source: KUAI JING CAO SU. Ref: 6.

791 3-O-Caffeoylshikimic acid
$C_{16}H_{16}O_8$ MW: 336.30 Property: mp 224-5°C (dec). Source: WU LOU ZI. Ref: 6.

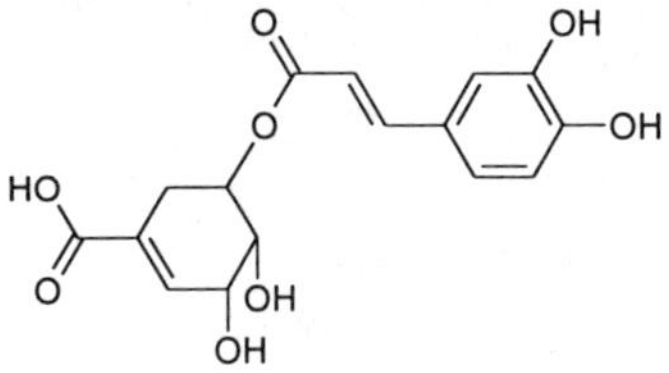

792 3-O-Caffeoyl-4-O-sinapoylquinic acid
$C_{27}H_{28}O_{13}$ MW: 560.52 Source: ZHI ZI. Ref: 2, 626.

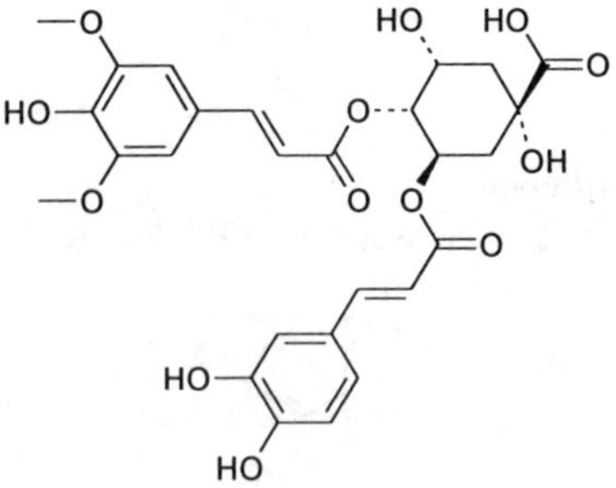

793 6'-O-Caffeylerigeroside

$C_{20}H_{20}O_{11}$ MW: 436.38 Property: light yellow amorphous, mp 154-6°C. Source: DUO SHE FEI PENG. Ref: 415.

794 Calacone

$C_{15}H_{24}O$ MW: 220.36 Source: BAI CHANG. Ref: 6.

795 α-Calacorene

$C_{15}H_{20}$ MW: 200.33 Source: DU SONG SHI, ZHANG MU. Ref: 6.

796 γ-Calacorene

$C_{15}H_{20}$ MW: 200.33 Source: DU SONG SHI, PI JIU HUA. Ref: 6.

797 Calamendiol

$C_{15}H_{24}O_2$ MW: 236.36 Property: mp 168°C. Source: BAI CHANG. Ref: 6.

798 trans-Calamenene

$C_{15}H_{22}$ MW: 202.34 Source: HUO XIANG, ZHANG MU. Ref: 2, 6.

799 cis-Calamenene

$C_{15}H_{22}$ MW: 202.34 Source: HUO XIANG, ZHANG MU. Ref: 2, 6.

800 Calarene

$C_{15}H_{24}$ MW: 204.36 Property: bp 120-3°C/13mm. Source: GAN SONG. Ref: 6.

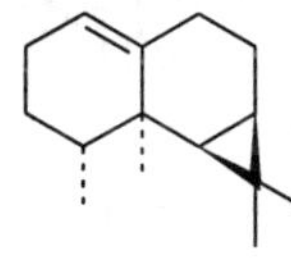

801 Calarenol

$C_{15}H_{24}O$ MW: 220.36 Property: bp 120-5°C/0.1mm. Source: GAN SONG. Ref: 6.

802 Callistephin

$C_{21}H_{21}O_{10}$•Cl MW: 433.40•35.45 Source: NAN TIAN ZHU ZI, QIU MU GUA. Ref: 6.

803 Calliterpenone

$C_{20}H_{32}O_3$ MW: 320.48 Property: mp 153-5°C. Source: DA YE ZI ZHU. Ref: 6.

804 Calliterpenone monoacetate
$C_{22}H_{34}O_4$ MW: 362.51 Property: mp 124°C. Source: DA YE ZI ZHU. Ref: 6.

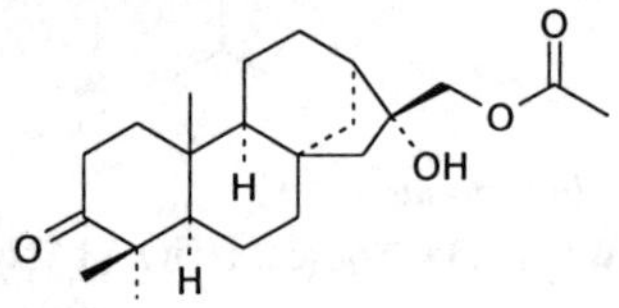

805 Calotropagenin
$C_{23}H_{32}O_6$ MW: 404.51 Property: mp 238-50°C. Source: LIAN SHENG GUI ZI HUA. Ref: 6.

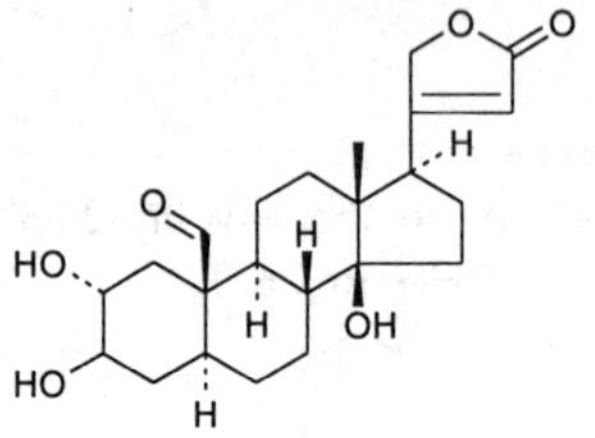

806 Calotropin
CAS: 2513-4-1 $C_{30}H_{42}O_8$ MW: 530.66 Property: mp 221°C (dec). Source: LIAN SHENG GUI ZI HUA. Ref: 1, 5, 6.

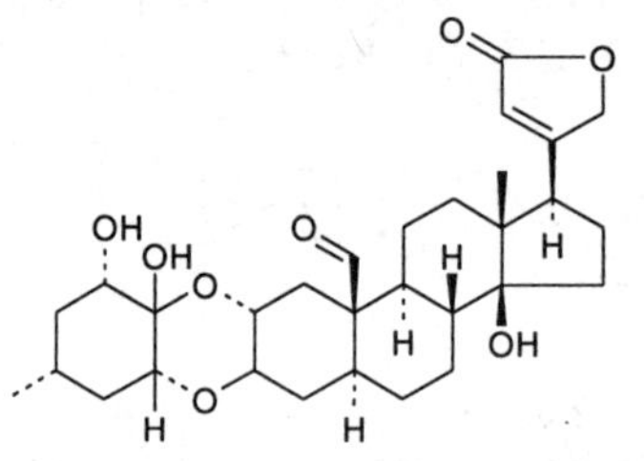

807 Calycanthine
$C_{22}H_{26}N_4$ MW: 346.48 Property: mp (+): 250-1°C, (±): 253-8°C. Source: LA MEI HUA. Ref: 1, 6.

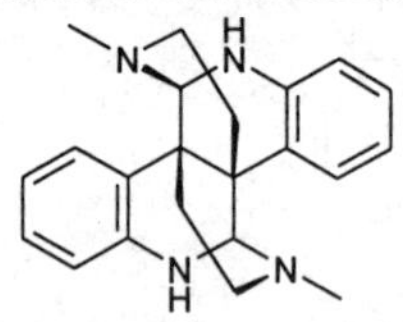

808 Calycine
$C_{23}H_{31}NO_3$ MW: 369.51 Property: mp 205°C. Source: NIU ER FENG ZHI YE. Ref: 6.

809 Camaroside
4',5-dihydroxy-3,7-dimethoxyflavone-4'-O-β-D-glucopyranoside. $C_{23}H_{24}O_{11}$ MW: 476.44 Property: light yellow rabdiod crystal, mp 252-4°C. Source: MA YING DAN. Ref: 253.

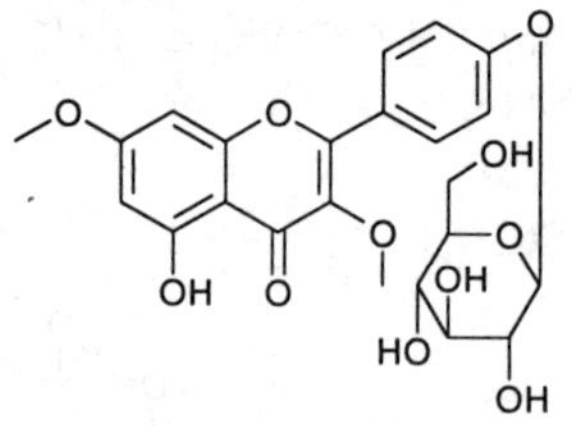

810 Camelliagenin A
Camellia sapogenol I; Dihydropriverogenin A; Theasapogenol D. $C_{30}H_{50}O_4$ MW: 474.73 Property: mp 282-3°C, 290-3°C. Source: CHA ZI XIN, ZHEN ZHU CAI (ZHEN ZHU YE). Ref: 6.

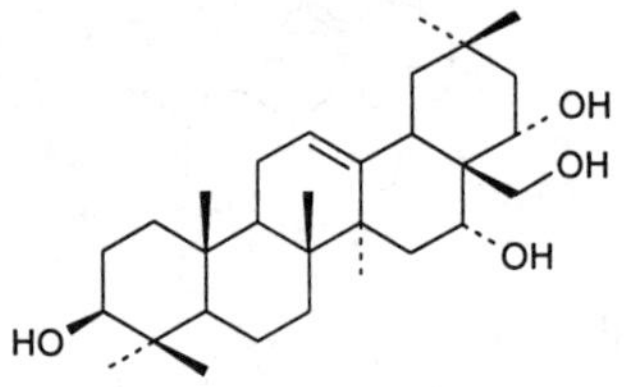

811 Camelliagenin B
$C_{30}H_{48}O_5$ MW: 490.73 Property: mp 200-5°C, 195-204°C. Source: CHA ZI XIN. Ref: 6.

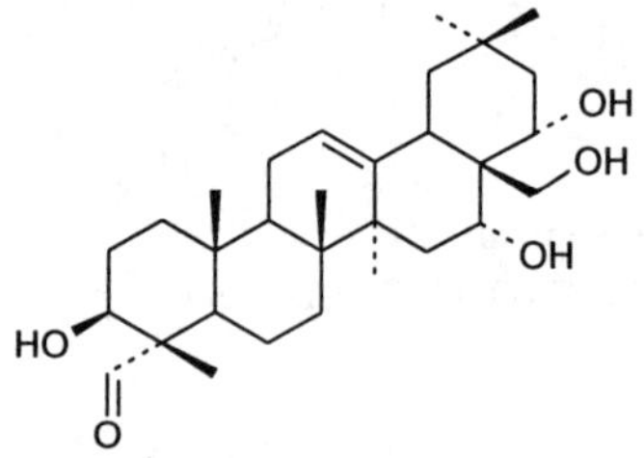

812 Camelliagenin C
Theasapogenol C. $C_{30}H_{50}O_5$ MW: 490.73 Property: mp 262-3°C, 280-3°C. Source: CHA ZI XIN, ZHEN ZHU CAI (ZHEN ZHU YE). Ref: 6.

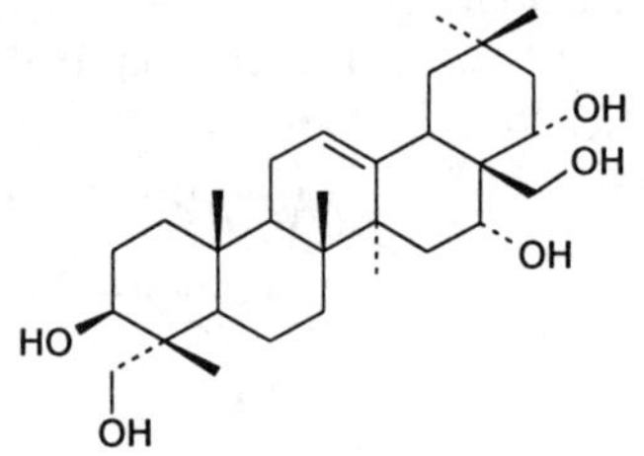

813 Camelliagenin D

$C_{30}H_{48}O_6$ MW: 504.71 Property: mp 250-8°C. Source: CHA ZI XIN, ZHEN ZHU CAI (ZHEN ZHU YE). Ref: 6.

814 Camelliagenin E

Theasapogenol E. $C_{30}H_{48}O_6$ MW: 504.71 Property: mp 237.5-9°C. Source: CHA ZI XIN, ZHEN ZHU CAI (ZHEN ZHU YE). Ref: 6.

815 Camellianin A

Apigenin-5-O-α-L-rhamnosyl-(1→4)-6"-acetyl-β-D-glucoside. $C_{29}H_{32}O_{15}$ MW: 620.57 Property: colorless acicular crystal (methanol), mp 196-7°C. Source: CHA YE. Ref: 636.

816 Camellianin B

Apigenin-5-O-α-L-rhamnosyl-(1→4)-β-D-glucoside. Property: colorless acicular crystal (methanol), mp 328-30°C. Source: CHA YE. Ref: 636.

816b Camellin

$C_{18}H_{30}O_7$ MW: 358.44 Source: CHA ZI XIN, SHAN CHAI HUA. Ref: 6.

817 Campesterol

$C_{28}H_{48}O$ MW: 400.69 Source: CHAN SU, CU LIU GUO (SHA JI), GAN DI HUANG, GUA LOU, HUANG BAI, HUANG QIN, LU HUI, REN SHEN. Ref: 2.

818 Δ[7]-Campesterol

$C_{27}H_{44}O$ MW: 384.65 Source: GUA LOU. Ref: 2.

819 Campesteryl ferulate

$C_{38}H_{56}O_4$ MW: 576.87 Source: MI PI KANG. Ref: 6.

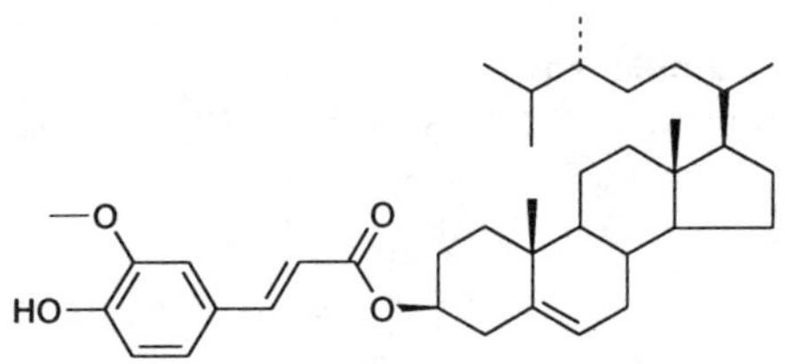

820 Campesteryl-D-glucoside

$C_{35}H_{60}O_5$ MW: 560.87 Source: DONG FANG GOU JI. Ref: 6.

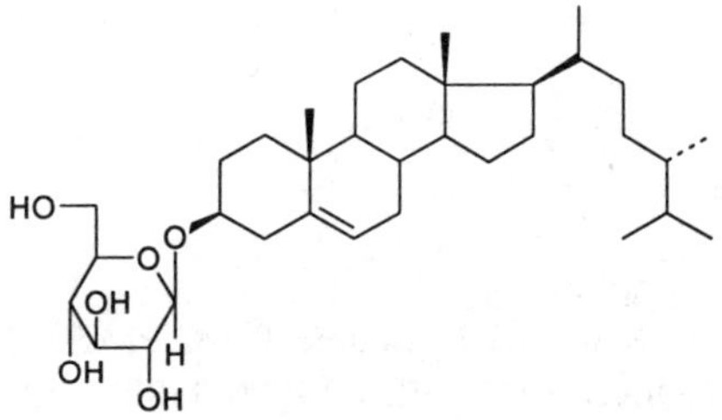

821 Campesteryl-D-glucoside-6'-palmitate

$C_{51}H_{90}O_6$ MW: 799.28 Source: DONG FANG GOU JI. Ref: 6.

822 Campesteryl palmitate
$C_{44}H_{78}O_2$ MW: 639.11 Source: DONG FANG GOU JI. Ref: 6.

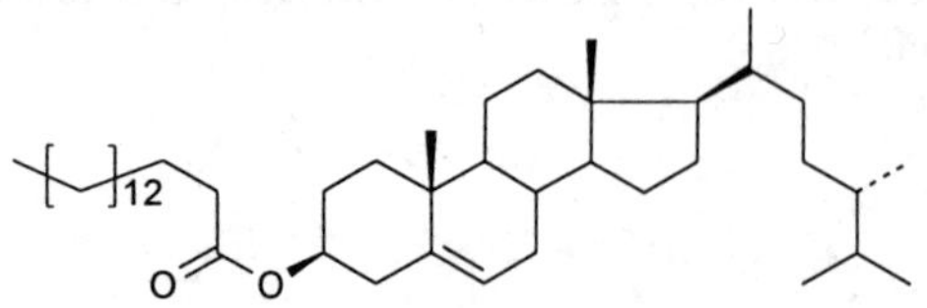

823 Camphene
$C_{10}H_{16}$ MW: 136.24 Property: mp (+) 51°C, bp 160-2°C, (-) 51-2°C, bp 158-60°C. Source: BO HE, CHAI HU, DANG GUI, GAN JIANG, JIN JIE, LIAN QIAO, MU XIANG, QIANG HUO, QING HAO, SHENG JIANG, WU WEI ZI, XI XIN, YU XING CAO, ZI SU, etc. Ref: 2, 6.

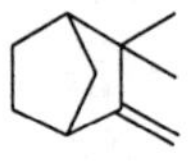

824 Campherenol
$C_{15}H_{26}O$ MW: 222.37 Source: LU HUI. Ref: 2.

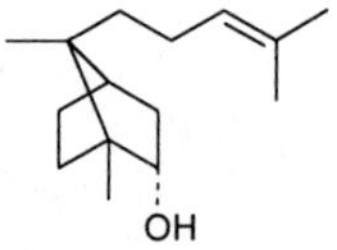

825 Campherenone
$C_{15}H_{24}O$ MW: 220.36 Source: ZHANG MU. Ref: 6.

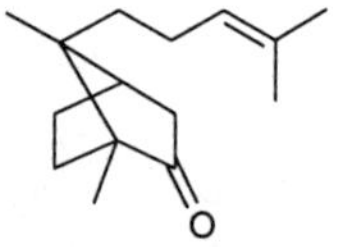

826 Camphor
$C_{11}H_{20}O$ MW: 168.28 Source: BING PIAN, LIAN QIAO, QING HAO, SHENG JIANG. Ref: 1, 2.

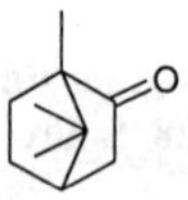

827 α-Camphorene
$C_{20}H_{32}$ MW: 272.48 Property: bp 190-2°C/12mm. Source: ZHANG MU. Ref: 6.

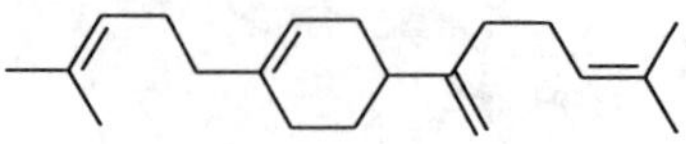

828 γ-Camphorene
$C_{20}H_{32}$ MW: 272.48 Property: bp 176-8°C/4.5mm. Source: ZHANG MU. Ref: 6.

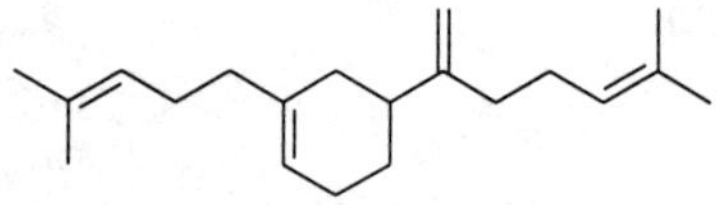

829 Camphoric acid
$C_9H_{14}O_4$ MW: 186.21 Source: DANG GUI. Ref: 2.

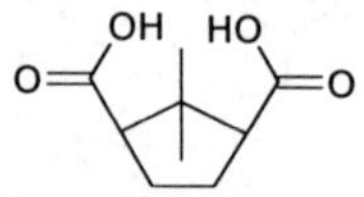

830 Camptothecin(e)
CAS: 7689-03-4 $C_{20}H_{16}N_2O_4$ MW: 348.36 Property: mp 264-7°C (dec). Source: XI SHU. Ref: 1, 5, 6.

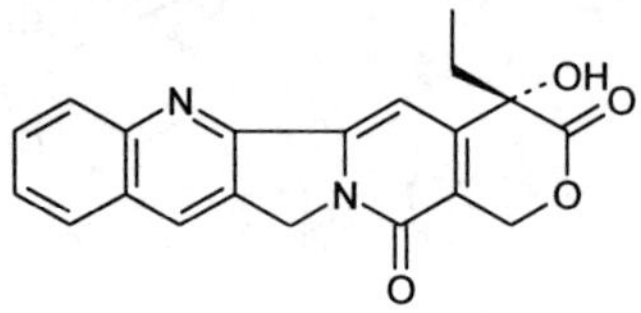

831 Canadine
$C_{20}H_{21}NO_4$ MW: 339.39 Property: mp (+): 132°C, (-): 134°C. Source: YAN HU SUO. Ref: 1, 6.

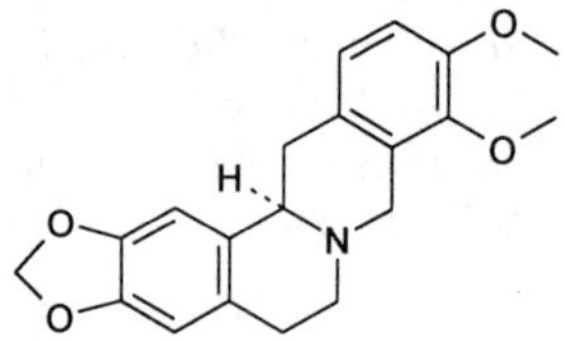

832 Canaline
$C_4H_{10}N_2O_3$ MW: 134.14 Property: mp 214°C. Source: CI HUAI HUA, DAO DOU, DI YANG QUE, MU XU. Ref: 6.

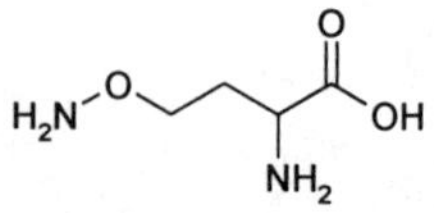

833 Canavalia gibberellin I
$C_{19}H_{24}O_7$ MW: 364.40 Property: mp 244-6°C. Source: DAO DOU. Ref: 6.

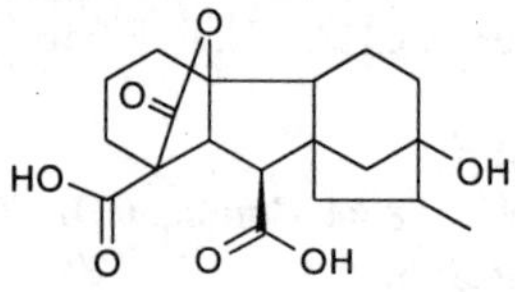

834 Canavalia gibberellin II
$C_{19}H_{24}O_6$ MW: 348.40 Property: mp 213-4°C. Source: DAO DOU. Ref: 6.

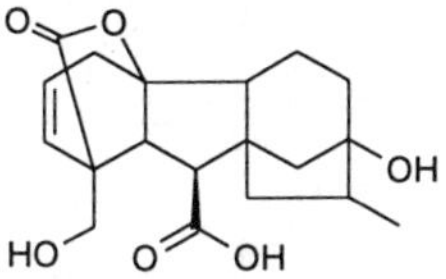

835 Canavanine
$C_5H_{12}N_4O_3$ MW: 176.18 Source: HUANG QI. Ref: 2.

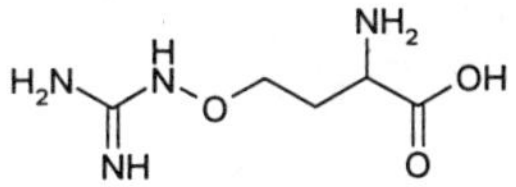

836 N-Candicine
$C_{11}H_{18}NO$ MW: 180.27 Property: mp 279-80°C. Source: HUANG BAI. Ref: 1, 2.

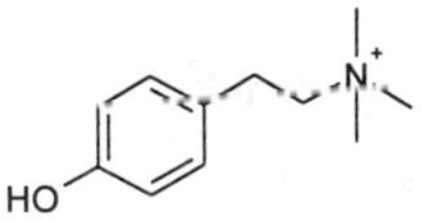

837 Cannabichromenic acid
$C_{22}H_{30}O_4$ MW: 358.48 Source: MA YE. Ref: 6.

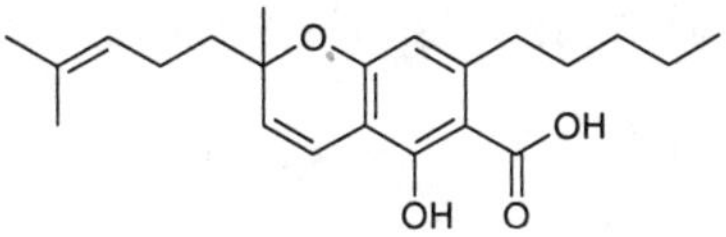

838 Cannabidiol
$C_{21}H_{30}O_2$ MW: 314.47 Property: mp 66-7°C. Source: MA HUA. Ref: 1, 6.

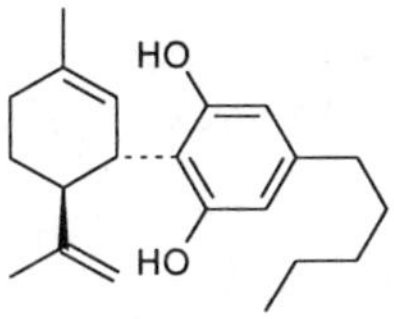

839 Cannabidiolic acid
$C_{22}H_{30}O_4$ MW: 358.48 Property: mp 43-7°C (dec). Source: MA YE, MA HUA. Ref: 6.

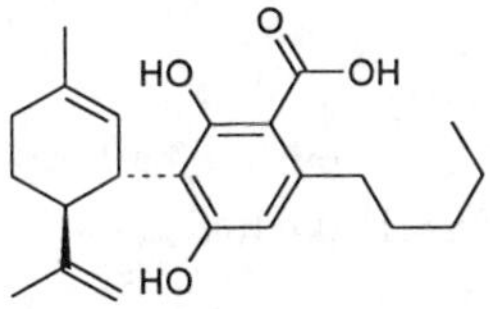

840 Cannabigerol
$C_{21}H_{32}O_2$ MW: 316.49 Property: mp 51-3°C. Source: MA HUA. Ref: 6.

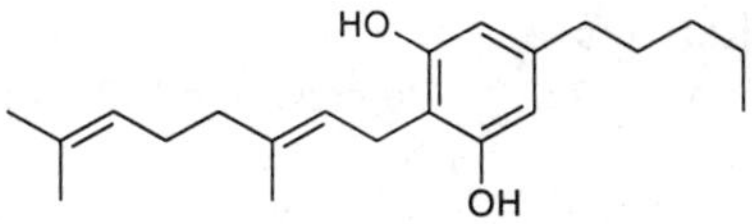

841 Cannabinol
CAS: 521-35-7 $C_{21}H_{26}O_2$ MW: 310.44 Property: mp 76-7°C. Source: HUO MA REN, MA HUA. Ref: 1, 5, 6.

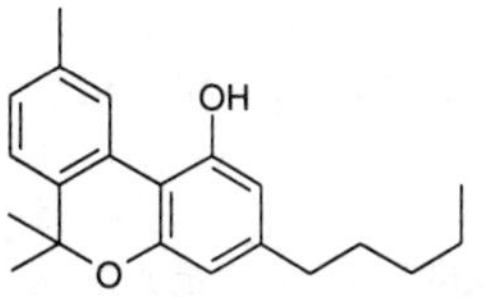

842 Cannabinolic acid
$C_{22}H_{26}O_4$ MW: 354.45 Source: MA YE. Ref: 6.

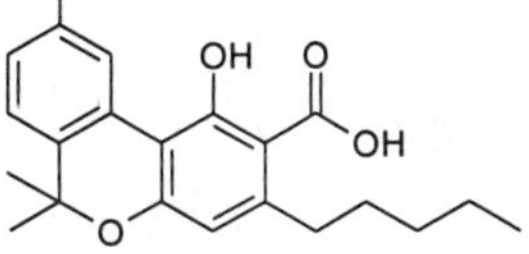

843 Cannabiscitrin
$C_{21}H_{20}O_{13}$ MW: 480.39 Property: mp 220°C (210°C soften). Source: YANG MEI SHU PI. Ref: 6.

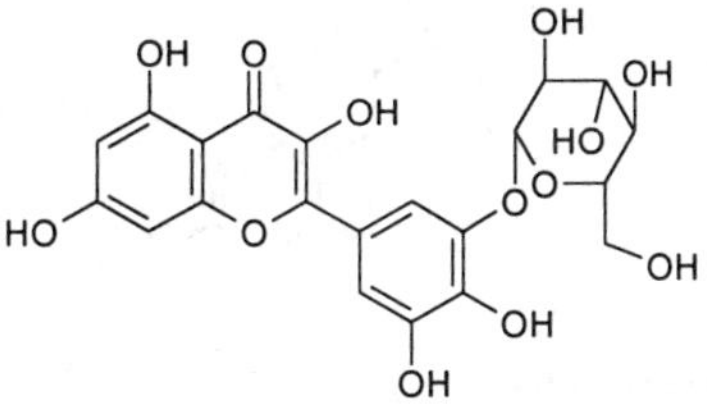

844 Cantharidin
$C_{10}H_{12}O_4$ MW: 196.20 Property: mp 218°C. Source: BAN MAO, GE SHANG TING CHANG, HONG NIANG ZI, QING NIANG ZI. Ref: 4, 6.

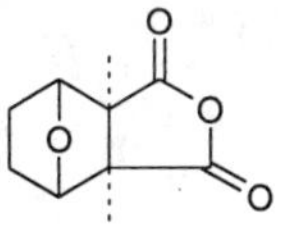

845 Canthaxanthin
$C_{40}H_{70}O_2$ MW: 5830 Property: mp 218°C. Source: HAI XIA, JIN YU. Ref: 6.

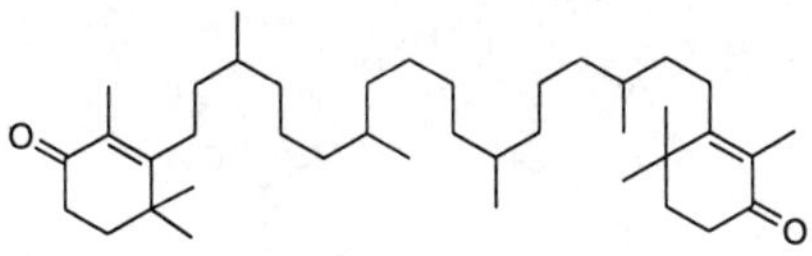

846 Canthin-6-one
$C_{14}H_8N_2O$ MW: 220.23 Property: mp 159-60°C. Source: KU SHU PI. Ref: 1, 12.

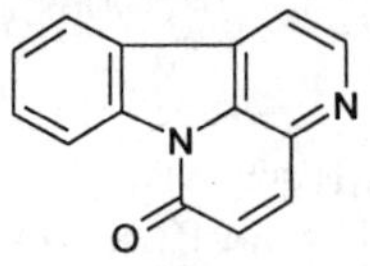

847 Cantleyine
Source: MAO ZHU MA QIAN. Ref: 576.

848 Caohuoside B
Source: YIN YANG HUO. Ref: 635.

849 Caohuoside C
Source: YIN YANG HUO. Ref: 635.

850 Caohuoside D
Source: YIN YANG HUO. Ref: 635.

851 Capauridine
$C_{21}H_{25}NO_5$ MW: 371.44 Property: mp 208°C. Source: JU HUA HUANG LIAN. Ref: 1, 6.

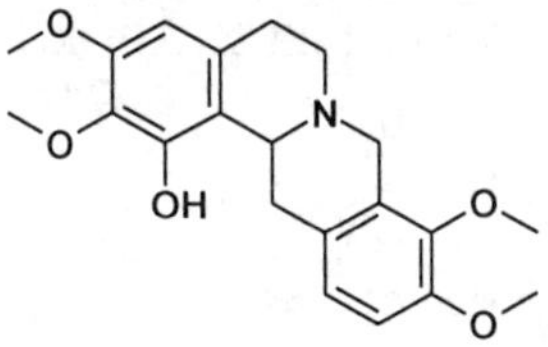

852 Capaurimine
$C_{20}H_{23}NO_5$ MW: 357.41 Property: mp 212°C. Source: JU HUA HUANG LIAN. Ref: 6.

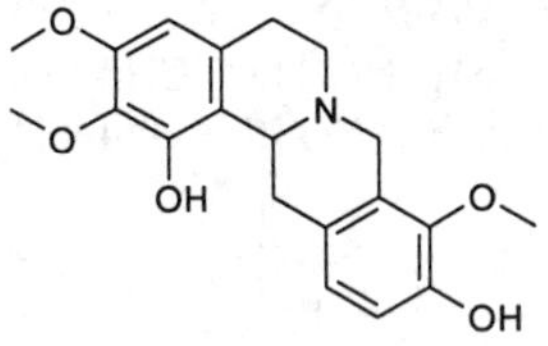

853 Capaurine
$C_{21}H_{25}NO_5$ MW: 371.44 Property: mp 164°C. Source: JU HUA HUANG LIAN. Ref: 1, 6.

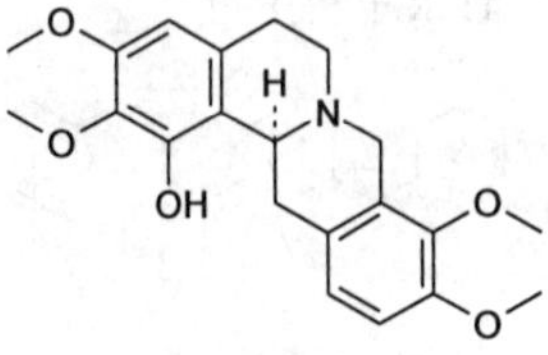

854 Capillanol
$C_{12}H_{14}O$ MW: 174.24 Source: YIN CHEN HAO. Ref: 2.

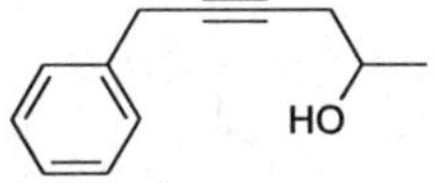

855 Capillarin
$C_{13}H_{10}O_2$ MW: 198.22 Source: YIN CHEN HAO. Ref: 2.

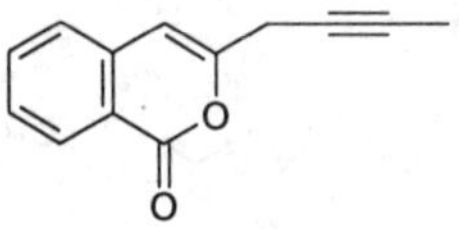

856 Capillarisin
$C_{16}H_{12}O_7$ MW: 316.27 Property: mp 226-8°C. Source: YIN CHEN HAO. Ref: 1, 2.

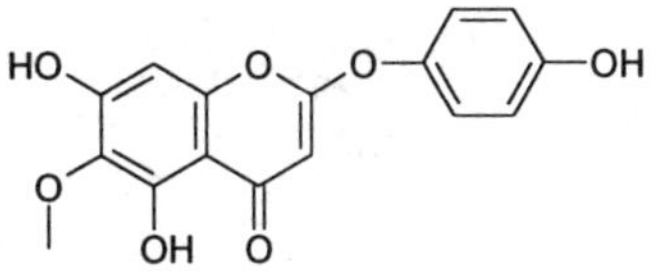

857 Capillartemisin A
$C_{19}H_{26}O_4$ MW: 318.42 Source: YIN CHEN HAO. Ref: 2.

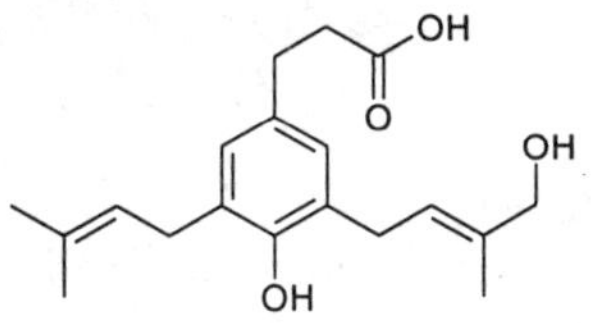

858 Capillartemisin B
$C_{19}H_{26}O_4$ MW: 318.42 Source: YIN CHEN HAO. Ref: 2.

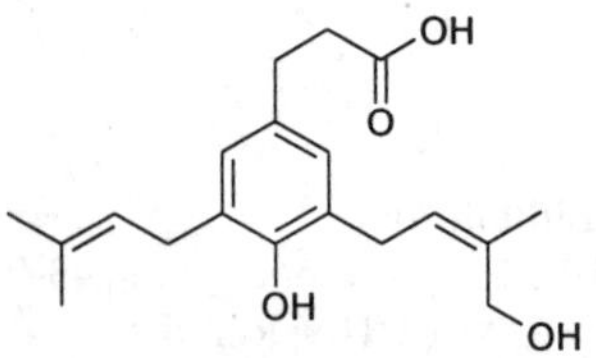

859 Capillene
$C_{12}H_{10}$ MW: 154.21 Property: bp 124°C/4mm. Source: YIN CHEN HAO. Ref: 2, 6.

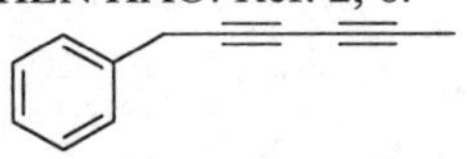

860 Capillin
CAS: 495-74-9 $C_{12}H_8O$ MW: 168.20 Property: mp 81°C. Source: YIN CHEN HAO. Ref: 1, 2, 4.

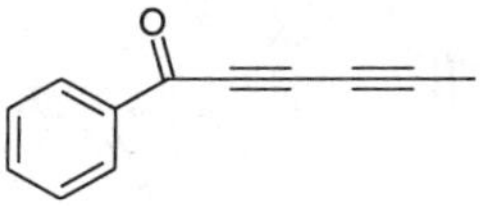

861 Capillon(e)
$C_{12}H_{12}O$ MW: 172.23 Property: mp 69-70°C. Source: YIN CHEN HAO. Ref: 2, 6.

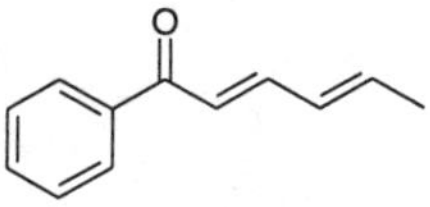

862 Capitasterone
$C_{29}H_{44}O_7$ MW: 504.67 Property: mp 234-5°C. Source: CHUAN NIU XI. Ref: 6.

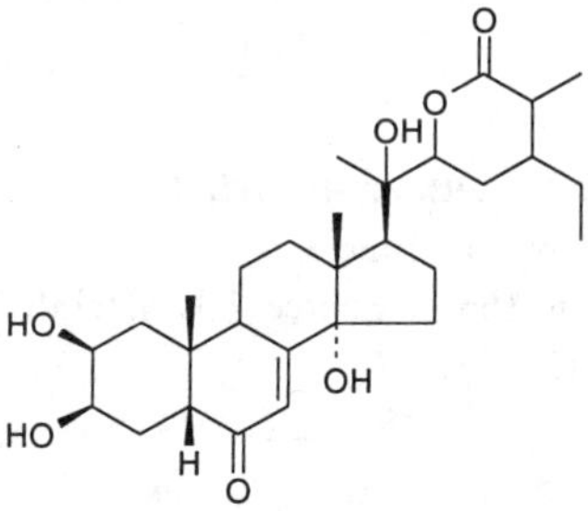

863 Capric acid
$C_{10}H_{20}O_2$ MW: 172.27 Source: BING LANG, CU LIU GUO (SHA JI), GUA LOU, LU HUI, YU XING CAO. Ref: 2.

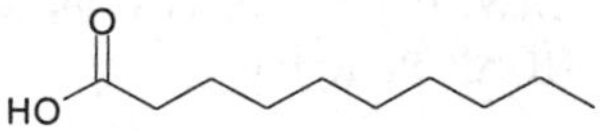

865 Caproic acid
$C_6H_{12}O_2$ MW: 116.16 Source: CHAI HU, CU LIU GUO (SHA JI), DANG SHEN, XI YANG SHEN. Ref: 2.

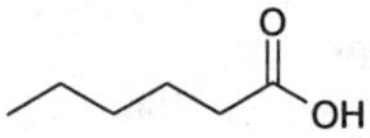

866 Caprylic acid
$C_8H_{16}O_2$ MW: 144.22 Source: BAI GUO, CHAI HU, CU LIU GUO (SHA JI), DANG SHEN, FU LING, GAN DI HUANG, XI YANG SHEN. Ref: 2.

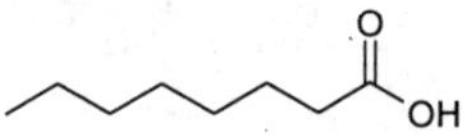

867 Capsaicin(e)
Styptysat. CAS: 7553-53-9 $C_{18}H_{27}NO_3$ MW: 305.42 Property: mp 64-5°C. Source: LA JIAO. Ref: 4, 15.

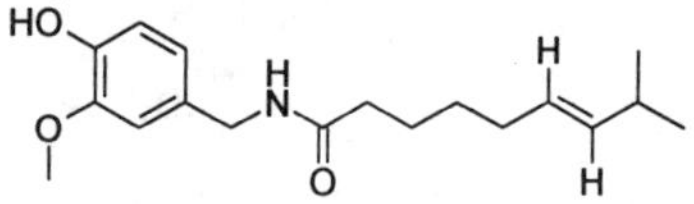

868 Capsanthin
$C_{40}H_{56}O_3$ MW: 584.89 Property: mp175-6°C. Source: LA JIAO. Ref: 15.

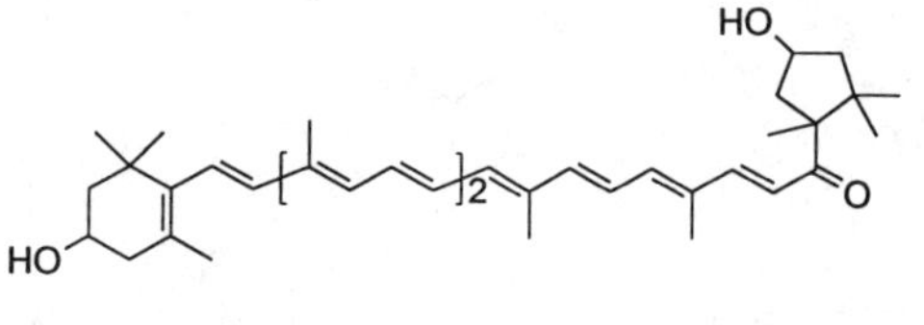

869 Capsicosin
$C_{57}H_{94}O_{29}$ MW: 1243.37 Source: LA JIAO. Ref: 15.

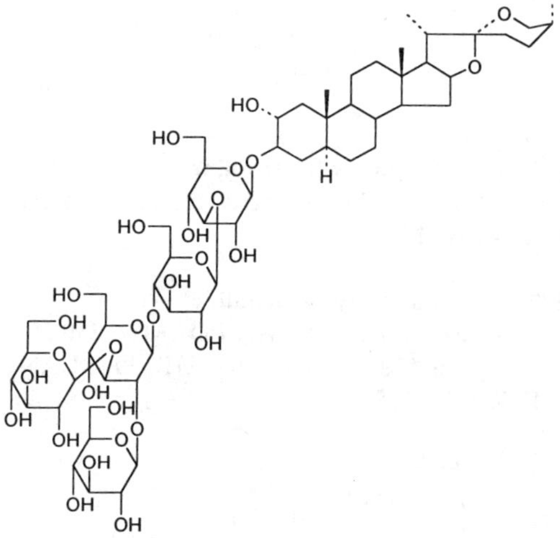

870 Capsularin
$C_{22}H_{36}O_8$ MW: 428.53 Property: mp 175-6°C. Source: HUANG MA YE. Ref: 6.

871 Capsularol
$C_{41}H_{70}O_{11}$ MW: 739.01 Property: mp 204-5°C. Source: HUANG MA YE. Ref: 6.

872 Capsularone
Property: mp 258-60°C. Source: HUANG MA YE. Ref: 6.

873 Carabrone
$C_{15}H_{20}O_3$ MW: 248.32 Property: mp (+): 90-1°C, (±): 89-91°C. Source: HE SHI, TIAN MING JING. Ref: 1, 6.

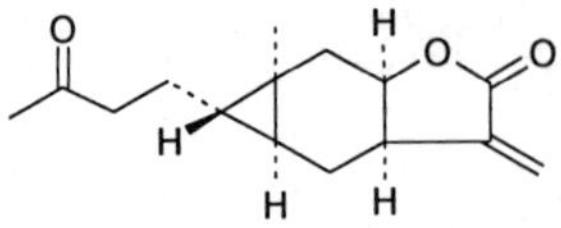

874 3-Caraneol
$C_{10}H_{18}O$ MW: 154.25 Source: SHENG JIANG. Ref: 2.

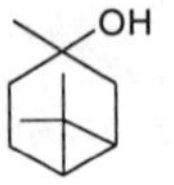

875 2-Caraneol
$C_{10}H_{18}O$ MW: 154.25 Source: SHENG JIANG. Ref: 2.

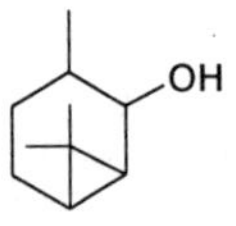

876 1-Carbobutoxy-β-carboline
Carbobutoxycarboline. Property: mp 95°C. Source: YUAN ZHI. Ref: 538.

877 1-Carboethoxy-β-carboline
Carboethoxycarboline, $C_{14}H_{12}N_2O_2$ MW: 240.26 Property: mp 123°C. Source: KU SHU PI, YUAN ZHI. Ref: 12, 538.

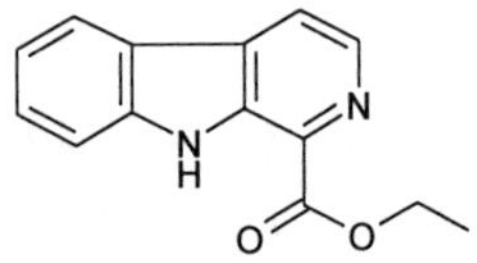

878 β-Carboline-1-propionic acid
$C_{14}H_{12}N_2O_2$ MW: 240.26 Source: KU SHU PI. Ref: 12.

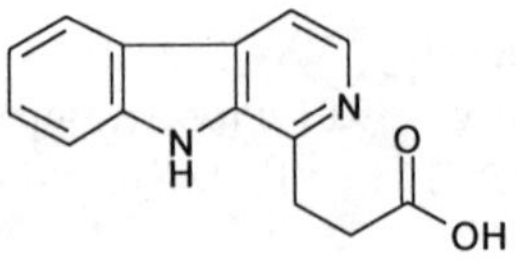

879 1-(β-Carbolin-1-yl)-4-(4,8-dimethoxy-β-carbolin-1-yl)-2-methoxy-butan-1-one
$C_{29}H_{26}N_4O_4$ MW: 494.55 Source: KU SHU PI. Ref: 12.

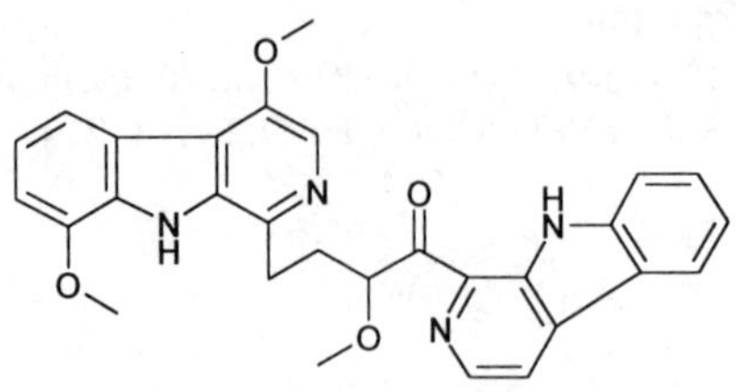

880 1-(β-Carbolin-1-yl)-3-(4,8-dimethoxy-β-carbolin-1-yl) propan-1-one
$C_{27}H_{22}N_4O_3$ MW: 450.50 Source: KU SHU PI. Ref: 12.

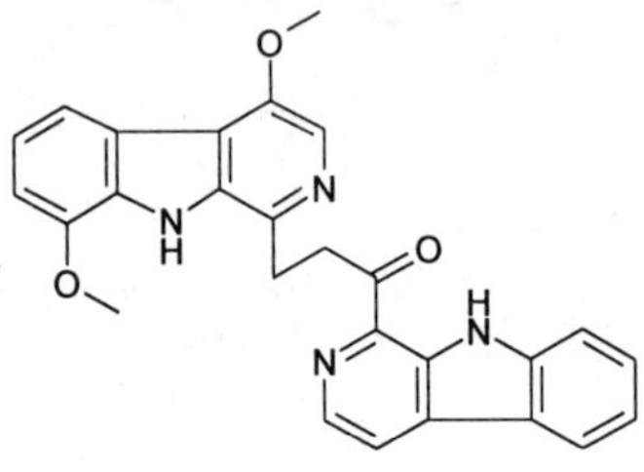

881 1-Carbomethoxy-β-carboline
Carbomethoxycarboline. $C_{13}H_{10}N_2O_2$ MW: 226.24 Property: mp 166°C. Source: KU SHU PI, YUAN ZHI. Ref: 12, 538.

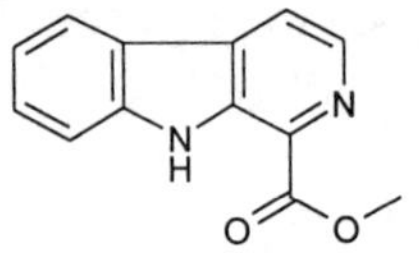

882 S-(2-Carboxyethyl)-L-cysteine
$C_6H_{11}NO_4S$ MW: 193.22 Property: mp 218°C. Source: HE HUAN PI. Ref: 6.

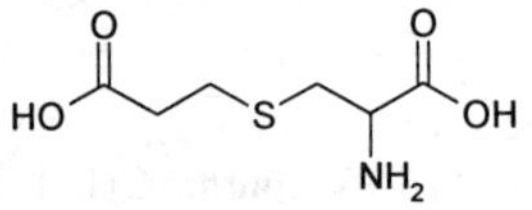

883 5-Carboxy-7-glucosyloxy-2-methyl-benzopyran-γ-one
$C_{17}H_{18}O_{10}$ MW: 382.33 Source: DA HUANG. Ref: 2.

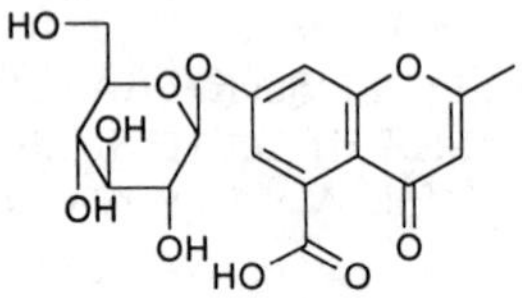

884 5-Carboxy-7-hydroxy-2-methyl-benzo-pyran-γ-one
$C_{11}H_8O_5$ MW: 220.18 Source: DA HUANG. Ref: 2.

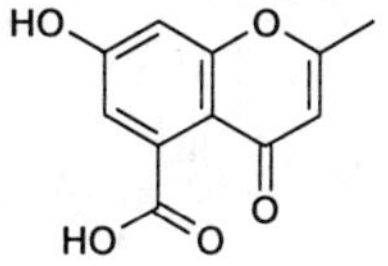

885 3-Carboxy-4-hydroxy-phenoxy glucoside
$C_{13}H_{16}O_9$ MW: 316.27 Source: HUANG LIAN. Ref: 2.

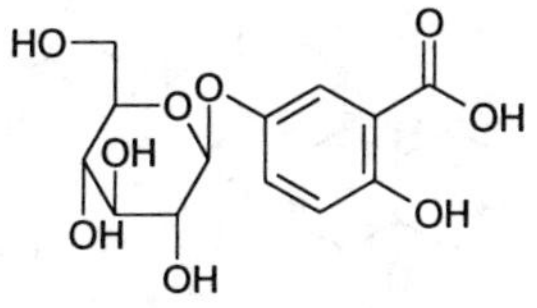

886 16-Carboxytotarol
$C_{20}H_{28}O_3$ MW: 316.44 Source: LUO HAN SONG YE. Ref: 6.

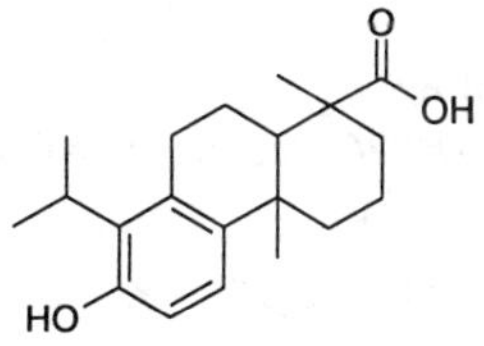

887 Cardamonin
$C_{16}H_{14}O_4$ MW: 270.29 Property: mp 207°C. Source: CAO DOU KOU, DA CAO KOU. Ref: 6.

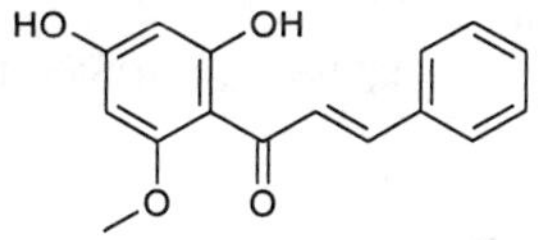

888 Cardanol
Anacardol. Source: DU XIAN ZI. Ref: 6.

889 Δ^3-Carene
Carene-3. $C_{10}H_{16}$ MW: 136.24 Property: bp (+): 170°C, (-): 166-7°C/685mm. Source: HOU PO, JIU LI XIANG, LIAN QIAO, SHENG JIANG. Ref: 2, 11.

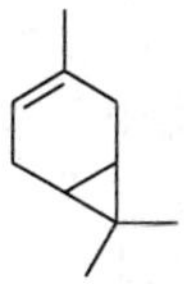

890 Carene-4
$C_{10}H_{16}$ MW: 136.24 Source: JU PI, QIANG HUO. Ref: 2.

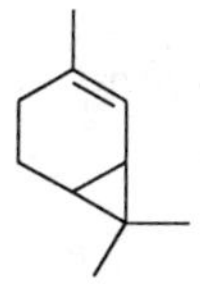

891 (±)-Car-3-ene-2,5-dione
$C_{10}H_{12}O_2$ MW: 164.21 Source: XI XIN. Ref: 2.

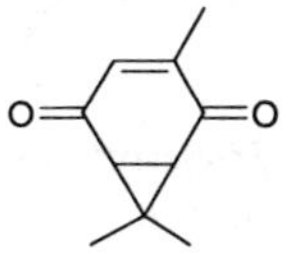

892 Carmichaeline
Chuan-Wu-base B. $C_{22}H_{35}NO_4$ Source: FU ZI. Ref: 2.

893 Carnosine
$C_9H_{14}N_4O_3$ MW: 226.24 Property: mp L (+): 246-50°C, D (-): 260°C (dec). Source: GOU ROU, XIA TIAN GAO, MO GU, MAN LI YU, QING WA, XIA TIAN GAO. Ref: 6.

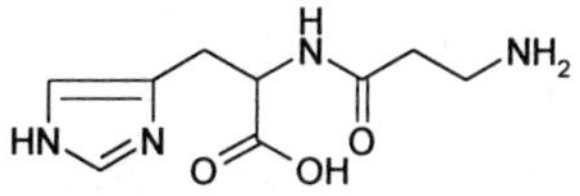

894 Carnosol
$C_{20}H_{26}O_4$ MW: 330.43 Property: mp 221-6°C. Source: MI DIE XIANG. Ref: 6.

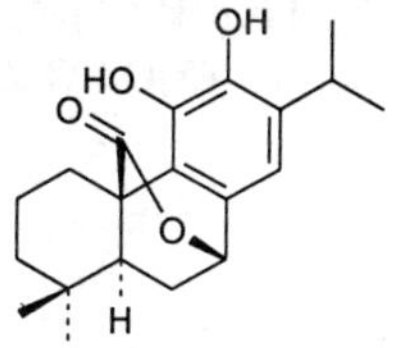

895 β-Carotene
$C_{40}H_{56}$ MW: 536.89 Property: mp 184°C. Source: LA JIAO, LU HUI. Ref: 2, 15.

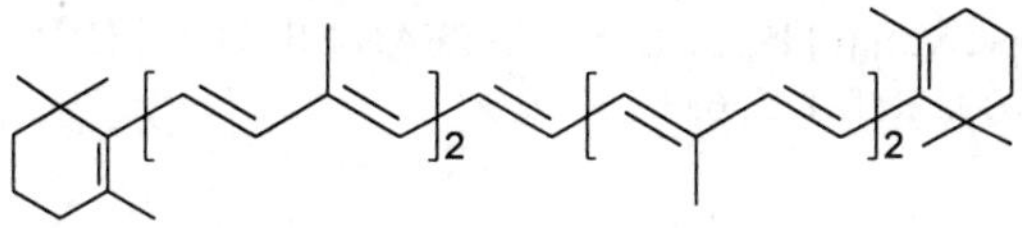

896 γ-Carotene
$C_{40}H_{56}$ MW: 536.89 Property: mp 154°C. Source: FAN MU GUA. Ref: 6.

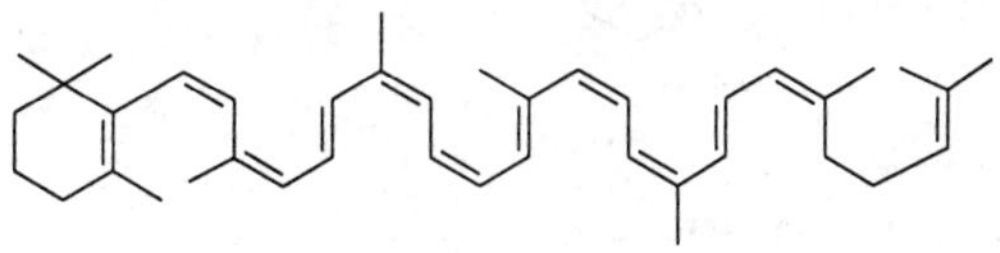

897 ζ-Carotene
$C_{40}H_{60}$ MW: 540.92 Property: mp 38-42°C. Source: FAN MU GUA. Ref: 6.

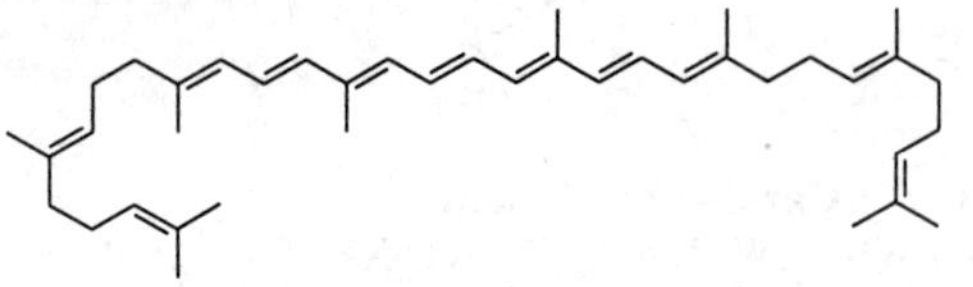

898 ε-Carotene
$C_{40}H_{56}$ MW: 536.89 Property: mp 199-201°C. Source: HU LUO BO. Ref: 6.

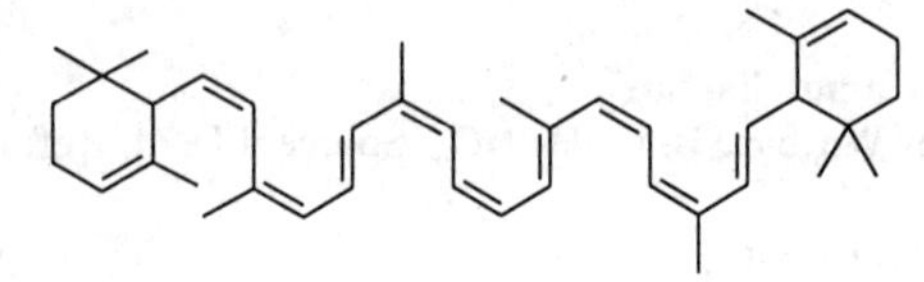

901 α-Carotene-5,6-epoxide
$C_{40}H_{56}O$ MW: 552.89 Source: TU SI ZI. Ref: 6.

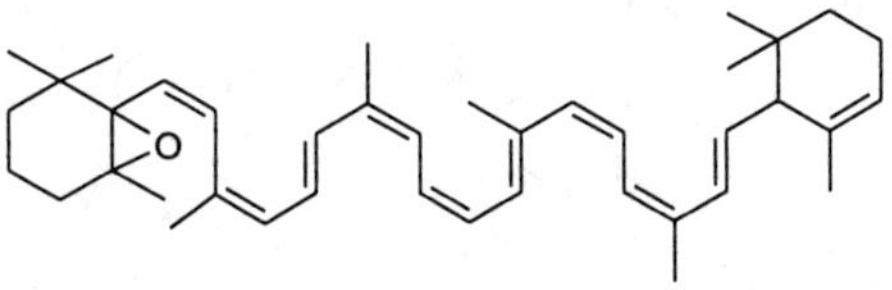

902 Carotol
$C_{15}H_{26}O$ MW: 222.37 Property: bp (+): 126°C/2.5mm. Source: HU LUO BO ZI, HE SHI, HE SHI FENG. Ref: 6.

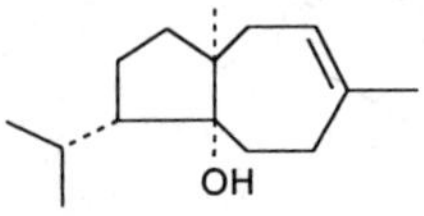

903 Carpaine
CAS: 72362-02-8 $C_{28}H_{50}N_2O_4$ MW: 478.72 Property: mp 119-20°C. Source: FAN MU GUA, HU LU BA. Ref: 1, 5, 6.

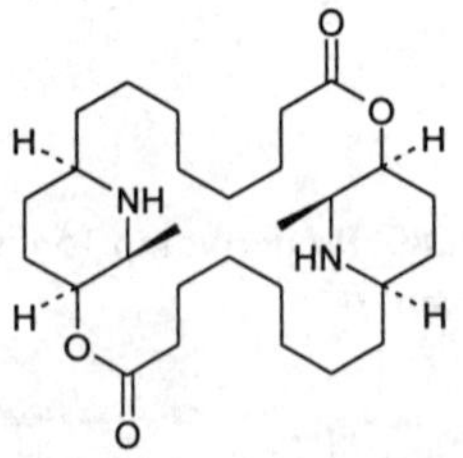

904 Carpesia lactone
$C_{15}H_{20}O_3$ MW: 248.32 Property: bp 195°C/4mm. Source: HE SHI, TIAN MING JING. Ref: 1, 6.

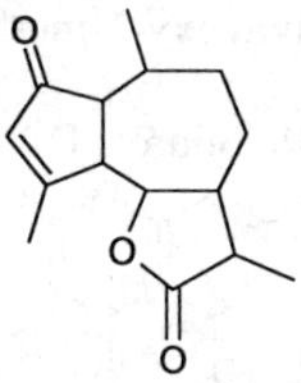

905 Carpesterol
$C_{37}H_{54}O_4$ MW: 562.84 Property: mp 248°C. Source: HUANG GUO QIE. Ref: 6.

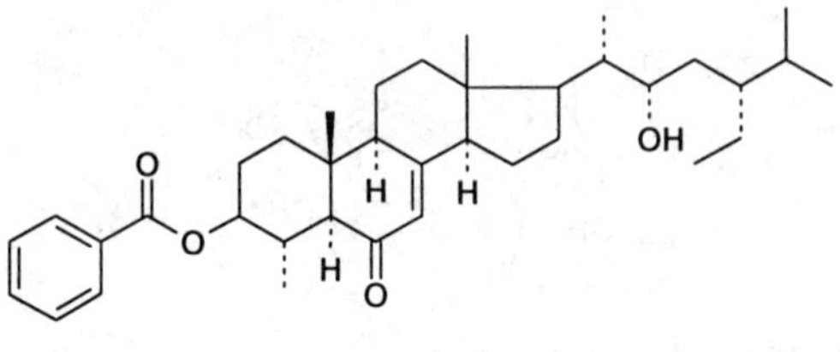

906 Carposide
Source: FAN MU GUA. Ref: 6.

907 Carthamidin
$C_{15}H_{12}O_6$ MW: 288.26 Source: HONG HUA. Ref: 2.

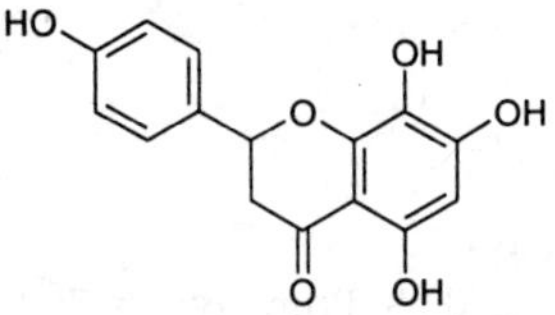

908 Carthamin
$C_{21}H_{22}O_{11}$ MW: 450.40 Source: HONG HUA. Ref: 2.

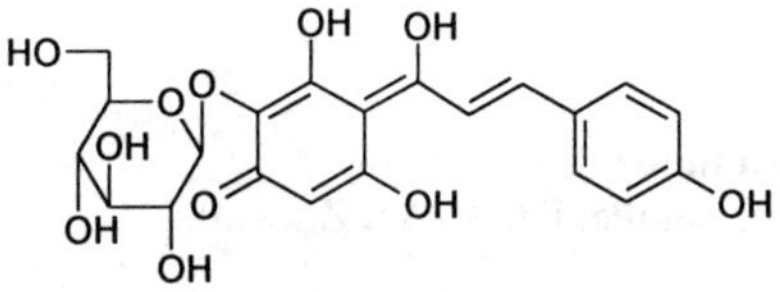

909 Carthamone
$C_{21}H_{20}O_{11}$ MW: 448.39 Source: HONG HUA. Ref: 2.

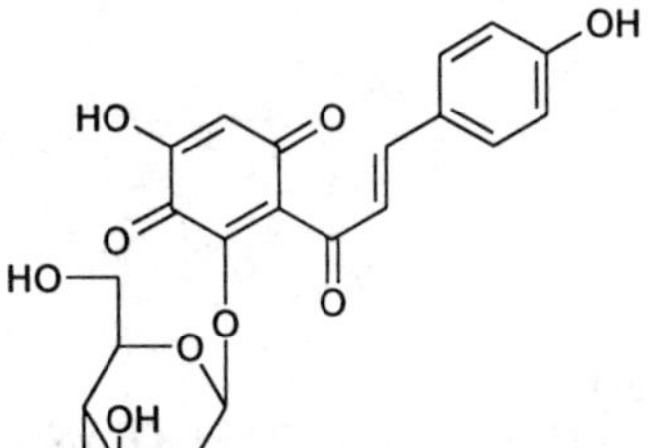

910 Carvacrol
2-p-Cymenol; 2-Hydroxy-p-cymene; Isopropyl-O-cresol; Isothymol. $C_{10}H_{14}O$ MW: 150.22 Property: bp 237-8°C. Source: DANG GUI, JIN YIN HUA, JU PI. Ref: 1, 2.

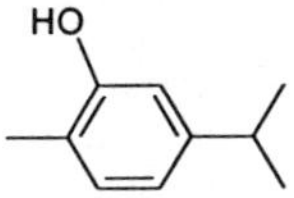

911 Carvacrol acetate
$C_{12}H_{16}O_2$ MW: 192.26 Property: bp 245-8°C. Source: SHI XIANG ROU. Ref: 6.

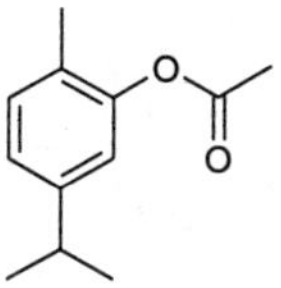

912 cis-Carveol
$C_{10}H_{16}O$ MW: 152.24 Source: QING HAO. Ref: 1, 2.

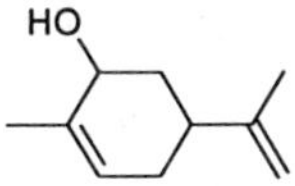

913 trans-Carveol
$C_{10}H_{16}O$ MW: 152.24 Source: QING HAO. Ref: 1.

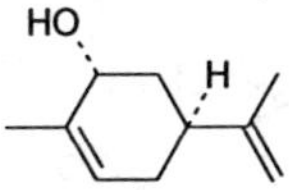

914 Carvomenthol
$C_{10}H_{20}O$ MW: 156.27 Property: bp (+): 101.8°C/14mm. Source: CHOU SHAN YANG. Ref: 6.

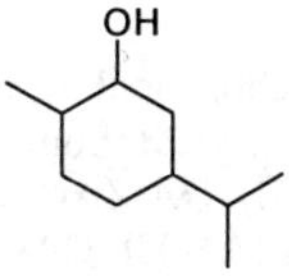

915 Carvone
Carvol. $C_{10}H_{14}O$ MW: 150.22 Property: bp 230°C/755mm, 91°C/5-6mm. Source: CHAI HU, QIANG HUO, YIN CHEN HAO. Ref: 1, 2.

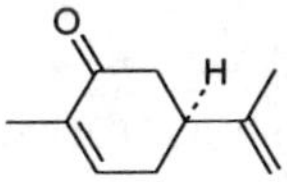

916 Caryophyllene
$C_{15}H_{24}$ MW: 204.36 Property: bp 129-30°C/14mm. Source: BING PIAN, HOU PO, HUO XIANG, JIN JIE, QING HAO, REN SHEN, SAN QI, SHENG JIANG, WU WEI ZI,XI YANG SHEN, YIN CHEN HAO, YU XING CAO. Ref: 1, 2.

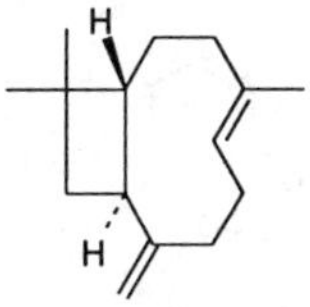

917 β-Caryophyllene
Property: bp (-): 118-9°C/9.7mm. Source: JIU LI XIANG. Ref: 11.

918 Caryophyllene epoxide
Caryophyllene oxide. $C_{15}H_{24}O$ MW: 220.36 Source: YIN CHEN HAO. Ref: 2.

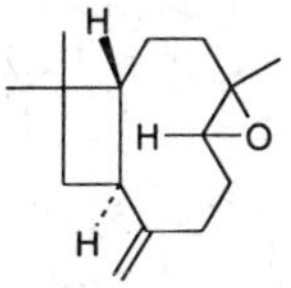

919 Caryoptoside
Source: XIAN SHENG MA XIAN HAO. Ref: 579.

920 Cassiaside
$C_{21}H_{22}O_9$ MW: 418.40 Source: JUE MING ZI. Ref: 2.

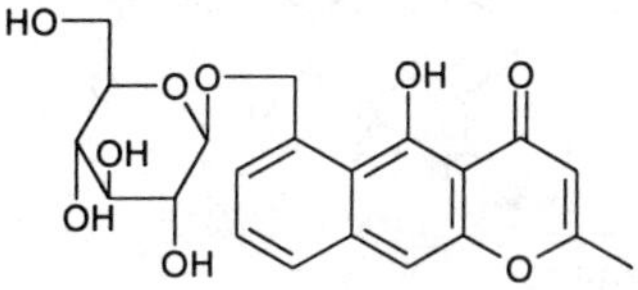

921 Cassyfiline
$C_{19}H_{19}NO_5$ MW: 341.37 Property: mp 217-9°C (dec). Source: WU YE TENG. Ref: 6.

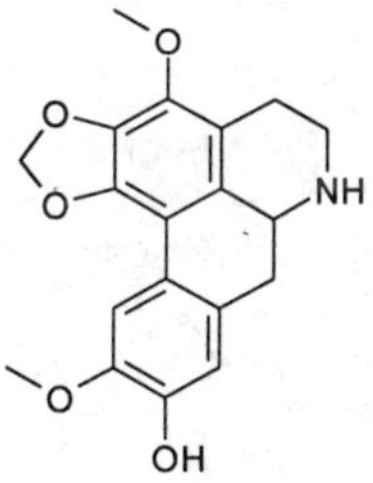

922 Cassythidine
$C_{19}H_{17}NO_5$ MW: 339.35 Property: mp 206-7°C. Source: WU YE TENG. Ref: 6.

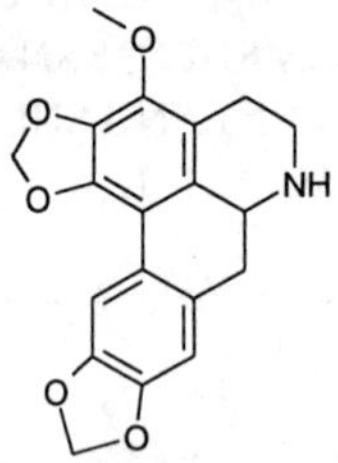

923 Castalagin
$C_{41}H_{26}O_{26}$ MW: 934.65 Property: light yellow amorphous powder, easy soluble in MeOH, Me_2CO and H_2O. Source: TAO JIN NIANG. Ref: 429.

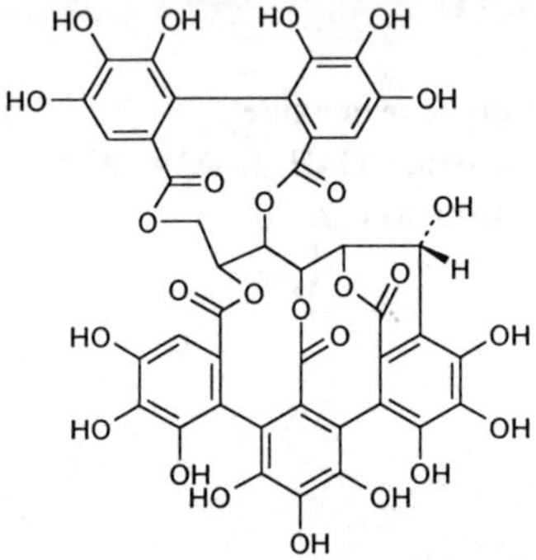

924 Casticin
$C_{19}H_{18}O_8$ MW: 374.35 Property: mp 186-7°C. Source: MAN JING ZI. QING HAO. Ref: 2, 562.

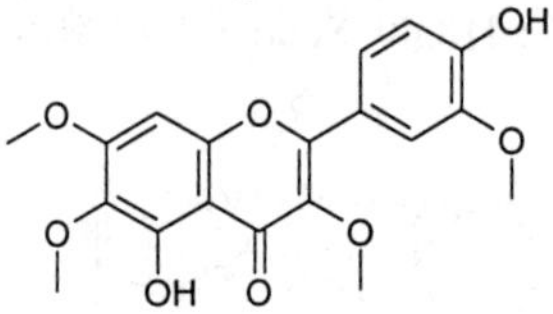

925 Casuariin
$C_{34}H_{24}O_{22}$ MW: 784.56 Property: brownish amorphous powder, easy soluble in MeOH and Me_2CO. Source: TAO JIN NIANG. Ref: 429.

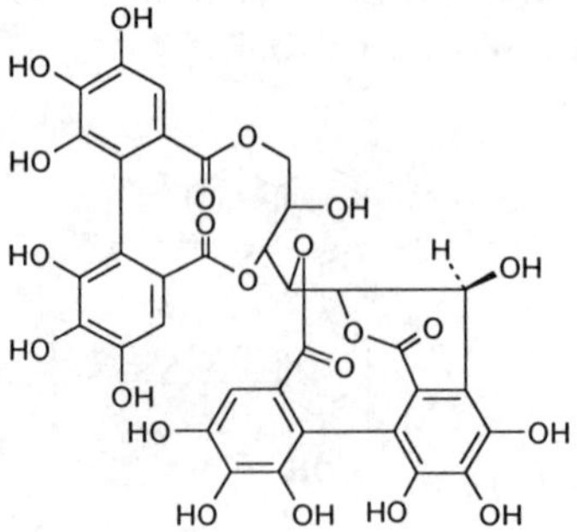

926 Catalpalactone
$C_{15}H_{14}O_4$ MW: 258.28 Property: mp 105-6°C/110-1°C. Source: ZI MU. Ref: 6.

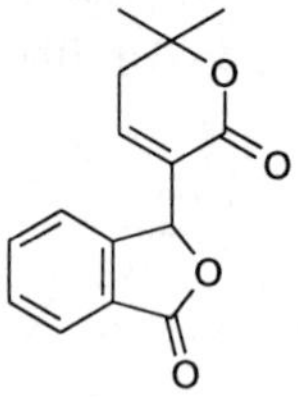

927 Catalpol
Catalpinoside. $C_{15}H_{22}O_{10}$ MW: 362.34 Property: mp 207-9°C (dec). Source: GAN DI HUANG, TONG MU. Ref: 1, 2.

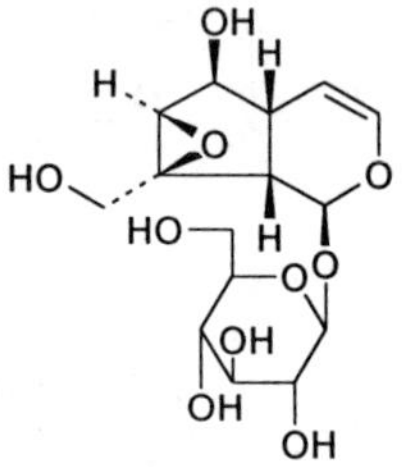

928 Catalposide
Catalpin. $C_{22}H_{26}O_{12}$ MW: 482.45 Source: ZI SHI, ZI YE. Ref: 1, 6.

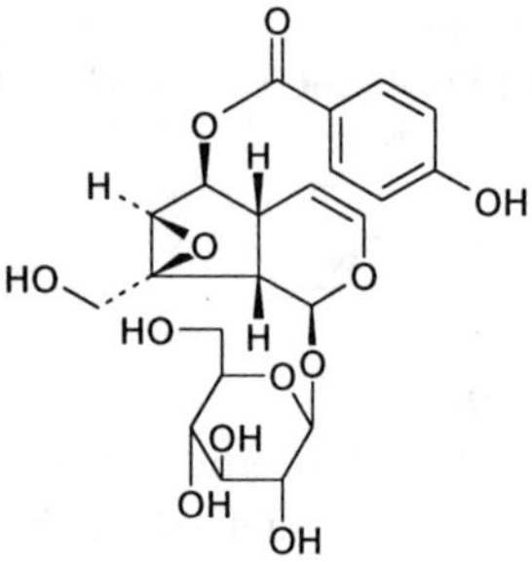

929 Catechin
Catechinic acid, Catechuic acid, Cyanidol. CAS: 154-23-4 $C_{15}H_{14}O_6$ MW: 290.28 Source: BING LANG, CU LIU GUO (SHA JI), DA ZAO, KUN MING SHAN HAI TANG, XIAN HE CAO. Ref: 1, 2, 6, 612.

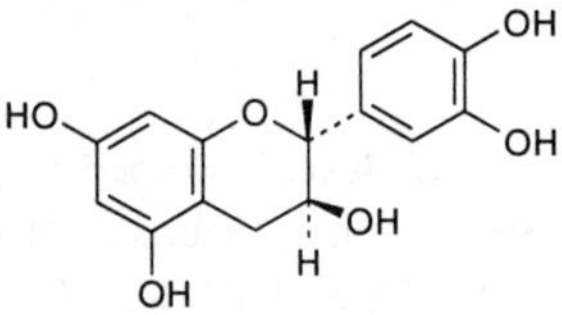

930 2R,3R-Catechin
Source: YUN NAN HONG DOU SHAN (bark). Ref: 563.

931 (+)-Catechin-5-O-glucoside
$C_{21}H_{24}O_{11}$ MW: 452.42 Source: DA HUANG. Ref: 2.

932 (+)-Catechin-pentaacetate
$C_{25}H_{24}O_{11}$ MW: 500.46 Source: BAI GUO. Ref: 2.

933 Catechol
$C_6H_6O_2$ MW: 110.11 Property: mp 105°C, bp 240°C. Source: DA ZAO. Ref: 1, 2.

934 Catharanthamine
$C_{47}H_{56}N_4O_9$ MW: 820.99 Source: CHANG CHUN HUA. Ref: 2.

935 Catharanthine
(+)-Catharanthine. CAS: 2468-21-5 $C_{21}H_{24}N_2O_2$ MW: 336.44 Property: mp (+): 126-8°C. Source: CHANG CHUN HUA. Ref: 1, 2, 5.

936 Catharine
$C_{46}H_{54}N_4O_{10}$ MW: 822.96 Source: CHANG CHUN HUA. Ref: 2.

937 Catharosine
$C_{22}H_{28}N_2O_4$ MW: 384.48 Source: CHANG CHUN HUA. Ref: 2.

938 Caudatin
$C_{27}H_{40}O_7$ MW: 476.62 Property: mp 158-60°C/190-5°C. Source: BAI SHOU WU. Ref: 6.

939 Caudoside
$C_{30}H_{44}O_9$ MW: 548.68 Property: mp 249-52°C. Source: YANG JIAO AO ZI. Ref: 6.

940 Caudostroside
$C_{30}H_{44}O_9$ MW: 548.68 Source: YANG JIAO AO ZI. Ref: 6.

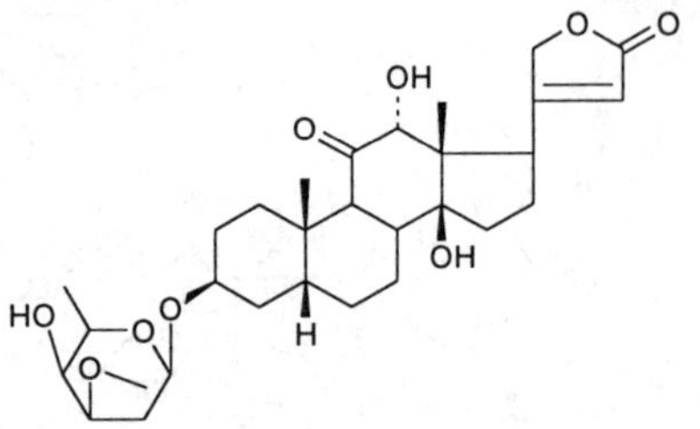

941 Cauloside A
$C_{35}H_{56}O_8$ MW: 604.83 Property: mp 228°C (dec). Source: HONG MAO QI. Ref: 6.

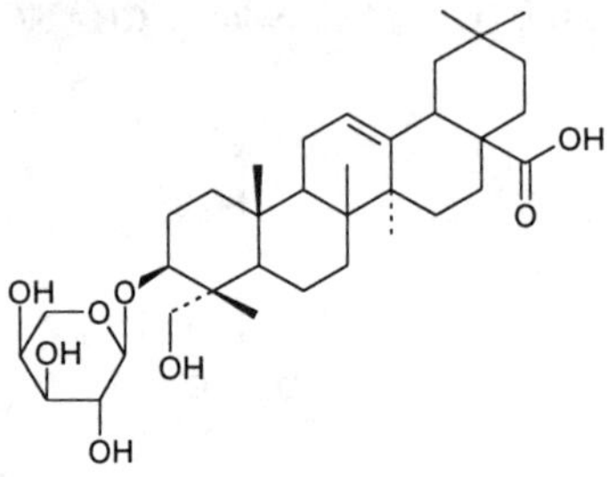

942 Cauloside B
$C_{35}H_{56}O_9$ MW: 620.83 Source: HONG MAO QI. Ref: 6.

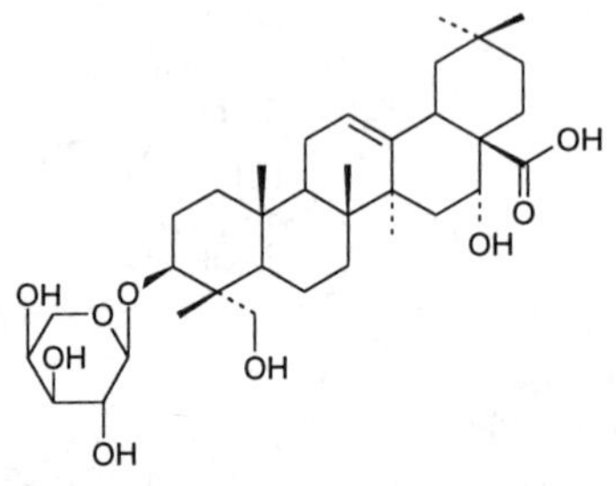

943 Cauloside C
$C_{41}H_{66}O_{13}$ MW: 766.98 Property: mp 252-5°C (dec). Source: HONG MAO QI. Ref: 6.

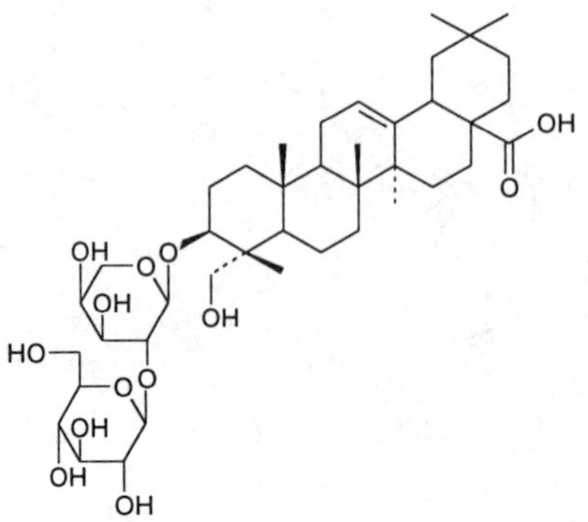

944 Cauloside D
$C_{53}H_{86}O_{22}$ MW: 1075.26 Source: HONG MAO QI. Ref: 6.

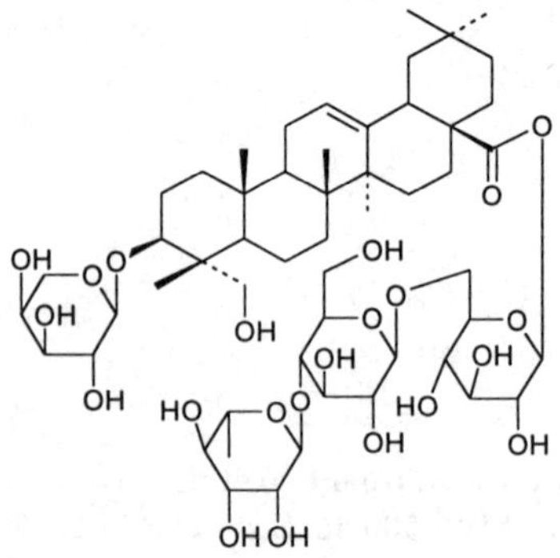

945 Cavincine sulfate
Source: CHANG CHUN HUA. Ref: 2.

946 Cayratinin
$C_{42}H_{47}O_{26}$•Cl 935.83•35.45 MW: 971.28 Source: WU LIAN MEI. Ref: 6.

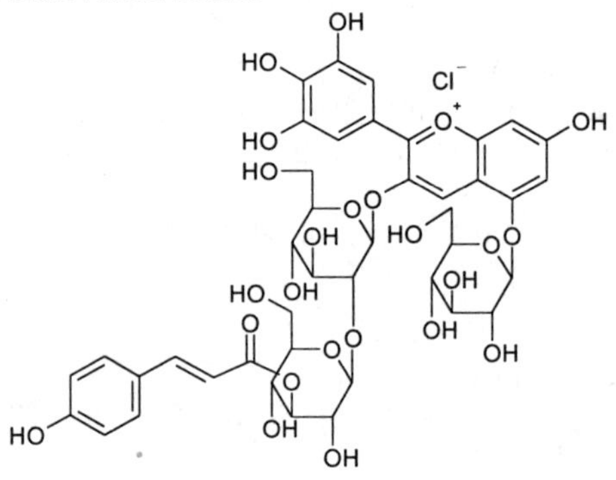

947 Ceanothic acid
$C_{30}H_{46}O_5$ MW: 486.70 Source: SUAN ZAO REN. Ref: 2.

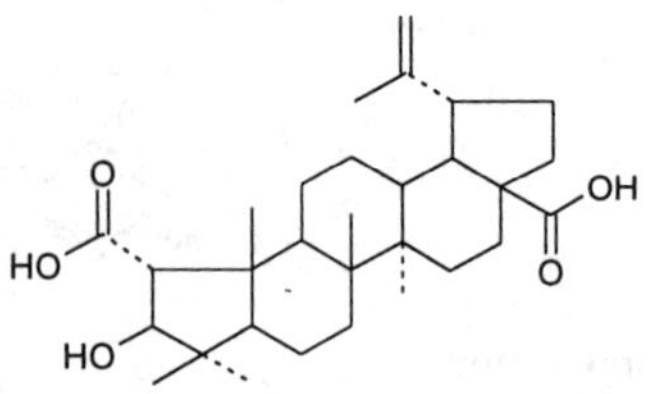

948 α-Cedrene
$C_{15}H_{24}$ MW: 204.36 Source: DANG GUI. Ref: 2.

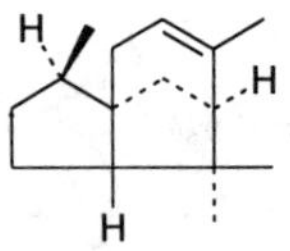

949 β-Cedrene
$C_{15}H_{24}$ MW: 204.36 Source: DU HUO, SHENG JIANG. Ref: 2.

950 Cedrol
$C_{15}H_{26}O$ MW: 222.37 Source: REN SHEN. Ref: 2.

951 Celabenzine
$C_{23}H_{29}N_3O_2$ MW: 379.51 Source: LEI GONG TENG. Ref: 2.

952 Celacinnine
$C_{25}H_{31}N_3O_2$ MW: 405.54 Source: LEI GONG TENG. Ref: 2.

953 Celafurine
$C_{21}H_{27}N_3O_3$ MW: 369.47 Source: LEI GONG TENG. Ref: 2.

954 Celallocinnine
$C_{25}H_{31}N_3O_2$ MW: 405.54 Source: LEI GONG TENG. Ref: 2.

955 Celastrine B
$C_{35}H_{40}O_7$ MW: 572.70 Property: amorphous powder, mp 69-70°C. Source: CI NAN SHE TENG. Ref: 384.

956 Celastrol
$C_{29}H_{38}O_4$ MW: 450.62 Property: mp red crystal, 205°C (dec). Source: LEI GONG TENG, NAN SHE TENG GEN. Ref: 1, 6.

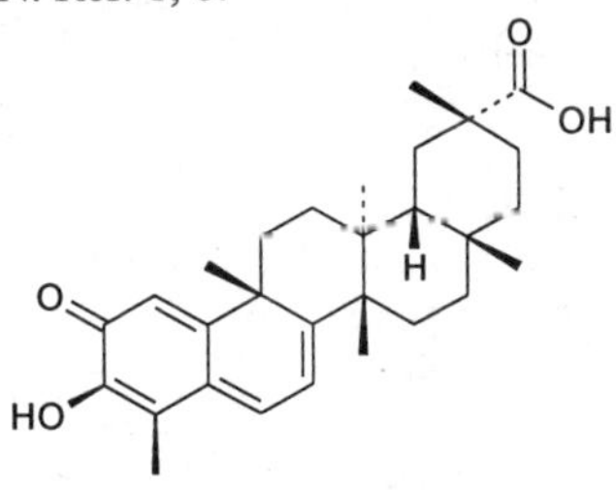

957 Celaxanthin
$C_{40}H_{54}O$ MW: 550.88 Property: mp 209-10°C. Source: CI NAN SHE TENG. Ref: 6.

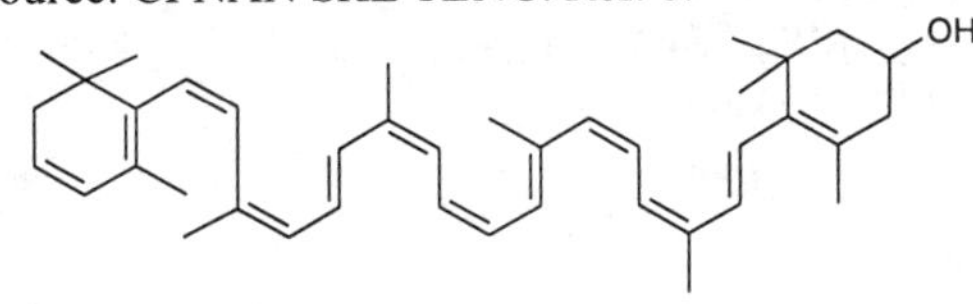

958 Celebroside
$C_{40}H_{75}NO_9$ MW: 714.05 Source: GAN DI HUANG. Ref: 2.

959 Celerin
$C_{15}H_{16}O_4$ MW: 260.29 Source: HAN QIN. Ref: 19.

960 Celeroin
$C_{14}H_{14}O_5$ MW: 262.26 Source: HAN QIN. Ref: 19.

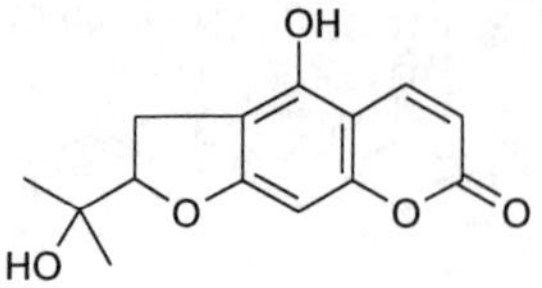

961 Celeroside
$C_{20}H_{24}O_{10}$ MW: 424.41 Source: HAN QIN. Ref: 19.

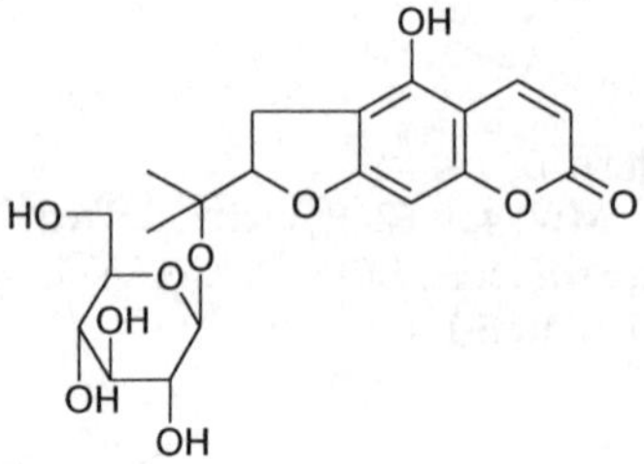

962 Cellobiose
$C_{12}H_{22}O_{11}$ MW: 342.30 Property: mp 225°C (dec). Source: PI HAN CAO. Ref: 6.

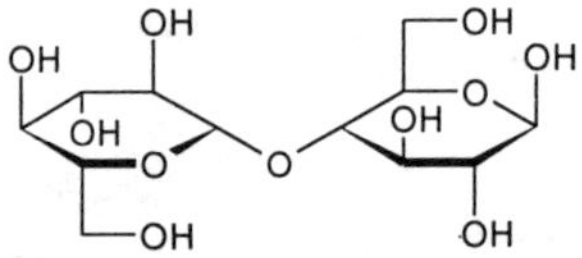

963 Cembrene
$C_{20}H_{34}$ MW: 274.49 Property: mp 58-9°C. Source: HAI SONG ZI. Ref: 6.

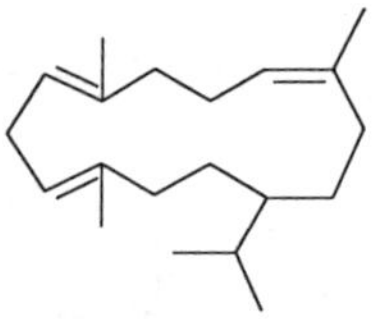

964 Centaur X
$C_{19}H_{22}O_4$ MW: 314.38 Property: mp 54-6°C. Source: QI ZHOU YI ZHI HAO. Ref: 6.

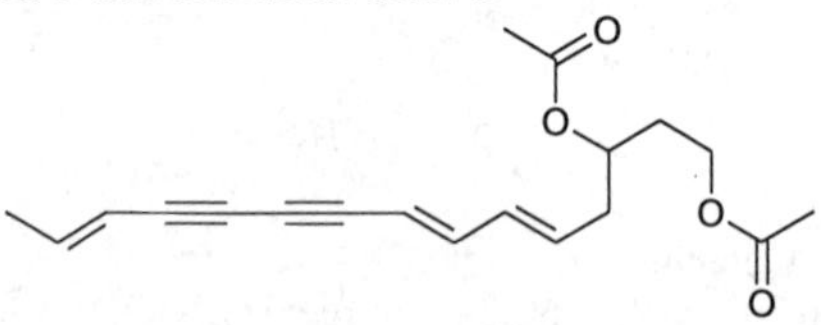

965 Centellose
Source: JI XUE CAO. Ref: 6.

966 Cephalin
Source: LU RONG. Ref: 2.

967 Cephalofortuneine
$C_{20}H_{27}NO_5$ MW: 361.44 Source: SAN JIAN SHAN. Ref: 2.

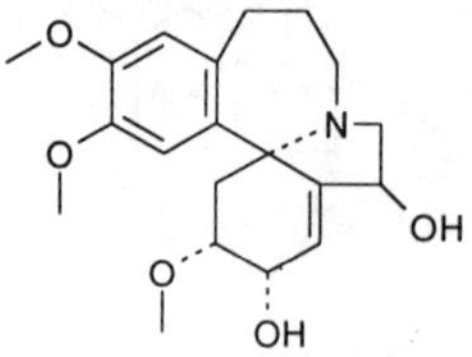

968 Cephalotaxinamide
$C_{18}H_{19}NO_5$ MW: 329.36 Source: SAN JIAN SHAN. Ref: 20.

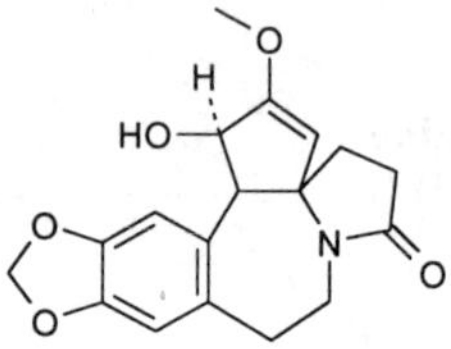

969 Cephalotaxine
CAS: 71610-00-9 $C_{18}H_{21}NO_4$ MW: 315.37 Property: mp 134-7°C. Source: SAN JIAN SHAN. Ref: 1, 4, 5, 20.

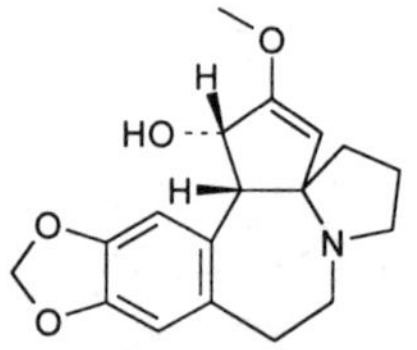

970 Cephalotaxinone
$C_{18}H_{19}NO_4$ MW: 313.36 Source: SAN JIAN SHAN. Ref: 20.

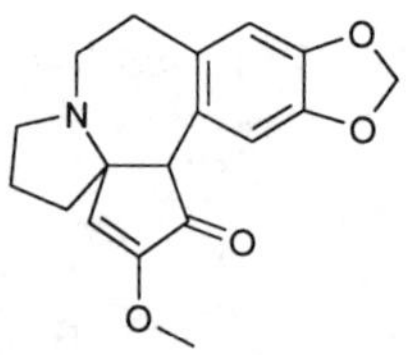

971 Cepharamine
$C_{19}H_{23}NO_4$ MW: 329.40 Property: mp 186-7°C. Source: BAI YAO ZI. Ref: 6.

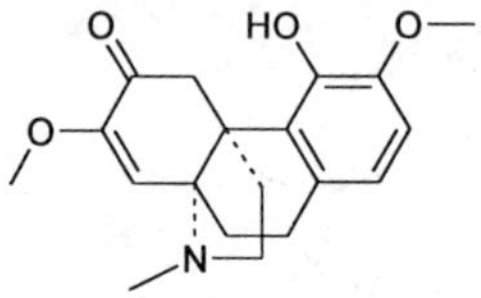

972 Cepharanoline
$C_{36}H_{36}N_2O_6$ MW: 592.70 Property: mp 270°C (dec). Source: BAI YAO ZI. Ref: 6.

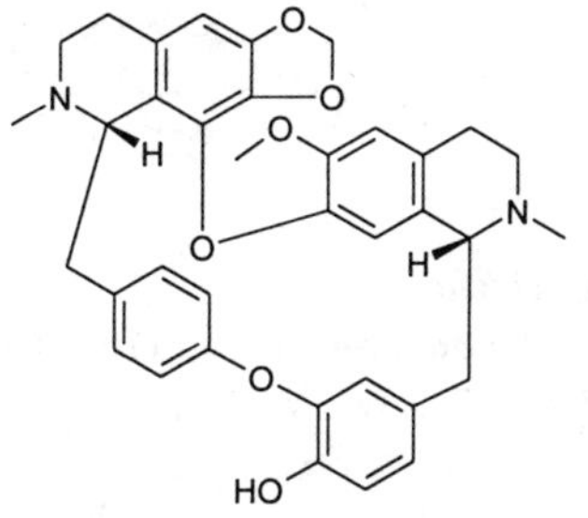

973 Cepharanthine
CAS: 481-49-2 $C_{37}H_{38}N_2O_6$ MW: 606.73 Property: mp 145-55°C. Source: BAI YAO ZI, DI BU RONG. Ref: 1, 4, 5, 6.

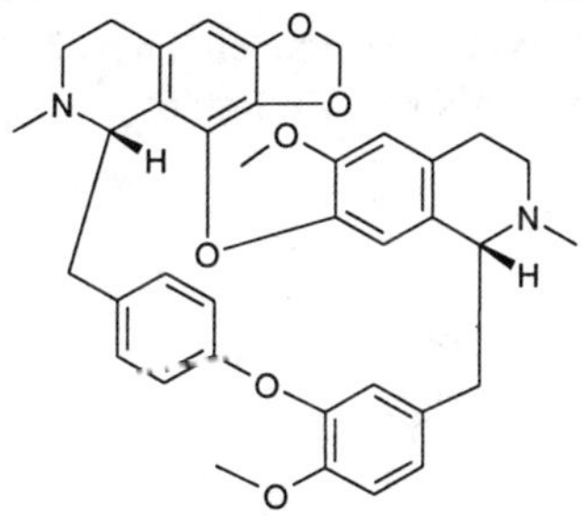

974 Ceramide
Ceramide aminoethyl phosphoric acid. Source: LU RONG. Ref: 2.

975 Cerberin
Veneniferin; Monoacetylneriifolin. $C_{32}H_{48}O_9$ MW: 576.73 Property: mp 212-5°C. Source: HUANG HUA JIA ZHU TAO, NIU XIN QIE ZI. Ref: 1, 6.

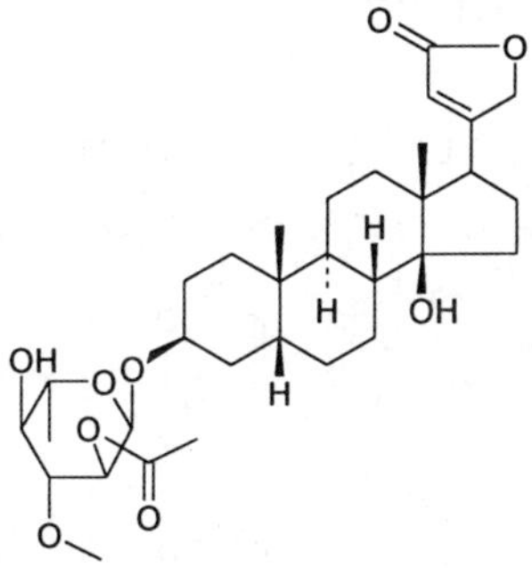

976 Cerberoside
$C_{42}H_{66}O_{18}$ MW: 858.8 Property: mp 187.5-8.5°C(197-201°C). Source: HUANG HUA JIA ZHU TAO, NIU XIN QIE ZI. Ref: 6.

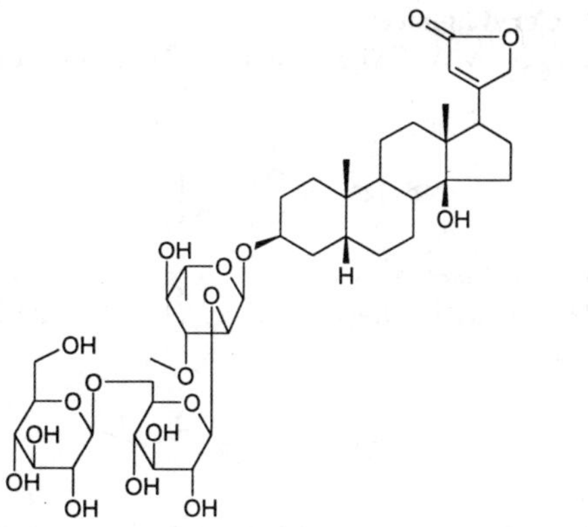

977 Cernoside
$C_{39}H_{32}O_{14}$ MW: 724.68 Property: mp 225-30°C (dec). Source: PU DI WU GONG. Ref: 6.

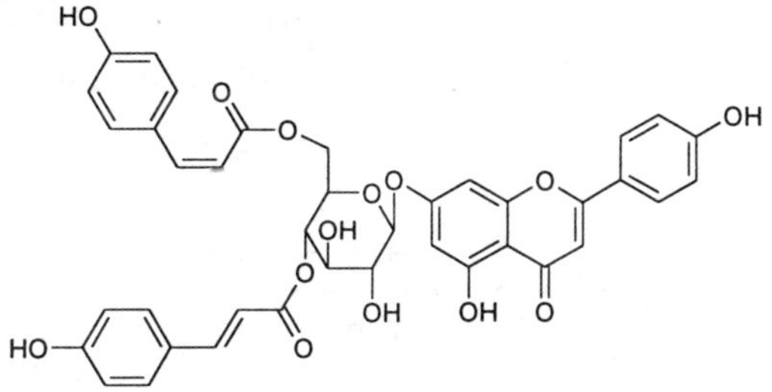

978 Cernuine
$C_{16}H_{26}N_2O$ MW: 262.40 Property: mp 106°C. Source: PU DI WU GONG. Ref: 6.

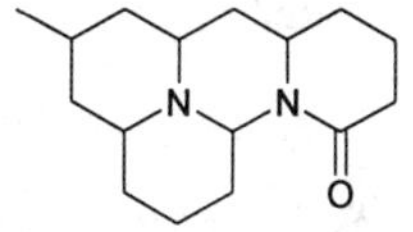

979 Cerotic acid
$C_{26}H_{52}O_2$ MW: 396.70 Property: colorless acicular crystal. Source: GUA LOU, JIN QUE GEN. Ref: 2, 455.

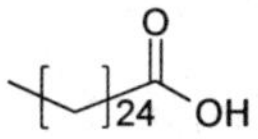

980 Ceryl alcohol
$C_{25}H_{54}O$ MW: 382.72 Source: YIN YANG HUO. Ref: 2.

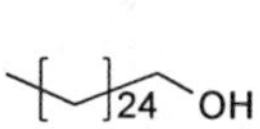

981 Ceryl cerotate
$C_{52}H_{104}O_2$ MW: 761.41 Property: mp 82-4°C. Source: CHONG BAI LA. Ref: 6.

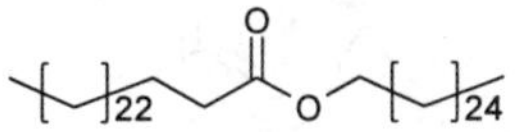

982 Ceryl lignocerate
$C_{50}H_{100}O_2$ MW: 733.35 Source: CHONG BAI LA. Ref: 6.

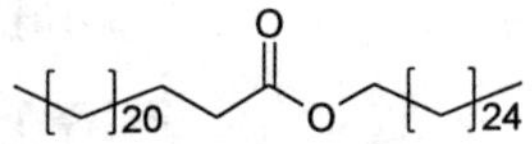

983 Ceryl montanate
$C_{54}H_{108}O_2$ MW: 789.46 Source: CHONG BAI LA. Ref: 6.

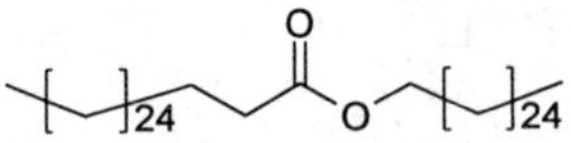

984 5α,14α-Cevanine-3β,20β-dihydroxy-6-one
$C_{27}H_{43}NO_3$ MW: 429.65 Property: colorless crystal (acetone), mp 181-3oC, $[\alpha]_D^{10}$ -48.76° (c=0.035, chloroform). Source: ZHE BEI MU. Ref: 233.

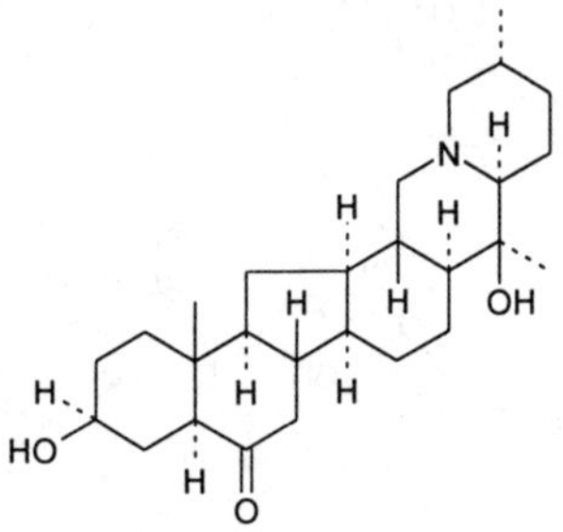

985 Chalepensin
$C_{16}H_{14}O_3$ MW: 254.29 Property: mp 80-90°C. Source: CHOU CAO. Ref: 6.

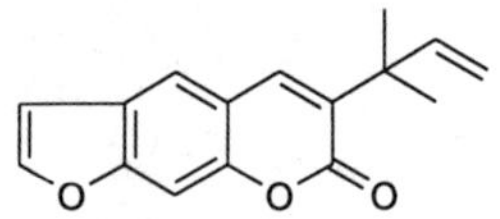

986 Chamazulene
Dimethulene. $C_{14}H_{16}$ MW: 184.28 Property: bp 161°C/12mm. Source: MU JU, WU YAO, YI ZHI HAO. Ref: 1, 6.

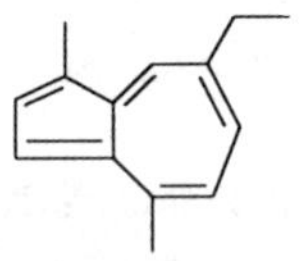

987 Chamigrene
$C_{15}H_{24}$ MW: 204.36 Source: DANG GUI. Ref: 2.

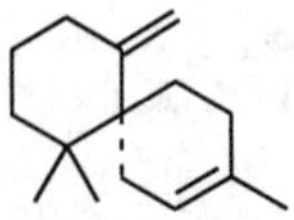

988 α-Chamigrene
$C_{16}H_{26}$ MW: 218.39 Source: WU WEI ZI. Ref: 2.

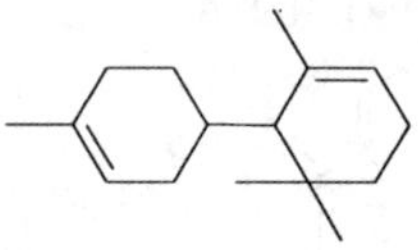

989 β-Chamigrene
$C_{15}H_{24}$ MW: 204.36 Property: bp 110-3°C/13mm. Source: BAI ZHI JIE, WU WEI ZI. Ref: 2, 6.

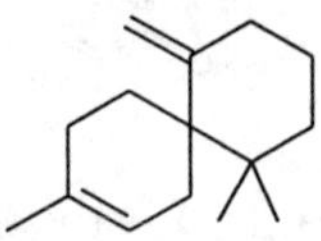

990 Chanoclavine
$C_{17}H_{22}N_2O$ MW: 270.38 Property: mp 220-2°C (dec). Source: QIAN NIU ZI. Ref: 6.

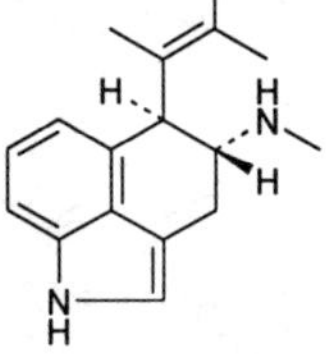

991 Chaohuoside A
7-O-β-D-glucopyranosyl-anhydroicaritin-3-O-β-D-(3,6-O-diacetyl)-glucopyranosyl-(1→3)-α-L-(4-O-acetyl)-rhamnopyranoside. $C_{45}H_{56}O_{23}$ MW: 964.93 Property: yellow powder, mp 144-5.5°C, $[\alpha]_D^{18}$ -86° (c=0.01, methanol). Source: CHAO XIAN YIN YANG HUO. Ref: 357.

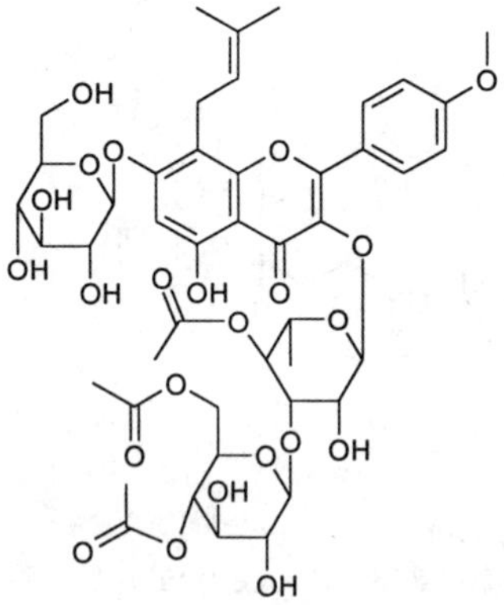

992 Chaparrinone
CAS: 2261-34-3 $C_{20}H_{26}O_7$ MW: 378.43 Property: mp 236-48°C. Source: CHU BAI PI. Ref: 1, 5, 6.

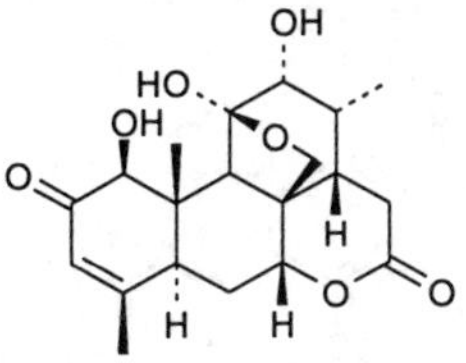

993 Chasmanine
Property: mp 90-1°C. Source: HUANG MAO WU TOU. Ref: 513.

994 Chaulmoogric acid
$C_{18}H_{32}O_2$ MW: 280.45 Property: mp (+): 68.5°C, (±): 68.5°C, bp (+): 247-8°C/20mm. Source: DA FENG ZI. Ref: 6.

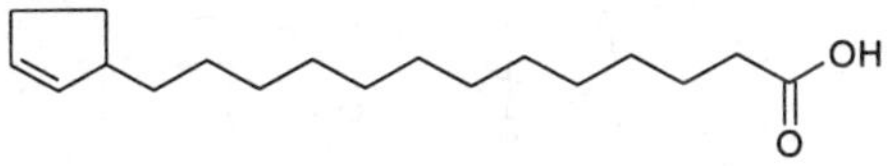

995 Chavibetol
$C_{10}H_{12}O_2$ MW: 164.21 Property: mp 8.5°C, bp 254-5°C. Source: JU JIANG YE. Ref: 6.

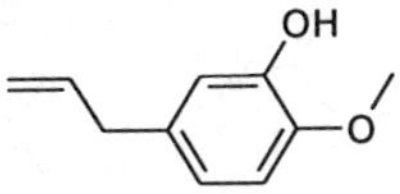

996 Chavicine
$C_{17}H_{19}NO_3$ MW: 285.35 Property: bp 245-60°C/0.25mm. Source: HU JIAO. Ref: 6.

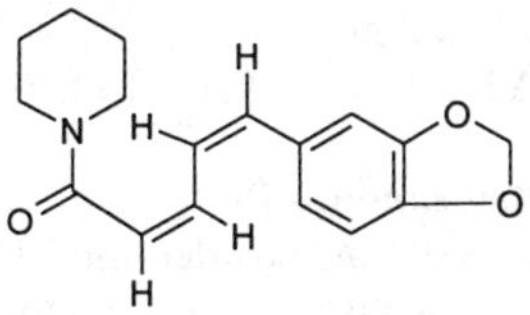

997 Chavicol
$C_9H_{10}O$ MW: 134.18 Property: mp 16°C, bp 237°C. Source: DING XIANG, JU JIANG YE. Ref: 6.

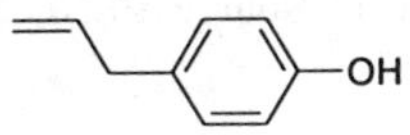

998 Chebulagic acid
$C_{41}H_{32}O_{28}$ MW: 972.7 Property: mp >240°C. Source: AN MO LE, CAO YUAN LAO GUAN, HE ZI, YOU GAN MU PI, YOU GAN YE. Ref: 6.

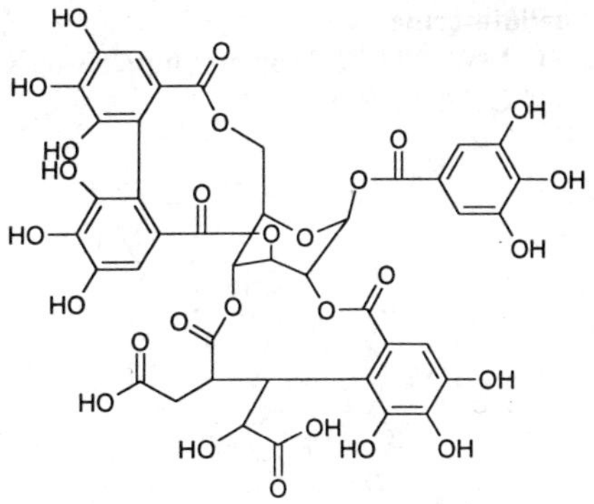

999 Chebulinic acid
$C_{41}H_{34}O_{28}$ MW: 974.71 Property: mp 234°C. Source: AN MO LE, HE ZI, YOU GAN MU PI, YOU GAN YE. Ref: 6.

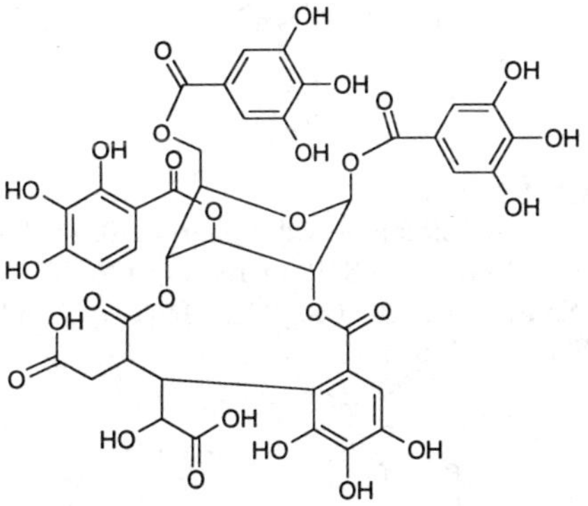

1000 Cheilanthifoline
$C_{19}H_{19}NO_4$ MW: 325.37 Property: mp (-): 178-80 °C. Source: BIAN FU GE GEN, HE BAO MU DAN GEN, ZI HUA YU DENG CAO (LIE BAO ZI JING). Ref: 6.

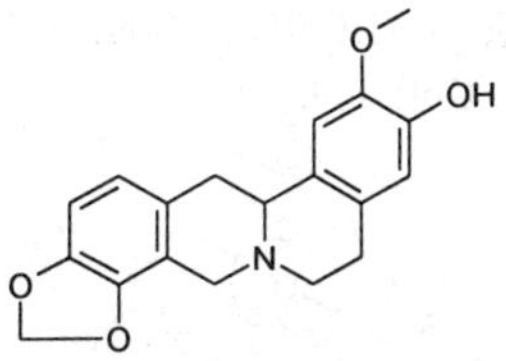

1001 Chelerythrine
$C_{21}H_{18}NO_4$ MW: 348.38 Source: BAI QU CAI, BO LUO HUI, FEI LONG ZHANG XUE, HE BAO MU DAN GEN, HE QING HUA, LI CHUN HUA, XI GUO JIAO HUI XIANG. Ref: 6.

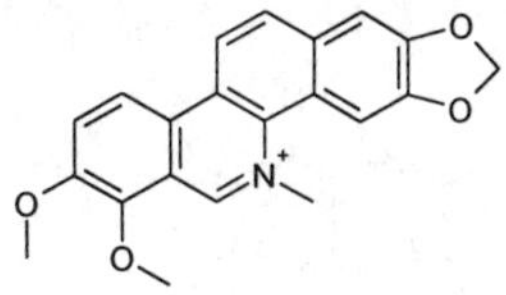

1002 Chelidimerine
$C_{43}H_{36}N_2O_9$ MW: 724.77 Property: mp 258-60°C. Source: BAI QU CAI. Ref: 6.

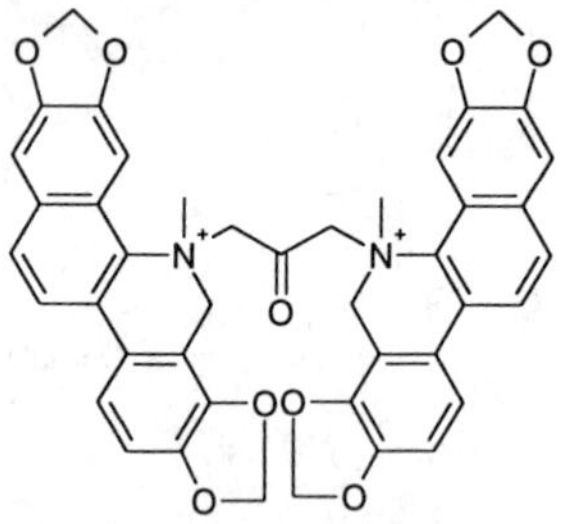

1003 Chelidonic acid
$C_7H_4O_6$ MW: 184.11 Property: mp 262°C. Source: BAI QU CAI, LING LAN, XIAO BAI BU. Ref: 6.

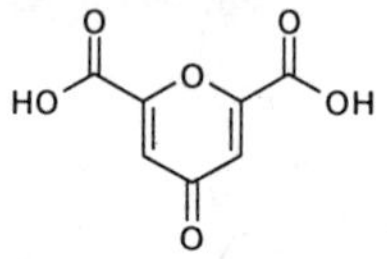

1004 Chelidonine
Diphyline; D-Chelidonine; Stylophorin. 30343-76-0 $C_{20}H_{19}NO_5$ MW: 353.38 Property: mp 136-40°C, bp 220°C. Source: BAI QU CAI, HE QING HUA, YE YING SU. Ref: 4, 6, 590.

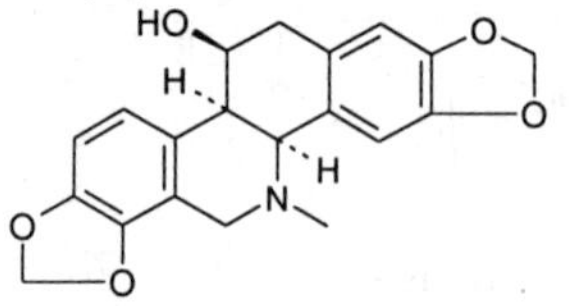

1005 Cheliensisin A
5α-acetoxy-goniothalamin oxide. $C_{15}H_{14}O_5$ MW: 274.28 Property: white prismatic crystal, mp 152-3°C, $[\alpha]_D^{24}$ +293.45° (c=1.31,CHCl$_3$). Source: HONG JING GE NA XIANG. Ref: 419.

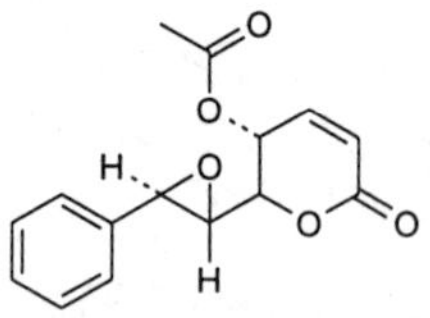

1006 Chelilutine
$C_{22}H_{20}NO_5$ MW: 378.41 Source: BAI QU CAI, HE BAO MU DAN GEN, HE QING HUA. Ref: 6.

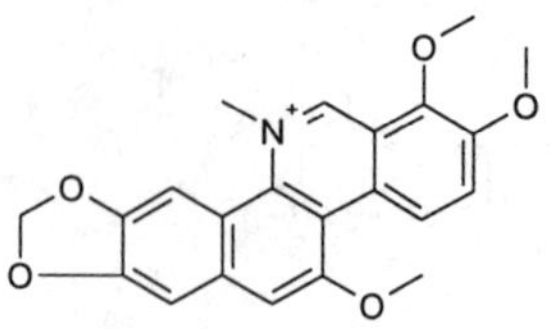

1007 Chelirubine
$C_{21}H_{16}NO_5$ MW: 362.37 Source: BAI QU CAI, HE BAO MU DAN GEN, HE QING HUA. Ref: 6.

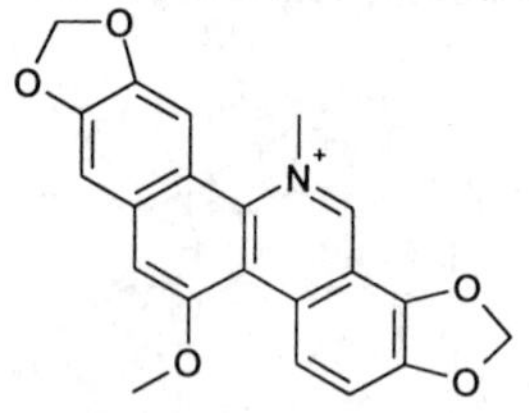

1008 Chenodeoxycholic acid
$C_{24}H_{40}O_4$ MW: 392.58 Source: NIU HUANG, XIONG DAN. Ref: 2.

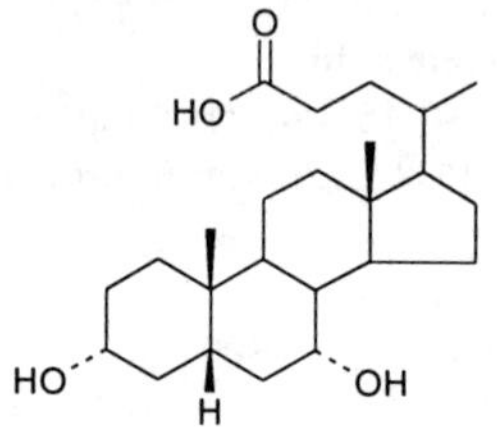

1009 Chicoric acid
$C_{22}H_{18}O_{12}$ MW: 474.38 Property: mp 206°C. Source: JU QU. Ref: 6.

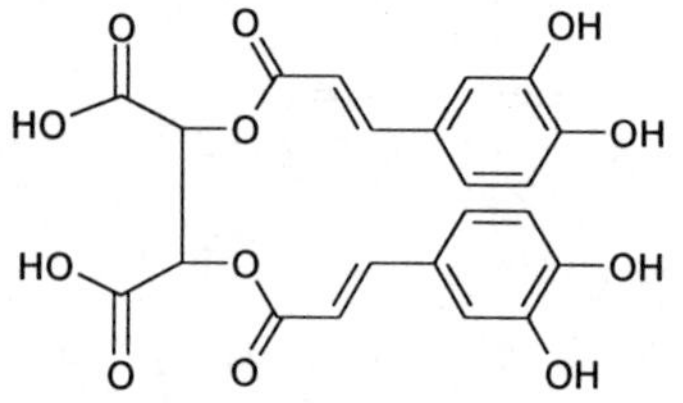

1010 Chikusaikoside I
Source: XIAO YE HEI CHAI HU. Ref: 598.

1011 Chikusetsu saponin Ib
Property: white crystalline powder, mp 233-5°C, $[\alpha]_D^{20}$ -21.7°(c=0.1, MeOH). Source: TAI BAI HU MU. Ref: 462.

1012 Chikusetsu saponin Iva
Property: mp 214-6°C. Source: PENG XIAN XUE DAN. Ref: 554.

1013 Chimaphilin
$C_{12}H_{10}O_2$ MW: 186.21 Property: mp 113.5-4.5°C. Source: LU SHOU CAO. Ref: 6.

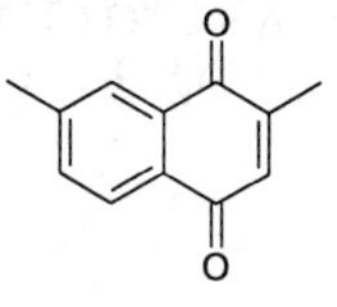

1014 Chimonanthine
$C_{22}H_{26}N_4$ MW: 346.48 Property: mp 188-9°C. Source: LA MEI HUA. Ref: 6.

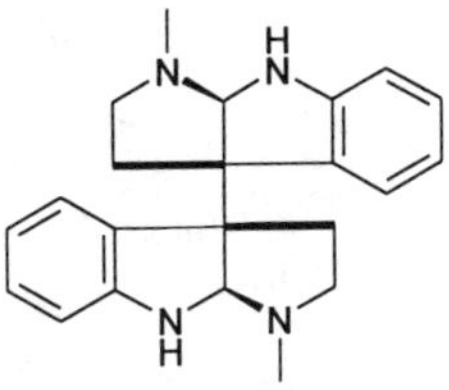

1015 Chinenoside
(25S)-24-O-β-D-glucopyranosyl-3β,24β-dihydroxy-5α-spirost-3-O-α-arabinopyranosyl-(1→6)-β-D-glucopyranoside. $C_{44}H_{70}O_{19}$ MW: 902 Property: white amorphous powder, mp 219-21°C. Source: XIE BAI. Ref: 409.

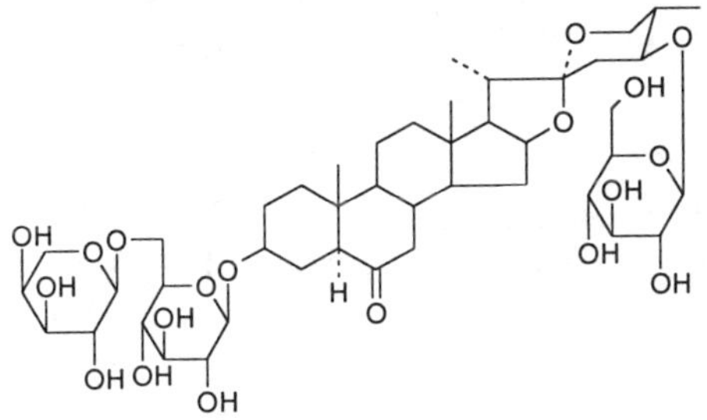

1016 Chinensin
$C_{21}H_{16}O_6$ MW: 364.36 Property: mp 220-1°C. Source: DA JIN NIU CAO. Ref: 6.

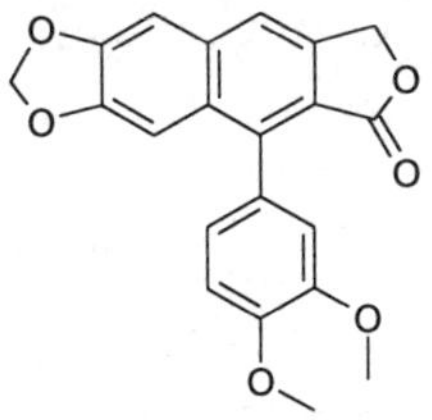

1017 Chinensinaphthol
$C_{21}H_{16}O_7$ MW: 380.36 Property: mp 285-6°C. Source: DA JIN NIU CAO. Ref: 6.

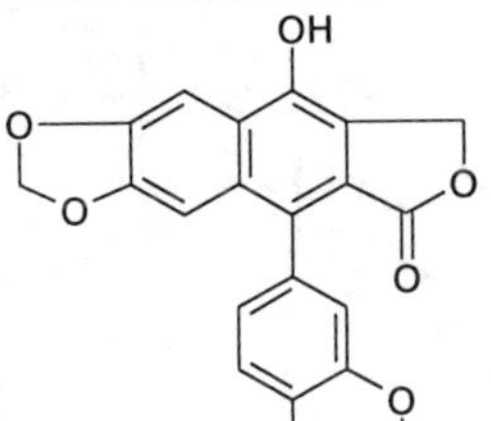

1018 Chinensinaphthol methyl ether
$C_{22}H_{18}O_7$ MW: 394.38 Property: mp 257-8°C. Source: DA JIN NIU CAO. Ref: 6.

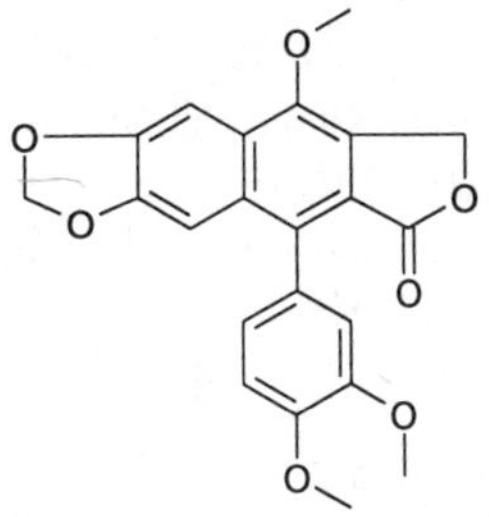

1019 Chinpeimine
$C_{27}H_{43}NO_2$ Source: CHUAN BEI MU. Ref: 2.

1020 Chisulactone
$C_{21}H_{20}O_6$ MW: 368.39 Property: mp 108-10°C. Source: DA JIN NIU CAO. Ref: 6.

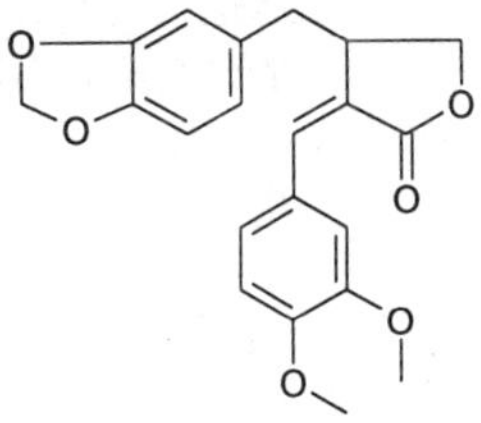

1021 Chitin
$C_{36}H_{58}O_{21}$ MW: 826.85 Source: FU LING, JIU XIANG CHONG, WEN GE, XIE KE, ZHANG LANG, ZHEN MO. Ref: 6.

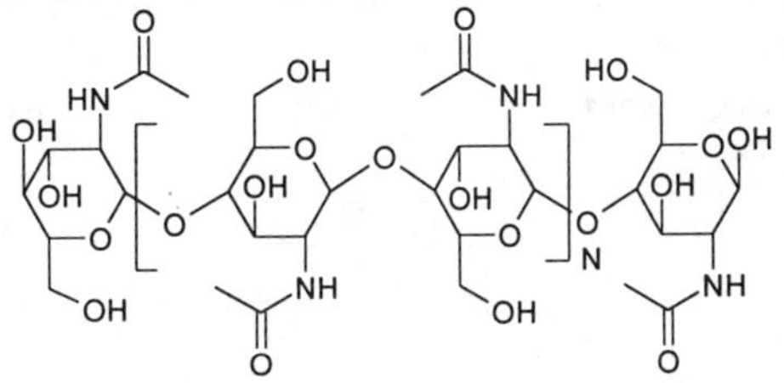

1022 26-Chloro-26-deoxycryptogenin
$C_{27}H_{41}ClO_3$ MW: 449.08 Property: mp 149-51°C. Source: YU ER QI. Ref: 6.

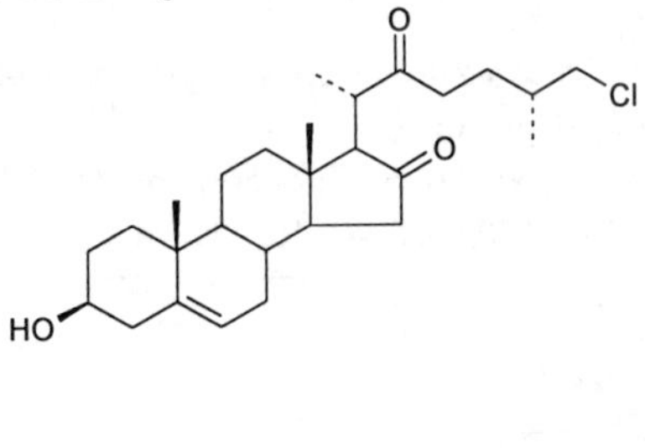

1023 Chlorogenic acid
3-Caffeoylquinid acid; Caffeotamic acid. CAS: 327-97-9 $C_{16}H_{18}O_9$ MW: 354.32 Property: mp 110°C. Source: CU LIU GUO (SHA JI), DU ZHONG, GUANG YE DING GONG TENG, JIAN DI PU GONG YING, JIN YIN HUA, MA QIAN ZI, SHAN ZHA, YIN CHEN HAO, YU XING CAO, ZHI ZI. Ref: 2, 4, 585, 602, 638.

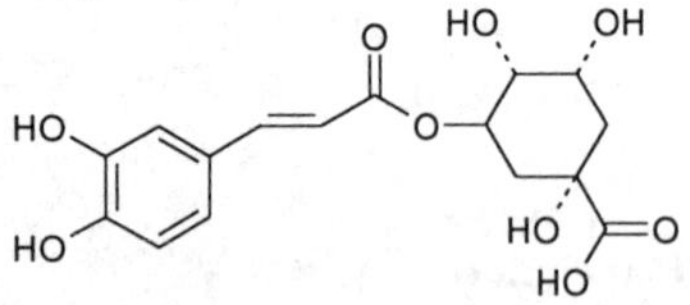

1024 Chlorogenin
$C_{27}H_{44}O_4$ MW: 432.65 Property: mp 273-6°C. Source: DONG YI HAO JIAN MA, DUAN YE LONG SHE LAN, FAN MA, JI LI GEN, JIAN MA, WU CI FAN MA, XIA YE LONG SHE LAN, YIN BIAN LONG SHE LAN. Ref: 6,10.

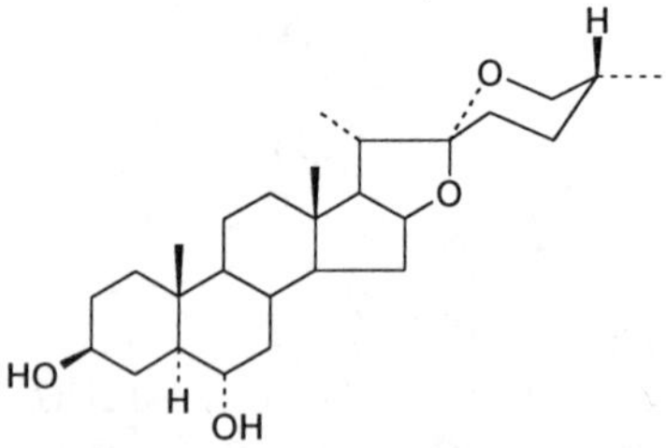

1025 2-(4-Chloro-3-hydroxybut-1-ynyl)-5-(penta-1,3-diynyl) thiophene
$C_{13}H_9ClOS$ MW: 248.73 Source: MO HAN LIAN. Ref: 6.

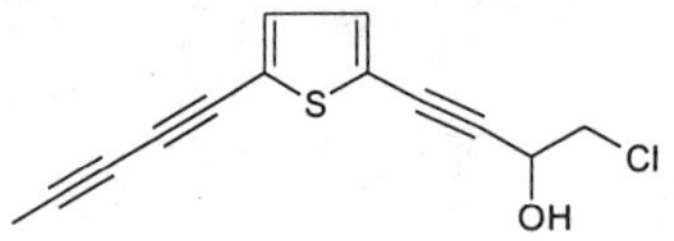

1026 8-(3-Chloro-2-hydroxy-3-methylbutyloxy-psoralen
Source: YUN NAN QIANG HUO. Ref: 558.

1027 5-Chloro-2-(octa-2,4,6-triynylidene)-5,6-dihydro-2H-pyran
$C_{13}H_9ClO$ MW: 216.67 Property: mp 73°C. Source: DA YE BAI TOU WENG. Ref: 6.

1028 3-Chloroplumbagin
$C_{11}H_7ClO_3$ MW: 222.63 Source: BAI HUA DAN. Ref: 6.

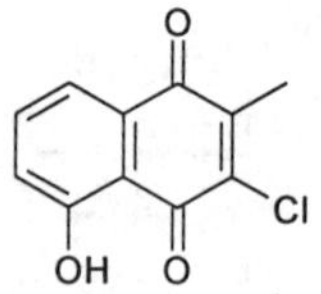

1029 5β-Cholanic acid
$C_{24}H_{40}O_2$ MW: 360.59 Property: mp 164°C. Source: XIANG SI ZI. Ref: 6.

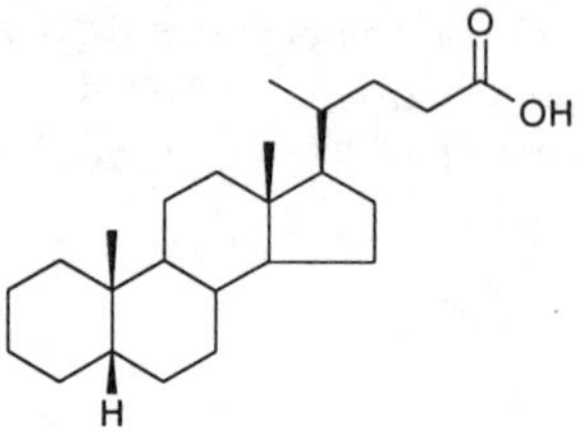

1030 Cholest-4-ene-3-one
$C_{19}H_{28}O$ MW: 272.43 Source: SHE XIANG. Ref: 2.

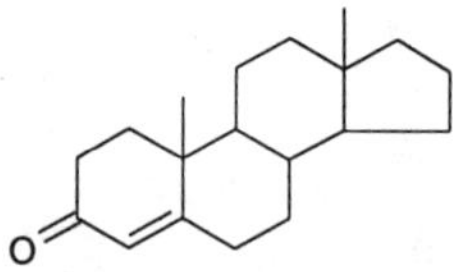

1031 Cholesterol
$C_{27}H_{46}O$ MW: 386.67 Source: CHAN SU, LU HUI, LU RONG, QUAN XIE, SHE XIANG, etc. Ref: 2.

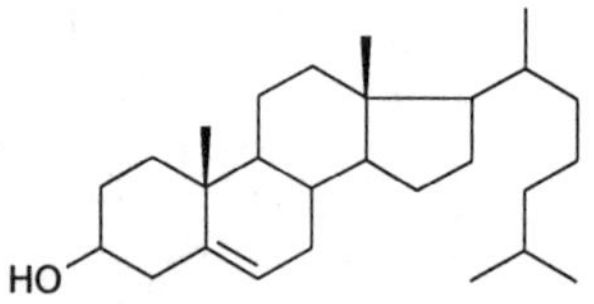

1032 Cholesteryl ferulate
$C_{37}H_{54}O_4$ MW: 562.84 Source: MI PI KANG. Ref: 6.

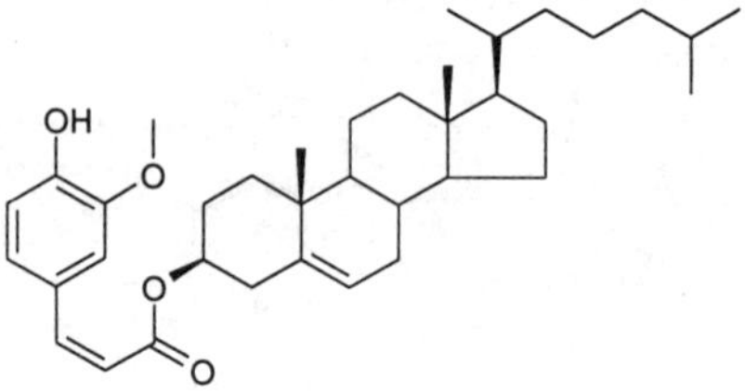

1033 Cholic acid
$C_{24}H_{40}O_5$ MW: 408.58 Source: NIU HUANG, XIONG DAN. Ref: 2.

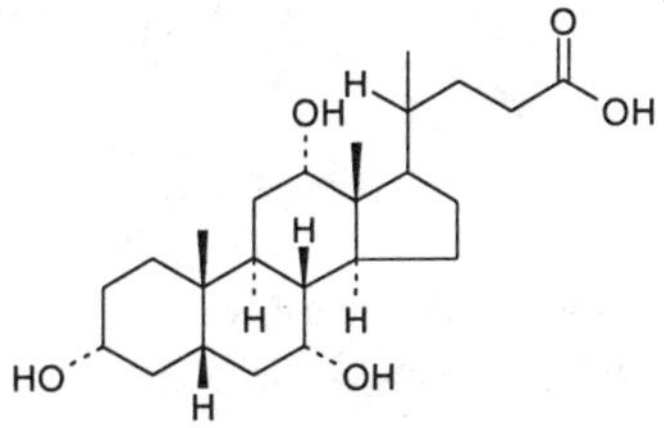

1034 Choline
Source: BAN XIA, CHUAN XIONG, DANG GUI, DANG SHEN, FU LING, HUANG QI, REN SHEN, ZHI MU. Ref: 2.

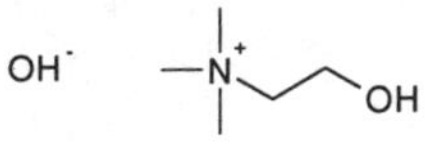

1035 Chondroitin sulfuric acid
Source: LU RONG. Ref: 2.

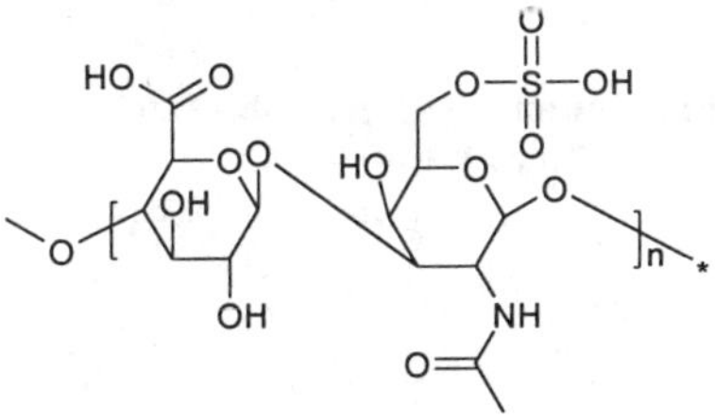

1036 Chrysanthemaxanthin
$C_{40}H_{56}O_3$ MW: 584.89 Property: mp 184-5°C. Source: QIAN LI GUANG, YE JU. Ref: 6.

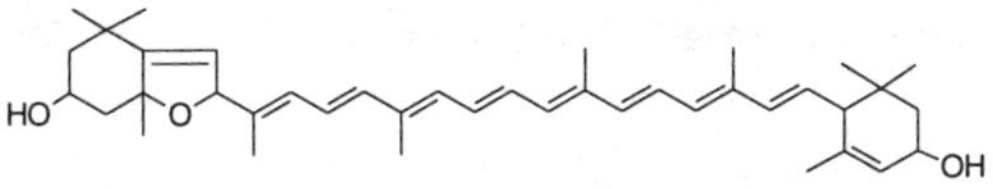

1037 Chrysanthemin
$C_{21}H_{21}O_{11}$•Cl MW: 449.39•35.45 Property: mp 205°C (dec). Source: BAI FAN DOU, DI YU, DU JUAN HUA, HEI DA DOU PI, JU HUA, LING MU, QIU MU GUA, TOU GU CAO, YE JU, YE JU HUA. Ref: 6.

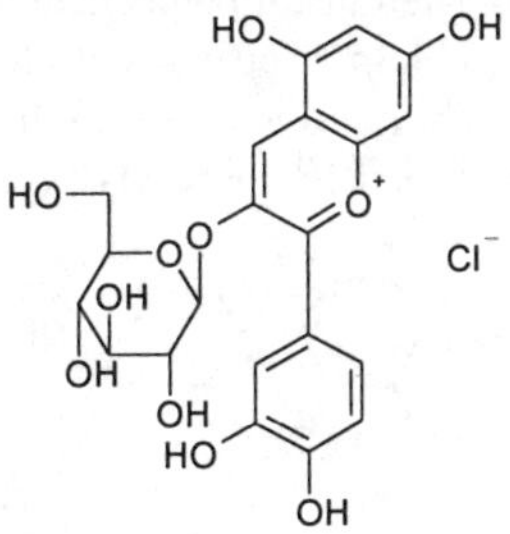

1038 Chrysanthemol
$C_{15}H_{26}O_2$ MW: 238.37 Property: white crystal, mp 144-6°C, $[\alpha]_D^{20}$ +5.8° (chloroform). Source: YE JU HUA. Ref: 90.

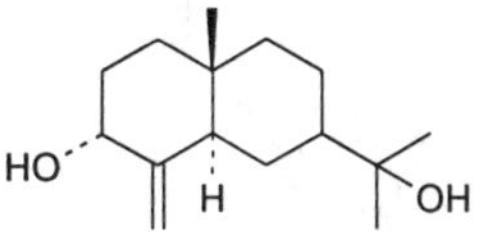

1039 Chrysanthenone
$C_{10}H_{14}O$ MW: 150.22 Property: bp 105-14°C/44mm. Source: JU HUA. Ref: 6.

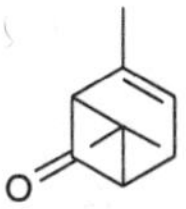

1040 Chrysanthetriol
$C_{15}H_{26}O_3$ MW: 254.37 Property: colorless oleaginous viscose liquid, $[\alpha]_D^{20}$ -31.8° (c=0.3, chloroform). Source: YE JU HUA. Ref: 222.

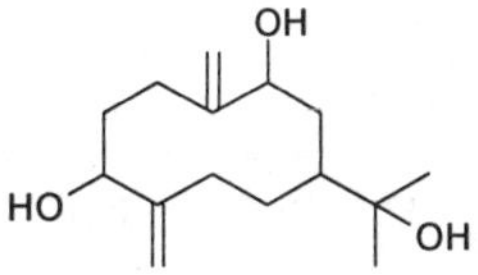

1041 Chrysarobin
$C_{15}H_{12}O_3$ MW: 240.26 Source: JUE MING ZI, LI LA GEN. Ref: 6, 627.

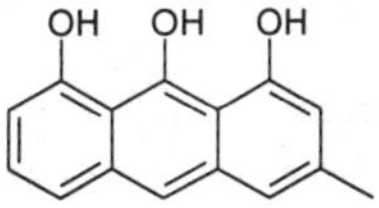

1042 Chrysergonic acid
Source: MAI JIAO. Ref: 6.

1043 Chrysin
5,7-dihydroxy-2-phenyl 4H-1-Benzopyran-4-one. CAS: 481-74-3 $C_{15}H_{10}O_4$ MW: 254.24 Property: yellow granular crystal (MeOH), mp 266-8°C. Source: FENG JIAO, HUANG QIN. Ref: 2, 5, 463.

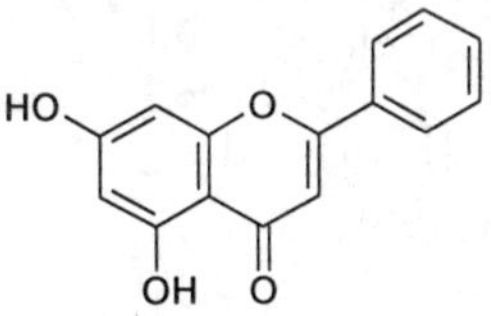

1044 Chrysoeriol
$C_{16}H_{12}O_6$ MW: 300.27 Source: QING HAO. Ref: 2.

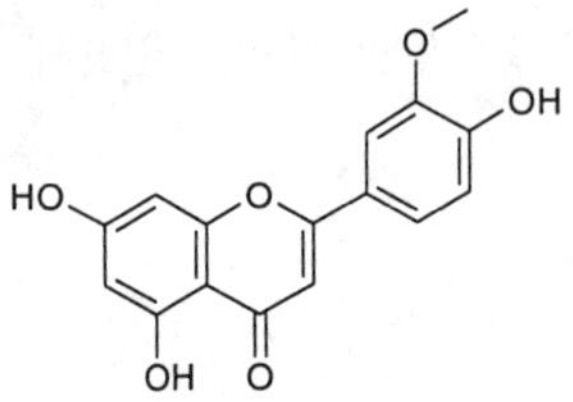

1045 Chrysoeriol-7-apio-glucoside
Graveobioside B. $C_{27}H_{30}O_{15}$ MW: 574.53 Property: mp 214-6°C. Source: HAN QIN. Ref: 6.

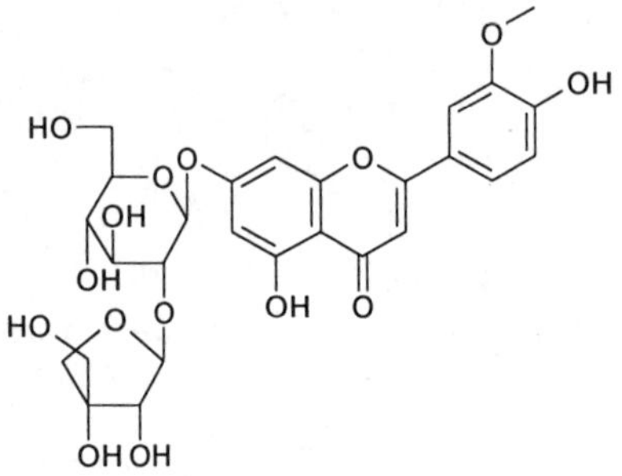

1046 Chrysograyanin
$C_{18}H_{16}O_8$ MW: 360.32 Property: mp 245-7°C. Source: JIN QIAN KU YE CAO. Ref: 6.

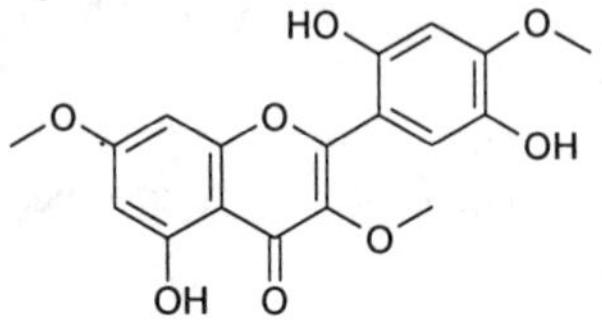

1047 Chrysophanein
Chrysophanol-1-O-β-D-glucopyranoside; Chrysophanol-1-monoglucoside. Property: mp 245°C. Source: DA HUANG, NIU ER DA HUANG, SUAN MO. Ref: 2, 6.

1048 Chrysophanol
Chrysophanic acid; 3-Methylchrysazin. CAS: 481-74-3 $C_{15}H_{10}O_4$ MW: 254.24 Property: mp 196-201°C (sublimation). Source: CHUAN XIONG, DA HUANG, HE SHOU WU, HU ZHANG, NIU XI, JUE MING ZI, LU HUI, TIAN SHAN DA HUANG. Ref: 2, 4, 582, 608, 627.

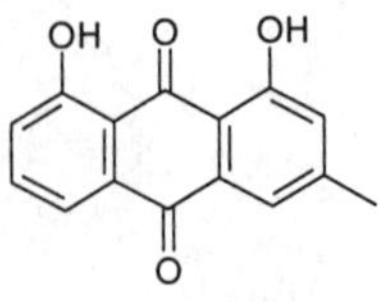

1049 Chrysophanic acid anthrone
$C_{15}H_{12}O_3$ MW: 240.26 Source: HE SHOU WU, JUE MING ZI. Ref: 2.

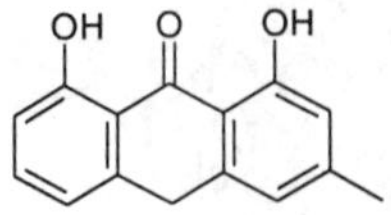

1050 Chrysophanol diglucoside
Source: DA HUANG. Ref: 2.

1051 Chrysophanol glucoside
$C_{21}H_{20}O_9$ MW: 416.39 Source: LU HUI. Ref: 2.

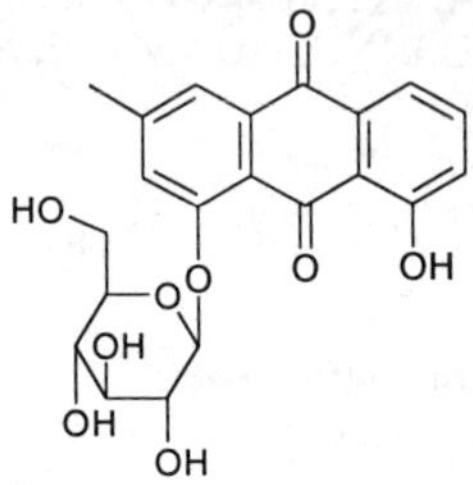

1052 Chrysophanol-1-β-gentiobioside
Source: JUE MING ZI. Ref: 2.

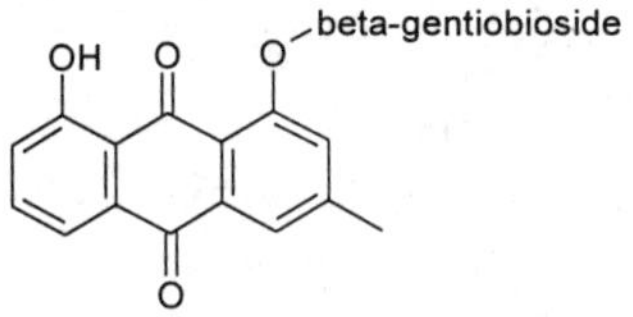

1053 Chrysophanol-8-O-β-D-glucopyranoside
$C_{21}H_{20}O_9$ MW: 416.39 Source: DA HUANG, TIAN SHAN DA HUANG. Ref: 2, 608.

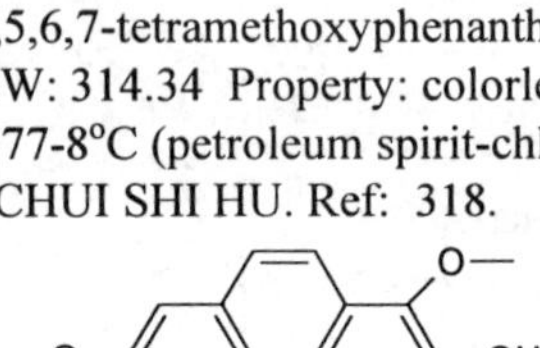

1054 Chrysotoxene
2-hydroxy-1,5,6,7-tetramethoxyphenanthrene. $C_{18}H_{18}O_5$ MW: 314.34 Property: colorless lamellar crystal, mp 177-8°C (petroleum spirit-chloroform). Source: GU CHUI SHI HU. Ref: 318.

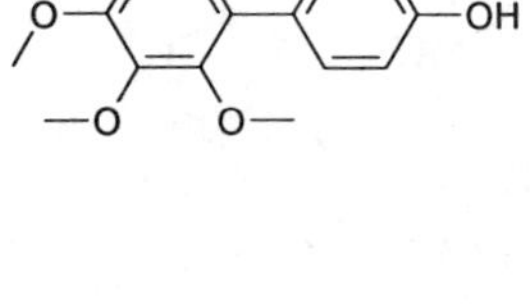

1055 Chrysotoxine
4-hydroxy-3,5,3',4'-tetramethoxybibenzyl. $C_{18}H_{22}O_5$ MW: 318.37 Property: colorless needle(n-hexane-chloroform), mp 97-8 °C. Source: GU CHUI SHI HU. Ref: 318, 351.

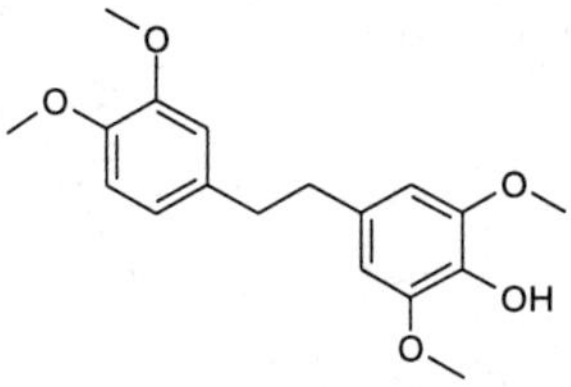

1056 Chuanbeinone
$C_{26}H_{41}NO_2$ MW: 399.62 Source: CHUAN BEI MU, NING XIA BEI MU. Ref: 2, 271.

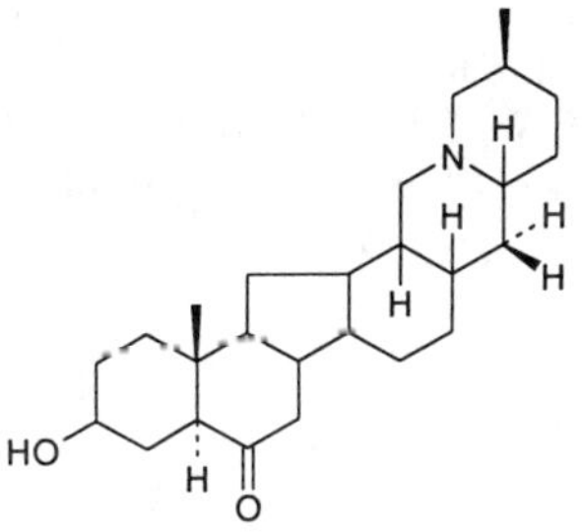

1057 Chuan-wu-base A
$C_{27}H_{37}NO_6$ Source: FU ZI. Ref: 2.

1058 Chuanxiongol
$C_{13}H_{14}O_3$ MW: 218.25 Source: CHUAN XIONG. Ref: 2.

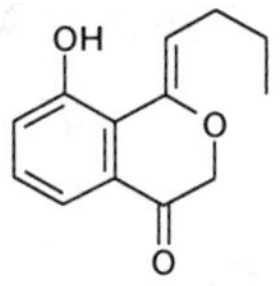

1059 Chuanxiongzine
Tetramethyl-pyrazine. CAS: 1124-11-4 $C_8H_{12}N_2$ MW: 136.20 Source: CHUAN XIONG, MA HUANG. Ref: 2, 4.

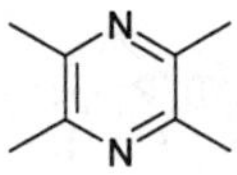

1060 Cichoriin
$C_{15}H_{16}O_9$ MW: 340.29 Property: mp 215-20°C. Source: JU QU. Ref: 6.

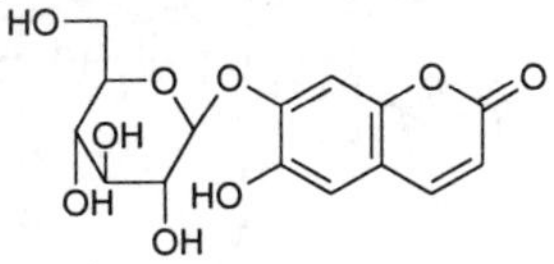

1061 Cicutol
$C_{14}H_{18}O$ MW: 202.30 Property: mp 66°C. Source: DU QIN GEN. Ref: 6.

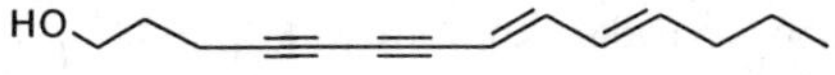

1062 Cicutoxin
$C_{15}H_{20}O_2$ MW: 232.33 Property: mp 54°C. Source: DU QIN GEN. Ref: 6.

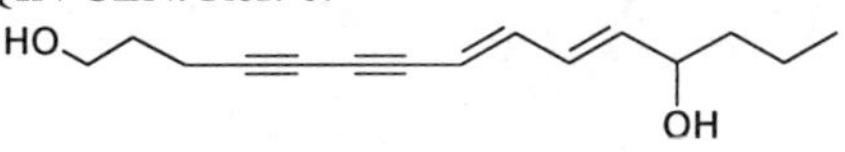

1063 Cimicifugenol
$C_{30}H_{48}O$ MW: 424.72 Property: mp 112-3°C. Sourcc: SAN MIAN DAO, YE SHENG MA. Ref: 6.

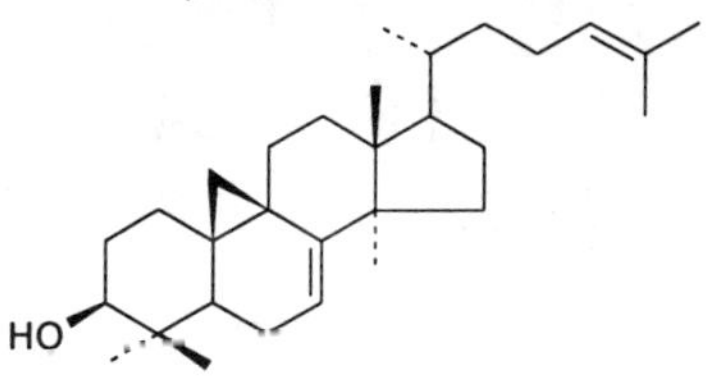

1064 Cimicifugin
Source: FANG FENG. Ref: 2.

1065 Cimicifugoside
$C_{37}H_{54}O_{11}$ MW: 674.84 Property: mp 237-8°C. Source: YE SHENG MA. Ref: 6.

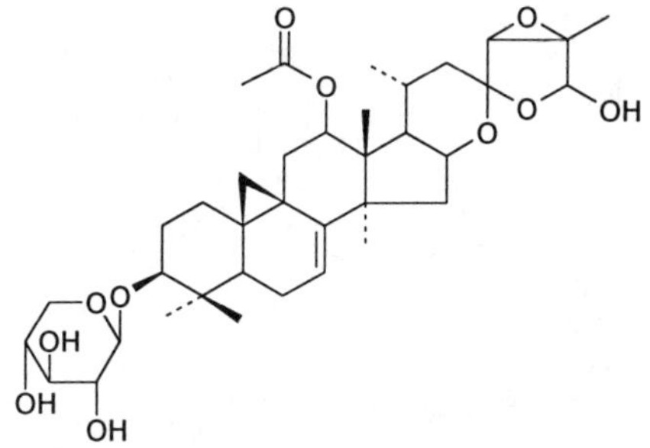

1066 Cimidahurine
3,4-Dihydroxy-β-phenethanol-3-O-β-D-galacto-pyranoside. $C_{14}H_{20}O_8$ MW: 316.31 Property: white amorphous powder, mp 78-80°C, $[\alpha]_D^{17}$ -51.2° (c=0.15, methanol). Source: XING AN SHENG MA. Ref: 294.

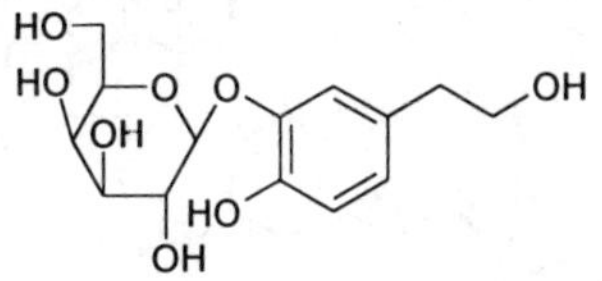

1067 Cimidahurinine
3,4-Dihydroxy-β-phenethanol-3-O-β-D-glucopyranoside. $C_{14}H_{20}O_8$ MW: 316.31 Property: white amorphous powder, mp 86-90°C, $[\alpha]_D^{17}$ -45.6° (c = 0.07, methanol). Source: XING AN SHENG MA. Ref: 294.

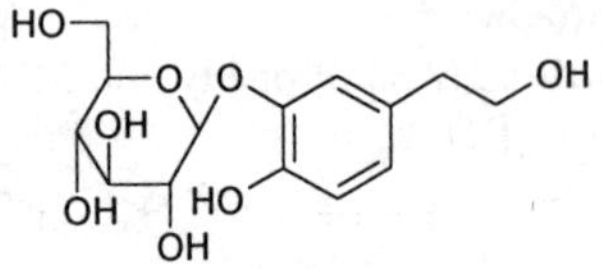

1068 Cimigenoside
$C_{34}H_{54}O_9$ MW: 606.80 Property: mp 261-4°C. Source: YE SHENG MA. Ref: 6.

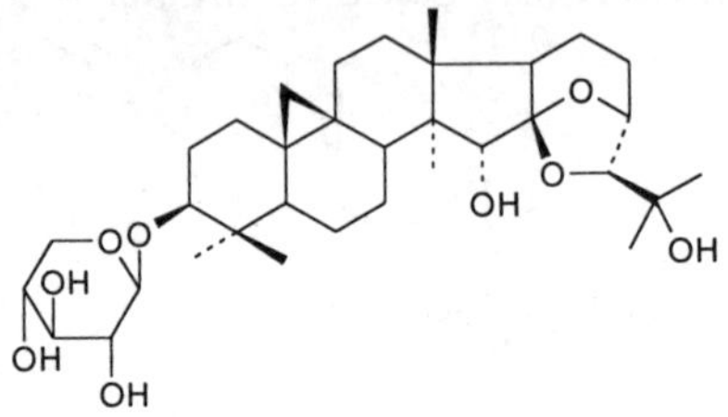

1069 Cimiside A
$C_{35}H_{56}O_{10}$ MW: 636.83 Property: colorless acicular crystal, mp 262-4°C, $[\alpha]_D^{15}$ -36.8° (c=0.063, $CHCl_3$-CH_3OH (1:1)). Source: XIN GAN SHENG MA. Ref: 282.

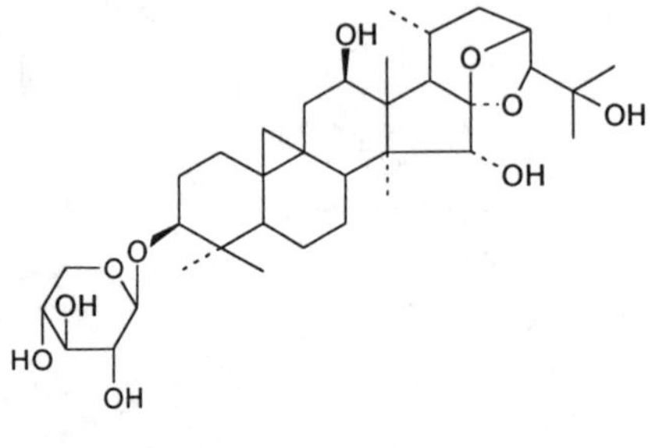

1070 Cimiside B
$C_{40}H_{64}O_{13}$ MW: 752.95 Property: white amorphous powder, $[\alpha]_D^{15}$ -15.3° (c=0.072, $CHCl_3$-CH_3OH (1:1)). Source: XING AN SHENG MA. Ref: 282.

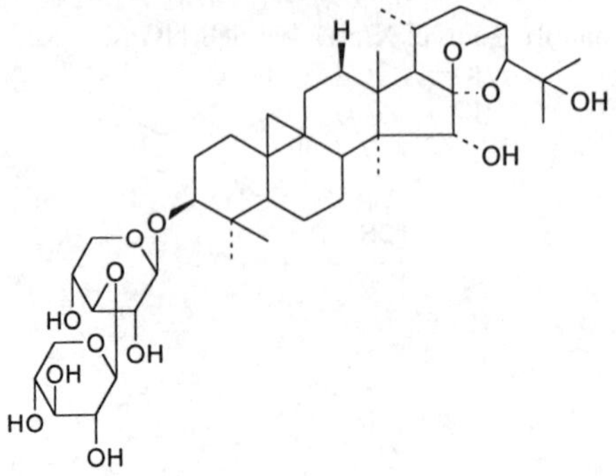

1071 Cimiside E
25-Anhydrocimicigenol-3-O-β-D-xylopyranoside (23R,24S). $C_{35}H_{54}O_8$ MW: 602.82 Property: colorless acicular crystal, mp >300°C, $[\alpha]_D^{19}$ +31.4° (c=0.058, chloroform-methanol (1:1)). Source: SHENG MA. Ref: 304.

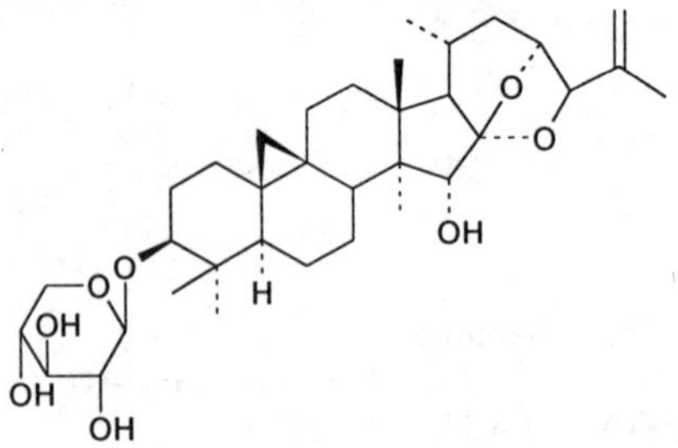

1072 Cimiside F
$C_{36}H_{58}O_{10}$ MW: 650.86 Property: white powder, mp 107-10°C, $[\alpha]_D^{29}$ 0° (c=0.075, methanol). Source: SHENG MA. Ref: 320.

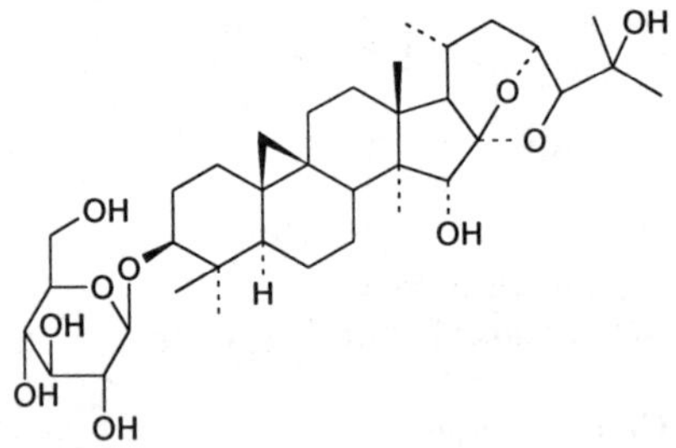

1073 Cinchamidine
Hydrocinchonidine. $C_{19}H_{24}N_2O$ MW: 296.42 Source: JIN JI LE. Ref: 6.

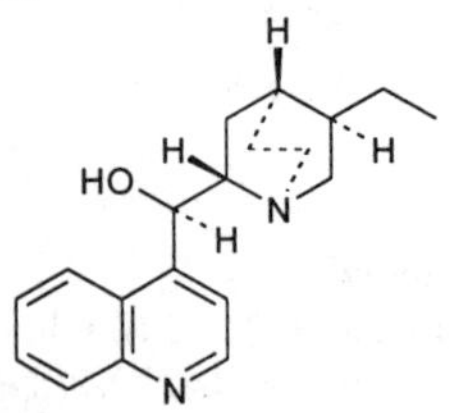

1074 Cincholic acid
$C_{30}H_{46}O_5$ MW: 486.70 Property: mp 265-8°C (dec). Source: SHUI TUAN HUA. Ref: 6.

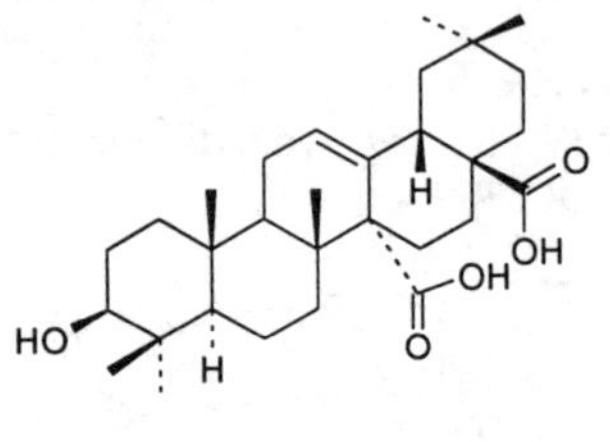

1075 Cinchonamine
$C_{19}H_{24}N_2O$ MW: 296.42 Property: mp 186°C.
Source: JIN JI LE. Ref: 6.

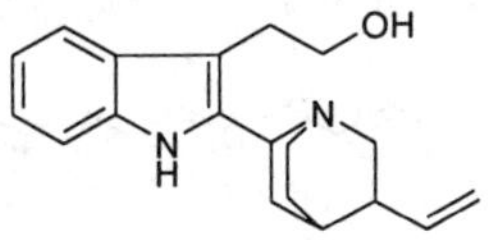

1076 Cinchonic acid
$C_{10}H_7NO_2$ MW: 173.17 Property: mp 253-4°C.
Source: SHE XIANG CAO. Ref: 6.

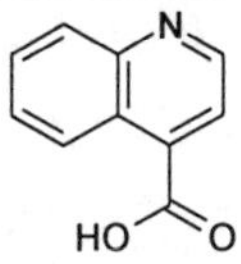

1077 Cinchonicine
$C_{19}H_{22}N_2O$ MW: 294.40 Property: mp 58-60°C.
Source: JIN JI LE. Ref: 6.

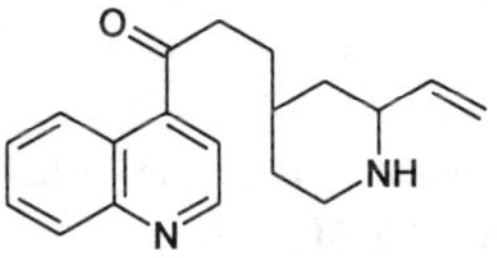

1078 Cinchonidine
$C_{19}H_{22}N_2O$ MW: 294.40 Property: mp 210.5°C.
Source: JIN JI LE. Ref: 6.

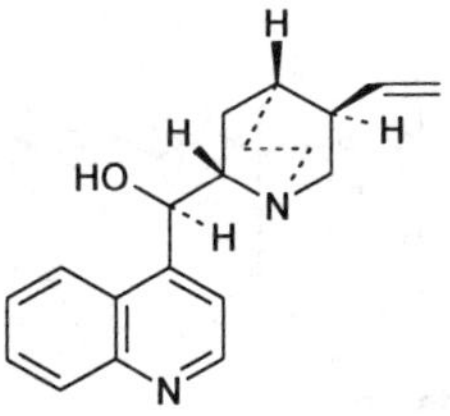

1079 Cinchonine
$C_{19}H_{22}N_2O$ MW: 294.40 Property: mp 255°C.
Source: JIN JI LE. Ref: 6.

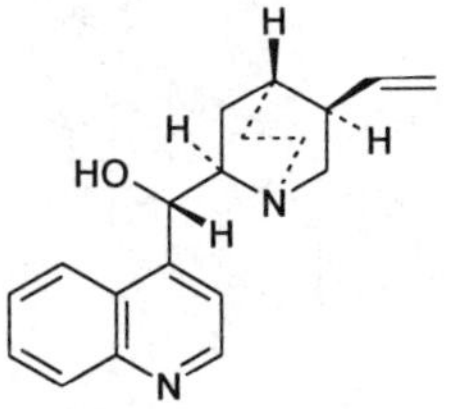

1080 Cinchotannic acid
$C_{14}H_{16}O_9$ MW: 328.28 Source: JIN JI LE. Ref: 6.

1081 Cinchotine
$C_{19}H_{24}N_2O$ MW: 296.42 Property: mp 268-9°C.
Source: JIN JI LE. Ref: 6.

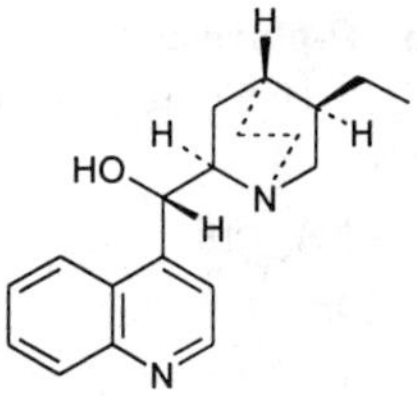

1082 1, 4-Cineole
$C_{10}H_{18}O$ MW: 154.25 Source: HOU PO. Ref: 2.

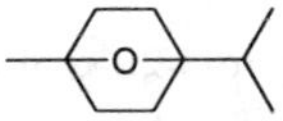

1083 1, 8-Cineole
$C_{10}H_{18}O$ MW: 154.25 Source: DONG LING CAO, GAN JIANG, QING HAO, SHENG JIANG, XI XIN. Ref: 2.

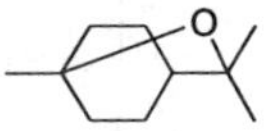

1084 Cinnamic acid
trans-Cirnnamic acid. CAS: 621-82-9 $C_9H_8O_2$ MW: 148.16 Property: mp 132-4°C. Source: DI GU PI, GAN DI HUANG, MA HUANG, ROU GUI. Ref: 2, 4.

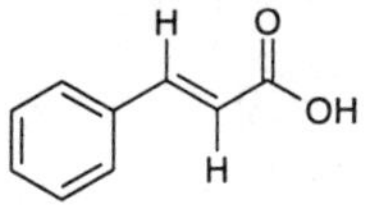

1085 Cinnamic alcohol
$C_9H_{10}O$ MW: 138.18 Property: mp 33°C, bp 258°C.
Source: SHUI XIAN HUA. Ref: 6.

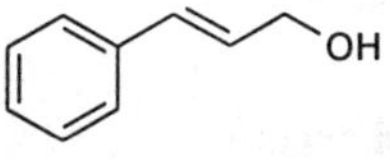

1086 Cinnamic aldehyde
C_9H_8O MW: 132.16 Source: GUI ZHI, HUO XIANG. Ref: 2.

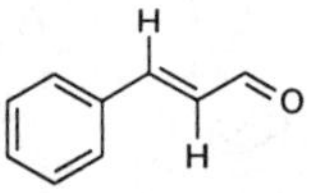

1087 2-O-Cinnamoyl-glucogallin
$C_{22}H_{22}O_{11}$ MW: 462.41 Source: DA HUANG.
Ref: 2.

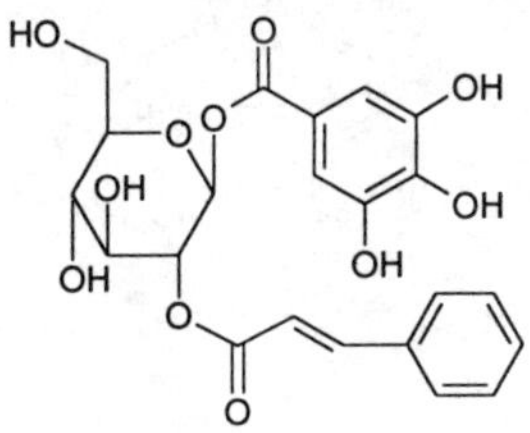

1088 2-Cinnamoyl-glucose
$C_{15}H_{18}O_7$ MW: 310.31 Source: DA HUANG. Ref: 2.

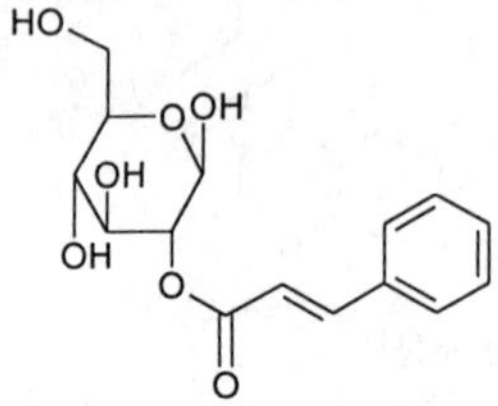

1089 12-O-Cinnamoyl-20-O-ikemaoyl sarcostin
$C_{37}H_{50}O_8$ MW: 622.81 Property: mp 158-63°C. Source: BAI SHOU WU. Ref: 6.

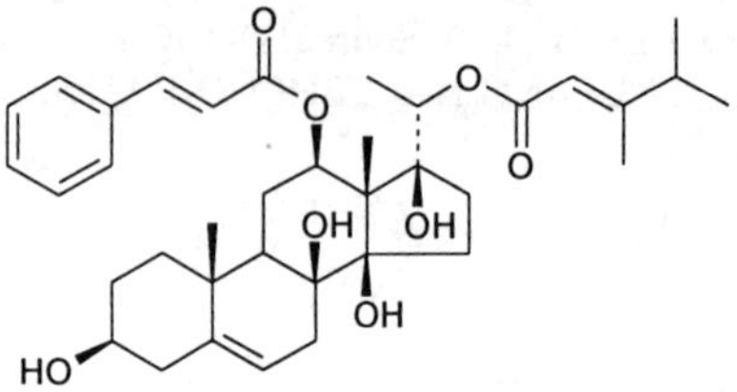

1090 12-O-Cinnamoyl-20-O-tigloyl sarcostin
$C_{35}H_{46}O_8$ MW: 594.75 Source: BAI SHOU WU. Ref: 6.

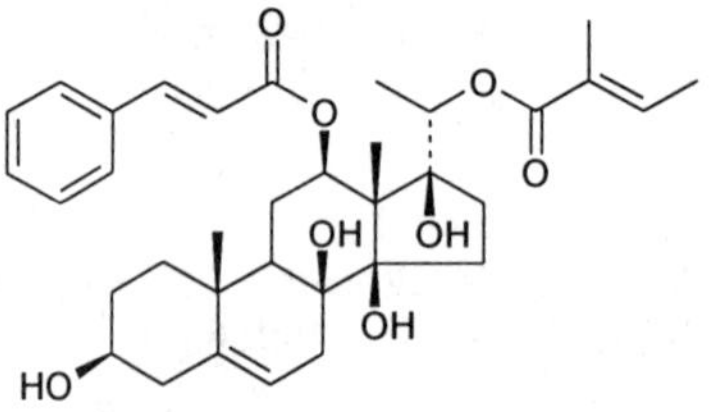

1091 Cinnamyl acetate
$C_{11}H_{12}O_2$ MW: 176.22 Property: bp 141°C/18mm. Source: ROU GUI. Ref: 6.

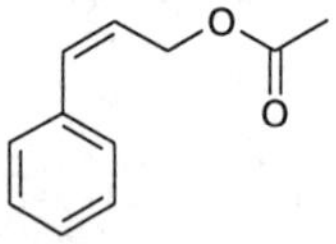

1092 Cinnamyl benzoate
$C_{16}H_{14}O_2$ MW: 238.29 Property: bp 209°C/12mm. Source: AN XI XIANG. Ref: 6.

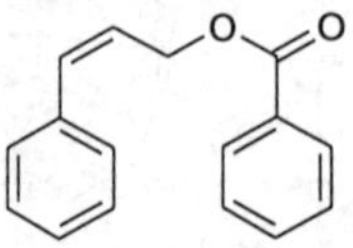

1093 Cinnamyl cinnamate
$C_{18}H_{16}O_2$ MW: 264.33 Property: mp 44°C. Source: AN XI XIANG. Ref: 6.

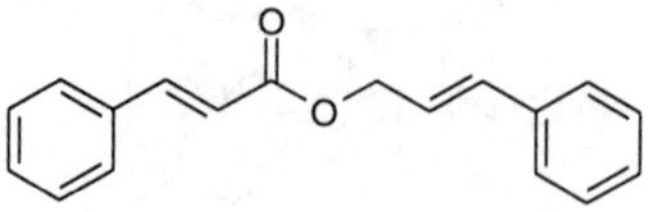

1094 Cinobufagin
$C_{26}H_{34}O_6$ MW: 442.56 Source: CHAN SU. Ref: 2, 617.

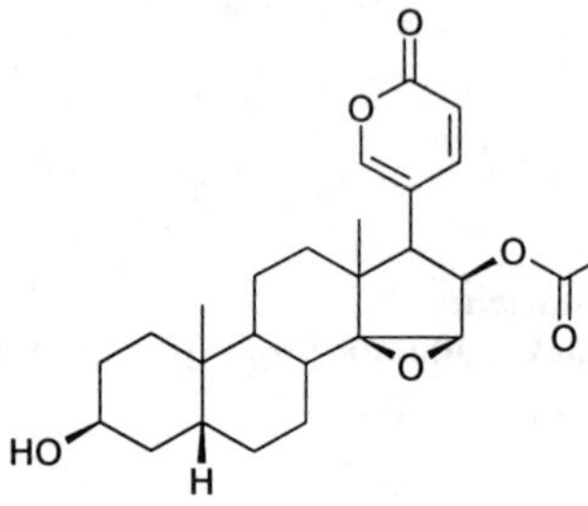

1095 Cinobufagin-3-hydrogen suberate
$C_{34}H_{46}O_9$ MW: 598.74 Source: CHAN SU. Ref: 2, 6.

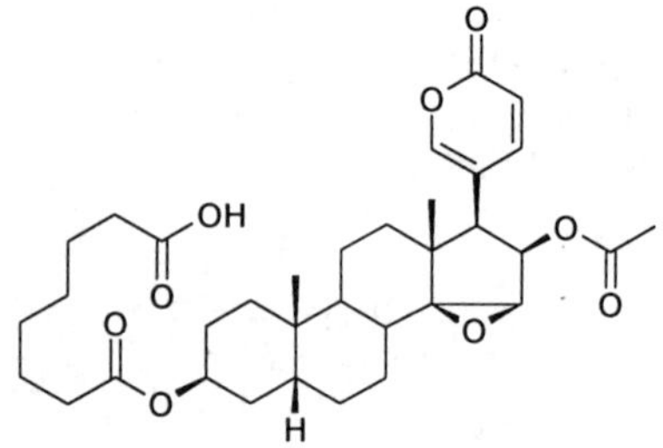

1096 Cinobufaginol
$C_{26}H_{34}O_7$ MW: 458.56 Source: CHAN SU. Ref: 2, 6.

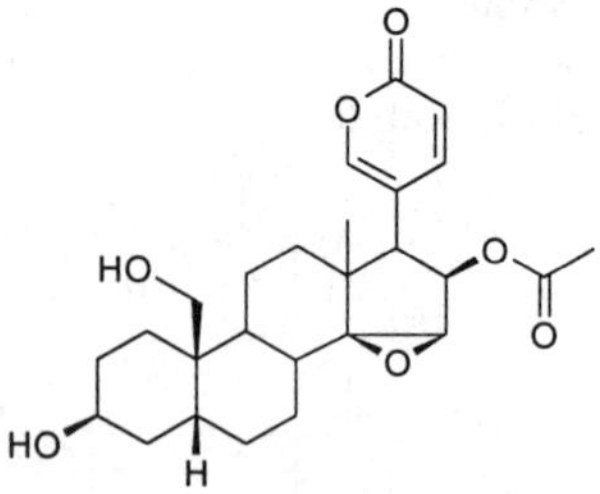

1097 Cinobufotalidin
$C_{24}H_{34}O_6$ Source: CHAN SU. Ref: 2.

1098 Cinobufotalin

$C_{26}H_{34}O_7$ MW: 458.56 Source: CHAN SU. Ref: 2.

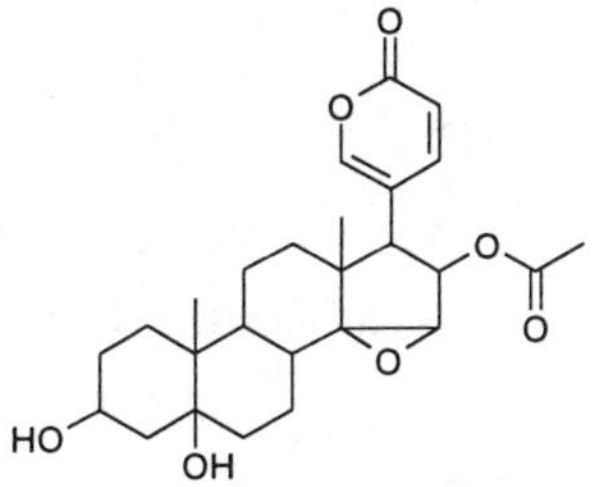

1099 Cinobufotenine

Bufotenine. $C_{12}H_{16}N_2O$ MW: 204.27 Source: CHAN SU. Ref: 2.

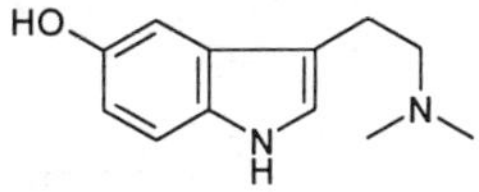

1100 Cinobufotoxin

$C_{40}H_{58}N_4O_{10}$ MW: 754.93 Source: CHAN SU. Ref; 2.

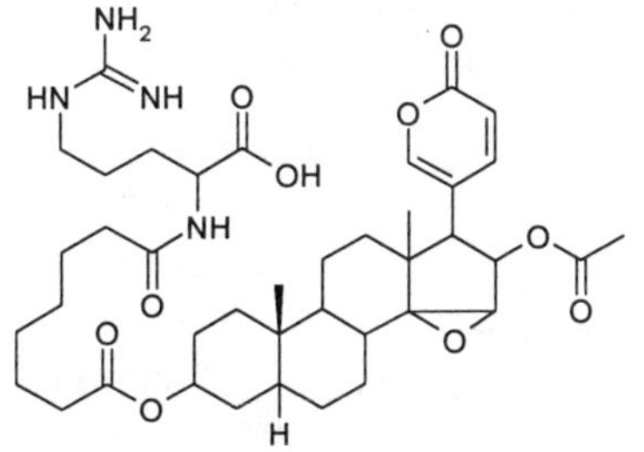

1101 Cirsilineol

$C_{18}H_{16}O_7$ MW: 344.32 Source: YIN CHEN HAO, QING HAO. Ref: 2.

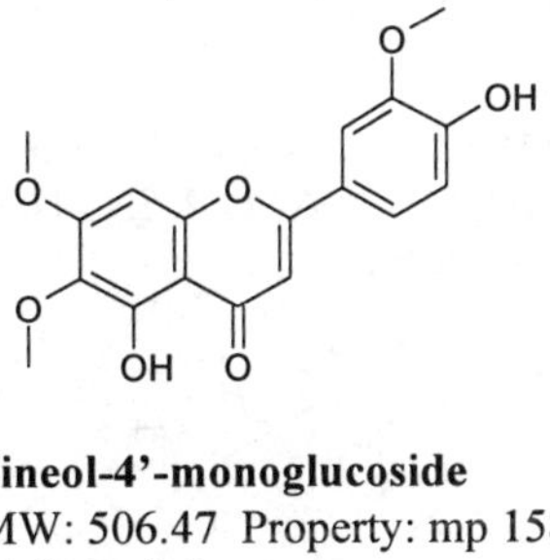

1102 Cirsilineol-4'-monoglucoside

$C_{24}H_{26}O_{12}$ MW: 506.47 Property: mp 158-9°C. Source: KU AO. Ref: 6.

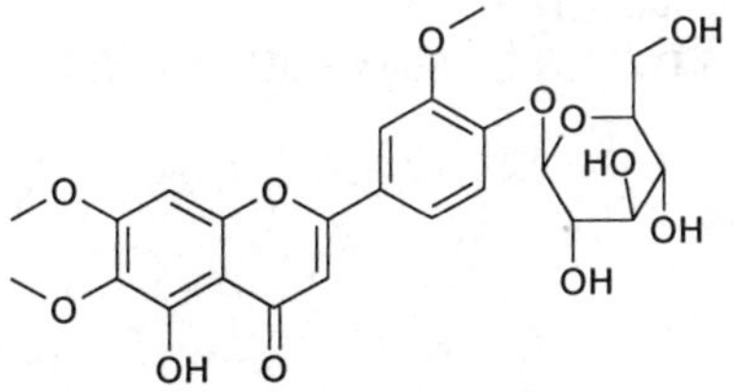

1103 Cirsiliol

$C_{17}H_{14}O_7$ MW: 330.30 Source: QING HAO. Ref: 2.

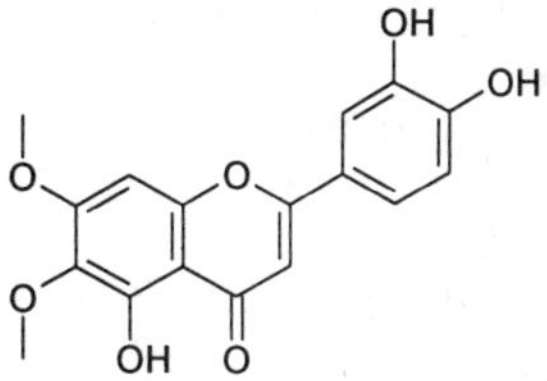

1104 Cirsiliol-4'-monoglucoside

$C_{23}H_{24}O_{12}$ MW: 492.44 Property: mp 215-7°C. Source: KU AO. Ref: 6.

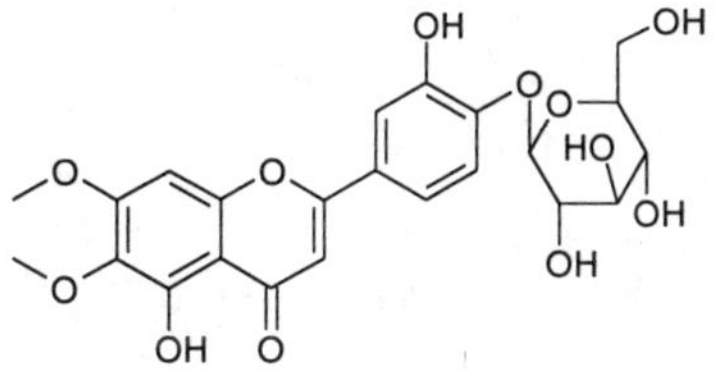

1105 Cirsimaritin

$C_{17}H_{14}O_6$ MW: 314.30 Source: QING HAO, YIN CHEN HAO. Ref: 2.

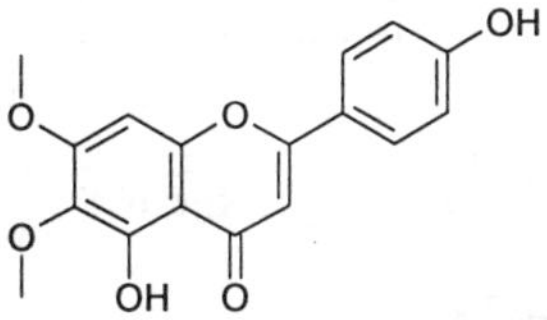

1106 Cissamine

Cyclanoline. $C_{20}H_{24}NO_4$ MW: 342.42 Source: FANG JI, XI SHENG TENG, ZHU SHA LIAN. Ref: 2, 4, 6.

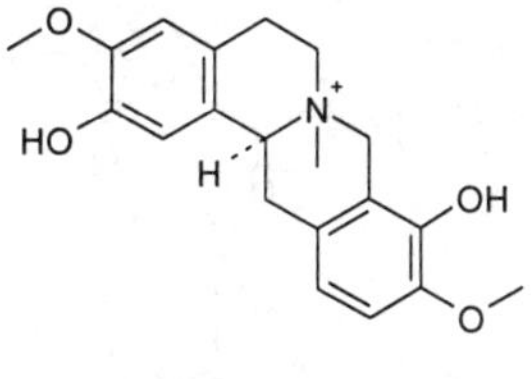

1107 Cissampareine

Methylwarifteine. CAS: 32728-54-4 $C_{37}H_{38}N_2O_6$ MW: 606.73 Property: mp 239-40°C (dec). Source: XI SHENG TENG. Ref: 5, 6.

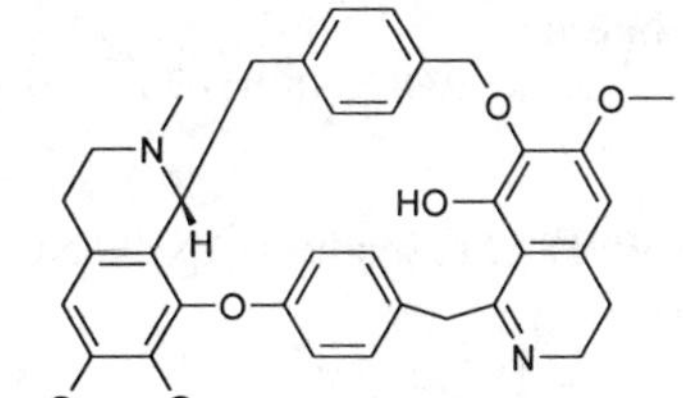

1108 Cistachlorin
Source: ROU CONG RONG. Ref: 628

1109 Cistanin
Source: ROU CONG RONG. Ref: 628.

1110 Cistanoside A
Source: GAN DI HUANG. Ref: 2, 628.

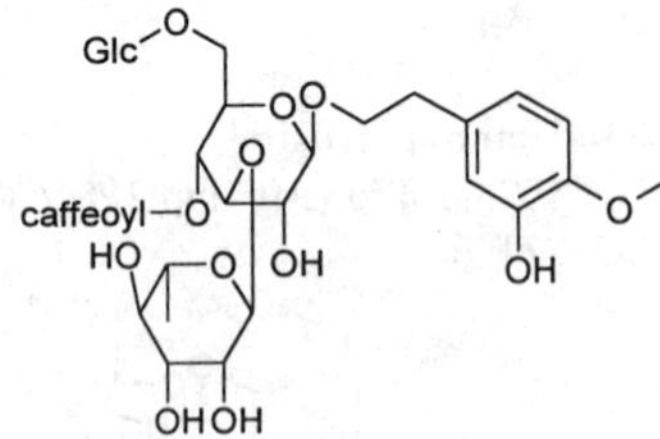

1111 Cistanoside B
Source: ROU CONG RONG. Ref: 628.

1112 Cistanoside C
Source: ROU CONG RONG. Ref: 628.

1113 Cistanoside D
Source: ROU CONG RONG. Ref: 628.

1114 Cistanoside E
Source: ROU CONG RONG. Ref: 628.

1115 Cistanoside F
$C_{21}H_{30}O_{13}$ MW: 490.47 Source: GAN DI HUANG. Ref: 2.

1116 Cistanoside G
Source: ROU CONG RONG. Ref: 628.

1117 Cistanoside I
Source: ROU CONG RONG. Ref: 628.

1118 Citral
$C_{10}H_{16}O$ MW: 152.24 Source: GAN JIANG, WU WEI ZI. Ref: 2.

1119 (E)-Citral
$C_{10}H_{16}O$ MW: 152.24 Source: SHENG JIANG. Ref: 2.

1120 (Z)-Citral
$C_{10}H_{16}O$ MW: 152.24 Source: SHENG JIANG. Ref: 2.

1121 Citraurin α
$C_{30}H_{40}O_2$ MW: 432.65 Property: mp 153°C. Source: DAI DAI HUA. Ref: 6.

1122 Citraurin β
$C_{30}H_{40}O_2$ MW: 432.65 Property: mp 146-7°C. Source: DAI DAI HUA. Ref: 6.

1123 Citreorosein
$C_{15}H_{10}O_6$ MW: 286.24 Source: HU ZHANG. Ref: 2.

1124 Citric acid
$C_6H_8O_7$ MW: 192.13 Source: CU LIU GUO (SHA JI), MA HUANG, PU HUANG, REN SHEN, SHAN ZHA, TIAN MA. Ref: 2.

1125 Citronellal
$C_{10}H_{18}O$ MW: 154.25 Source: JU PI. Ref: 2.

1126 Citronellol
$C_{10}H_{20}O$ MW: 156.27 Property: bp 222°C. Source: JIN YIN HUA, JIU LI XIANG, JU PI, SHENG JIANG, WU WEI ZI. Ref: 6, 11.

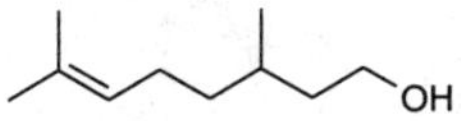

OH

1127 Citronellyl acetate
$C_{12}H_{22}O_2$ MW: 198.31 Source: SHENG JIANG, WU WEI ZI. Ref: 2.

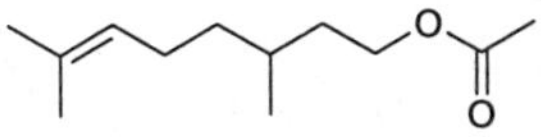

1128 Citropten
Limettin. CAS: 487-06-9 $C_{11}H_{10}O_4$ MW: 206.20 Property: mp 147.5°C. Source: FO SHOU (FO SHOU GAN), NING MENG, XIANG YUAN, XIANG YUAN YE. Ref: 5, 6.

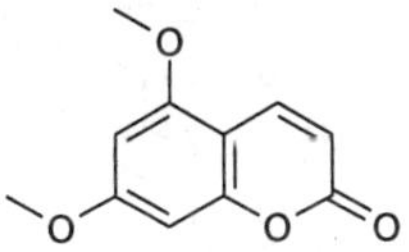

1129 Citrostadienol
$C_{30}H_{50}O$ MW: 426.73 Property: mp 162-4°C. Source: SHUI LONG GU. Ref: 6.

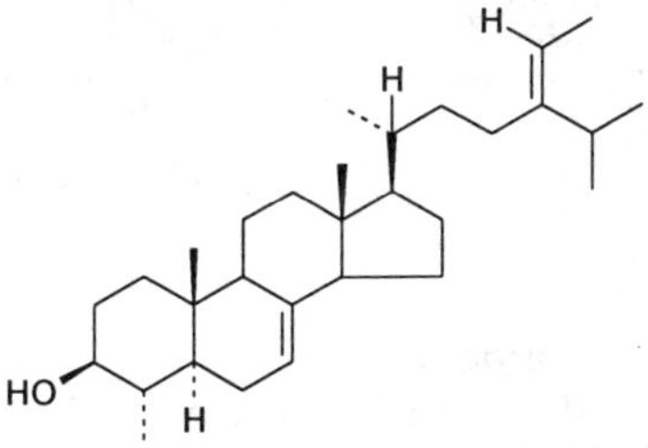

1130 Citrulline
$C_6H_{13}N_3O_3$ MW: 175.19 Property: mp 222°C. Source: DONG GUA ZI, HU TAO REN, KU GUA, MO GU, MU XU, NAN GUA, SHI ZI, SI GUA, TIAN HUA FEN, XI GUA. Ref: 2, 6.

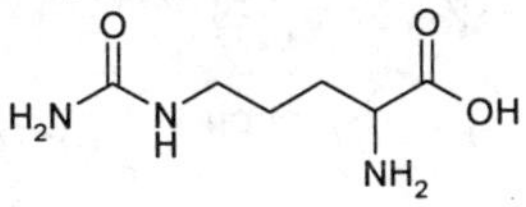

1131 Citrusin B
Source: DU ZHONG. Ref: 2.

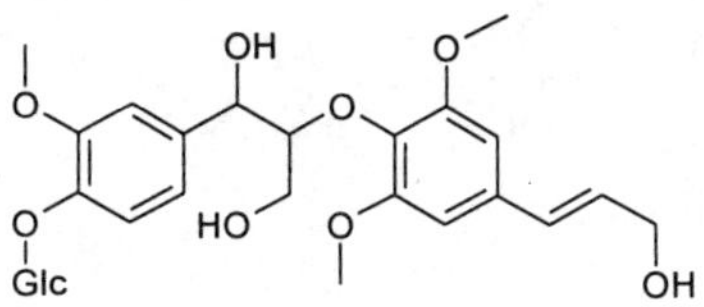

1132 Civetone
$C_{17}H_{30}O$ MW: 250.43 Property: mp 32.5°C, bp 342 °C/742mm. Source: LING MAO XIANG. Ref: 6.

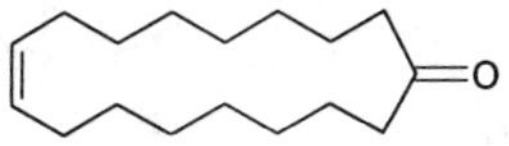

1133 Clausenamide
$C_{18}H_{19}NO_3$ MW: 297.36 Property: white acicular crystal (methanol), mp 239-40°C. Source: HUANG PI YE. Ref: 72.

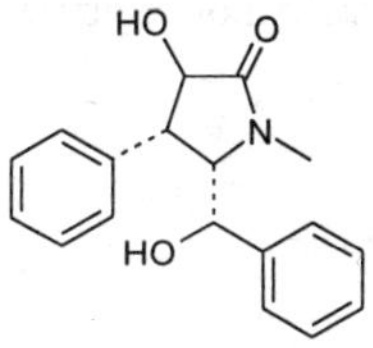

1134 Clausenidin
$C_{19}H_{20}O_5$ MW: 328.37 Property: mp 135-6°C. Source: SHAN HUANG PI. Ref: 6.

1135 Clausenin
$C_{14}H_{12}O_5$ MW: 260.25 Property: mp 156-7°C. Source: SHAN HUANG PI. Ref: 6.

1136 Clavatine
$C_{16}H_{25}NO_2$ MW: 263.38 Property: mp 212-3°C. Source: SHEN JIN CAO. Ref: 6.

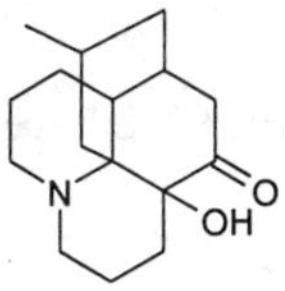

1137 Clavatol
$C_{28}H_{50}O_4$ MW: 450.71 Property: mp 277-9°C. Source: SHEN JIN CAO. Ref: 6.

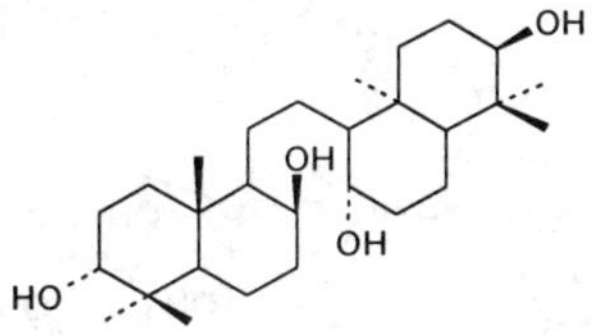

1138 Clavolonine
$C_{16}H_{25}NO_2$ MW: 263.38 Property: mp 238°C. Source: SHEN JIN CAO. Ref: 6.

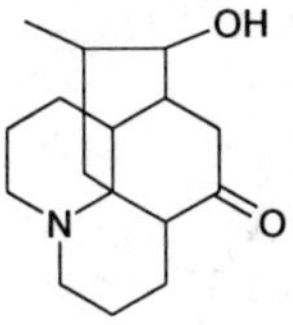

1139 Clavorubin
$C_{16}H_{10}O_8$ MW: 330.25 Source: MAI JIAO. Ref: 6.

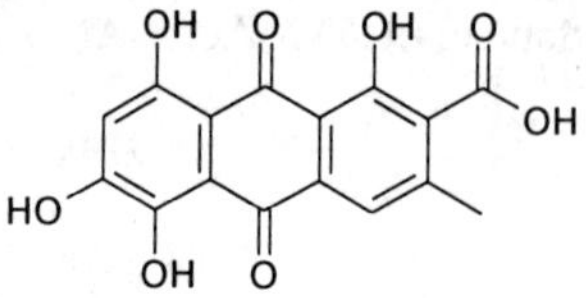

1140 Clematis prosapogenin, Cp7a
$C_{47}H_{76}O_{17}$ MW: 913.12 Property: white powdere, $[\alpha]_D^{20}$ -18° (c=0.8, methanol). Source: CI QIU. Ref: 457.

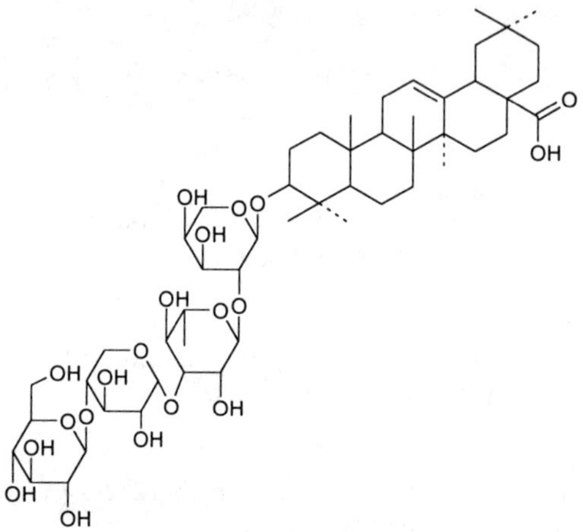

1141 Clematoside A
$C_{81}H_{132}O_{43}$ MW: 1793.93 Source: WEI LING XIAN. Ref: 6.

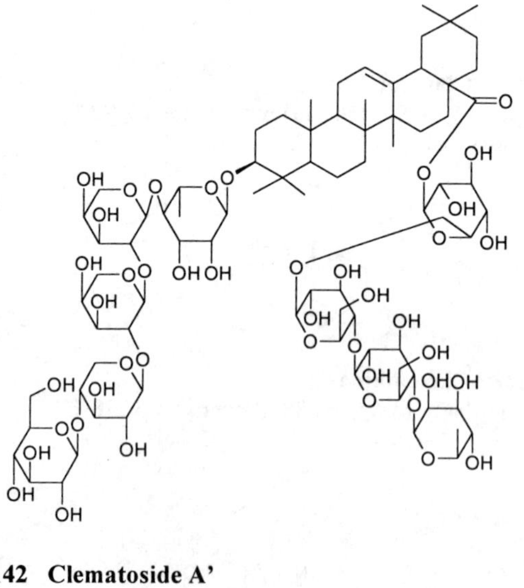

1142 Clematoside A'
$C_{57}H_{92}O_{24}$ MW: 1161.35 Property: mp 176-9°C. Source: WEI LING XIAN. Ref: 6.

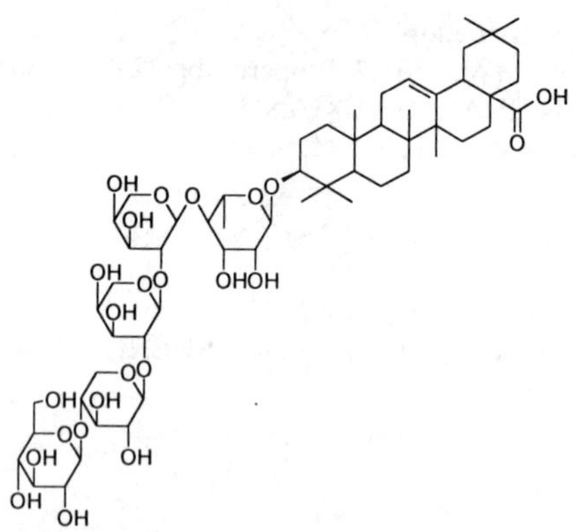

1143 Clematoside B
$C_{87}H_{142}O_{48}$ MW: 1955.07 Property: mp 200-2°C. Source: WEI LING XIAN. Ref: 6.

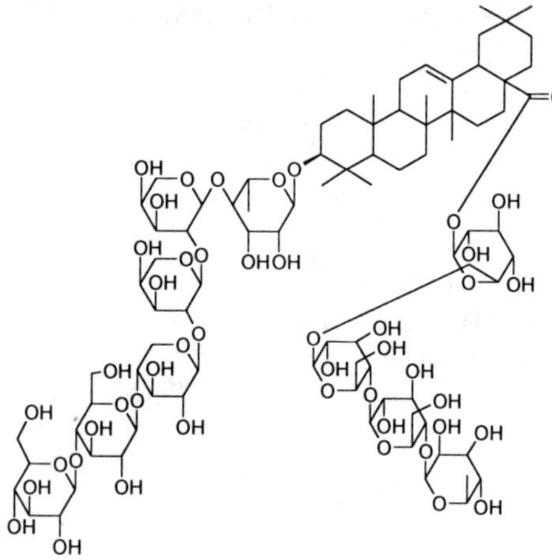

1144 Clematoside C
$C_{93}H_{152}O_{52}$ MW: 2102.22 Property: mp 213-5°C. Source: WEI LING XIAN. Ref: 6.

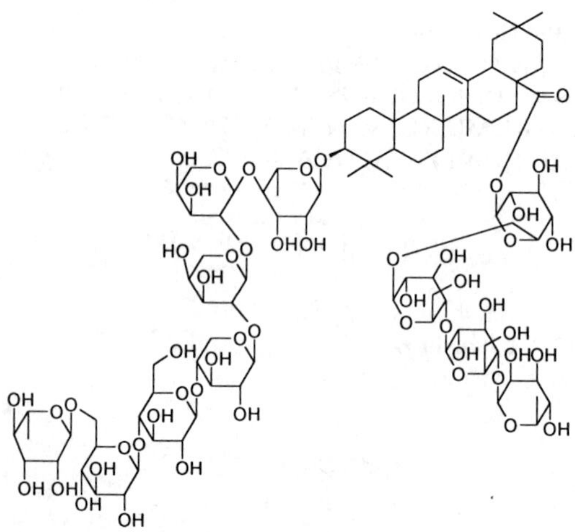

1145 Cleomin
$C_6H_{11}NOS$ MW: 145.22 Property: mp 52°C. Source: BAI HUA CAI ZI. Ref: 6.

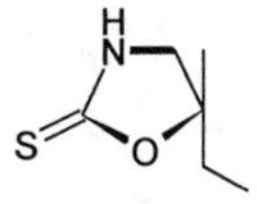

1146 Clerodendrin
Property: mp 215°C (dec). Source: CHOU WU TONG. Ref: 6.

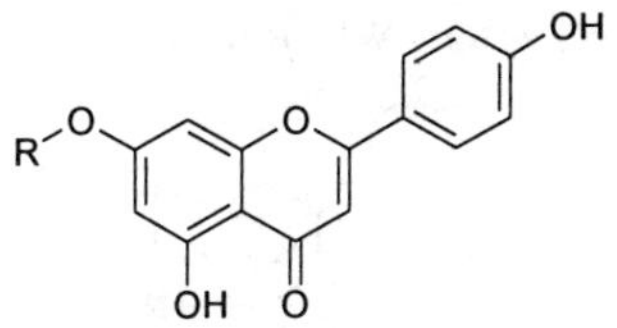

1147 Clerodendrin A
$C_{34}H_{48}O_{11}$ MW: 632.76 Source: CHOU WU TONG. Ref: 6.

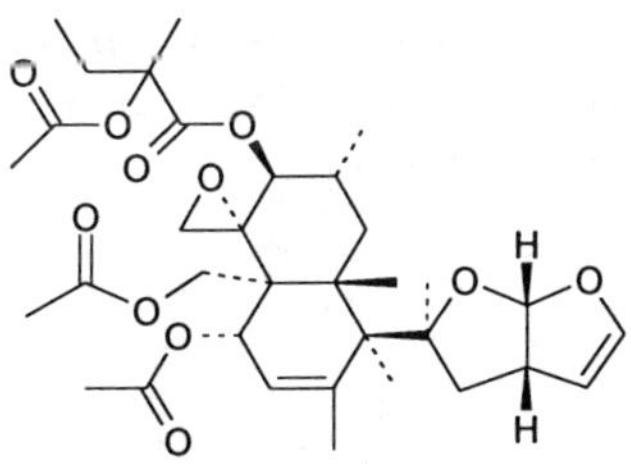

1148 Clerodin
$C_{20}H_{30}O_5$ MW: 350.46 Property: mp 161-2°C (dec). Source: GUI DENG LONG. Ref: 6.

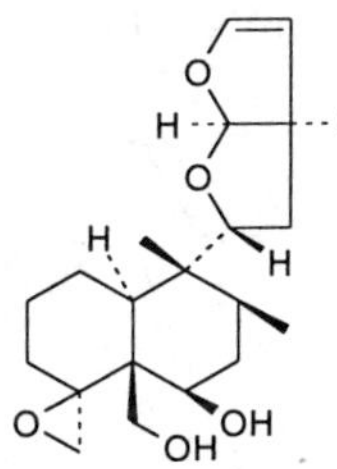

1149 Clerodolone
$C_{30}H_{48}O_3$ MW: 456.72 Property: mp 282-4°C. Source: GUI DENG LONG, CHOU WU TONG GEN. Ref: 6.

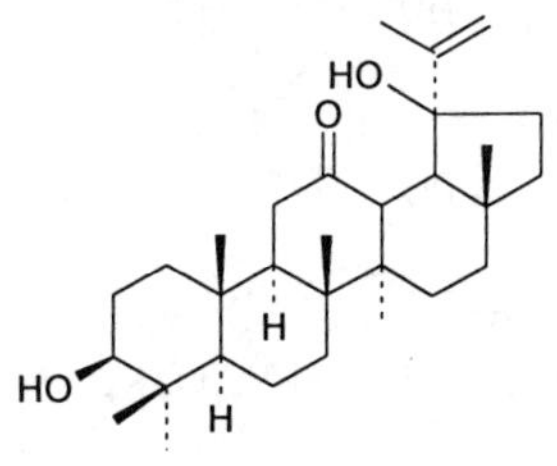

1150 Clerodone
$C_{30}H_{50}O$ MW: 426.73 Property: mp 260°C. Source: GUI DENG LONG, CHOU WU TONG GEN. Ref: 6.

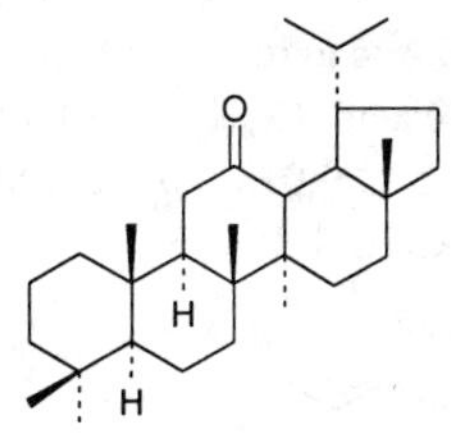

1151 Clerosterol
$C_{29}H_{48}O$ MW: 412.71 Property: mp 147°C. Source: GUI DENG LONG, CHOU WU TONG GEN. Ref: 6.

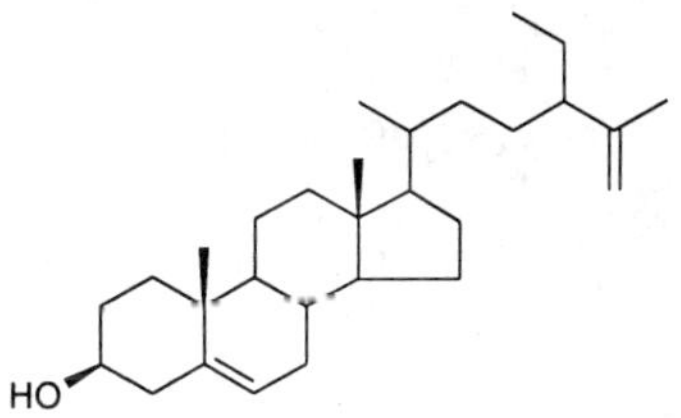

1152 Clinodiside A
3-O-β-D-Glucopyranosyl (1→6)-[β-D-glucopyranosyl(1→4)](β-D-glucopyranosyl-olean-11,13(18)-diene-3β,16β,23,28-tetrol. $C_{48}H_{78}O_{19}$ MW: 959.15 Property: white granular crystal, mp 249-51°C. Source: FENG LUN CAI. Ref: 224.

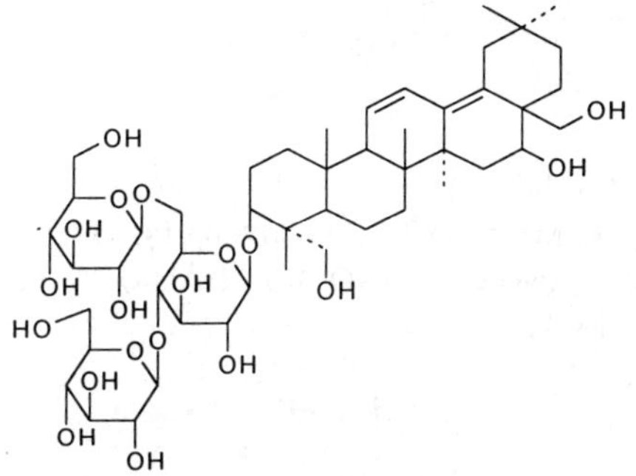

1153 Clivorine
$C_{21}H_{31}NO_7$ MW: 409.48 Property: mp 148-50°C. Source: HU LU QI. Ref: 6.

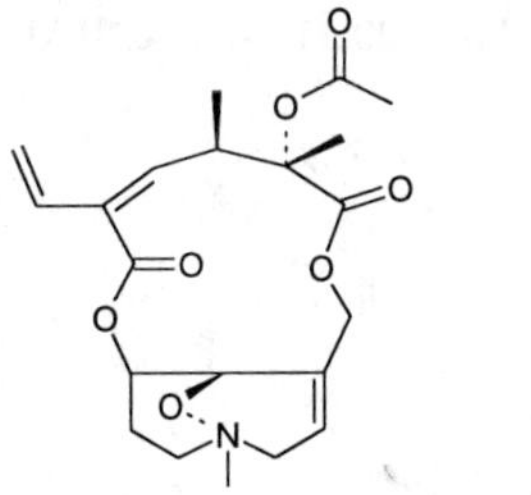

1154 Clovene
$C_{15}H_{24}$ Source: WU WEI ZI. Ref: 2.

1155 Clupanodonic acid
Docosa-pentenoic acid. $C_{18}H_{28}O_2$ MW: 276.42
Property: bp 174-5°C/0.018-0.02mm. Source: HAI REN CAO, SHI CHUN. Ref: 6.

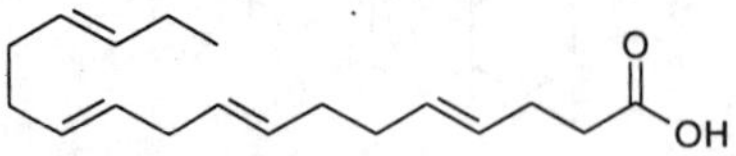

1156 Cluytyl ferulate
$C_{38}H_{66}O_4$ MW: 586.95 Source: HOU PI SHU. Ref: 6.

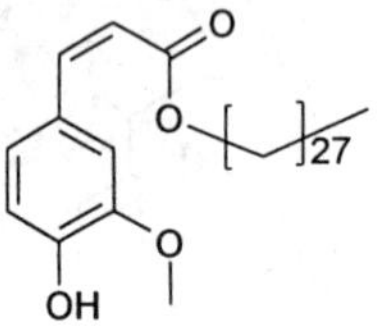

1157 Cnidiadin
$C_{18}H_{20}O_5$ MW: 316.36 Property: mp 144-5°C.
Source: SHE CHUANG ZI. Ref: 6.

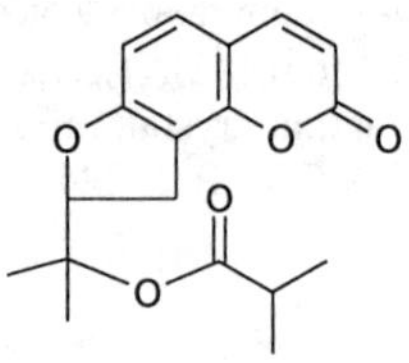

1158 Cnidilide
$C_{12}H_{18}O_2$ MW: 194.28 Property: bp 145-6°C/2.5mm.
Source: DANG GUI, GAO BEN, HAN QIN.
Ref: 6, 18, 19.

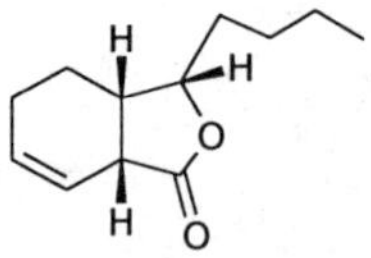

1159 Cnidilin
$C_{17}H_{16}O_5$ MW: 300.31 Source: BAI ZHI. Ref: 2.

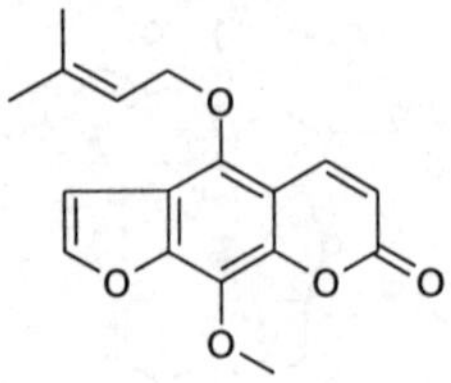

1160 Cnidium lactone
$C_{12}H_{18}O_2$ MW: 194.28 Source: CHUAN XIONG.
Ref: 2.

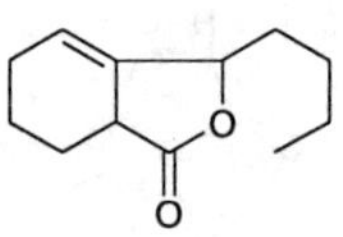

1161 Cocculidine
$C_{18}H_{23}NO_2$ MW: 285.39 Property: mp 86-7°C.
Source: HENG ZHOU WU. Ref: 6.

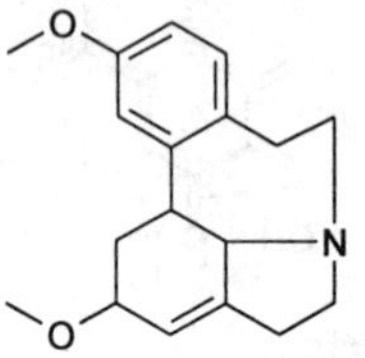

1162 Cocculine
$C_{17}H_{21}NO_2$ MW: 271.36 Property: mp 217-8°C.
Source: HENG ZHOU WU YAO. Ref: 6.

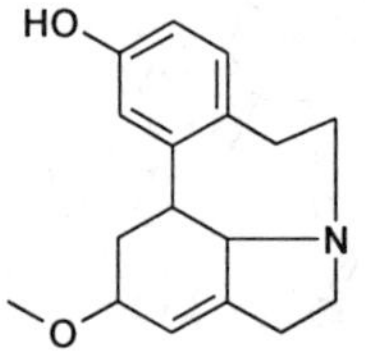

1163 Cocculolidine
$C_{15}H_{17}NO_3$ MW: 259.31 Property: mp 144-6°C.
Source: QING TAN XIANG. Ref: 6.

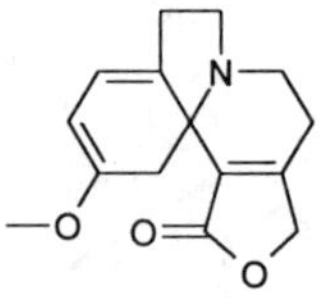

1164 Coclaurine
$C_{17}H_{19}NO_3$ MW: 285.35 Property: mp (-): 220-1°C.
Source: HENG ZHOU WU YAO. Ref: 6.

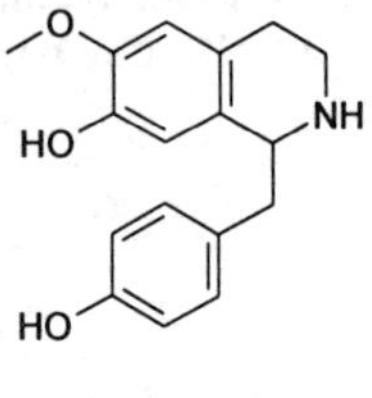

1165 Coclifoline
Source: HENG ZHOU WU YAO. Ref: 6.

1166 Coclobine
$C_{37}H_{38}N_2O_6$ MW: 606.73 Source: FANG JI. Ref: 6.

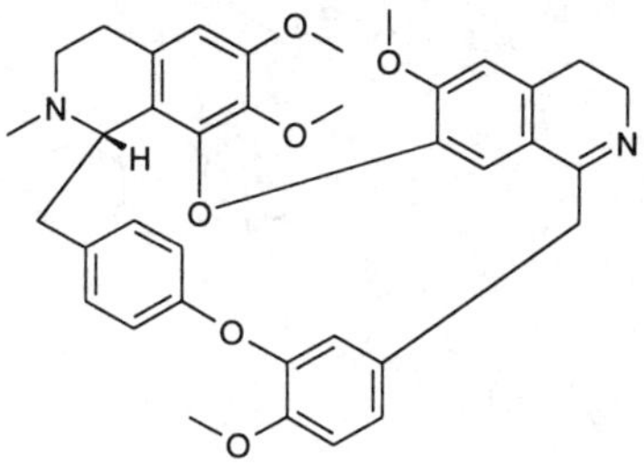

1167 Cocositol
$C_6H_{12}O_6$ MW: 180.16 Property: mp 353°C (dec). Source: YE ZI PI. Ref: 6.

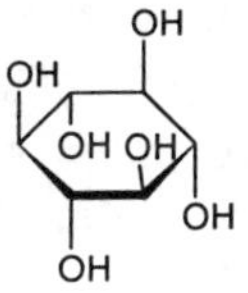

1168 Codamine
$C_{20}H_{25}NO_4$ MW: 343.43 Property: mp (+): 126-7°C, (-): 127-8°C, (±): 106-8°C. Source: YA PIAN. Ref: 6.

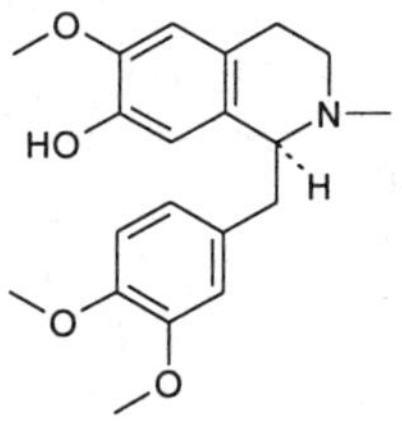

1169 Codeine
$C_{18}H_{21}NO_3$ MW: 299.37 Property: mp 155°C. Source: BAI YAO ZI,YA PIAN, YING SU, YING SU KE. Ref: 6.

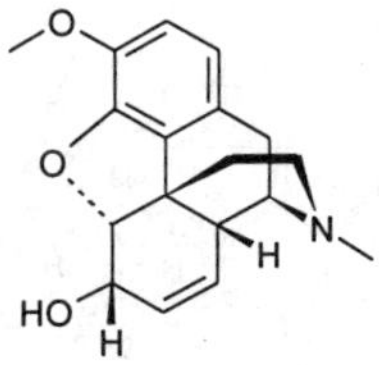

1170 Codonolactone
$C_{15}H_{20}O_3$ MW: 248.32 Source: DANG SHEN. Ref: 2.

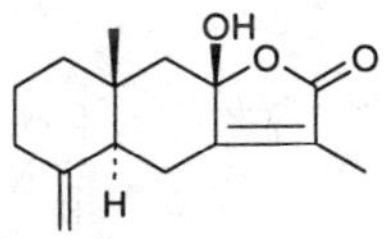

1171 Codopiloic acid
$C_5H_5NO_3$ MW: 127.10 Source: DANG SHEN. Ref: 2.

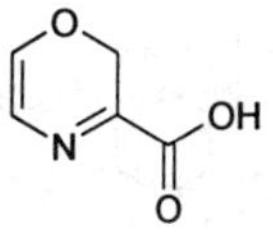

1172 Coenzyme I
$C_{21}H_{31}N_7O_{14}P_2$ MW: 667.47 Source: YUAN CAN ZI. Ref: 6.

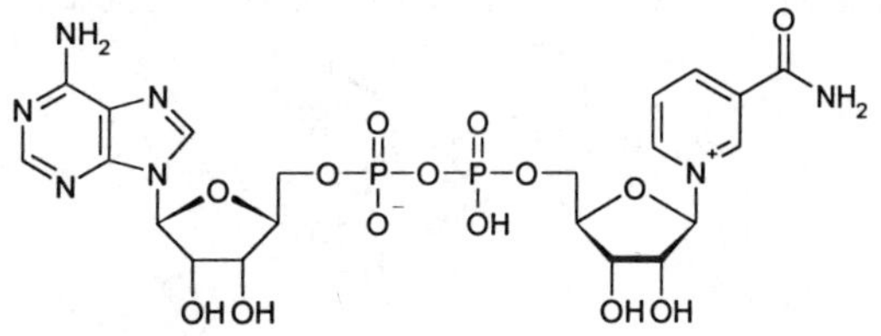

1173 Coenzyme II
$C_{21}H_{27}N_7O_{17}P_3$ MW: 742.41 Source: YUAN CAN ZI. Ref: 6.

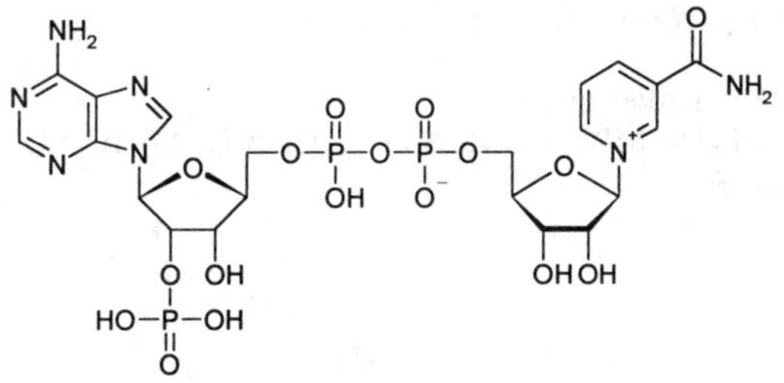

1174 Coetsoidin A
$C_{22}H_{26}O_6$ MW: 386.45 Property: colorless column crystal, mp 180-1°C. Source: JIA XI ZHUI XIANG CHA CAI. Ref: 132.

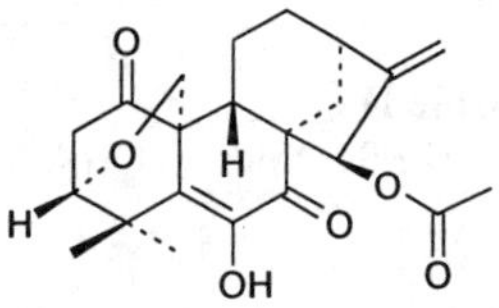

1175 Coixenolide
CAS: 290-43-1 $C_{38}H_{70}O_4$ MW: 590.98 Source: YI YI REN. Ref: 5, 6.

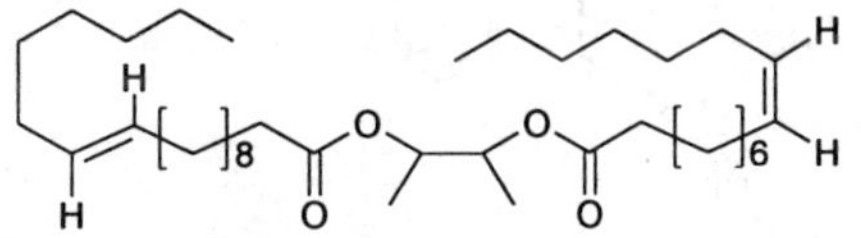

1176 Coixol
CAS: 53-91-2 $C_8H_7NO_3$ MW: 165.15 Property: mp 151-3°C. Source: BAI MAO GEN, LU GEN, YI YI REN, YI YI GEN. Ref: 4, 6.

1177 Colchicine
$C_{22}H_{25}NO_6$ MW: 399.45 Property: mp 142-50°C, 155-7°C. Source: BAI HE, GUANG CI GU, CAO BEI MU, XUAN CAO GEN, LI LU. Ref: 4, 5, 6.

1178 Coleonolic acid
Source: SAN YE SHU WEI CAO. Ref: 570.

1179 Collagen
Source: NIU CH, YANG PI, CI WEI PI, HUANG MING JIAO, SHE TUI. Ref: 6.

1180 Collettinside I
$C_{33}H_{52}O_8$ MW: 576.78 Source: CHA RUI SHU YU. Ref: 10.

1181 Collettinside II
$C_{39}H_{62}O_{12}$ MW: 722.92 Source: CHA RUI SHU YU. Ref: 10.

1182 Collettinside III
$C_{45}H_{72}O_{16}$ MW: 869.07 Source: CHA RUI SHU YU. Ref: 10.

1183 Collettinside IV
$C_{45}H_{72}O_{17}$ MW: 885.07 Source: CHA RUI SHU YU. Ref: 10.

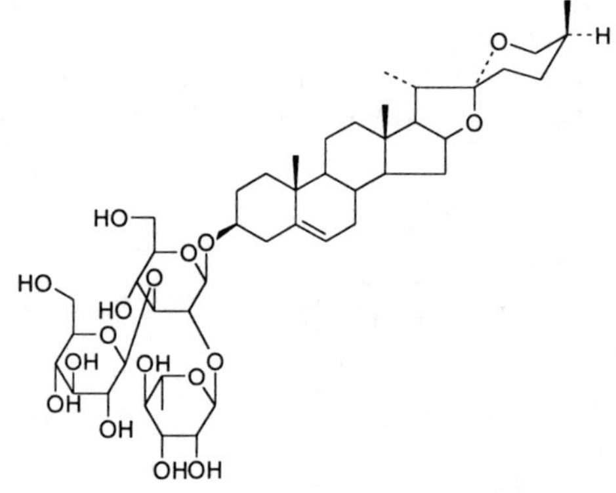

1184 α-Colubrine
$C_{22}H_{24}N_2O_3$ MW: 364.45 Source: MA QIAN ZI. Ref: 2.

1185 β-Colubrine
$C_{22}H_{24}N_2O_3$ MW: 364.45 Source: MA QIAN ZI. Ref: 2, 542.

1186 Columbamine
$C_{20}H_{20}NO_4$ MW: 338.39 Source: HUANG LIAN, YAN HU SUO. Ref: 2.

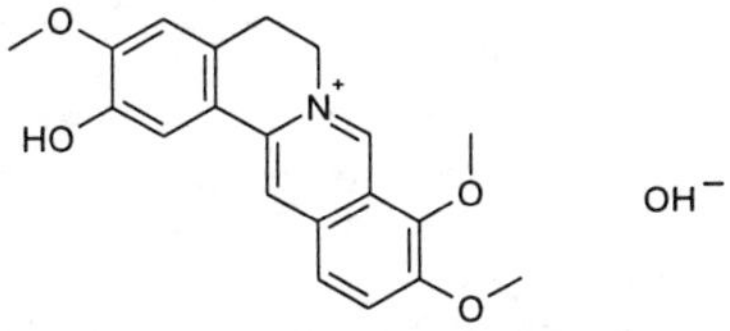

1187 Columbianadin
$C_{19}H_{20}O_5$ MW: 328.37 Source: DU HUO, ZHONG CHI MAO DANG GUI. Ref: 2, 344

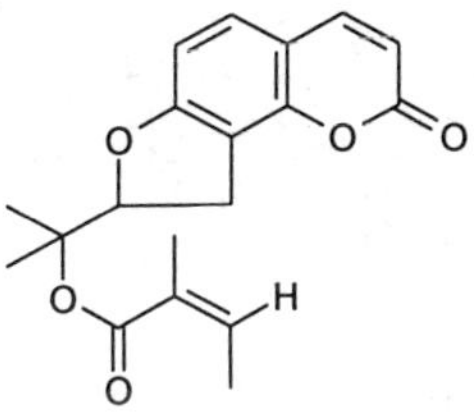

1188 Columbianetin
Dihydrooroselol. $C_{14}H_{14}O_4$ MW: 246.27 Property: mp 164-6°C. Source: DU HUO, QIANG HUO, SHE CHUANG ZI. Ref: 2, 6, 500.

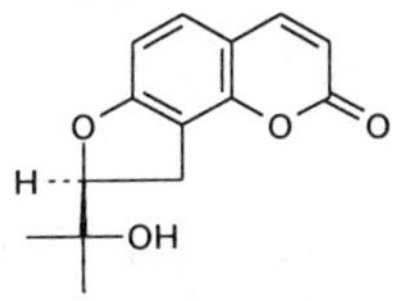

1189 Columbianetin acetate
$C_{16}H_{16}O_5$ MW: 288.30 Source: DU HUO. Ref: 2.

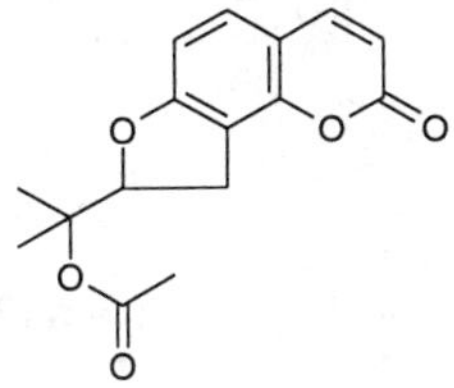

1190 Columbin
$C_{20}H_{22}O_6$ MW: 358.39 Property: mp 192-5°C (dec). Source: JIN GUO LAN, MIAN GEN TENG. Ref: 6.

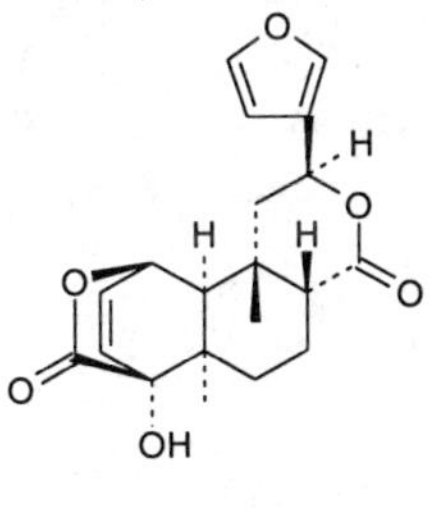

1191 Commiferin
$C_{15}H_{20}O_3$ MW: 248.32 Property: mp 170°C. Source: MO YAO. Ref: 6.

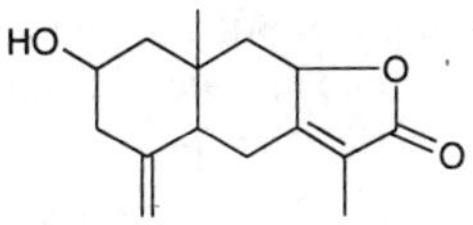

1192 α-Commiphoric acid
$C_{14}H_{18}O_4$ MW: 250.30 Property: mp 201°C. Source: MO YAO. Ref: 6.

1193 β-Commiphoric acid
$C_{14}H_{18}O_4$ MW: 250.30 Property: mp 205°C. Source: MO YAO. Ref: 6.

1194 γ-Commiphoric acid
$C_{17}H_{22}O_5$ MW: 306.36 Property: mp 169-72°C. Source: MO YAO. Ref: 6.

1195 Commiphorinic acid
$C_{28}H_{36}O_8$ MW: 500.59 Property: mp 135°C. Source: MO YAO. Ref: 6.

1196 Commisterone
$C_{27}H_{44}O_7$ MW: 480.65 Property: mp 146-51°C. Source: LU SHUI CAO (II). Ref: 6.

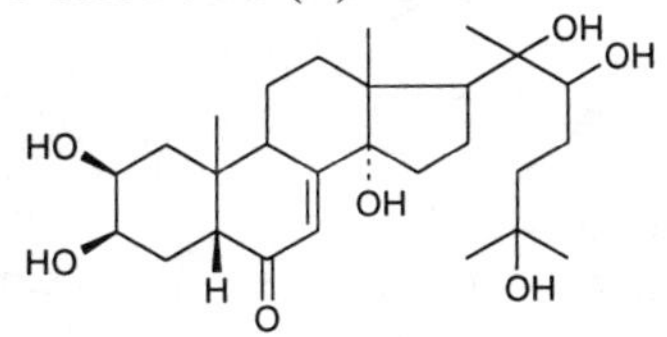

1197 Comosimine
$C_{20}H_{22}O_4$ MW: 326.40 Source: SAN JIAN SHAN. Ref: 2.

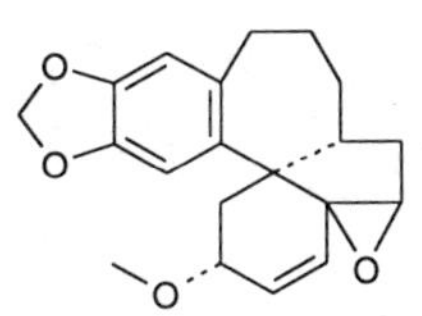

1198 Complanatine
$C_{16}H_{27}NO$ MW: 249.40 Property: mp 169°C. Source: GUO JIANG LONG. Ref: 6.

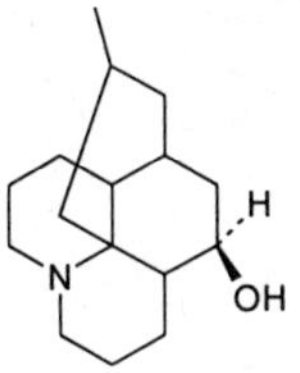

1199 Complanatuside
Glucoside-rhamnocitrin-3,4'-O-β-D-diglucoside. $C_{28}H_{32}O_{16}$ MW: 624.56 Property: light yellow acicular crystal, mp 279-80°C, easy soluble in 50% ethanol, hardly soluble in water, insoluble in ether, chloroform and acetic ester, $[\alpha]_D^{19}$ -50.83° (c=0.02, DMSO). Source: SHA YUAN ZI. Ref: 99.

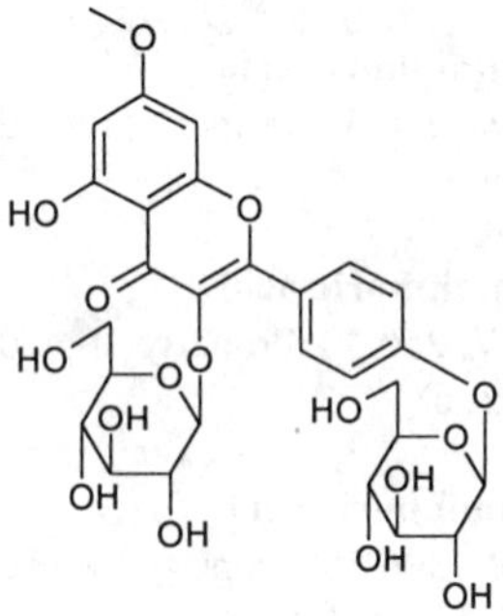

1200 Conamine
$C_{22}H_{36}N_2$ MW: 328.55 Property: mp 130°C. Source: ZHI XIE MU PI. Ref: 6.

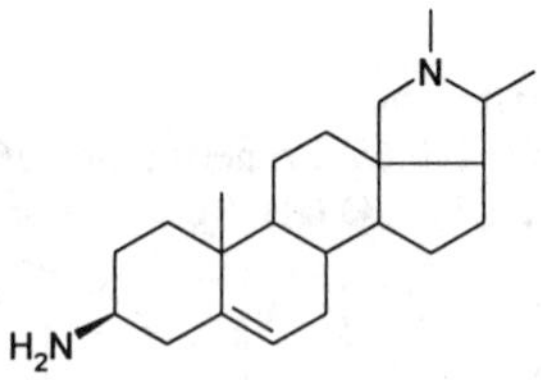

1201 Concuressine
$C_{24}H_{40}N_2$ MW: 356.60 Property: mp 86.5-7.5°C. Source: ZHI XIE MU PI. Ref: 6.

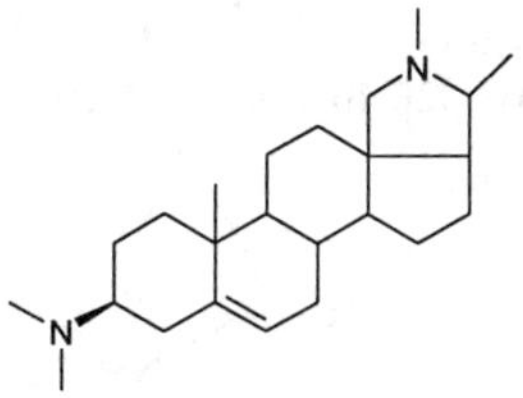

1202 Conessidine
$C_{22}H_{34}N_2$ MW: 326.53 Property: mp 123°C. Source: ZHI XIE MU PI. Ref: 6.

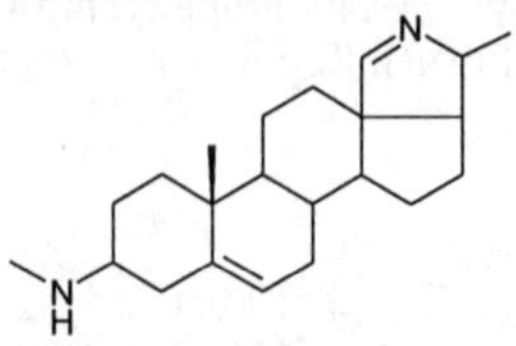

1203 Conessimine
$C_{23}H_{38}N_2$ MW: 342.57 Property: mp 100°C, bp 230°C/1.8mm. Source: ZHI XIE MU PI. Ref: 6.

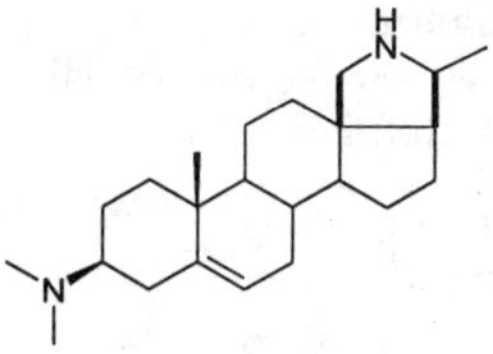

1204 Conessine
Neriine; Roquessine; Wrightine. $C_{24}H_{40}N_2$ MW: 356.60 Property: mp 123-8°C. Source: ZHI XIE MU PI. Ref: 4, 6.

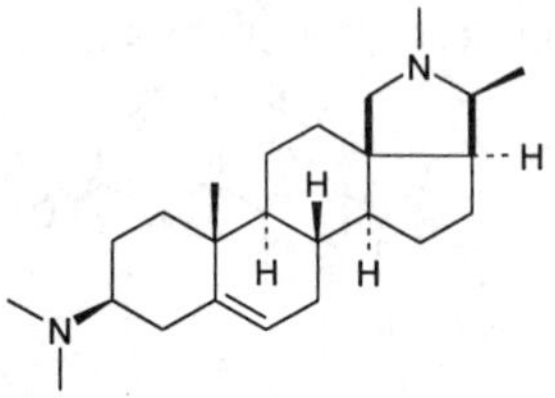

1205 Conferol
$C_{24}H_{30}O_4$ MW: 382.50 Source: A WEI. Ref: 6.

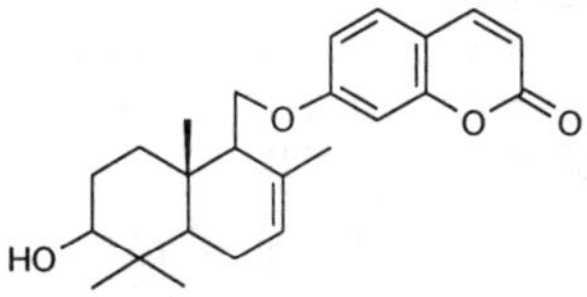

1206 Conferone
$C_{24}H_{28}O_4$ MW: 380.49 Property: mp 142-2.5°C. Source: A WEI. Ref: 6.

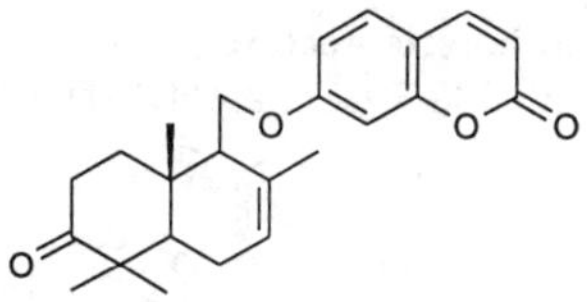

1207 Confertifolin
$C_{15}H_{22}O_2$ MW: 234.34 Property: mp 152°C. Source: SHUI LIAO. Ref: 6.

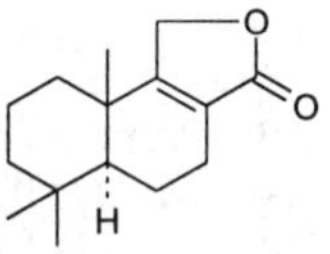

1208 Coniferin
$C_{16}H_{22}O_8$ MW: 342.35 Source: DU ZHONG. Ref: 2.

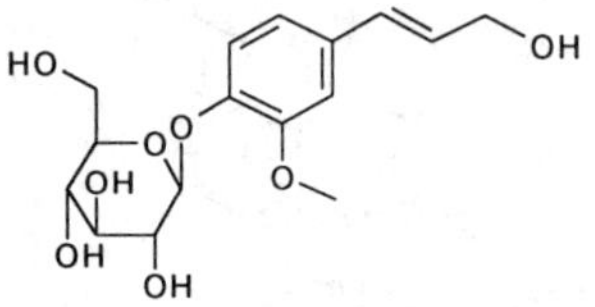

1209 Coniferyl benzoate
$C_{17}H_{16}O_4$ MW: 281.31 Property: mp 158-9°C. Source: AN XI XIANG. Ref: 6.

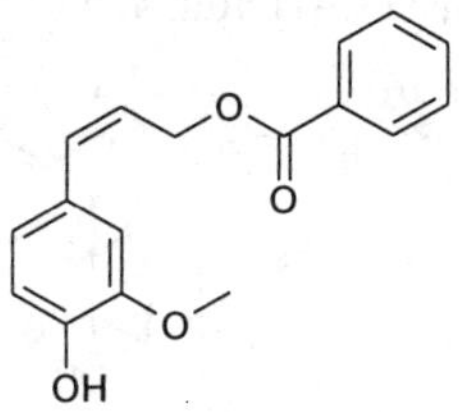

1210 Coniferyl cinnamate
$C_{19}H_{18}O_4$ MW: 310.35 Source: AN XI XIANG. Ref: 6.

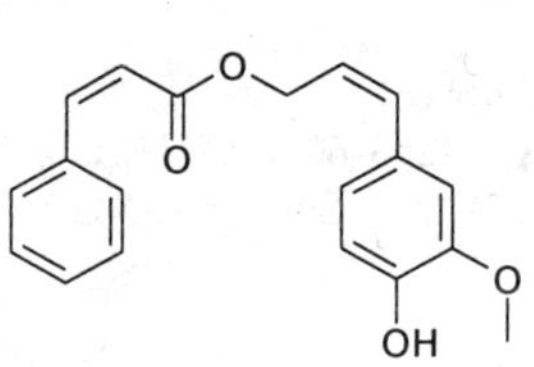

1211 Coniferyl diangelate
$C_{21}H_{26}O_5$ MW: 358.44 Property: bp 130°C/0.01mm. Source: HONG TOU CAO. Ref: 6.

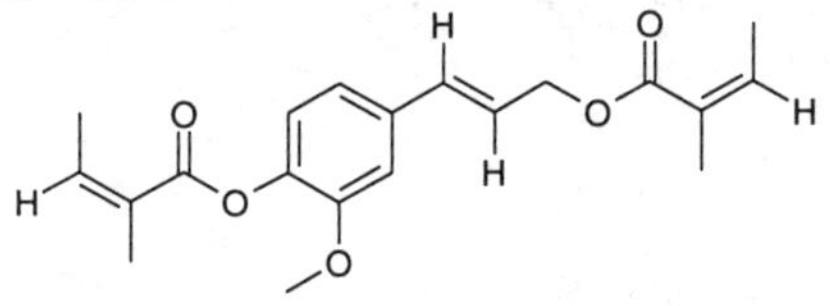

1212 Coniine
$C_8H_{17}N$ MW: 127.23 Source: BAN XIA. Ref: 2.

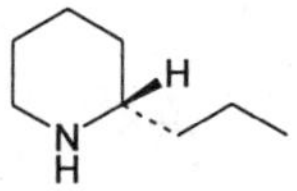

1213 Conimine
$C_{22}H_{36}N_2$ MW: 328.55 Property: mp 134°C. Source: ZHI XIE MU PI. Ref: 6.

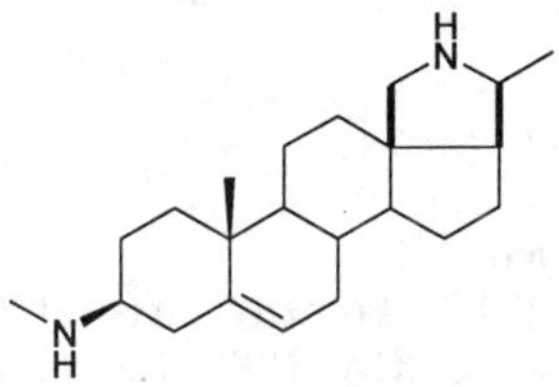

1214 Coniselin
$C_{21}H_{20}O_8$ MW: 400.39 Property: white acicular crystal, mp 119-120°C. Source: XIN JIANG GAO BEN. Ref: 333.

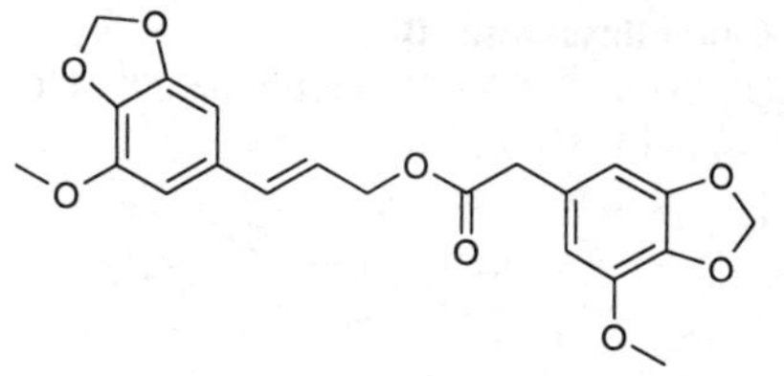

1215 Conkurchine
$C_{21}H_{32}N_2$ MW: 312.50 Property: mp 153°C. Source: ZHI XIE MU PI. Ref: 6.

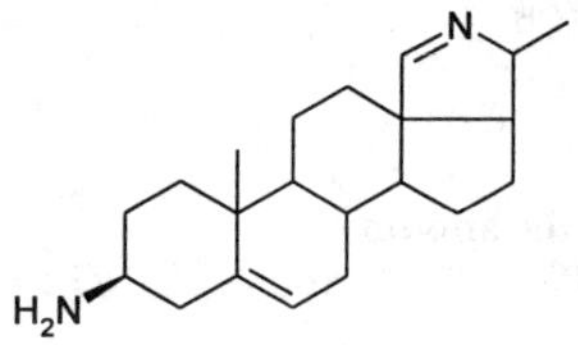

1216 Conquinamine
$C_{19}H_{24}N_2O_2$ MW: 312.42 Property: mp 121°C. Source: JIN JI LE. Ref: 6.

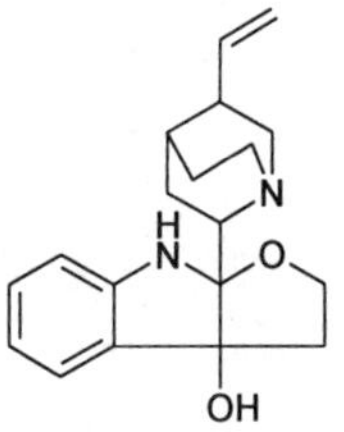

1217 Convallamarin
Source: YU ZHU. Ref: 6.

1218 Convallarin
Source: YU ZHU. Ref: 6.

1219 Convallasaponin A
$C_{32}H_{52}O_9$ MW: 580.77 Property: mp 238-40°C. Source: LING LAN. Ref: 6.

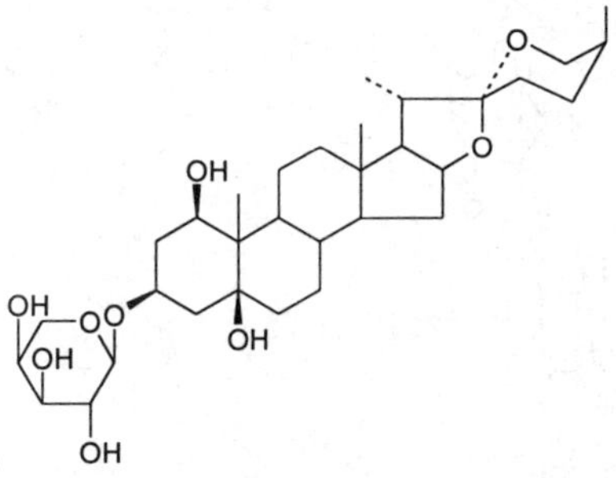

1220 Convallasaponin B
$C_{32}H_{52}O_{10}$ MW: 596.77 Property: mp 273-4°C. Source: LING LAN Ref: 6.

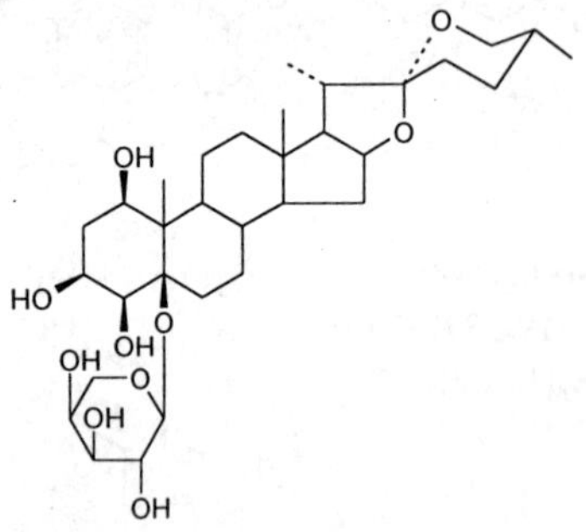

1221 Convallasaponin C
$C_{44}H_{72}O_{16}$ MW: 857.05 Source: LING LAN. Ref: 6.

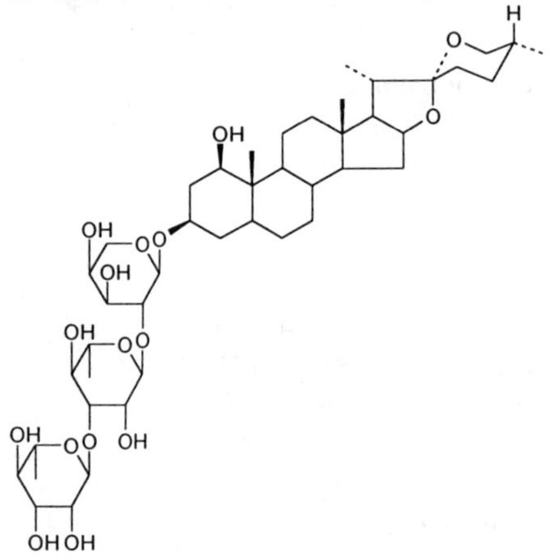

1222 Convallasaponin D
$C_{50}H_{82}O_{21}$ MW: 1019.20 Property: mp 264-5°C. Source: LING LAN. Ref: 6.

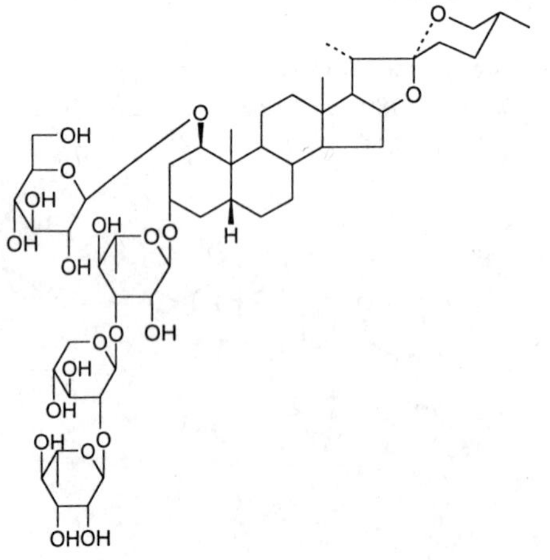

1223 Convallatoxin
Convallaton; Corglykon. CAS: 508-75-8 $C_{29}H_{42}O_{10}$ MW: 550.65 Property: mp 235-42°C. Source: FU SHOU CAO, LING LAN. Ref: 4, 6.

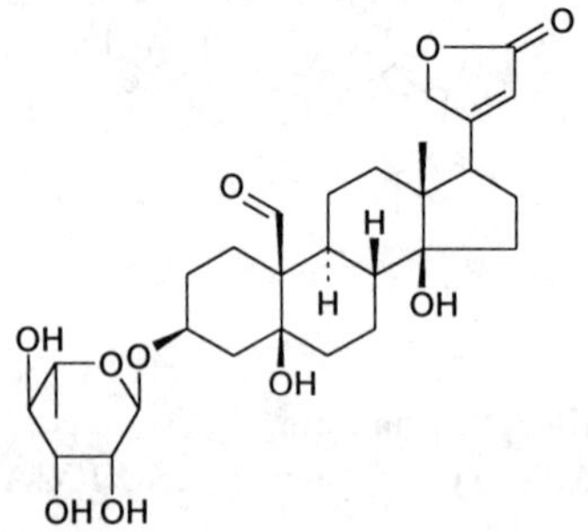

1224 Convallatoxol
Perconval. CAS: 3253-62-1 $C_{29}H_{44}O_{10}$ MW: 552.67 Property: mp 171-5°C. Source: LING LAN. Ref: 4, 6.

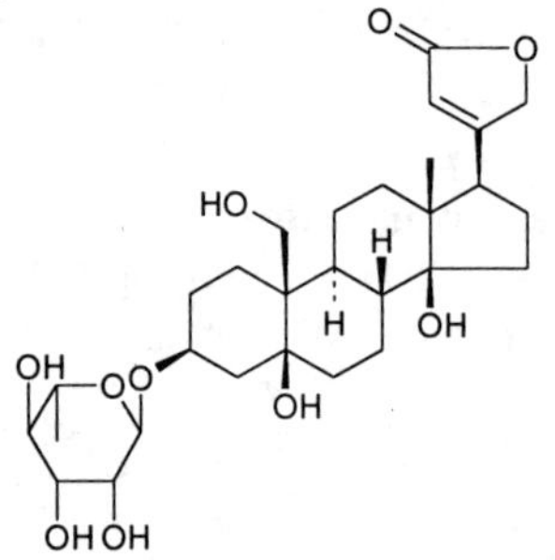

1225 Convalloside
Bogoroside. $C_{35}H_{52}O_{15}$ MW: 712.80 Property: mp 201-4°C. Source: LING LAN. Ref: 4, 6.

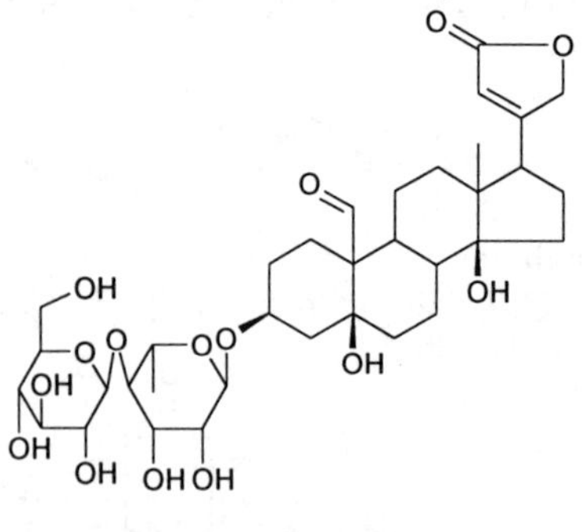

1226 Copadiene
$C_{15}H_{22}$ MW: 202.34 Property: bp (+): 130-40°C/1mm. Source: XIANG FU. Ref: 6.

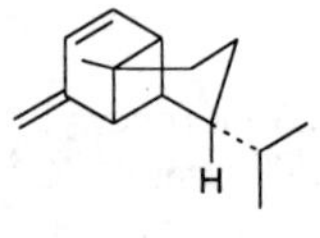

1227 α-Copaene
$C_{15}H_{24}$ MW: 204.36 Source: CHAI HU, DU HUO, HOU PO, QIANG HUO, QING HAO, SAN QI, SHENG JIANG. Ref: 2.

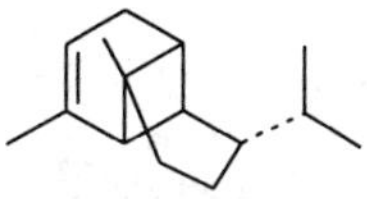

1228 Coprocholic acid
$C_{27}H_{46}O_5$ MW: 450.66 Property: mp 180-2°C. Source: CHEN DONG CAI LU ZHI. Ref: 6.

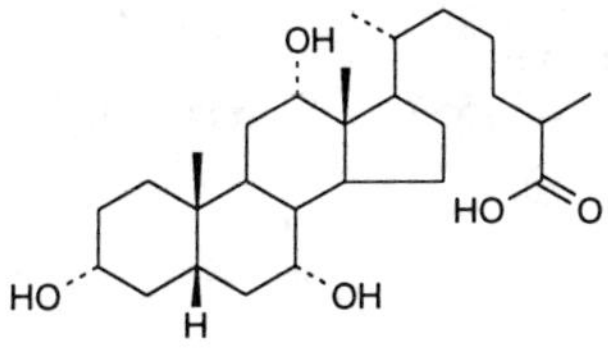

1229 Coptisine
$C_{19}H_{14}NO_4$ MW: 320.33 Source: HUANG LIAN, YAN HU SUO. Ref: 2.

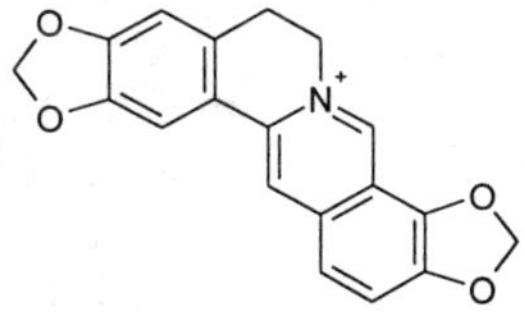

1230 Corchoritin
$C_{12}H_{18}O_3$ MW: 210.28 Property: mp 218-20°C. Source: HUANG MA ZI. Ref: 6.

1231 Corchorol
$C_{22}H_{38}O_9$ MW: 446.54 Property: mp 184°C. Source: HUANG MA YE. Ref: 6.

1232 Corchoroside A
$C_{29}H_{42}O_9$ MW: 534.65 Property: mp 188-90°C. Source: FU SHOU CAO, GUI ZHU TANG JIE, HUANG MA ZI. Ref: 4, 6.

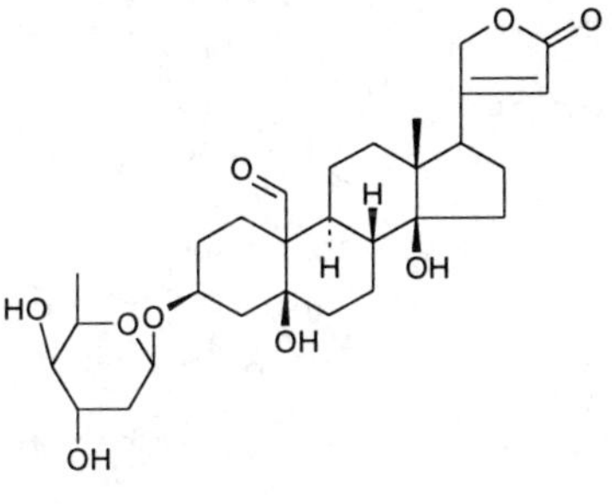

1233 Corchorosol A
$C_{29}H_{44}O_9$ MW: 536.67 Property: mp 199-201°C. Source: HUANG MA YE. Ref: 6.

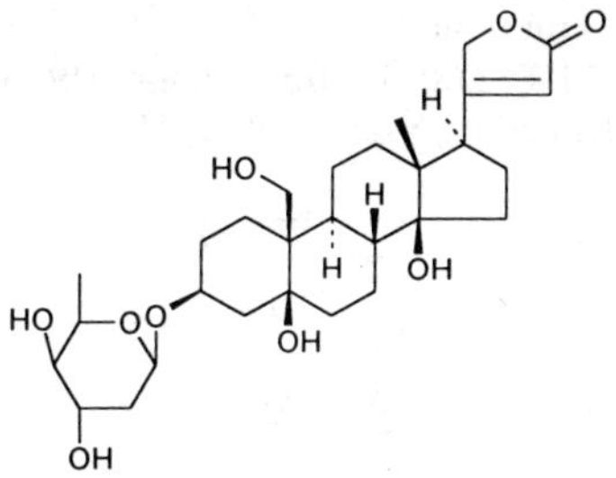

1234 Cordarine
Source: YU XING CAO. Ref: 6.

1235 Cordycepic acid
$C_7H_{12}O_6$ MW: 192.17 Source: DONG CHONG XIA CAO. Ref: 2.

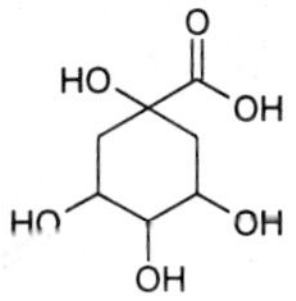

1236 Cordycepin
$C_{10}H_{13}N_5O_3$ MW: 251.25 Property: mp 225-6°C. Source: DONG CHONG XIA CAO. Ref: 6.

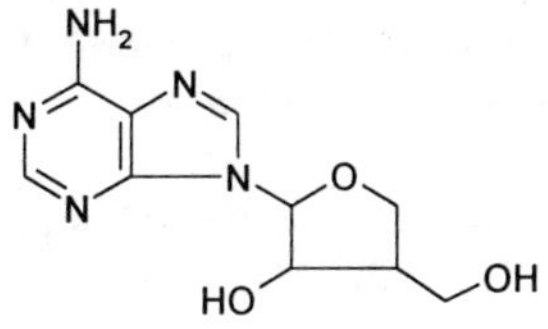

1237 Cordylagenin
$C_{27}H_{44}O_4$ MW: 432.65 Property: mp (-): 216°C. Source: JIAN YE TIE SHU YE. Ref: 6.

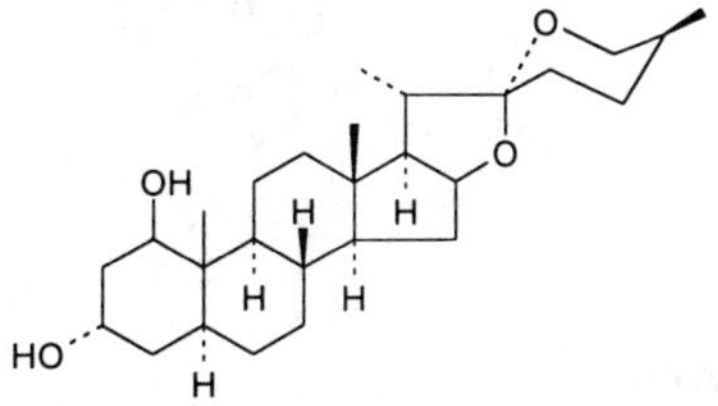

1238 Coreximine
$C_{19}H_{21}NO_4$ MW: 327.38 Property: mp (-): 262°C, (±): 233-4.0°C. Source: ZI HUA YU DENG CAO (LIE BAO ZI JING), YA PIAN. Ref: 6.

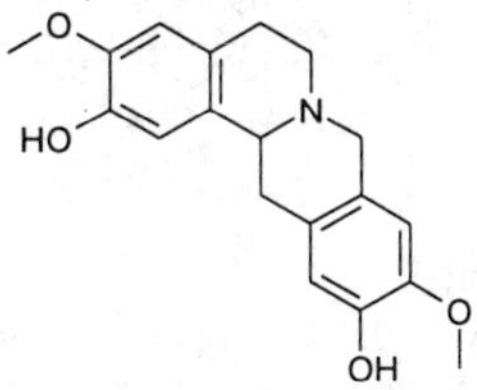

1239 Coriamyrtin
$C_{15}H_{18}O_5$ MW: 278.31 Property: mp 229-30°C.
Source: MA SANG YE. Ref: 4, 6, 413.

1240 Corilgin
$C_{27}H_{22}O_{18}$ MW: 634.47 Property: mp 204-5°C.
Source: AN MO LE, HE ZI, YOU GAN MU PI, YOU GAN YE. Ref: 6.

1241 Coriose
$C_7H_{14}O_7$ MW: 210.19 Property: mp 169-71°C.
Source: MA SANG YE. Ref: 6.

1242 Cornigerine
$C_{21}H_{21}NO_6$ MW: 383.40 Property: mp 268-70°C.
Source: CAO BEI MU. Ref: 6.

1243 Cornin
Verbenalin. $C_{17}H_{24}O_{10}$ MW: 388.37 Property: mp 182.2-2.8°C. Source: MA BIAN CAO, SHAN ZHU YU. Ref: 2, 6.

1244 Cornuside
$C_{34}H_{50}O_{20}$ MW: 778.77 Property: white amorphous powder, mp 135-8°C, $[\alpha]_D^{16.5}$ -83.7° (c=0.2, methanol).
Source: SHAN ZHU YU. Ref: 247.

1245 Cornusiin A
$C_{68}H_{52}O_{43}$ MW: 1557.15 Source: SHAN ZHU YU.
Ref: 2.

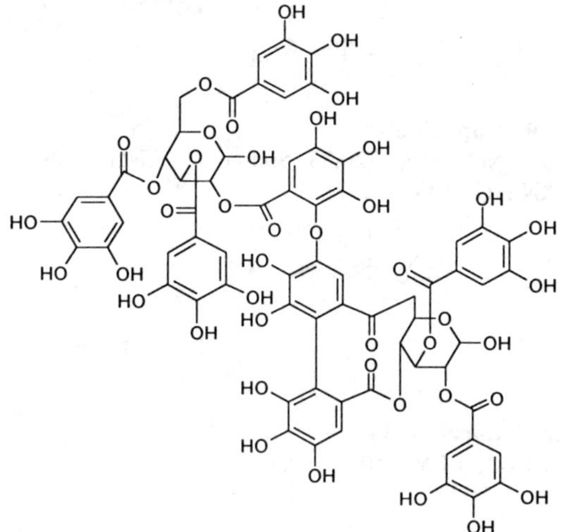

1246 Cornusiin B
$C_{48}H_{30}O_{30}$ MW: 1086.76 Source: SHAN ZHU YU.
Ref: 2.

1247 Cornusiin C
$C_{34}H_{24}O_{22}$ MW: 784.56 Source: SHAN ZHU YU. Ref: 2.

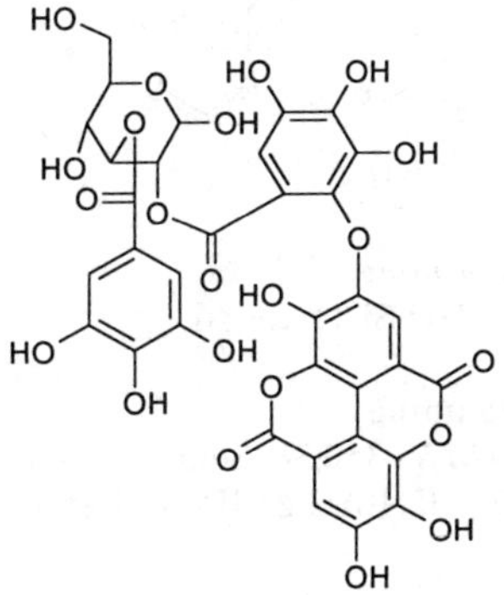

1248 Cornusiin G
$C_{75}H_{56}O_{48}$ MW: 1725.25 Source: SHAN ZHU YU. Ref: 2.

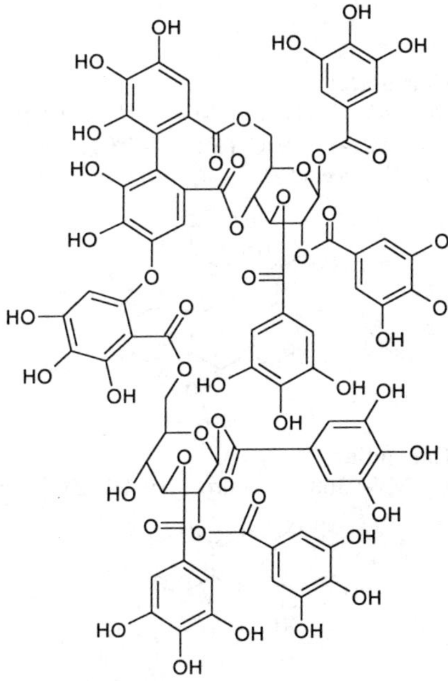

1249 α-Corocalene
$C_{15}H_{20}$ MW: 200.33 Source: PI JIU HUA. Ref: 6.

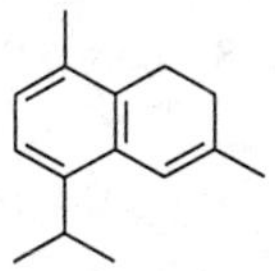

1250 Coroglaucigenin
$C_{23}H_{34}O_5$ MW: 390.52 Property: mp 249°C. Source: LIAN SHENG GUI ZI HUA. Ref: 6.

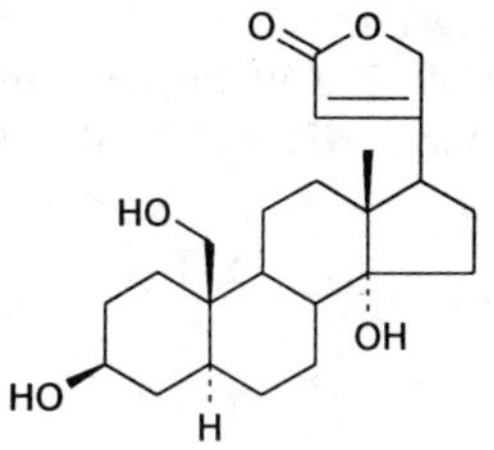

1251 Coronaric acid
Source: XI XIAN. Ref: 2.

1252 Coronaridine
$C_{21}H_{26}N_2O_2$ MW: 338.45 Source: CHANG CHUN HUA. Ref: 2.

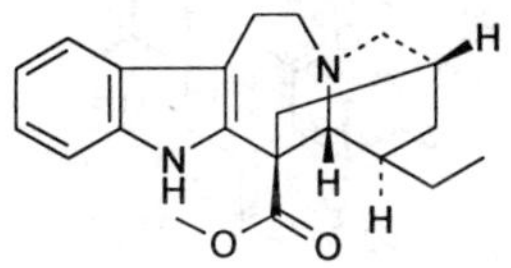

1253 Corosolic acid
Property: mp 242-5°C. Source: CU YE XUAN GOU ZI. Ref: 420.

1254 Corossoline
$C_{35}H_{64}O_6$ MW: 580.90 Property: white amorphous solid, $[\alpha]_D^{25}$ +19° (c=0.2, MeOH). Source: JIN PING GE NA XIANG. Ref: 420.

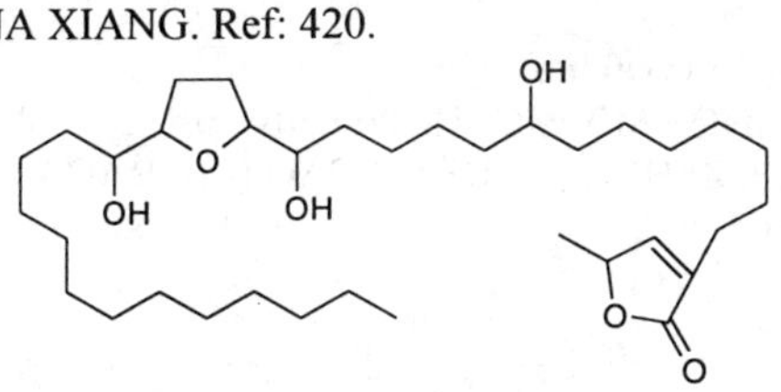

1255 Corotoxigenin
$C_{23}H_{32}NO_5$ MW: 388.51 Property: mp 221°C. Source: LIAN SHENG GUI ZI HUA. Ref: 6.

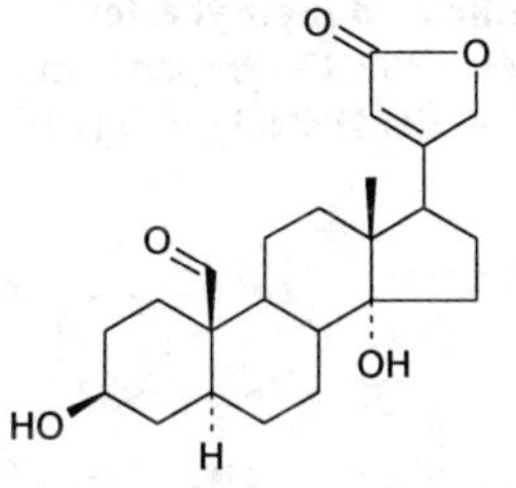

1256 Corticosterone
$C_{22}H_{32}O_4$ MW: 360.50 Property: mp 177-9°C. Source: NIU SHEN. Ref: 6.

1257 Cortisone
17-Hydroxy-11-dehydrocorticosterone. $C_{22}H_{30}O_5$ MW: 374.48 Property: mp 230-1°C. Source: NIU SHEN, ZI HE CHE. Ref: 6.

1258 (+)-Corybulbine
$C_{21}H_2NO_4$ MW: 355.44 Source: YAN HU SUO. Ref: 2.

1259 Corycavine
$C_{21}H_{21}NO_5$ MW: 367.41 Property: mp (±): 218-9°C. Source: ZI HUA YU DENG CAO (LIE BAO ZI JING). Ref: 6.

1260 Corydalic acid methyl ester
$C_{22}H_{23}NO_6$ MW: 397.43 Property: mp 140-1°C. Source: ZI HUA YU DENG CAO (LIE BAO ZI JING). Ref: 6.

1261 (+)-Corydaline
CAS: 518-69-4 $C_{22}H_{27}NO_4$ MW: 369.46 Property: mp (+): 135°C. Source: YAN HU SUO. Ref: 2, 4.

1262 Corydalmine
Source: YAN HU SUO. Ref: 6.

1263 Corydamine
$C_{20}H_{18}N_2O_4$ MW: 350.38 Source: ZI HUA YU DENG CAO (LIE BAO ZI JING). Ref: 6.

1264 Corydin(e)
CAS: 476-69-7 $C_{20}H_{23}NO_4$ MW: 341.41 Property: mp (+): 149°C, (-): 149°C, (±): 165-7°C. Source: YAN HU SUO. Ref: 5, 6.

1265 Corylidin
$C_{20}H_{16}O_7$ MW: 368.35 Source: BU GU ZHI. Ref: 2.

1266 Corylifolin
$C_{20}H_{20}O_4$ MW: 324.38 Source: BU GU ZHI. Ref: 2.

1267 Corylifolinin
Isobavachalcone. CAS: 20784-50-3 $C_{20}H_{20}O_4$ MW: 324.38 Property: mp 154-6°C, 166-7°C. Source: BU GU ZHI. Ref: 4.

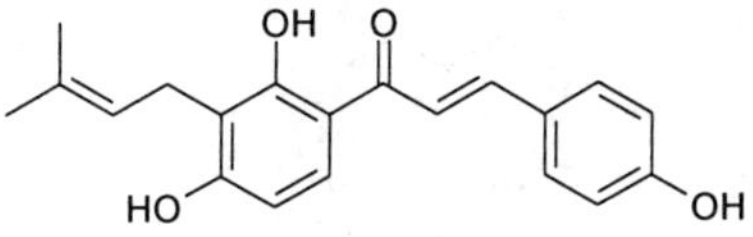

1268 Corylin
$C_{20}H_{16}O_4$ MW: 320.35 Source: BU GU ZHI. Ref: 2.

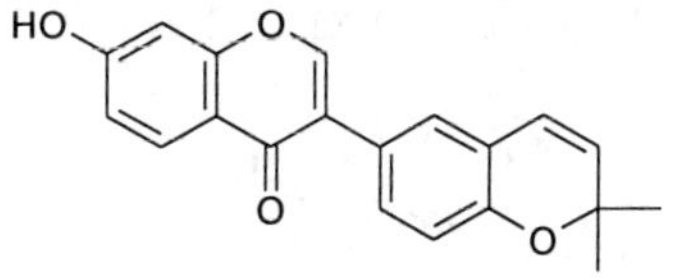

1269 Corylinal
$C_{16}H_{10}O_5$ MW: 282.26 Source: BU GU ZHI. Ref: 2, 630.

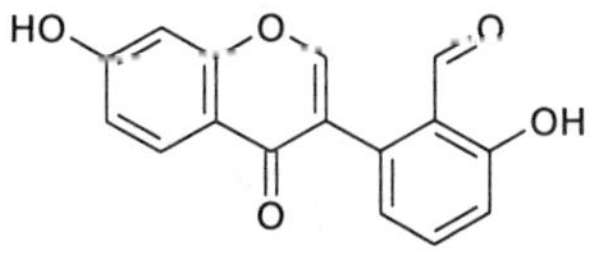

1270 Corynantheine
$C_{22}H_{26}N_2O_3$ MW: 366.46 Source: GOU TENG. Ref: 2.

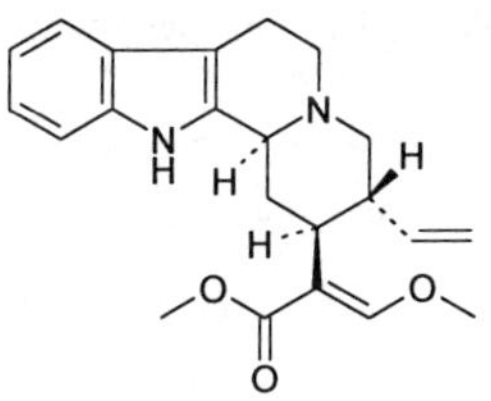

1271 Corynoline
$C_{21}H_{21}NO_5$ MW: 367.41 Property: mp 216-7°C. Source: ZI HUA YU DENG CAO (LIE BAO ZI JING). Ref: 6.

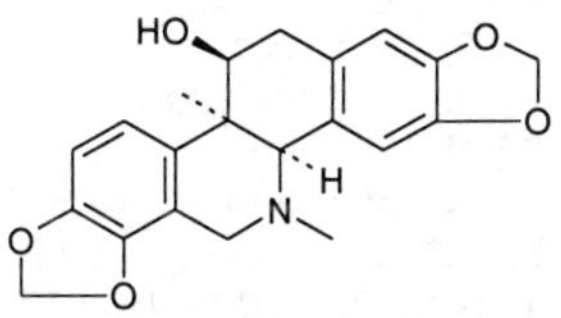

1272 Corynoloxin(e)
$C_{21}H_{19}NO_5$ MW: 365.39 Property: mp 209-10°C. Source: ZI HUA YU DENG CAO (LIE BAO ZI JING). Ref: 6.

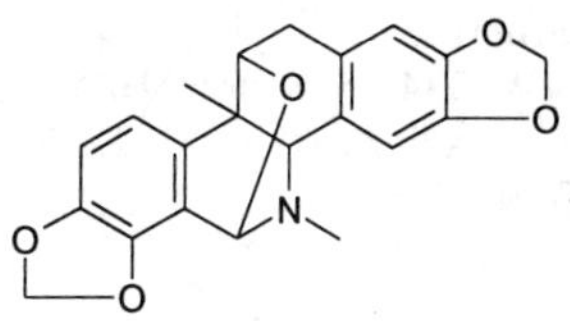

1273 Corynoxeine
$C_{22}H_{26}N_2O_4$ MW: 382.46 Property: mp 212-4°C. Source: GOU TENG. Ref: 2, 6.

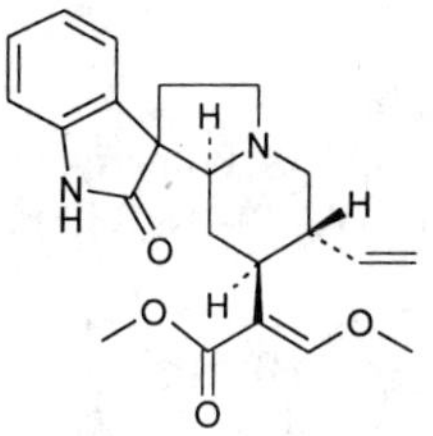

1274 Corynoxine
$C_{22}H_{28}N_2O_4$ MW: 384.48 Property: mp 166-8°C. Source: GOU TENG. Ref: 2, 6.

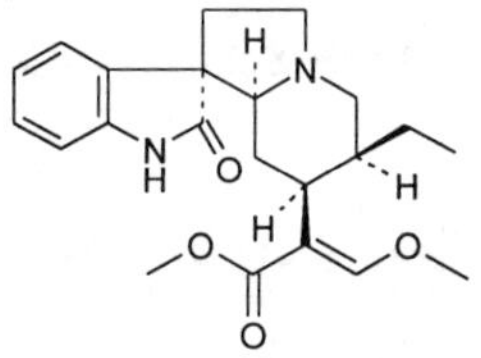

1275 Corynoxine B
$C_{22}H_{28}N_2O_4$ MW: 384.48 Source: GOU TENG, DA YE GOU TENG. Ref: 2, 6.

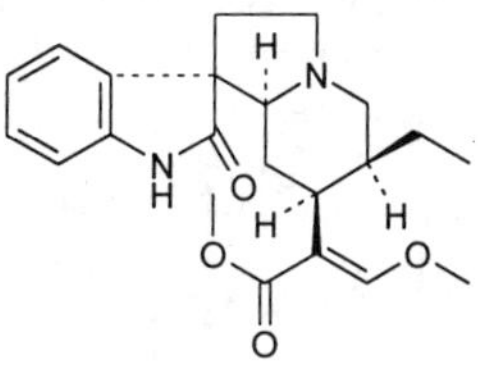

1276 Corypalmine
Tetrahydrojatrorrhizine. $C_{20}H_{23}NO_4$ MW: 341.41 Property: mp (+): 235-6°C, (-): 230°C, (±): 215-7°C. Source: HUANG BAI, TU HUANG LIAN, YAN HU SUO, ZI HUA YU DENG CAO (LIE BAO ZI JING). Ref: 6.

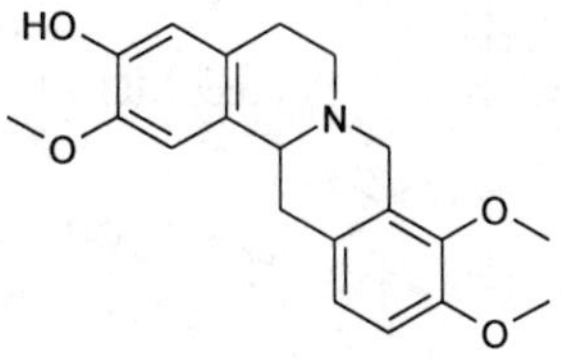

1277 Corysamine
$C_{20}H_{16}NO_4$ MW: 334.35 Source: BAI QU CAI, JU HUA HUANG LIAN, ZI HUA YU DENG CAO (LIE BAO ZI JING). Ref: 6.

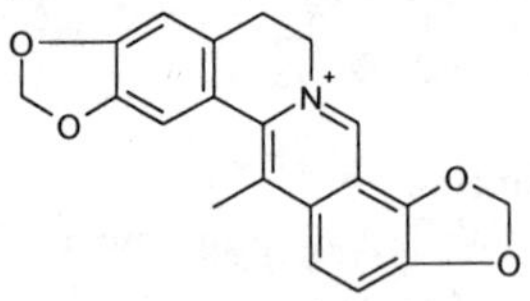

1278 Corytuberine
$C_{19}H_{21}NO_4$ MW: 327.38 Property: mp (+): 240°C, (±): 242°C. Source: YA PIAN. Ref: 6.

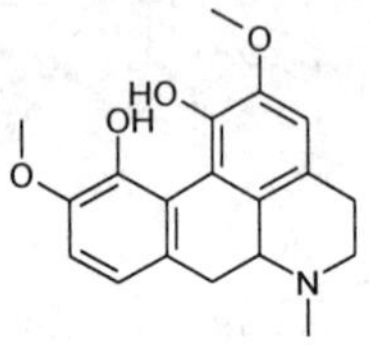

1279 Cosmosiin
$C_{21}H_{20}O_{10}$ MW: 432.39 Source: XIAN HE CAO. Ref: 2.

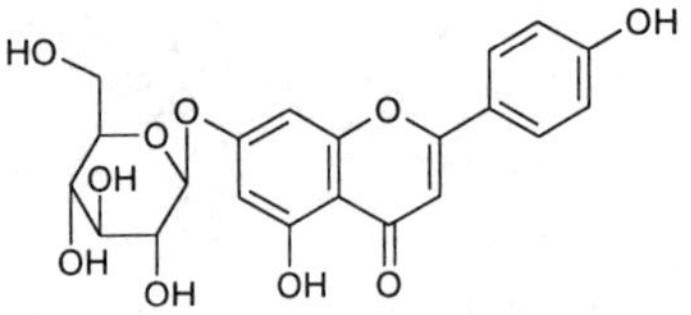

1280 Costaclavine
$C_{16}H_{20}N_2$ MW: 240.35 Property: mp 182-4°C. Source: MAI JIAO. Ref: 6.

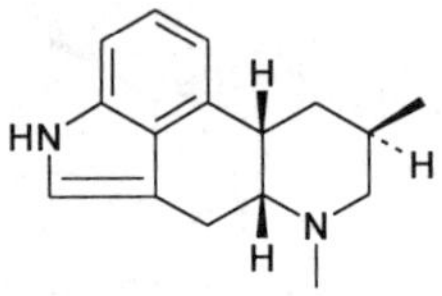

1281 β-Costene
$C_{15}H_{24}$ Source: MU XIANG. Ref: 2.

1282 α-Costene
$C_{15}H_{24}$ Source: MU XIANG. Ref: 2.

1283 Costic acid
$C_{16}H_{24}O_2$ MW: 248.37 Source: MU XIANG. Ref: 2.

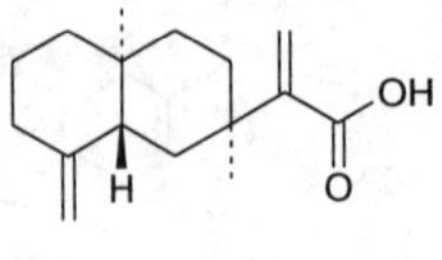

1284 Costol
$C_{15}H_{24}O$ MW: 220.36 Property: bp (+): 145°C /0.5mm. (±): 90°C/0.2mm. Source: MU XIANG, MU BIE GEN. Ref: 6.

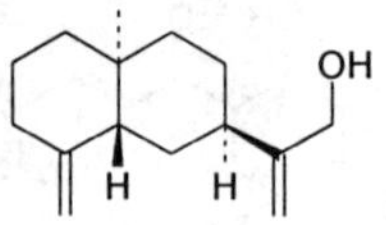

1285 Costunolide
CAS: 553-21-9 $C_{15}H_{20}O_2$ MW: 232.33 Property: bp (+): 105-6°C. Source: MU XIANG. Ref: 2, 5.

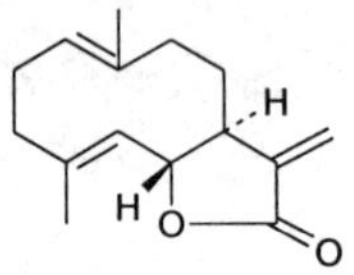

1286 Costuslactone
$C_{15}H_{24}O_2$ MW: 236.36 Source: MU XIANG. Ref: 2.

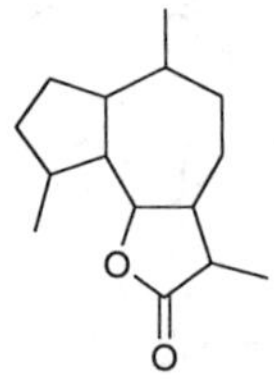

1287 Cotarnine
$C_{12}H_{15}NO_4$ MW: 237.26 Property: mp 132-3°C. Source: YA PIAN. Ref: 6.

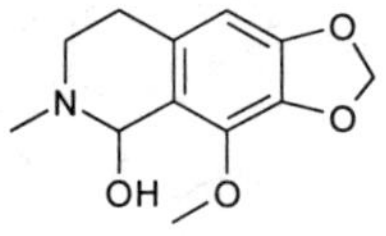

1288 m-Coumaric acid
$C_9H_8O_3$ MW: 164.16 Property: mp 193°C. Source: NING MENG GEN. Ref: 6.

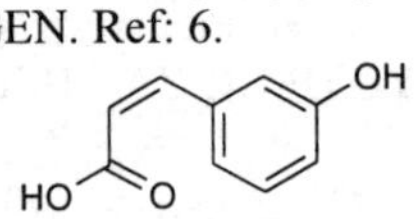

1289 o-Coumaric acid
trans-o-Hydroxycinnamic acid. $C_9H_8O_3$ MW: 164.16 Property: mp 217°C (dec). Source: PEI LAN, NING MENG YE, NING MENG GEN, HUI XIANG JING YE, YANG CONG, CHOU MU XU GEN, PI HAN CAO. Ref: 6.

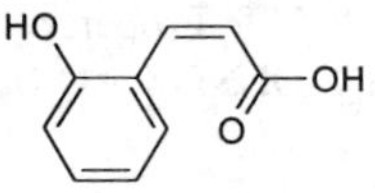

1290 p-Coumaric acid
E-p-Hydroxy-cinnamic acid. $C_9H_8O_3$ MW: 164.16 Property: mp 171°C (dec). Source: LU HUI, MA HUANG, NAN FANG TU SI ZI. Ref: 2, 589.

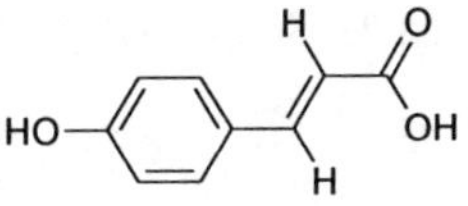

1291 o-Coumaric acid-β-D-glucoside
$C_{15}H_{18}O_8$ MW: 326.31 Property: mp 241°C. Source: PI HAN CAO. Ref: 6.

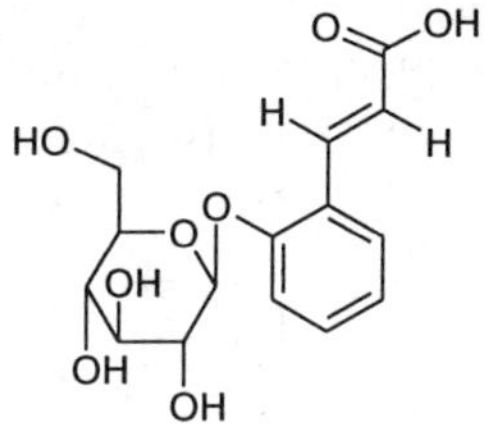

1292 Coumarin
$C_9H_6O_2$ MW: 146.15 Source: GUI ZHI, QING HAO, HUANG JIN FENG. Ref: 2, 548.

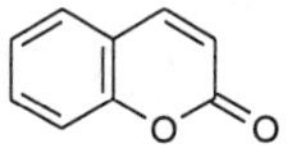

1293 Coumarinic acid
$C_9H_8O_3$ MW: 164.16 Source: PI HAN CAO. Ref: 6.

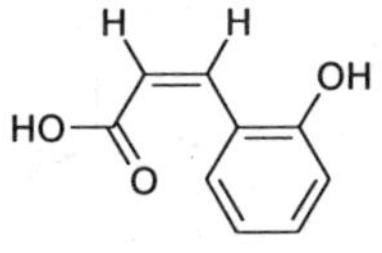

1294 Coumarinic acid-β-D-glucoside
$C_{15}H_{18}O_8$ MW: 326.31 Property: mp 216°C. Source: MAO XIANG HUA, PI HAN CAO. Ref: 6.

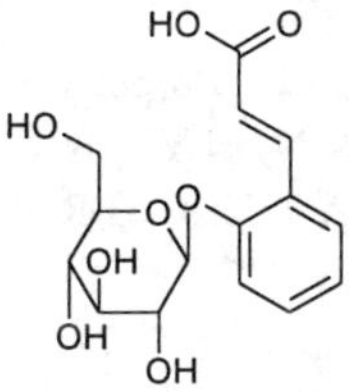

1295 Coumarone
C_8H_6O MW: 118.14 Property: bp 174°C. Source: JIU JIE CHA, SHUI HUANG YANG MU. Ref: 6.

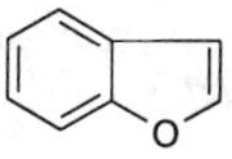

1296 6-O-p-Coumaroylajugol
Source: GAN DI HUANG. Ref: 2.

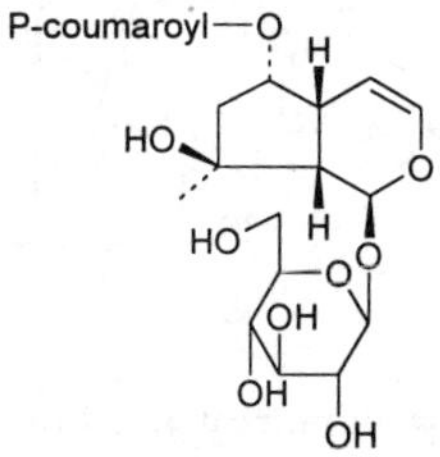

1297 2''-O-p-Coumaroylaloesin
Source: LU HUI. Ref: 2.

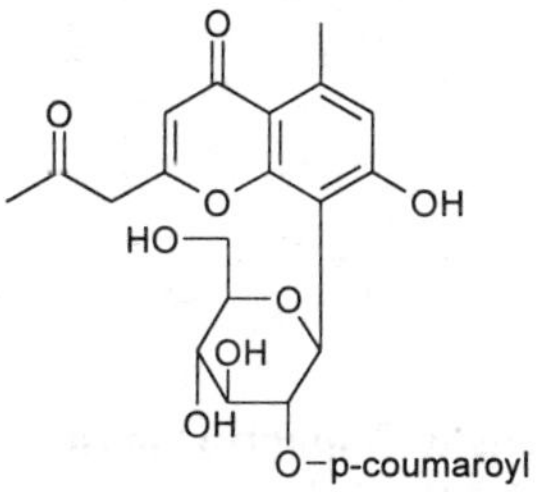

1298 6''-O-p-Coumaroylaloesin
Source: LU HUI. Ref: 2.

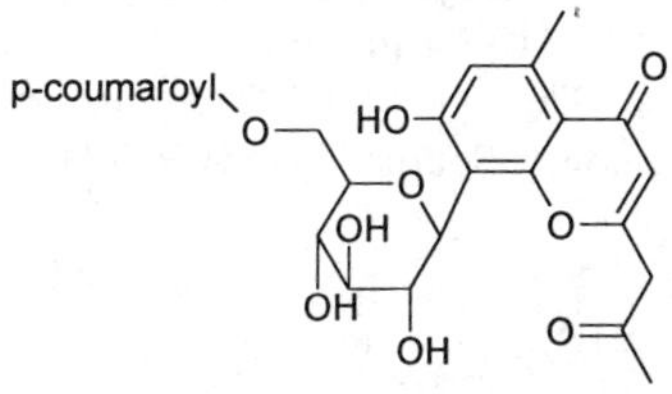

1299 3-O-cis-p-Coumaroyl alphitolic acid
$C_{40}H_{56}O_6$ MW: 632.89 Source: DA ZAO. Ref: 2.

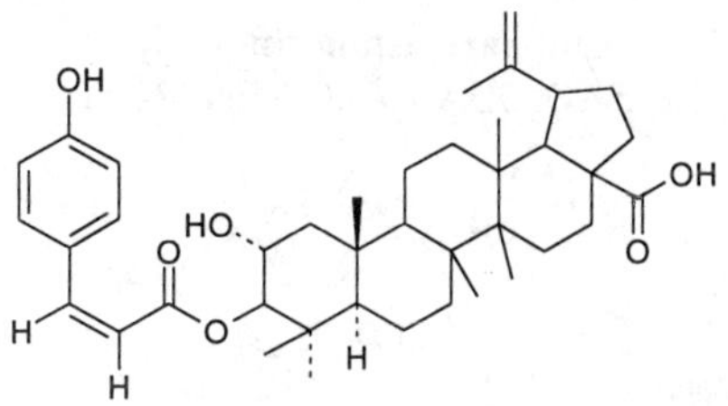

1300 6''-O-p-Coumaroylgenipingentiobioside
$C_{32}H_{40}O_{17}$ MW: 696.67 Source: ZHI ZI. Ref: 2, 626.

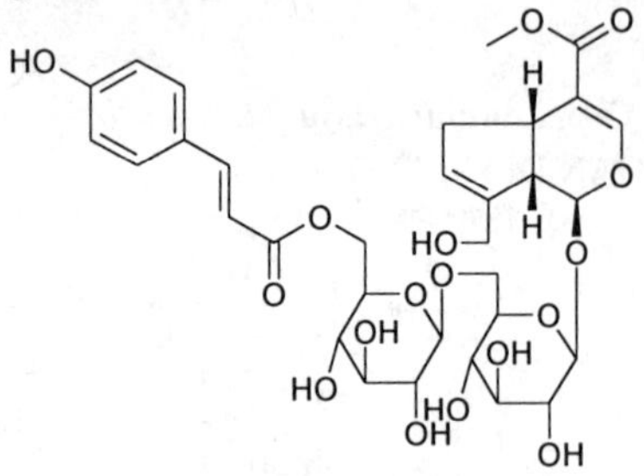

1301 3-O-cis-p-Coumaroyl maslinic acid
$C_{39}H_{54}O_6$ MW: 618.86 Source: DA ZAO. Ref: 2.

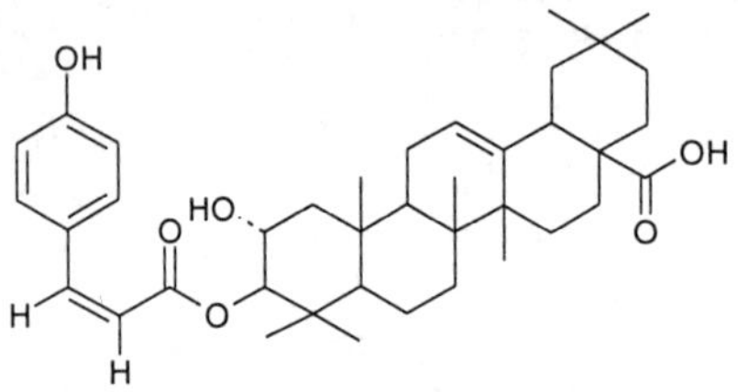

1302 3-O-trans-p-Coumaroyl maslinic acid
$C_{39}H_{54}O_6$ MW: 618.86 Source: WU LING ZHI. Ref: 637.

1303 1-(p-Coumaroyl)-α-L-rhamnopyranose
$C_{15}H_{18}O_7$ MW: 310.31 Property: colorless prismatic crystal, mp 81-3°C and 188-90°C (chloroform-methanol-acetone). Source: DONG BEI HE SHI. Ref: 48.

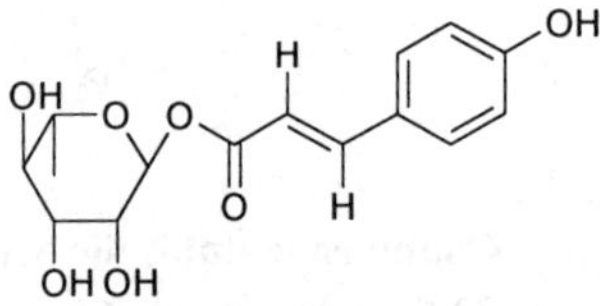

1304 6'''-p-Coumaroylspinosin
Source: DA ZAO, SUAN ZAO REN. Ref: 2.

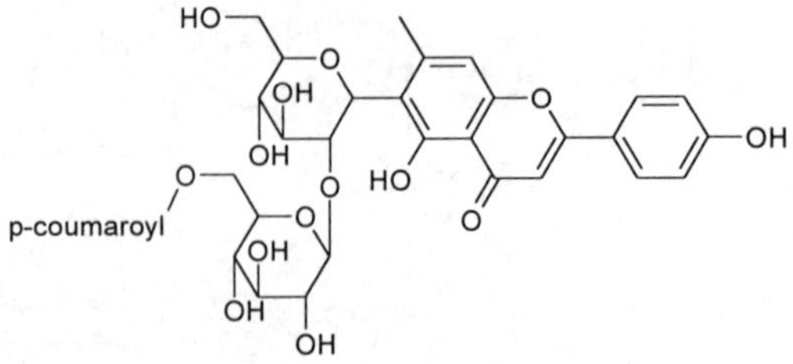

p-coumaroyl

1305 3-O-cis-p-Coumaroyltormentic acid
Source: WU LING ZHI. Ref: 637.

1306 3-O-trans-p-Coumaroyltormentic acid
Source: WU LING ZHI. Ref: 637.

1307 Coumestrol
$C_{15}H_8O_5$ MW: 268.23 Source: GE GEN. Ref: 2.

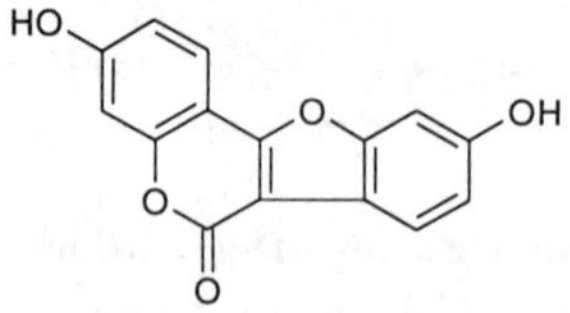

1308 Coumurrayin
$C_{16}H_{18}O_4$ MW: 274.32 Property: mp 157°C. Source: JIU LI XIANG, YUN QIAN HU. Ref: 6, 11, 177.

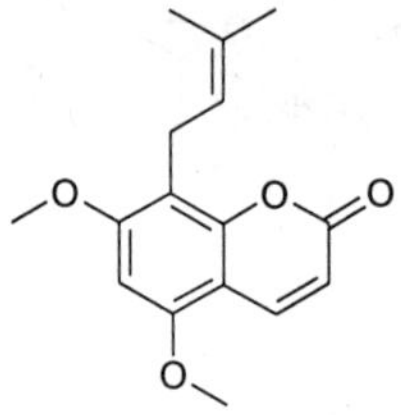

1309 Crassicauline A
Source: DIAN XI WU TOU. Ref: 618.

1310 Crategolic acid
$C_{30}H_{48}O_4$ MW: 472.71 Property: mp 263-5°C. Source: SHAN ZHA, SHAN ZHA YE. Ref: 6.

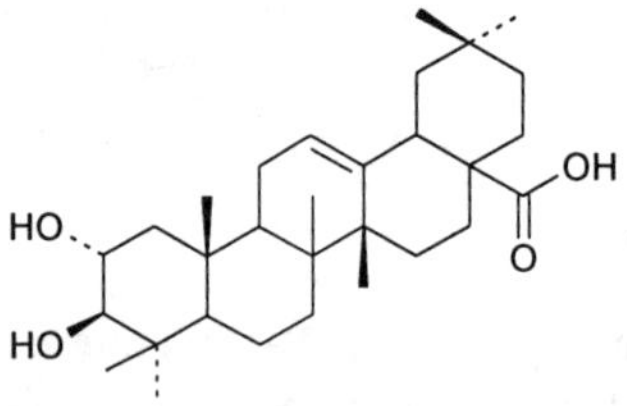

1311 Creatine
$C_5H_{10}NO_2$ MW: 130.15 Property: mp 303°C. Source: GOU ROU, GOU XIN, LI YU, NIU XUE, QING WA, XIA TIAN GAO, XIANG ROU. Ref: 6.

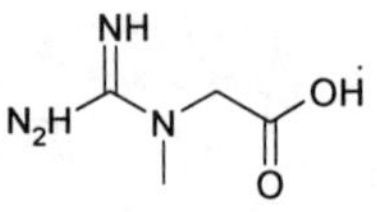

1312 Creatine phosphoric acid
$C_4H_{10}N_3O_5P$ MW: 211.12 Source: QING WA, LI YU. Ref: 6.

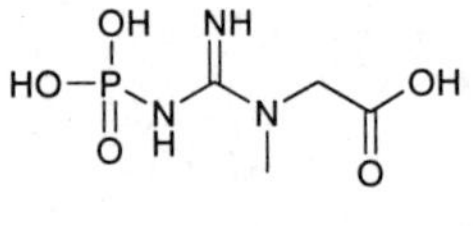

1313 Creatinine

$C_4H_7N_3O$ MW: 113.12 Property: mp 260°C (dec). Source: MO GU, NIU XUE, REN NIAO. Ref: 6.

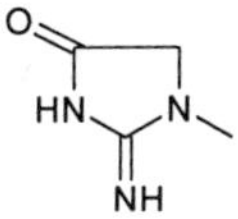

1314 Crenulatin

Δ^1-Isopentenyl-3-O-β-D-glucopyranoside. $C_{11}H_{20}O_6$ MW: 248.28 Property: colorless little prismatic crystal, mp 118-20°C (acetone), $[\alpha]_D^{20}$ -26.76° (c=1.1, ethanol). Source: DA HUA HONG JING TIAN. Ref: 218.

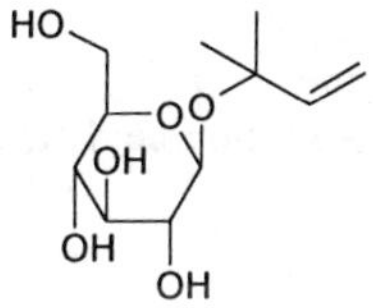

1315 m-Cresol

C_7H_8O MW: 108.14 Property: mp 11-2°C, bp 202°C. Source: MO YAO, SANG YE. Ref: 6.

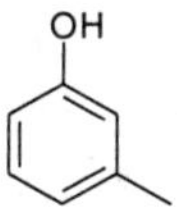

1316 O-Cresol

C_7H_8O MW: 108.14 Source: DANG GUI. Ref: 2.

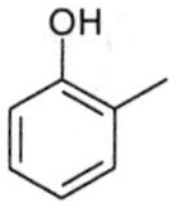

1317 p-Cresol

C_7H_8O MW: 108.14 Property: mp 34°C. Source: DANG GUI, DU HUO. Ref: 2.

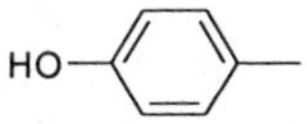

1318 Croalbidine

$C_{18}H_{29}NO_7$ MW: 371.43 Property: mp 208-9°C. Source: HUANG HUA DI DING. Ref: 6.

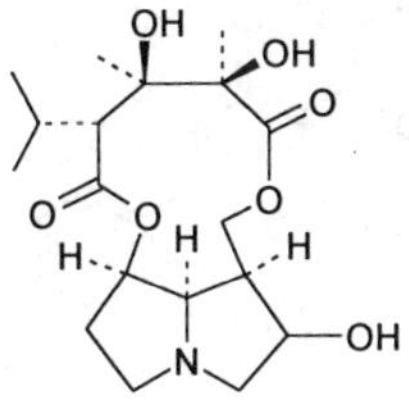

1319 Crocetin

α-Crocetin. $C_{20}H_{24}O_4$ MW: 328.41 Property: mp trans-: 285°C. Source: ZHI ZI. Ref: 2, 4.

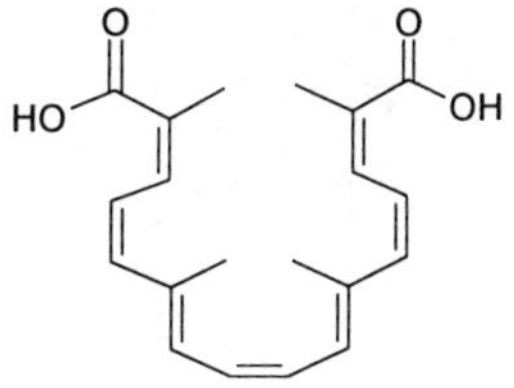

1320 Crocetin dimethyl ester

$C_{22}H_{28}O_4$ MW: 356.47 Property: mp cis-: 141°C, trans-: 222.5°C. Source: JIU BI YING (BAI MU XIANG), ZANG HONG HUA. Ref: 6.

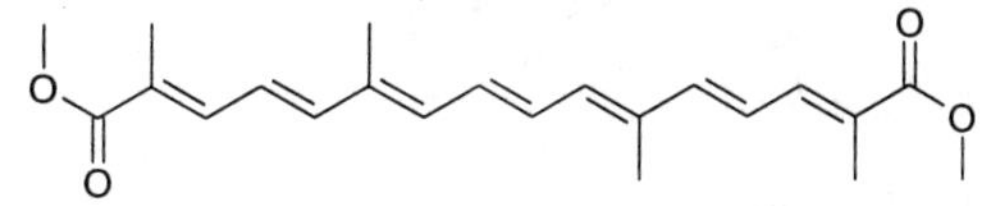

1321 Crocin

$C_{44}H_{64}O_{24}$ MW: 976.99 Source: ZHI ZI. Ref: 2.

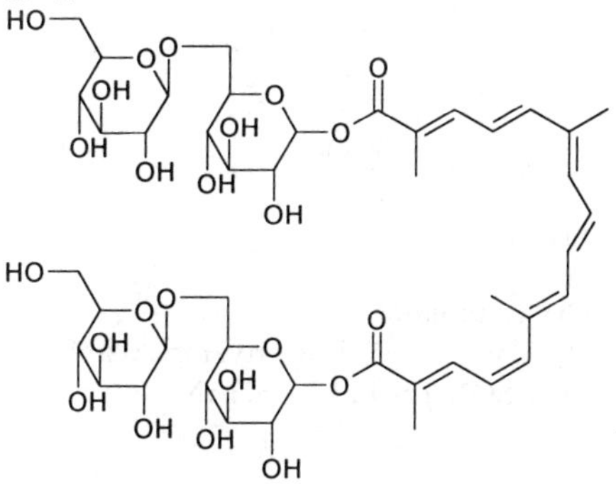

1322 Croomionidine

$C_{24}H_{42}N_2$ MW: 358.62 Property: crystal, mp 150-152°C, $[\alpha]_D^{25}$ -120°(c=0.15, MeOH). Source: JIN GANG DA. Ref: 261.

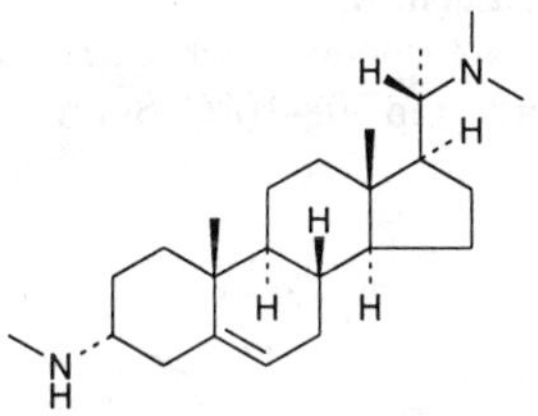

1323 Crotonic acid

$C_4H_6O_2$ MW: 86.09 Source: BA DOU. Ref: 2.

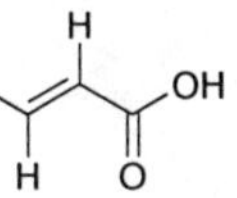

1324 Crotonoside
2-Hydroxy-6-aminopurine-9-β-D-ribofuranoside. $C_{10}H_{13}N_5O_5$ MW: 283.25 Source: BA DOU. Ref: 2.

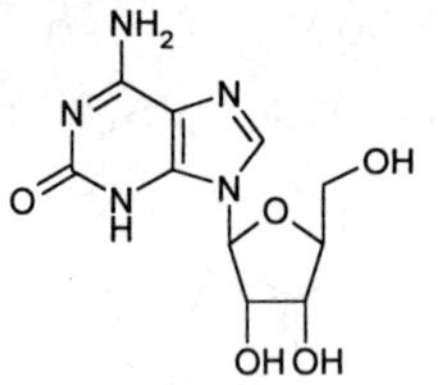

1325 Croweacin
$C_{11}H_{12}O_3$ MW: 192.22 Source: XI XIN. Ref: 2.

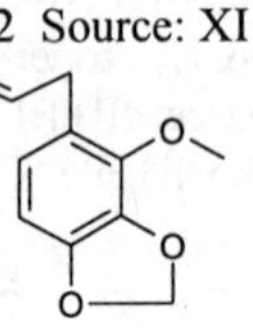

1326 Cryptogenin
$C_{28}H_{44}O_4$ MW: 444.66 Property: mp 187-9°C. Source: YU ER QI. Ref: 6.

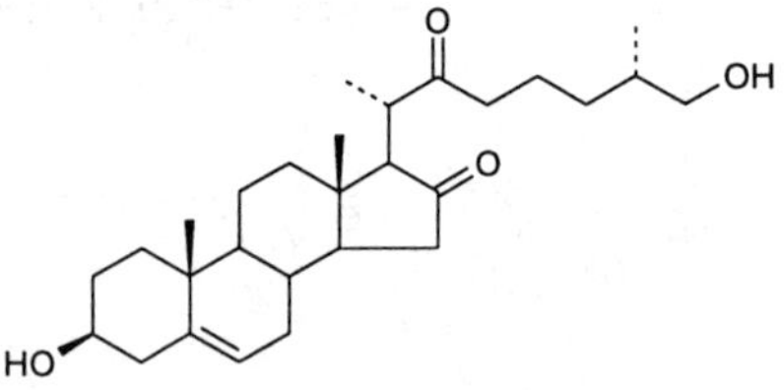

1327 Cryptojaponol
$C_{21}H_{30}O_3$ MW: 330.47 Property: mp 204-5°C. Source: DU SONG SHI, LIU SHAN. Ref: 6.

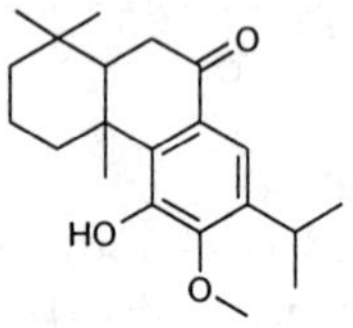

1328 Cryptomerin A
Hinokiflavone 4'''-methylether. $C_{31}H_{20}O_{10}$ MW: 552.50 Property: mp 308-10°C. Source: LIU SHAN. Ref: 6.

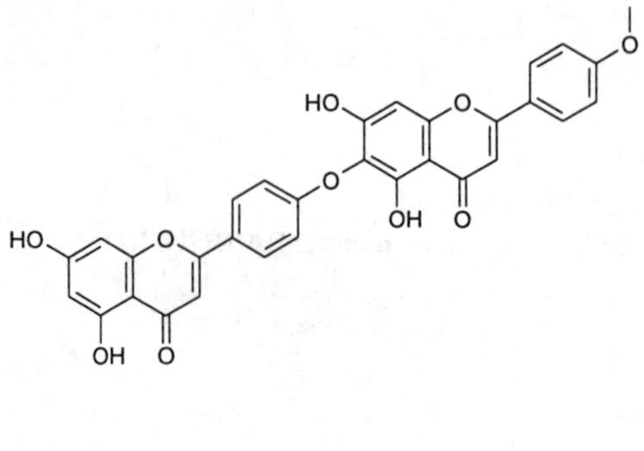

1329 Cryptomerin B
Hinokiflavone 4''',7''-dimethylether. $C_{32}H_{22}O_{10}$ MW: 566.53 Property: mp 302-3°C (dec). Source: LIU SHAN. Ref: 6.

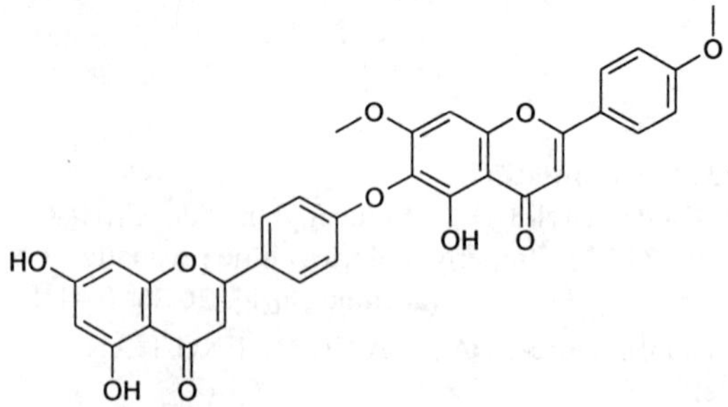

1330 Cryptomerion
$C_{15}H_{22}O$ MW: 218.34 Source: LIU SHAN. Ref: 6.

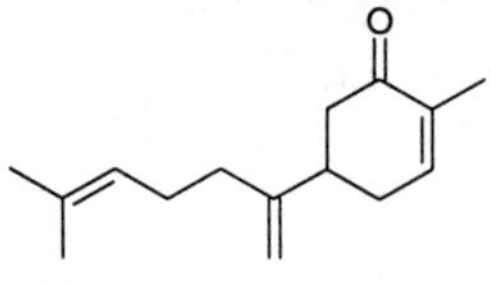

1331 Cryptone
$C_9H_{14}O$ MW: 138.21 Property: bp (-): 98-100°C /10mm. (±): 103°C/17mm. Source: HU JIAO. Ref: 6.

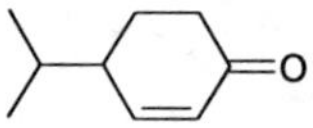

1332 Cryptopimaric acid
$C_{20}H_{30}O_2$ MW: 302.46 Property: mp 171-3°C. Source: LIU SHAN. Ref: 6.

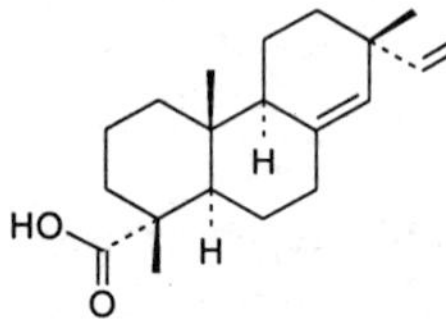

1333 Cryptopine
Cryptocavine. $C_{21}H_{23}NO_5$ MW: 369.42 Property: mp 221-3°C. Source: BAI QU CAI, HE BAO MU DAN GEN, HE QING HUA, JU HUA HUANG LIAN, YA PIAN, YING SU KE. Ref: 6.

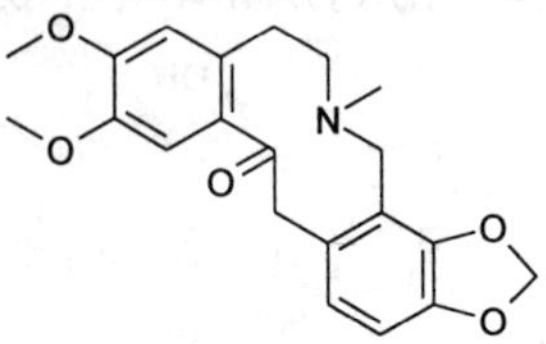

1334 Cryptotanshinone
$C_{19}H_{20}O_3$ MW: 296.37 Property: mp 191°C. Source: DAN SHEN. Ref: 2.

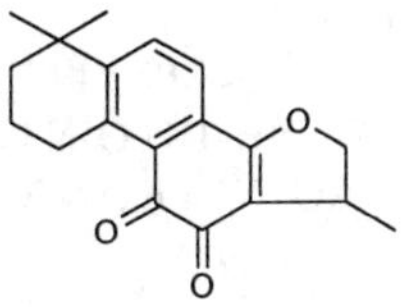

1335 Cryptoxanthin
$C_{40}H_{56}O$ MW: 552.89 Property: mp 169°C. Source: GOU QI ZI. Ref: 2.

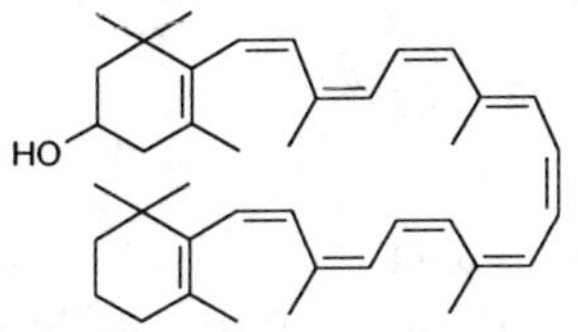

1336 Cryptoxanthin monoepoxide
$C_{40}H_{56}O_2$ MW: 568.89 Property: mp 154°C. Source: FAN MU GUA. Ref: 6.

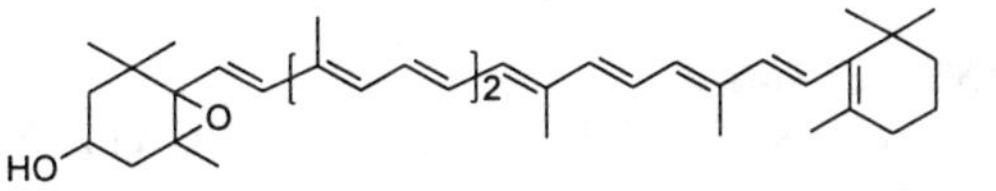

1337 Crysoeriol
$C_{16}H_{12}O_6$ MW: 300.27 Source: SAN JIAN SHAN. Ref: 2.

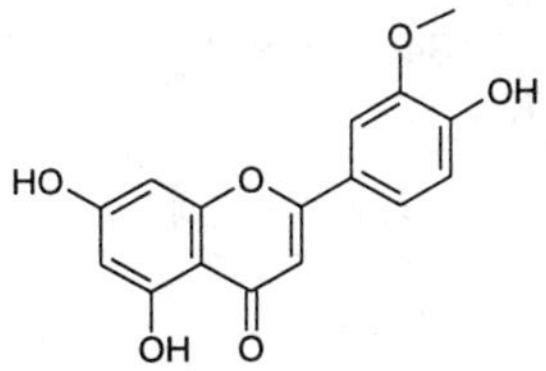

1338 Cubeben camphor
$C_{15}H_{26}O$ MW: 222.37 Property: mp 61-2°C. Source: BI CHENG QIE. Ref: 6.

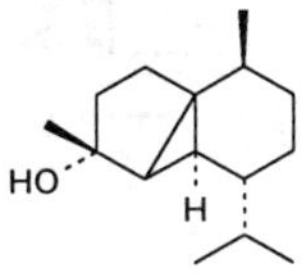

1339 α-Cubebene
$C_{14}H_{22}$ MW: 190.33 Source: CHAI HU, SHENG JIANG. Ref: 2.

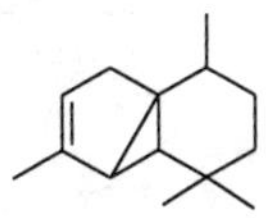

1340 Cubebin
$C_{20}H_{20}O_6$ MW: 356.38 Property: mp 131-2°C. Source: BI CHENG QIE. Ref: 6.

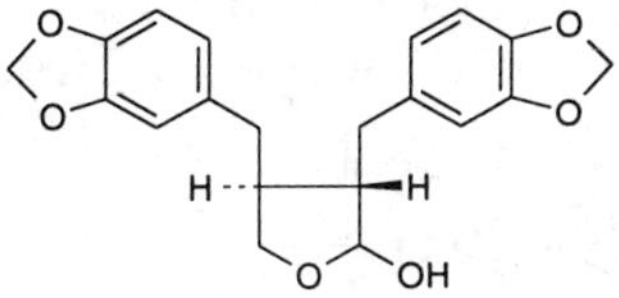

1341 Cubebinolide
$C_{20}H_{18}O_6$ MW: 354.36 Property: mp (+): 64-5°C, (-): 64-5°C, (±): 108°C. Source: BI CHENG QIE. Ref: 6.

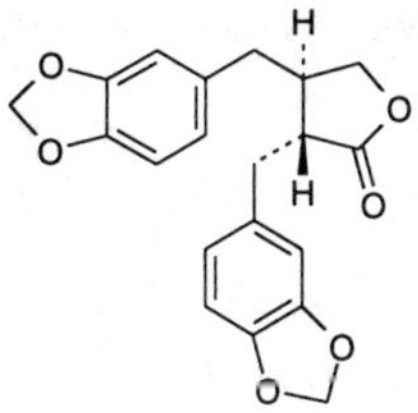

1342 Cuchiloside
$C_{19}H_{28}O_{11}$ MW: 432.43 Source: MA QIAN ZI. Ref: 2.

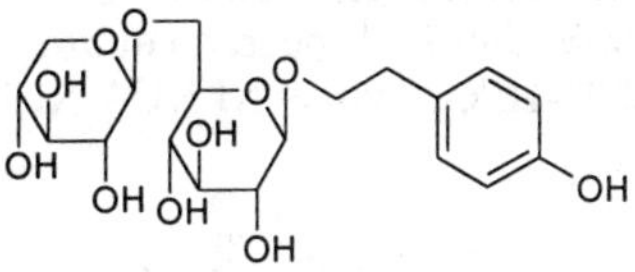

1343 Cucurbitacin A
$C_{32}H_{46}O_9$ MW: 574.72 Property: mp 207-8°C. Source: HUANG GUA. Ref: 6.

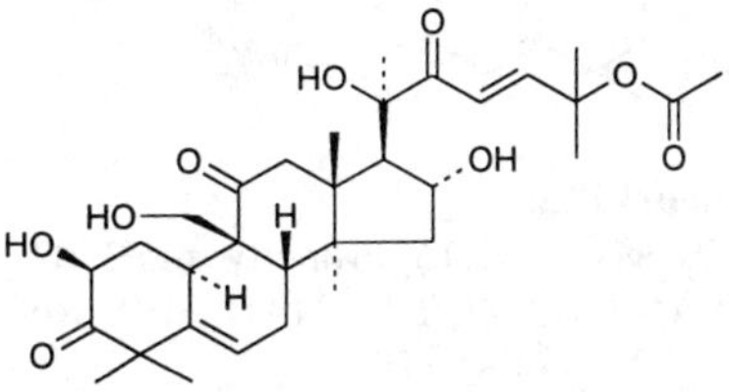

1344 Cucurbitacin B
Amarin; Fabacei II. CAS: 6199-67-3 $C_{32}H_{46}O_8$ MW: 558.72 Property: mp 178-86°C. Source: HU LU, HUANG GUA, GUA DI, GUA LOU, YANG JIAO AO ZI. Ref: 4, 5, 6, 532.

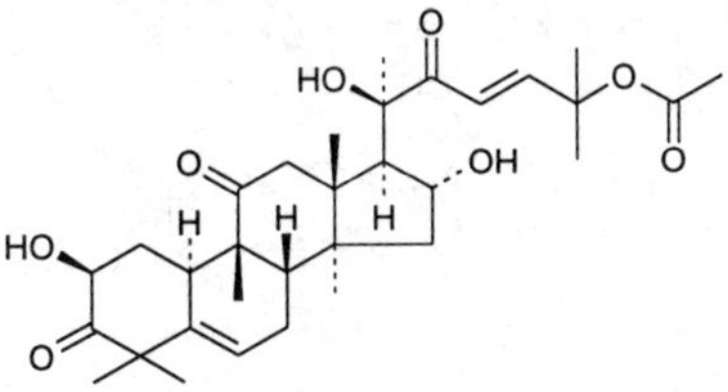

1345 Cucurbitacin C
$C_{32}H_{48}O_8$ MW: 560.73 Property: mp 207-7.5°C. Source: HUANG GUA. Ref: 6.

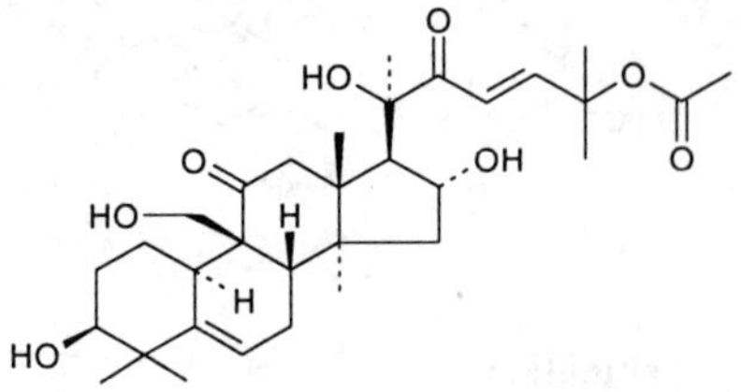

1346 Cucurbitacin D
Elatericin. CAS: 3877-86-9 $C_{30}H_{44}O_7$ MW: 516.68 Property: mp 149-53°C (dec). Source: HUANG GUA. Ref: 5, 6.

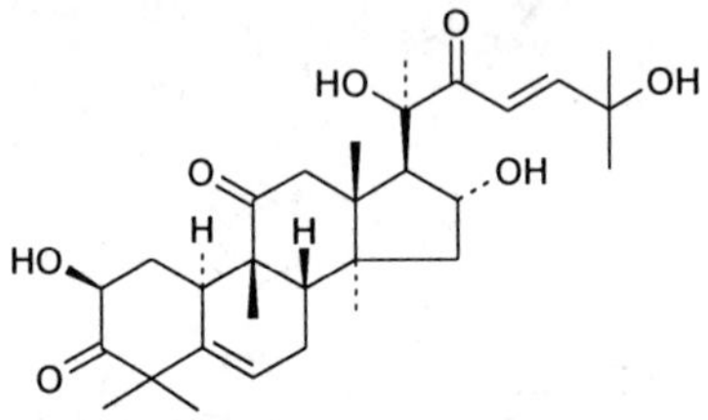

1347 Cucurbitacin F-25-acetate
$C_{32}H_{48}O_8$ MW: 560.73 Property: colorless acicular crystal, mp208-10°C, Source: XI HUA XUE DAN. Ref: 33.

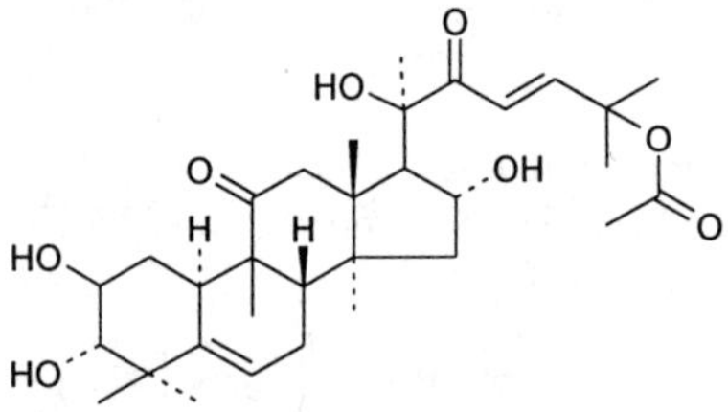

1348 Cucurbitine
$C_5H_{10}N_2O_2$ MW: 130.15 Property: mp 260°C (dec). Source: NAN GUA ZI, TAO NAN GUA. Ref: 6.

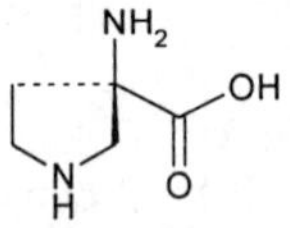

1349 Cudranin
$C_{14}H_{12}O_4$ MW: 244.25 Property: mp 202°C. Source: SANG ZHI. Ref: 6.

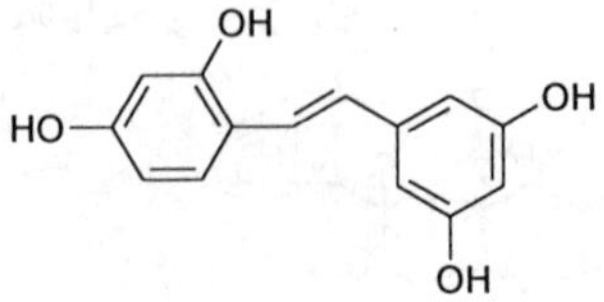

1350 Cuhuoside
Source: YIN YANG HUO. Ref: 635.

1351 Cumaldehyde
Cuminaldehyde. $C_{10}H_{12}O$ MW: 148.21 Property: bp 235-6°C. Source: AN YE, DU QIN GEN, HUANG HUA HAO, MO YAO, XI YE AN YE. Ref: 6.

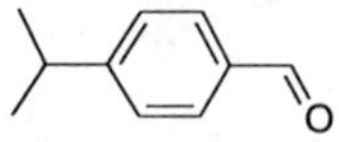

1352 Cumic acid
$C_{10}H_{12}O_2$ MW: 164.21 Source: ZI SU. Ref: 2.

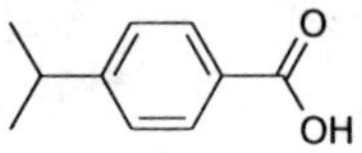

1353 Cumic alcohol
$C_{10}H_{14}O$ MW: 150.22 Property: bp 246°C. Source: HUA JIAO. Ref: 6.

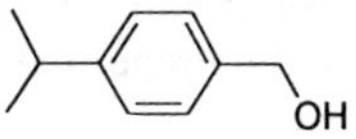

1354 Cumulene
$C_{10}H_{10}O_2$ MW: 162.19 Source: QI ZHOU YI ZHI. Ref: 6.

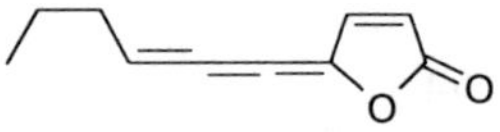

1355 Cuparene
$C_{15}H_{22}$ MW: 202.34 Source: FANG FENG, SAN QI, WU WEI ZI. Ref: 2.

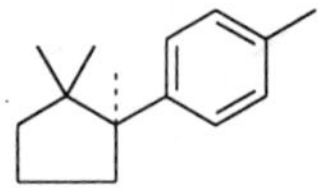

1356 α-Cuparenol
$C_{15}H_{22}O$ MW: 218.34 Property: mp 73°C. Source: BAI ZHI JIE. Ref: 6.

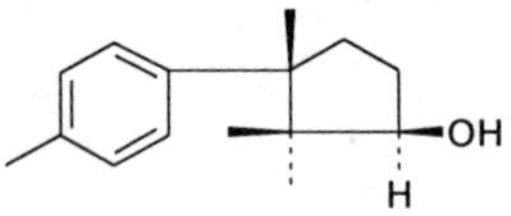

1357 β-Cuparenol
$C_{15}H_{22}O$ MW: 218.34 Source: BAI ZHI JIE. Ref: 6.

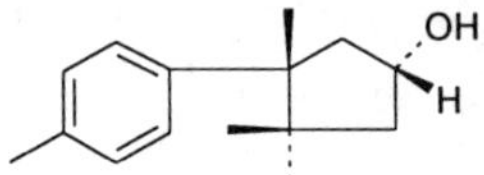

1358 γ-Cuparenol
$C_{15}H_{22}O$ MW: 218.34 Property: bp 110°C/0.5mm. Source: BAI ZHI JIE. Ref: 6.

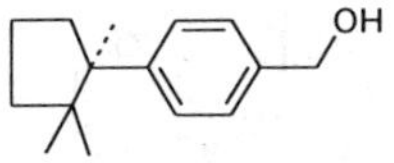

1359 α-Cuparenone
$C_{15}H_{20}O$ MW: 216.33 Property: mp (+): 52-3°C. Source: BAI ZHI JIE. Ref: 6.

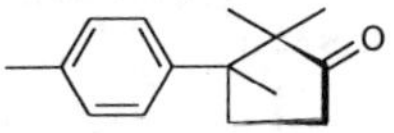

1360 β-Cuparenone
$C_{15}H_{20}O$ MW: 216.33 Property: bp 114-5°C /0.8mm. Source: BAI ZHI JIE. Ref: 6.

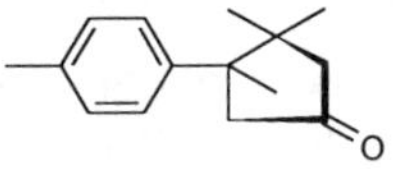

1361 Cupreine
Hydroxycinchonine. $C_{19}H_{22}NO_2$ MW: 310.40 Property: mp 198°C. Source: JIN JI LE. Ref: 6.

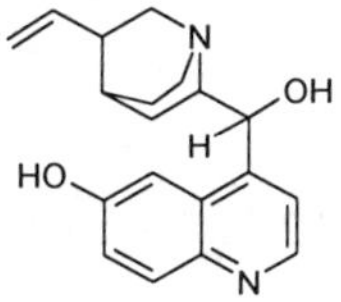

1362 α-Cuprenene
$C_{15}H_{24}$ MW: 204.36 Property: bp 140-1°C. Source: BAI ZHI JIE. Ref: 6.

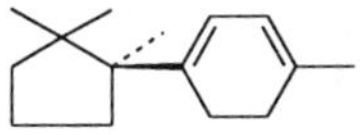

1363 γ-Cuprenene
$C_{15}H_{24}$ MW: 204.36 Property: bp 140-1°C. Source: BAI ZHI JIE. Ref: 6.

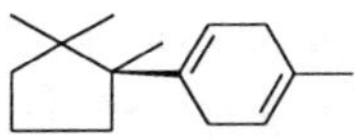

1364 Cupressuflavone
$C_{30}H_{18}O_{10}$ MW: 538.47 Property: mp >360°C. Source: CE BAI YE. Ref: 6.

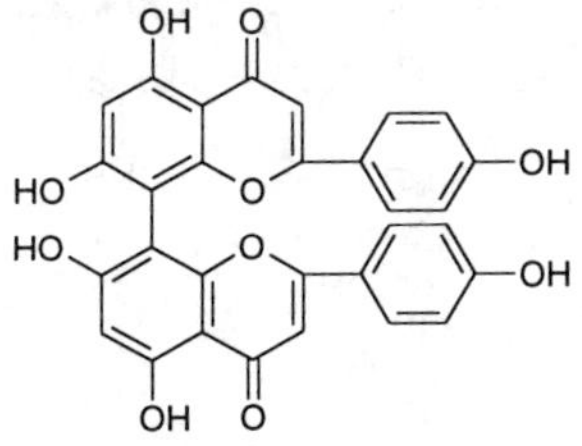

1365 Curcolone
$C_{15}H_{18}O_3$ MW: 246.31 Source: PENG E SHU. Ref: 6.

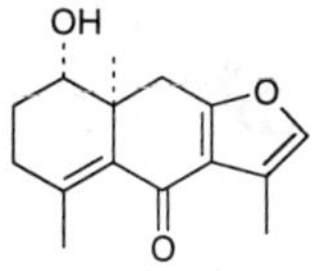

1366 Curculigine B
$C_{19}H_{26}Cl_2O_{11}$ MW: 501.32 Property: colorless acicular crystal (CH_3COCH_3), mp 202-5°C, $[\alpha]_D^{18}$-33.6° (c=0.15, methanol). Source: XIAN MAO. Ref: 227.

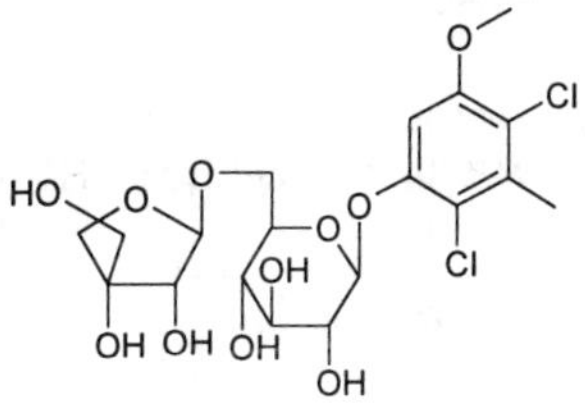

1367 Curculigine C
$C_{19}H_{25}Cl_3O_{11}$ MW: 535.76 Property: colorless acicular crystal, mp 178-81°C, $[\alpha]_D^{18}$-38.94° (c=0.94, methanol). Source: XIAN MAO. Ref: 227.

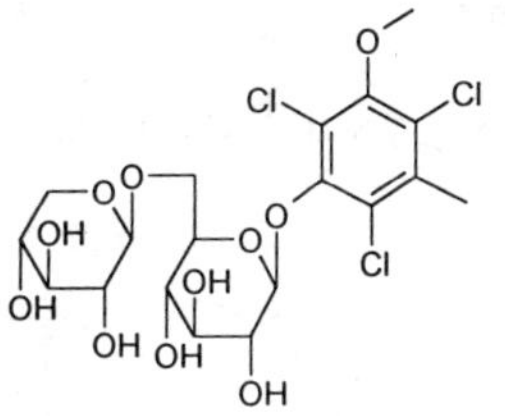

1368 Curculigoside B
$C_{21}H_{24}O_{11}$ MW: 452.42 Property: colorless acicular crystal, mp 219-22°C. Source: XIAN MAO. Ref: 227.

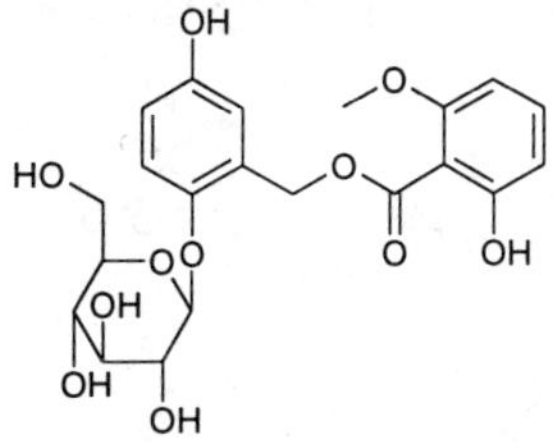

1369 Curcumadiol
$C_{15}H_{26}O_2$ MW: 238.37 Property: mp 145-5.5°C. Source: PENG E SHU. Ref: 6.

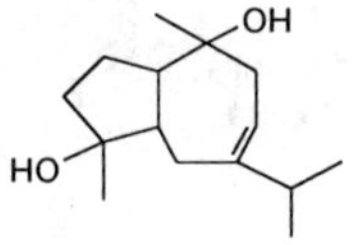

1370 α-Curcumene
$C_{15}H_{22}$ MW: 202.34 Source: DANG SHEN, GAN JIANG, SHENG JIANG, XI YANG SHEN. Ref: 2.

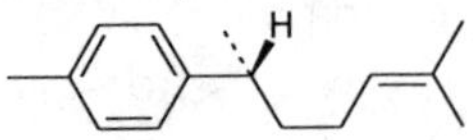

1371 β-Curcumene
$C_{15}H_{24}$ MW: 204.36 Property: bp (+): 98-100°C/2.2mm, (-): 142°C/19mm. Source: YU JIN. Ref: 6.

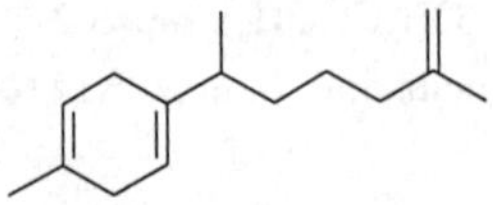

1372 Curcumenether
$C_{15}H_{22}O$ MW: 218.34 Source: BAI ZHI JIE. Ref: 6.

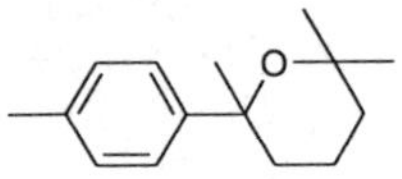

1373 Curcumenol
Property: mp 118.5-9.5°C. Source: PENG E SHU. Ref: 6.

1374 Curcumin
$C_{21}H_{20}O_6$ MW: 368.39 Property: mp 183°C. Source: BAI CHANG, YU JIN, JIANG HUANG, PENG E SHU. Ref: 6.

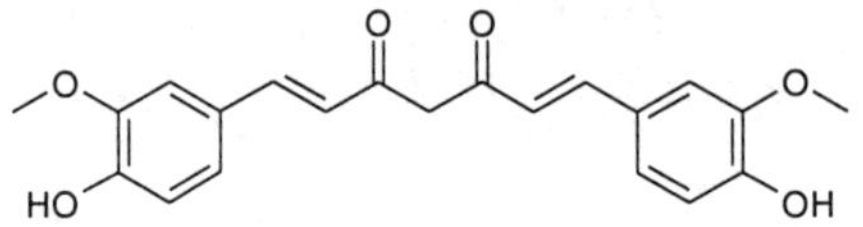

1375 Curcumol
CAS: 4871-97-0 $C_{15}H_{24}O_2$ MW: 236.36 Property: mp 141-4°C. Source: PENG E SHU. Ref: 4, 5, 6.

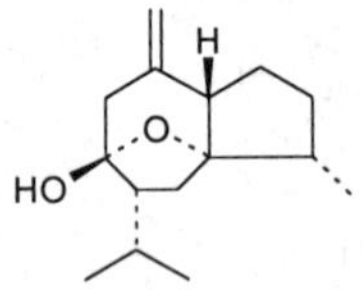

1376 Curdione
CAS: 13657-68-6 $C_{15}H_{24}O_2$ MW: 236.36 Property: mp 61-2°C. Source: PENG E SHU. Ref: 4, 5, 6.

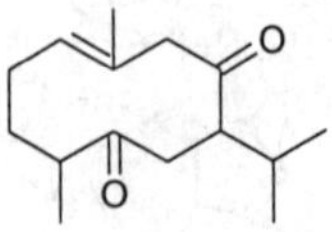

1377 Curzerene
Isofuranogermacrene. $C_{15}H_{20}O$ MW: 216.33 Source: PENG E SHU, SHUI CAI. Ref: 6.

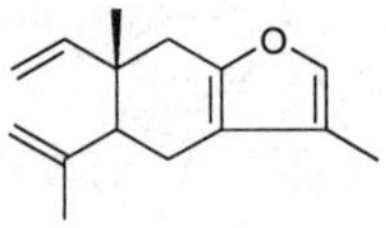

1378 Curzerenone
$C_{15}H_{18}O_2$ MW: 230.31 Property: bp 104°C/3mm. Source: SHUI CAI. Ref: 6.

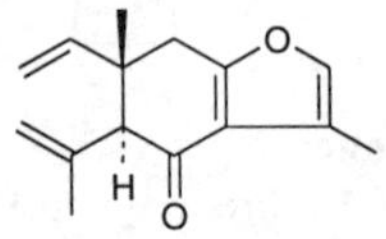

1379 Cuscohygrine
$C_{15}H_{24}N_2O$ MW: 224.35 Property: bp 169-70°C /23mm. Source: MAN TUO LUO GEN, MAN TUO LUO YE, PAO NANG CAO, SAI LANG DANG, SAN FEN SAN, TIAN XIAN ZI, ZANG QIE. Ref: 6.

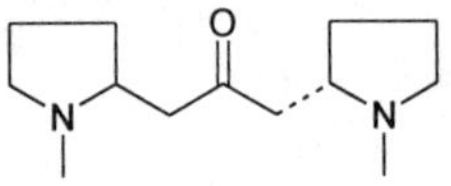

1380 Cyanidin
$C_{15}H_{11}O_6$ MW: 287.25 Source: CHOU MO LI. Ref: 6.

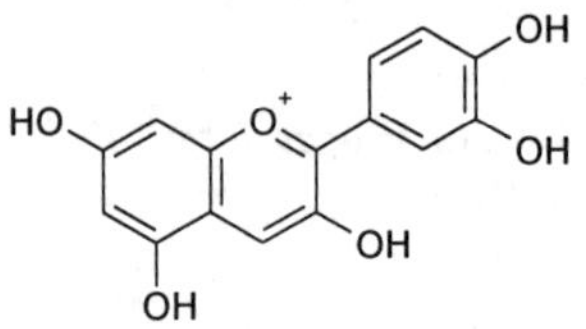

1381 Cyanidin-3-(6-p-coumaroyl-β-D-gluco-side) 5-β-D-glucoside
Source: ZI SU. Ref: 2.

1382 Cyanidin-3-gentiobioside
$C_{27}H_{31}O_{16}$ MW: 611.54 Source: YI ZHI HUANG HUA. Ref: 6.

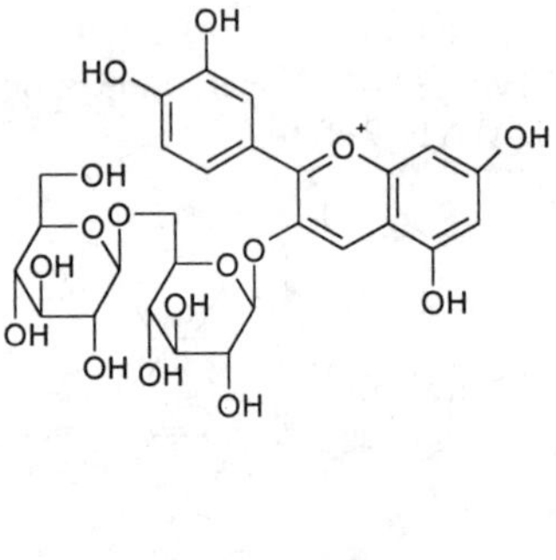

1383 Cyanidin-3-monogalactoside
Idaein. $C_{20}H_{19}O_{11}$ MW: 435.37 Property: mp 210°C (dec). Source: HUANG LU ZHI YE, QIAN QU CAI, QIU MU GUA. Ref: 6.

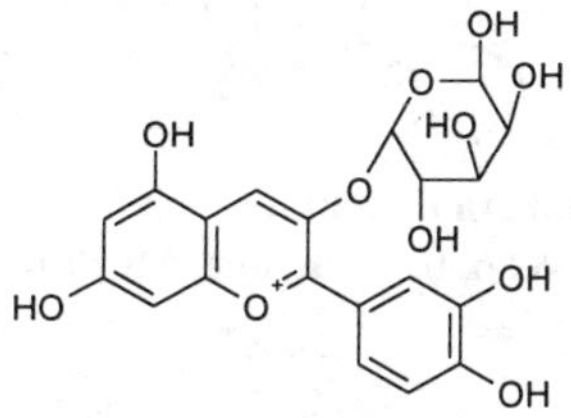

1384 Cyanidin monoglycoside
Cyrysanthemin. Source: FENG XIAN GEN, HUANG LU ZHI YE, HUANG MA YE, SHI JUN ZI. Ref: 6.

1385 Cyanidin-3-rutinoside
Cyanidin rhamno-glucoside. $C_{27}H_{31}O_{15}$ MW: 595.54 Source: MO PAN CAO, YE DONG QING QUO. Ref: 6.

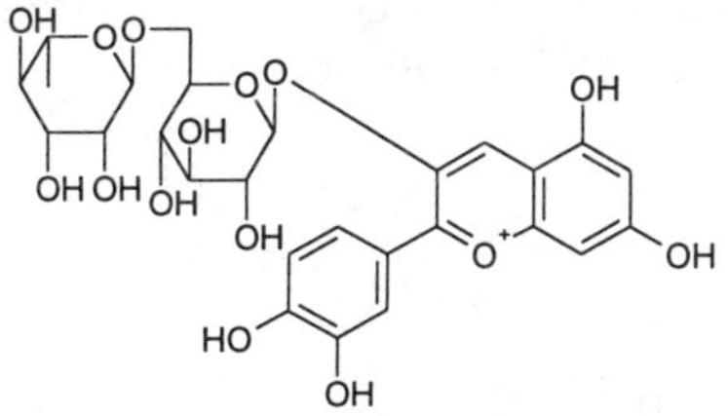

1386 Cyanidin-3-rutinoside-5-glucoside
$C_{34}H_{43}O_{19}$ MW: 755.71 Source: MU FU RONG HUA. Ref: 6.

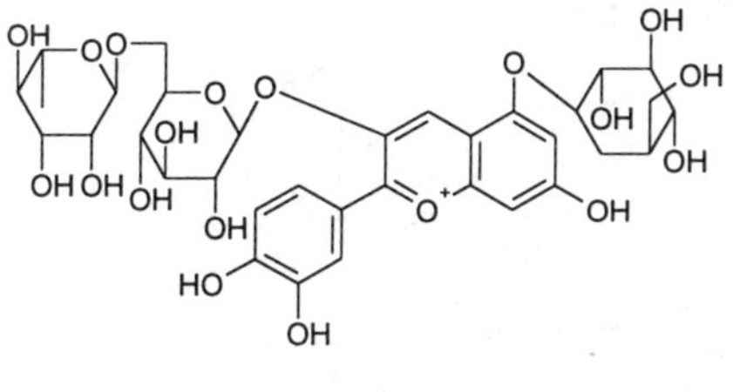

1387 Cyanidin-3-sophoroside-5-glucoside
$C_{34}H_{43}O_{21}$ MW: 787.71 Source: FU SANG HUA. Ref: 6.

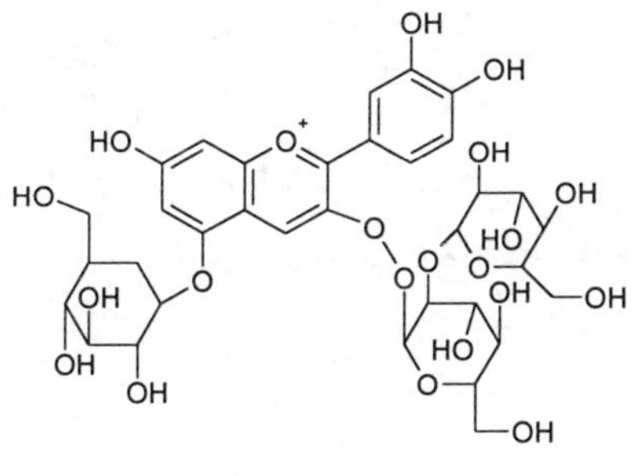

1388 Cyanidin-3-xylosyl-glucoside
$C_{26}H_{29}O_{15}$ MW: 581.51 Source: BU XUE CAO. Ref: 6.

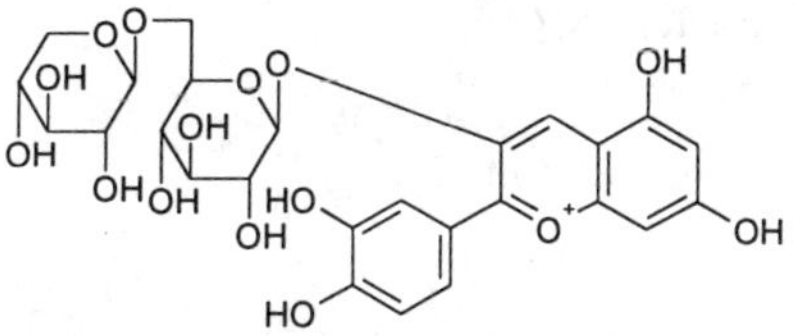

1389 Cyanin
Cyanidin diglucoside; Cyanidin 3,5-diglucoside. $C_{27}H_{31}O_{16}$ MW: 611.54 Property: mp 205°C (dec). Source: BAI FAN DOU, DI YU, DU JUAN HUA, MAO SHU, MEI GUI HUA, MU FU RONG HUA, YU JIN XIANG. Ref: 6.

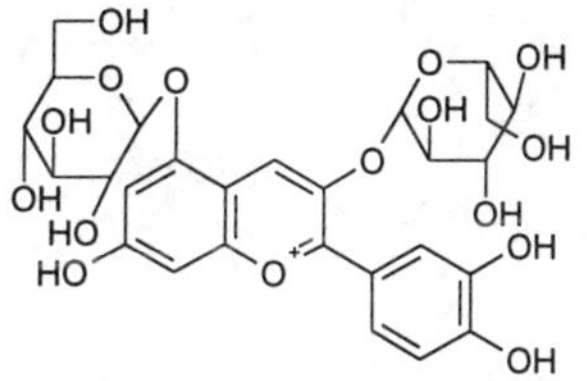

1390 1-Cyano-2-hydroxy methylprop-1-ene-3-ol
$C_5H_7NO_2$ MW: 113.12 Source: JIA KU GUA. Ref: 6.

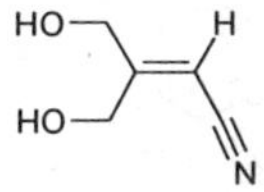

1391 1-Cyano-2-hydroxy methylprop-2-ene-1-ol
$C_5H_7NO_2$ MW: 113.12 Source: JIA KU GUA. Ref: 6.

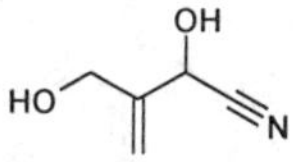

1392 Cyanophoric glycoside
Source: BIAN DOU, BAI GUO, JIU JIE CHA, SHI NAN YE, TAO YE, WEN PO, YING TAO. Ref: 6.

1393 Cyasterone
$C_{29}H_{44}O_8$ MW: 520.67 Property: mp 164-6°C. Source: BAI MAO XIA KU CAO, CHUAN NIU XI, YU ER QI. Ref: 6.

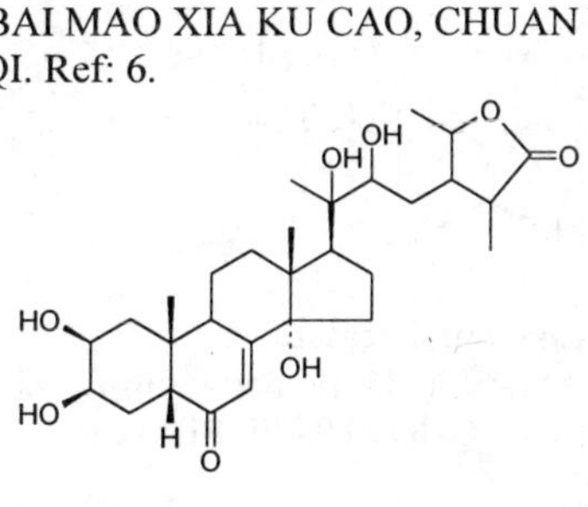

1394 Cycasin
CAS: 14901-08-7 $C_8H_{16}N_2O_7$ MW: 252.23 Property: mp 154°C (dec). Source: FENG WEI JIAO YE, TIE SHU GUO. Ref: 5, 6.

1395 Cycleaneonine
$C_{38}H_{42}N_2O_6$ MW: 622.77 Property: slightly yellow crystalline powder, mp 96-7°C, $[\alpha]_D^{16}$ +376.8° (c=0.501, chloroform). Source: LUN HUAN TENG. Ref: 104.

1396 Cycleanine
CAS: 518-94-5 $C_{38}H_{42}NO_6$ MW: 622.77 Property: mp 268-73°C. Source: BAI YAO ZI, DI BU RONG, SI CHUAN LUN HUAN TENG. Ref: 5, 6, 274.

1397 Cycloartanol
$C_{31}H_{56}O$ MW: 444.79 Property: mp 101-2°C. Source: HUO YANG LE, SHUI LONG GU, DOU YOU. Ref: 6.

1398 Cycloartanol acetate
$C_{33}H_{48}O_2$ MW: 486.83 Property: mp 132-3°C. Source: MANG GUO SHU PI. Ref: 6.

1399 Cycloartanol ferulate
$C_{41}H_{64}O_4$ MW: 620.96 Source: MI PI KANG. Ref: 6.

1400 Cycloartenol
$C_{31}H_{54}O$ MW: 442.78 Property: mp 115°C. Source: DOU YOU, GAN PI, HUO YANG LE, SHI CHUN, YA PIAN, YAN CAO. Ref: 6.

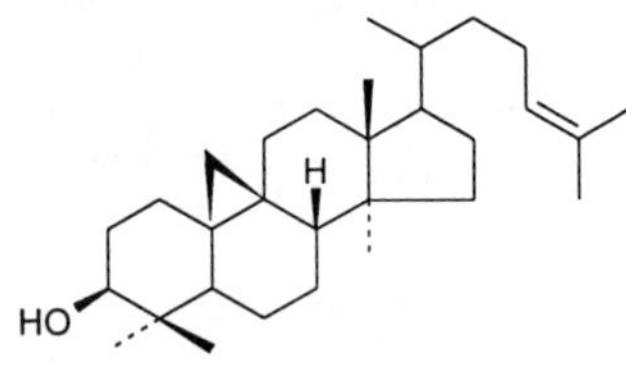

1401 Cycloartenone
$C_{31}H_{52}O$ MW: 454.79 Property: mp 109°C. Source: YA PIAN. Ref: 6.

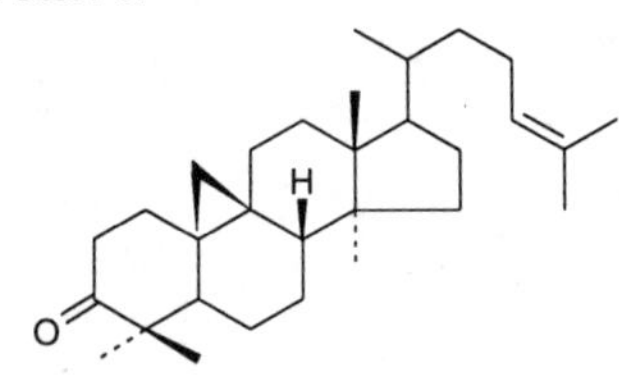

1402 Cycloartenyl ferulate
Oryzanol A. $C_{41}H_{62}O_4$ MW: 618.95 Source: MI PI KANG. Ref: 6.

1403 Cycloastragenol
$C_{30}H_{50}O_5$ MW: 490.73 Source: HUANG QI. Ref: 2.

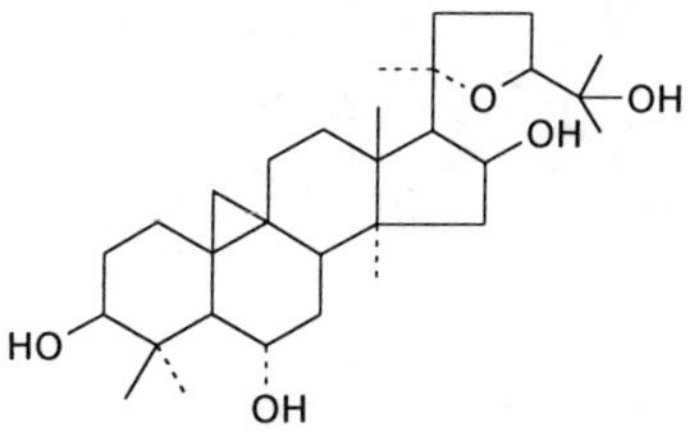

1404 Cyclocaric acid B
3-Oxo-2α,23-Dihydroxyolean-12-en-28-oic acid. $C_{30}H_{46}O_5$ MW: 486.70 Property: white granular crystal, mp 258-60°C (MeOH). Source: QING QIAN LIU. Ref: 493.

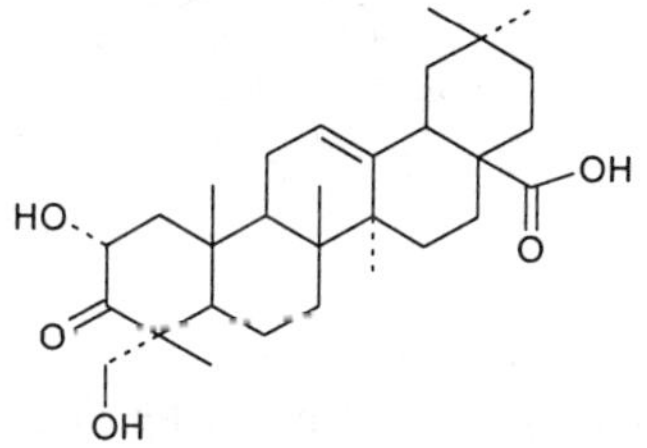

1405 Cyclocarioside I
20,24-Epoxy-dammarane-(3β,12β,20*S*,24*R*.)-12-O-β-D-quinovopyranosyi-25-hydroxy-3-O-α-L-arabinofuranoside. $C_{41}H_{70}O_{12}$ MW: 755.01 Property: white powdery crystal, mp 143-4°C. Source: QING QIAN LIU. Ref: 338.

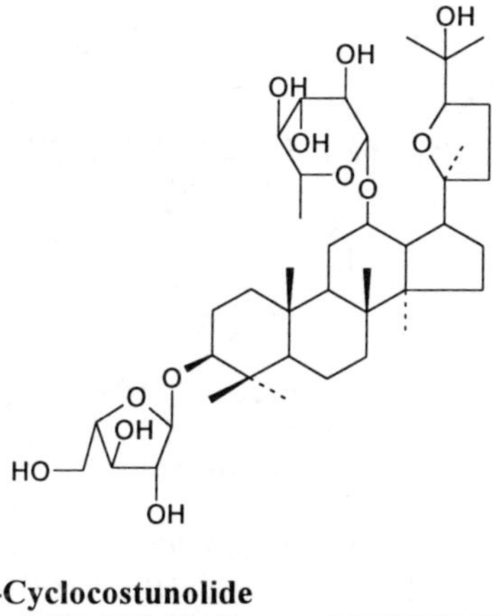

1406 α-Cyclocostunolide
$C_{15}H_{20}O_2$ MW: 232.33 Source: MU XIANG. Ref: 2.

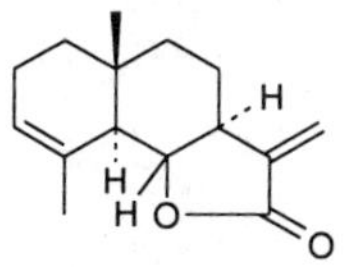

1407 β-Cyclocostunolide
Source: MU XIANG. Ref: 2.

1408 20(R)-21, 24-Cyclo-3β,25-dihydroxyl-dammar-23(24)-en-21-one
$C_{30}H_{48}O_3$ MW: 456.72 Source: QI YE DAN. Ref: 2.

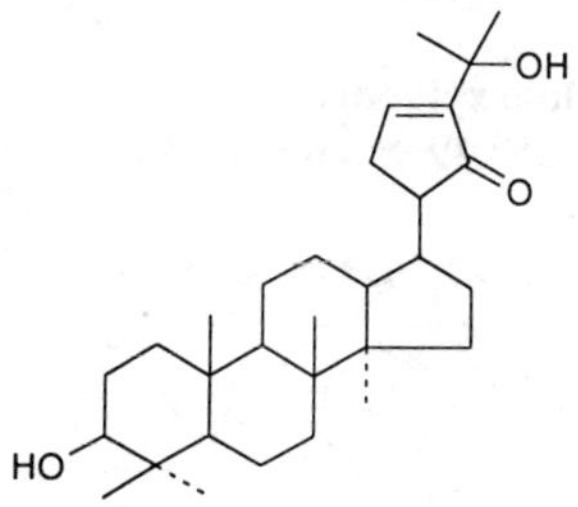

1409 Cyclododecanone
$C_{12}H_{22}O$ MW: 182.31 Source: SAN QI. Ref: 2.

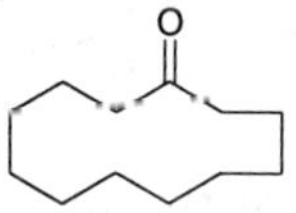

1410 Cycloeucalenol
$C_{31}H_{54}O$ MW: 442.78 Property: mp 138-9°C. Source: BA WANG BIAN. Ref: 6.

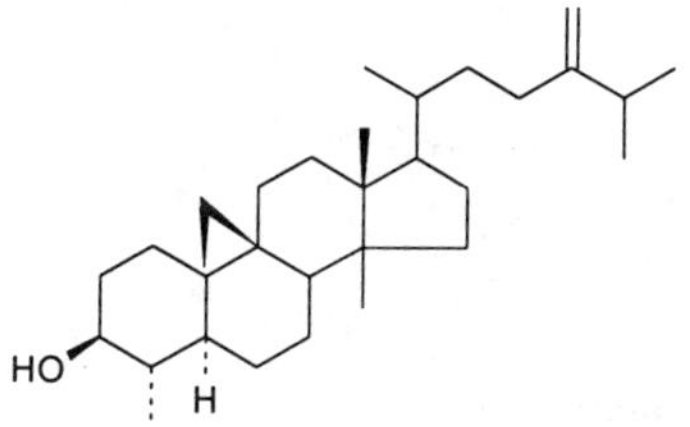

1411 Cycloheterophyllin
$C_{30}H_{30}O_7$ MW: 502.57 Source: BO LUO MI. Ref: 6.

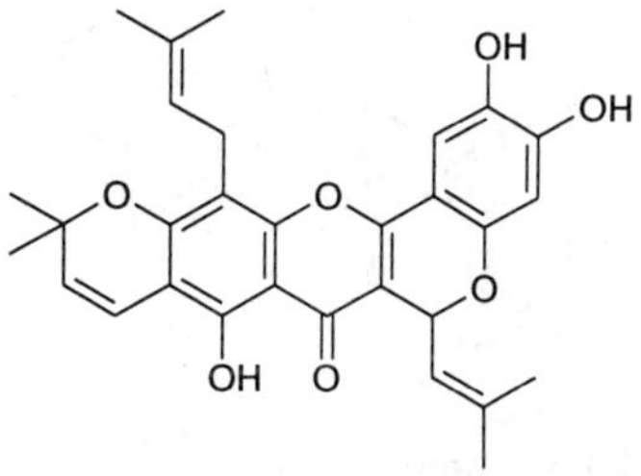

1412 Cyclohexanone pedunculosyl-3,23-O-acetal
Source: SI JI QING. Ref: 527.

1413 2-Cyclohexyl decane
$C_{16}H_{32}$ MW: 224.43 Source: DU HUO. Ref: 2.

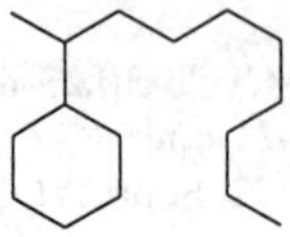

1414 3-Cyclohexyldodecane
$C_{18}H_{36}$ MW: 252.49 Source: XI YANG SHEN. Ref: 2.

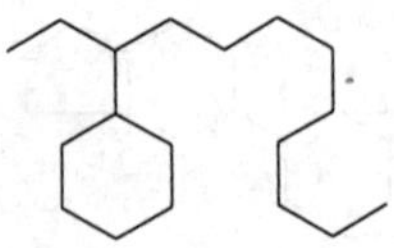

1415 2-(p-Cyclohexyl-phenoxy)ethanol
$C_{14}H_{20}O_2$ MW: 220.31 Source: WU WEI ZI. Ref: 2.

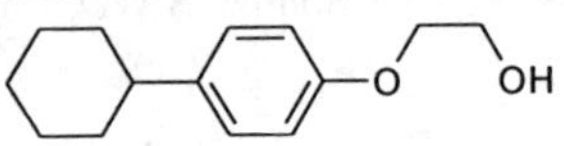

1416 Cyclokoreanine B
$C_{28}H_{50}N_2O$ MW: 430.72 Property: mp 235-6°C. Source: HUANG YANG MU YE. Ref: 6.

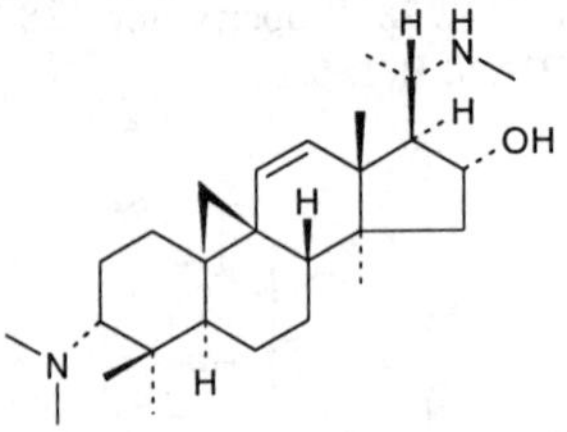

1417 Cyclolaudenol
$C_{32}H_{56}O$ MW: 456.80 Property: mp 125°C. Source: SHUI LONG GU, YA PIAN. Ref: 6.

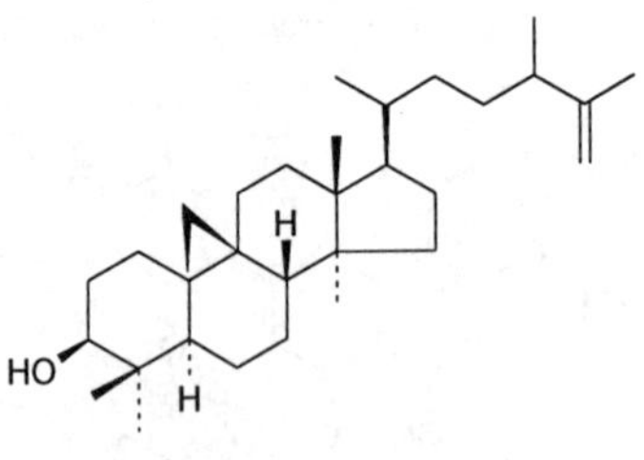

1418 Cyclolaudenone
$C_{32}H_{54}O$ MW: 454.79 Source: YA PIAN. Ref: 6.

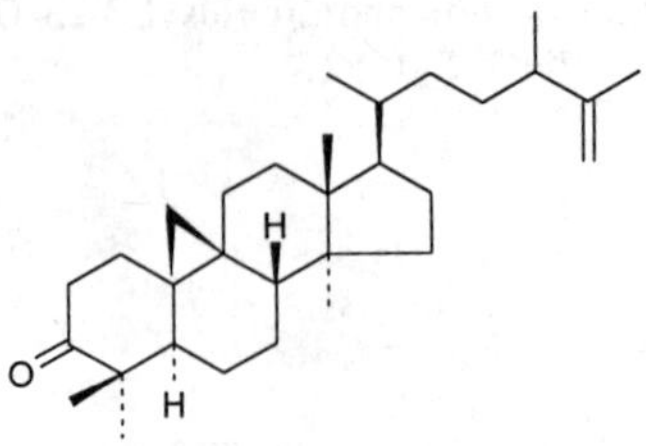

1419 Cyclomahanimbine
$C_{23}H_{25}NO$ MW: 331.46 Source: JIU LI XIANG. Ref: 11.

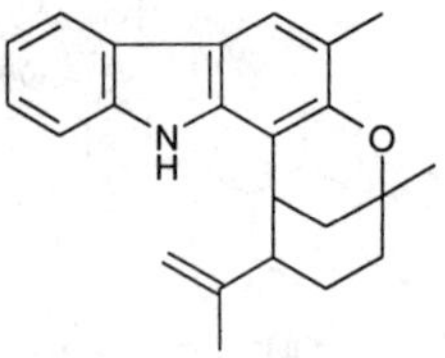

1420 Cyclomulberrin
$C_{25}H_{24}O_6$ MW: 420.47 Property: mp 231-2°C. Source: SANG BAI PI, SANG ZHI. Ref: 6.

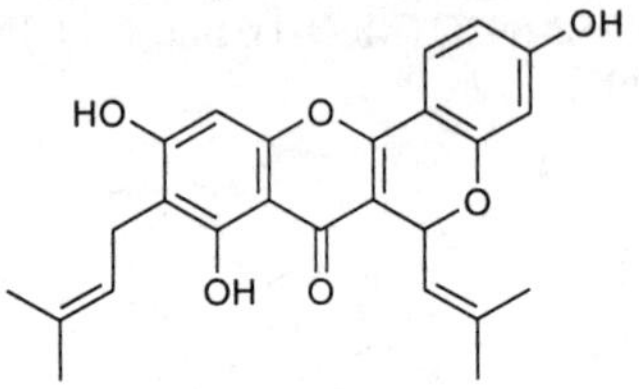

1412 Cyclomulberrochromene
$C_{25}H_{22}O_6$ MW: 418.45 Property: mp 233-4°C. Source: SANG BAI PI, SANG ZHI. Ref: 6.

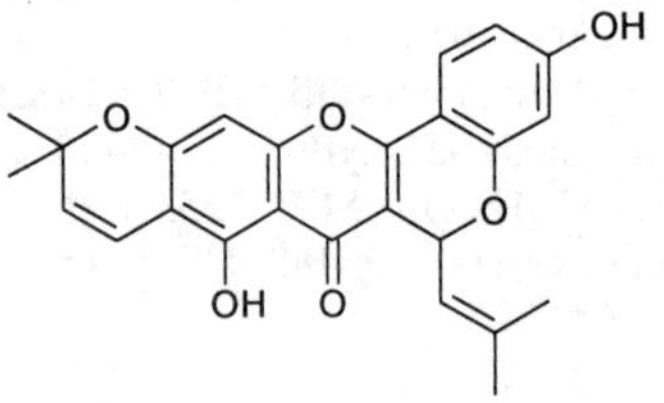

1422 (+)-Cyclo-olivil
$C_{20}H_{24}O_7$ MW: 376.41 Source: DU ZHONG. Ref: 2.

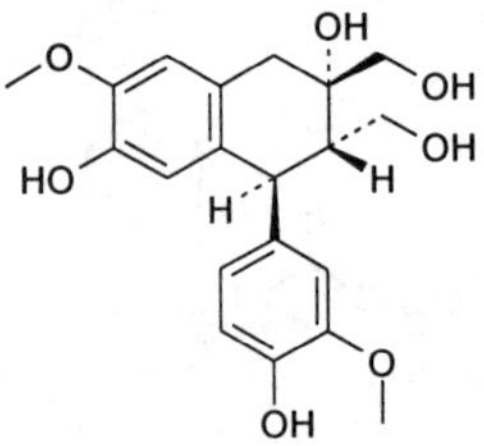

1423 5-cis-Cyclopentadecen-1-one
$C_{15}H_{26}O$ MW: 222.37 Source: SHE XIANG. Ref: 2.

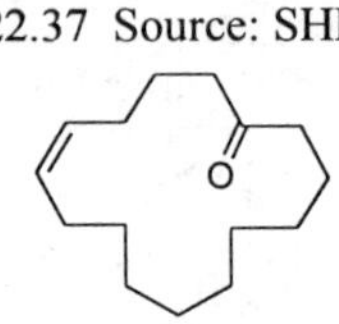

1424 Cyclopiloselloidone
$C_{18}H_{22}O_3$ MW: 286.37 Source: MAO DA DING CAO. Ref: 6.

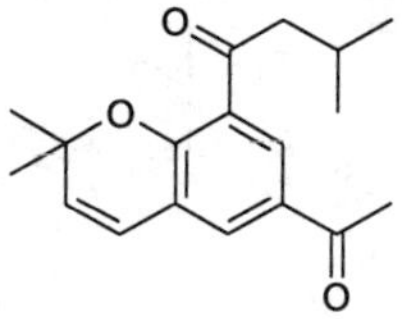

1425 Cyclo-(D-seryl-L-tyrosyl)
$C_{12}H_{14}N_2O_4$ MW: 250.26 Property: white acicular crystal, mp 256-9°C, $[\alpha]_D^{19}$+18.4° (c=1.09). Source: CHUAN SHAN JIA. Ref: 110.

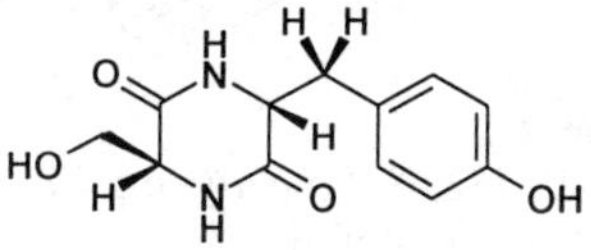

1426 Cyclotetradecan-1-one
$C_{14}H_{26}O$ MW: 210.36 Source: SHE XIANG. Ref: 2.

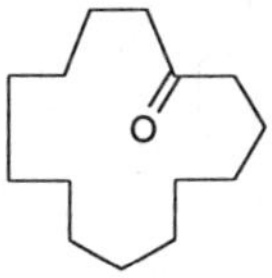

1427 5-cis-Cyclotetradecen-1-one
$C_{14}H_{24}O$ MW: 208.35 Source: SHE XIANG. Ref: 2.

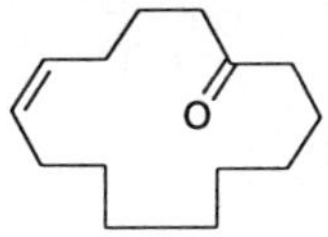

1428 Cyclovirobuxine D
$C_{27}H_{48}N_2O$ MW: 416.70 Property: mp 221-4°C. Source: HUANG YANG MU YE. Ref: 6.

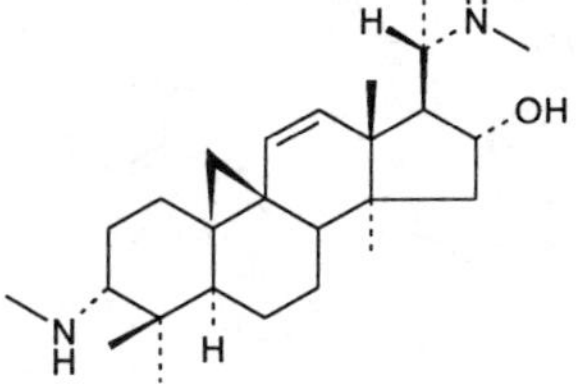

1429 Cylindrin
$C_{31}H_{52}O$ MW: 440.76 Property: mp 269-70°C. Source: BAI MAO GEN, DAN ZHU YE, MAO CAO YE, SUI GU ZI. Ref: 6.

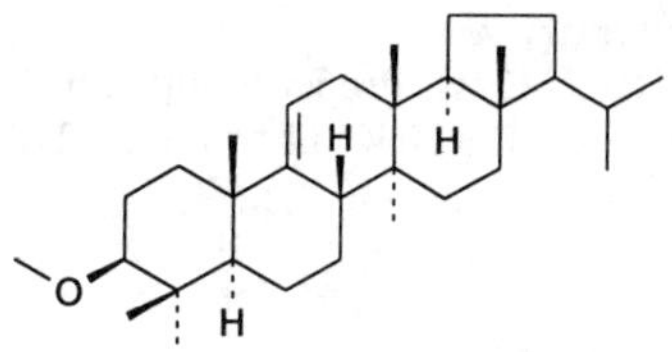

1430 Cymarin
CAS: 508-77-0 $C_{30}H_{44}O_9$ MW: 548.68 Property: mp 148°C, 185-7°C. Source: FU SHOU CAO, LUO BU MA. Ref: 4, 5, 6.

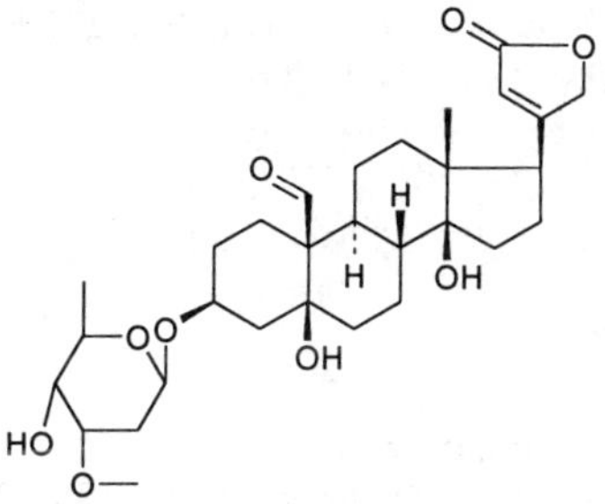

1431 Cymarol
$C_{30}H_{46}O_9$ MW: 550.70 Property: mp 240-3°C. Source: FU SHOU CAO. Ref: 6.

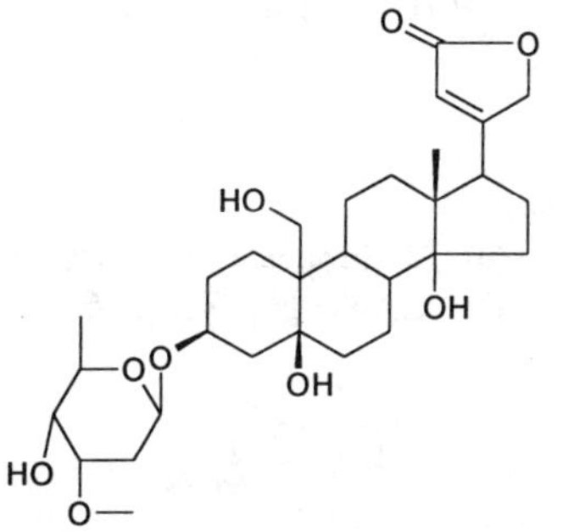

1432 p-Cymene
$C_{10}H_{14}$ MW: 134.22 Source: DONG LING CAO, DU HUO, GAN JIANG, HOU PO, HUO XIANG, JIN JIE, JU PI, LIAN QIAO, QIANG HUO, SHENG JIANG, WU WEI ZI, XI XIN, YIN CHEN HAO. Ref: 2.

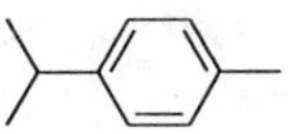

1433 p-Cymene-α-ol
$C_{10}H_{14}O$ MW: 150.22 Source: XI XIN. Ref: 2.

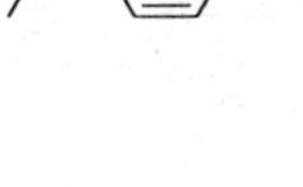

1434 Cynanester A
$C_{35}H_{60}O_2$ MW: 512.87 Property: mp 156-8°C (acetone). Source: E RONG TENG. Ref: 212.

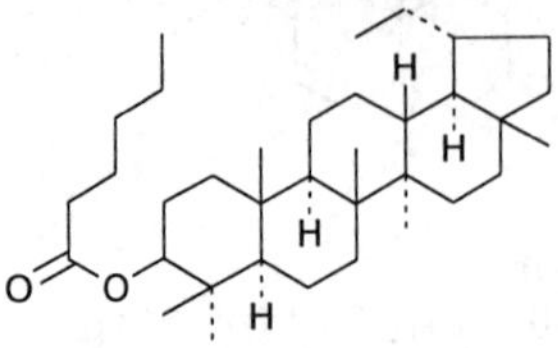

1435 Cynarin
$C_{25}H_{24}O_{12}$ MW: 516.46 Property: mp 227-8°C. Source: HUANG WAN. Ref: 6.

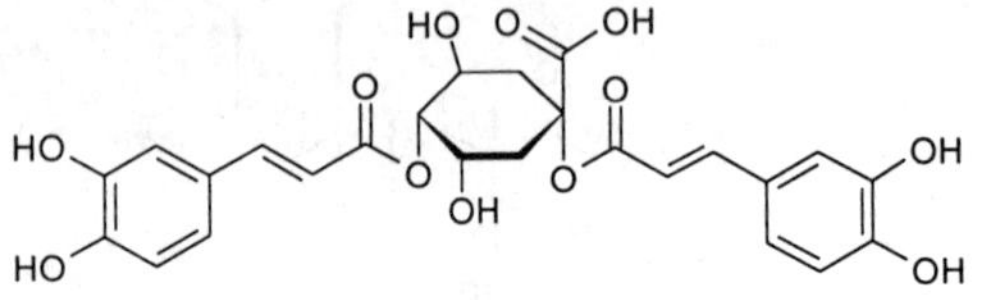

1436 Cynthiaxanthin
$C_{40}H_{52}O_2$ MW: 564.86 Property: mp 188-90°C. Source: HAI XIA. Ref: 6.

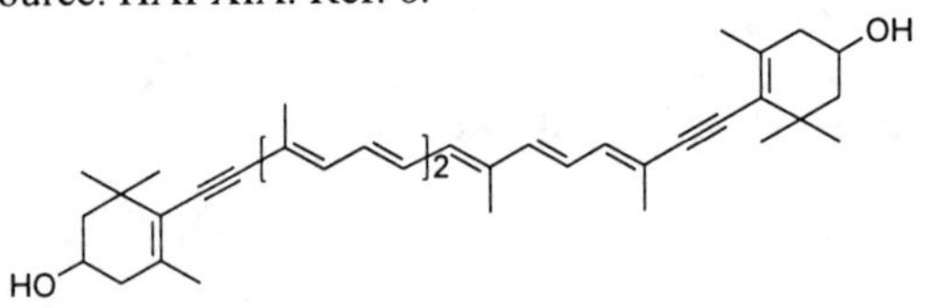

1437 Cyperene
$C_{15}H_{24}$ MW: 204.36 Property: bp 104°C/5mm. Source: SAN QI, XIANG FU. Ref: 2, 6.

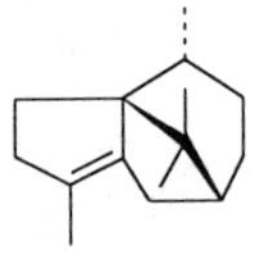

1438 Cyperol
$C_{15}H_{24}O$ MW: 220.36 Property: bp 147-50°C/8mm. Source: XIANG FU. Ref: 6.

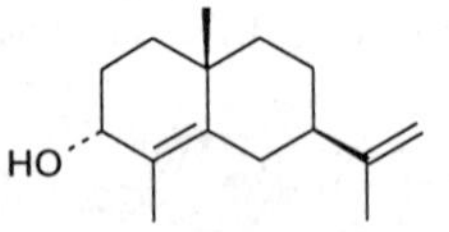

1439 Cyperolone
$C_{15}H_{24}O_2$ MW: 236.36 Property: mp 41-2°C, bp 120°C/0.1mm. Source: XIANG FU. Ref: 6.

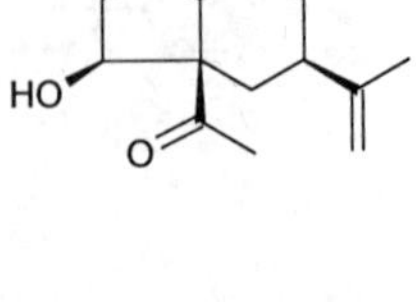

1440 α-Cyperone
$C_{15}H_{22}O$ MW: 218.34 Property: bp (+): 177°C, (±): 128-9°C/2.8mm. Source: XIANG FU. Ref: 6.

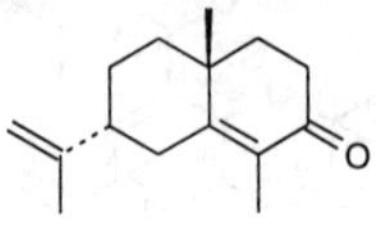

1441 β-Cyperone
$C_{15}H_{22}O$ MW: 218.34 Property: bp 175-6°C. Source: XIANG FU. Ref: 6.

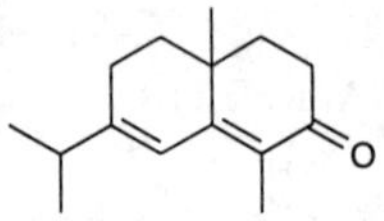

1442 Cyprinol
$C_{27}H_{48}O_5$ MW: 452.68 Property: mp 242-4°C. Source: LI YU DAN. Ref: 6.

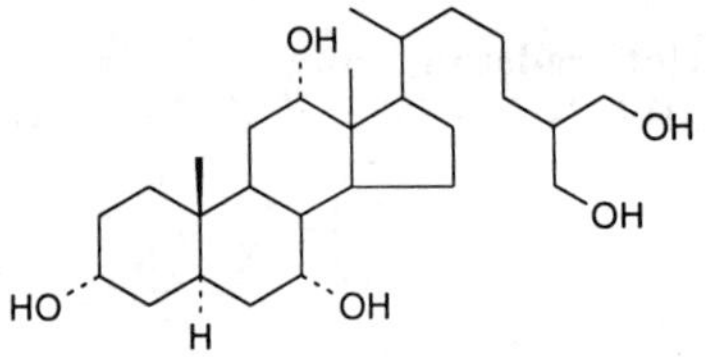

1443 5β-Cyprinol
$C_{26}H_{46}O_5$ MW: 438 .65 Source: QING WA DAN. Ref: 6.

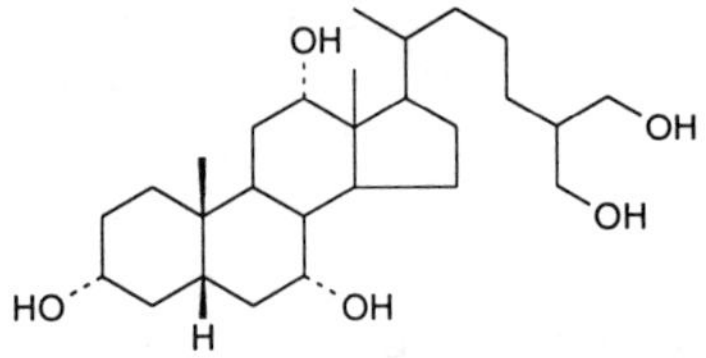

1444 Cyrtomin
$C_{17}H_{16}O_6$ MW: 316.31 HUN JI TOU. Source: HUN JI TOU. Ref: 6.

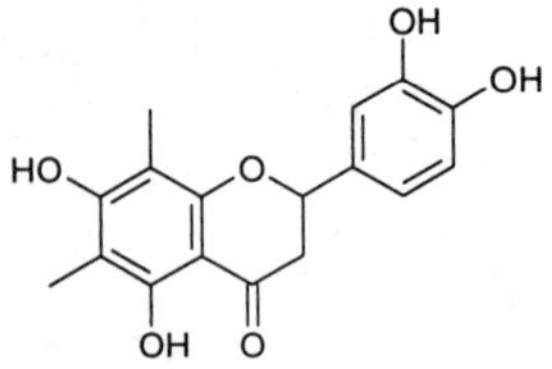

1445 Cystathionine
$C_7H_{14}N_3O_8S_2$ MW: 254.33 Property: mp L(+): 312°C (dec). Source: MO GU. Ref: 6.

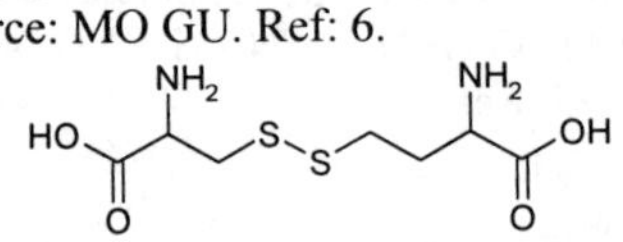

1446 Cytidylic acid A
$C_9H_{16}N_3O_8P$ MW: 323.20 Property: mp 238-9°C. Source: GOU QI YE. Ref: 6.

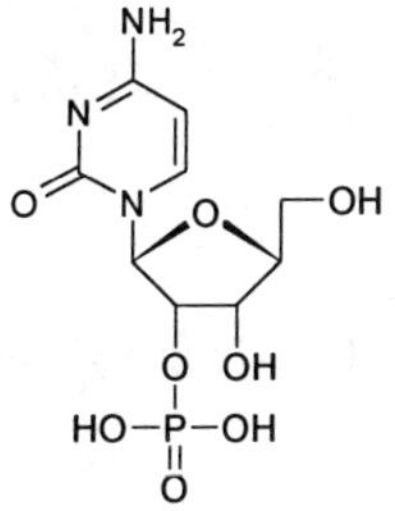

1447 Cytidylic acid B
$C_9H_{14}N_3O_8P$ MW: 323.20 Property: mp 233-4°C. Source: GOU QI YE. Ref: 6.

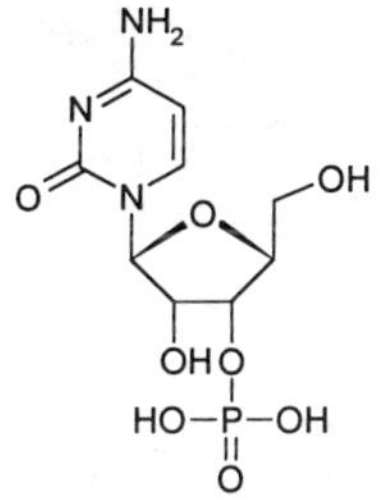

1448 Cytisine
CAS: 485-35-8 $C_{11}H_{14}N_2O$ MW: 190.25 Property: mp (+): 155°C, (±): 147°C. Source: GAO SHAN HUANG, KU DOU ZI, KU SHEN SHI, MU MA DOU, YE JUE MING, ZI TENG ZI. Ref: 4, 6, 593.

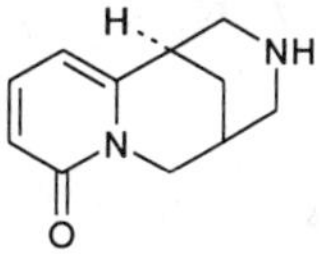

1449 Daechualkaloid A
$C_7H_9NO_2$ MW: 139.16 Source: DA ZAO. Ref: 2.

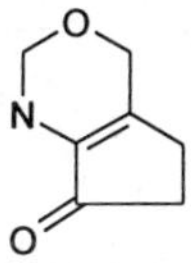

1450 Daidzein
Daizeol. CAS: 486-66-8 $C_{15}H_{10}O_4$ MW: 254.24 Source: GE GEN. Ref: 2, 4.

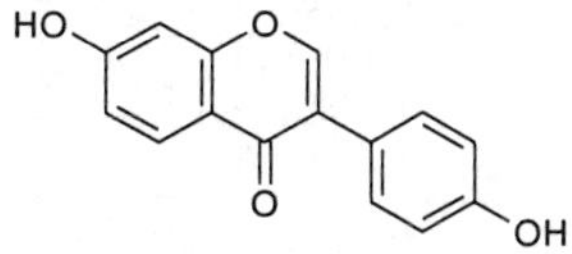

1451 Daidzein 4',7-diglucoside
$C_{27}H_{30}O_{14}$ MW: 578.53 Source: GE GEN. Ref: 2.

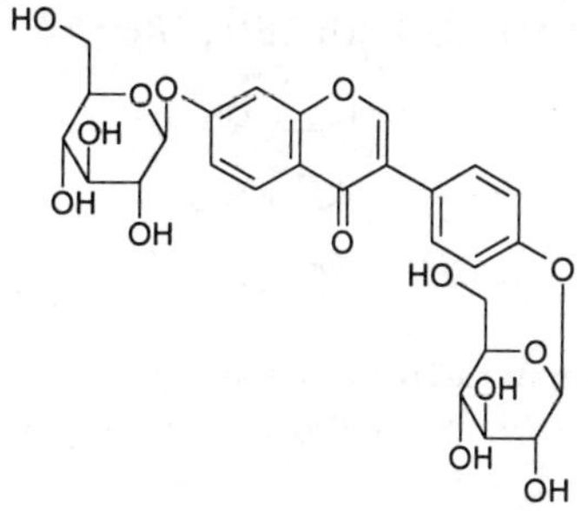

1452 Daidzin
$C_{21}H_{20}O_9$ MW: 416.39 Source: GE GEN. Ref: 2.

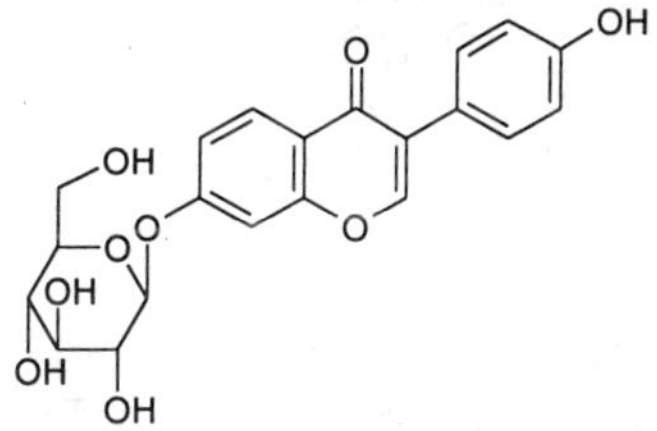

1453 Dalbergenone
$C_{16}H_{14}O_3$ MW: 254.29 Property: mp 114-6°C. Source: JIANG ZHEN XIANG. Ref: 6.

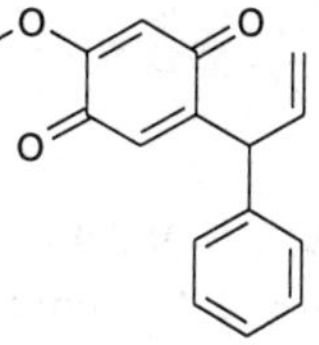

1454 Dalbergichromene
$C_{16}H_{14}O_5$ MW: 254.29 Property: mp 99-100°C. Source: JIANG ZHEN XIANG. Ref: 6.

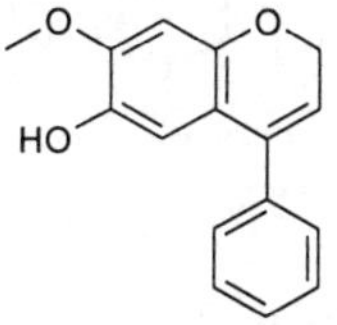

1455 Dalbergin
$C_{16}H_{12}O_4$ MW: 268.27 Property: mp 210°C. Source: JIANG ZHEN XIANG. Ref: 6.

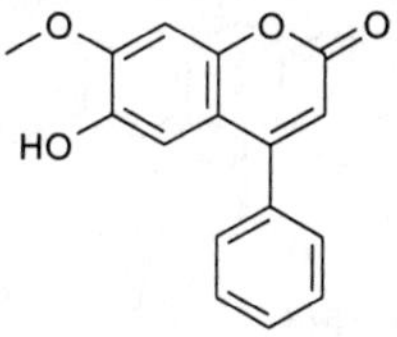

1456 Dambonitol
$C_9H_{18}O_6$ MW: 222.24 Property: mp 210°C. Source: JIA ZHU TAO, LUO SHI TENG. Ref: 6.

1457 Dammara-20,24-dien-3β-ol
$C_{30}H_{50}O$ MW: 426.73 Property: mp 136-8°C. Source: WU YUE CHA. Ref: 6.

1458 Dammardienyl acetate
$C_{32}H_{52}O_2$ MW: 468.77 Property: mp 148-9°C. Source: PEI LAN, TU MU XIANG. Ref: 6.

1459 Dammar-24-ene-3β,20-diol
$C_{30}H_{52}O_2$ MW: 444.75 Property: mp 142-4°C. Source: MANG GUO SHU PI. Ref: 6.

1460 Damnacanthal
$C_{16}H_{10}O_5$ MW: 282.26 Property: mp 208°C. Source: HU CI, TU LIAN QIAO. Ref: 6.

1461 Damnacanthol
$C_{16}H_{12}O_5$ MW: 284.27 Property: mp 288°C. Source: HU CI. Ref: 6.

1462 Damnidin
$C_{17}H_{16}O_5$ MW: 300.31 Property: mp 180°C. Source: HU CI. Ref: 6.

1463 Damsin
Dihydroambrosin. CAS: 1216-42-8 $C_{15}H_{20}O_3$ MW: 248.32 Property: mp 109-11°C, 124-5°C. Source: TUN CAO. Ref: 4.

1464 Damsinic acid
CAS: 22844-19-5 $C_{15}H_{22}O_3$ MW: 250.34 Property: mp 112-3°C. Source: TUN CAO. Ref: 4.

1465 Danmelittoside
Source: GAN DI HUANG. Ref: 2.

1466 Danshen spiroketallactone
$C_{17}H_{16}O_3$ MW: 268.32 Property: white acicular crystal, mp 203-5°C. Source: DAN SHEN. Ref: 38.

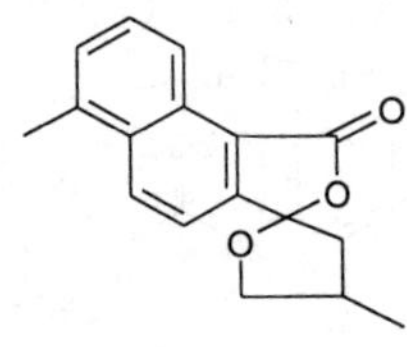

1467 Danshensuan B
$C_{37}H_{34}O_{16}$ MW: 734.67 Source: DAN SHEN. Ref: 2.

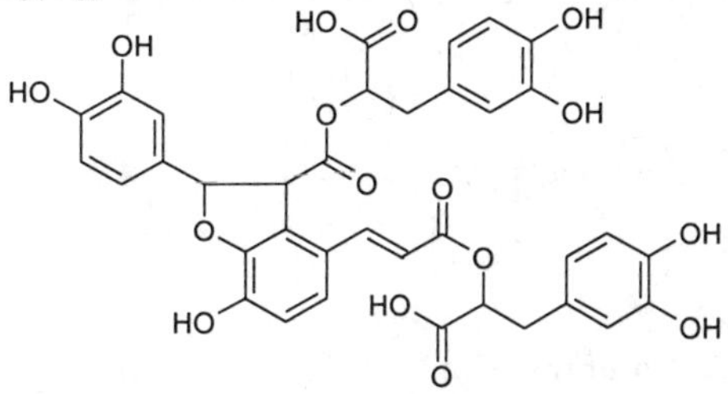

1468 Danshenxinkun D
$C_{21}H_{20}O_4$ MW: 336.39 Property: pink acicular crystal, mp 178-80°C. Source: DAN SHEN. Ref: 34.

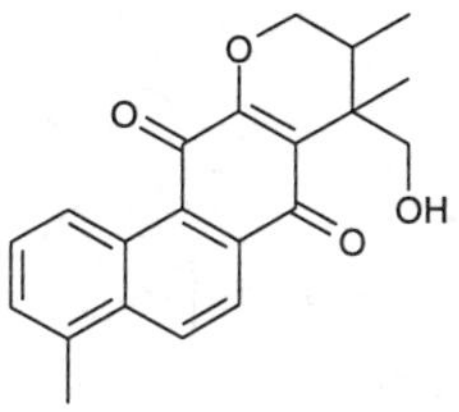

1469 Daphneolone
$C_{17}H_{18}O_3$ MW: 270.33 Source: RUI XIANG GEN. Ref: 6.

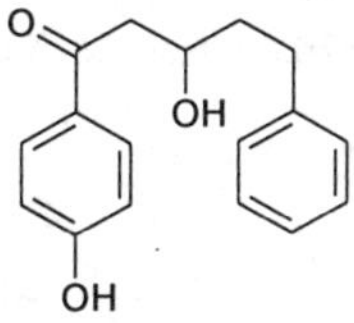

1470 Daphnetin
CAS: 486-35-1 $C_9H_6O_4$ MW: 178.15 Property: mp 257-8°C, 263-4°C. Source: LANG DU, QIAN JIN ZI, RUI XIANG HUA. Ref: 4, 6, 556.

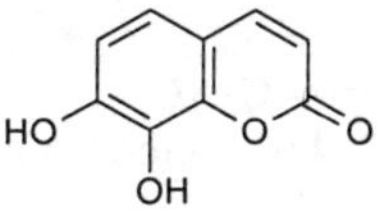

1471 Daphnetin-8-glucoside
$C_{15}H_{16}O_9$ MW: 340.29 Property: mp 223-4°C. Source: RUI XIANG HUA. Ref: 6.

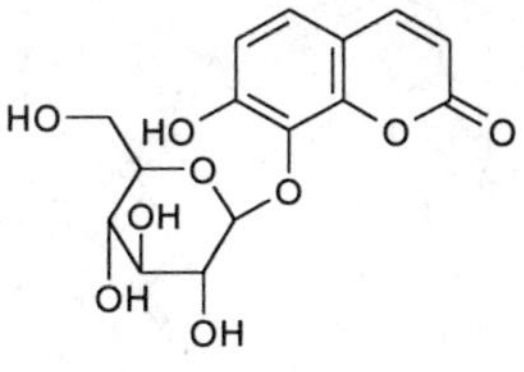

1472 Daphnetin-7-methyl ether
$C_{10}H_8O_4$ MW: 192.17 Property: mp 175.5°C. Source: BA XIAN HUA. Ref: 6.

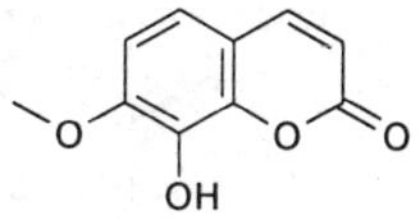

1473 Daphnetin-8-methyl ether
$C_{10}H_8O_4$ MW: 192.17 Property: mp 185°C. Source: BA XIAN HUA. Ref: 6.

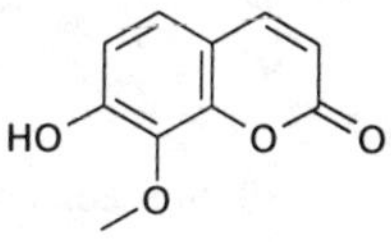

1474 Daphnicadine
$C_{21}H_{31}NO_2$ MW: 329.49 Property: mp 221-2°C. Source: NIU ER FENG ZI. Ref: 6.

1475 Daphnicaline
$C_{21}H_{29}NO_2$ MW: 327.47 Source: NIU ER FENG ZI. Ref: 6.

1476 Daphnicamine
$C_{22}H_{37}NO_2$ MW: 347.55 Property: mp 285-7°C. Source: NIU ER FENG ZI. Ref: 6.

1477 Daphnin
Daphnetin-7-glucoside. $C_{15}H_{16}O_9$ MW: 340.29 Property: mp 215°C (dec). Source: RUI XIANG HUA, SU MI. Ref: 6.

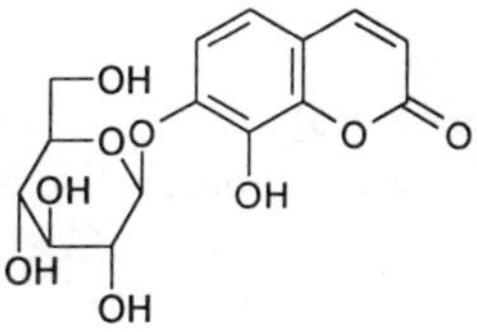

1478 Darutin bitter
Source: XI XIAN. Ref: 6.

1479 Dasycarpamin
$C_{17}H_{21}NO_4$ MW: 303.36 Property: mp 149°C. Source: BAI XIAN PI. Ref: 6.

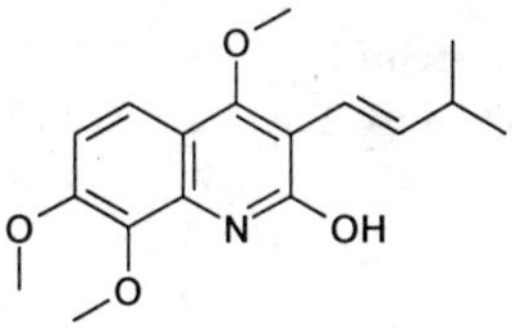

1480 Datumetelin
$C_{29}H_{40}O_5$ MW: 468.64 Source: YANG JIN HUA. Ref: 2.

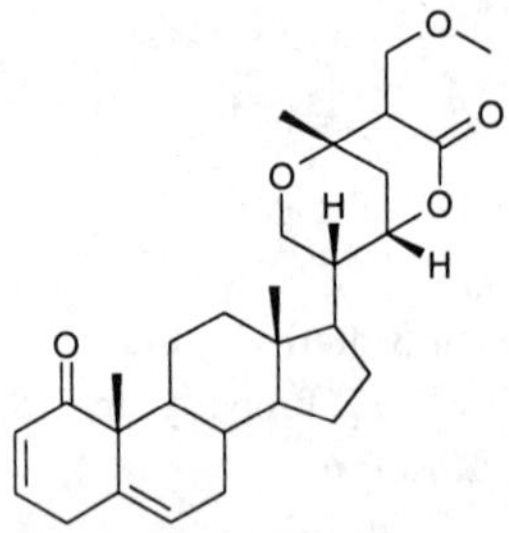

1481 Datumetine
$C_{17}H_{23}NO_2$ MW: 273.38 Source: YANG JIN HUA. Ref: 2.

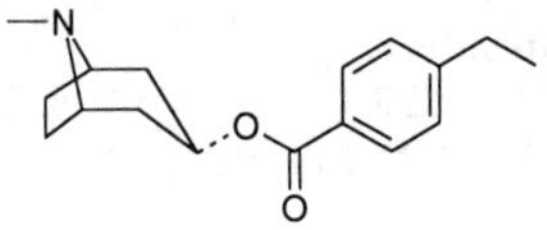

1482 Daturametelin A
$C_{34}H_{48}O_9$ MW: 600.76 Source: YANG JIN HUA. Ref: 2.

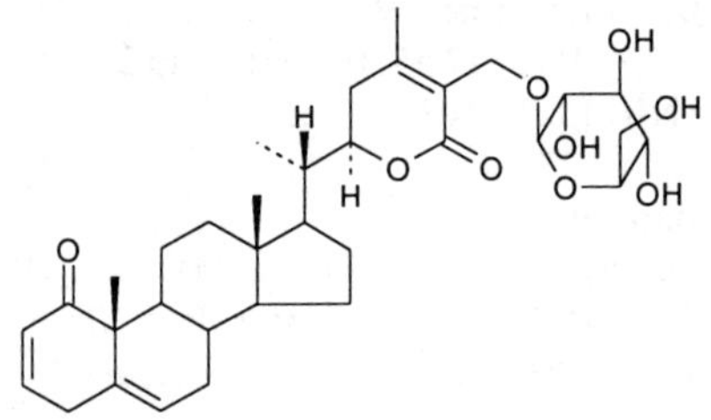

1483 Daturametelin B
$C_{34}H_{48}O_{10}$ MW: 616.76 Source: YANG JIN HUA. Ref: 2.

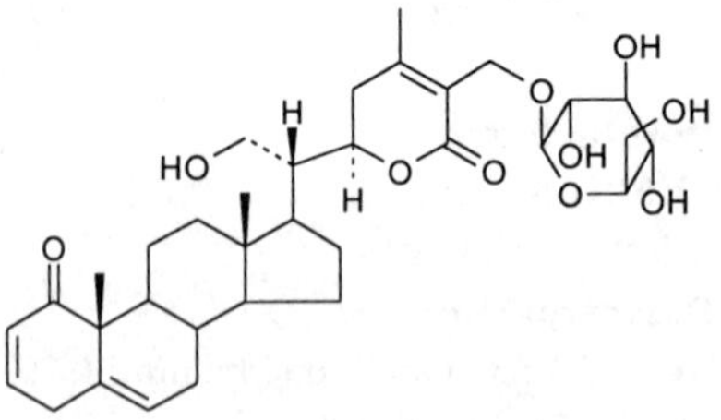

1484 Daturametelin C
$C_{29}H_{40}O_5$ MW: 48.64 Source: YANG JIN HUA. Ref: 2.

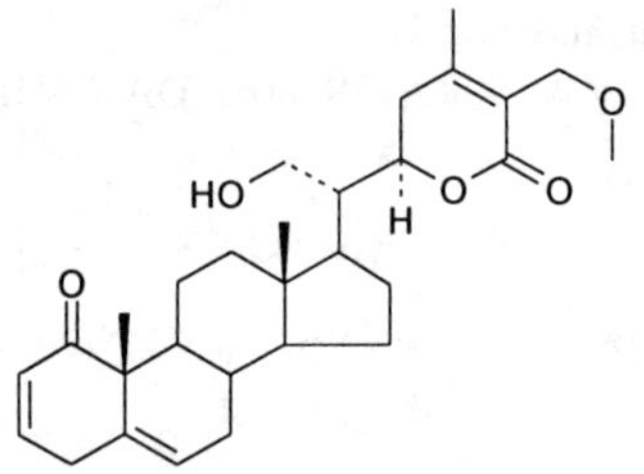

1485 Daturametelin D
Source: YANG JIN HUA. Ref: 2.

1486 Daturametelin E
$C_{29}H_{42}O_8S$ MW: 550.72 Source: YANG JIN HUA. Ref: 2.

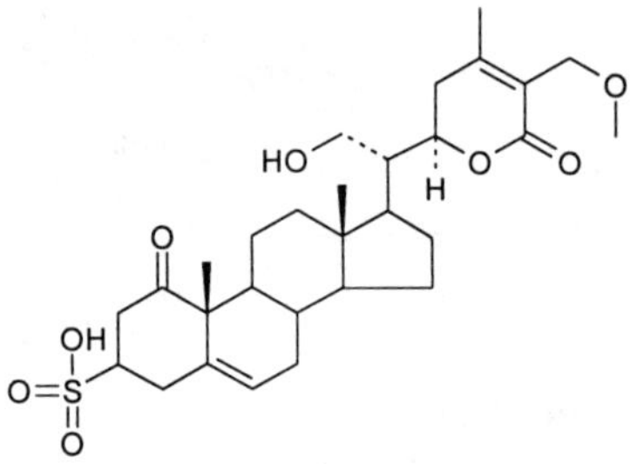

1487 Daturametelin F
$C_{27}H_{36}O_8S$ MW: 520.65 Source: YANG JIN HUA. Ref: 2.

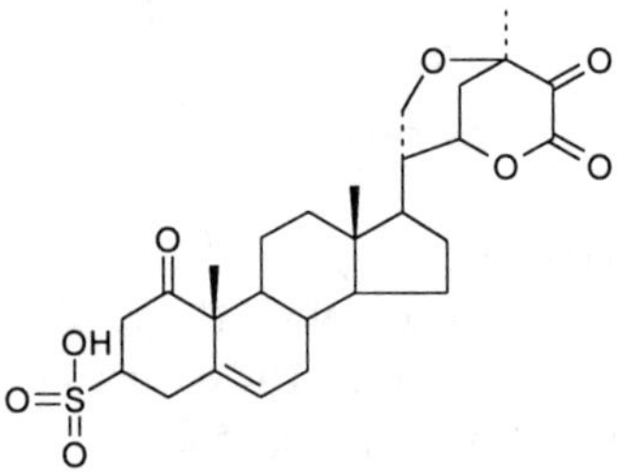

1488 Daturametelin G-AC
$C_{42}H_{56}O_{14}$ MW: 784.91 Source: YANG JIN HUA. Ref: 2.

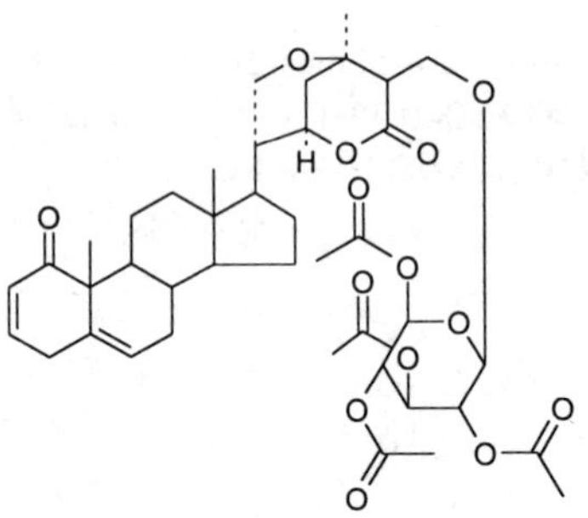

1489 Daturic acid
$C_{17}H_{34}O_2$ MW: 270.46 Property: mp 60-1°C. Source: SHU MI. Ref: 6.

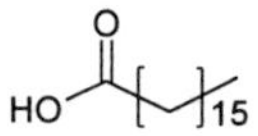

1490 Daturilin
$C_{28}H_{36}O_4$ MW: 436.60 Source: YANG JIN HUA. Ref: 2.

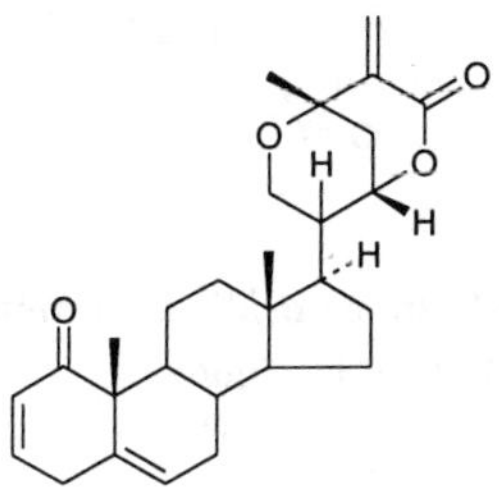

1491 Daturilinol
$C_{28}H_{38}O_5$ MW: 454.61 Source: YANG JIN HUA. Ref: 2.

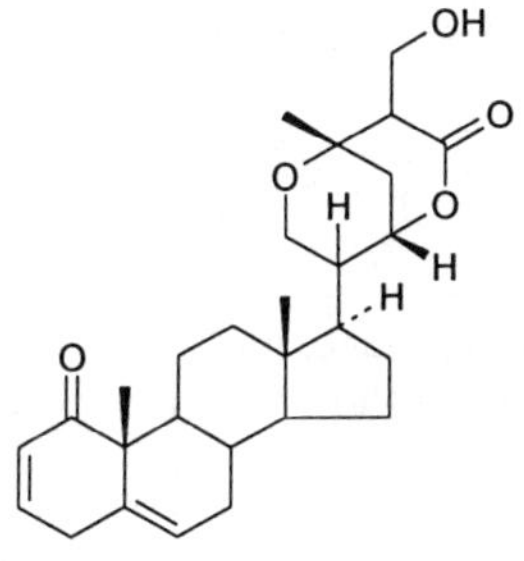

1492 Daucene
$C_{15}H_{24}$ MW: 204.36 Property: bp 96°C/4mm. Source: HE SHI. Ref: 6.

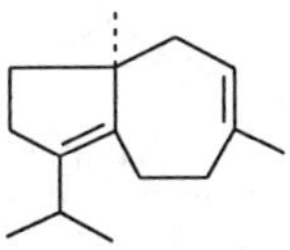

1493 Daucic acid
$C_7H_8O_7$ MW: 204.14 Source: HE SHI FENG. Ref: 6.

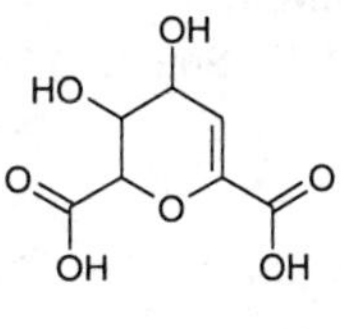

1494 Daucine
$C_{11}H_{18}N_2$ MW: 178.28 Property: bp 240-50°C. Source: HU LUO BO ZI, HE SHI FENG. Ref: 6.

1495 Daucol
$C_{15}H_{27}O_2$ MW: 239.38 Property: mp 113-5°C, bp 124-32°C/2mm. Source: HU LUO BO ZI, HE SHI, HE SHI FENG. Ref: 6.

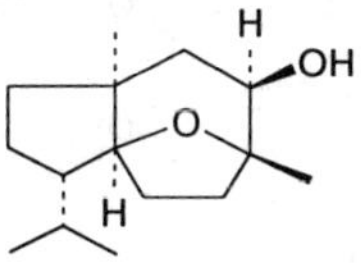

1496 Daucosterol
Eleutheroside A. $C_{35}H_{60}O_6$ MW: 576.86 Property: white powder, mp 295°C. Source: BAI JIANG, BAI TOU WENG, BAN XIA, BU GU ZHI, CAO CONG RONG, CHUAN XIN LIAN, CI WU JIA, DAN SHEN, DONG BEI CI REN SHEN, FANG FENG, GAN DI HUANG, GE GEN, JIN QUE GEN, MAO LIAN HAO, PU GONG YING, REN SHEN, ROU CONG RONG, RUAN ZAO MI HOU TAO, SAN QI, SUAN ZAO REN, SUAN ZAO REN, TIAN MA, TUN XING GUO, YA DAN ZI, etc. Ref: 2, 440, 447, 450, 454, 455, 471, 474, 502, 556, 580, 582, 585, 594, 596, 614, 622.

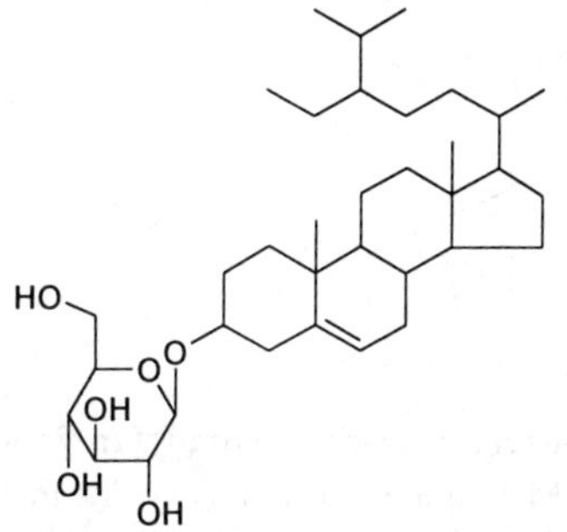

1497 Dauricine
CAS: 524-17-4 $C_{38}H_{44}N_2O_6$ MW: 624.78 Property: mp 115°C. Source: BIAN FU GE, BIAN FU GE GEN. Ref: 4, 6.

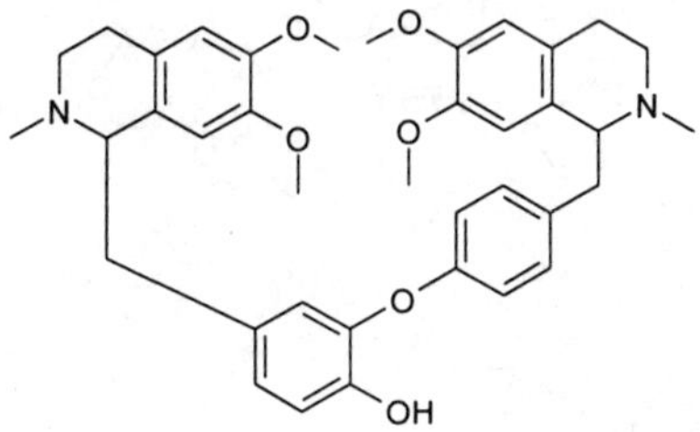

1498 Dauricinoline
$C_{37}H_{42}N_2O_6$ MW: 610.76 Source: BIAN FU GE GEN. Ref: 6.

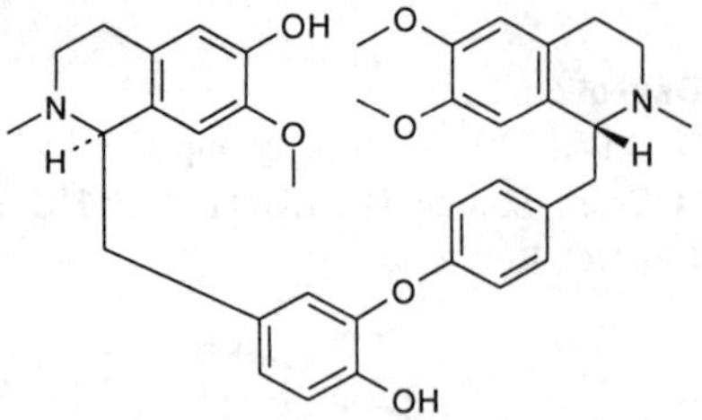

1499 Dauricoline
$C_{36}H_{40}N_2O_6$ MW: 596.73 Source: BIAN FU GE GEN. Ref: 6.

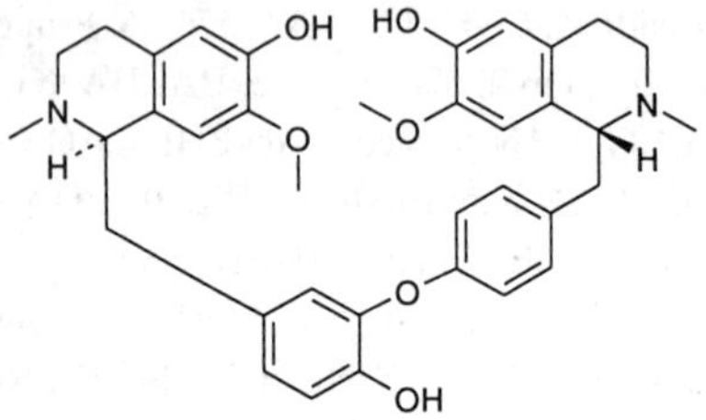

1500 Daurinoline
$C_{37}H_{42}N_2O_6$ MW: 610.76 Source: BIAN FU GE GEN. Ref: 6.

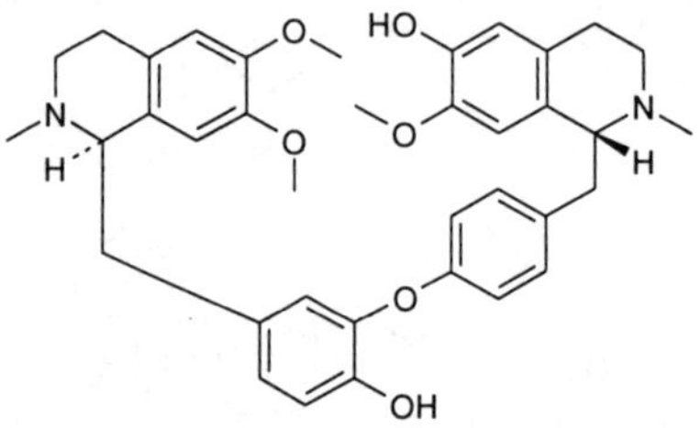

1501 2-Deacetoxy-5-decinnamoyl taxinine J
$C_{28}H_{40}O_9$ MW: 520.63 Property: white massive crystal, mp 178-80°C, $[\alpha]_D^{12}$ +112.93° (c=0.058, chloroform). Source: YUN NAN HONG DOU SHAN. Ref: 296.

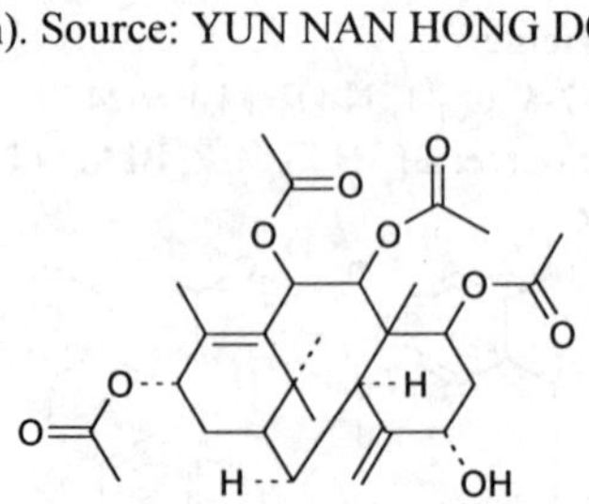

1502 Deacetoxyvinblastine
$C_{43}H_{54}N_4O_7$ MW: 738.93 Source: CHANG CHUN HUA. Ref: 2.

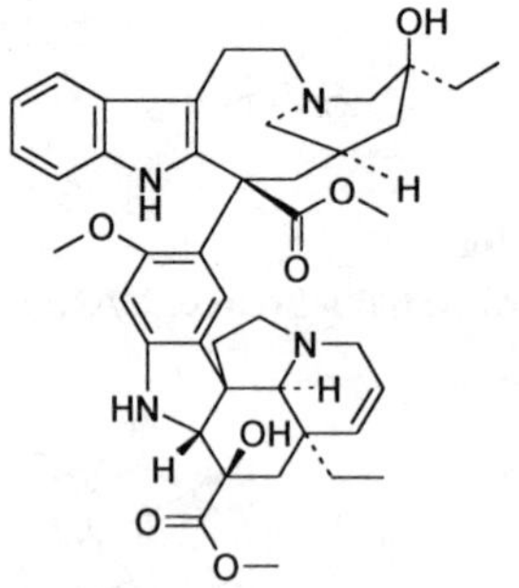

1503 Deacetyl asperulosidic acid methyl ester
$C_{17}H_{24}O_{11}$ MW: 404.37 Source: ZHI ZI. Ref: 2, 626.

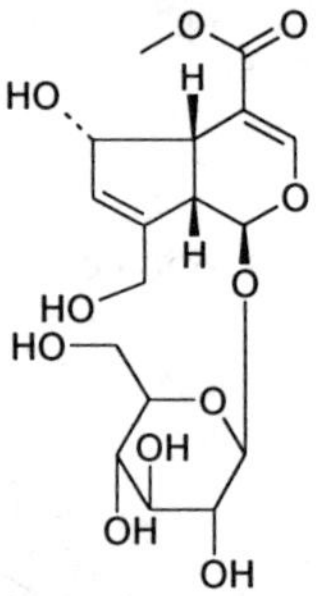

1504 10-Deacetyl baccatin III
Source: YUN NAN HONG DOU SHAN. Ref: 316, 563.

1505 Deacetylmatricrin
$C_{15}H_{18}O_4$ MW: 262.31 Property: mp 123-5°C, 143-6°C. Source: YANG SHI CAO, YI ZHI HAO. Ref: 6.

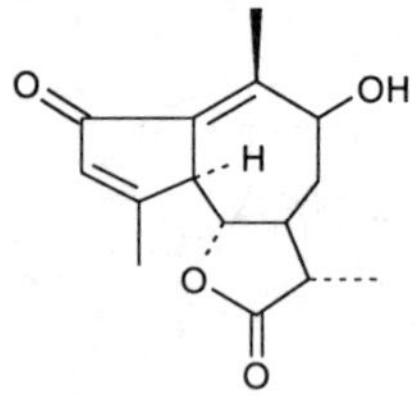

1506 Deacetylnomilin
$C_{25}H_{30}O_8$ MW: 458.51 Source: YOU HE. Ref: 6.

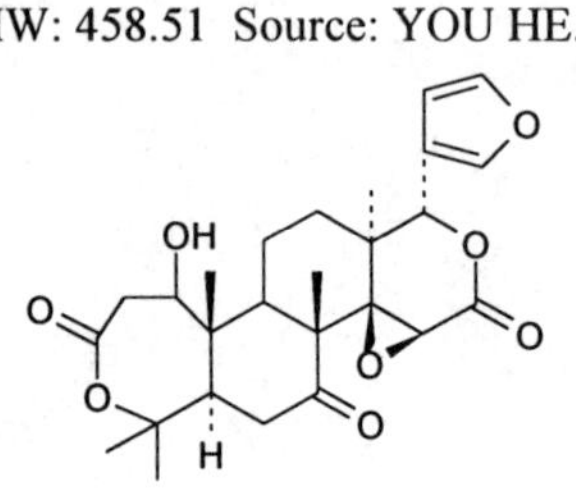

1507 Deacetyloleandrin
$C_{30}H_{46}O_8$ MW: 534.70 Property: mp 235-8°C. Source: JIA ZHU TAO. Ref: 6.

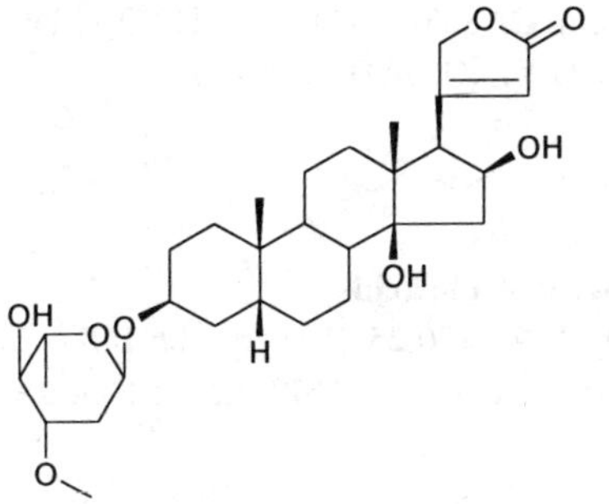

1508 O-Deacetylpachysandrine B
$C_{30}H_{52}N_2O$ MW: 456.76 Property: mp 184-5°C. Source: XUE SHAN LIN. Ref: 6.

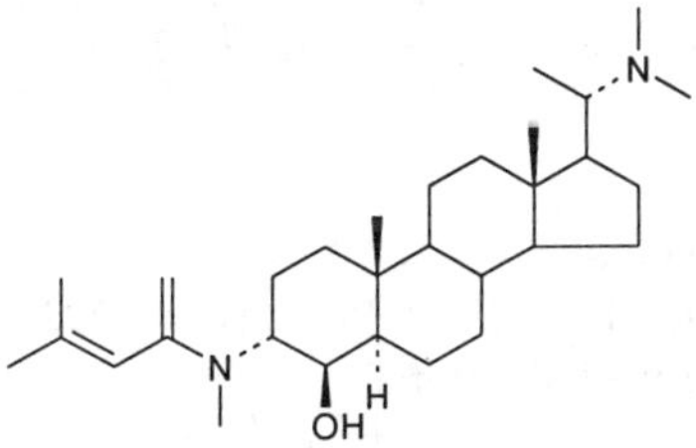

1509 Deacetylpicraline 3,4,5-trimethoxybenzoat
$C_{31}H_{34}N_2O_8$ MW: 562.63 Property: white acicular crystal, mp 222°C, $[\alpha]_D^{17}$ -185° (c=0.052, chloroform). Source: JI GU CHANG SHAN. Ref: 42.

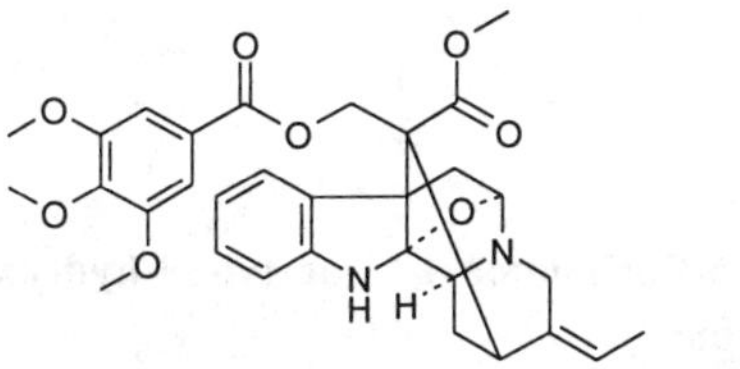

1510 10-Deacetyl taxinine B
$C_{35}H_{42}O_{10}$ MW: 622.72 Property: colorless thin acicular crystal, mp 245-8°C. Source: DONG BEI HONG DOU SHAN. Ref: 291.

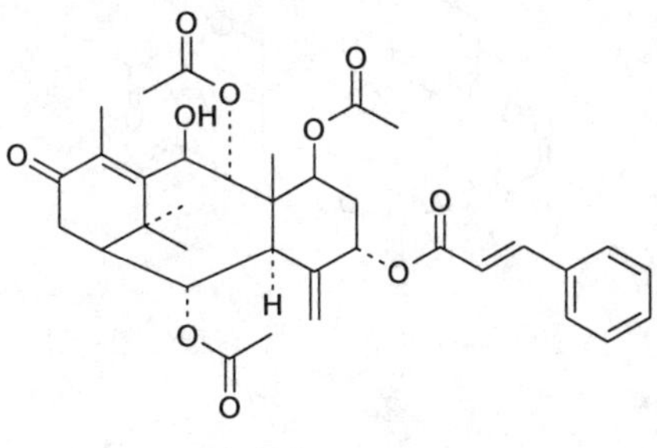

1511 Deacetylturraeanthin
$C_{30}H_{48}O_4$ MW: 472.71 Property: mp 202-6°C. Source: KU LIAN PI. Ref: 6.

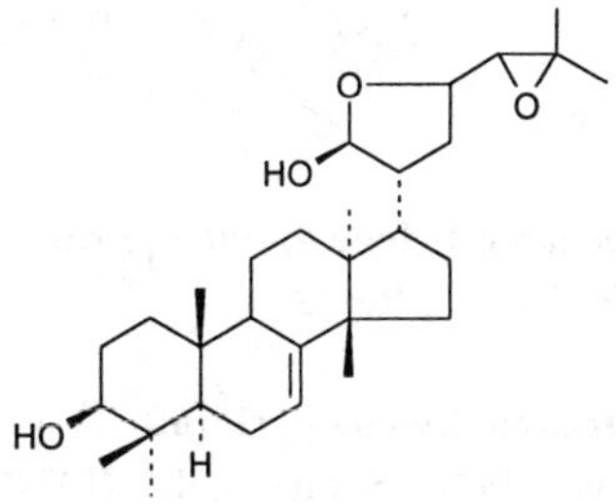

1512 Deacylmetaplexigenin
$C_{21}H_{32}O_6$ MW: 380.48 Source: LUO MO, BAI SHOU WU. Ref: 6.

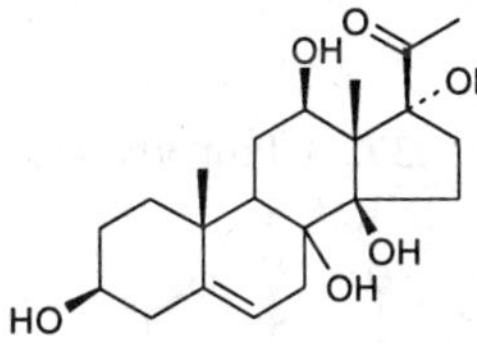

1513 Debilic acid
$C_{18}H_{13}NO_7$ MW: 355.31 Property: mp >350°C (dec). Source: JI SHI TENG GUO. Ref: 6.

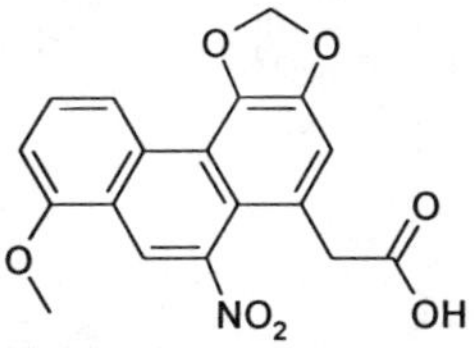

1514 Debilon(e)
9-Hydroxy-$\Delta^{1(10)}$-aristolen-2-one. $C_{15}H_{22}O_2$ MW: 234.34 Property: mp 135°C. Source: GAN SONG. Ref: 6.

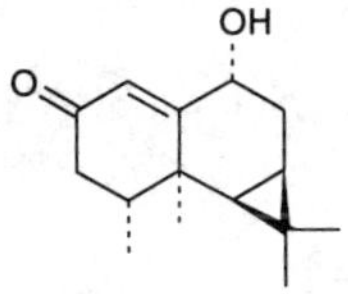

1515 (E,E)-2,4-Decadienal
$C_{10}H_{16}O$ MW: 152.24 Source: XING REN. Ref: 2.

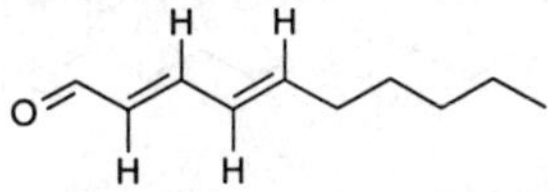

1516 Decaffeoylacteoside
Source: ROU CONG ROUN. Ref: 628.

1517 γ-Decalactone
$C_8H_{14}O_2$ MW: 142.20 Source: CHAI HU. Ref: 2.

1518 2,6-Decamethylene dihydropyran
Source: SHE XIANG. Ref: 2.

1519 2,6-Decamethylene pyridine
$C_{15}H_{23}N$ MW: 217.36 Source: SHE XIANG. Ref: 2.

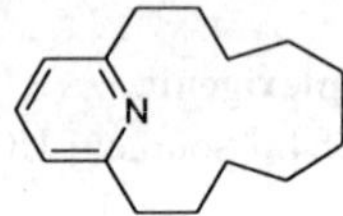

1520 Decamine
$C_{26}H_{31}NO_5$ MW: 437.54 Property: mp 223-4°C. Source: ZI WEI YE. Ref: 6.

1521 Decanal
Capric aldehyde. $C_{10}H_{20}O$ MW: 156.27 Source: DONG LING CAO, GAN JIANG, JU PI, YU XING CAO. Ref: 2.

1522 Decane
$C_{10}H_{22}$ MW: 142.29 Source: SHAN ZHA. Ref: 2.

1523 Decanoic acid
$C_{10}H_{20}O_2$ MW: 172.27 Source: GAN DI HUANG. Ref: 2.

1524 γ-Decanolactone
$C_{10}H_{18}O_2$ MW: 170.25 Source: XING REN. Ref: 2.

1525 Decanoylacetaldehyde
Houttuynin. CAS: 3018-41-0 $C_{12}H_{22}O_2$ MW: 198.31 Source: YU XING CAO. Ref: 2, 4.

1526 Decen-4-oic acid
$C_{10}H_{18}O_2$ MW: 170.25 Property: bp 148-50°C/13mm. Source: SAN ZUAN FENG. Ref: 6.

1527 cis-4-Decenoic acid
$C_{10}H_{18}O_2$ MW: 170.25 Source: ZHEN CAI. Ref: 6.

1528 Decinine
$C_{26}H_{31}NO_5$ MW: 437.54 Property: mp 222-4°C. Source: ZI WEI YE. Ref: 6.

1529 5-Decinnamoyl-11-acetyl-19-hydroxyl taxagifine
$C_{30}H_{40}O_{14}$ MW: 624.64 Property: white massive crystal, mp 209-10°C, $[\alpha]_D^{14}$ -12.1° (chloroform). Source: YUN NAN HONG DOU SHAN. Ref: 296.

1530 Decodine
$C_{25}H_{29}O_5$ MW: 423.51 Property: mp 193-7°C. Source: ZI WEI YE. Ref: 6.

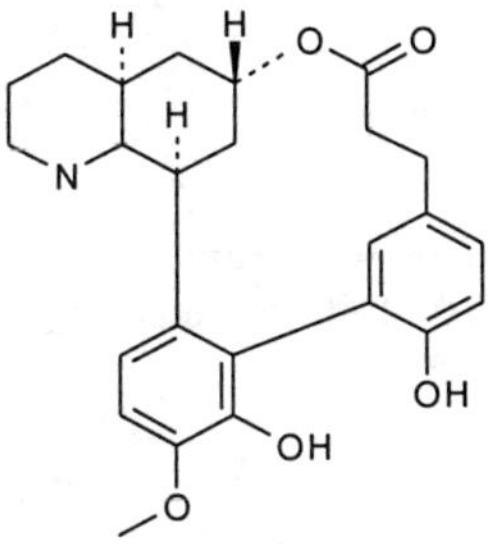

1531 Decoyl vanillylamide
$C_{16}H_{25}NO_3$ MW: 279.38 Source: LA JIAO. Ref: 6.

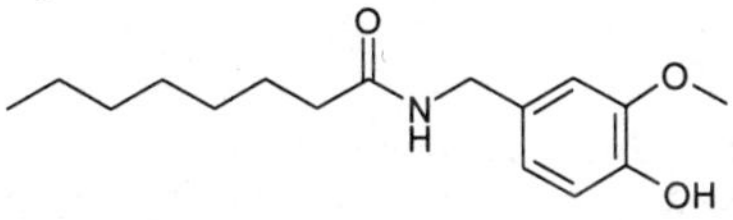

1532 Decursin
$C_{19}H_{20}O_5$ MW: 328.37 Property: mp 110-1°C. Source: TU DANG GUI (II). Ref: 6.

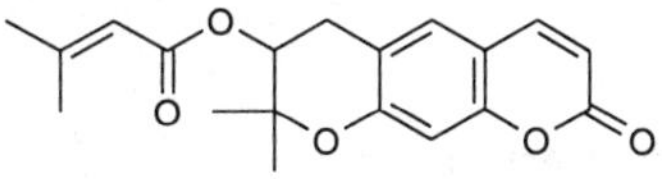

1533 Decursinol
$C_{14}H_{14}O_4$ MW: 246.27 Property: mp 176-7°C. Source: TU DANG GUI (II). Ref: 6.

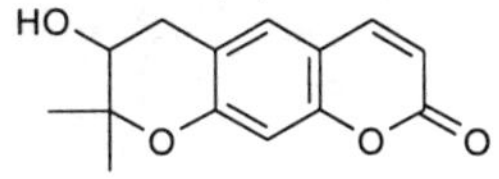

1534 n-Decyl acetate
$C_{12}H_{24}O_2$ MW: 200.32 Property: mp -15.05°C, bp 244°C. Source: HEI MA YI. Ref: 6.

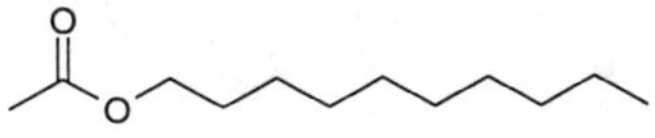

1535 Deglucocheirotoxin
$C_{29}H_{42}O_{10}$ MW: 550.65 Property: mp 188-91°C. Source: LING LAN. Ref: 6.

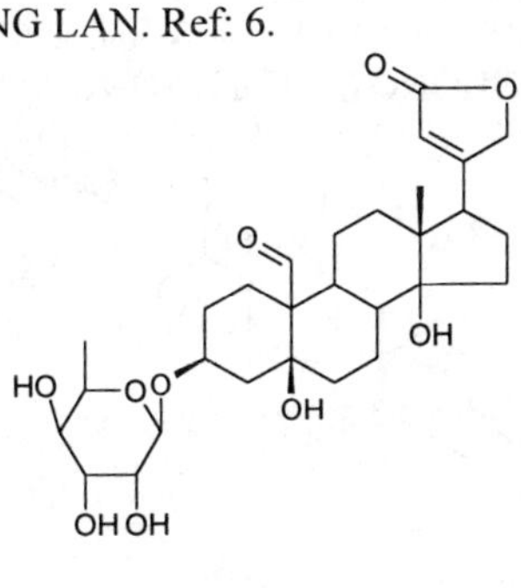

1536 Deguelin
$C_{23}H_{22}O_6$ MW: 394.43 Property: mp 171°C. Source: HUI YE GEN, YU TENG. Ref: 6.

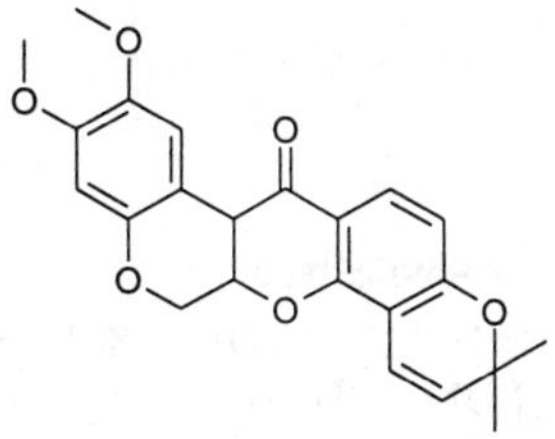

1537 Dehydroagastol
19(4→3)Abeo-11,14-dihydroxy-12-methoxy-abieta-8,11,13,15-tetraen-7-one. $C_{21}H_{26}O_4$ MW: 342.44 Property: yellow green acicular crystal, mp 159-61 °C, soluble in hexane, chloroform and methanol. Source: HUO XIANG. Ref: 210.

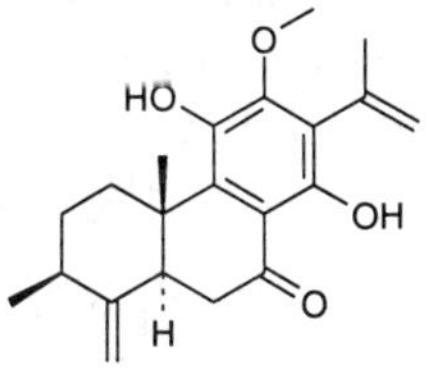

1538 6,7-Dehydroartemisinic acid
$C_{15}H_{20}O_2$ MW: 232.33 Source: QING HAO. Ref: 2.

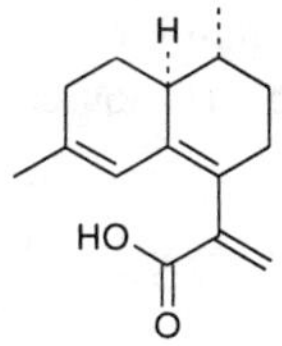

1539 Dehydroascorbic acid
$C_8H_{10}O_6$ MW: 202.17 Property: mp 196°C (dec). Source: HUI XIANG JING YE, JIANG MANG, MA BO. Ref: 6.

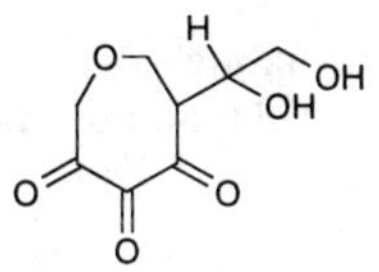

1540 Dehydrobaimuxinol
$C_{15}H_{24}O_2$ MW: 236.36 Property: colorless acicular crystal, mp 136-8 °C, $[\alpha]_D^{26}$ +25° (c=1.6, chloroform). Source: BAI MU XIANG. Ref: 13, 58.

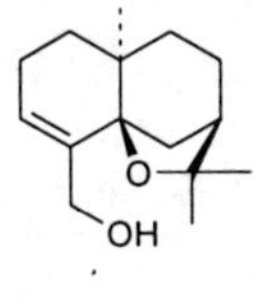

1541 Dehydrobufotenine
$C_{12}H_{14}N_2O$ MW: 202.26 Source: CHAN SU. Ref: 2.

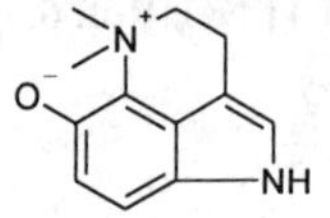

1542 7-Dehydrocholesterol
$C_{27}H_{40}O$ MW: 384.65 Property: mp 142-3°C, 150°C. Source: SHUI LONG GU. Ref: 6.

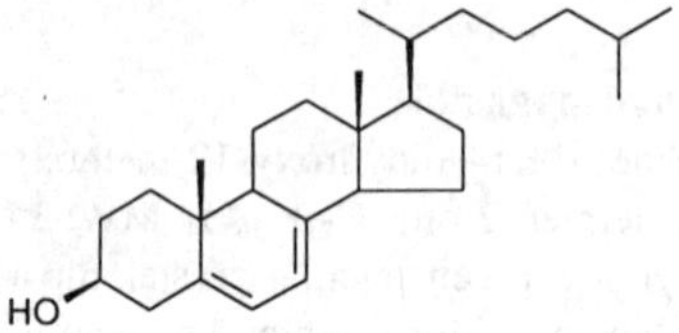

1543 11-Dehydrocorticosterone
$C_{21}H_{28}O_4$ MW: 344.45 Property: mp 183-3.5°C. Source: NIU SHEN, ZI HE CHE. Ref: 6.

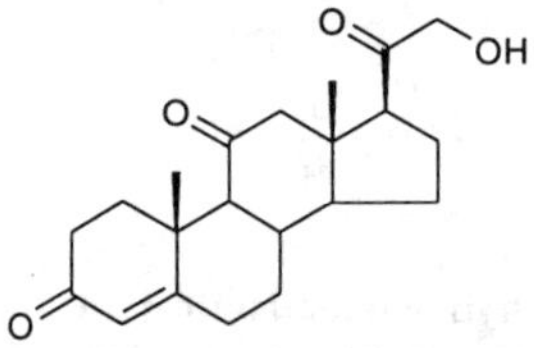

1544 Dehydrocorybulbine
$C_{21}H_{22}NO_4$ MW: 352.41 Source: YAN HU SUO. Ref: 2.

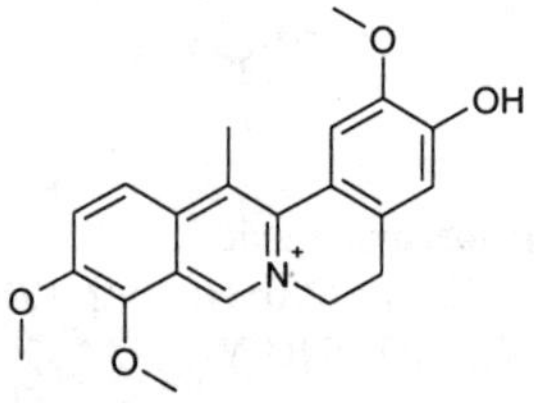

1545 Dehydrocorydaline
$C_{22}H_{24}NO_4$ MW: 366.44 Source: YAN HU SUO. Ref: 2.

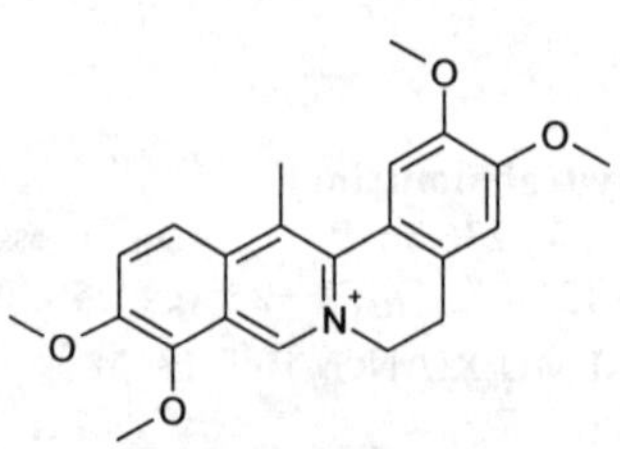

1546 Dehydrocorydalmine
$C_{20}H_{20}NO_4$ MW: 338.39 Source: YAN HU SUO. Ref: 6.

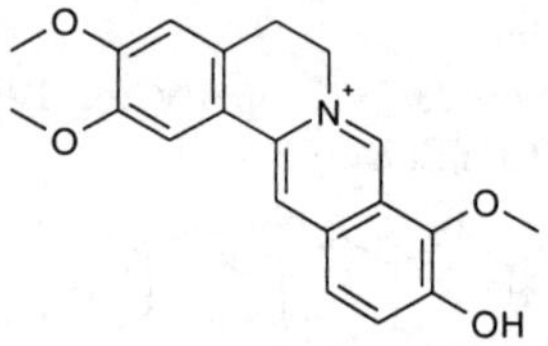

1547 Dehydrocostus lactone
$C_{15}H_{18}O_2$ MW: 230.31 Property: mp 60.5°C. Source: MU XIANG. Ref: 2, 6.

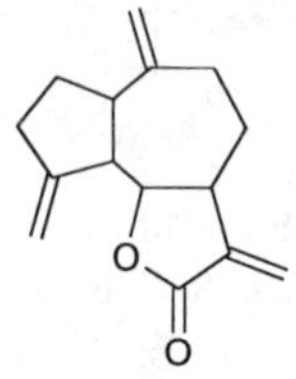

1548 Dehydro-α-curcumene
$C_{15}H_{20}$ MW: 200.33 Source: BAI ZHI JIE. Ref: 6.

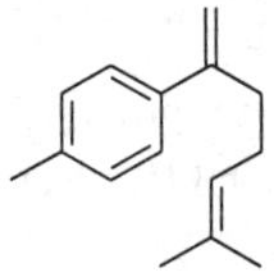

1549 Dehydrocurdione
$C_{15}H_{22}O_2$ MW: 234.34 Source: PENG E SHU, JIANG HUANG. Ref: 6, 640.

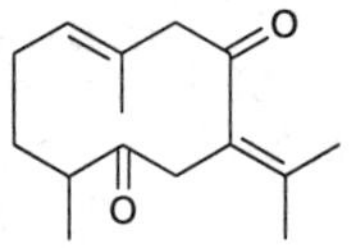

1550 Dehydrodiconiferyl alcohol 4,γ'-di-O-β-D-glucopyranoside
Source: DU ZHONG. Ref: 2

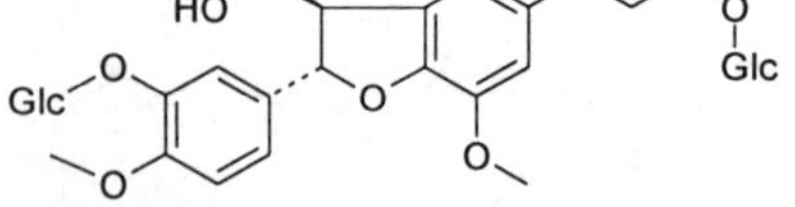

1551 Dehydroeburicoic acid
$C_{31}H_{48}O_3$ MW: 468.73 Property: mp 286-8°C. Source: A LI HONG (LUO YE SONG XUN). Ref: 6.

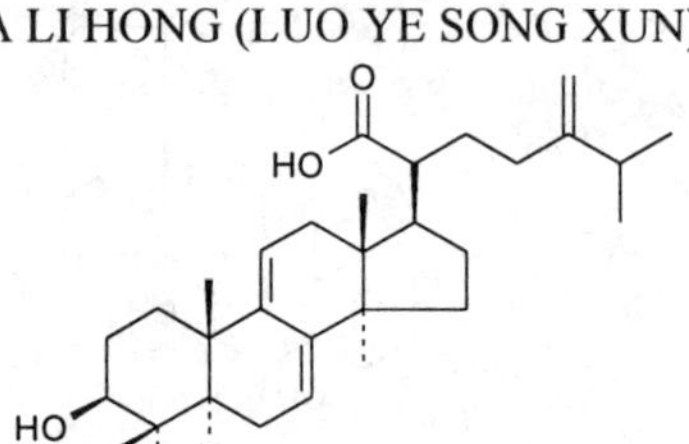

1552 Dehydroeburiconic acid
$C_{31}H_{46}O_3$ MW: 466.71 Property: mp 240-2°C. Source: A LI HONG (LUO YE SONG XUN). Ref: 6.

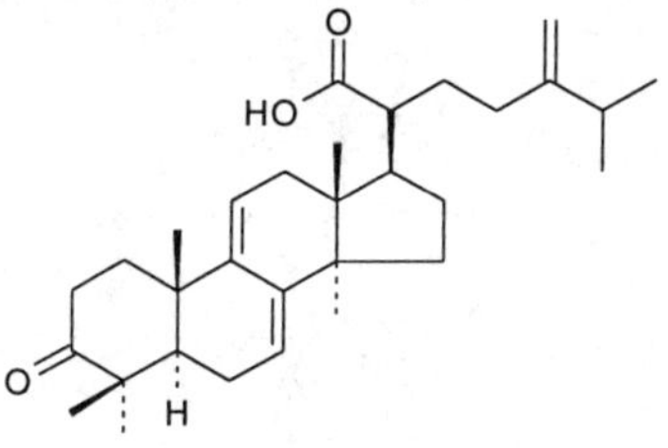

1553 Dehydrofalcarinol
$C_{18}H_{26}O$ MW: 258.41 Source: YIN CHEN HAO. Ref: 2.

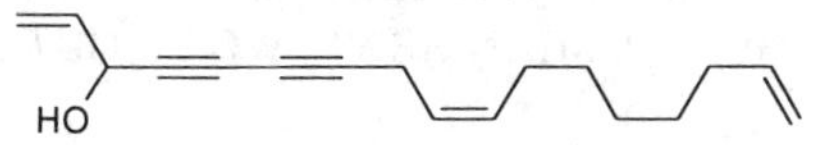

1554 Dehydrofalcarinone
$C_{18}H_{24}O$ MW: 256.39 Source: YIN CHEN HAO. Ref: 2.

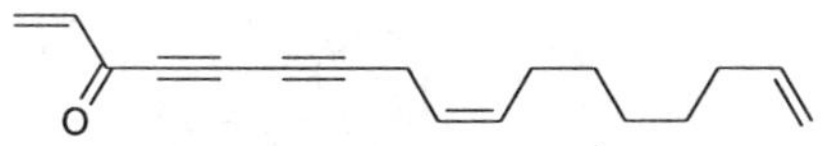

1555 Δ6-Dehydroferruginol
$C_{20}H_{28}O$ MW: 284.45 Source: DU SONG SHI. Ref: 6.

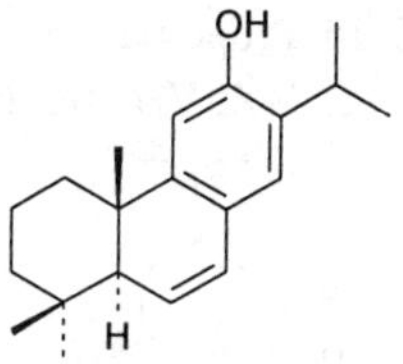

1556 10-Dehydrogingerdione
$C_{21}H_{30}O_4$ MW: 346.47 Source: SHENG JIANG. Ref: 2.

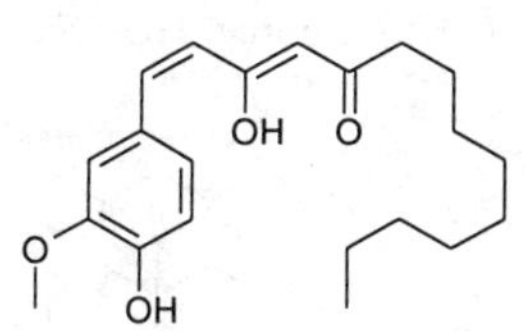

1557 6-Dehydrogingerdione
$C_{17}H_{22}O_4$ MW: 290.36 Source: SHENG JIANG. Ref: 2.

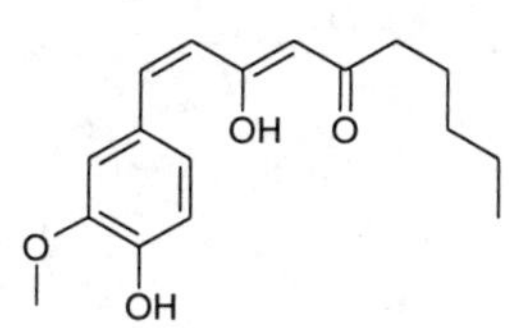

1558 10-Dehydrohecogenin
$C_{26}H_{38}O_3$ MW: 398.59 Source: DUAN YE LONG SHE LAN, FAN MA, WU CI FAN MA. Ref: 10.

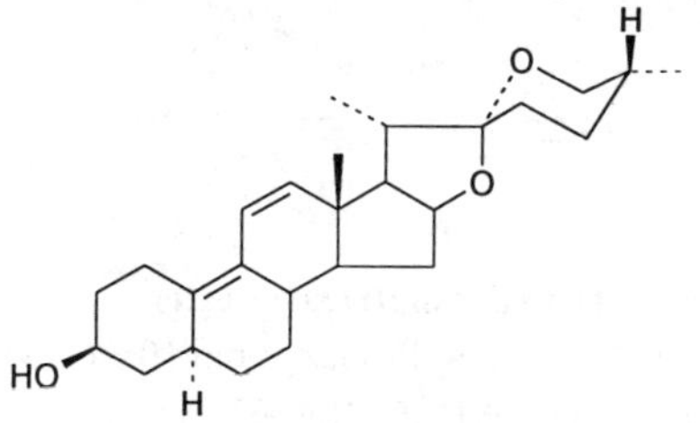

1559 Dehydrojinkoheremol
$C_{15}H_{24}O$ MW: 220.36 Source: CHEN XIANG. Ref: 13.

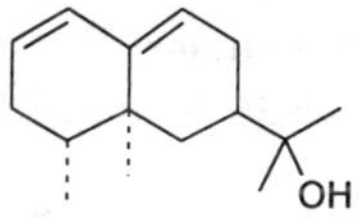

1560 Dehydrolindestrenolide
$C_{15}H_{16}O_2$ MW: 228.29 Property: mp 111-3°C. Source: WU YAO. Ref: 6.

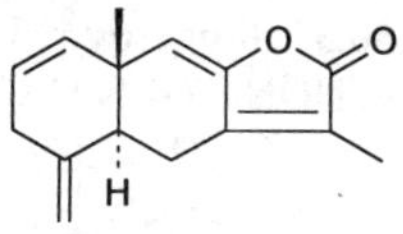

1561 Dehydrologanin
$C_{17}H_{24}O_{10}$ MW: 388.37 Source: CHANG CHUN HUA, SHAN ZHU YU. Ref: 2, 639.

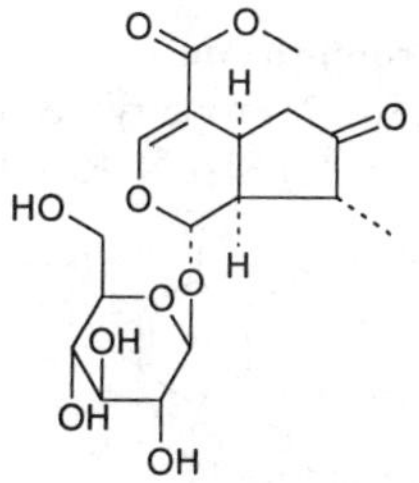

1562 3,4-Dehydrolycopen-16-al
$C_{40}H_{52}O$ MW: 548.86 Source: KU QIE. Ref: 6.

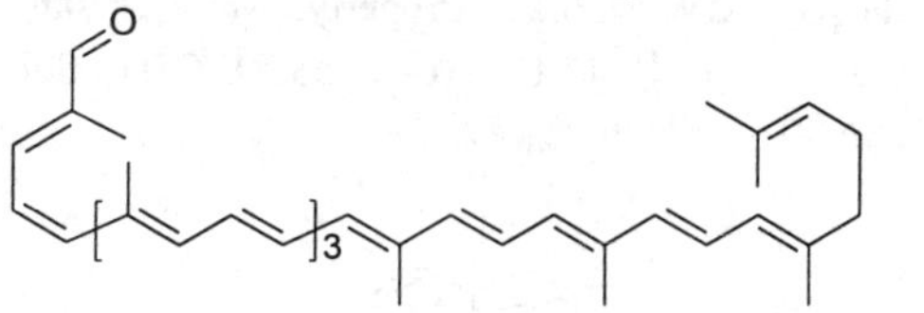

1563 Dehydromatricaria ester
$C_{11}H_8O_2$ MW: 172.19 Property: mp 114-5°C. Source: AI YE, QI ZHOU YI ZHI HAO. Ref: 6.

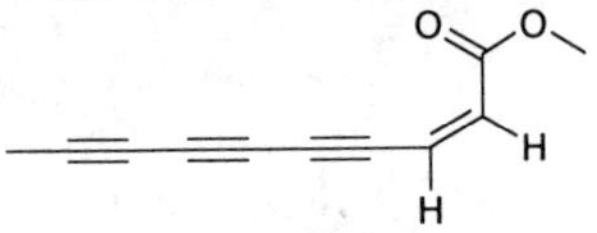

1564 trans-Dehydromatricaria ester
$C_{11}H_8O_2$ MW: 172.19 Property: mp 105°C. Source: DA YE BAI TOU WENG. Ref: 6.

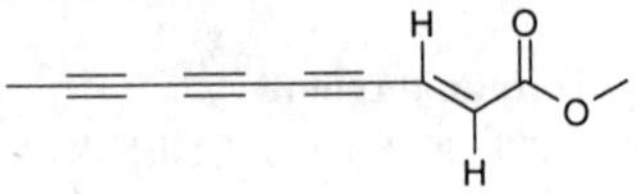

1565 7,11-Dehydromatrine
$C_{15}H_{22}N_2O$ MW: 246.36 Source: KU SHEN. Ref: 2.

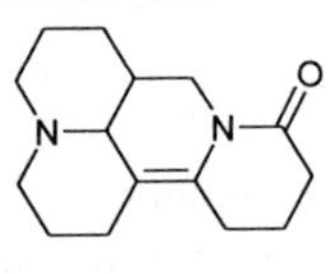

1566 Dehydromiltirone
$C_{19}H_{20}O_2$ MW: 280.37 Property: red acicular crystal, mp 45-6°C. Source: HONG GEN CAO. Ref: 102.

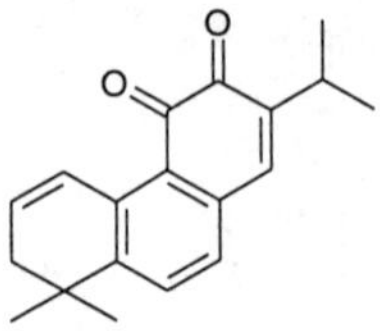

1567 Δ1-Dehydromiltirone
$C_{19}H_{20}O_2$ MW: 280.37 Property: red oleaginous substance. Source: DAN SHEN. Ref: 116.

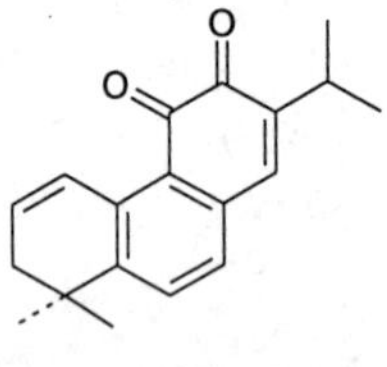

1568 Dehydromorroniaglycone
$C_{11}H_{14}O_5$ MW: 226.23 Property: white crystal, mp 119-20°C, $[\alpha]_D^{21}$ -47.17° (c=0.053, EtOH). Source: SHAN ZHU YU. Ref: 479.

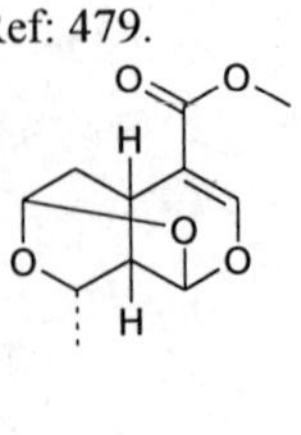

1569 7,8–dehydropenstemoside
$C_{17}H_{24}O_{11}$ MW: 404.37 Property: colorless powder, mp 119-20°C. Source: DU YI WEI. Ref: 381.

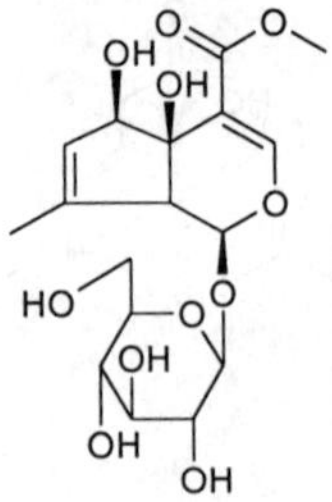

1570 Dehydropodophyllotoxin
$C_{22}H_{18}O_8$ MW: 410.38 Property: mp 275-6°C. Source: GUI JIU, SHAN HE YE, WO ER QI. Ref: 6, 279.

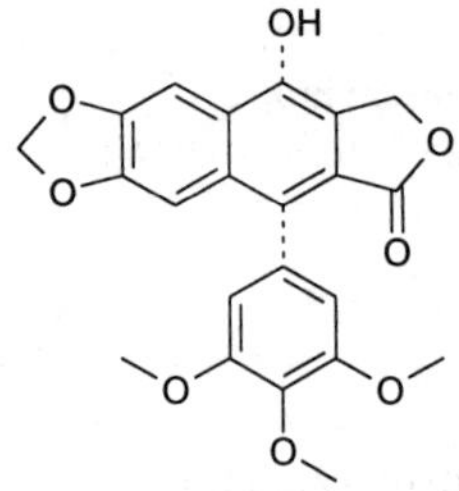

1571 Dehydroshikimic acid
$C_7H_8O_5$ MW: 172.14 Property: mp 150-2°C, 201-2°C. Source: HE ZI, HE ZI YE. Ref: 6.

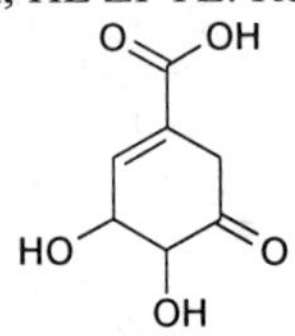

1572 7-Dehydrosigmasterol
$C_{29}H_{50}O$ MW: 414.72 Source: HUANG BAI. Ref: 2.

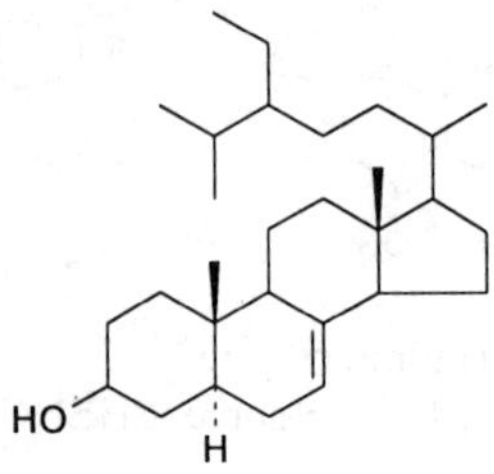

1573 Δ7-Dehydrosophoramine
$C_{15}H_{18}N_2O$ MW: 242.32 Source: HUANG BAI. Ref: 2.

1574 Δ1-Dehydrotanshinone
$C_{19}H_{16}O_3$ MW: 292.34 Property: dark red acicular crystal, mp 147-8°C. Source: DAN SHEN. Ref: 116.

1575 1-Dehydroxy-baccatin
$C_{37}H_{46}O_{13}$ MW: 698.77 Property: colorless crystal, mp 220-1°C. Source: MEI LI HONG DOU SHAN. Ref: 139.

1576 Dehydroxy-15-O-methylcimigenol
$C_{31}H_{48}O_4$ MW: 484.73 Property: mp 222-3°C. Source: SAN MIAN DAO. Ref: 6.

1577 Delamide
$C_{13}H_{16}N_2O_4$ MW: 357.41 Source: FU ZI. Ref: 16.

1578 Delavaine
$C_{20}H_{23}NO_5$ MW: 357.41 Property: mp 149-50°C. Source: DI BU RONG. Ref: 6.

1579 Delavine
$C_{27}H_{45}NO_2$ MW: 415.67 Source: CHUAN BEI MU. Ref: 2.

1580 Delavinone
$C_{27}H_{43}NO_2$ MW: 413.65 Source: CHUAN BEI MU. Ref: 2.

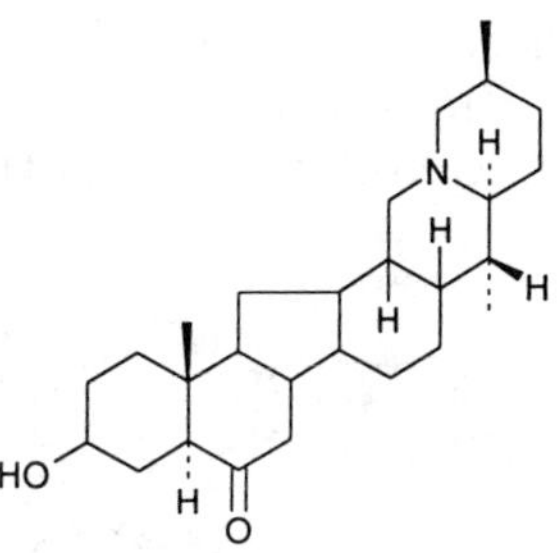

1581 Delbruine
Source: FU ZI. Ref: 16.

1582 Delbruline
Source: FU ZI. Ref: 16.

1583 Delbrusine
Source: FU ZI. Ref: 16.

1584 Delcosine
$C_{24}H_{39}NO_7$ MW: 453.58 Property: mp 203-4°C.
Source: FEI YAN CAO, XIAO CAO WU. Ref: 6, 16.

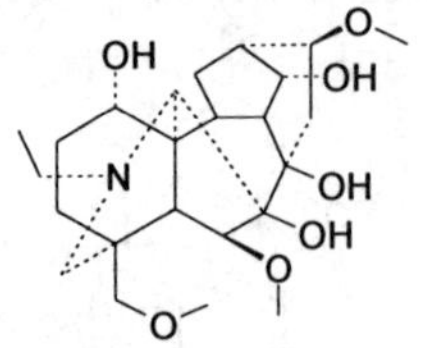

1585 Delgrandine
Source: FU ZI. Ref: 16.

1586 Delphatine
Source: FU ZI. Ref: 16.

1587 Delphin
Delphinidin-3,5-diglucoside. $C_{27}H_{31}O_{17}$ MW: 627.54
Source: BAI FAN DOU, FEI YAN CAO, MU XU, QIE ZI, YA ZHI CAO. Ref: 6.

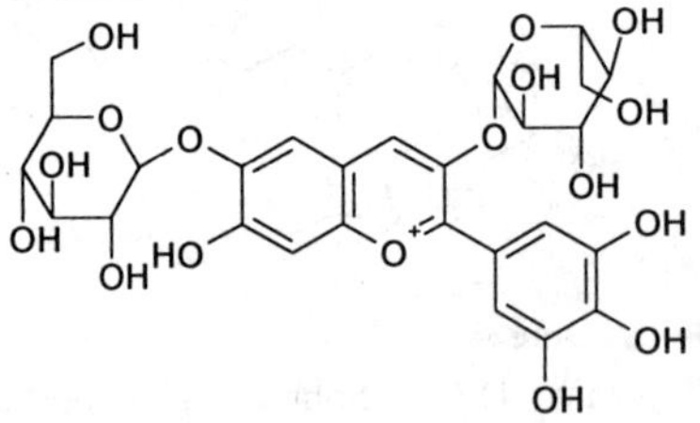

1588 Delphinidin
Delphinidol. $C_{15}H_{11}O_7$ MW: 323.25 Source: BU XUE CAO, FENG XIAN HUA, PU TAO, TAO ER QI. Ref: 6.

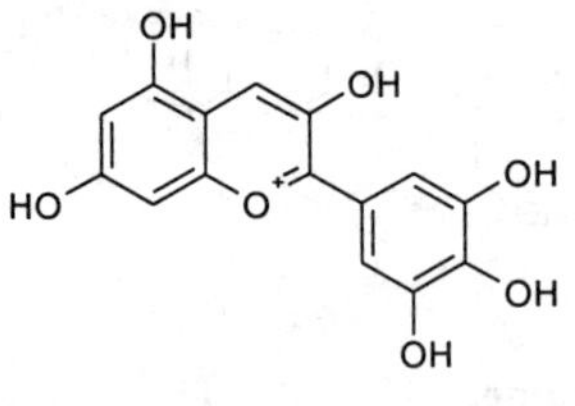

1589 Delphinidin-3-arabinoside
$C_{20}H_{19}O_{11}$ MW: 435.37 Source: ZI WEI HUA. Ref: 6.

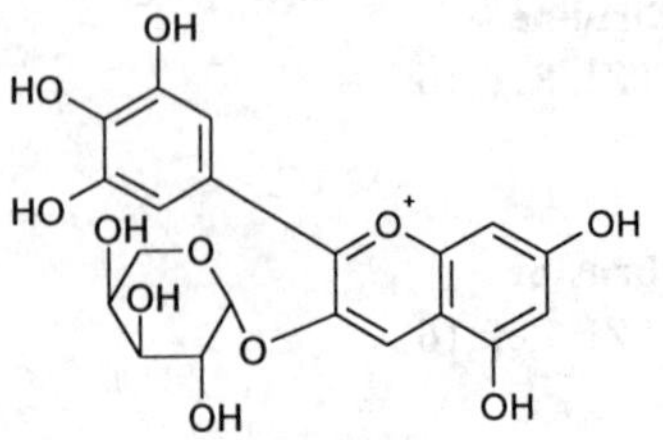

1590 Delphinidin-3-di-caffeoyl rutinosido-5-glucoside
Source: JIE GENG. Ref: 6.

1591 Delphinidin-3-diglucoside
$C_{27}H_{31}O_{17}$ MW: 627.54 Source: SHUI HULU. Ref: 6.

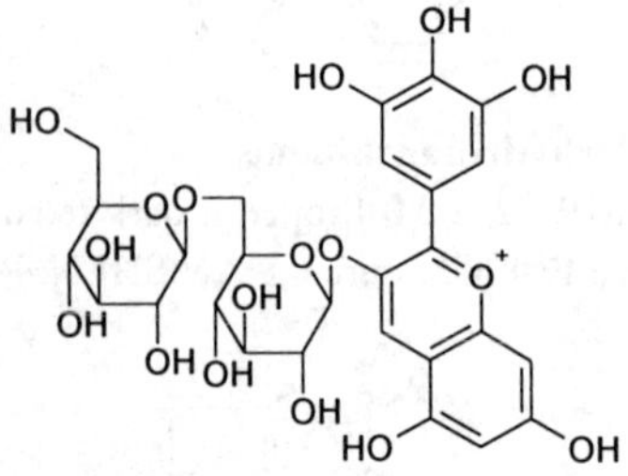

1592 Delphinidin-monoglucoside
Source: HUANG LU ZHI YE. Ref: 6.

1593 Delphinidin-3-monoglucoside
$C_{21}H_{21}O_{12}$ MW: 465.39 Source: BAI FAN DOU, HEI DA DOU PI, QIE ZI. Ref: 6.

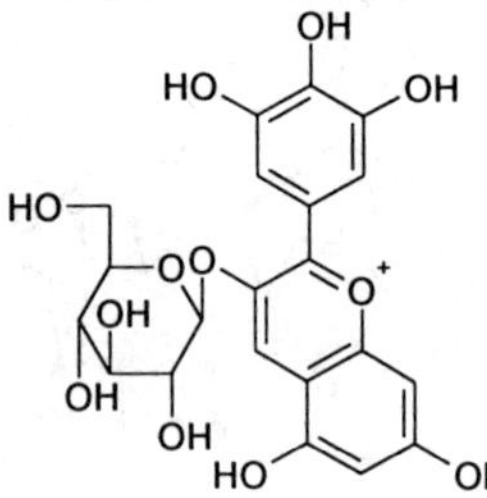

1594 Delsemine A
Source: FU ZI. Ref: 16.

1595 Delsemine B
Source: FU ZI. Ref: 16.

1596 Delsoline
$C_{25}H_{41}NO_7$ MW: 467.61 Property: mp 213-6.5°C.
Source: FEI YAN CAO. Ref: 6.

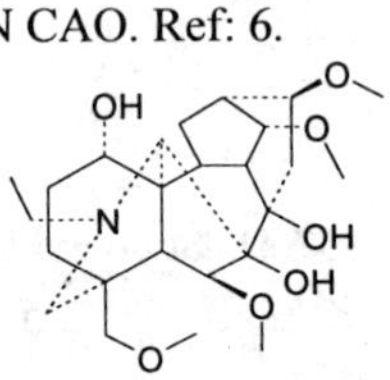

1597 Deltaline
$C_{28}H_{43}NO_7$ MW: 505.66 Source: FU ZI. Ref: 16.

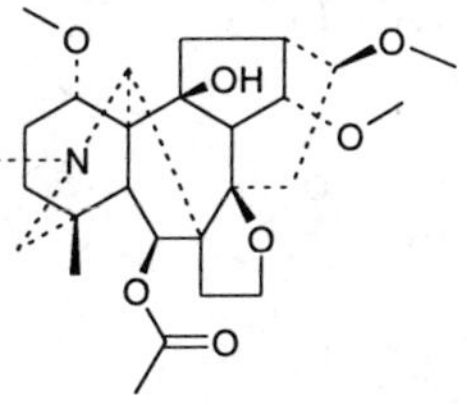

1598 Deltamine
$C_{26}H_{41}NO_6$ MW: 463.62 Source: FU ZI. Ref: 16.

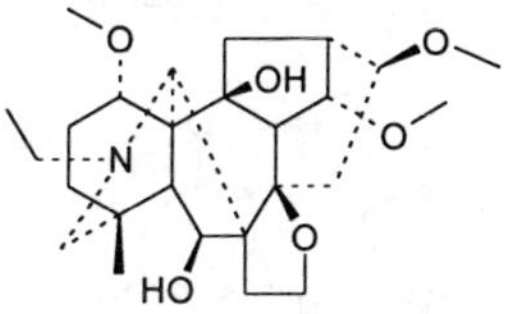

1599 Deltoin
$C_{19}H_{20}O_5$ MW: 328.37 Source: FANG FENG, YUN QIAN HU. Ref: 2, 177.

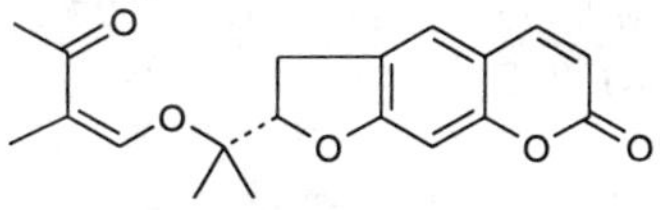

1600 Deltonin(e)
$C_{45}H_{72}O_{17}$ MW: 885.07 Property: mp 290-2°C. Source: SHAN YAO, XIAO HUA DUN YE SHU YU (fresh rhizome). Ref: 6, 10.

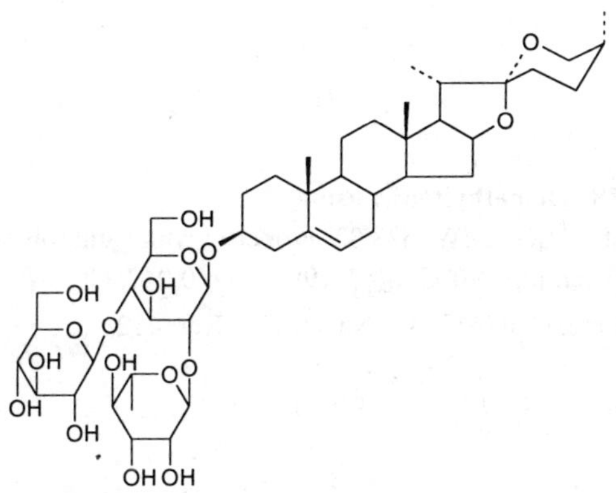

1601 Deltoside
$C_{51}H_{82}O_{23}$ MW: 1063.21 Source: XIAO HUA DUN YE SHU YU (fresh rhizome). Ref: 10.

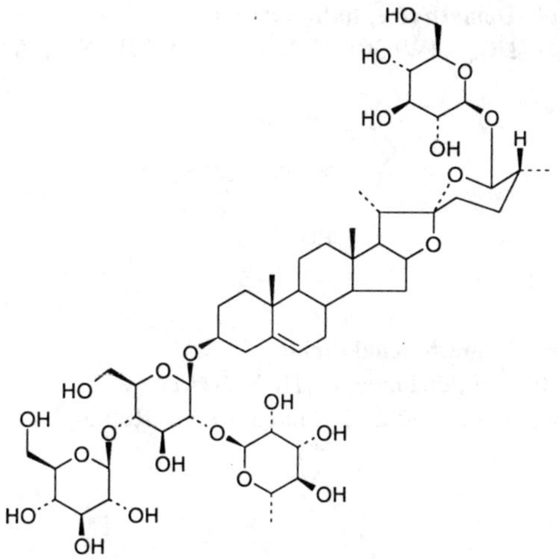

1602 Demethoxyaschantin
Source: WANG CHUN MU LAN. Ref: 543.

1603 6-Demethoxycapillarisin
$C_{15}H_{12}O_6$ MW: 288.26 Source: YIN CHEN HAO. Ref: 2.

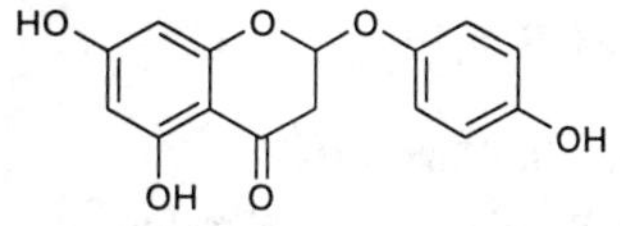

1604 Demethoxycurcumin
$C_{19}H_{16}O_4$ MW: 308.34 Property: mp 218-22°C. Source: YU JIN. Ref: 6.

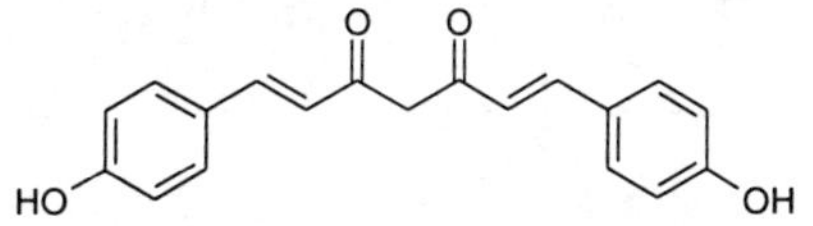

1605 6-Demethoxy-4'-methoxylcapillarisin
$C_{16}H_{14}O_6$ MW: 302.29 Source: YIN CHEN HAO. Ref: 2.

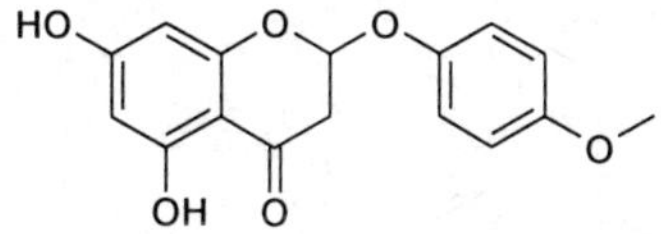

1606 N-Demethyl-acronycine
$C_{19}H_{17}NO_3$ MW: 307.35 Source: JIU LI XIANG. Ref: 11.

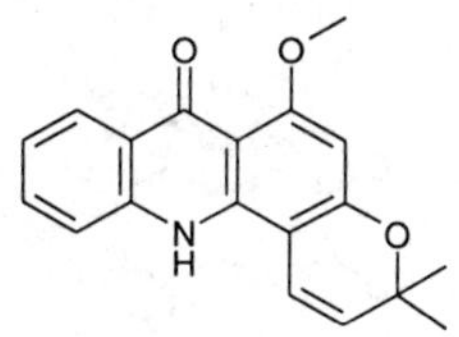

1607 Demethylcephalotaxinoen
$C_{17}H_{19}NO_4$ MW: 301.35 Source: SAN JIAN SHAN. Ref: 2.

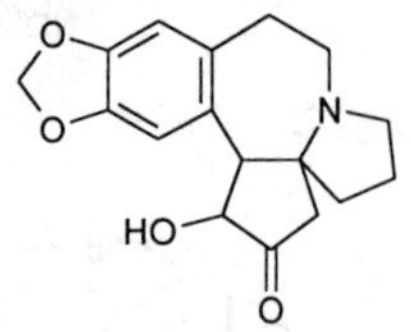

1608 Demethylcoclaurine
Cnetine; Higenamine. $C_{16}H_{17}NO_3$ MW: 271.32 Property: mp 260-2°C. Source: FU ZI. Ref: 2, 4.

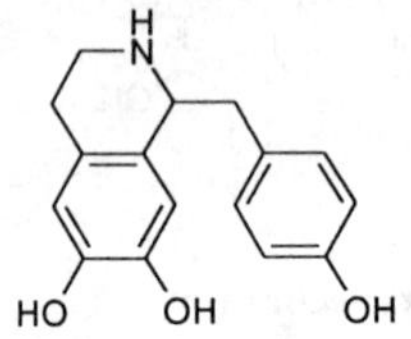

1609 Demethyldelavaine A
Source: FU ZI. Ref: 16.

1610 Demethyldelavaine B
Source: FU ZI. Ref: 16.

1611 8-Demethylfarrerol
$C_{16}H_{14}O_5$ MW: 286.29 Property: mp 267-70°C. Source: MAN SHAN HONG. Ref: 6, 507.

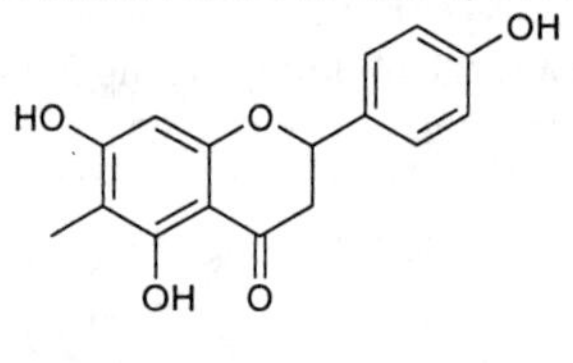

1612 Demethylfuropinnarin
$C_{16}H_{14}O_4$ MW: 270.29 Source: QIANG HUO. Ref: 2, 325.

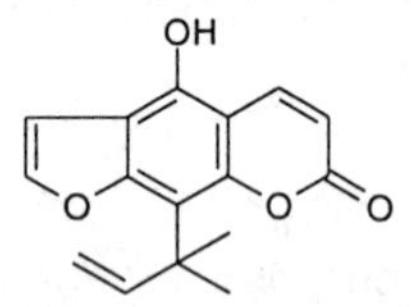

1613 9-Demethylhomolycorine
$C_{17}H_{19}NO_4$ MW: 301.35 Property: mp 213-4°C Source: SHI SUAN. Ref: 6.

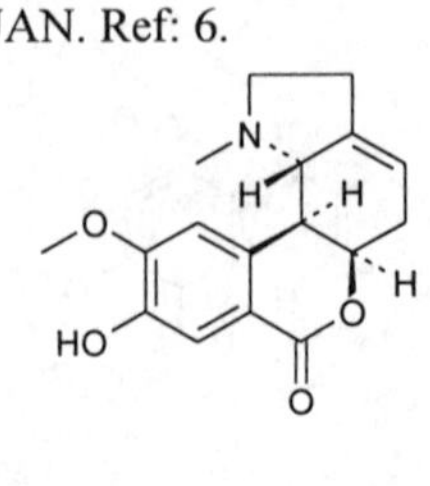

1614 Demethylnobiletin
$C_{20}H_{20}O_8$ MW: 388.38 Property: mp 144°C. Source: A ER TAI ZI WAN. Ref: 6.

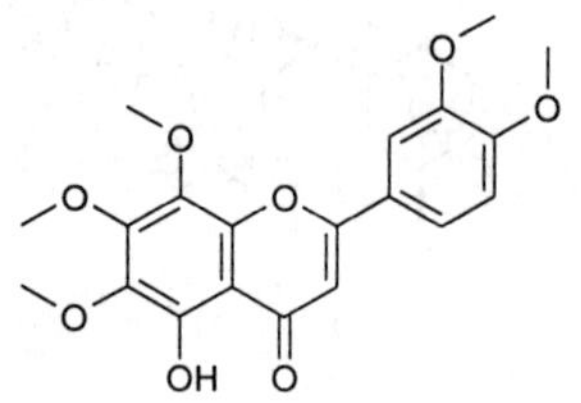

1615 N-Demethyl-noracronycine
$C_{18}H_{15}NO_3$ MW: 293.33 Source: JIU LI XIANG. Ref: 11.

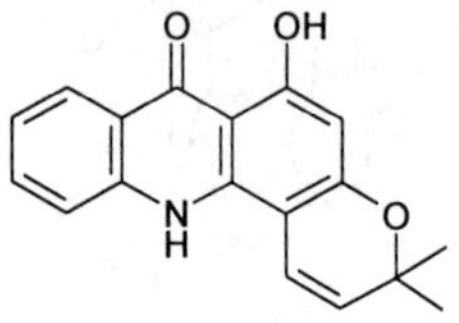

1616 d-Demethyl pseudoephedrine
$C_9H_{13}NO$ MW: 151.21 Property: mp 77°C. Source: MA HUANG. Ref: 6.

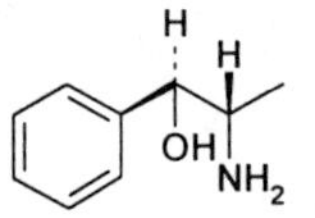

1617 7-Demethylsuberosin
$C_{14}H_{14}O_3$ MW: 230.27 Source: BAI ZHI. Ref: 2.

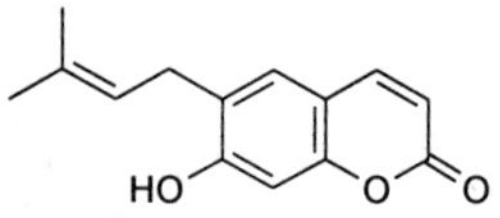

1618 Demethylteuicausine
$C_{40}H_{44}N_4O_3$ MW: 628.82 Property: white amorphous powder, mp 190°C, $[\alpha]_D^{13}$ -198.5° (c= 0.047, $CHCl_3$). Source: CHUAN SHAN CHENG. Ref: 412.

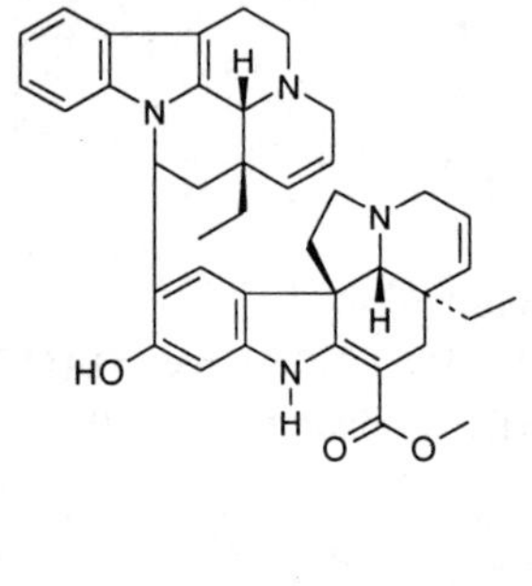

1619 Demethylwedelolactone
$C_{15}H_{10}O_7$ MW: 302.24 Source: MO HAN LIAN. Ref: 6.

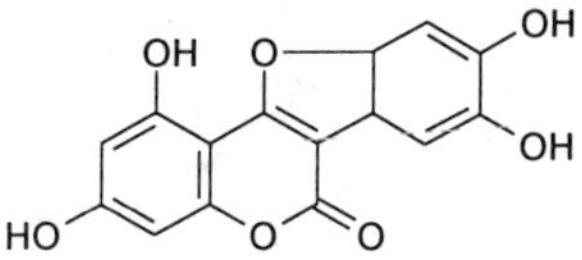

1620 Demethylwedelolactone-7-glucoside
$C_{21}H_{18}O_{12}$ MW: 462.37 Source: MO HAN LIAN. Ref: 6.

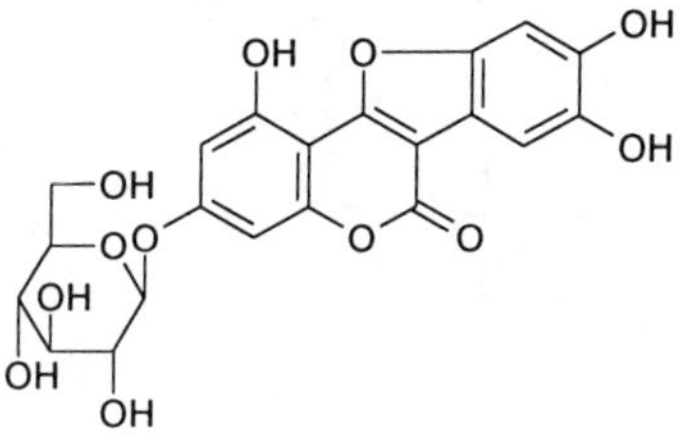

1621 Dencichine
$C_5H_8N_2O_5$ MW: 176.13 Source: SAN QI. Ref: 2.

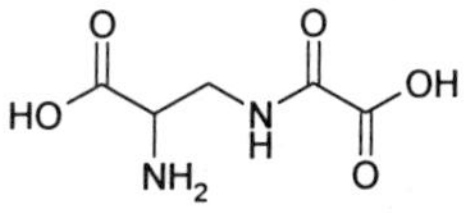

1622 Dendramine
$C_{16}H_{25}NO_3$ MW: 279.38 Property: mp 186-8°C. Source: SHI HU. Ref: 6.

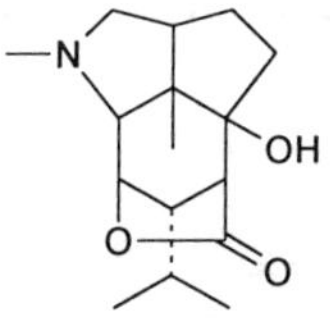

1623 Dendrin(e)
$C_{19}H_{29}NO_4$ MW: 335.45 Property: mp 191-2°C. Source: SHI HU. Ref: 6.

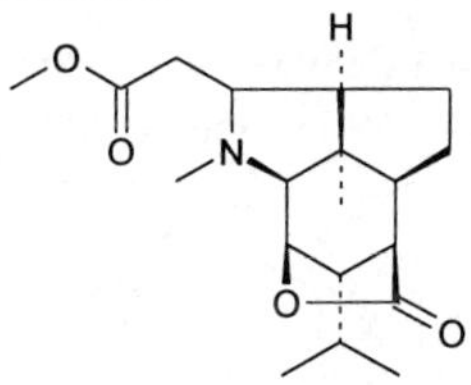

1624 Dendrobine
$C_{16}H_{25}NO_2$ MW: 263.38 Property: mp 135-6°C. Source: SHI HU. Ref: 6.

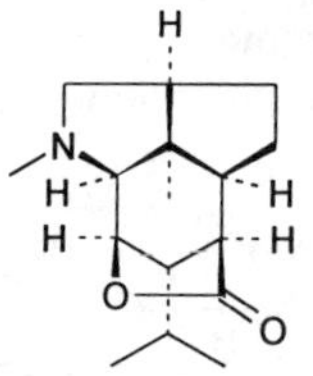

1625 Dendrolasin
$C_{15}H_{22}O$ MW: 218.34 Property: bp 148-50°C /16mm. Source: TAN XIANG. Ref: 6.

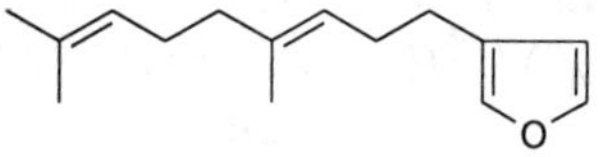

1626 Dendroxine
$C_{17}H_{25}NO_3$ MW: 291.39 Property: mp 114-5°C. Source: SHI HU. Ref: 6.

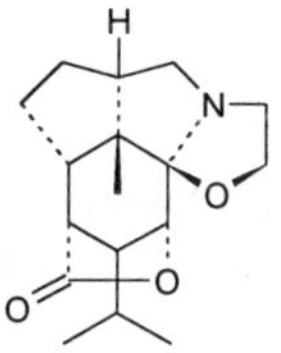

1627 Dentatin
$C_{20}H_{22}O_4$ MW: 326.40 Property: mp 95-6°C. Source: YE HUANG PI. Ref: 6.

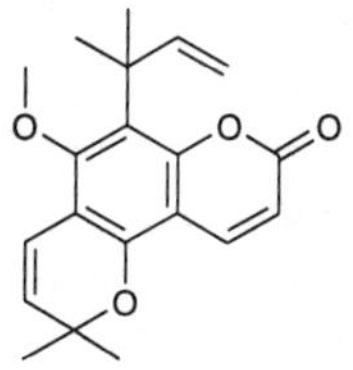

1628 (-)-Denudatin B
$C_{21}H_{24}O_5$ MW: 356.42 Property: colorless oleaginous substance, $[\alpha]_D^{15}$ -76.4° (c=0.11, $CHCl_3$). Source: HAI FENG TENG. Ref: 267.

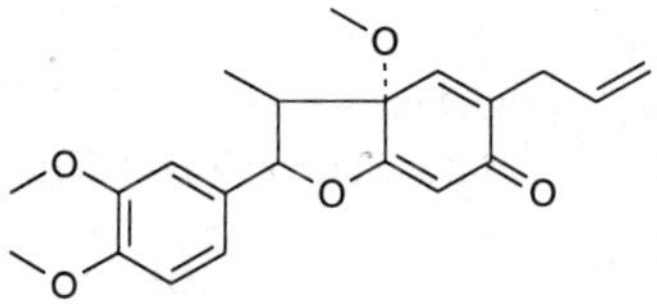

1629 Denudatine
$C_{22}H_{35}NO_2$ MW: 345.53 Source: FU ZI. Ref: 16.

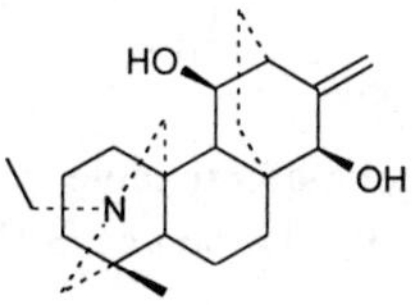

1630 11-Deoxojervine
$C_{27}H_{41}NO_2$ MW: 411.63 Property: mp 237-8°C. Source: LI LU. Ref: 6.

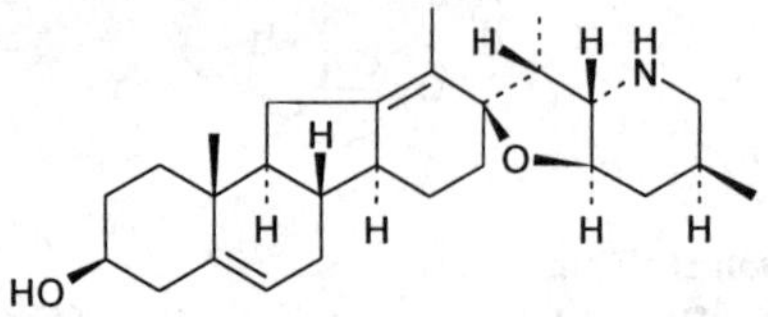

1631 Deoxyaconitine
$C_{33}H_{45}NO_{10}$ MW: 615.73 Source: FU ZI. Ref: 16.

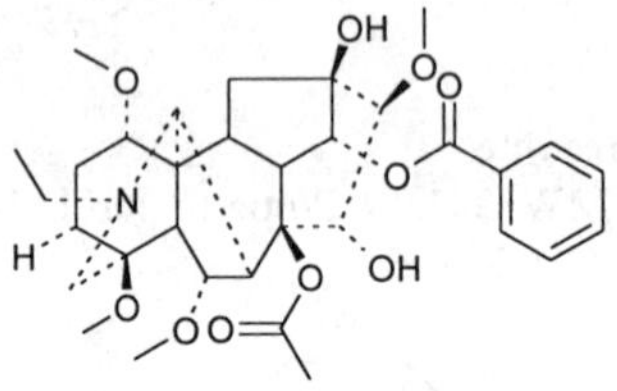

1632 Deoxyandrographolide
$C_{20}H_{30}O_4$ MW: 334.46 Source: CHUAN XIN LIAN. Ref: 2.

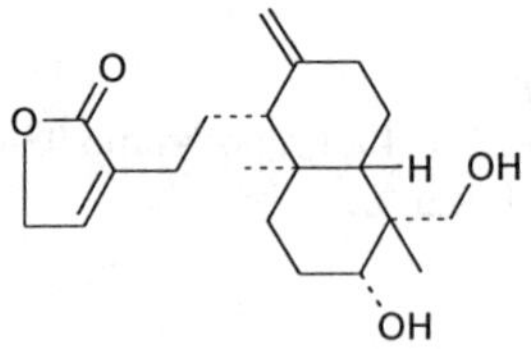

1633 Deoxycamptothecine
$C_{20}H_{16}N_2O_3$ MW: 332.36 Property: mp 171-2°C. Source: XI SHU. Ref: 6.

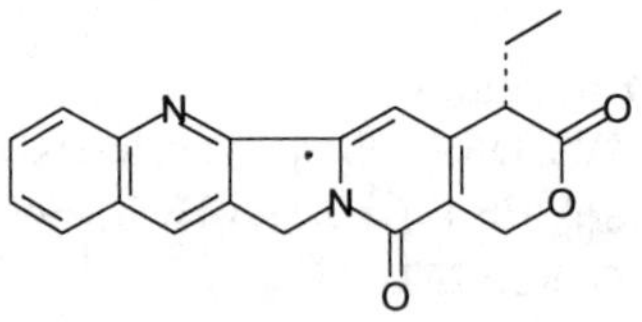

1634 Deoxycapillartemisin
$C_{19}H_{26}O_3$ MW: 302.42 Source: YIN CHEN HAO. Ref: 2.

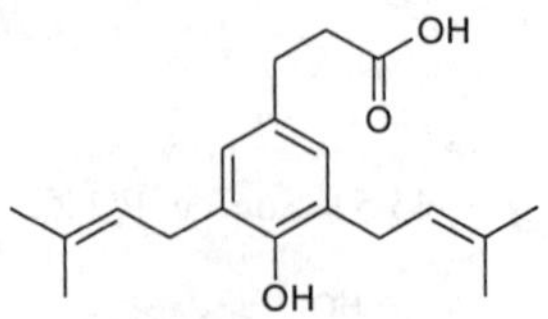

1635 7-Deoxycephalofortuneine
$C_{20}H_{27}NO_4$ MW: 345.44 Source: SAN JIAN SHAN. Ref: 2.

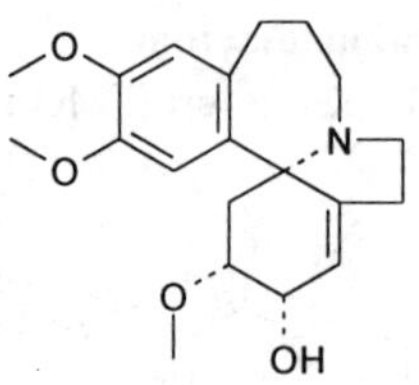

1636 Deoxycholic acid
$C_{24}H_{40}O_4$ MW: 392.58 Source: NIU HUANG, XIONG DAN. Ref: 2.

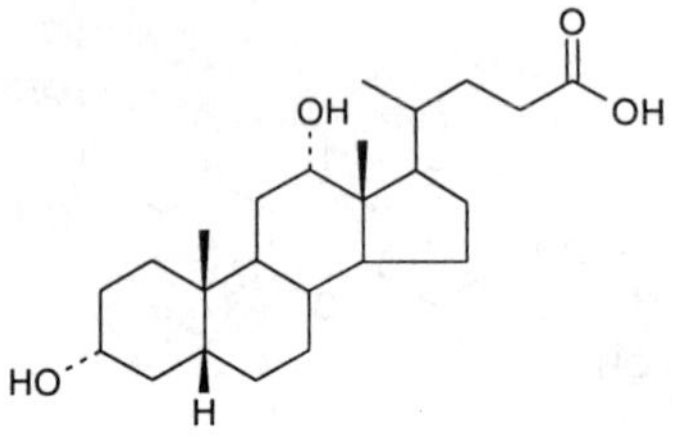

1637 Deoxycorticosterone
11-Deoxycorticosterone. $C_{21}H_{30}O_3$ MW: 330.47 Property: mp 141-2°C. Source: NIU SHEN, ZI HE CHE. Ref: 6.

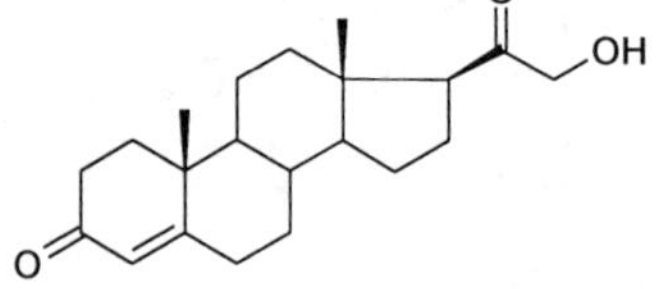

1638 14-Deoxy-11,12-didehydroandrographolide
$C_{20}H_{28}O_4$ MW: 332.44 Source: CHUAN XIN LIAN. Ref: 2.

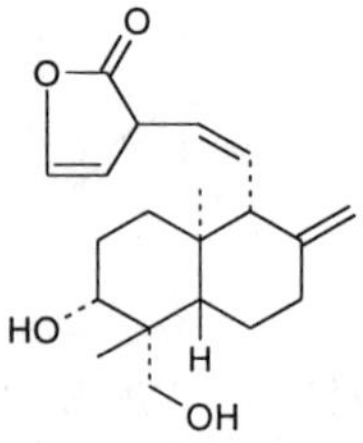

1639 8-Deoxy-14-dehydro-aconosine
$C_{22}H_{33}NO_3$ MW: 359.51 Source: FU ZI. Ref: 16.

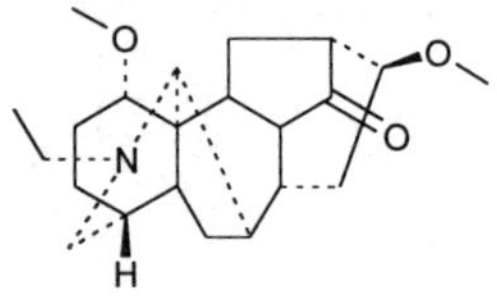

1640 Deoxyelephantopin
$C_{19}H_{20}O_6$ MW: 344.37 Property: mp >320°C. Source: KU DI DAN. Ref: 5, 6.

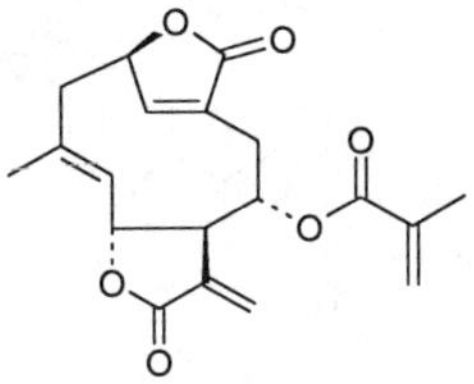

1641 1-Deoxyeucommiol
$C_9H_{16}O_3$ MW: 172.23 Source: DU ZHONG. Ref: 2.

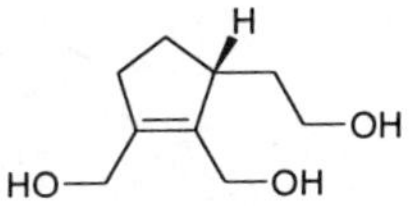

1642 11-Deoxyglycyrrhetinic acid
$C_{30}H_{48}O_3$ MW: 456.72 Source: GAN CAO. Ref: 2.

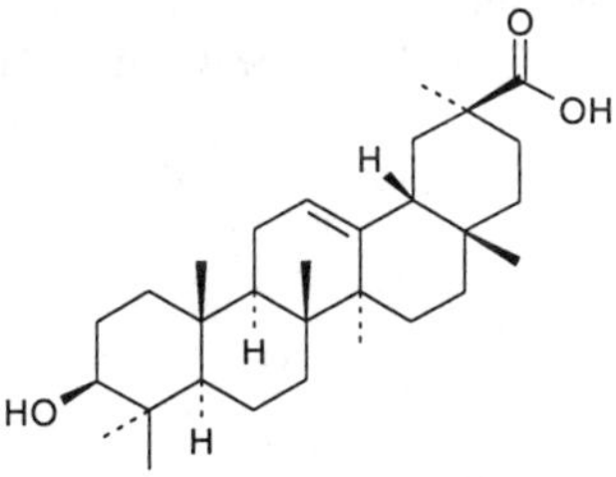

1643 Deoxyharringtonine
$C_{28}H_{37}NO_8$ MW: 515.61 Source: SAN JIAN SHAN. Ref: 2, 5.

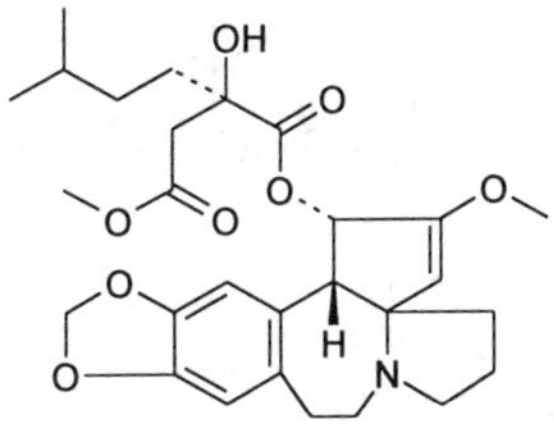

1644 Δ3,5-Deoxyneotigogenin
$C_{27}H_{40}O_3$ MW: 412.62 Source: CHA RUI SHU YU, FEN BEI SHU YU. Ref: 10.

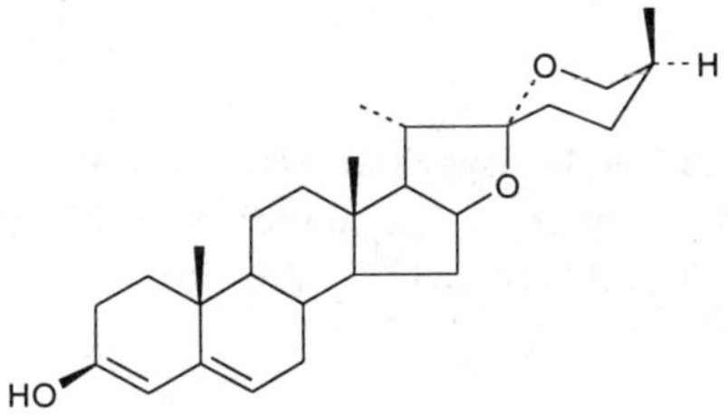

1645 14-Deoxy-11-oxoandrographolide
$C_{20}H_{28}O_5$ MW: 348.44 Property: mp 98-100°C. Source: CHUAN XIN LIAN, JI XING ZI. Ref: 2, 6.

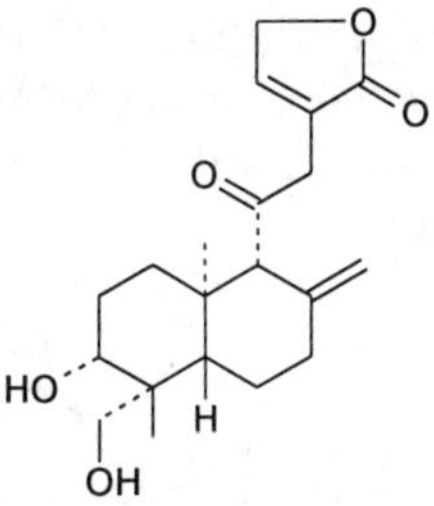

1646 Deoxypeganine
$C_{11}H_{12}N_2$ MW: 172.23 Property: mp 87-8°C. Source: LUO TUO PENG. Ref: 6.

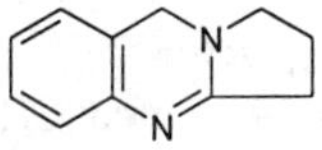

1647 6-Deoxypseudoanisatin
$C_{15}H_{22}O_5$ MW: 282.34 Property: white acicular crystal (acetic ester), mp 235-7°C, $[\alpha]_D^{25}$ +15.5° (c=1.406, ethanol). Source: HONG HUI XIANG, MIN NAN BA JIAO GUO. Ref: 100, 315.

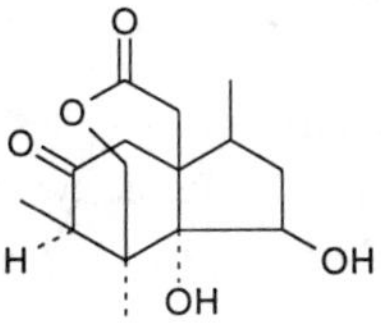

1648 Deoxyschisandrin
$C_{24}H_{32}O_6$ MW: 416.52 Source: WU WEI ZI. Ref: 2.

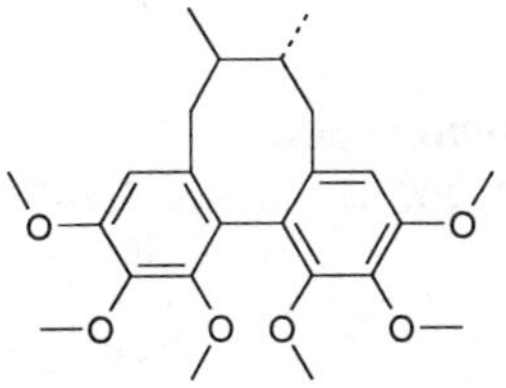

1649 Deoxyshikonin
$C_{16}H_{16}O_4$ MW: 272.30 Source: ZI CAO. Ref: 2.

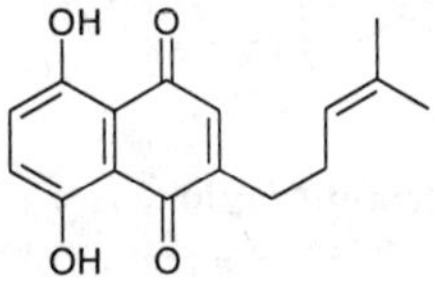

1650 $\Delta^{3,5}$-Deoxytigogenin
$C_{27}H_{40}O_3$ MW: 412.62 Source: CHA RUI SHU YU, CHAI HUANG JIANG, CHUNG LONG SHU YU, DUN YE SHU YU, FEN BEI SHU YU, FU ZHOU SHU YU, HUANG SHAN YAO, MIAN BI XIE, SHU KUI YE, XIAN XI SHU YU, XIAO HUA DUN YE SHU YU. Ref: 10.

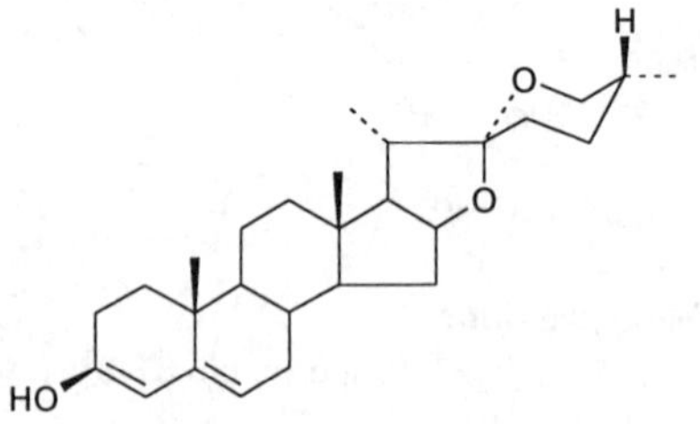

1651 Deoxy-$\Delta^{3,5}$-tigogenin
$C_{26}H_{38}O_2$ MW: 382.59 Source: CHUAN SHAN LONG. Ref: 6.

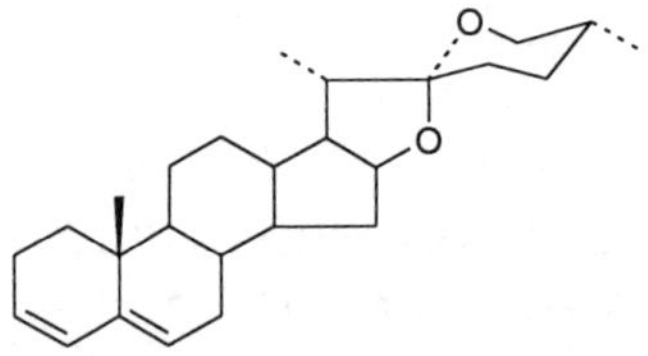

1652 Deoxyvasicinone
$C_{11}H_{10}N_2O$ MW: 186.22 Property: mp 109-10°C. Source: LUO TUO PENG, LUO TUO PENG ZI. Ref: 6.

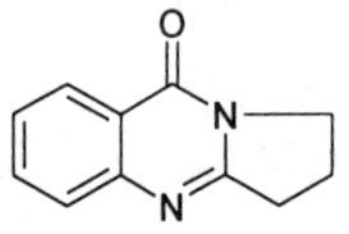

1653 Desacetylbufotalin
$C_{24}H_{34}O_5$ MW: 402.54 Source: CHAN SU. Ref: 2, 6.

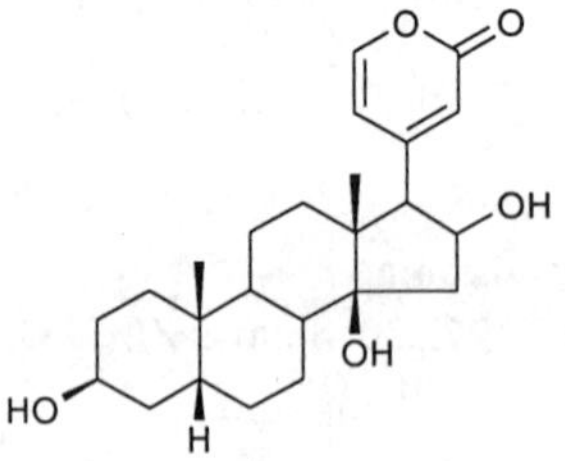

1654 Desacetylcinobufagin
$C_{24}H_{32}O_5$ MW: 400.52 Source: CHAN SU. Ref: 2, 6.

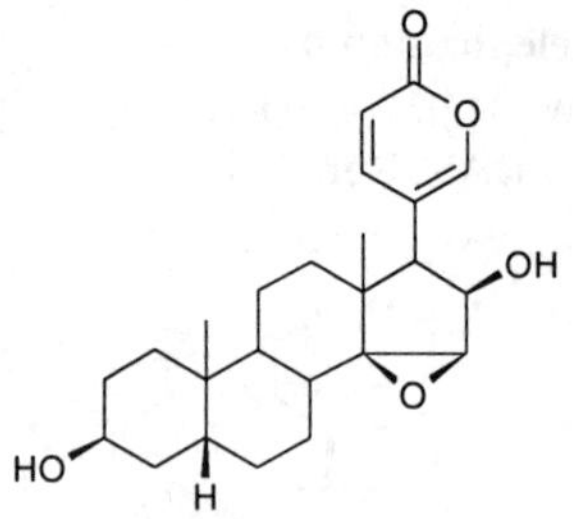

1655 Desacetyl cinobufotalin
$C_{24}H_{32}O_6$ MW: 416.52 Source: CHAN SU. Ref: 2, 6.

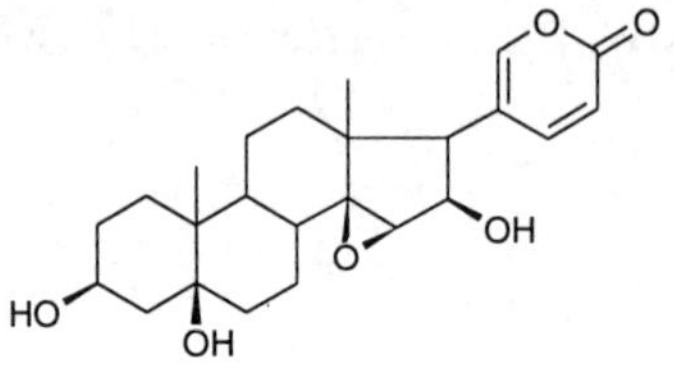

1656 Desapidinol
$C_{11}H_{14}O_4$ MW: 210.23 Source: GUAN ZHONG. Ref: 6.

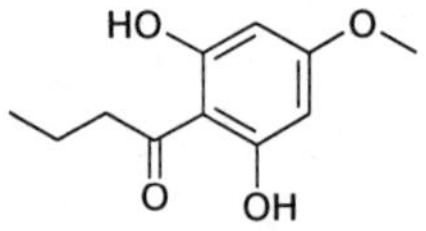

1657 Desgalactotigonin
$C_{50}H_{82}O_{22}$ MW: 1035.20 Source: ZHI MU. Ref: 2.

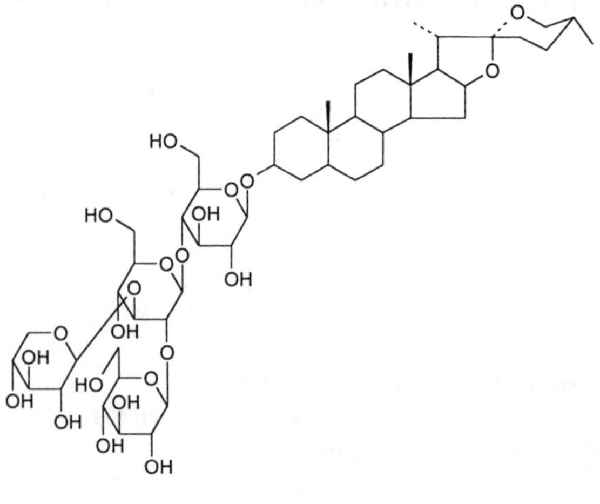

1658 28-Desglucosyl-chikusetsusaponin
Property: white crystalline powder, mp 232 °C (dec). Source: TAI BAI SONG MU. Ref: 462.

1659 N-Desmethoxyhumantenine
$C_{20}H_{24}N_2O_2$ MW: 324.43 Property: mp 238-40°C, $[\alpha]_D$ -188.5°. Source: HU MAN TENG. Ref: 14.

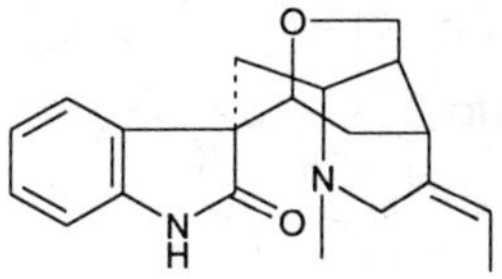

1660 N-Desmethoxyrankinidine
$C_{19}H_{22}N_2O_2$ MW: 310.40 Property: mp 258-60°C, $[\alpha]_D$ -169.2°. Source: HU MAN TENG. Ref: 14.

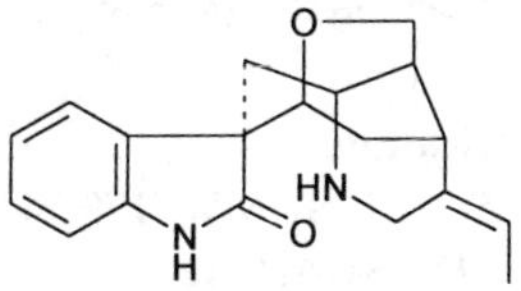

1661 Desmethylanhydroicaritin
MW: 354 Property: yellow powder, mp 208-10°C. Source: WAN SHAN YIN YANG HUO. Ref: 465.

1662 Desmethylanhydroicaritin-3-O-α-L-rhamnopyranosyl-(1→2)-α-L-rhamnopyranoside
Source: WAN SHAN YIN YANG HUO. Ref: 574

1663 Des-O-methylicariin
$C_{33}H_{42}O_{15}$ MW: 678.69 Property: mp 235-7°C. Source: YIN YANG HUO GEN. Ref: 6.

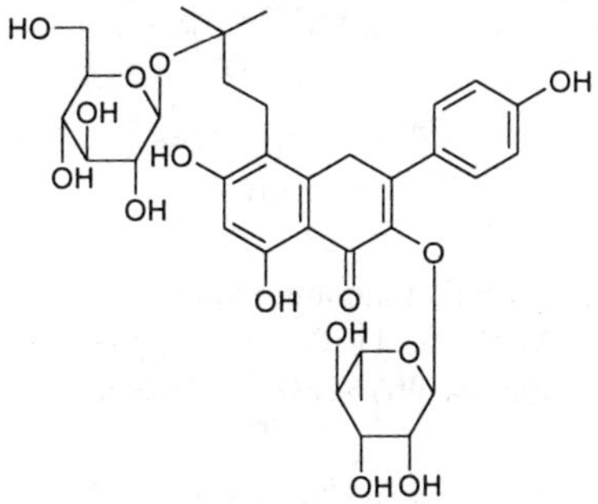

1664 Desmethyl tangeretin
Gardenin B. Source ZHI ZI, Ref: 626.

1665 Desmodilactoe
$C_8H_{13}NO_3$ MW: 171.20 Property: colorless massive crystal, mp 84-85°C, $[\alpha]_D^{18}$-16.4° (c=0.11, MeOH). Source: GUANG JIN QIAN CAO. Ref: 260.

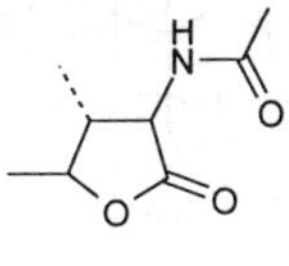

1666 Desmodimine
$C_{12}H_{15}NO_4$ MW: 237.26 Property: colorless gummy substance. Source: GUANG JIN QIAN CAO. Ref: 260.

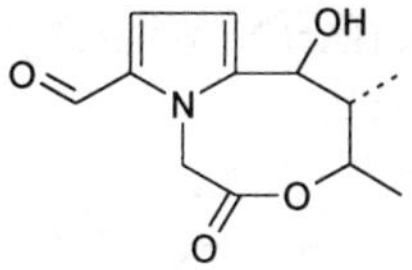

1667 Desmosflavone I
5-Hydroxy-7-methoxy-6,8-dimethyflavone. $C_{17}H_{14}O_5$ MW: 298.30 Property: orange sandy crystal (chloroform), mp 197-8°C. Source: JIA YING ZHUA. Ref: 312.

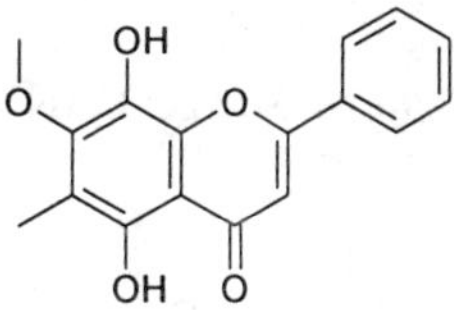

1668 Desoxodehydrocyclopiloselloidone
$C_{18}H_{22}O_2$ MW: 270.37 Source: MAO DA DING CAO. Ref: 6.

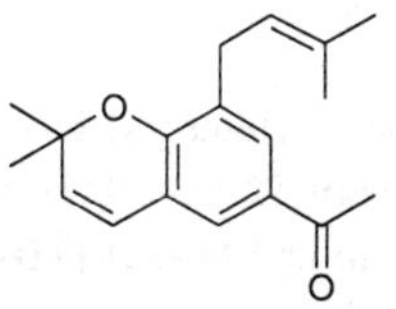

1669 16-Desoxybarringtogenol C
$C_{30}H_{50}O_4$ MW: 474.73 Property: mp 288-90.5°C. Source: SUO LUO ZI. Ref: 6.

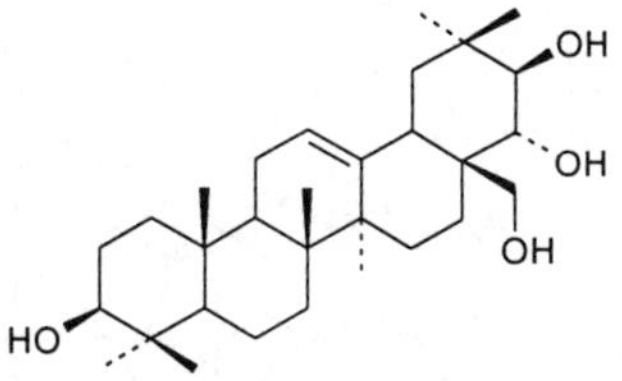

1670 Desoxyrhaponticin
$C_{21}H_{24}O_8$ MW: 404.42 Source: DA HUANG, TIAN SHAN DA HUANG. Ref: 2, 609.

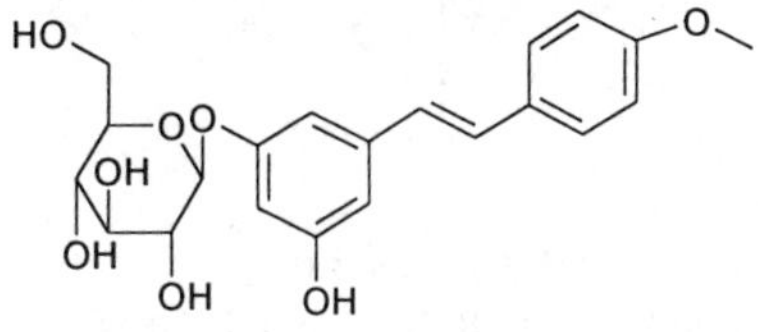

1671 12,13-Di-acetoxyl-1,4,6,11-eudesmanetetrol

$C_{19}H_{32}O_8$ MW: 388.46 Property: colorless acicular crystal, mp 145-7°C, $[\alpha]_D^{22}$ -2.56° (c=0.391, $CHCl_3$). Source: YU NAN HAN XIAO. Ref: 426.

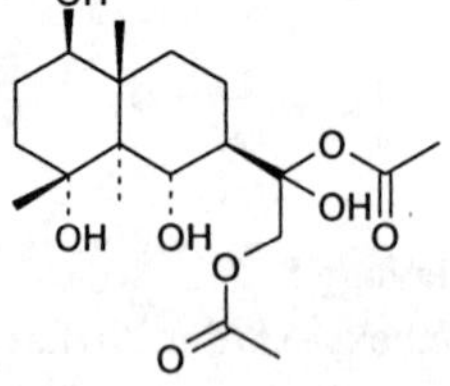

1672 3-5-Diacetoxy-1-(4-hydroxy-3, 5-dimethoxyphenyl)-7-(4-hydroxy-3-methoxyphenyl) heptane

$C_{26}H_{34}O_9$ MW: 490.56 Source: GAN JIANG, SHENG JIANG. Ref: 2.

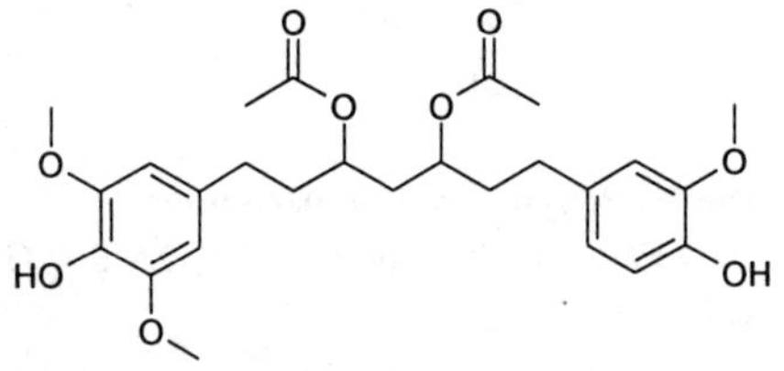

1673 3-O-α(2',4'-O-Diacetyl)-L-arabinopyranosyl-3β-hydroxyolean-12-ene-28,29-dioicacid-28-O-[α-L-rhamnopyranosyl-(1→4)-β-D-glucopyranosyl-(1→6)-β-D-glucopyranosyl] ester

$C_{57}H_{88}O_{25}$ MW: 1173.32 Property: white powder (methanol), mp 206-10°C, $[\alpha]_D^{20}$ +2.37° (c=0.1, methanol). Source: YI YE LIANG WANG CHA. Ref: 216.

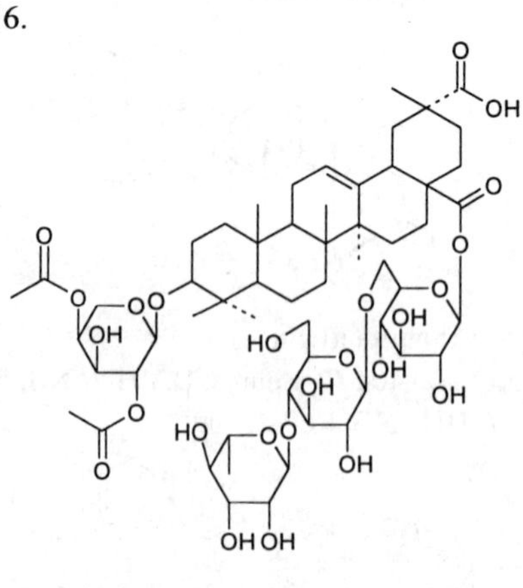

1674 4',6''-Diacetyl puerarin

$C_{25}H_{26}O_{11}$ MW: 502.48 Source: GE GEN. Ref: 2.

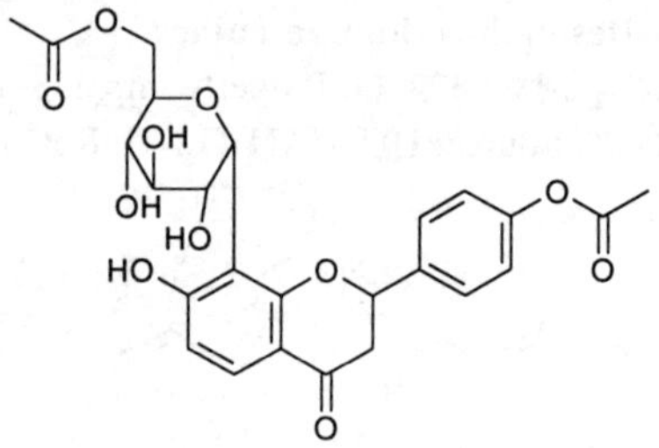

1675 Diallyl tetrasulfide

$C_6H_{10}S_4$ MW: 210.40 Source: DA SUAN. Ref: 2.

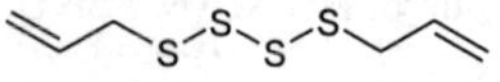

1676 Diallyl trisulfide

CAS: 2050-87-5 $C_6H_{10}S_3$ MW: 178.34 Property: bp 87-8°C. Source: DA SUAN. Ref: 4.

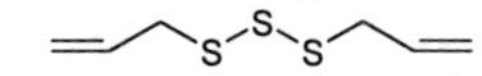

1677 2,3-Diaminobutyric acid

$C_4H_{10}N_2O_2$ MW: 118.14 Source: HUANG JING, MO GU. Ref: 6.

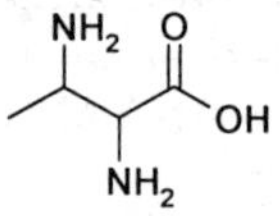

1678 2,4-Diaminobutyric acid

$C_4H_{10}N_2O_2$ MW: 118.14 Property: mp 205°C (dec). Source: HUANG JING, MO GU. Ref: 6.

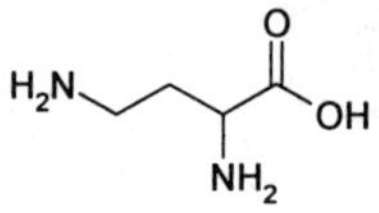

1680 α,β-Diaminopropionic acid

$C_3H_8N_2O_2$ MW: 104.11 Property: mp (-): 193°C, (±): 110-20°C. Source: WANG GUA ZI. Ref: 6.

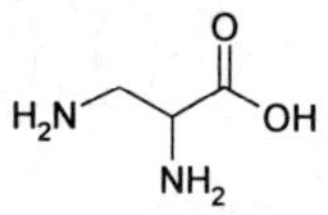

1681 Dibenzoylgaimol

$C_{35}H_{42}O_9$ MW: 606.72 Property: mp 192-7°C. Source: LUO MO. Ref: 6.

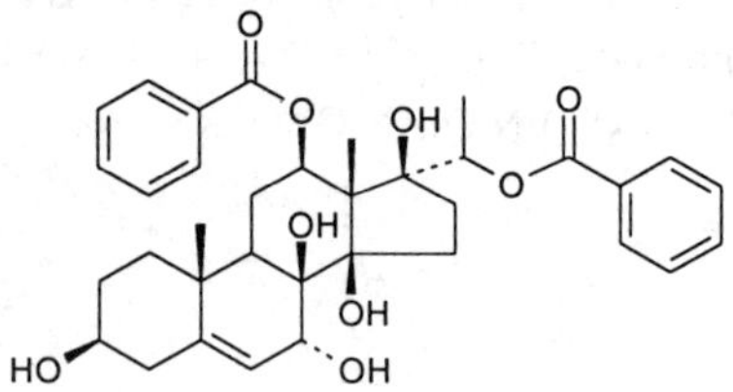

1682 Di-n-butyl oxalate
$C_{10}H_{18}O_4$ MW: 202.25 Source: REN SHEN. Ref: 2.

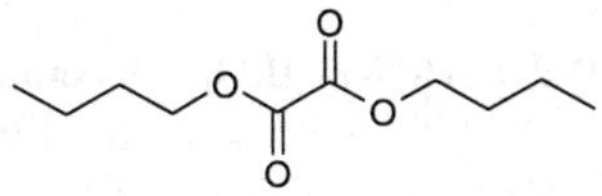

1683 Dibutyl phthalate
Source: NIU XI. Ref: 582.

1684 3,4-Dicaffeoyl-5-(3-hydroxy-3-methyl) glutaroyl quinic acid
$C_{31}H_{32}O_{16}$ MW: 660.59 Source: ZHI ZI. Ref: 2, 626.

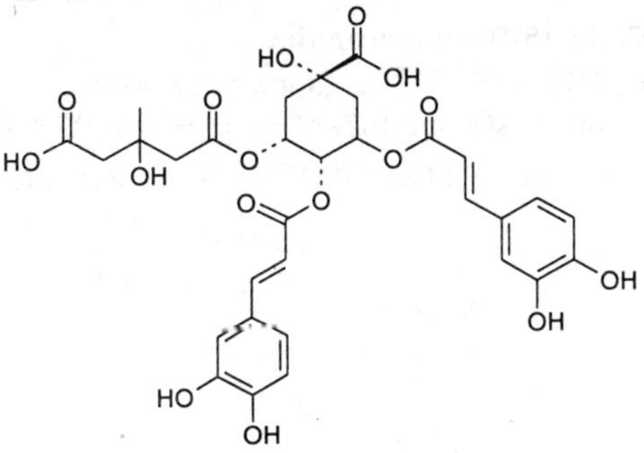

1685 3,5-Di-O-caffeoyl-4-O-(3-hydroxy-3-methyl)glutaroylquinic acid
$C_{31}H_{32}O_{16}$ MW: 660.59 Source: ZHI ZI. Ref: 2, 626.

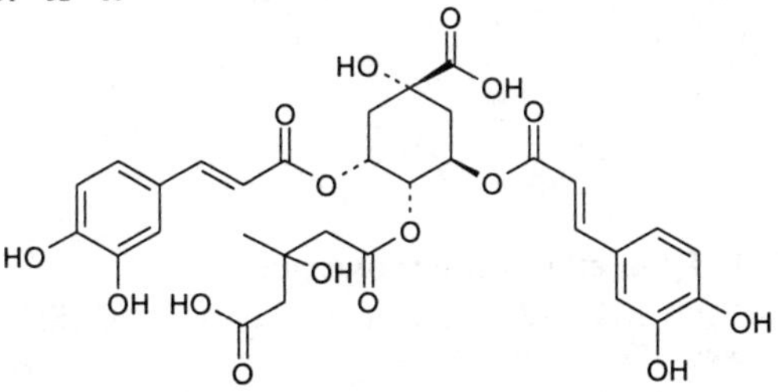

1686 1,4-Dicaffeoylquinic acid
$C_{25}H_{24}O_{12}$ MW: 516.46 Property: mp 229-30°C. Source: CANG ER. Ref: 6.

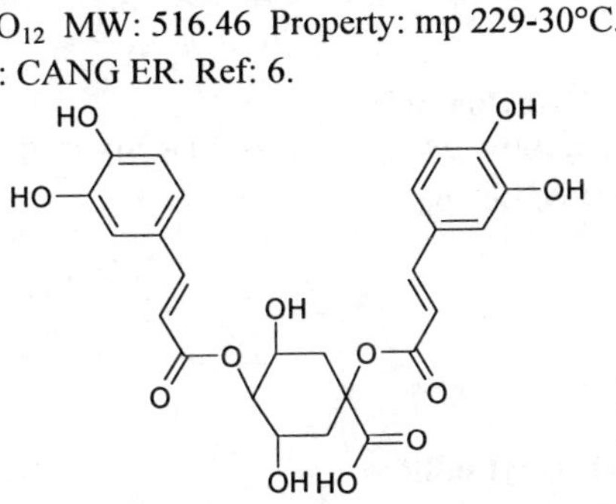

1687 3,4-Di-O-caffeoylquinic acid
$C_{26}H_{26}O_{12}$ MW: 530.49 Source: ZHI ZI. Ref: 2, 626.

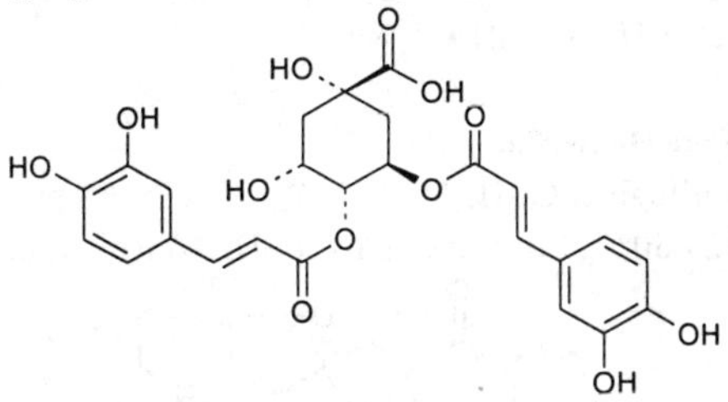

1688 Dicapryl phthalate
$C_{24}H_{38}O_4$ MW: 390.57 Source: SAN QI. Ref: 2.

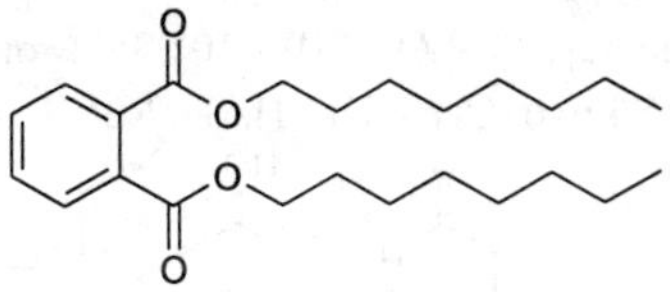

1689 2,4-Dichloro-6-aminopyridine
$C_5H_4Cl_2N_2$ MW: 163.01 Property: mp 271°C. Source: KU SHU PI. Ref: 6.

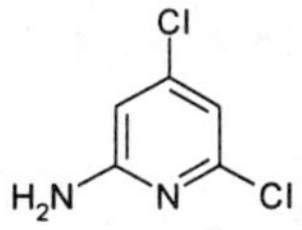

1690 2',2'-N,N-Dichloromethyltetrandrine
$C_{40}H_{46}Cl_2N_2O_2{\bullet}2Cl^-$ MW: 721.73•70.90 Source: FANG JI. Ref: 2.

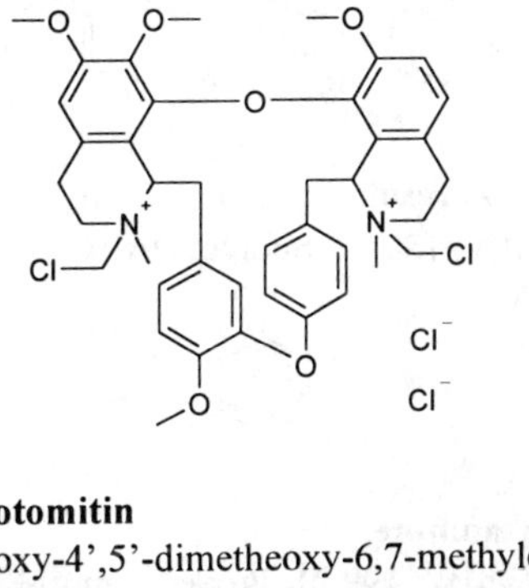

1691 Dichotomitin
5,3'-Dihvdroxy-4',5'-dimetheoxy-6,7-methylene-dioxyisoflavone. $C_{18}H_{14}O_8$ MW: 358.31 Property: light yellow rhomboid crystal, mp 249-51°C. Source: BAI HUA SHE GAN. Ref: 69.

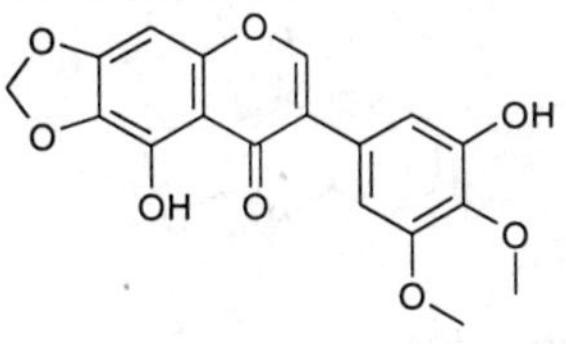

1692 Dichroidine
$C_{18}H_{25}N_3O_3$ MW: 331.42 Property: mp 212-3°C. Source: CHANG SHAN. Ref: 6.

1693 α-Dichroine
Isofebrifugine. $C_{16}H_{19}N_3O_3$ MW: 301.35 Property: mp 129-30°C. Source: CHANG SHAN. Ref: 4, 6.

1694 β-Dichroine
Febrivugine. $C_{16}H_{19}N_3O_3$ MW: 301.35 Property: mp 139-40°C. Source: CHANG SHAN. Ref: 4, 5.

1695 γ-Dichroine
$C_{16}H_{21}N_3O_3$ MW: 303.36 Property: mp 160-1°C. Source: CHANG SHAN. Ref: 4, 6.

1696 Dicoumarin
Dicoumarol. CAS: 66-76-2 $C_{19}H_{12}O_6$ MW: 336.30 Property: mp 288-9°C. Source: HONG CHE ZHOU CAO, MU XU, PI HAN CAO. Ref: 4, 5, 6.

1697 2,3-Dicresol
$C_8H_{10}O$ MW: 122.17 Source: DANG GUI. Ref: 2.

1698 Dictamnine
$C_{12}H_9NO_2$ MW: 199.21 Property: mp 132°C. Source: BAI XIAN PI, CHU YE HUA JIAO PI, YAN JIAO CAO, ZHU YE JIAO GEN. Ref: 6.

1699 Dictamnolide
$C_{28}H_{30}O_9$ Source: HUANG BAI. Ref: 2.

1700 Dictysine
Source: FU ZI. Ref: 16.

1701 O,N-Dideacyl-N-methylpachysandrine A
$C_{25}H_{46}N_2O$ MW: 390.66 Property: mp 126-50°C. Source: XUE SHAN LIN. Ref: 6.

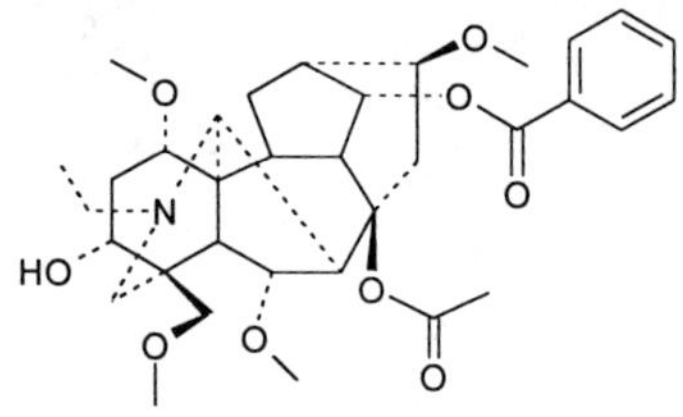

1702 13,15-Dideoxyaconitine
$C_{34}H_{47}NO_9$ MW: 613.32 Property: colorless rhomboid crystal, mp 167-9°C, $[\alpha]_D^{25}$ +16.4° (c=0.07, ethanol). Source: SONG PAN WU TOU. Ref: 107.

1703 1,1-Diethoxy-n-nonane
$C_{13}H_{28}O_2$ MW: 216.37 Source: CU LIU GUO (SHA JI). Ref: 2.

1704 1,1-Diethoxy-n-tetradecane
$C_{18}H_{38}O_2$ MW: 286.50 Source: CU LIU GUO (SHA JI). Ref: 2.

1705 Diethylphthalate
$C_{12}H_{14}O_4$ MW: 222.24 Property: bp 295°C. Source: SHUI QIN. Ref: 6.

1706 Diethyl sulfide
$C_4H_{10}S$ MW: 90.19 Source: SHENG JIANG. Ref: 2.

1707 Difengpin
4-allyl-2,6-dimethoxyphenyol cinnamate. $C_{20}H_{20}O_4$ MW: 324.38 Property: colorless granular crystal, mp 153-5°C (petroleum spirit-acetic acid). Source: DI FENG PI. Ref: 354.

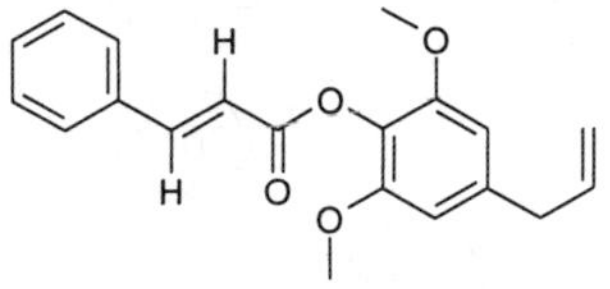

1708 Diffractaic acid
$C_{20}H_{22}O_7$ MW: 374.39 Property: mp 189-90°C. Activity: an inhibitor of tumor promoter-induced Epstein-Barr virus activation. Source: SONG LUO. Ref: 6.

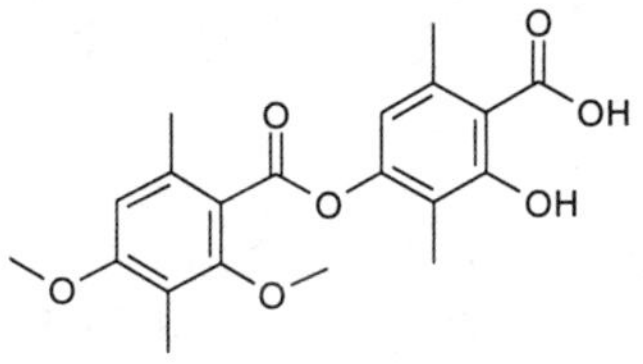

1709 5,5'-Di-α-furaldehyde dimethyl ether
Source: JIN QIAO MAI. Ref: 594.

1710 Difurocurcumenone
Source: JIANG HUANG. Ref: 640.

1711 m-Digallic acid
$C_{14}H_{10}O_9$ MW: 322.23 Property: mp 268-70°C (dec). Source: MANG GUO. Ref: 6.

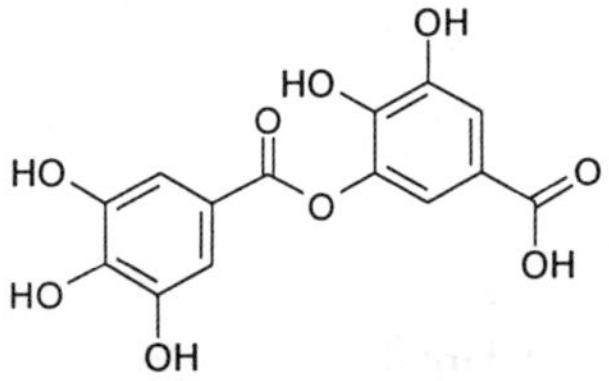

1712 1,6-Digalloyl-2-cinnamoyl-glucose
$C_{29}H_{26}O_{15}$ MW: 614.52 Source: DA HUANG. Ref: 2.

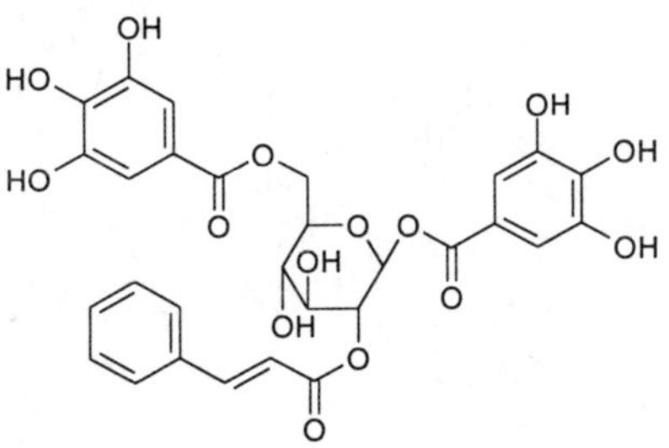

1713 1,6-Di-O-galloyl-glucose
$C_{20}H_{20}O_{14}$ MW: 484.37 Source: DA HUANG. Ref: 2.

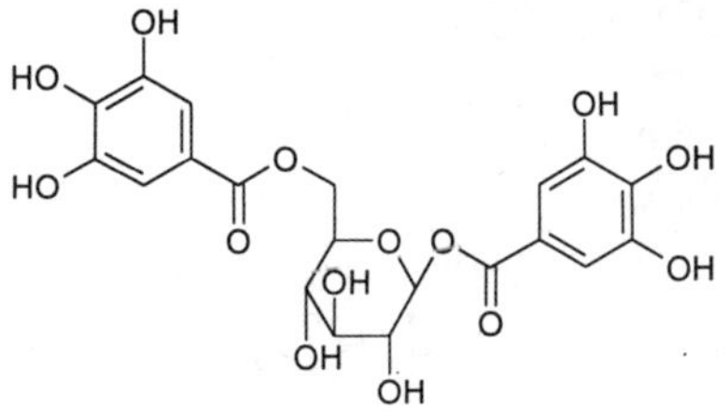

1714 3,6-Digalloylglucose
$C_{20}H_{20}O_{14}$ MW: 484.37 Property: mp 185°C (dec). Source: AN MO LE, CAO YUAN LAO GUAN CAO, QUAN SHEN, YOU GAN YE, YOU GAN MU PI. Ref: 6.

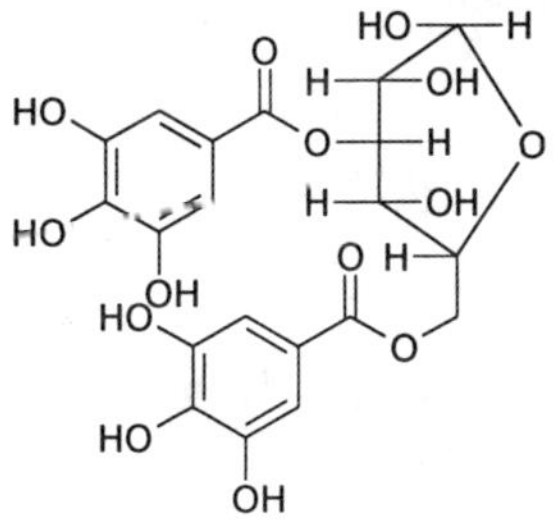

1715 2,3-Di-O-galloyl-D-glucose
$C_{20}H_{20}O_{14}$ MW: 484.37 Source: SHAN ZHU YU. Ref: 2.

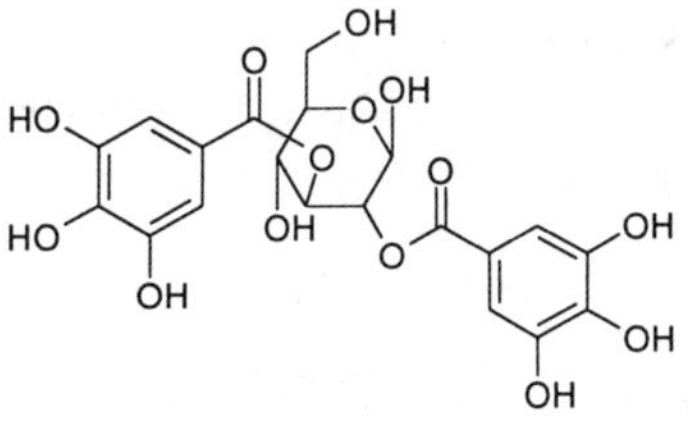

1716 Digitalis glycoside
Source: HUANG JING. Ref: 6.

1717 Digitonide
$C_{30}H_{44}O_7$ MW: 516.68 Source: CU LIU GUO (SHA JI). Ref: 2.

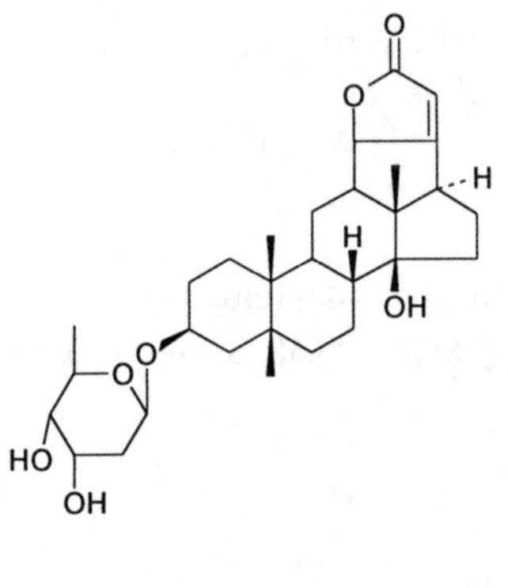

1718 Digitoxigenin
$C_{24}H_{36}O_4$ MW: 388.55 Property: mp 253°C. Source: FU SHOU CAO. Ref: 6.

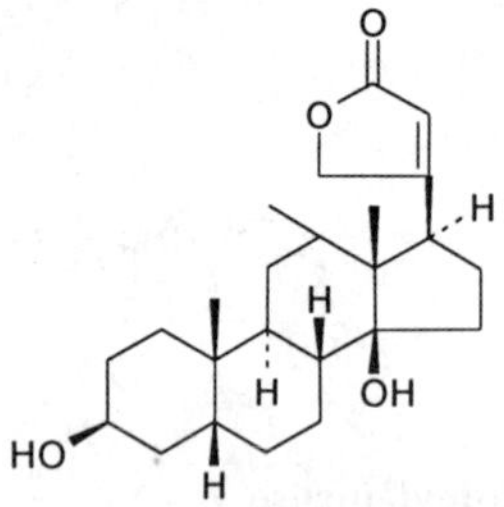

1719 Digitoxose
$C_6H_{12}O_4$ MW: 148.16 Property: mp 110-2°C. Source: LUO MO ZI. Ref: 6.

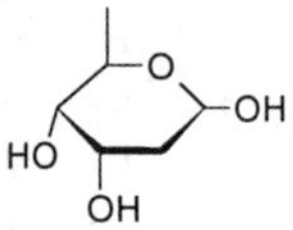

1720 6,8-Di-C-glucosyl-2(R)-naringenin
Source: DA ZAO. Ref: 2.

1721 6,8-Di-C-glucosyl-2(S)-naringenin
Source: DA ZAO. Ref: 2.

1722 Dihydroagarofuran
$C_{15}H_{26}O$ MW: 222.37 Property: bp 135°C/8mm. Source: CHEN XIANG. Ref: 6, 13.

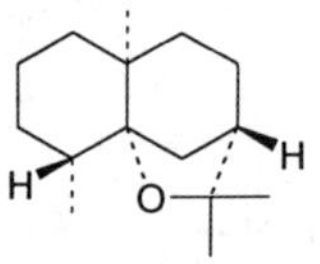

1723 Dihydrobaicalin
$C_{21}H_{20}O_{11}$ MW: 448.39 Source: HUANG QIN. Ref: 2.

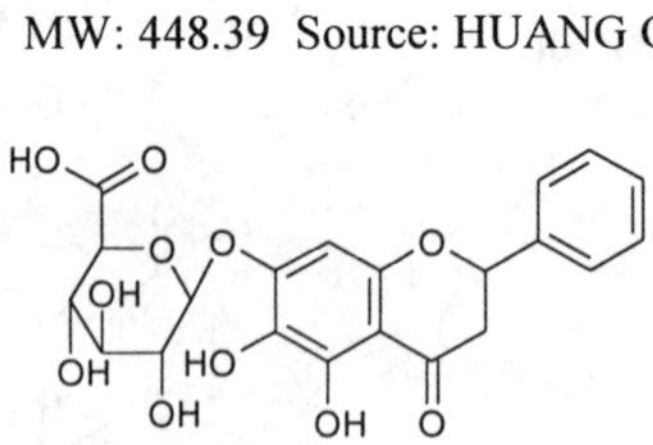

1724 3α-Dihydrocadambine
$C_{27}H_{34}N_2O_{10}$ MW: 546.58 Source: GOU TENG. Ref: 2.

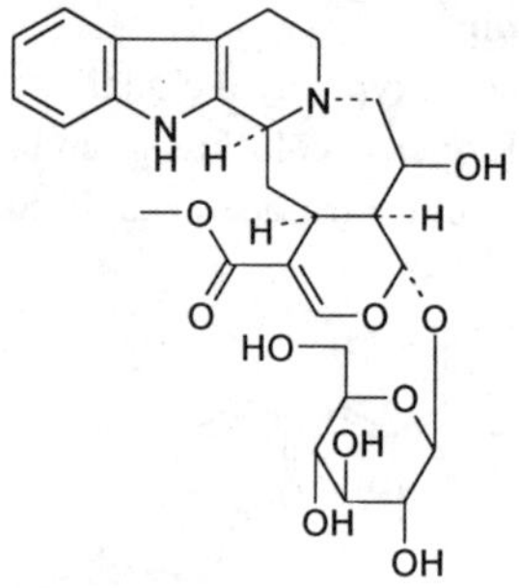

1725 Dihydrocapsacine
$C_{18}H_{29}NO_3$ MW: 307.44 Source: LA JIAO. Ref: 6, 15.

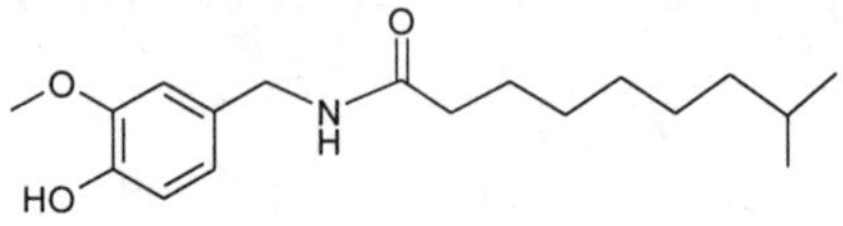

1726 Dihydrocarveol
$C_{10}H_{18}O$ MW: 154.25 Source: GAN DI HUANG. Ref: 2.

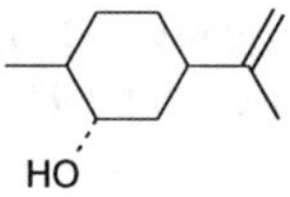

1727 Dihydrocarveol acetate
$C_{12}H_{14}O_2$ MW: 190.24 Source: JIU LI XIANG. Ref: 11.

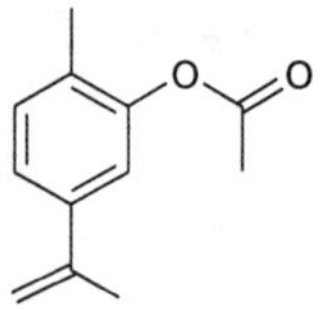

1728 Dihydrocatalpol
$C_{15}H_{24}O_{10}$ MW: 364.35 Source: GAN DI HUANG. Ref: 2.

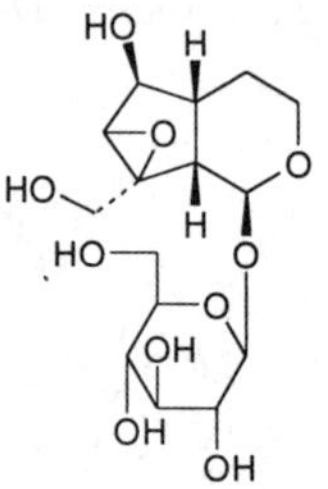

1729 Dihydrochelerythrine

$C_{21}H_{19}NO_4$ MW: 349.39 Property: mp 160-5°C. Source: FEI LONG ZHANG XUE. Ref: 6.

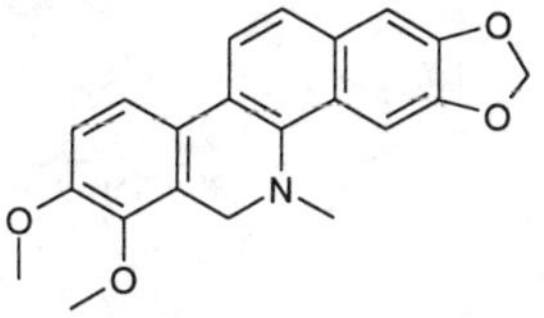

1730 Dihydroconcuressine

$C_{24}H_{42}N_2$ MW: 358.62 Property: mp 93-4°C. Source: ZHI XIE MU PI. Ref: 6.

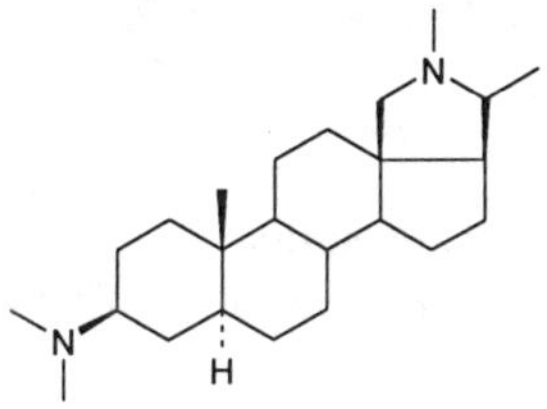

1731 Dihydroconessine

$C_{24}H_{42}N_2$ MW: 358.42 Property: mp 190-1°C. Source: ZHI XIE MU PI. Ref: 6.

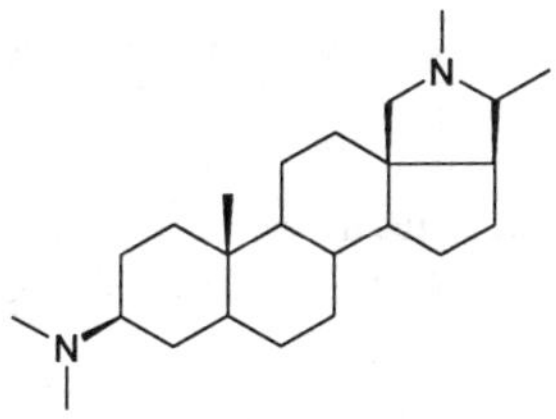

1732 Dihydrocorynantheine

$C_{22}H_{28}N_2O_3$ MW: 368.48 Source: GOU TENG. Ref: 2.

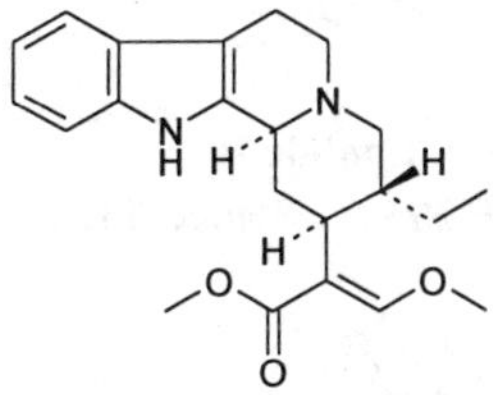

1733 Dihydrocucurbitacin F

$C_{30}H_{48}O_7$ MW: 520.71 Property: mp 155-7°C. Source: LUO GUO DI, PENG XIAN XUE DAN. Ref: 6, 554.

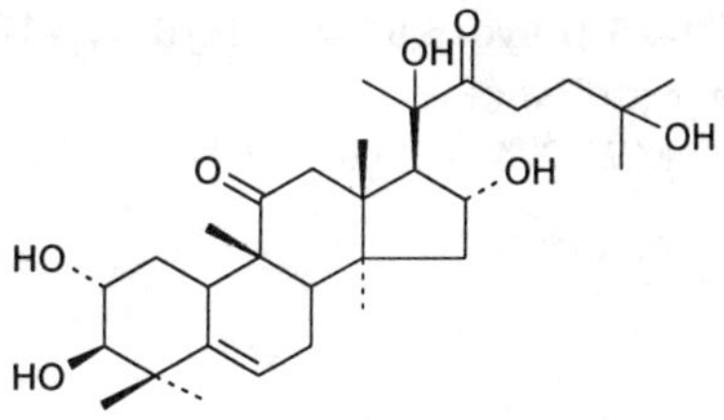

1734 Dihydrocucurbitacin F-25-acetate

$C_{32}H_{50}O_8$ MW: 562.75 Property: mp 266-8°C. Source: LUO GUO DI, PENG XIAN XUE DAN. Ref: 6, 554.

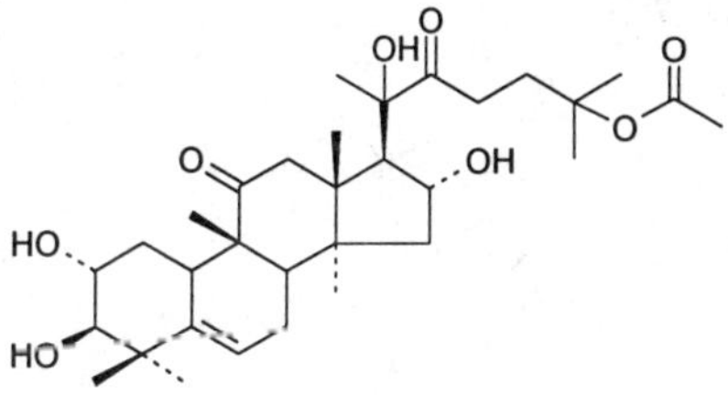

1735 Dihydrocyperaquinone

$C_{14}H_{12}O_4$ MW: 244.25 Property: mp 113-4°C. Source: PIAO FU CAO. Ref: 6.

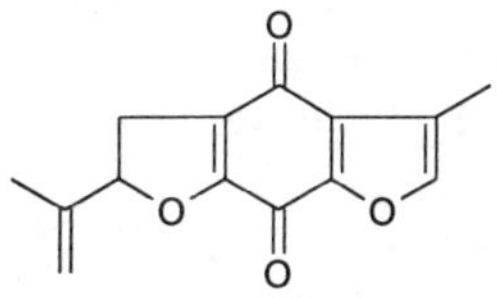

1736 Dihydrodehydrocostus lactone

$C_{15}H_{20}O_2$ MW: 232.33 Source: MU XIANG. Ref: 2.

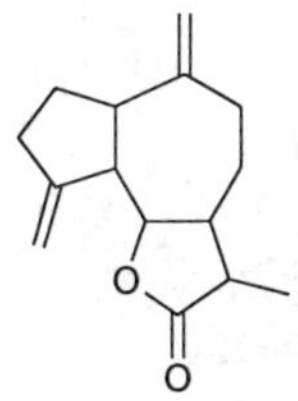

1737 (Z)-4,5-Dihydro-6,7-trans-dihydroxy-3-butylidene phthalide

$C_{12}H_{16}O_4$ MW: 224.26 Source: CHUAN XIONG. Ref: 2.

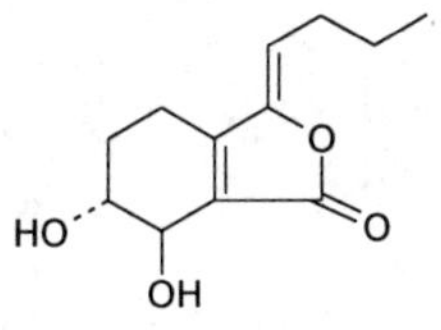

1738 (Z)-4,5-Dihydro-6,7-cis-dihydroxy-3-butylidene phthalide
$C_{12}H_{16}O_4$ MW: 224.26 Source: CHUAN XIONG. Ref: 2.

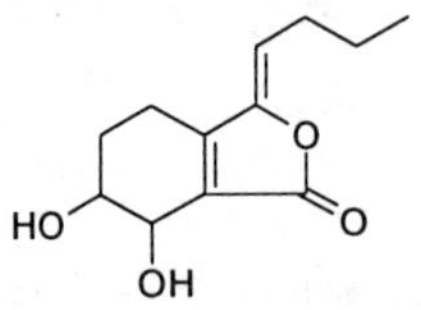

1739 (Z')-3,8-Dihydro-6,6',7,3'α-diligustilide
$C_{24}H_{30}O_4$ MW: 382.50 Source: CHUAN XIONG. Ref: 2.

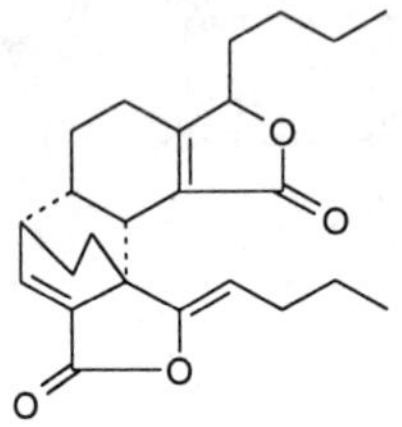

1740 7,8-Dihydroergosterol
Source: CHA YE. Ref: 6.

1741 22,23-Dihydroergosterol
Source: CHA YE. Ref: 6.

1742 5,6-Dihydroergosterol
$C_{28}H_{46}O$ MW: 398.68 Property: mp 176-7°C. Source: CHA YE. Ref: 6.

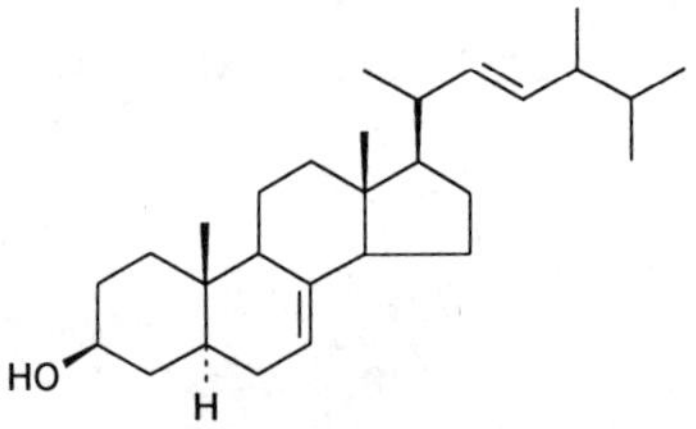

1743 22,23-Dihydroergosterol
$C_{28}H_{44}O$ MW: 396.66 Property: mp 152-3°C. Source: MU ER. Ref: 6.

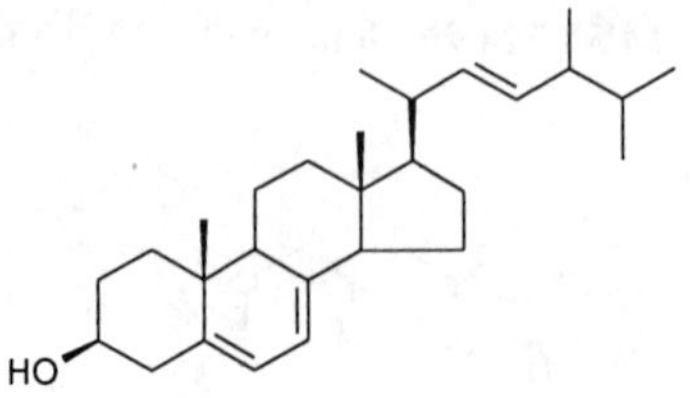

1744 Dihydrofisetin
$C_{15}H_{12}O_6$ MW: 288.26 Property: mp (+): 228-9°C, (-): 228°C, (±): 228-9°C. Source: JI CAI. Ref: 6.

(+):

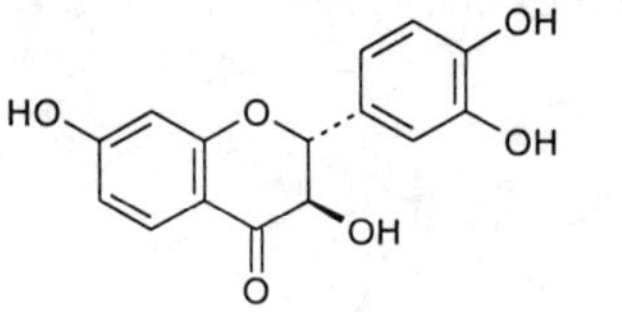

(-):

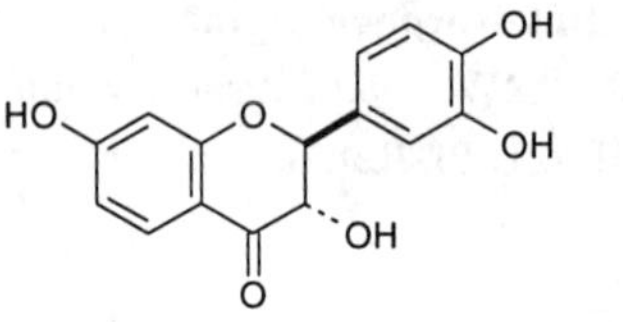

1745 Dihydrofoliamenthin
$C_{26}H_{38}O_{12}$ MW: 542.59 Source: SHUI CAI, SHUI CAI GEN. Ref: 6.

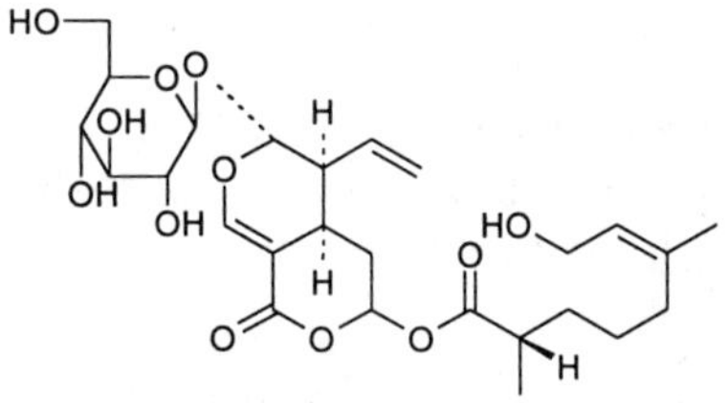

1746 β-Dihydrofucosterol
$C_{29}H_{50}O$ MW: 414.72 Source: ZE QI. Ref: 6.

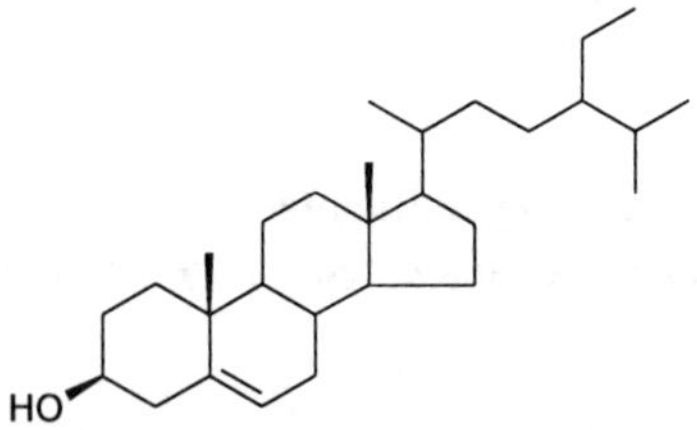

1747 Dihydrofukinolide
$C_{22}H_{32}O_6$ MW: 392.50 Source: FENG DOU CAI. Ref: 6.

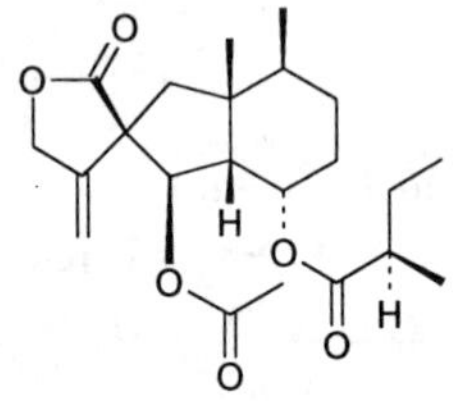

1748 Dihydroharman
$C_{12}H_{12}N_2$ MW: 184.24 Source: SHA ZAO SHU PI. Ref: 6.

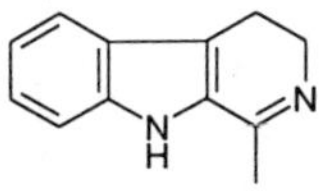

1749 Dihydro-β-ionone
$C_{13}H_{22}O$ MW: 194.32 Property: bp 126-9°C/12mm. Source: GUI HUA. Ref: 6.

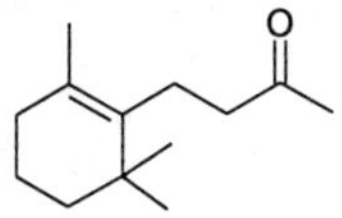

1750 Dihydroisoalantolactone
$C_{15}H_{22}O_2$ MW: 234.34 Property: mp 171-2°C. Source: TU MU XIANG. Ref: 6.

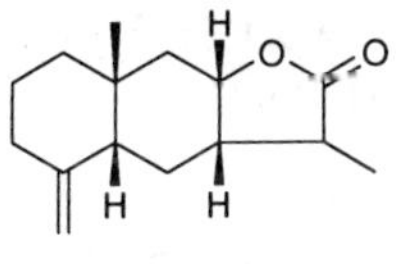

1751 Dihydroisocucurbitacin-β-25-acetate
$C_{32}H_{48}O_8$ MW: 560.73 Property: colorless acicular crystal, mp 235-7°C. Source: DA BAO CHI BO. Ref: 425.

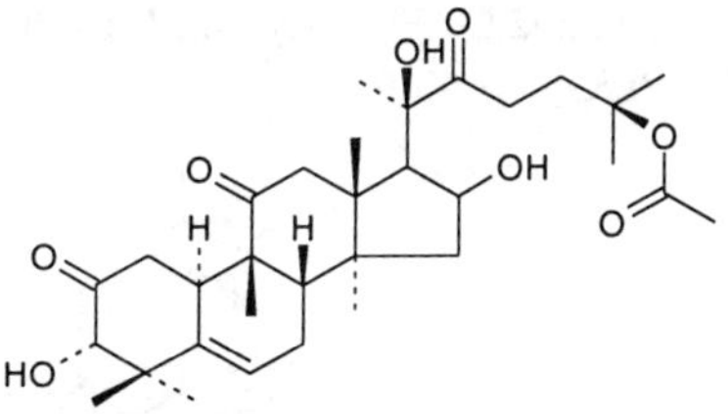

1752 Dihydroisomorellin
$C_{33}H_{38}O_7$ MW: 546.67 Property: mp 167°C. Source: TENG HUANG. Ref: 6.

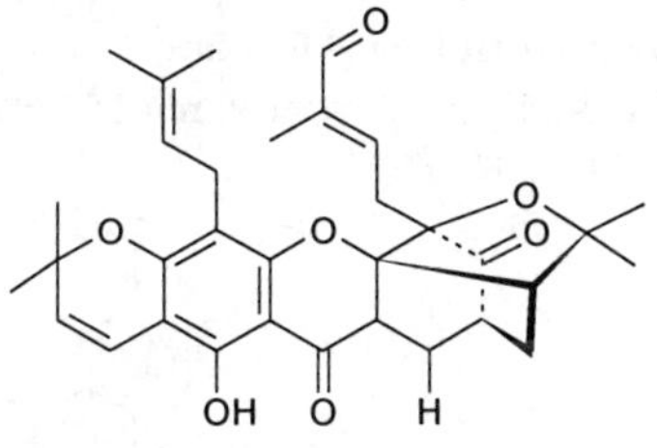

1753 Dihydroisotanshinone I
$C_{18}H_{16}O_3$ MW: 280.33 Source: DAN SHEN. Ref: 2.

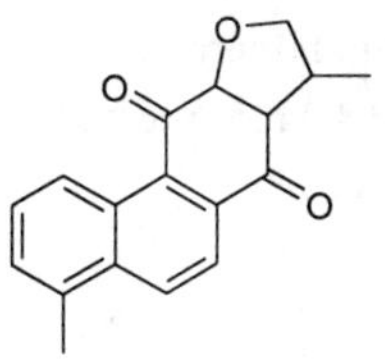

1755 Dihydrokaempferol
$C_{15}H_{12}O_6$ MW: 288.26 Property: mp 247-9°C. Source: SANG ZHI, ZHI YU ZI. Ref: 6, 391.

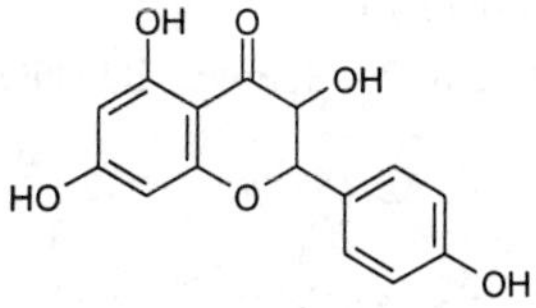

1756 Dihydrokaranone
$C_{15}H_{22}O$ MW: 218.34 Source: BAI MU XIANG, CHEN XIANG. Ref: 13.

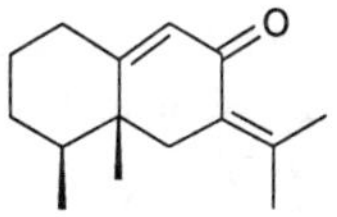

1757 Dihydrokoumine
$C_{20}H_{24}N_2O$ MW: 308.43 Source: HU MAN TENG. Ref: 14.

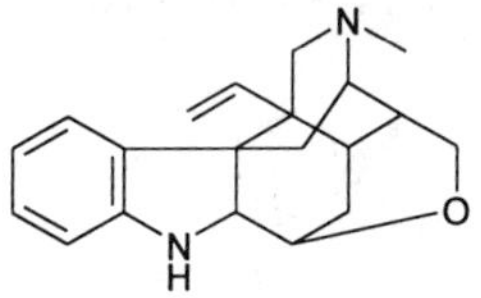

1758 Dihydromorin
$C_{15}H_{12}O_7$ MW: 304.26 Property: mp 226-8°C. Source: SANG ZHI. Ref: 6.

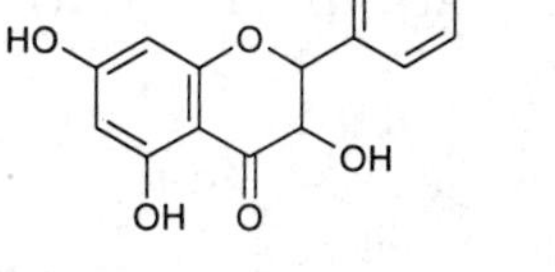

1759 Dihydromyricetin
$C_{15}H_{12}O_8$ MW: 320.26 Property: white acicular crystal, mp 245-6°C. Source: TENG CHA, ZHI YU ZI. Ref: 391, 466.

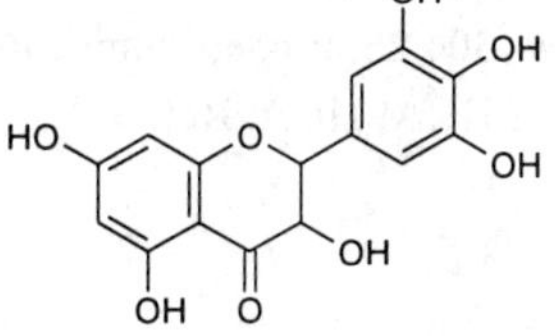

1760 Dihydronepetalactone

$C_{10}H_{16}O_2$ MW: 168.24 Source: JIA JING JIE, MU TIAN LIAO. Ref: 6.

1761 Dihydrooroxylin A

$C_{16}H_{14}O_5$ MW: 286.29 Source: HUANG QIN. Ref: 2.

1762 Dihydroperilla alcohol

$C_{10}H_{18}O$ MW: 154.25 Source: ZI SU. Ref: 2.

1763 Δ2,4 Dihydrophthalic anhydride

$C_8H_6O_3$ MW: 150.14 Source: DANG GUI. Ref: 2.

1764 Dihydroquercetin

$C_{15}H_{12}O_7$ MW: 304.26 Property: mp (+): 240-2°C. Source: BA DAN XING REN, BAI HUA YING SHAN HONG, MAN SHAN HONG, YING SHAN HONG. Ref: 6.

1765 Dihydrorobinetin

$C_{15}H_{12}O_7$ MW: 304.26 Property: mp 246°C, 225-6°C. Source: CI HUAI HUA. Ref: 6.

1766 Dihydrosanguinarine

$C_{20}H_{15}NO_4$ MW: 333.35 Property: mp 191°C. Source: JU HUA HUANG LIAN, YING SU KE. Ref: 6.

1767 Dihydrosecurinine

$C_{13}H_{17}NO_2$ MW: 219.29 Property: mp 58-60°C. Source: YI YE QIU. Ref: 6.

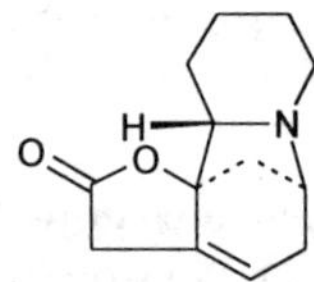

1768 Dihydro-β-sitosteryl ferulate

$C_{39}H_{60}O_4$ MW: 592.91 Property: mp 156-7°C. Source: MI PI KANG. Ref: 6.

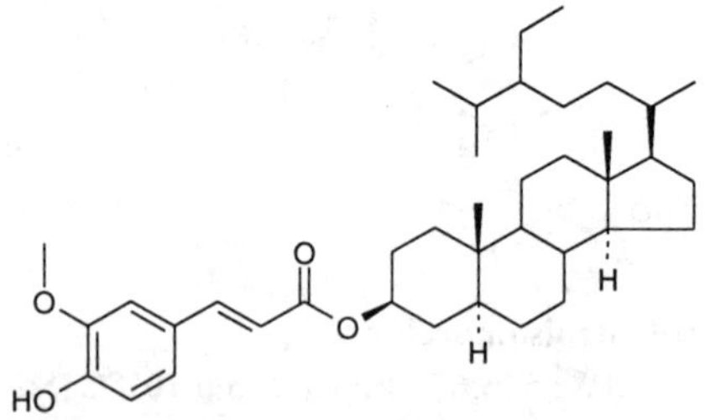

1769 Dihydro-γ-sitosteryl ferulate

$C_{39}H_{60}O_4$ MW: 592.91 Property: mp 155-6°C. Source: MI PI KANG. Ref: 6.

1770 Dihydrositsirikine
$C_{21}H_{28}N_2O_3$ MW: 356.47 Source: CHANG CHUN HUA. Ref: 2.

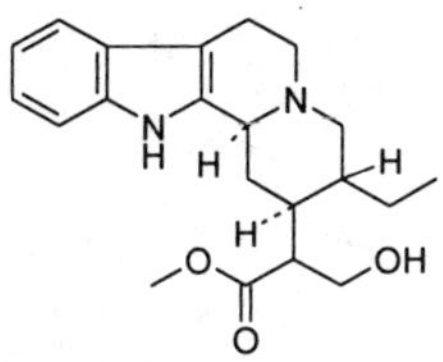

1771 22-Dihydrostigmast-4-en-3,6-dione
$C_{29}H_{44}O_2$ MW: 424.67 Property: mp 170-1°C. Source: LING. Ref: 6.

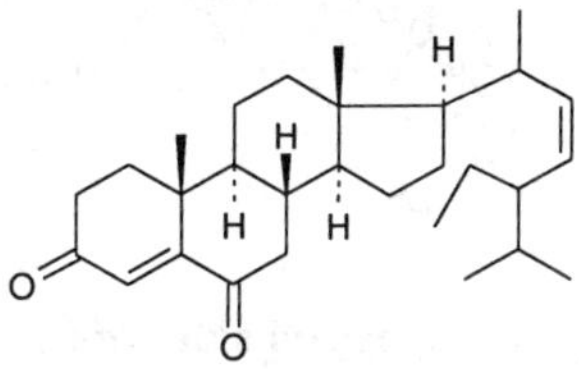

1772 22-Dihydrostigmasterol
$C_{30}H_{52}$ MW: 412.75 Source: MU XIANG. Ref: 2.

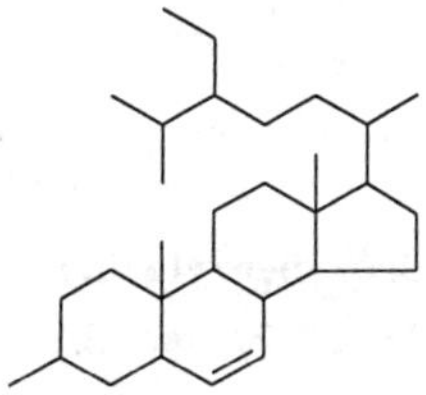

1773 22,23-Dihydrostigmasterol
$C_{29}H_{50}O$ MW: 414.72 Property: mp 135.5-6.0°C. Source: ZI TENG. Ref: 6.

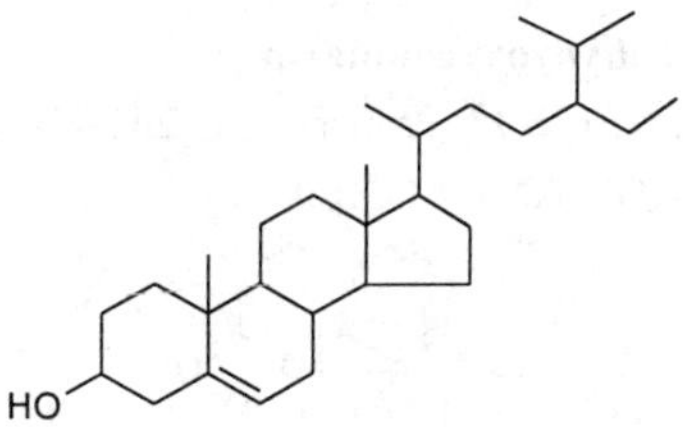

HO

1774 Dihydrotanshinone I
$C_{18}H_{14}O_3$ MW: 278.31 Source: DAN SHEN. Ref: 2.

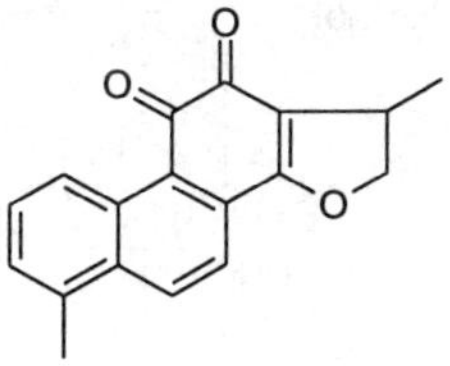

1775 Dihydro-valepotriate
$C_{23}H_{34}O_8$ MW: 438.52 Property: mp 62-3°C. Source: ZHI ZHU XIANG. Ref: 6.

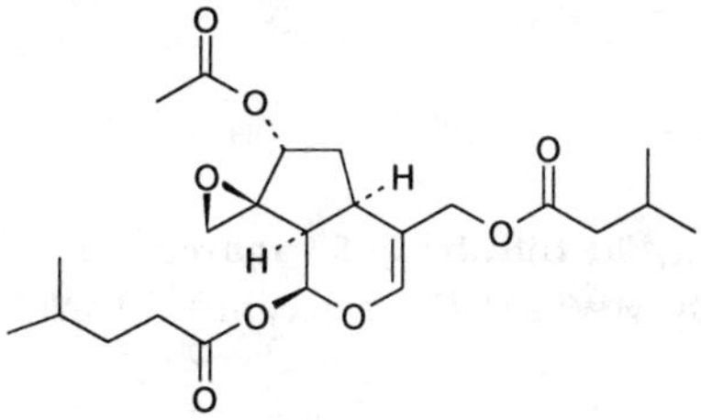

1776 Dihydroverticillatine
$C_{25}H_{29}NO_5$ MW: 423.51 Property: mp 258-9°C. Source: ZI WEI YE. Ref: 6.

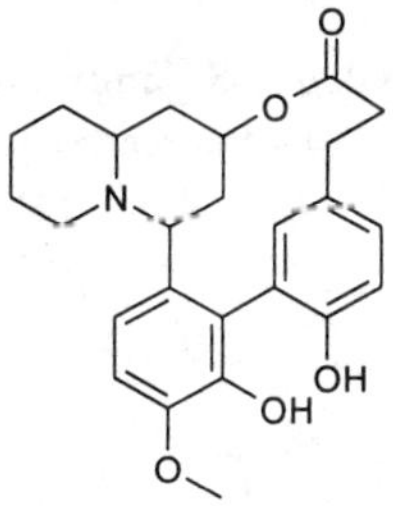

1777 Dihydrovindolinine
$C_{21}H_{26}N_2O_2$ MW: 338.45 Source: CHANG CHUN HUA. Ref: 2.

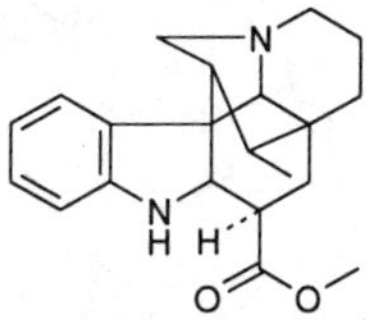

1778 6,12-Dihydroxy-5,8,11,13-abietetraene-7-one
$C_{20}H_{26}O_3$ MW: 314.43 Source: DU SONG SHI. Ref: 6.

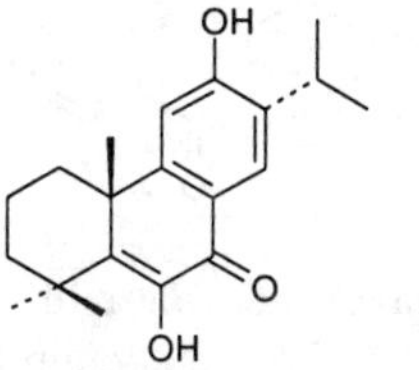

1779 Dihydroxyacetone
$C_3H_6O_3$ MW: 90.08 Source: CU. Ref: 6.

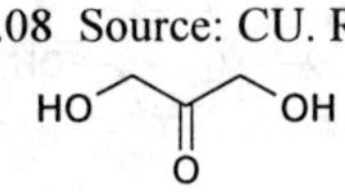

1780 2,4-Dihydroxyacetophenone
$C_8H_8O_3$ MW: 152.15 Source: DANG GUI. Ref: 2.

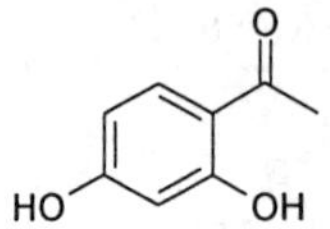

1781 3α,17α-Dihydroxy-5β-androstane
$C_{19}H_{32}O_2$ MW: 292.47 Source: SHE XIANG. Ref: 2.

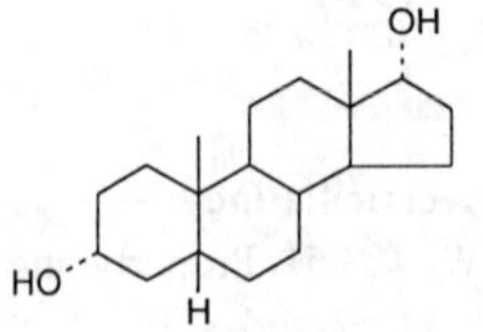

1782 3α,17-Dihydroxy-5β-androstane
$C_{19}H_{32}O_2$ MW: 292.47 Source: SHE XIANG. Ref: 2.

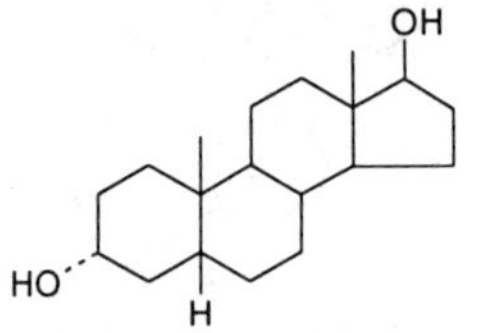

1783 3β,17α-Dihydroxy-5α-androstane
$C_{19}H_{32}O_2$ MW: 292.47 Source: SHE XIANG. Ref: 2.

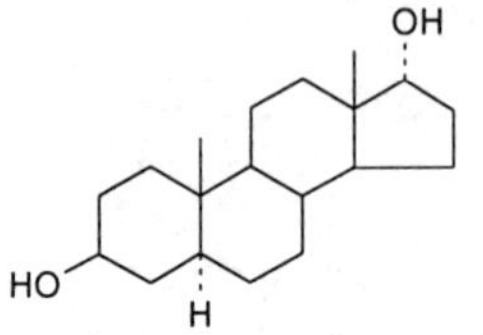

1784 1,8-Dihydroxy-anthraquinone
$C_{14}H_8O_4$ MW: 240.22 Property: mp 193°C. Source: WANG JIANG NAN. Ref: 6.

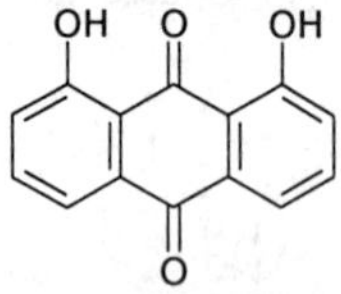

1785 3,4-Dihydroxybenzoic acid
$C_7H_6O_4$ MW: 154.12 Property: mp 199°C. Source: BAN XIA, HUANG JING YE. Ref: 6.

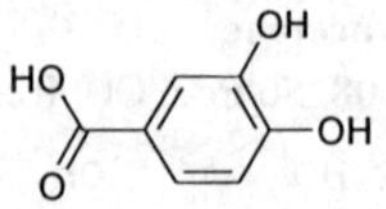

1786 3,5-Dihydroxybenzoic acid
$C_7H_6O_4$ MW: 154.12 Property: mp 232-3°C. Source: ZE QI. Ref: 6.

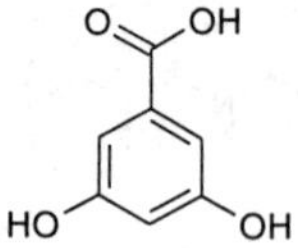

1787 3,4-Dihydroxybenzyl alcohol-4-glucoside
$C_{13}H_{18}O_8$ MW: 302.28 Source: YE LI ZHI YE. Ref: 6.

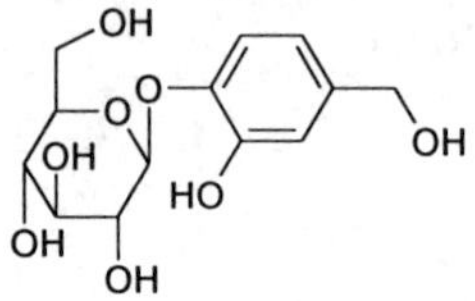

1788 3,4-Dihydroxybenzyl aldehyde
$C_7H_6O_3$ MW: 138.12 Source: BAN XIA, TIAN MA. Ref: 2.

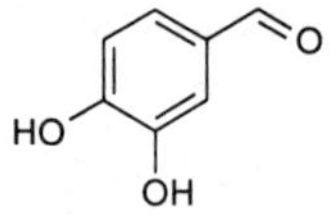

1789 4,4'-Dihydroxybenzyl ether
$C_{14}H_{14}O_3$ MW: 230.27 Source: BAN XIA, TIAN MA. Ref: 2.

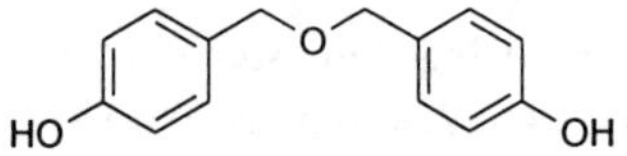

1790 6,7-Dihydroxycoumarin
$C_9H_6O_4$ MW: 178.15 Property: mp 242-8°C (dec). Source: MAO YAN CAO. Ref: 6.

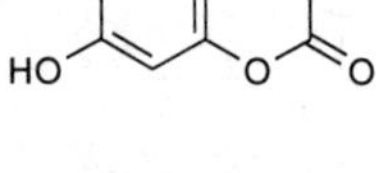

1791 3,4-Dihydroxydihydgaroaroiuran
$C_{16}H_{28}O_2$ MW: 252.40 Property: mp 176°C. Source: CHEN XIANG. Ref: 6.

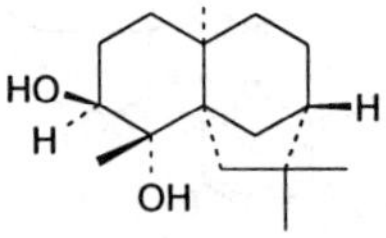

1792 3,4-Dihydroxydihydroagarofuran
$C_{15}H_{26}O_3$ MW: 254.37 Source: CHEN XIANG. Ref: 13.

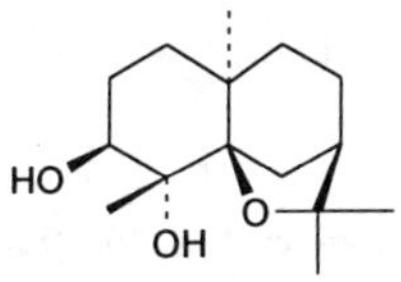

1793 1,6-Dihydroxy-2,4-dimethoxyanthraqui-none V
$C_{16}H_{12}O_6$ MW: 300.27 Property: yellow acicular crystal, mp 205-7°C. Source: BA JI TIAN. Ref: 228.

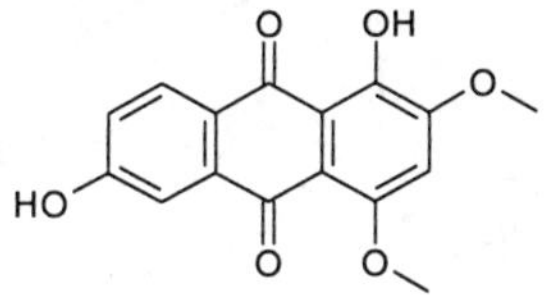

1794 5,8-Dihydroxy-6,7-dimethoxyflavone
$C_{17}H_{14}O_6$ MW: 314.30 Source: HUANG QIN. Ref: 2.

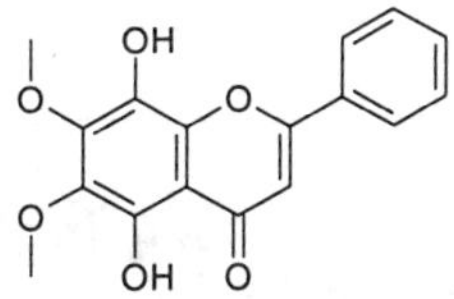

1795 2',4'-Dihydroxy-5,6-dimethoxyisoflavane
Source: HUANG QI. Ref: 2.

1796 1,6-Dihydroxy-3,7-dimethoxy xanthone
$C_{15}H_{12}O_6$ MW: 288.26 Source: YUAN ZHI. Ref: 2.

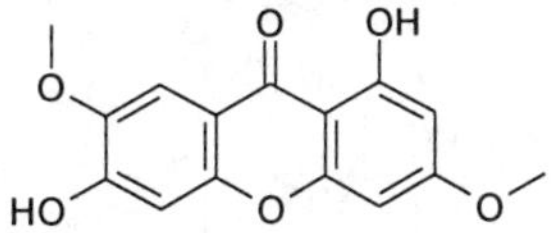

1797 1,3-Dihydroxy-4,5-dimethoxyxanthone
$C_{15}H_{12}O_6$ MW: 288.26 Property: mp 274-5°C. Source: ZHANG YA CAI. Ref: 6.

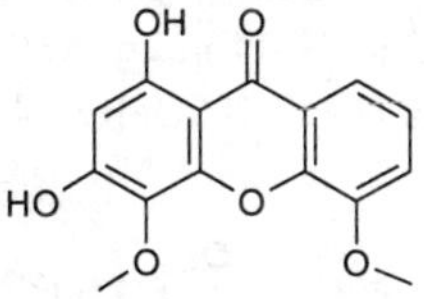

1798 1,3-Dihydroxy-4,5-dimethoxyxanthone-1-O-β-D-glucopyranoside
$C_{21}H_{22}O_{11}$ MW: 450.40 Property: mp 269-74°C (dec). Source: ZHANG YA CAI. Ref: 6.

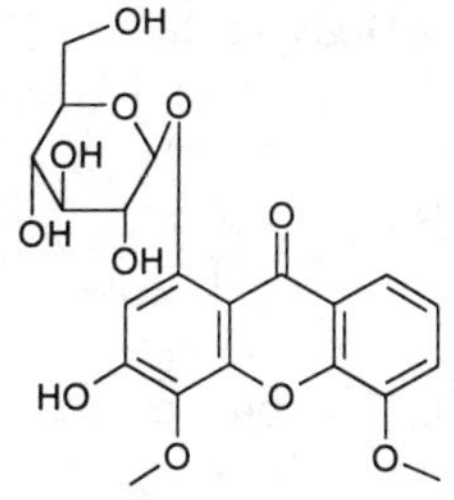

1799 1,3-Dihydroxy-4,5-dimethoxyxanthone-3-O-β-D-glucopyranoside
$C_{21}H_{22}O_{11}$ MW: 450.40 Property: mp 264-6°C. Source: ZHANG YA CAI. Ref: 6.

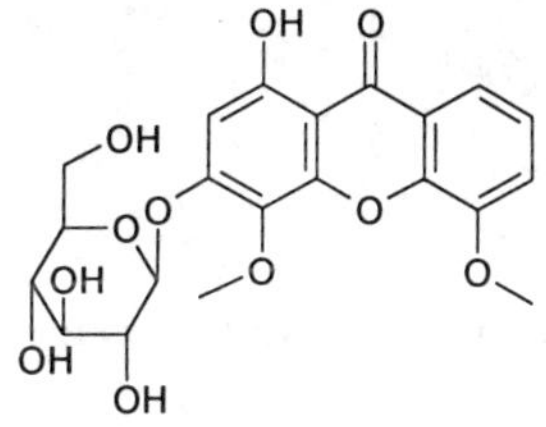

1800 1,3-dihydroxy-6,7-dimethylxanthone-1-O-β-D-glucoside
$C_{21}H_{22}O_9$ MW: 418.48 Property: light yellow massive crystal, mp 262-5°C. Source: HE SHOU WU. Ref: 292.

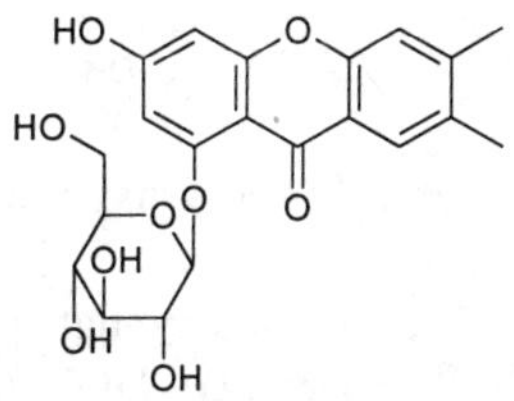

1801 4,4'-Dihydroxydiphenyl methane
$C_{13}H_{12}O_2$ MW: 200.24 Source: TIAN MA. Ref: 2.

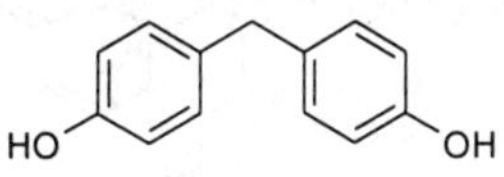

1802 Dihydroxyevocarpine
Source: WU ZHU YU. Ref: 2.

1804 4',7-Dihydroxy flavone
$C_{15}H_{10}O_4$ MW: 254.24 Source: BAI CI HUA, GAN CAO. Ref: 2, 561.

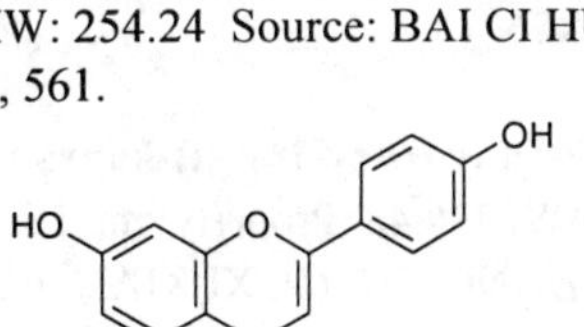

1805 5,4'-Dihydroxyflavone-6-C-β-D-glycosylrhamnoside-7-O-glycoside
Property: mp 194-6°C. Source: HUANG JING. Ref: 6.

1806 5,6-Dihydroxy-7-O-glucoside-flavone
$C_{21}H_{20}O_{10}$ MW: 432.39 Source: HUANG QIN. Ref: 2.

1807 1,8-Dihydroxy-4-hydroxymethyl anthraquinone
$C_{15}H_{10}O_5$ MW: 270.24 Source: LEI GONG TENG. Ref: 2.

1808 5,8-dihydroxy-7-(4-hydroxy-5-methylcoumarin-3)-coumarin
$C_{19}H_{17}O_7$ MW: 352.30 Property: light pink granular crystal, mp >300°C. Source: DA DING CAO. Ref: 141.

1809 16β,17-Dihydroxy-kaurane
$C_{20}H_{34}O_2$ MW: 306 Property: white powder crystal (methanol), mp 195-7°C. Source: MAO GENG XI XIAN. Ref: 476.

1810 16,17-Dihydroxy-16β-(l)-kauran-19-oic acid
$C_{20}H_{32}O_4$ MW: 336.48 Property: mp 260-2°C. Source: TU DANG GUI (I), XI XIAN. Ref: 2, 6.

1812 3β,23-Dihydroxy-lup-20(29)-ene-28-O-β-D-glucopyranosyl(1→6)-β-D-glucopyranoside
Source: BAI TOU WENG. Ref: 2.

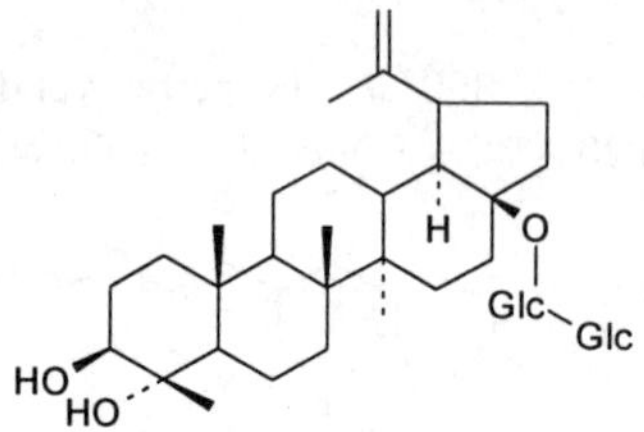

1813 3β,23-Dihydroxy-lup-20(29)-ene-28-O-α-L-rhamnopyranosyl-(1→4)-β-D-glucopyranosyl (1→6)-β-D-glucopyranoside
Source: BAI TOU WENG. Ref: 2.

1814 5α,9α-Dihydroxymatrine
$C_{15}H_{24}N_2O_3$ MW: 280.37 Source: XI XIAN. Ref: 2.

1815 3-(α,4-dihydroxy-3-methoxybenzyl)-4-(hydroxy-3-methoxybenzyl) tetrahydrofuran
$C_{20}H_{24}O_6$ MW: 360.41 Property: yellow colloid. Source: YU NAN HAN XIAO. Ref: 426.

1816 2',6'-Dihydroxy-4'-methoxychalcone
$C_{16}H_{14}O_4$ MW: 270.29 Property: mp 161-2°C. Source: ZHEN CAI. Ref: 6.

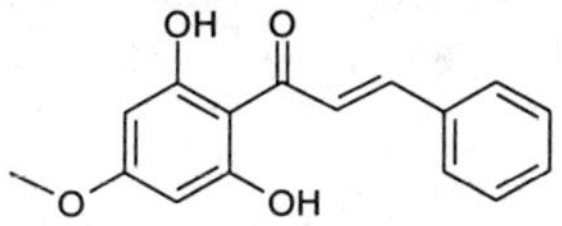

1817 4',5-Dihydroxy-7-methoxy flavone
$C_{16}H_{12}O_5$ MW: 284.27 Property: mp 293°C. Source: MI DIE XIANG. Ref: 6.

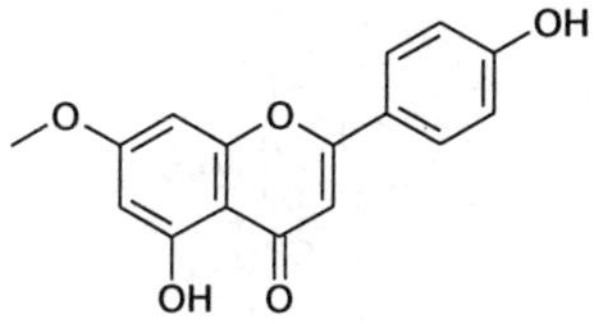

1818 7,3'-Dihydroxy-4'-methoxy flavone
Source: BAI CI HUA. Ref: 561.

1819 7,6'-Dihydroxy-3'-methoxy isoflavone
$C_{16}H_{12}O_5$ MW: 284.27 Property: light yellow crystal (Me_2CO), mp 250-2°C. Source: TU FU LING. Ref: 416.

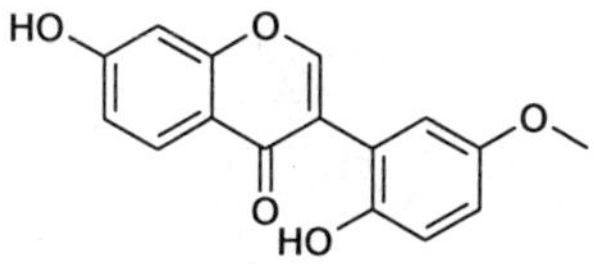

1820 4,7-Dihydroxy-5-methoxyl-6-methyl-8-formyl-flavan
$C_{18}H_{18}O_5$ MW: 314.34 Property: light yellow rhomboid crystal 137-9°C. Source: JIA YIN ZHAO. Ref: 121.

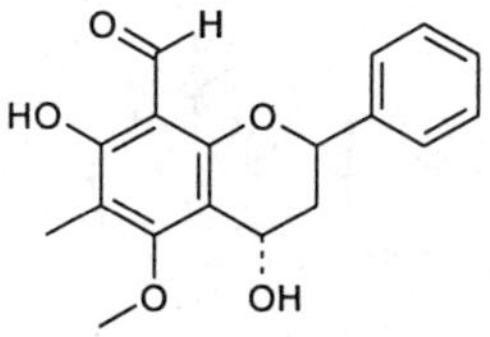

1821 3,8-dihydroxy-4-methoxy-2-oxo-2H-1-benzopyran-5-carboxylic acid
$C_{11}H_8O_7$ MW: 252.18 Property: light yellow acicular crystal, mp277-9°C. Source: DA DING CAO. Ref: 141.

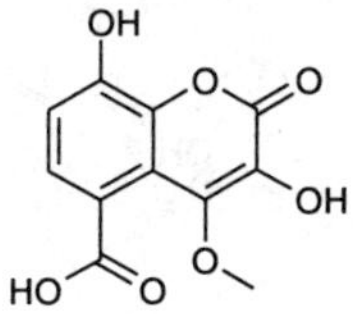

1822 2-(3',5'-Dihydroxy-4'-methoxyphenyl)-3-methoxy-5-hydroxy benzofuran
$C_{16}H_{14}O_6$ MW: 302.29 Property: colorless acicular, mp 219-21°C. Source: XIAO YE MAI MA TENG. Ref: 193.

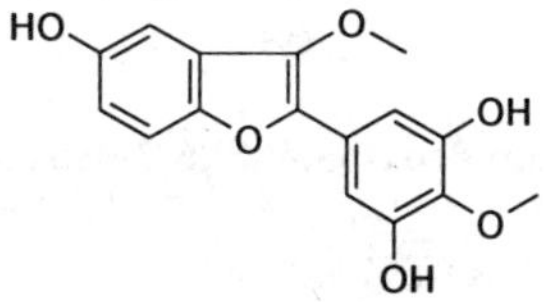

1823 3,5-Dihydroxy-4'-methoxystilbene
Property: mp 167-9°C. Source: TIAN SHAN DA HUANG. Ref: 609.

1824 1,3-Dihydroxy-2-methoxy xanthone
$C_{14}H_{10}O_5$ MW: 258.23 Property: colorless acicular crystal (chloroform-methanol), 162-4°C. Source: HUANG HUA YUAN ZHI. Ref: 382.

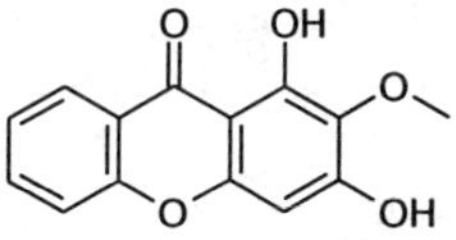

1825 1,7-Dihydroxy-3-methoxy xanthone
$C_{14}H_{10}O_5$ MW: 258.23 Source: YUAN ZHI. Ref: 2.

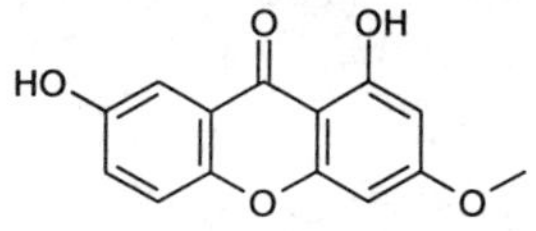

1826 1,8-Dihydroxy-3-methyl-9-anthrone
$C_{15}H_{12}O_3$ MW: 240.26 Property: mp 206-8°C. Source: NIU ER DA HUANG. Ref: 6.

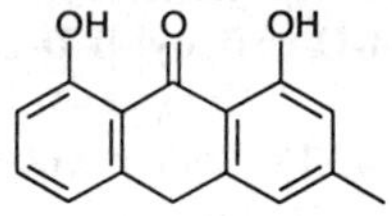

1827 1,7-Dihydroxy-2,3-methylenedioxyxanthone
$C_{14}H_8O_6$ MW: 272.22 Property: colorless acicular crystal (chloroform-methanol), mp 224-6°C. Source: HUANG HUA YUAN ZHI. Ref: 345.

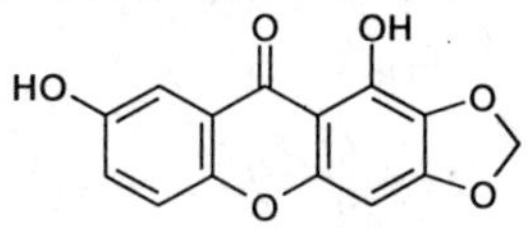

1828 9,12-Dihydroxy-15-nonadecenoic acid
$C_{19}H_{36}O_4$ MW: 328.50 Source: CU LIU GUO (SHA JI). Ref: 2.

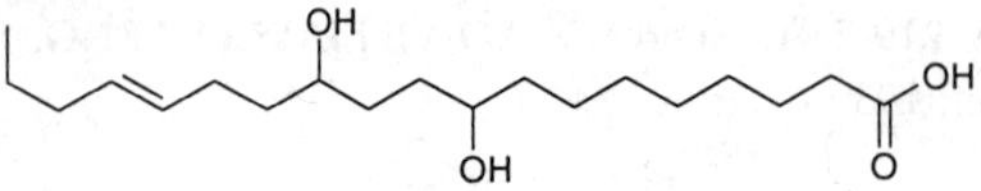

1829 3',5'-Dihydroxy-3,4',5',6,7-pentamethoxy flavone
Source: ZHI ZI. Ref: 626.

1830 3,4-Dihydroxy-phenylethyl alcohol glucoside
$C_{14}H_{20}O_8$ MW: 316.31 Source: HUANG LIAN. Ref: 2.

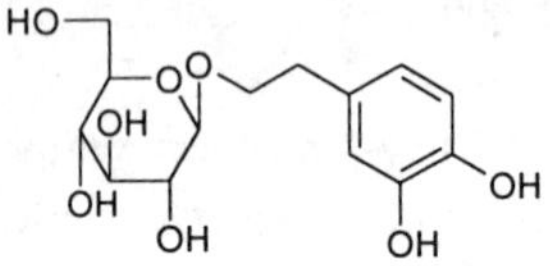

1831 3,4-Dihydroxyphenylethylamine
$C_8H_{11}NO_2$ MW: 153.18 Source: SHAN YAO. Ref: 2.

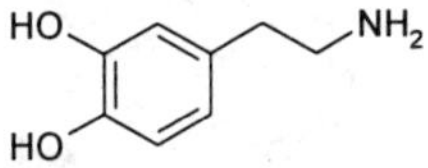

1832 5,8-Dihydroxy-2-(2-phenylethyl) chromone
$C_{17}H_{14}O_4$ MW: 282.30 Property: colorless lump crystal, mp 159-60°C. Source: BAI MU XIANG, CHEN XIANG. Ref: 13.

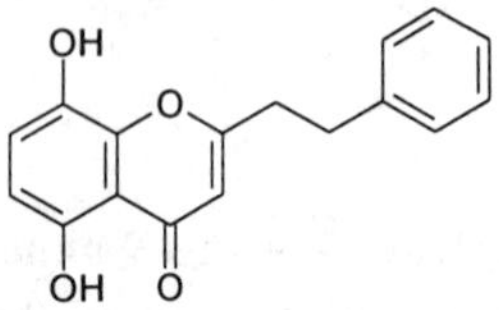

1833 3,4-Dihydroxy-β-phenethyl-O-β-D-glucopyranosyl(1→3)-4-O-caffeoyl-β-D-glucopyranoside
$C_{29}H_{36}O_{16}$ MW: 153.18 Source: GAN DI HUANG. Ref: 2.

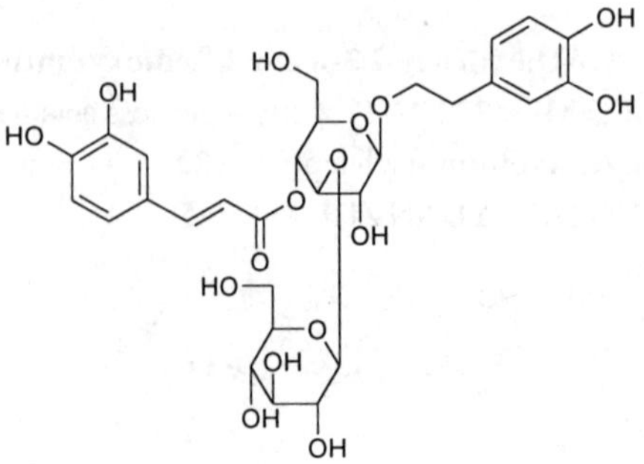

1834 3,4-Dihydroxy-β-phenethyl-O-β-D-glucopyranosyl(1→3)-O-α-L-rhmnopyranosy1(1→6)-4-O-caffeoyl-β-D-glucopyranoside
$C_{35}H_{46}O_{20}$ MW: 786.74 Source: GAN DI HUANG. Ref: 2.

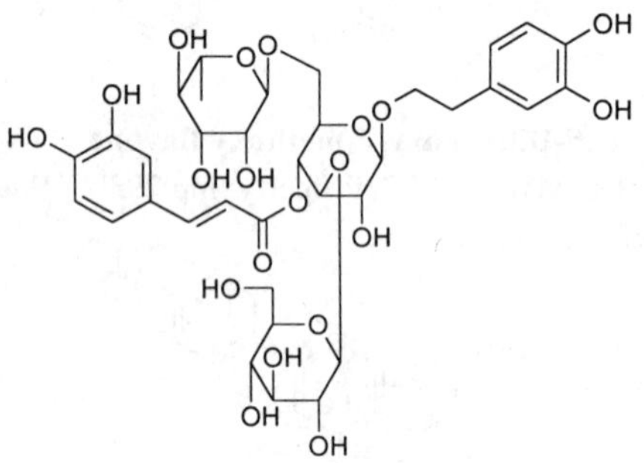

1835 3,4-Dihydroxy-β-phenethyl-O-α-L-rhamnopyranosyl(1→3)-O-β-D-galactopyranosyl(1→6)-4-O-caffeoyl-β-D-glucopyranoside
$C_{35}H_{46}O_{20}$ MW: 786.74 Source: GAN DI HUANG. Ref: 2.

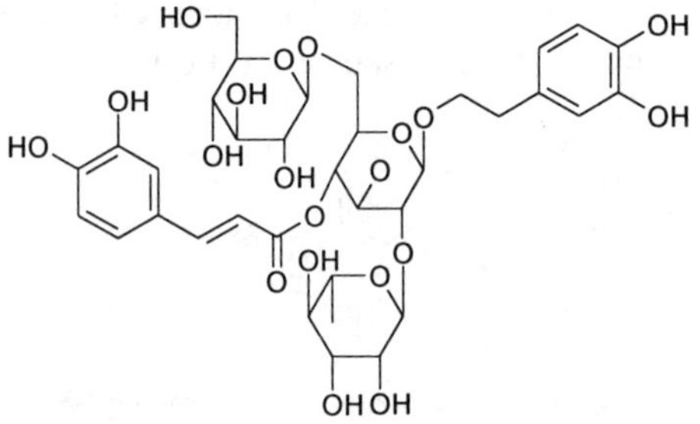

1836 15α,20β-Dihydroxy-Δ4-pregnen-3-one
$C_{21}H_{32}O_3$ MW: 332.49 Source: HONG HUA. Ref: 2.

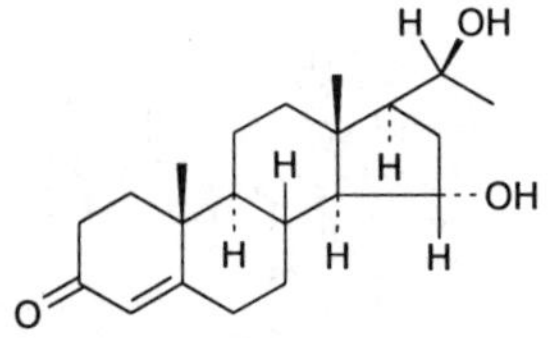

1837 3,4-Dihydroxyrottlerin
$C_{30}H_{28}O_{10}$ MW: 548.55 Property: mp 200°C. Source: LU SONG QIU MAO. Ref: 6.

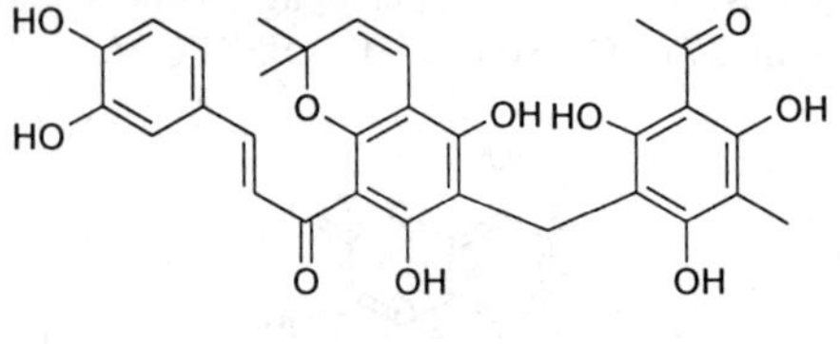

1848 5,8-Dihydroxy-7,3',4'-trimethoxyflavone

1838 Dihydroxyrutaecarpine

$C_9H_{17}N_3O$ MW: 303.37 Source: WU ZHU YU. Ref: 2.

1839 (1R)-1,11α-Dihydroxy-3,4-seco-lupa-4(23), 20(29)-diene-3,28-dioic acid 3,11-lactone 28-O-α-L-rhamnopyranosyl(1→4)-β-D-glucopyranosyl (1→6)-β-D-glucopyranoside

$C_{48}H_{74}O_{19}$ Property: white acicular crystal, mp 232-47°C, $[\alpha]_D^{14}$ +11.7° (c=0.5, MeOH). Source: WU GENG WU JIA YE. Ref: 469.

1840 3,5-Dihydroxy-6,7,3',4'-tetramethoxyflavone

$C_{19}H_{18}O_8$ MW: 374.35 Source: QING HAOV. Ref: 2.

1841 5,4'-Dihydroxy-3,3',6,7-tetra-methoxyflavone

$C_{19}H_{18}O_8$ MW: 374.35 Property: mp 183-4°C. Source: MU JU. Ref: 6.

1842 5',5'-Dihydroxy-6,7,2',3'-tetramethoxy flavone

Source: ZHI ZI. Ref: 626.

1843 5,7-Dihydroxy-6,8,2',3'-tetramethoxyflavone

$C_{19}H_{18}O_8$ MW: 374.35 Source: HUANG QIN. Ref: 2.

1844 3,4-Dihydroxy-6,7,3',4'-tetramethoxyflavonol

$C_{19}H_{20}O_7$ MW: 360.37 Source: QING HAO. Ref: 2.

1845 (24Z)-3β,27-Dihydroxy-7,24-titucalladien-21-al

$C_{30}H_{48}O_3$ MW: 456.72 Source: KU SHU PI. Ref: 12.

1846 2,5-Dihydroxytoluene

Homoquinol; 2-Methyl-hydroquinone; Methylquinol; Piroline; Pyrolin; Toluhydroquinone; Toluquinol. CAS: 95-71-6 $C_7H_8O_2$ MW: 124.14 Property: mp 124-5°C. Source: LU XIAN CAO. Ref: 6.

1847 5,2'-Dihydroxy-6,7,8-trimethoxyflavone

$C_{18}H_{16}O_7$ MW: 344.32 Source: HUANG QIN. Ref: 2.

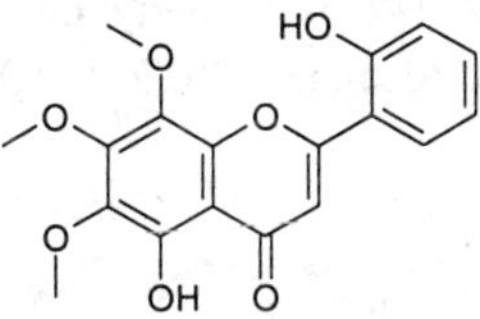

1848 5,8-Dihydroxy-7,3',4'-trimethoxyflavone

Property: mp 208-13°C. Source: JIN LONG DAN CAO. Ref: 604.

1849 1,6-Dihydroxy-3,5,7-trimethoxy xanthone
$C_{16}H_{14}O_7$ MW: 318.29 Source: YUAN ZHI. Ref: 2.

1850 2α,19α-Dihydroxy ursolic acid
Tormentic acid. $C_{30}H_{48}O_5$ MW: 488.71 Property: light yellow crystalline powder, mp 265-9°C, 273°C, 288-9°C, $[\alpha]_D^{15}$ -17.3° (c=0.2, pyridine). Source: CU YE XUAN GOU ZI, DA HONG PAO, QIANG WEI GEN, SHAN DI XIANG CHA CAI, TUN XING GUO, WU LING ZHI. Ref: 6, 447, 592, 595, 606, 637.

1851 3',4'-Dihydroxywogonin
Source: ZHI ZI. Ref: 626.

1852 4'-Dihydroxywogonin
Source: ZHI ZI. Ref: 626.

1853 3,3'-diiodothyronine
$C_{15}H_{13}I_2NO_4$ MW: 525.08 Source: NIU YE. Ref: 6.

1854 Diiodotyrosine
$C_9H_9INO_3$ MW: 432.99 Property: mp (+): 202°C (dec), (-): 213°C (dec), (±): 202°C (dec). Source: NIU YE. Ref: 6.

1855 1,5-Di-isobutyl-3,3-dimethyl[3,1,0]cyclo-hexadione
$C_{16}H_{26}O_2$ MW: 250.38 Source: DANG SHEN. Ref: 2.

1856 Diisocapryl phthalate
$C_{24}H_{38}O_4$ MW: 390.57 Source: SAN QI. Ref: 2.

1857 4,4'-Diketo-3-hydroxy-β-carotene
$C_{40}H_{52}O_3$ MW: 580.86 Source: JIN YU. Ref: 6.

1858 (Z,Z')-Diligustilide
$C_{24}H_{28}O_4$ MW: 380.49 Source: CHUAN XIONG. Ref: 2.

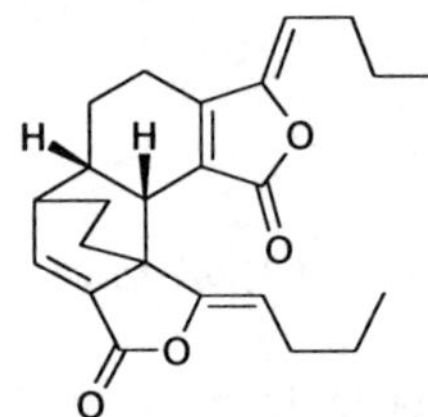

1859 (Z)-6,8'7,3'-Diligustilide
$C_{24}H_{26}O_4$ MW: 378.47 Source: CHUAN XIONG. Ref: 2.

1860 Dill-apiol
$C_{12}H_{14}O_4$ MW: 222.24 Property: mp 29.5°C, bp 185°C. Source: DA YE XIANG RU, HUI XIANG GEN, SHI LUO ZI. Ref: 6.

1861 7β,12-Dimethoxy-8,11,13-abietatrien-11-ol
$C_{22}H_{34}O_3$ MW: 346.51 Source: DU SONG SHI. Ref: 6.

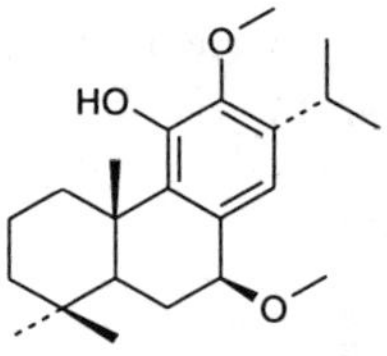

1862 2,4-Dimethoxybenzaldehyde
$C_9H_{10}O_3$ MW: 166.18 Property: mp 71°C, bp 165°C/10mm. Source: XIANG GEN QIN. Ref: 6.

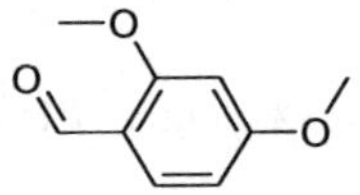

1863 2,6-Dimethoxy-p-benzoquinone
$C_8H_8O_4$ MW: 168.15 Source: CI WU JIA, QIN PI. Ref: 2.

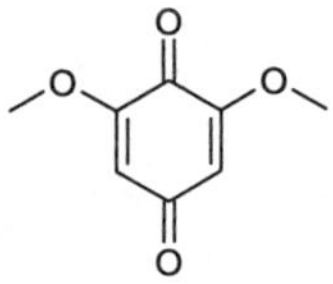

1864 4,5-Dimethoxycanthin-6-one
$C_{16}H_{12}N_2O_3$ MW: 280.29 Property: yellowish needle crystal, mp 148-9°C. Source: KU SHU PI. Ref: 6, 12.

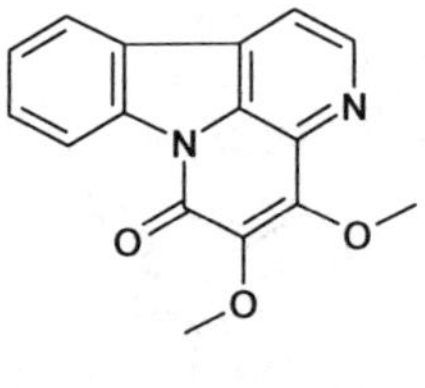

1865 6,7-Dimethoxy coumarin
$C_{11}H_{10}O_4$ MW: 206.20 Source: GE GEN, LIAN QIAO, YIN CHEN HAO. Ref: 2, 642.

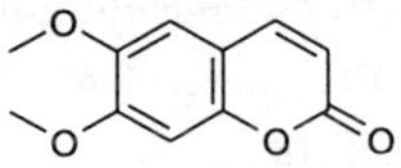

1866 2,3-Dimethoxy-9,10-dihydroxy-N-methyl-tetrahydroproto-berberine quaternary salt
$C_{20}H_{24}NO_4$ MW: 342.42 Property: white crystal, mp 242-5°C. Source: HAI NAN QING NIU DAN. Ref: 408.

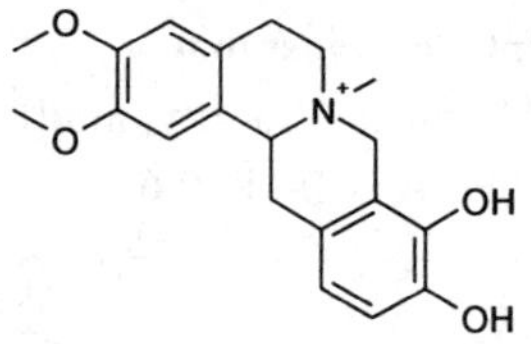

1867 2,2'-Dimethoxy-3,3'-dihydroxy-5,5'-oxygen-6,6'-biphenylformic anhydride
$C_{16}H_{10}O_8$ MW: 330.25 Property: white powder, mp 296.5-8.0 °C. Source: DA JI (a). Ref: 360.

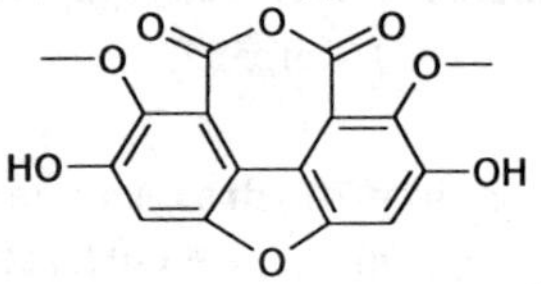

1868 2,3-Dimethoxyellagic acid
$C_{16}H_{10}O_8$ MW: 330.25 Source: BA WANG BIAN. Ref: 6.

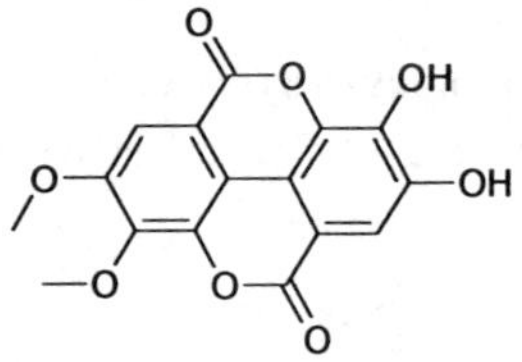

1869 6,14-Dimethoxyforesticine
$C_{26}H_{43}NO_6$ MW: 465.64 Property: white powder, $[\alpha]_D^{18}$ +27.2° (c= 0.31, EtOH). Source: BAI HOU WU TOU. Ref: 483.

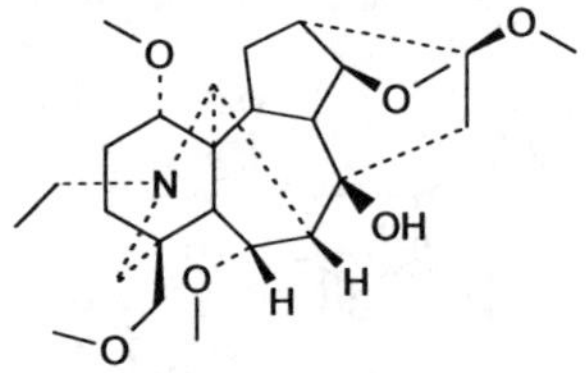

1870 3,5-Dimethoxy-4-glucosyloxy-phenyl-propenyl alcohol
$C_{17}H_{24}O_9$ MW: 372.38 Source: CANG ZHU. Ref: 2.

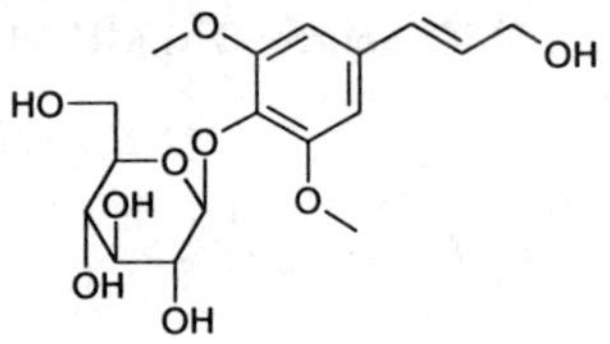

1871 6,6'-Dimethoxygossypol
$C_{32}H_{38}O_8$ MW: 550.65 Property: mp 181-4°C. Source: MIAN HUA GEN. Ref: 6.

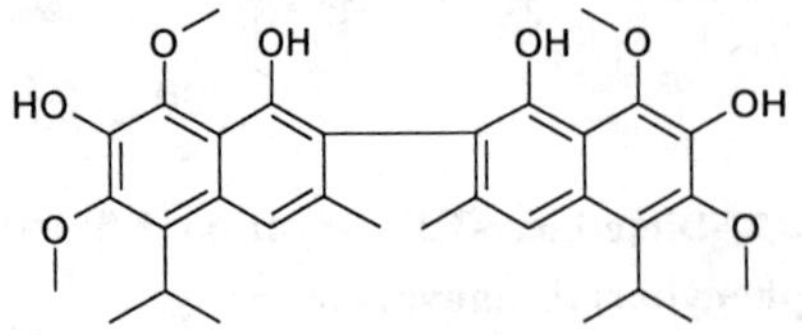

1872 3,5-Dimethoxy-4-hydroxybenzoic acid
Source: SHE PU TAO. Ref: 552.

1873 6,8-Dimethoxy-7-hydroxycoumarin
$C_{11}H_{10}O_5$ MW: 222.20 Source: QING HAO. Ref: 2.

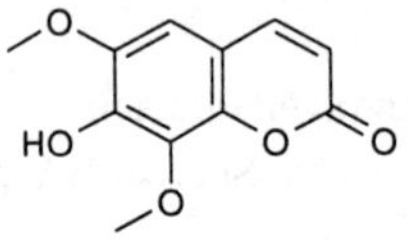

1874 5,6-Dimethoxy-7-hydroxycoumarin
$C_{11}H_{10}O_5$ MW: 222.20 Source: QING HAO. Ref: 2.

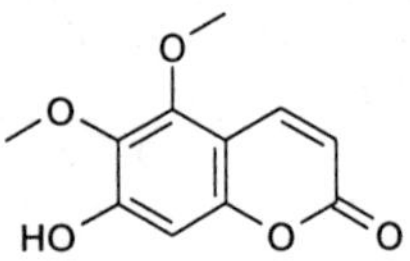

1875 4,8-Dimethoxy-1-(2-methoxyethyl)-β-carboline
$C_{16}H_{18}N_2O_3$ MW: 286.33 Source: KU SHU PI. Ref: 12.

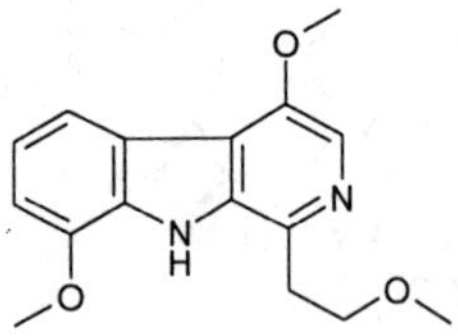

1876 5,8-Dihydroxy-2-[2-(4'-methoxyphenyl) ethyl]chromone
$C_{18}H_{16}O_5$ MW: 312.33 Property: colorless acicular crystal, mp 172-80°C. Source: BAI MU XIANG. Ref: 13.

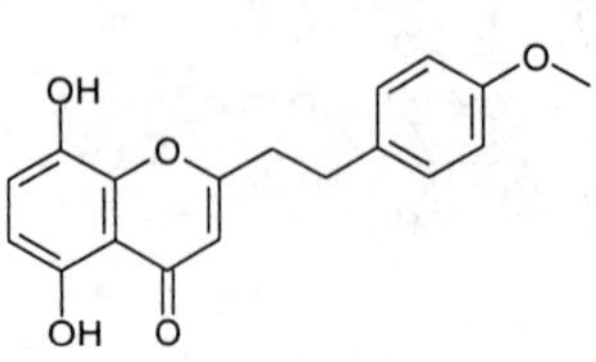

1877 6,7-Dimethoxy-2-[2-(4'-methoxyphenyl) ethyl]chromone
$C_{20}H_{20}O_5$ MW: 340.38 Property: colorless acicular crystal, mp 88-90°C. Source: BAI MU XIANG, CHEN XIANG. Ref: 13.

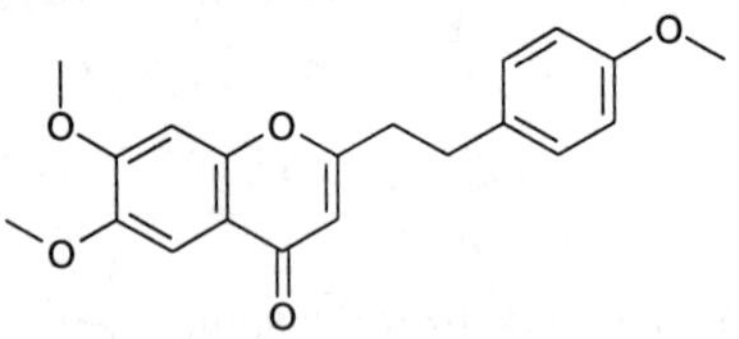

1878 5,6-Dimethoxy-8-(3'-methyl-2'-oxobutyl) coumarin
$C_{16}H_{18}O_5$ MW: 290.32 Source: JIU LI XIANG. Ref: 11.

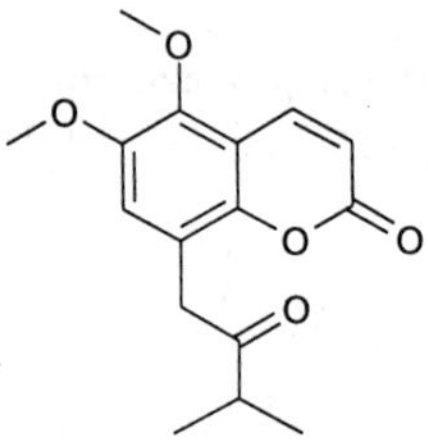

1879 5,7-Dimethoxy-8-(2'-oxo-3'-methylbutyl) coumarin
$C_{16}H_{18}O_5$ MW: 290.32 Source: JIU LI XIANG. Ref: 11.

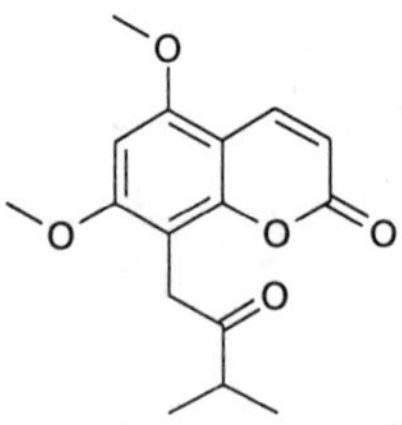

1881 6,7-Dimethoxy-2-(2-phenylethyl) chromone
$C_{19}H_{18}O_4$ MW: 310.35 Property: colorless acicular crystal, mp 118-20°C. Source: BAI MU XIANG, CHEN XIANG. Ref: 13.

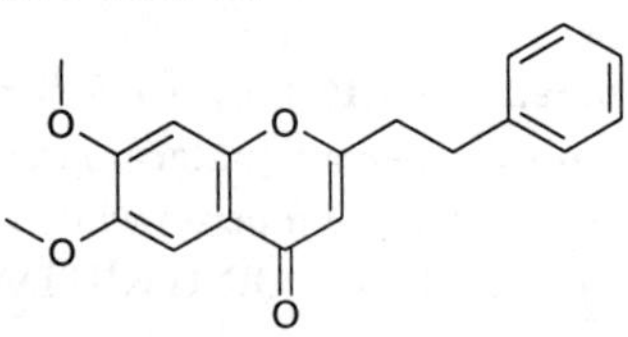

1882 9,10-Dimethoxy-pterocarpane-3-O-β-D-glucoside
$C_{23}H_{28}O_{10}$ MW: 464.47 Source: HUANG QI. Ref: 2.

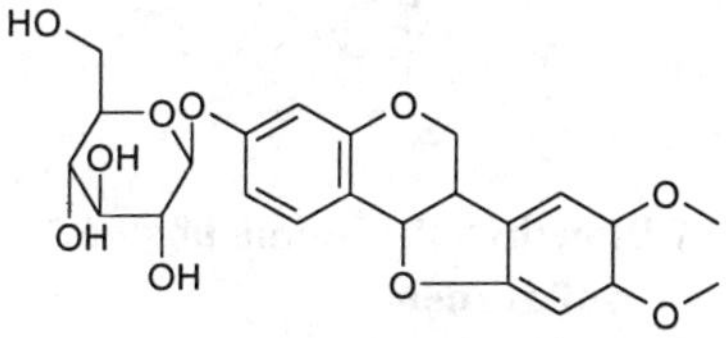

1883 2,6-Dimethoxyquinone
$C_8H_8O_4$ MW: 168.15 Property: mp 260°C. Source: CHU BAI PI. Ref: 6.

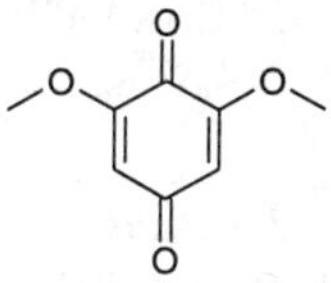

1884 3,5-Dimethoxystilbene
$C_{16}H_{16}O_2$ MW: 240.30 Source: HAI SONG ZI. Ref: 6.

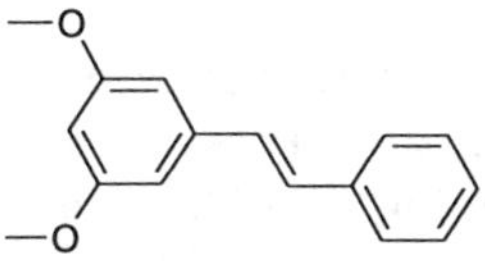

1885 3,5-Dimethoxytoluene
$C_9H_{12}O_2$ MW: 152.19 Source: XI XIN. Ref: 2.

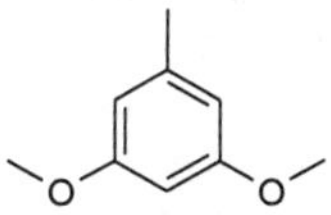

1886 4,9-Dimethoxy-1-vinyl-β-carboline
$C_{15}H_{14}N_2O_3$ MW: 254.29 Source: KU SHU PI. Ref: 12.

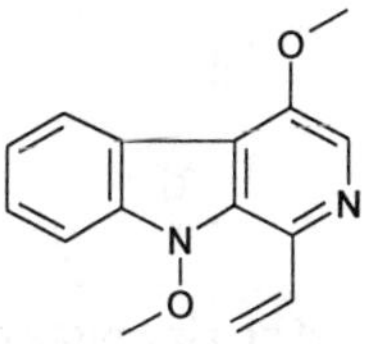

1887 3',4'-Dimethoxywogonin
Source: ZHI ZI. Ref: 626.

1888 2,8-Dimethyl-5-acetyl-bicyclo[5,3,0] decadiene-1,8
$C_{14}H_{20}O$ MW: 204.31 Source: SAN QI. Ref: 2.

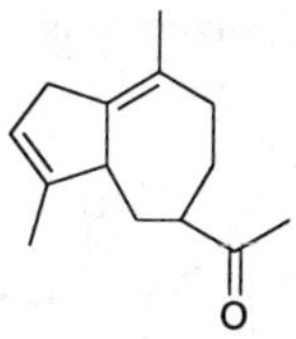

1889 β,β-Dimethylacryloylshikonin
$C_{21}H_{22}O_6$ MW: 370.41 Property: mp 116-7°C. Source: ZI CAO. Ref: 2, 5.

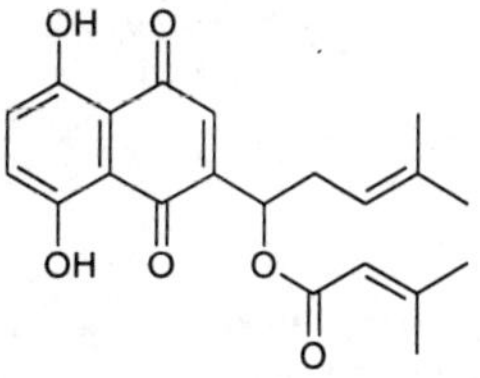

1890 3-(1,1-Dimethyl allyl)herniarin
$C_{15}H_{16}O_3$ MW: 244.29 Property: mp 126-8°C. Source: CHOU CAO. Ref: 6.

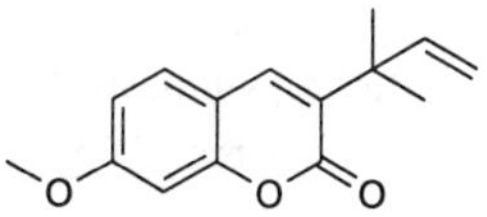

1891 3,3-Dimethyl allyl p-propenyl phenyl ether
$C_{14}H_{22}O$ MW: 206.33 Source: BA JIAO HUI XIANG. Ref: 6.

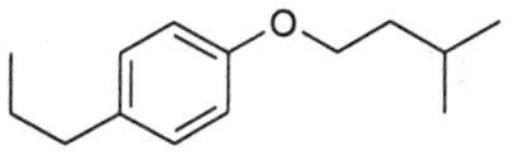

1892 Dimethyl azelate
$C_{11}H_{20}O_4$ MW: 216.28 Source: DANG GUI. Ref: 2.

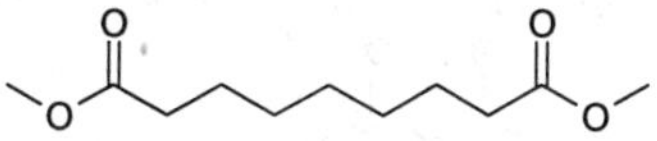

1893 1,2-Dimethyl-benzene
C_8H_{10} MW: 106.17 Source: SHAN ZHA. Ref: 2.

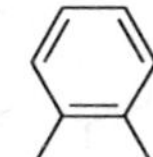

1894 α,α-Dimethyl-benzene methanol
$C_9H_{12}O$ MW: 136.20 Source: SAN QI. Ref: 2.

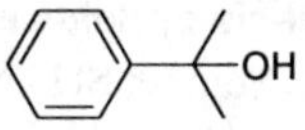

1895 3,4-Dimethylbenzoic acid
$C_9H_{10}O_2$ MW: 150.18 Property: mp 166°C. Source: MU TIAN LIAO. Ref: 6.

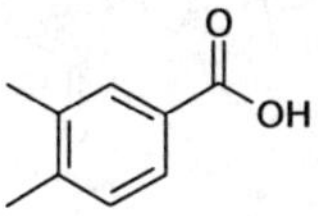

1896 3,5-Dimethyl-butyl-benzene
$C_{12}H_{18}$ MW: 162.27 Source: SHAN ZHA. Ref: 2.

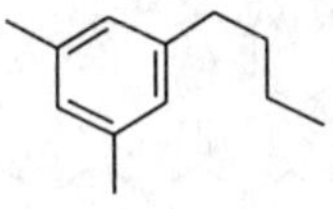

1897 Dimethyl camphorate
$C_{13}H_{22}O_4$ MW: 242.32 Source: DANG GUI. Ref: 2.

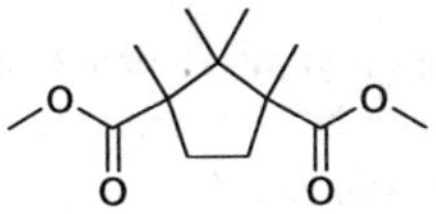

1898 24,24-Dimethyl-5α-cholesta-8-en-3β-ol
$C_{29}H_{50}O$ MW: 414.72 Source: QI YE DAN. Ref: 2.

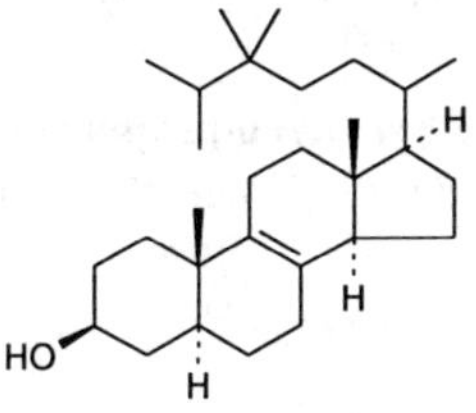

1899 7,7''-Di-O-methylcupressu-flavone
$C_{32}H_{22}O_{10}$ MW: 566.53 Property: mp >300°C. Source: CE BAI YE. Ref: 6.

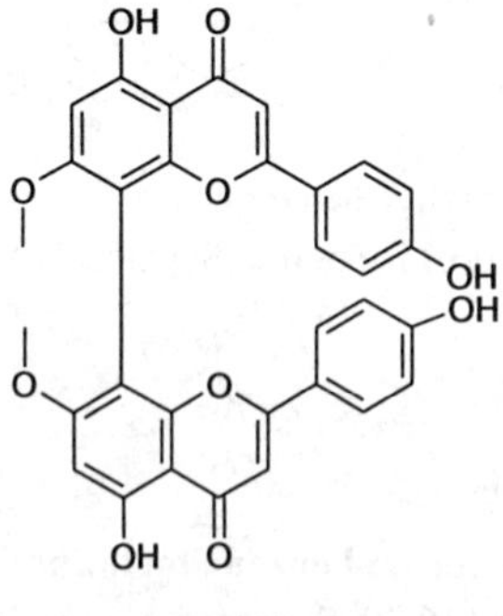

1900 1,4-Dimethyl-cis-cyclohexane
C_8H_{16} MW: 112.22 Source: SHAN ZHA. Ref: 2.

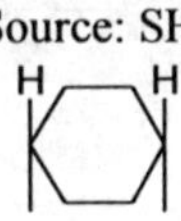

1901 1,6-Dimethyl-cis-cyclohexane
C_8H_{16} MW: 112.22 Source: SHAN ZHA. Ref: 2.

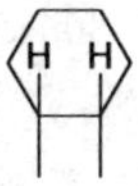

1902 3',14-Dimethyl-4',11-dimethoxy-5,7-dihydroxybenzoflavanone
Source: LANG DU. Ref: 556.

1903 Dimethyl disulfide
$C_2H_6S_2$ MW: 94.20 Property: mp -98°C, bp 110°C. Source: DA SUAN, JIU CAI. Ref: 6.

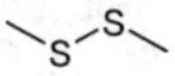

1904 4,6-Dimethyl dodecane
$C_{14}H_{30}$ MW: 198.40 Source: ROU CONG RONG[1]. Ref: 2.

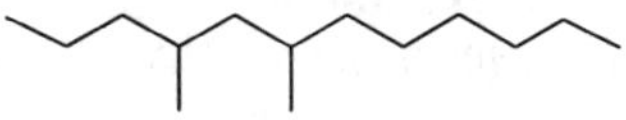

1905 3,4-Di-O-methylellagic acid
$C_{16}H_{10}O_8$ MW: 330.25 Property: mp >300°C. Source: WU JIU MU GEN PI. Ref: 6.

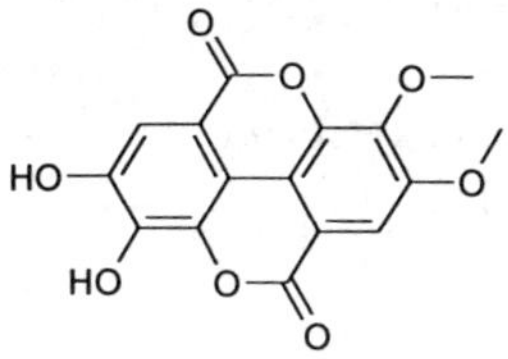

1906 Dimethyl ether of phloroacetophenone
$C_{10}H_{12}O_4$ MW: 196.20 Property: mp 85-8°C. Source: AI NA XIANG. Ref: 6.

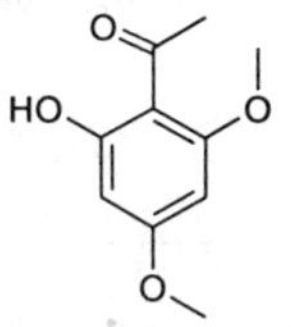

1907 N,N-Dimethyl glycine methyl ester
$C_5H_{11}NO_2$ MW: 117.15 Source: ROU CONG RONG. Ref: 2.

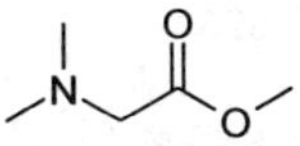

1908 2,3-Dimethyl-heptane
C_9H_{20} MW: 128.26 Source: SHAN ZHA. Ref: 2.

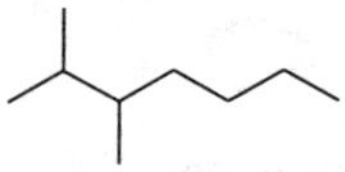

1909 4-(1,5-Dimethyl-1,4-hexadienyl)-1-methyl-cyclohexene
$C_{14}H_{22}$ MW: 190.33 Source: WU WEI ZI. Ref: 2.

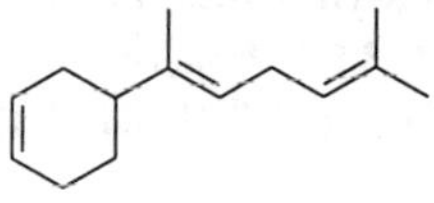

1910 1-(1,5-Dimethyl-4-hexenyl)-4-methyl benzene
$C_{15}H_{28}$ MW: 208.39 Source: SHENG JIANG. Ref: 2.

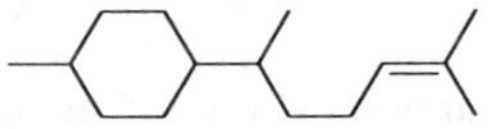

1911 2,5-Dimethyl-7-hydroxy chromone
$C_{11}H_{10}O_3$ MW: 190.20 Property: mp 220-2°C. Source: HU ZHANG, REN SHEN, TAIN SHAN DA HUANG. Ref: 2, 609.

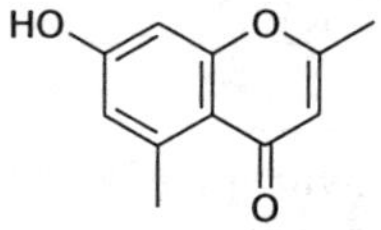

HO O O

1912 1,6-Dimethyl-4-isopropyl-7,8-dihydro-naphthalene
$C_{15}H_{20}$ MW: 200.33 Source: ZHANG MU. Ref: 6.

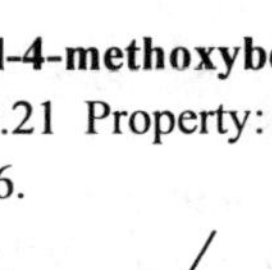

1913 3,5-Dimethyl-4-methoxybenzoic acid
$C_{10}H_{12}O_3$ MW: 180.21 Property: mp 145°C. Source: FAN XIE YE. Ref: 6.

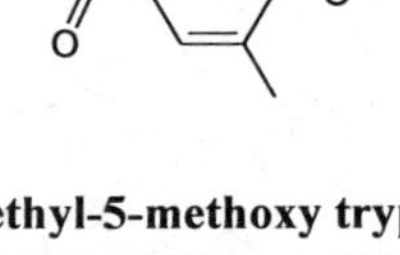

HO O O

1914 N,N-Dimethyl-5-methoxy tryptamine
$C_{13}H_{18}N_2O$ MW: 218.30 Source: WU ZHU YU. Ref: 2.

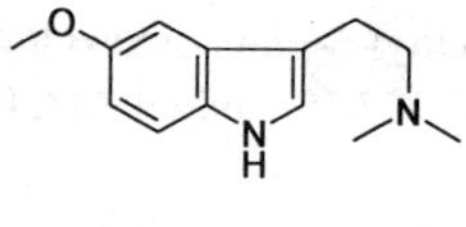

O N H N

1915 1,1-Dimethyl-2-(3-methyl-1,3-butadiene)cyclo-propane
$C_{10}H_{16}$ MW: 136.24 Source: BAI ZHI. Ref: 2.

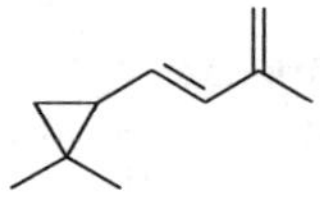

1916 2,2-Dimethyl-3-methylenebicyclo[2,2,1] heptane
$C_{10}H_{16}$ MW: 136.24 Source: WU WEI ZI. Ref: 2.

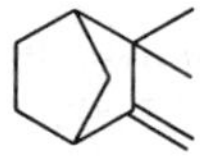

1917 1,8-Dimethyl-4-(1-methylenyl)-spiro(4,5) dec-7-ene
$C_{15}H_{24}$ MW: 204.36 Source: WU WEI ZI. Ref: 2.

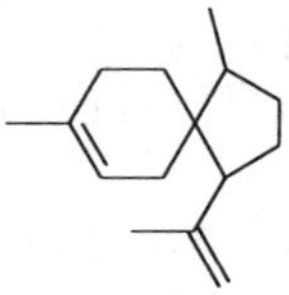

1918 2,6-Dimethyl-6-(4-methyl-3-pentenyl) biscyclo[3,1,1]hept-2-ene
$C_{15}H_{24}$ MW: 204.36 Source: SHENG JIANG. Ref: 2.

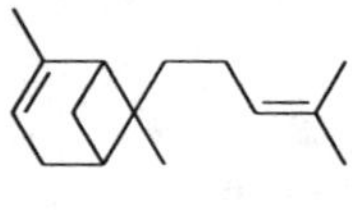

1919 3,7-Dimetyl-1,5,7-octatrien-3-ol
$C_{10}H_{16}O$ MW: 152.24 Source: CHA YE. Ref: 6.

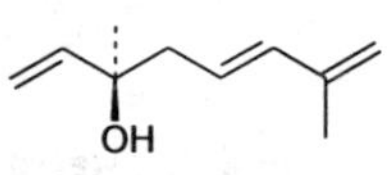

OH

1920 3,7-Dimethyl-7-octenal
$C_{10}H_{18}O$ MW: 154.25 Source: JU PI. Ref: 2.

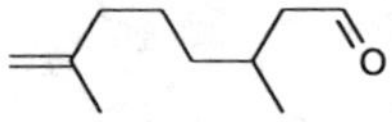

O

1921 3,4-Dimethyl-5-phenyloxazolidine
$C_{11}H_{15}NO$ MW: 177.25 Source: MA HUANG. Ref: 2.

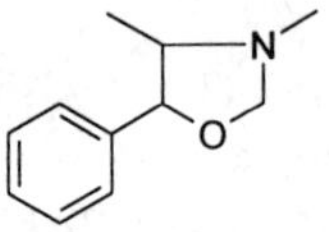

1922 Dimethyl phthalate
$C_{10}H_{10}O_4$ MW: 194.19 Source: DANG GUI. Ref: 2.

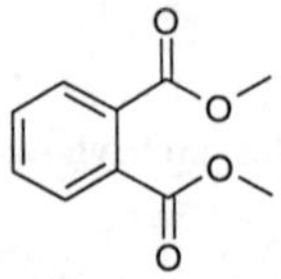

1923 Dimethyl-β-propiothetin
$C_5H_{11}O_2S{\bullet}Cl$ MW: 135.21•35.45 Source: SHI CHUN. Ref: 6.

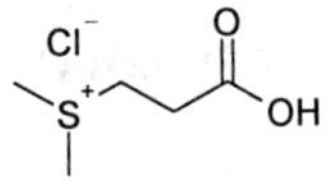

1924 Dimethyl sebacate
$C_{12}H_{22}O_4$ MW: 230.31 Source: DANG GUI. Ref: 2.

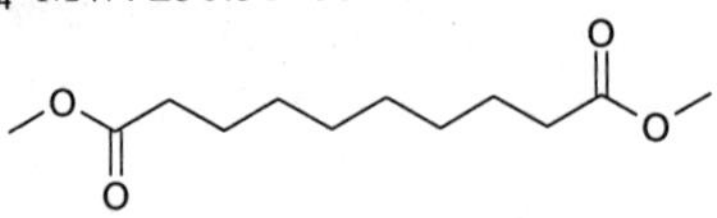

1925 Dimetyl sulfide
C_2H_6S MW: 62.13 Property: bp 37.5-8.0°C. Source: DA SUAN, SHUI SONG. Ref: 6.

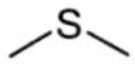

1926 Dimethyl sulfone
$C_2H_6O_2S$ MW: 94.13 Source: MU ZEI. Ref: 2.

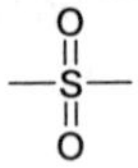

1927 5,6-Dimethyl-3a,4,7,7a-tetrahydro-1,3-Isoben-zofurandione
$C_{10}H_{12}O_3$ MW: 180.21 Source: DU HUO. Ref: 2.

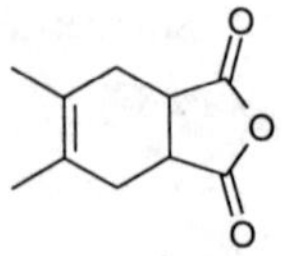

1928 Dimethyl tetrasulfide
$C_2H_6S_4$ MW: 158.33 Source: JIU CAI. Ref: 6.

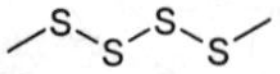

1929 Dimethyl trisulfide
$C_2H_6S_3$ MW: 126.26 Source: DA SUAN. Ref: 2.

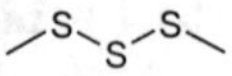

1930 N,N-Dimethyltryptamine
$C_{12}H_{16}N_2$ MW: 188.27 Property: mp 48-9°C. Source: HONG MU JI CAO, LU ZHU GEN, PAI QIAN CAO. Ref: 6.

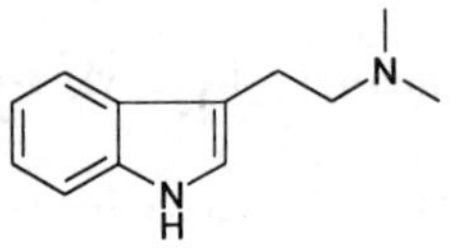

1931 N,N-Dimethyltryptamine-methohydroxide
$C_{13}H_{19}N_2$ MW: 203.31 Source: LU ZHU GEN. Ref: 6.

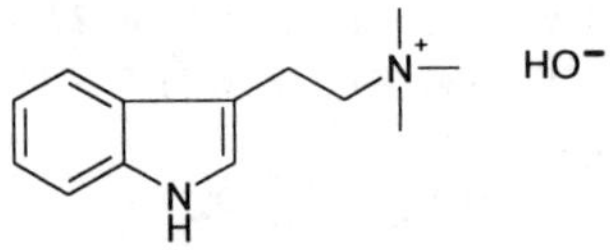

1932 N,N-Dimethyltryptamine-Nb-oxide
$C_{12}H_{16}N_2O$ MW: 204.27 Source: HONG MU JI CAO, PAI QIAN CAO. Ref: 6.

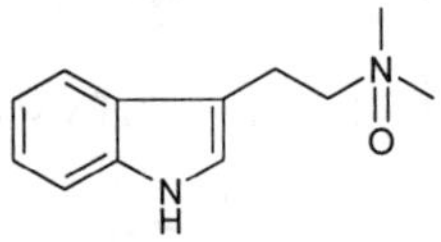

1933 2,4-Dimethyl-undecane
$C_{13}H_{28}$ MW: 184.37 Source: SHAN ZHA. Ref: 2.

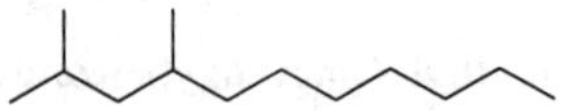

1934 3,6-Dimethyl-undecane
$C_{13}H_{28}$ MW: 184.37 Source: ROU CONG RONG. Ref: 2.

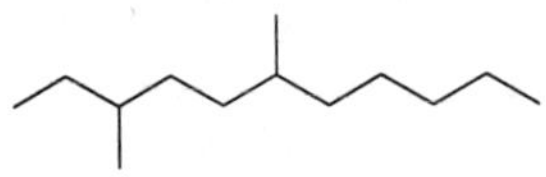

1935 Dioctyl phthalate
Source: GUANG XI XUE JIE. Ref: 616.

1936 3-O-α-(3',4'-O-Dioic-acetyl)-L-arabino-pyranosyl-3β-hydroxylean-12-ene-28,29-dioic acid-28-O-[α-L-rhamnopyranosyl-(1→6)-β-D-glycopyranosyl-(1→4)-β-D-glycopyranosyl] ester
$C_{57}H_{88}O_{25}$ MW: 1173.32 Property: white powder, mp 203-5°C, $[\alpha]_D^{25}$ -3.47° (c=0.1, methanol). Source: YI YE LIANG WANG CHA. Ref: 187.

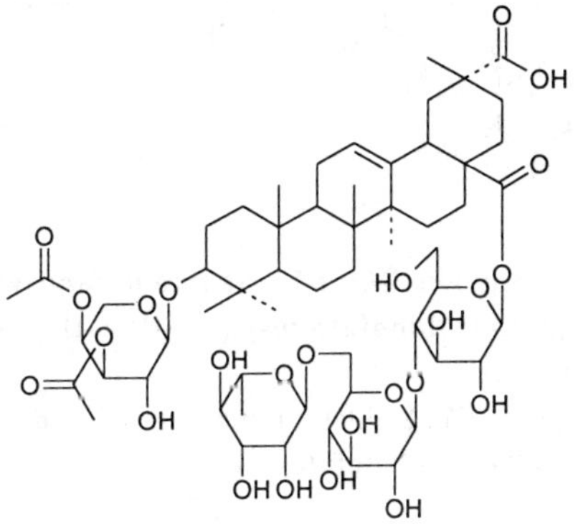

1937 α:α-Diolein
$C_{39}H_{72}O_5$ MW: 621.01 Property: mp 25°C, 21.5°C. Source: MANG GUO HE. Ref: 6.

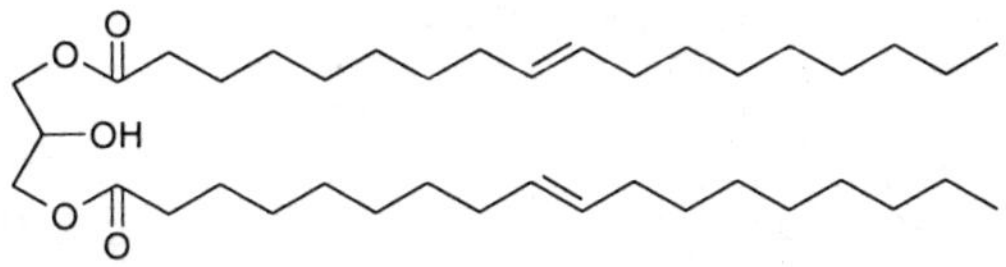

1938 α:β-Diolein
$C_{39}H_{72}O_5$ MW: 621.01 Source: MANG GUO HE. Ref: 6.

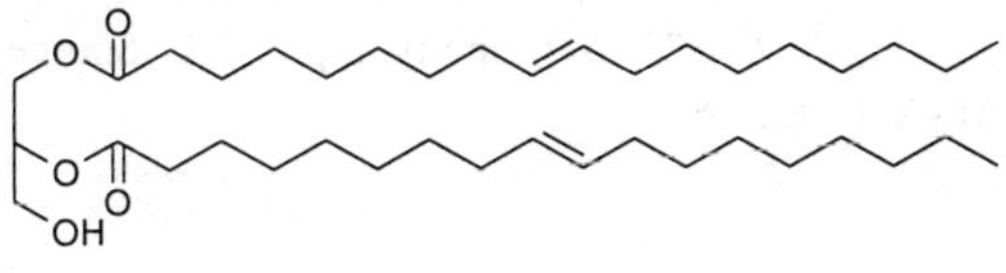

1939 Diosbulbin A
$C_{20}H_{24}O_7$ MW: 376.41 Property: mp 265°C. Source: HUANG YAO ZI. Ref: 6, 641.

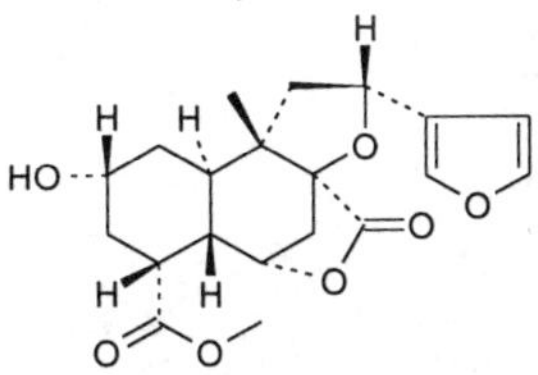

1940 Diosbulbin B
$C_{19}H_{20}O_6$ MW: 344.37 Property: mp 285°C (dec). Source: HUANG YAO ZI. Ref: 6, 641.

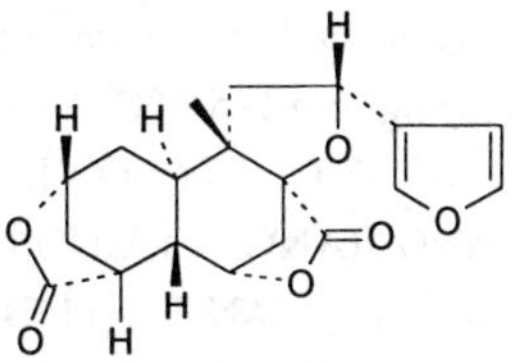

1941 Diosbulbin C
$C_{19}H_{22}O_7$ MW: 362.38 Property: mp 247-50°C (dec). Source: HUANG YAO ZI. Ref: 6, 641.

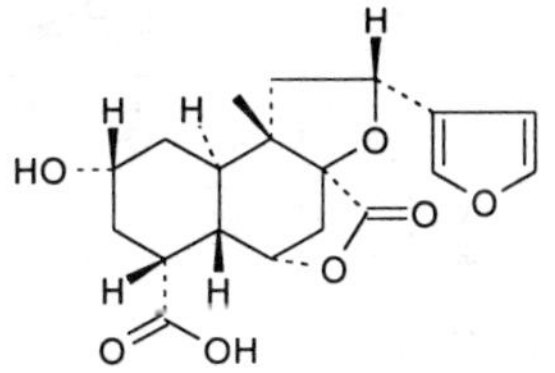

1942 Dioscin
CAS: 19057-60-4 $C_{45}H_{72}O_{16}$ MW: 869.07 Property: mp 288°C. Source: BAI YAO ZI, BEI XIE, CHUAN SHAN LONG, FU ZHOU SHU YU (dried rhizome), SHAN YAO, SHU KUI YE (dried rhizome), ZAO XIU. Ref: 4, 10.

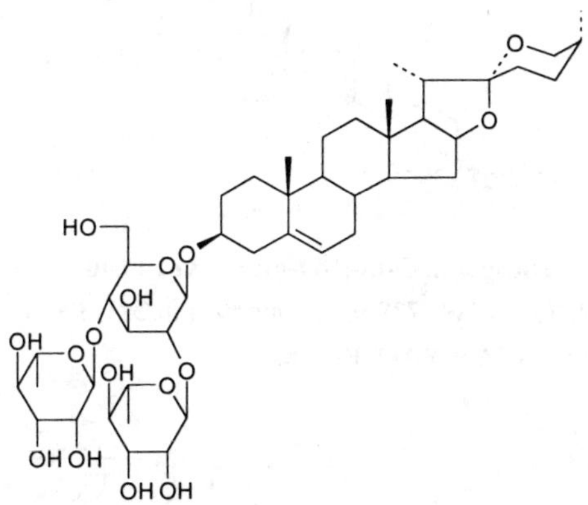

1943 Dioscorine
$C_{13}H_{19}NO_2$ MW: 221.30 Property: mp 55°C. Source: BAI SHU LANG. Ref: 6.

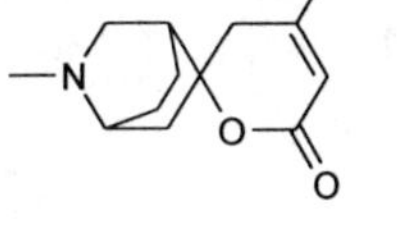

1945 Diosgenin

Δ^5-Sapogenin. $C_{27}H_{42}O_3$ MW: 414.63 Property: mp 205-6°C, 189-92°C, 196-8°C, 204-5°C, 199-202°C, from moldy source plant, both mp and content of sapogenin decreasing, mp 195-6°C, 176-8°C, 186-94°C, 194-5°C, 180-92°C. Source: CHA RUI SHU YU, CHAI HUANG JIANG, CHUNG LONG SHU YU, DUN YE SHU YU, FANG JI YE BA QIA, FEN BEI SHU YU, FU ZHOU SHU YU, HUANG SHAN YAO, MIAN BI XIE, SHU KUI YE, XIAN XI SHU YU, XIAO HUA DUN YE SHU YU. Ref: 10.

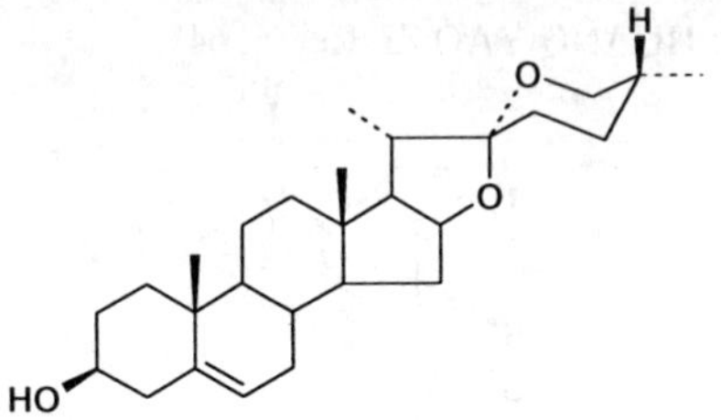

1946 Diosgenin acetate

$C_{29}H_{44}O_4$ MW: 456.67 Source: FANG JI YE BA QIA, FEN BEI SHU YU. Ref: 10.

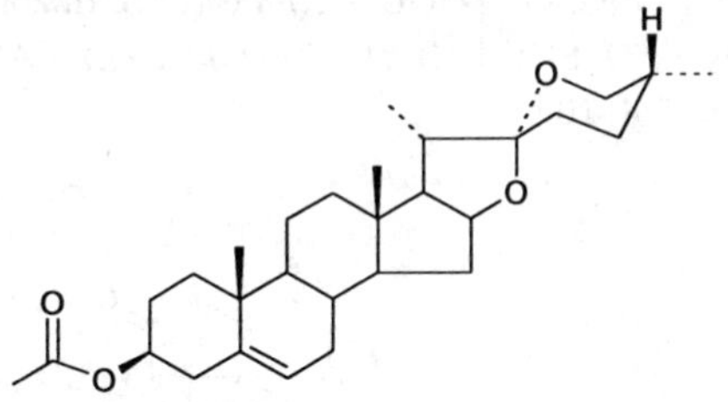

1947 Diosgenin-3-di-β-O-glucopyranoside

$C_{39}H_{62}O_{13}$ MW: 738.92 Property: mp 271-3°C. Source: SHAN YAO. Ref: 6.

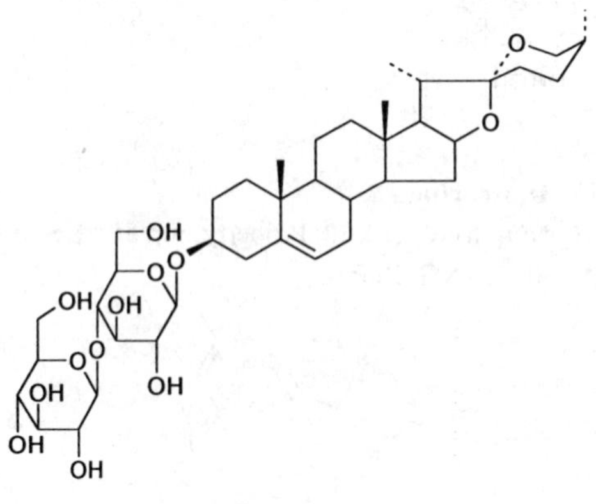

1948 Diosgenin-dioglucoside

$C_{39}H_{62}O_{13}$ MW: 738.92 Source: DUN YE SHU YU (fresh rhizome). Ref: 10.

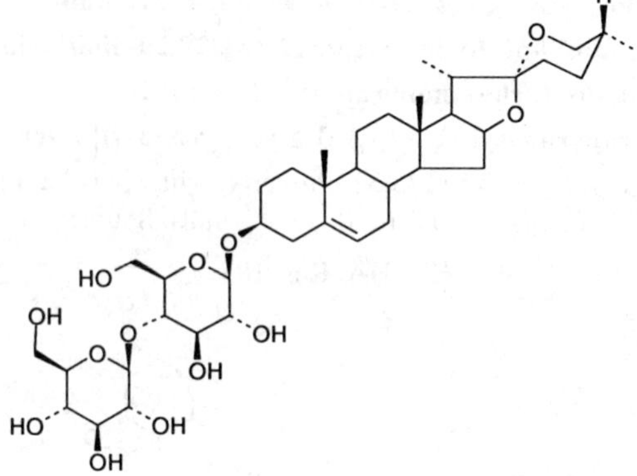

1949 Diosgenin-3-O-α-L-rhamno pyranosyl-(1→2)[α-L-arabinofuranosyl(1→4)]-β-D-gluco-pyranoside

$C_{44}H_{70}O_{16}$ MW: 855.04 Property: mp 276-8°C (dec). Source: ZAO XIU. Ref: 6.

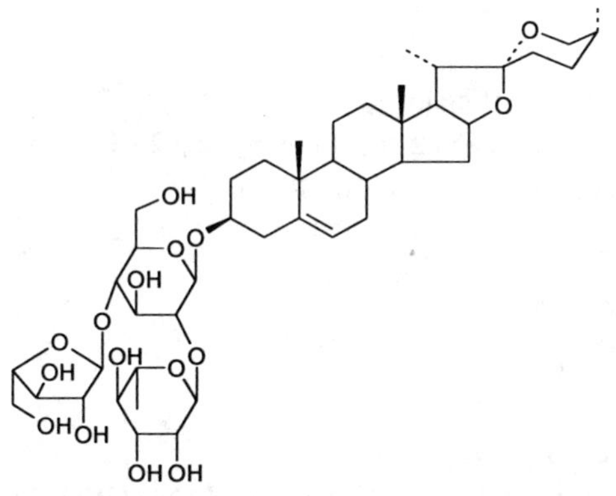

1950 Diosgenin-3-O-β-D-glucopyranoside

$C_{33}H_{52}O_8$ MW: 576.78 Property: mp 274°C. Source: ZAO XIU. Ref: 6.

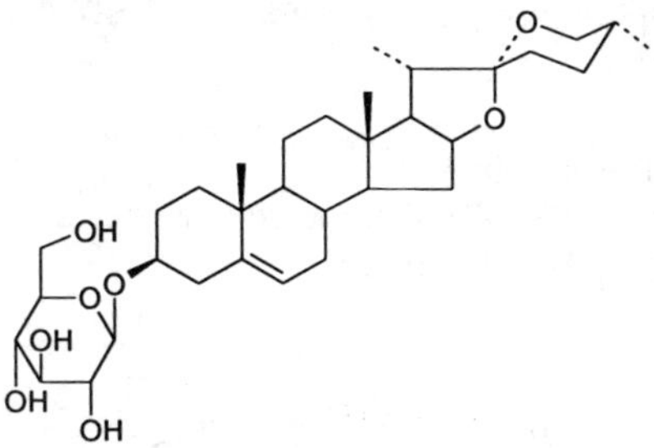

1951 Diosgenin palmitate

$C_{43}H_{72}O_4$ MW: 653.05 Source: CHA RUI SHU YU, FEN BEI SHU YU. Ref: 10.

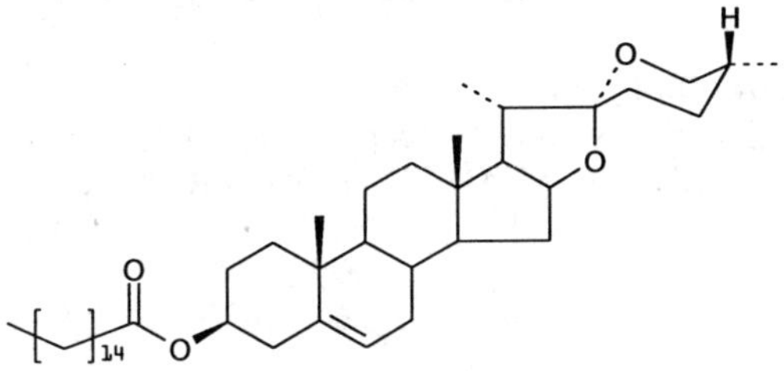

1952 Diosgenin-3-α-L-rhamnopyranosyl-β-D-glucopyranoside

$C_{39}H_{62}O_{12}$ MW: 722.92 Source: ZAO XIU. Ref: 6.

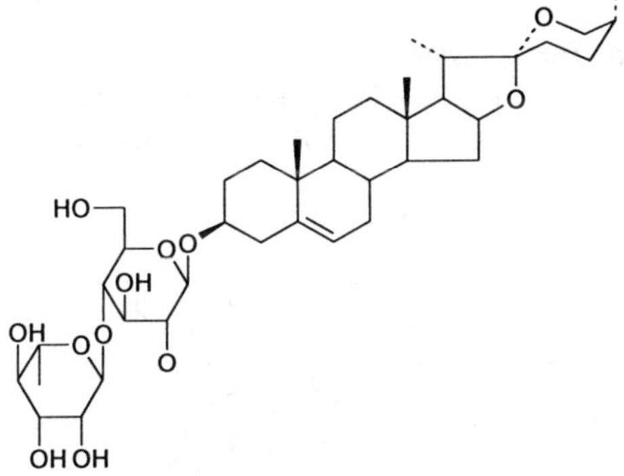

1953 Diosgenin tetraglycoside

$C_{51}H_{82}O_{20}$ MW: 1015.21 Property: mp 203-6°C (dec). Source: ZAO XIU. Ref: 6.

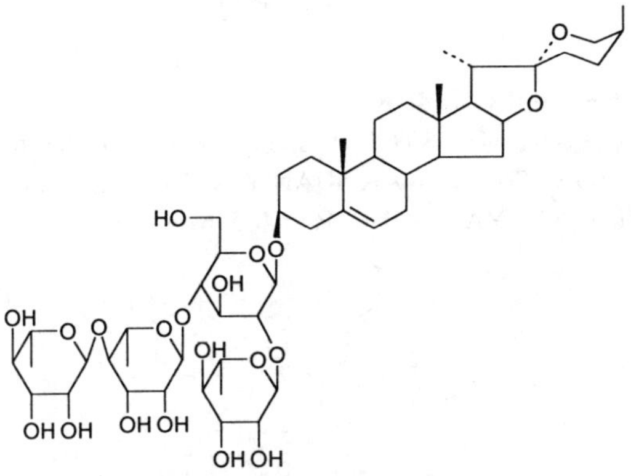

1954 Diosmetin

5,7,3'-Trihydroxy-4'-methoxyflavone. $C_{16}H_{12}O_6$ MW: 300.27 Property: mp 253-5°C. Source: BAI CI HUA, JIAN DI PU GONG YING, MENG GU SHAN LUO BO. Ref: 6, 561, 602.

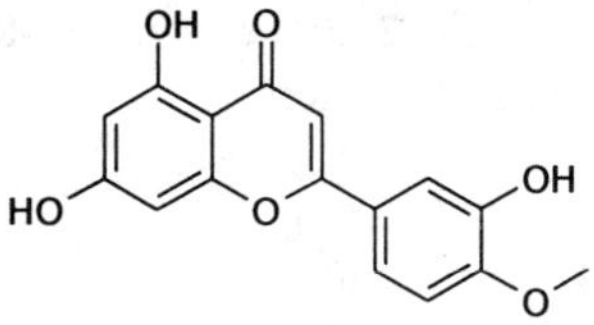

1955 Diosmin

$C_{28}H_{32}O_{15}$ MW: 608.56 Property: mp 278-80°C. Source: BA XIAN CAO, BAI CI HUA YE, FEI LONG ZHANG XUE, FO SHOU (FO SHOU GAN), JI CAI, JI CAI ZI, MI DIE XIANG, NING MENG, RU DI JIN NIU, YING BU BO. Ref: 6.

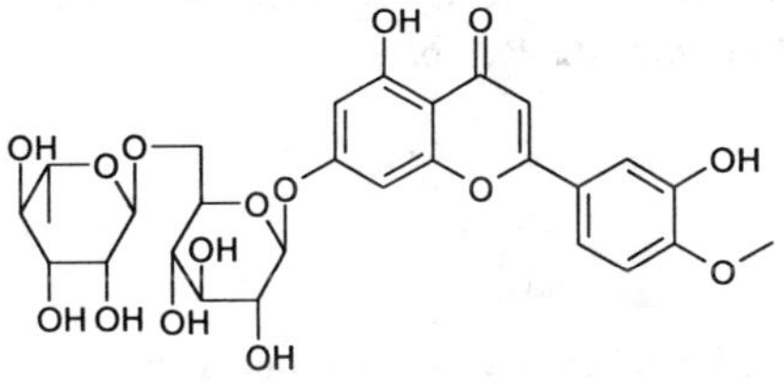

1956 3,24-Dioxofridelan-29-oic acid

$C_{30}H_{48}O_4$ MW: 472.71 Source: LEI GONG TENG. Ref: 2.

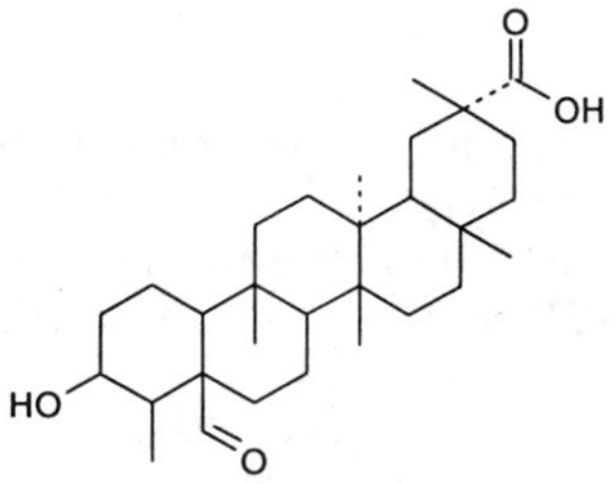

1957 3,24-Dioxo-fridelan-29-oic acid

$C_{30}H_{46}O_4$ MW: 470.70 Property: colorless acicular crystal, mp 294°C. Source: LEI GONG TENG. Ref: 60.

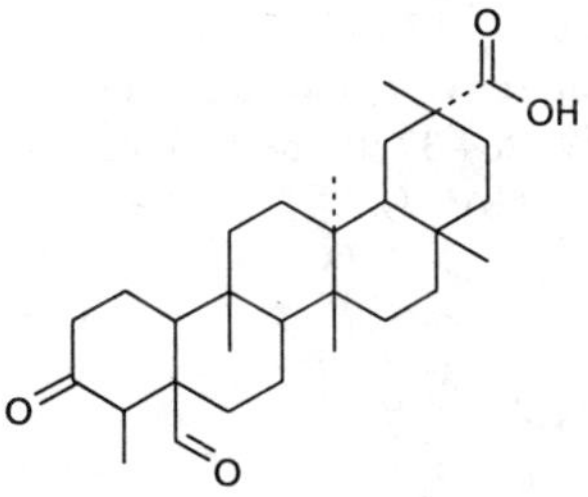

1958 3,4-Dioxymethylene-5-methoxy-1-(1-oxopropyl)benzene
$C_{11}H_{12}O_4$ MW: 208.22 Property: mp 87-8°C, 91-2°C. Source: SHA QIAN HU. Ref: 6.

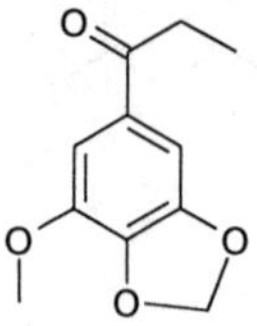

1959 Dipentene
$C_{10}H_{16}$ MW: 136.24 Property: bp 178°C. Source: DA YE XIANG RU, FENG XIANG SHU YE (b), GANG SONG, HAI SONG ZI, HU SUI ZI, HUI XIANG, LU DOU LE HUA, MO YAO, RU XIANG, YA ER QIN, ZHI ZHU XIANG. Ref: 6.

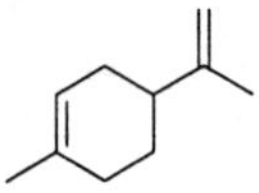

1960 2,3-Diphenyl-2-cyclopropen-1-one
$C_{15}H_{10}O$ MW: 206.25 Source: DU HUO. Ref: 2.

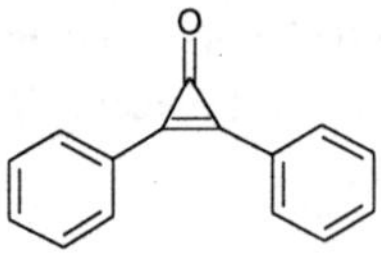

1961 2,2'-Di-(2-phenylethyl)-8,6'-dihydroxy-5,5'-bichromone (AH11)
$C_{34}H_{26}O_6$ MW: 530.58 Property: light dark-yellow powder, mp 239-42°C. Source: CHEN XIANG. Ref: 13.

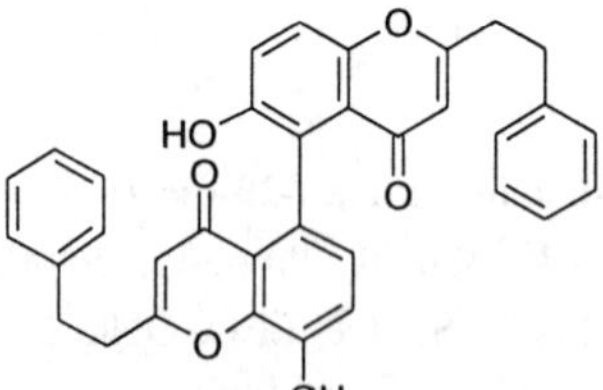

1962 1,7-Diphenylhept-4-en-3-one
$C_{19}H_{20}O$ MW: 264.37 Property: colorless oleaginous liquid. Source: GAO LIANG JIANG. Ref: 435.

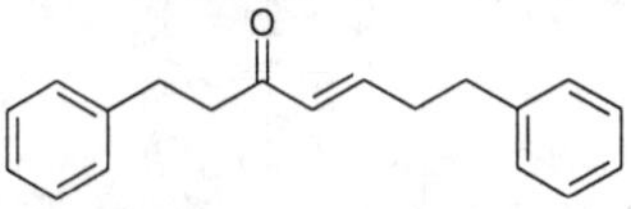

1963 1,3-Diphenylpropane-1,2-diol-3-one
$C_{15}H_{14}O_3$ MW: 242.28 Source: LUO HUA SHENG. Ref: 6.

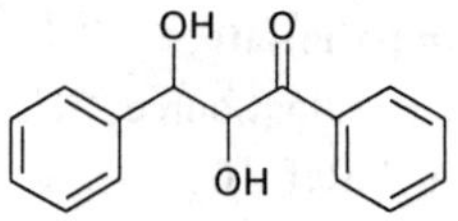

1964 Diphyllin
$C_{21}H_{16}O_7$ MW: 380.36 Property: mp 291°C. Source: JUE CHUANG, SHAN HE YE, WO ER QI. Ref: 6, 279.

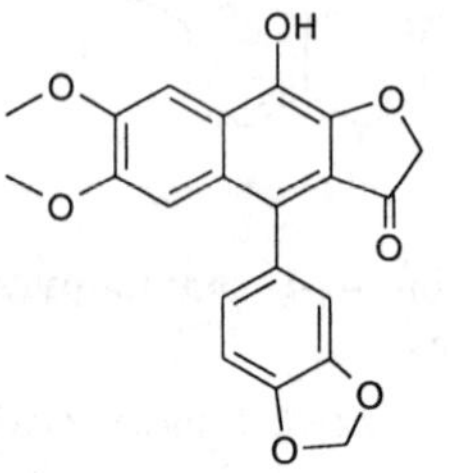

1965 Diphylloside A
$C_{38}H_{48}O_{20}$ MW: 824.79 Property: yellow powder, mp 204-6°C. Source: WAN SHAN YIN YANG HUO. Ref: 465.

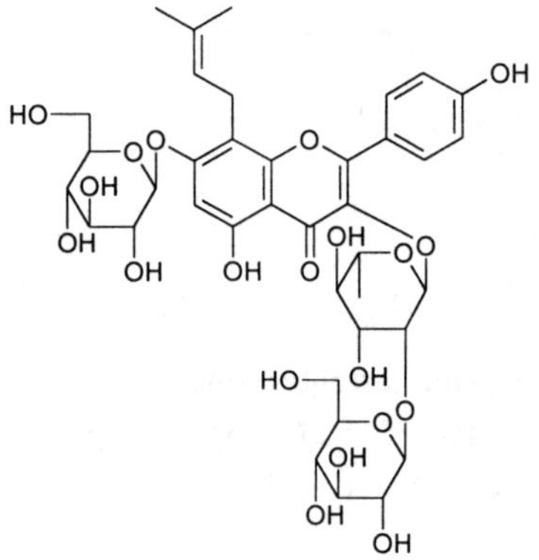

1966 Diphylloside B
$C_{38}H_{48}O_{19}$ MW: 808.79 Property: yellow powder, mp 187-9°C. Source: WAN SHAN YIN YANG HUO, CU MAO YIN YANG HUO. Ref: 465, 624.

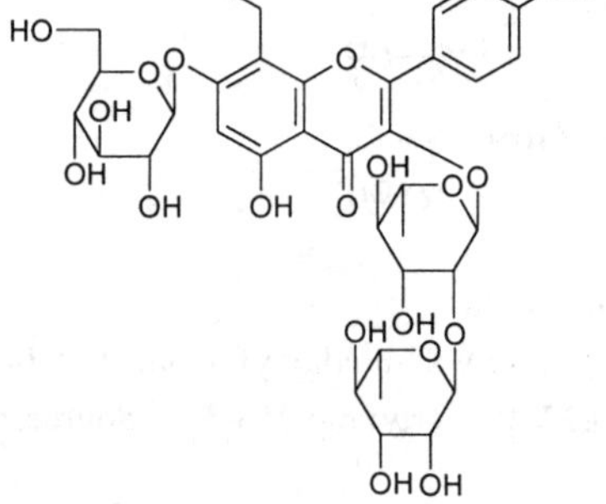

1967 Dipiperitylmagnolol
$C_{38}H_{50}O_2$ MW: 538.82 Source: DU HUO. Ref: 2.

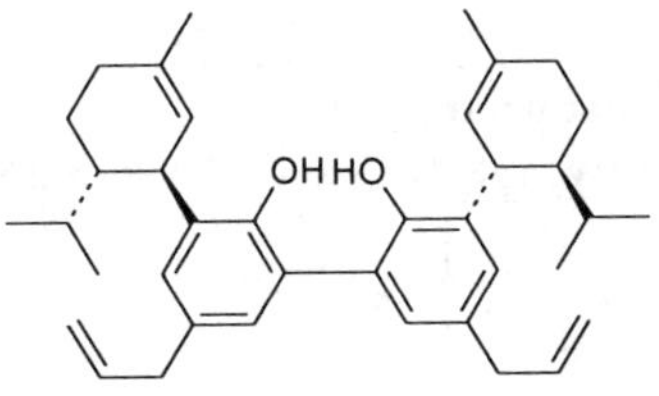

OH HO

1968 Dipropyl disulfide
$C_6H_{14}S_2$ MW: 150.31 Source: DA SUAN. Ref: 2.

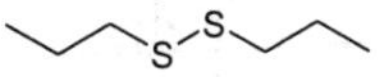

1969 Dipterocarpol
$C_{36}H_{60}O_2$ MW: 524.88 Source: BING PIAN. Ref: 2.

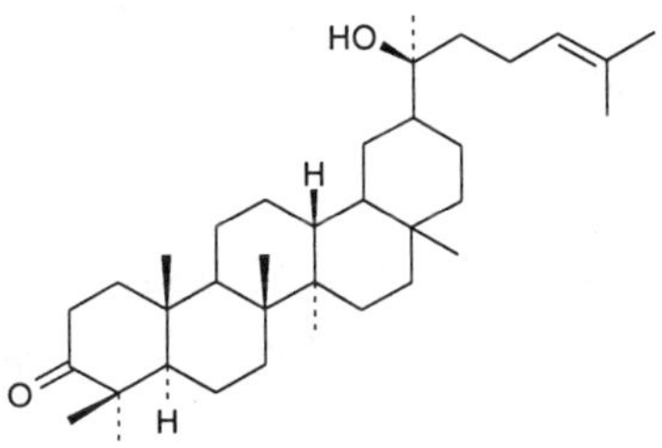

1970 Disacoside B
Source: JIN YIN HUA. Ref: 638.

1971 Disinomenine
$C_{38}H_{44}N_2O_8$ MW: 656.78 Property: mp 222°C.
Source: BIAN FU GE, QING FENG TENG. Ref: 6.

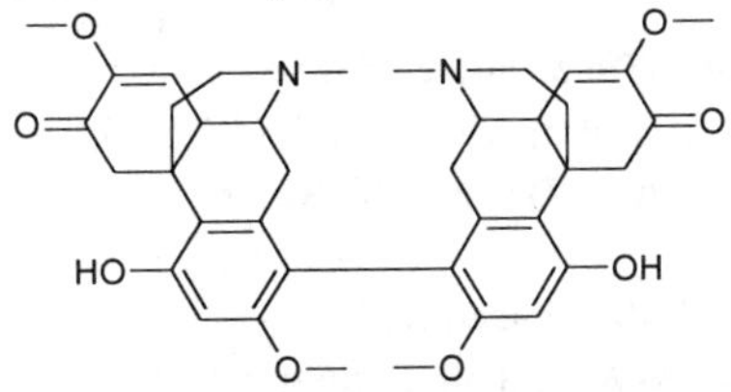

1972 Dispegatrine
$C_{40}H_{48}N_4O_4{\bullet}2Cl^-$ MW: 648.85•70.90 Property: colorless square crystal, mp >280°C(d), $[\alpha]_D^{23}$ +230° (c=0.1, methanol). Source: HAI NAN LUO FU MU. Ref: 46.

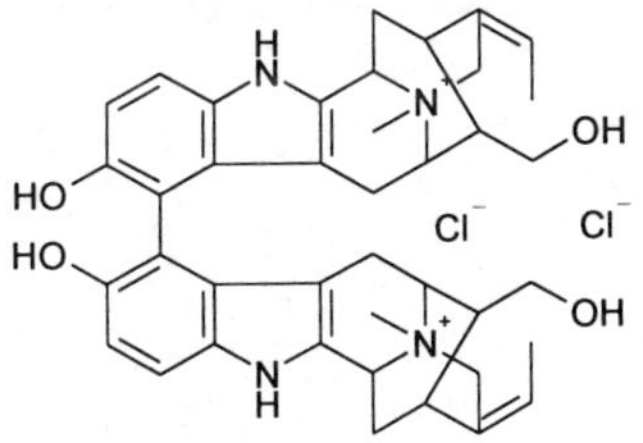

1973 Ditamine
$C_{16}H_{19}NO_2$ MW: 257.34 Property: mp 75°C. Source: XIANG PI MU. Ref: 6.

1974 2,6-Ditertbutyl-4-methyl phenol
$C_{15}H_{24}O$ MW: 220.36 Source: REN SHEN, SAN QI, XI YANG SHEN. Ref: 2.

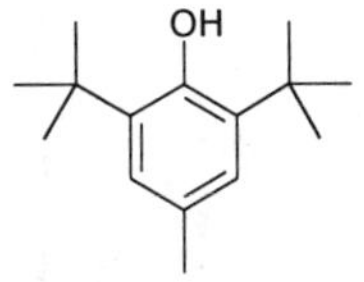

1975 Ditertbutyl phthalate
$C_{16}H_{22}O_4$ MW: 278.35 Source: SAN QI. Ref: 2.

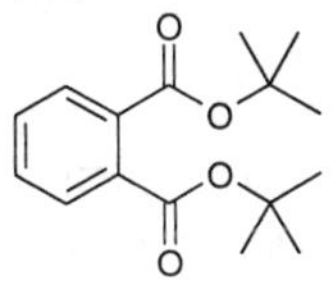

1976 Dithiocyclopentene
$C_3H_4S_2$ MW: 104.19 Source: DA SUAN. Ref: 2.

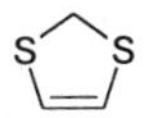

1977 l-3α,6β-Ditigloyloxytropane
$C_{18}H_{29}NO_4$ MW: 323.44 Source: MAN TUO LUO GEN. Ref: 6.

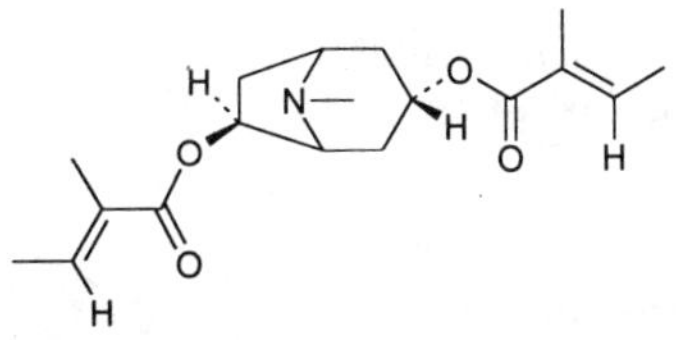

1978 Divaricoside
$C_{31}H_{48}O_8$ MW: 548.72 Property: mp 220-3°C.
Source: YANG JIAO AO ZI. Ref: 4, 6.

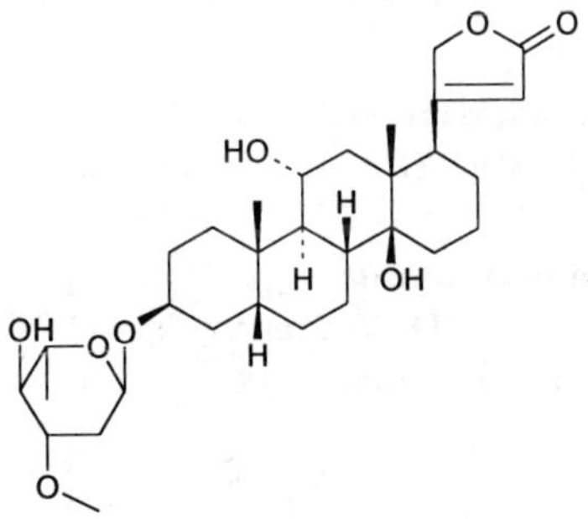

1979 Divinyl sulfide
C_4H_6S MW: 86.16 Source: DA SUAN. Ref: 2.

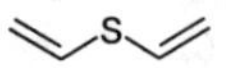

1980 Divostroside
$C_{31}H_{48}O_8$ MW: 548.72 Property: mp 225-31°C. Source: YANG JIAO AO ZI. Ref: 6.

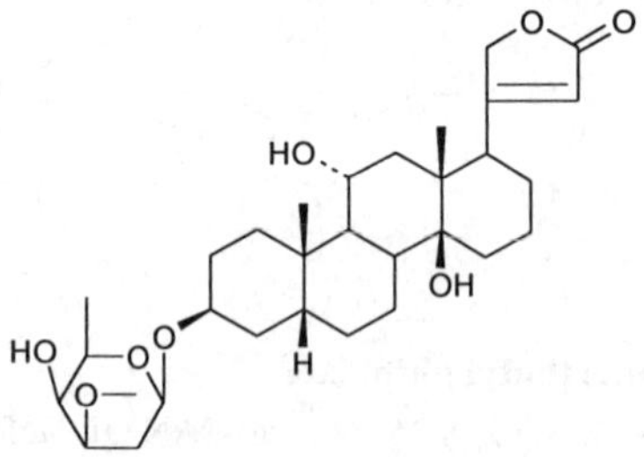

1981 Docosandioic acid
$C_{22}H_{42}O_4$ MW: 370.58 Property: mp 124.2-4.4°C. Source: LIN BEI ZI, QI ZI. Ref: 6.

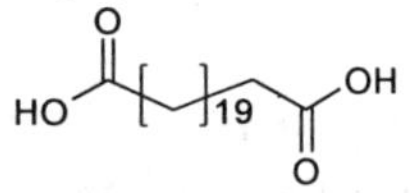

1982 Docosane
$C_{22}H_{46}$ MW: 310.61 Source: DANG SHEN, SAN QI. Ref: 2.

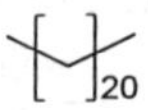

1983 1,22-Docosanediol
Source: MU JIN PI. Ref: 519.

1984 Docosanic acid
$C_{22}H_{44}O_2$ MW: 340.59 Source: BU GU ZHI, GAN DI HUANG, QIANG HUO. Ref: 2.

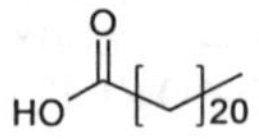

1985 Docosanyl ferulate
Source: GUANG XI XUE JIE. Ref: 616.

1986 Docosyl caffeate
$C_{31}H_{52}O_4$ MW: 488.76 Property: mp 115°C. Source: SHAN DOU GEN. Ref: 6, 408.

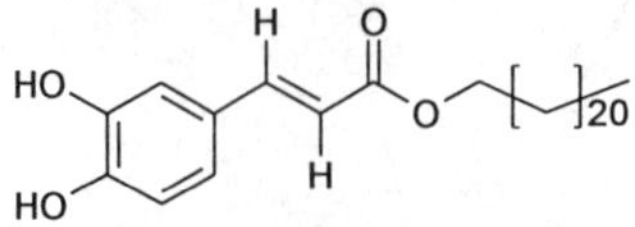

1987 Docosyl hexylate
Source: SHA REN. Ref: 518.

1988 γ-Dodecalactone
$C_{12}H_{22}O_2$ MW: 198.31 Source: XING REN. Ref: 2.

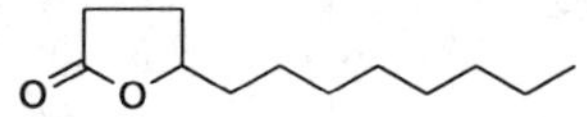

1989 Dodecane
$C_{12}H_{26}$ MW: 170.34 Source: REN SHEN, XI YANG SHEN. Ref: 2.

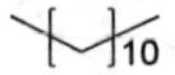

1990 Dodecanoic acid
$C_{12}H_{24}O_2$ MW: 200.32 Source: BING LANG. Ref: 2.

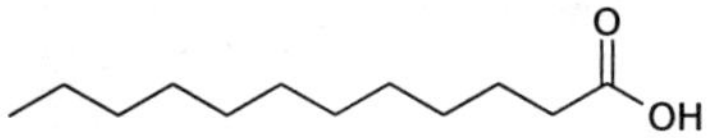

1991 Dodecanol
$C_{12}H_{26}O$ MW: 186.34 Source: DANG GUI. Ref: 2.

1992 Dodecenoic acid
$C_{12}H_{22}O_2$ MW: 198.31 Property: bp 165-8°C/8mm. Source: BING LANG, FU LING, YANG RU. Ref: 2, 6.

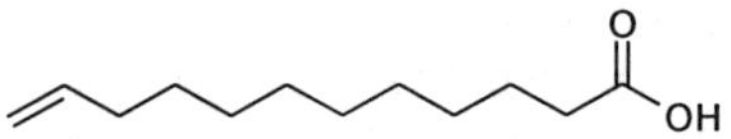

1993 cis-4-Dodecenoic acid
Linderic acid. Property: mp 1-1.3°C, bp 170-2.0°C /13mm. Source: ZHEN CAI. Ref: 6.

1994 n-Dodecyl acetate
$C_{14}H_{28}O_2$ MW: 228.38 Property: bp 150.5-1.5°C /15mm. Source: HEI MA YI. Ref: 6.

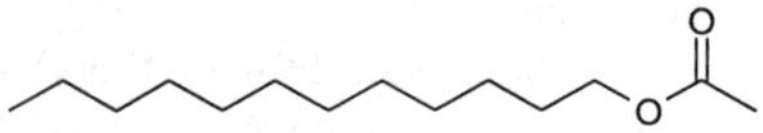

1995 Dodecyl isopropyl ether
$C_{15}H_{32}O$ MW: 228.42 Source: DU HUO. Ref: 2.

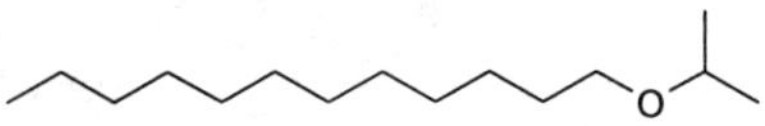

1996 Doederleinic acid
7(β)-Oxa-bicyclo-[4,1,0]-hept-3-ene-3-carboxylic acid-5(β)-hydroxy. $C_7H_8O_4$ MW: 156.14 Property: white granular powder, mp 185-6°C, $[\alpha]_D^{10}$ -13.8° (c= 0.2, EtOH). Source: DA YE CAI. Ref: 484.

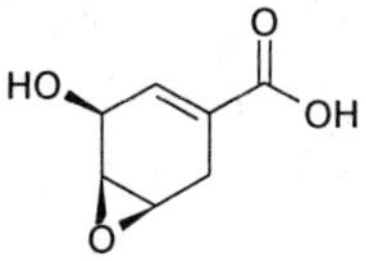

1997 Dolineone
$C_{19}H_{12}O_6$ MW: 336.30 Property: mp 233-5°C. Source: DI GUA ZI. Ref: 6.

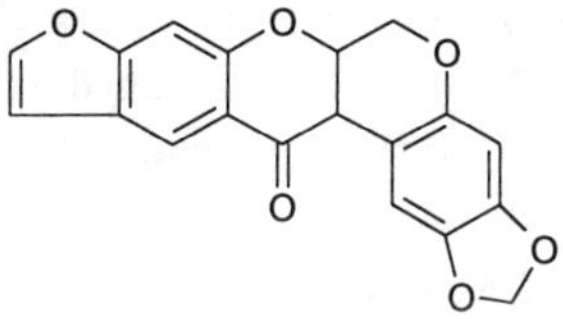

1998 Domesticine
$C_{19}H_{19}NO_4$ MW: 325.37 Property: mp 115-7°C. Source: NAN TIAN ZHU ZI, NAN TIAN ZHU GEN, NAN TIAN ZHU GENG. Ref: 4, 6.

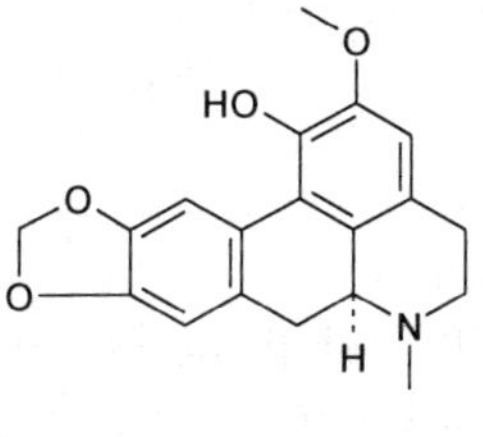

1999 Dongnoside C
$C_{50}H_{82}O_{22}$ MW: 1035.20 Source: DONG YI HAO JIAN MA, precipitate from fermented juice. Ref: 10.

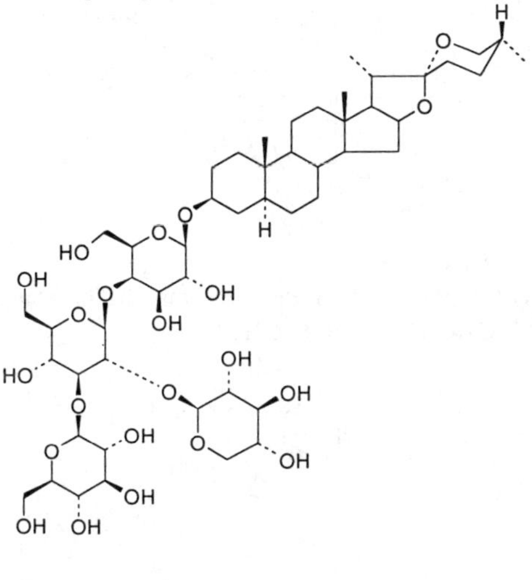

2000 Dongnoside D
$C_{55}H_{90}O_{26}$ MW: 1167.31 Source: DONG YI HAO JIAN MA. Ref: 10.

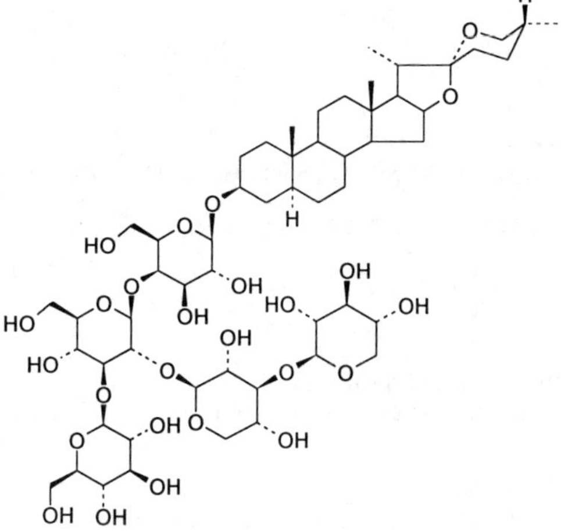

2001 Dongnoside E
$C_{56}H_{92}O_{26}$ MW: 1181.34 Source: DONG YI HAO JIAN MA. Ref: 10.

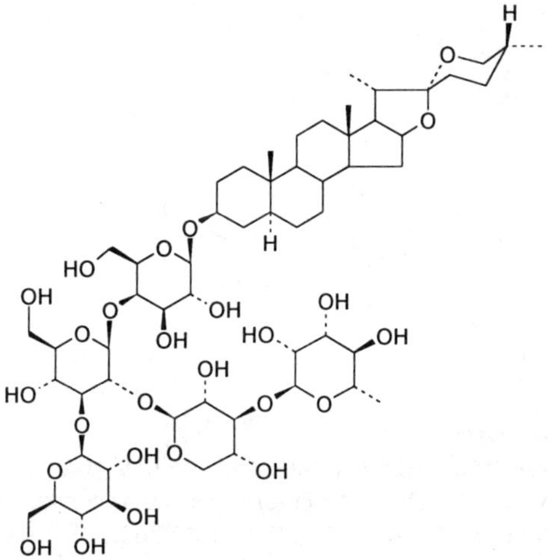

2002 Dopa
L-3,4-Dihydroxyphenylalanine. $C_9H_{11}NO_4$ MW: 197.19 Property: mp (-): 283°C, (±): 271-2°C (dec). Source: CAN DOU YE, CAN DOU KE, LI DOU, MA CHI XIAN, XU SUI ZI JING ZHONG BAI ZHI. Ref: 6.

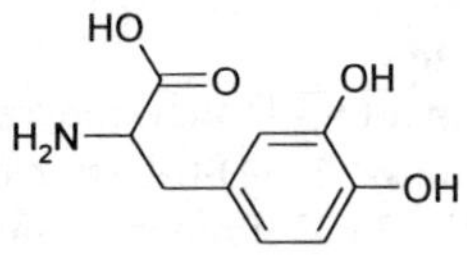

2003 Dopamine
$C_8H_{11}NO_2$ MW: 153.18 Source: MA CHI XIAN, XIANG JIAO. Ref: 6.

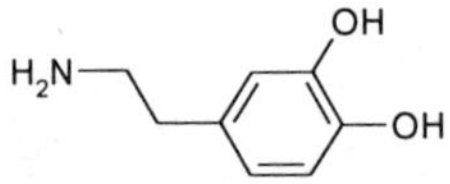

2004 Doradexanthin
$C_{40}H_{54}O_3$ MW: 582.87 Source: LI YU PI. Ref: 6.

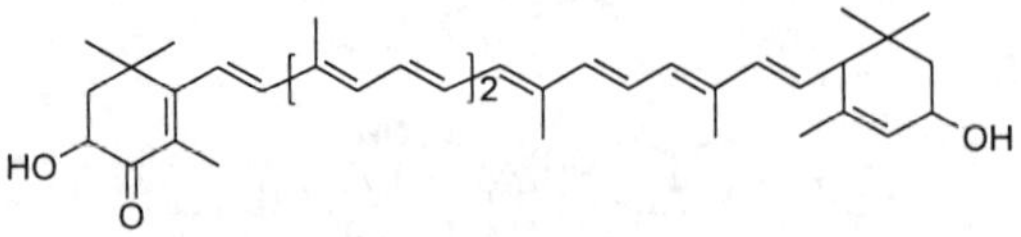

2005 Dotriacontanic acid
Source: HUI BAO HAO. Ref: 503.

2006 Dregeoside B
12,20-Di-O-isovaleryl-tomentogenin-3-O-α-L-oleandropyranosyl-(1→4)-O-α-L-oleandropyranoside. $C_{45}H_{76}O_{13}$ MW: 825.10 Property: white powder, mp 123-6°C, $[\alpha]_D^{20}$ +38.5° (c=0.25, methanol). Source: KU SHENG. Ref: 165.

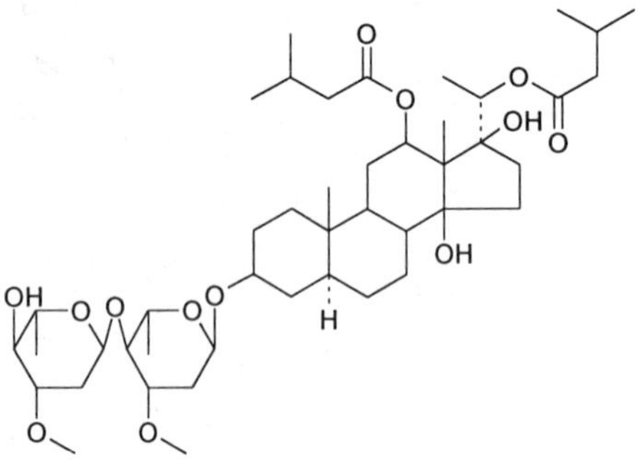

2007 Dresigenin B
20-O-(2-methylbutyryl)-tomentogenin. $C_{26}H_{44}O_6$ MW: 452.64 Property: colorless acicular crystal, mp 232-235°C. Source: KU YING. Ref: 363.

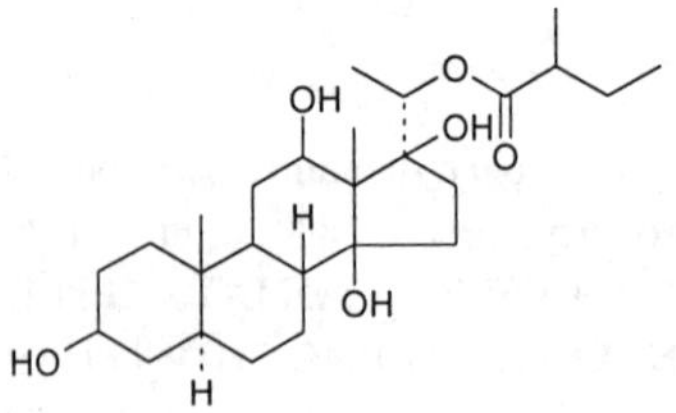

2008 Dresioside I
Dihydrosarcostin 3-O-β-D-thevetopyranosyl(1→4)-β-D-oleandropyranosyl(1→4)-β-D-cymaropyrano-side. $C_{42}H_{72}O_{16}$ MW: 833.03 Property: white amorphous powder, mp 151-4°C. Source: KU YING. Ref: 363.

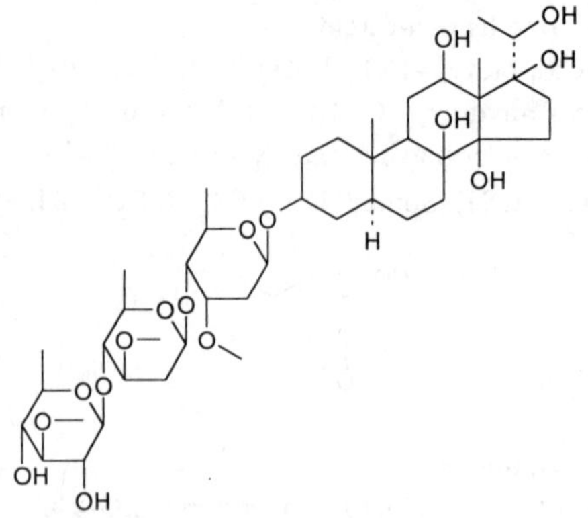

2009 Drevodein I
C/D cis 5α-H,3β,8β,14β,17β tetrahydroxy-12β-O-isovaleryl-20-O-isovaleryl-pregnane. $C_{31}H_{52}O_8$ MW: 552.76 Property: prismatic crystal, mp 235-8°C, $[\alpha]_D^{25}$ +34.5° (c=0.15 MeOH). Source: KU SHENG. Ref: 134.

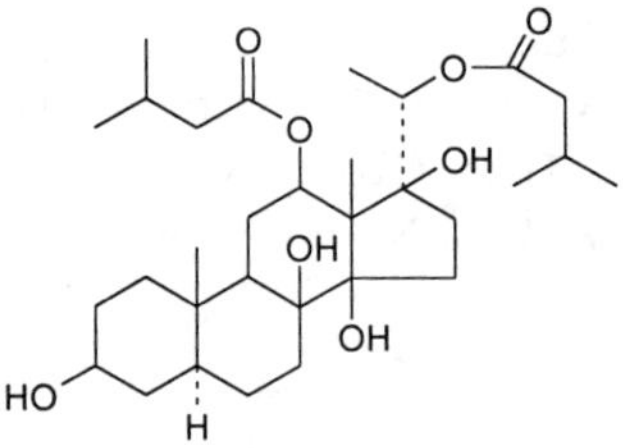

2010 Drevodein II
C/D cis 5α-H,3β,14β,17β trihydroxy-12β-O-acetyl-20-O-benzoyl-pregnane. $C_{30}H_{42}O_7$ MW: 514.67 Property: prismatic crystal, mp 235-7°C, $[\alpha]_D^{25}$ +36.5° (c=0.52, MeOH). Source: KU SHENG. Ref: 134.

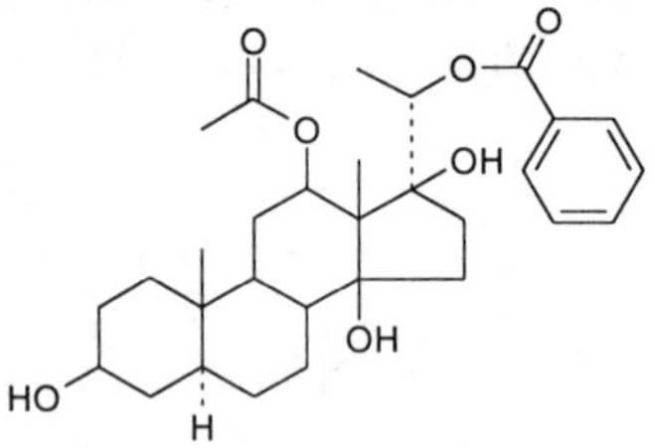

2011 Droserone
$C_{11}H_8O_4$ MW: 204.18 Property: mp 181°C. Source: MAO GAO CAI. Ref: 6, 621.

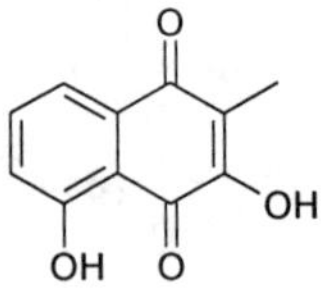

2012 Drupacine
$C_{18}H_{21}NO_5$ MW: 331.37 Source: SAN JIAN SHAN. Ref: 2.

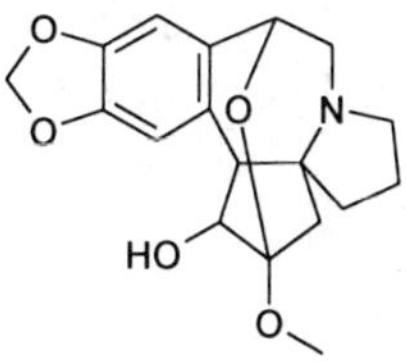

2013 Dryobalanone
$C_{30}H_{50}O_3$ MW: 458.73 Source: BING PIAN. Ref: 2.

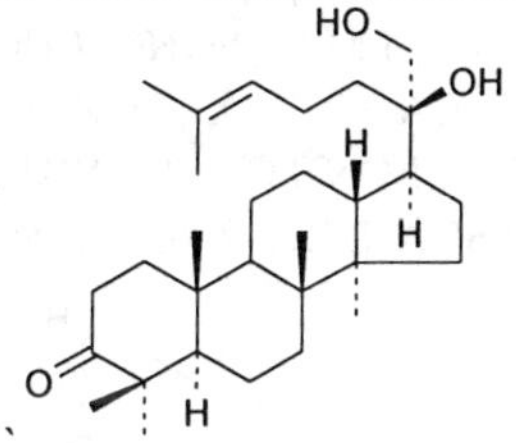

2014 Ducheside A
3'-O-methyl-ellagic acid-4-O-β-D-xylopyranoside. $C_{20}H_{16}O_{12}$ MW: 448.34 Property: light yellow powder, mp >360°C, $[\alpha]_D^{18}$ -11.3° (c=0.035, methanol). Source: SHE MEI. Ref: 368.

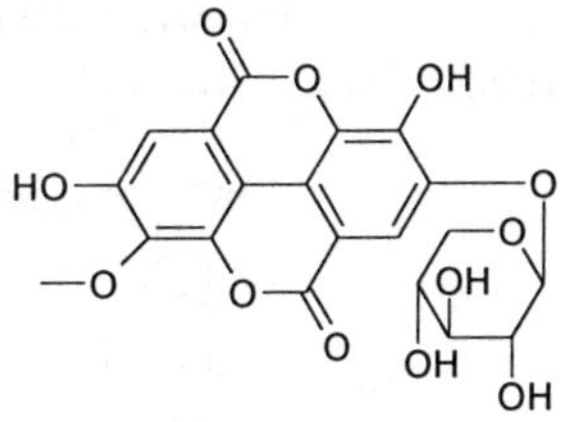

2015 Ducheside B
3'-O-methyl-ellagic acid-4-O-α-L-arabinofuranoside. $C_{19}H_{14}O_{12}$ MW: 434.32 Property: light yellow powder, mp >360°C, $[\alpha]_D^{19}$ -126.5° (c=0.027, methanol). Source: SHE MEI. Ref: 368.

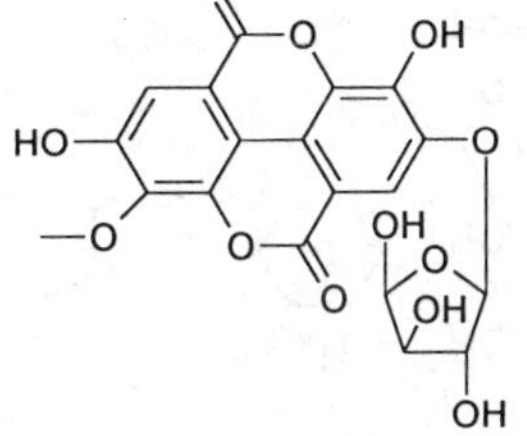

2016 Dulcitol
$C_6H_{14}O_6$ MW: 182.17 Property: mp 188.5°C, bp 275-80°C/1mm. Source: FU FANG TENG, GUI JIAN YU, HAI HONG DOU, LEI GONG TENG, SI MIAN MU, SUO LA MU. Ref: 2, 6.

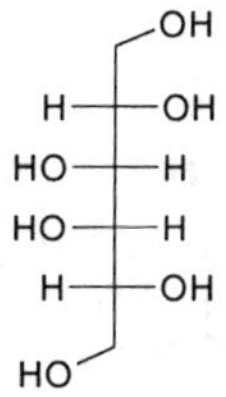

2017 Ebelin lactone
$C_{30}H_{46}O_3$ MW: 454.70 Property: mp 182-5°C. Source: SUAN ZAO REN. Ref: 2.

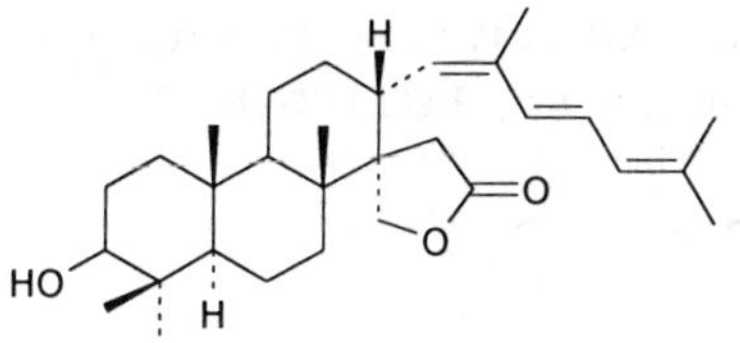

2018 Ebracteolatanolide A
$C_{20}H_{28}O_4$ MW: 332.44 Property: white acicular crystal, mp 210°C. Source: YUE XIAN DA JI. Ref: 404.

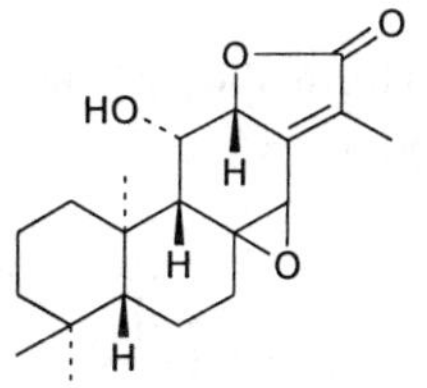

2019 Ebracteolatanolide B
$C_{20}H_{30}O_5$ MW: 350.46 Property: white acicular crystal, mp 218°C. Source: YUE XIAN DA JI. Ref: 404.

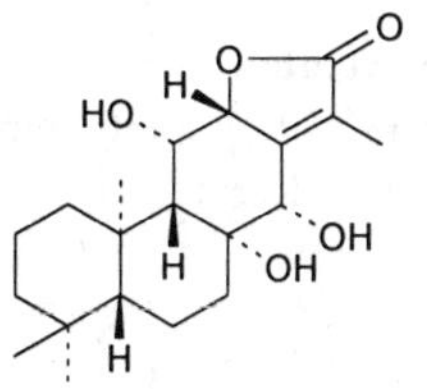

2020 Eburical
$C_{31}H_{50}O_2$ MW: 454.74 Source: A LI HONG. Ref: 6.

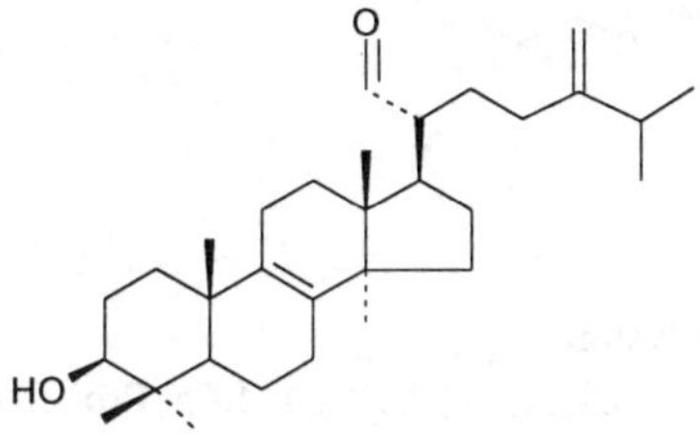

2021 Eburicodiol
$C_{31}H_{52}O_2$ MW: 456.76 Source: A LI HONG. Ref: 6.

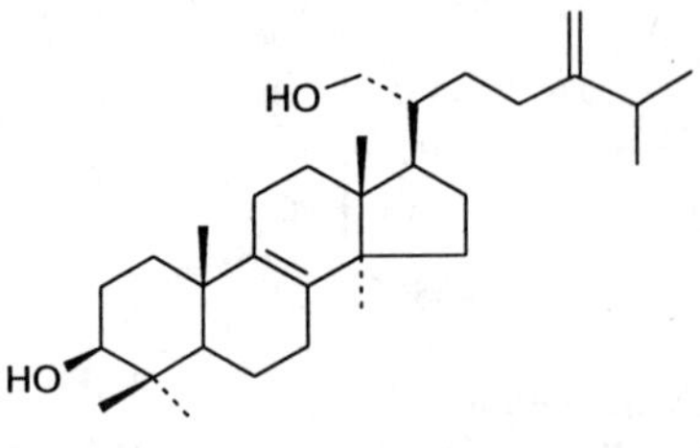

2022 Eburicoic acid
$C_{31}H_{50}O_3$ MW: 470.74 Property: mp 292-3°C. Source: A LI HONG, FU LING. Ref: 2.

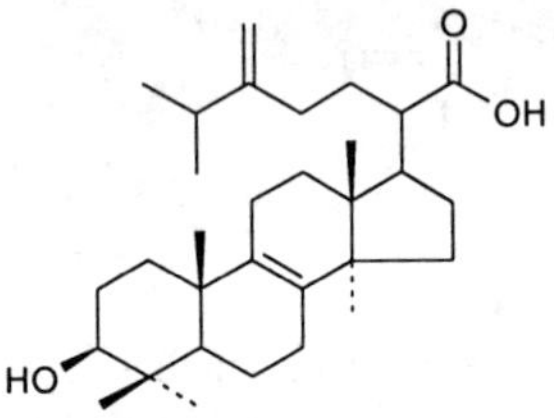

2023 Eburicol
$C_{31}H_{52}O$ MW: 440.76 Property: mp 158-9°C. Source: A LI HONG. Ref: 6.

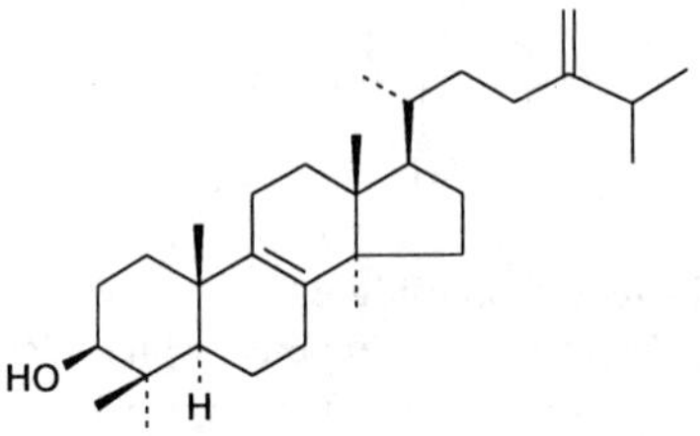

2024 Eburicyl acetate
$C_{33}H_{54}O_2$ MW: 482.80 Property: mp 142-3°C. Source: A LI HONG. Ref: 6.

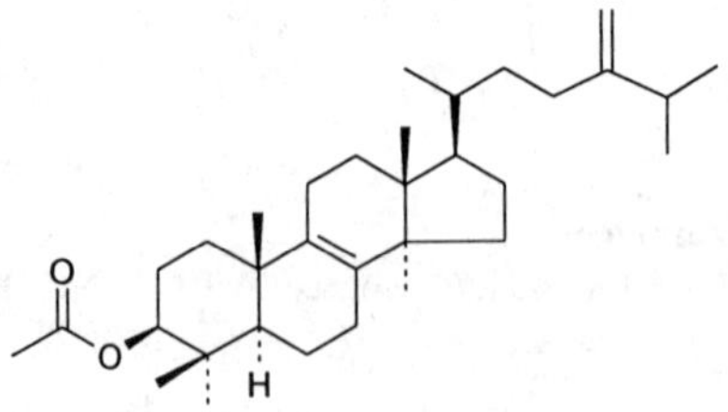

2025 Ecdysone
α-Ecdysone. $C_{27}H_{44}O_6$ MW: 464.65 Property: mp 242°C. Source: GUAN ZHONG, LUO YAN CAO, SHUI LONG GU, YUAN CAN E. Ref: 6.

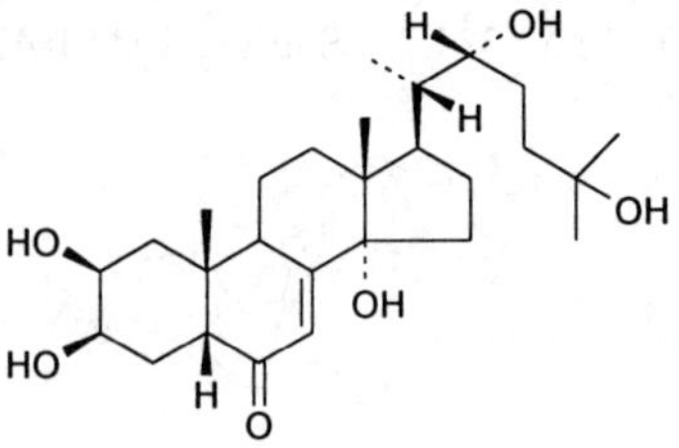

2026 Ecdysterone
β-Ecdysone. $C_{27}H_{44}O_7$ MW: 480.65 Property: mp 237.5-9.5°C. Source: BAI MAO XIA KU, GUAN ZHONG, NIU XI, JI MAO SONG, LUO HAN SONG YE, LUO YAN CAO, NIU XI, QI ZHOU LOU LU, SANG YE, SHUI LONG GU, TU NIU XI, WA WEI, YU ER QI, ZI SHAN. Ref: 2, 6, 194, 580, 582.

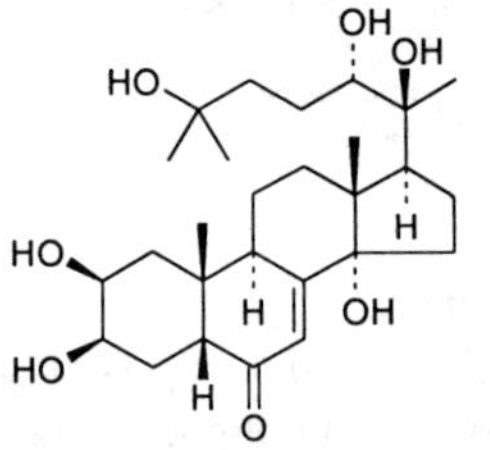

2027 Ecdysterone-3-O-β-D-glucopyranoside
$C_{32}H_{52}O_{12}$ MW: 628.76 Property: white powder. Source: QI ZHOU LOU LU. Ref: 444.

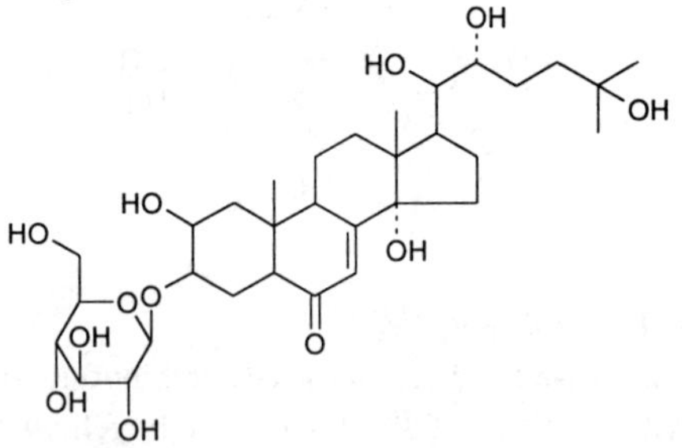

2028 Echinacoside
Source: GAN DI HUANG, ROU CONG RONG. Ref: 2, 628.

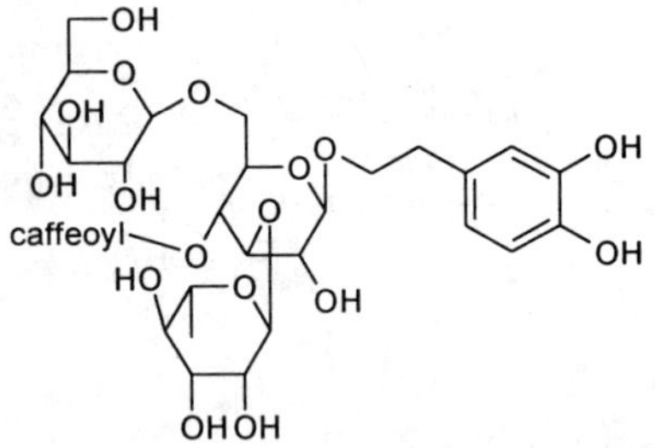

2029 Echinatine

$C_{15}H_{25}NO_5$ MW: 299.37 Property: mp 109-10°C. Source: GOU SHI HUA, YAO YONG DAO TI HU. Ref: 6.

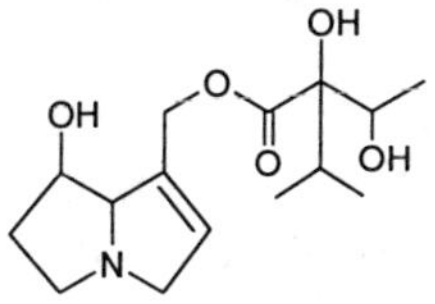

2030 Echinenone

$C_{40}H_{54}O$ MW: 550.88 Property: mp 192-3°C. Source: HAI XIA. Ref: 6.

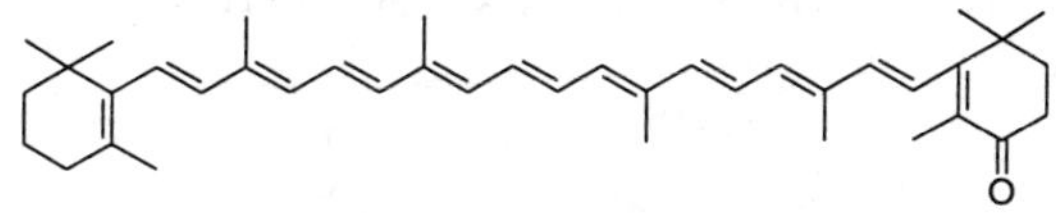

2031 Echinine

$C_{11}H_{13}NO_2$ MW: 191.23 Source: LOU LU. Ref: 6.

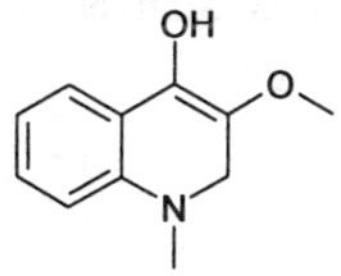

2032 Echinopsine

CAS: 83-54-5 $C_{10}H_9NO$ MW: 159.19 Property: mp α: 152°C, β: 135°C. Source: LOU LU. Ref: 4, 6.

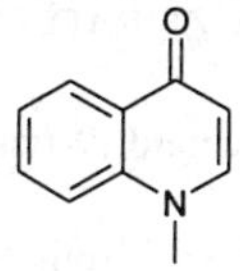

2033 Echinorine

$C_{11}H_{12}NO$ MW: 174.24 Source: LOU LU. Ref: 6.

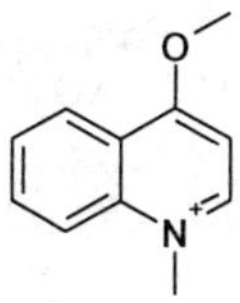

2034 Echitamidine

$C_{21}H_{26}N_2O_3$ MW: 354.45 Property: mp 244°C (dec). Source: DAI YAO XIAO DENG TAI, XIANG PI MU. Ref: 6, 270.

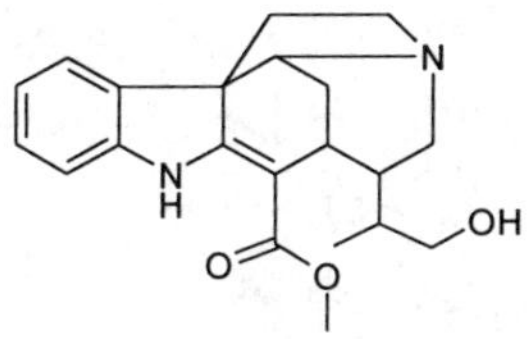

2035 Echitamine

$C_{22}H_{29}N_2O_4$ MW: 385.49 Source: XIANG PI MU. Ref: 6.

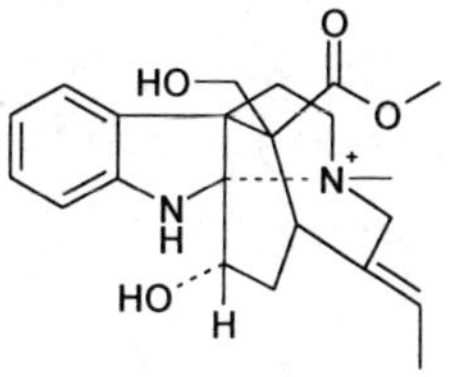

2036 Ecliptasaponin

$C_{36}H_{58}O_9$ MW: 634.86 Property: white powder, mp 240-3°C. Source: HAN LIAN CAO. Ref: 392.

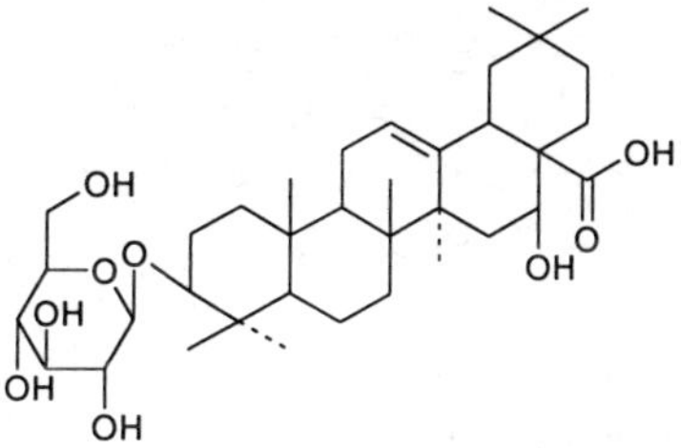

2037 Ecliptasaponin A

3β,16α-dihydroxyolean-12-ene-28-oic acid-3-O-β-D-glucopyranoside. $C_{36}H_{58}O_9$ MW: 634.86 Property: white acicular crystal, mp 237-8°C (methanol). Source: HAN LIAN CAO. Ref: 349.

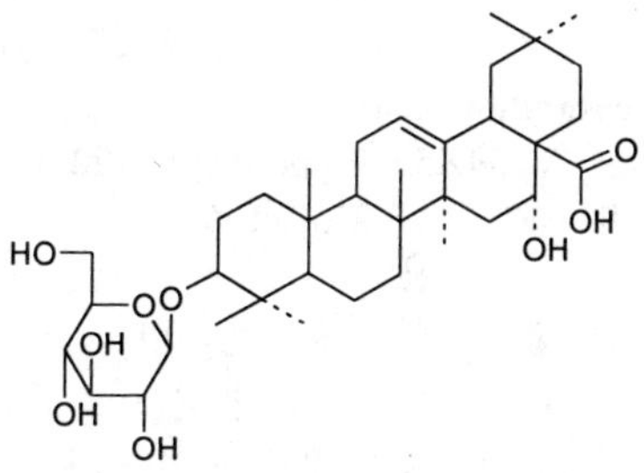

2038 Ecliptasaponin B

3β-O-(β-D-glucopyranosyl(1-4)-β-D-glucopyranosyl-16α-hydroxyolean-12-ene-28-oic acid-28-O-β-D-glucopyranoside. $C_{48}H_{78}O_{19}$ MW: 959.15 Property: white acicular crystal, mp 220-1°C (methanol). Source: HAN LIAN CAO. Ref: 349.

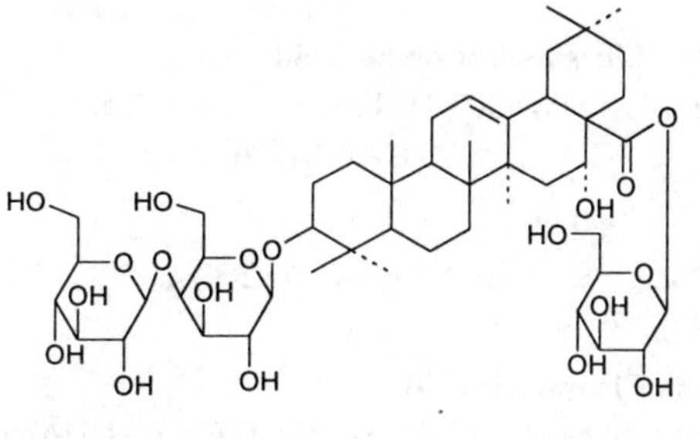

2039 Edulinine
$C_{16}H_{21}NO_4$ MW: 291.35 Property: mp 140-2°C. Source: CHOU CAO. Ref: 6.

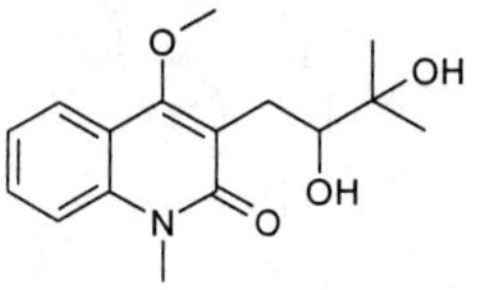

2040 Edultin
Cnidimine. $C_{21}H_{22}O_7$ MW: 386.41 Source: SHE CHUANG ZI. Ref: 6.

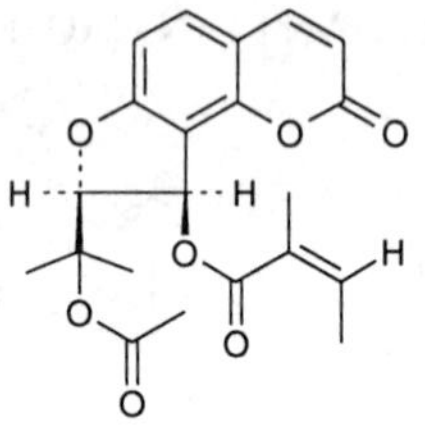

2041 Egomaketone
$C_{10}H_{12}O_2$ MW: 164.21 Property: bp 124-6°C/20mm. Source: BAI SU ZI. Ref: 6.

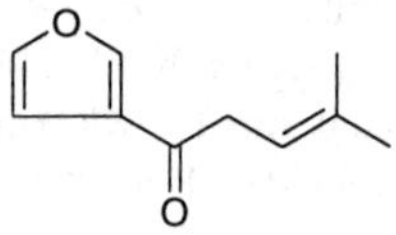

2042 Eicosandioic acid
$C_{20}H_{38}O_4$ MW: 342.52 Property: mp 122-3°C. Source: LIN BEI ZI, QI ZI. Ref: 6.

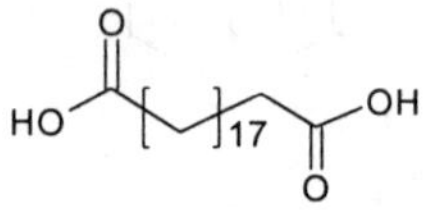

2043 Eicosane
$C_{20}H_{42}$ MW: 282.56 Source: DONG CHONG XIA CAO, REN SHEN, ROU CONG RONG, SAN QI. Ref: 2.

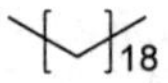

2044 Eicosanetetraenoic acid
$C_{20}H_{32}O_2$ MW: 304.48 Property: mp -49.5°C. Source: NIU GAN, ZI CAI. Ref: 6.

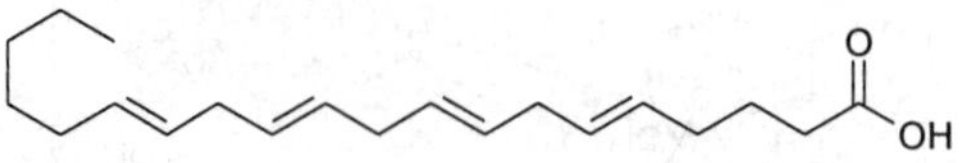

2045 Eicosanoic acid
$C_{20}H_{40}O_2$ MW: 312.54 Source: GAN DI HUANG, GUANG JIN QIAN CAO, QIANG HUO, XING REN. Ref: 2, 260.

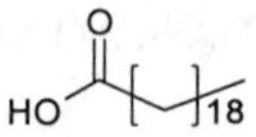

2046 Eicosanol
$C_{20}H_{42}O$ MW: 298.56 Property: mp 65.5°C, bp 220°C/3mm. Source: KU CAO (I). Ref: 6.

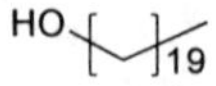

2047 11-Eicosenoic acid
$C_{20}H_{38}O_2$ MW: 310.52 Source: QIANG HUO. Ref: 2.

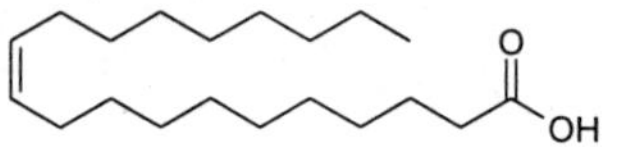

2048 Eicosyl ferulate
$C_{30}H_{50}O_4$ MW: 474.73 Source: YA MA ZI. Ref: 6.

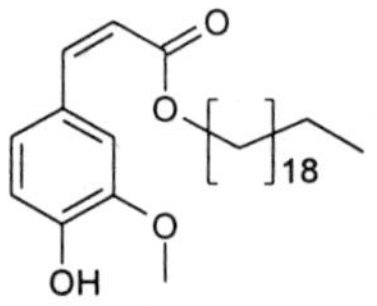

2049 α-Elaeostearic acid (9-cis,11-trans,13-trans)
α-Eleostearic acid. Property: mp 49.0-49.2°C. Source: BI MA YE, KU GUA ZI, PAO TONG GUO. Ref: 6.

2050 β-Elaeostearic acid (9-trans,11-trans,13-trans)
Property: mp 71.0-71.5°C. Source: BI MA YE, KU GUA ZI, PAO TONG GUO. Ref: 6.

2051 Elaidic acid
$C_{18}H_{34}O_2$ MW: 282.47 Property: mp 44.5°C. Source: DENG LONG CAO, HU TAO YE. Ref: 6.

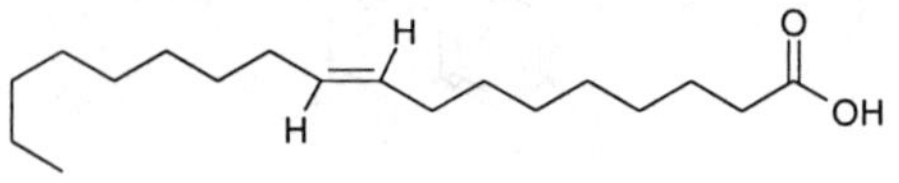

2052 Elaterin
$C_{32}H_{46}O_8$ MW: 558.72 Property: mp 234°C. Source: GUA DI, SI GUA ZI. Ref: 6.

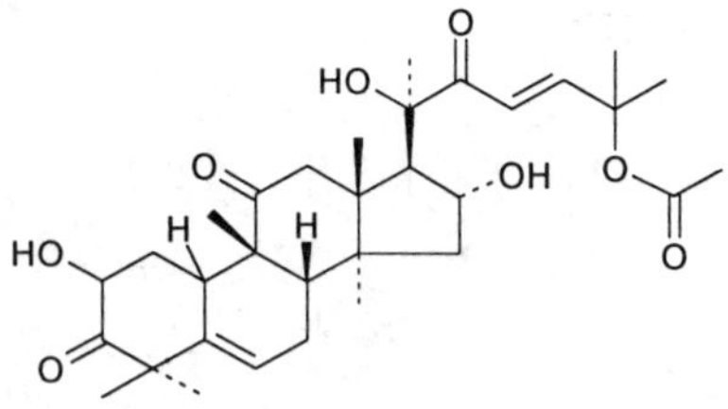

2053 Elatine
$C_{39}H_{52}N_2O_{10}$ MW: 708.86 Property: mp 233-5°C.
Source: FEI YAN CAO. Ref: 6.

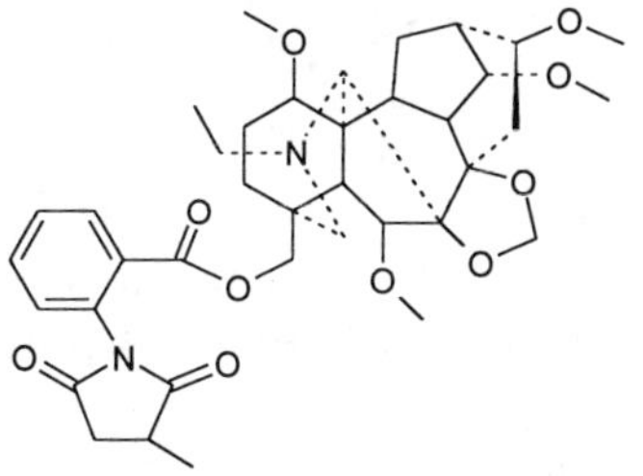

2054 Eleagnine
$C_{12}H_{14}N_2$ MW: 186.26 Property: mp 180-1.5°C.
Source: LU ZHU GEN, SHA ZAO SHU PI. Ref: 6.

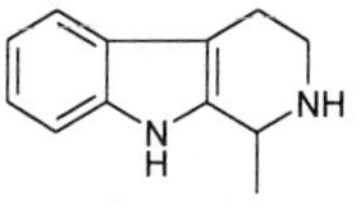

2055 Elegansamine
$C_{29}H_{36}N_2O_6$ MW: 508.62 Property: mp 172-3°C.
Source: GOU WEN. Ref: 13.

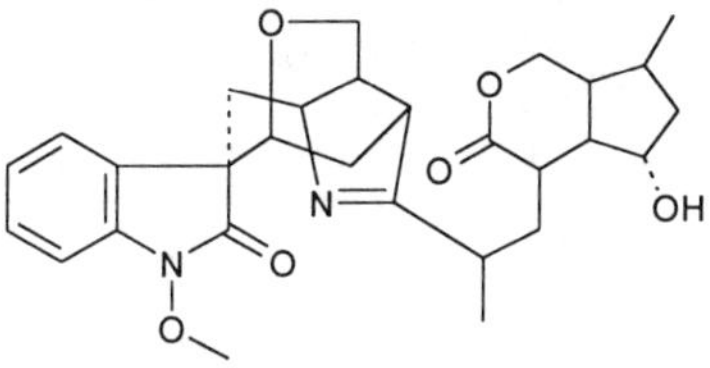

2056 β-Elemene
CAS: 515-13-9 $C_{15}H_{24}$ MW: 204.36 Property: bp 117-24°C/15.5mm. Source: BING PIAN, CHAU HU, DONG LING CAO, DU HUO, HUO XIANG, JIN JIE, QING HAO, REN SHEN, SAN QI, SHENG JIANG, WU WEI ZI, YIN CHEN HAO, etc. Ref: 2, 5.

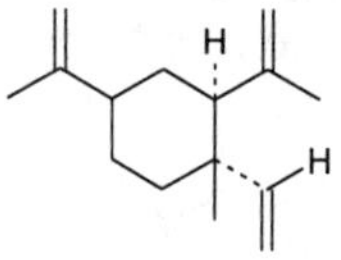

2057 γ-Elemene
Source: QING HAO, REN SHEN, SAN QI, SHENG JIANG. Ref: 2.

2058 δ-Elemene
$C_{15}H_{24}$ MW: 204.36 Property: bp 107°C/10mm.
Source: REN SHEN. Ref: 2.

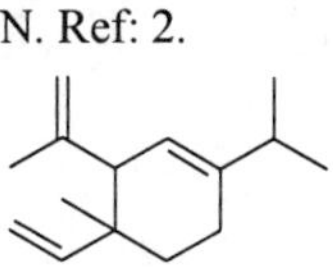

2059 Elemicin
$C_{12}H_{16}O_3$ MW: 208.26 Property: bp 144-7°C/10mm.
Source: SHAN ZHU YU, XI XIN, ZI SU. Ref: 2.

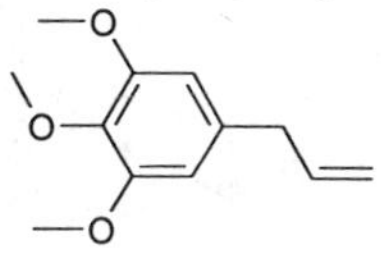

2060 Elemol
$C_{15}H_{26}O$ MW: 222.37 Property: mp 52.5-3.5°C.
Source: CANG ZHU, HOU PO, SHENG JIANG.
Ref: 2.

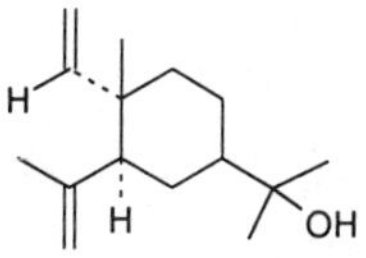

2061 α-Eleostearin
$C_{57}H_{92}O_6$ MW: 873.37 Source: TONG YOU. Ref: 6.

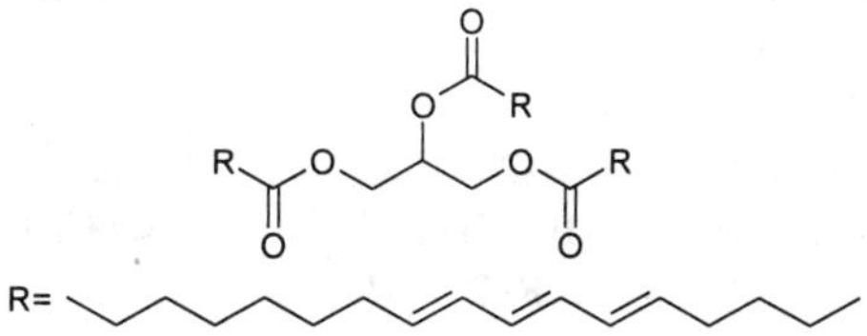

2062 Eleutheroside B1
7-Hydroxy-6,8-dimethoxycoumarin glucoside.
$C_{17}H_{20}O_{10}$ MW: 384.34 Property: mp 218°C. Source: WU JIA PI. Ref: 6.

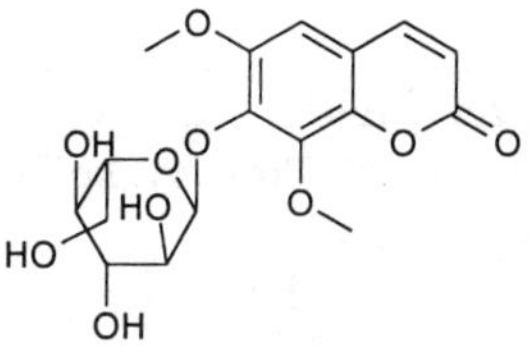

2063 Eleutheroside I
$C_{41}H_{66}O_{11}$ MW: 734.98 Source: WU JIA YE. Ref: 6.

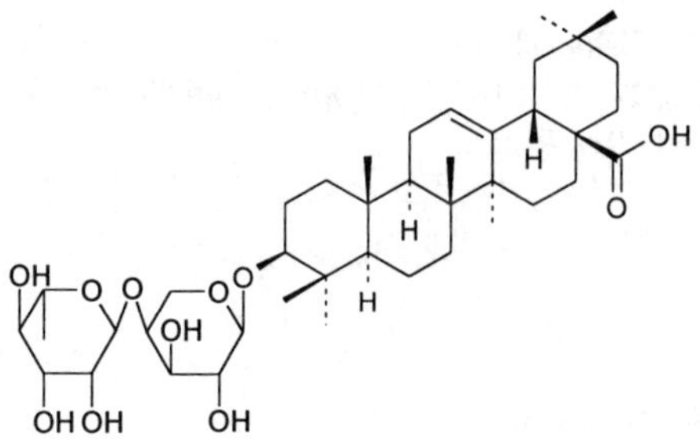

2064 Eleutheroside K
$C_{41}H_{66}O_{11}$ MW: 734.98 Source: WU JIA YE. Ref: 6.

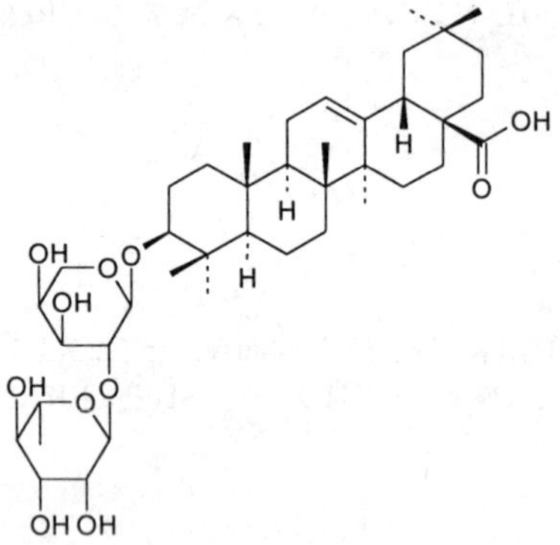

2065 Eleutheroside L
Source: WU JIA YE. Ref: 6.

2066 Eleutheroside M
Source: WU JIA YE. Ref: 6.

2067 Ellagic acid
CAS: 476-66-4 $C_{14}H_6O_8$ MW: 302.20 Property: mp >360°C. Source: SHU ZHANG LAO GUAN CAO, XIAN HE CAO, etc. Ref: 6, 71.

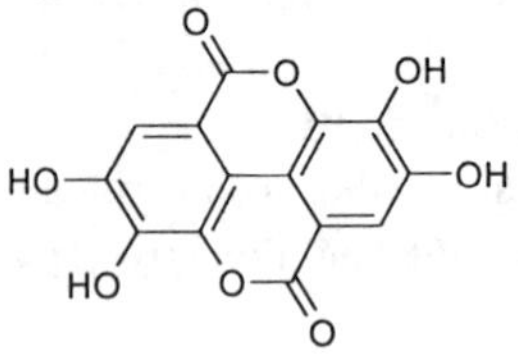

2068 Elsholtzia ketone
$C_{10}H_{14}O_2$ MW: 166.22 Property: bp 210°C. Source: BAN BIAN SU. Ref: 6.

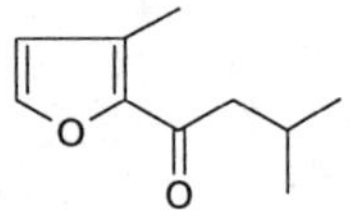

2069 Elsholtzidiol
$C_{10}H_{16}O_3$ MW: 184.24 Property: mp 58-9°C. Source: XIANG RU. Ref: 6.

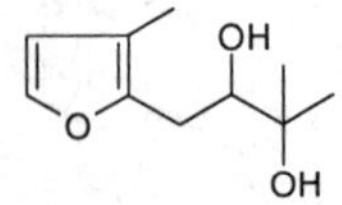

2070 Elymoclavine
$C_{16}H_{18}N_2O$ MW: 254.33 Property: mp 250-2°C. Source: MAI JIAO, QIAN NIU ZI. Ref: 6.

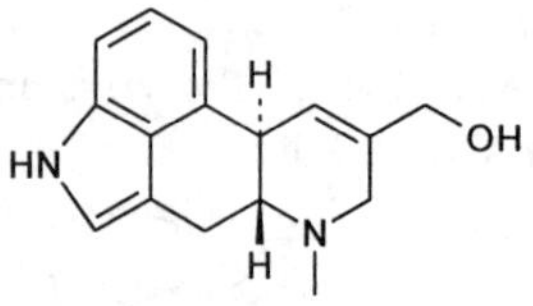

2071 Embelin
$C_{17}H_{26}O_4$ MW: 294.39 Property: mp 143°C. Source: DA HONG PAO, MA GUI HUA, WEI LING XIAN. Ref: 6.

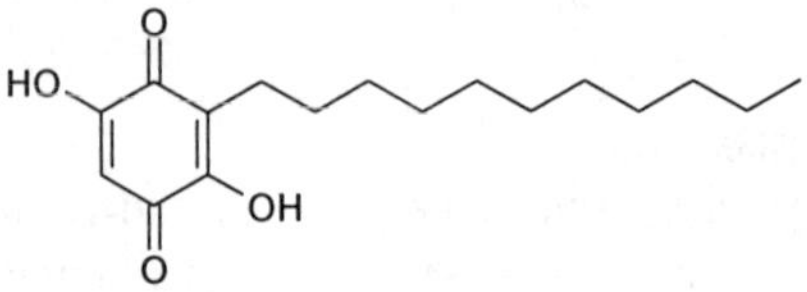

2072 Embinin
$C_{29}H_{34}O_{14}$ MW: 606.59 Property: mp 181°C. Source: HU DIE HUA, YUAN WEI. Ref: 6.

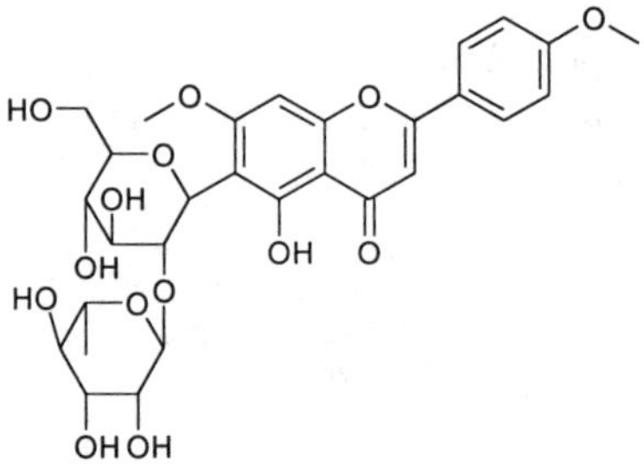

2073 Emodin
CAS: 518-82-1 $C_{15}H_{10}O_5$ MW: 270.24 Property: orange red prismatic crystal, mp 250-7°C. Source: BAI HE HUA, CHAO XIAN YIN YANG HUO, DA HUANG, HE SHOU WU, HU ZHANG, JUE MING ZI, TIAN SHAN DA HUANG. Ref: 2, 4, 458, 511, 608.

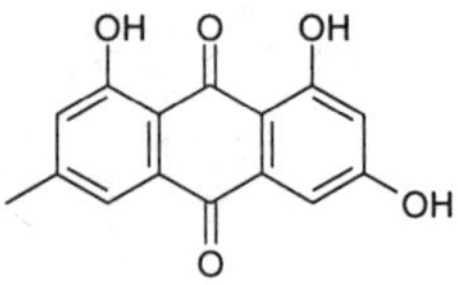

2074 Emodin anthrone
$C_{15}H_{12}O_4$ MW: 256.26 Property: mp 236°C. Source: JUE MING ZI. Ref: 2, 6.

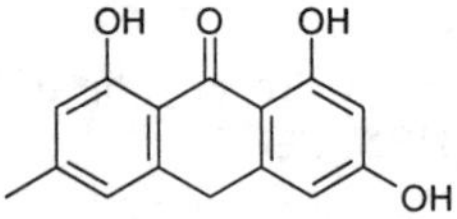

2075 Emodin-1-O-β-D-glucopyranoside

$C_{21}H_{20}O_{10}$ MW: 432.39 Source: DA HUANG. Ref: 2.

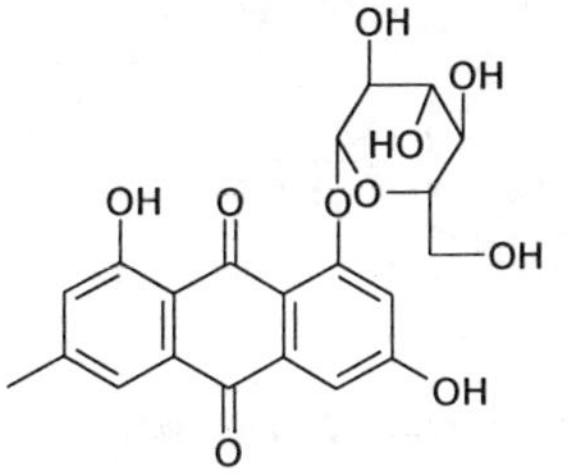

2077 Emodin-6-glucoside

$C_{21}H_{20}O_{10}$ MW: 432.39 Source: JUE MING ZI. Ref: 2.

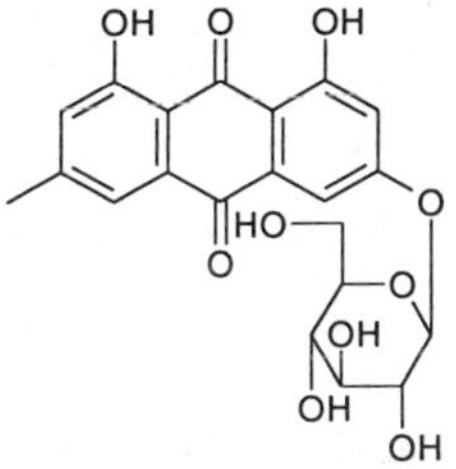

2078 Emodin-1-monomethyl ether

$C_{16}H_{12}O_5$ MW: 284.27 Property: mp 301-3°C. Source: NIU XI XI, HE SHOU WU, HU ZHANG, YE JIAO TENG. Ref: 6.

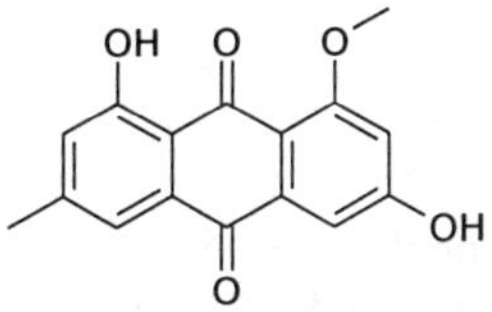

2079 Emodin-3-monomethyl ether

$C_{16}H_{12}O_5$ MW: 284.27 Property: mp 206-7°C. Source: NIU XI XI, HE SHOU WU, HU ZHANG, YE JIAO TENG. Ref: 6.

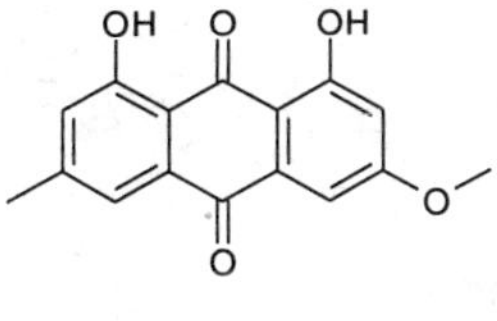

2080 Enanthic acid

$C_7H_{14}O_2$ MW: 130.19 Source: DANG SHEN. Ref: 2.

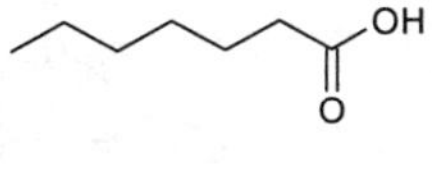

2081 5-Ene-methyl-cholate-3-O-β-D-glucopyranoside

$C_{31}H_{50}O_5$ MW: 550.74 Property: white lamellar crystal, mp 201-5°C, soluable in methanol. Source: SAN LENG. Ref: 497.

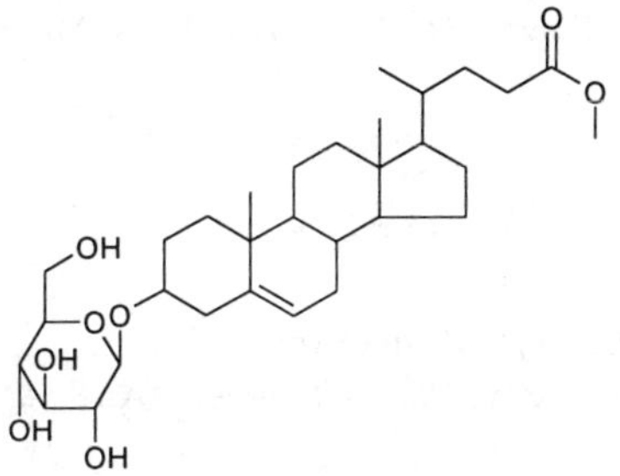

2082 5-Ene-methyl-cholate-3-O-β-D-glucuronopyranosyl-(14)-α-L- rhamnopyranoside

$C_{37}H_{58}O_{13}$ MW: 710.8 Property: white amorphous powder, mp 215-9°C, soluable in methanol. Source: SAN LENG. Ref: 497.

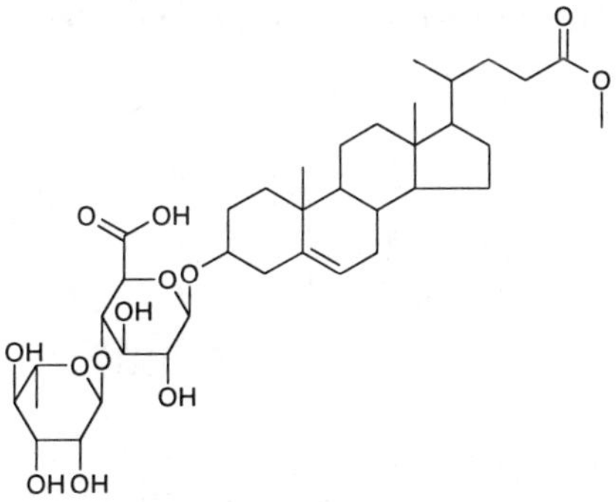

2083 3-Ene-nonanone-2

$C_9H_{16}O$ MW: 140.23 Source: SAN QI. Ref: 2.

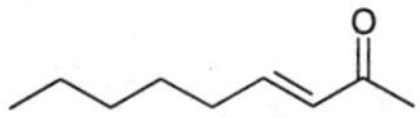

2084 Entagenic acid

$C_{30}H_{48}O_5$ MW: 488.71 Property: mp 310-5°C. Source: KE TENG ZI. Ref: 6.

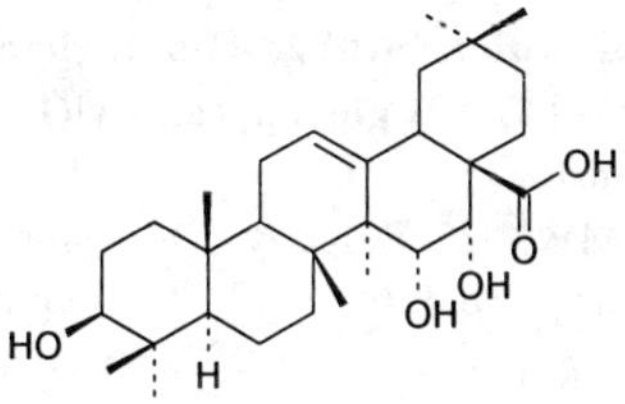

2085 Ephedine

$C_8H_{18}N_2O_3$ Property: mp 87°C. Source: MA HUANG. Ref: 2, 6.

2086 Ephedrine
CAS: 299-42-3 $C_{10}H_{15}NO$ MW: 165.24 Property: mp 34°C. Source: HUANG HUA REN, MA HUANG. Ref: 4.

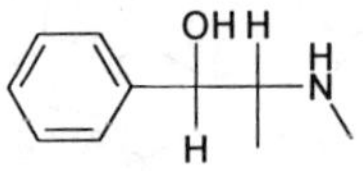

2087 (4S,5R) Ephedroxane
$C_{11}H_{13}NO_2$ MW: 191.23 Source: MA HUANG. Ref: 2.

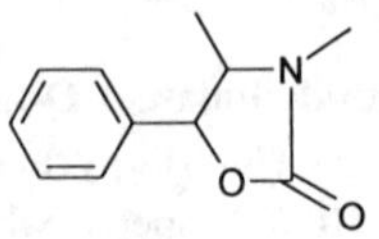

2088 Epialisol A
$C_{30}H_{50}O_5$ MW: 490.73 Source: ZE XIE. Ref: 6.

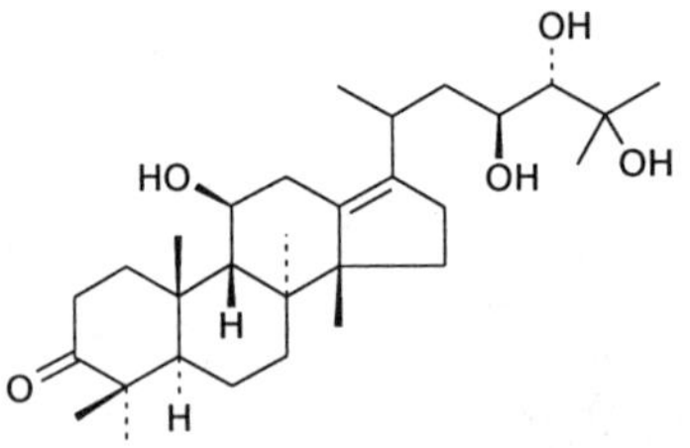

2089 Epi-α-amyrin
$C_{30}H_{50}O$ MW: 426.73 Source: MI DIE XIANG. Ref: 6.

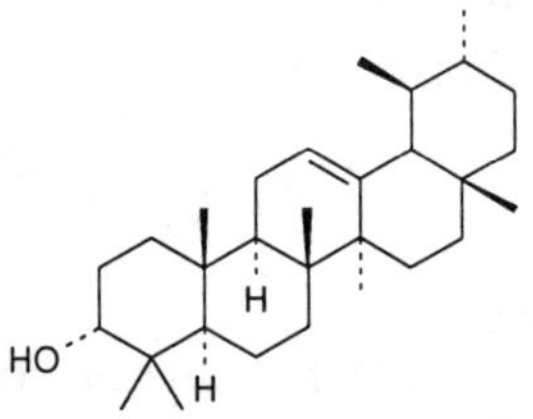

2090 3-Epibetulinic acid 28-O-α-L-rhamnopyranosyl (1→4)-β-D-glucopyranosyl(1→6)-β-D-glucopyranoside
$C_{48}H_{78}O_{17}$ MW: 925 Property: white powder, mp 208-10°C, $[\alpha]_D^{20}$ -38.7° (c=0.4, MeOH). Source: CI REN SHEN. Ref: 467.

2091 Epicatechin
Epicatechol. CAS: 490-46-0 $C_{15}H_{14}O_6$ MW: 290.28 Property: mp (+) 245°C (dec), (-) 245°C (dec), (±) 224-6°C (dec). Source: BAI GUO YE, CHI ZI SHU, DA HUANG, HAI ER CHA, SHAN ZHA, etc. Ref: 2, 6, 433.

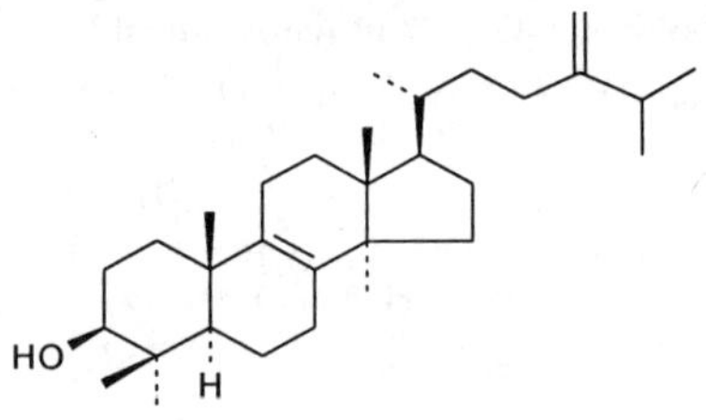

2092 (-)-Epicatechin-3-O-gallate
$C_{22}H_{18}O_{10}$ MW: 442.38 Source: DA HUANG. Ref: 2.

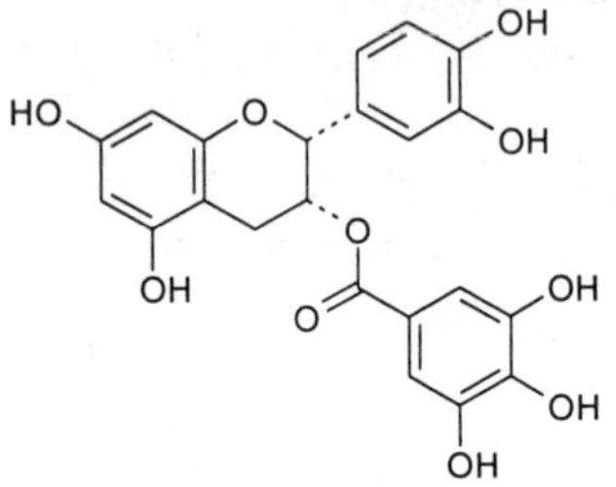

2093 (-)-Epicatechin-pentaacetate
$C_{25}H_{24}O_{11}$ MW: 500.46 Source: BAI GUO. Ref: 2.

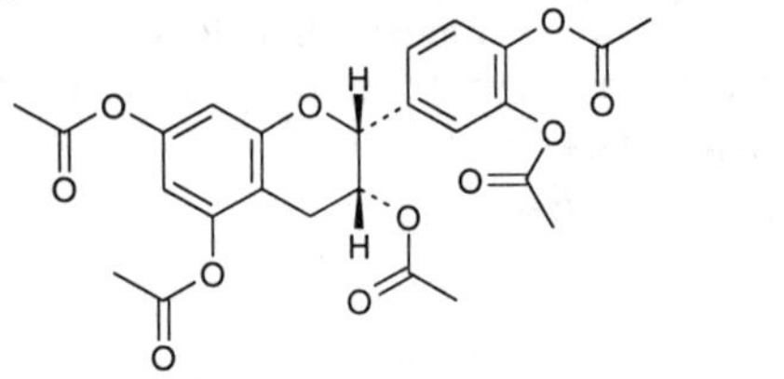

2094 2-Epicephalofortuneine
$C_{20}H_{27}NO_5$ MW: 361.44 Property: white crystal, mp 80-3°C, $[\alpha]_D^{32}$ + 12.1° (c=0.15, chloroform). Source: SAN JIAN SHAN. Ref: 2, 27.

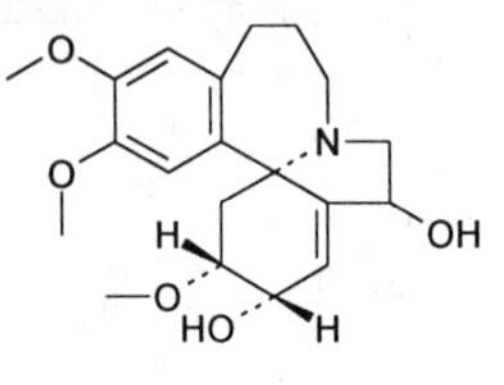

2095 3-Epiconamine
$C_{22}H_{36}N_2$ MW: 328.55 Property: mp 95-100°C. Source: ZHI XIE MU PI. Ref: 6.

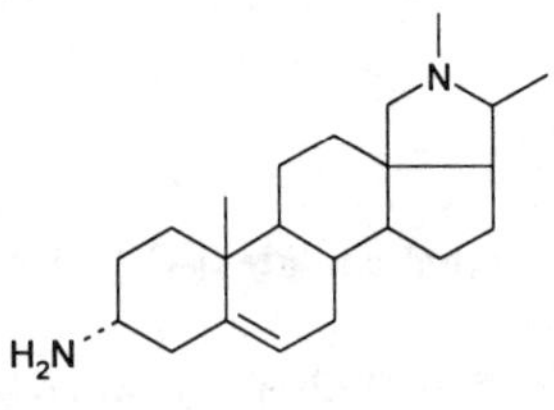

2096 (+)-14-Epicorynoline
$C_{21}H_{21}NO_5$ MW: 367.41 Source: ZI HUA YU DENG CAO (LIE BAO ZI JING). Ref: 6.

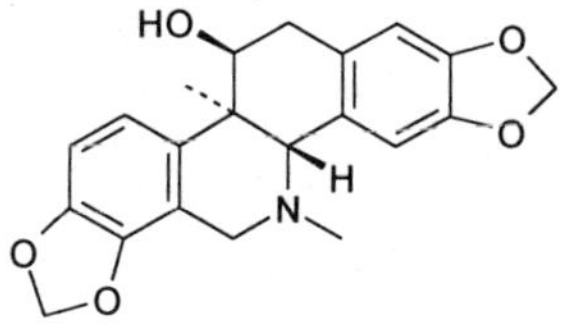

2097 Epicurzerenone
$C_{15}H_{18}O_2$ MW: 230.31 Source: PENG E SHU. Ref: 6.

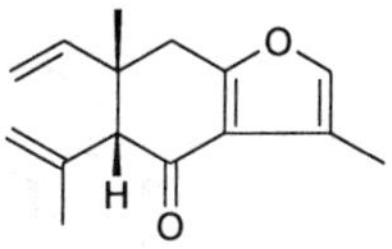

2098 Epideoxyarteannuin B
$C_{15}H_{20}O_2$ MW: 232.33 Source: QING HAO. Ref: 2.

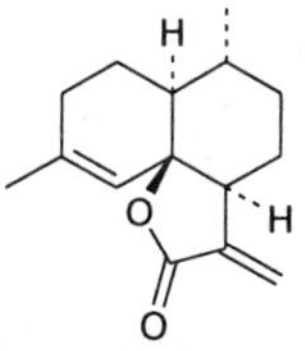

2099 Epideoxyloganic acid
Source: ROU CONG RONG. Ref: 826.

2100 (-)-10-Epi-γ-eudesmol
$C_{15}H_{26}O$ MW: 222.37 Source: CHEN XIANG. Ref: 13.

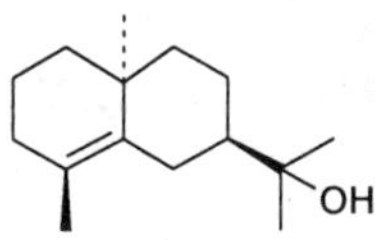

2101 3-Epifortuneine
$C_{20}H_{25}NO_3$ MW: 327.43 Source: SAN JIAN SHAN. Ref: 2.

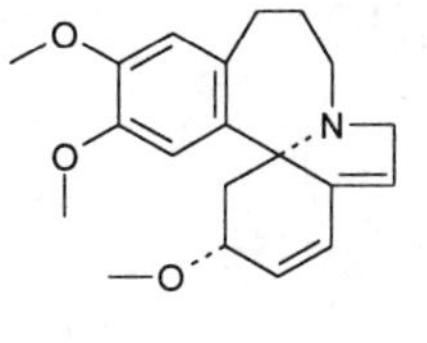

2102 Epifriedelanol
Friedelan-3β-ol. $C_{30}H_{52}O$ MW: 428.75 Property: colorless acicular crystal, mp 283.5-5.0°C. Source: DIAO JING CAO, DONG FENG CAI, DUO SUI SHI KE YE, GUI JIAN YU, HUO XIANG, HUO YANG LE, JI XUE TENG, KU DI DAN, LONG YAN YE, NAN ZHU YE, QIU FENG MU, XI YUAN TENG, YU DAI GEN, ZI WAN. Ref: 6, 505, 596.

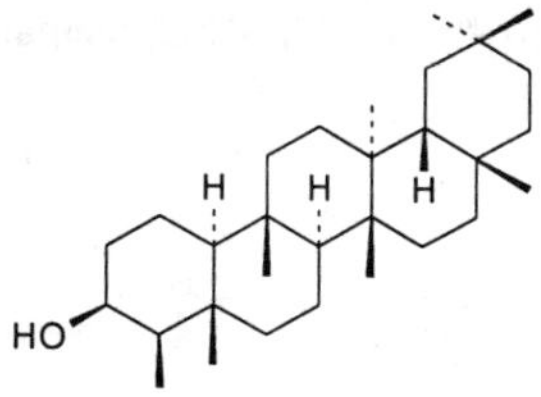

2103 Epifriedelanol acetate
$C_{32}H_{54}O_2$ MW: 470.79 Property: mp 282-5°C. Source: QIU FENG MU, YU DAI GEN. Ref: 6.

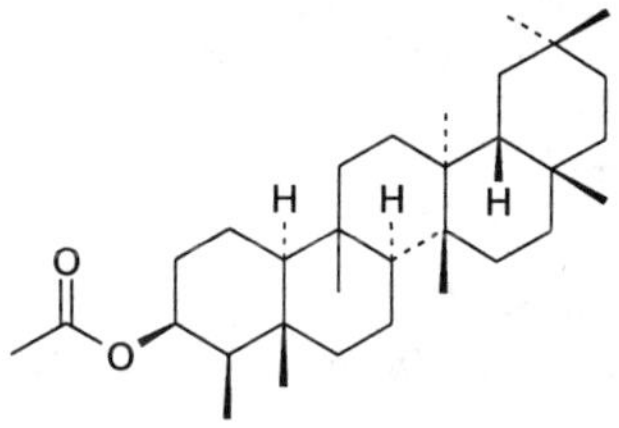

2104 Epifriedelin
MW: 428 Property: colorless acicular crystal, mp 257-9°C, $[\alpha]_D^{28}$ +14.1°C (c=0.07, $CHCl_3$). Source: TUN XING GUO. Ref: 447.

2105 2-Epigalanthamine
$C_{17}H_{21}NO_3$ MW: 287.36 Property: mp 190°C. Source: SHI SUAN. Ref: 6.

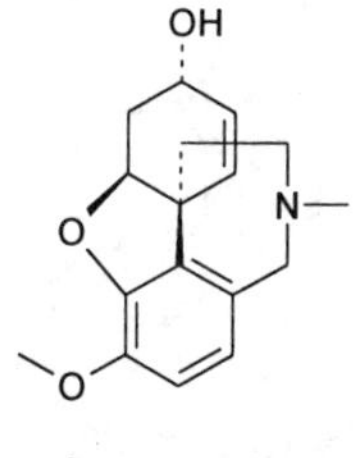

2106 l-Epigallocatechin
$C_{15}H_{14}O_7$ MW: 306.27 Property: mp 227°C. Source: CHA YE, KUN MING SHAN HAI TANG. Ref: 6, 612.

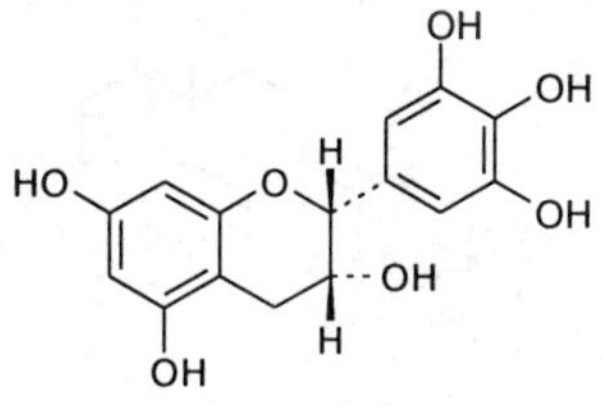

2107 Epigeoside

Catechin-3-O-α-L-rhamnopyranosyl-(1→4)-β-D-glucopyranosyl-(1→6)-β-D-glucopyranoside.

$C_{33}H_{44}O_{20}$ MW: 760.71 Property: colorless powder, mp 165-8°C, $[\alpha]_D^{20}$ -32.5° (c=1.05, methanol). Source: SI MAO TENG. Ref: 208.

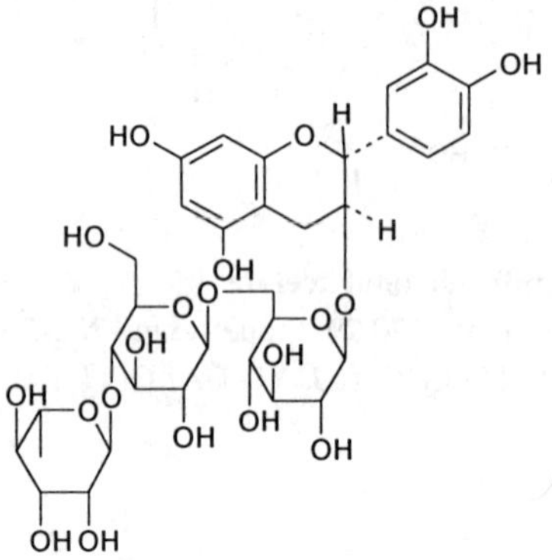

2108 Epigomisin O

$C_{23}H_{28}O_7$ MW: 416.48 Source: WU WEI ZI. Ref: 2.

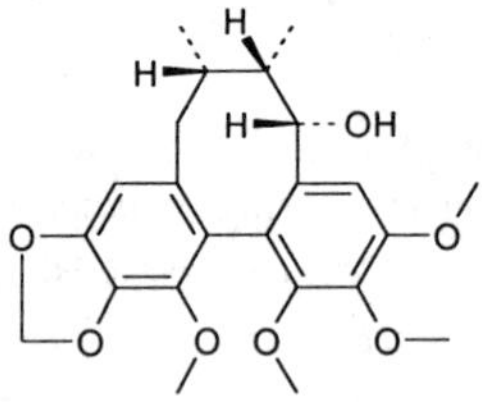

2109 Epiguaipyridine

$C_{15}H_{21}N$ MW: 215.34 Source: HUO XIANG. Ref: 2, 6.

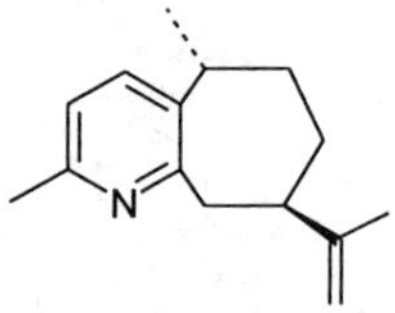

2110 Epiheteroconessine

$C_{25}H_{44}N_2$ MW: 372.64 Property: mp 148-50°C. Source: ZHI XIE MU PI. Ref: 6.

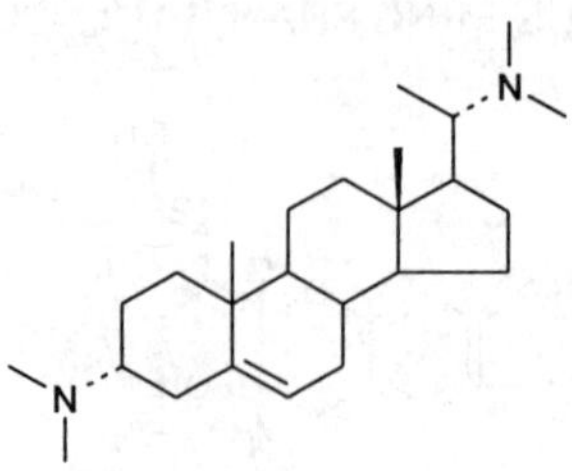

2111 4-Epiisocembrol

$C_{20}H_{34}O$ MW: 290.49 Source: HAI SONG ZI. Ref: 6.

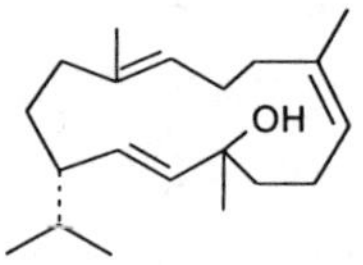

2112 3-Epikatonic acid

$C_{30}H_{48}O_3$ MW: 456.72 Source: LEI GONG TENG. Ref: 2, 60.

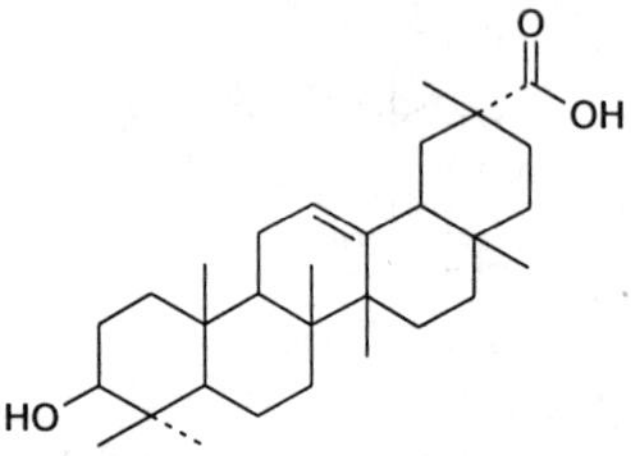

2113 8-Epiloganic acid

$C_{16}H_{24}O_{10}$ MW: 376.36 Source: GAN DI HUANG, ROU CONG RONG, DI HUANG. Ref: 2, 502, 628.

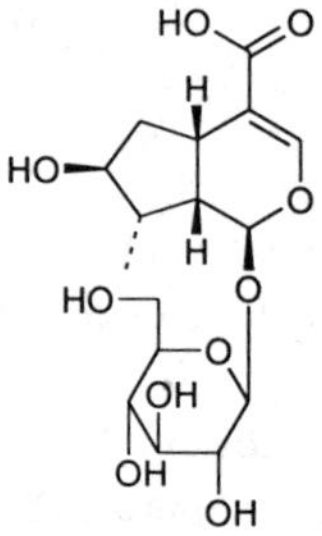

2114 Epimedin A

$C_{39}H_{50}O_{19}$ MW: 822.82 Source: YIN YANG HUO. Ref: 2.

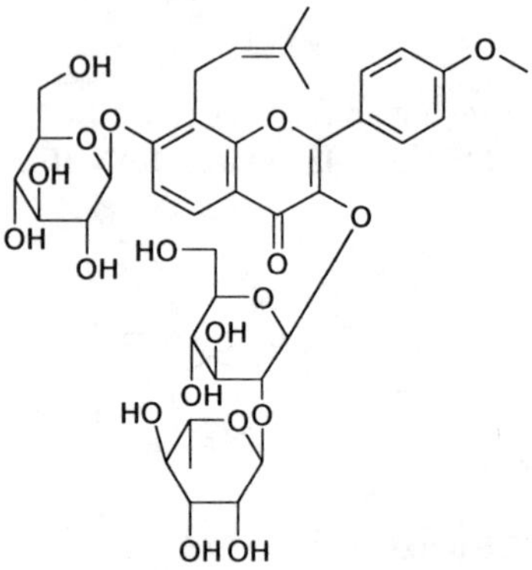

2115 Epimedin B
$C_{38}H_{48}O_{18}$ MW: 792.80 Source: CHUAN E YIN YANG HUO, YIN YANG HUO. Ref: 2, 567.

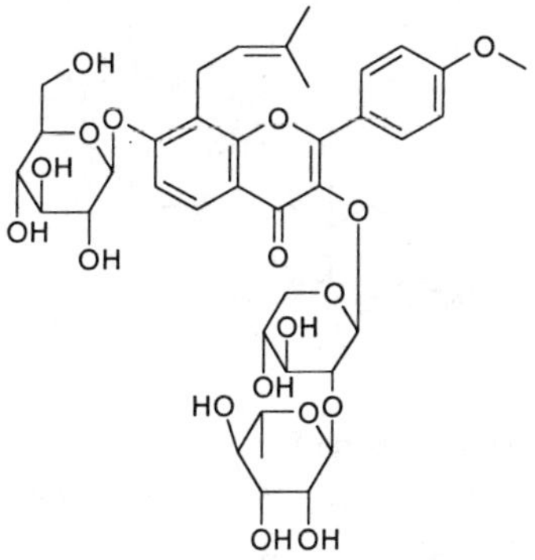

2116 Epimedin C
$C_{39}H_{50}O_{17}$ MW: 790.82 Source: CHUAN E YIN YANG HUO, CU MAO YIN YANG HUO, YIN YANG HUO. Ref: 2, 567, 624.

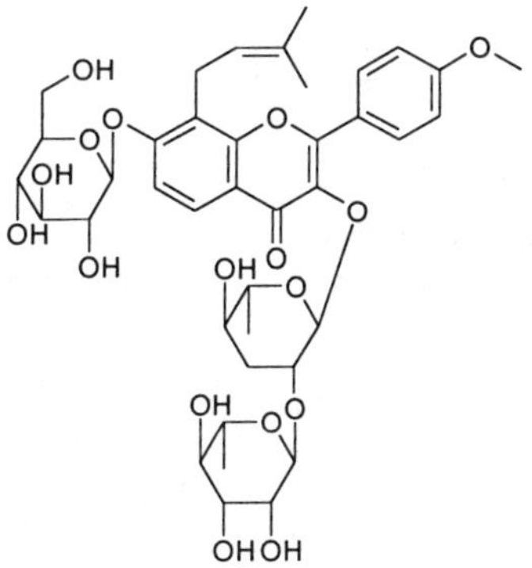

2117 Epimedin K
Source: CHAO XIAN YIN YANG HUO. Ref: 635.

2118 Epimedoicarisoside A
Source: CHAO XIAN YIN YANG HUO. Ref: 635.

2119 Epimedokoreanin A
Source: CHAO XIAN YIN YANG HUO. Ref: 635.

2120 Epimedokoreanin B
Source: CHAO XIAN YIN YANG HUO. Ref: 635.

2121 Epimedokoreanin C
Source: CHAO XIAN YIN YANG HUO. Ref: 635.

2122 Epimedokoreanin D
5,7,3',4'-tetrahydroxy-5'-prenylflavone. $C_{20}H_{18}O_6$ MW: 354.35 Property: yellow acicular, mp 213-215 °C. Source: CHAO XIAN YIN YANG HUO. Ref: 342.

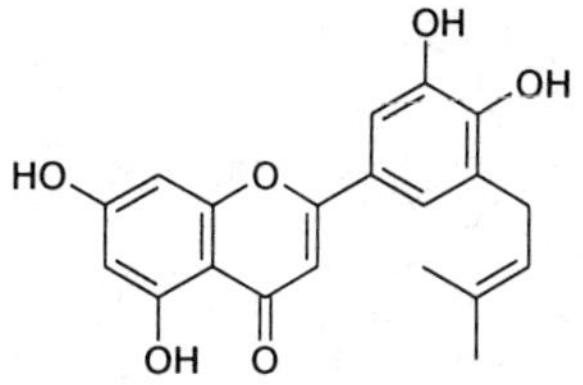

2123 Epimedokoreanone A
Source: CHAO XIAN YIN YANG HUO. Ref: 635.

2124 Epimedokoreanoside I
Source: YIN YANG HUO. Ref: 2.

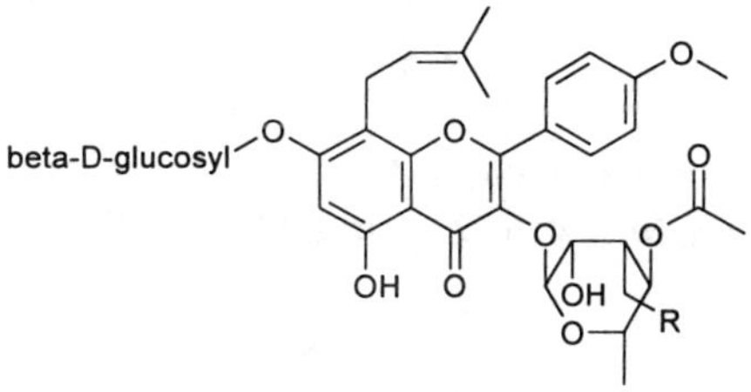

R=Acetyl-β-glucosyl

2125 Epimedokoreanoside II
Source: YIN YANG HUO. Ref: 2.

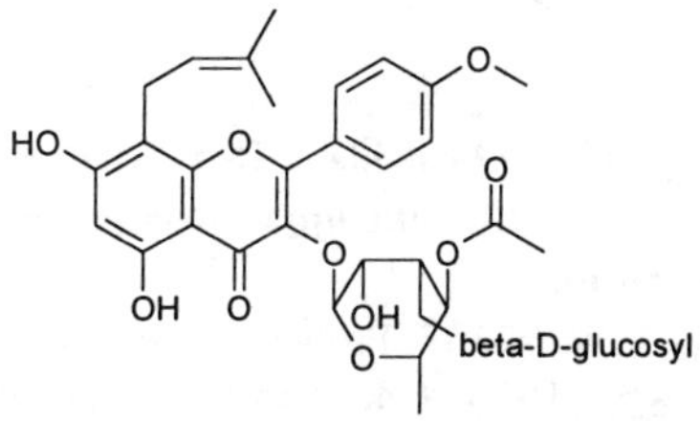

2126 Epimedoside A
$C_{32}H_{38}O_{15}$ MW: 662.65 Source: CU MAO YIN YANG HUO, CHUAN E YIN YANG HUO, YIN YANG HUO. Ref: 2, 112, 514, 567, 624.

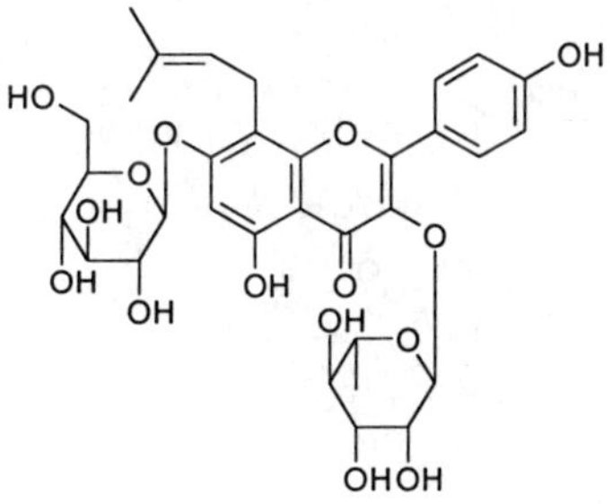

2127 Epimedoside C
$C_{26}H_{30}O_{11}$ MW: 329.44 Source: YIN YANG HUO. Ref: 2, 112.

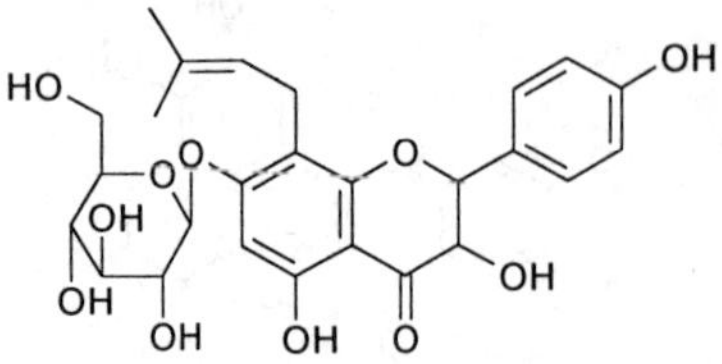

2128 3-Epimethylschelhammericine B
$C_{20}H_{27}NO_3$ MW: 329.44 Source: SAN JIAN SHAN. Ref: 2, 27.

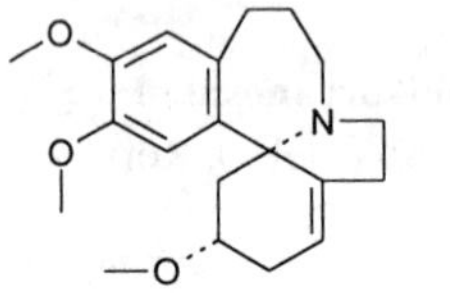

2129 3-Epioleanolic acid
$C_{30}H_{48}O_3$ MW: 456.72 Source: SU HE XIANG. Ref: 6.

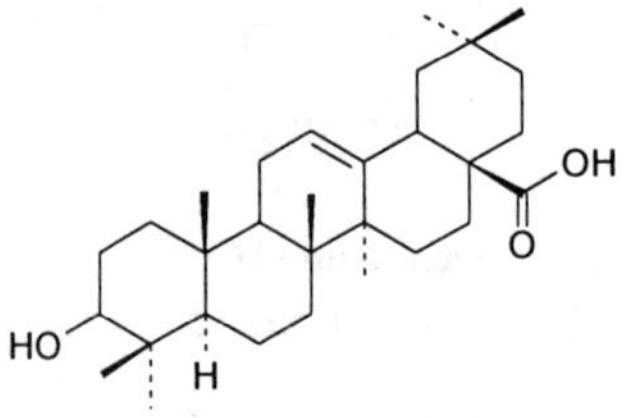

2130 3-Epi-oleanolic acid-28-O-α-L-rhamnopyranosyl (1→4)-β-D-glucopyranosyl(1→6)-β-D-glucopyranoside
$C_{48}H_{78}O_{17}$ MW: 927.15 Property: white powder, mp 207-9°C, $[\alpha]_D^{20}$ -15° (c=0.4, methanol). Source: CI REN SHEN. Ref: 370.

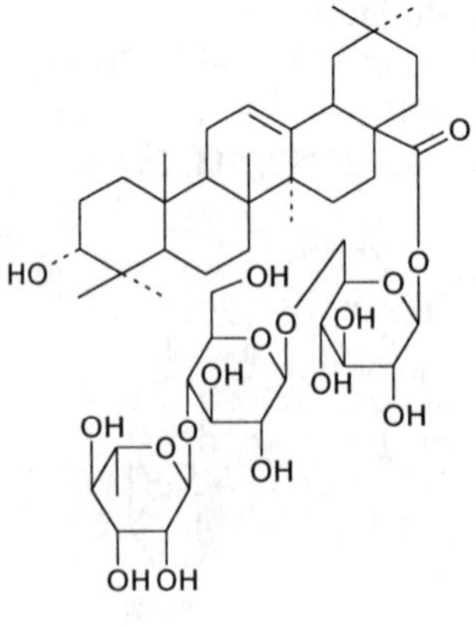

2131 Epipachysamine A
$C_{26}H_{46}N_2O$ MW: 402.67 Property: mp 203-5°C. Source: XUE SHAN LIN. Ref: 6.

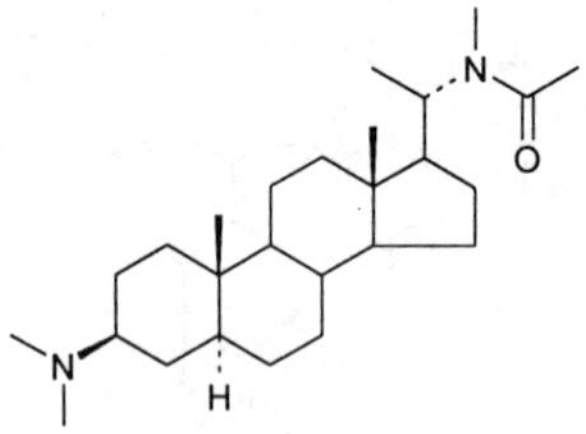

2132 Epipachysamine B
$C_{29}H_{45}N_3O$ MW: 451.70 Property: mp 260-2°C. Source: XUE SHAN LIN. Ref: 6.

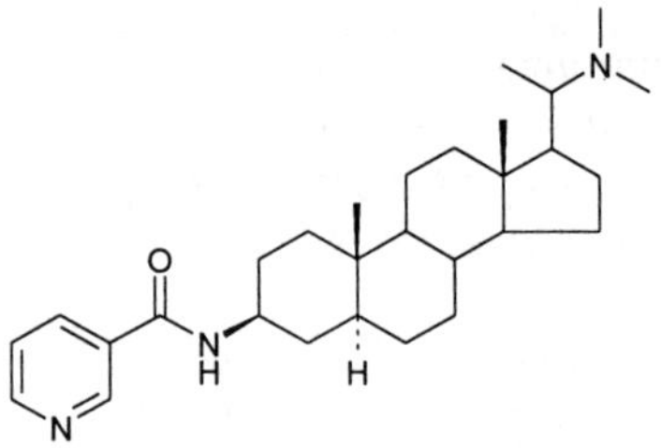

2133 Epipachysamine C
$C_{25}H_{46}N_2$ MW: 374.66 Source: XUE SHAN LIN. Ref: 6.

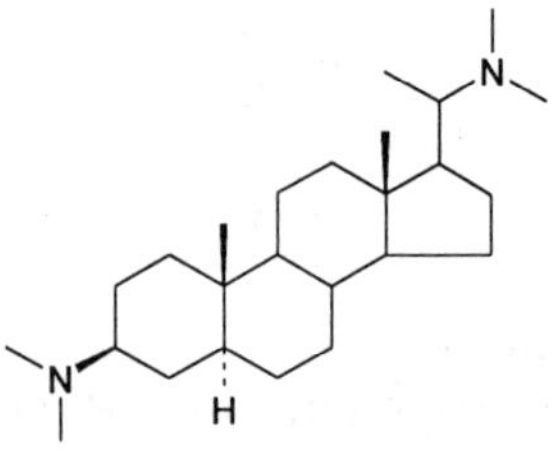

2134 Epipachysamine D
$C_{30}H_{46}N_2O$ MW: 450.71 Property: mp 245-8°C. Source: XUE SHAN LIN. Ref: 6.

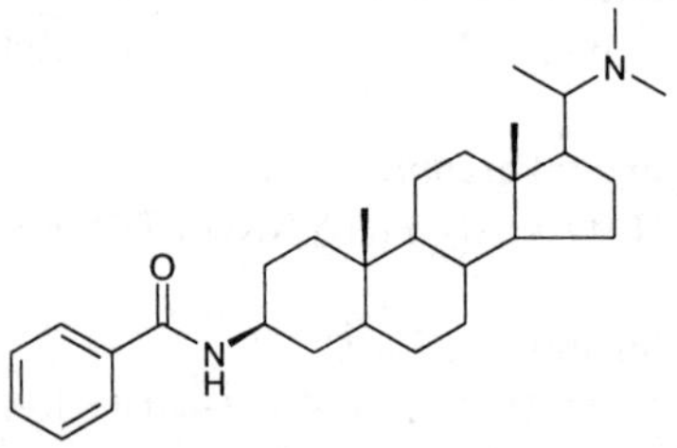

2135 Epipachysamine E
$C_{28}H_{48}N_2O$ MW: 428.71 Property: mp 210-2°C. Source: XUE SHAN LIN. Ref: 6.

2136 Epipachysamine F
$C_{23}H_{42}N_2$ MW: 346.60 Property: mp 250-3°C. Source: XUE SHAN LIN. Ref: 6.

2137 Epipachysandrine A
$C_{30}H_{46}N_2O_2$ MW: 466.71 Property: mp >295°C. Source: XUE SHAN LIN. Ref: 6.

2138 7-Epiphlomiol
$C_{17}H_{26}O_{13}$ MW: 438.39 Source: MENG GU CAO SU. Ref: 561.

2139 (+)-Epipinoresinol
$C_{20}H_{22}O_6$ MW: 358.39 Source: DU ZHONG. Ref: 2.

2140 Epiquinidine
$C_{20}H_{24}N_2O_2$ MW: 324.43 Property: mp 113°C . Source: JIN JI LE. Ref: 6.

2141 Epiquinine
$C_{20}H_{24}N_2O_2$ MW: 324.43 Source: JIN JI LE. Ref: 6.

2142 Epirockogenin
$C_{27}H_{44}O_4$ MW: 432.65 Source: FAN MA, JIAN MA. Ref: 10.

2143 12-Epirockogenin
$C_{28}H_{46}O_4$ MW: 446.68 Property: mp 218°C. Source: TAN XIANG. Ref: 6.

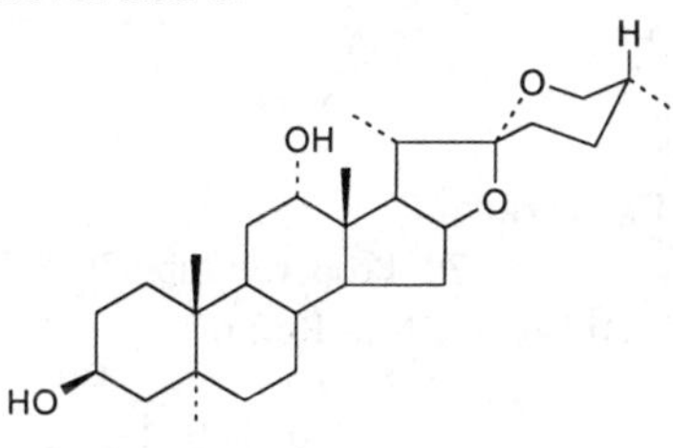

2144 Epi-β-santalene
$C_{15}H_{24}$ MW: 204.36 Source: TAN XIANG. Ref: 6.

2145 16-Episarpagine

$C_{19}H_{22}N_2O_2$ MW: 310.40 Property: acicular crystal, mp 300°C, (decomposition) $[\alpha]_D^{30}$ +34.7° (c=0.085, ethanol). Source: JI GU CHANG SHAN. Ref: 42.

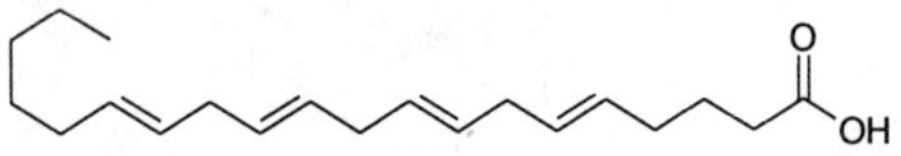

2146 Epi-sarsasapogenin

$C_{27}H_{44}O_3$ MW: 416.65 Property: 204-6°C, $[\alpha]_D^{29}$ -49.6° (c=0.31, $CHCl_3$). Source: CHA RUI SHU PIN, CHA RUI SHU YU. Ref: 10, 24.

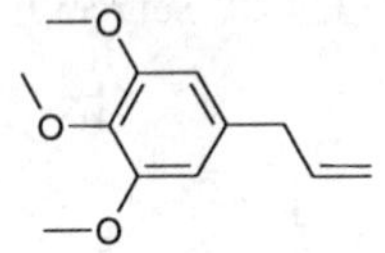

2147 3-Epischelhammericine

$C_{19}H_{23}NO_3$ MW: 313.40 Source: SAN JIAN SHAN. Ref: 2, 27.

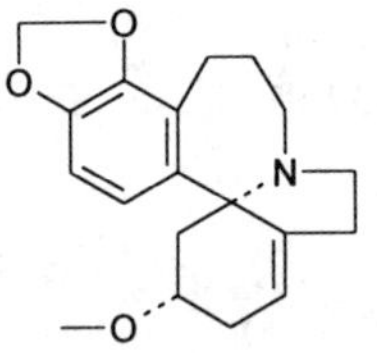

2148 21-Episerratenediol

$C_{30}H_{50}O_2$ MW: 442.73 Property: mp 303-8°C. Source: QIAN CENG TA. Ref: 6, 109.

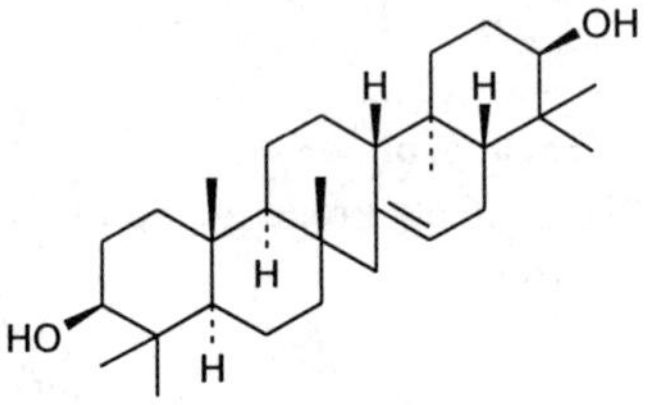

2149 21-Episerratriol

$C_{29}H_{48}O_3$ MW: 444.70 Property: mp 330-3°C. Source: PU DI WU GONG. Ref: 6.

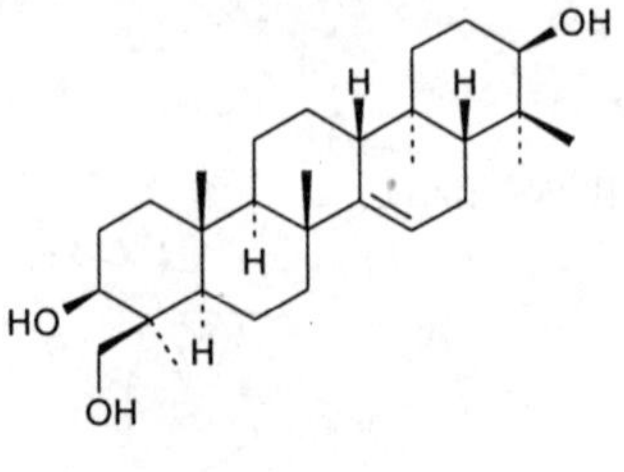

2150 Epishyobunone

$C_{15}H_{24}O$ MW: 220.36 Source: BAI CHANG. Ref: 6.

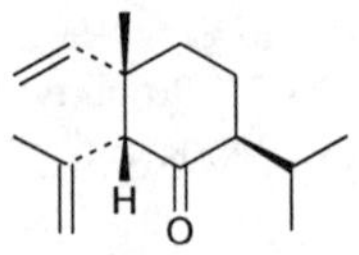

2151 Epismilagenin

$C_{27}H_{44}O_3$ MW: 416.65 Source: BEI XIE, CHA RUI SHU YU, CHUNG LONG SHU YU, DUN YE SHU YU, FU ZHOU SHU YU, SHU KUI YE. Ref: 10, 24.

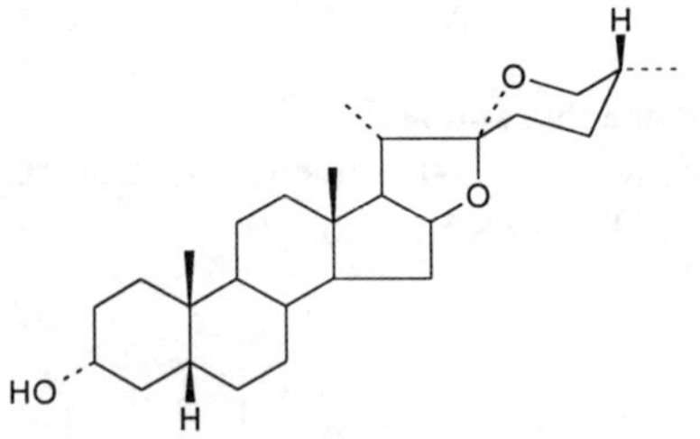

2151 Epistephanine

$C_{37}H_{38}N_2O_6$ MW: 606.73 Property: mp 202°C. Source: QIAN JIN TENG. Ref: 6.

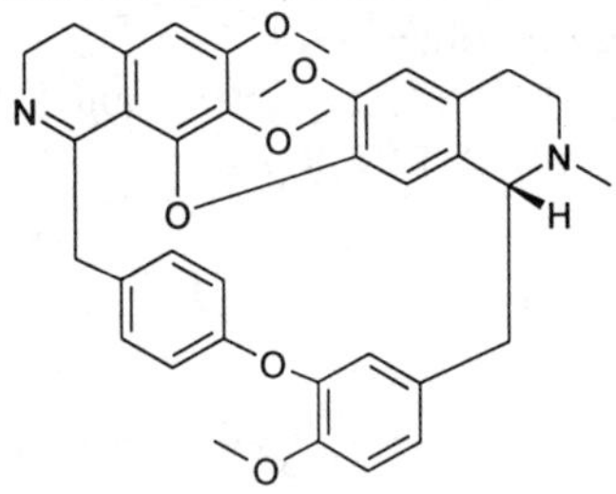

2153 16-Epi-voacarpine

$C_{21}H_{24}N_2O_4$ MW: 368.44 Property: mp 162-5°C (dec), $[\alpha]_D$ +42.3°. Source: GOU WEN. Ref: 13.

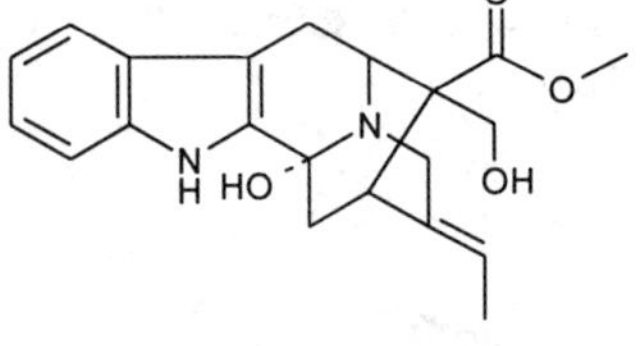

2154 Epiwilsonine

$C_{20}H_{25}NO_4$ MW: 343.43 Source: SAN JIAN SHAN. Ref: 2.

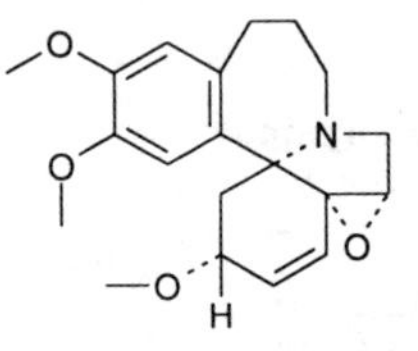

2155 Epmedin B
MW: 808 Property: yellow powder, mp 170-3°C. Source: WAN SHAN YIN YANG HUO. Ref: 465.

2156 Epmedin C
MW: 822 Property: yellow powder, mp 178-81°C. Source: WAN SHAN YIN YANG HUO. Ref: 465.

2157 13,14-Epoxide 9,11,12-hydroxytriptolide
$C_{20}H_{26}O_7$ MW: 378.43 Property: colorless filiform crystal, mp 268-270°C. Source: LEI GONG TENG. Ref: 256.

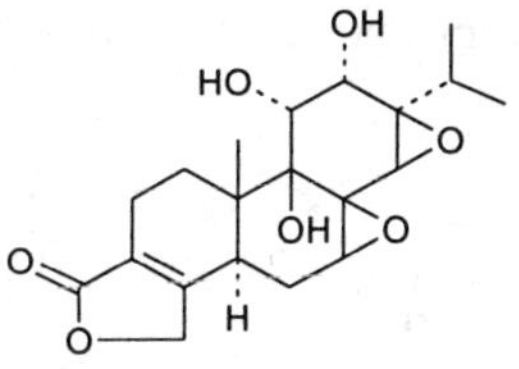

2158 Epoxyarteannuinic acid
$C_{15}H_{22}O_3$ MW: 250.34 Source: QING HAO. Ref: 2.

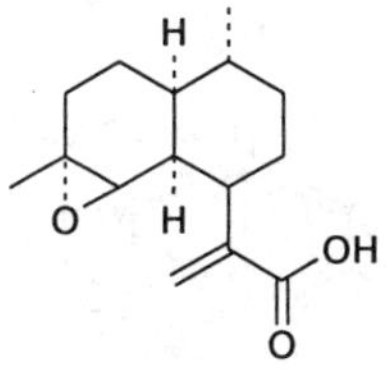

2159 20R,24R-Epoxy-25-dammaren-3-one
$C_{30}H_{48}O_2$ MW: 440.72 Property: colorless acicular crystal (MeOH), mp 225°C, $[\alpha]_D^{21.5}$ +57°(c=1.0, $CHCl_3$). Source: XIANG GANG JIAN MU. Ref: 422.

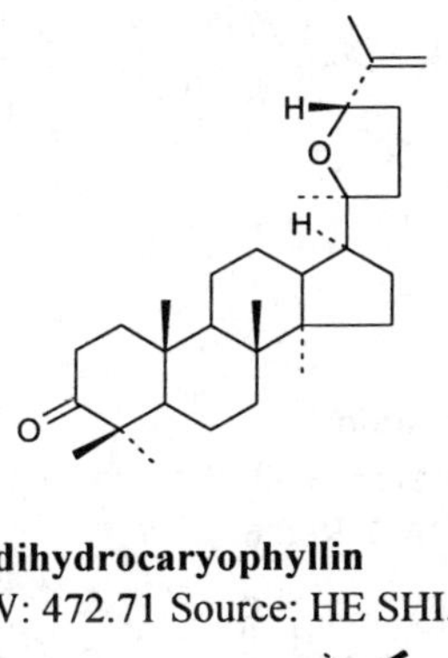

2160 Epoxydihydrocaryophyllin
$C_{30}H_{48}O_4$ MW: 472.71 Source: HE SHI. Ref: 6.

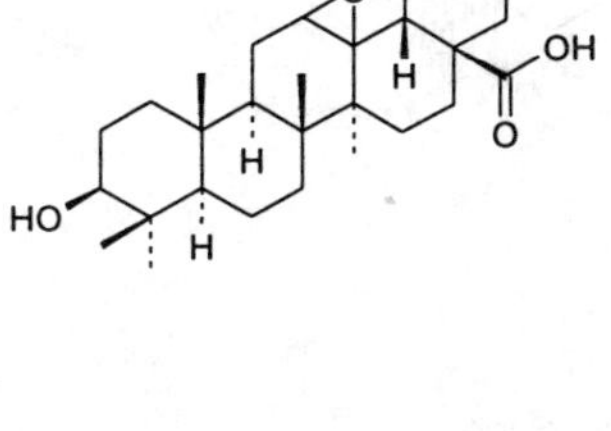

2161 (Z)-6,7-Epoxy-6,7-dihydroligustilide
$C_{12}H_{14}O_3$ MW: 206.24 Source: CHUAN XIONG. Ref: 2.

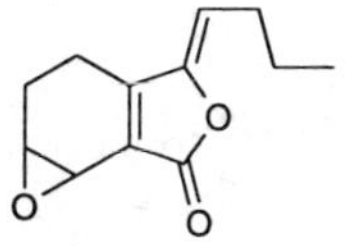

2162 Epoxydihydrolinalool
$C_{10}H_{20}O_2$ MW: 172.27 Source: XING ZI. Ref: 6.

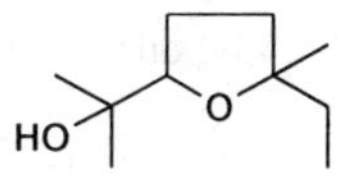

2163 3α,4α-Epoxyfilicane
$C_{30}H_{50}O$ MW: 426.73 Property: mp 229-31°C. Source: ZHU ZONG CAO. Ref: 6.

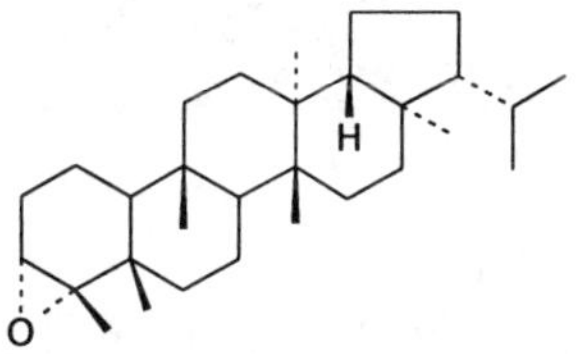

2164 (-)-1,10-Epoxy-guaia-11-ene
$C_{15}H_{24}O$ MW: 220.36 Source: CHEN XIANG. Ref: 13.

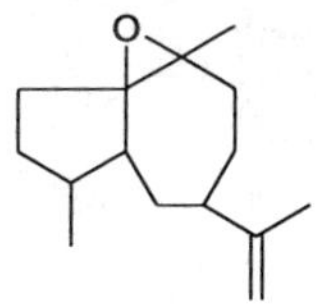

2165 Epoxyguaine
$C_{15}H_{24}O$ MW: 220.36 Property: bp 102-4°C/1mm. Source: XIANG FU. Ref: 6.

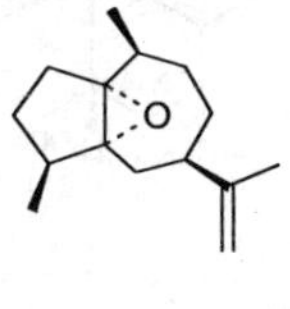

2166 (E)-8β,17-Epoxylabd-12-ene-15,16-dial
$C_{20}H_{30}O_3$ MW: 318.46 Source: GAN JIANG, SHENG JIANG. Ref: 2.

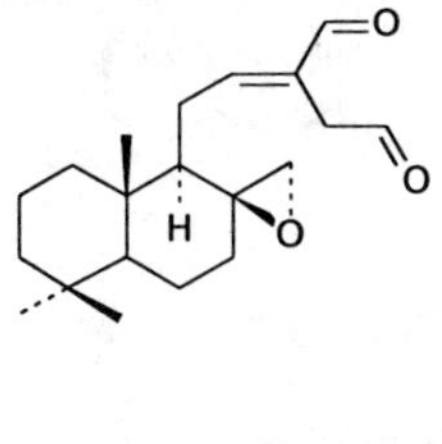

2167 (+)-1,5-Epoxy-nor-ketoguaia-11-ene
$C_{14}H_{20}O_2$ MW: 220.31 Source: CHEN XIANG. Ref: 13.

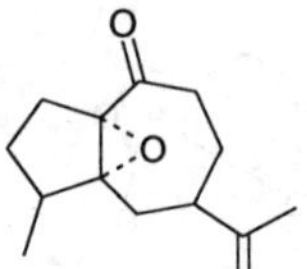

2168 5β,6β-Epoxyphysalin B
$C_{28}H_{30}O_{10}$ MW: 526.55 Source: TIAN PAO ZI. Ref: 6.

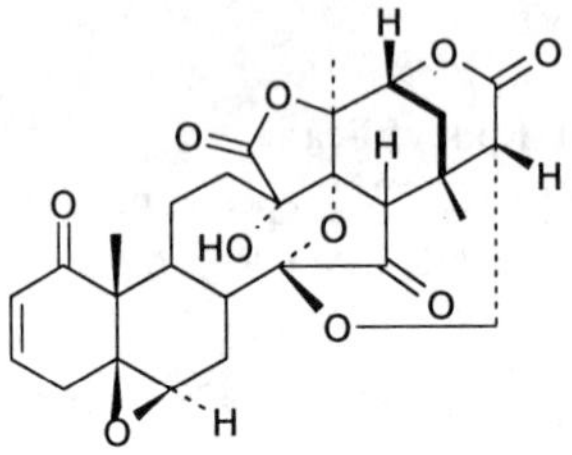

2169 Equisetrin
$C_{27}H_{30}O_{16}$ MW: 610.53 Property: mp 195-6°C. Source: WEN JING. Ref: 6.

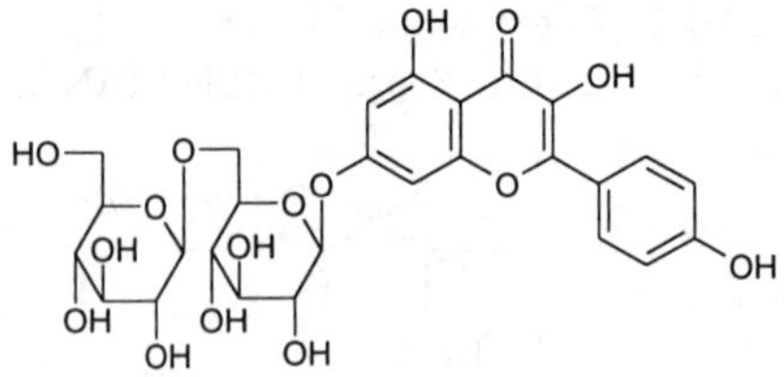

2170 Eremofukinone
$C_{15}H_{24}O$ MW: 220.36 Property: bp 75-110°C/0.15mm. Source: FENG DOU CAI. Ref: 6.

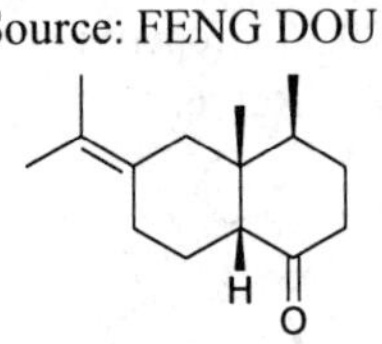

2171 Eremophilene
$C_{15}H_{24}$ MW: 204.36 Property: bp 129.5°C/13mm. Source: DU HUO, FENG DOU CAI, XIE CAO. Ref: 2.

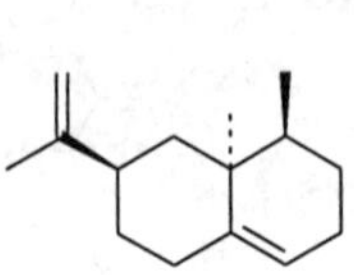

2172 Ergochrysin
$C_{31}H_{28}O_{14}$ MW: 624.56 Property: mp 285°C (dec). Source: MAI JIAO. Ref: 6.

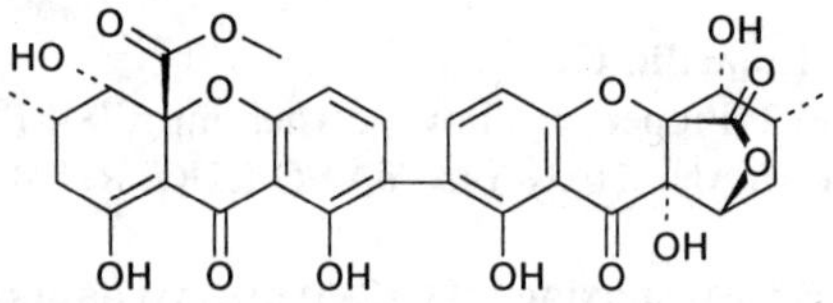

2173 Ergocornine
CAS: 564-36-3 $C_{31}H_{39}N_5O_5$ MW: 561.69 Property: mp 181-4°C (dec). Source: MAI JIAO. Ref: 5, 6.

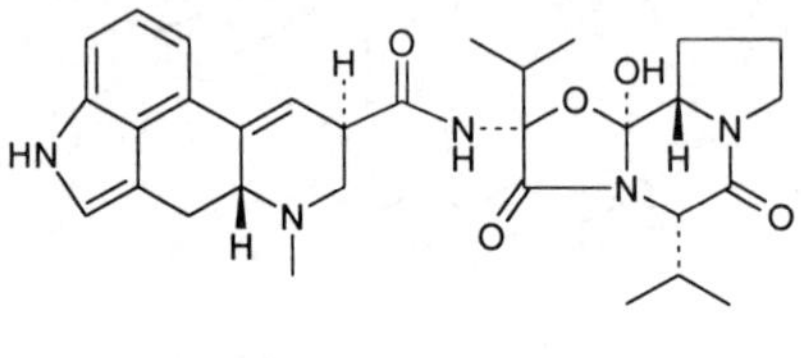

2174 Ergocorninine
$C_{31}H_{41}N_5O_5$ MW: 563.70 Property: mp 228°C (dec). Source: MAI JIAO. Ref: 6.

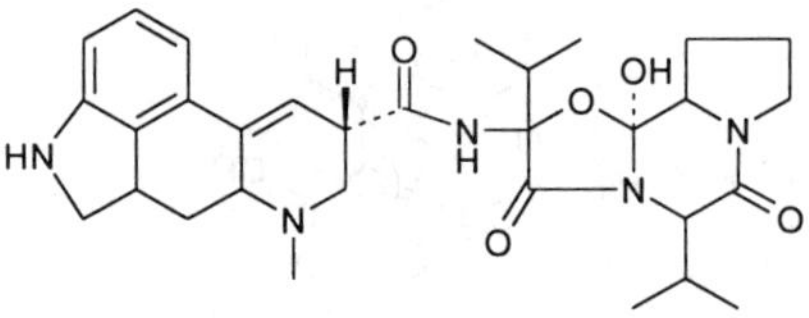

2175 Ergocristine
$C_{35}H_{39}N_5O_5$ MW: 609.73 Property: mp 165-70°C (dec). Source: MAI JIAO. Ref: 6.

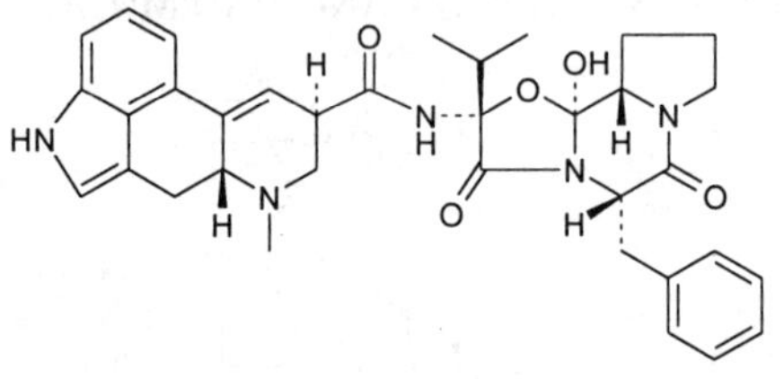

2176 Ergocristinine
$C_{35}H_{39}N_5O_5$ MW: 609.73 Property: mp 214°C (dec). Source: MAI JIAO. Ref: 6.

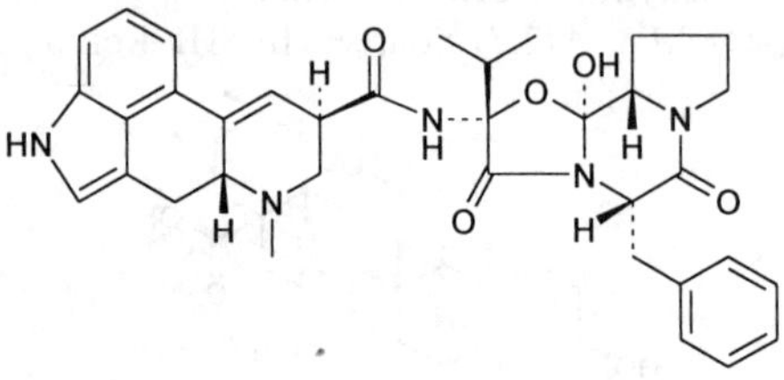

2177 Ergoflavine
$C_{30}H_{26}O_{14}$ MW: 610.53 Property: mp 350°C (dec). Source: MAI JIAO. Ref: 6.

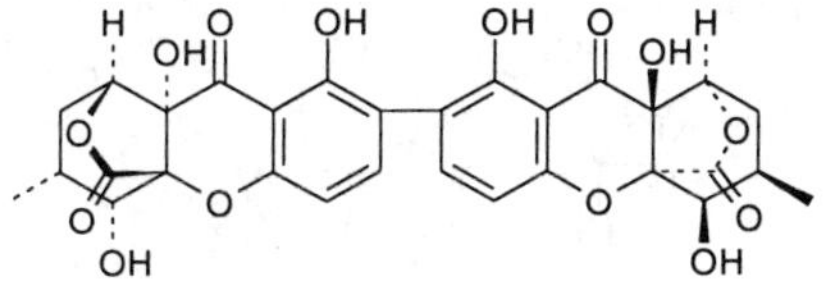

2178 Ergokryptine
Ergocryptine; α-Ergokryptine. $C_{32}H_{41}N_5O_5$ MW: 575.71 Property: mp 212-4°C. Source: MAI JIAO. Ref: 5, 6.

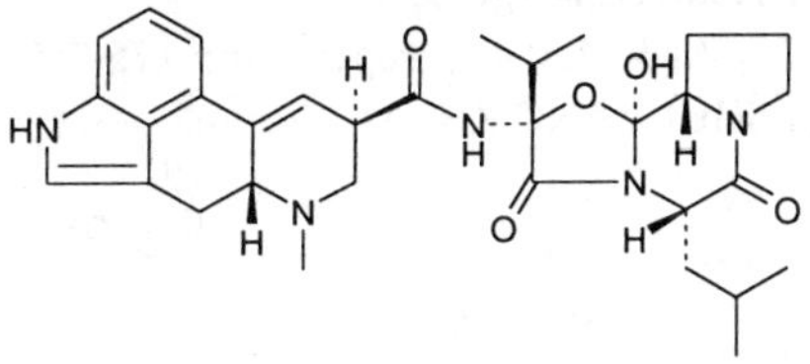

2179 Ergokryptinine
$C_{32}H_{41}N_5O_5$ MW: 575.71 Property: mp 240-2°C (dec). Source: MAI JIAO. Ref: 6.

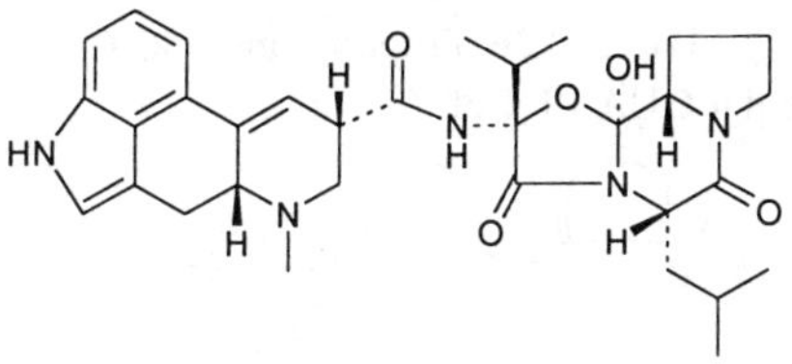

2180 Ergolide
$C_{17}H_{22}O_5$ MW: 306.36 Property: white acicular crystal, mp 169-70°C, $[\alpha]_D$ +133° (c=1.26, CH_2Cl_2). Source: SHUI CHAO YANG. Ref: 430.

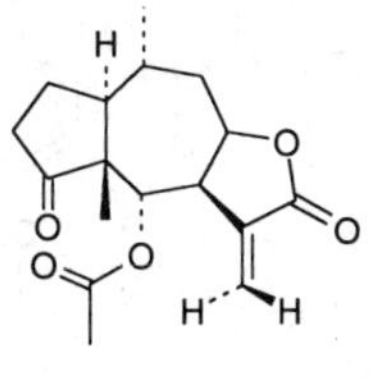

2181 Ergometrine
Ergobasine; Ergolkinine; Ergonetrine; Ergonovine; Ergosteterine; Ergotrane. CAS: 60-79-7 $C_{19}H_{23}N_3O_2$ MW: 325.41 Property: mp 162°C. Source: MAI JIAO. Ref: 4.

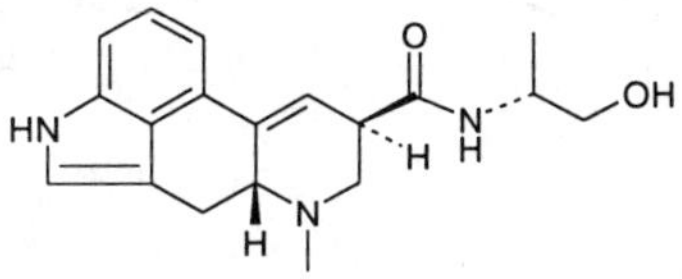

2182 Ergometrinine
$C_{19}H_{23}N_3O_2$ MW: 325.41 Property: mp (+): 195-7°C (dec). Source: MAI JIAO. Ref: 6.

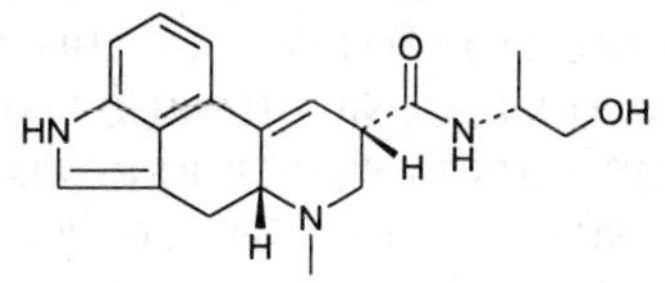

2183 Ergosecalinine
$C_{24}H_{28}N_4O_4$ MW: 436.52 Property: mp 217°C (dec). Source: MAI JIAO. Ref: 6.

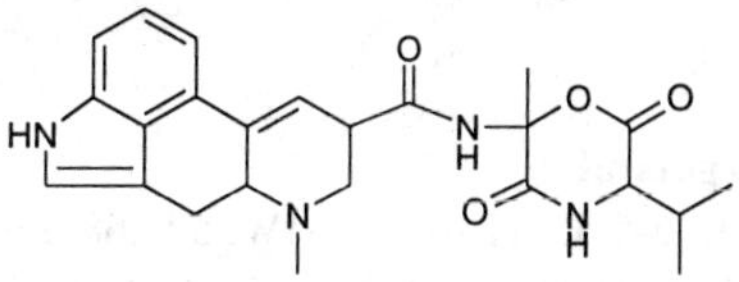

2184 Ergosine
$C_{30}H_{37}N_5O_5$ MW: 547.66 Property: mp 228°C (dec). Source: MAI JIAO. Ref: 6.

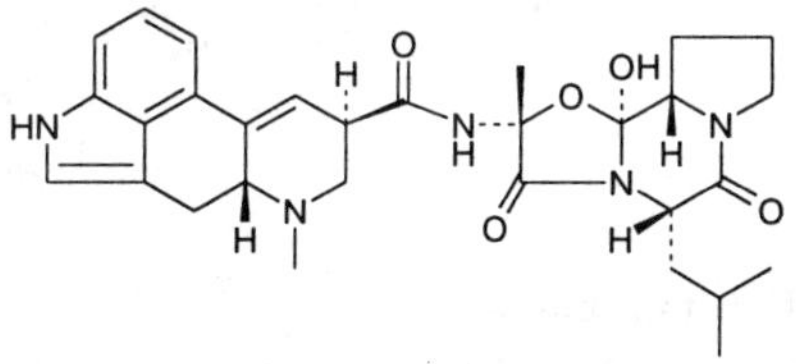

2185 Ergosinine
$C_{30}H_{37}N_5O_5$ MW: 547.66 Property: mp 228°C (dec). Source: MAI JIAO. Ref: 6.

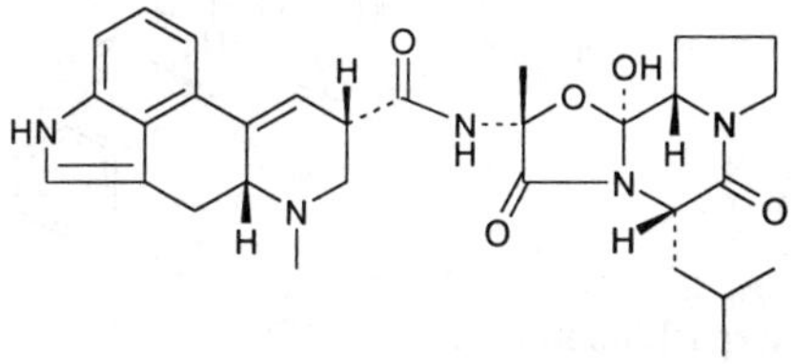

2186 Ergosta-5,24(28)-dien-3β-ol
$C_{28}H_{46}O$ Property: colorless lamellar crystal, mp 139.5-41°C(methanol-chloroform). Source: TOU JIE HAI MIAN. Ref: 459.

2187 Ergosta-4,6,8(14),22-tetraen-3-one
$C_{28}H_{40}O$ MW: 392.63 Property: mp 114-5°C. Source: A LI HONG, LING, ZHU LING. Ref: 2, 6.

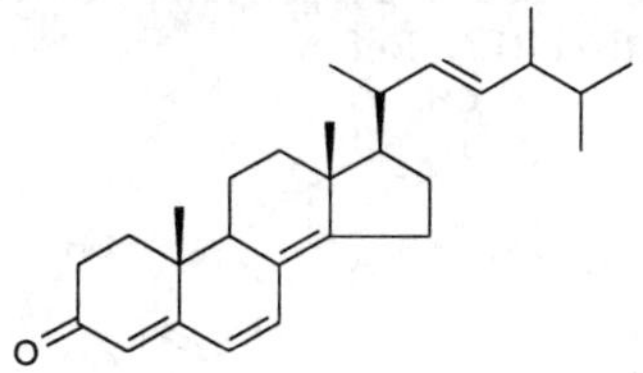

2188 Ergosterol
$C_{28}H_{44}O$ MW: 396.66 Property: mp 163°C. Source: A LI HONG, BAI QU CAI, DONG CHONG XIA CAO, FU LING, JI CONG, JIAO TUO LUO, LING ZHI CAO, MA PUO, MAI JIAO, MU RE, NIU HUANG, QIN MOU, SANG HUANG, SONG XUN, TENG DU ZHONG, XIANG XUN, YUAN CAN SHA, ZHU LING. Ref: 2, 6, 587.

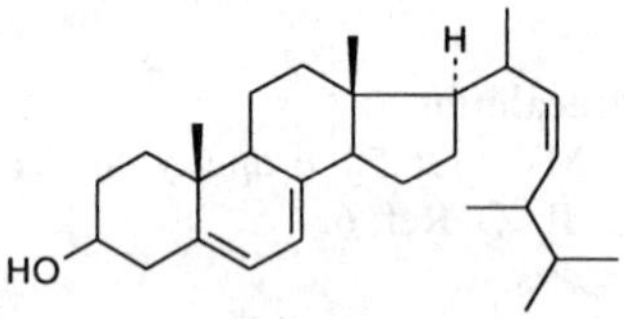

2189 Ergotamine
CAS: 113-15-5 $C_{33}H_{35}N_5O_5$ MW: 581.68 Property: mp 212-4°C (dec). Source: MAI JIAO. Ref: 4.

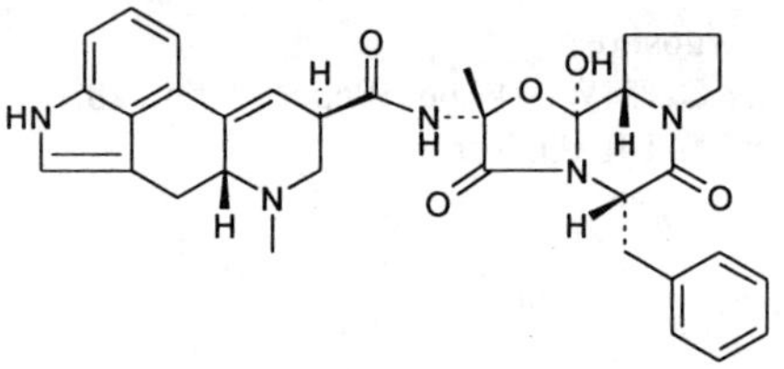

2190 Ergotaminine
$C_{33}H_{35}N_5O_5$ MW: 581.68 Property: mp 252°C (dec). Source: MAI JIAO. Ref: 6.

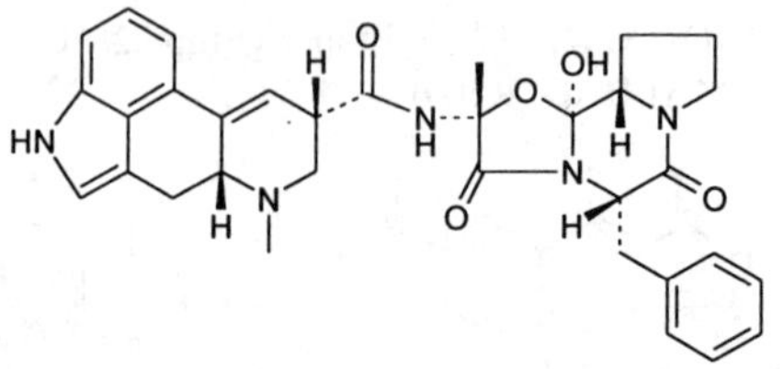

2191 Ergothioneine
$C_9H_{15}N_3O_2S$ MW: 229.30 Property: mp 290°C (dec). Source: MAI JIAO. Ref: 6.

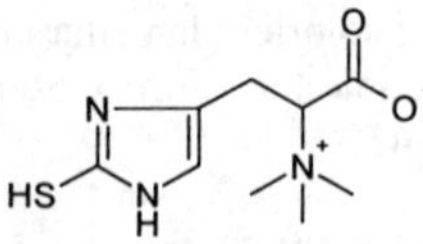

2192 Eriodictyol
$C_{15}H_{12}O_6$ MW: 288.26 Property: mp 267°C. Source: BA DAN XING REN. Ref: 6.

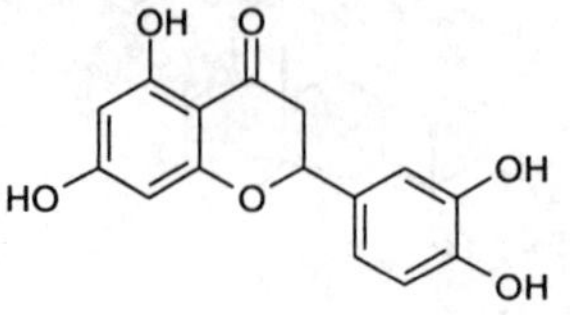

2193 Eriodictyol-7,3-diglucoside
$C_{27}H_{32}O_{17}$ MW: 628.55 Source: SHAN ZHA. Ref: 2.

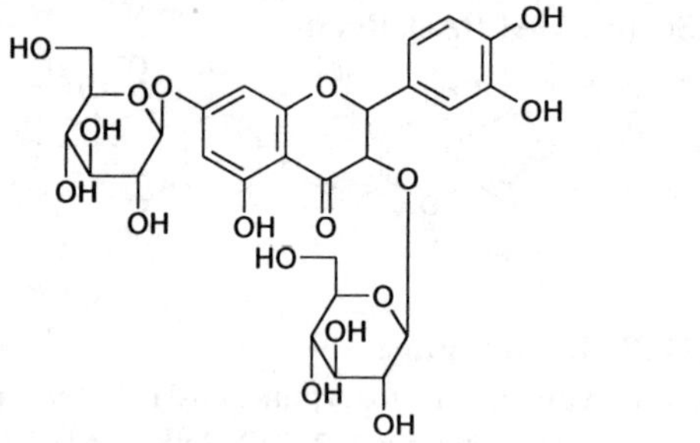

2194 Eriodictyol-7-glucoside
$C_{21}H_{22}O_{11}$ MW: 450.40 Property: mp 175-7°C. Source: SHUI YANG ZHI YE . Ref: 6.

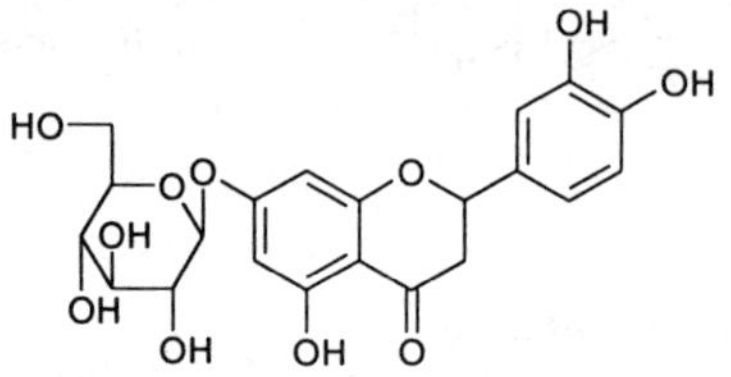

2195 Erosnine
$C_{18}H_8O_6$ MW: 320.26 Property: mp 350°C (dec). Source: DI GUA ZI. Ref: 6.

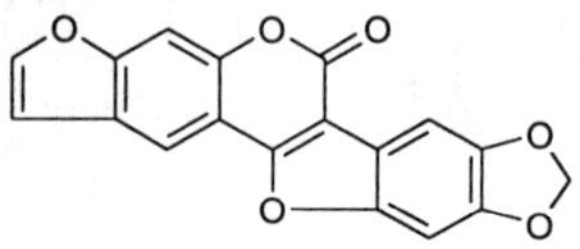

2196 Erosone
$C_{20}H_{16}O_6$ MW: 352.35 Property: mp 218°C. Source: DI GUA ZI. Ref: 6.

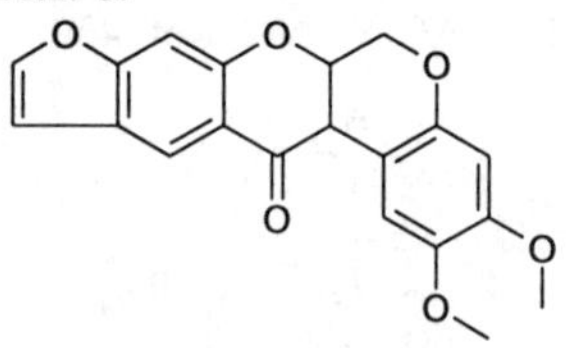

2197 Erucic acid
$C_{22}H_{42}O_2$ MW: 338.58 Property: mp 33.5-4.0°C; bp 241-3°C/5mm. Source: HAN LIAN HUA, LAI FU ZI, TING LI ZI, YUN TAI ZI. Ref: 6.

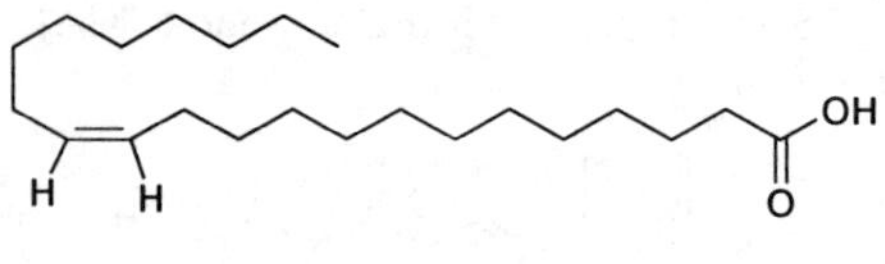

2198 Erychroside
$C_{34}H_{50}O_{13}$ MW: 666.77 Source: GUI ZHU TANG JIE. Ref: 6.

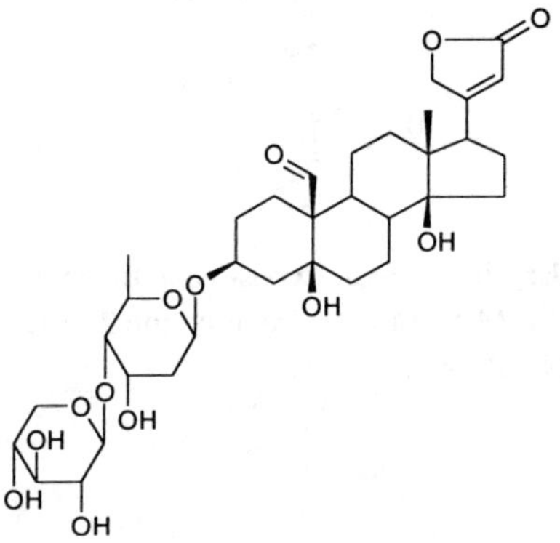

2199 Erychrozol
$C_{34}H_{52}O_{13}$ MW: 668.79 Source: GUI ZHU TANG JIE. Ref: 6.

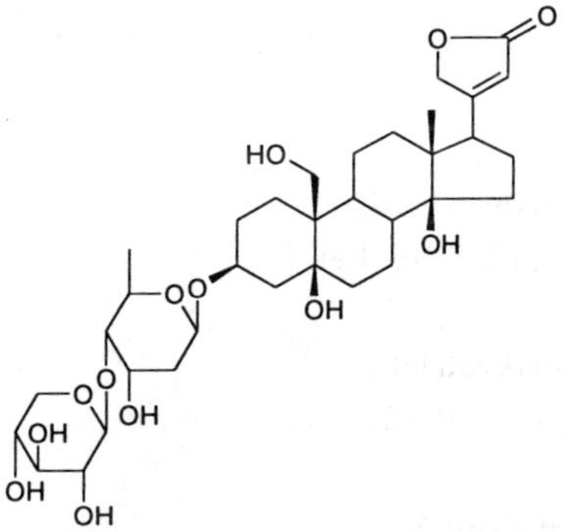

2200 Erycibelline
2β,7β-Dihydroxynortropane. $C_7H_{13}NO_2$ MW: 143.19 Source: WA MAI DING GONG TENG. Ref: 68.

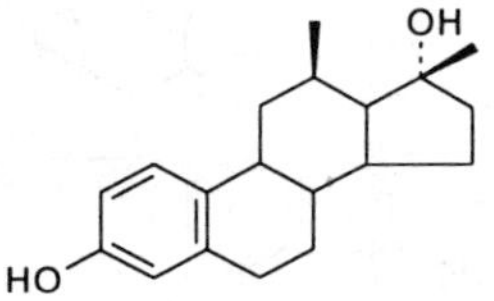

2201 Erycordine
$C_{35}H_{54}O_{14}$ MW: 698.81 Source: GUI ZHU TANG JIE. Ref: 6.

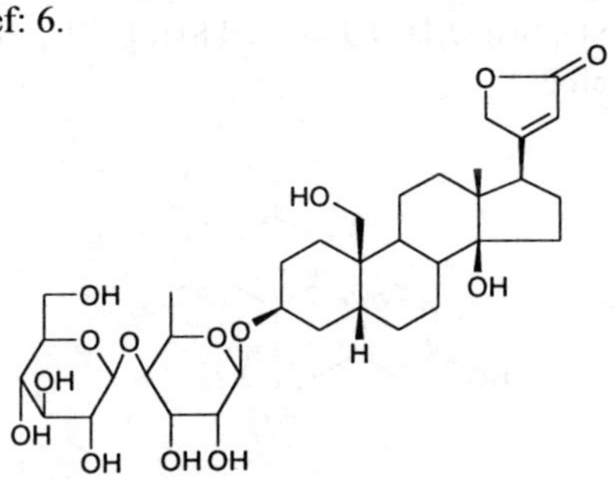

2202 Erysimoside
$C_{35}H_{52}O_{14}$ MW: 696.80 Property: mp 170-3°C. Source: GUI ZHU TANG JIE, HUANG MA ZI, TANG JIE. Ref: 6.

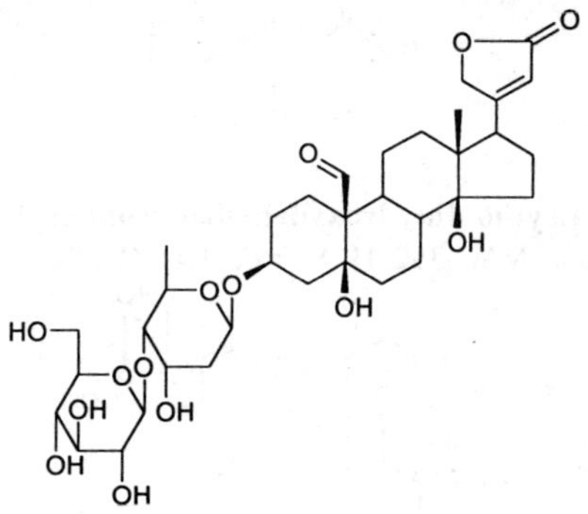

2203 Erysimosol
$C_{35}H_{54}O_{14}$ MW: 698.81 Source: GUI ZHU TANG JIE. Ref: 6.

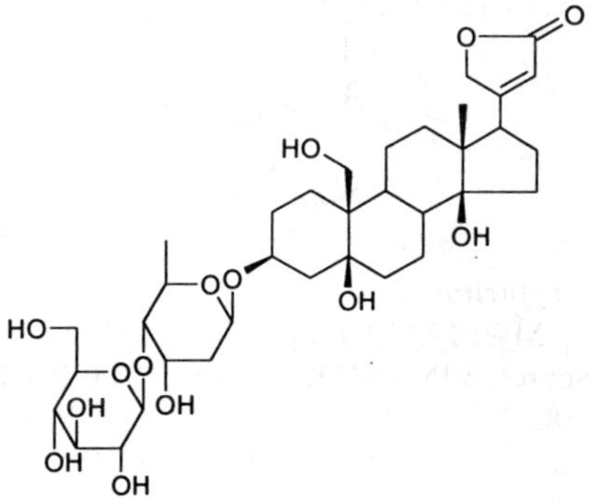

2204 Erysodine
$C_{18}H_{21}NO_3$ MW: 299.37 Property: mp 204-5°C. Source: QIAO MU CI TONG. Ref: 6.

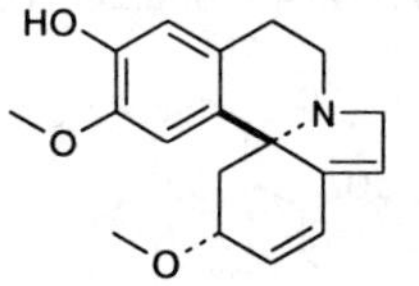

2205 Erysopine
$C_{17}H_{19}NO_3$ MW: 285.35 Property: mp 242-3°C. Source: QIAO MU CI TONG. Ref: 6.

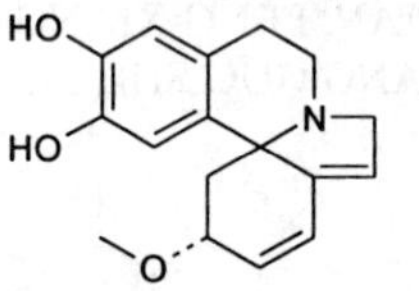

2206 Erysovine
$C_{18}H_{21}NO_3$ MW: 299.81 Property: mp 178-9°C. Source: QIAO MU CI TONG. Ref: 6.

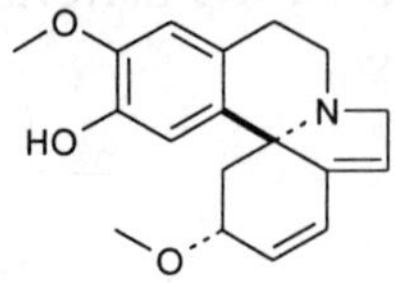

2207 Erytho-dihydroxydehydrodiconiferyl alcohol
$C_{20}H_{24}O_8$ MW: 392.41 Source: DU ZHONG. Ref: 2.

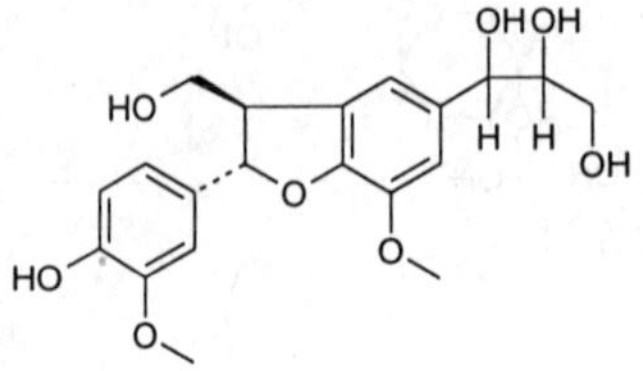

2208 Erythraline
$C_{18}H_{19}NO_3$ MW: 297.36 Property: mp 106-7°C. Source: HAI TONG PI. Ref: 6.

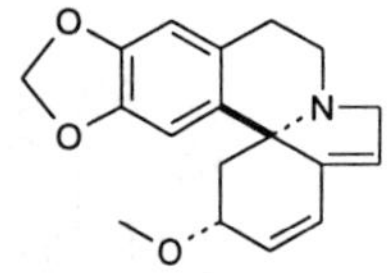

2209 Erythritol
$C_4H_{10}O_4$ MW: 122.12 Property: mp 121.5°C; bp 329-31°C. Source: YING SU KE, ZHANG YE BAN XIA. Ref: 6, 586.

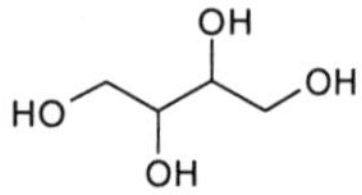

2210 Erythroculine
$C_{20}H_{25}NO_4$ MW: 343.43 Source: HENG ZHOU WU YAO. Ref: 6.

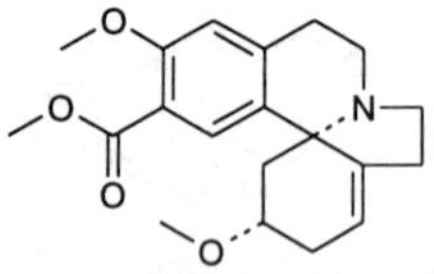

2211 Erythrodiol
$C_{30}H_{50}O_2$ MW: 442.73 Property: mp 215-7°C. Source: BING PIAN, FENG XIANG JI SHENG, BING PIAN, MANG GUO SHU PI, Ref: 2.

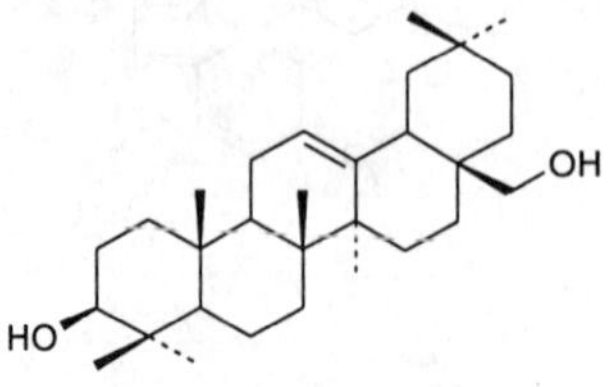

2212 (+)-Erythro-guaiacylglycerol
$C_{10}H_{14}O_5$ MW: 214.22 Source: DU ZHONG. Ref: 2.

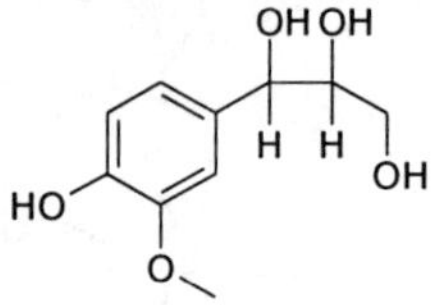

2213 Erythro-β-hydroxy-L-aspartic acid
$C_4H_7NO_5$ MW: 149.10 Property: mp 210°C. Source: ZI YUN YING ZI. Ref: 6.

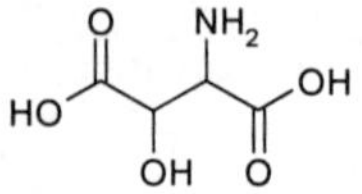

2214 Erythro-2,3-octadecane-diol
$C_{18}H_{38}O_2$ MW: 286.50 Source: ZHI. Ref: 6.

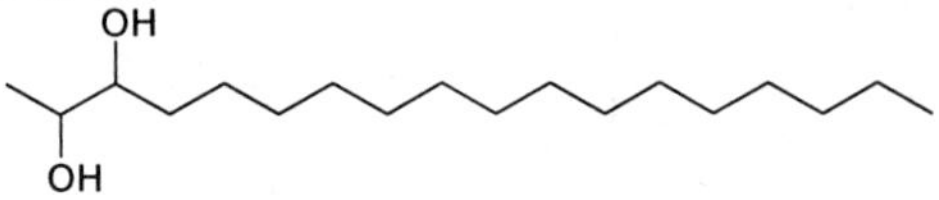

2215 Erythropoietin
Source: ZI HE CHE. Ref: 6.

2216 Erythrotriol
Source: MU CHUAN JIN PI. Ref: 519.

2217 α-Estradiol
$C_{19}H_{26}O_2$ MW: 286.42 Property: mp 223°C. Source: LU RONG, SHE XIANG, SUAN SHI LIOU, ZI HE CHE. Ref: 2.

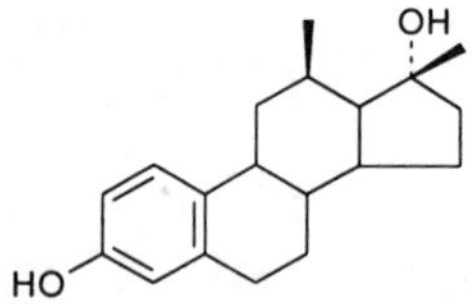

2218 β-Estradiol
$C_{19}H_{26}O_2$ MW: 286.42 Property: mp 178°C. Source: LU RONG, SHE XIANG, SUAN SHI LIOU, ZI HE CHE. Ref: 2.

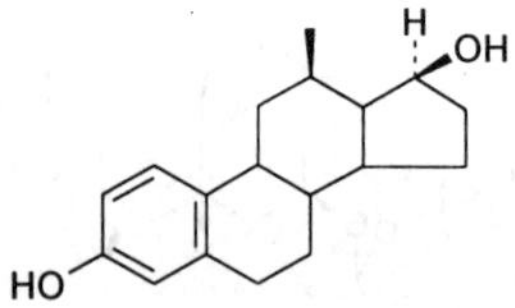

2219 Estragole
$C_{10}H_{12}O$ MW: 148.21 Property: bp 215-6°C. Source: HUA JIAO, HUI XIANG, QIAN HU, SHUI HUI XIANG, XI XIN. Ref: 2, 6.

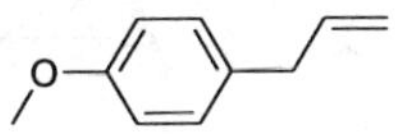

2220 Estriol
Theelol. $C_{18}H_{24}O_3$ MW: 288.39 Property: mp 282-3°C. Source: ZI HE CHE. Ref: 5, 6.

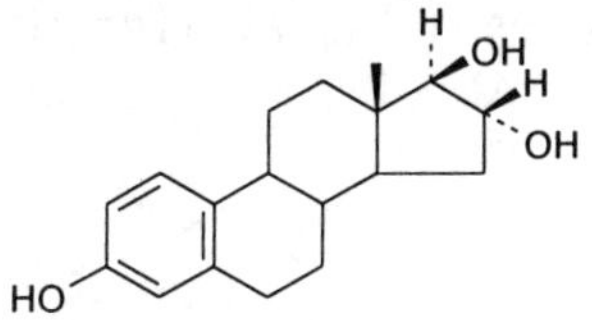

2221 Estrogen
Source: REN NIAO, SAN XIAO CAO. Ref: 6.

2222 Estrone
Oestrone. $C_{18}H_{22}O_2$ MW: 270.37 Property: mp 254°C, 256°C, 259°C. Source: SUAN SHI LIU, WU LOU ZI, ZI HE CHE. Ref: 6.

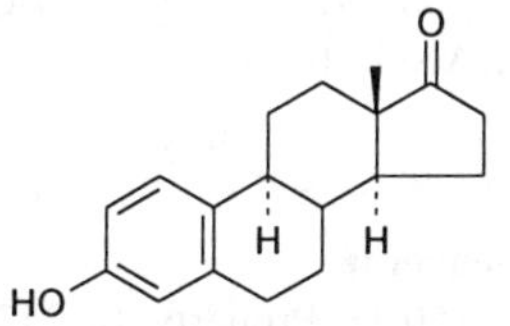

2223 Ethanedioic acid
Source: JIAO TUO LUO. Ref: 587.

2224 Ethanolamine
C_2H_7NO MW: 61.08 Property: bp 171°C. Source: XI JIAO. Ref: 6.

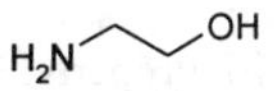

2225 2-(Ethenylbutadiynyl)-5-(propyny)-thiophene
$C_{13}H_8S$ MW: 196.27 Source: MO LI HUA. Ref: 6.

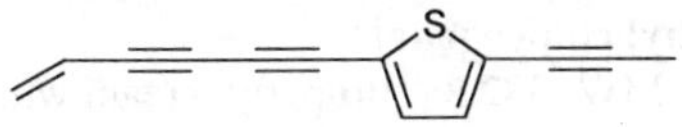

2226 2-(5-Ethenyl-5-methyl-2-tetrahydrofuranyl)-6-methyl-5-hepten-3-one
$C_{15}H_{24}O_2$ MW: 236.36 Source: WU WEI ZI. Ref: 2.

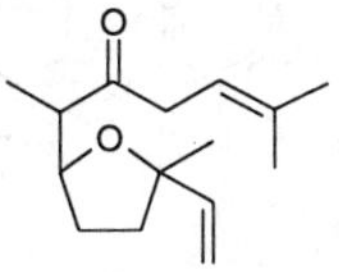

2227 4-Ethenyl-2,2,4-trimethyl-3-(1-methyl-ethenyl)-cyclohexane-methanol
$C_{15}H_{26}O$ MW: 222.37 Source: SHENG JIANG. Ref: 2.

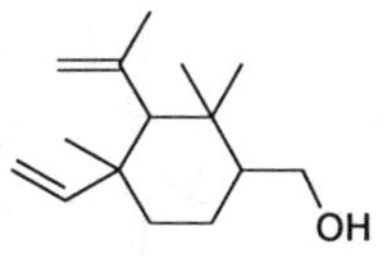

2228 9-Ethoxy-aristololactam
$C_{19}H_{15}NO_5$ MW: 337.34 Source: MIAN MAO MA DOU LING. Ref: 127.

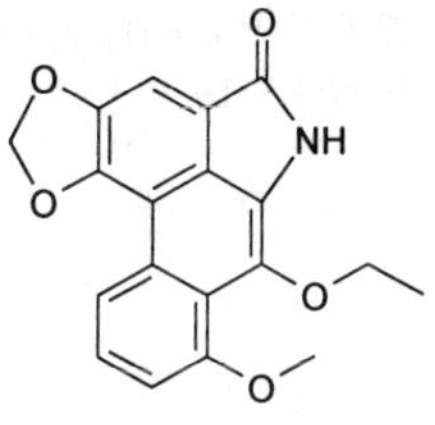

2229 9-Ethoxy-aristololactone
$C_{19}H_{14}O_6$ MW: 338.32 Source: MIAN MAO MA DOU LING. Ref: 127.

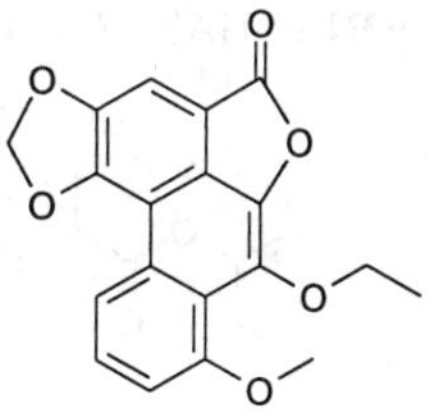

2230 8-β-Ethoxy atractylenolide III
$C_{18}H_{26}O_3$ MW: 290.41 Source: BAI ZHU. Ref: 2.

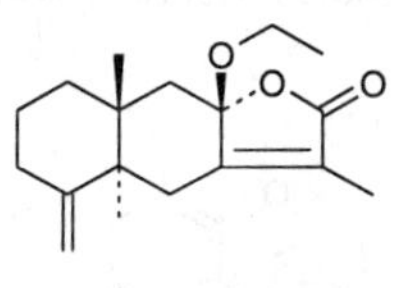

2231 4-Ethoxycarbonyl-2-quinolone
$C_{12}H_{11}NO_3$ MW: 217.23 Property: colorless acicular crystal, mp 208-9°C. Source: YA DAN ZI. Ref: 2, 156.

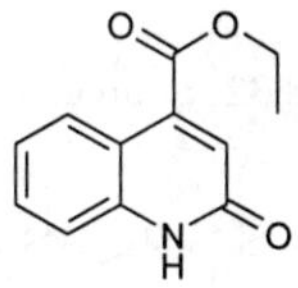

2232 Ethoxydihydroisomorellin
$C_{35}H_{42}O_8$ MW: 590.72 Property: mp 143°C. Source: TENG HUANG. Ref: 6.

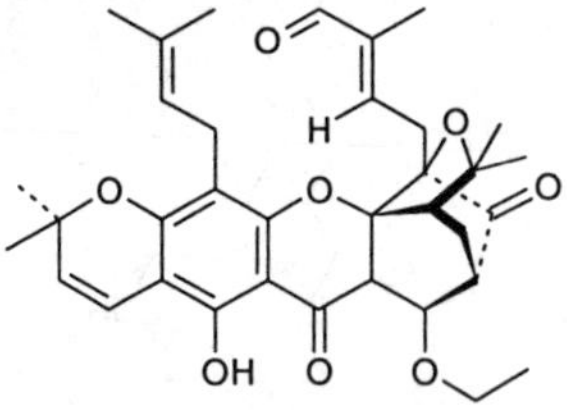

2233 2-(1-Ethoxy-2-hydroxy) propyl-4-methoxyphenol (I)
$C_{12}H_{18}O_4$ MW: 226.27 Property: colorless liquid. Source: YANG HONG SHAN. Ref: 371.

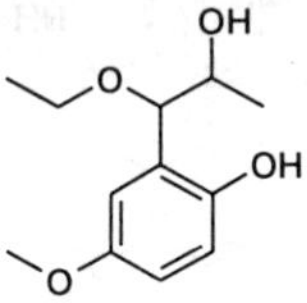

2234 2-(1-Ethoxy-2-hydroxy)propyl-4-methoxyphenol-2-methyl- butyrate(II)
$C_{17}H_{26}O_5$ MW: 310.39 Property: colorless liquid. Source: YANG HONG SHAN. Ref: 371.

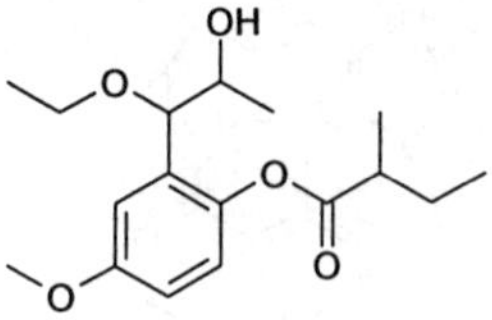

2235 7β-Ethoxy-12-methoxy-8,11,13-abietatrien-11-ol
$C_{23}H_{36}O_3$ MW: 360.54 Source: DU SONG SHI. Ref: 6.

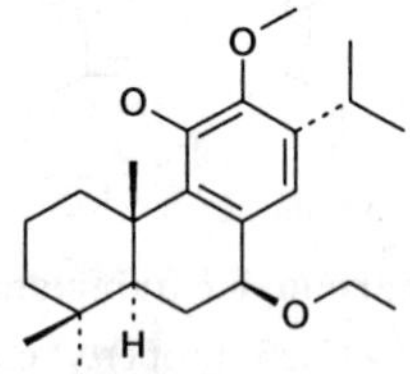

2236 4-Ethoxy methyl phenyl-4'-hydroxy benzyl ether
$C_{16}H_{18}O_3$ MW: 258.32 Source: TIAN MA. Ref: 2.

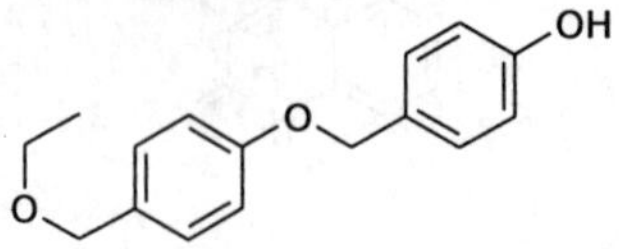

2237 16-Ethoxystrychnine
$C_{22}H_{24}N_2O_3$ MW: 364.45 Property: mp 224-5°C. Source: LU SONG GUO. Ref: 6.

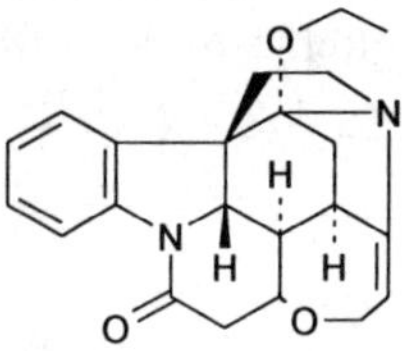

2238 Ethyl acetate
$C_4H_8O_2$ MW: 88.11 Property: bp 77.1°C. Source: JIU, SHENG JIANG. Ref: 2.

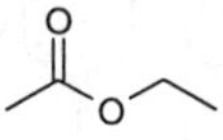

2239 Ethyl aldehyde
Acetaldehyde. C_2H_4O MW: 44.05 Source: HAI JIU CAI, NIU BANG GEN. Ref: 6.

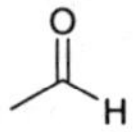

2240 Ethylamine
C_2H_7N MW: 45.08 Property: bp 16.6°C. Source: LING MAO XIANG. Ref: 6.

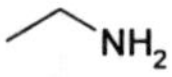

2241 Ethyl benzoate
$C_9H_{10}O_2$ MW: 150.18 Property: bp 212.9°C. Source: XUAN CAO GEN. Ref: 6.

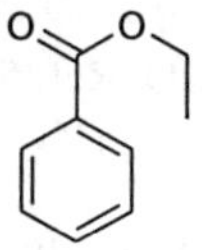

2242 Ethyl butyrate
$C_6H_{12}O_2$ MW: 116.16 Property: bp 119.9°C. Source: JIU. Ref: 6.

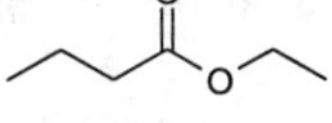

2243 Ethyl chlorogenate
$C_{18}H_{22}O_9$ MW: 382.37 Property: cream white acicular crystal (acetone), mp 106-10°C. Source: XI NAN REN DONG. Ref: 439.

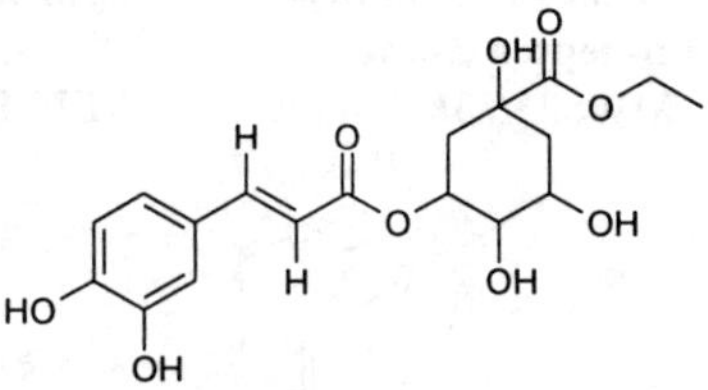

2244 24α-Ethyl-5α-cholestan-3β-ol
$C_{29}H_{52}O$ MW: 416.74 Source: QI YE DAN. Ref: 2.

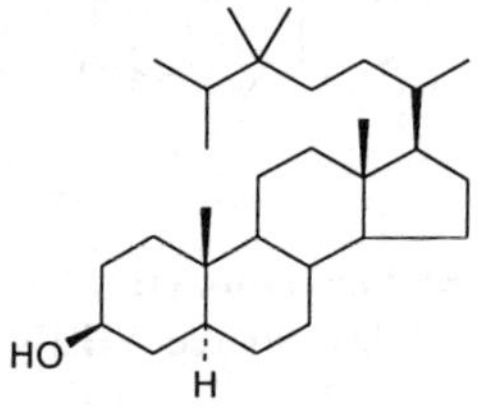

2245 (24S)-Ethylcholesta-5,22,25-trans-3β-ol
$C_{29}H_{46}O$ MW: 410.69 Property: mp 152-3°C. Source: CHOU MO LI, SHUI HU MAN. Ref: 6.

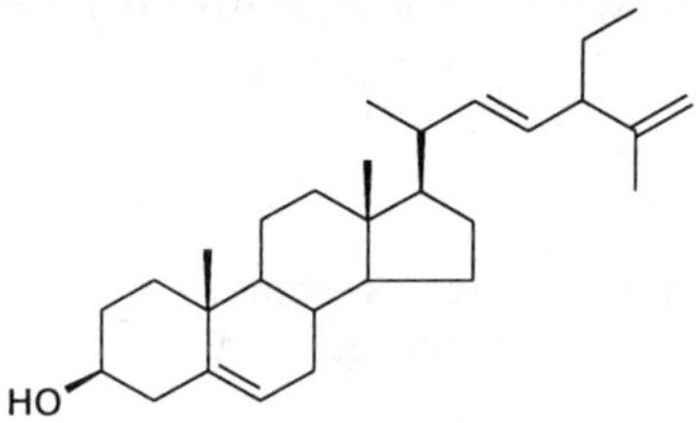

2246 Ethyl cinnamate
$C_{11}H_{12}O_2$ MW: 176.22 Property: bp cis: 125°C /12mm. trans-: 271°C. Source: SHAN NAI. Ref: 6.

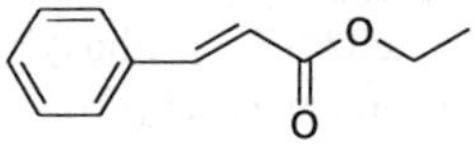

2247 Ethyl-cyclohexane
C_8H_{16} MW: 112.22 Source: SHAN ZHA. Ref: 2.

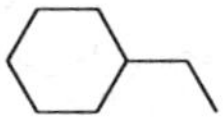

2248 1-Ethyl-4,8-dimethoxy-β-carboline
$C_{15}H_{16}N_2O_2$ MW: 256.31 Source: KU SHU PI. Ref: 12.

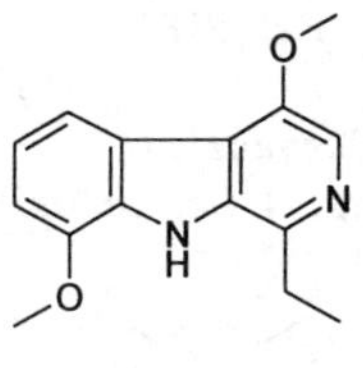

2249 3-Ethyl-2,3-dimethyl-pentane
C_9H_{20} MW: 128.26 Source: SHAN ZHA. Ref: 2.

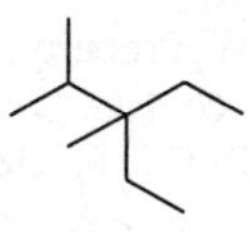

2250 Ethyl-α-D-fructofuranoside
$C_8H_{16}O_6$ MW: 208.21 Source: DANG SHEN. Ref: 2.

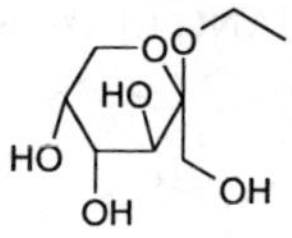

2251 Ethyl-α-D-galactoside
Eleutheroside C. $C_8H_{16}O_6$ MW: 208.21 Property: mp 142°C. Source: CI WU JIA, WU JIA PI. Ref: 2, 6.

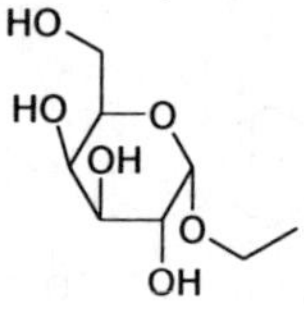

2252 1-Ethyl-β-D-galactoside
$C_8H_{16}O_6$ MW: 208.21 Source: GAN DI HUANG. Ref: 2.

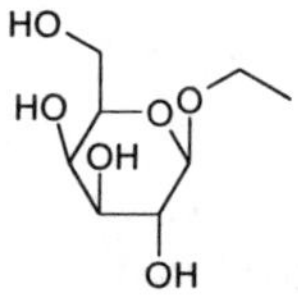

2253 Ethyl gallate
Source: SHE PU TAO. Ref: 552.

2254 Ethyl geranate
$C_{12}H_{20}O_2$ MW: 196.29 Property: bp 110-20°C. Source: YUN XIANG CAO. Ref: 6.

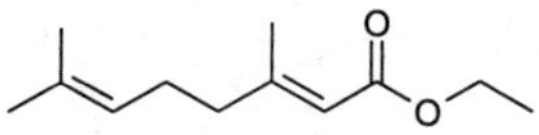

2255 Ethyl heptadecanoate
$C_{19}H_{38}O_2$ MW: 298.51 Source: CHUAN XIONG. Ref: 2.

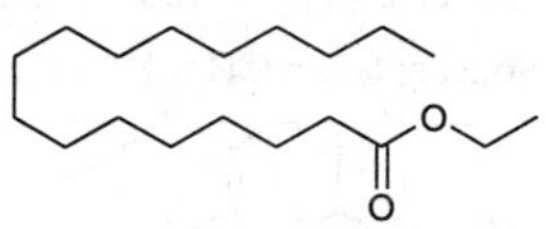

2256 24-Ethylidene lophenol
$C_{30}H_{50}O$ MW: 426.73 Property: mp 162-4°C. Source: GAN ZHE. Ref: 6.

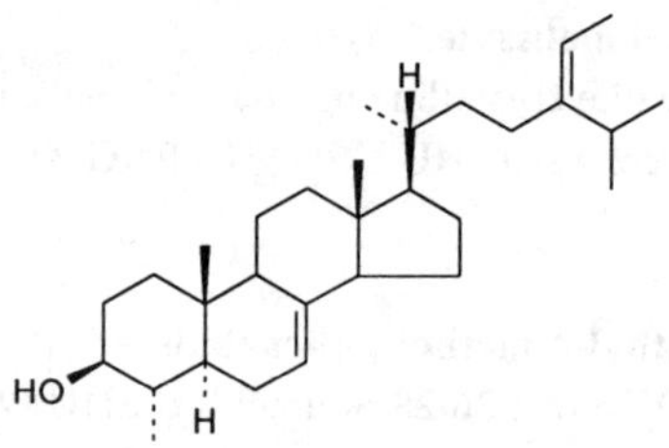

2257 trans-3-Ethylidene-2-pyrrolidone
C_6H_9NO MW: 111.14 Property: mp 172-4°C. Source: JU HUA HUANG LIAN. Ref: 6.

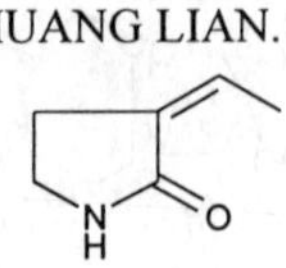

2258 Ethyl isoheptadecanoate
$C_{19}H_{38}O_2$ MW: 298.51 Source: CHUAN XIONG. Ref: 2.

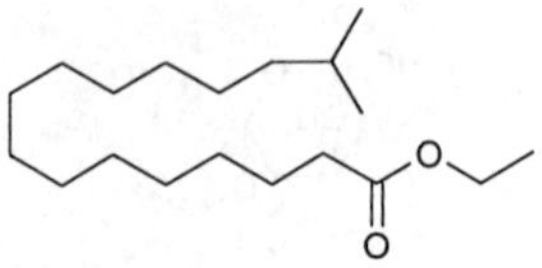

2259 Ethyl isooctadecanoate
$C_{20}H_{40}O_2$ MW: 312.54 Source: CHUAN XIONG. Ref: 2.

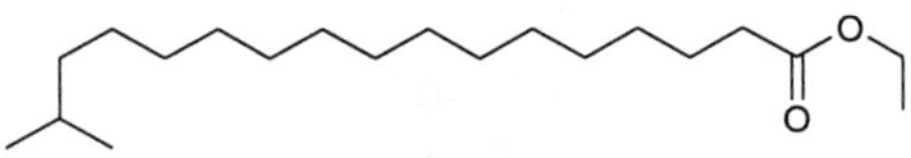

2260 Ethyl isopropyl sulfide
$C_5H_{12}S$ MW: 104.22 Source: SHENG JIANG. Ref: 2.

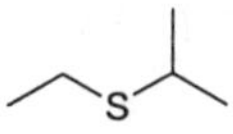

2261 Ethyl laurate
$C_{14}H_{28}O_2$ MW: 228.38 Source: BAI ZHI. Ref: 2.

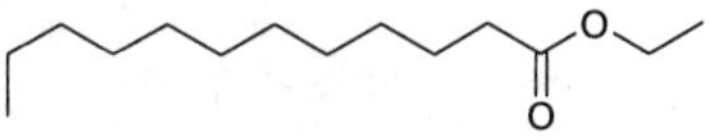

2262 Ethylleptol B
$C_{17}H_{24}O_4$ MW: 292.38 Property: light yellow oleaginous substances, $[\alpha]_D^{10}$ +3.26° (c=0.307, CH_3COCH_3). Source: SAN CHA KU. Ref: 393.

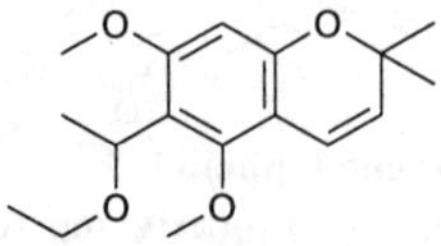

2263 Ethyl melissate
Property: white crystalline powder (ethanol), mp 89-90°C. Source: XIAO HUA SUAN TENG ZI. Ref: 437.

2264 1-Ethyl-4-methoxy-β-carboline
$C_{14}H_{14}N_2O$ MW: 226.28 Source: KU SHU PI.Ref: 12.

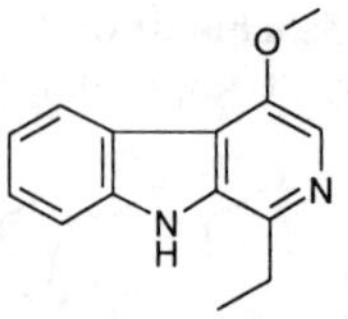

2265 Ethyl-p-methoxycinnamate
$C_{12}H_{14}O_3$ MW: 206.24 Source: SHAN NAI. Ref: 6.

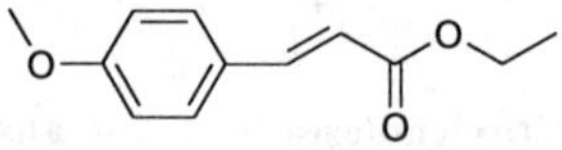

2266 1-Ethyl-2-methyl-benzene
C_9H_{12} MW: 120.20 Source: SHAN ZHA. Ref: 2.

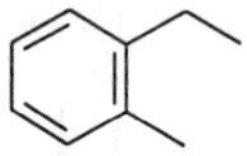

2267 5-Ethyl-2-methyl-heptane
$C_{10}H_{22}$ MW: 142.29 Source: SHAN ZHA. Ref: 2.

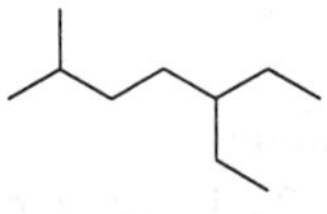

2268 Ethylnotopterol
5-{(2E,5E)-3,7-dimethyl-7-[(1-ethoxy)-ethoxy-2,5-octadienyloxy]} psoralen. $C_{23}H_{26}O_5$ MW: 328.26 Property: colorless ropy substance. Source: QIANG HUO. Ref: 325.

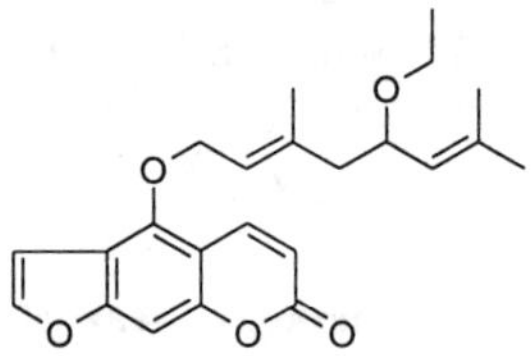

2269 Ethyl octacosate
Source: SHA REN. Ref: 518.

2270 Ethyl octadecanoate
$C_{20}H_{40}O_2$ MW: 312.54 Source: CHUAN XIONG. Ref: 2.

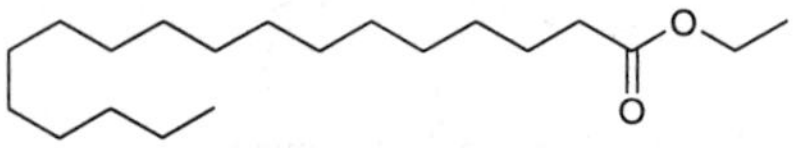

2271 Ethyl palmitate
$C_{18}H_{36}O_2$ MW: 284.49 Property: mp α: 24°C, β: 19.3 °C. Source: CHUAN XIONG, DANG SHEN, JIN YIN HUA, SAN QI. Ref: 2, 6, 638.

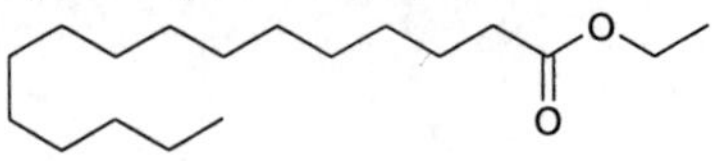

2272 Ethyl pentadecanoate
$C_{17}H_{34}O_2$ MW: 270.46 Source: CHUAN XIONG. Ref: 2.

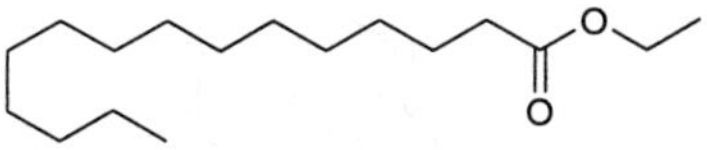

2273 p-Ethyl phenol
$C_8H_{10}O$ MW: 122.17 Source: DANG GUI. Ref: 2.

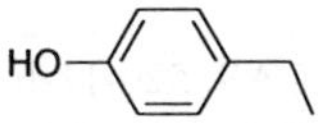

2274 o-Ethyl phenol
$C_8H_{10}O$ MW: 122.17 Source: DANG GUI. Ref: 2.

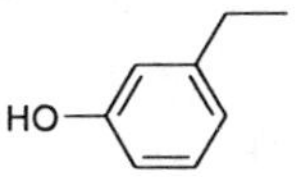

2275 Ethyl propionate
$C_5H_{10}O_2$ MW: 102.13 Source: SHENG JIANG. Ref: 2.

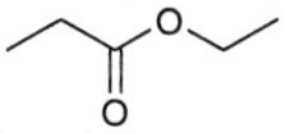

2276 4-Ethyl resorcinol
$C_8H_{10}O_2$ MW: 138.17 Source: DANG GUI. Ref: 2.

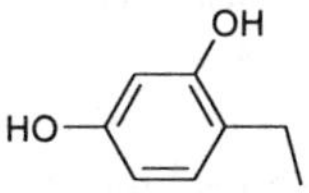

2277 Eucalyptin
$C_{19}H_{18}O_5$ MW: 326.35 Property: mp 198.5-200°C. Source: AN YE, NING MENG AN YE. Ref: 6.

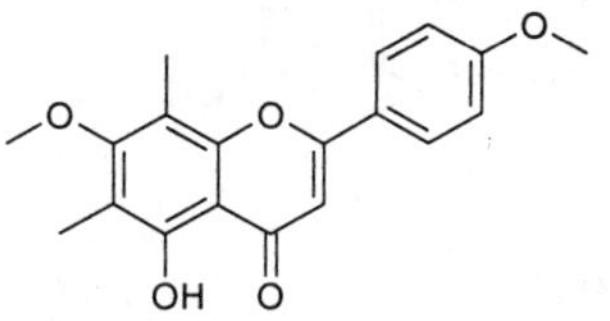

2278 Eucalyptole
Cineole. Source: LUO LE, TU QIANG HUO. Ref: 6.

2279 Eucarvone
$C_{10}H_{14}O$ MW: 150.22 Property: bp 99-100°C/22mm. Source: XI XIN. Ref: 2.

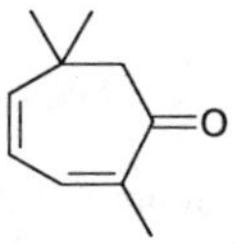

2280 Eucommin A
$C_{27}H_{34}O_{12}$ MW: 550.56 Source: DU ZHONG. Ref: 2.

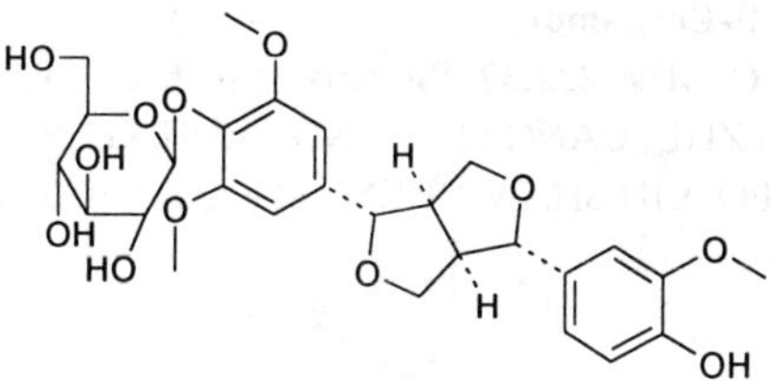

2281 Eucommiol
$C_9H_{16}O_4$ MW: 188.23 Source: DU ZHONG. Ref: 2.

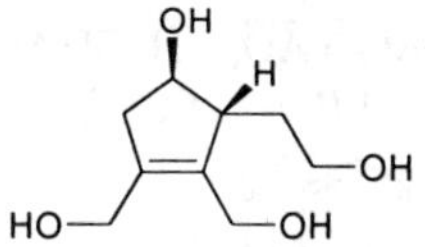

2282 Eucommioside
$C_{15}H_{26}O_9$ MW: 350.37 Source: DU ZHONG. Ref: 2.

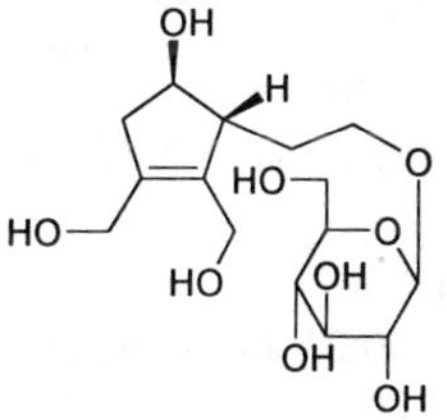

2283 Eucommioside-II
$C_{15}H_{26}O_9$ MW: 350.37 Source: DU ZHONG. Ref: 2.

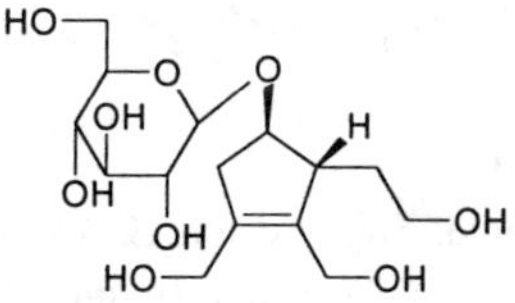

2284 Eudesmin
$C_{22}H_{26}O_6$ MW: 386.45 Property: mp 107-8°C. Source: XIN YI. Ref: 6.

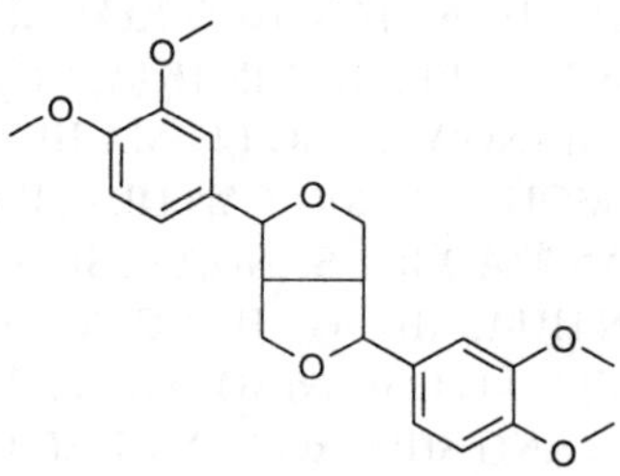

2285 α-Eudesmol
$C_{15}H_{26}O$ MW: 222.37 Property: mp 75°C; bp 156°C/10mm. Source: CANG ZHU, HOU PO. Ref: 6.

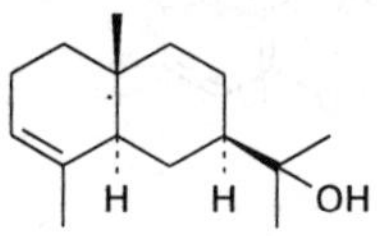

2286 β-Eudesmol
$C_{15}H_{26}O$ MW: 222.37 Property: mp 76°C. Source: CANG ZHU, CANG SU, FANG FENG, GAN SONG, HOU PO, LIU SHAN, SHENG JIANG. Ref: 2, 6.

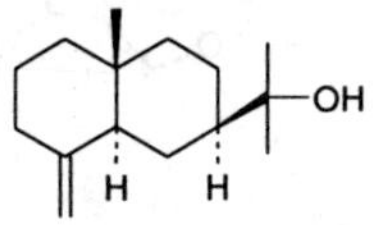

2287 Eugeniin
Source: BAI SHAO YAO, CHI SHAO YAO. Ref: 2.

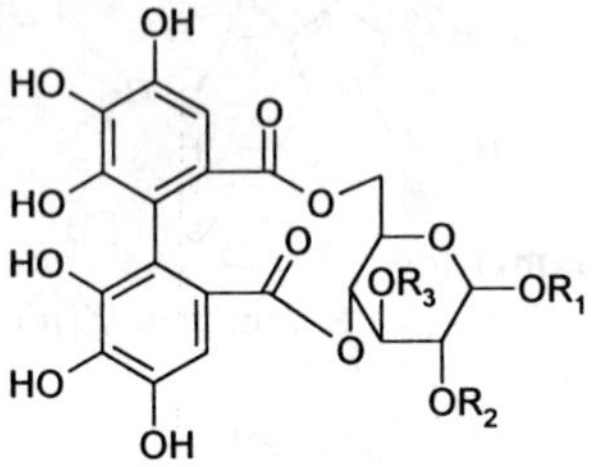

R1=β-galloyl R2,R3=galloyl

2288 Eugenitin
$C_{12}H_{12}O_4$ MW: 220.23 Property: mp 162°C. Source: DING XIANG. Ref: 6.

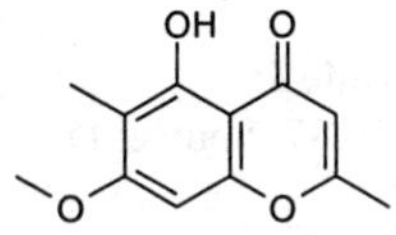

2289 Eugenol
Coryophyllic acid; Eugenic acid. CAS: 97-53-0 $C_{10}H_{12}O_2$ MW: 164.21 Property: mp -9°C, bp 254-5°C. Source: BAI CHANG, CHA SHU, CHAI HU, DA LIANG JIANG, DING XIANG, DU HENG, FEI LONG ZHANG XUE, GAO LIANG JIANG, GUI PI, HOU ZHANG, HUA LIAN, HUO XIANG, HUO XIANG, JIA JING JIE, JIN YIN HUA, JIU LI XIANG, JU JIANG YE, LUO LE, MA HUA, MEI GUI HUA, MOU YAO, MU LAN HUA, PAN SHI LIU YE, SAN TIAO JIN, SANG YE, SHI CHUN, SHUI XIAN HUA, XIANG ZHANG, XIANG ZHANG YE, XIAO CAO NIAO, XIN YI, XI XIN, XUE MAI, YANG SHI CAO, YIN CHEN GAO, YIN CHEN HAO, YIN XIANG PI, YIN XIANG YE, YUE GUI ZI, ZHANG MU, ZI SU, ZI SU YE.
Ref: 2, 4, 11, 638.

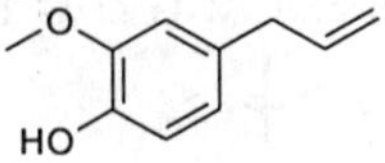

2290 Eugenone
$C_{13}H_{16}O_5$ MW: 252.27 Property: mp 97-8°C. Source: DING XIANG. Ref: 6.

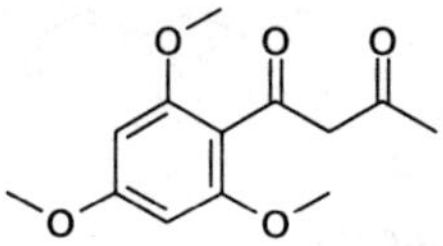

2291 Eupafolin
6-Methoxyluteolin. CAS: 520-11-6 $C_{16}H_{12}O_7$ MW: 316.27 Source: LI ZHI CAO. Ref: 5.

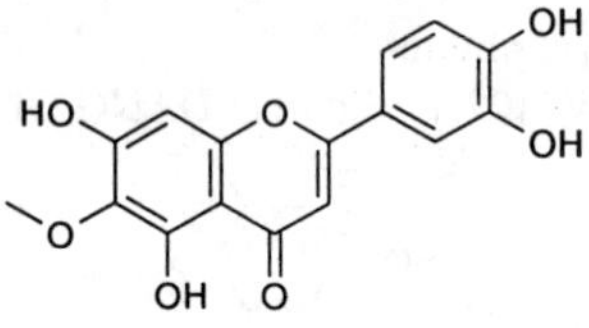

2292 Eupafolin-7-glucoside
$C_{22}H_{22}O_{12}$ MW: 478.41 Property: mp 252-6°C (dec). Source: LI ZHI CAO. Ref: 6.

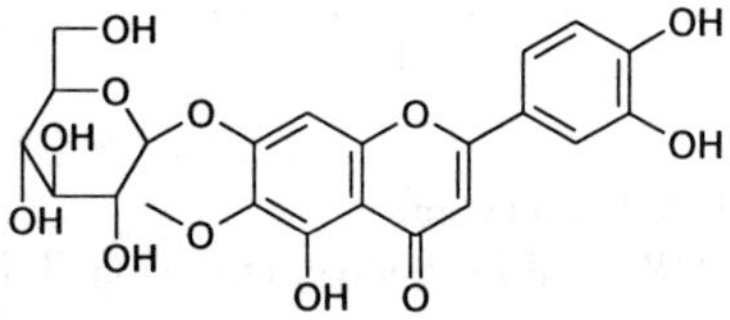

2293 Eupalitin
$C_{17}H_{14}O_7$ MW: 330.30 Source: YIN CHEN HAO. Ref: 2.

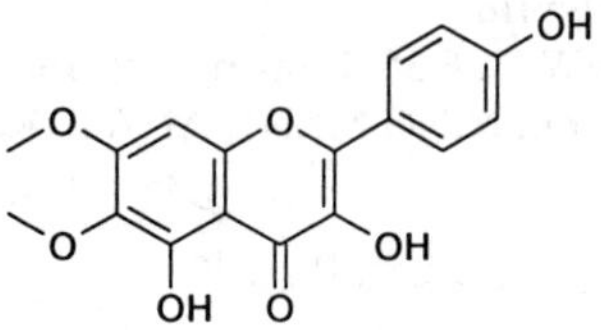

2294 Euparin
$C_{13}H_{12}O_3$ MW: 216.24 Property: mp 121-2°C. Source: CHENG GAN SHENG MA, PEI LIAN. Ref: 6.

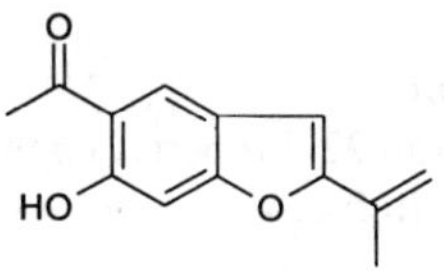

2295 d-Eupatene
Property: bp 9.2-4°C. Source: FEI JI CAO. Ref: 6.

2296 l-Eupatene
Property: bp 106°C/5mm. Source: FEI JI CAO. Ref: 6.

2297 Eupatolin
$C_{23}H_{24}O_{12}$ MW: 492.44 Property: mp 200-1°C. Source: PEI LAN. Ref: 6.

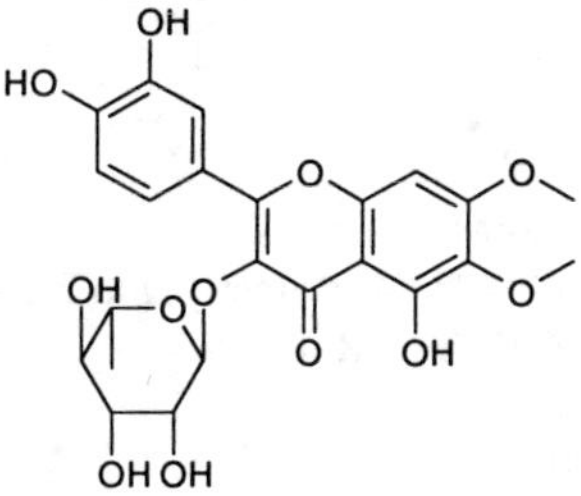

2298 Eupatolitin
$C_{17}H_{14}O_8$ MW: 346.30 Source: QING HAO, YIN CHEN HAO. Ref: 2.

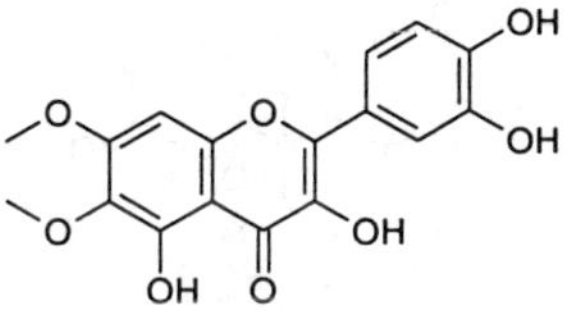

2299 Eupatoriopicrin
$C_{20}H_{26}O_6$ MW: 362.43 Property: mp 157-61°C. Source: PEI LAN. Ref: 6.

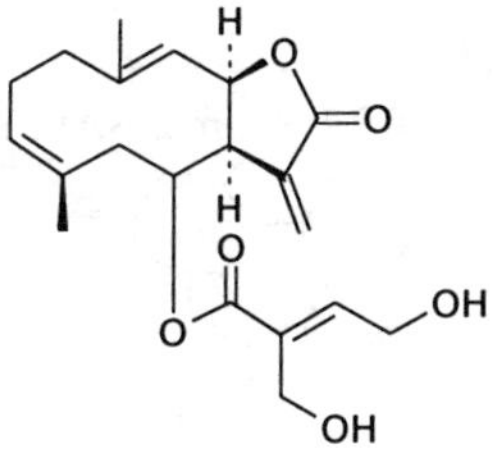

2300 Euphobiasteroid
5,10-Diacetyl-6,20-epoxy-3-phenyl-acetyllathyrol. $C_{32}H_{40}O_8$ MW: 552.67 Property: mp 199.5°C. Source: QIAN JIN ZI. Ref: 6.

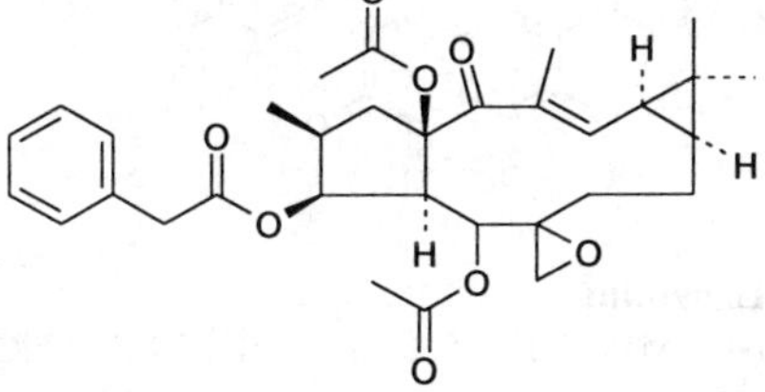

2301 Euphol
Euphadienol. $C_{30}H_{50}O$ MW: 426.73 Property: mp 116°C. Source: BA WANG BIAN, GAN SUI, HUO YANG LE, XI YE DA JI. Ref: 6.

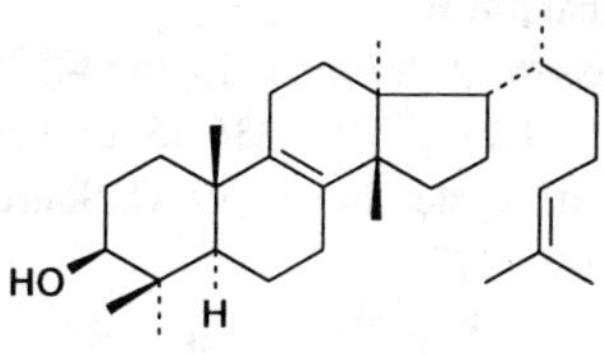

2302 Euphorbetin
$C_{18}H_{10}O_8$ MW: 354.28 Source: QIAN JIN ZI. Ref: 6.

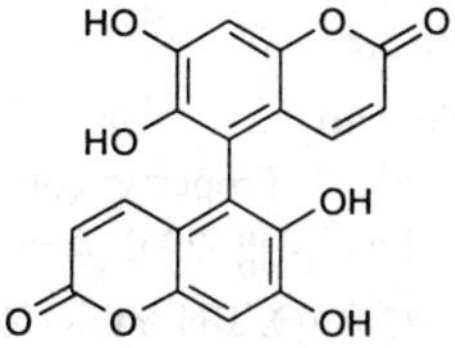

2303 Euphorbia A
$C_{16}H_{10}O_5$ MW: 282.26 Property: mp 217°C. Source: DA JI (a). Ref: 6.

2304 Euphorbia B
$C_{15}H_8O_5$ MW: 268.23 Property: mp 224°C. Source: DA JI (a). Ref: 6.

2305 Euphorbia C
Property: mp 283°C. Source: DA JI (a). Ref: 6.

2306 Euphorbol
α-Euphorbol. $C_{31}H_{52}O$ MW: 440.76 Property: mp 127-8°C. Source: BA WANG BIAN, GAN SUI, HUO YANG LE. Ref: 6.

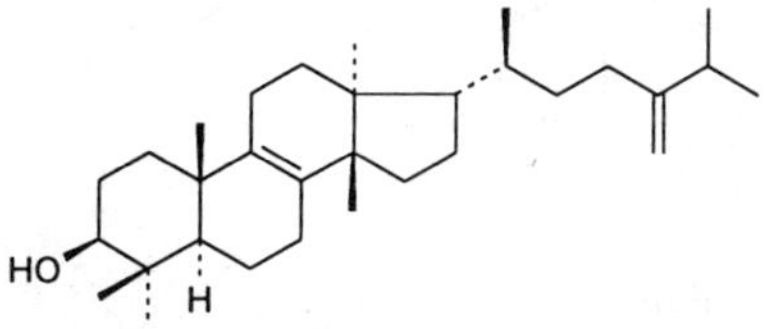

2307 Euphorbon
$C_{37}H_{58}O_{12}$ MW: 694.87 Property: mp 67-8°C. Source: DA JI (a), GAN SUI. Ref: 6.

2308 Eurycarpin A
7,2',4'-trihydroxy-(3,3-dimethylally) isoflavone $C_{20}H_{18}O_5$ MW: 338.36 Property: light yellow powder (methanol), mp 85-7 °C. Source: HUANG GAN CAO. Ref: 379.

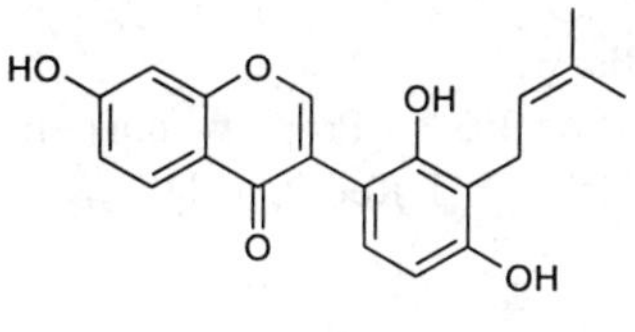

2309 Eurycarpin B
7,2'-dihydroxy-6'',6''-dimethylpyrano-(2'',3'':4',3') isoflavone. $C_{20}H_{16}O_5$ MW: 336.35 Property: light yellow acicular crystal, mp 227-9 °C. Source: HUANG GAN CAO. Ref: 379.

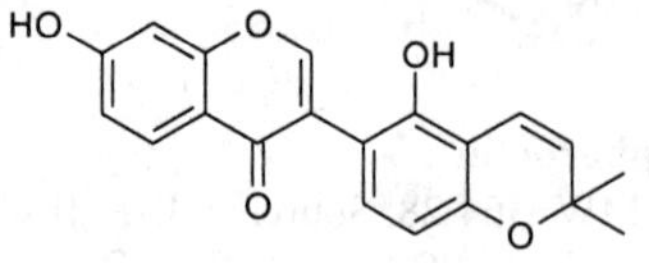

2310 Euscaphic acid
$C_{30}H_{48}O_5$ MW: 488.71 Property: colorless powder crystal, mp 269-71°C, $[\alpha]_D^{18}$ -22.4° (c=0.05, pyridine). Source: DA HONG PAO, JIN YING ZI, SAN YE SHU WEI CAO, TUN XING GUO. Ref: 447, 570, 592, 643.

2311 Evernic acid
$C_{17}H_{16}O_7$ MW: 332.31 Property: mp 169.6-70.1°C. Source: XIAO LA BA. Ref: 6.

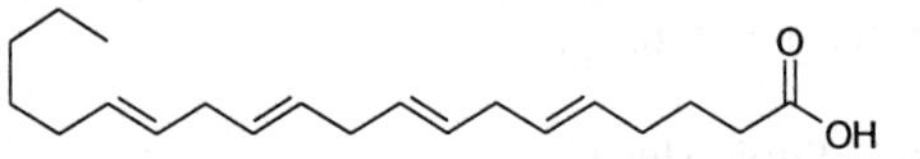

2312 Evocarpine
$C_{23}H_{33}NO$ MW: 339.53 Note: evocarpine is a mixture, the following structure is its main component. Source: WU ZHU YU. Ref: 2.

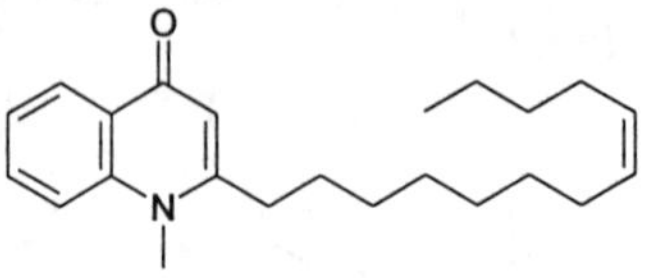

2313 Evoden
$C_{10}H_{16}$ MW: 136.24 Source: WU ZHU YU. Ref: 6.

2314 Evodiamide
$C_{19}H_{21}N_3O$ MW: 307.40 Source: WU ZHU YU. Ref: 2, 347.

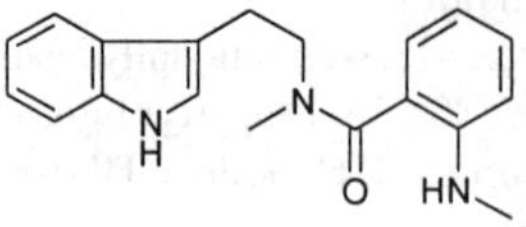

2315 Evodiamine
$C_9H_{17}N_3O$ MW: 303.37 Property: mp (+): 270-2°C. Source: WU ZHU YU. Ref: 2, 6, 347.

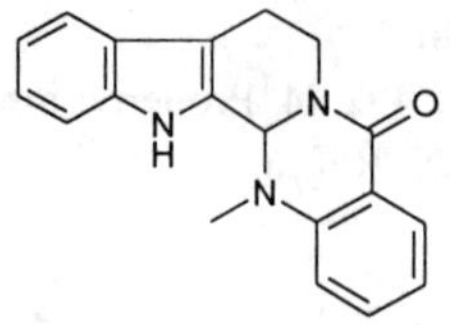

2317 Evodinone
$C_{26}H_{32}O_9$ MW: 488.54 Property: mp 295-7°C (dec). Source: WU ZHU YU. Ref: 6.

2318 Evodol
$C_{26}H_{28}O_9$ MW: 484.51 Property: mp 280-1°C. Source: WU ZHU YU. Ref: 2.

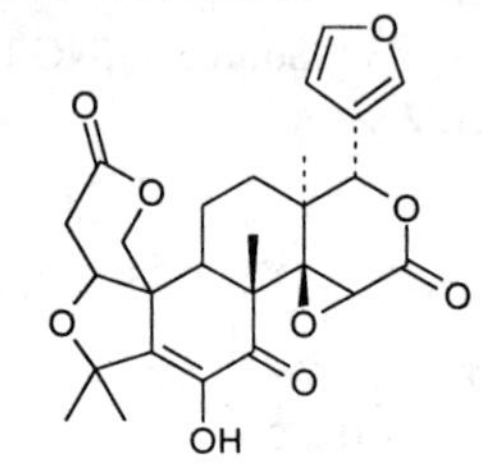

2319 Evogin
$C_{24}H_{28}O_8$ MW: 444.49 Property: mp 279-81°C (dec). Source: WU ZHU YU. Ref: 6.

2320 Exaltolide
$C_{15}H_{28}O_2$ MW: 240.39 Source: BAI ZHI. Ref: 2.

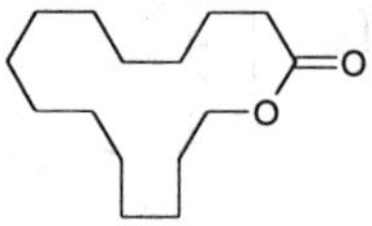

2321 Exoticin
$C_{23}H_{26}O_{10}$ MW: 462.46 Property: mp 124-5°C. Source: JIU LI XIANG. Ref: 6, 11.

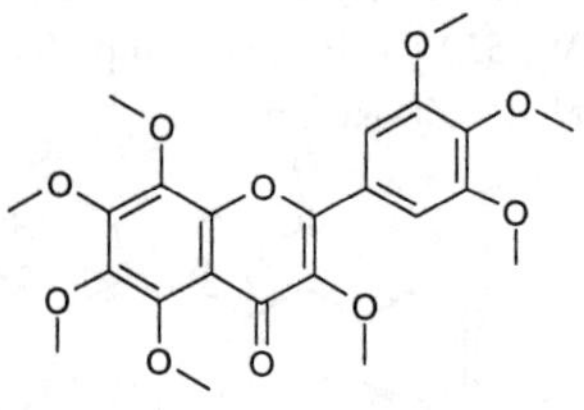

2322 Exozoline
$C_{22}H_{25}NO$ MW: 319.45 Source: JIU LI XIANG. Ref: 11.

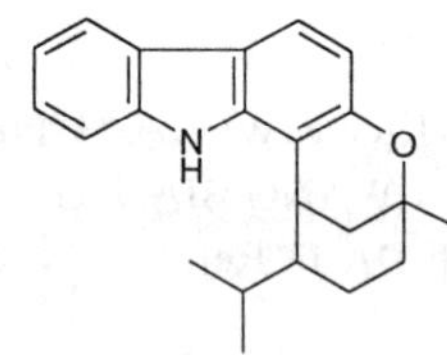

2324 γ-Fagarine
$C_{13}H_{11}NO_3$ MW: 229.24 Property: mp 142°C. Source: BAI XIAN PI, CHOU CAO, ZHU YE JIAO GEN. Ref: 6.

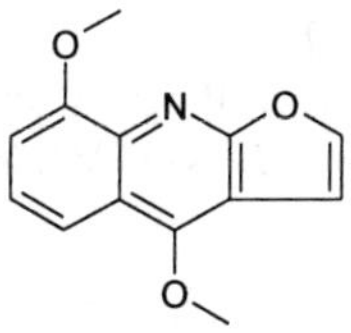

2325 Falcarindiol
$C_{17}H_{24}O_2$ MW: 260.38 Source: FANG FENG, LI JIANG QIAN HU, LONG YAN DU HUO, SONG YE FANG FENG. Ref: 2, 549, 557, 571.

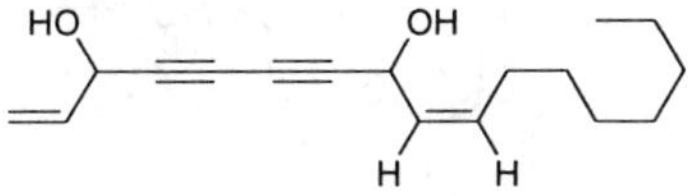

2326 Falcarinol
$C_{17}H_{24}O$ MW: 244.38 Source: FANG FENG. Ref: 2.

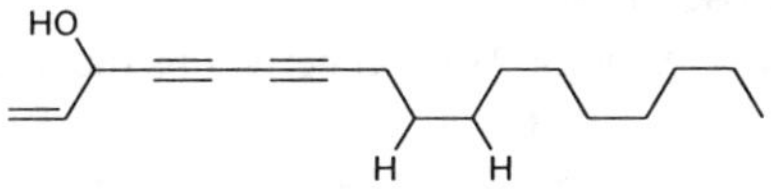

2327 Fallacinol
$C_{16}H_{12}O_6$ MW: 300.27 Source: HU ZHANG. Ref: 2.

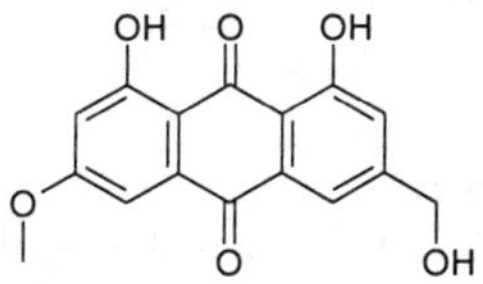

2328 Fangchinoline
Demethyltetrandrine; Hanfangichin B. CAS: 436-77-1 $C_{37}H_{40}N_2O_6$ MW: 608.74 Property: mp 237-8°C (in acetone), mp 177-9°C (in CH_3OH). Source: FANG JI, FEN FANG JI, RU LAN. Ref: 2, 4, 5, 44.

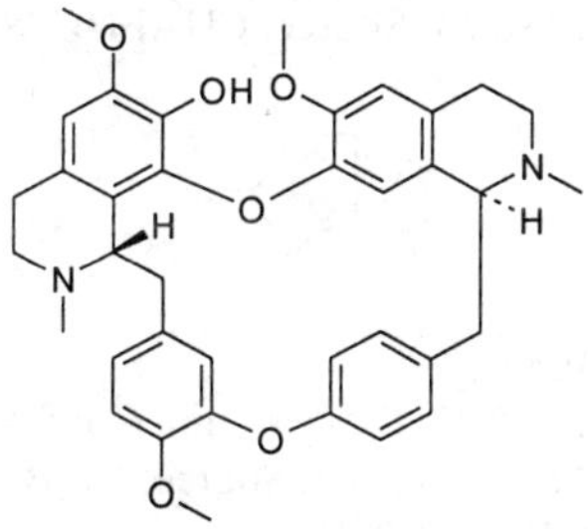

2329 Faradiol
$C_{29}H_{48}O_2$ MW: 428.70 Property: mp 236-7°C. Source: KUAN DONG HUA. Ref: 6.

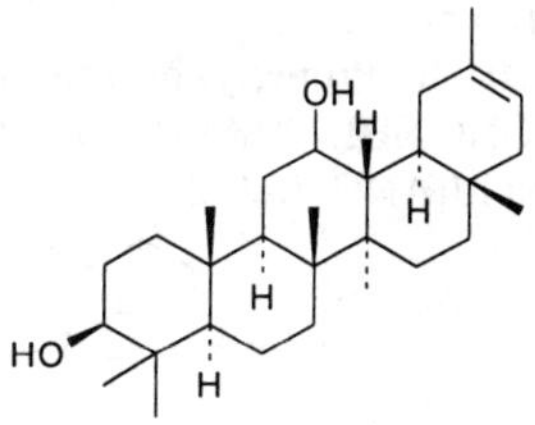

2330 Farcarineiol
$C_{17}H_{24}O_2$ MW: 260.38 Property: brown oleaginous substance. Source: QIANG HUO. Ref: 452.

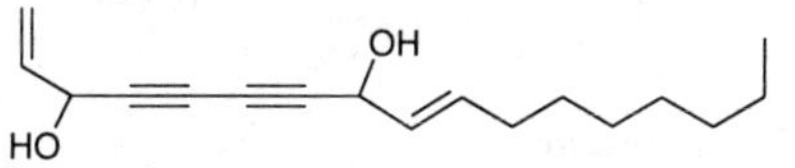

2331 Farfaratin
$C_{23}H_{34}O_5$ MW: 390.52 Property: white hyaloid crystal, mp 100-1°C. Source: KUAN DONG HUA. Ref: 145.

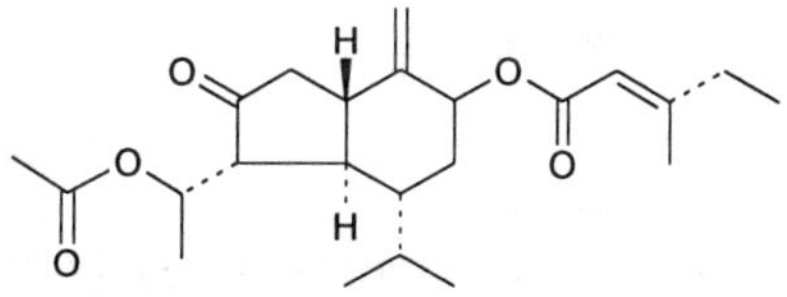

2332 Farfugin A
$C_{15}H_{18}O$ MW: 214.31 Source: LIAN PENG CAO. Ref: 6.

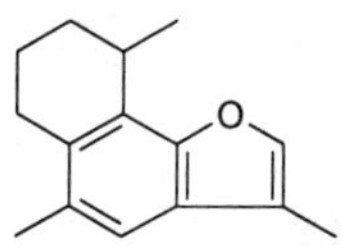

2333 Farfugin B
$C_{15}H_{18}O$ MW: 214.31 Source: LIAN PENG CAO. Ref: 6.

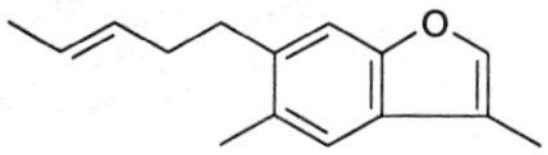

2334 Fargesin
$C_{21}H_{22}O_6$ MW: 370.41 Property: mp 139°C. Source: XIN YI. Ref: 6, 543.

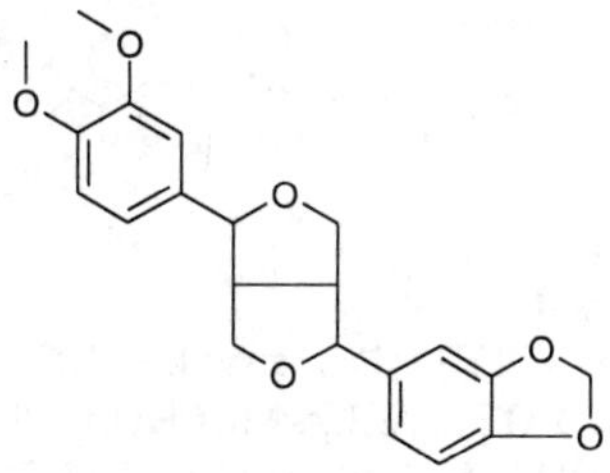

2335 α-Farnesene
$C_{15}H_{24}$ MW: 204.36 Property: bp 128-30°C/12mm. Source: DU SONG SHI, CHAI HU, JU PI, MU JU, PI PA YE, SHENG JIANG. Ref: 2.

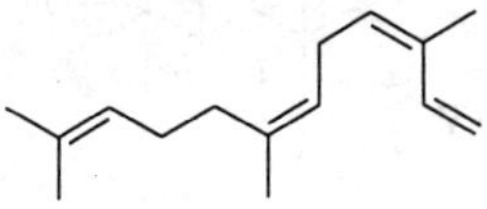

2336 (E)(E)-α-Farnesene
$C_{15}H_{24}$ MW: 204.36 Source: GAN JIANG. Ref: 2.

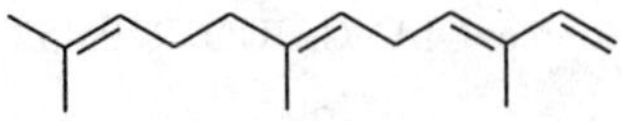

2337 β-Farnesene
$C_{15}H_{24}$ MW: 204.36 Property: bp 121-2°C/9mm. Source: CHAN CHU DAN, HUO XIANG, MA HUA, PI PA YE, REN SHEN, SHENG JIANG, TAN XIANG, XI YANG SHEN. Ref: 2.

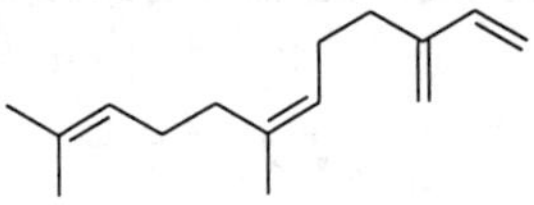

2338 Farnesiferol A
$C_{24}H_{30}O_4$ MW: 382.50 Property: mp (-): 155°C, (±): 152-6°C. Source: A WEI. Ref: 6.

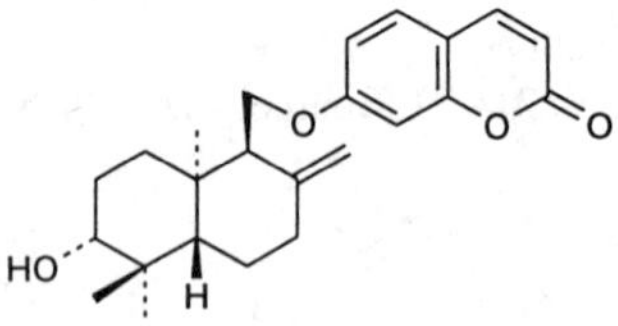

2339 Farnesiferol B
$C_{24}H_{30}O_4$ MW: 382.50 Property: mp 112.5-3.5°C. Source: A WEI. Ref: 6.

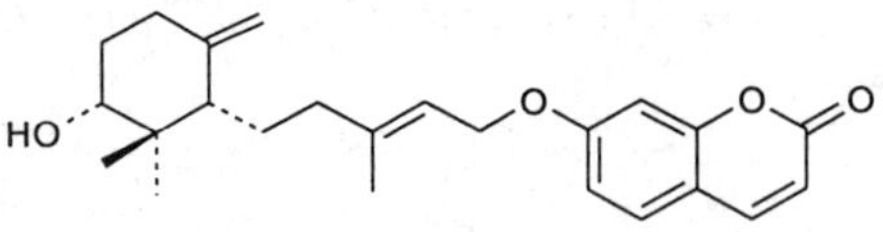

2340 Farnesiferol C
$C_{24}H_{30}O_4$ MW: 382.50 Property: mp 83.5-4.5°C. Source: A WEI. Ref: 6.

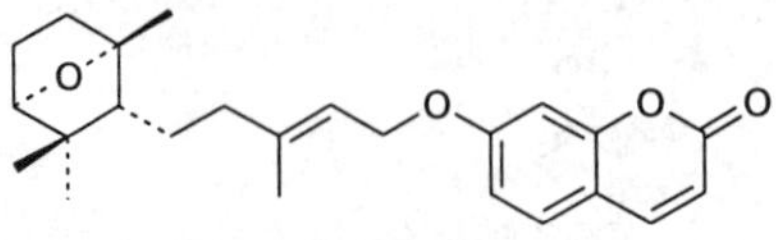

2341 Farnesol
$C_{15}H_{26}O$ MW: 222.37 Property: bp 160°C/10mm. Source: DAI DAI HUA, LA MEI HUA, PI PA YE, PU TI SHU HUA, SHENG JIANG. Ref: 2, 6.

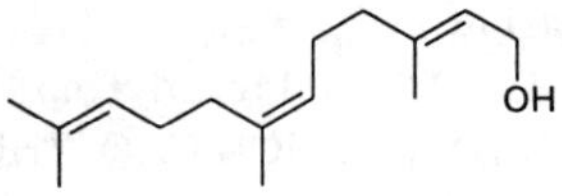

2342 Farnesyl acetate
$C_{17}H_{28}O_2$ MW: 264.41 Property: bp 169-70°C/10mm. Source: QING HAO, MU HAO. Ref: 6.

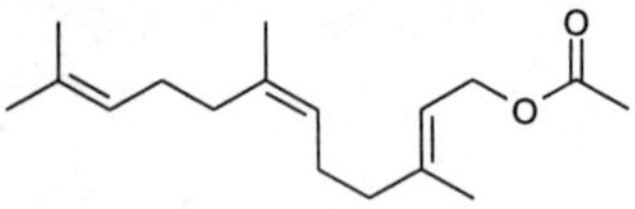

2343 Farrerol
$C_{17}H_{16}O_5$ MW: 300.31 Property: mp (±): 223-4°C. Source: MAN SHAN HONG. Ref: 4, 6.

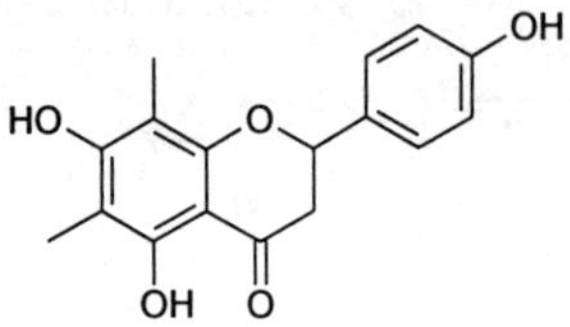

2344 Fawcettiine
$C_{18}H_{29}NO_3$ MW: 307.44 Property: mp 166-7°C. Source: SHEN JIN CAO. Ref: 6.

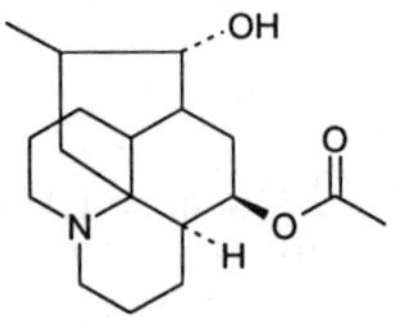

2345 α-Fenchene
$C_{10}H_{16}$ MW: 136.24 Property: bp (+): 155-6°C, (-): 153-4°C/720mm, (±): 154-6°C. Source: XIE CAO. Ref: 6.

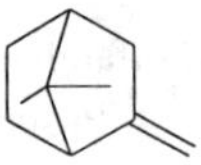

2346 β-Fenchene
$C_{10}H_{16}$ MW: 136.24 Source: CHAI HU, SHENG JIANG. Ref: 2.

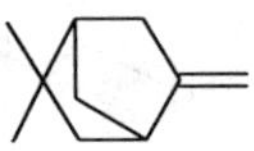

2347 Fenchone
$C_{11}H_{18}$ MW: 150.27 Property: mp (+): 5.5°C, (-): 6°C; bp (±): 72-3°C/12mm. Source: CE BAI YE, HUI XIANG, XIA KU CAO. Ref: 6.

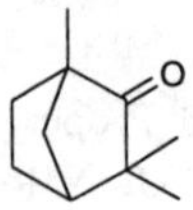

2348 Fenchyl alcohol
$C_{10}H_{18}O$ MW: 154.25 Property: bp 200°C. Source: GANG SONG, SHENG JIANG. Ref: 2.

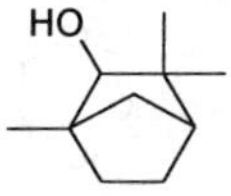

2349 Fenfangjine A
$C_{38}H_{42}N_2O_7$ MW: 638.77 Source: FANG JI. Ref: 2.

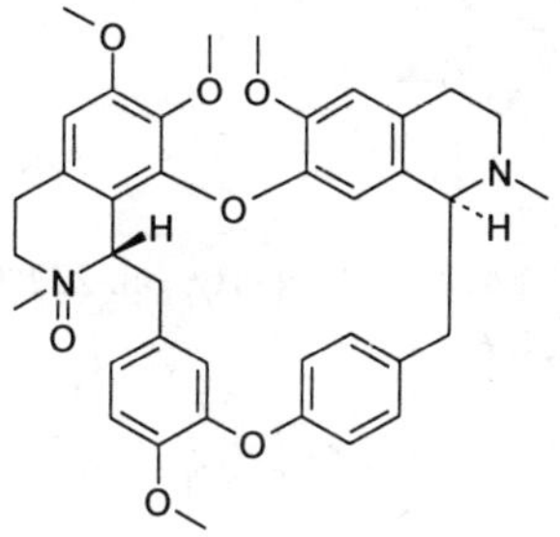

2350 Fenfangjine D
Source: FANG JI. Ref: 2.

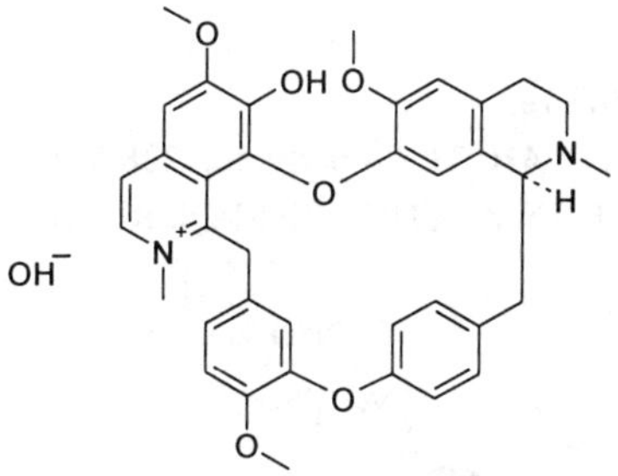

2351 Fernene
$C_{30}H_{50}$ MW: 410.73 Property: mp 170-1°C. Source: GUAN ZHONG, TIE SI QI. Ref: 6.

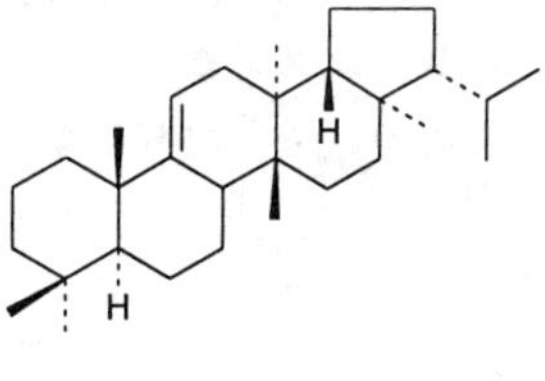

2352 7-Fernene
$C_{30}H_{50}$ MW: 410.73 Property: mp 208.5-9.5°C. Source: TIE SI QI. Ref: 6.

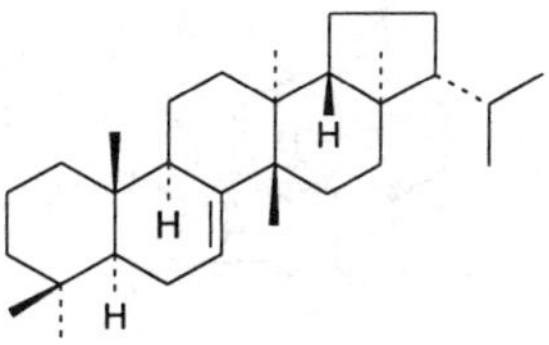

2353 9-(11)-Fernene
Fernene. Property: mp 170-1°C. Source: SHUI LONG GU. Ref: 6.

2354 Fernenol
$C_{30}H_{50}O$ MW: 426.73 Property: mp 194°C. Source: AI YE, LONG XUCAO (II), MAO CAO YE. Ref: 6.

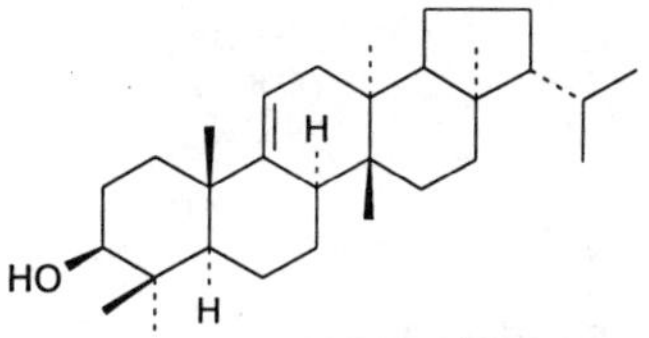

2355 Ferruginol
$C_{20}H_{30}O$ MW: 286.46 Property: mp 57-9°C; bp 175°C/0.3mm. Source: DAN SHEN, DU SONG SHI, SANYE SHU WEI CAO. Ref: 6, 116, 182.

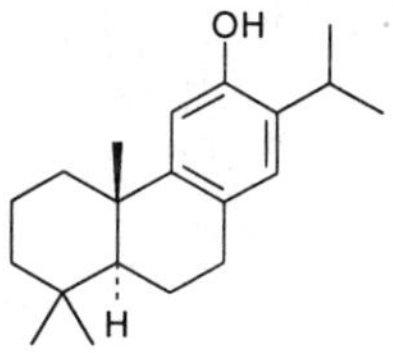

2356 Ferulic acid
CAS: 1135-24-6 $C_{10}H_{10}O_4$ MW: 194.19 Property: mp 173-8°C. Source: A WEI, CHA XIONG, CHUAN XIONG, DANG GUI, DI XIAO GUA, HUANG LIAN, HUI XIANG JIN YE, JIAN DO PU GONG YING, LAI FU, LAO SHU GUA, MAO GENG XI XIAN, MI PI KANG, MU ZEI, NING MENG, NING MENG GEN, NING MENG YE, QIANG HUO, SHEN JIN CAO, SHENG MA, SUAN ZAO REN, XIA TIAN WE, XIAO JIE JIN CAO, XIN BAI PI, YANG CONG. Ref: 2, 4, 456, 476, 500, 507, 512, 601, 602.

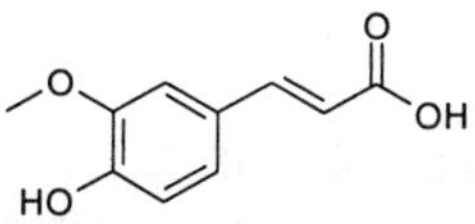

2357 6-O-Z-Feruloylajugol
Source: GAN DI HUANG. Ref: 2.

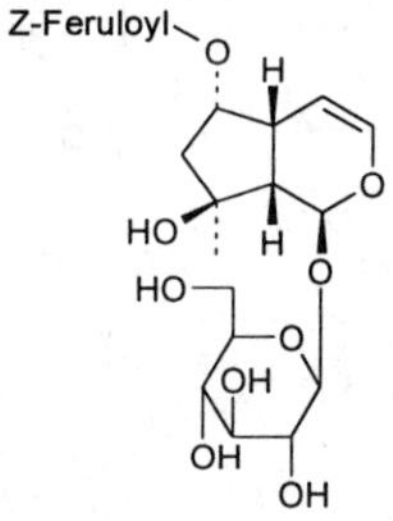

2358 6-O-E-Feruloylajugol
Source: GAN DI HUANG. Ref: 2.

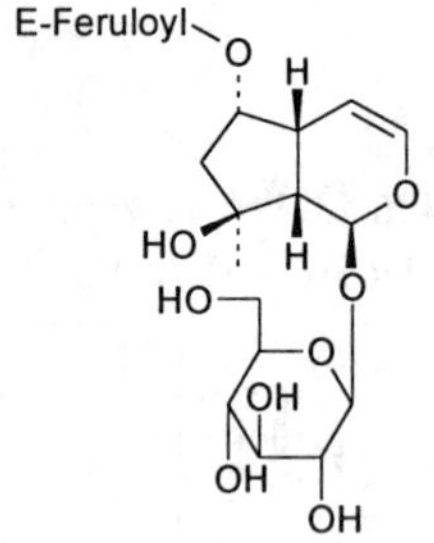

2359 2"-O-Feruloylaloesin
Source: LU HUI. Ref: 2.

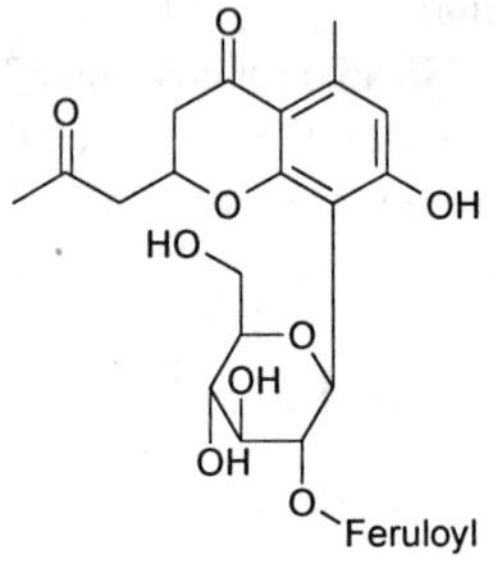

2360 6'-O-trans-Feruloylnodakenin
Source: QIANG HUO. Ref: 566.

2361 3-O-Feruloylquinic acid
$C_{17}H_{22}O_9$ MW: 370.36 Property: mp 196-7°C.
Source: DI SHAO GUA, XIANG RI KUI YE. Ref: 6.

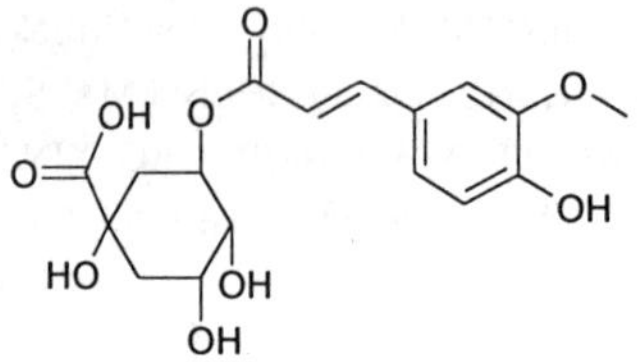

2362 6'''-Feruloylspinosin
Source: DA ZAO, SUAN ZAO REN. Ref: 2.

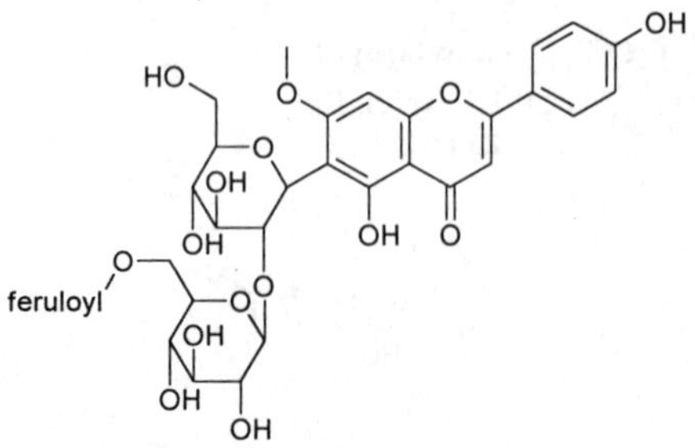

2363 Fetidine
$C_{40}H_{46}N_2O_8$ MW: 682.82 Property: mp (+): 132-5°C.
Source: MA WEI LIAN. Ref: 6.

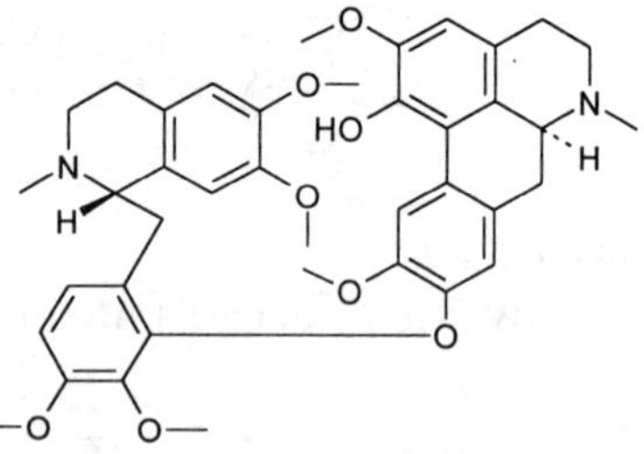

2364 Filicenal
$C_{30}H_{48}O$ MW: 424.72 Property: mp 272°C. Source: TIE SI QI. Ref: 6.

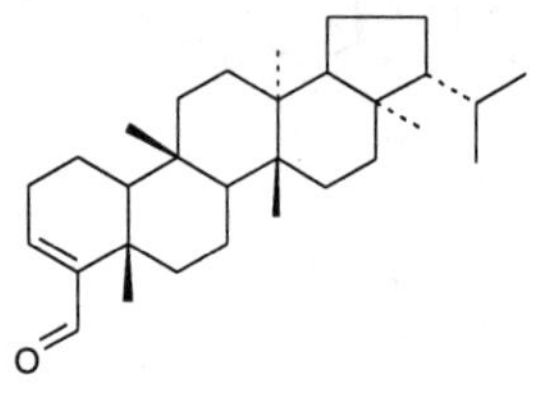

2365 Filicene
$C_{30}H_{50}$ MW: 410.73 Property: mp 228.5-9.5°C.
Source: GUAN ZHONG, TIE SI QI. Ref: 6.

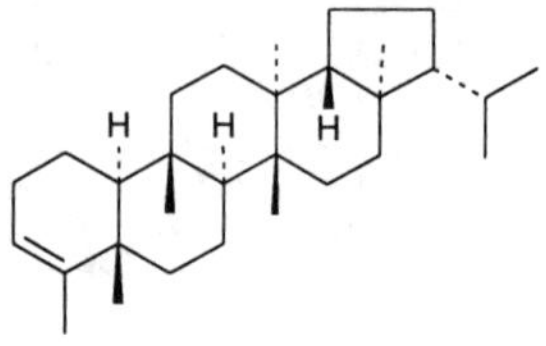

2366 Filicinic acid
$C_8H_{10}O_3$ MW: 154.17 Property: mp 215°C (dec).
Source: GUAN ZHONG. Ref: 6.

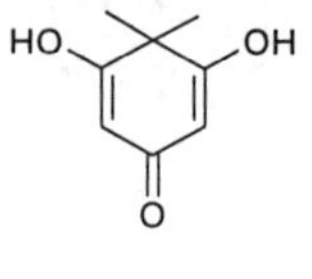

2367 Finitin
$C_{15}H_{20}O_3$ MW: 248.32 Property: mp 153-5°C.
Source: DONG BEI HUI HAO. Ref: 6.

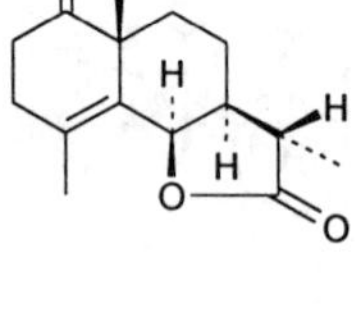

2368 Fisetin

$C_{15}H_{10}O_6$ MW: 286.24 Property: mp 350°C. Source: HAI ER CHA, HUANG LIAN YA, LIN BEI ZI, YE QI SHU YE. Ref: 6.

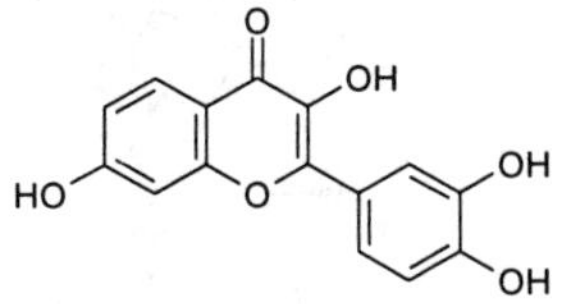

2369 Fistucacidin

$C_{15}H_{14}O_6$ MW: 290.28 Property: mp 245-7°C. Source: PO LUO MEN ZAO JIA. Ref: 6.

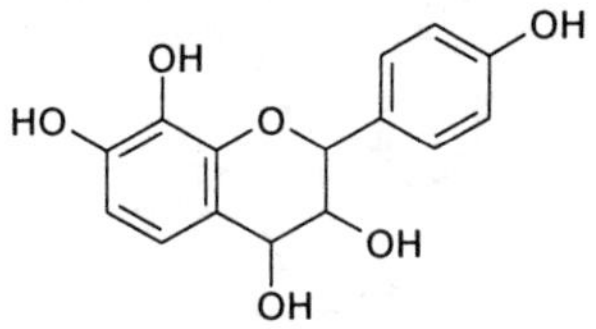

2370 Flavanol

$C_{15}H_{14}O_2$ MW: 226.28 Property: mp 119°C. Source: CI MI, CHA SHU GEN. Ref: 6.

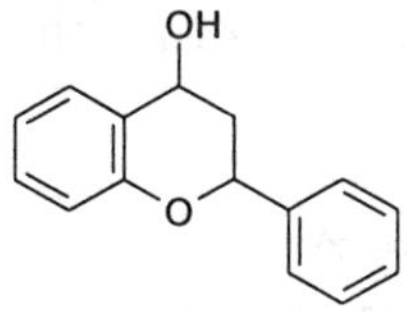

2371 Flavaspidic acid

$C_{24}H_{30}O_8$ MW: 446.50 Property: mp α: 92°C/150°C β: 156°C. Source: GUAN ZHONG. Ref: 6.

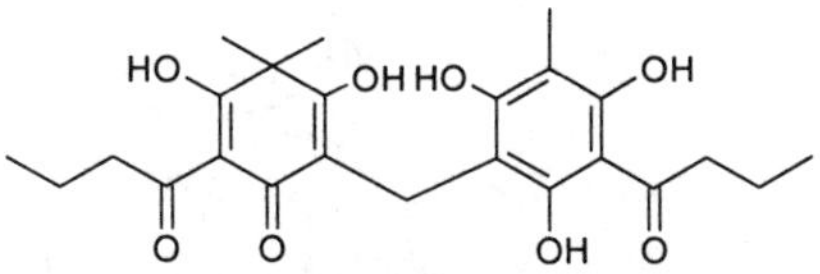

2372 Flavaspidinin

$C_{23}H_{30}O_8$ MW: 434.49 Property: mp 211-12°C. Source: GUAN ZHONG. Ref: 6.

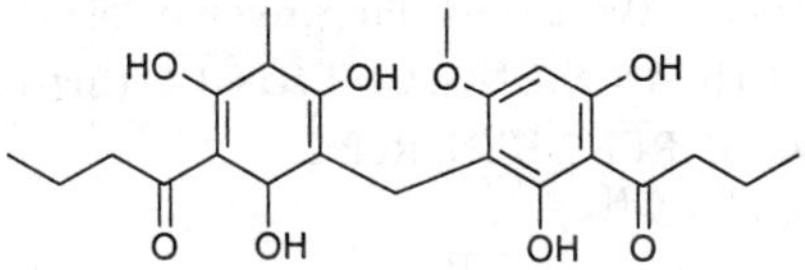

2373 Flavin adenine dinucleotide

$C_{27}H_{35}N_9O_{15}P_2$ MW: 787.58 Source: QING WA, YUAN CAN ZI. Ref: 6.

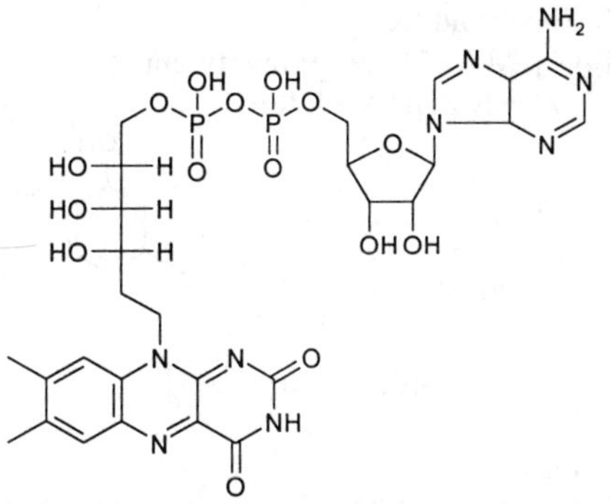

2374 Flavin mononucleotide

$C_{17}H_{21}N_4O_9P$ MW: 456.58 Source: YUAN CAN ZI, ZHANG LANG. Ref: 6.

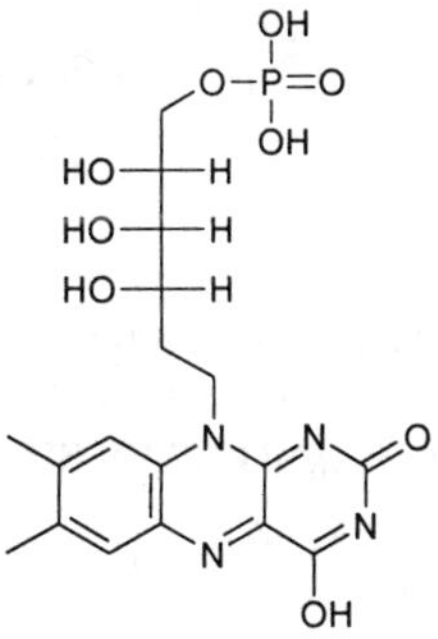

2375 Flavocommelin

$C_{28}H_{32}O_{15}$ MW: 608.56 Property: mp 216-7°C. Source: YA ZHI CAO. Ref: 6.

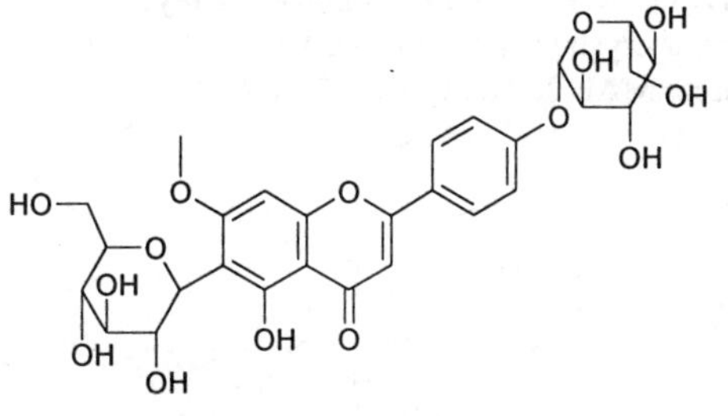

2376 Flavone

$C_{15}H_{10}O_2$ MW: 222.25 Property: mp 97°C. Source: WU LOU ZI. Ref: 6.

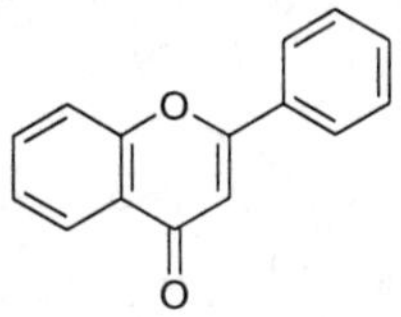

2377 Flavonoid IX
$C_{26}H_{28}O_{14}$ MW: 564.50 Property: mp 244-7°C. Source: ZHEN ZHU MEI. Ref: 6.

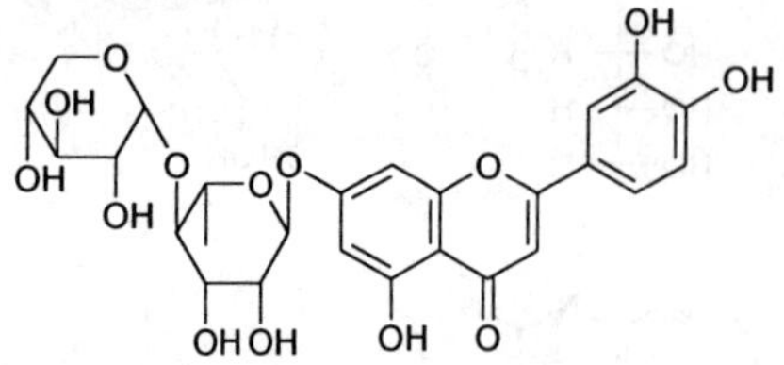

2378 Flavonol
$C_{15}H_{10}O_3$ MW: 238.25 Property: mp 169-70°C. Source: BAI GUO YE, BAI QU CAI, CHA SHU GEN. Ref: 6.

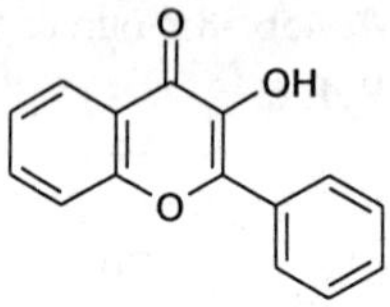

2379 Flavoxanthin
$C_{40}H_{56}O_3$ MW: 584.89 Property: mp 184°C. Source: DA BAI DING CAO, JIN ZHAN JU, PU GONG YING, QIAN LI GUANG, WAN SHOU JU. Ref: 6.

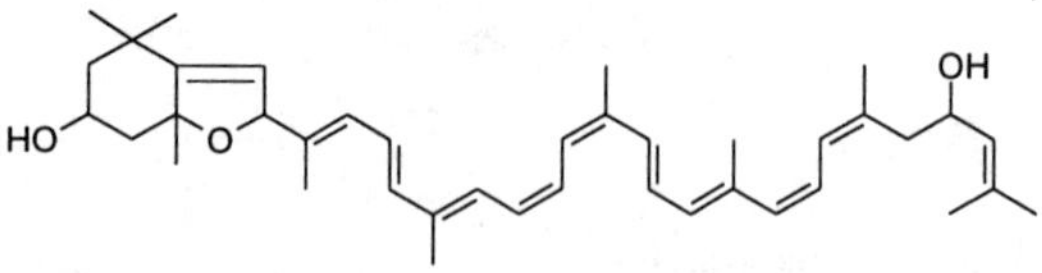

2380 Flemiphilippinin C
$C_{26}H_{26}O_6$ MW: 434.49 Property: light yellow acicular crystal (methanol-water), mp 143-5°C. Source: MAN XING QIAN JIN BA. Ref: 179.

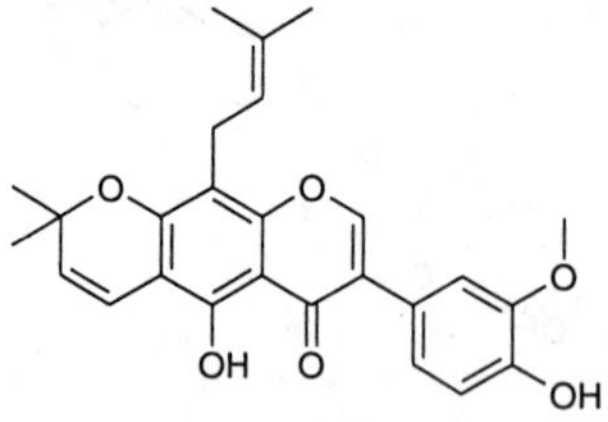

2381 Flemiphilippinin D
$C_{25}H_{28}O_6$ MW: 424.50 Property: white solid, mp 161-3°C, $[\alpha]_D^{25}$ -15.2° (c=0.5, ethanol). Source: MAN XING QIAN JIN BA. Ref: 179.

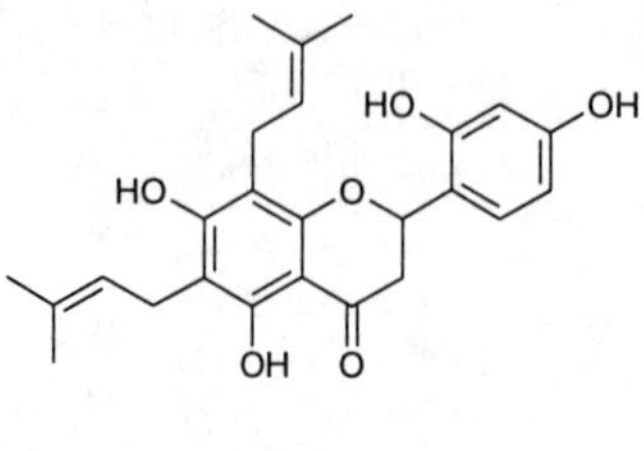

2382 Fluorocarpamine
$C_{20}H_{22}N_2O_3$ MW: 338.41 Source: CHANG CHUN HUA. Ref: 2.

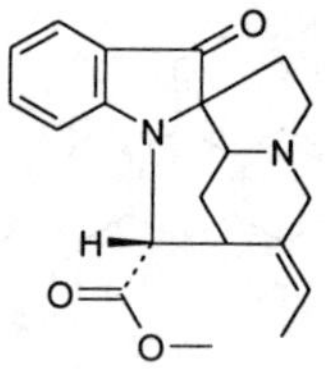

2383 Fluorocarpamine-N-oxide
$C_{20}H_{24}N_2O_4$ MW: 356.43 Source: CHANG CHUN HUA. Ref: 2.

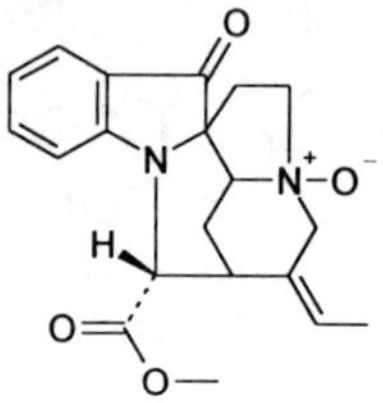

2384 Foeniculin
Quercetin-3-arabinoside. Source: HUI XIANG JING YE. Ref: 6.

2385 Foliamenthin
$C_{26}H_{36}O_{12}$ MW: 540.57 Property: mp 194-6°C. Source: SHUI CAI, SHUI CAI GEN. Ref: 6.

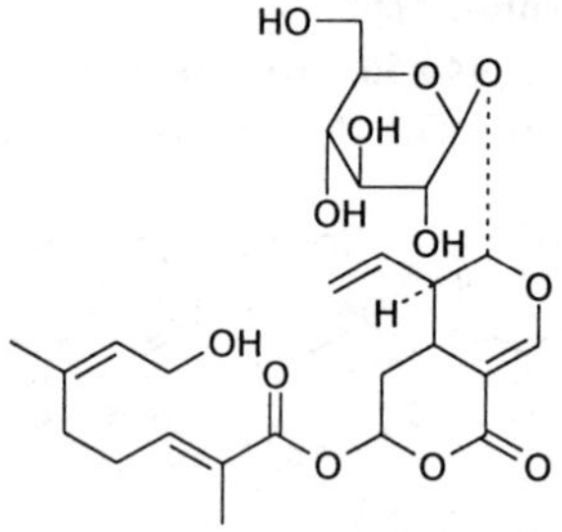

2386 Folic acid
$C_{19}H_{19}N_7O_6$ MW: 441.41 Property: mp 250°C (dec). Source: CHUAN XIONG, CU LIU GUO (SHA JI), HUANG QI, REN SHEN. Ref: 2.

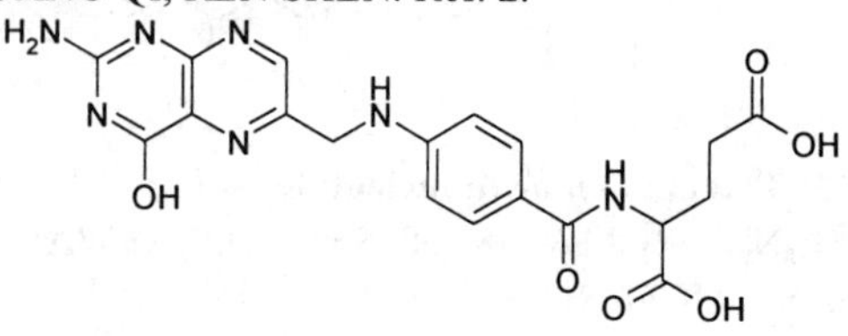

2387 Folinic acid
$C_{21}H_{24}NO_7$ MW: 472.46 Property: mp 248-50°C. Source: BA JIAO HUI XIANG, BE CAI, CAN DOU YE, CU LIU GUO, DANG GUI, FENG MI, FENG RU, HEI DA DOU, HEI DA DOU YE, HEI ZHI MA, HONG CHE ZHOU CAO, HONG CHE ZHOU CAO, HUANG QI, LI ZHI, LIN QIN, MANG GUO, MOU GU, NIU RU, PU GONG YING, SANG YE, YE DONG QING GUO. Ref: 6.

2388 Fordimine
$C_{16}H_{20}N_2O_2$ MW: 256.35 Property: acicular crystal, mp 149-50°C (dec). Source: HUA NAN MA WEI SHAN. Ref: 95.

2389 Formaldehyde
CH_2O MW: 30.03 Property: mp -92°C; bp -21°C. Source: CU, NIU BANG GEN, YANG SHI CAO. Ref: 6.

2390 Formic acid
CH_2O_2 MW: 46.03 Property: mp 8.4°C, bp 100.5°C. Source: BAI GUO, PU HUANG. Ref: 2.

2391 Formononetin
$C_{16}H_{12}O_4$ MW: 268.27 Property: mp 257°C. Source: CI GUO GAN CAO, GAN CAO, GE GEN, HUANG QI, HONG CHE ZHOU CAO, KU SHEN, MU XU. Ref: 2, 243, 372, 379.

2392 Formononetin-7-glucoside
$C_{22}H_{22}O_9$ MW: 430.42 Source: GE GEN. Ref: 2.

2393 1-Formyl-β-carboline
$C_{12}H_8N_2O$ MW: 196.21 Property: orange crystal, mp 200-2°C. Source: KU SHU PI. Ref: 12.

2394 N-Formylcorydamine
$C_{21}H_{18}N_2O_5$ MW: 378.39 Property: mp 159.5-60.5°C. Source: ZI HUA YU DENG CAO. Ref: 6.

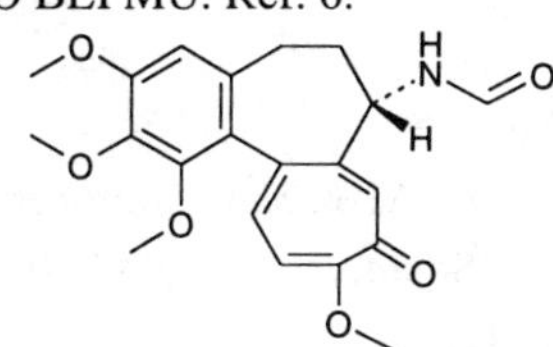

2395 N-Formyl-N-deacetylcolchicine
$C_{21}H_{23}NO_6$ MW: 385.42 Property: mp 264-6°C. Source: CAO BEI MU. Ref: 6.

2396 14-Formyldihydroxyrutaecarpine
$C_{19}H_{15}N_3O_2$ MW: 317.35 Source: WU ZHU YU. Ref: 2.

2397 Formylharman
N_9-Formylharman. Property: mp 178°C. Source: YUAN ZHI. Ref: 538.

2398 1-Formyl-4-methoxy-β-carboline
$C_{13}H_{10}N_2O_2$ MW: 226.24 Property: yellowish needle crystal, mp 209-10°C. Source: KU SHE PI. Ref: 12.

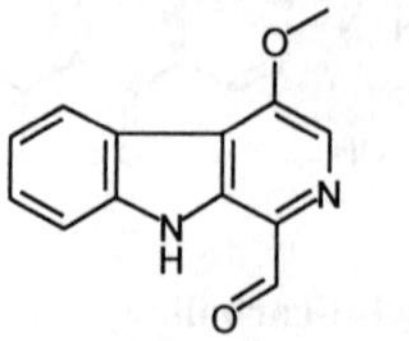

2399 Forrestiin A
$C_{20}H_{26}O_4$ MW: 330.43 Property: acicular crystal, $[\alpha]_D^{19}$ +105.6° (c=0.71, chloroform). Source: YUAN BAN JIANG HUA. Ref: 322.

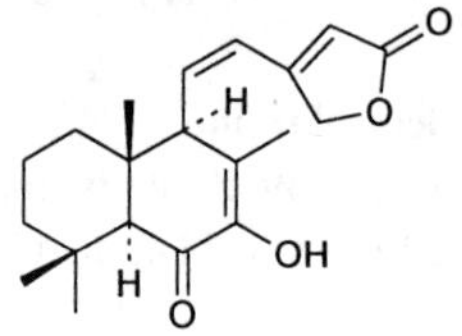

2400 Forsythiaside
Source: GAN DI HUANG. Ref: 2.

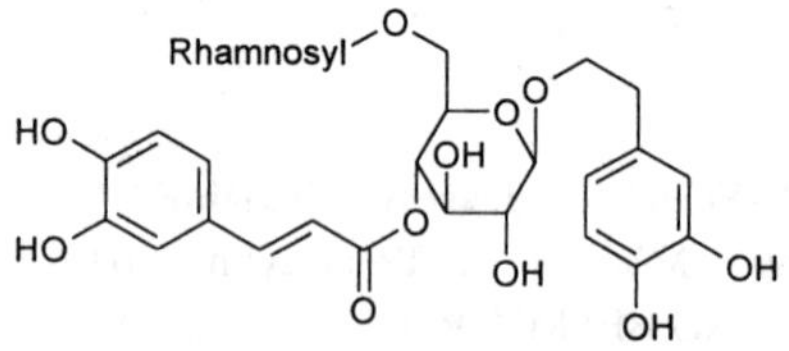

2401 Forsythin
Phillyrin. $C_{27}H_{34}O_{11}$ MW: 534.57 Property: mp α: 155°C, β: 185°C. Source: LIAN QIAO JING YE, LIAN QIAO. Ref: 2.

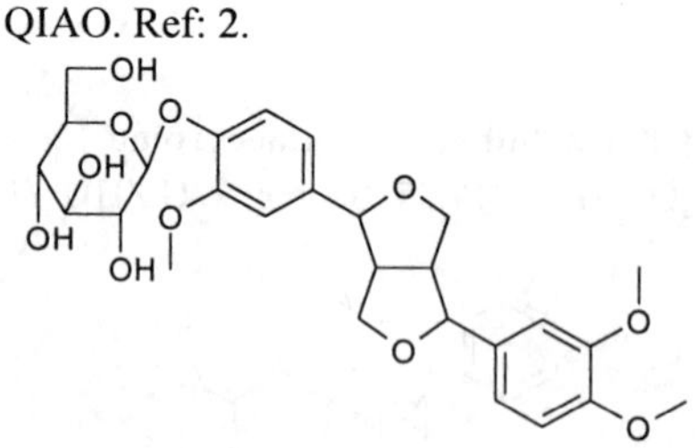

2402 Forsythol
Source: LIAN QIAO. Ref: 2.

2403 Forsythoside A
$C_{29}H_{36}O_{15}$ MW: 624.60 Source: LIAN QIAO. Ref: 2.

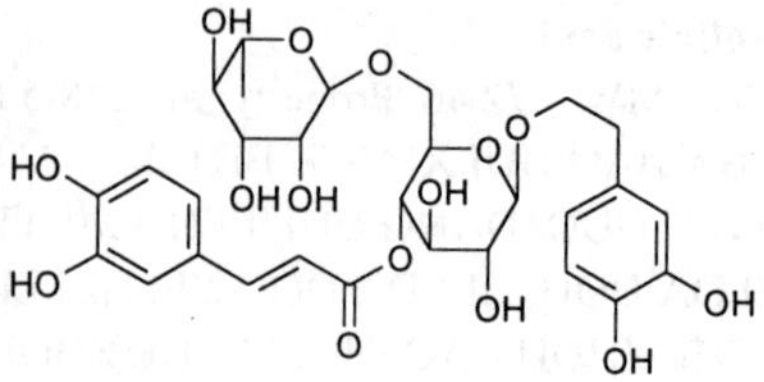

2404 Forsythoside B
$C_{35}H_{46}O_{18}$ MW: 754.75 Source: LIAN QIAO. Ref: 2.

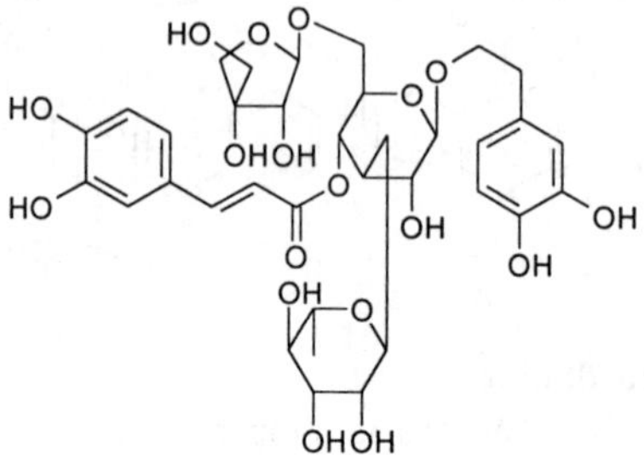

2405 Fortuneine
$C_{20}H_{25}NO_3$ MW: 327.43 Source: SAN JIAN SHAN. Ref: 2.

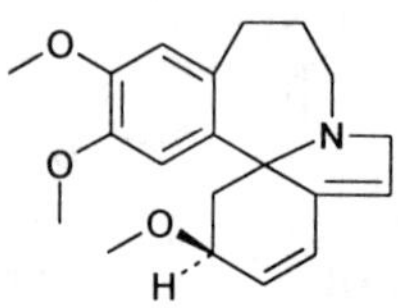

2406 Fortunellin
$C_{28}H_{32}O_{14}$ MW: 592.56 Property: mp 214-6°C. Source: JIN JU. Ref: 6.

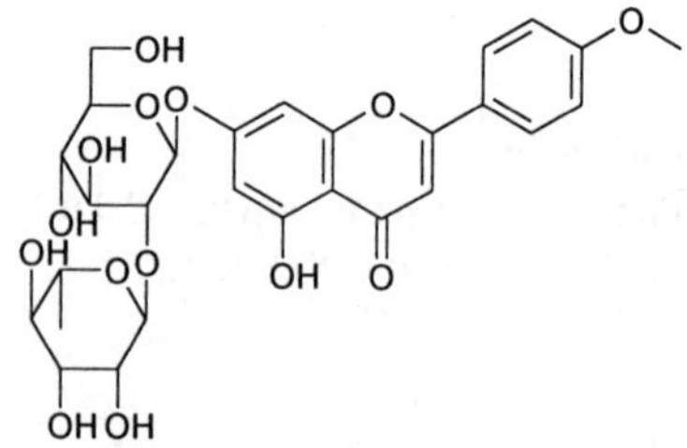

2407 Frangufoline
$C_{31}H_{42}N_4O_4$ MW: 534.70 Property: mp 244°C. Source: MIAN ZAO. Ref: 6.

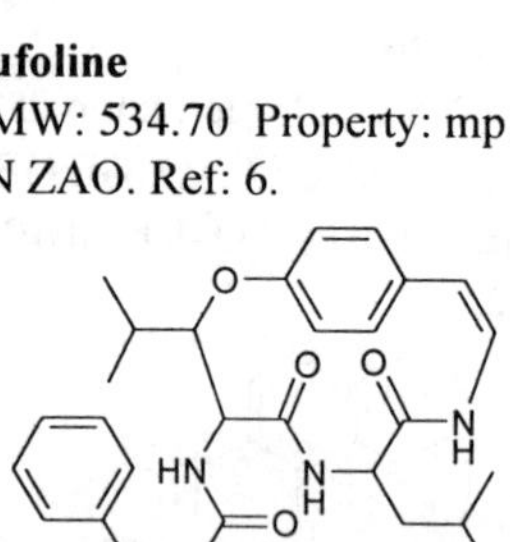

2408 Frangulanine

$C_{28}H_{44}N_4O_4$ MW: 500.69 Property: mp 275-7°C. Source: QIN PI. Ref: 6.

2409 Fraxetin

$C_{10}H_8O_5$ MW: 208.17. Property: mp 228°C. Source: QIN PI. Ref: 2.

2410 Fraxin

$C_{16}H_{18}O_{10}$ MW: 370.32 Property: mp 205°C. Source: QIN PI. Ref: 2.

2411 Fraxinellone

$C_{14}H_{16}O_3$ MW: 232.28 Property: mp 108-10°C, 120°C. Source: BAI XIAN PI, KU LIAN PI. Ref: 6.

2412 Friedelan-1,3-dion-24-al

$C_{30}H_{46}O_3$ MW: 454.70 Source: SUO LA MU. Ref: 6.

2413 Friedelan-1,3-dion-7α-ol

$C_{30}H_{48}O_3$ MW: 456.72 Source: SUO LA MU. Ref: 6.

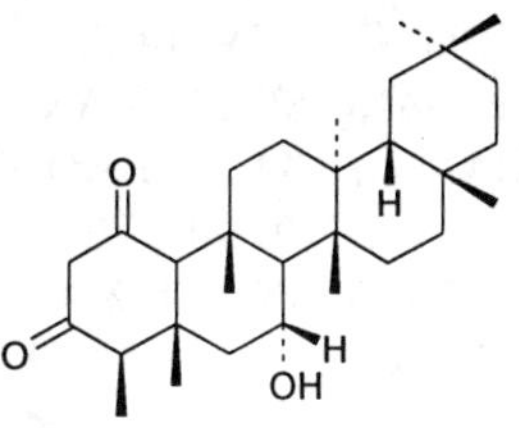

2414 Friedelanol

$C_{30}H_{52}O$ MW: 428.75 Property: mp 302-4°C. Source: DIAO JING CAO. Ref: 6.

2415 Friedelan-3α-ol

Friedelinol, Friedelan-3β-ol. Property: mp 263-5°C. Source: HUO YANG LE, JIN LONG DAN CAO, QIU FENG MU. Ref: 6.

2416 Friedelan-3α-yl acetate

$C_{32}H_{52}O_3$ MW: 484.77 Property: mp 317-9°C. Source: QIU FENG MU. Ref: 6.

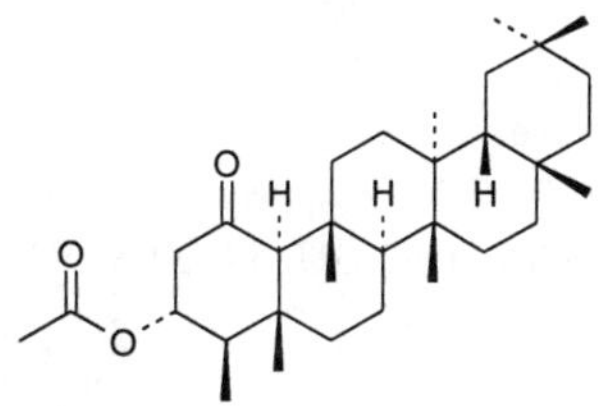

2417 1-Friedelen 3-one

$C_{30}H_{48}O$ MW: 424.72 Property: mp 262-3°C. Source: SUO LA MU. Ref: 6.

2418 Friedelin
$C_{30}H_{50}O$ MW: 426.73 Property: colorless thin acicular crystal, mp 257-64°C, $[\alpha]_D^{28}$ -14.1° (c=0.07, $CHCl_3$). Source: DANG SHEN, BIAN TAO, CHI NAN, HUO XIANG, HUI BAO HAO, MAO LIAN HAO, MENG GU LI, QUE MEI TENG, TUN XING GUO, XIAO SHE ZI WAN. Ref: 2, 447, 474, 503, 505, 515, 550, 572, 600, 611.

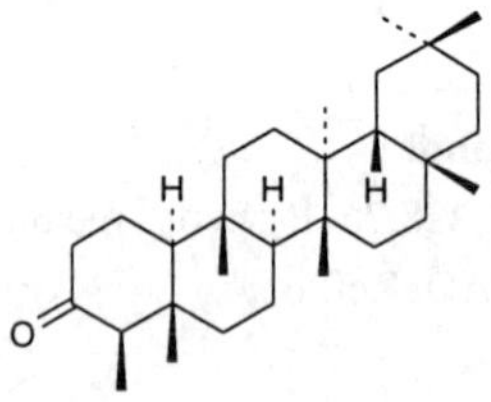

2419 Fritimine
$C_{38}H_{62}N_2O_3$ Property: mp 167°C. Source: CHUAN BEI MU. Ref: 2.

2420 Fritiminine
$C_{27}H_{39}NO_3$ Property: mp 258-60°C. Source: CHUAN BEI MU. Ref: 2.

2421 Fructose
$C_6H_{12}O_6$ MW: 180.16 Property: mp L(+): 101-3°C, D(-): 102-4°C (dec). Source: REN SHEN. Ref: 2.

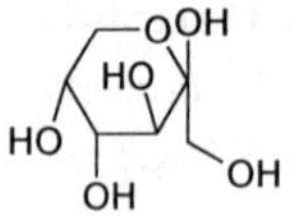

2422 Fucosterol
$C_{29}H_{48}O$ MW: 412.71 Property: mp 124°C. Source: KUN BU, SHUI LONG GU, YE ZI YOU. Ref: 6.

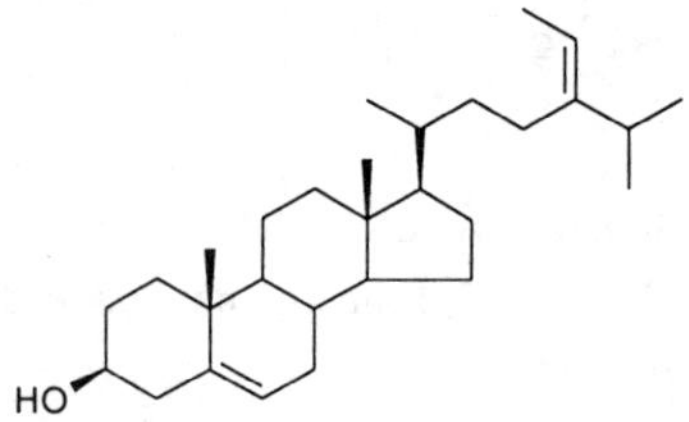

2423 Fukinanolide
$C_{15}H_{22}O_2$ MW: 234.34 Property: mp 80.5-0.6°C. Source: FENG DOU CAI. Ref: 6.

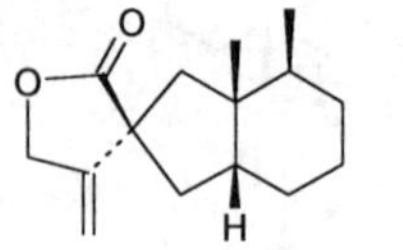

2424 Fukinolic acid
$C_{22}H_{22}O_{11}$ MW: Source: FENG DOU CAI. Ref: 6.

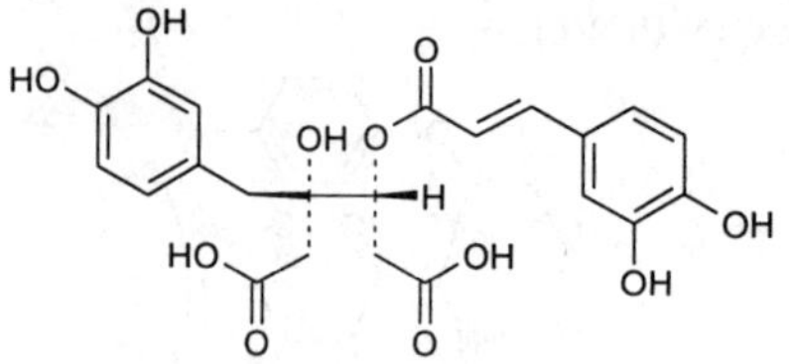

2425 Fukinolide
$C_{22}H_{30}O_6$ MW: 390.48 Property: mp 101-2°C. Source: FENG DOU CAI. Ref: 6.

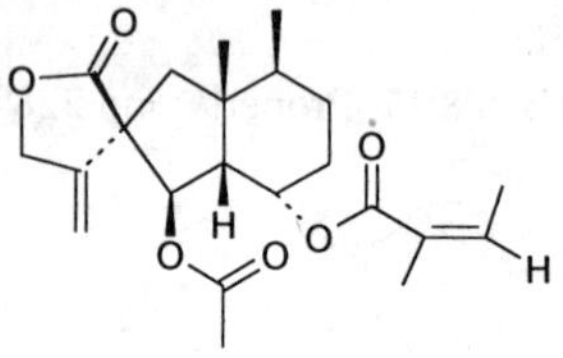

2426 S-Fukinolide
$C_{21}H_{28}O_6S$ MW: 408.52 Property: mp 207°C. Source: FENG DOU CAI. Ref: 6.

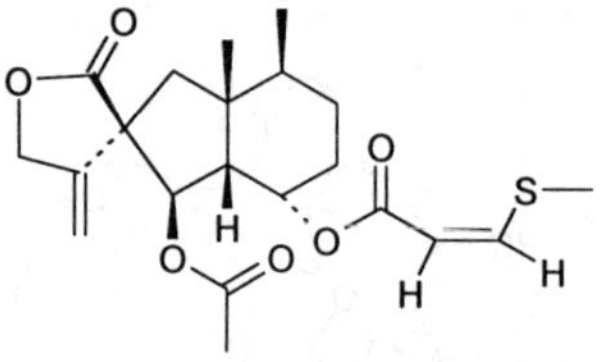

2427 Fukinone
$C_{15}H_{24}O$ MW: 220.36 Property: bp 97°C/0.8mm. Source: FENG DOU CAI. Ref: 6.

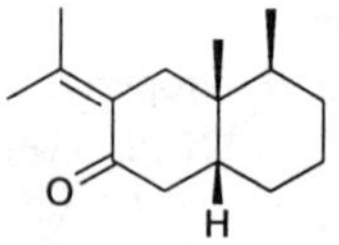

2428 Fukugiside
$C_{36}H_{30}O_{16}$ MW: 718.63 Property: mp 242-3°C (dec). Source: SHAN ZHU ZI. Ref: 6.

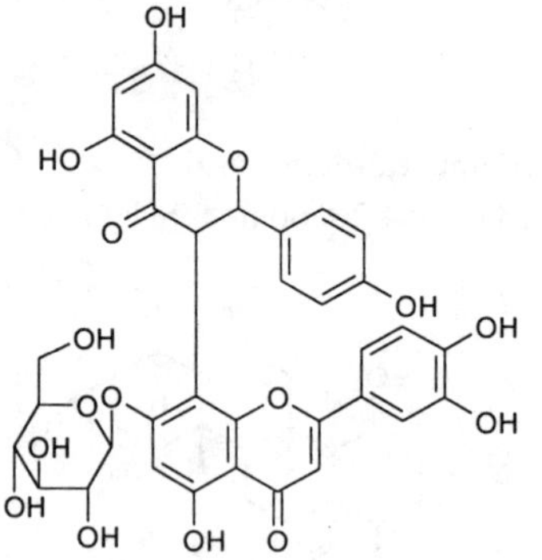

2429 Fukujusone
$C_{21}H_{32}O_4$ MW: 348.49 Property: mp 224-7°C. Source: FU SHOU CAO. Ref: 6.

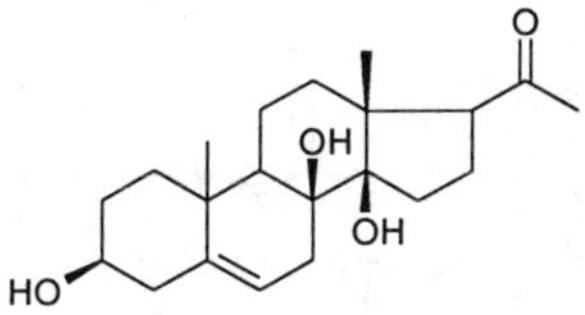

2430 Fukujusonorone
$C_{20}H_{26}O_3$ MW: 314.43 Property: mp 88-90°C. Source: FU SHOU CAO. Ref: 6.

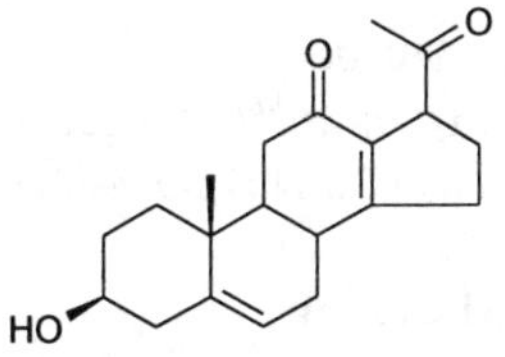

2431 Fulyotomentoside A
$C_{58}H_{94}O_{26}$ MW: 1207.38 Property: white thin acicular crystal, mp 215-7°C, $[\alpha]_D^{27.5}$ -14.9°(c=0.98, MeOH). Source: HUANG HE MAO REN DONG. Ref: 126.

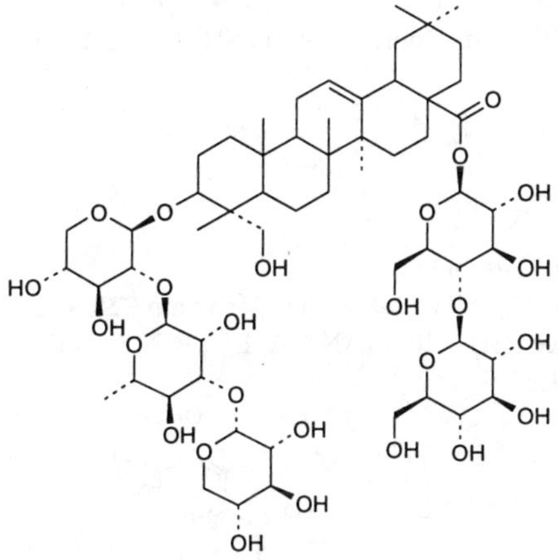

2432 Fumaric acid
Allomaleic acid; Boketic acid. CAS: 110-17-8
$C_4H_4O_4$ MW: 116.07 Source: MA HUANG, MU ZEI, REN SHEN, YI MU CAO. Ref: 2, 4, 411.

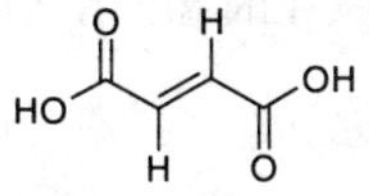

2433 Fumarprotocetraric acid
$C_{22}H_{16}O_{12}$ MW: 472.37 Property: mp 250-60°C. Source: JIN SHUA BA, SHI RUI. Ref: 6.

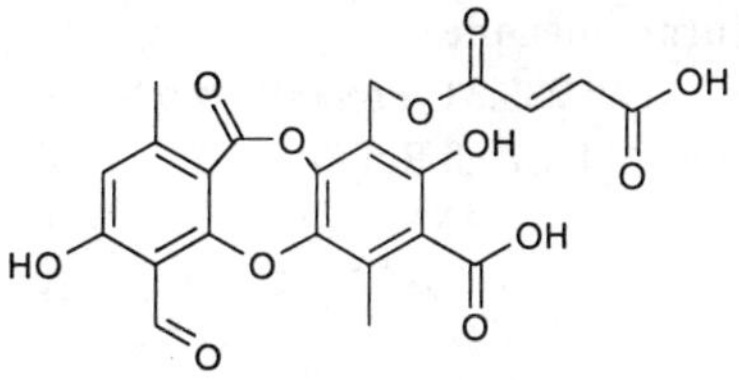

2434 α-Funebrene
C_5H_{24} MW: 204.36 Source: BAI SHU YE, DU HUO. Ref: 2.

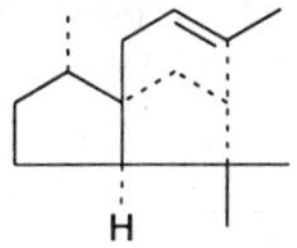

2435 Fungisterol
$C_{28}H_{48}O$ MW: 400.69 Property: mp 152°C. Source: XIANG XUN. Ref: 6.

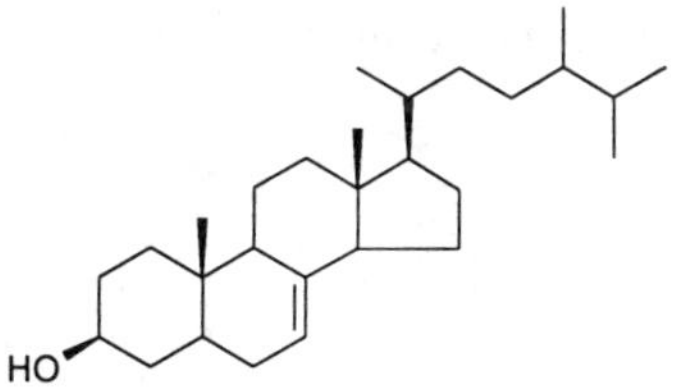

2436 2-Furaldehyde
Furfural. C_5HO_2 MW: 96.09 Property: bp 162°C. Source: CANG ZHU, HONG CHE ZHOU CAO, LUO LE, SHAN ZHU YU, SHI CHUN, SHUI SONG, YANG SHI, YIN CHEN GAO, YIN CHEN HAO, ZE XIE, ZI CAI. Ref: 2.

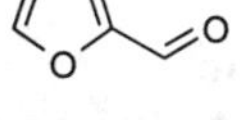

2437 2-Furancarboxylic acid
$C_5H_4O_3$ MW: 112.09 Source: DANG SHEN. Ref: 2.

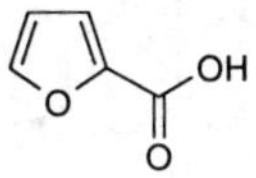

2438 Furanodiene
$C_{15}H_{20}O$ MW: 216.38 Property: mp 44-5.0°C. Source: PENG E SHU. Ref: 6.

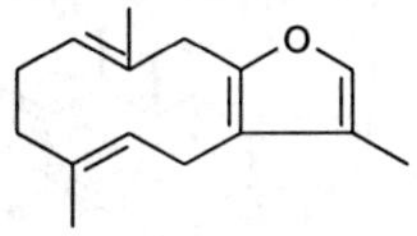

2439 Furanodienone
$C_{15}H_{18}O_2$ MW: 230.31 Property: mp 89.5-90.5°C. Source: PENG E SHU. Ref: 6.

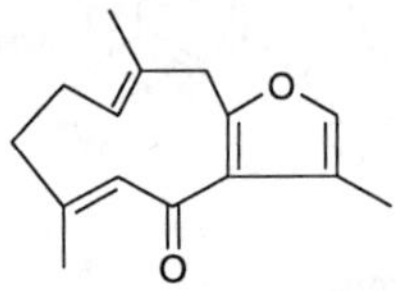

2440 Furanoeremophilane
$C_{15}H_{22}O$ MW: 218.34 Property: bp 148°C/16mm. Source: FENG DOU CAI. Ref: 6.

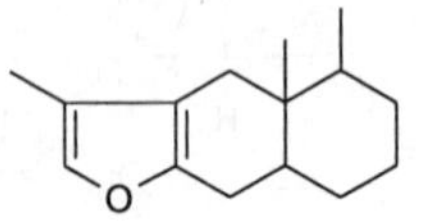

2441 Furanoeremophilane-6β,10β-diol
$C_{15}H_{22}O_3$ MW: 250.34 Property: mp 122°C. Source: LIAN PENG CAO. Ref: 6.

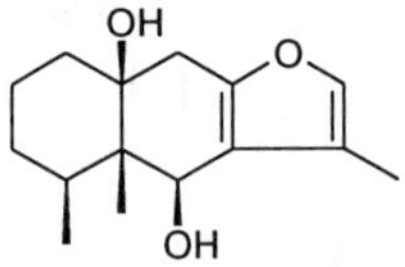

2442 Furanofukinol
$C_{15}H_{22}O_3$ MW: 250.34 Property: mp 178-80°C (dec). Source: FENG DOU CAI. Ref: 6.

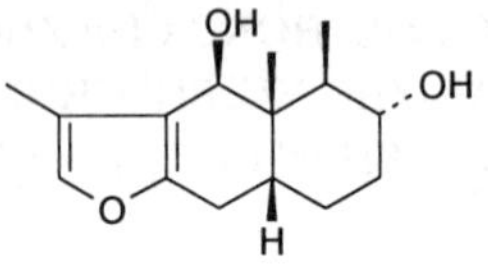

2443 Furanojaponin
$C_{20}H_{28}O_3$ MW: 316.44 Property: bp110-30°C/5×10^{-5}mm. Source: FENG DOU CAI. Ref: 6.

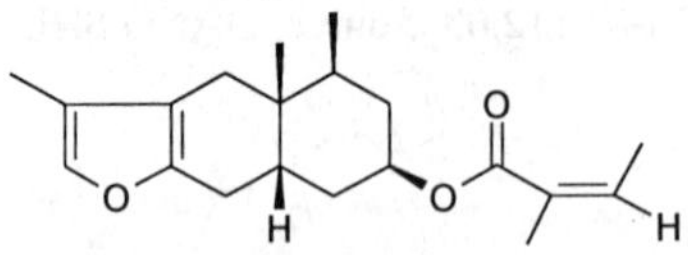

2444 10α-H-Furanoligularenone
$C_{15}H_{18}O_2$ MW: 230.31 Property: mp 95°C. Source: HU LU QI. Ref: 6.

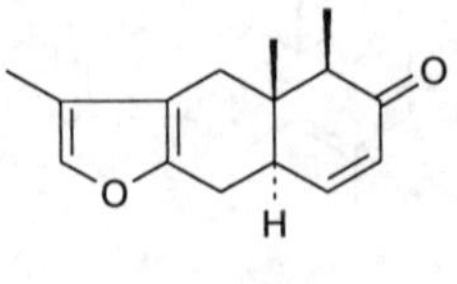

2445 S-Furanopetasitin
$C_{25}H_{34}O_5S$ MW: 446.61 Property: mp 107-8°C. Source: FENG DOU CAI. Ref: 6.

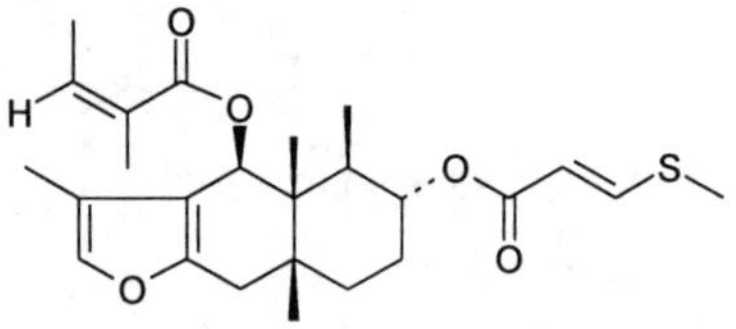

2446 Furano-phenanthra-quinone pigments
Source: DAN SHEN. Ref: 6.

2447 Furfuraldehyde
Furfural. Property: bp 162°C. Source: HONG CHE ZHOU CAO, YIN CHEN HAO. Ref: 6.

2448 Furfuryl alcohol
$C_5H_6O_2$ MW: 98.10 Property: bp 170-1°C. Source: CHA YE, SHUI SONG. Ref: 6.

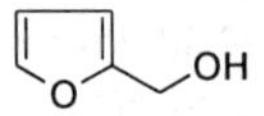

2449 cis-1-(2-Furyl)-4-(2-thienyl)-1-buten-3-yne
$C_{12}H_8OS$ MW: 200.26 Property: bp 100-10°C/0.3mm. Source: YANG SHI CAO. Ref: 6.

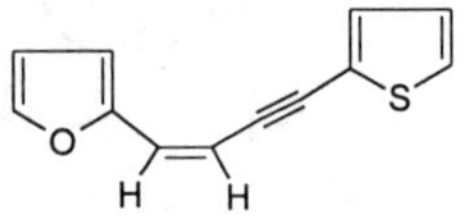

2450 Fustin (+)
$C_{15}H_{12}O_6$ MW: 288.26 Property: mp 228-9°C. Source: HUANG LIAN YA, LIN BEI ZI, YE QI SHU YE. Ref: 6.

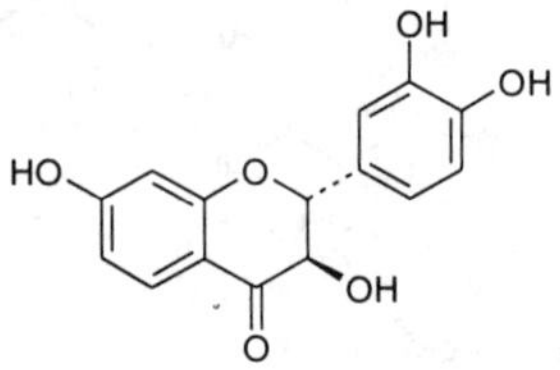

2451 Fustin (-)
$C_{15}H_{12}O_6$ MW: 288.26 Property: mp 228°C. Source: HUANG LIAN YA, LIN BEI ZI, YE QI SHU YE. Ref: 6.

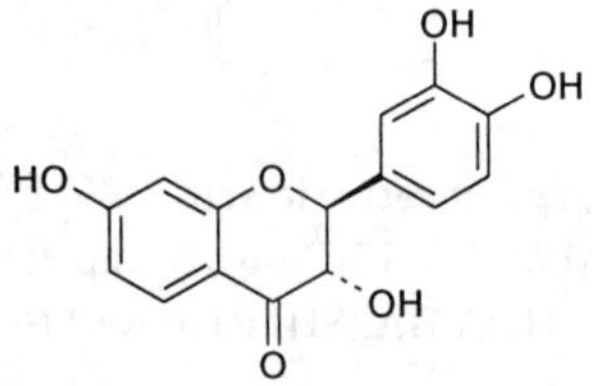

2452 Futoamide
$C_{18}H_{23}NO_3$ MW: 301.39 Property: mp 128-30°C. Source: HAI FENG TENG, SHAN JU. Ref: 6, 75.

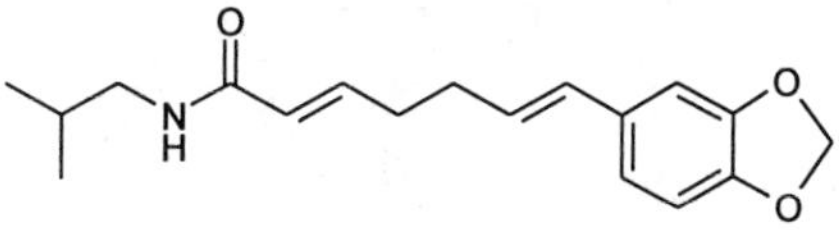

2453 Futoenone
$C_{20}H_{20}O_5$ MW: 340.38 Property: mp 197°C. Source: HAI FENG TENG. Ref: 6.

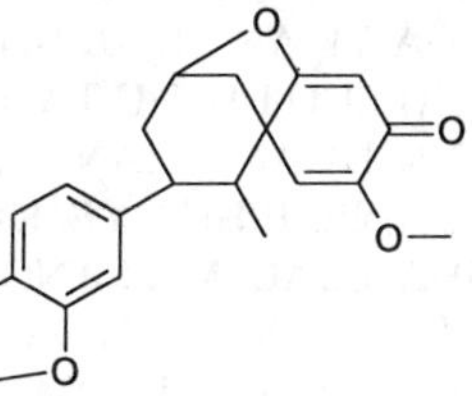

2454 Futoquinol
$C_{21}H_{22}O_5$ MW: 354.41 Property: mp 97-8°C. Source: HAI FENG TENG. Ref: 6.

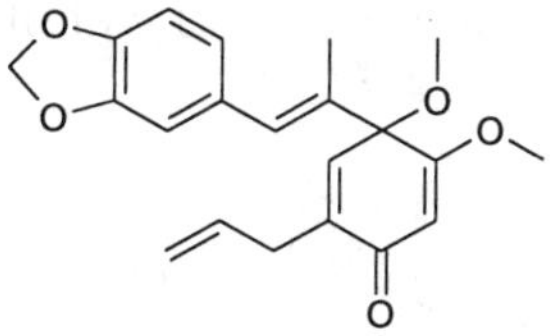

2455 Futoxide
$C_{18}H_{18}O_8$ MW: 362.34 Property: mp 150-1°C. Source: HAI FENG TENG. Ref: 6.

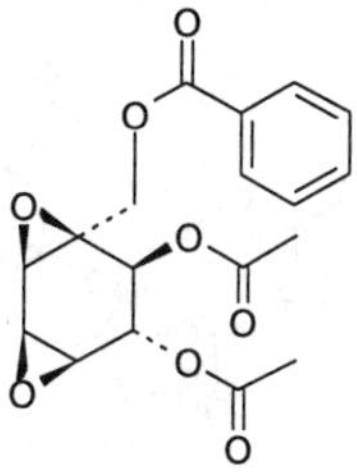

2456 Fuziline
$C_{24}H_{39}NO_7$ MW: 453.27 Property: colorless powder, $[\alpha]_D^{26}$ +10.8° (c=1.564, $CHCl_3$). Source: E ZHANG YE FU ZI. Ref: 461.

2457 Gadoleiic acid
$C_{22}H_{42}O_2$ MW: 338.58 Property: mp cis: 23.0-3.5°C, bp 170°C/0.1mm. Source: LUO HUA SHENG YOU. Ref: 6.

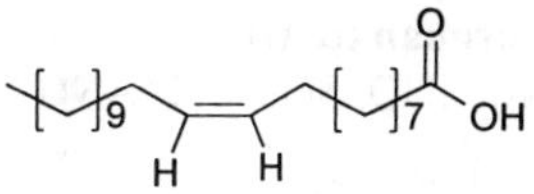

2458 Gagaminin
$C_{36}H_{43}NO_8$ MW: 617.75 Property: mp 166-9°C. Source: LUO MO. Ref: 6.

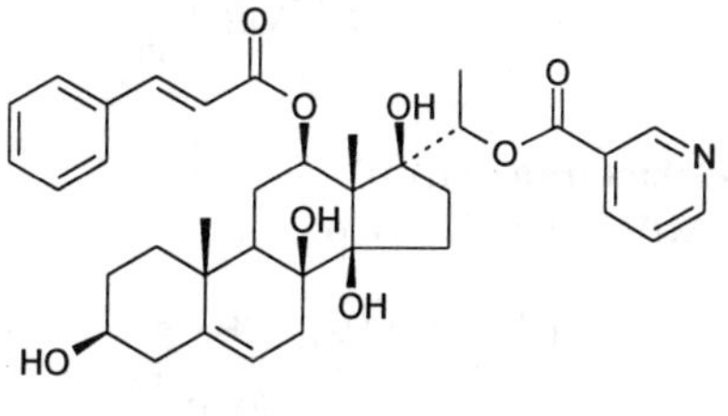

2459 Galacitiol
$C_6H_{14}O_6$ MW: 182.17 Property: mp 188-90°C, bp 275-80°C/1mm. Source: JIAO TUO LUO. Ref: 587.

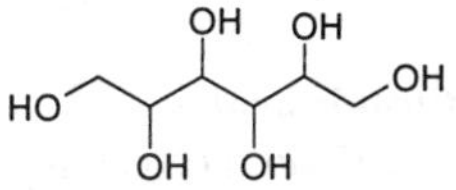

2461 Galactitol
$C_6H_{14}O_6$ MW: 182.17 Property: mp 188-90°C, bp 275-80°C/1mm. Source: DI JING, DU ZHONG, WU YE TENG. Ref: 2.

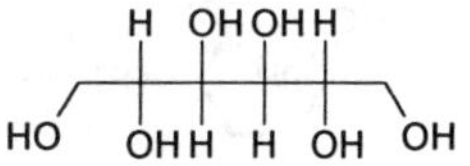

2462 L-Galactoheptulose
$C_7H_{14}O_7$ MW: 210.19 Property: mp 110-5°C (dec). Source: MU XU. Ref: 6.

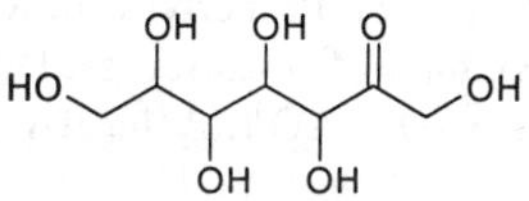

2463 3-O-β-D-Galactopyranosyl(1→2)-β-D-glucuronopyranosyl gypsoside
Property: white powder, mp 225-7°C. Source: DA BAO CHI BO. Ref: 425.

2464 Galactosamine
$C_6H_{13}NO_5$ MW: 179.17 Property: mp D(-): 185°C. Source: LU RONG, MAN YU, YE YU. Ref: 2.

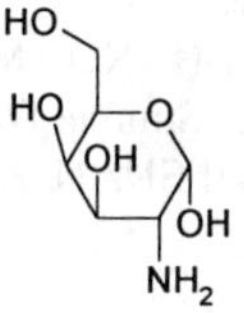

2465 Galacturonan (α-D)
Source: MANG GUO. Source: MANG GUO. Ref: 6.

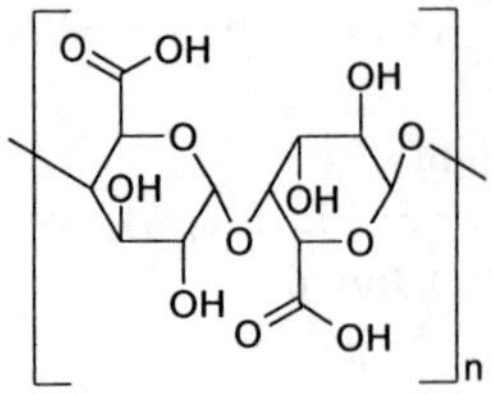

2466 Galacturonan (β-D)
Source: MANG GUO. Ref: 6.

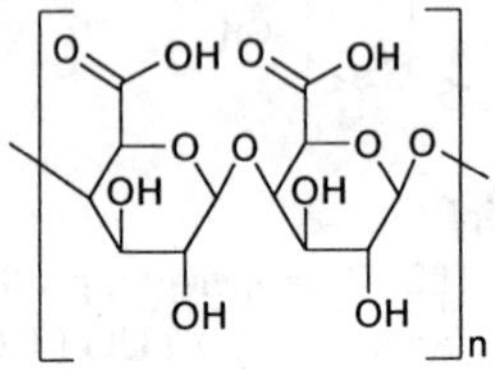

2467 D-Galacturonic acid
$C_7H_{12}O_6$ MW: 192.17 Property: mp α: 156-9°C (dec), mp β: 160°C (dec). Source: CHUN, FEN TUAN HUA, HAI DAI (DA YE ZAO), KU GUA, LUO LE ZI, MU MIAN HUA, YE YU, YU SHU SHU. Ref: 6.

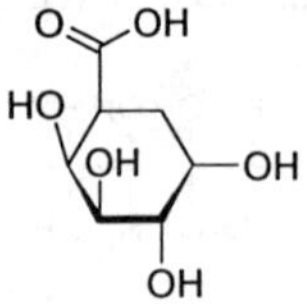

2468 Galangin
4H-1-benzopyran-4-one,3,5,7-trihydroxy-2-phenyl. $C_{15}H_{10}O_5$ MW: 270.24 Property: yellow acicular crystal (MeOH), mp 214-6°C. Source: DA LIANG JIANG, FENG JIAO, GAO LIANG JIANG. Ref: 6, 463.

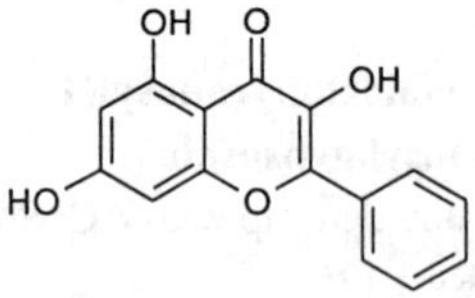

2469 Galangol
Source: GAO LIANG JIANG. Ref: 6.

2470 Galanthamine
Jikon; Lycoremine. $C_{17}H_{21}NO_3$ MW: 287.36 Property: mp 126-7°C. Source: DA YI ZHI JIAN, SHUI XIAN GEN, SHI SUAN. Ref: 4, 6.

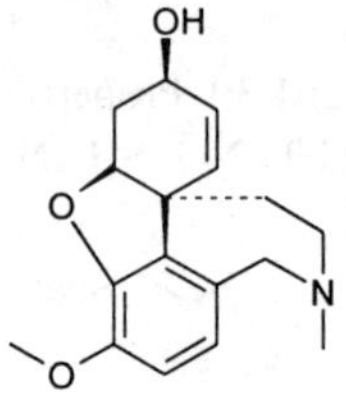

2471 Gallic acid
CAS: 149-91-7 $C_7H_6O_5$ MW: 170.12 Property: mp 253-40°C (dec). Source: BAI HUA QIA HU, CAO YUAN LAO GUAN CAO, CU LIU GUO (SHA JI), DA HUANG, DA YE AN YE, DI JIN CAO, HAI ER CHA, HE ZI, HU LUO BU, HU TAO YE, HUA XIANG SHU YE, HUANG LIAN YA, HUANG LU, HUANG LU ZHI YE, JI HUA YE, KUAN DONG HUA, LAO GUAN CAO, MA SANG YE, MANG GUO, MEI GUI HUA, MOU SHI ZI, MU DAN PI, PANSHI LIU GAN, PIAN XU, QIAN NIU ZI, QIAN QU LAI, QUAN SHEN, SHAN ZHU YU, SHAN ZHU YU, SHI LIU PI, SHUI JIE GU DAN, WU JIU YE, XI PAN LIAN, XIAN HE CAO, XIANG SI ZI, YAN FU ZI, YAN MOU LE, YE XIA ZHU, YOU GAN MU PI, YOU GAN YE, ZI WEI HUA, etc. Ref: 2, 4, 5, 6, 283, 297.

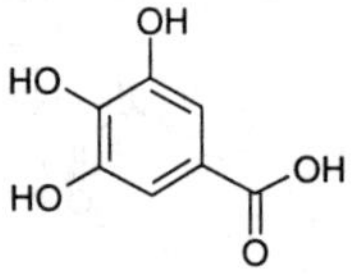

2472 Gallic acid-3-O-(6'-O-galloy)-glucoside
$C_{20}H_{20}O_{14}$ MW: 484.37 Source: DA HUANG. Ref: 2.

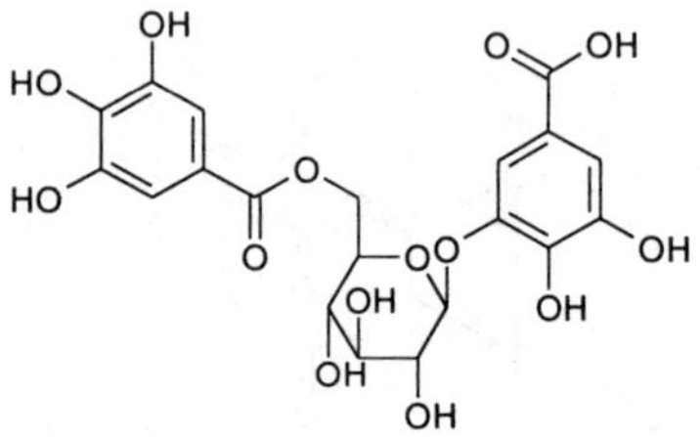

2473 Gallic acid-4-O-(6'-O-galloyl)-glucoside
$C_{20}H_{20}O_{14}$ MW: 484.37 Source: DA HUANG. Ref: 2.

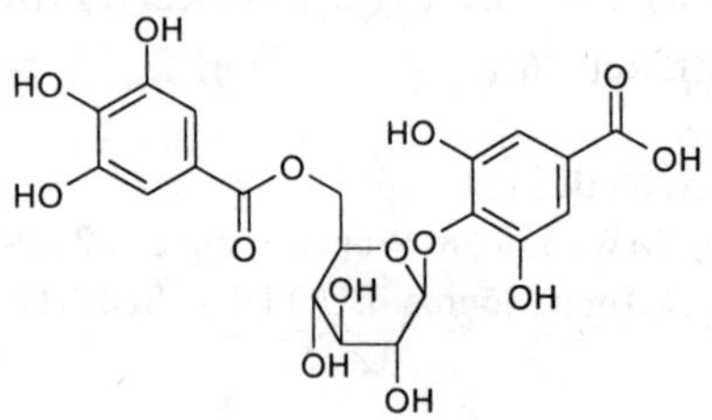

2474 Gallocatechin
$C_{15}H_{14}O_7$ MW: 306.27 Property: mp (+): 185-8°C, (-): 218°C(edc). Source: BAI GUO YE. Ref: 6.

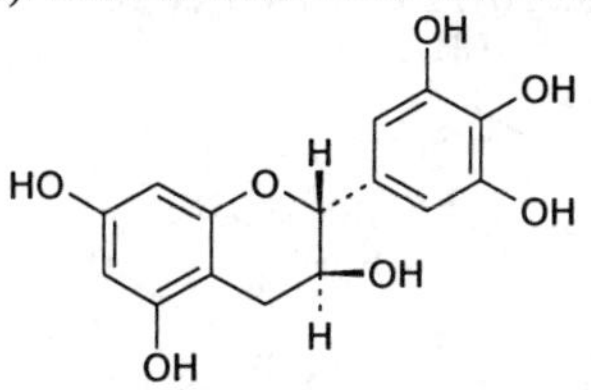

2475 Gallocatechin-(4α→8)epicatechin
Property: mp 223-7°C. Source: KUN MING SHAN HAI TANG. Ref: 612.

2476 (+)-Gallocatechin-hexacetate
$C_{27}H_{26}O_{13}$ MW: 558.50 Source: BAI GUO. Ref: 2.

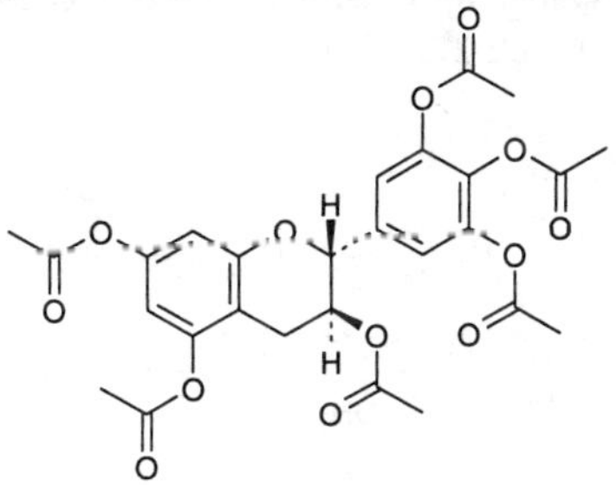

2477 1-Galloyl-2-cinnamoyl-glucose
$C_{22}H_{22}O_{11}$ MW: 462.41 Source: DA HUANG. Ref: 2.

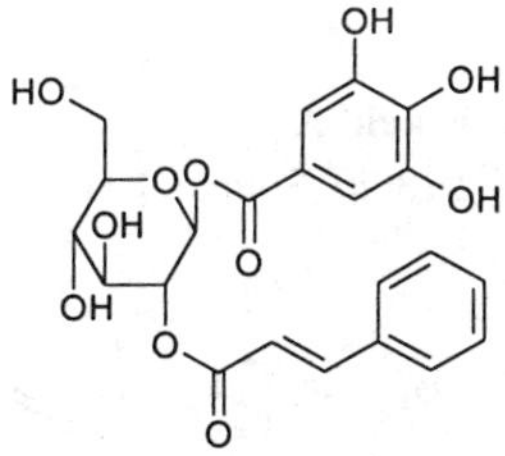

2478 Galloylepicatechin
$C_{22}H_{18}O_{10}$ MW: 442.38 Property: mp 253°C. Source: CHA YE, TAO GEN. Ref: 6.

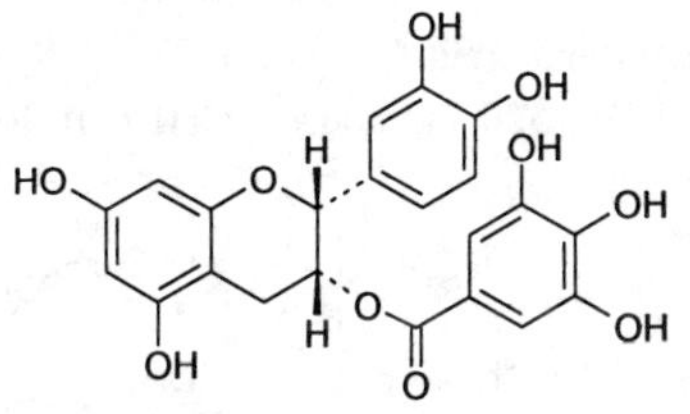

2479 Galloyl-l-epigallocatechol
$C_{22}H_{18}O_{11}$ MW: 458.38 Property: mp 215-6°C. Source: CHA YE. Ref: 6.

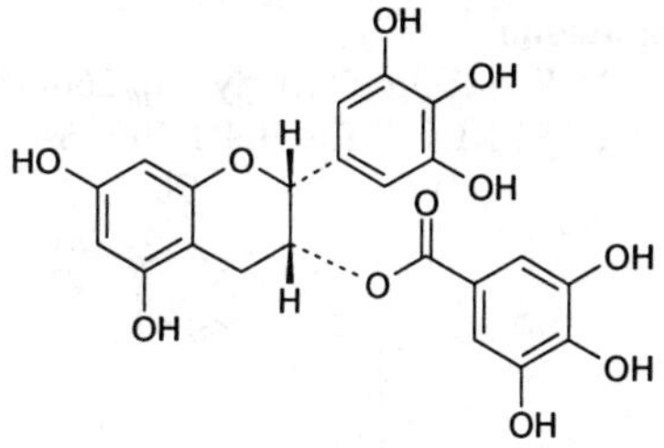

2480 1-Galloyl glucose
$C_{13}H_{16}O_{10}$ MW: 332.27 Property: mp 212°C (dec). Source: DA HUANG. Ref: 6.

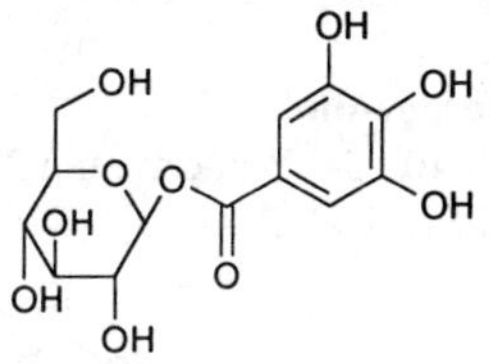

2481 6-O-Galloyl-glucose
$C_{13}H_{16}O_{10}$ MW: 332.27 Property: mp 166°C (dec). Source: CAO YUAN LAO, DA HUANG, GUAN CAO, ZUAN SHUN. Ref: 2.

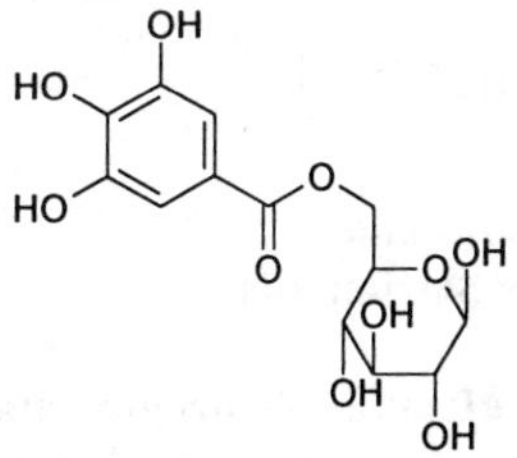

2482 1-O-Galloyl-glycerol
$C_{10}H_{12}O_7$ MW: 244.20 Source: DA HUANG. Ref: 2.

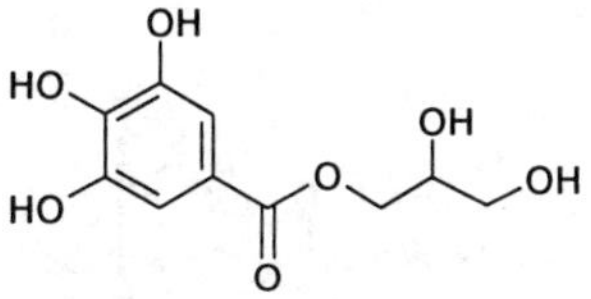

2483 1-O-Galloylpedunculagin
Source: BAI SHAO YAO. Ref: 2.

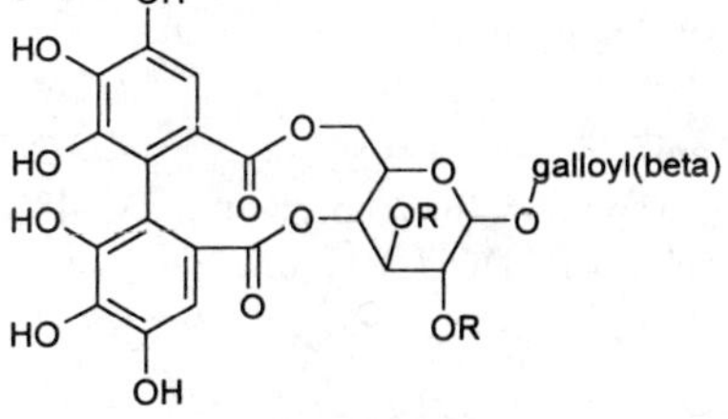

R=(S)HHDP

2484 Galuteolin
$C_{21}H_{20}O_{11}$ MW: 448.39 Property: mp 260-3°C. Source: LIAN ZI XIN, WEN JING. Ref: 6.

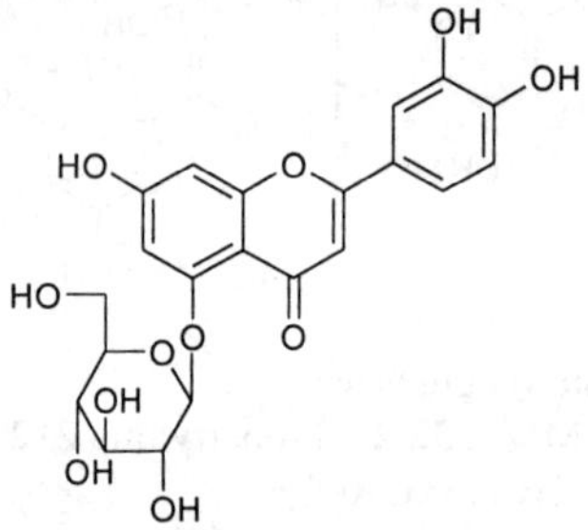

2485 Gamabufogenin
$C_{24}H_{34}O_5$ MW: 402.54 Property: mp 261-3°C (dec). Source: CHAN SU. Ref: 2.

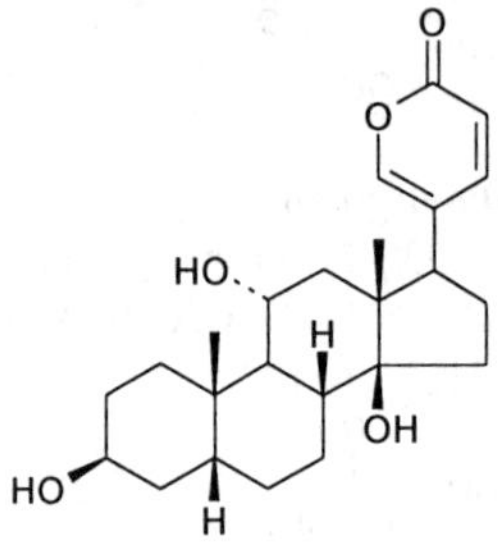

2486 Gamabufotalin
Source: CHAN SU. Ref: 618.

2487 Gamabufotalin-3-hydrogen suberate
$C_{32}H_{46}O_8$ MW: 558.72 Source: CHAN SU. Ref: 6.

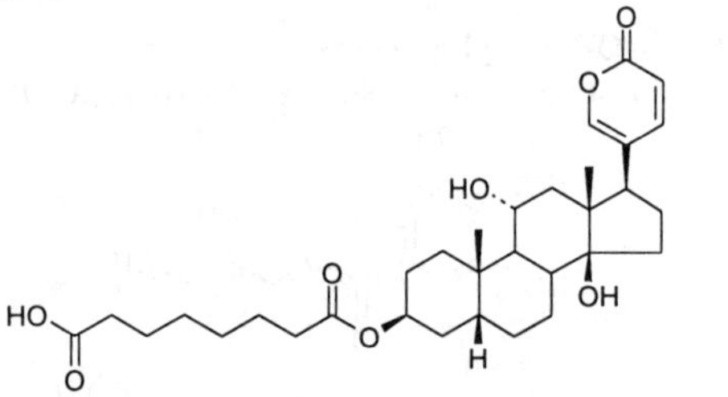

2488 Gamabufotalininol
$C_{26}H_{36}O_6$ MW: 444.57 Property: mp 263-5°C. Source: CHAN PI. Ref: 6.

2489 Gamatin
$C_{19}H_{12}O_6$ MW: 336.36 Property: mp 233-4°C. Source: SHUI LIU DOU. Ref: 6.

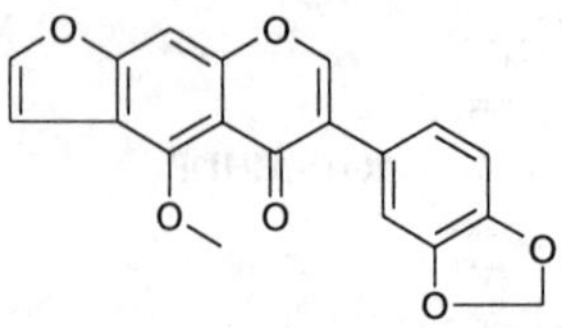

2490 Gambirine
$C_{22}H_{30}N_2O_4$ MW: 386.50 Property: mp 163-5°C (dec). Source: HAI ER CHA. Ref: 6.

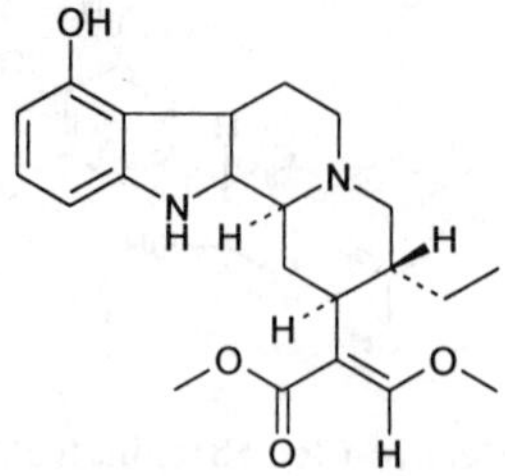

2491 Gancaoning P-3'-nethylether
3,5,7,4'-Tetrahydroxy-3'-methoxy-6-isoprenyl flavone. $C_{21}H_{20}O_7$ MW: 384.39 Property: yellow lamellar crystal. mp 160-2°C. Source: WU LA ER GAN CAO. Ref: 275.

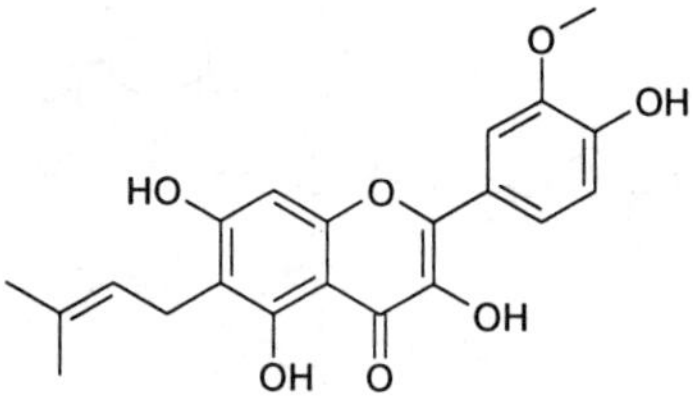

2492 Gandiflorc acid
$C_{20}H_{30}O_3$ MW: 318 Property: white massive crystal (acetone), mp 220-2°C. Source: MAO GENG XI XIAN. Ref: 476.

2493 Ganoderic acid A
$C_{30}H_{46}O_7$ MW: 518.70 Source: CHI ZHI. Ref: 188, 387.

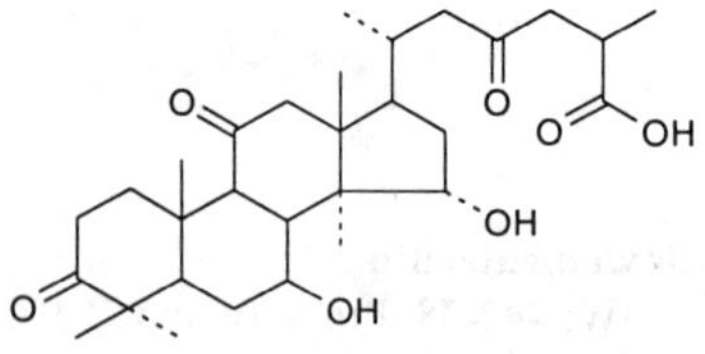

2494 Ganoderic acid C
$C_{30}H_{48}O_7$ MW: 520.71 Source: CHI ZHI. Ref: 387.

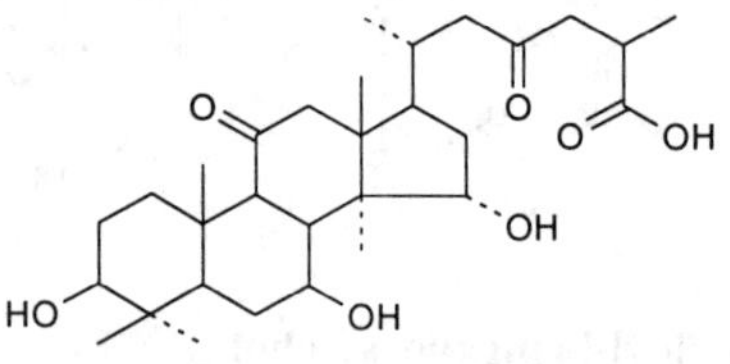

2495 Ganoderic acid DM
$C_{30}H_{44}O_4$ MW: 468.68 Property: light yellow acicular crystal (chloroform-methanol), mp 203-5°C. Source: CHI ZHI. Ref: 387.

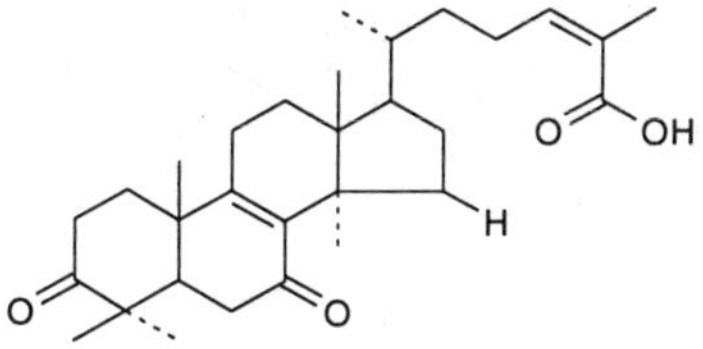

2496 Ganoderic acid MA
$C_{30}H_{48}O_5$ MW: 488.71 Source: CHI ZHI. Ref: 387.

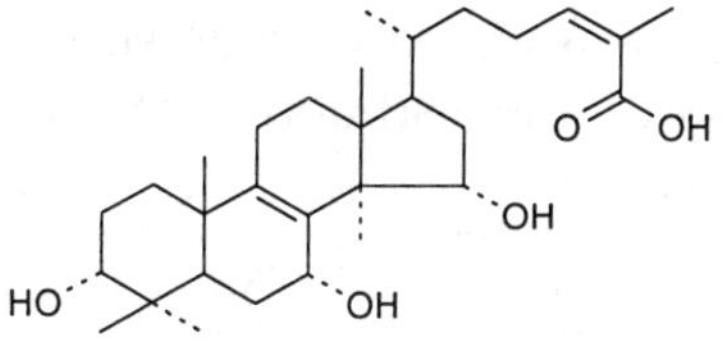

2497 Ganoderiol D
$C_{30}H_{48}O_5$ MW: 488.71 Source: CHI ZHI. Ref: 387.

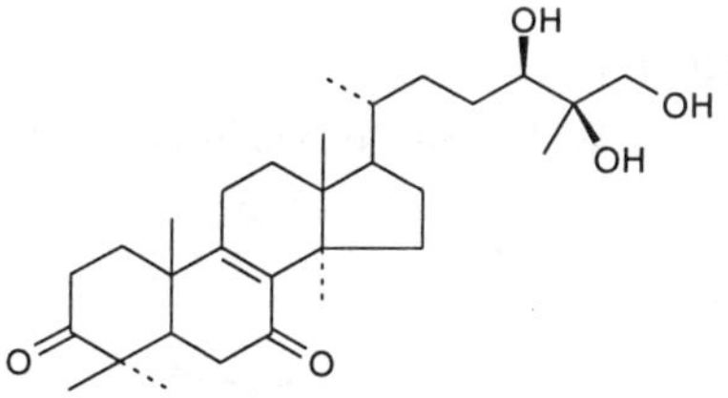

2498 Ganoderpurine III
$C_{11}H_{17}N_5O$ MW: 233.28 Property: oleaginous substance, mp 151-2°C. Source: BAO GAI LING ZHI. Ref: 164.

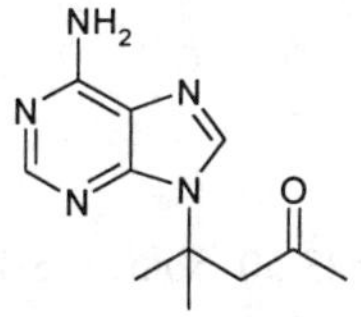

2499 Ganoine I
$C_{11}H_{17}NO_2$ MW: 195.26 Property: oleaginous liquid. Source: BAO GAI LING ZHI. Ref: 164.

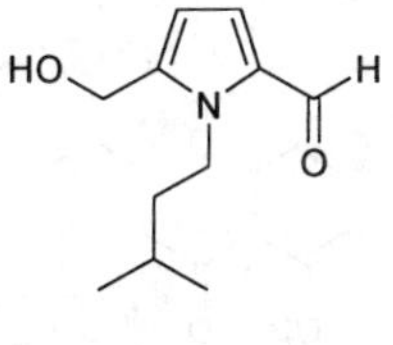

2500 Ganoine II
$C_{14}H_{15}NO_2$ MW: 229.28 Source: BAO GAI LING ZHI. Ref: 164.

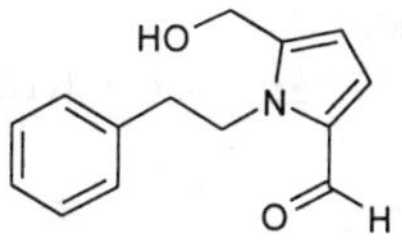

2501 Ganolactone
$C_{27}H_{36}O_6$ MW: 456.58 Property: white acicular crystal, mp 294-6°C, $[\alpha]_D^{20}$ +6° (c=0.1148, chloroform). Source: CHI ZHI. Ref: 350.

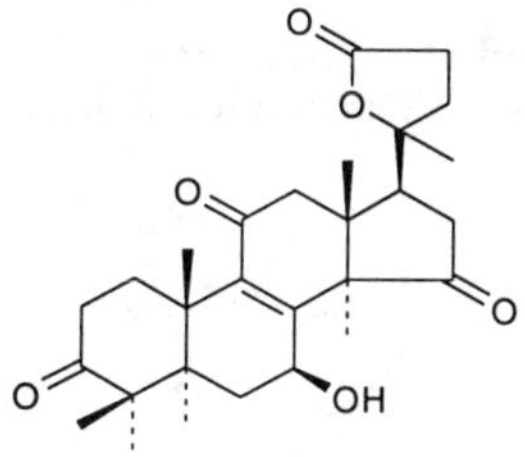

2502 Ganosporelactone A
$C_{30}H_{40}O_7$ MW: 512.65 Property: white acicular crystal, mp 238-40°C, $[\alpha]_D^{13}$ +74.5° (c=0.057, chloroform). Source: CHI ZHI. Ref: 192.

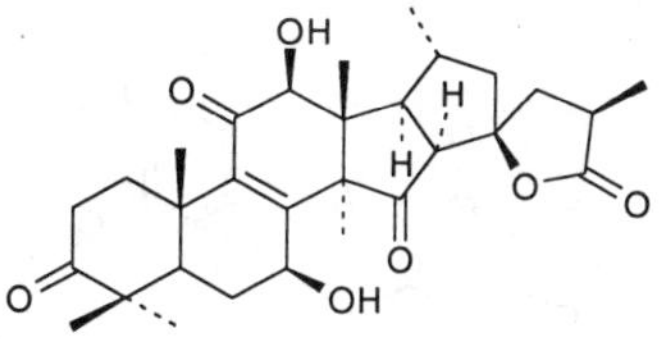

2503 Ganosporelactone B
$C_{30}H_{42}O_7$ MW: 514.67 Property: white acicular crystal, mp 235-7°C, $[\alpha]_D^{12}$ +68.8° (c=0.083, chloroform). Source: CHI ZHI. Ref: 192.

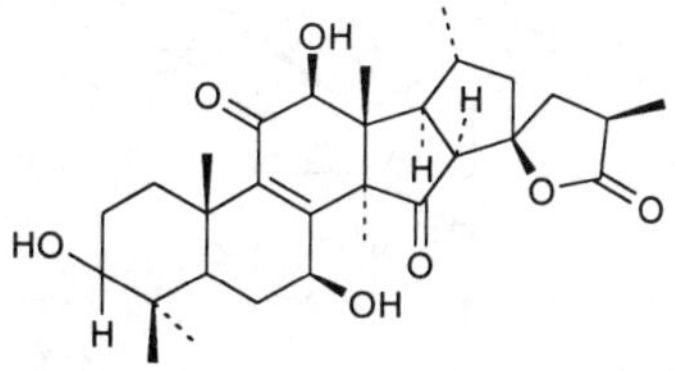

2504 Ganosporeric acid A (1)
$C_{30}H_{38}O_8$ MW: 526.63 Property: yellow acicular crystal, mp 115-8°C, $[\alpha]_D^{28}$ +48° (c=0.1, chloroform). Source: CHI ZHI. Ref: 188.

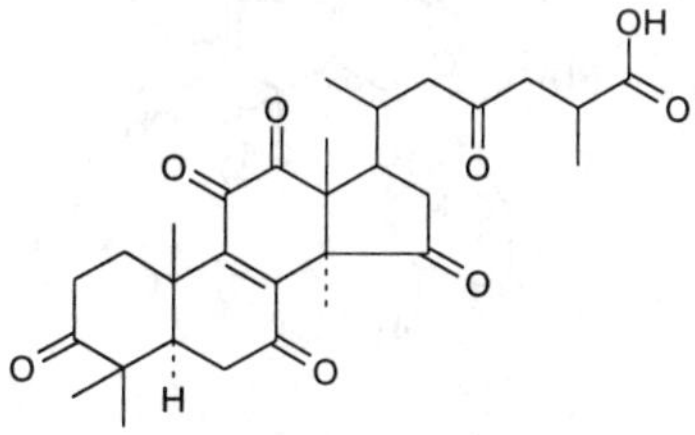

2505 Garbanzol
$C_{15}H_{12}O_5$ MW: 272.26 Source: HUI HUI DOU. Ref: 6.

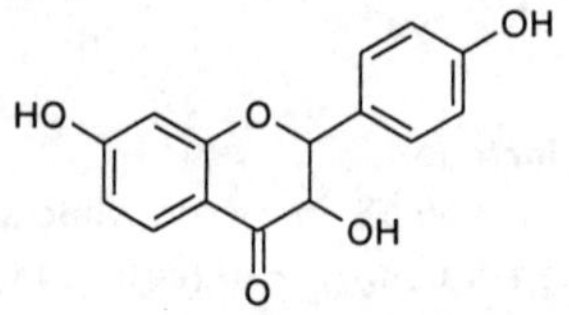

2506 Gardendiol
$C_{11}H_{16}O_4$ MW: 212.25 Source: SHAN ZHI ZI. Ref: 317.

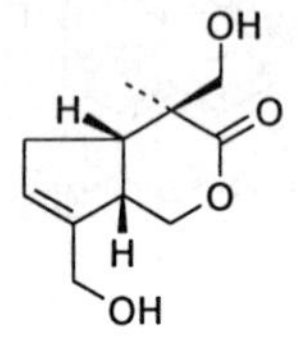

2507 Gardenin
$C_{21}H_{22}O_9$ MW: 418.40 Property: mp 163-4°C. Source: ZHI ZI, YI ZHI HAO. Ref: 2, 33.

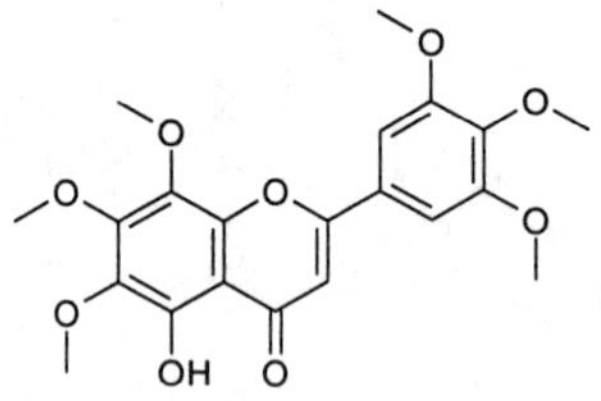

2508 Gardenone
$C_{13}H_{22}O_3$ MW: 226.32 Source: SHAN ZHI ZI. Ref: 317.

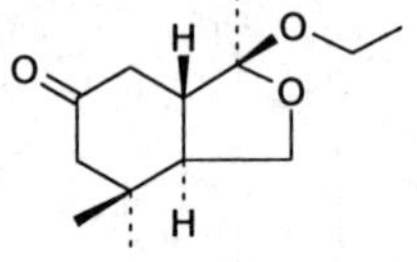

2509 Gardenoside
$C_{17}H_{24}O_{11}$ MW: 404.37 Property: mp 118-20°C. Source: ZHI ZI. Ref: 2.

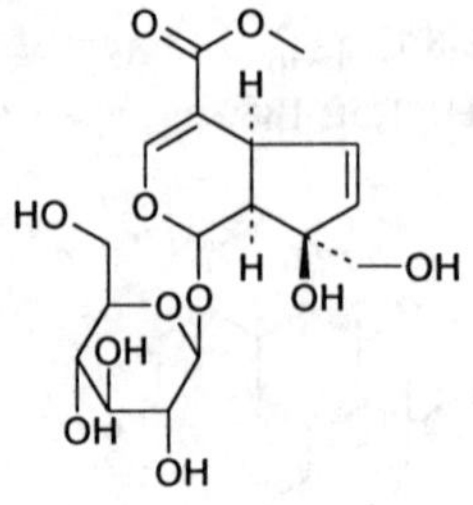

2510 Gardoside
$C_{16}H_{22}O_{10}$ MW: 374.35 Source: ZHI ZI. Ref: 2.

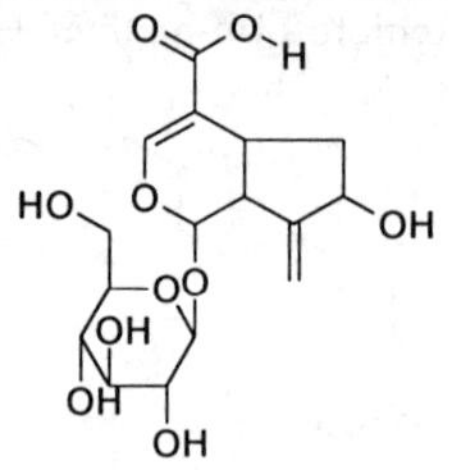

2511 Gastrodin
4-(β-D-glucopyranosyloxy) benzyl alcohol. CAS: 62499-27-8 $C_{13}H_{18}O_7$ MW: 286.28 Property: mp 96-8°C, 145-8°C. Source: SHAN HU LAN, TIAN MA. Ref: 4, 280.

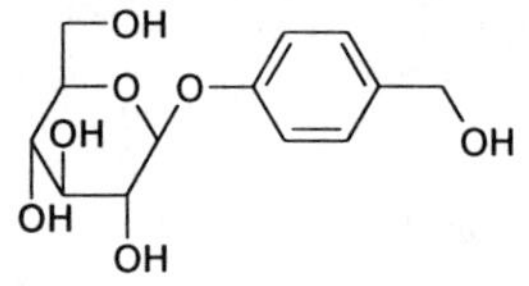

2512 GB-1
$C_{30}H_{22}O_{11}$ MW: 558.50 Source: SHAN ZHU ZI. Ref: 6.

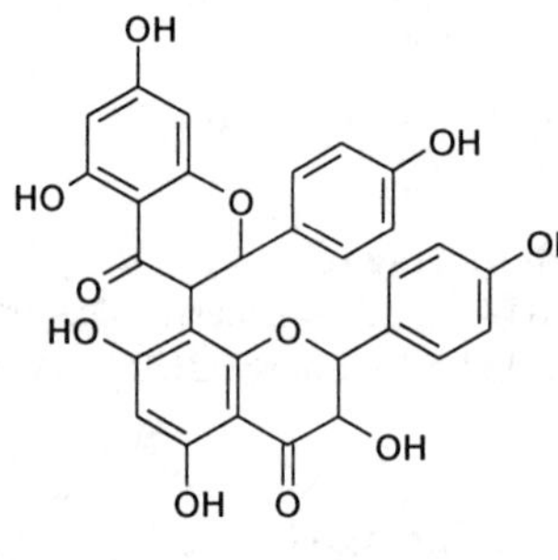

2513 GB-1a
$C_{30}H_{22}O_{10}$ MW: 542.50 Source: SHAN ZHU ZI. Ref: 6.

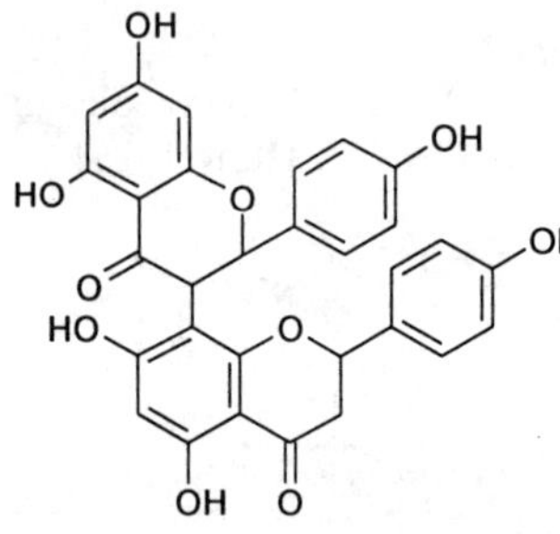

2514 GB-2

$C_{30}H_{22}O_{12}$ MW: 574.50 Source: SHAN ZHU ZI. Ref: 6.

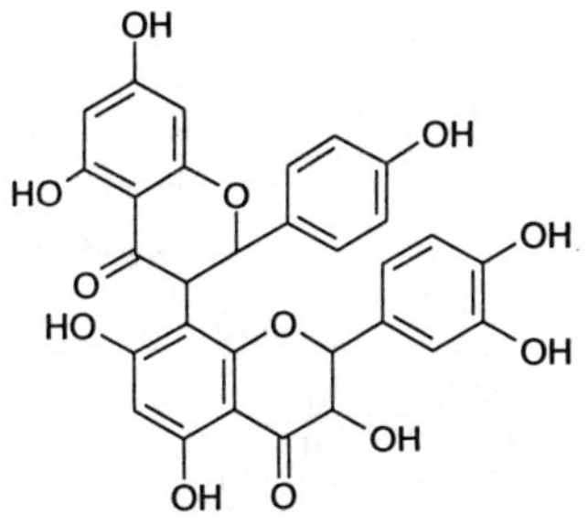

2515 GB-2a

$C_{30}H_{22}O_{11}$ MW: 558.50 Source: SHAN ZHU ZI. Ref: 6.

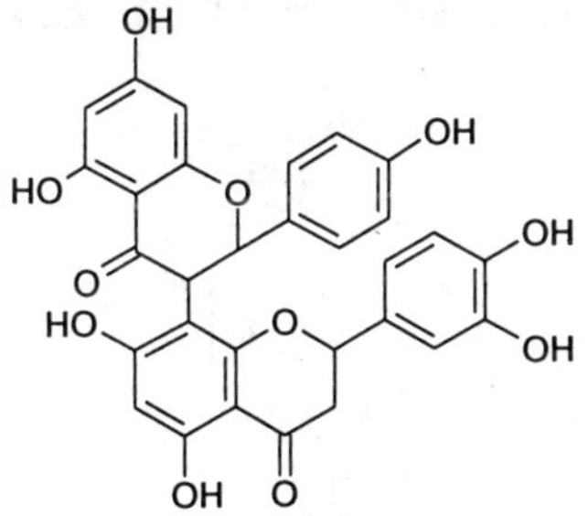

2516 Gedunin

$C_{28}H_{34}O_7$ MW: 482.58 Property: mp 157°C, 218°C. Source: KU LIAN PI. Ref: 6.

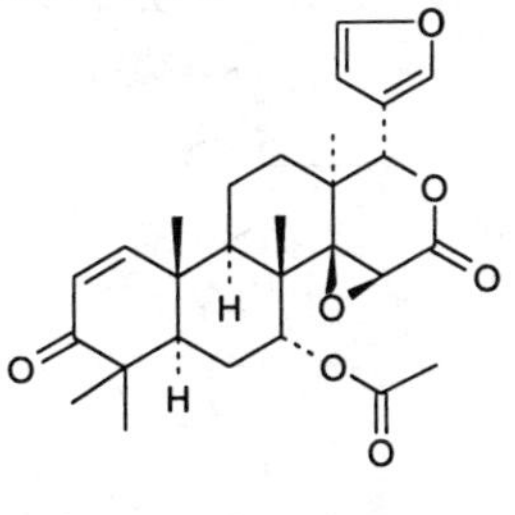

2517 Gein

Geoside. $C_{21}H_{30}O_{11}$ MW: 458.47 Property: mp 146-7°C; bp 183-4°C. Source: SHUI YANG MEI (I), SHUI YANG MEI GEN (I). Ref: 6.

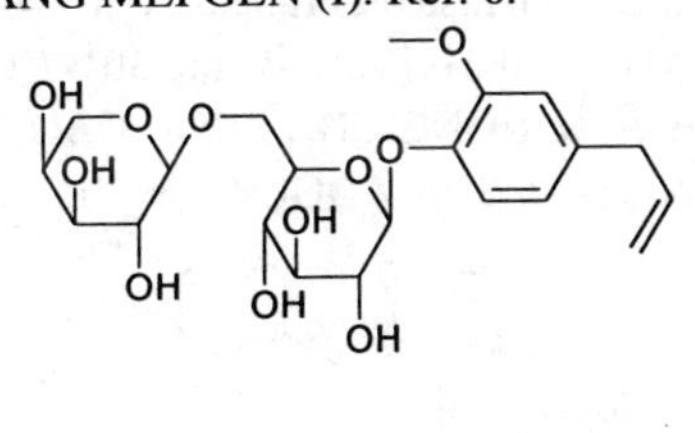

2518 Geissoschizine methyl ether

$C_{21}H_{26}N_2O_3$ MW: 354.45 Source: GOU TENG. Ref: 2.

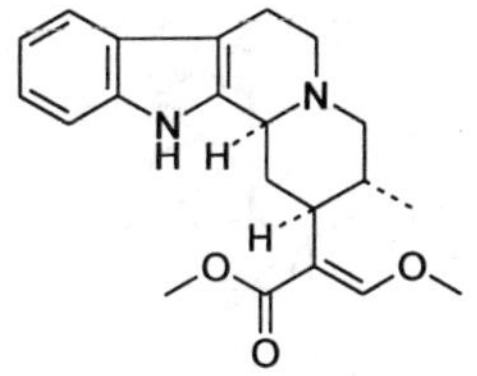

2519 Gelsamydine

$C_{29}H_{36}N_2O_6$ MW: 508.62 Property: mp194-6°C, $[\alpha]_D$ -126.9°. Source: GOU MAN. Ref: 14.

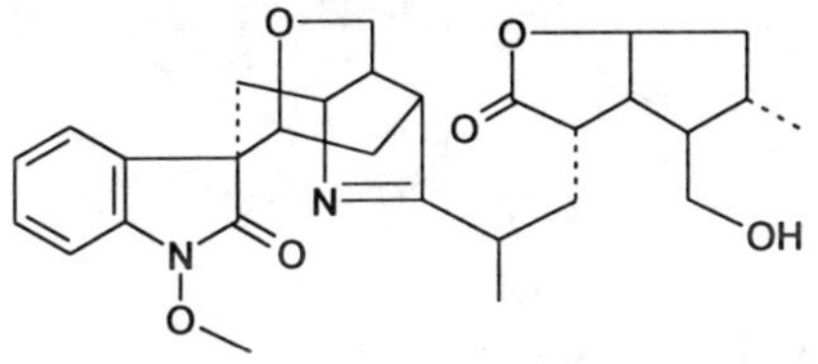

2520 Gelsedine

$C_{19}H_{24}N_2O_3$ MW: 328.41 Property: mp 172.5-174°C. Source: HU MAN TENG. Ref: 14.

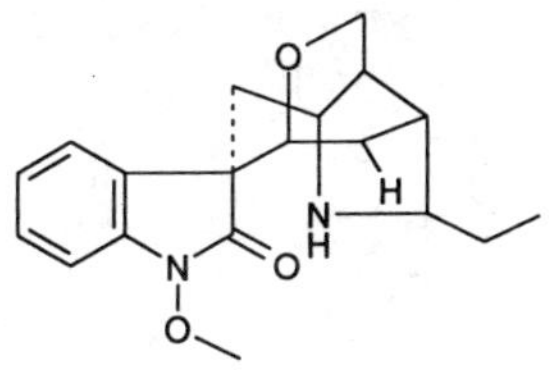

2521 Gelselegine

$C_{20}H_{26}N_2O_4$ MW: 358.44 Property: mp 167-8 °C, $[\alpha]_D$ -30°. Source: HOU MAN. Ref: 14.

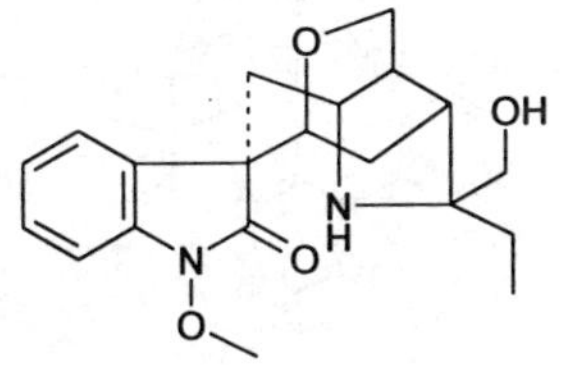

2522 Gelsemamide

$C_{20}H_{24}N_2O_3$ MW: 340.43 Property: mp 183-4°C, $[\alpha]_D$ +228.3°. Source: GOU MAN. Ref: 14.

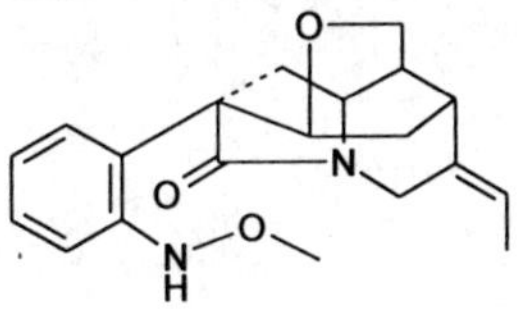

2523 Gelsemine
Kiuminine. $C_{20}H_{22}N_2O_2$ MW: 322.41 Property: mp 178°C. Source: GOU WEN. Ref: 5, 6, 14.

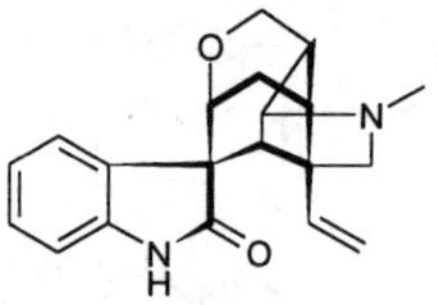

2524 Gelsemine N-oxide
$C_{20}H_{22}N_2O_3$ MW: 338.41 Property: amorphous, $[\alpha]_D$ -16.9°. Source: GOU MAN. Ref: 14.

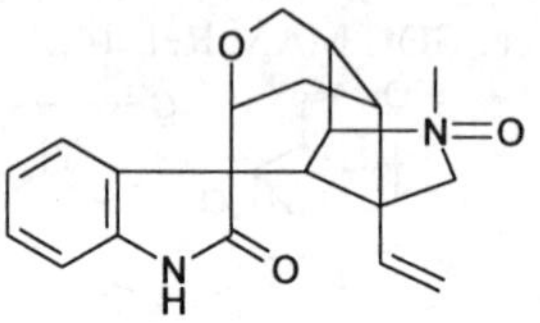

2525 Gelsemoxonine
$C_{19}H_{22}N_2O_5$ MW: 358.40 Property: powder, $[\alpha]_D$ -188.5°. Source: GOU MAN. Ref: 14.

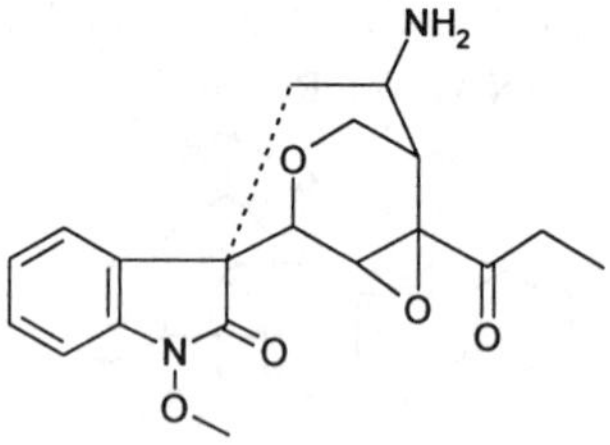

2526 Gelsevirine
$C_{21}H_{24}N_2O_3$ MW: 352.44 Property: oil, $[\alpha]_D$ -4.5°. Source: GOU MAN. Ref: 14.

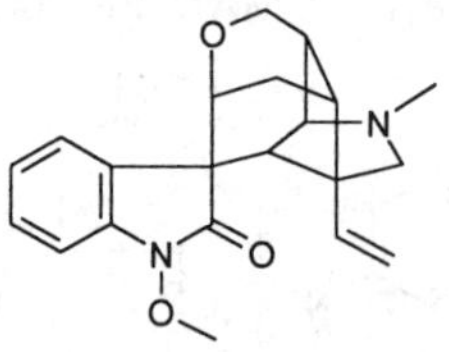

2527 Genipin
$C_{11}H_{16}O_5$ MW: 228.25 Source: DU ZHONG. Ref: 2.

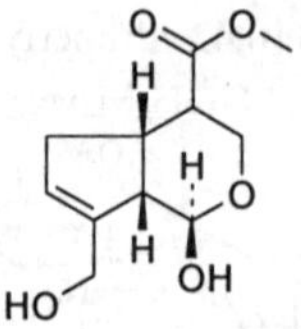

2528 Genipingentiobioside
$C_2H_{34}O_{15}$ MW: 550.52 Property: mp 193-5°C(C_2H_5OH), 227-9°C. Source: SHUI ZHI, ZHI ZI. Ref: 2.

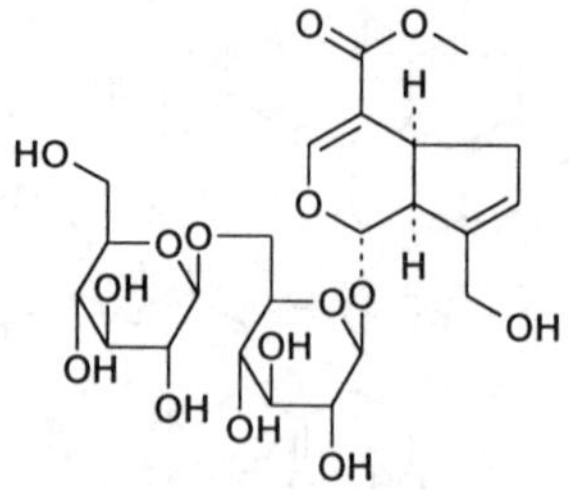

2529 Geniposide
$C_{17}H_{24}O_{10}$ MW: 388.37 Property: mp 163-4°C. Source: DU ZHONG, GAN DI HUANG, MA YING DAN, SHUI ZHI, SHUI ZHI YE, ZHI ZI, ZHI ZI YE. Ref: 2, 234.

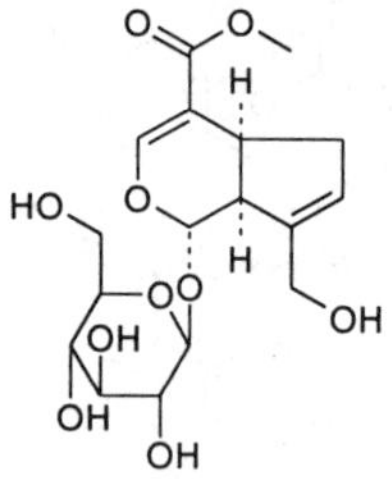

2530 Geniposidic acid
$C_{16}H_{22}O_{10}$ MW: 374.35 Source: DU ZHONG, ROU CONG RONG, ZHI ZI. Ref: 2, 628.

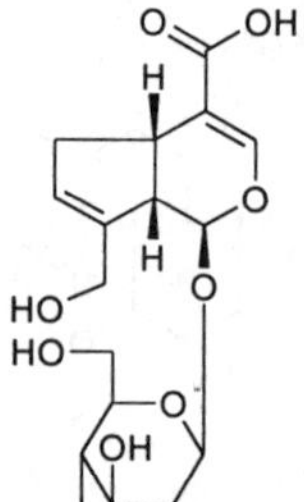

2531 Genistein
5,7,4'-Genistein; Genisteol; Prunetol. CAS: 446-72-0 $C_{15}H_{10}O_5$ MW: 270.24 Property: mp 301-2°C (dec). Source: GE GEN, HONG CHE ZHOU CAO, HUI DA DOU, HUAI JIAO, SHAN DOU GEN. Ref: 2, 4, 5.

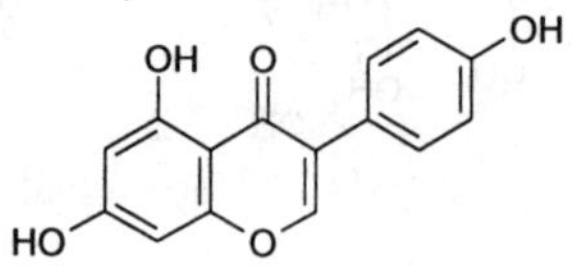

2532 Genistin
$C_{21}H_{20}O_{10}$ MW: 432.39 Property: mp 254-6°C. Source: HEI DA DOU. Ref: 6.

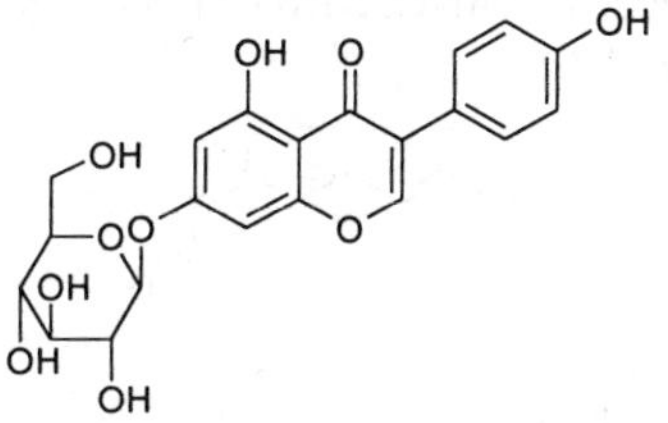

2533 Genkdaphin
$C_{20}H_{16}O_7$ MW: 368.35 Property: colorless acicular crystal, mp 118-9.5°C, $[\alpha]_D$ -64.8° (c=0.5, chloroform). Source: YUAN HUA. Ref: 175.

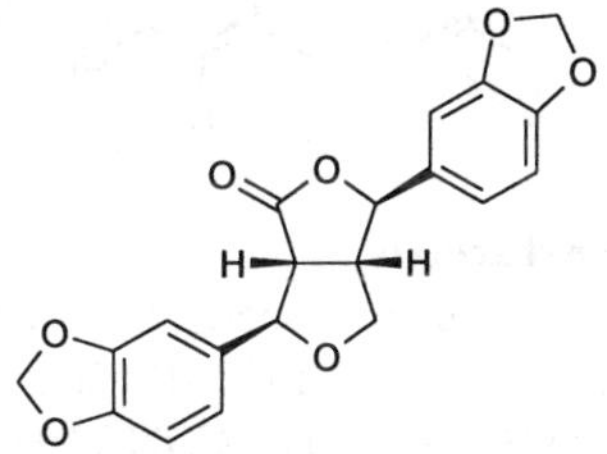

2534 Genkwanin
$C_{16}H_{12}O_5$ MW: 284.27 Property: mp 286°C. Source: YUAN HUA, YING TAO, YIN CHEN HAO. Ref: 2.

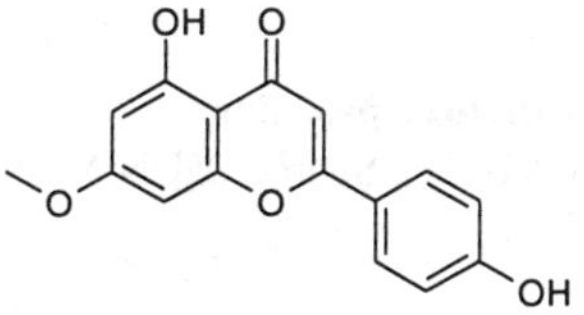

2535 Gentialutine
$C_9H_{11}NO$ MW: 149.19 Property: mp 129-30°C. Source: QIN JIAO, SHUI CAI. Ref: 6.

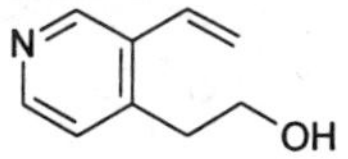

2536 Gentianaine
$C_6H_7NO_3$ MW: 141.13 Property: mp 149-50°C. Source: QIN JIAO. Ref: 6.

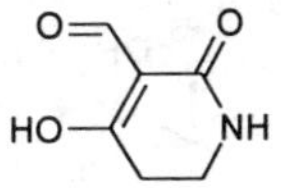

2537 Gentianidine
$C_9H_9NO_2$ MW: 163.18 Property: mp 131-2°C. Source: LONG DAN, QIN JIAO, SHUI CAI. Ref: 2.

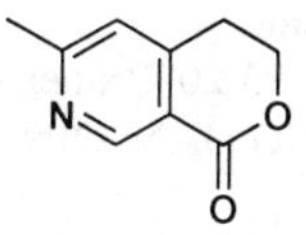

2538 Gentianine
$C_{10}H_9NO_2$ MW: 175.19 Property: mp 82-3°C. Source: BAI HUA LONG DAN, HU LU BA, LONG DAN, QIN JIAO, SHUI CAI. Ref: 2, 4.

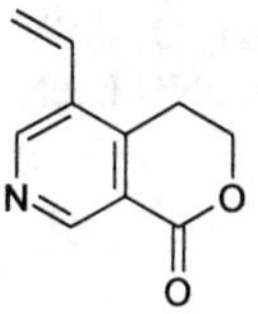

2539 Gentianol
$C_{10}H_{11}NO_3$ MW: 193.20 Source: LONG DAN. Ref: 2.

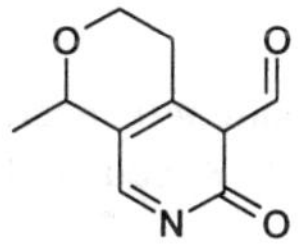

2540 Gentianose
$C_{18}H_{32}O_{16}$ MW: 504.45 Property: mp 209°C. Source: LONG DAN. Ref: 2.

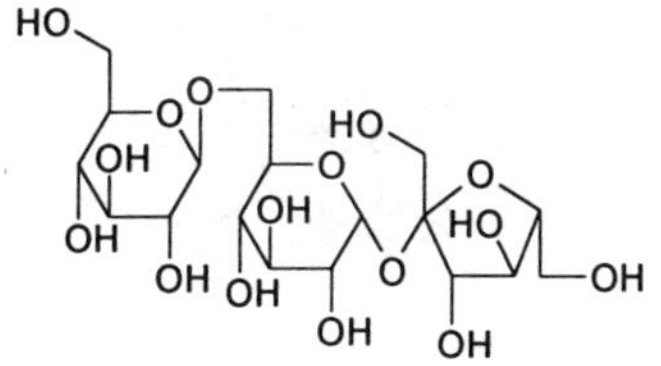

2541 Gentiatibetine
$C_9H_{11}NO_2$ MW: 165.19 Property: mp 161°C. Source: SHUI CAI GEN. Ref: 6.

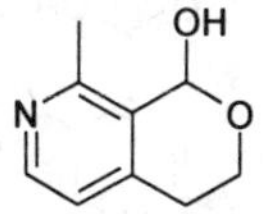

2542 Gentiobiose
$C_{12}H_{22}O_{11}$ MW: 342.30 Property: mp α: 85.5-6.0°C, β: 190-5°C. Source: ZANG HONG HUA. Ref: 6.

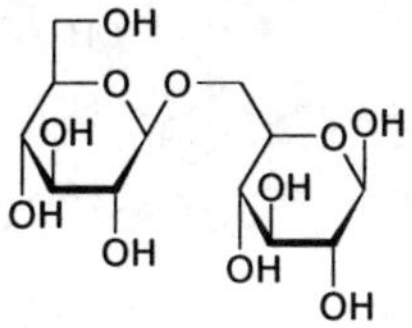

2543 Gentioflavine
$C_{10}H_{11}NO_3$ MW: 193.20 Property: mp 218-20°C (dec). Source: LONG DAN, QIN JIAO. Ref: 2.

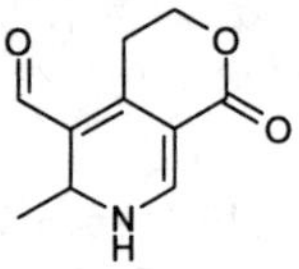

2544 Gentiopicrin
Gentiopicroside. $C_{16}H_{20}O_9$ MW: 356.33 Property: mp 122°C. Source: LONG DAN, QIN JIAO. Ref: 2.

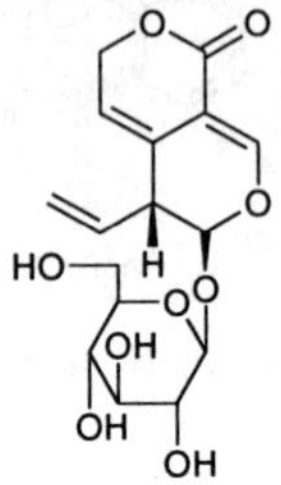

2545 Gentiopicroside tetraacetate
$C_{24}H_{28}O_{13}$ MW: 524.48 Source: LONG DAN. Ref: 2.

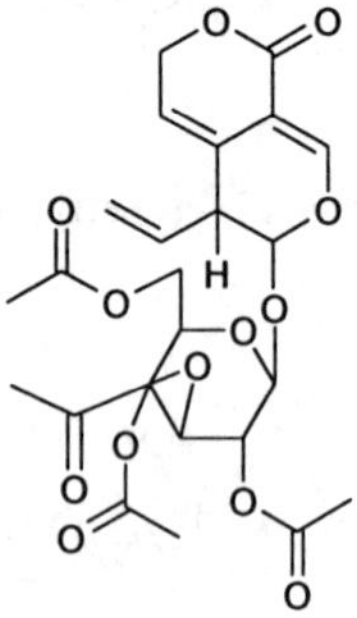

2546 Gentisic acid
$C_7H_6O_4$ MW: 154.12 Property: mp 204.5-5°C. Source: HUI XIANG JING YE, LAI FU, NING MENG GEN, NING MENG YE. Ref: 6.

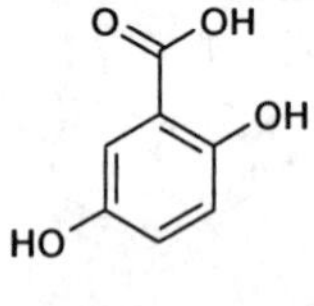

2547 Gentisin
$C_{14}H_{10}O_5$ MW: 258.23 Property: mp 266-7°C. Source: ZHANG YA CAI. Ref: 6.

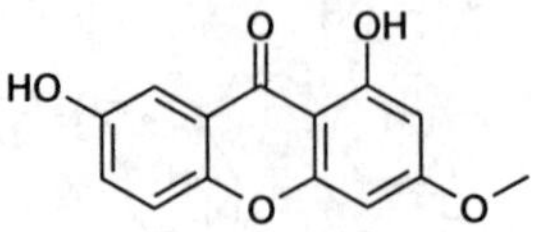

2548 Geranial
$C_{10}H_{16}O$ MW: 152.24 Property: bp 226-8°C. Source: CHA YE, GAN JIANG, JU ZI, JU ZI PI, LIAN QIAO, SHENG JIANG, XING ZI, YUN XIANG CAO. Ref: 2, 6.

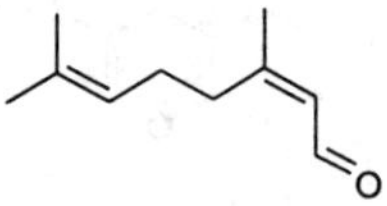

2549 Geraniol
Lemonol. CAS: 106-24-1 $C_{10}H_{18}O$ MW: 154.25 Property: mp 230°C. Source: CHAI HU, GAN JIANG, JIN YIN HUA, JIU LI XIANG, SHENG JIANG, WU WEI ZI. Ref: 2, 4, 11, 638.

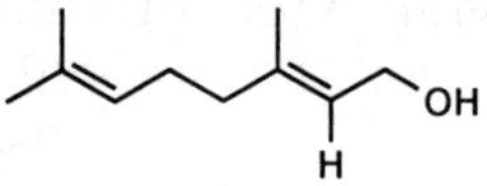

2550 Geranyl acetate
$C_{12}H_{20}O_2$ MW: 196.29 Property: bp 242-5°C/764 mm. Source: HE SHI, HU LUO BO ZI, NING MENG, SHENG JIANG, TU XIANG RU, YE XIANG MAO, YIN CHEN HAO. Ref: 6.

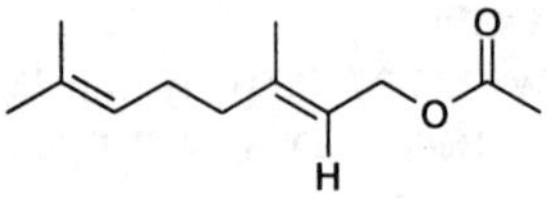

2551 8-Geranyloxy psoralen
Property: mp 51-3°C. Source: YUN NAN QIANG HUO. Ref: 551.

2552 Germacranolide
$C_{17}H_{22}O_4$ MW: 290.36 Source: YUE GUI ZI. Ref: 6.

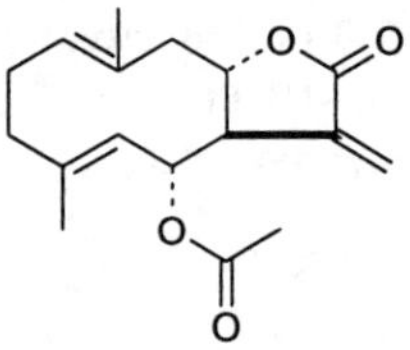

2553 Germacra-1(10),4,7(11)-trien-9α-ol
$C_{15}H_{24}O$ MW: 220.36 Property: bp 62-3°C/13mm. Source: XI XIN. Ref: 6.

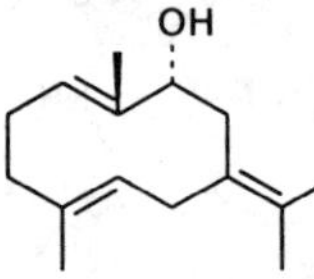

2554 Germacrene B

$C_{15}H_{24}$ MW: 204.36 Source: CHEN ZI PI. Ref: 6.

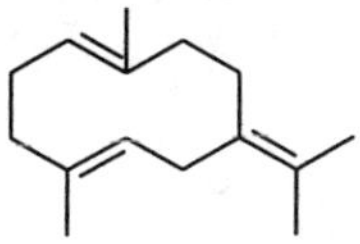

2555 Germacrene D

$C_{15}H_{24}$ MW: 204.36 Source: CHEN ZI PI. Ref: 6.

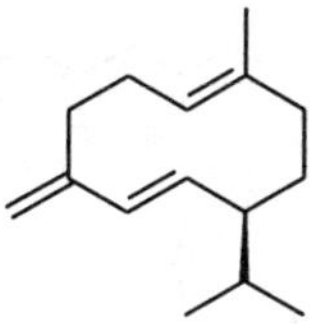

2556 Germacrone 1-cis, 5-cis

$C_{15}H_{22}O$ MW: 218.34 Property: bp-: 100°C/1mm. Source: MAN SHAN HONG. Ref: 6.

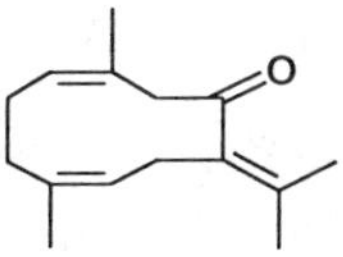

2557 Germacrone 1-cis, 5-trans

$C_{15}H_{22}O$ MW: 218.34 Property: bp-: 100°C/1mm. Source: MAN SHAN HONG. Ref: 6.

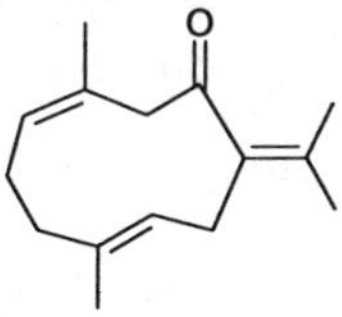

2558 Germanicol

$C_{30}H_{50}O$ MW: 426.73 Property: mp 176-7°C. Source: SHAN WO JU. Ref: 6.

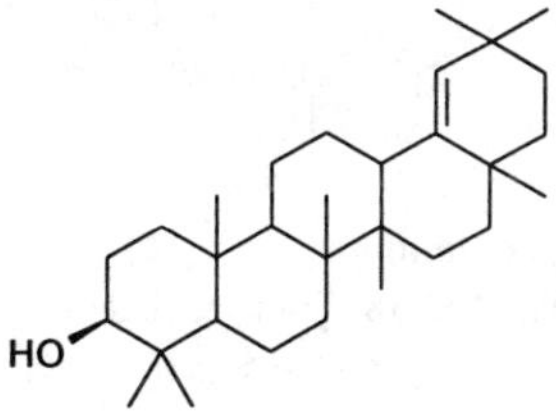

2559 Germerine

$C_{37}H_{59}NO_{11}$ MW: 693.88 Property: mp 193-5°C (dec). Source: LI LU. Ref: 6.

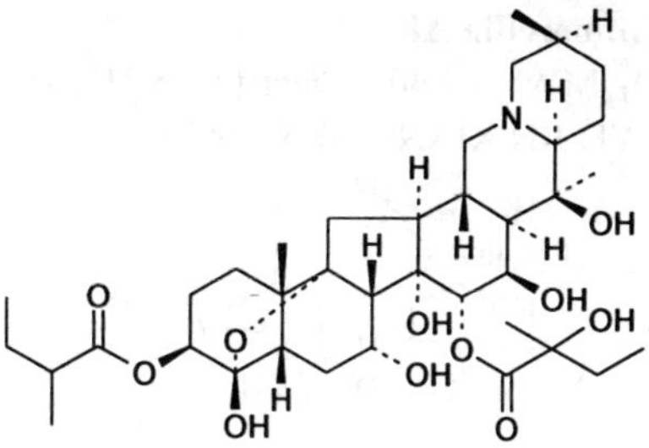

2560 Gertiopicrin

Geatiopicroside. CAS: 20831-76-9 $C_{16}H_{20}O_9$ MW: 356.32 Source: LONG DAN. Ref: 4.

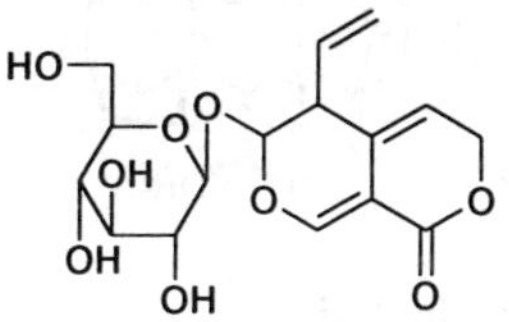

2561 Gibberellin A1

$C_{19}H_{24}O_6$ MW: 348.40 Property: mp 255-8°C (dec). Source: YU JIN XIANG, YU JIN XIANG GEN. Ref: 6.

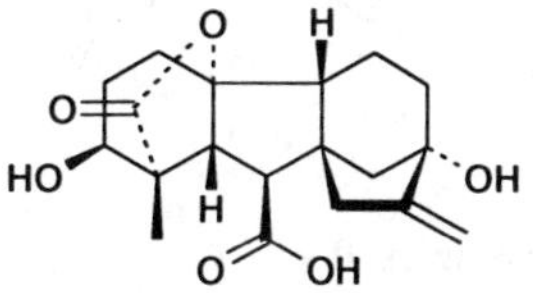

2562 Gibberellin A3

$C_{19}H_{22}O_6$ MW: 346.38 Property: mp 235°C (dec). Source: QIAN NIU ZI. Ref: 6.

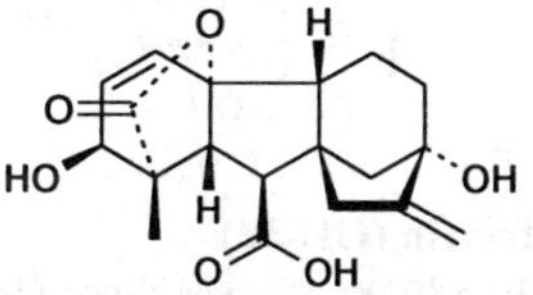

2563 Gibberellin A5

$C_{19}H_{22}O_5$ MW: 330.38 Property: mp 260-1°C (dec). Source: QIAN NIU ZI, YU JIN XIANG GEN. Ref: 6.

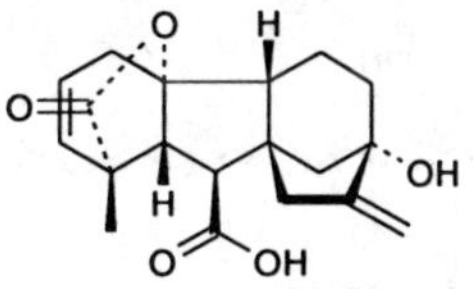

2564 Gibberellin A8
$C_{19}H_{24}O_7$ MW: 364.40 Property: mp 210-5°C (dec). Source: YU JIN XIANG GEN. Ref: 6.

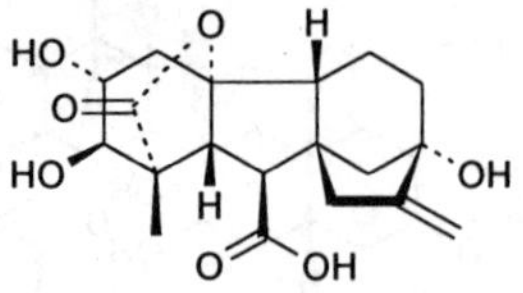

2565 Gibberellin A9
$C_{19}H_{24}O_4$ MW: 316.40 Property: mp 208-11°C. Source: YU JIN XIANG GEN. Ref: 6.

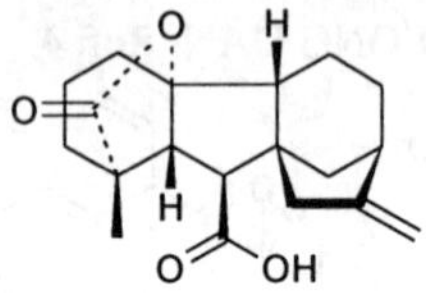

2566 Gibberellin A13
$C_{20}H_{26}O_7$ MW: 378.43 Property: mp 194-6°C (dec). Source: YU JIN XIANG GEN. Ref: 6.

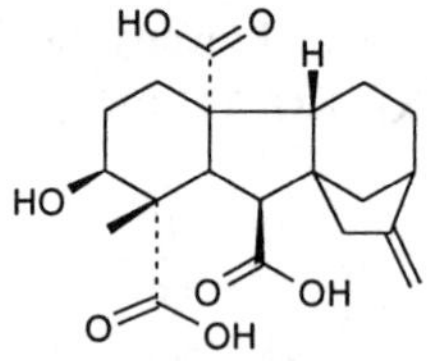

2567 Gibberellin A20
$C_{19}H_{24}O_5$ MW: 332.40 Source: QIAN NIU ZI, WAN DOU. Ref: 6.

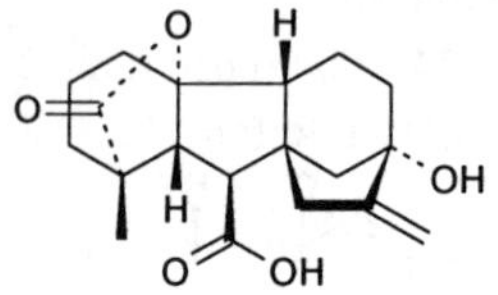

2568 Gigantriocin (GL-32)
$C_{35}H_{64}O_6$ MW: 580.90 Property: mp 69-71°C, $[\alpha]_D^{25}$ +18° ($CHCl_3$). Source: JIN PING GE NA XIANG. Ref: 420.

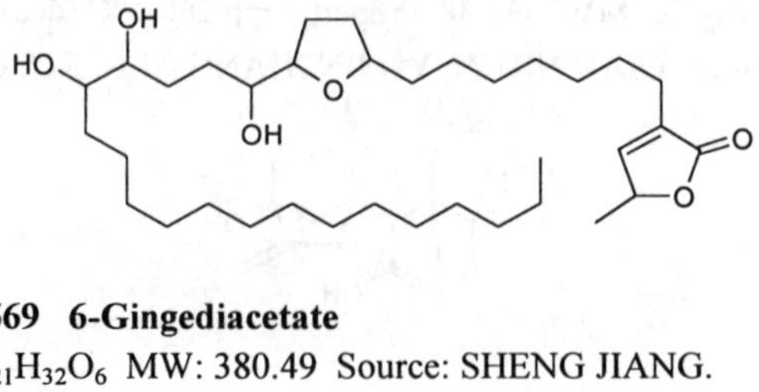

2569 6-Gingediacetate
$C_{21}H_{32}O_6$ MW: 380.49 Source: SHENG JIANG. Ref: 2.

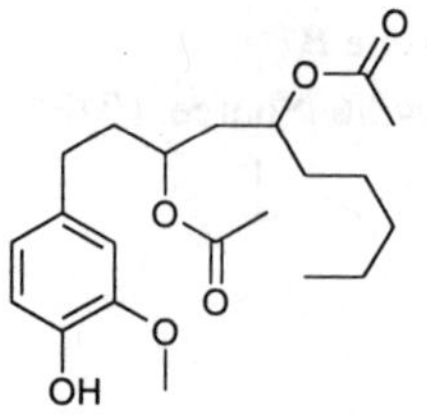

2570 6-Gingediol
$C_{17}H_{28}O_4$ MW: 296.41 Source: SHENG JIANG. Ref: 2.

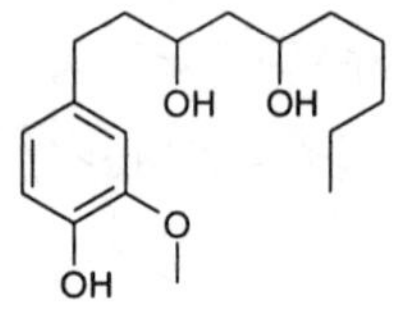

2571 10-Gingediol
$C_{21}H_{36}O_4$ MW: 352.52 Source: SHENG JIANG. Ref: 2.

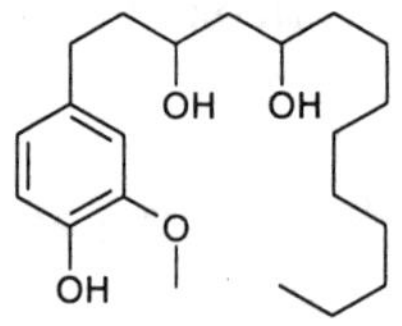

2572 8-Gingediol
$C_{19}H_{32}O_4$ MW: 324.46 Source: SHENG JIANG. Ref: 2.

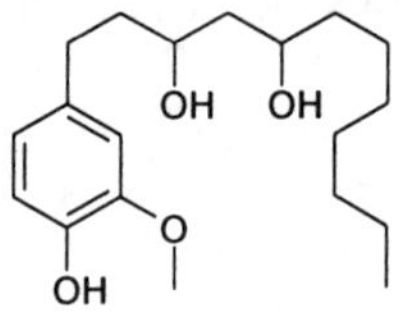

2573 Gingerdione
$C_{17}H_{24}O_4$ MW: 292.38 Source: GAN JIANG. Ref: 2.

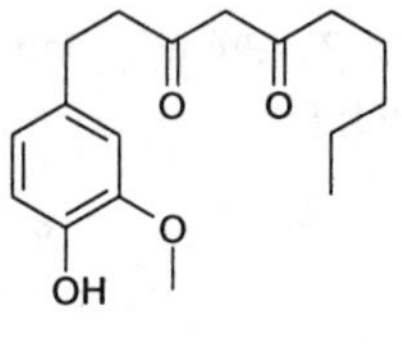

2574 6-Gingerdione
$C_{17}H_{24}O_4$ MW: 292.38 Source: GAN JIANG. Ref: 2.

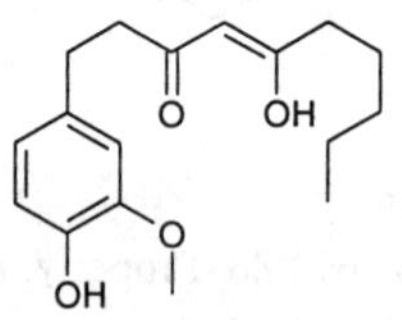

2575 10-Gingerdione
$C_{21}H_{32}O_4$ MW: 348.49 Source: GAN JIANG. Ref: 2.

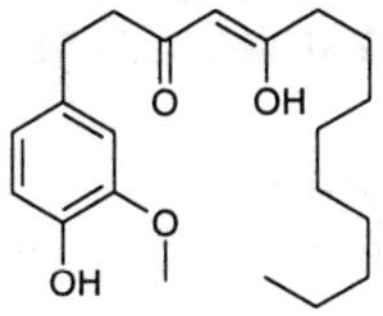

O OH
OH

2576 Gingerenone A
Dehydroxytetrahydrocurcumin. $C_{20}H_{22}O_5$ MW: 342.40 Source: GAN JIANG, SHENG JIANG. Ref: 2.

O
OH
OH

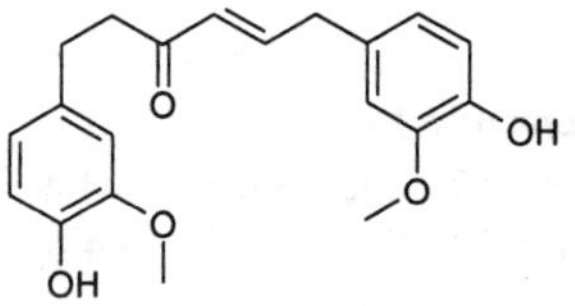

2577 Gingerenone B
$C_{22}H_{26}O_6$ MW: 386.45 Source: GAN JIANG, SHENG JIANG. Ref: 2.

O
HO OH

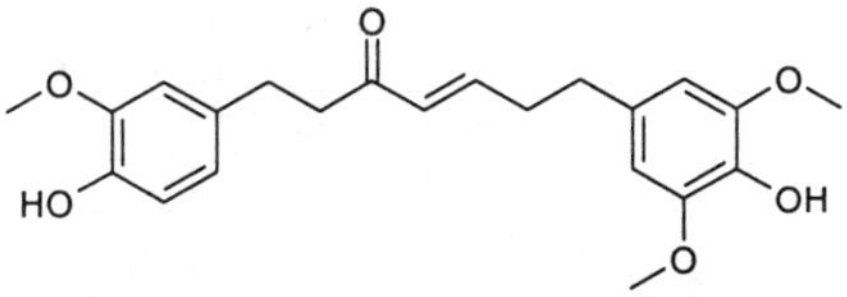

2578 Gingerenone-C
$C_{20}H_{22}O_4$ MW: 326.40 Source: GAN JIANG, SHENG JIANG. Ref: 2.

O
HO OH

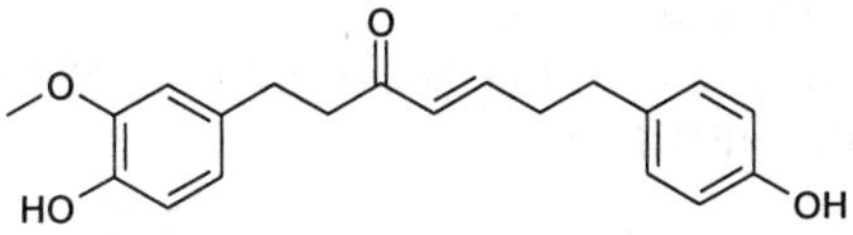

2580 Gingerol
$C_{17}H_{26}O_4$ MW: 294.39 Property: bp 277-9°C/6mm. Source: GAN JIANG, SHENG JIANG. Ref: 2, 6.

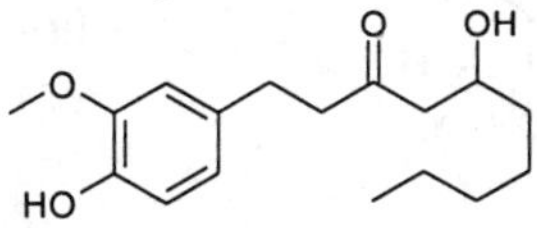

O OH
HO

2581 4-Gingerol
$C_{15}H_{22}O_4$ MW: 266.34 Source: GAN JIANG, SHENG JIANG. Ref: 2.

O OH
OH

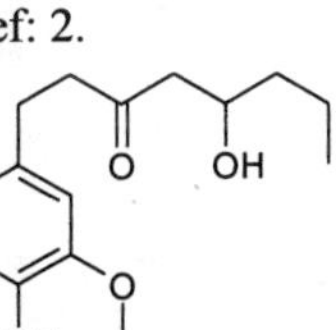

2582 10-Gingerol
$C_{21}H_{34}O_4$ MW: 350.50 Source: GAN JIANG. Ref: 2.

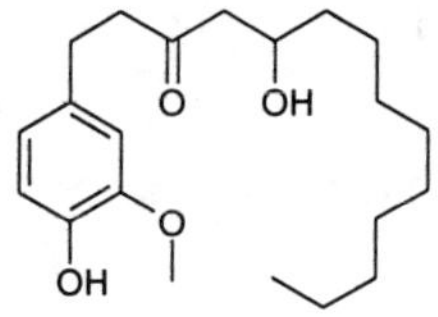

O OH
OH

2583 8-Gingerol
$C_{19}H_{30}O_4$ MW: 322.45 Source: GAN JIANG. Ref: 2.

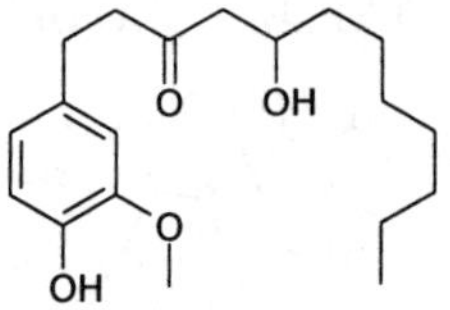

O OH
OH

2584 12-Gingerol
$C_{23}H_{38}O_4$ MW: 378.56 Source: GAN JIANG. Ref: 2.

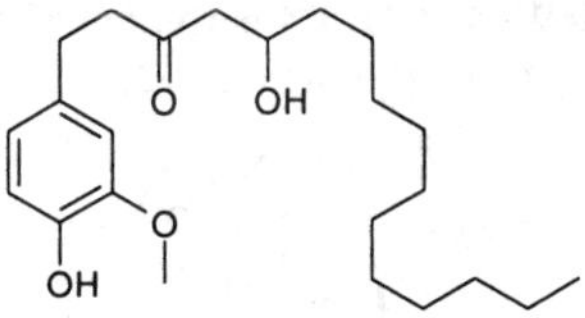

O OH
OH

2585 Ginkgetin
$C_{32}H_{22}O_{10}$ MW: 566.53 Property: yellow powder mp 330°C (dec). Source: BAI GUO, BAI GUO YE, CHAO XIAN YIN, SAN JIAN SHAN, YANG HUO. Ref: 2, 442.

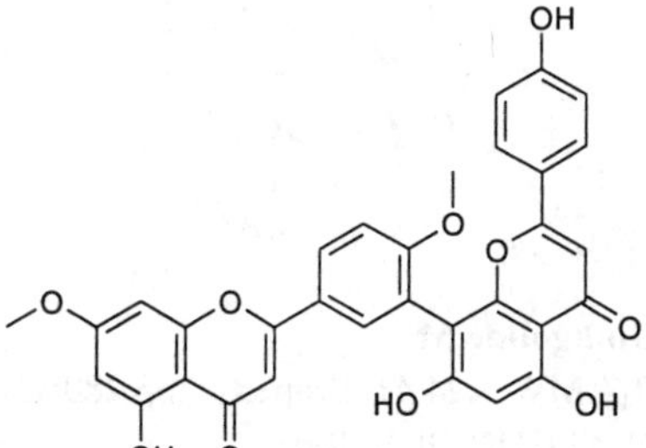

OH
O O
O
HO OH
OH O

2586 Ginkgol
$C_{21}H_{34}O$ MW: 302.50 Source: BAI GUO. Ref: 2.

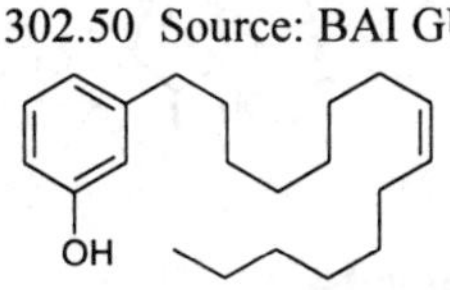

OH

2587 Ginkgolic acid
$C_{22}H_{34}O_3$ MW: 346.51 Property: mp 41-3°C. Source: BAI GUO. Ref: 4.

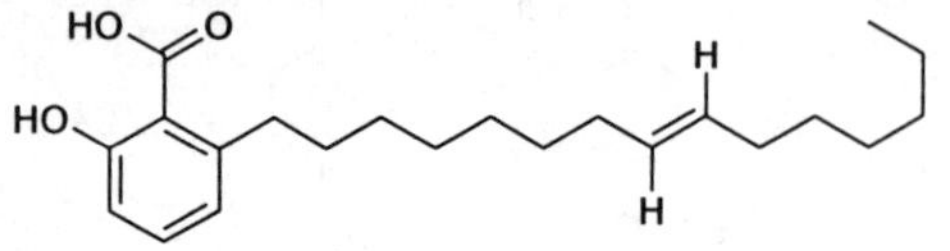

2588 Ginkgolide A
$C_{20}H_{24}O_9$ MW: 408.41 Property: mp ≈300°C. Source: BAI GUO YE, BAI GUO GEN. Ref: 6.

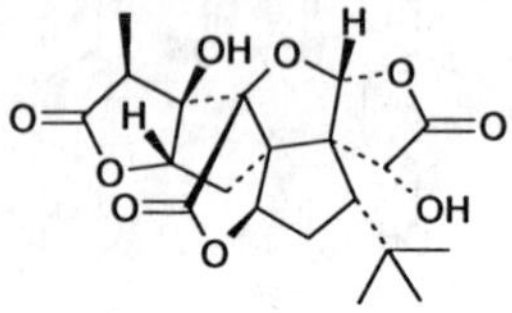

2589 Ginkgolide B
$C_{20}H_{24}O_{10}$ MW: 424.41 Property: mp ≈300°C. Source: BAI GUO YE, BAI GUO GEN. Ref: 6.

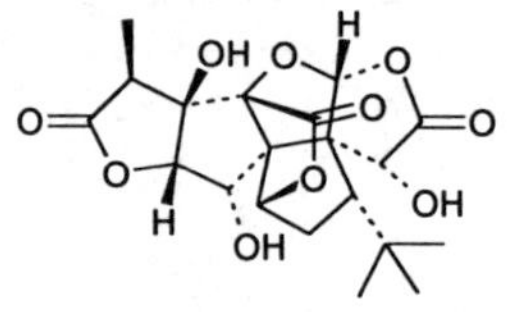

2590 Ginkgolide C
$C_{20}H_{24}O_{11}$ MW: 440.41 Property: mp ≈300°C. Source: BAI GUO YE, BAI GUO GEN. Ref: 6.

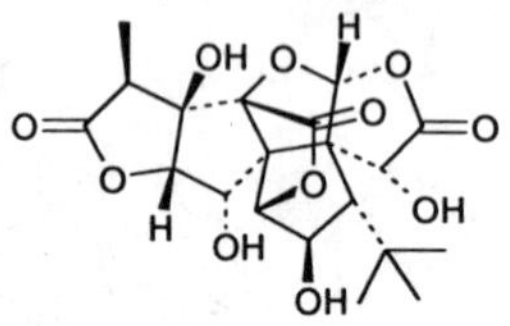

2591 Ginkgolide M
$C_{20}H_{24}O_{10}$ MW: 424.41 Property: mp 280°C (dec). Source: BAI GUO GEN. Ref: 6.

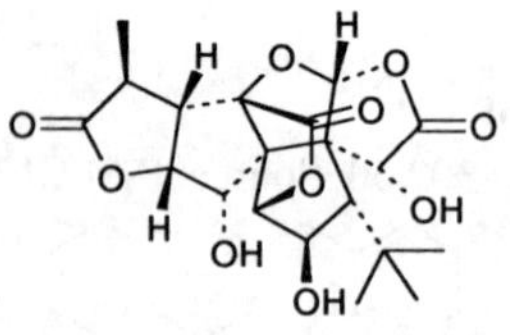

2592 Ginsenoside-F2
Property: white powder, $[\alpha]_D^{20}$ +20.0° (c=0.50, MeOH). Source: XI YANG SHEN, YU YE SAN QI. Ref: 135, 451.

2593 Ginsenoside-F11
Property: white crystal, $[\alpha]_D^{20}$ -13.0° (c=1.0, MeOH). Source: XI YANG SHEN. Ref: 451.

2594 Ginsenoside-Fh1
Property: white powder, $[\alpha]_D^{20}$ +19.0° (c=0.9, MeOH). Source: XI YANG SHEN. Ref: 451.

2595 Ginsenoside-Fh2
Property: white powder, mp 217-20°C, $[\alpha]_D^{20}$ +20.5° (c=0.93, MeOH). Source: XI YANG SHEN. Ref: 451.

2596 Ginsenoside-La
$C_{42}H_{70}O_{13}$ MW: 783.02 Property: white powder (methanol), mp 179-80°C, $[\alpha]_D^{20}$ -18.4° (pyridine-d_5). Source: REN SHEN. Ref: 155.

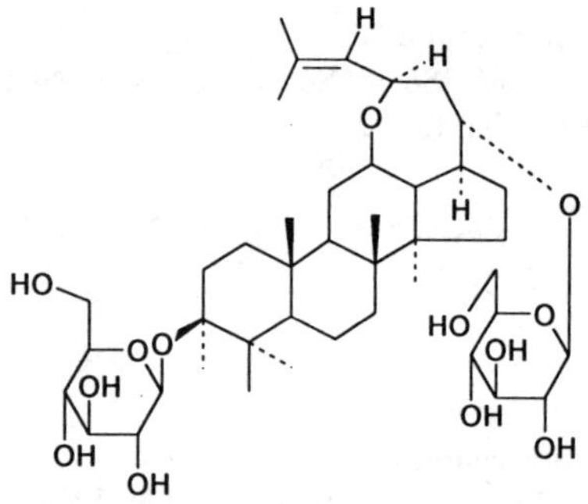

2597 Ginsenoside R0
$C_{48}H_{76}O_{19}$ MW: 957.13 Source: REN SHEN, XI YANG SHEN. Ref: 2.

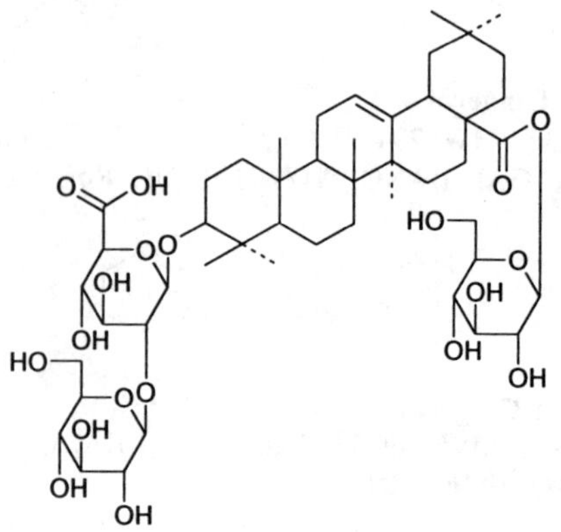

2598 Ginsenoside-Ra0
20(S)-Protopanaxadiol 3-O-β-D-glucopyranosyl-(1→2)-β-D-glucopyranosyl-(1→2)-β-D-glucopyranoside, 20-O-β-D-glucopyranosyl-(1→2)-β-D-glucopynoside. $C_{60}H_{102}O_{28}$ MW: 1271.47 Property: white acicular crystal, mp 192-3°C. Source: REN SHEN, XI YANG SHEN. Ref: 2, 87.

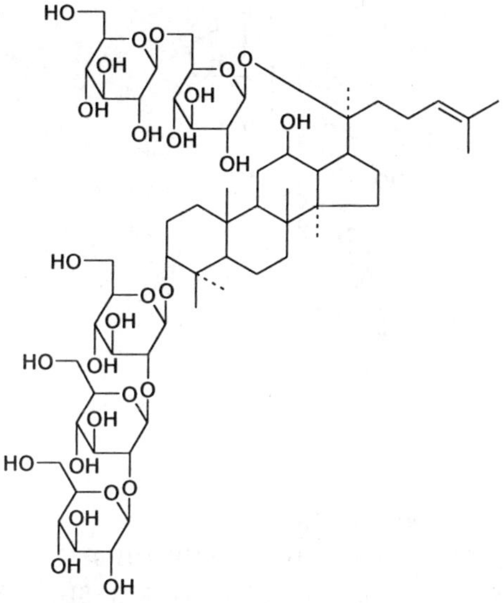

2599 Ginsenoside Ra1
Source: REN SHEN. Ref: 2.

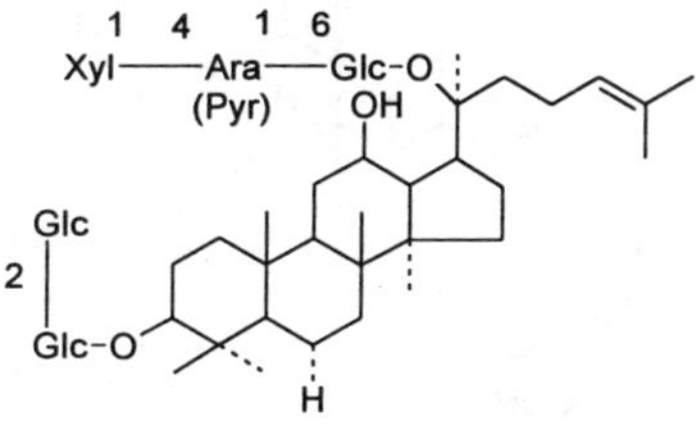

2600 Ginsenoside Ra2
Source: REN SHEN. Ref: 2.

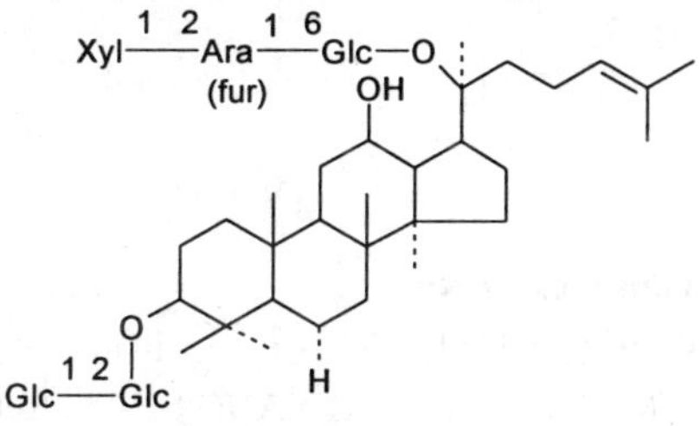

2601 Ginsenoside Ra_3
Source: REN SHEN. Ref: 2.

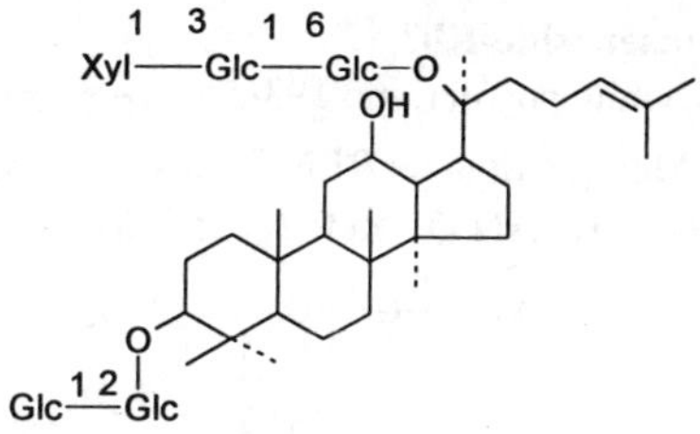

2602 Ginsenoside-Rb1
Sanchinoside E_1. CAS: 41753-43-9 $C_{54}H_{92}O_{32}$ MW: 1109.32 Property: white powder, mp 197-8°C. Source: HUI GUO JIAO GU LAN, REN SHEN, SAN QI, XI YANG SHEN, YU YE SAN QI. Ref: 4, 87, 135, 329, 613.

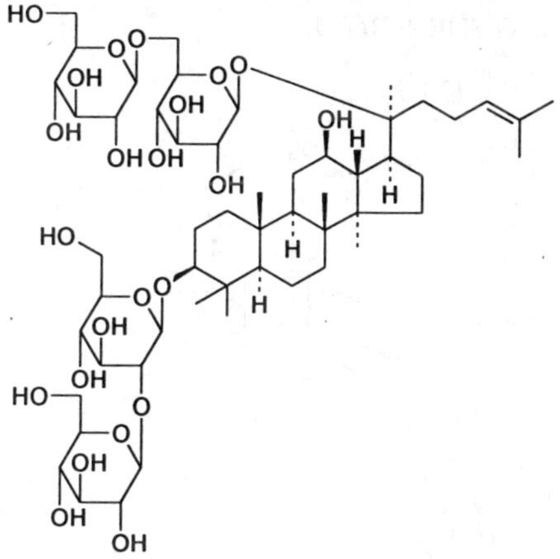

2603 Ginsenoside-Rb2
CAS: 11021-13-9 $C_{53}H_{90}O_{22}$ MW: 1079.30 Property: white powder, mp 200-3°C, $[\alpha]_D^{20}$ +12.3° (c=0.92, MeOH). Source: REN SHEN, XI YANG SHEN. Ref: 4, 87, 451.

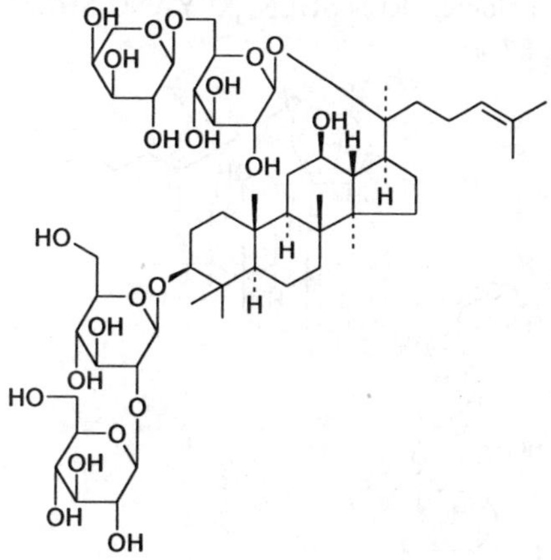

2604 Ginsenoside-Rb3
Property: white powder, mp 193-5°C, $[\alpha]_D^{20}$ +19.4° (c=1.00, MeOH). Source: REN SHEN, XI YANG SHEN, YU YE SAN QI. Ref: 2, 135, 451.

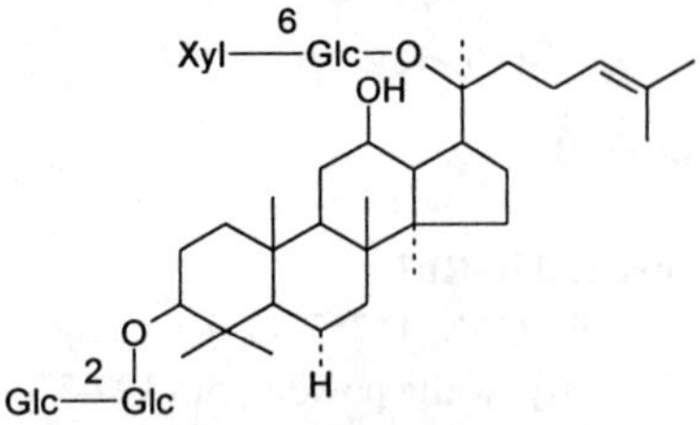

2605 Ginsenoside-Rc
CAS: 11021-14-0 $C_{53}H_{90}O_{22}$ MW: 1079.24 Source: XI YANG SHEN. Ref: 4.

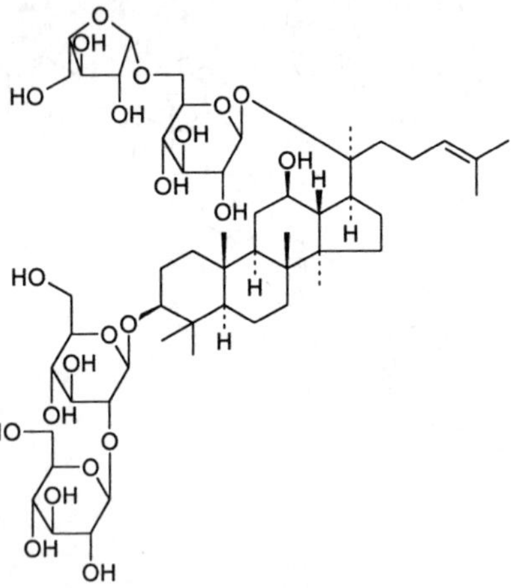

2606 Ginsenoside-Rd
CAS: 52705-93-9 $C_{48}H_{82}O_{18}$ MW: 947.18 Property: white powder, mp 206-9°C, $[\alpha]_D^{20}$ +19.2° (c=0.40, MeOH). Source: REN SHEN, XI YANG SHEN. Ref: 4, 87, 451.

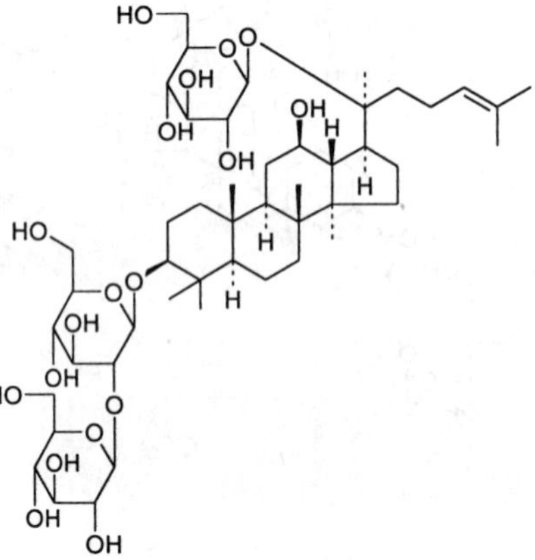

2607 Ginsenoside-Re
Chikusetsusaponin Ivc. CAS: 52286-59-6 $C_{48}H_{82}O_{18}$ MW: 947.18 Property: coloeless acicular crystal, mp 201-3°C, $[\alpha]_D^{20}$ -1.5° (c=0.52, MeOH). Source: REN SHEN, XI YANG SHEN. Ref: 4, 87, 451, 613.

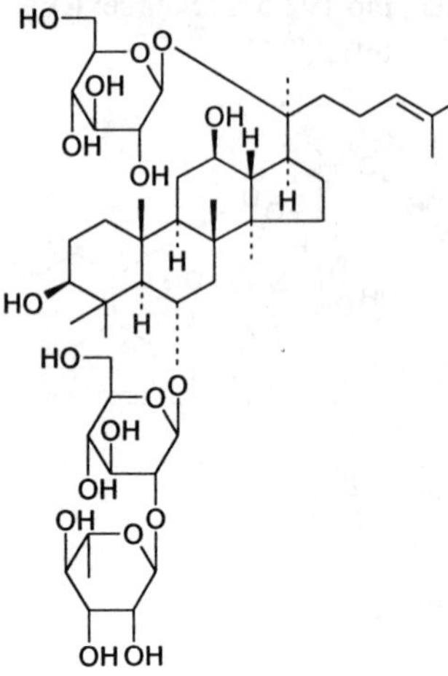

2608 Ginsenoside-Rf
CAS: 52286-58-5 $C_{42}H_{72}O_{14}$ MW: 801.03 Property: white powder, mp 197-8°C. Source: REN SHEN, XI YANG SHEN. Ref: 4, 87.

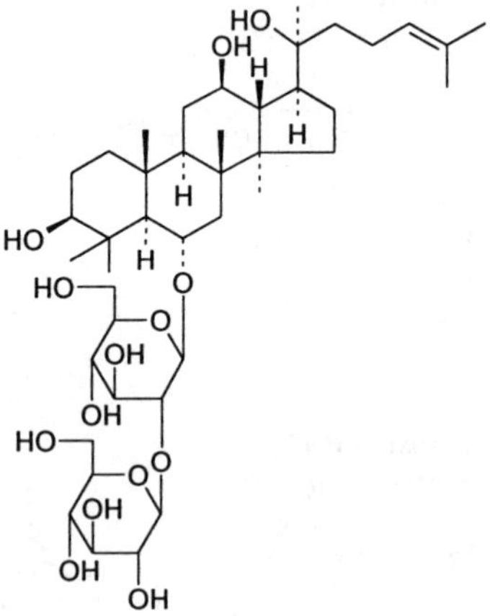

2609 Ginsenoside-Rg
Property: white powder, mp 194-5°C, $[\alpha]_D^{20}$ +26.0° (c=0.30, MeOH). Source: XI YANG SHEN. Ref: 451.

2610 Ginsenoside-Rg1
CAS: 22427-39-0 $C_{42}H_{72}O_{14}$ MW: 801.03 Property: mp 194-6.5°C. Source: REN SHEN, XI YANG SHEN. Ref: 4, 87.

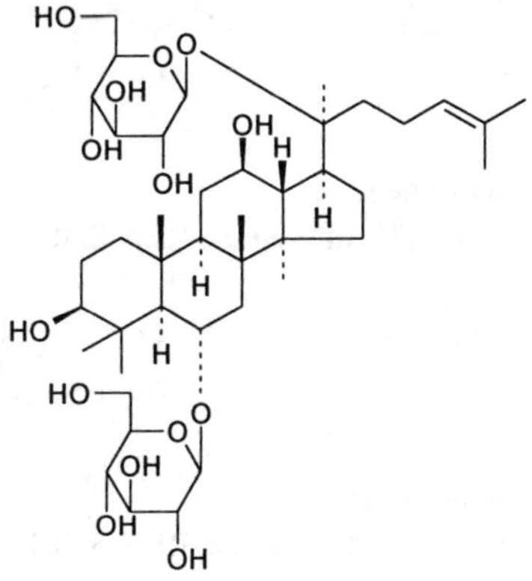

2611 20-(R)-Ginsenoside-Rg2
Source: REN SHEN, XI YANG SHEN. Ref: 2

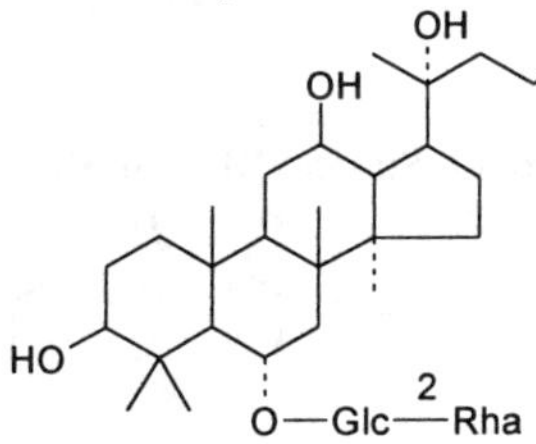

2612 (20R)-Ginsenoside-Rg3
Source: QI YE DAN, REN SHEN, XI YANG SHEN. Ref: 2.

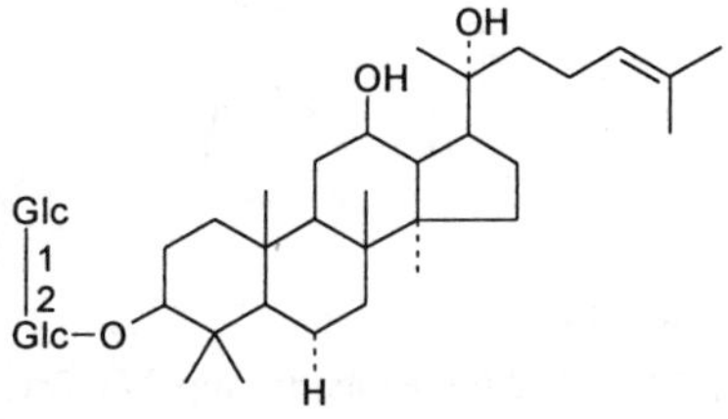

2613 20(S)-Ginsenoside-Rg3
Source: REN SHEN. Ref: 2.

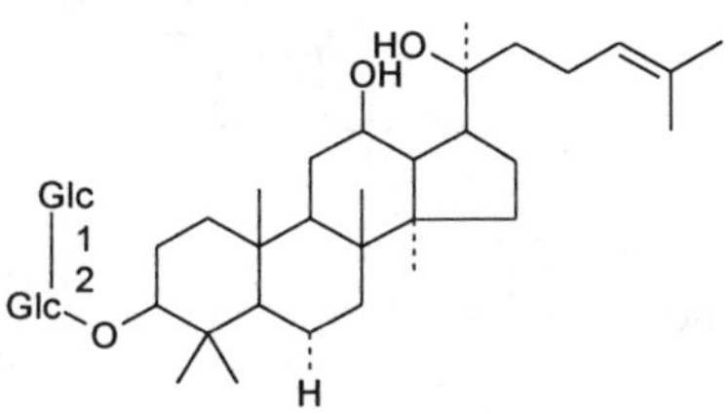

2614 Ginsenoside-Rh1
Source: REN SHEN, SAN QI, XI YANG SHEN. Ref: 2, 28, 87.

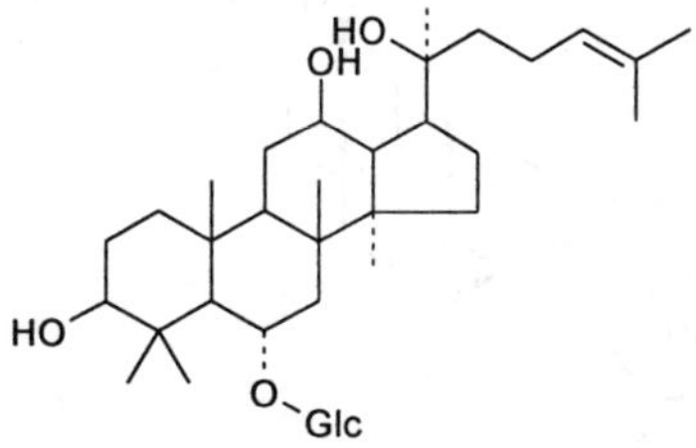

2615 20(R)-Ginsenoside-Rh1
Source: REN SHEN. Ref: 2.

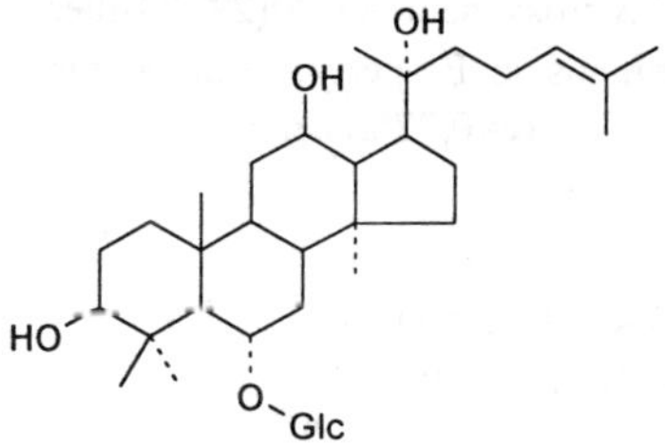

2616 20(S)-Ginsenoside-Rh1
Source: SAN QI. Ref: 2.

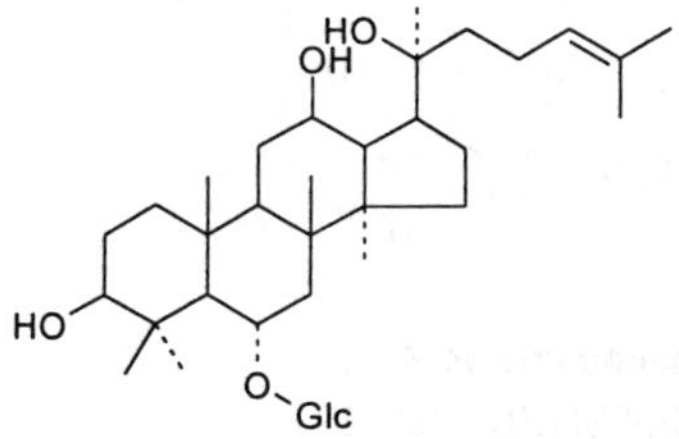

2617 20(R)-Ginsenoside-h2
$C_{36}H_{62}O_8$ MW: 622.89 Source: REN SHEN. Ref: 2.

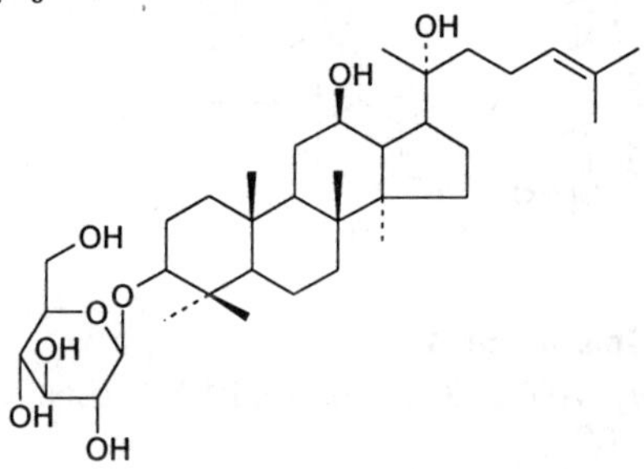

2618 20(R)-Ginsenoside-Rh2
Property: white powder, mp 288-90°C, $[\alpha]_D^{27}$ +21.1° (c=0.61, methanol). Source:REN SHEN. Ref: 84.

2619 20(S)-Ginsenoside-Rh2
$C_{36}H_{62}O_8$ MW: 622.89 Source: REN SHEN. Ref: 2.

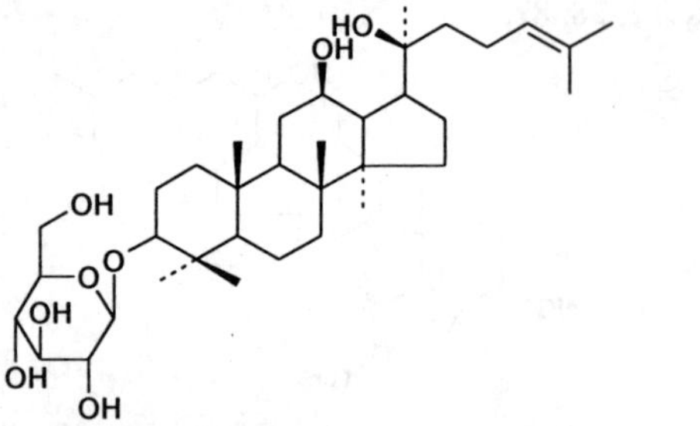

2620 Ginsenoside-Rh3
3β,12β-Dihydroxy-dammar-20(22),24-diene-3-O-β-D-glucopyranoside. Property: white powder, mp 255-7°C, $[\alpha]_D^{27}$ +7.0° (c=0.778, methanol). Source: REN SHEN. Ref: 84.

2621 Ginsenoside-Rs1
Source: REN SHEN. Ref: 2.

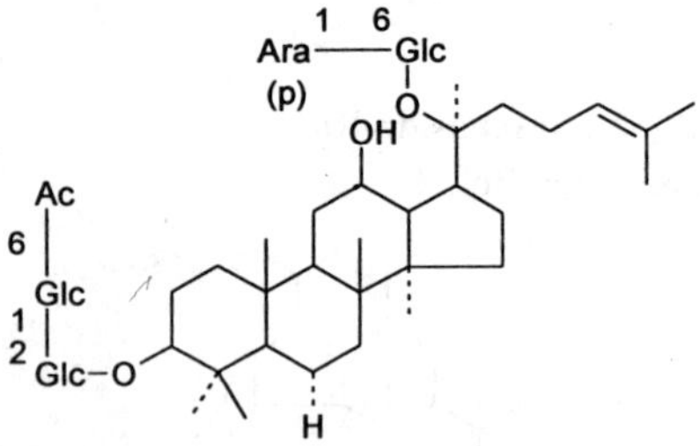

2622 Ginsenoside-Rs2
Source: REN SHEN. Ref: 2.

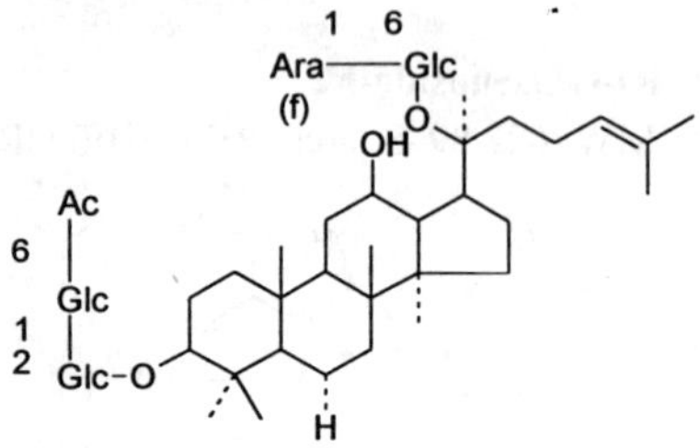

2623 Ginsenoyne A
$C_{17}H_{22}O_2$ MW: 258.36 Source: REN SHEN. Ref: 2.

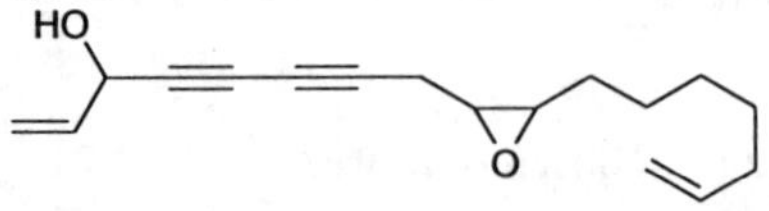

2624 Ginsenoyne B
$C_{17}H_{23}ClO_2$ MW: 294.82 Source: REN SHEN. Ref: 2.

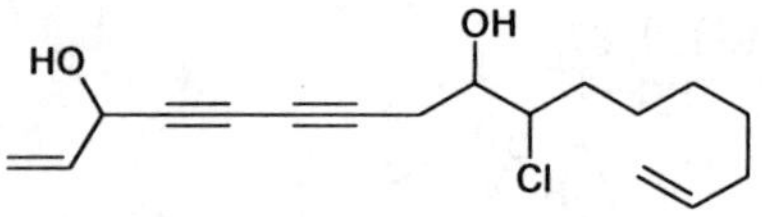

2625 Ginsenoyne C
$C_{17}H_{24}O_3$ MW: 276.38 Source: REN SHEN. Ref: 2.

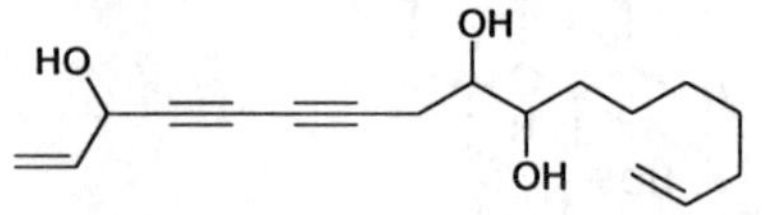

2626 Ginsenoyne D
$C_{17}H_{26}O_2$ MW: 262.40 Source: REN SHEN. Ref: 2.

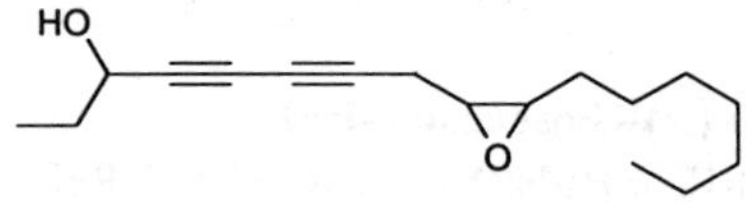

2627 Ginsenoyne E
$C_{18}H_{24}O$ MW: 256.39 Source: REN SHEN. Ref: 2.

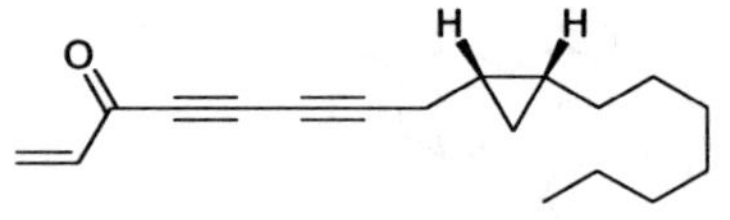

2628 Girinimbine
$C_{18}H_{17}NO$ MW: 263.34 Source: NEN YE JIU LI XIANG, YUAN DONG JIU LI XIANG. Ref: 11.

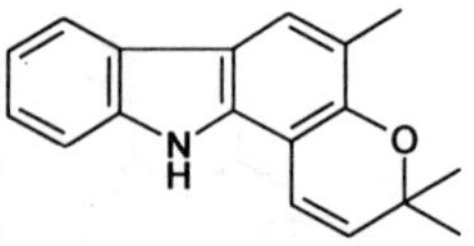

2629 Gitogenin
$C_{27}H_{44}O_4$ MW: 432.65 Property: mp 271-2°C. Source: DA YU BIAO HUA, FAN MA, HU LU BA, JI LI GEN. Ref: 6, 10.

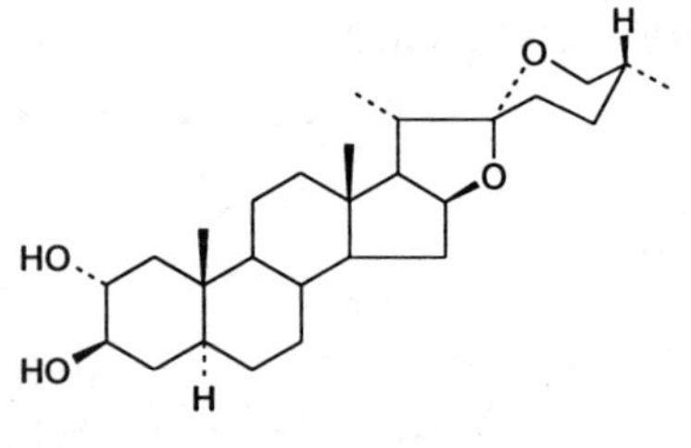

2630 Gitoxigenin
$C_{23}H_{34}O_5$ MW: 390.52 Property: mp 220-5°C. Source: JIA ZHU TAO. Ref: 6.

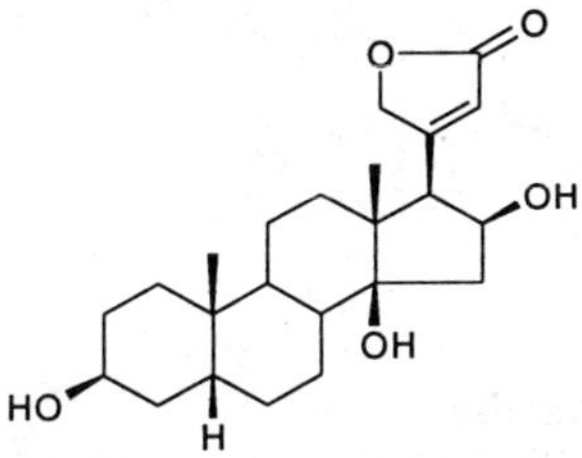

2631 Glabranine
$C_{20}H_{18}O_4$ MW: 322.36 Source: GAN CAO. Ref: 2.

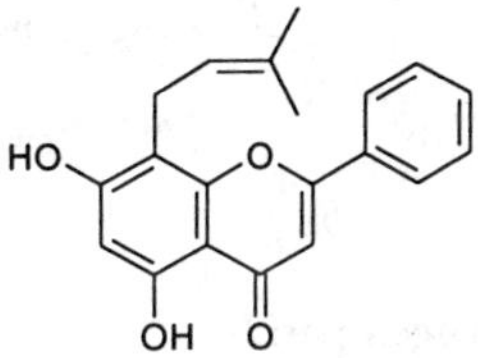

2632 Glabredelphinine
$C_{22}H_{33}NO_6$ MW: 407.51 Property: white acicular crystal, mp 201-3°C. Source: ZHAN MAO CUI QUE HUA. Ref: 157.

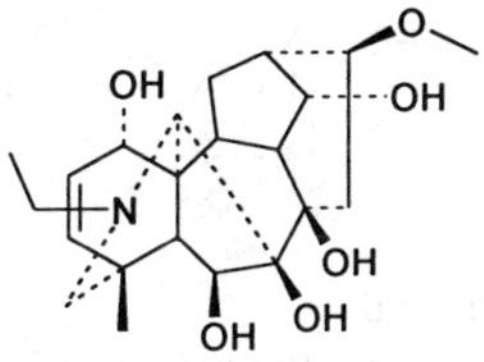

2633 Glabrene
$C_{20}H_{18}O_4$ MW: 322.36 Source: GAN CAO. Ref: 2.

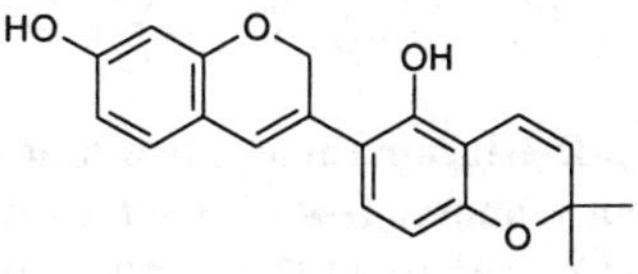

2634 Glabridin
$C_{16}H_{14}O_5$ MW: 286.29 Source: GAN CAO. Ref: 2.

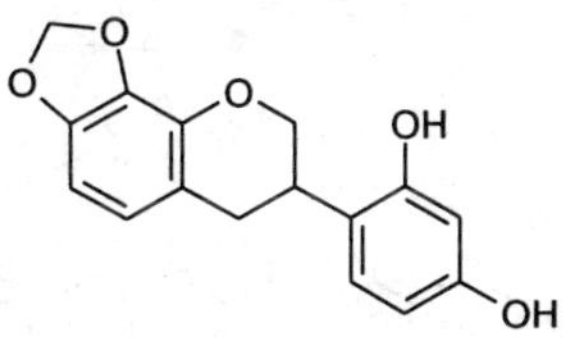

2635 Glabrol
$C_{25}H_{26}O_4$ MW: 390.48 Source: HUANG GAN CAO, GAN CAO. Ref: 2, 591.

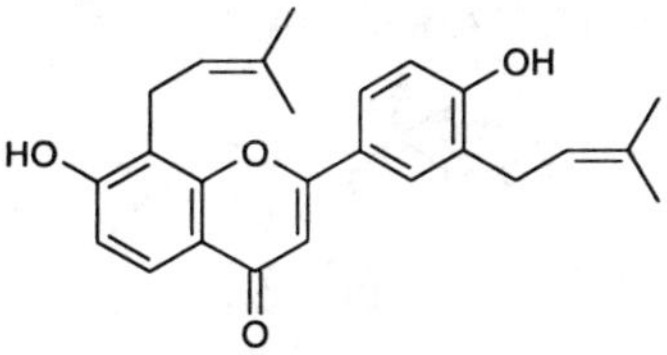

2636 Glabrone
$C_{20}H_{16}O_5$ MW: 336.35 Source: GAN CAO. Ref: 2.

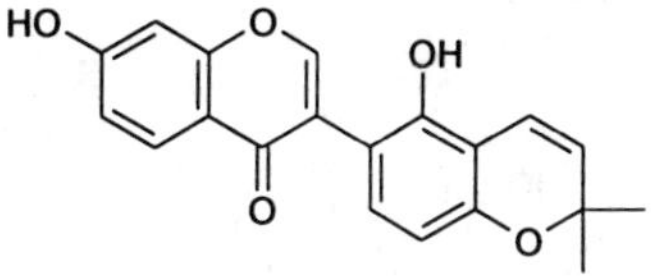

2637 Glanolactone
$C_{20}H_{30}O_3$ MW: 318.46 Source: GAN JIANG, SHENG JIANG. Ref: 2.

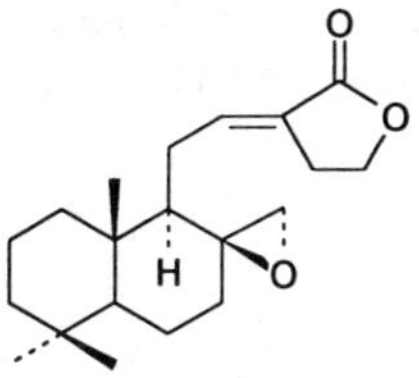

2638 Glaucine
CAS: 475-81-0 $C_{21}H_{25}NO_4$ MW: 355.44 Property: mp 120°C. Source: YAN HU SUO, YING SU. Ref: 4, 56.

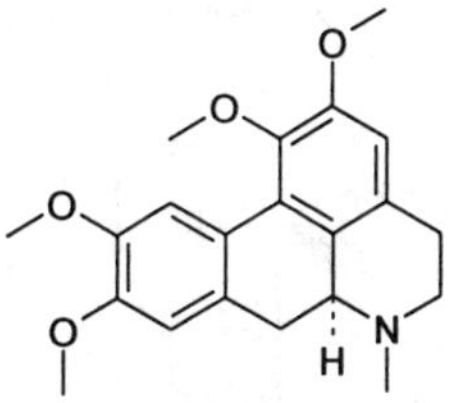

2639 Glaudine
$C_{22}H_{25}NO_6$ MW: 398.46 Property: mp 103-5°C. Source: YA PIAN. Ref: 6.

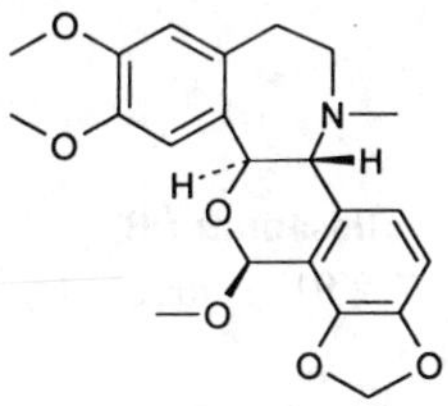

2640 Gloeosteretriol

$C_{17}H_{30}O_3$ MW: 282.43 Property: colorless prismatic crystal, mp 205-6°C, $[\alpha]_D^{22}$ +5.6° (c= 0.115, methanol). Source: YU ER. Ref: 214.

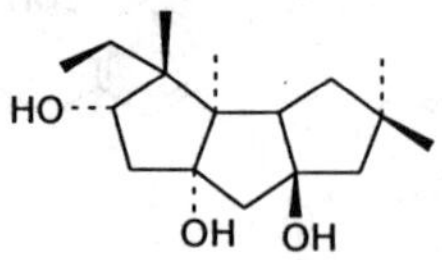

2641 Glucobrassicin

$C_{16}H_{19}N_2O_9S_2$ MW: 447.47 Source: DA QING YE, GAN LAN. Ref: 2.

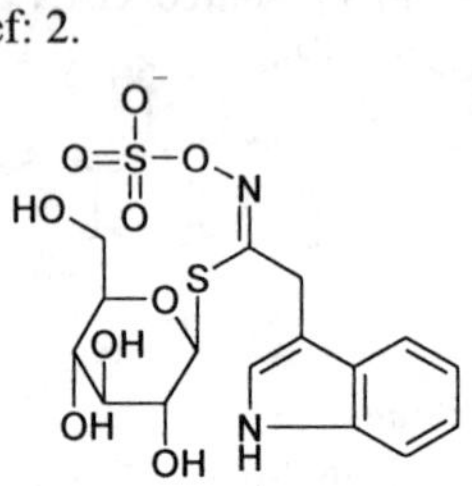

2642 Glucobrassicin-1-Sulfonate

$C_{16}H_{19}N_2O_{12}S_3$ MW: 527.53 Source: DA QING YE. Ref: 2, 6.

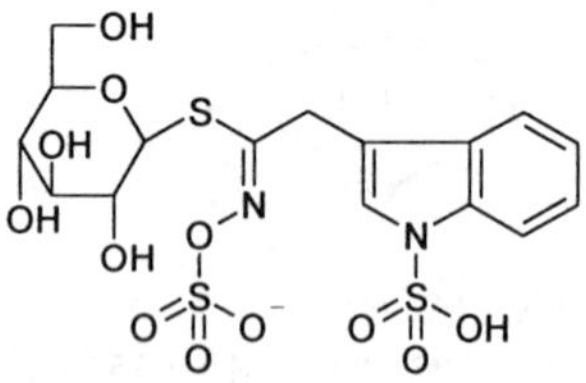

2643 Glucoconvallasaponin A

$C_{38}H_{62}O_{14}$ MW: 742.91 Source: LING LAN. Ref: 6.

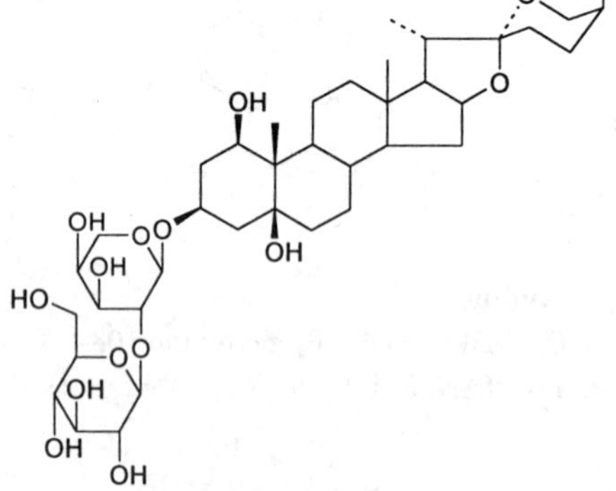

2644 Glucoconvallasaponin B

$C_{38}H_{62}O_{15}$ MW: 758.91 Source: LING LAN. Ref: 6.

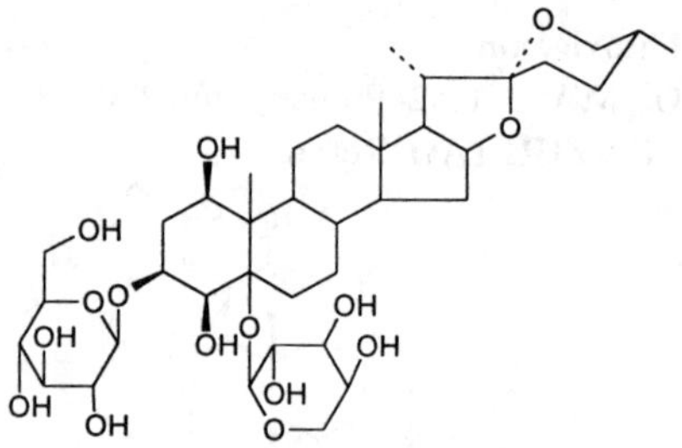

2645 Glucogallin

$C_{13}H_{16}O_{10}$ MW: 332.27 Property: mp α: 179-81°C, β: 207°C. Source: AN MO LE, DA HUANG, HE ZI, YOU GAN MU PI, YOU GAN YE. Ref: 6.

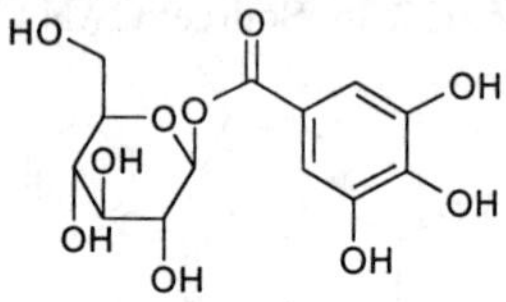

2646 1-β-Glucogeniposide

$C_{17}H_{26}O_{10}$ MW: 390.39 Source: ZHI ZI. Ref: 2.

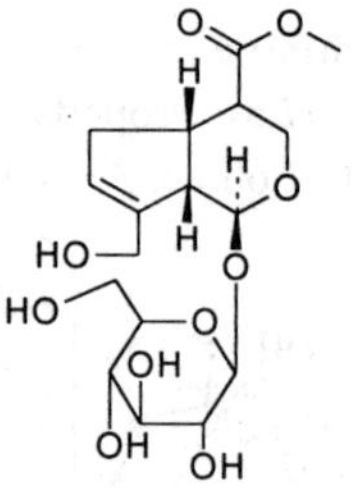

2647 Gluconic acid

$C_6H_{12}O_7$ MW: 196.16 Property: mp 125-6°C. Source: HE YE. Ref: 6.

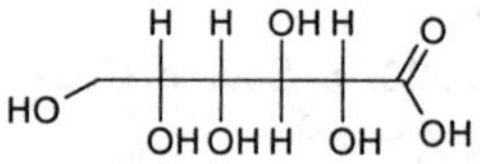

2648 3-O-β-D-Glucopyranosyl betulinic acid-28-O-β-D-glucopyranosyl(1→6)-β-D-glucopyranoside

$C_{48}H_{78}O_{18}$ MW: 941.13 Property: white powder, mp 204-6°C, $[\alpha]_D^{20}$ -16.9° (c=0.5, methanol). Source: CIRENSHEN. Ref: 370.

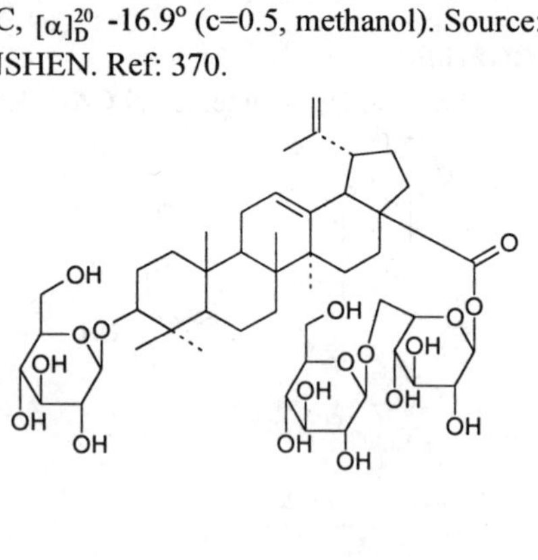

2649 26-O-β-D-Glucopyranosyl-3β,26-dihydroxy choleslen-16,22-dioxo-3-O-α-L-rhamnopyranosyl-(1→2)-β-D-glucopyranoside

$C_{45}H_{74}O_{18}$ MW: 903.08 Property: white powder (MeOH), mp 225-6°C. Source: BAI HE. Ref: 418.

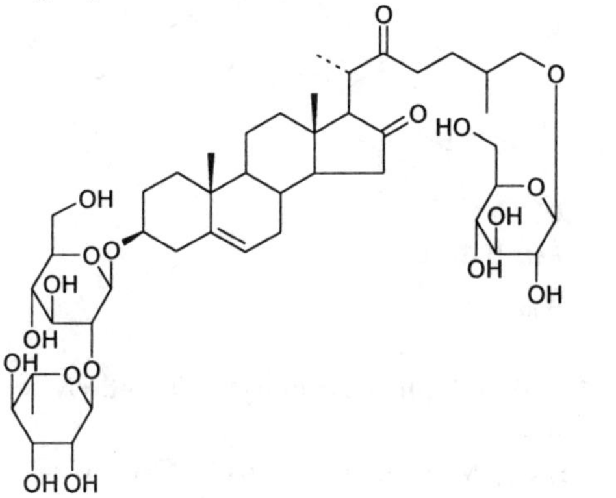

2650 26-O-β-D-Glucopyranosyl-3β,26-dihydroxy-5-choleslen-16,22-dioxo-3-O-α-L-rhamnopyranosyl(1→2)-β-D-glucopyranoside

$C_{45}H_{72}O_{18}$ MW: 901.06 Property: white powder (MeOH), mp 208-9°C. Source: BAI HE. Ref: 418.

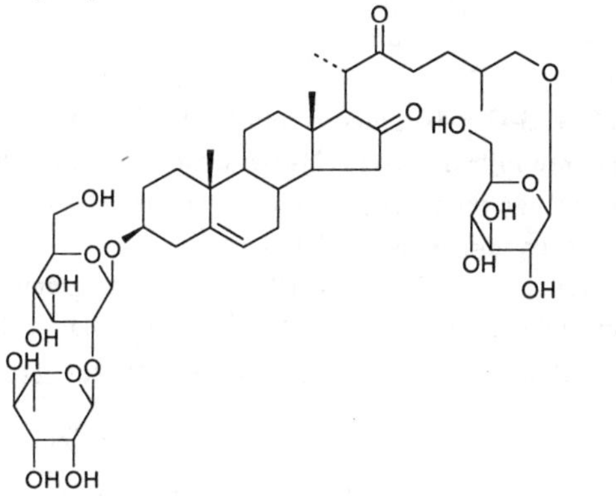

2651 28-O-β-D-Glucopyranosyl(1→6)-β-D-glucopyranosyl ester of 3-O-[β-D-glucopyranosyl (1→4)] [α-L-rhamnopyranosyl(1→3)]-β-D-glucopyrano-syl(1→3)-α-L-rhamno-pyranosyl(1→2)-α-arabi-nopyranosyl-hederagenin

$C_{71}H_{116}O_{36}$ MW:1545.69 Property: white powder, mp 224-227°C, $[\alpha]_D^{21}$ -17.4°(c=0.25, MeOH). Source: CHUAN XU DUAN. Ref: 265.

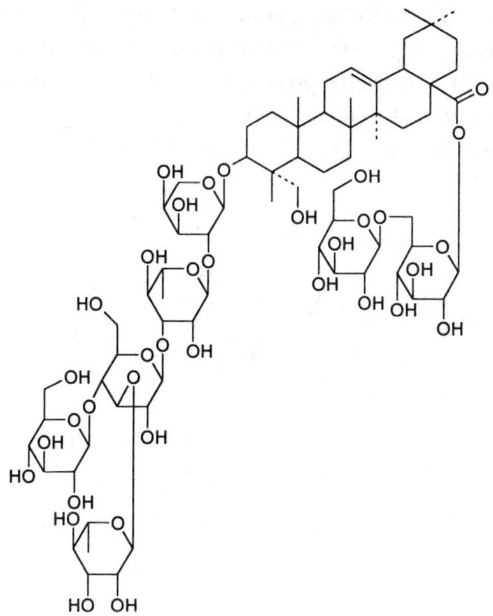

2652 28-O-β-D-Glucopyranosyl(1→6)-β-D-glucopyranosyl ester of 3-O-[β-D-xylopyranosyl (1→4)-β-D-glucopyranosyl(1→4)] [α-L-rhamnopyranosyl (1→3)]-β-D-glucopyranosyl (1→3)-α-L-rhamnopyranosyl (1→2)-α-arabinopyranosyl-hederagenin

$C_{76}H_{124}O_{40}$ MW: 1677.81 Property: white powder, mp 236-40°C (methanol-acetic ester), $[\alpha]_D^{21}$ -21.8° (c=0.24, methanol). Source: CHUAN XU DUAN. Ref: 249.

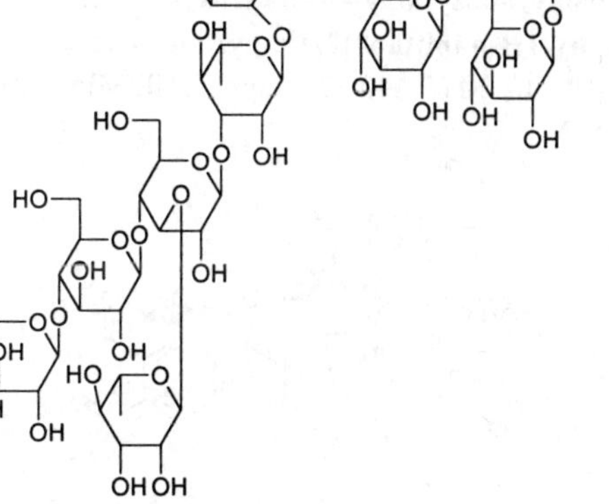

2653 1-[(β-D-Glucopyranosyl-(1→6)-O-β-D-glucopyranosyl-(1→3)-O-β-D-glucopyranosyl-(1→6)-O-β-D-glucopyranosyl) oxy] -8-hydroxy-3-methyl-9,10-anthraquinone
$C_{39}H_{50}O_{24}$ MW: 902.82 Source: JUE MING ZI. Ref: 2.

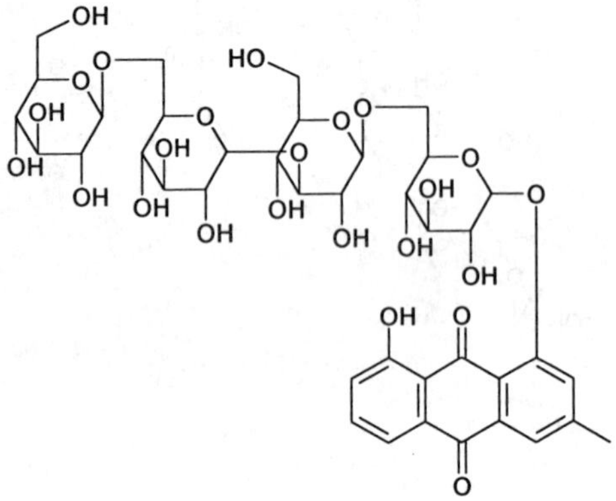

2654 1-[(β-D-Glucopyranosyl-(1→3)-O-β-D-glucopyranosyl-(1→6)-O-β-D-glucopyranosyl) oxy]-8-hydroxy-3-methyl-9,10-anthraquinone
$C_{33}H_{40}O_{19}$ MW: 740.68 Source: JUE MING ZI. Ref: 2.

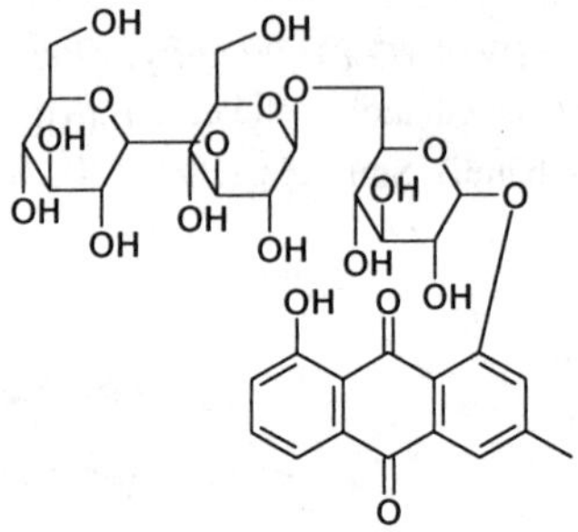

2655 9-[(β-D-Glucopyranosyl-(1→6)-O-β-D-glucopyranosyl)oxy]-10-hydroxy-7-methoxy-3-methy-1H-naphthol [2,3-c]pyran-1-one
$C_{28}H_{34}O_{15}$ MW: 610.57 Source: JUE MING ZI. Ref: 2.

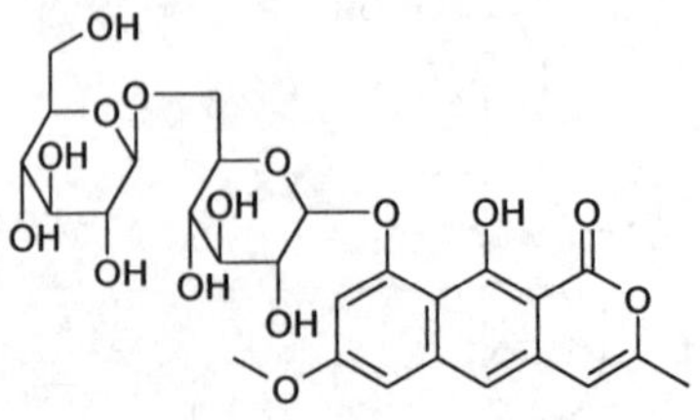

2656 (25s)-26-O-β-D-Glucopyranosyl-22-hydroxy-5β-furostane-3β,26-diol 3-O-β-D-glucopyranosyl(1→2)-O-β-D-galactopyranoside
Source: ZHI MU. Ref: 2.

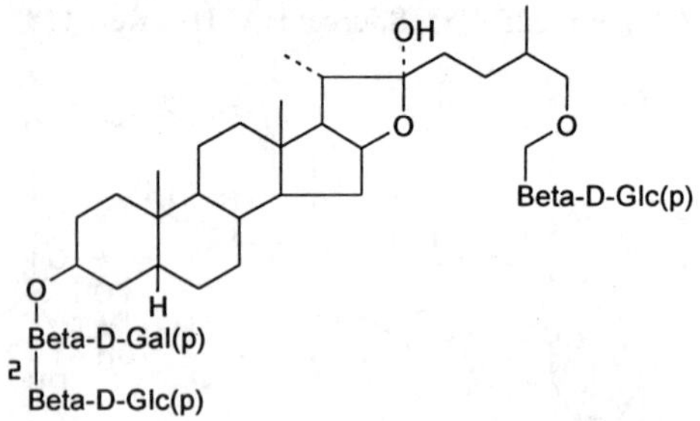

Beta-D-Glc(p)
Beta-D-Gal(p)
Beta-D-Glc(p)

2657 4'-O-β-Glucopyranosyl-5-O-methylvisamminol
$C_{22}H_{28}O_{10}$ MW: 452.46 Source: FANG FENG. Ref: 2.

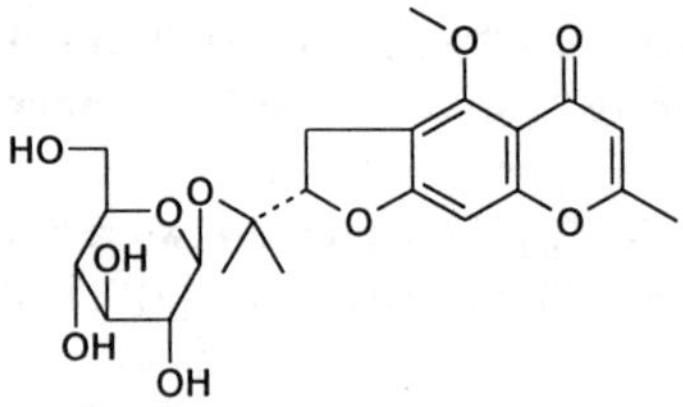

2658 3-O-β-D-Glucopyranosyl(1→3)-α-L-rhamnopyranosyl(1→2)-α-L-arabinopyranosyl hederagenin 28-O-β-D-glucopyranosyl(1→6)-β-D-glucopyranosyl ester (VII)
$C_{59}H_{96}O_{27}$ MW: 1237.41 Property: white granular crystal (methanol), mp 218-20°C, $[\alpha]_D^{21}$ -3.3° (c=0.3, pyridine). Source: CHUAN XU DUAN. Ref: 211.

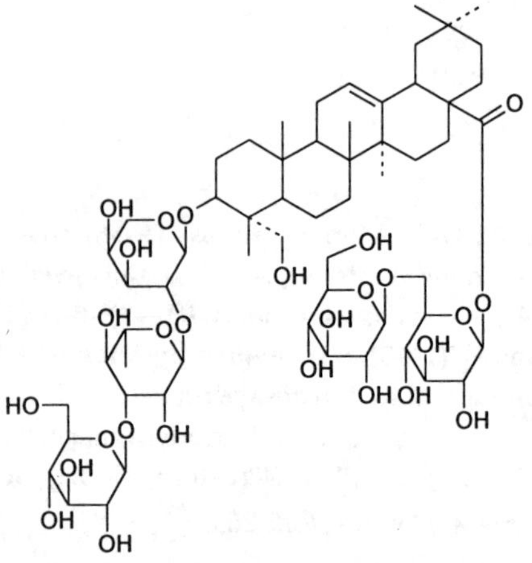

2659 3-O-[β-D-Glucopyranosyl(1→4)][α-L-rhamnopyranosyl(1→3)]-β-D-glucopyranosyl (1→3)-α-L-rhamnopyranosyl(1→2)-α-arabino-pyranosyl-hederagenin

$C_{59}H_{96}O_{26}$ MW:1221.41 Property: white powder, mp 239-243°C, $[\alpha]_D^{21}$ -12.3°(c=0.28, MeOH). Source: CHUAN XU DUAN. Ref: 265.

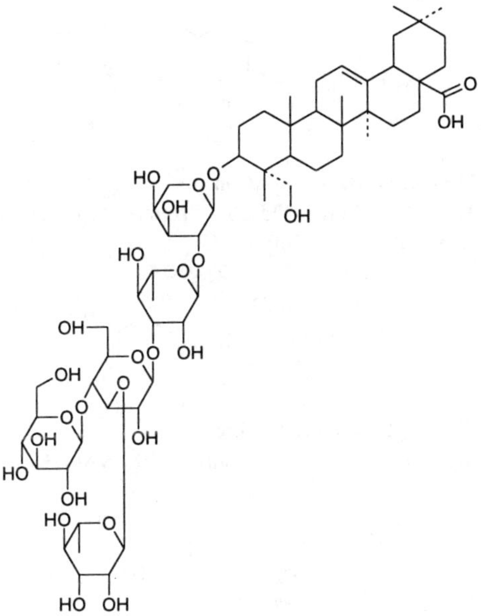

2661 2-(β-D-Glucopyranosyloxy)-8-hydroxy-1-methoxy-3-methyl-9,10-anthraquinone

$C_{22}H_{22}O_{10}$ MW: 446.41 Source: JUE MING ZI. Ref: 2.

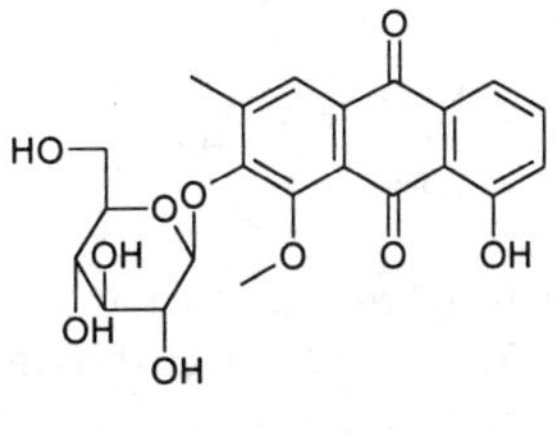

2662 2''-O-β-D-Glucopyranosylswertisin

$C_{28}H_{32}O_{15}$ MW: 608.56 Source: SUAN ZAO REN. Ref: 2.

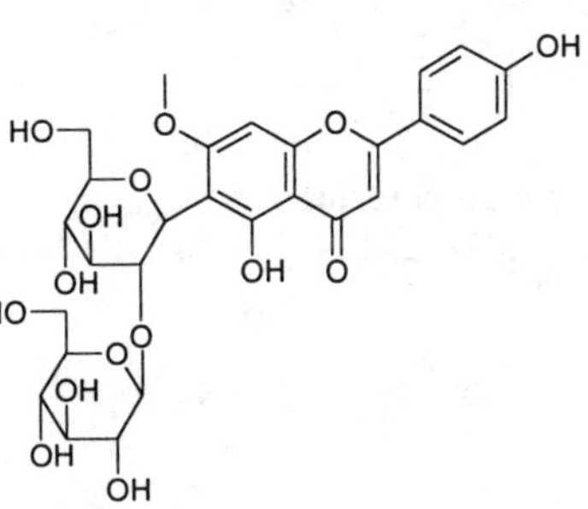

2663 3-O-β-D-Glucopyranosyl-5,9,4'-trihydroxy-8-methoxyflavone

$C_{22}H_{22}O_{11}$ MW: 462.41 Source: MA HUANG. Ref: 2.

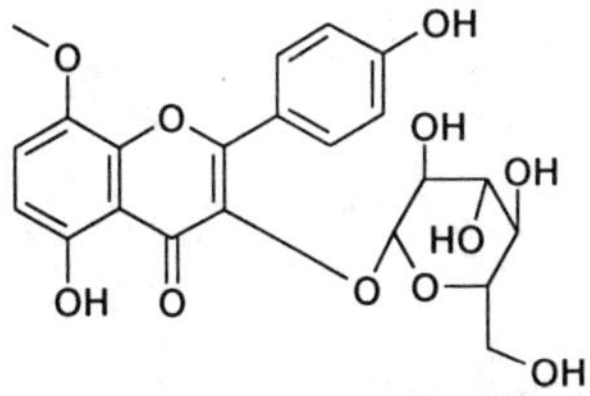

2664 Glucosamine

$C_6H_{13}NO_5$ MW: 179.17 Property: mp α: 88°C, β: 110°C (dec). Source: BAI FAO DOU, GAN DI HUANG, HAI SHEN CHANG, LING ZHI CAO, LU RONG, NOU NAO, YE JU. Ref: 2.

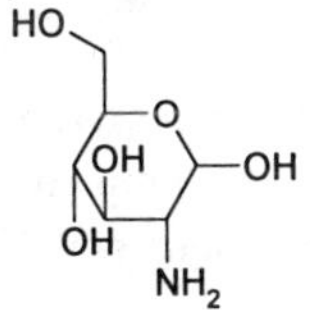

2665 20-Glucosylginsenoside Rf

Source: REN SHEN. Ref: 2.

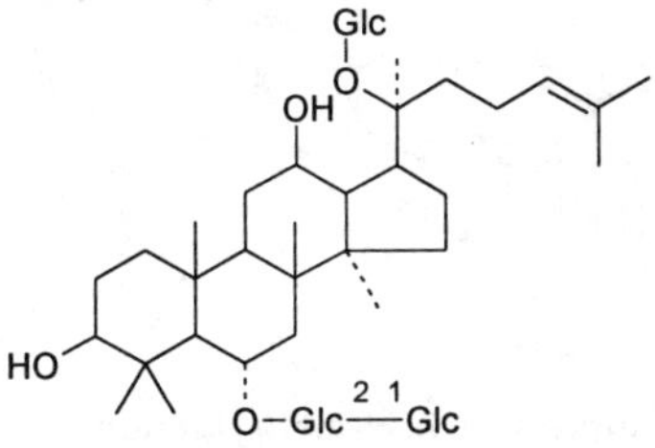

2666 o-(β-D-Glucosyloxy) hydrocinnamic acid

Melilotic acid glucoside. $C_{15}H_{20}O_8$ MW: 328.32 Source: PI HAN CAO. Ref: 6

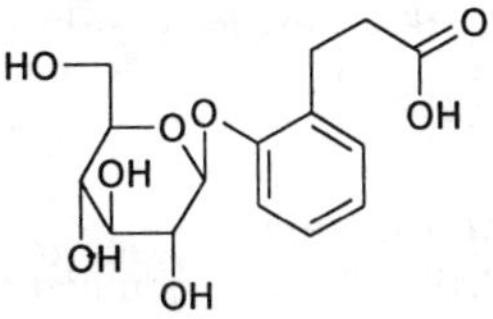

2667 Gluco-syringic acid

Property: mp 215-7°C. Source: QUE MEI TENG. Ref: 515

2668 Glucotropaeolin
$C_{14}H_{18}NO_8S_2{\bullet}K$ MW: 406.46•39.10 Source: HAN LIAN HUA. Ref: 6.

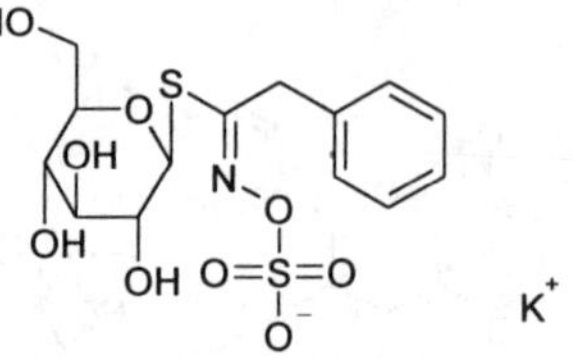

2669 Glucuronic acid
$C_6H_{10}O_7$ MW: 194.14 Source: HUANG QI, LU HUI, REN SHEN, etc. Ref: 2.

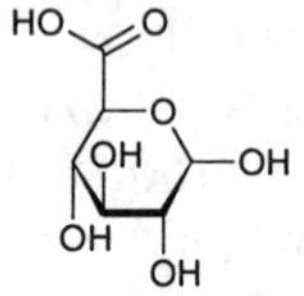

2670 3-O-β-D-Glucuronopyranosyl gypsogenin
$C_{36}H_{54}O_{10}$ MW: 646.83 Property: white lamellar crystal, mp 238-40°C. Source: SHAN KU GUA. Ref: 645.

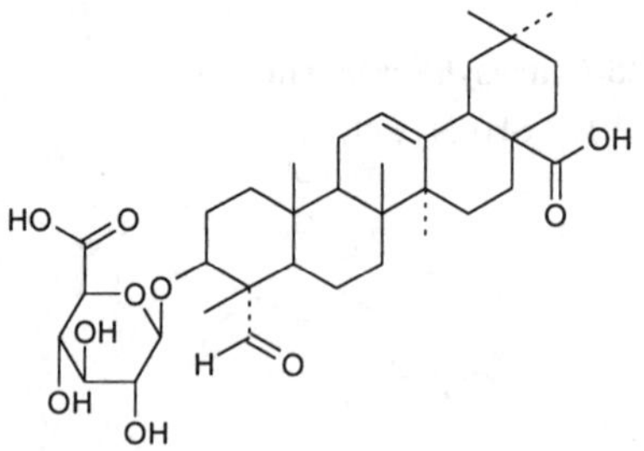

2671 l-Glutamic acid-γ-methylamide
$C_6H_{10}N_2O_5$ MW: 190.16 Source: CHA ZI XIN, YOU CHA GEN PI. Ref: 6.

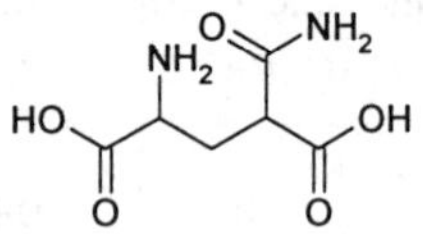

2673 γ-Glutamyl-alanine
$C_8H_{14}N_2O_5$ MW: 218.21 Property: mp 194-5°C (dec). Source: NIU NAO. Ref: 6.

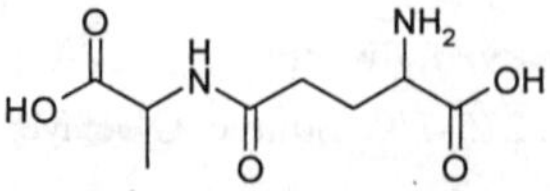

2674 γ-L-Glutamyl-L-β-aminoisobutyric acid
$C_9H_{16}N_2O_5$ MW: 232.24 Property: mp 156-8.5°C (dec). Source: NIU NAO. Ref: 6.

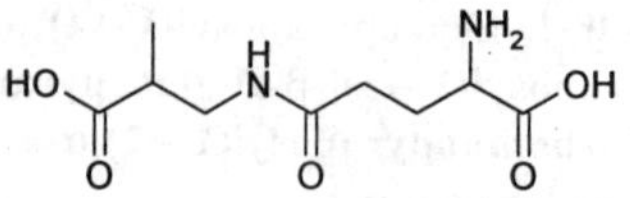

2675 γ-L-Glutamyl-L-glutamic acid
$C_{10}H_{16}N_2O_7$ MW: 276.25 Property: mp 191-2°C. Source: NIU NAO. Ref: 6.

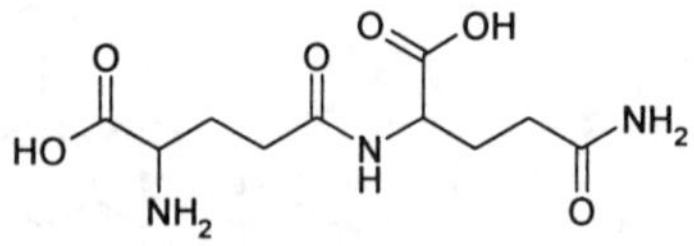

2676 γ-L-Glutamyl-glutamine
$C_{10}H_{17}N_3O_6$ MW: 275.26 Property: mp 191-2°C. Source: NIU NAO. Ref: 6.

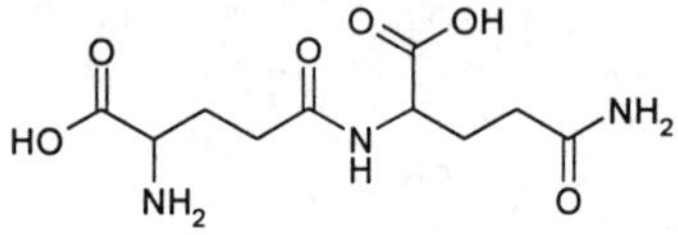

2677 γ-L-Glutamyl glycine
$C_7H_{12}N_2O_5$ MW: 204.18 Source: NIU NAO. Ref: 6.

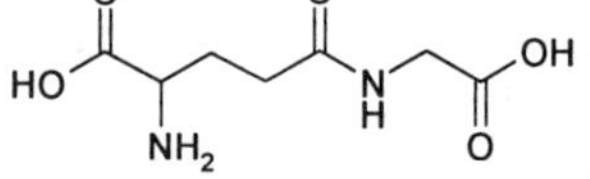

2678 γ-L-Glutamyl-L-phenylalanine
$C_{14}H_{18}N_2O_5$ MW: 294.31 Property: mp 164-74°C (dec). Source: DI YANG QUE. Ref: 6.

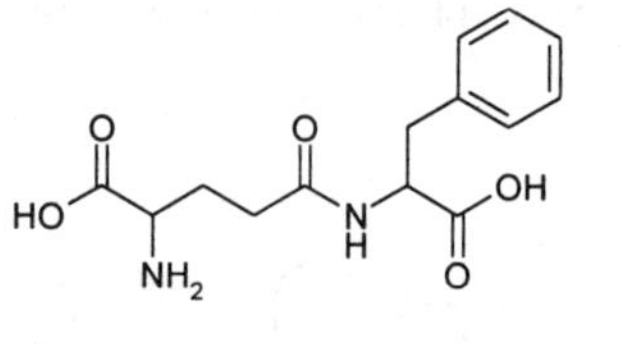

2679 γ-L-Glutamyl-S-(prop-1-enyl)cystein sulfoxide
$C_{11}H_{18}N_2O_6S$ MW: 306.34 Source: TAN XIANG. Ref: 6.

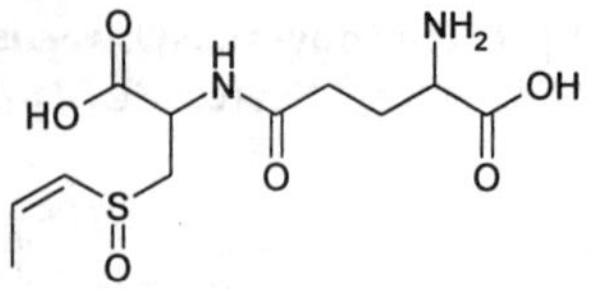

2680 γ-Glutamyl-serine
$C_8H_{14}N_2O_6$ MW: 234.21 Source: NIU NAO. Ref: 6.

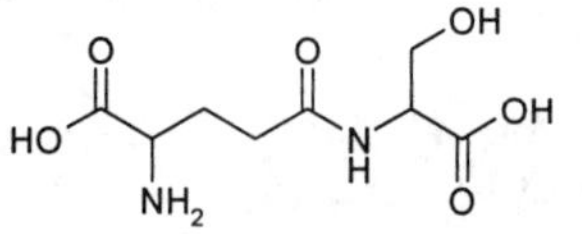

2681 γ-L-Glutamyl-L-tyrosine
$C_{14}H_{18}N_2O_6$ MW: 310.31 Property: mp 221-2°C (dec). Source: DI YANG QUE. Ref: 6.

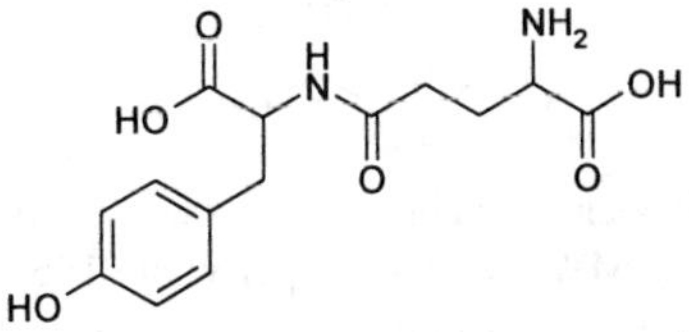

2682 γ-Glutamylvaline
$C_{10}H_{18}N_2O_5$ MW: 246.27 Property: mp 207°C. Source: NIU NAO. Ref: 6.

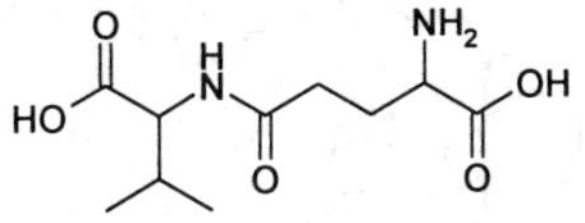

2683 Glutaric acid
$C_5H_8O_4$ MW: 132.12 Property: mp 97-8°C; bp 302-4°C. Source: NING MENG AN YE. Ref: 6.

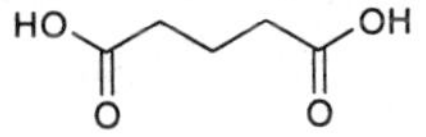

2684 Glutathione
$C_{10}H_{17}N_3O_6S$ MW: 307.33 Property: mp 190-2°C (dec). Source: MU LI ROU, XIAO BAI BU. Ref: 6.

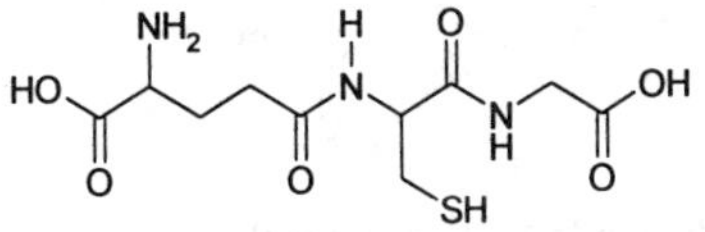

2685 Glutenol
Glut-5-en-3α-ol. $C_{30}H_{50}O$ MW: 426.73 Property: mp 203-5°C. Source: XI YE DA JI. Ref: 6.

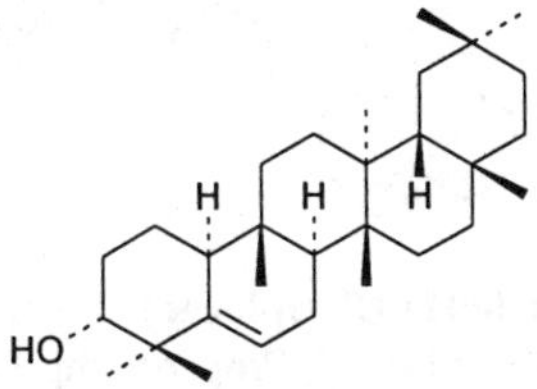

2687 Glutinic acid
$C_{20}H_{30}O_4$ MW: 338.49 Property: white acicular crystal, mp 119-20°C, easily soluble in acetone and pyridine. Source: NIAN YE YOU. Ref: 248.

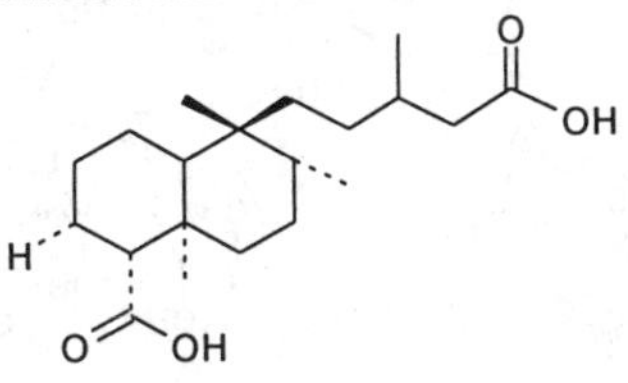

2688 Glutinol
Glutin-5-en-3β-ol. $C_{30}H_{50}O$ MW: 426.73 Property: mp 211°C. Source: BA WANG BIAN, CHI YANG, MENG GU LI. Ref: 6, 611.

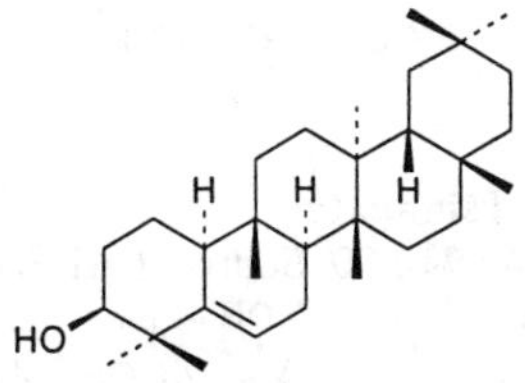

2689 Glutinone
$C_{30}H_{48}O$ MW: 424.72 Property: mp 245-6°C. Source: LONG XU CAO. Ref: 6.

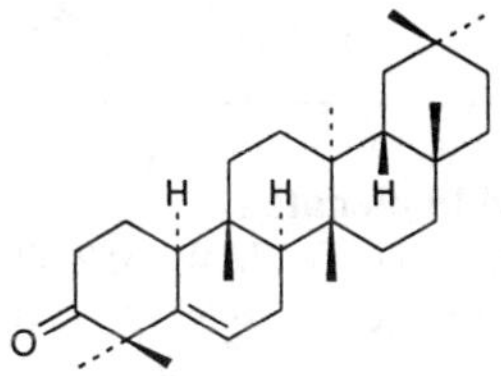

2690 Glutinoside
$C_{15}H_{23}ClO_{10}$ MW: 398.80 Source: GAN DI HUANG. Ref: 2.

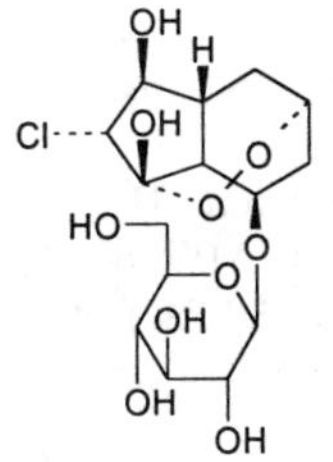

2691 D-Glyceric acid
$C_3H_6O_4$ MW: 106.08 Source: CAN DOU YE, CAN DOU JING, CAN DOU JIA KE, PU TAO TENG YE. Ref: 6.

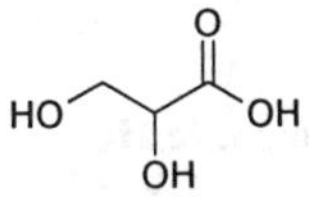

2692 Glyceride-1,3-dipalmito-2-sorbate
$C_{41}H_{74}O_6$ MW: 647.04 Property: colorless acicular crystal, mp 62-2.5°C (petroleum spirit-acetic ester). Source: DI SHAO GUA. Ref: 236.

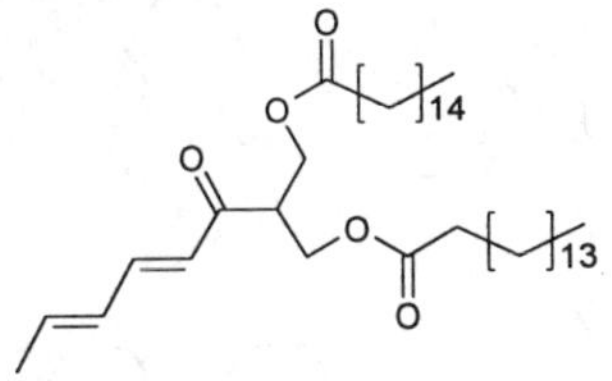

2693 Glycerol
Glycerin. $C_3H_8O_3$ MW: 92.10 Property: mp 20°C, bp 290°C (dec). Source: BAI YAO ZI, JIU, SHI LI ZI, SHI LIU GEN. Ref: 6.

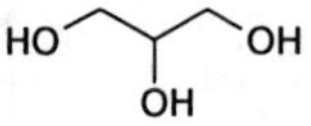

2694 Glycerol sinapate
$C_{36}H_{38}O_{15}$ MW: 710.70 Source: LAI FU ZI. Ref: 6.

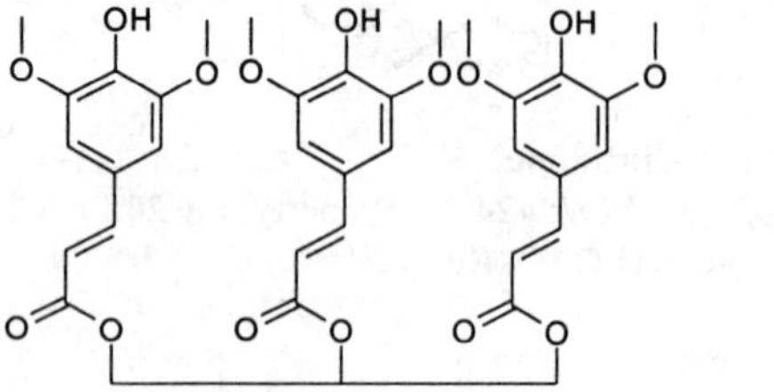

2695 Glyceryl linolenate I
Monolinolenin. $C_{21}H_{36}O_4$ MW: 352.52 Property: mp β: 15.7°C, β': -13.5°C. Source: YU ZHI ZI. Ref: 6.

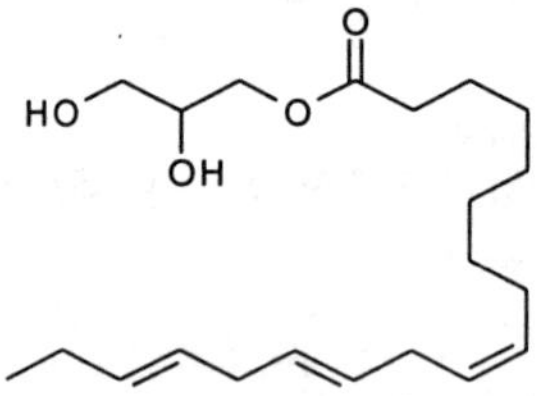

2696 Glyceryl linolenate II
Dilinolenin. $C_{39}H_{64}O_5$ MW: 612.94 Property: mp -12.3°C. Source: YU ZHI ZI. Ref: 6.

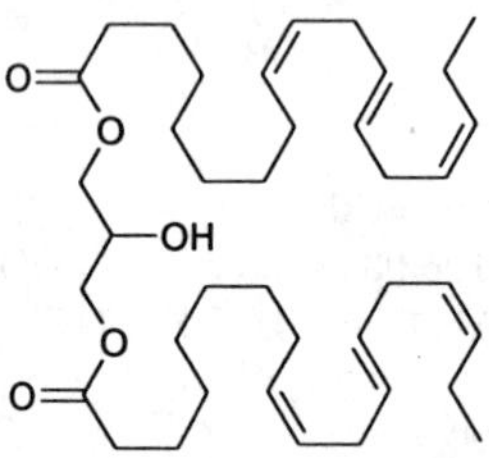

2697 Glyceryl linolenate III
Trilinolenin. $C_{57}H_{92}O_6$ MW: 873.37 Property: mp -23°C. Source: YU ZHI ZI. Ref: 6.

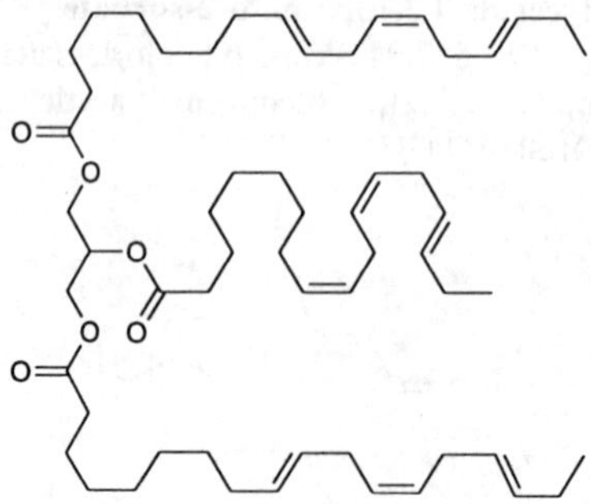

2698 Glycine
$C_2H_5NO_2$ MW: 75.07 Property: mp 262°C (dec). Source: LONG KUI. Ref: 6.

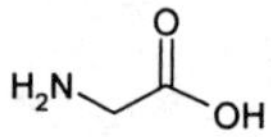

2699 Glycocholic acid
$C_{26}H_{43}NO_6$ MW: 465.64 Property: mp 165-8°C (anhydrous), mp 230-40°C (sodium salt). Source: NIU DAN. Ref: 6.

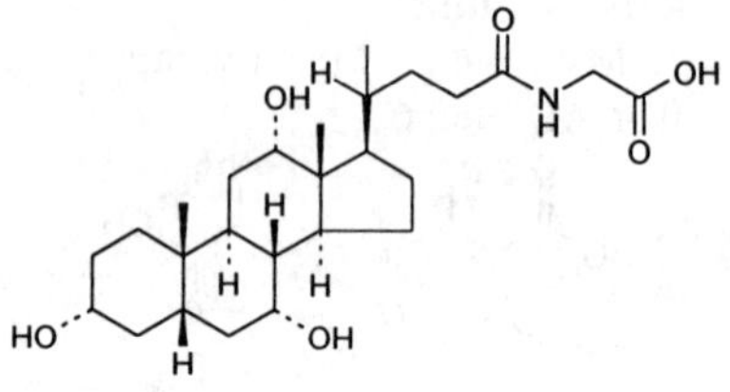

2700 Glycol
$C_2H_6O_2$ MW: 62.07 Property: mp -11.5°C, bp 197°C. Source: XI GUA. Ref: 6.

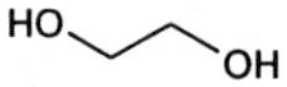

2701 Glycolic acid
$C_2H_4O_3$ MW: 76.05 Property: mp 80°C. Source: GAN ZHE, HAN QIN, MENG GU SHAN LUO BO. Ref: 6.

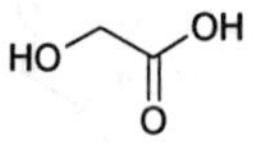

2702 Glycoside E (Periplocae)
$C_{27}H_{44}O_6$ MW: 464.65 Property: mp 239-40°C. Source: XIANG JIA PI. Ref: 6.

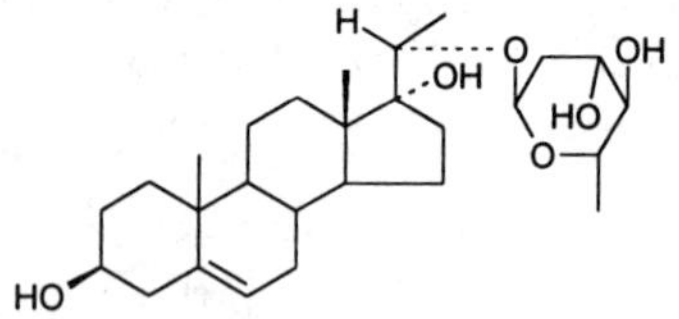

2704 Glycoside H1 (Periplocae)
$C_{56}H_{92}O_{24}$ MW: 1149.34 Property: mp 182°C. Source: XIANG JIA PI. Ref: 6.

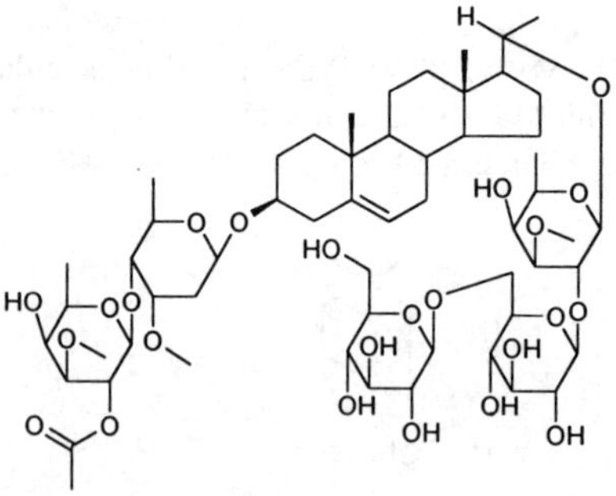

2705 Glycoside K (Periplocae)
$C_{40}H_{66}O_{16}$ MW: 802.96 Property: mp 240-1°C. Source: XIANG JIA PI. Ref: 6.

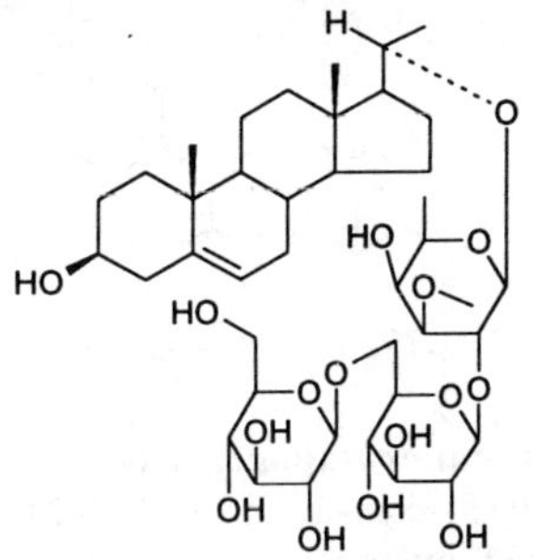

2706 Glycycoumarin
$C_{21}H_{20}O_6$ MW: 368.39 Source: GAN CAO. Ref: 2.

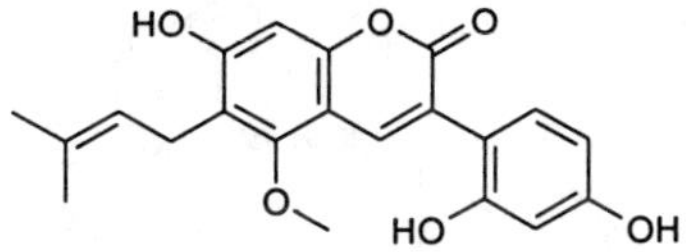

2707 Glycyrin
$C_{22}H_{22}O_6$ MW: 382.42 Source: GAN CAO. Ref: 2.

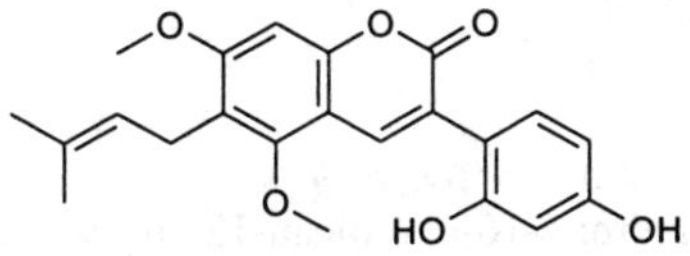

2708 Glycyrol
$C_{21}H_{18}O_6$ MW: 366.37 Property: mp 243.5-5.0°C. Source: GAN CAO. Ref: 2, 6.

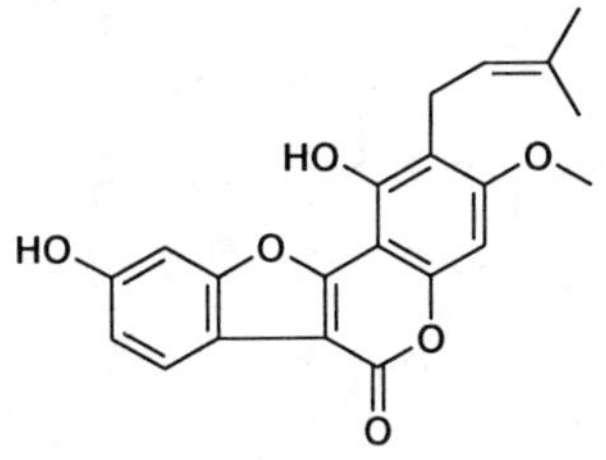

2709 Glycyroside
Formononetin-7-O-[D-apio-β-D-furanosyl(1→2)]-β-D-(glucopyranoside). $C_{27}H_{30}O_{13}$ MW: 562.53 Property: light yellow powder, mp 126-8°C. Source: HUANG GAN CAO. Ref: 133.

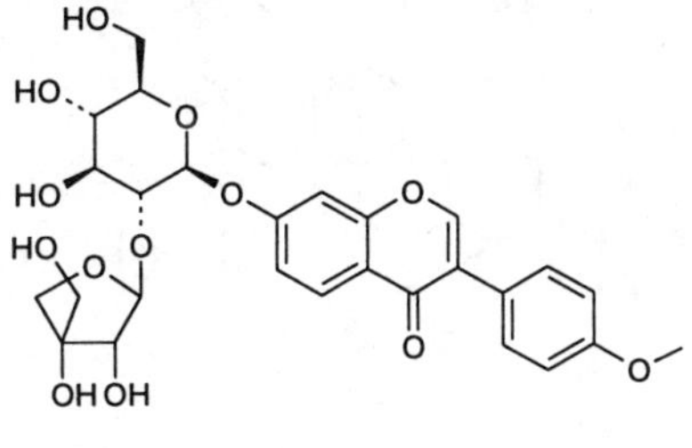

2710 Glycyrrhetic acid acetate
$C_{32}H_{48}O_5$ MW: 512.74 Source: GAN CAO. Ref: 2.

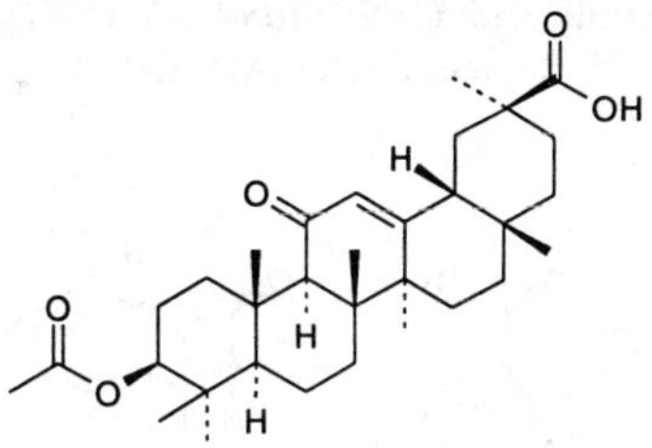

2711 Glycyrrhetinic acid
Biosone; Enoxolone; Glycyrrhetic acid; 18β-Glycyrrhetic acid; 18β-Glycyrrhetinic acid; Glycyrrhetin; Uralenic acid. CAS: 471-53-4 $C_{30}H_{46}O_4$ MW: 470.70 Property: mp 297-8°C. Source: GAN CAO. Ref: 4.

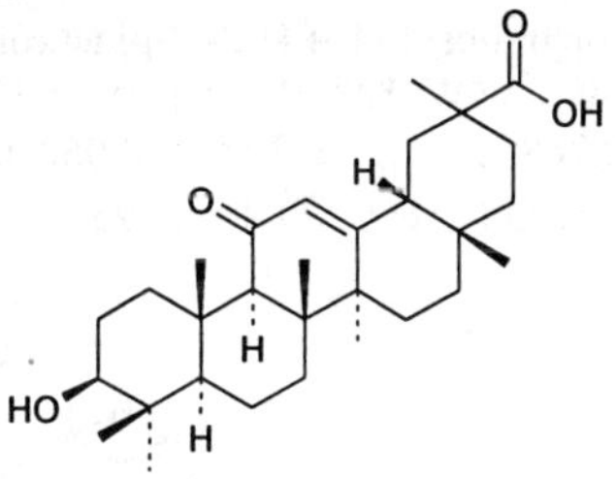

2712 Glycyrrhetol
$C_{30}H_{48}O_3$ MW: 456.72 Source: GAN CAO. Ref: 2.

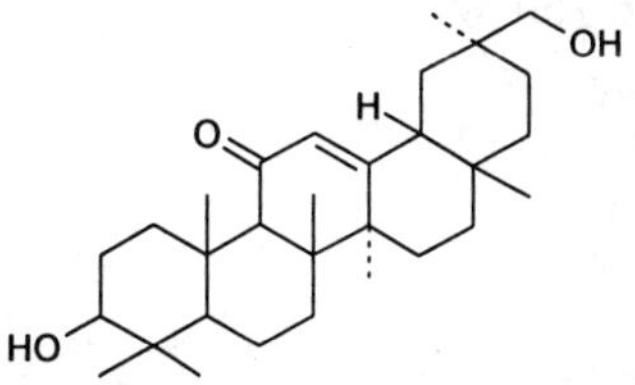

2713 Glycyrrhisoflavanone
$C_{21}H_{20}O_6$ MW: 368.39 Source: GAN CAO. Ref: 2.

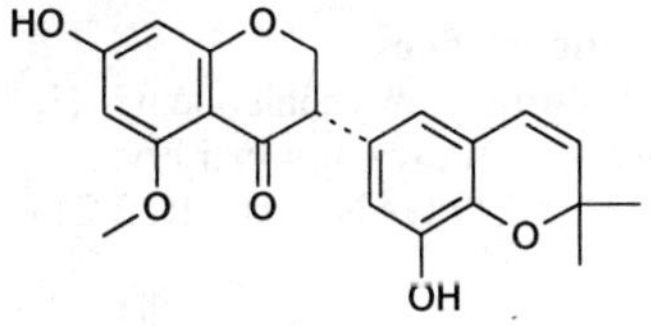

2714 Glycyrrhisoflavone
$C_{20}H_{18}O_6$ MW: 354.36 Source: GAN CAO. Ref: 2.

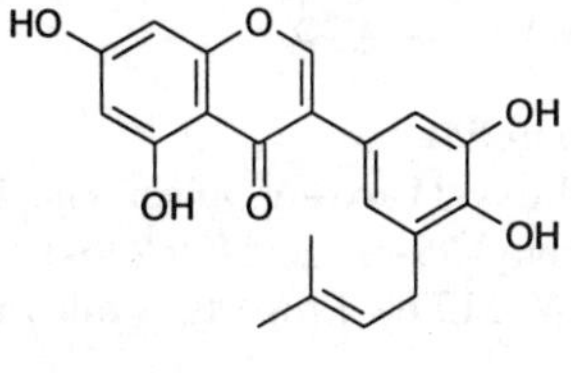

2715 Glycyrrhizic acid
Glycyrrhizin; Glycyrrhetinic acid glycyside; Glycyrrhizinic acid. CAS: 1405-86-3 $C_{42}H_{62}O_{16}$ MW: 822.95 Source: GAN CAO. Ref: 4.

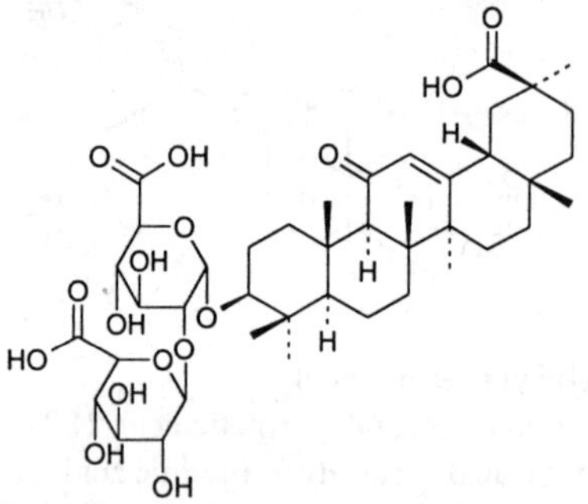

2716 Glyeurysaponin
3β-Hydroxy-11-oxo-olean-12-en-30-oic acid–3-O-β-D-glucuronopyranosyl-(1→4)-β-D-glucuronopyranoside. $C_{42}H_{62}O_{16}$ MW: 822.95 Property: white powder, mp 288°C, $[\alpha]_D^{18}$ +22.5° (c=0.062, methanol). Source: HUANG GAN CAO. Ref: 195.

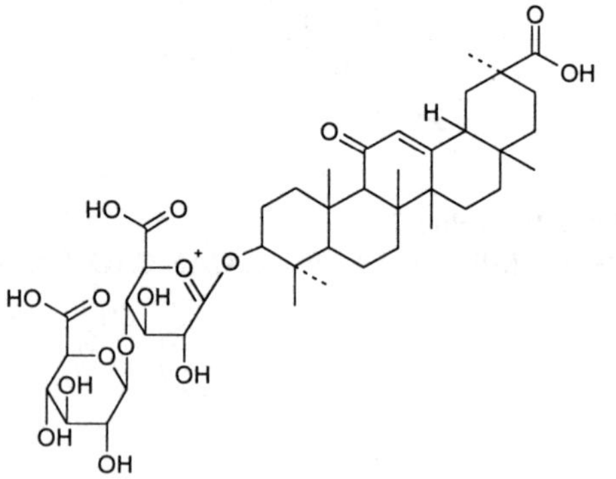

2717 Glyoxal
$C_2H_2O_2$ MW: 58.04 Source: SHENG JIANG. Ref: 2.

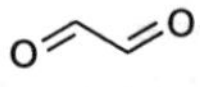

2718 Glypallichalcone
4-Hydroxy-2,4'-dimethoxychalcone. $C_{17}H_{16}O_4$ MW: 284.31 Property: yellow columnar crystal, mp 140-2°C. Source: CI GUO GAN CAO. Ref: 243.

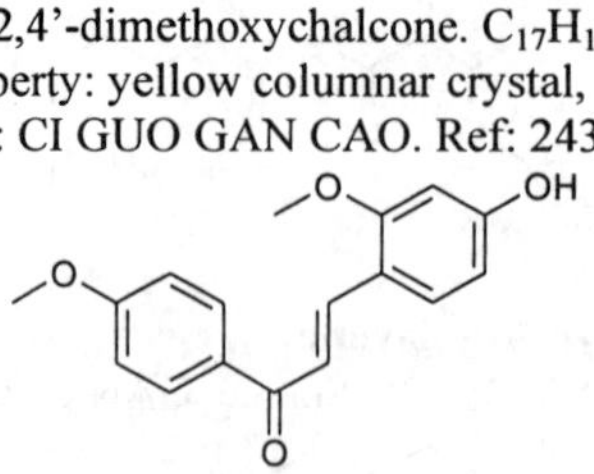

2719 Glyuranolide
3β,22α-digydroxy-11-oxo-Δ^{12}-olean-ene-27α-methoxy carbonyl-29-oic acid (29,22α-) lactone. $C_{31}H_{44}O_6$ MW: 512.68 Property: white rhomboid crystal, mp 301-3°C, $[\alpha]_D^{14}$ + 46.0° (c=0.087). Source: WU LA ER GAN CAO. Ref: 128.

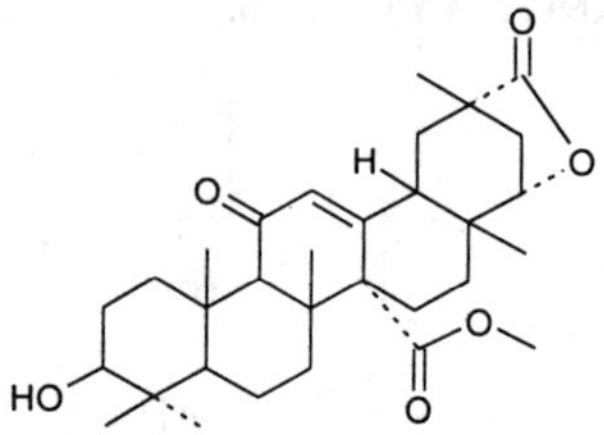

2720 Glyyunnanprosapogenin D
Oleana-11,13(18)-dien-29-oic acid,3β,21α-di-(O-β-D-glucuronic acid) pyranoside. $C_{42}H_{62}O_{17}$ MW: 838.95 Source: YUN NAN GAN CAO. Ref: 170.

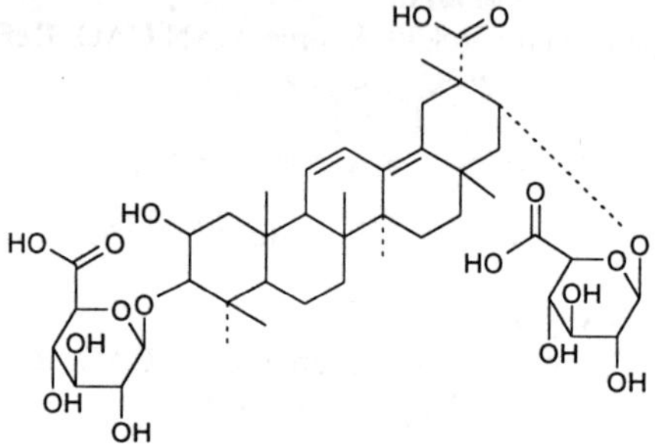

2721 Glyyunnansapogenin A
3β,24-Dihydroxy-16-oxo-olean-12-en-29-oic acid. $C_{30}H_{46}O_5$ MW: 486.70 Property: colorless crystal. Source: YUN NAN GAN CAO. Ref: 160.

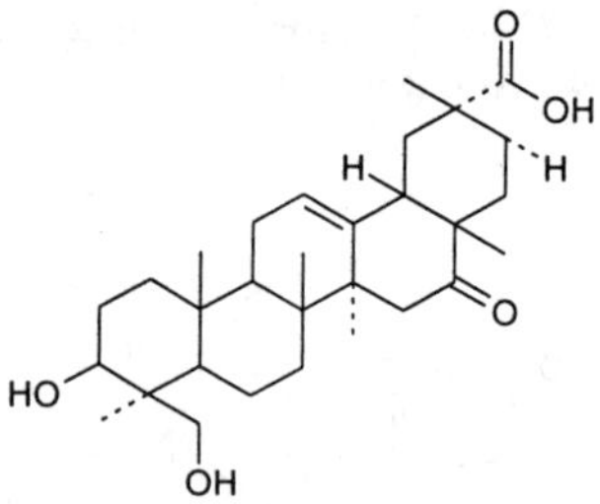

2722 Glyyunnansapogenin B
3β,21α,24-trihydroxy-olean-12-en-30-oic acid. $C_{30}H_{48}O_5$ MW: 500.73 Property: colorless crystal mp 287-9°C. Source: YUN NAN GAN CAO. Ref: 160.

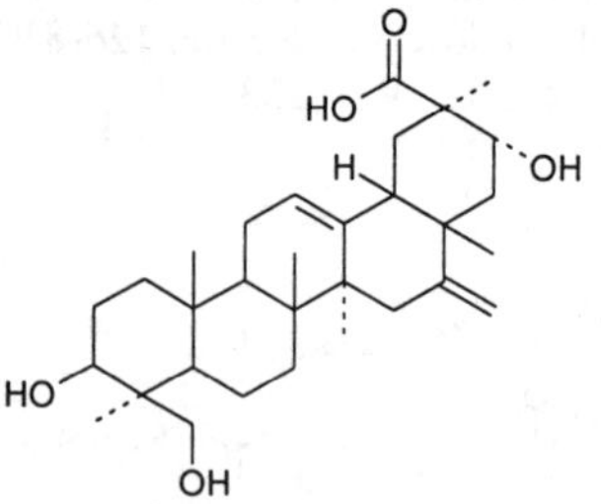

2723 Glyyunnansapogenin B1
$C_{30}H_{48}O_5$ MW: 488.71 Property: white acicular crystal, mp 303-5°C. Source: YUN NAN GAN CAO. Ref: 321.

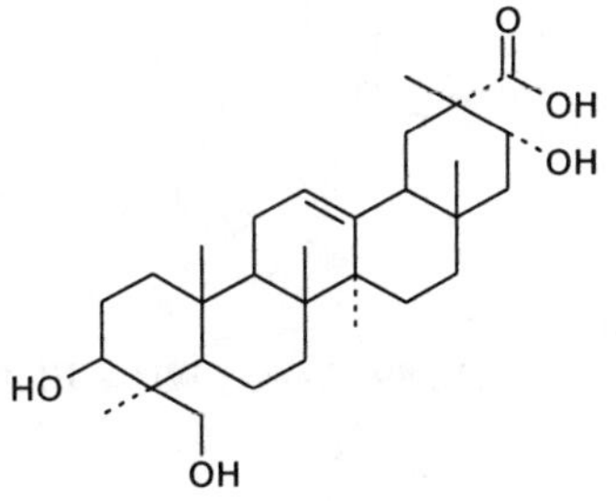

2724 Glyyunnansapogenin B2
$C_{30}H_{50}O_2$ MW: 442.73 Property: white powder, mp 224-8°C. Source: YUN NAN GAN CAO. Ref: 321.

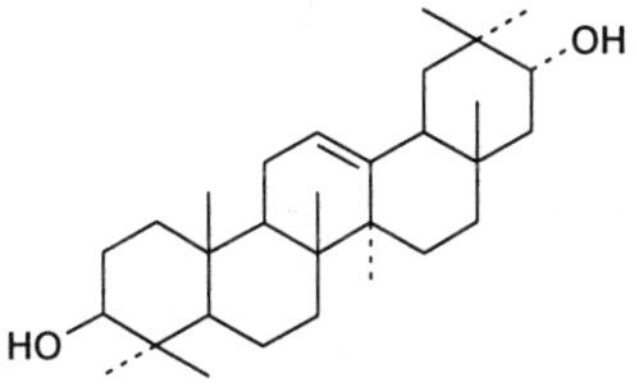

2725 Glyyunnansapogenin F
3β,24α-Dihydroxy-16-oxo-oleana-11,13(18)-dien-30-oic acid. $C_{30}H_{44}O_5$ MW: 484.68 Source: YUN NAN GAN CAO. Ref: 170.

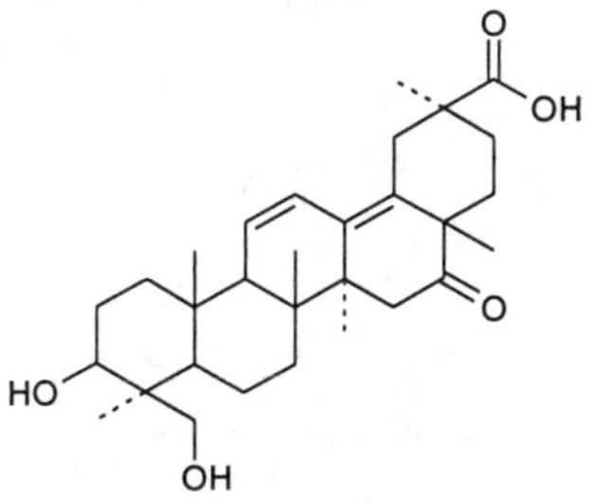

2726 Glyzaglabrin
$C_{16}H_{10}O_6$ MW: 298.25 Source: GAN CAO. Ref: 2.

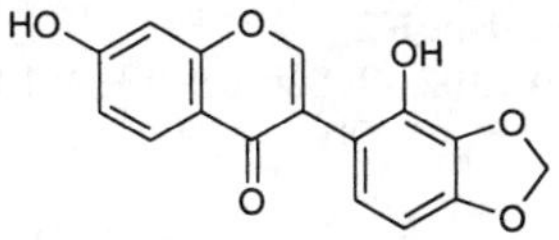

2727 Gmelofuran
$C_{15}H_{18}O_3$ MW: 246.31 Source: CHEN XIANG. Ref: 13.

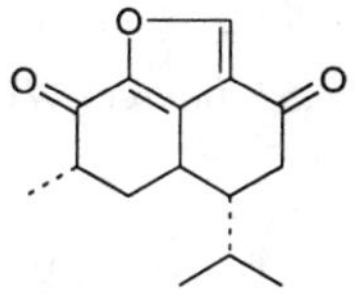

2728 Gnoscopine
$C_{24}H_{27}O_6$ MW: 425.49 Property: mp 232°C. Source: YA PIAN. Ref: 6.

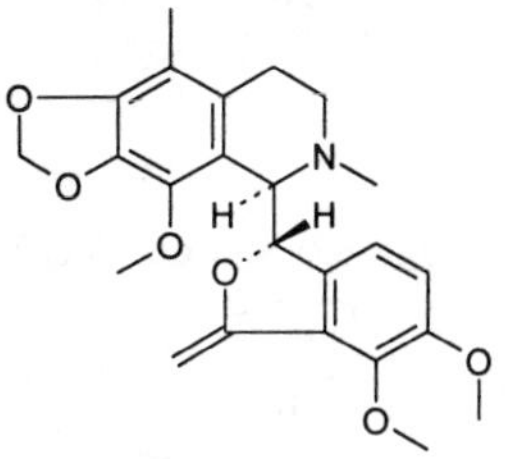

2729 Gomaline
$C_{20}H_{22}N_2O_3$ MW: 338.41 Source: CHANG CHUN HUA. Ref: 2.

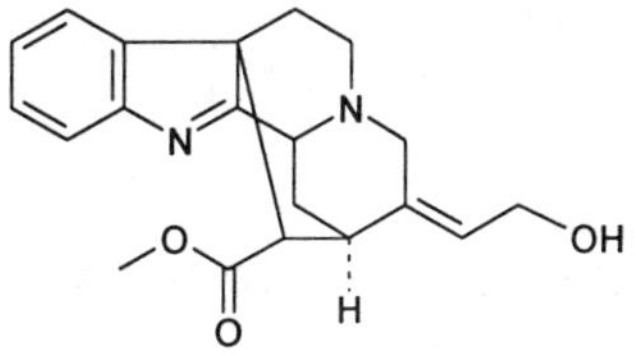

2730 Gomisin A
$C_{23}H_{28}O_7$ MW: 416.48 Source: REN SHEN, WU WEI ZI. Ref: 2.

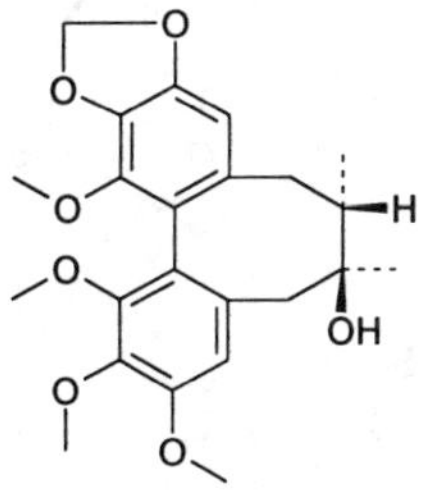

2731 Gomisin B
Source: WU WEI ZI. Ref: 2.

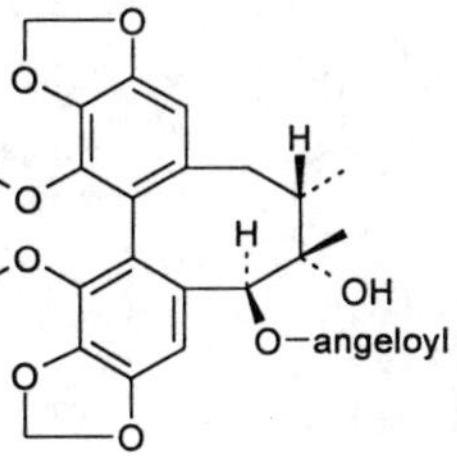

2732 Gomisin C
$C_{29}H_{32}O_8$ MW: 508.57 Source: WU WEI ZI. Ref: 2.

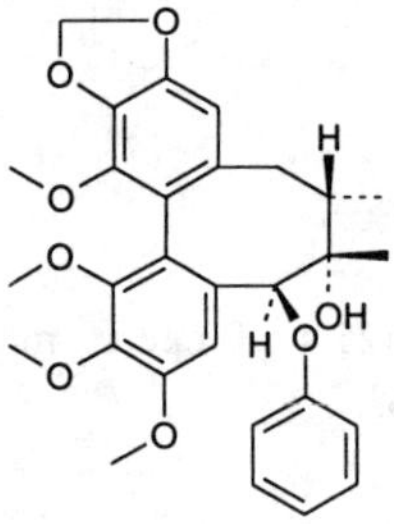

2733 Gomisin D
$C_{29}H_{38}O_{10}$ MW: 546.62 Source: WU WEI ZI. Ref: 2.

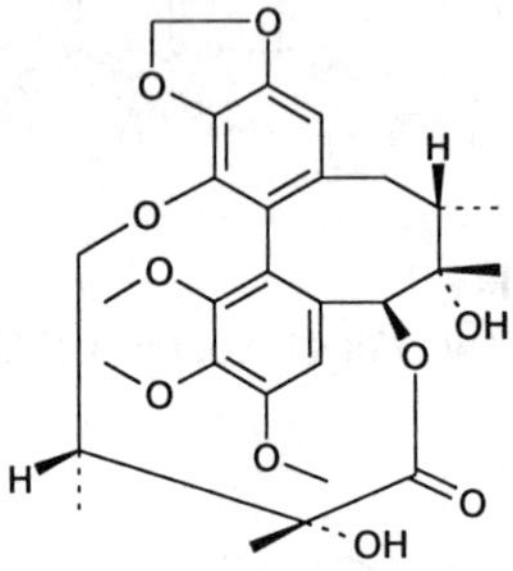

2734 Gomisin E
$C_{28}H_{34}O_9$ MW: 514.58 Source: WU WEI ZI. Ref: 2.

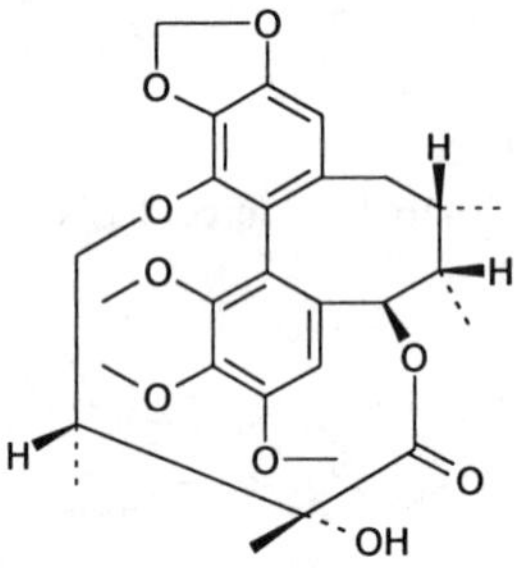

2735 Gomisin F
Source: WU WEI ZI. Ref: 2.

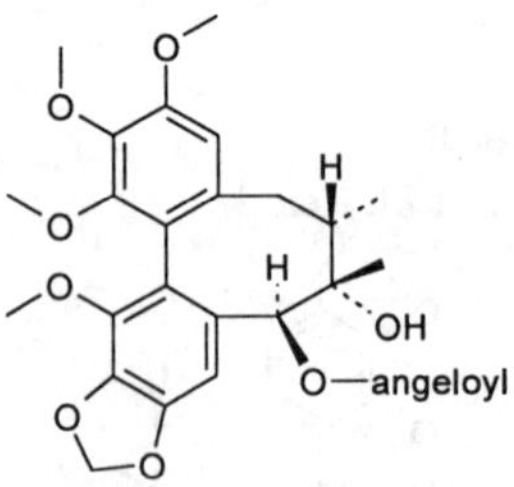

O—angeloyl

2736 Gomisin G
$C_{29}H_{32}O_8$ MW: 508.57 Source: WU WEI ZI. Ref: 2.

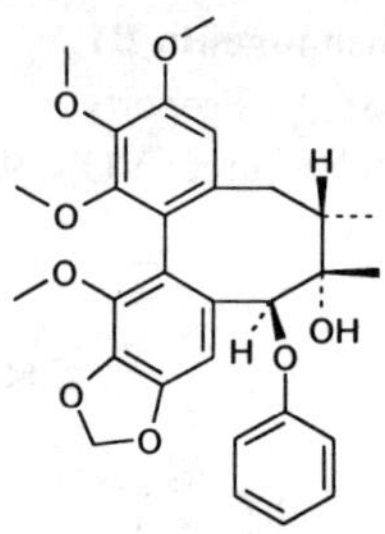

2737 Gomisin H
$C_{23}H_{30}O_7$ MW: 418.49 Source: WU WEI ZI. Ref: 2.

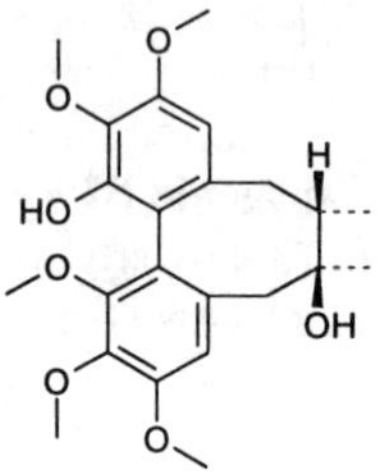

2738 Gomisin J
$C_{22}H_{28}O_6$ MW: 388.46 Source: WU WEI ZI. Ref: 2.

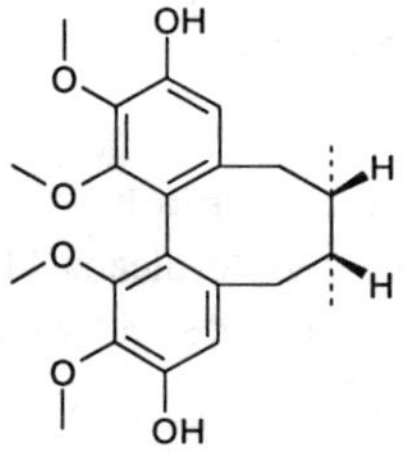

2739 (-)-Gomisin K1
$C_{23}H_{30}O_6$ MW: 402.49 Source: WU WEI ZI. Ref: 2.

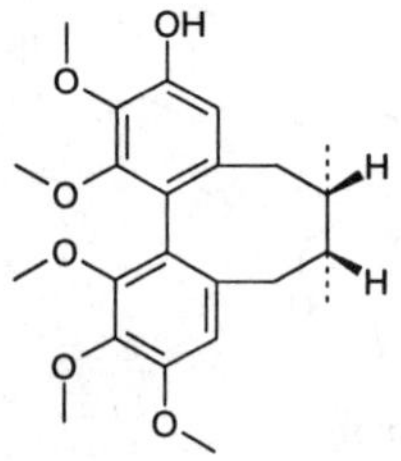

2740 (+)-Gomisin K2
$C_{23}H_{30}O_6$ MW: 402.49 Source: WU WEI ZI. Ref: 2.

methyl(ax.)
methyl(eq.)

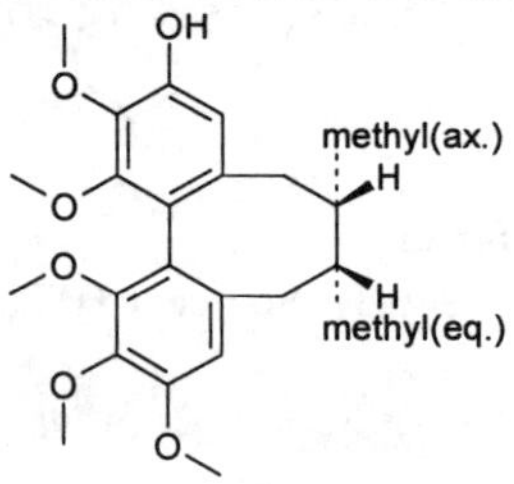

2741 (+)-Gomisin K3

$C_{23}H_{30}O_6$ MW: 402.49 Source: WU WEI ZI. Ref: 2.

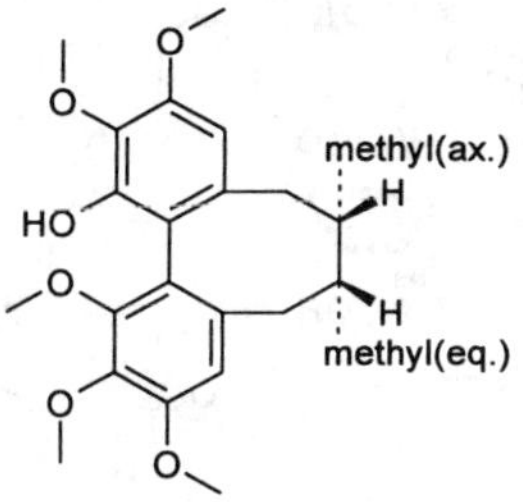

2742 (-)-Gomisin L1

$C_{22}H_{26}O_6$ MW: 386.45 Source: WU WEI ZI. Ref: 2.

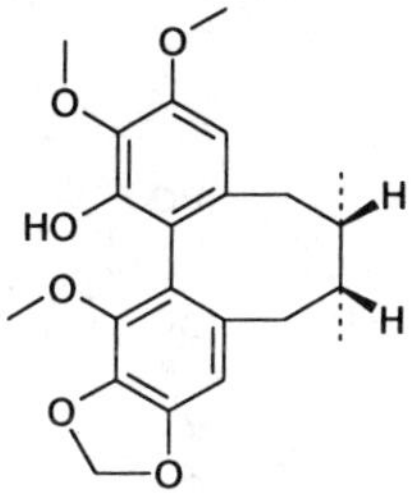

2743 (-)-Gomisin L2

$C_{22}H_{26}O_6$ MW: 386.45 Source: WU WEI ZI. Ref: 2.

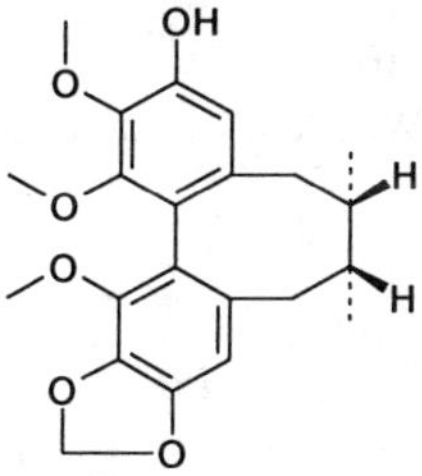

2744 (±)-Gomisin M1

$C_{22}H_{26}O_6$ MW: 386.45 Source: WU WEI ZI. Ref: 2.

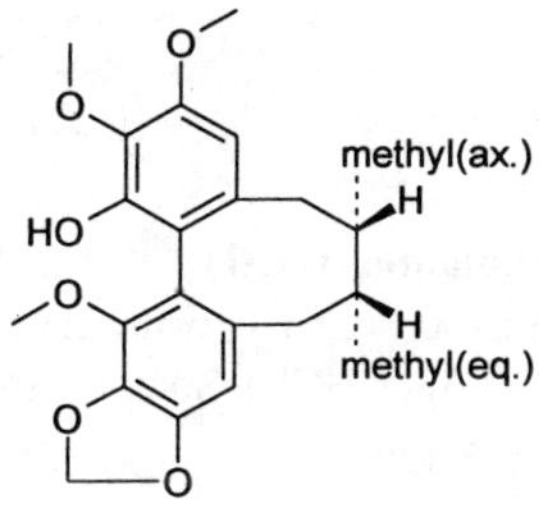

2745 (+)-Gomisin M2

$C_{22}H_{26}O_6$ MW: 386.45 Source: WU WEI ZI. Ref: 2.

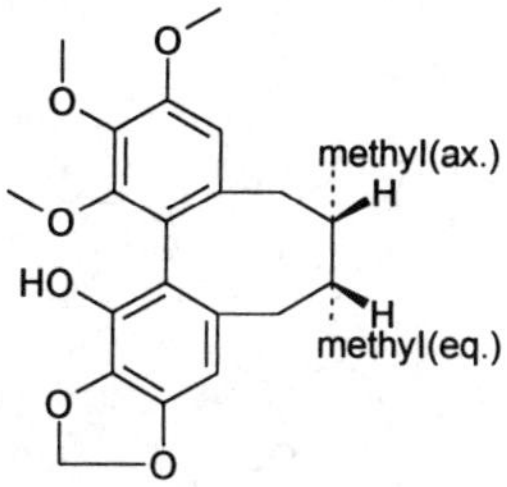

2746 Gomisin N

$C_{23}H_{28}O_6$ MW: 400.48 Source: WU WEI ZI, REN SHEN. Ref: 2.

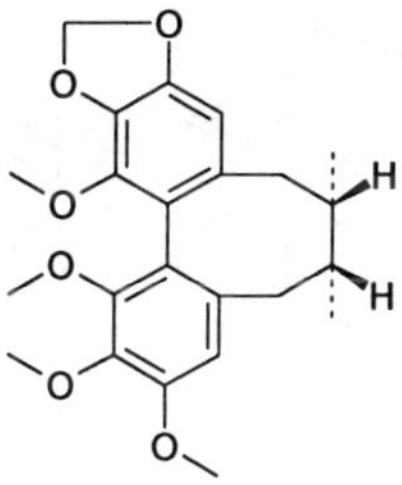

2747 Gomisin O

$C_{23}H_{28}O_7$ MW: 416.48 Source: HONG HUA WU WEI ZI, WU WEI ZI. Ref: 2, 39.

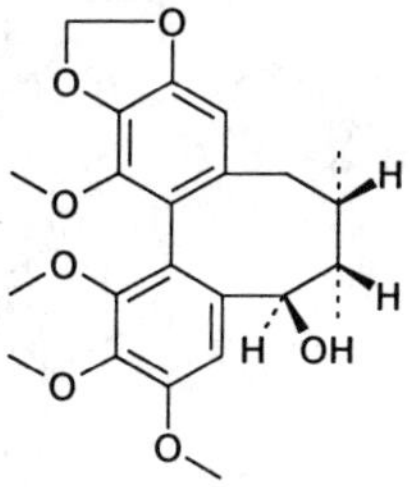

2748 Gomisin R

$C_{22}H_{24}O_7$ MW: 400.43 Source: WU WEI ZI. Ref: 2.

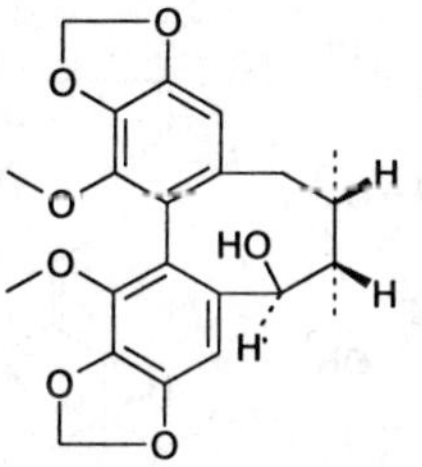

2749 Gomisin S

$C_{24}H_3O_7$ MW: 432.52 Source: WU WEI ZI. Ref: 2.

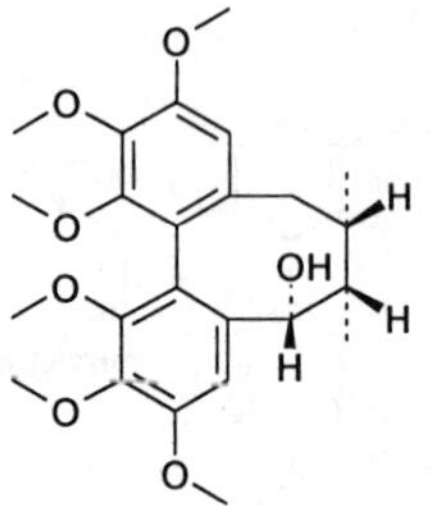

2750 Gomisin T

$C_{23}H_{30}O_6$ MW: 402.49 Source: WU WEI ZI. Ref: 2.

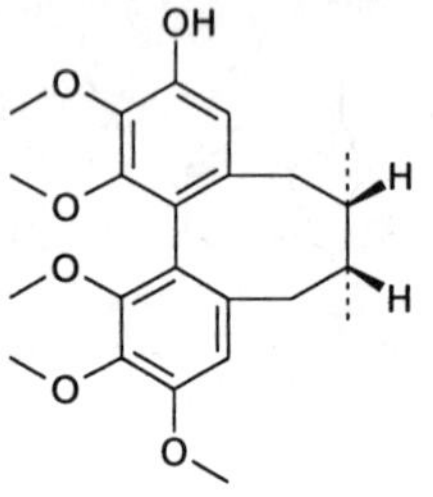

2751 Gomphernin I

$C_{24}H_{26}N_2O_{13}$ MW: 550.48 Source: QIAN RI HONG. Ref: 15.

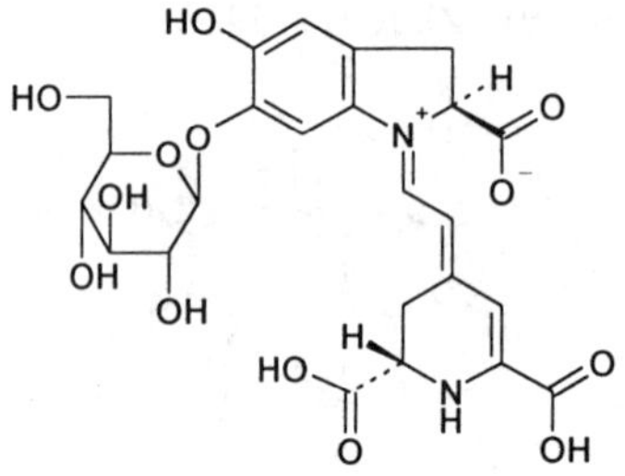

2752 Gomphernin II

$C_{24}H_{26}N_2O_{13}$ MW: 550.48 Source: QIAN RI HONG. Ref: 15.

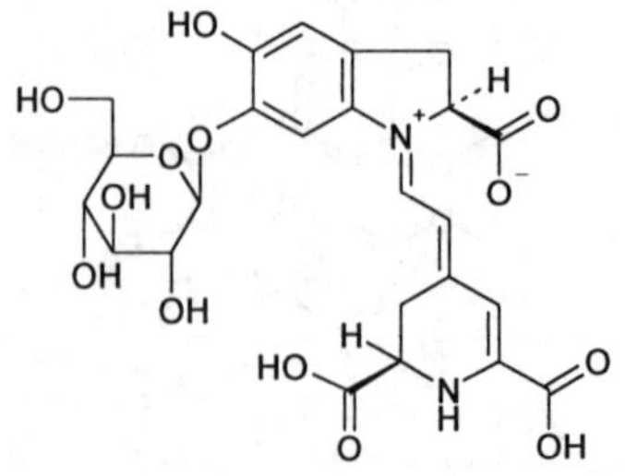

2753 Gomphernin III

$C_{33}H_{32}N_2O_{15}$ MW: 696.63 Source: QIAN RI HONG. Ref: 6, 15.

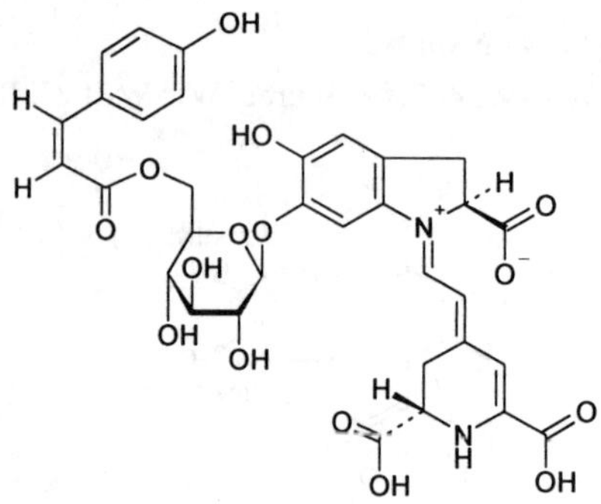

2754 Gomphernin V

$C_{34}H_{34}N_2O_{16}$ MW: 726.65 Source: QIAN RI HONG. Ref: 6, 15.

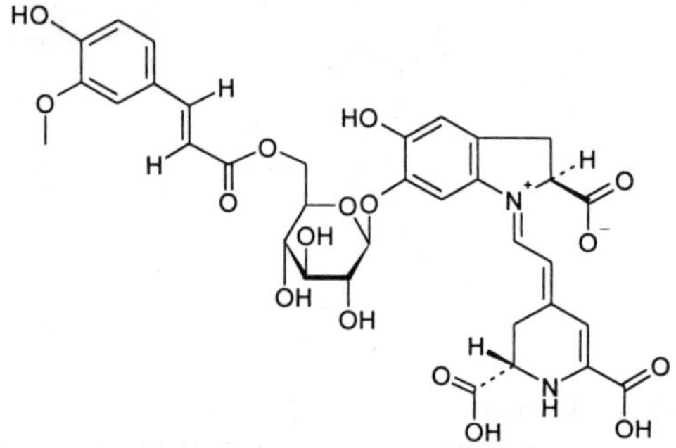

2755 Gomphernin VI

$C_{33}H_{32}N_2O_{15}$ MW: 696.63 Source: QIAN RI HONG. Ref: 6, 15.

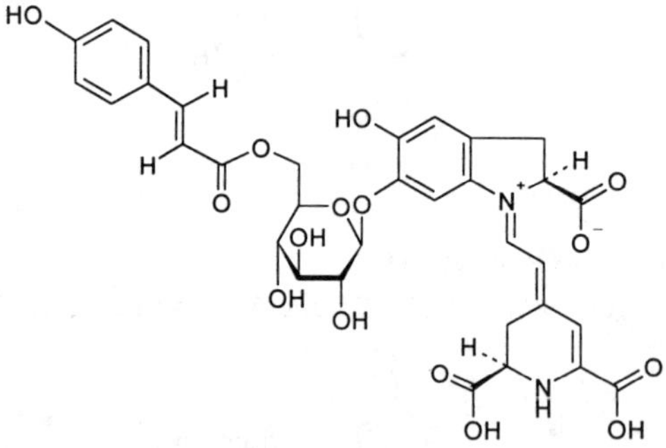

2756 Goniothalamin (GL-1)

$C_{13}H_{12}O_2$ MW: 200 Property: white crystal, mp 85°C, $[\alpha]_D^{25}$ +170° (c=1.38, $CHCl_3$). Source: JIN PING GE NA XIANG. Ref: 420.

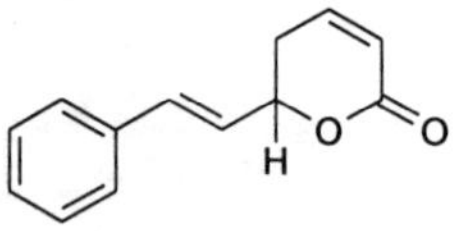

2757 Goshuynic acid
$C_{14}H_{24}O_2$ MW: 224.35 Source: WU ZHU YU. Ref: 6.

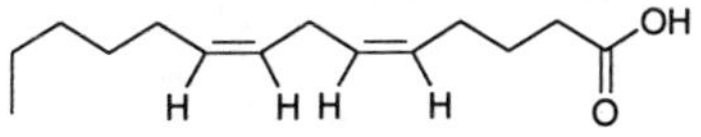

2758 Goshuyuamide-I
$C_{19}H_{19}N_3O$ MW: 305.38 Source: WU ZHU YU. Ref: 2, 347.

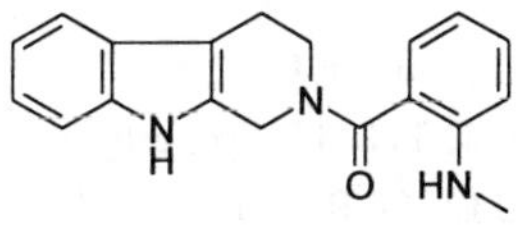

2759 Goshuyuamide-II
$C_{19}H_{17}N_3O_2$ MW: 319.37 Source: WU ZHU YU. Ref: 2.

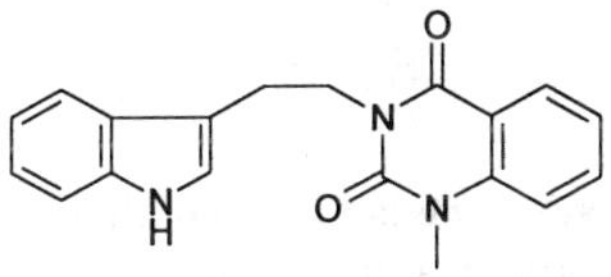

2760 Gossypetin
$C_{15}H_{10}O_8$ MW: 318.24 Property: mp 311-3°C. Source: BAI HUA YING SHAN HONG, FEI CAI, MAN SHAN, XIAO YE PI PA, YING SHAN HONG, ZHAO SHAN BAI. Ref: 6.

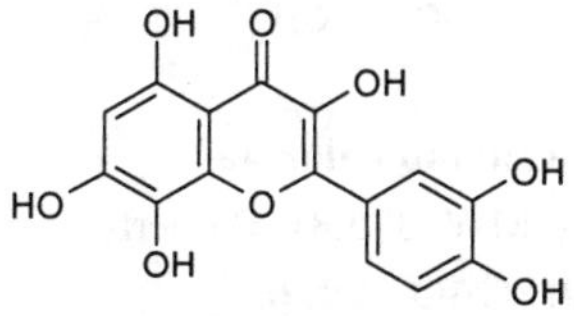

2761 Gossypetin-3-β-D-(2-O-β-D-glucopyranosidoglucopyranoside)-8-β-D-glucopyranoside
Source: MU ZEI. Ref: 2.

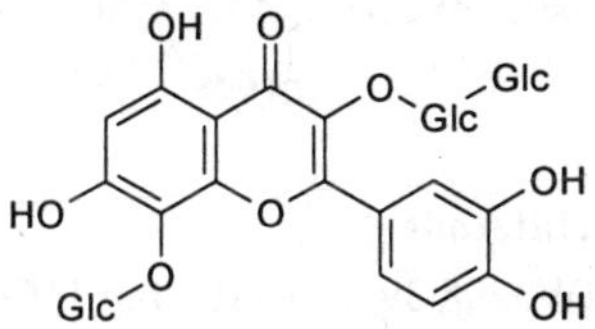

2762 Gossypetin hexamethyl ether
$C_{21}H_{22}O_8$ MW: 402.40 Property: mp 159-61°C/170-1°C. Source: JI CAI. Ref: 6.

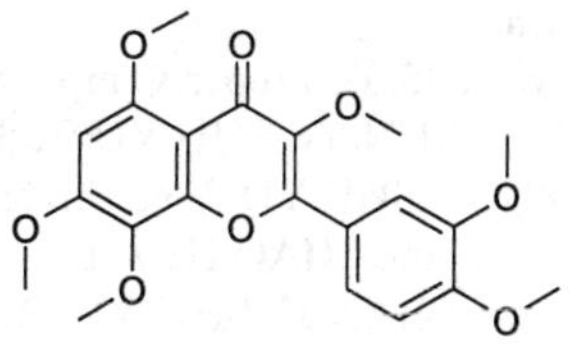

2763 Gossypetin-7-methylether
$C_{16}H_{12}O_8$ MW: 332.27 Source: DI YANG QUE. Ref: 6.

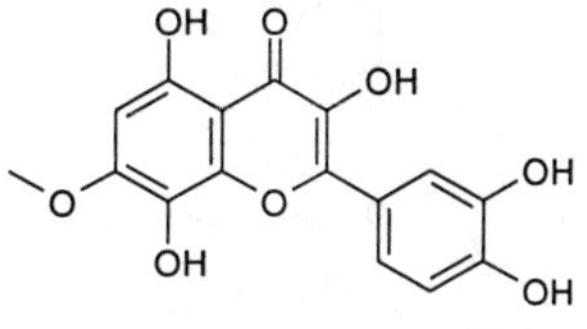

2764 Gossypin
$C_{21}H_{20}O_{13}$ MW: 480.39 Property: mp 230°C (dec). Source: FEI CAI, MO PAN CAO. Ref: 6.

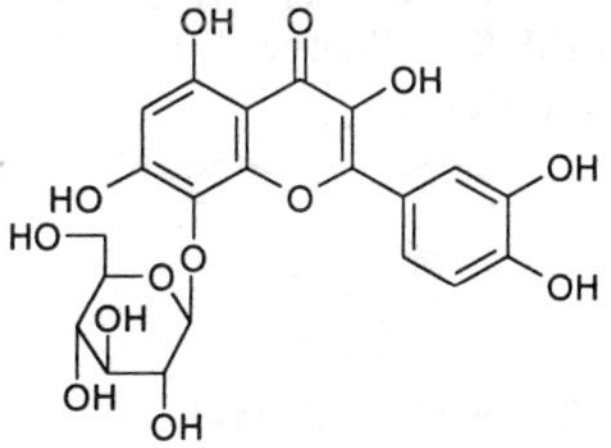

2765 Gossypitrin
$C_{21}H_{20}O_{13}$ MW: 480.39 Property: mp 252°C. Source: MU ZEI, ME PAN CAO, WEN JING. Ref: 2.

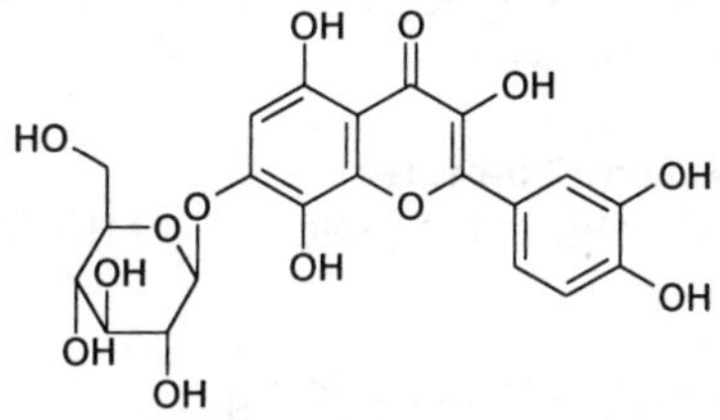

2766 Gossypol
CAS: 303-45-7 $C_{30}H_{30}O_8$ MW: 518.57 Property: mp 184°C, 199°C, 214°C. Source: DI TANG HUA, MIAN ZI YOU. Ref: 4, 5, 6.

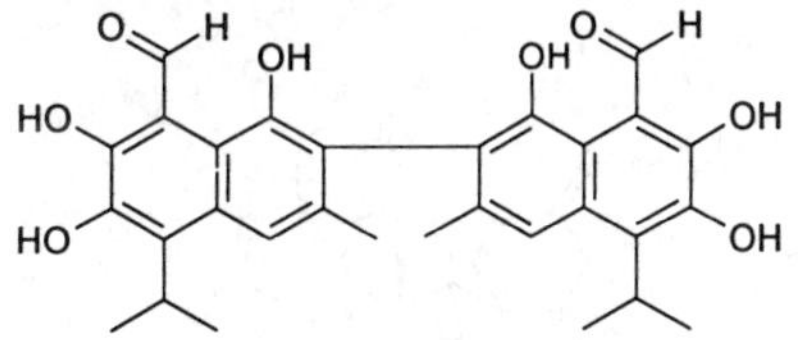

2767 Gracillin
$C_{45}H_{72}O_{17}$ MW: 885.07 Property: mp 290-3°C. Source: BEI XIE, DUN YE SHU YU fresh or dried rhizome, FU ZHOU SHU YU dried rhizome, SHU KUI YE dried rhizome, XIAO HUA DUN YE SHU YU fresh rhizome, XIAN XI SHU YU. Ref: 6, 10, 15.

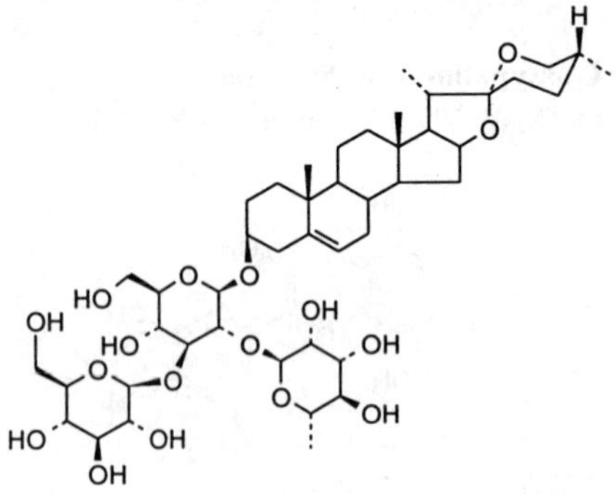

2768 Gramine
Donaxine. CAS: 87-52-5 $C_{11}H_{14}N_2$ MW: 174.25 Property: mp138-9°C. Source: JI HUA YE, LU ZHU GEN, MAI YA. Ref: 4, 6.

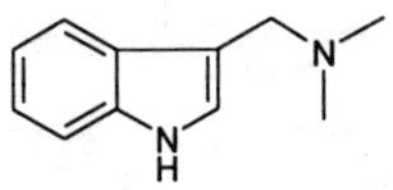

2769 Gramine methohydroxide
$C_{12}H_{17}N_2$ MW: 189.28 Source: LU ZHU GEN. Ref: 6.

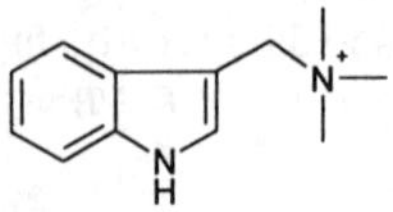

2770 Gramine Nb-oxide
$C_{11}H_{14}N_2O$ MW: 190.25 Source: LU ZHU GEN. Ref: 6.

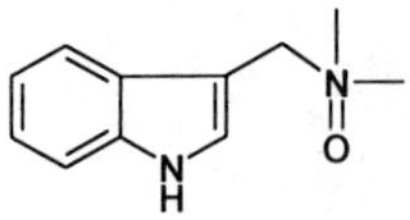

2771 Graucin A
$C_{26}H_{30}O_{10}$ MW: 502.52 Source: WU ZHU YU. Ref: 2.

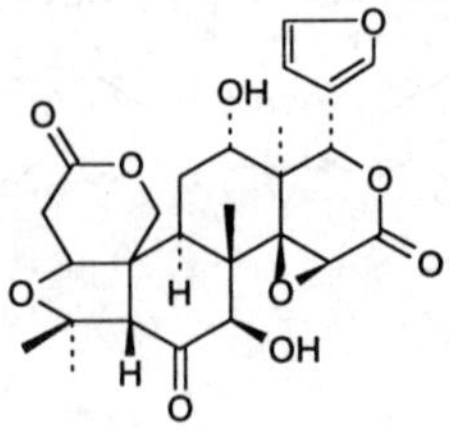

2772 Gravacridonechlorine
$C_{19}H_{18}ClNO_5$ MW: 359.81 Property: mp 254-7°C. Source: CHOU CAO. Ref: 6.

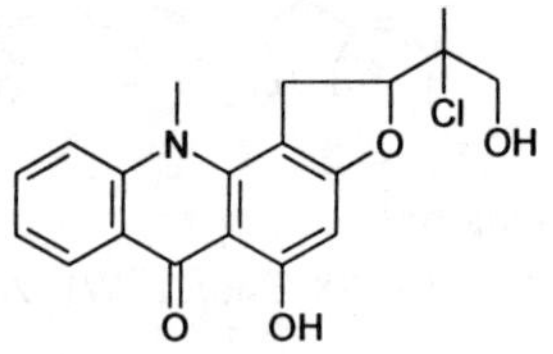

2773 Gravacridonediol
$C_{19}H_{19}NO_5$ MW: 341. 37 Property: mp 224-7°C. Source: CHOU CAO. Ref: 6.

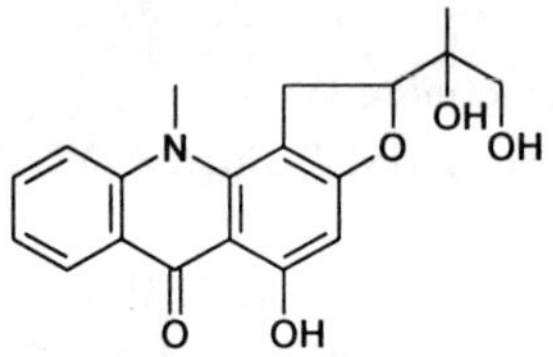

2774 Gravacridonediol monomethyl ether
$C_{20}H_{21}NO_5$ MW: 355.39 Property: mp 219-21°C. Source: CHOU CAO. Ref: 6.

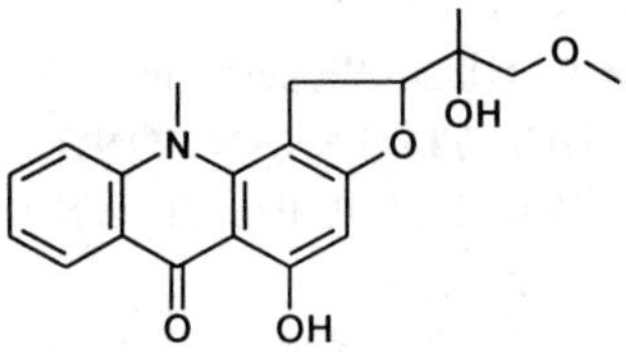

2775 Gravacridonolchlorine
$C_{19}H_{18}ClNO_5$ MW: 375.81 Property: mp 233-7°C. Source: CHOU CAO. Ref: 6.

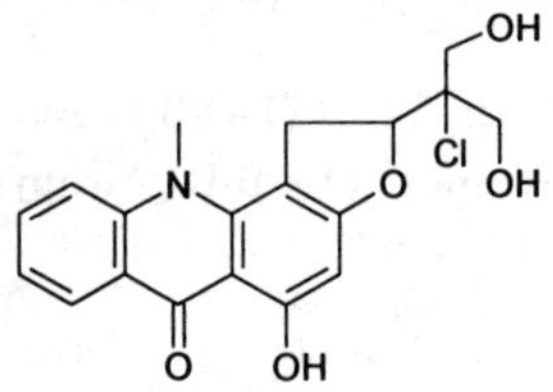

2776 Gravelliferone
$C_{19}H_{22}O_3$ MW: 298.39 Property: mp 116-8°C. Source: CHOU CAO. Ref: 6.

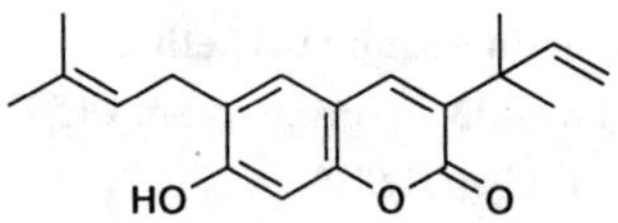

2777 Gravelliferone methyl ether
$C_{20}H_{24}O_3$ MW: 312.41 Property: mp 70-2°C. Source: CHOU CAO. Ref: 6.

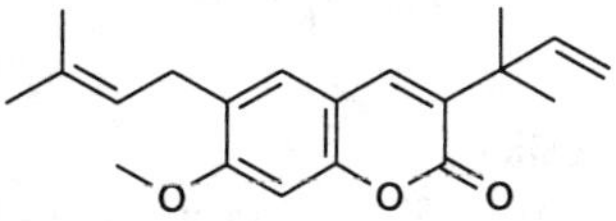

2778 Graveobioside A
Luteolin-7-apio-glucoside. Property: mp 251-2°C. Source: HAN QIN. Ref: 6.

2780 Graveoline
$C_{17}H_{13}NO_3$ MW: 279.30 Property: mp 204-5°C. Source: CHOU CAO. Ref: 6.

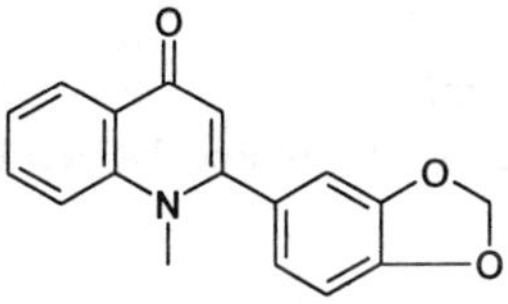

2781 Graveolinine
$C_{17}H_{15}NO_3$ MW: 281.31 Property: mp 115-6°C. Source: CHOU CAO. Ref: 6.

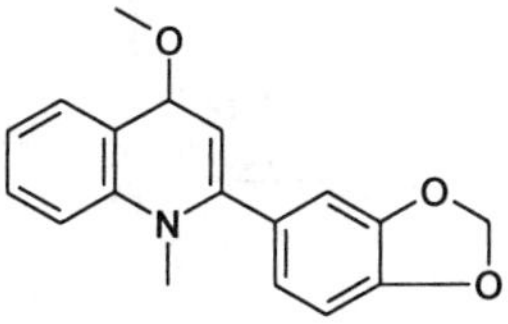

2782 Guaiacol
$C_7H_8O_2$ MW: 124.14 Property: mp 32°C, bp 205°C. Source: AN YE, DANG GUI, LIANG YE HUAPI, SANG YE, WU HUA GUO YE. Ref: 2.

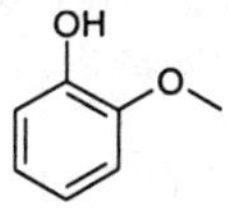

2783 (-)-Guaia-1 (10), 11-dien-15-al
$C_{15}H_{22}O$ MW: 218.34 Source: CHEN XIANG. Ref: 13.

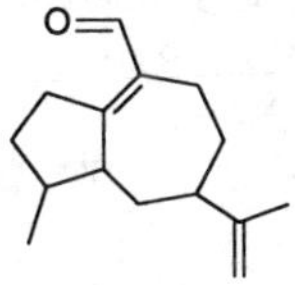

2784 (-)-Guaia-1 (11), 11-dien-15-al
$C_{15}H_{24}O$ MW: 220.36 Source: CHEN XIANG. Ref: 13

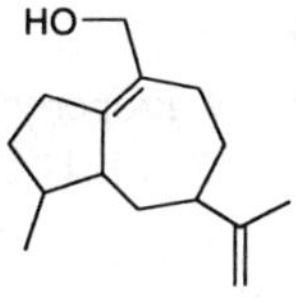

2785 (-)-Guaia-1 (10), 11-dien-15-carboxylic acid
$C_{15}H_{22}O_2$ MW: 234.34 Source: CHEN XIANG. Ref: 13.

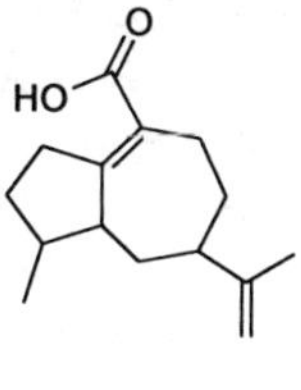

2786 (-)-Guaia-1 (10),11-dien-15,2-olide
$C_{16}H_{24}O_2$ MW: 248.37 Source: CHEN XIANG. Ref: 13.

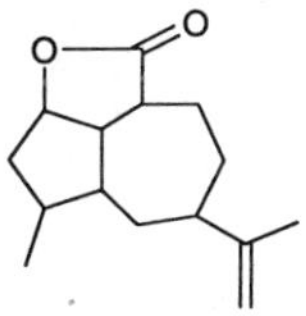

2787 (+)-Guaia-1 (10),11-dien-9-one
$C_{15}H_{22}O$ MW: 218.34 Source: CHEN XIANG. Ref: 13.

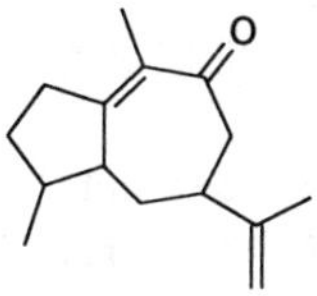

2788 α-Guaiene
$C_{15}H_{24}$ MW: 204.36 Property: 78-9°C/2.5mm. Source: HUO XIANG, REN SHEN, SAN QI. Ref: 2.

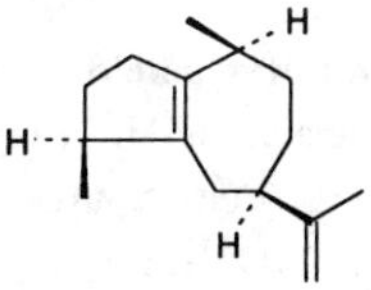

2789 δ-Guaiene
$C_{15}H_{24}$ MW: 204.36 Property: bp 118°C/8mm. Source: HUO XIANG, SAN QI. Ref: 2.

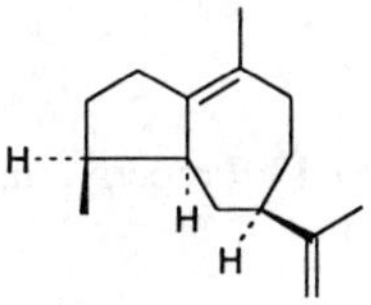

2790 Guaijaverin

$C_{21}H_{20}O_{11}$ MW: 448.39 Property: mp 256°C. Source: DIAO GAN MA, FAN SHI LIU GAN, FAN SHI LIU YE. Ref: 6.

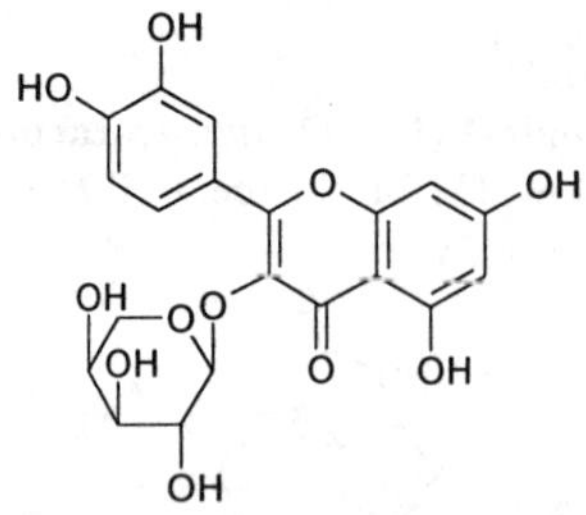

2791 Guaiol

$C_{15}H_{26}O$ MW: 222.37 Property: mp 91°C, bp 288°C. Source: AN YE, DU HUO, HOU PO, NING MENG, QIANG HUO. Ref: 2.

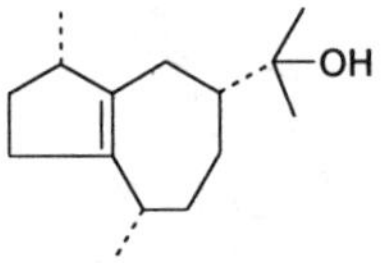

2792 Guanidine

CH_5N_3 MW: 59.07 Source: GUI GAI, QIU YIN, SHUI NIU JIAO. Ref: 6.

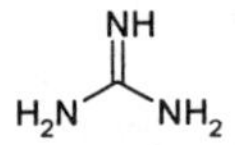

2793 4-Guanidino-1-butanol

$C_5H_{13}N_3O$ MW: 131.18 Source: YI MU CAO. Ref: 6.

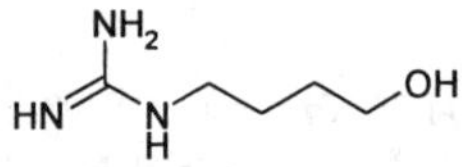

2794 γ-Guanidinobutyric acid

4-Guanidino-butyric acid. $C_5H_{11}N_3O_2$ MW: 145.16 Property: mp 276-8°C (dec). Source: WANG GUA ZI, WEI NAO, YI MU CAO. Ref: 6.

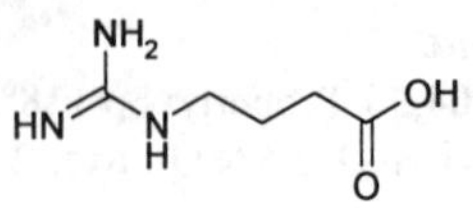

2795 Guanine

$C_5H_5N_5O$ MW: 151.13 Property: mp >300°C. Source: QIU YIN. Ref: 6.

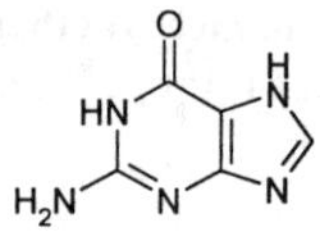

2796 Guanosine

$C_{10}H_{13}N_5O_5$ MW: 283.25 Property: mp 230-5°C (dec). Source: BAN XIA, MAI JIAO. Ref: 2.

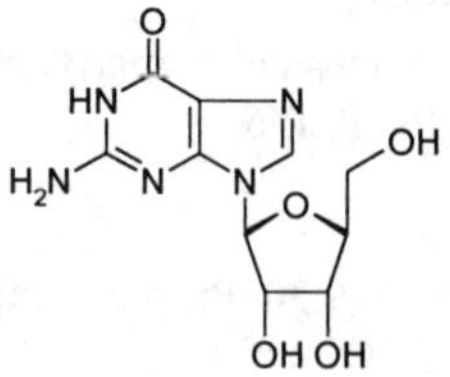

2797 Guidongnin

Property: mp 233-4°C. Source: DONG LING CAO. Ref: 501.

2798 α-Guriunene

$C_{15}H_{24}$ MW: 204.36 Property: bp 114-6°C/10mm. Source: BAI ZHI, HUO XIANG, HE SHI, REN SHEN, SAN QI, SHUI CAI. Ref: 2.

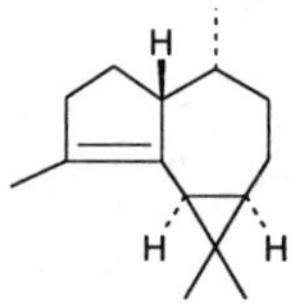

2799 β-Guriunene

1(10)-Aristolene. $C_{15}H_{24}$ MW: 204.36 Property: 120-3°C/13mm. Source: GAN SONG, HUO XIANG, REN SHEN, XI YANG SHEN, HUO XIANG. Ref: 2.

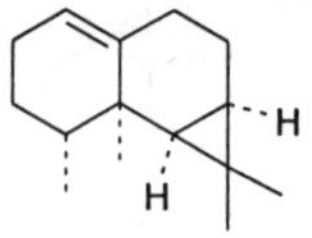

2800 α-Guttiferin

$C_{27}H_{32}O_6$ MW: 452.55 Property: mp 113-5°C. Source: TENG HUANG. Ref: 6.

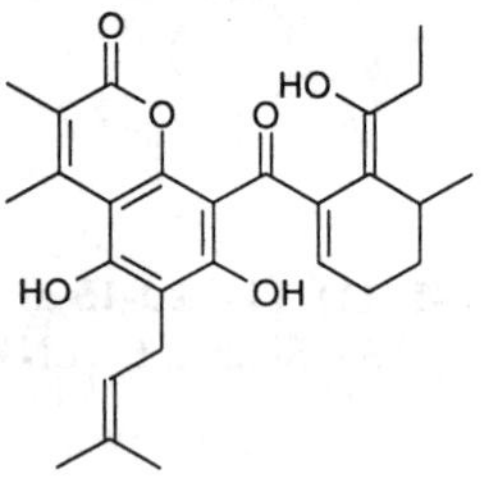

2801 Guvacine
$C_6H_9NO_2$ MW: 127.14 Property: mp 285°C (dec). Source: BING LANG. Ref: 6.

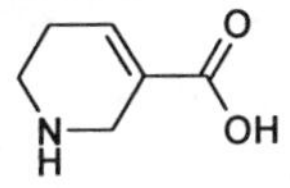

2802 Guvacoline
$C_7H_{11}NO_2$ MW: 14.17 Property: mp 27°C, bp 114°C/14mm. Source: BING LANG. Ref: 2.

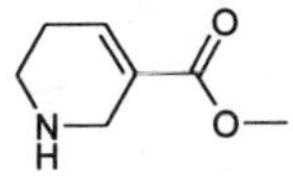

2803 Gycomoside I
1β,3β,12β,20(S),26-pentahydroxy-dammer-24(25)-en-20(S)-O-β-D-glucopyranosyl-(1→6)-β-D-glucopyranoside $C_{42}H_{72}O_{15}$ MW: 817.03 Property: colorless acicular crystal, mp 196-7°C, $[\alpha]_D^{22}$ + 18.56° (c= 1.67, MeOH). Source: BIAN GUO JIAO GU LAN. Ref: 266.

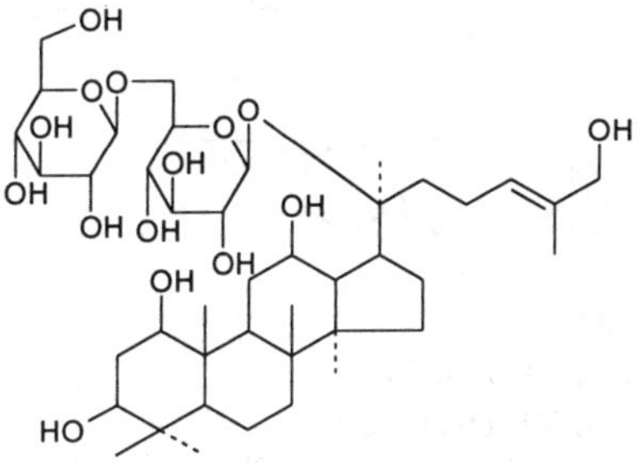

2804 Gycomoside II
1β,3β,12β,20(S)-tetrahydroxy-dammer-24(25)-en-3-O-β-D-glucopyranosyl-20(S)-O-β-D-glucopyranosyl-(1→6)-β-D-glucopyranoside $C_{48}H_{82}O_{19}$ MW: 963.18 Property: white powder, mp 195-7°C, $[\alpha]_D^{22}$ +21.05°(c=0.57, MeOH). Source: BIAN GUO JIAO GU LAN. Ref: 266.

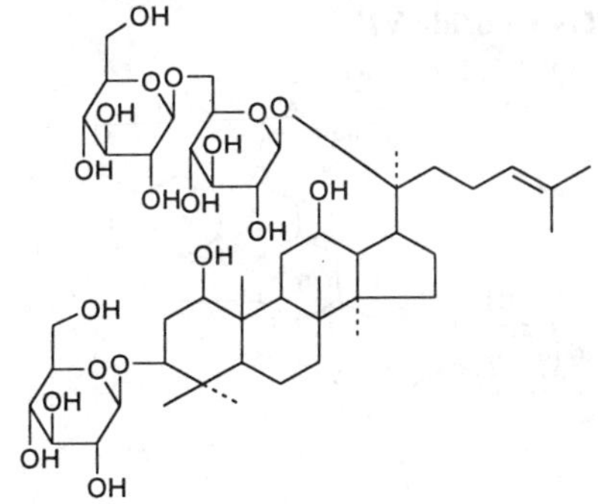

2805 Gycomoside III
1β,3β,12β,20(S),26-pentahydroxy-dammer-24(25)-en-20(S)-O-β-D-glucopyranoside. $C_{36}H_{62}O_{10}$ MW: 654.89 Property: light yellowder powder, mp 178-80°C, $[\alpha]_D^{22}$ +23.73°(c=0.59, MeOH). Source: BIAN GUO JIAO GU LAN. Ref: 266.

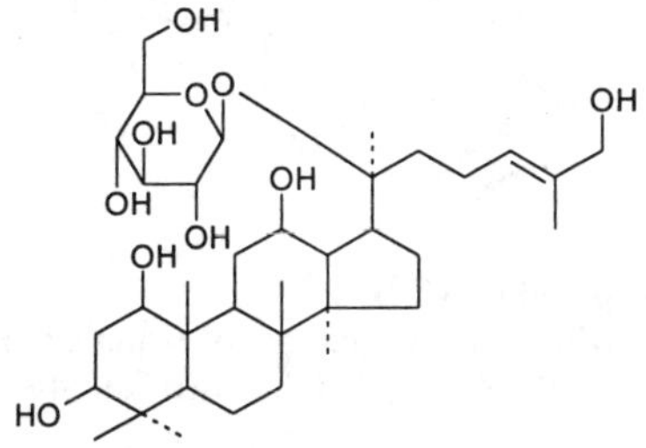

2806 Gycomoside IV
1β,3β,12β,20(S),26-pentahydroxy-dammer-24(25)-en-3-O-β-D-glucopyranosyl-20(S)-O-β-D-glucopyranosyl (1→6)-β-D-glucopyranoside $C_{48}H_{82}O_{20}$ MW: 979.18 Property: white powder, mp 207-9°C, $[\alpha]_D^{22}$ +12.96° (c=1.08, MeOH). Source: BIAN GUO JIAO GU LAN. Ref: 266.

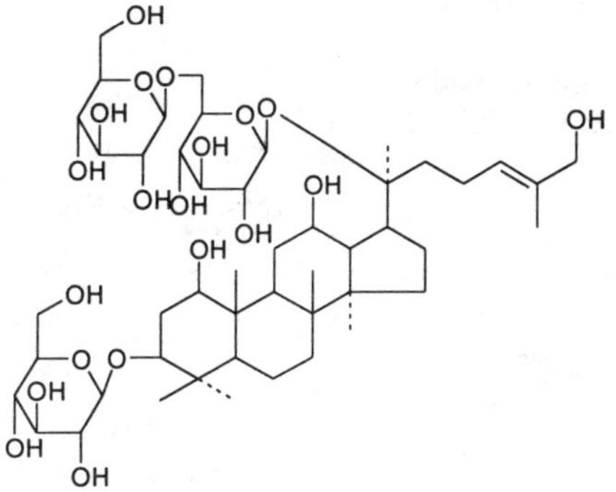

2807 Gylongiposide I
$C_{46}H_{76}O_{16}$ MW: 885.11 Property: white crystalline powder, mp 219.5-20 °C, $[\alpha]_D^{20}$ -1.7° (c=1.0, methanol). Source: CHANG GENG JIAO GU LAN . Ref: 390.

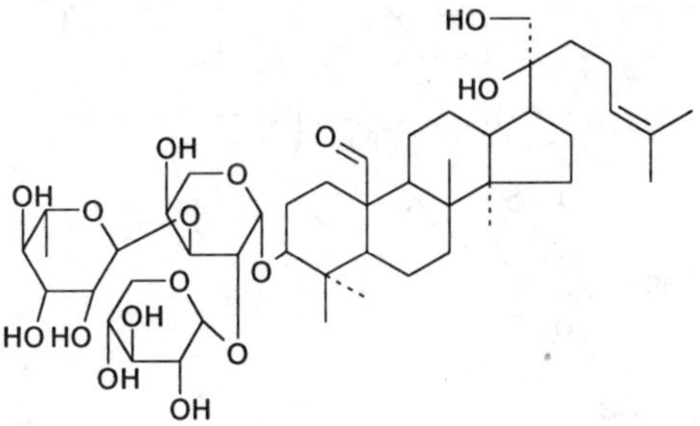

2808 Gymnaconitine
$C_{34}H_{47}NO_8$ MW: 597.76 Property: white acicular crystal, mp 110-1°C, $[\alpha]_D^{17}$ +18.2°. Source: LU RUI WU TOU. Ref: 52.

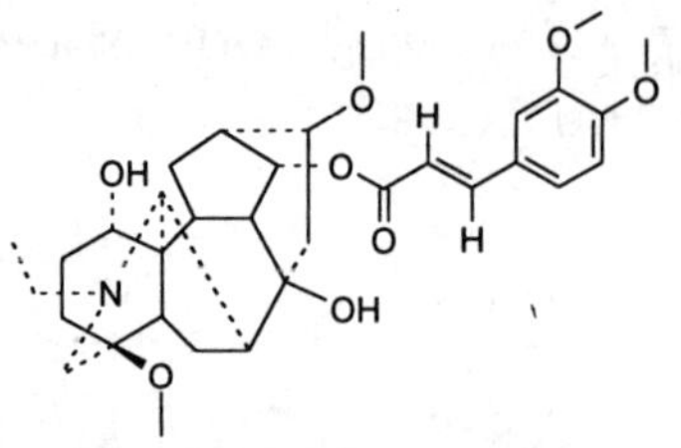

2809 Gypenoide XVII
Property: white powder (methanol-water), mp 157-9°C. Source: REN SHEN HUA LEI. Ref: 446.

2810 Gypenoside I
Source: QI YE DAN. Ref: 2.

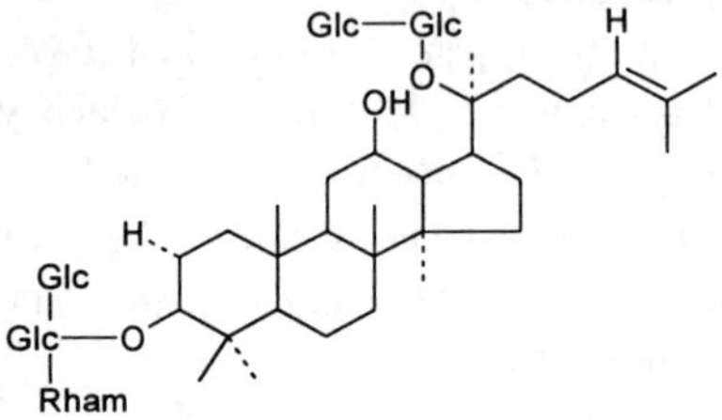

2811 Gypenoside II
Source: QI YE DAN. Ref: 2.

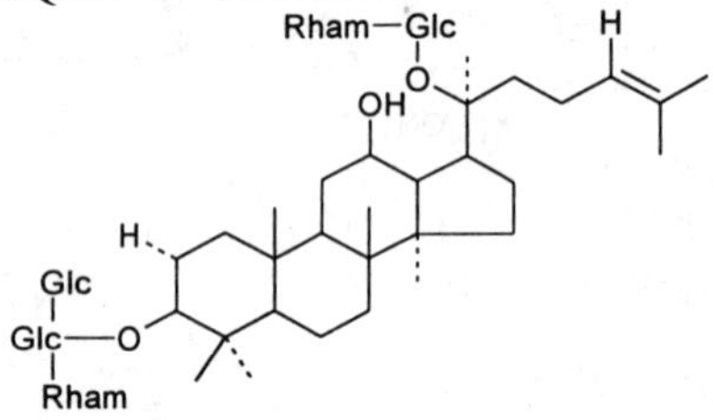

2812 Gypenoside III
$C_{54}H_{92}O_{23}$ MW: 1109.32 Source: QI YE DAN. Ref: 2.

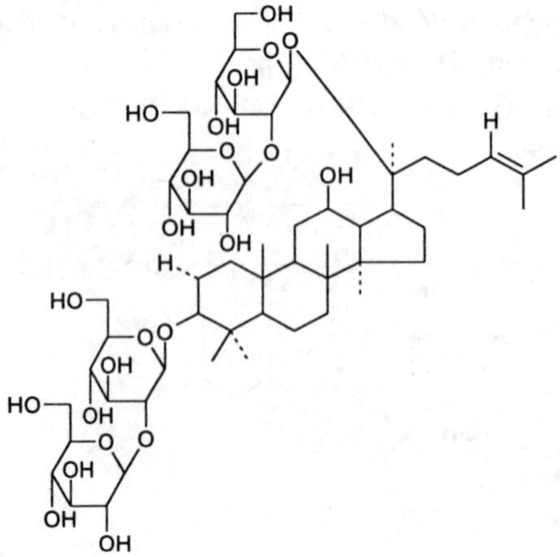

2813 Gypenoside IV
$C_{52}H_{90}O_{22}$ MW: 1079.32 Source: QI YE DAN. Ref: 2.

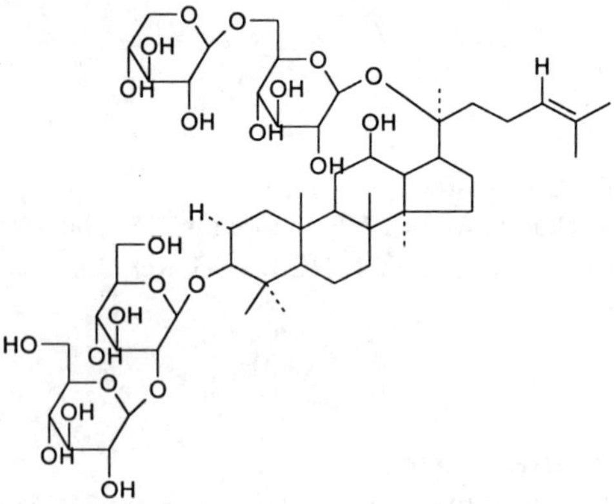

2814 Gypenoside V
Source: QI YE DAN. Ref: 2.

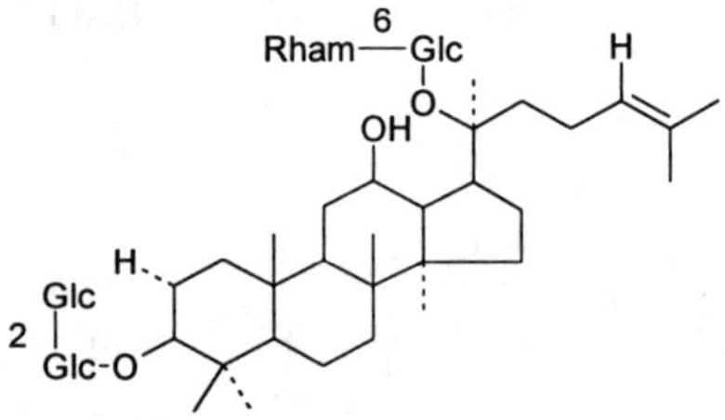

2815 Gypenoside VI
Source: QI YE DAN. Ref: 2.

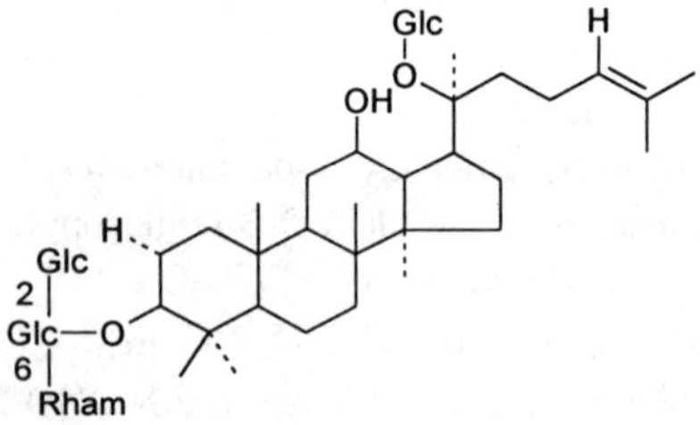

2816 Gypenoside VII
Source: QI YE DAN. Ref: 2.

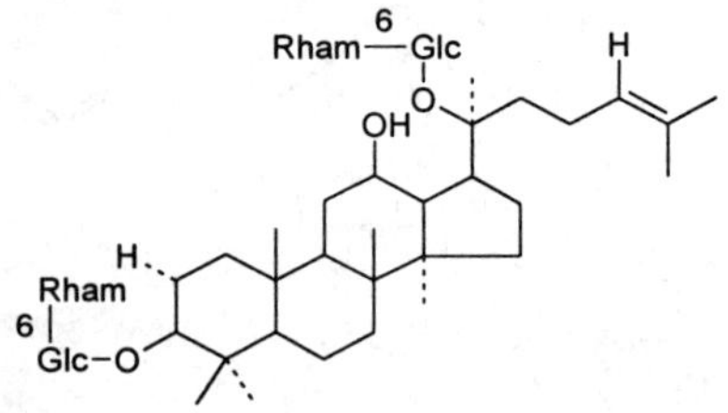

2817 Gypenoside VIII
Source: QI YE DAN. Ref: 2.

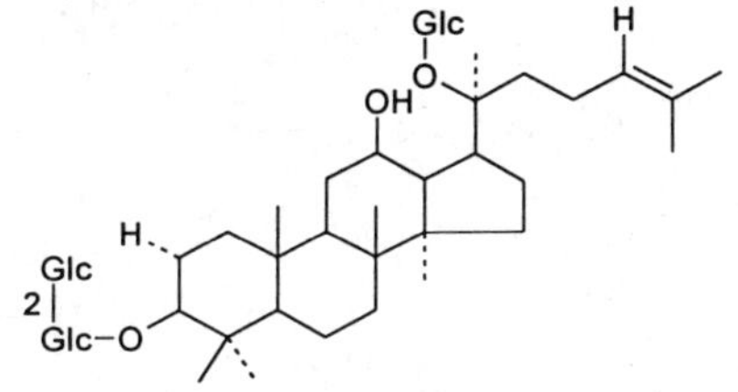

2818 Gypenoside IX
Source: QI YE DAN. Ref: 2.

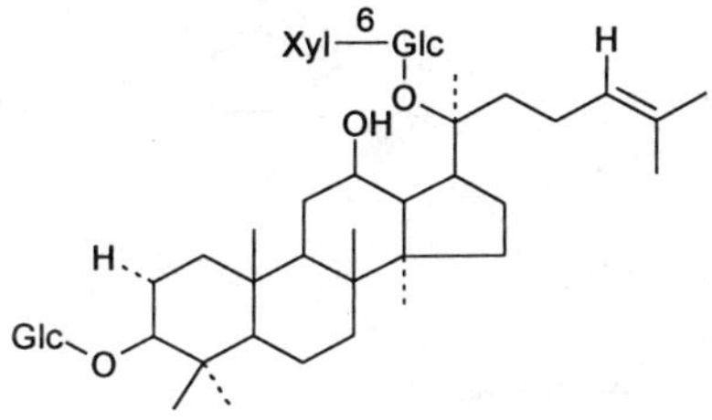

2819 Gypenoside X
Source: QI YE DAN. Ref: 2.

2820 Gypenoside XI
Source: QI YE DAN. Ref: 2.

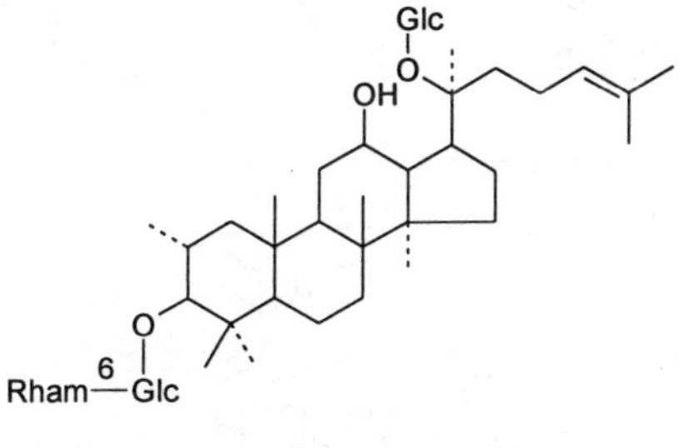

2821 Gypenoside XII
Source: QI YE DAN. Ref: 2.

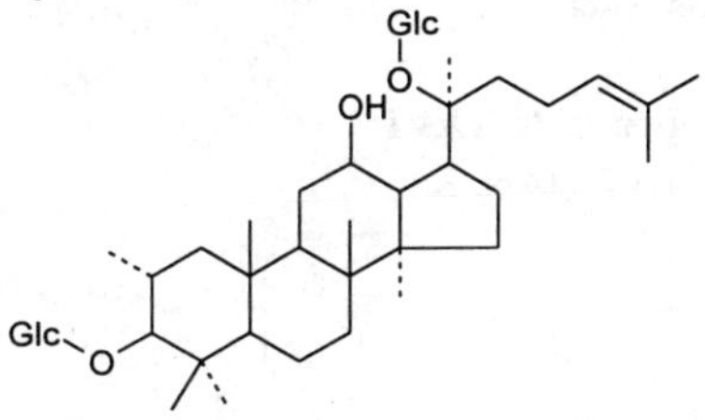

2822 Gypenoside XIII
Source: QI YE DAN. Ref: 2.

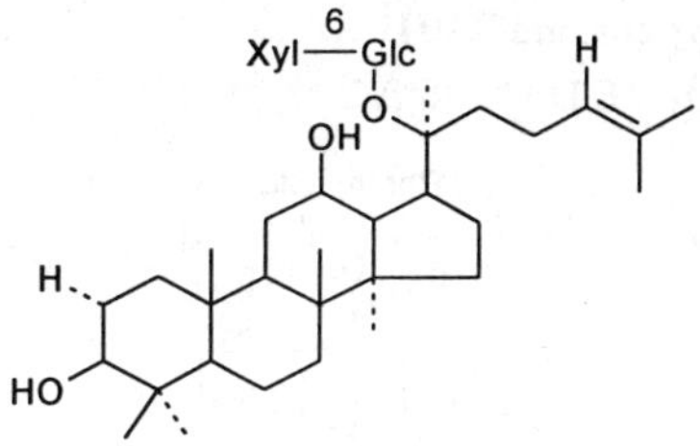

2823 Gypenoside XIV
Source: QI YE DAN. Ref: 2.

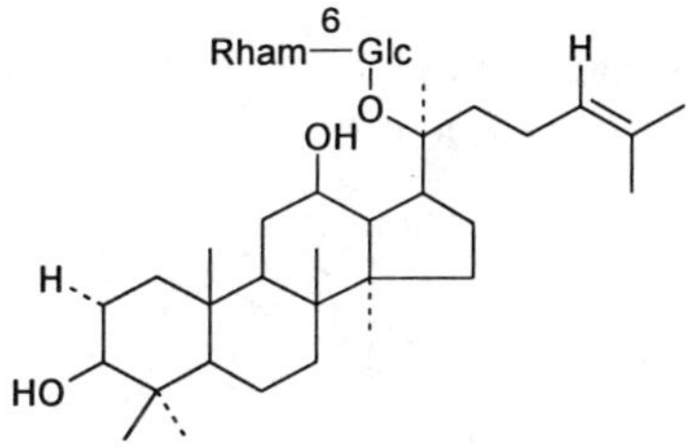

2824 Gypenoside XV
Source: QI YE DAN. Ref: 2.

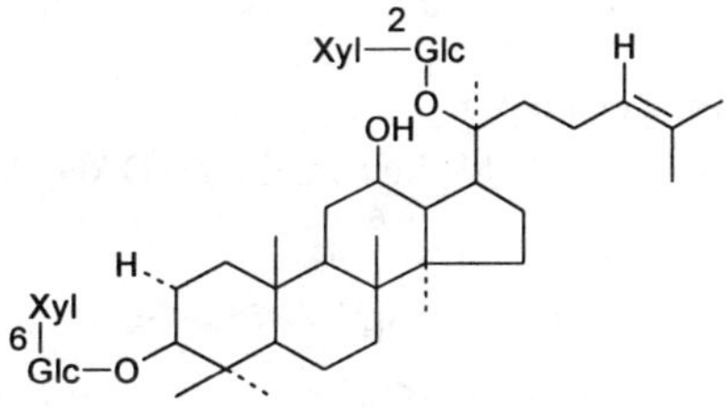

2825 Gypenoside XVI
Source: QI YE DAN. Ref: 2.

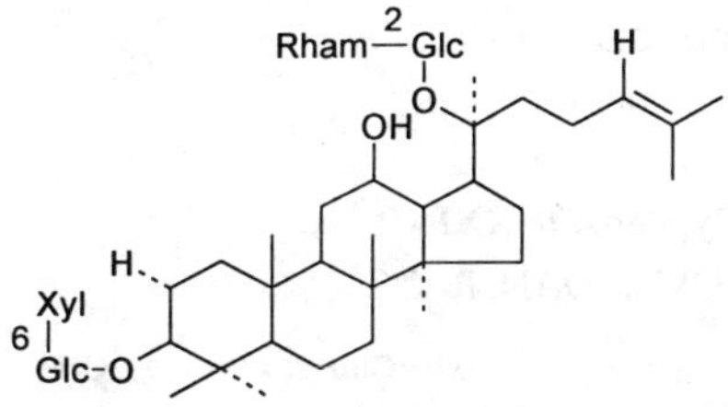

2826 Gypenoside XVII
Source: QI YE DAN. Ref: 2.

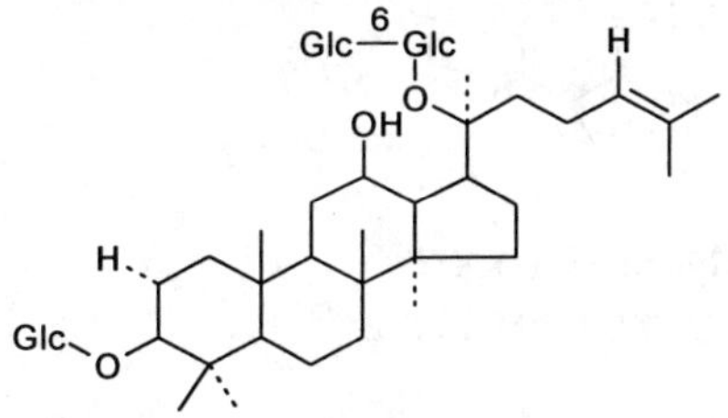

2827 Gypenoside XVIII

Source: QI YE DAN. Ref: 2.

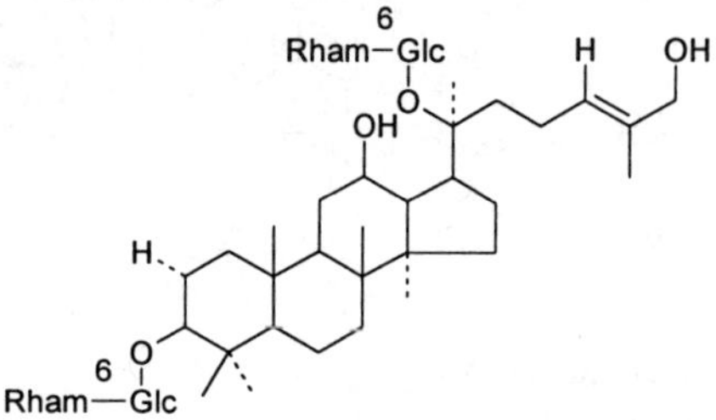

2828 Gypenoside XIX

Source: QI YE DAN. Ref: 2.

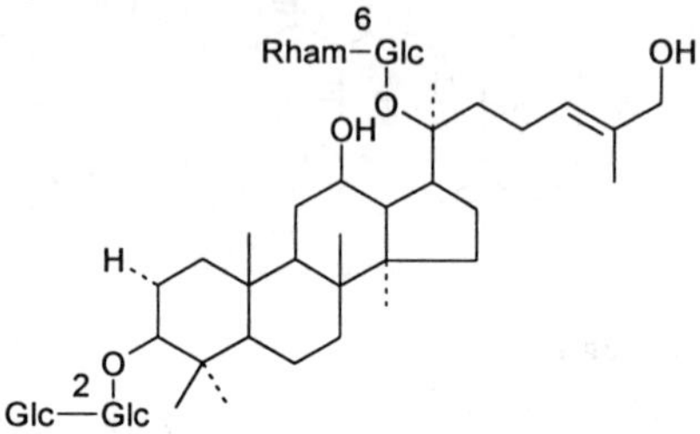

2829 Gypenoside XX

$C_{35}H_{62}O_4$ MW: 546.88 Source: QI YE DAN. Ref: 2.

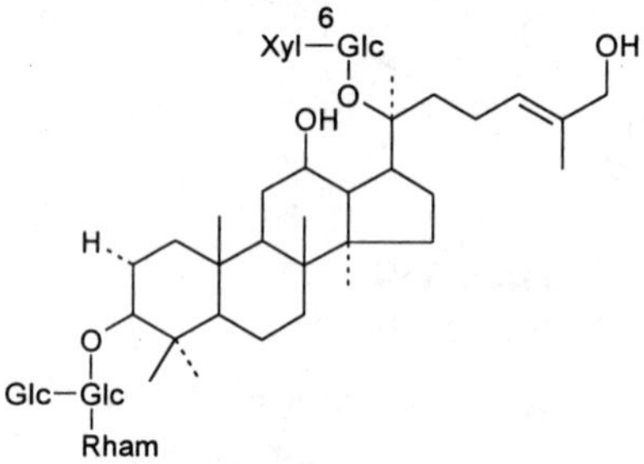

2830 Gypenoside XXI

Source: QI YE DAN. Ref: 2.

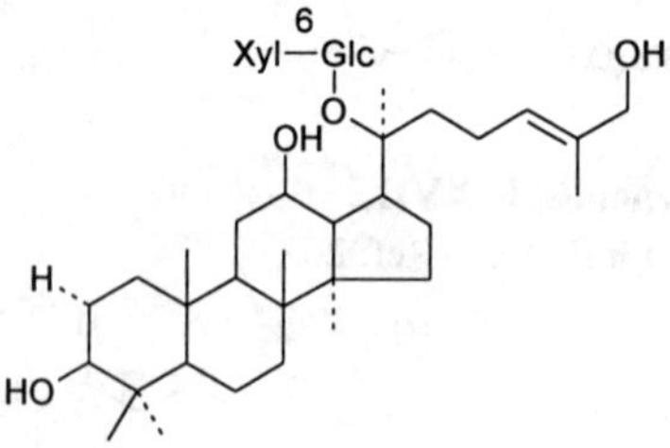

2831 Gypenoside XXII

Source: QI YE DAN. Ref: 2.

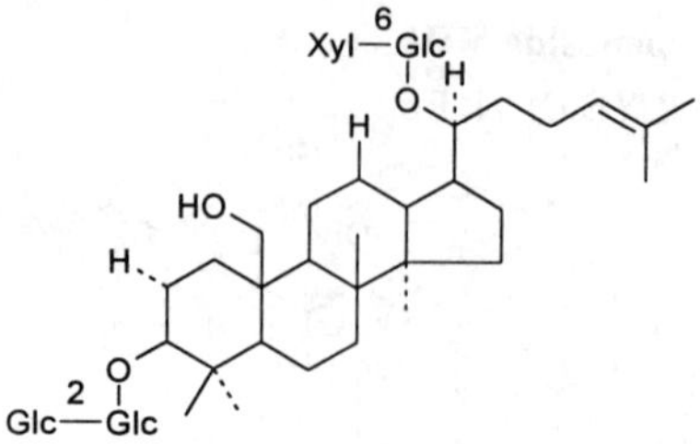

2832 Gypenoside XVIII

Source: QI YE DAN. Ref: 2.

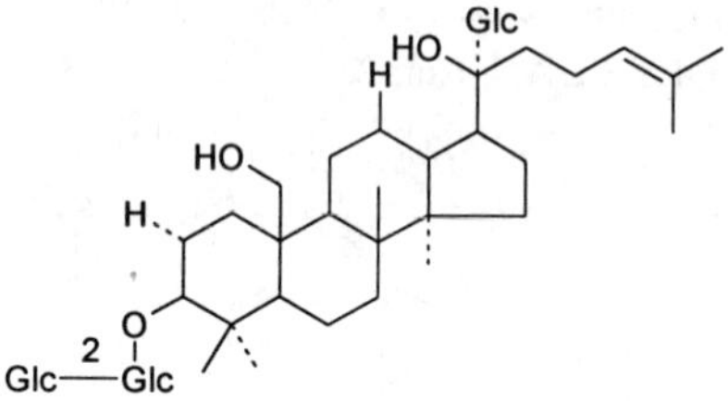

2833 Gypenoside XXIV

Source: QI YE DAN. Ref: 2.

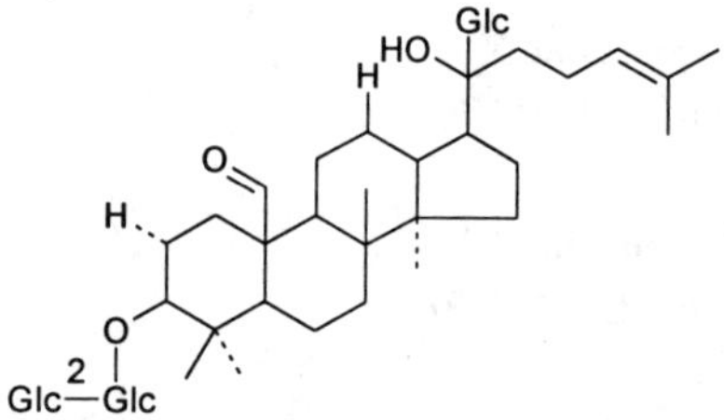

2834 Gypenoside XXV

Source: QI YE DAN. Ref: 2.

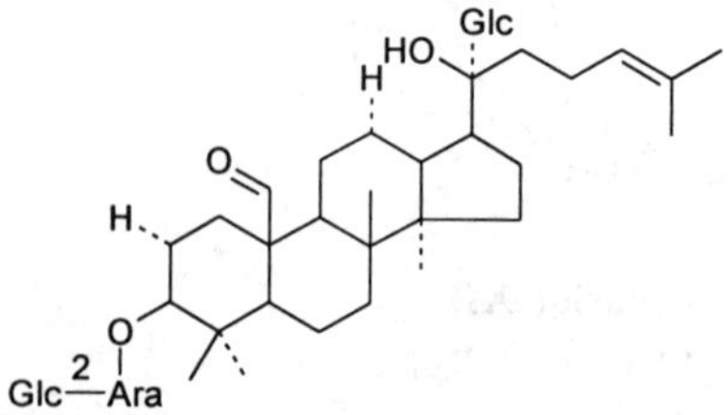

2835 Gypenoside XXVI

Source: QI YE DAN. Ref: 2.

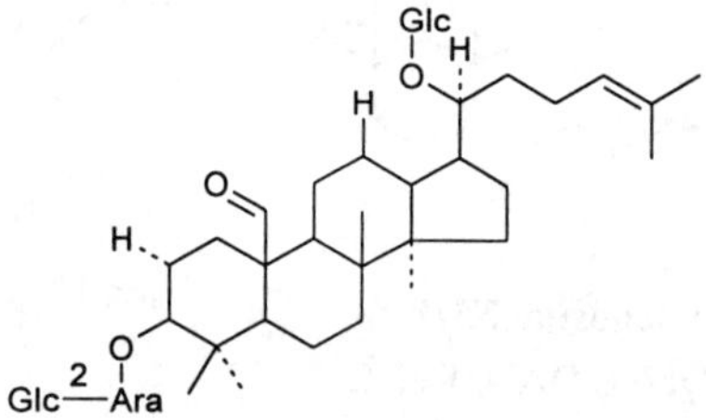

2836 Gypenoside XXVII
Source: QI YE DAN. Ref: 2.

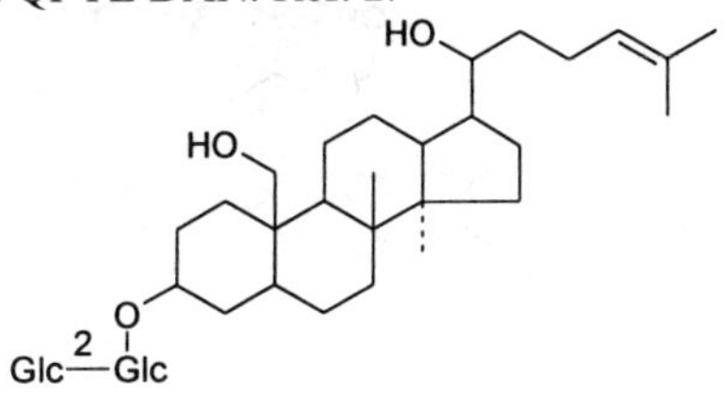

2837 Gypenoside XXVIII
Source: QI YE DAN. Ref: 2.

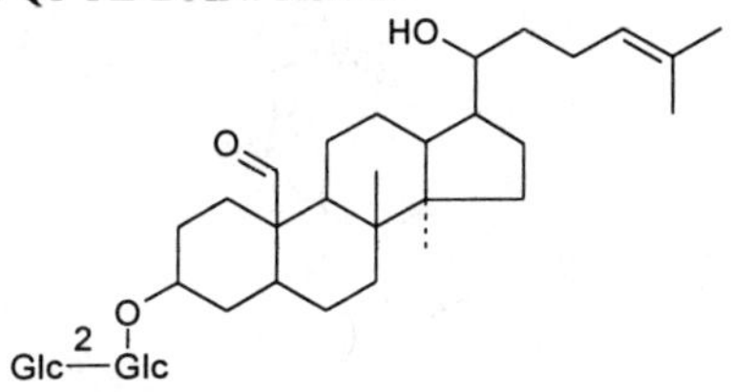

2838 Gypenoside XXIX
Source: QI YE DANV. Ref: 2.

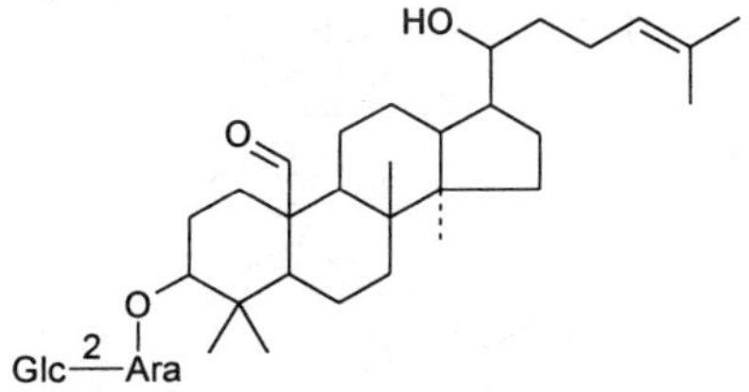

2839 Gypenoside XXX
Source: QI YE DAN. Ref: 2.

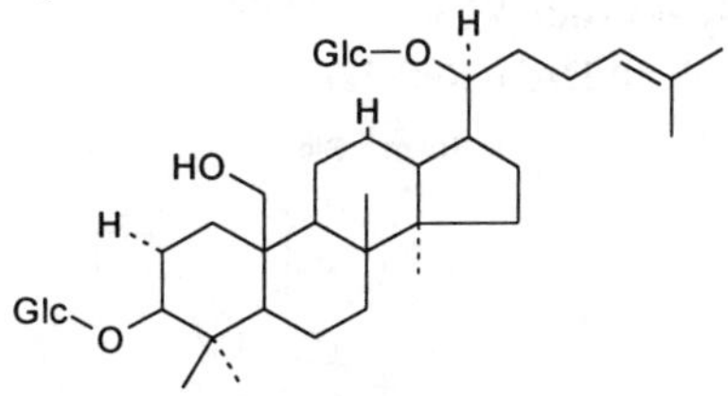

2840 Gypenoside XXXI
Source: QI YE DAN. Ref: 2.

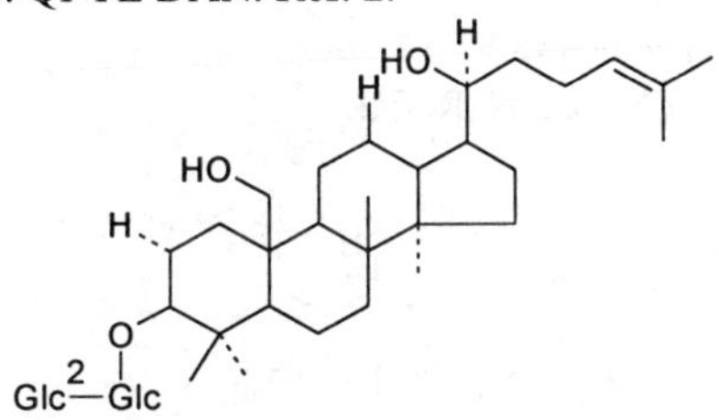

2841 Gypenoside XXXII
Source: QI YE DAN. Ref: 2.

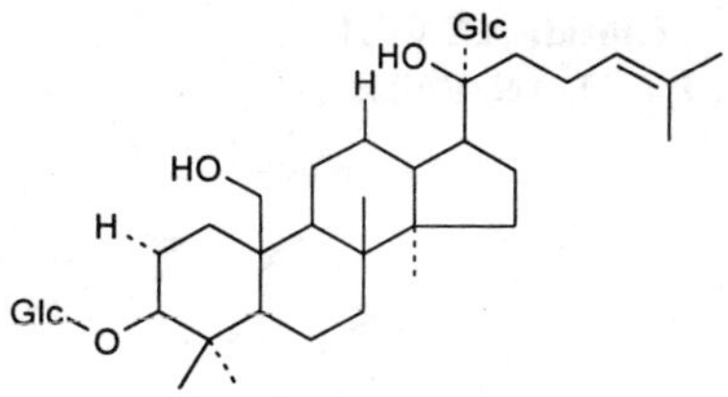

2842 Gypenoside XXVIII
Source: QI YE DAN. Ref: 2.

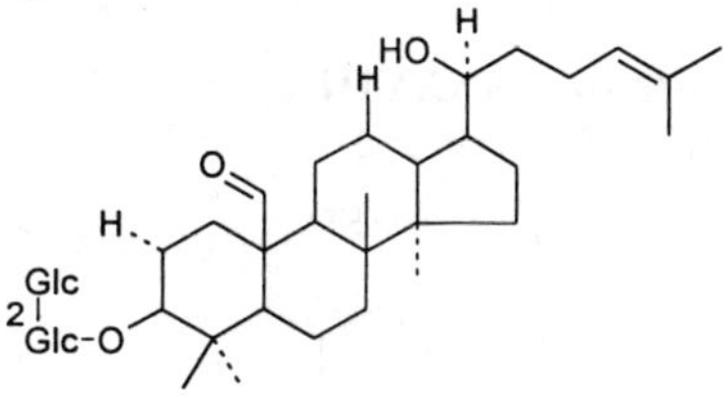

2843 Gypenoside XXXIV
Source: QI YE DANV. Ref: 2.

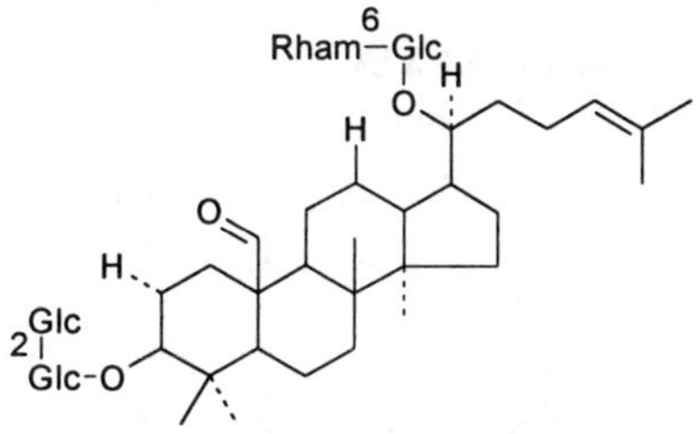

2844 Gypenoside XXXV
Source: QI YE DAN. Ref: 2.

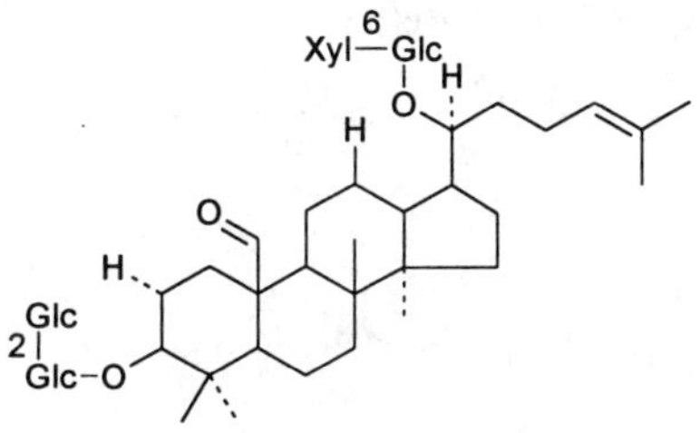

2845 Gypenoside XXXVI
Source: QI YE DAN. Ref: 2.

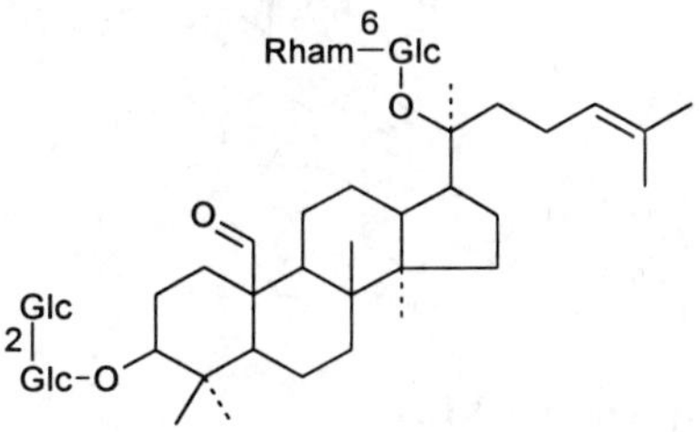

2846 Gypenoside XXXVII
Source: QI YE DAN. Ref: 2.

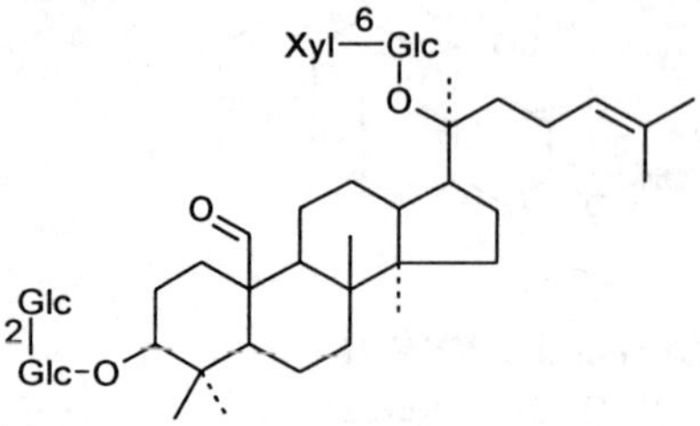

2847 Gypenoside XXXVIII
Source: QI YE DAN. Ref: 2.

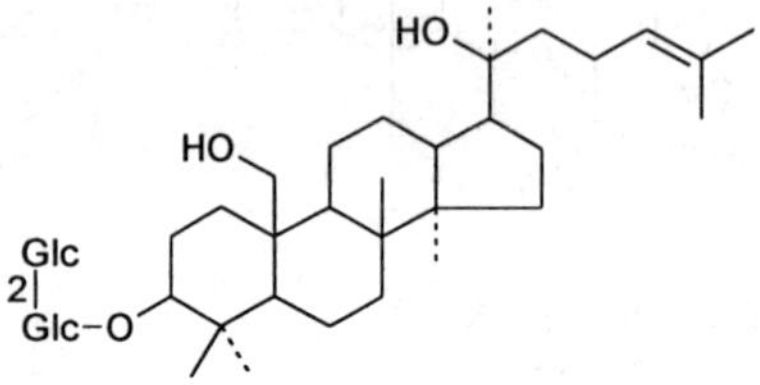

2848 Gypenoside XXXIX
Source: QI YE DAN. Ref: 2.

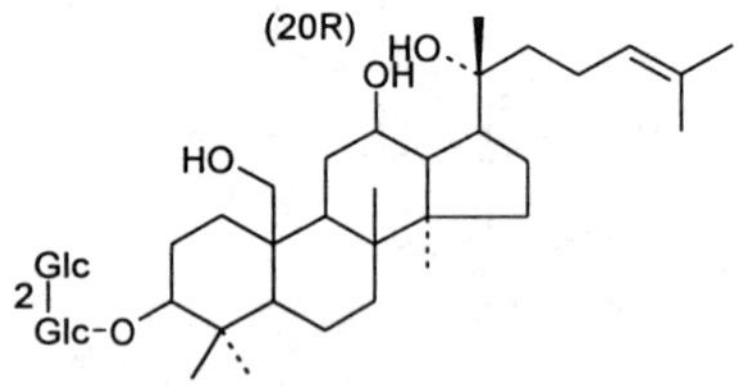

2849 Gypenoside XL
Source: QI YE DAN. Ref: 2.

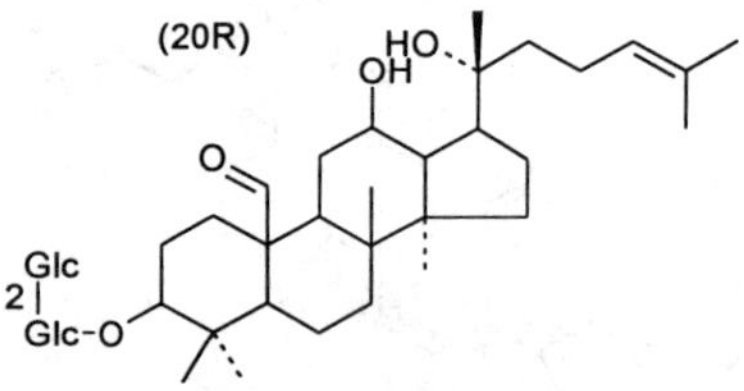

2850 Gypenoside XLI
$C_{32}H_{56}O_3$ MW: 488.80 Source: QI YE DAN. Ref: 2.

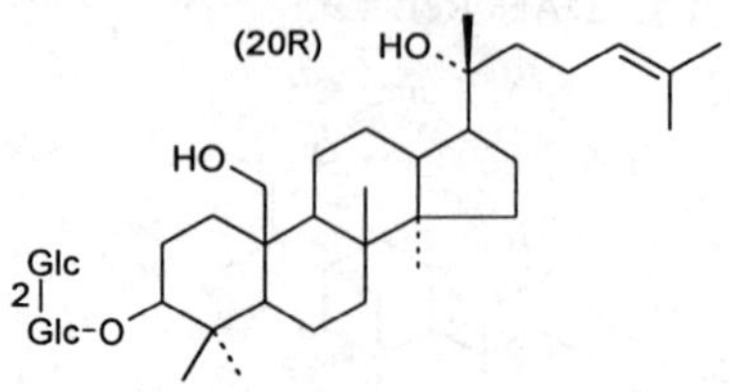

2851 Gypenoside XLII
Source: HUI GUO JIAO GU LAN, QI YE DAN. Ref: 2, 329.

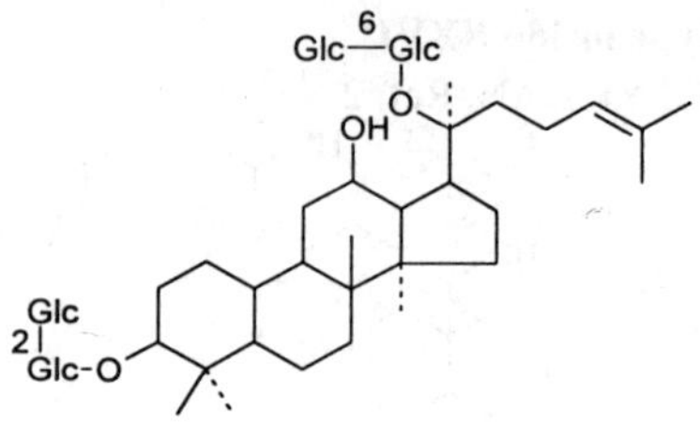

2852 Gypenoside XLIII
Source: QI YE DAN. Ref: 2.

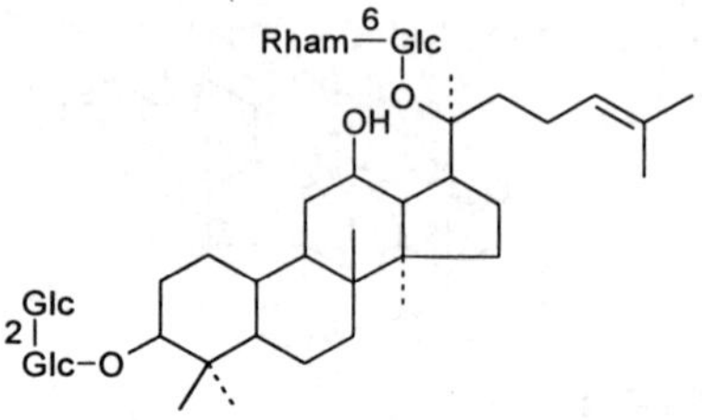

2853 Gypenoside XLIV
$C_{32}H_{56}O_3$ MW: 488.80 Source: HUI GUO JIAO GU LAN, QI YE DAN. Ref: 2, 329.

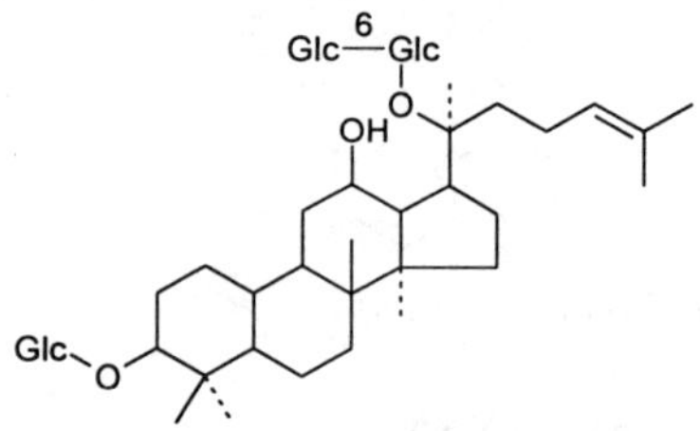

2854 Gypenoside XLV
Source: QI YE DAN. Ref: 2.

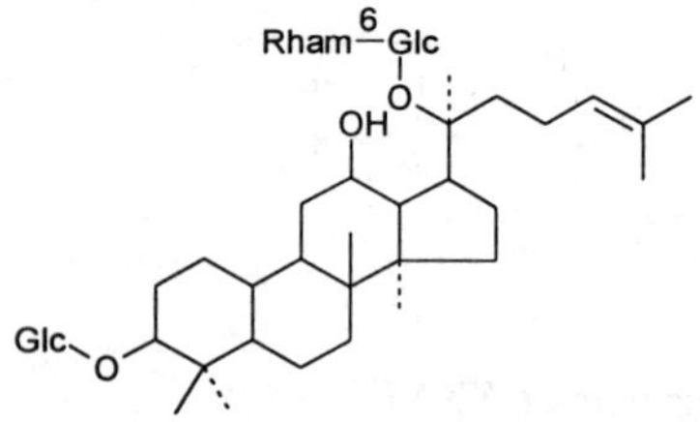

2855 Gypenoside XLVI
Source: QI YE DAN. Ref: 2.

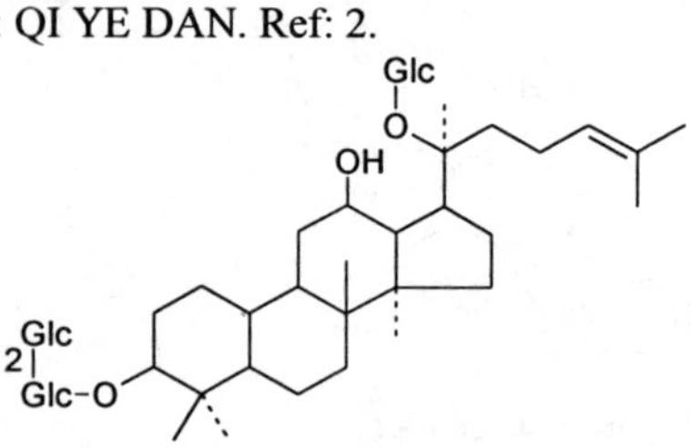

2856 Gypenoside XLVII
Source: QI YE DAN. Ref: 2.

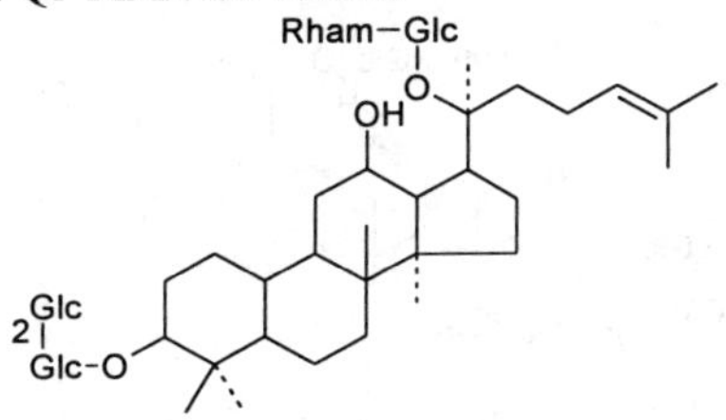

2857 GypenosideXLVIII
Source: QI YE DAN. Ref: 2.

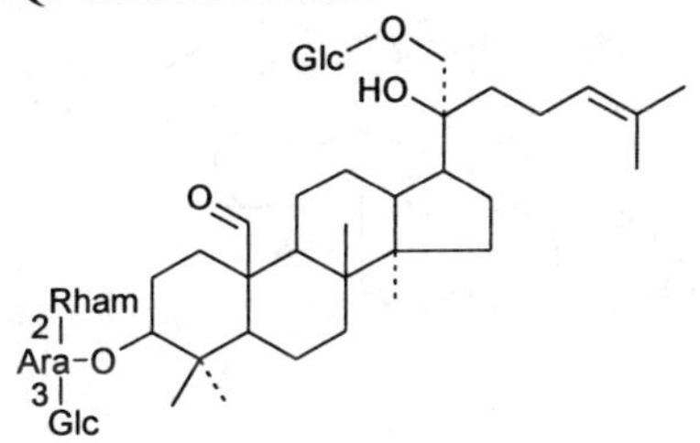

2858 Gypenoside XLIX
Source: QI YE DAN. Ref: 2.

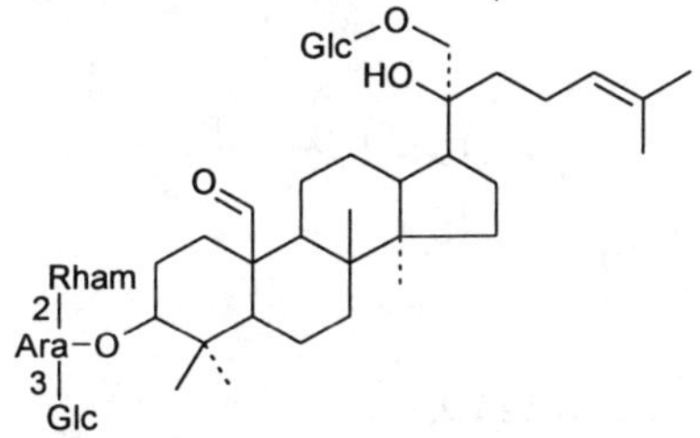

2859 Gypenoside L
Source: QI YE DAN. Ref: 2.

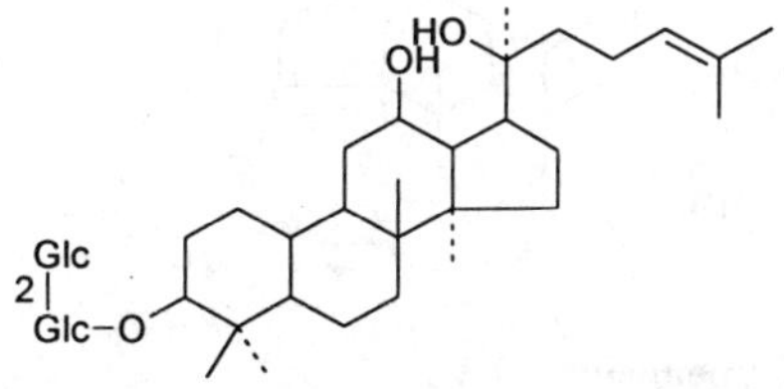

2860 Gypenoside LI
Source: QI YE DAN. Ref: 2.

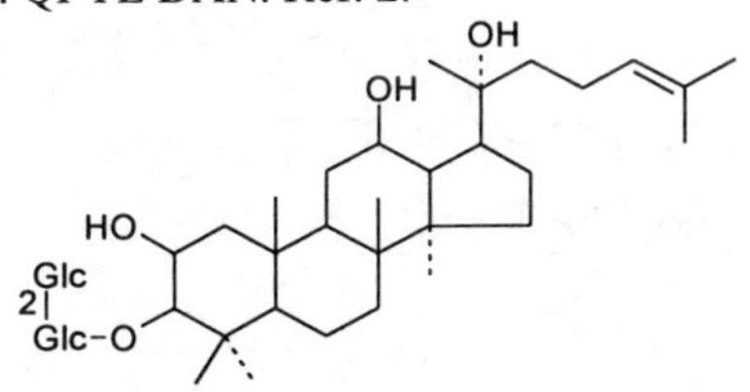

2861 Gypenoside LII
Source: QI YE DAN. Ref: 2.

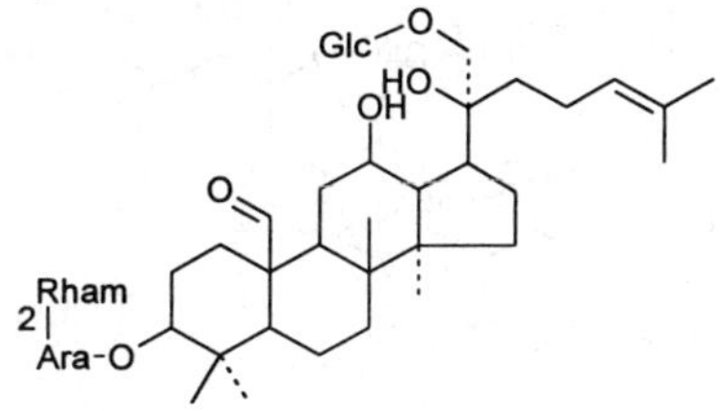

2862 Gypenoside LIII
Source: QI YE DAN. Ref: 2.

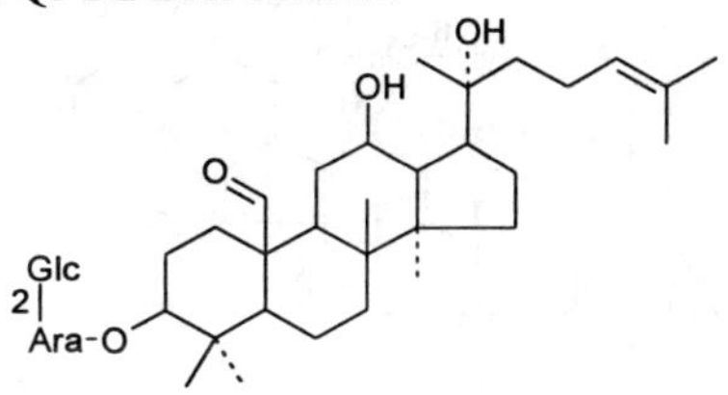

2863 Gypenoside LIV
Source: QI YE DAN. Ref: 2.

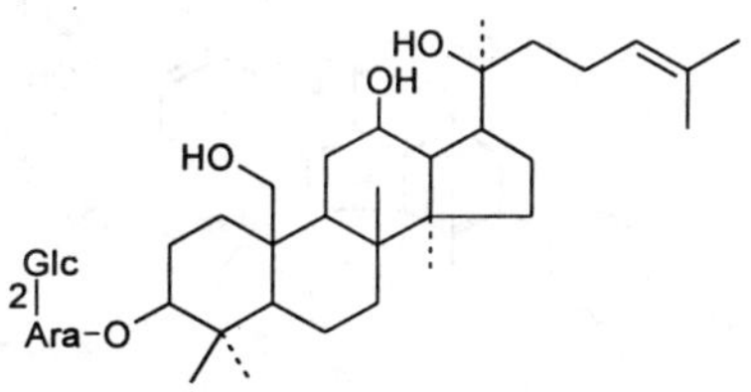

2864 Gypenoside LV
Source: QI YE DAN. Ref: 2.

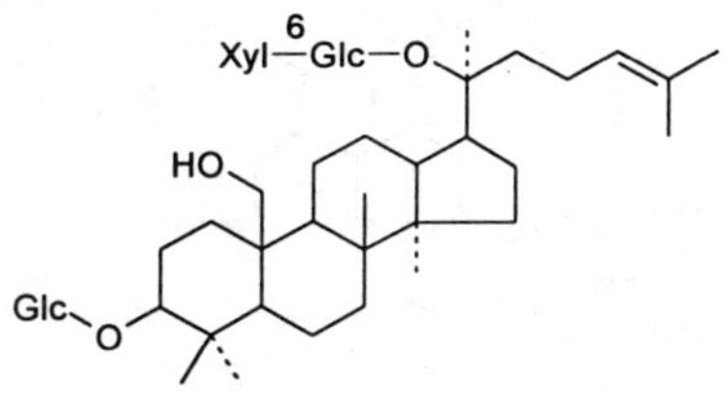

2865 Gypenoside LVI
Source: QI YE DAN. Ref: 2.

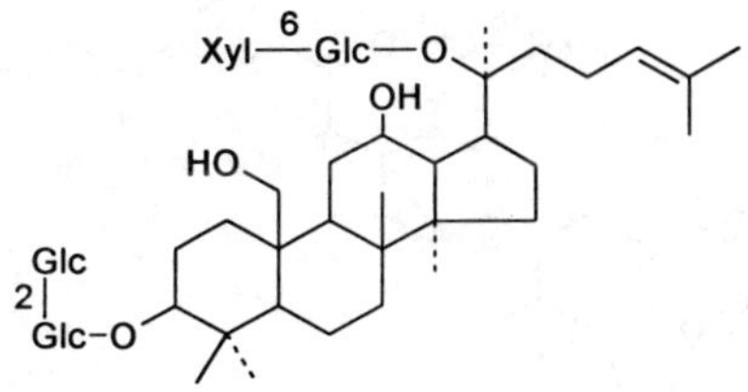

2866 Gypenoside LVII
Source: QI YE DAN. Ref: 2.

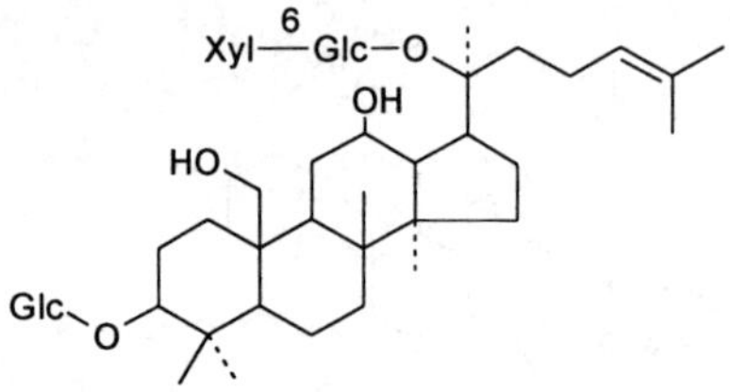

2867 Gypenoside LVIII
Source: QI YE DAN. Ref: 2.

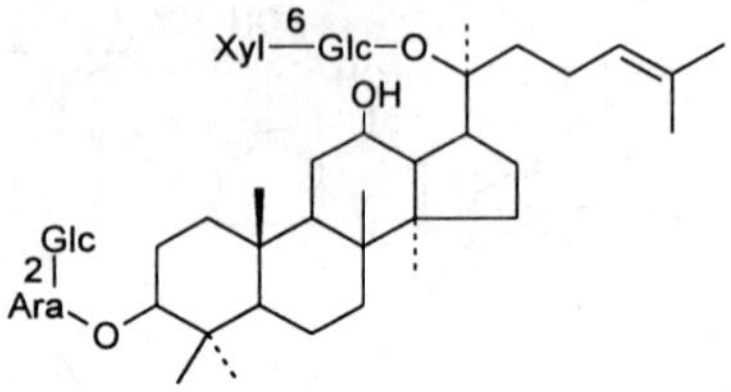

2868 Gypenoside LIX
Source: QI YE DAN. Ref: 2.

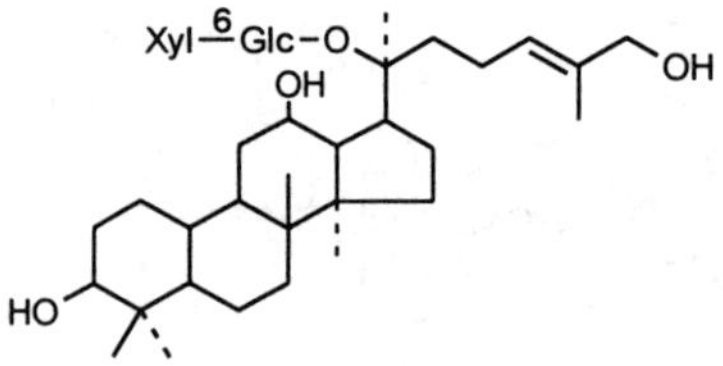

2869 Gypenoside LX
Source: QI YE DAN. Ref: 2.

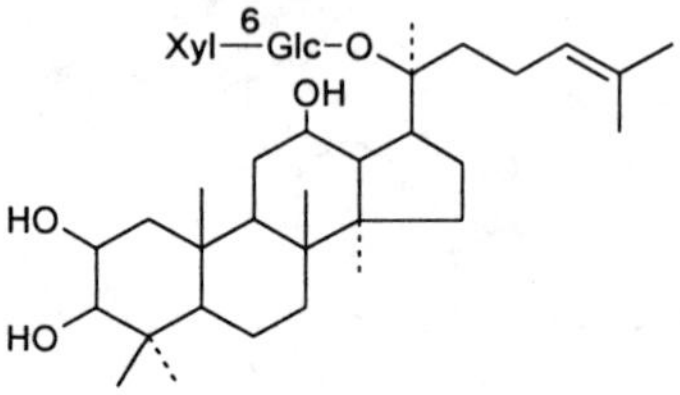

2870 Gypenoside LXI
Source: QI YE DAN. Ref: 2.

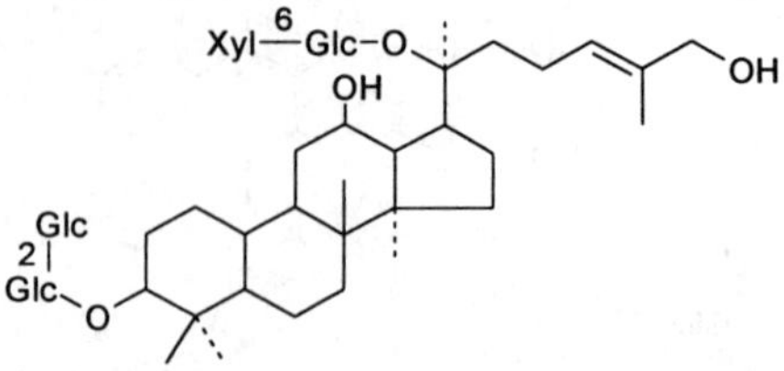

2871 Gypenoside LXII
Source: QI YE DAN. Ref: 2.

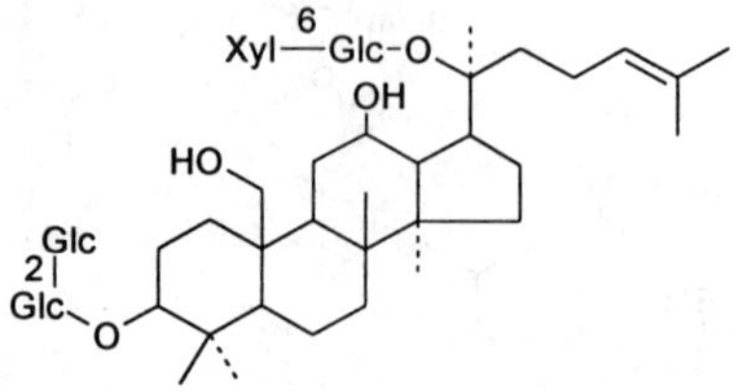

2872 Gypenoside LXIII
Source: QI YE DAN. Ref: 2.

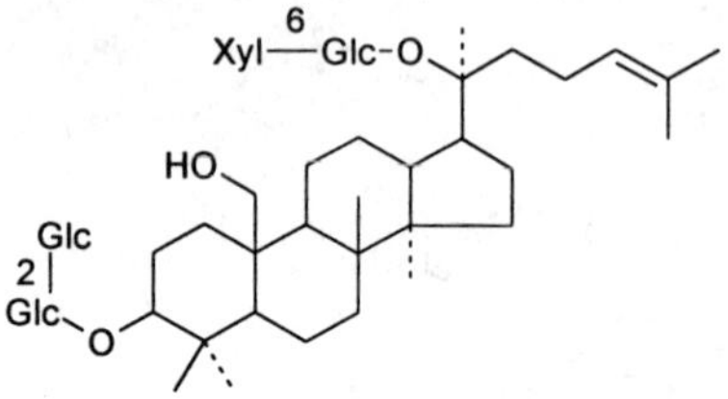

2873 Gypenoside LXIV
Source: QI YE DAN. Ref: 2.

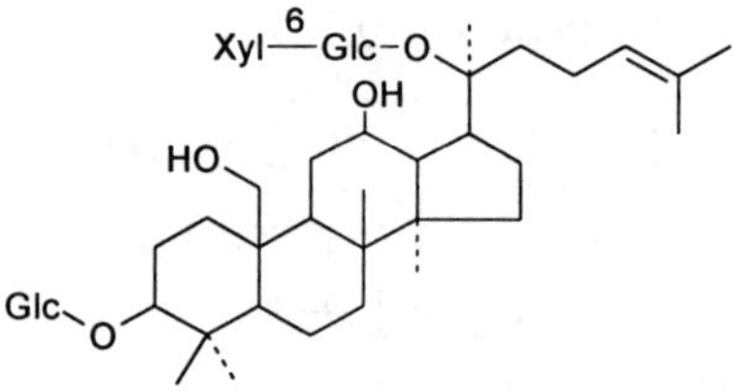

2874 Gypenoside LXV
Source: QI YE DAN. Ref: 2.

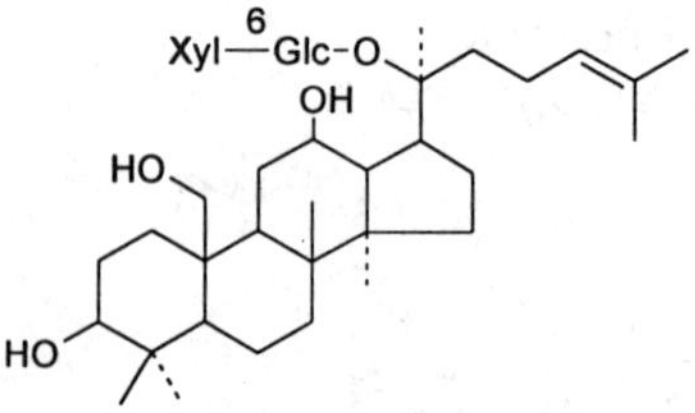

2875 Gypenoside LXVI
Source: QI YE DAN. Ref: 2.

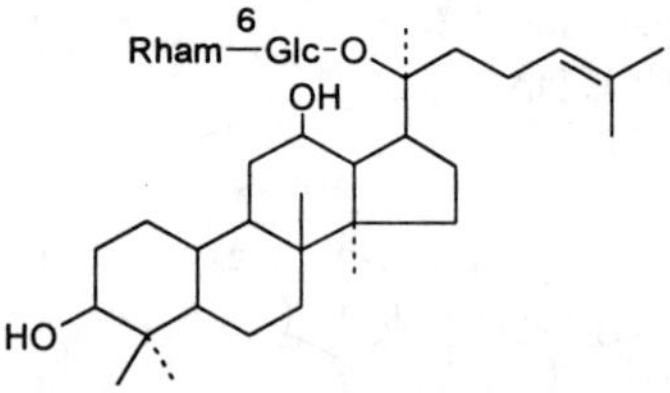

2876 Gypenoside LXVII
Source: QI YE DAN. Ref: 2.

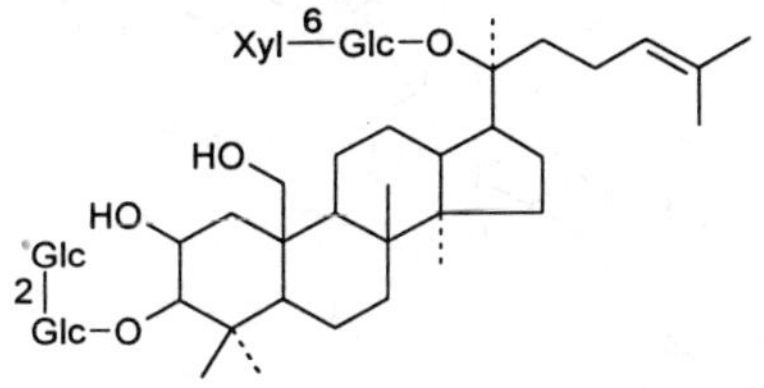

2877 Gypenoside LXVIII
Source: QI YE DAN. Ref: 2.

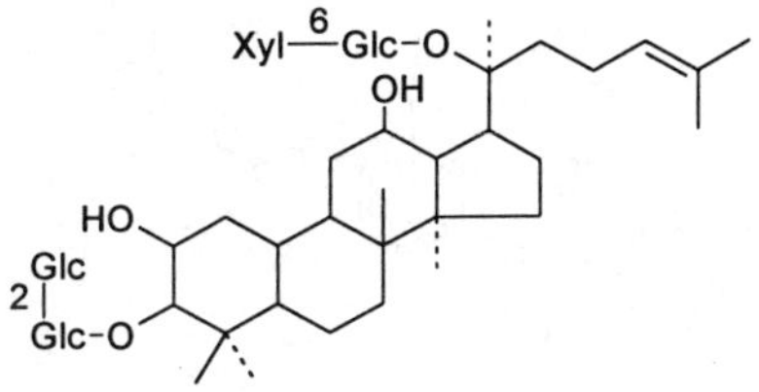

2878 Gypenoside LXIX
Source: QI YE DAN. Ref: 2.

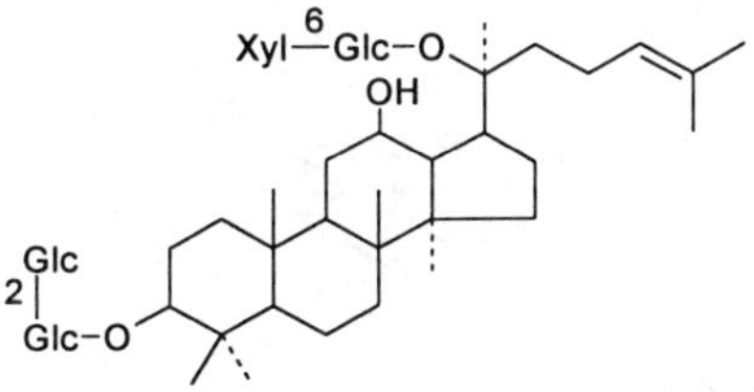

2879 Gypenoside LXX
Source: QI YE DAN. Ref: 2.

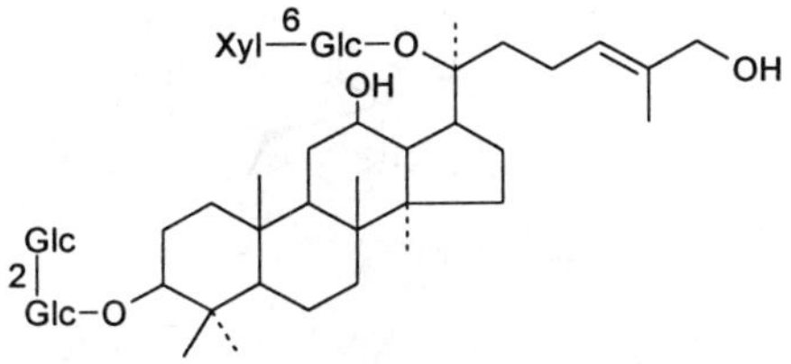

2880 Gypenoside LXXI
Source: QI YE DAN. Ref: 2.

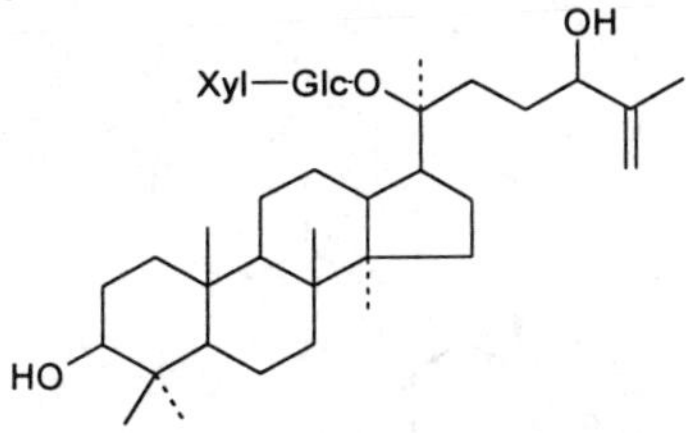

2881 Gypenoside LXXII
Source: QI YE DAN. Ref: 2.

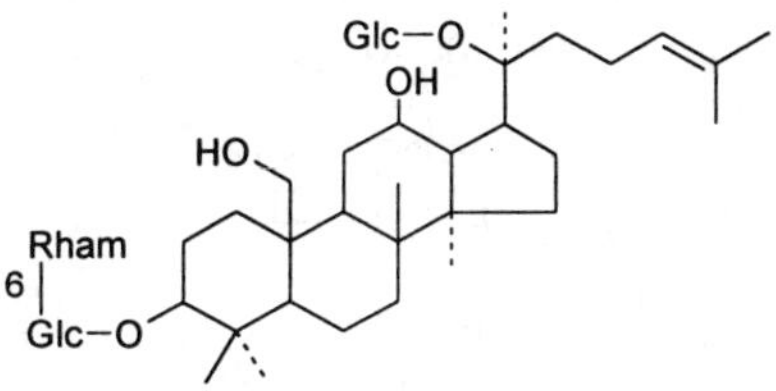

2882 Gypenoside LXXIII
Source: QI YE DAN. Ref: 2.

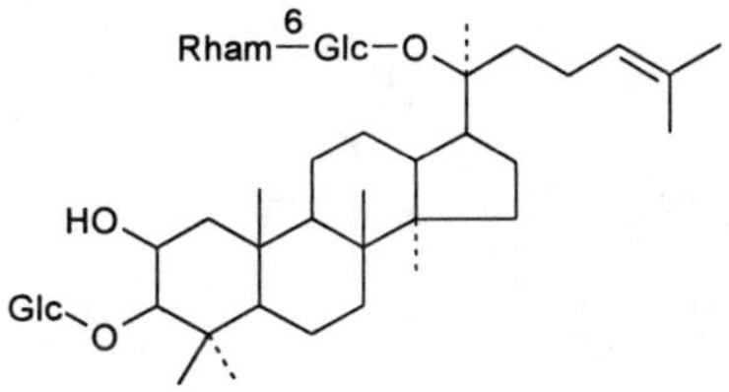

2883 Gypenoside LXXIV
Source: QI YE DAN. Ref: 2.

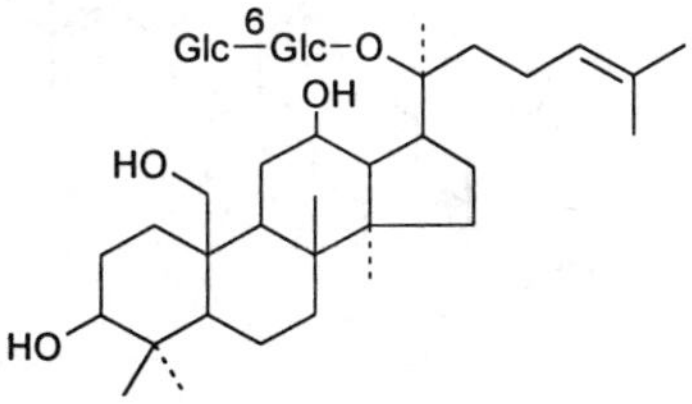

2884 Gypenoside LXXV
Source: QI YE DAN. Ref: 2.

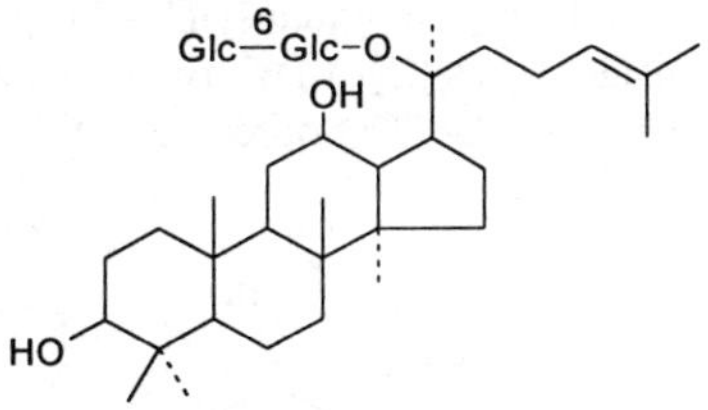

2885 Gypenoside LXXVI
Source: QI YE DAN. Ref: 2.

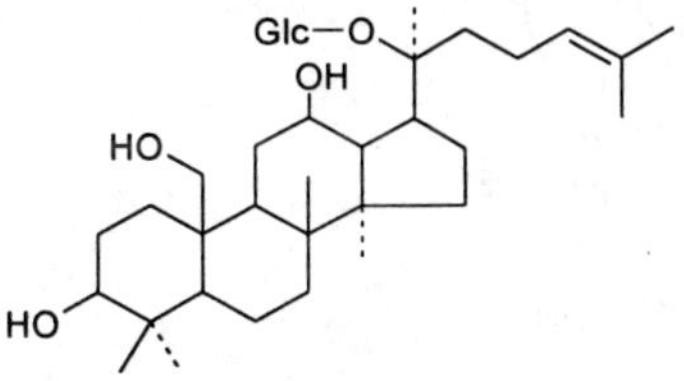

2886 Gypenoside LXXVII
Source: QI YE DAN. Ref: 2.

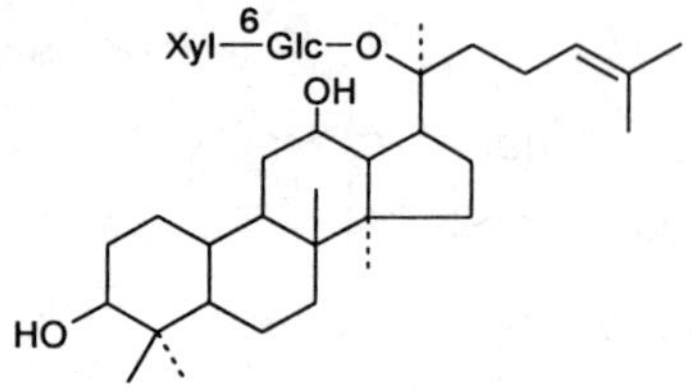

2887 Gypenoside LXXVIII
Source: QI YE DAN. Ref: 2.

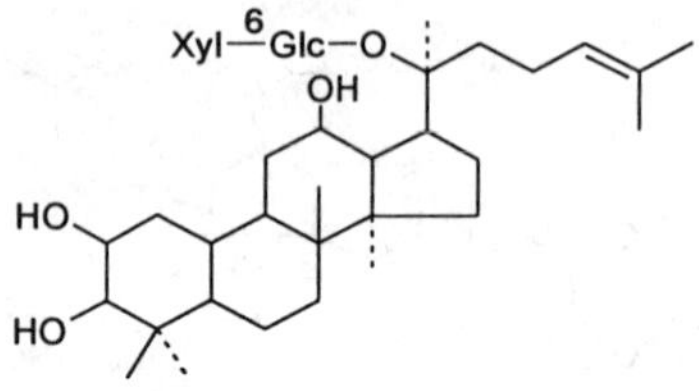

2888 Gypenoside LXXIX
Source: QI YE DAN. Ref: 2.

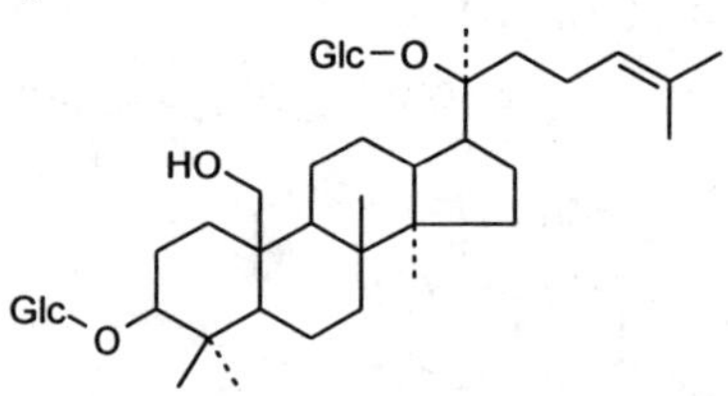

2889 Gypentonoside A
[20S]-3β,20-dihydroxy-24-dammaren-12,23-dione-3-O-[α-L-rhamnopyranosyl(1→2)-[α-L-rhamnopyranosyl(1→3)]-α-L-rhamnopyranosyl(1→6)]-β-D-glucopyranoside. $C_{54}H_{88}O_{21}$ MW: 1073.29 Property: white powder, mp 272-4°C. Source: QI YE DAN.
Ref: 364.

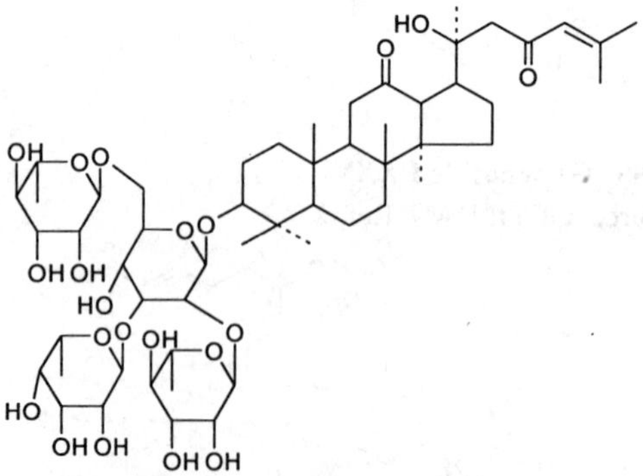

2890 Gypsogenin
$C_{30}H_{46}O_4$ MW: 470.70 Property: mp 274°C. Source: YIN CHAI HU. Ref: 6.

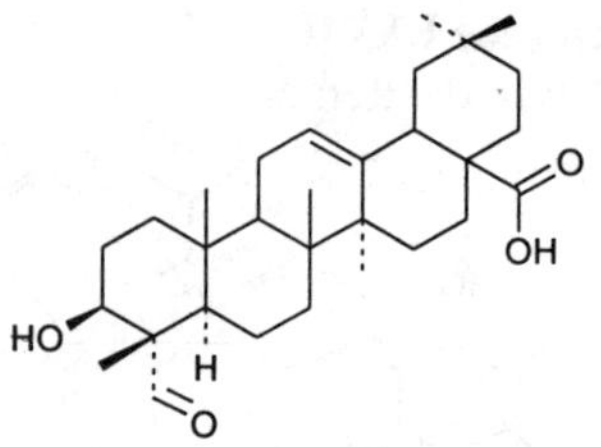

2891 Gyrophoric acid
$C_{24}H_{20}O_{10}$ MW: 468.42 Property: mp 220°C (dec). Source: SHI HUA. Ref: 6.

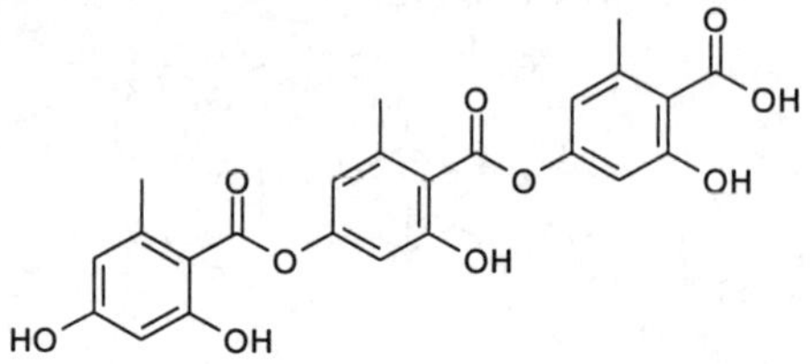

2892 Haemanthidine
$C_{17}H_{19}NO_5$ MW: 317.34 Property: mp 189-90°C. Source: GAN FENG CAO, SHI SUAN. Ref: 6.

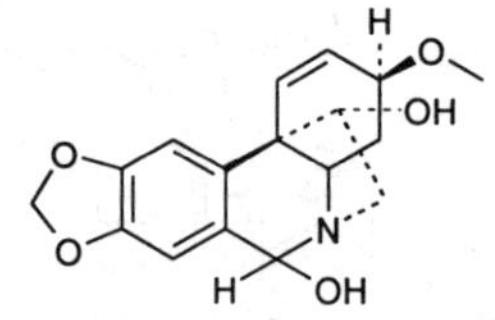

2893 Hainanensine
CAS: 64761-48-4 $C_{19}H_{18}O_4$ MW: 310.35 Property: mp 266-8°C. Source: *Cephalotaxus hainanensis* Li, etc. Ref: 5.

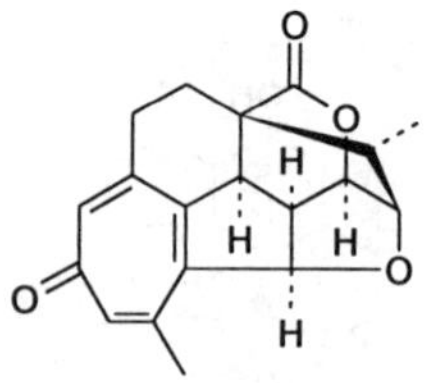

2894 Hainangenin
$C_{27}H_{44}O_5$ MW: 448.65 Source: JIAN MA, WU CI FAN MA. Ref: 10.

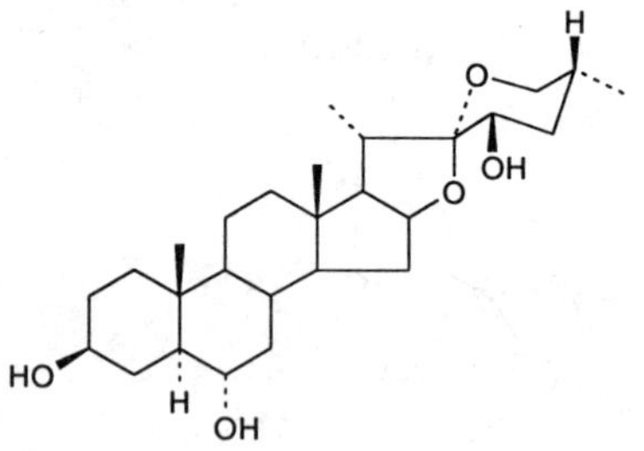

2895 Hainanmurpanin
$C_{17}H_{18}O_6$ MW: 318.33 Source: JIU LI XIANG.
Ref: 11.

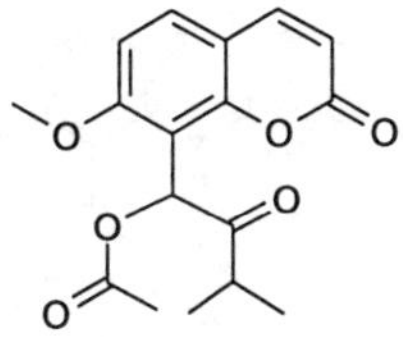

2896 Hainanolide
$C_{20}H_{20}O_4$ MW: 324.38 Source: SAN JIAN SHAN.
Ref: 2.

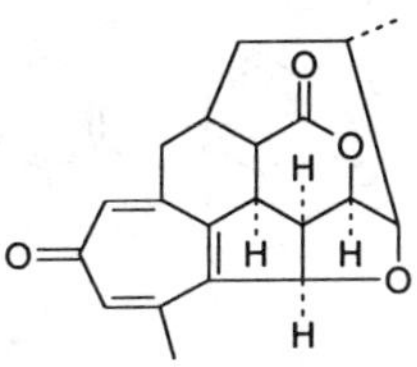

2897 Hainanolidol
$C_{19}H_{20}O_4$ MW: 312.37 Source: SAN JIAN SHAN.
Ref: 2.

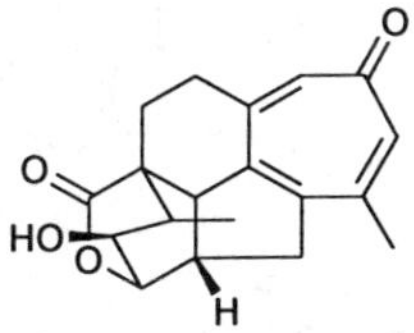

2898 Hamaudol
$C_{15}H_{16}O_5$ MW: 276.29 Source: FANG FENG. Ref: 2.

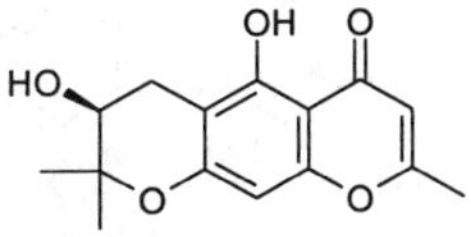

2899 Hancinol
Rel-(7S,8S,1'R,3'S,4'R)-1'-allyl-7-(3,4-dimethoxyphenyl)-4'-hydroxy-5'-methoxy-8-methyl-2'-oxobicyclo[3.2.1]oct-5'-ene. $C_{22}H_{28}O_5$ MW: 372.47
Source: SHAN JU. Ref: 75.

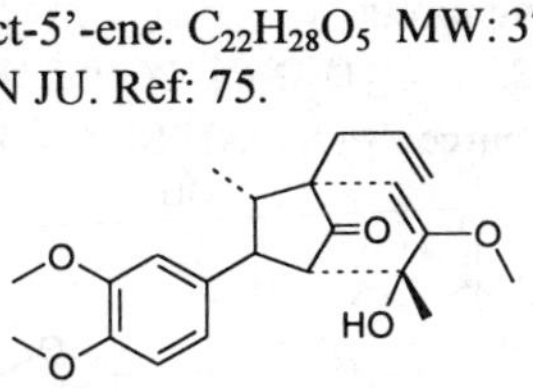

2900 Hancinone D
$C_{21}H_{22}O_5$ MW: 354.41 Property: white crystal (hexane), mp 96-7°C, $[\alpha]_D^{14}$ 0°(c=0.3 $CHCl_3$). Source: SHAN JU, ZHANG YE HU JIAO. Ref: 130, 191.

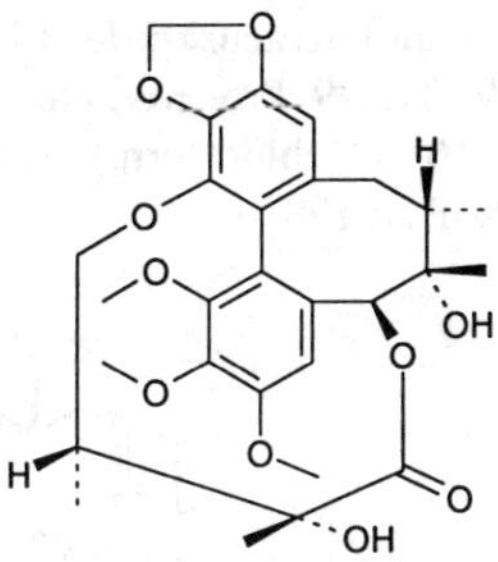

2901 Hancockinol
25,26-Dinor-9,13-dimethyllup-5-en-3-ol. Property: 221-3°C. Source: LIU YE BAI QIAN. Ref: 510.

2902 Hancockinol Ia
$C_{30}H_{50}O$ MW: 426.73 Property: colorless acicular crystal (chloroform), mp 223-5°C, $[\alpha]_D^{20}$ +16.19° (c=0.77, chloroform). Source: HUA BEI BAI QIAN.
Ref: 198.

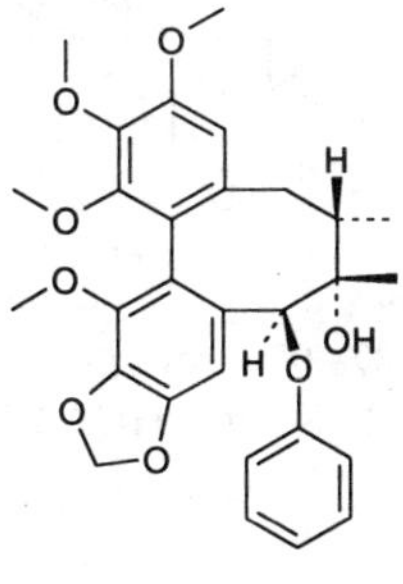

2903 Hancogenin B
$C_{21}H_{28}O_7$ MW: 392.45 Property: colorless acicular crystal (acetone), mp 202-3°C. Source: HUA BEI BAI QIAN. Ref: 237.

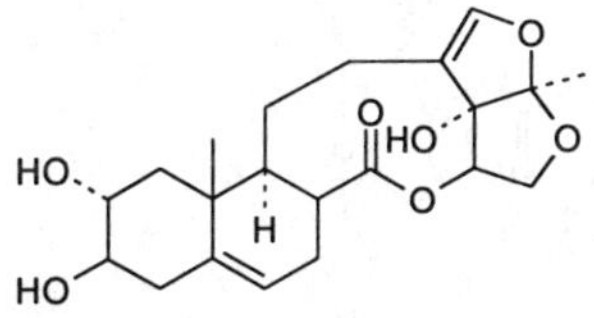

2904 Hancolupenol Iia
$C_{30}H_{50}O$ MW: 426.73 Property: colorless acicular crystal, mp 184-5°C (chloroform), $[\alpha]_D^{29}$ +14.9° (c=0.3, chloroform). Source: HUA BEI BAI QIAN.
Ref: 198.

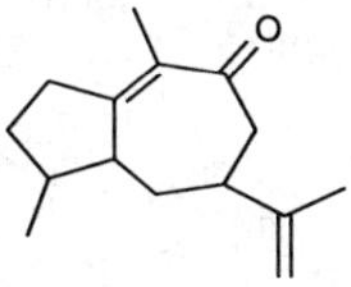

2905 Hancolupenol octacosanate IId
$C_{59}H_{104}O_2$ MW: 845.49 Property: amorphous powder, mp 99-101°C (chloroform). Source: HUA BEI BAI QIAN. Ref: 198.

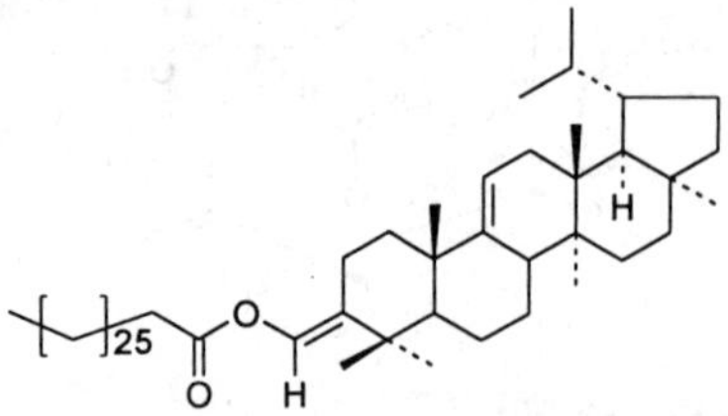

2906 Hancolupenone IIc
$C_{30}H_{48}O$ MW: 424.72 Property: colorless acicular crystal, mp 228-9.5°C (chloroform), $[\alpha]_D^{29}$ +14.9° (c=0.2, chloroform). Source: HUA BEI BAI QIAN. Ref: 198.

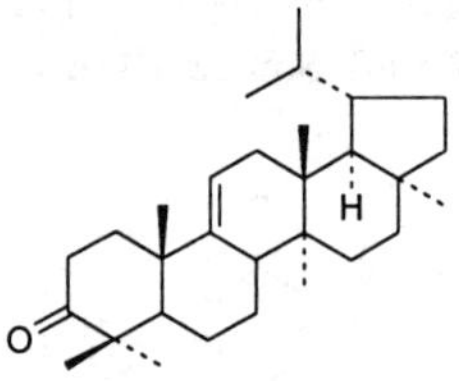

2907 Hancoside A
$C_{44}H_{62}O_{18}$ MW: 878.97 Property: white powder, mp 185-7°C (methanol). Source: HUA BEI BAI QIAN. Ref: 237.

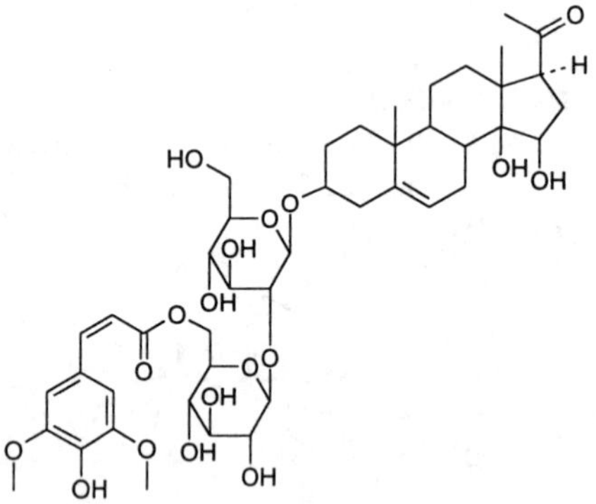

2908 Hanfangchin C
$C_{32}H_{42}N_2O_6$ Source: FANG JI. Ref: 2.

2909 Harmaline
$C_{13}H_{14}N_2O$ MW: 214.27 Property: mp 250°C (dec). Source: LUO TUO PENG, LUO TUO PENG ZI. Ref: 6.

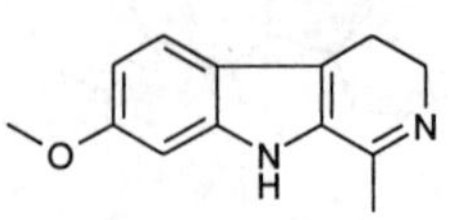

2910 Harman
$C_{12}H_{10}N_2$ MW: 182.23 Source: GOU TENG, YUAN ZHI. Ref: 2, 539.

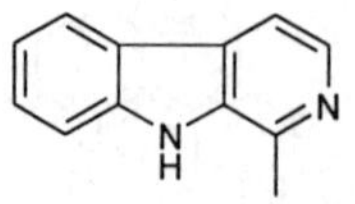

2911 Harmine
Banisterine; Leucuharmine; Telepathine; Yageine. CAS: 442-51-3 $C_{13}H_{12}N_2O$ MW: 212.25 Property: mp 257-9°C. Source: LUO TUO PENG ZI, SHAN YOU MA. Ref: 4, 6.

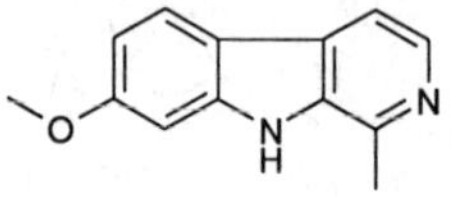

2912 Harmol
$C_{12}H_{10}N_2O$ MW: 198.23 Property: mp 321°C. Source: CU LIU GUO (SHA JI), LUO TUO PENG ZI, JI LI GEN, SHA ZAO. Ref: 6.

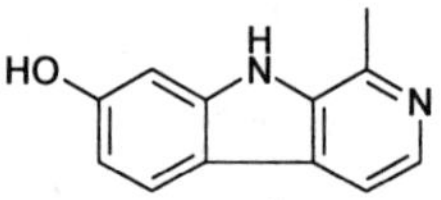

2913 Harpagideacetate
$C_{17}H_{26}NO_{10}$ MW: 390.39 Source: DU ZHONG. Ref: 2.

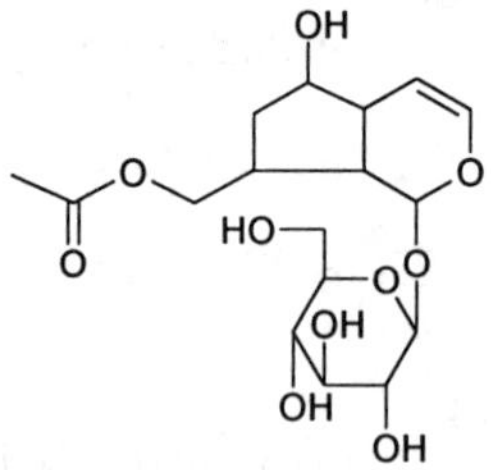

2914 Harringtonine
CAS: 26833-85-2 $C_{28}H_{37}NO_9$ MW: 531.61 Property: mp 73-5°C. Source: SAN JIAN SHAN. Ref: 4.

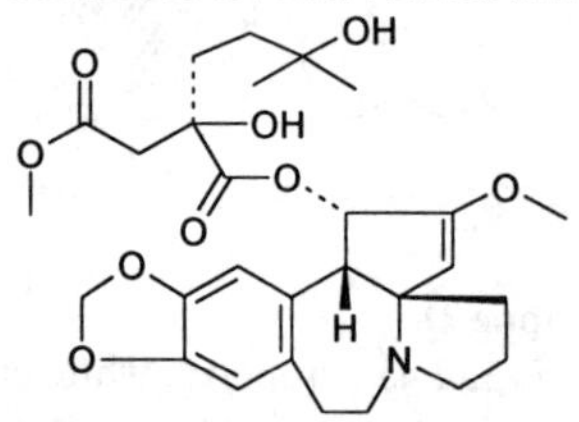

2915 Hasubanonine
$C_{21}H_{27}NO_5$ MW: 373.45 Property: mp 116-7°C. Source: QIAN JIN TENG. Ref: 6.

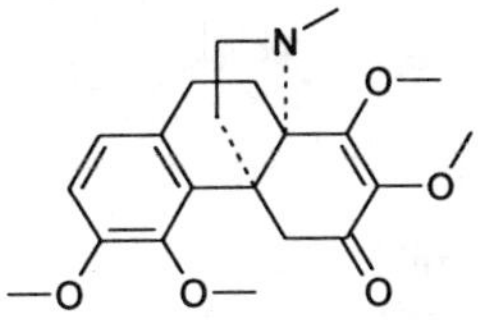

2916 Hautriwaic acid
$C_{20}H_{28}O_4$ MW: 332.44 Property: mp 183-4°C. Source: CHE SANG ZI YE. Ref: 6.

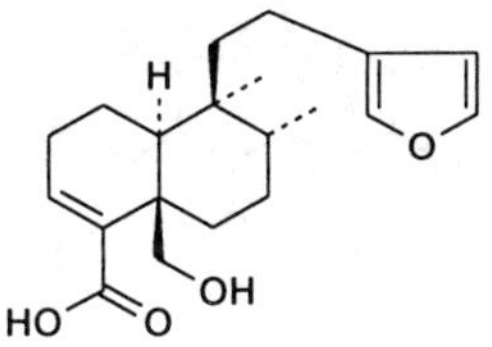

2917 Hayatidine
$C_{37}H_{40}N_2O_6$ MW: 608.74 Property: mp 179-80°C. Source: XI SHENG TENG. Ref: 6.

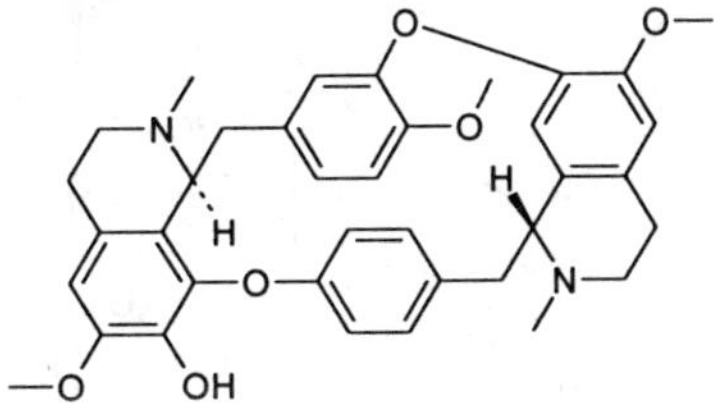

2918 Hayatine
$C_{36}H_{38}N_2O_6$ MW: 594.71 Property: mp 281°C (dec), (±): 303°C (dec). Source: XI SHENG TENG. Ref: 4.

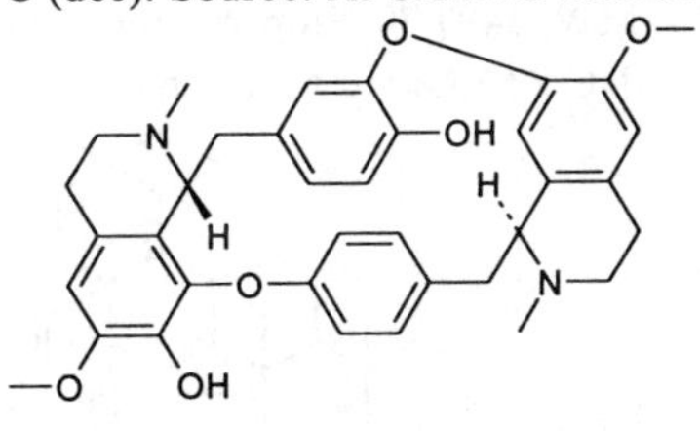

2919 Hayatinine
$C_{37}H_{40}N_2O_6$ MW: 608.74 Property: mp 231-2°C. Source: XI SHENG TENG. Ref: 6.

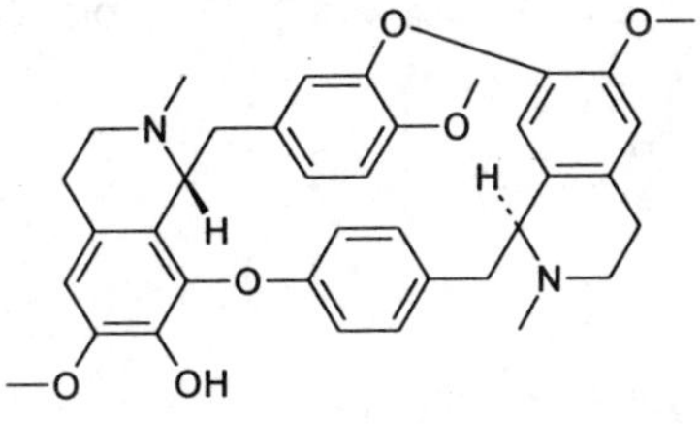

2920 Hecogenin
$C_{27}H_{42}O_4$ MW: 430.63 Property: mp 265°C. Source: DONG YI HAO JIAN MA, DUAN YE LONG SHE LAN, FAN MA, JIAN MA, WEN ZHU, WU CI FAN MA, XIA YE LONG SHE LAN, YIN BIAN LONG SHE LAN. Ref: 6, 10.

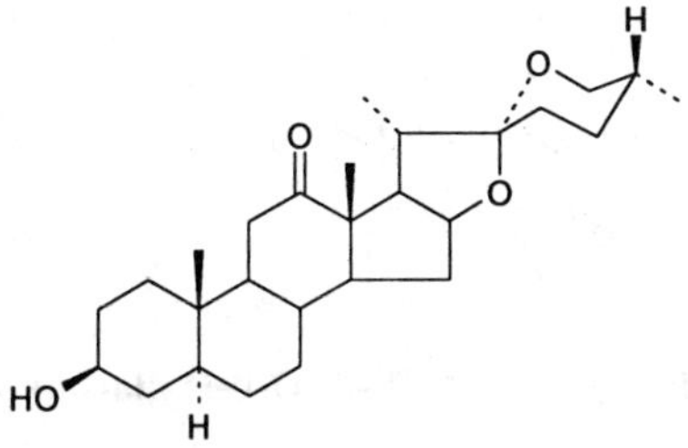

2921 Hederagenin
$C_{30}H_{48}O_4$ MW: 472.71 Property: mp 332-4°C. Source: BAI JIANG, BAI TOU WENG, GUAN MU TONG, JIN YIN HUA, WEI LING XIAN. Ref: 2, 6, 638.

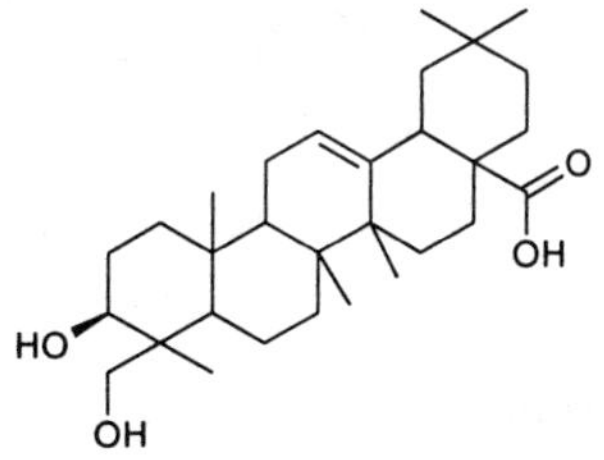

2922 Hederin
Property: mp 256°C. Source: CHANG CHUN TENG, JIN YIN HUA. Ref: 6, 638.

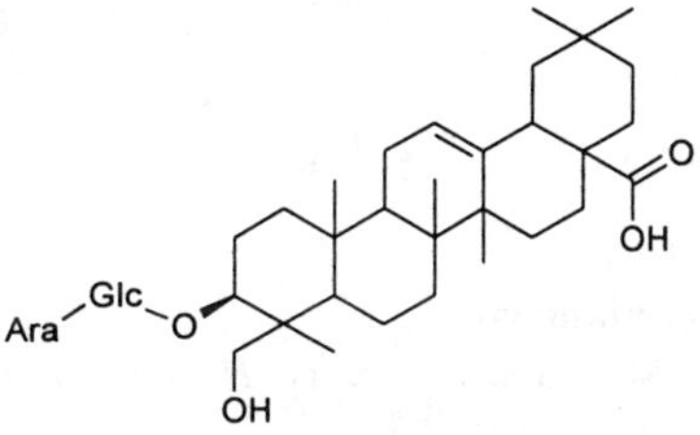

2923 Hedychenone
$C_{20}H_{26}O_2$ MW: 298.43 Property: mp 135-6°C. Source: TU LIANG JIANG, YUAN BAN JIANG HUA. Ref: 6, 322.

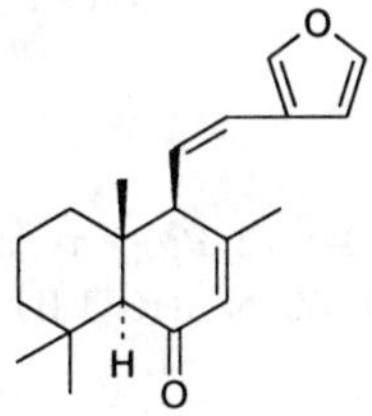

2924 Hedyoside
$C_{20}H_{30}O_{11}$ MW: 446.46 Property: white powder, $[\alpha]_D$ -26.3° (c=0.049, methanol). Source: HUANG MAO ER CAO. Ref: 40.

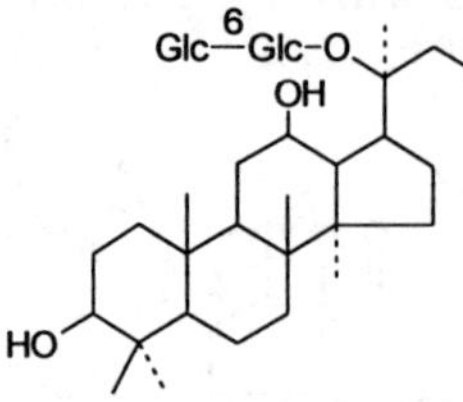

Glc—6—Glc—O OH HO

2925 Hedyotol C4'',4'''-di-O-β-D-glucopyranoside
$C_{43}H_{56}O_{21}$ MW: 908.91 Source: DU ZHONG. Ref: 2.

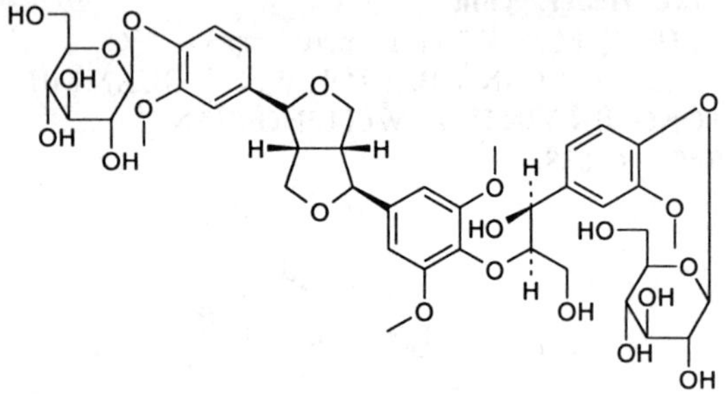

2926 Helenalin
$C_{15}H_{18}O_4$ MW: 262.21 Source: *Arnica longifolia* Eaton; *Balduina angustifolia* (Pursh) Robins; etc. Ref: 4.

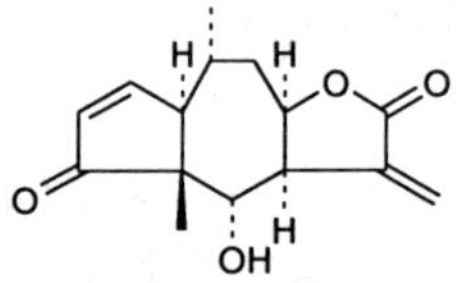

2927 Heleniamarin
$C_{17}H_{22}O_3$ MW: 306.36 Source: *Helenium amarum* (Rafin.) H. Rock. Ref: 4.

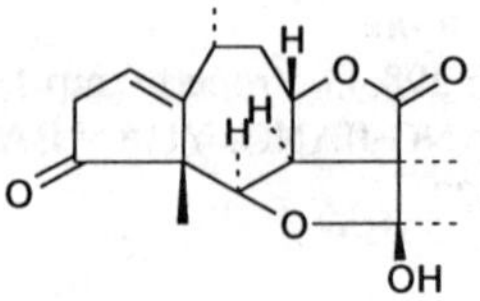

2928 Helenien
$C_{72}H_{116}O_4$ MW: 1045.72 Property: mp 92°C. Source: KONG QUE CAO, WAN SHOU JU. Ref: 6.

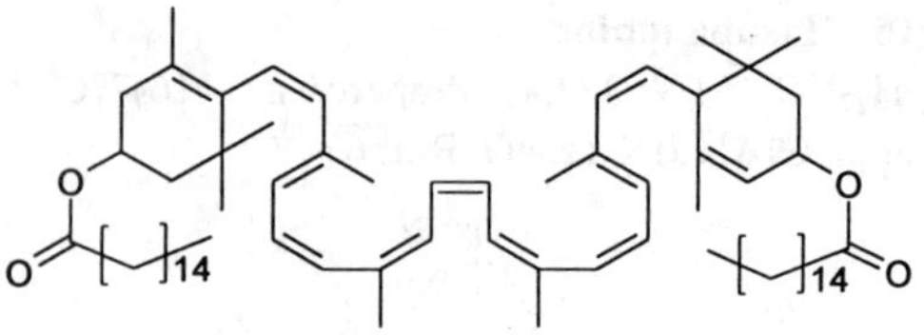

2929 Heliangine
$C_{20}H_{28}O_6$ MW: 364.44 Property: mp 227-9°C. Source: XIANG RI KUI YE. Ref: 6.

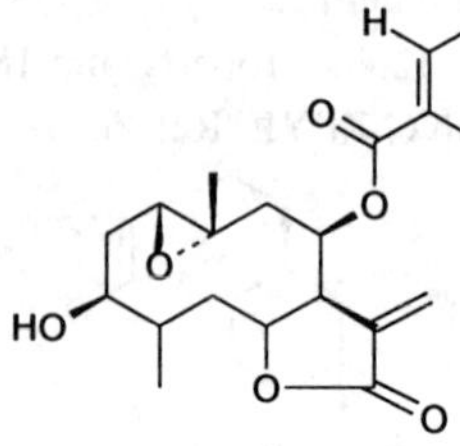

2930 Helianthoside B
$C_{58}H_{94}O_{25}$ MW: 1191.38 Source: XIANG RI KUI HUA. Ref: 6.

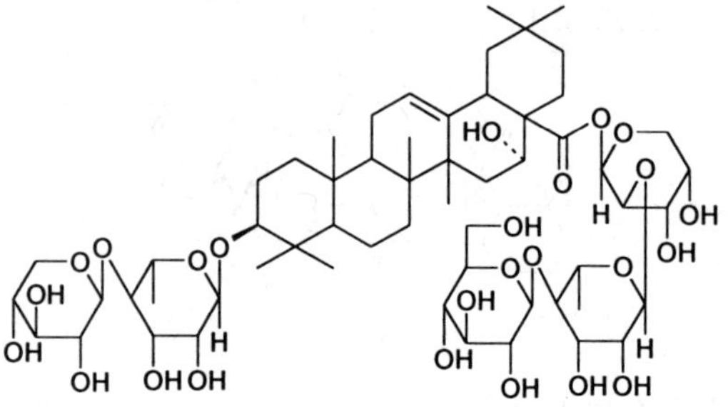

2931 Helianthoside C
$C_{71}H_{116}O_{33}$ MW: 1497.70 Property: mp 215-7°C. Source: XIANG RI KUI HUA. Ref: 6.

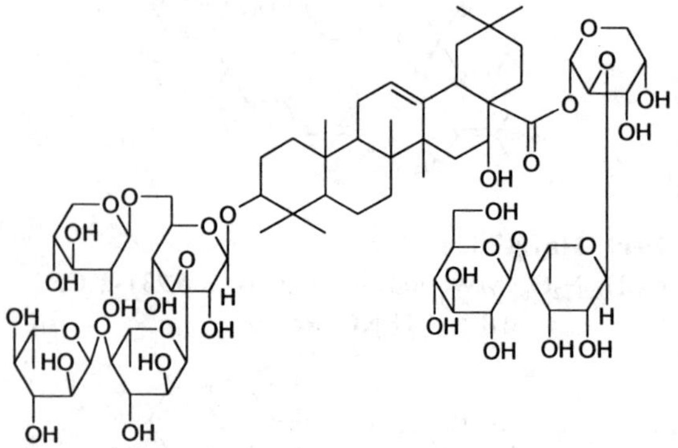

2932 Heliosupine

$C_{20}H_{31}NO_7$ MW: 397.47 Property: mp 148-9°C. Source: YAO YONG DAO TI HU. Ref: 6.

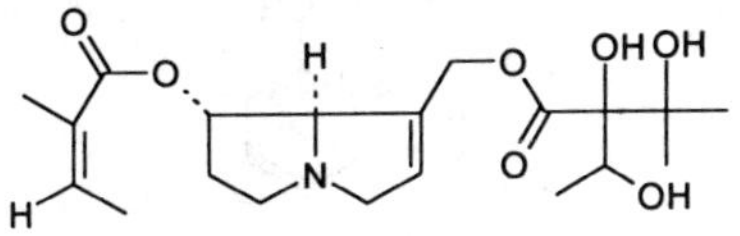

2933 Heliosupine N-oxide

$C_{20}H_{31}NO_8$ MW: 413.47 Property: mp 165°C (dec). Source: YAO YONG DAO TI HU. Ref: 6.

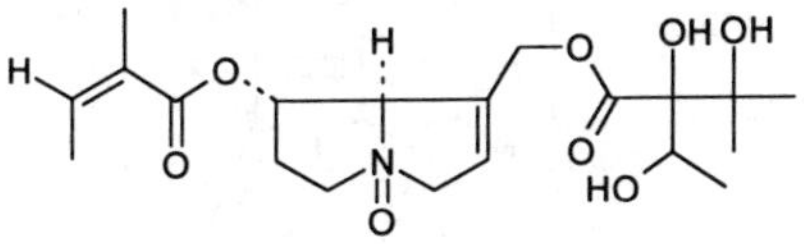

2934 Heliotridine viridiflorate N-oxide

Echinatine N-oxide. $C_{15}H_{25}NO_6$ MW: 315.37 Source: YAO YONG DAO TI HU. Ref: 6.

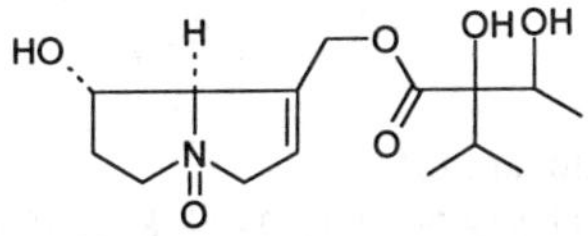

2935 Heliotrine

CAS: 303-33-3 $C_{16}H_{27}NO_5$ MW: 313.40 Property: mp 125-6°C. Source: YAO YONG DAO TI HU, YAO YONG DAO TI HU. Ref: 5.

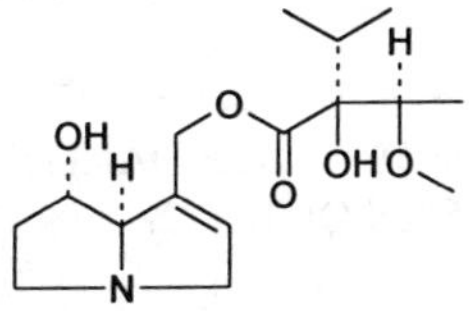

2936 Helioxanthin

$C_{20}H_{12}O_6$ MW: 348.32 Property: mp 240-1°C. Source: DA JIN NIU CAO. Ref: 6.

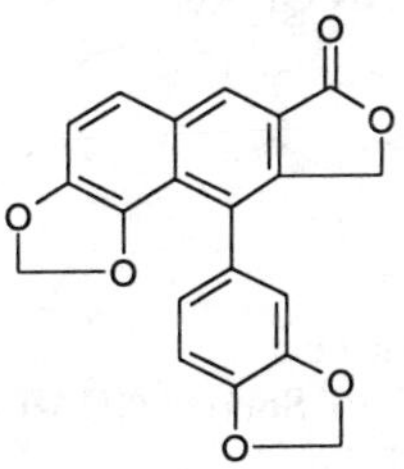

2937 Hellebrigenin β-D-glucoside

$C_{30}H_{42}O_{11}$ MW: 578.66 Source: *Urginea altissima* Baker. Ref: 5.

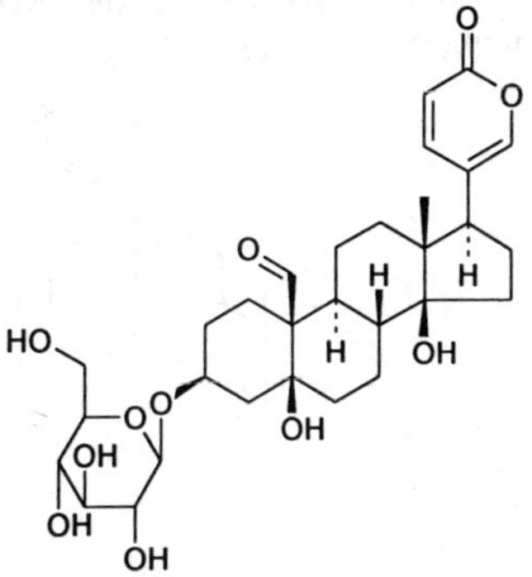

2938 Hellebrin

Hellebrigenin glucorhamnoside. CAS: 13289-18-4 $C_{36}H_{52}O_{15}$ MW: 724.81 Property: mp 283-4°C. Source: *Helleborus niger* L. etc. Ref: 5.

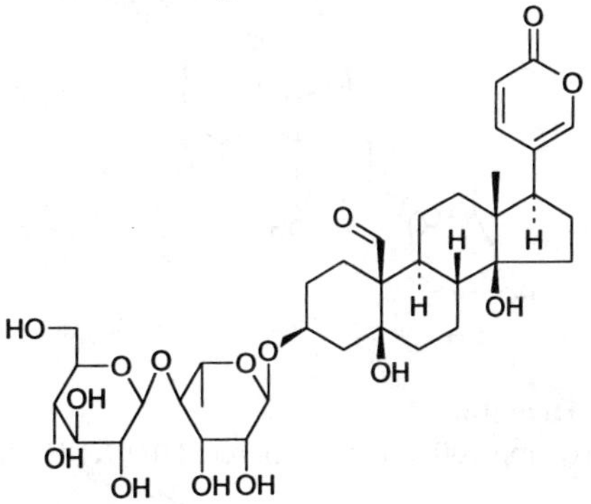

2939 Helminthosporin

$C_{15}H_{10}O_5$ MW: 270.24 Source: LU HUI. Ref: 2.

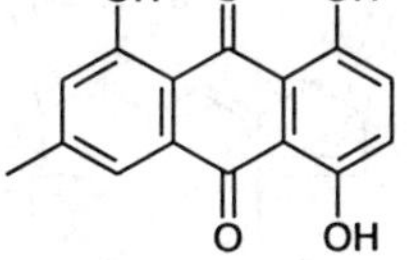

2940 Heloniogenin

$C_{27}H_{42}O_4$ MW: 430.63 Property: mp 212-3°C. Source: LEI GONG QI. Ref: 6.

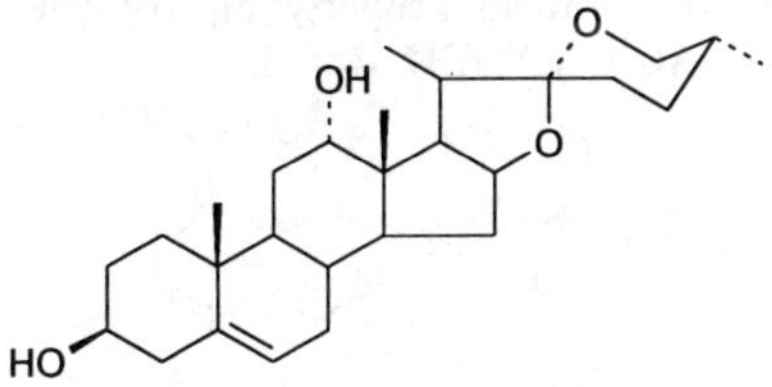

2941 Helveticoside
Alleoside A; Erysimin; Erysimotoxin. CAS: 630-64-8
$C_{29}H_{42}O_9$ MW: 534.65 Property: mp 153-7°C.
Source: GUI ZHU TANG JIE, HUANG MA ZI, TING LI ZI, TANG JIE. Ref: 5, 6.

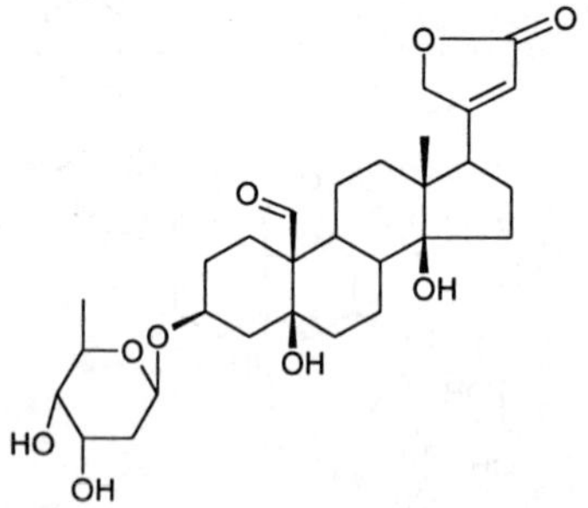

2942 Helveticosol
$C_{29}H_{44}O_9$ MW: 536.67 Property: mp 147-52°C.
Source: GUI ZHU TANG JIE. Ref: 6.

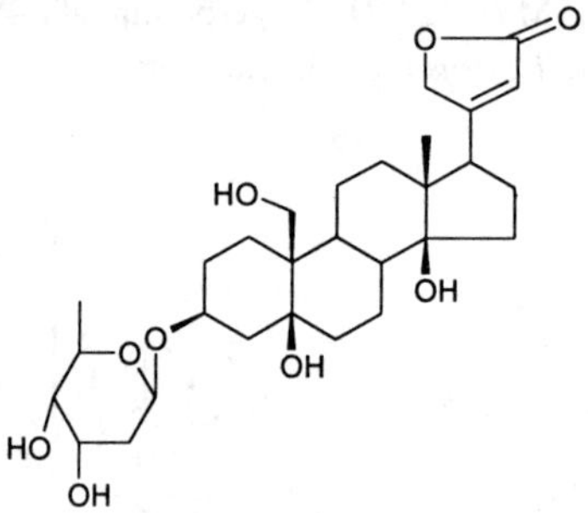

2943 Hematin
Property: mp 200°C (dec). Source: NIU XUE. Ref: 6.

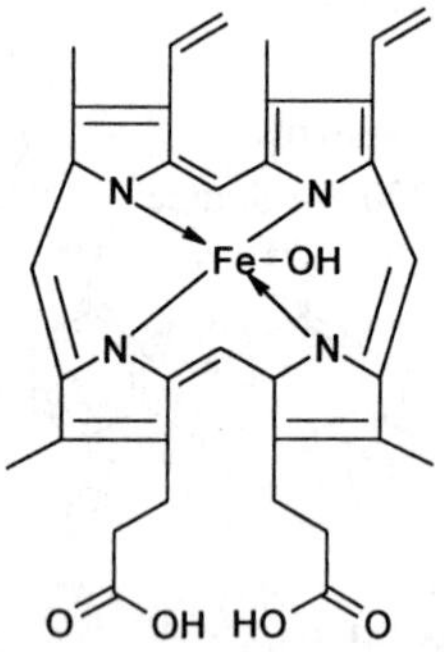

2944 Hemerocallin
$C_{26}H_{22}O_6$ MW: 430.46 Property: mp 266-9°C.
Source: XUAN CAO GEN. Ref: 6.

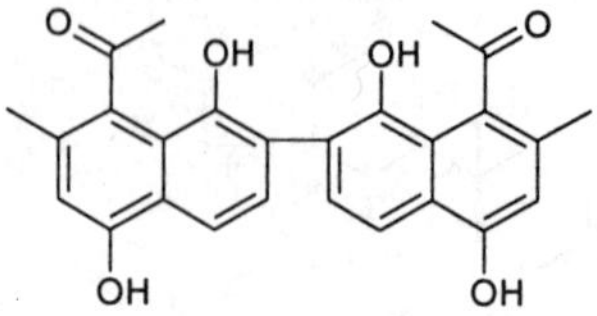

2945 Hemigossypol
$C_{15}H_{16}O_4$ MW: 260.29 Source: MIAN HUA GEN. Ref: 6.

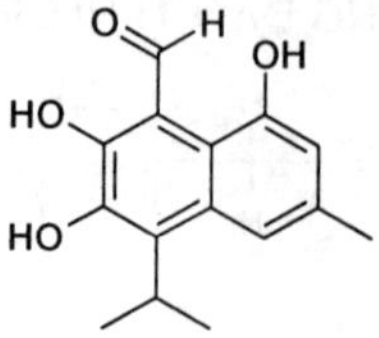

2946 Hemin
Source: CU LIU GUO (SHA JI). Ref: 6.

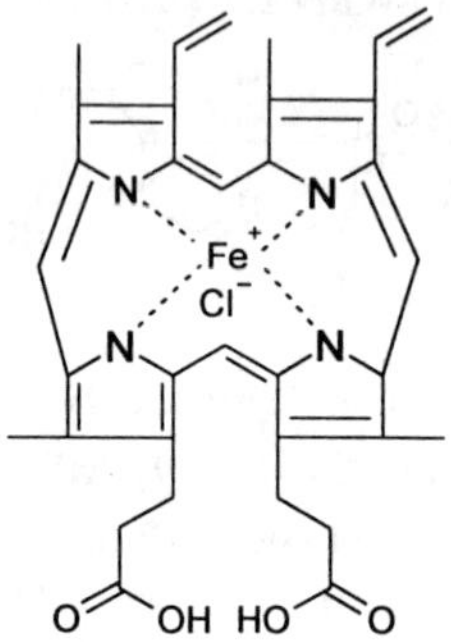

2947 Hemsloside G1
Source: PENG XIAN XUE DAN. Ref: 554.

2948 Hemsloside H1
Source: PENG XIAN XUE DAN. Ref: 554.

2949 Hemsloside Ma1
Source: PENG XIAN XUE DAN. Ref: 554.

2950 Heneicosane
$C_{21}H_{44}$ MW: 296.58 Source: DANG SHEN, ROU CONG RONG, SAN QI. Ref: 2.

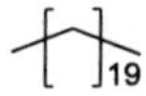

2951 Heneicosanic acid
$C_{21}H_{42}O_2$ MW: 326.57 Source: DANG SHEN, ROU CONG RONG, SAN QI. Ref: 2.

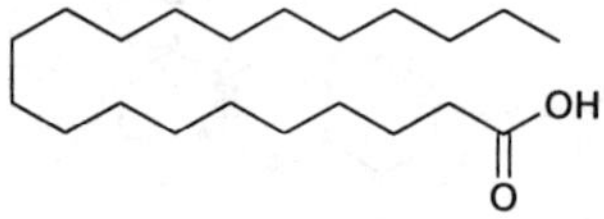

2952 Hentriacontane
$C_{31}H_{64}$ MW: 436.86 Source: GUA LOU, YIN YANG HUO. Ref: 2.

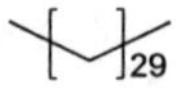

2953 Hentriacontanol-6
$C_{31}H_{64}O$ MW: 452.86 Source: PU HUANG. Ref: 2.

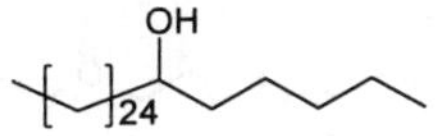

2954 Hentriacontic acid
$C_{31}H_{62}O_2$ MW: 466.84 Source: DI GU PI. Ref: 2.

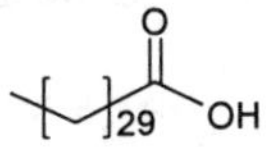

2955 n-Heptacosane
$C_{27}H_{56}$ MW: 380.75 Source: GUA LOU, GUANG XI XUE JIE. Ref: 2, 616.

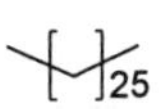

2956 Heptacosanol
Source: MAO GENG XI XIAN. Ref: 476.

2957 Heptacosyl heptacosanate
$C_{54}H_{108}O_2$ MW: 789.46 Source: CHONG BAI LA. Ref: 6.

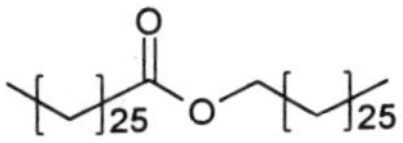

2958 Heptacosyl melissate
$C_{57}H_{114}O_2$ MW: 831.54 Source: CHONG BAI LA. Ref: 6.

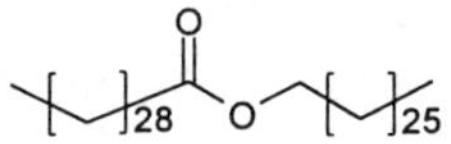

2959 8(E)-Heptadeca-1,8-dien-4,6-diyn-3,10-diol
$C_{19}H_{28}O_2$ MW: 288.43 Source: FANG FENG. Ref: 2.

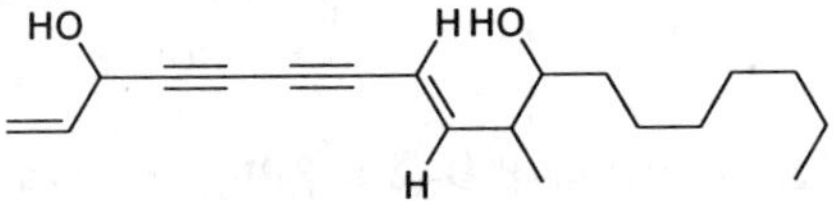

2960 Heptadeca-1-en-4,6-dihy-3,9-diol
$C_{17}H_{26}O_2$ MW: 262.40 Source: FANG FENG. Ref: 2.

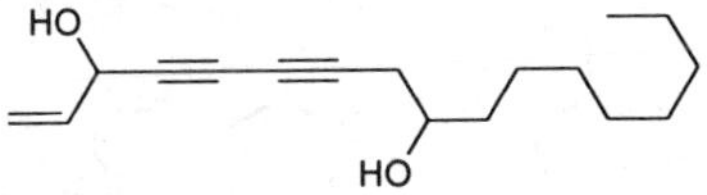

2961 Heptadecane
$C_{17}H_{36}$ MW: 240.48 Source: DANG SHEN, REN SHEN, ROU CONG RONG, SAN QI. Ref: 2.

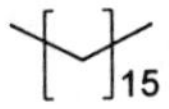

2962 Heptadecanoic acid
$C_{17}H_{34}O_2$ MW: 270.46 Source: GAN DI HUANG, XI YANG SHEN. Ref: 2.

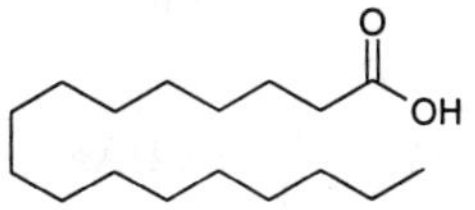

2963 1-Heptadecanol
$C_{17}H_{36}O$ MW: 256.48 Source: BAI ZHI, REN SHEN. Ref: 2.

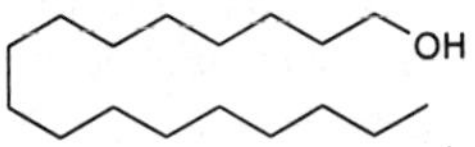

2964 Heptadec-1,7,9-trien-11,13,15-triyne
$C_{17}H_{18}$ MW: 222.33 Property: mp 18°C. Source: AI YE. Ref: 6.

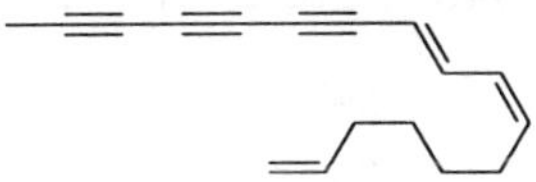

2965 γ-Heptalactone
$C_7H_{12}O_2$ MW: 128.17 Source: CHAI HU. Ref: 2.

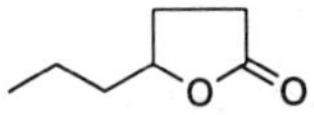

2966 3,3',4',5,5',6,7-Heptamethoxyflavone
$C_{22}H_{24}O_9$ MW: 432.43 Property: mp 156-7°C. Source: JIU LI XIANG. Ref: 6, 11.

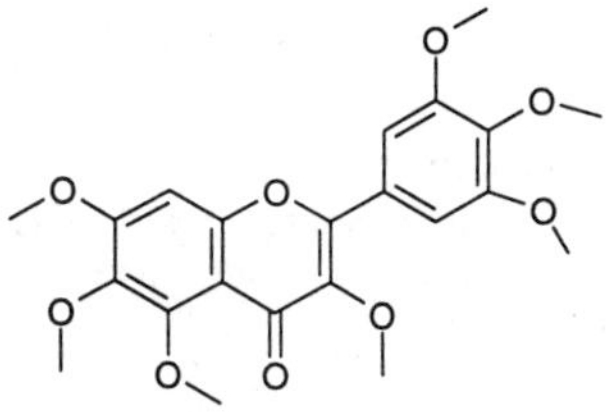

2967 3,3',4',5',5,7,8-Heptamethoxyflavone
$C_{22}H_{24}O_9$ MW: 432.43 Source: JIU LI XIANG. Ref: 11.

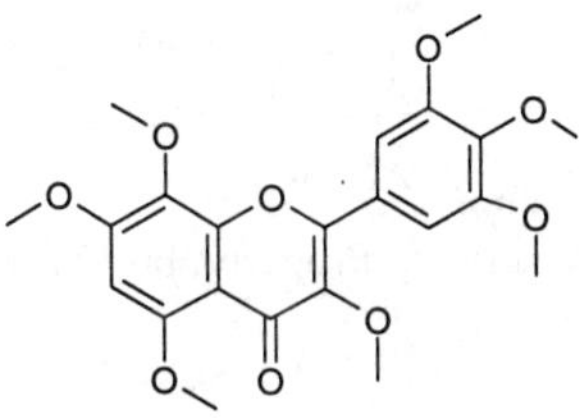

2968 Heptanal
$C_7H_{14}O$ MW: 114.19 Source: QIANG HUO. Ref: 2.

2969 Heptane
C_7H_{16} MW: 100.21 Source: SHAN ZHA, SHENG JIANG. Ref: 2.

2970 Heptanoic acid
Heptylic acid. $C_7H_{14}O_2$ MW: 130.19 Source: CHAI HU, SAN QI, XI YANG SHEN. Ref: 2, 6.

2971 2-Heptanol
$C_7H_{16}O$ MW: 116.21 Source: GAN JIANG, SHENG JIANG. Ref: 2.

2972 α-Heptenal
$C_7H_{12}O$ MW: 112.17 Property: bp 165-7°C. Source: CHA YE. Ref: 6.

2973 β-Heptenal
$C_7H_{12}O$ MW: 112.17 Property: bp 151°C. Source: CHA YE. Ref: 6.

2974 2-Heptenic acid
$C_7H_{12}O_2$ MW: 128.17 Source: CHAI HU. Ref: 2.

2975 5-Hepten-6-methyl-2-one
$C_8H_{14}O$ MW: 126.20 Source: SHENG JIANG. Ref: 2.

2976 β-Heptenol
$C_7H_{14}O$ MW: 114.19 Property: bp 177-9°C. Source: CHA YE. Ref: 6.

2977 γ-Heptenol
$C_7H_{14}O$ MW: 114.19 Property: bp (cis&trans): 81-3 °C/19mm, (trans): 170-1°C. Source: CHA YE. Ref: 6.

2978 Heptyl ethyl ether
$C_9H_{20}O$ MW: 144.26 Property: bp 166.6°C. Source: WEN PO. Ref: 6.

2979 Heraclenin
$C_{16}H_{14}O_5$ MW: 286.29 Property: mp (+): 111°C, (-): 106.5-8.0°C, (±): 113-4.5°C. Source: GOU JU HE. Ref: 6.

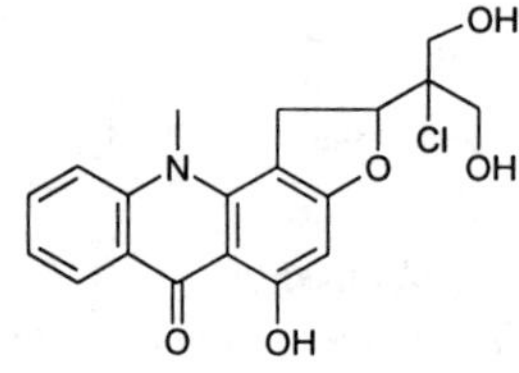

2980 Heraclenol
Property: mp 115-7°C. Source: YUN NAN QIANG HUO. Ref: 551.

2981 Heramandiol
$C_{14}H_{14}O_5$ MW: 262.26 Property: white acicular crystal, mp 148-50°C, $[\alpha]_D$ +122.5° (chloroform). Source: ZHONG CHI MAO DANG GUI. Ref: 344.

2982 Herbacetin
$C_{15}H_{10}O_7$ MW: 302.24 Source: MA HUANG. Ref: 2.

2983 Herbacetin-3-β-D-(2-O-β-D-glucopyranosidoglucopyranoside)-8-β-D-glucopyranoside
$C_{33}H_{40}O_{22}$ MW: 788.67 Source: MU ZEI. Ref: 2.

2984 Herbacetrin
Isoarticulatin. $C_{21}H_{20}O_{12}$ MW: 464.39 Source: MU ZEI, WEN JING. Ref: 2.

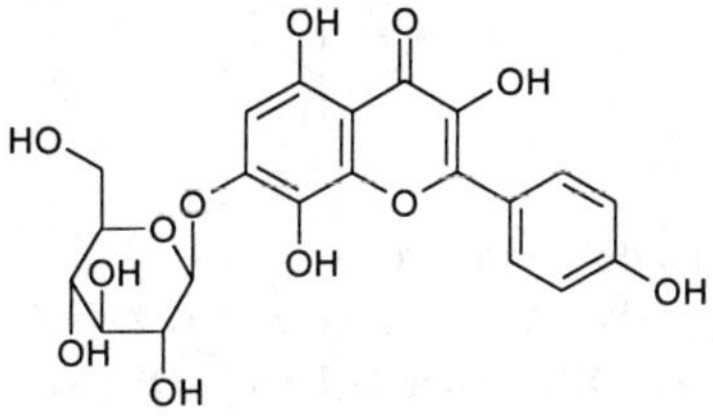

2985 Herbacin
$C_{21}H_{20}O_{12}$ MW: 464.39 Source: SHU KUI HUA. Ref: 6.

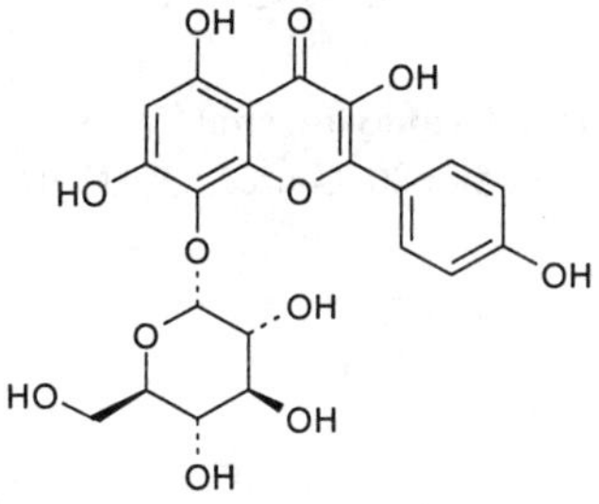

2986 Hernandezine
$C_{40}H_{46}N_2O_7$ MW: 666.82 Property: mp 192-3°C. Source: YING SHUI HUANG LIAN. Ref: 6.

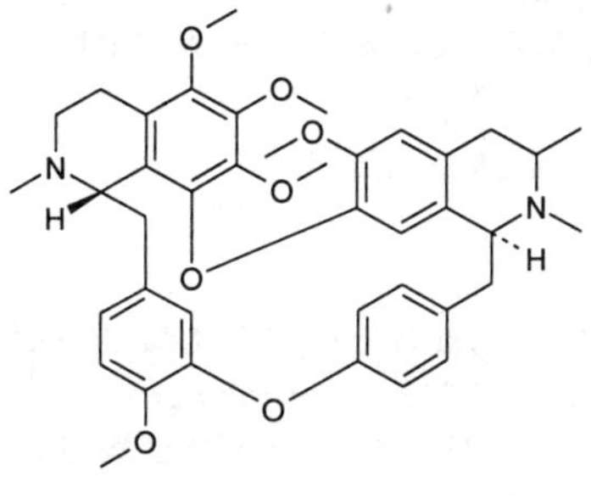

2987 Hernandifoline
$C_{29}H_{33}NO_9$ MW: 539.59 Source: RU LAN. Ref: 6.

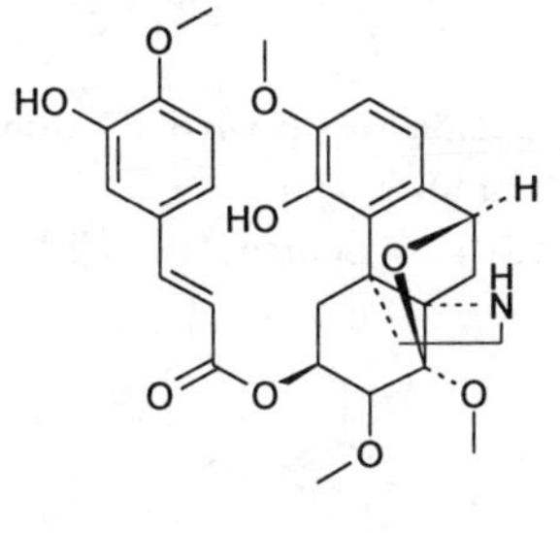

2988 Hernandine
$C_{19}H_{25}NO_6$ MW: 363.41 Source: RU LAN. Ref: 6.

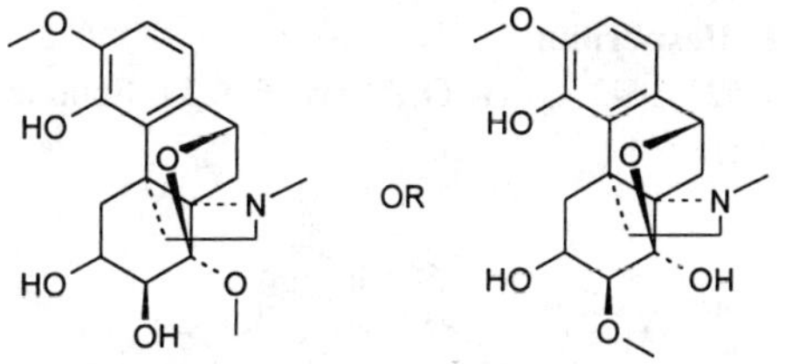

OR

2989 Hernandoline
$C_{19}H_{25}NO_6$ MW: 359.43 Source: RU LAN. Ref: 6.

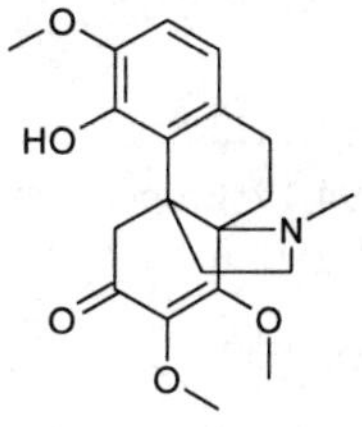

2990 Hernandolinol
$C_{19}H_{25}NO_6$ MW: 361. 44 Source: RU LAN. Ref: 6.

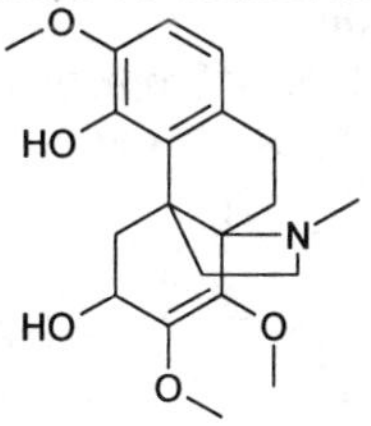

2991 Herniarin
$C_{10}H_8O_3$ MW: 176.17 Property: mp 117-8°C. Source: TING LI ZI, YA JIAO AI. Ref: 6.

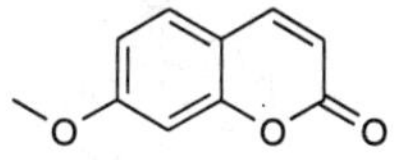

2992 Hesperetin
$C_{16}H_{14}O_6$ MW: 288.26 Source: JIN JIE. Ref: 2.

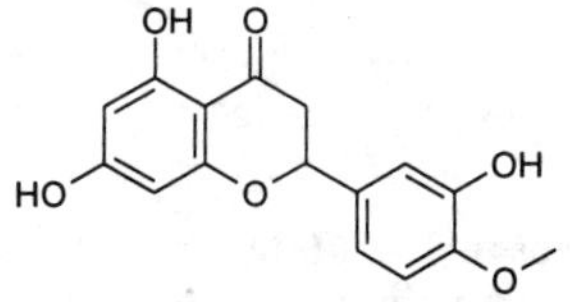

2993 Hesperetin-5-glucoside
$C_{22}H_{24}O_{11}$ MW: 464.43 Source: TAO GEN. Ref: 6.

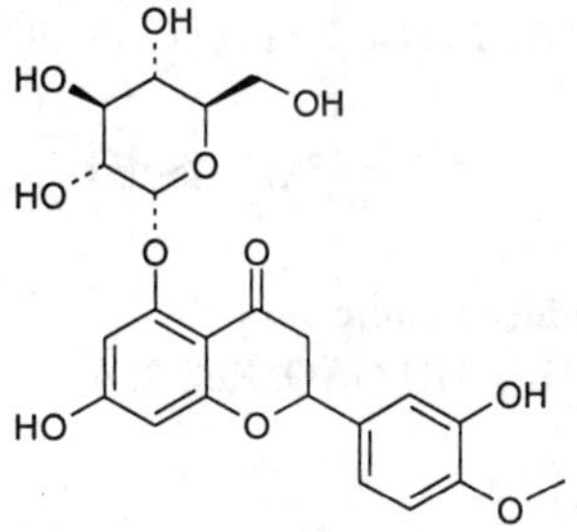

2994 Hesperidin
CAS: 520-26-3 $C_{28}H_{34}O_{15}$ MW: 610.57 Source: JIN JIE. Ref: 2, 4.

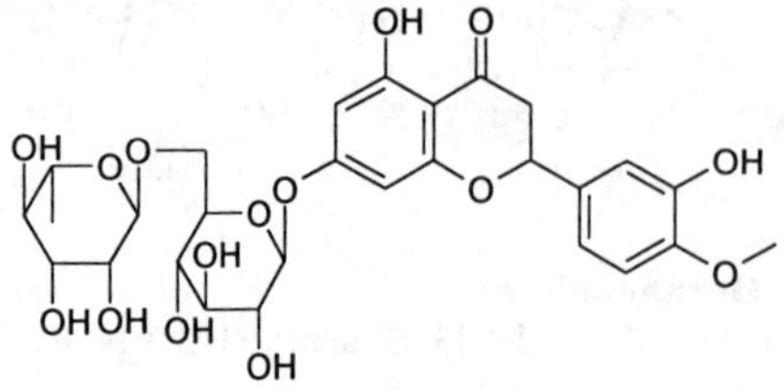

2995 Hespertitinic acid
$C_{10}H_{10}O_4$ MW: 194.19 Property: mp 238-40°C. Source: XIE CAO. Ref: 6.

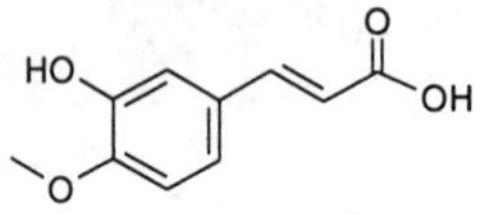

2996 Heteroauxin
$C_{10}H_9NO_2$ MW: 175.19 Property: mp 164-5°C. Source: YUAN CAN SHA. Ref: 6.

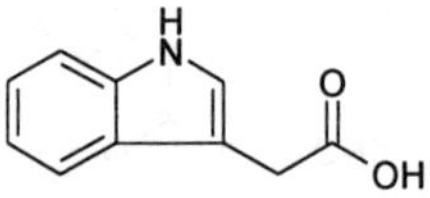

2997 Hexacosanoic acid
$C_{26}H_{52}O_2$ MW: 396.70 Property: mp 87.7-0.9°C. Source: CHONG BAI LA. Ref: 6.

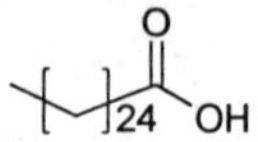

2998 Hexacosanol-1
$C_{26}H_{54}O$ MW: 382.72 Source: BAI GUO. Ref: 2.

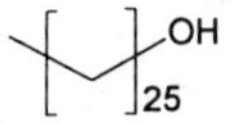

2999 Hexacosanyl ferulate
Source: GUANG XI XUE JIE. Ref: 616

3001 n-Hexacosanyl isovalerate
$C_{31}H_{62}O_2$ MW: 466.84 Source: GAN SONG. Ref: 6.

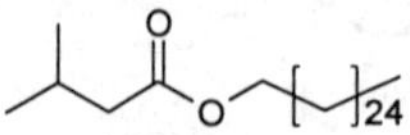

3002 Hexadecadienoic acid
Source: LU HUI, HU GAO. Ref: 2, 6.

3003 Hexadecane
$C_{16}H_{34}$ MW: 226.45 Source: REN SHEN, SAN QI, XI YANG SHEN. Ref: 2.

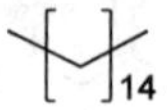

3004 Hexadecanoic acid
$C_{16}H_{32}O_2$ MW: 256.43 Source: BAI ZHI, CHAI HU, GUANG YE DING GONG TENG, QIANG HUO. Ref: 2, 585.

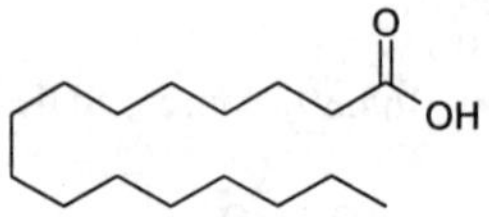

3005 20-Hexadecanoylingenol
$C_{36}H_{58}O_6$ MW: 586.86 Source: QIAN JIN ZI. Ref: 6.

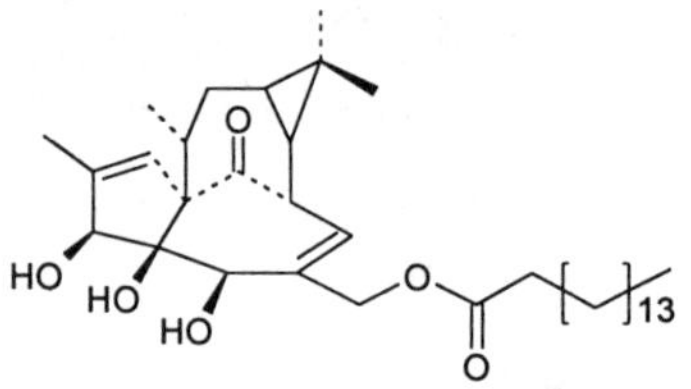

3006 2-(Hexa-2,4-diyn-1-ylidene)-1,6-dioxa-spiro[4,4]non-3-ene
$C_{15}H_{12}O_2$ MW: 224.26 Source: MU JU. Ref: 6.

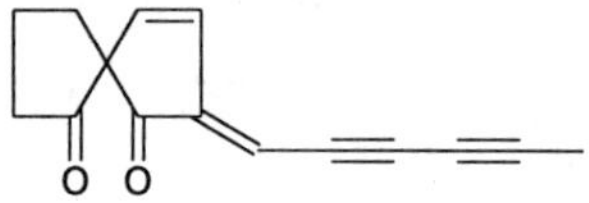

3007 4,4a,5,6,7,8-Hexahydro-4,4a-dimethyl-6-(1-methyl ethenyl)-2(3H)-naphthalene
$C_{15}H_{22}O$ MW: 218.34 Source: WU WEI ZI. Ref: 2.

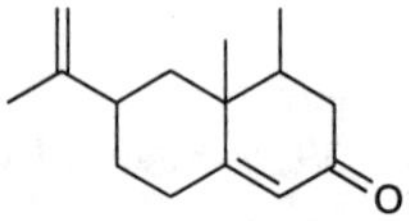

3008 1,2,4a,5,6,8a-Hexahydro-4,7-dimethyl-1-(1-methylethyl)-naphthalene
$C_{15}H_{24}$ MW: 204.36 Source: WU WEI ZI. Ref: 2.

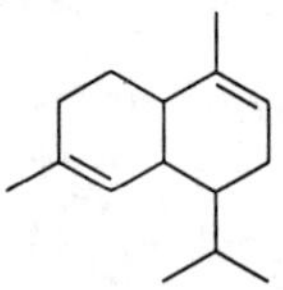

3009 1,3,4,5,6,7-Hexahydro-1,1,5,5-tetramethyl-2H-2,4-methanophthalene

$C_{15}H_{24}$ MW: 204.36 Source: WU WEI ZI. Ref: 2.

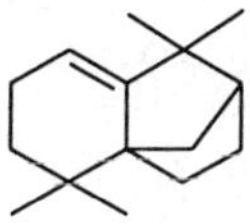

3010 1,2,3,3a,8,8a-Hexahydro-2,2,8-trimethyl-5,6-azulenedimethanol

$C_{15}H_{24}O_2$ MW: 236.36 Source: WU WEI ZI. Ref: 2.

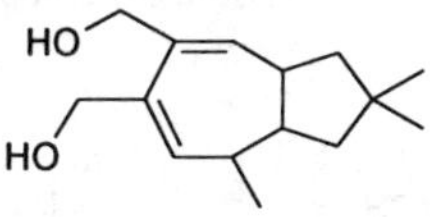

3011 5,6,7,8,3',4'-Hexamethoxyflavone

$C_{19}H_{18}O_8$ MW: 374.35 Source: JU PI. Ref: 2.

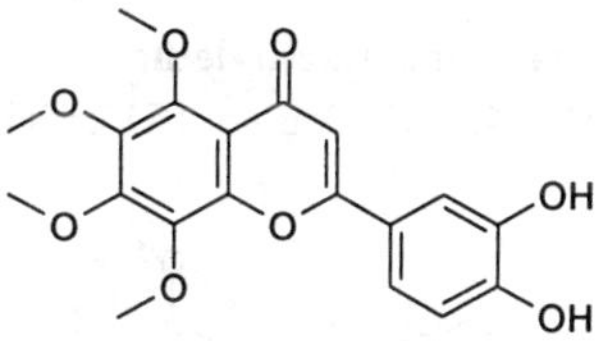

3012 Hexanac acid

$C_6H_{12}O_2$ MW: 116.16 Source: XI YANG SHEN. Ref: 2.

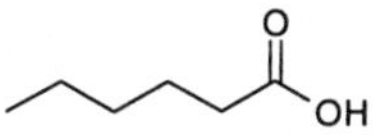

3013 Hexanal

$C_6H_{12}O$ MW: 100.16 Source: FANG FENG, QIANG HUO, XING REN. Ref: 2.

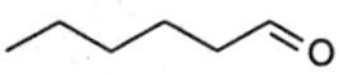

3014 Hexandraside E

Source: YIN YANG HUO. Ref: 623.

3015 Hexanol

$C_6H_{14}O$ MW: 102.18 Source: FANG FENG. Ref: 2.

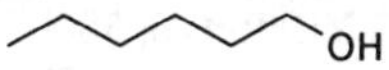

3016 (E)-2-Hexenal

$C_6H_{10}O$ MW: 98.15 Source: XING REN. Ref: 2.

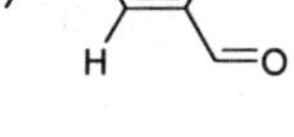

3017 1-Hexene

C_6H_{12} MW: 84.16 Source: JIN YIN HUA. Ref: 2.

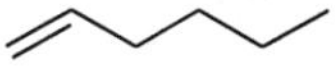

3018 trans-2-Hexenoic acid

$C_6H_{10}O_2$ MW: 114.15 Property: mp 36-7°C, bp 217°C. Source: NIU BANG GEN. Ref: 6.

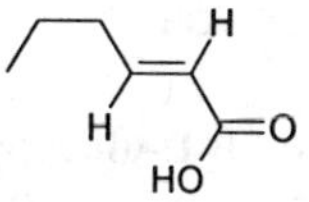

3019 trans-2-Hexenol

$C_6H_{12}O$ MW: 100.16 Property: mp 158-60°C. Source: XING ZI. Ref: 6.

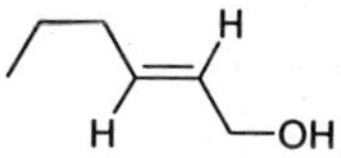

3020 β-Hexenol

cis-3-Hexen-1-ol; Leaf alcohol. $C_6H_{12}O$ MW: 100.16 Property: bp cis-: 156-7°C. Source: PI PA YE. Ref: 6.

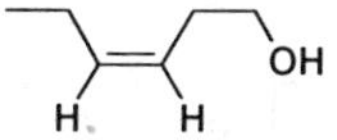

3021 γ-Hexenol

trans-3-Hexen-1-ol. $C_6H_{12}O$ MW: 100.16 Property: bp 153-6°C. Source: PI PA YE. Ref: 6.

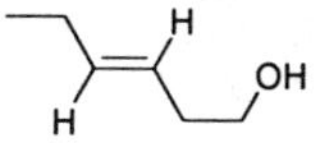

3022 (E)-2-Hexenyl-α-L-arabinopyranosyl-(1→2)-β-D-glucopyranoside

$C_{17}H_{30}O_{10}$ MW: 394.42 Source: DANG SHEN. Ref: 2.

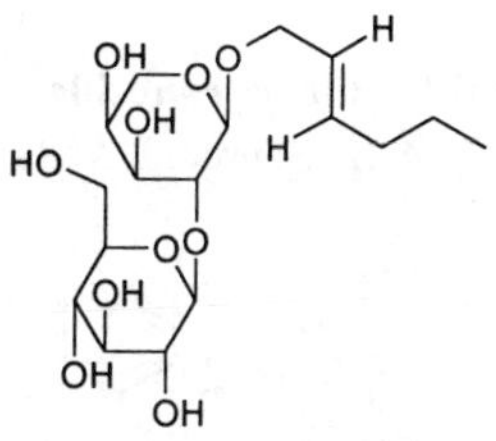

3023 2-Hexenyl benzoate

$C_{13}H_{16}O_2$ MW: 204.27 Source: CHA YE. Ref: 6.

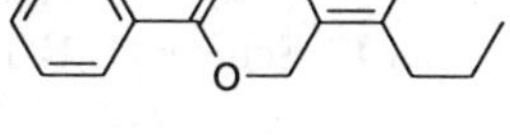

3024 (Z)-3-Hexenyl-β-D-glucopyranoside
$C_{12}H_{22}O_6$ MW: 262.31 Source: DANG SHEN. Ref: 2.

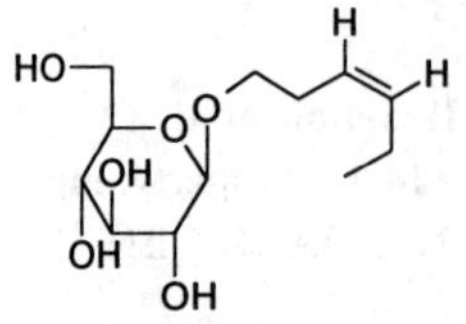

3025 (E)-2-Hexenyl-β-D-glucopyranoside
$C_{12}H_{22}O_6$ MW: 262.31 Source: DANG SHEN. Ref: 2.

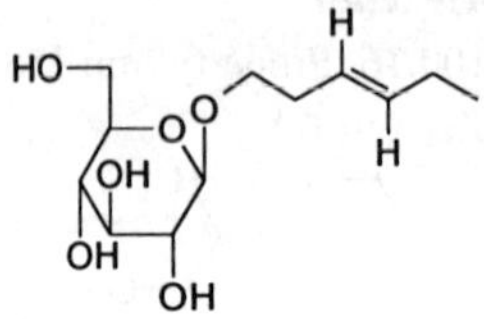

3026 (E)-2-Hexenyl-β-D-glucopyranosyl-(1→2)-β-D-glucopyranoside
$C_{18}H_{32}O_{11}$ MW: 424.45 Source: DANG SHEN. Ref: 2.

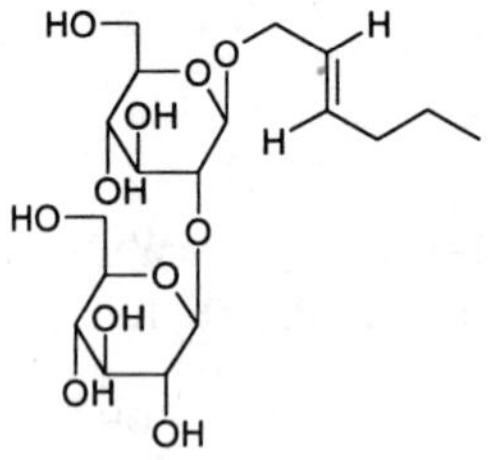

3027 Hexyl amine-1
$C_6H_{15}N$ MW: 101.19 Property: mp -19°C, bp 129-30°C/742mm. Source: MAI JIAO. Ref: 6.

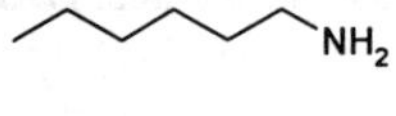

3028 n-Hexyl-β-D-glucopyranoside
$C_{12}H_{24}O_6$ MW: 264.32 Source: DANG SHEN. Ref: 2.

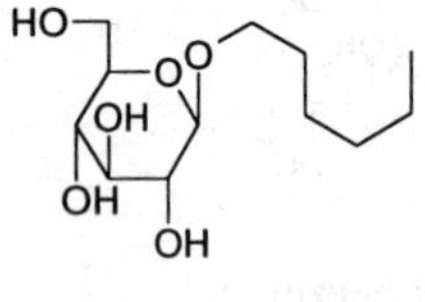

3029 Hexyl-β-D-glucopyranosyl(1→2)-β-D-glucopyranoside
$C_{18}H_{34}O_{11}$ MW: 426.47 Source: DANG SHEN. Ref: 2.

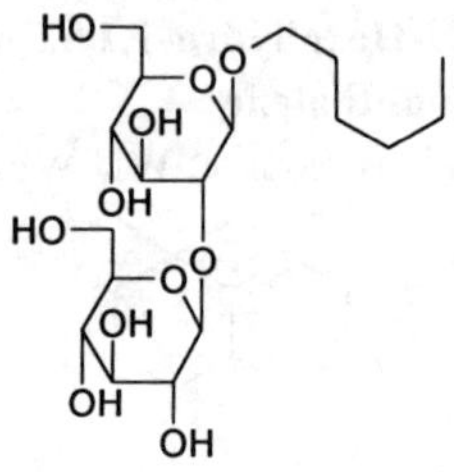

3030 Hexyl-β-D-glucopyranosyl(1→6)-β-D-glucopyranoside
$C_{18}H_{34}O_{11}$ MW: 426.47 Source: DANG SHEN. Ref: 2.

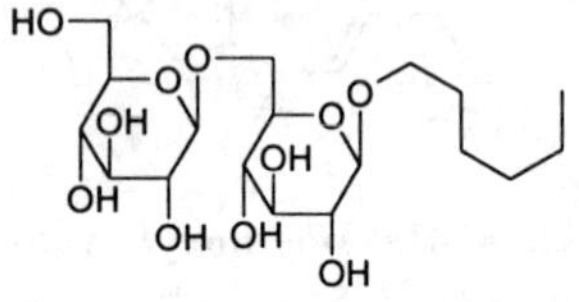

3031 Hibiscetin-heptamethylether
$C_{22}H_{24}O_9$ MW: 432.43 Source: JIU LI XIANG. Ref: 11.

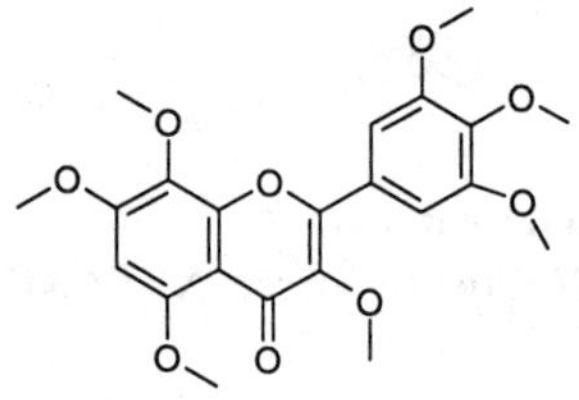

3032 Hinesol
$C_{15}H_{26}O$ MW: 222.37 Source: CANG ZHU. Ref: 2.

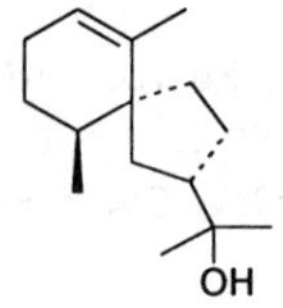

3033 Hinokiflavone
$C_{30}H_{18}O_{10}$ MW: 538.47 Property: mp 353-5°C (dec). Source: BAI SHU YE, CE BAI YE, DU SONG SHI, GUI YE, JI MAO SONG, JUAN BAI, LIU SHAN, LUO HAN SONG YE. Ref: 6, 580.

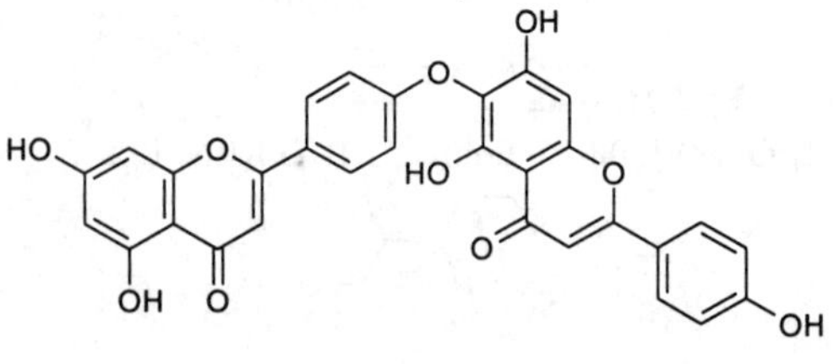

3034 Hippeastrine
$C_{18}H_{19}NO_5$ MW: 329.36 Property: mp 214-5°C. Source: SHI SUAN. Ref: 6.

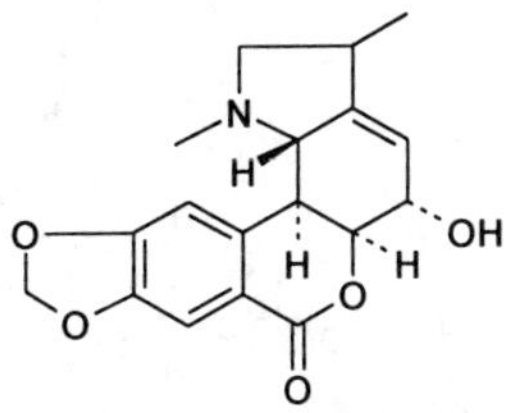

3035 Hippuric acid
$C_9H_9NO_3$ MW: 179.18 Property: mp 187°C. Source: REN NIAO. Ref: 6.

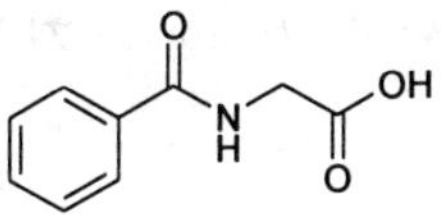

3036 Hirsuteine
$C_{22}H_{26}N_2O_3$ MW: 366.46 Property: mp 92-4°C. Source: GOU TENG. Ref: 2.

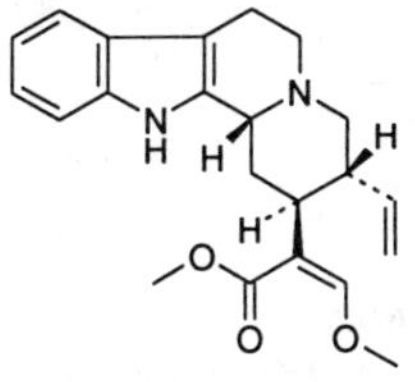

3037 Hirsutine
$C_{22}H_{28}N_2O_3$ MW: 368.48 Property: mp 101°C. Source: FENG XIANG SHU YE (a), GOU TENG. Ref: 2, 6.

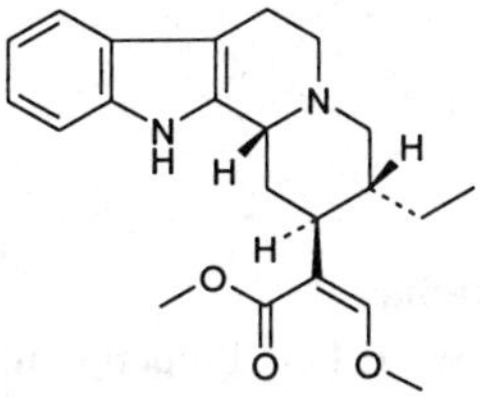

3038 Hispaglabridin A
$C_{21}H_{22}O_5$ MW: 354.41 Source: GAN CAO. Ref: 2.

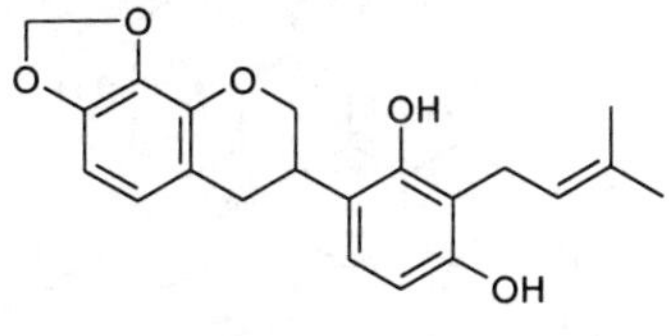

3039 Hispaglabridin B
$C_{25}H_{26}O_4$ MW: 390.48 Source: GAN CAO. Ref: 2.

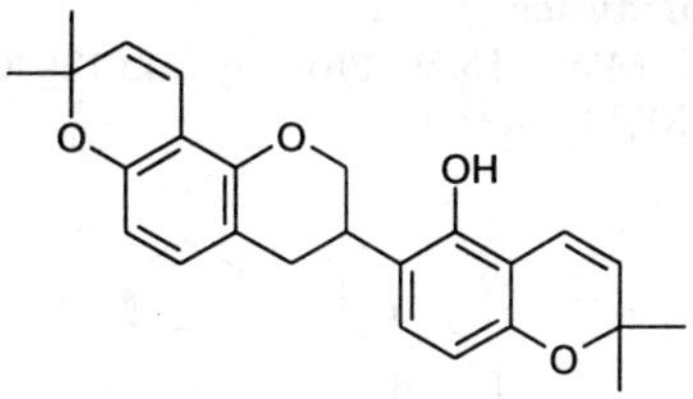

3040 Hispidulin
Dinatin. CAS: 1447-88-7 $C_{16}H_{12}O_6$ MW: 300.27 Property: mp 281-2°C. Source: CHANG GUAN JIA MO LI, CHOU MUO LI , LI ZHI CAO, YA PIAN. Ref: 5.

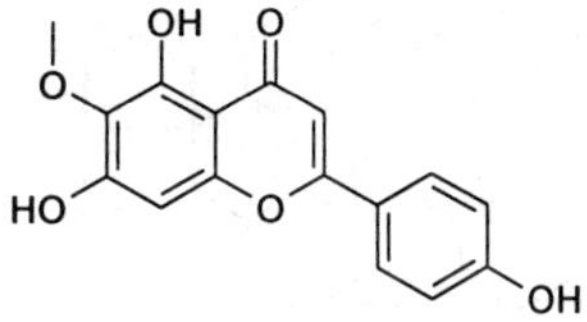

3041 Hispidulin-7-O-glucuronide
$C_{22}H_{20}O_{12}$ MW: 476.40 Property: mp 220-2°C. Source: JIN SI TAO GUO SHI. Ref: 6.

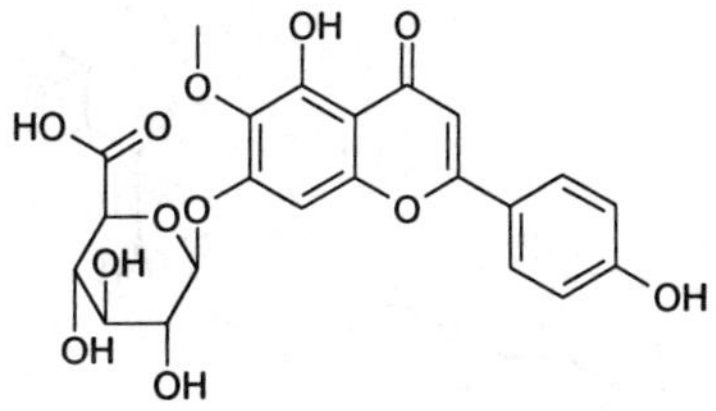

3042 Histamine
$C_5H_9N_3$ MW: 109.17 Property: mp 75-80°C, bp 167°C/0.8mm. Source: BAI QU CAI, CHUN, FENG DU, LI YU, LI YU, MAI JIAO, MAN LI YU, MIAN HUA, SAN XIAO CAO, WU GONG, YE DU ZHONG. Ref: 6.

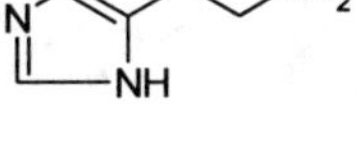

3043 Holadysamine
$C_{22}H_{35}NO$ MW: 329.53 Property: mp 173°C. Source: ZHI XIE MU PI. Ref: 6.

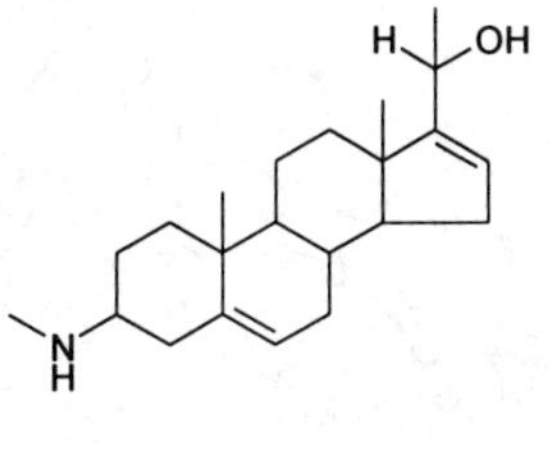

3044 Holadysine
$C_{21}H_{33}NO$ MW: 315.50 Property: mp 120°C. Source: ZHI XIE MU PI. Ref: 6.

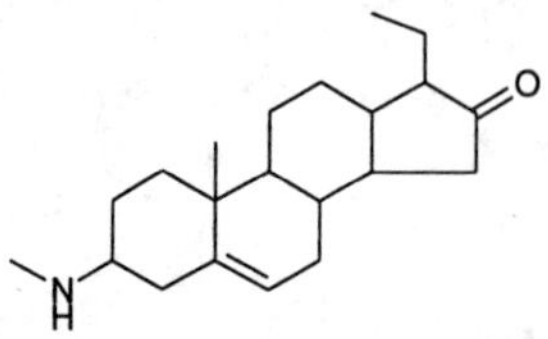

3045 Holafrine
$C_{29}H_{46}N_2O_2$ MW: 454.70 Property: mp 116-7°C. Source: ZHI XIE MU PI. Ref: 6.

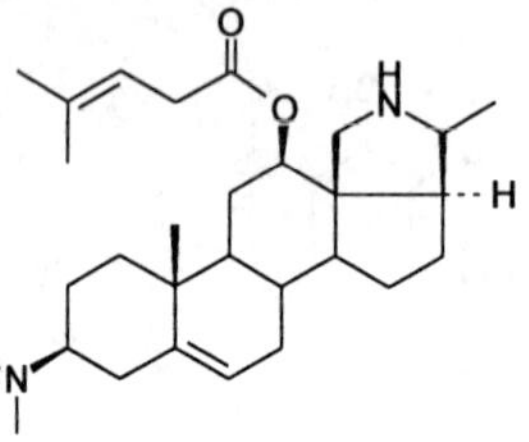

3046 Holantosine A
$C_{28}H_{47}NO_6$ MW: 493.69 Source: ZHI XIE MU PI. Ref: 6.

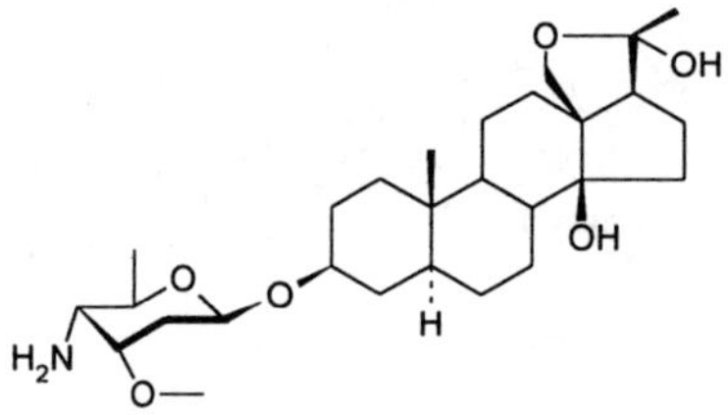

3047 Holantosine B
$C_{28}H_{45}NO_5$ MW: 475.67 Source: ZHI XIE MU PI. Ref: 6.

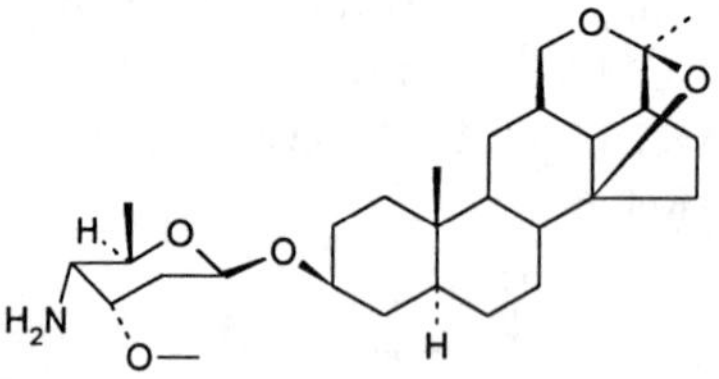

3048 Holantosine C
$C_{28}H_{47}NO_6$ MW: 493.69 Source: ZHI XIE MU PI. Ref: 6.

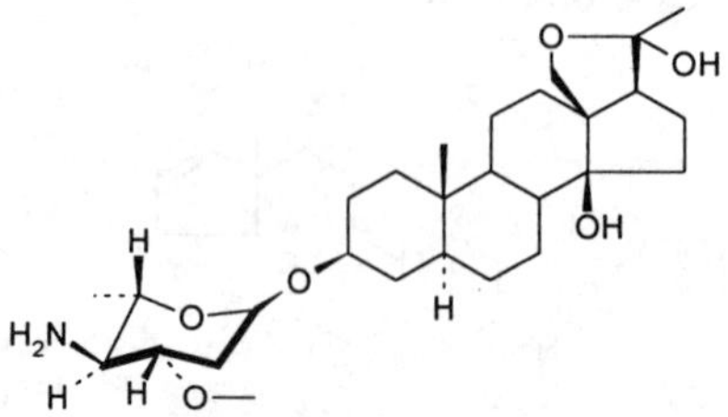

3049 Holantosine D
$C_{28}H_{45}NO_5$ MW: 475.67 Source: ZHI XIE MU PI. Ref: 6.

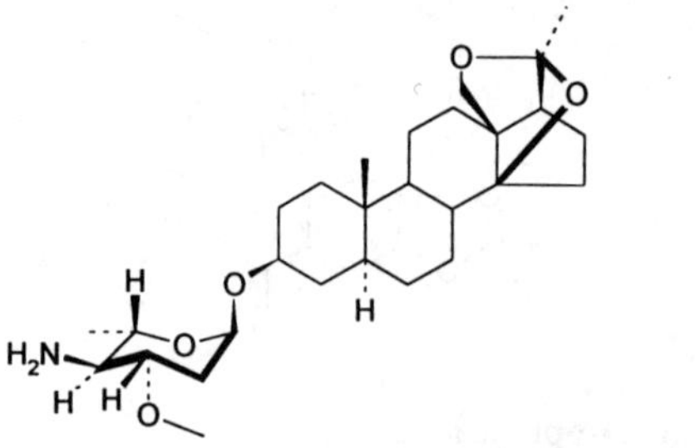

3050 Holarosine A
$C_{30}H_{47}NO_6$ MW: 517.71 Source: ZHI XIE MU PI. Ref: 6.

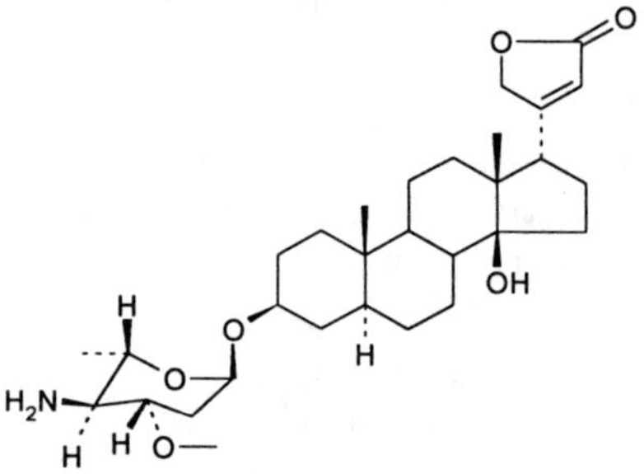

3051 Holarrhenine
$C_{24}H_{40}N_2O$ MW: 372.60 Property: mp 197-8°C. Source: ZHI XIE MU PI. Ref: 6.

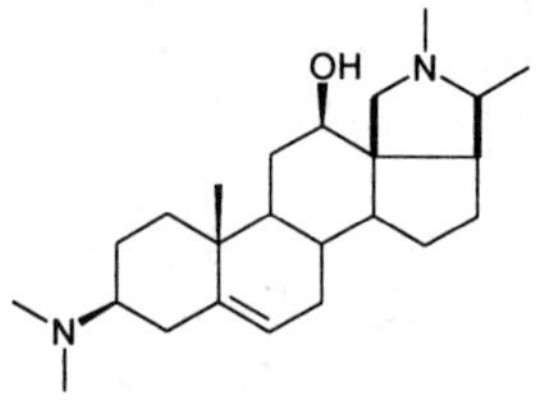

3052 Holarrhetine
$C_{29}H_{46}N_2O_2$ MW: 454.70 Property: mp 74-5°C. Source: ZHI XIE MU PI. Ref: 6.

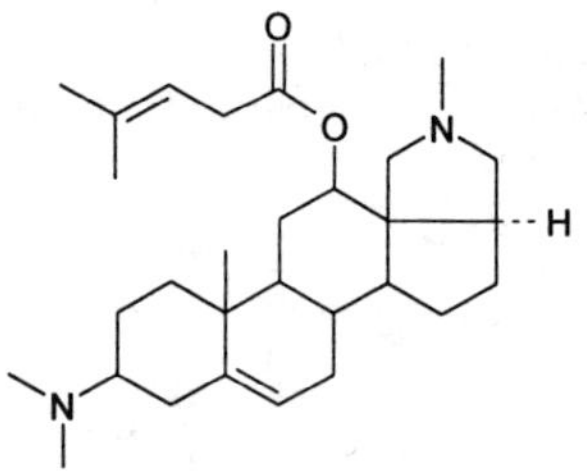

3053 Holarrhidine
$C_{21}H_{36}N_2O$ MW: 332.53 Property: mp 180-1°C. Source: ZHI XIE MU PI. Ref: 6.

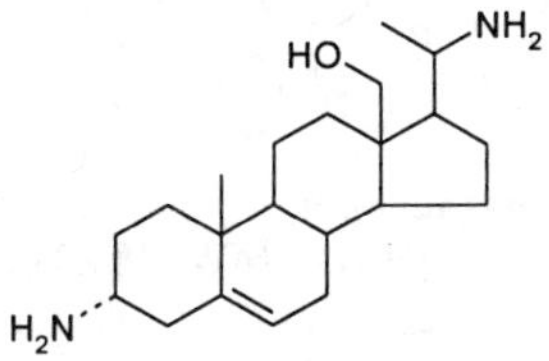

3054 Holarrhimine
$C_{21}H_{36}N_2O$ MW: 332.53 Property: mp 183°C. Source: ZHI XIE MU PI. Ref: 6.

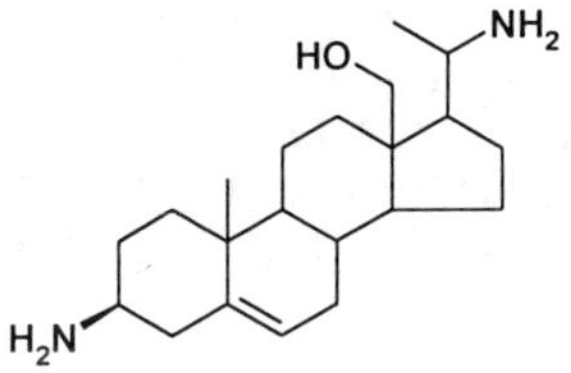

3055 Holarrhine
$C_{20}H_{38}N_2O_3$ Property: mp 240°C. Source: ZHI XIE MU PI. Ref: 6.

3056 Holonamine
$C_{21}H_{27}N_2O$ MW: 325.45 Property: mp 257-9°C. Source: ZHI XIE MU PI. Ref: 6.

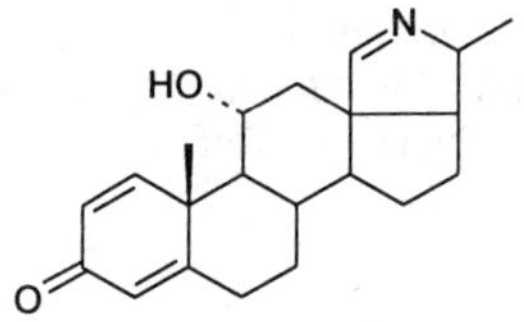

3057 Homoandrographolide
$C_{22}H_{32}O_4$ Source: CHUAN XIN LIAN. Ref: 2.

3058 Homoarbutin
$C_{13}H_{18}O_7$ MW: 286.28 Property: mp 192-3°C. Source: LU XIAN CAO. Ref: 6.

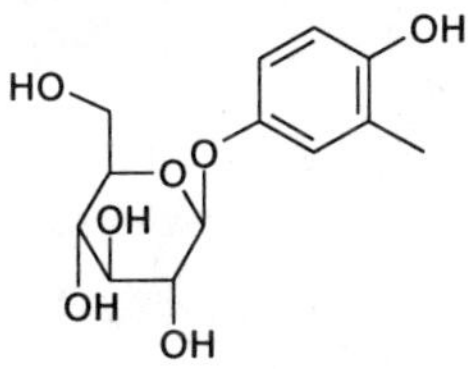

3059 Homoarecoline
$C_9H_{15}NO_2$ MW: 169.23 Source: BING LANG. Ref: 2.

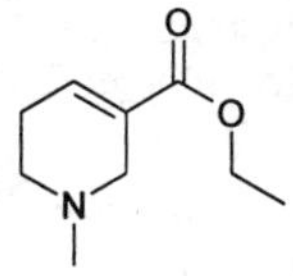

3060 Homoaromoline
$C_{37}H_{40}N_2O_6$ MW: 608.74 Property: mp 238-40°C. Source: BAI YAO ZI, YIN BU HUAN. Ref: 6.

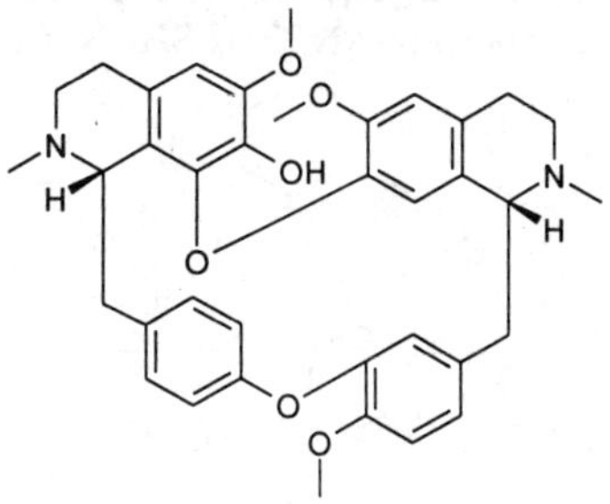

3061 Homochelidonine
α-Homochelidonine. $C_{21}H_{23}NO_5$ MW: 369.42 Property: mp 182°C. Source: BAI QU CAI. Ref: 6.

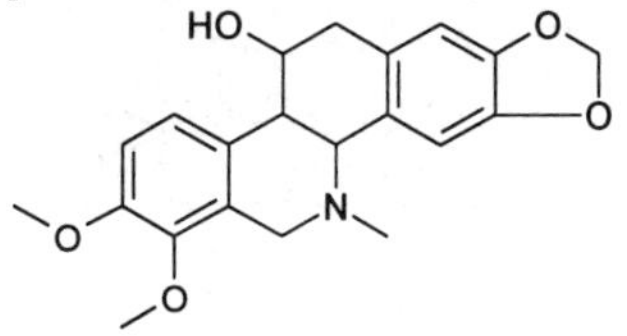

3062 Homocystine
$C_8H_{16}N_2O_4S_2$ MW: 268.36 Property: mp L(+): 281-4°C (dec), D(-): 281-4°C (dec), DL: 260-5°C (dec). Source: MO GU. Ref: 6.

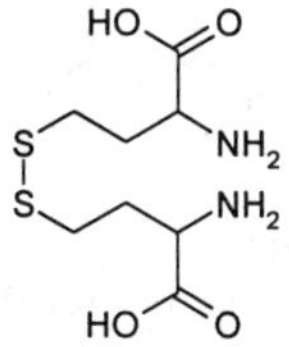

3063 Homofukinolide
$C_{25}H_{34}O_6$ MW: 430.55 Source: FENG DOU CAI. Ref: 6.

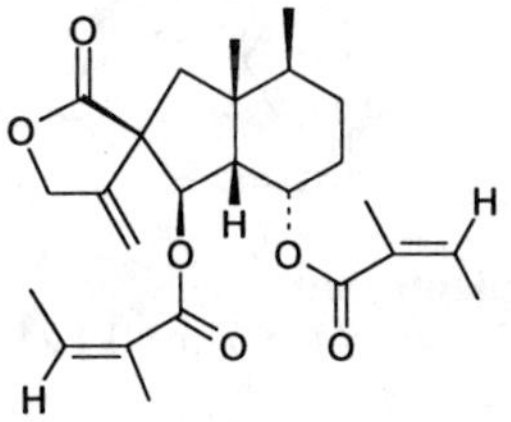

3064 Homogentisic acid
$C_8H_8O_4$ MW: 168.15 Source: BAN XIA. Ref: 2.

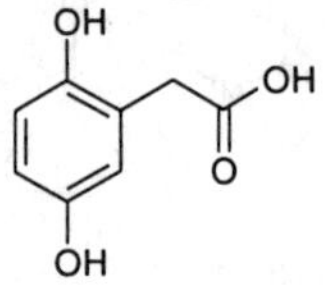

3065 Homoharringtonine
CAS: 26833-87-4 $C_{29}H_{39}NO_9$ MW: 545.64 Property: mp 144-6°C. Source: SAN JIAN SHAN. Ref: 2, 4.

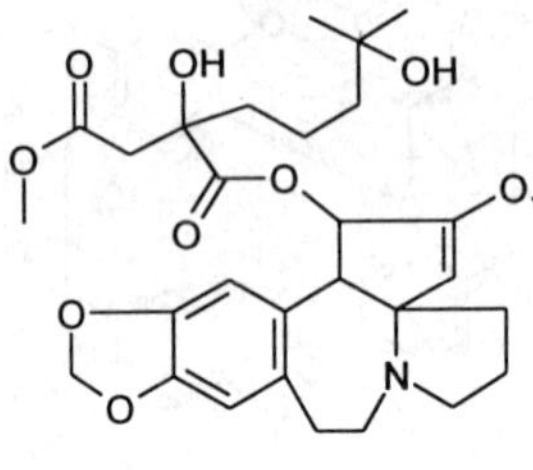

3066 Homolycorine
$C_{18}H_{21}NO_4$ MW: 315.37 Property: mp 175°C. Source: DA YI ZHI JIAN, SHI SUAN. Ref: 6.

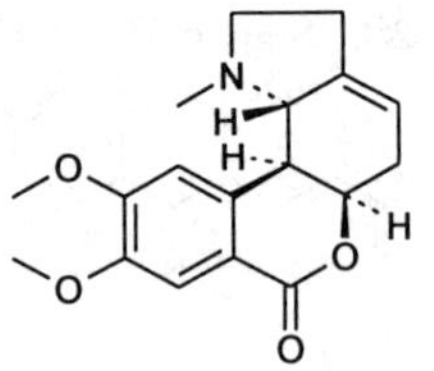

3067 Homomangiferin
$C_{20}H_{20}O_{12}$ MW: 452.38 Source: MANG GUO SHU PI. Ref: 6.

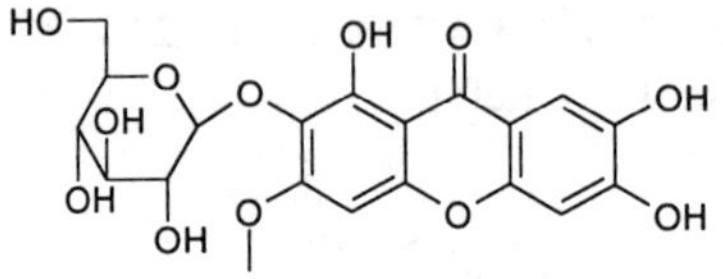

3068 Homonataloin
$C_{21}H_{22}O_{10}$ MW: 434.40 Source: LU HUI. Ref: 2

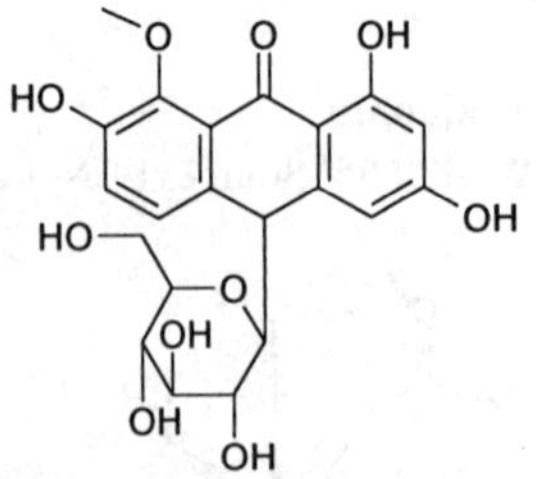

3069 Homoplantaginin
$C_{22}H_{22}O_{11}$ MW: 462.41 Source: LI ZHI CAO. Ref: 6.

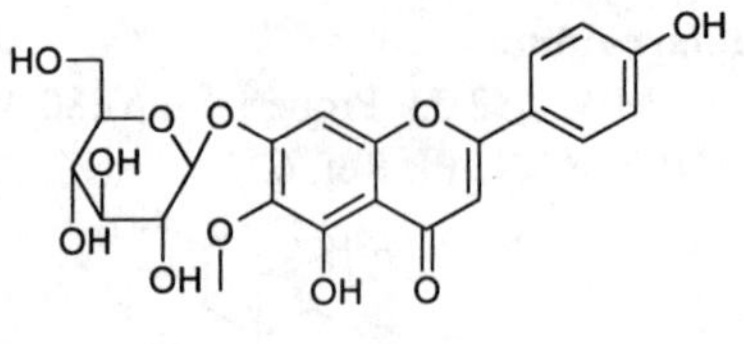

3070 Homopterocarpin
CAS: 606-91-7 $C_{17}H_{16}O_4$ MW: 284.31 Property: mp 83-5°C. Source: Pterocarpus indicus Willd. Ref: 5.

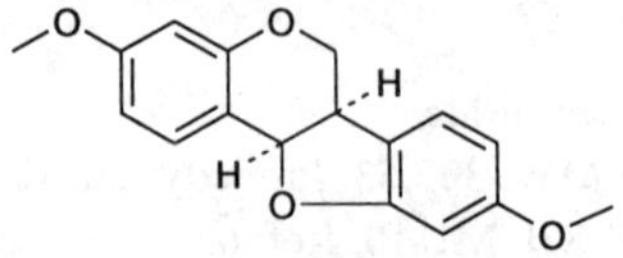

3071 L-Homoserine
$C_4H_9NO_3$ MW: 119.12 Property: mp (+): 203°C (dec). Source: AN YE, DAO DOU, HUANG JING, SAN YE SHU WEI CAO, ZI YUN YING ZI. Ref: 6, 182.

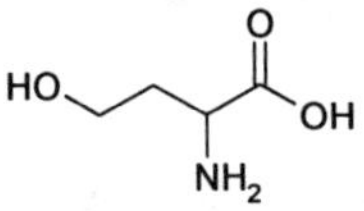

3072 sym-Homospermidine
$C_8H_{21}N$ MW: 159.28 Source: TAN XIANG. Ref: 6.

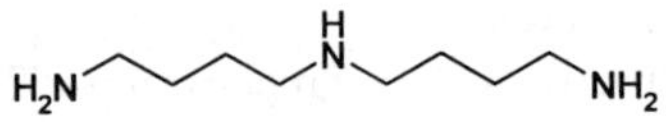

3073 Homostephanoline
$C_{20}H_{25}NO_5$ MW: 359.43 Property: mp 233°C. Source: QIAN JIN TENG. Ref: 6.

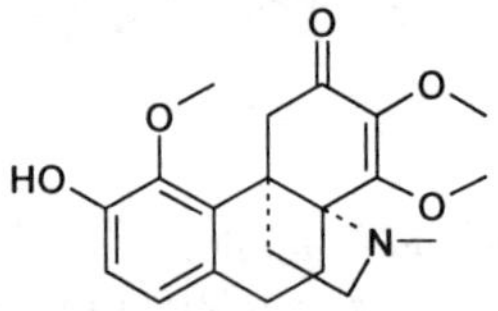

3074 Homothalicrine
$C_{37}H_{40}N_2O_6$ MW: 608.74 Property: mp 235-6°C (dec). Source: YAN GUO CAO. Ref: 6.

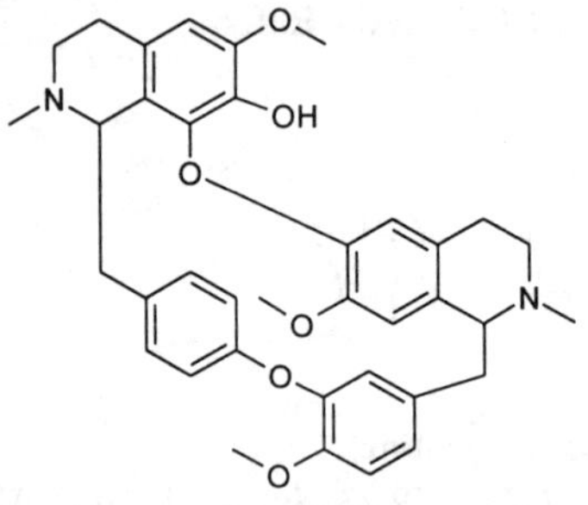

3075 Hongguanggenin
$C_{27}H_{44}O_5$ MW: 448.65 Source: JIAN MA. Ref: 10.

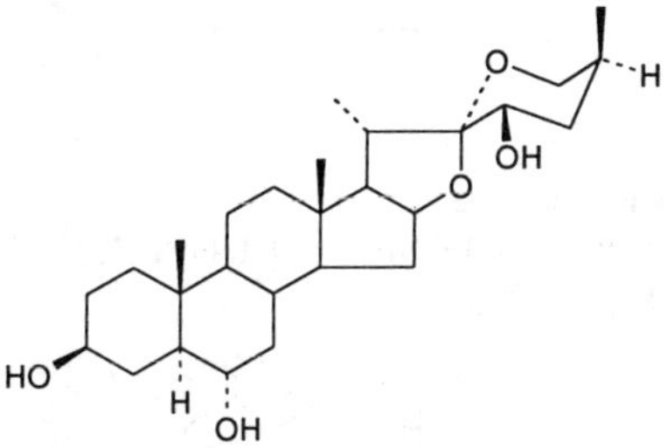

3076 Honokiol
$C_{18}H_{18}O_2$ MW: 266.34 Source: HOU PO. Ref: 2, 625.

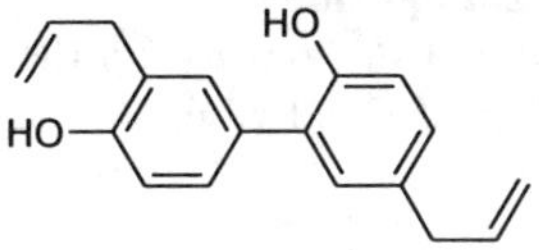

3077 Hopanol-29
$C_{30}H_{52}O$ MW: 428.75 Property: mp 242-4°C. Source: GUAN ZHONG. Ref: 6.

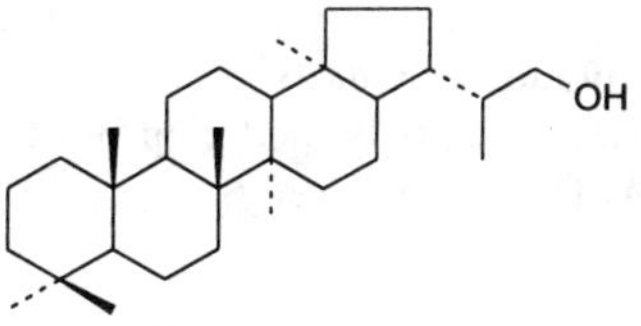

3078 Hopene II
$C_{30}H_{50}$ MW: 410.73 Property: mp 196-7°C. Source: TIE SI QI. Ref: 6.

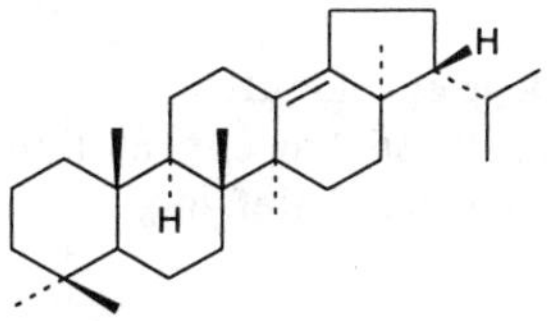

3079 22-(29)-Hopene
Diploptene; Hopene-b. $C_{30}H_{50}O$ MW: 410.73 Property: mp 210-1°C. Source: GUAN ZHONG, SHI WEI, SHUI LONG GU. Ref: 6.

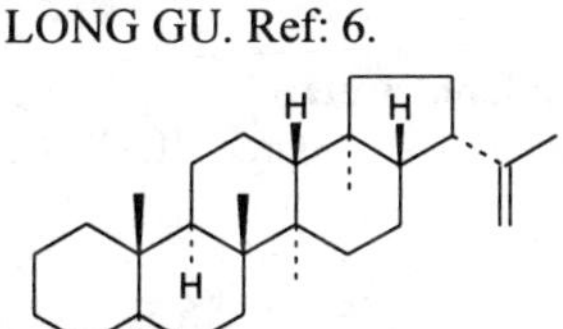

3080 Hordenine
N,N-Dimethyltyramine. $C_{10}H_{15}NO$ MW: 165.24 Property: mp 117°C, bp 173-4°C/11mm. Source: HONG MU JI CAO. Ref: 6.

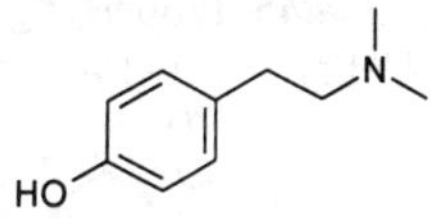

3081 Hovenine A
$C_{27}H_{42}N_4O_4$ MW: 486.66 Property: mp 215°C. Source: ZHI JU GEN. Ref: 6.

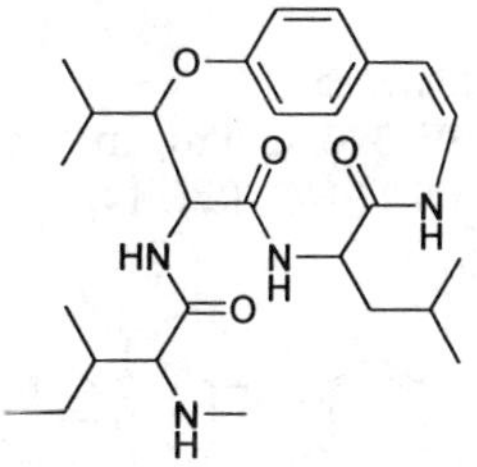

3082 Howiinol A, I
6S-(1R-Hydroxy-2R-cinnamyloxyphenethyl)5,6-dihydro-5S-hydroxy-2-pyrone. $C_{22}H_{20}O_6$ MW: 380.40 Property: white acicular crystal, mp 176-8°C, $[\alpha]_D$ +97.6° (c=0.087, chloroform). Source: HAI NAN GE NA XIANG. Ref: 410.

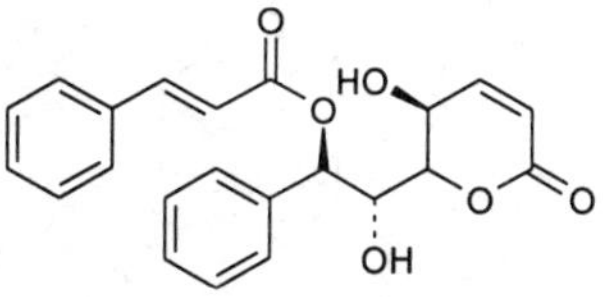

3083 Howiinol A, II
6S-(1S,2R-Epoxyphenethyl-5S-cinnamyloxy)5,6-dihydro-2-pyrone. $C_{22}H_{18}O_5$ MW: 362.40 Property: white acicular crystal, mp 176-8°C, $[\alpha]_D$ +97.6° (c=0.087, chloroform). Source: HAI NAN GE NA XIANG. Ref: 410.

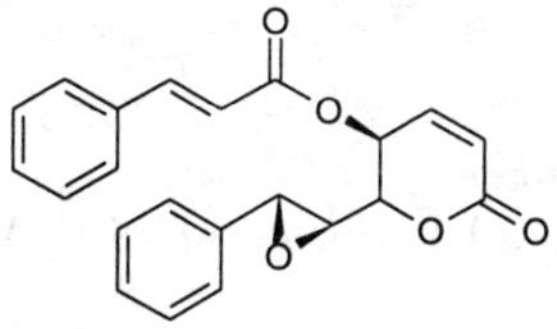

3084 Humantenidine
$C_{19}H_{22}N_2O_4$ MW: 342.40 Property: gem, $[\alpha]_D$ -123°. Source: HU MAN TENG. Ref: 14.

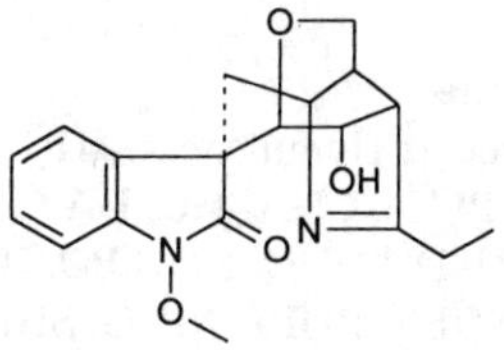

3085 Humantenine
$C_{21}H_{26}N_2O_3$ MW: 354.45 Property: gem, [α]$_D$ -142°. Source: HU MAN TENG. Ref: 14.

3086 Humantenirine
$C_{21}H_{26}N_2O_4$ MW: 370.45 Property: mp 168-9°C. Source: HU MAN TENG. Ref: 14.

3087 Humantenmine
Gelsenicine. $C_{19}H_{22}N_2O_3$ MW: 326.40 Property: mp 166-8°C, [α]$_D$ -147°. Source: HU MAN TENG. Ref: 14.

3088 Humuladienone
$C_{15}H_{22}O$ MW: 218.34 Source: PI JIU HUA. Ref: 6.

3089 Humulane
$C_{15}H_{30}$ MW: 210.41 Source: MAN SHAN HONG. Ref: 6.

3090 Humulene
α-Caryophyllene, α-Humulene. $C_{15}H_{24}$ MW: 204.36 Source: BING PIAN, CHAI HU, DA CAO KOU, DA YE XIANG RU, DU HUO, HOU PO, JI NING, LIAN JIANG, REN SHEN, SHI JI NING, SHI XIANG ROU, YIN CHEN HAO. Ref: 2, 6.

3091 β-Humulene
$C_{15}H_{24}$ MW: 204.36 Source: HUO XIANG, JIN JIE, REN SHEN. Ref: 2.

3092 Humulene epoxide I
$C_{15}H_{24}O$ MW: 220.36 Property: bp 104-5°C/105 mm. Source: BAI DOU KOU. Ref: 6.

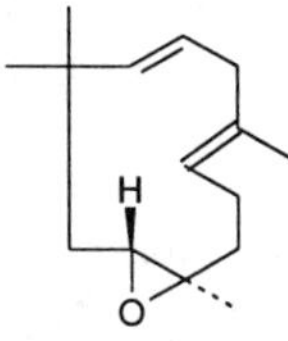

3093 Humulene epoxide II
$C_{15}H_{24}O$ MW: 220.36 Property: bp 105-6°C/1.5mm. Source: BAI DOU KOU. Ref: 6.

3094 Humulene epoxide III
$C_{15}H_{24}O$ MW: 220.36 Property: bp 120-30°C/15mm. Source: BAI DOU KOU. Ref: 6.

3095 α-Humulenol acetate
$C_{17}H_{26}O_2$ MW: 262.40 Source: JU PI (CHEN PI). Ref: 6.

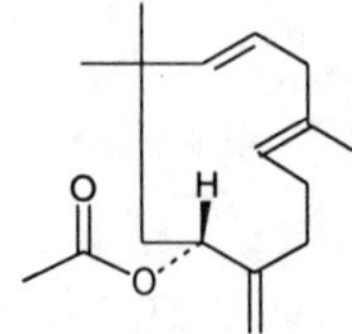

3096 Humulenone-II
$C_{15}H_{24}O$ MW: 220.36 Source: PI JIU HUA. Ref: 6.

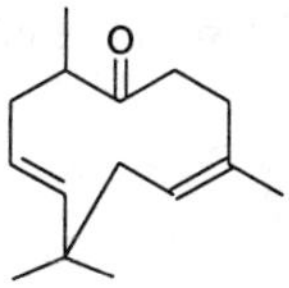

3097 Humulone
$C_{21}H_{30}O_5$ MW: 362.47 Property: mp 63-5°C. Source: LU CAO, PI JIU HUA. Ref: 6.

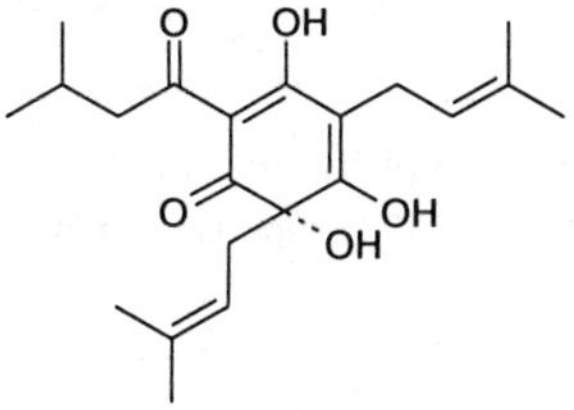

3098 Hupehemonoside
$C_{33}H_{53}NO_8$ MW: 591.79 Property: colorless amorphous powder, mp 206-8°C, $[\alpha]_D^{27}$ -48.3° (c=0.46, methanol). Source: HU BEI BEI MU. Ref: 206.

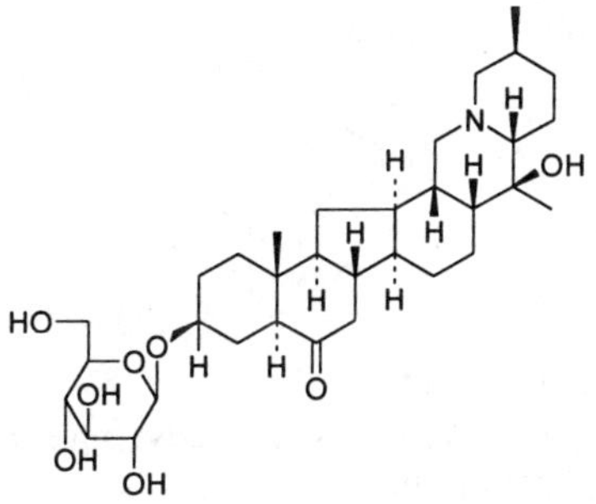

3098b Hupeheninoside
5α,14α-Cevanine-6α-hydroxyl-3α-β-D-glucoside. $C_{33}H_{55}NO_7$ MW: 577.81 Property: colorless prismatic crystal, mp 241-4°C, $[\alpha]_D^{20}$ -41° (c=0.16, methanol). Source: HU BEI BEI MU. Ref: 30.

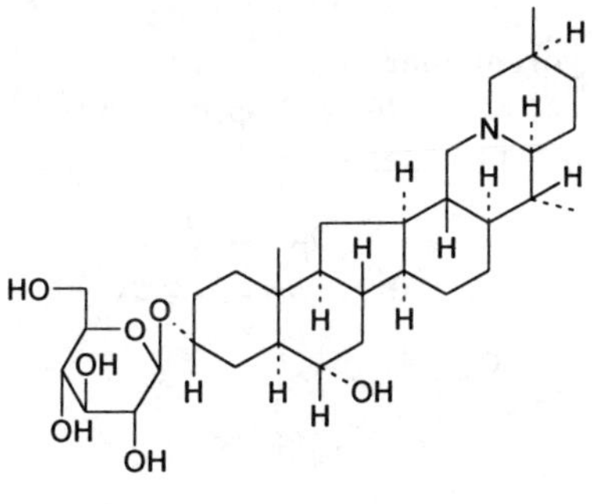

3099 Huperzinine
$C_{17}H_{22}N_2O$ MW: 270.38 Property: white thin acicular crystal, mp 251-3°C, $[\alpha]_D^{25}$-25.3° (c=0.1456, chloroform). Source: SHE ZU SHI SHAN. Ref: 108.

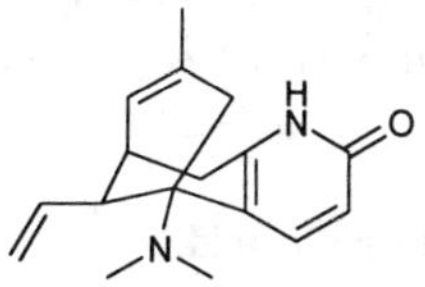

3100 D-Hurulon-14-en-3-ol
Source: XIAO SHE ZI WAN. Ref: 572.

3101 Hydnocarpic acid
$C_{16}H_{28}O_2$ MW: 252.40 Property: mp (+): 59-60°C, (±): 59-9.5°C. Source: DA FENG ZI. Ref: 6.

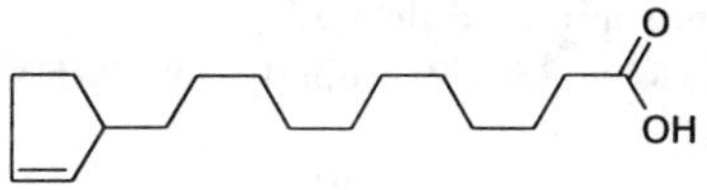

3102 Hydrangeic acid
$C_{15}H_{12}O_4$ MW: 256.26 Property: mp 181°C. Source: BA XIAN HUA. Ref: 6.

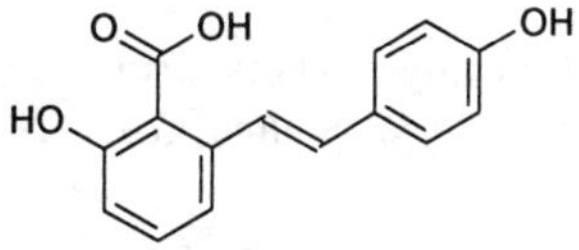

3103 Hydrangenol
$C_{15}H_{12}O_4$ MW: 256.26 Property: mp 181°C. Source: BA XIAN HUA. Ref: 6.

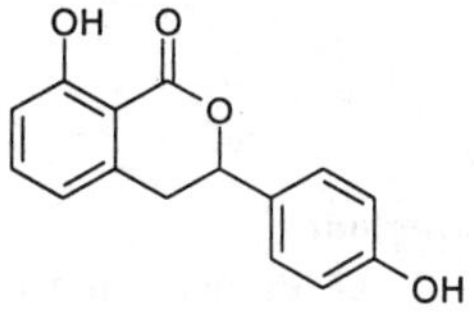

3104 Hydrocinnamic acid
$C_9H_{10}O_2$ MW: 150.18 Property: mp 48.5°C. Source: CHEN XIANG. Ref: 6.

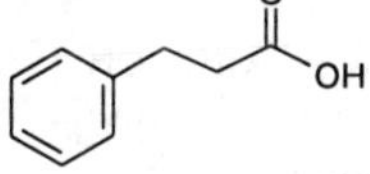

3105 Hydrocotarnine
$C_{12}H_{15}NO_3$ MW: 221.26 Property: mp 55-6°C. Source: YA PIAN. Ref: 6.

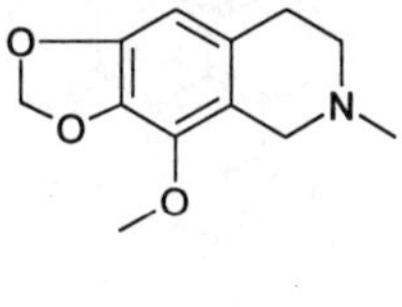

3106 Hydrocyanic acid
CHN MW: 27.03 Property: mp -13.3°C, bp 25.7°C. Source: BA DAN XING REN, CI NAN SHE TENG, DA CHAO CAI, HAI JIU CAI, LUO XIN FU, MANG GUO HE, MANG GUO YE, MU GUA, PI PA HE, SI GUA, WANG BU LIU XING, WU MEI, YING TAO, YU LI REN. Ref: 6.

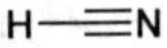

3107 Hydroginkgolic acid
$C_{22}H_{36}O_3$ MW: 348.53 Property: mp 92.5-3°C. Source: BAI GUO. Ref: 2.

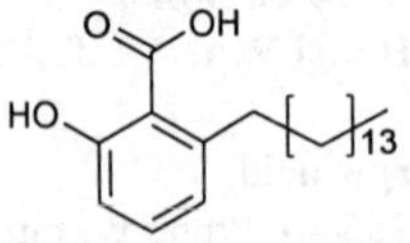

3108 Hydroginkgolinic acid
$C_{21}H_{34}O_3$ MW: 334.50 Property: mp 74-6°C. Source: BAI GUO. Ref: 6.

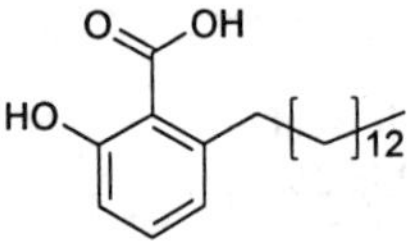

3109 18α-Hydroglycyrrhetic acid
$C_{29}H_{44}O_6$ MW: 488.67 Source: GAN CAO. Ref: 2.

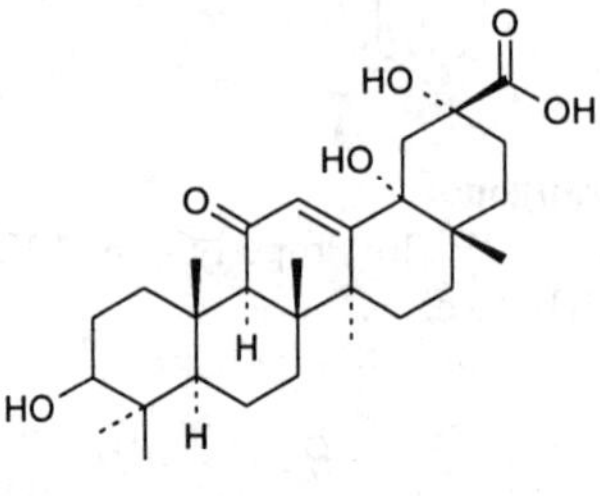

3110 α-Hydrojuglone
$C_{10}H_8O_3$ MW: 176.17 Property: mp 168-9°C. Source: HU TAO QING PI. Ref: 6.

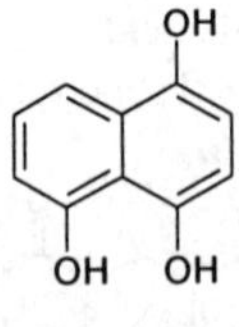

3111 β-Hydrojuglone
$C_{10}H_8O_3$ MW: 176.17 Property: mp 96-7°C. Source: HU TAO QING PI. Ref: 6.

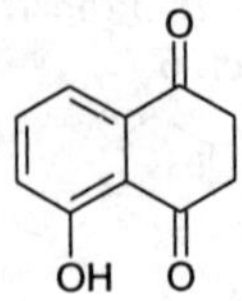

3112 α-Hydrojuglone glucoside
$C_{16}H_{18}O_8$ MW: 338.32 Property: mp 216°C (dec at 165°C). Source: HU TAO YE. Ref: 6.

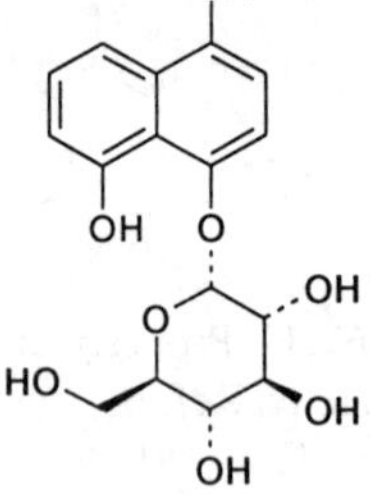

3113 1,2-Hydronaphthoquinone
$C_{10}H_8O_2$ MW: 160.17 Property: mp 60°C. Source: MAO GAO CAI. Ref: 6.

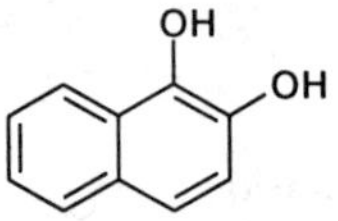

3114 1,4-Hydronaphthoquinone
$C_{10}H_8O_2$ MW: 160.17 Property: mp 175°C. Source: MAO GAO CAI. Ref: 6.

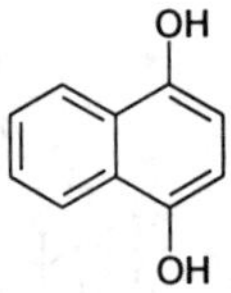

3115 Hydroquinidine
$C_{20}H_{26}N_2O_2$ MW: 326.44 Property: mp 168-9°C. Source: JIN JI LE. Ref: 6.

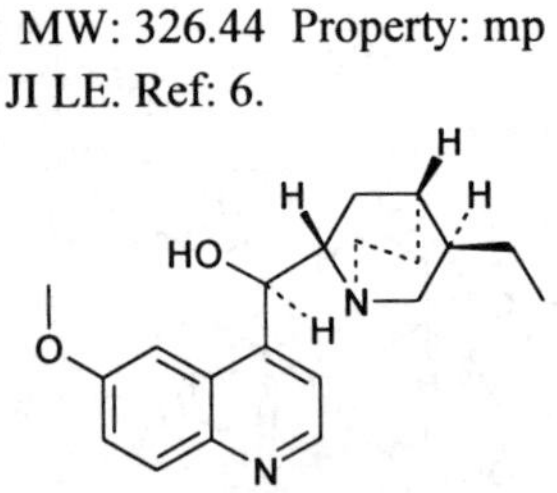

3116 Hydroquinine
$C_{20}H_{26}N_2O_2$ MW: 326.44 Property: mp 172.3°C. Source: JIN JI LE. Ref: 6.

3117 Hydroquinone
$C_6H_6O_2$ MW: 110.11 Property: mp 170.3°C. Source: JI SHI TENG GUO, MAN SHAN HONG, QIAN LI GUANG. Ref: 6.

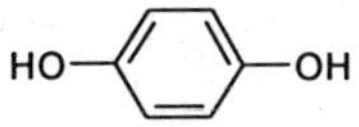

HO OH

3118 14-Hydroxy-abieta-8,11,13-trien-3-one
$C_{20}H_{28}O_2$ MW: 300.45 Source: LEI GONG TENG. Ref: 2.

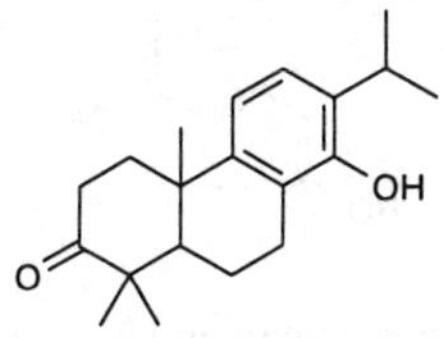

OH
O

3119 p-Hydroxy-acetophenone
$C_8H_8O_2$ MW: 136.15 Property: mp 109°C. Source: YIN CHEN HAO. Ref: 2, 6.

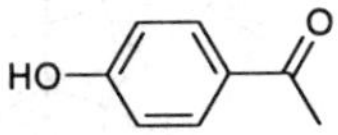

HO O

3120 (2R)-Hydroxy-4-(9-adenyl)butyric acid
$C_9H_{11}N_5O_3$ MW: 237.22 Source: XIANG XUN. Ref: 6.

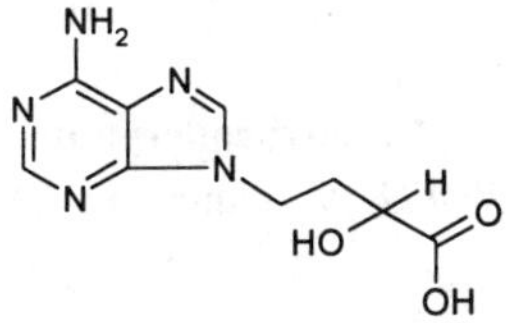

NH2 N N N N H O HO OH

3121 5-Hydroxyalizarin-methylether
$C_{15}H_{10}O_5$ MW: 270.24 Source: HU CI. Ref: 6.

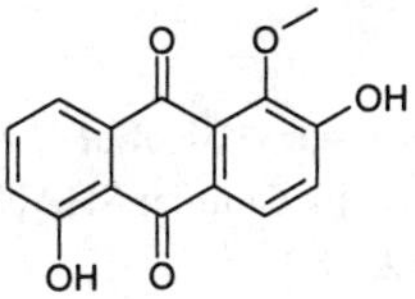

O OH OH O

3122 7-Hydroxyaloin
$C_{21}H_{22}O_{10}$ MW: 434.40 Source: LU HUI. Ref: 2.

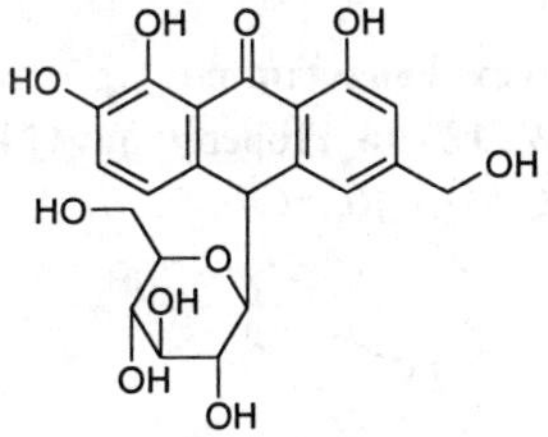

OH O OH HO OH HO O OH OH OH

3123 3α-Hydroxy-5β-androstan-17-one
$C_{19}H_{30}O_2$ MW: 290.45 Source: SHE XIANG. Ref: 2.

O HO H

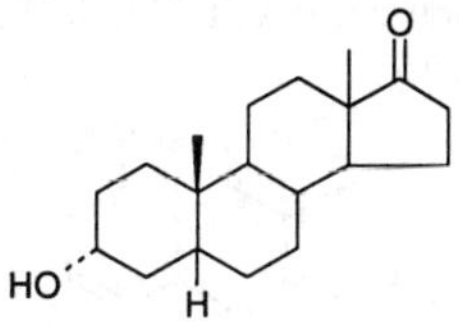

3124 3β-Hydroxy-5α-androstan-17-one
$C_{19}H_{30}O_2$ MW: 290.45 Source: SHE XIANG. Ref: 2.

O HO H

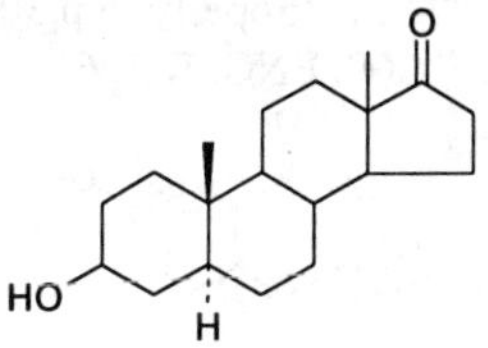

3125 3α-Hydroxy-androst-4-ene-17-one
$C_{19}H_{28}O_2$ MW: 288.43 Source: SHE XIANG. Ref: 2.

O HO

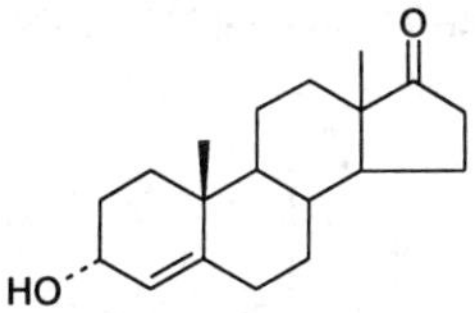

3126 3β-Hydroxy-androst-5-ene-17-one
$C_{19}H_{28}O_2$ MW: 288.43 Source: SHE XIANG. Ref: 2.

O HO

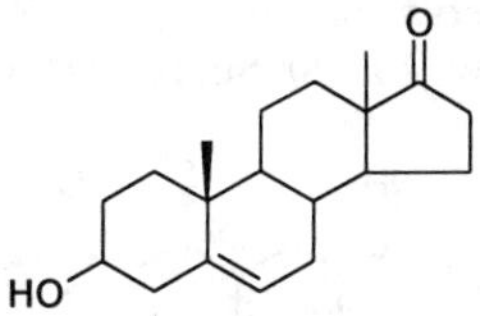

3127 3α-Hydroxy-5α-anodrostan-17-one
$C_{19}H_{30}O_2$ MW: 290.45 Source: SHE XIANG. Ref: 2.

O HO H

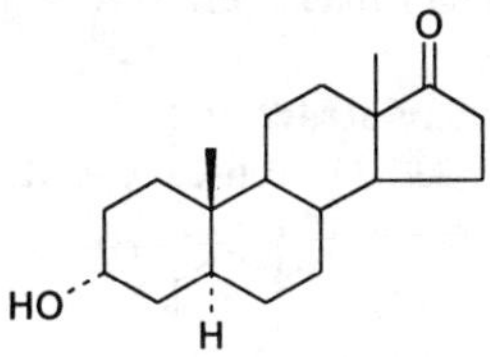

3128 α-Hydroxyanthraquinone
$C_{14}H_8O_3$ MW: 224.22 Property: mp 193°C (sublimation). Source: BA JI TIAN, WANG JIANG NAN. Ref: 6, 228.

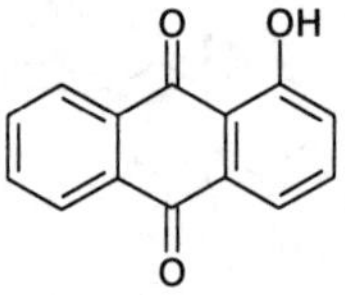

3129 2-Hydroxyanthraquinone
$C_{14}H_8O_3$ MW: 224.22 Property: mp 306°C, 320°C. Source: YANG JIAO TENG. Ref: 6.

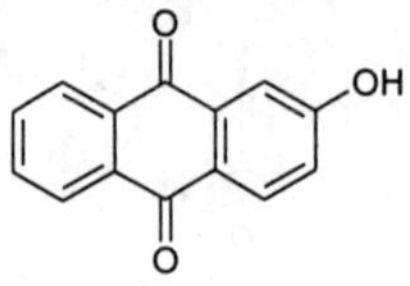

3130 1β-Hydroxyarbusculin A
$C_{15}H_{22}O_4$ MW: 266.34 Property: colorless acicular crystal, mp 194-6°C. Source: YU NAN HAN XIAO. Ref: 426.

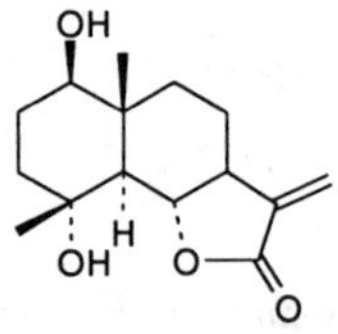

3131 γ-Hydroxyarginine
$C_6H_{14}N_4O_3$ MW: 190.20 Source: DA CHAO CAI. Ref: 6.

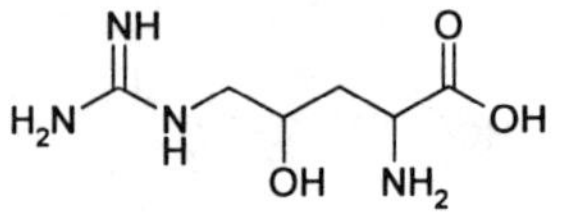

3132 7-Hydroxy-aristolochiac acid A
Source: MA DOU LING. Ref: 517.

3133 3β-Hydroxy-atractylon
$C_{15}H_{20}O_2$ MW: 232.33 Source: CANG ZHU. Ref: 2.

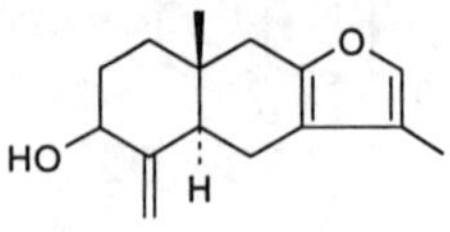

3134 p-Hydroxybenzaldehyde
$C_7H_6O_2$ MW: 122.12 Source: MU ZEI, PU HUANG, TIAN MA. Ref: 2.

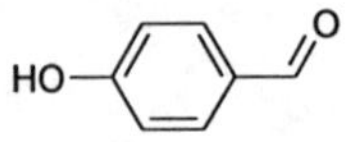

3135 m-Hydroxybenzoic acid
$C_7H_6O_3$ MW: 138.12 Source: MU ZEI. Ref: 2.

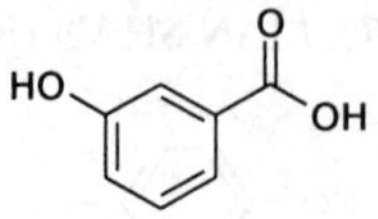

3136 p-Hydroxybenzoic acid
$C_7H_6O_3$ MW: 138.12 Source: JI MAO SONG, JIN QIAO MAI, MU ZEI, MA HUANG, MAN JING ZI. Ref: 2, 415, 544, 562, 594.

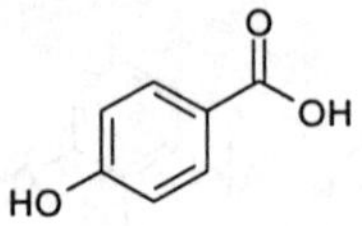

3137 6-O-p-Hydroxybenzoyl ajugol
Source: GAN DI HUANG. Ref: 2.

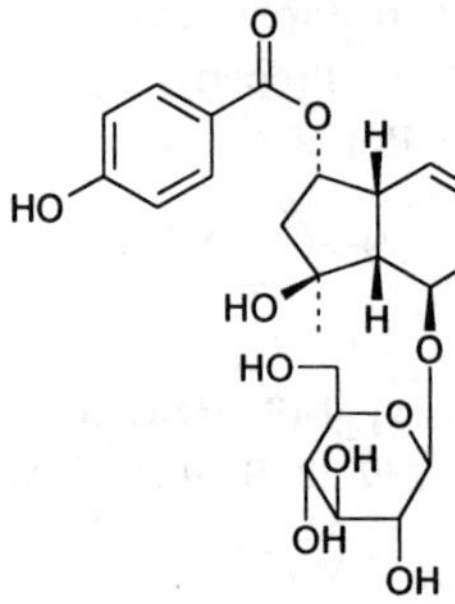

3138 p-Hydroxybenzoyl calleryanin
$C_{20}H_{22}O_{10}$ MW: 422.39 Source: YE LI ZHI YE. Ref: 6.

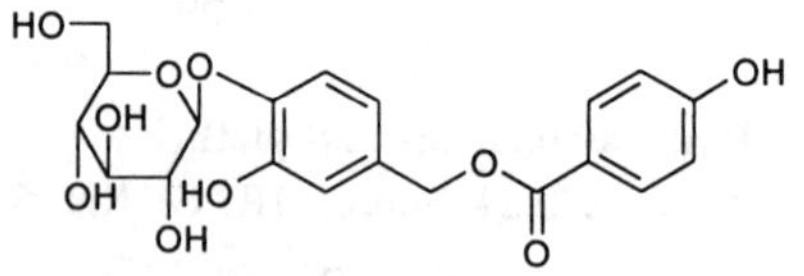

3139 p-Hydroxybenzyl alcohol
$C_7H_6O_2$ MW: 124.14 Source: SHAN HU LAN, TIAN MA. Ref: 2, 280.

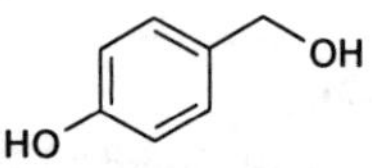

3140 4-Hydroxybenzylamine
C_7H_9NO MW: 123.16 Property: mp 114-5°C (dec). Source: QIAO MAI. Ref: 6.

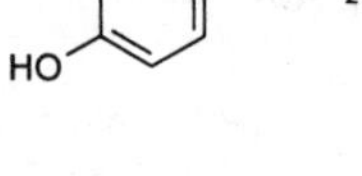

3141 p-Hydroxybenzyl ethyl ether
$C_9H_{12}O_2$ MW: 152.19 Source: TIAN MA. Ref: 2.

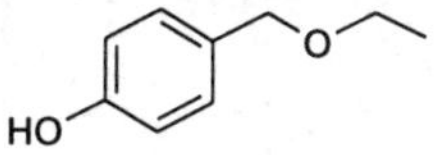

3142 4-Hydroxybenzyl methyl ether
$C_8H_{10}O_2$ MW: 138.17 Source: TIAN MA. Ref: 2.

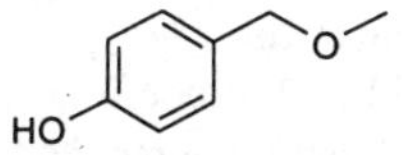

3143 4-(4'-Hydroxybenzyloxy)benzyl methyl ether
$C_{15}H_{16}O_3$ MW: 244.29 Source: TIAN MA. Ref: 2.

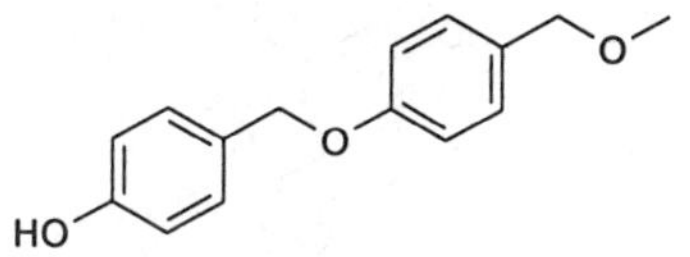

3144 7-Hydroxybiopterin
Ichthyopterin. $C_9H_{11}N_5O_4$ MW: 253.22 Property: mp >300°C (dec). Source: JIN YU, QING WA. Ref: 6.

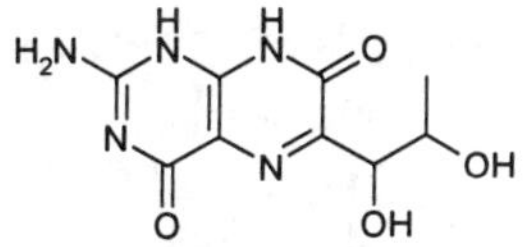

3145 7-Hydroxy-3,6-bis(tigloyloxy)tropane
$C_{18}H_{27}NO_5$ MW: 337.42 Source: MAN TUO LUO YE, MAN TUO LUO GEN. Ref: 6.

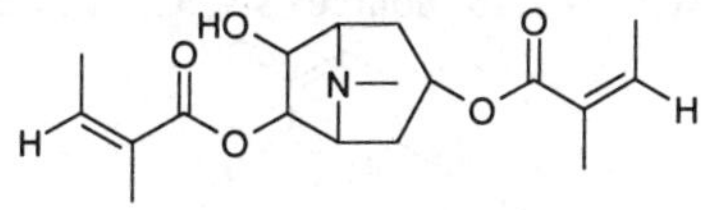

3146 (Z)-5-Hydroxy-3-butylidene-phthalide
$C_{12}H_{12}O_3$ MW: 204.23 Source: CHUAN XIONG. Ref: 2.

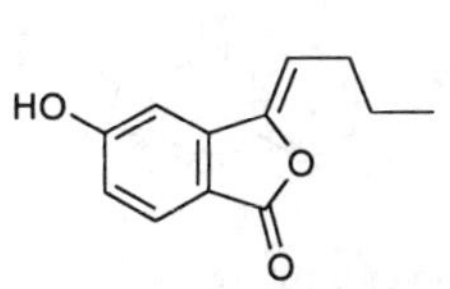

3147 7-Hydroxy-3-butylidene-phthalide
$C_{12}H_{12}O_3$ MW: 204.23 Source: CHUAN XIONG. Ref: 2.

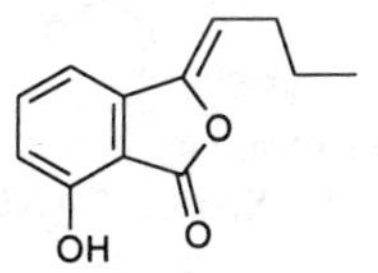

3148 7-Hydroxycadalenal
$C_{15}H_{16}O_2$ MW: 228.29 Property: mp 85°C. Source: LANG YU PI. Ref: 6.

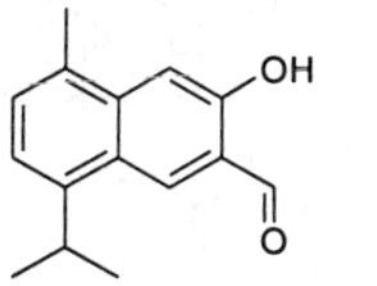

3149 Hydroxycamptothecin
$C_{20}H_{16}N_2O_5$ MW: 364.36 Property: mp 268-70°C. Source: XI SHU. Ref: 4.

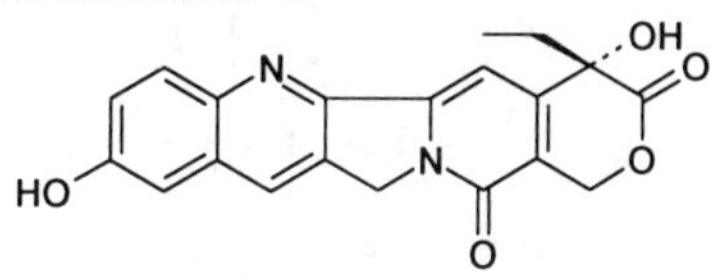

3150 18-Hydroxycamptothecin
$C_{20}H_{16}N_2O_5$ MW: 364.36 Property: yellow acicular crystal , mp 256-8°C, $[\alpha]_D^{11}$ -21.4° (c=0.11, pyridine). Source: XI SHU. Ref: 98.

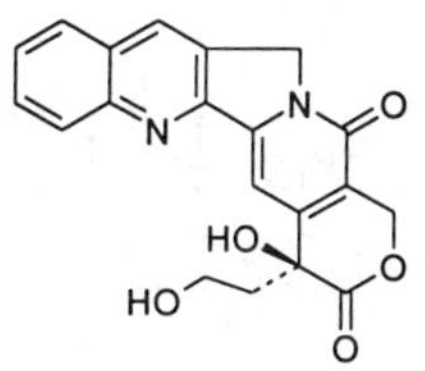

3151 11-Hydroxycephalotaxine
$C_{18}H_{21}NO_5$ MW: 331.37 Source: SAN JIAN SHAN. Ref: 2.

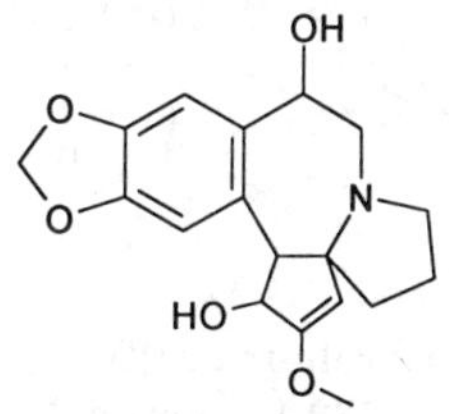

3152 4-Hydroxycephalotaxine
$C_{18}H_{21}NO_5$ MW: 331.37 Source: SAN JIAN SHAN. Ref: 2.

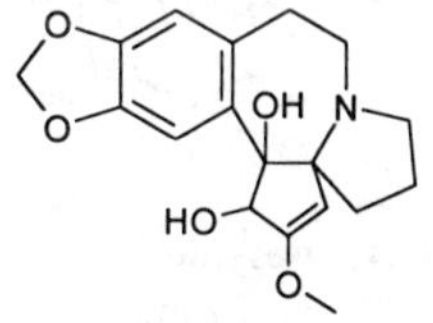

3153 Hydroxychelidonine
$C_{20}H_{17}NO_6$ MW: 367.36 Property: mp >285°C. Source: BAI QU CAI. Ref: 6.

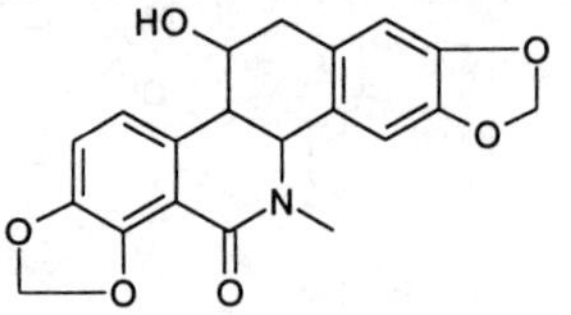

3154 7α-Hydroxycholesterol
$C_{28}H_{48}O_2$ MW: 416.69 Source: CHAN SU. Ref: 2.

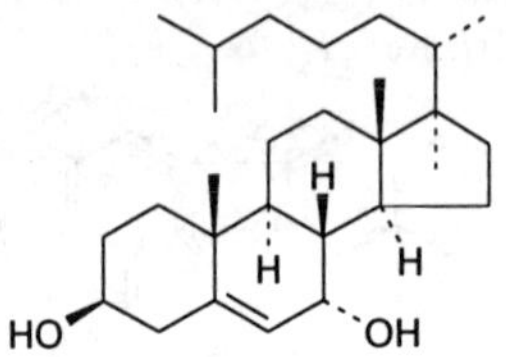

3155 3-O-p-Hydroxy-trans-cinnamoylmaslinic acid
$C_{39}H_{54}O_6$ MW: 618.86 Source: LI MU. Ref: 6.

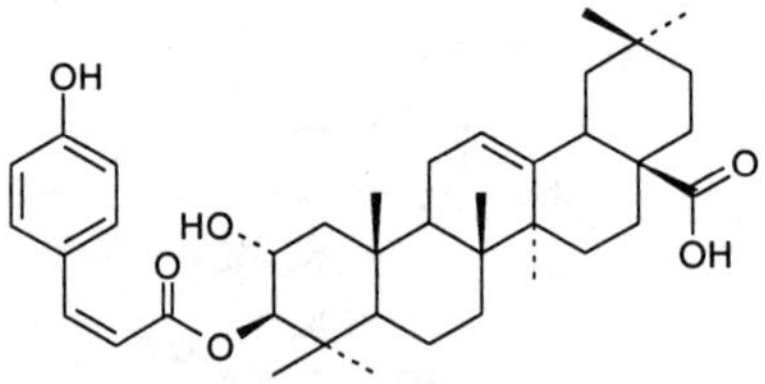

3156 16-Hydroxycolubrine (α)
$C_{22}H_{24}N_2O_4$ MW: 380.45 Source: MA QIAN ZI. Ref: 6.

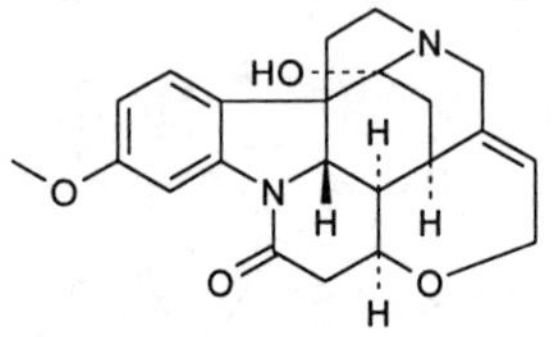

3157 16-Hydroxycolubrine (β)
$C_{22}H_{24}N_2O_4$ MW: 380.45 Source: MA QIAN ZI. Ref: 6.

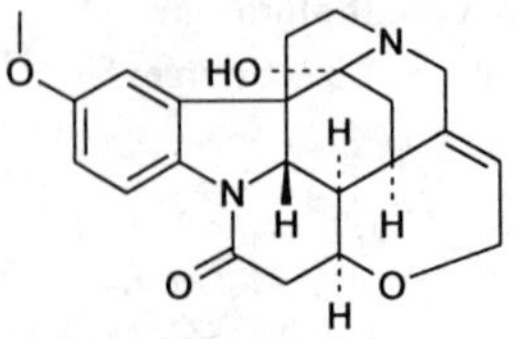

3158 7α-Hydroxyconessine
$C_{25}H_{41}NO$ MW: 371.61 Property: mp 176-8°C. Source: ZHI XIE MU PI. Ref: 6.

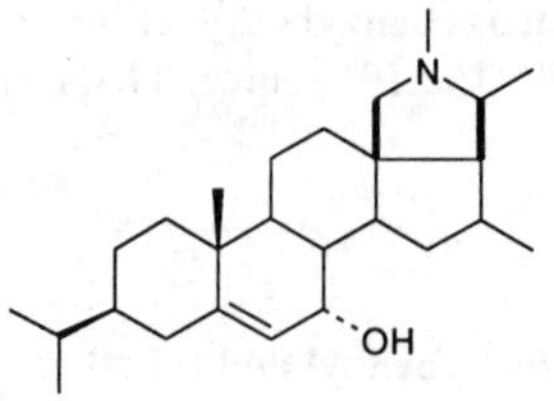

3159 Hydroxycoriatin
$C_{15}H_{20}O_7$ MW: 312.32 Property: white acicular crystal, mp 260°C (dec). Source: MA SANG. Ref: 413.

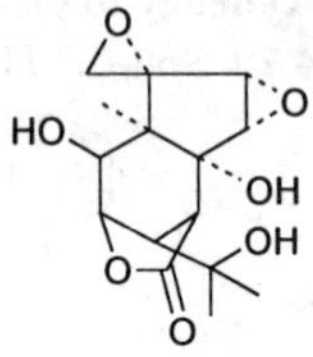

3160 17-Hydroxycorticosterone
$C_{22}H_{32}O_5$ MW: 376.50 Property: mp α: 220°C. Source: NIU SHEN, ZHI XIE MU PI. Ref: 6.

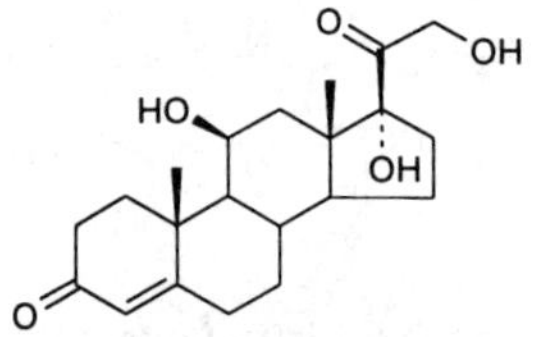

3161 3-Hydroxycoumarin
$C_9H_6O_3$ MW: 162.15 Source: SANG YE. Ref: 6.

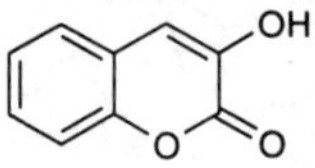

3162 4-Hydroxycoumarin
$C_9H_6O_3$ MW: 162.15 Source: SANG YE. Ref: 6.

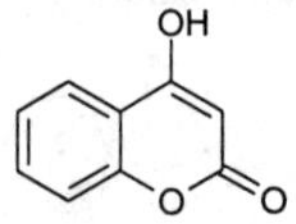

3163 5-Hydroxycoumarin
$C_9H_6O_3$ MW: 162.15 Source: SANG YE. Ref: 6.

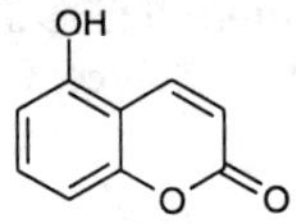

3164 6-Hydroxycoumarin
$C_9H_6O_3$ MW: 162.15 Source: SANG YE. Ref: 6.

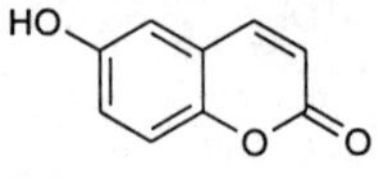

3165 26-Hydroxy-dammara-20,24-dien-3-one
$C_{30}H_{48}O_2$ MW: 440.72 Property: colorless acicular crystal (MeOH), mp 69°C, $[\alpha]_D^{21.5}$ +58° (c=1.0, $CHCl_3$). Source: XIANG GANG JIAN MU. Ref: 422.

3166 16β-Hydroxy-dammare-20(22),25-dien-3-one
$C_{30}H_{48}O_2$ MW: 440.72 Property: colorless acicular crystal (MeOH), mp 182°C, $[\alpha]_D^{21.5}$ +58° (c=1.0, $CHCl_3$). Source: XIANG GANG JIAN MU. Ref: 422.

3167 ω-Hydroxy-Δ2-decenoic acid
$C_{10}H_{18}O_3$ MW: 172.23 Property: mp trans: 64-5°C, cis: 74°C. Source: FENG RU. Ref: 6.

3168 6-Hydroxydendroxine
$C_{17}H_{25}NO_4$ MW: 307.39 Source: SHI HU. Ref: 6.

3169 24-Hydroxy-11-deoxyglycyrrhetic acid
$C_{29}H_{46}O_4$ MW: 458.69 Source: GAN CAO. Ref: 2.

3170 17-Hydroxy-11-desoxy-corticosterone
$C_{22}H_{32}O_4$ MW: 360.50 Property: mp 207-8°C. Source: NIU SHEN. Ref: 6.

3171 4-Hydroxydihydroagarofuran
$C_{15}H_{26}O_2$ MW: 238.37 Property: mp 130-1°C. Source: CHEN XIANG. Ref: 6, 13.

3172 19-(R)-Hydroxydihydrogelsemine
$C_{20}H_{24}N_2O_3$ MW: 340.43 Property: mp 230-2°C, $[\alpha]_D$ -20°. Source: HU MAN TENG. Ref: 14.

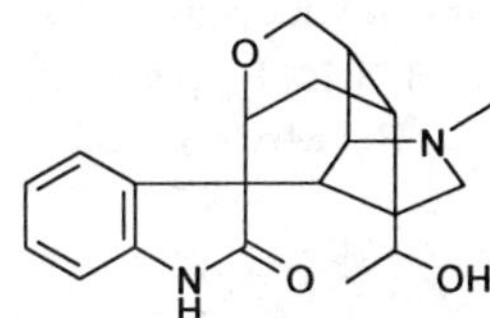

3173 19-(R)-Hydroxydihydrogelsevirine
$C_{21}H_{26}N_2O_4$ MW: 370.45 Property: mp 210-2°C, $[\alpha]_D$ -34°. Source: HU MAN TENG. Ref: 14.

3174 19-(S)-Hydroxydihydrogelsevirine
$C_{21}H_{26}N_2O_4$ MW: 370.45 Property: amorphous, $[\alpha]_D$ -68°. Source: HU MAN TENG. Ref: 14.

3175 19-(R)-Hydroxydihydrokoumine
$C_{20}H_{24}N_2O_2$ MW: 324.43 Property: mp 198-200°C, $[\alpha]_D$ -232.7°. Source: HU MAN TENG. Ref: 14.

3176 19-(S)-Hydroxydihydrokoumine
$C_{20}H_{24}N_2O_2$ MW: 324.43 Property: mp 270-2°C, $[\alpha]_D$ -184.6°. Source: HU MAN TENG. Ref: 14.

3177 7-Hydroxydihydromatatabiether
$C_{10}H_{18}O_2$ MW: 170.25 Source: MU TIAN LIAO. Ref: 6.

3178 20-Hydroxydihydrorankinidine
$C_{20}H_{26}N_2O_4$ MW: 358.44 Property: mp 173-4°C, $[\alpha]_D$ -165°. Source: HU MAN TENG. Ref: 14.

3179 7-Hydroxy-6,8-dimethoxy coumarin
Property: light yellow acicular crystal, mp 146-8°C. Source: MAO LIAN HAO. Ref: 474.

3180 4'-Hydroxy-2,6-dimethoxydihydrochal-cone
$C_{17}H_{18}O_4$ MW: 286.12 Property: white columnar crystal, mp 129-30°C(EtOH). Source: JIAN YE LONG XUE SHU. Ref:414.

3181 5-Hydroxy-4',7-dimethoxy-flavone
$C_{17}H_{14}O_5$ MW: 298.30 Source: MI DIE XIANG. Ref: 6.

3182 5-Hydroxy-7,8-dimethoxyflavone
$C_{17}H_{14}O_5$ MW: 298.30 Source: HUANG QIN. Ref: 2.

3183 2'-Hydroxy-3',4-dimethoxy-isoflavane-7-O-β-D-glucoside
$C_{23}H_{32}O_{10}$ MW: 468.51 Source: HUANG QI. Ref: 2.

3184 5-Hydroxy-8-(1',1'dimethylallyl) psoralen
$C_{16}H_{14}O_4$ MW: 270.29 Source: QIANG HUO. Ref: 2.

3185 12α-Hydroxydolineone
$C_{19}H_{12}O_7$ MW: 352.30 Property: mp 180-1°C. Source: DI GUA ZI. Ref: 6.

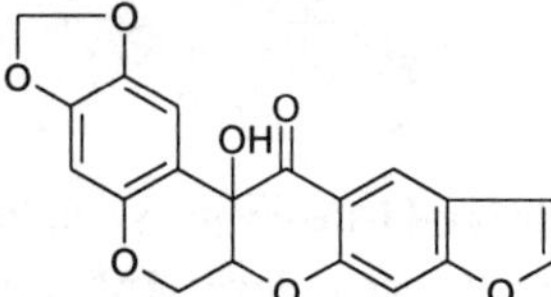

3186 Hydroxydroserone
Source: MAO GAO CAO. Ref: 621.

3187 5β-Hydroxyecdysterone
$C_{28}H_{47}O_8$ MW: 511.68 Property: mp 256°C. Source: SHUI LONG GU. Ref: 6.

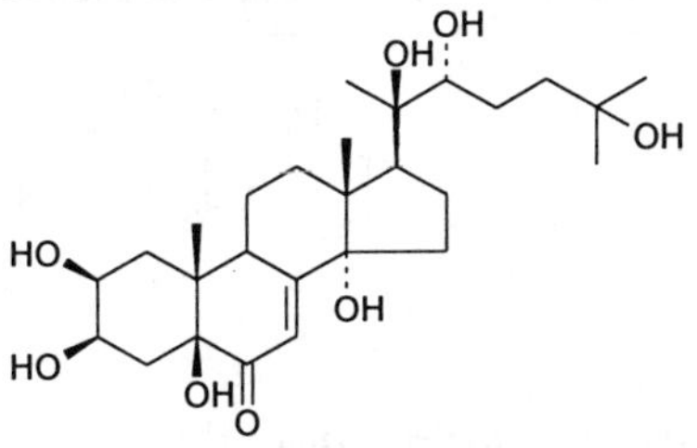

3188 6-Hydroxyeremophilenolide
$C_{15}H_{22}O_3$ MW: 250.34 Property: mp 208°C. Source: FENG DOU CAI. Ref: 6.

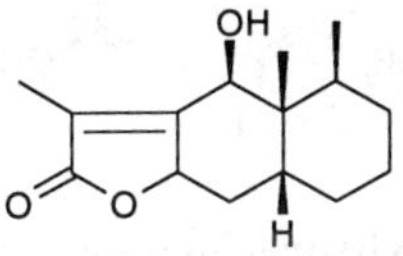

3189 22α-Hydroxyerythrodiol
$C_{30}H_{48}O_4$ MW: 472.71 Property: mp 279-82°C. Source: HU ZHI ZI. Ref: 6.

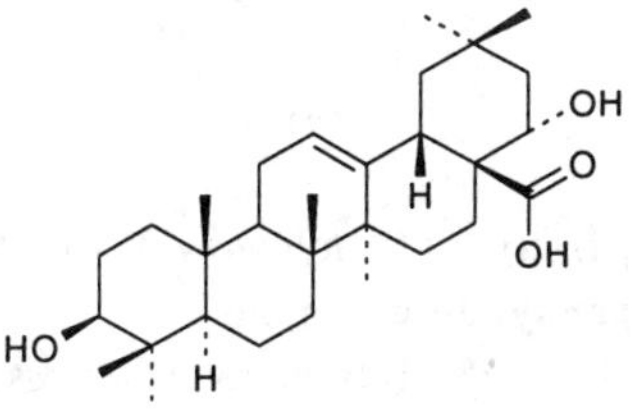

3190 6β-Hydroxy-7-α-ethoxy-16-acetoxyroyleanone
$C_{24}H_{34}O_7$ MW: 434.53 Property: yellow crystal, mp 184-5°C,. Source: XIAN WEN XIANG CHA CAI. Ref: 646.

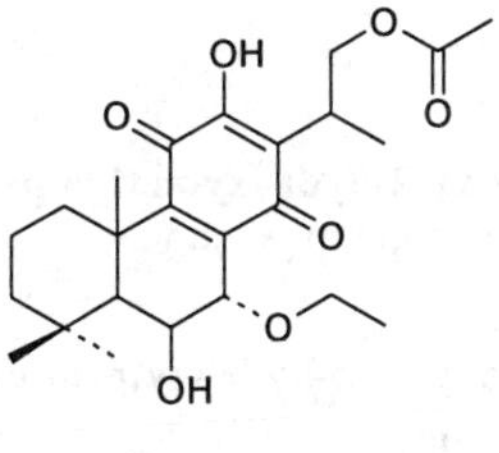

3191 Hydroxyevodiamine
$C_{19}H_{17}N_3O_2$ MW: 319.37 Source: WU ZHU YU. Ref: 2, 347.

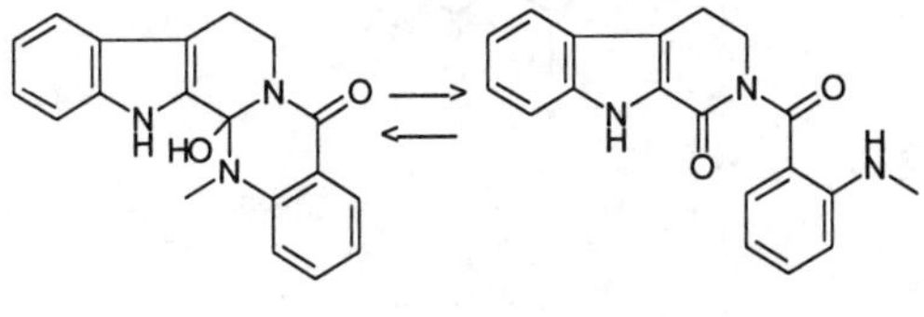

3192 12α-Hydroxyevodol
$C_{26}H_{28}O_{10}$ MW: 500.51 Source: WU ZHU YU. Ref: 2.

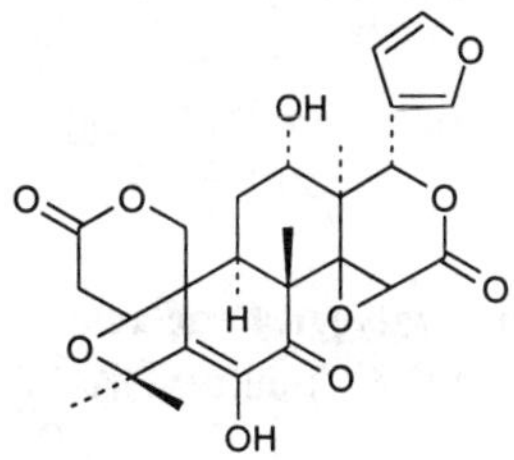

3193 10β-Hydroxyfuranoeremophilan-6β-yl 2'ξ-methylbutanoate
$C_{21}H_{32}O_3$ MW: 332.49 Source: LIAN PENG CAO. Ref: 6.

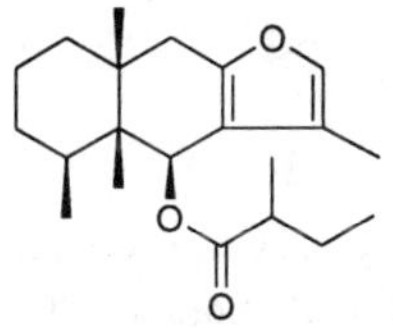

3194 14-Hydroxygelsedine
$C_{19}H_{24}N_2O_4$ MW: 344.41 Property: mp 214-6°C. Source: HU MAN TENG. Ref: 14.

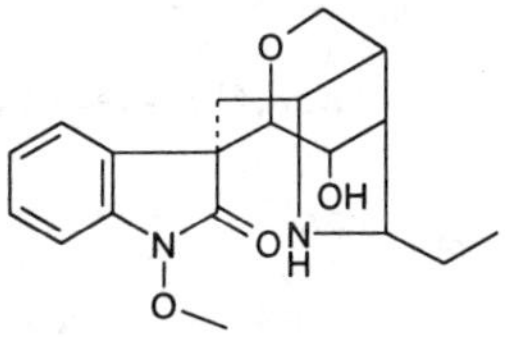

3195 Hydroxygenaiol-β-glucopyranoside
Source: ROU CONG RONG. Ref: 628.

3196 Hydroxygenkwanin
$C_{16}H_{12}O_6$ MW: 300.27 Property: mp 283-5°C. Source: YUAN HUA. Ref: 6.

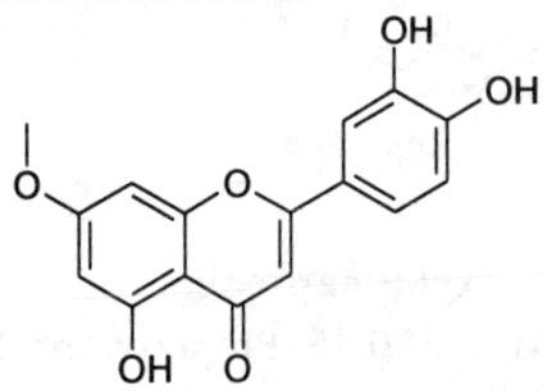

3197 3-Hydroxyglabrol
$C_{25}H_{28}O_5$ MW: 408.50 Source: GAN CAO. Ref: 2.

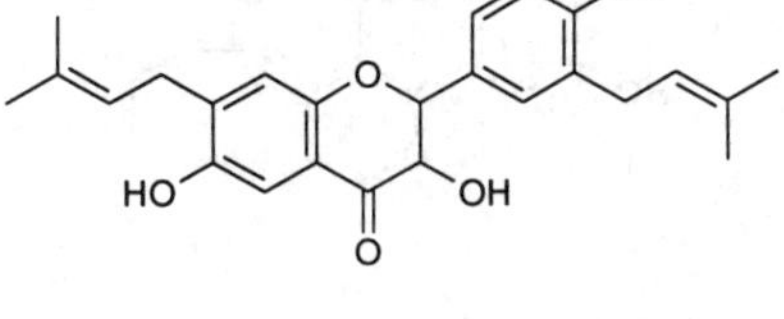

3198 γ-Hydroxy glutaminic acid
$C_5H_9NO_5$ MW: 163.13 Property: mp L-: 183-5°C. Source: XUAN CAO GEN. Ref: 6.

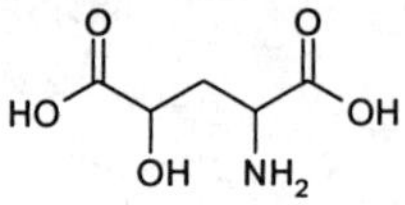

3199 24-Hydroxyglycyrrhetic acid
$C_{29}H_{44}O_5$ MW: 472.67 Source: GAN CAO. Ref: 2.

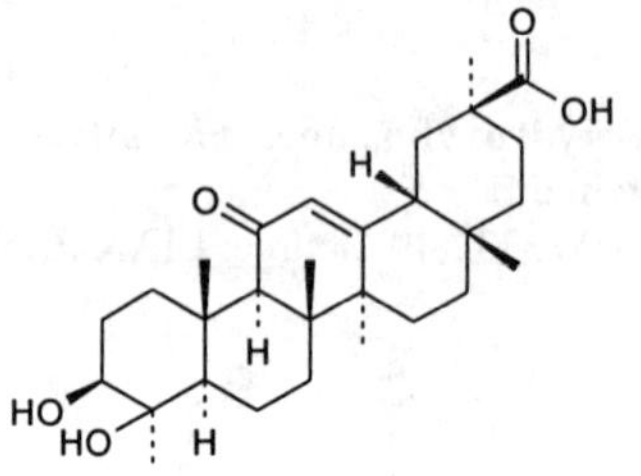

3200 13-Hydroxy-9,11-hexadecadienoic acid
$C_{16}H_{28}O_3$ MW: 268.40 Source: CU LIU GUO (SHA JI). Ref: 2.

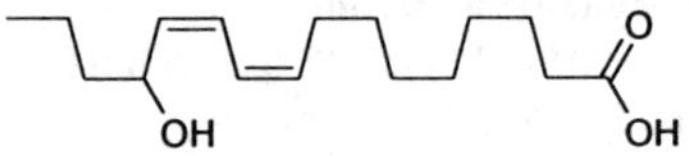

3201 5-Hydroxy-6,7,8,3',4',5'-hexamethoxy flavone
Source: ZHI ZI. Ref: 626.

3204 Hydroxyhopane
Diplopterol. $C_{30}H_{52}O$ MW: 428.75 Property: mp 254-6°C. Source: GUAN ZHONG. Ref: 6.

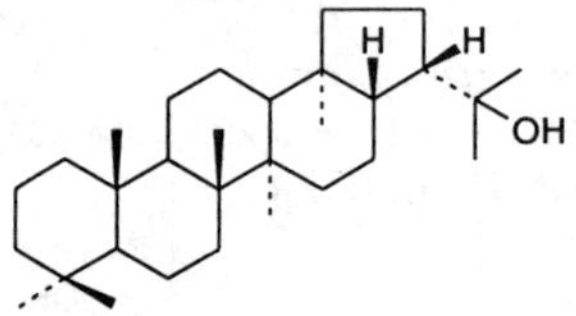

3205 11-Hydroxyhumantenine
$C_{21}H_{26}N_2O_4$ MW: 370.45 Property: mp 176-7°C, $[\alpha]_D$ -130°. Source: HU MAN TENG. Ref: 14.

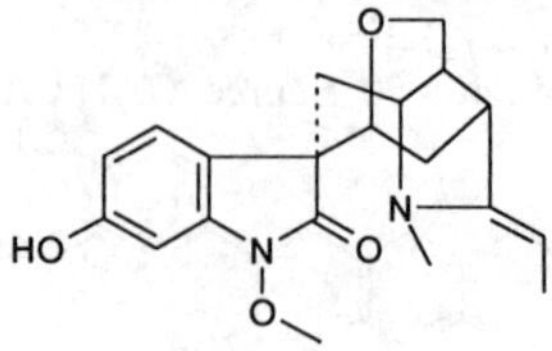

3206 15-Hydroxy-humantenine
$C_{21}H_{26}N_2O_4$ MW: 370.45 Property: mp213-5°C, $[\alpha]_D$ -82.2°. Source: HU MAN TENG. Ref: 14.

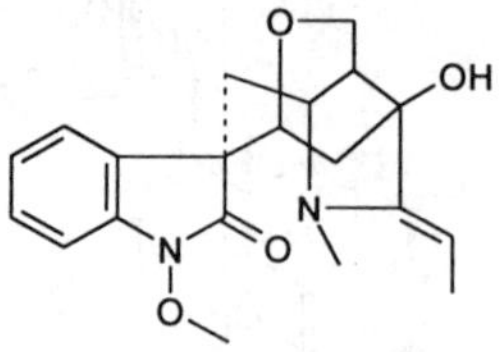

3207 α-Hydroxyhydrocaffeic acid
$C_9H_{10}O_5$ MW: 198.18 Source: MI DIE XIANG. Ref: 6.

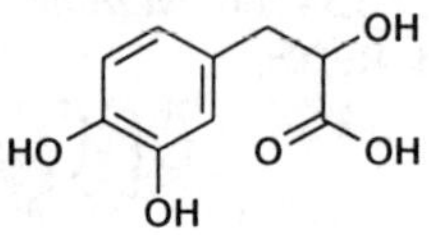

3208 o-Hydroxyhydrocinnamic acid
$C_9H_{10}O_3$ MW: 166.18 Property: mp 82-3°C. Source: PI HAN CAO. Ref: 6.

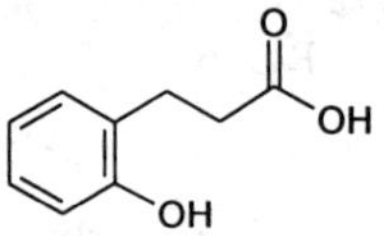

3209 5-Hydroxy-7-(4''-hydroxy-3''-methoxy-phenyl)-1-phenyl-3-heptanone
$C_{20}H_{24}O_4$ MW: 328.41 Property: colorless oleaginous liquid, $[\alpha]_D^{20}$ -13.9° (c=1.15, $CHCl_3$). Source: GAO LIANG JIANG. Ref: 435.

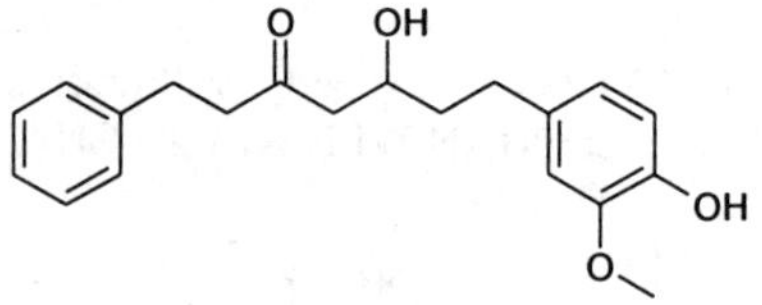

3210 5-Hydroxy-2-hydroxymethyl pyridine
Source: YE YING SU. Ref: 590.

3211 7-Hydroxy-2-(2-hydroxy)propyl-5-methyl-benzopyran-γ-one
$C_{13}H_{14}O_4$ MW: 234.25 Source: DA HUANG. Ref: 2.

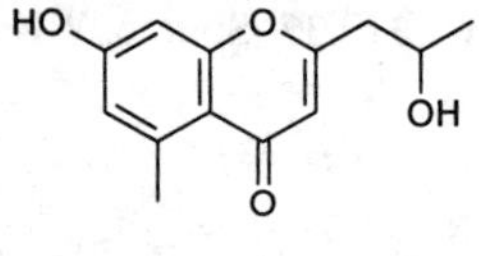

3212 21α-Hydroxyisoglabrolide
$C_{30}H_{44}O_5$ MW: 484.68 Source: GAN CAO. Ref: 2.

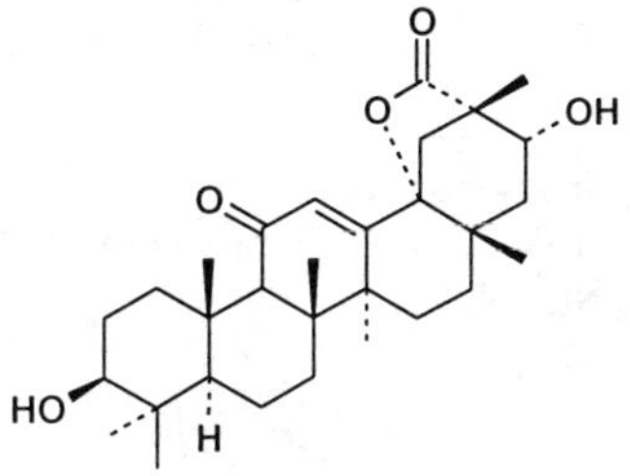

3213 5-Hydroxyisophthalic acid
$C_8H_6O_5$ MW: 182.13 Property: mp 284-5°C. Source: HUANG JING YE. Ref: 6.

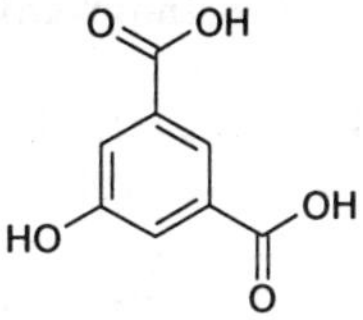

3214 Hydroxyisopiloselloidone
$C_{18}H_{24}O_4$ MW: 304.39 Source: MAO DA DING CAO. Ref: 6.

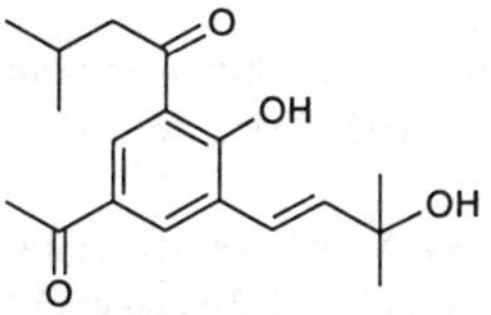

3215 β-Hydroxyisovalerylshikonin
$C_{21}H_{24}O_7$ MW: 388.42 Source: ZI CAO. Ref: 2.

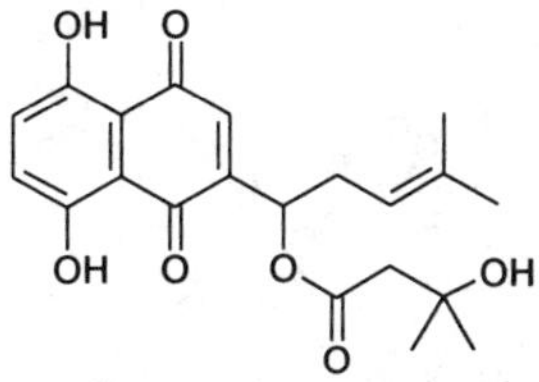

3216 6-Hydroxykaempferol-7-O-glucoside
$C_{21}H_{20}O_{12}$ MW: 464.39 Property: yellow acicular crystal. Source: HONG HUA. Ref: 644.

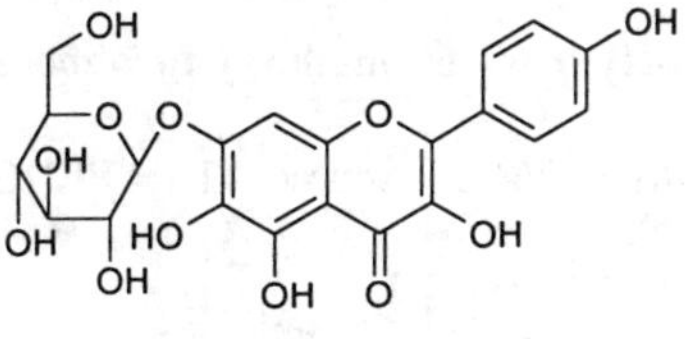

3217 (-)-17-Hydroxy-16β-kauran-19-oic acid
$C_{21}H_{34}O_3$ MW: 334.50 Source: XI XIAN. Ref: 2.

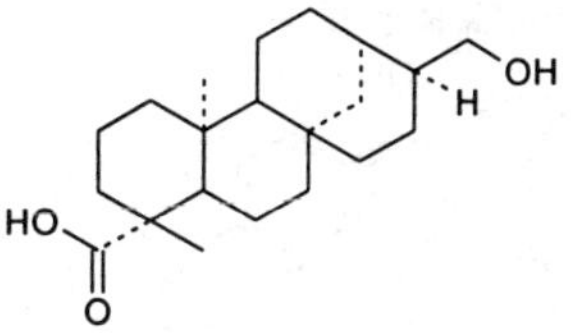

3218 3-Hydroxykynurenine
$C_{10}H_{12}NO_4$ MW: 224.22 Property: mp (-): 185-90°C, (±): 223°C (dec). Source: YUAN CAN ZI. Ref: 6.

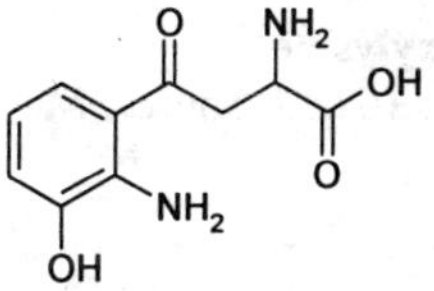

3219 3β-Hydoxylanosta-7,9(11),24-trien-21-oic acid
$C_{30}H_{46}O_3$ MW: 454.70 Property: mp 257-9°C. Source: FU LING. Ref: 2, 6.

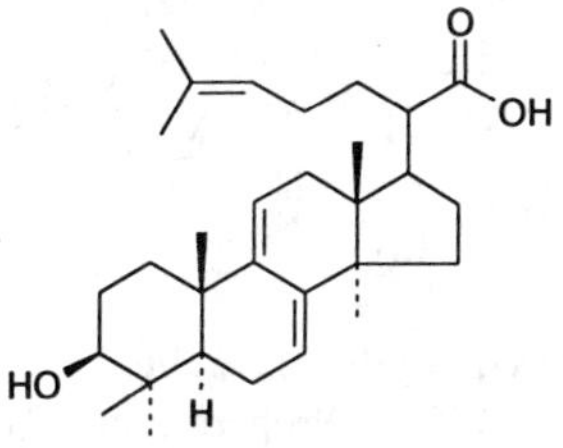

3220 12α-Hydroxylimonine
$C_{26}H_{30}O_9$ MW: 486.52 Source: WU ZHU YU. Ref: 2.

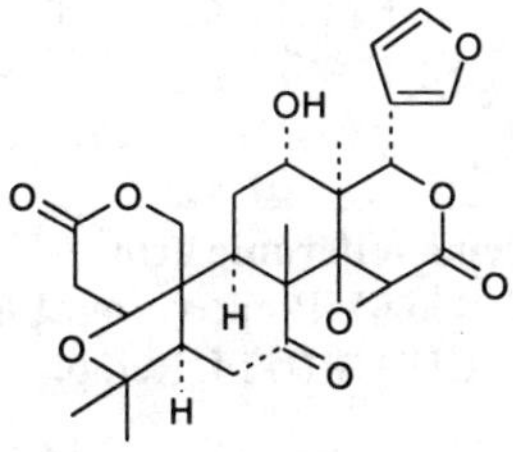

3221 6-Hydroxyluteolin
$C_{15}H_{12}O_7$ MW: 304.26 Property: mp 256°C. Source: CHOU MO LI, YI ZHI XIANG. Ref: 6.

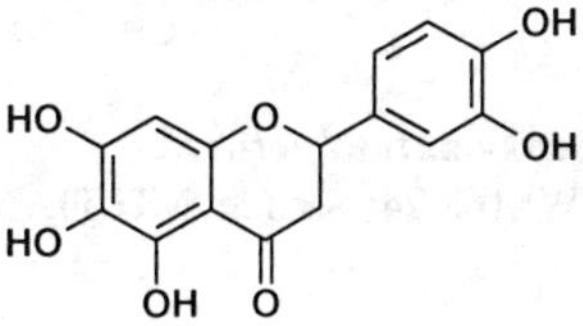

3222 8-Hydroxyluteolin-8-β-D-glucopranoside
$C_{21}H_{20}O_{12}$ MW: 464.39 Property: mp 269-71°C. Source: FU PING. Ref: 6.

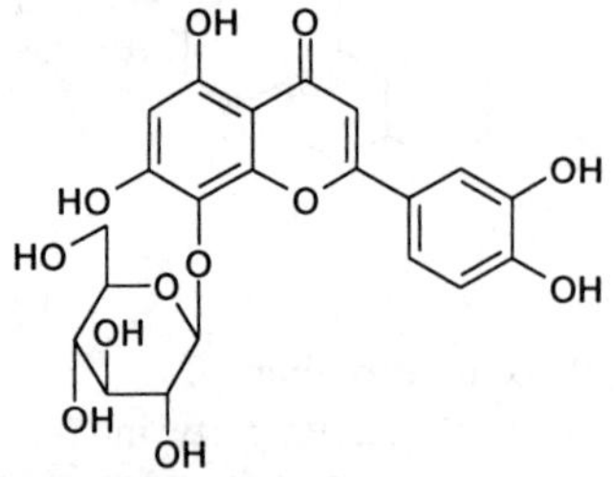

3223 δ-Hydroxylysine
$C_6H_{14}NO_3$ MW: 162.19 Source: MO GU. Ref: 6.

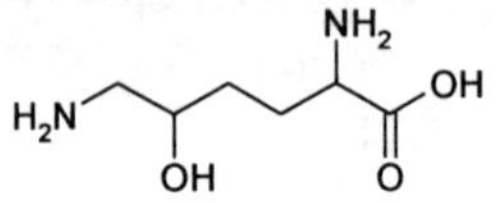

3224 p-Hydroxymandelonitril-glucoside
$C_{14}H_{17}NO_7$ MW: 311. 29 Source: GAO LIANG. Ref: 6.

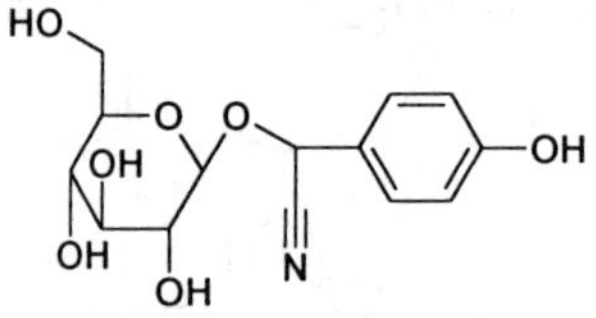

3225 Hydroxymangiferolic acid
$C_{29}H_{46}O_4$ MW: 458.69 Property: mp 201-4°C. Source: MANG GUO SHU PI. Ref: 6.

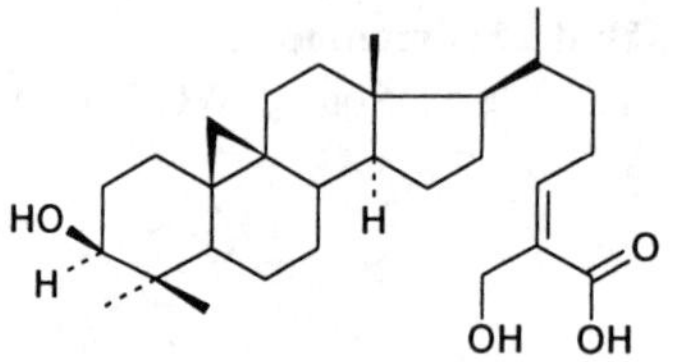

3226 Hydroxymangiferonic acid
$C_{29}H_{44}O_4$ MW: 456.67 Property: mp 190-2°C. Source: MANG GUO SHU PI. Ref: 6.

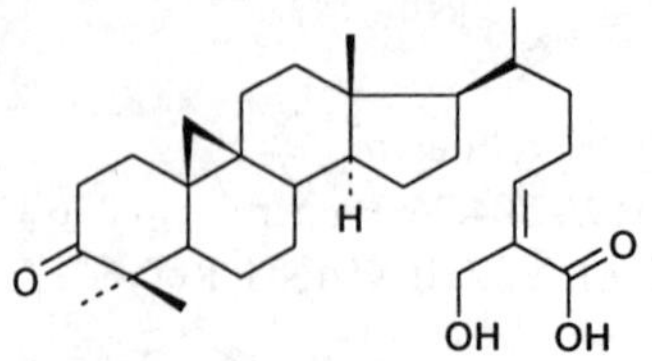

3227 5-Hydroxymatatabiether
$C_{10}H_{16}O_2$ MW: 168.24 Source: MU TIAN LIAO. Ref: 6.

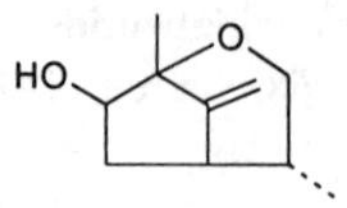

3228 5-Hydroxymatrine
$C_{15}H_{24}N_2O_2$ MW: 264.37 Property: mp 171°C. Source: KU SHEN. Ref: 6.

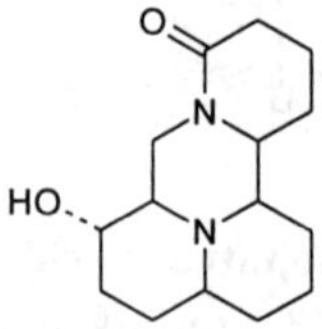

3229 11-Hydroxy-14-methoxy-abieta-8,11,13-trien-3-one
$C_{21}H_{30}O_3$ MW: 330.47 Source: LEI GONG TENG. Ref: 2.

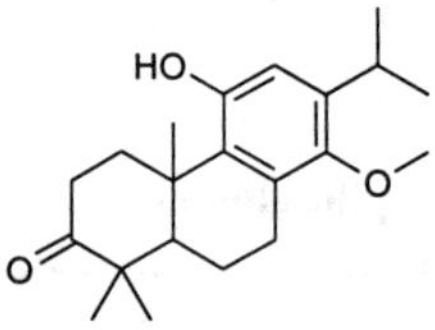

3230 p-Hydroxy-m-methoxy-benzonic acid
Source: QIANG HUO. Ref: 507.

3231 5-Hydroxy-4-methoxy-flavone-7-O-α-L-rhamnopyranosyl (1→6)[2-O-acetyl-β-D-gluco-pyranosyl (1→2)]-β-D-glucopyranoside
$C_{36}H_{44}O_{20}$ MW: 796.74 Property: white powder crystal, mp 246-8°C. Source: GAN JU. Ref: 388.

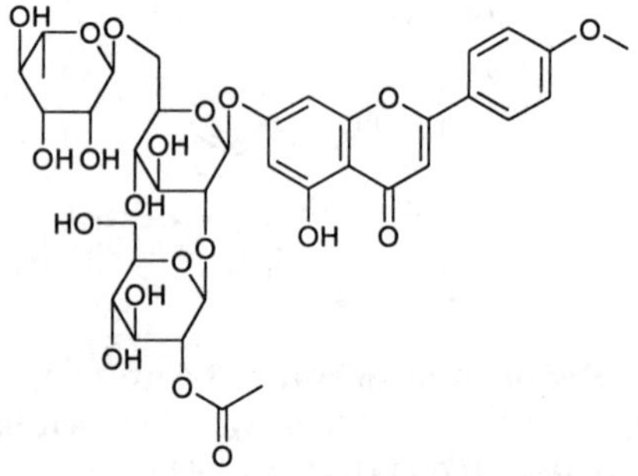

3232 10β-Hydroxy-6β-methoxy-furanoeremo-philane
$C_{16}H_{24}O_3$ MW: 264.37 Source: LIAN PENG CAO. Ref: 6.

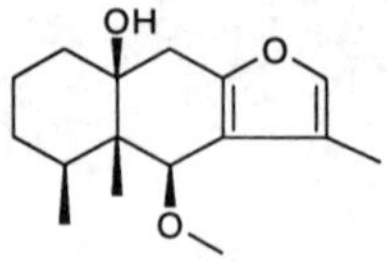

3233 6-Hydroxy-7-methoxy-8-glucosyloxy-3-(3-glucosyloxy-4-xylosylglucosyloxyphenyl)-4H-1-benzopyran-4-one

Source: GE GEN. Ref: 2.

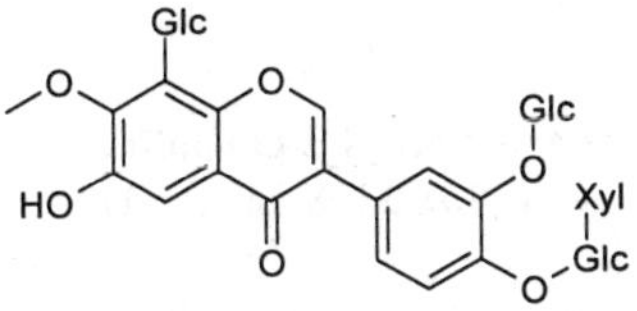

3234 6-Hydroxy-7-methoxy-3-(4'-hydroxy-benzyl) chromane

$C_{17}H_{18}O_4$ MW: 286.33 Property: colorless short columnar crystal, mp 195-7°C ($CHCl_3$). Source: JIAN YE LONG XUE SHU. Ref: 414.

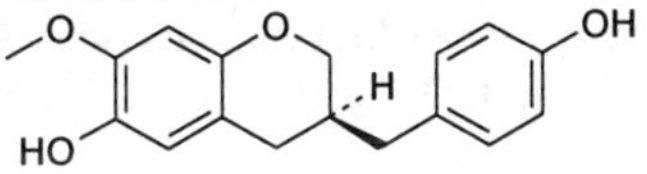

3235 3'-Hydroxy-4'-methoxyisoflavone-7-O-β-D-glucoside

$C_{22}H_{22}O_{10}$ MW: 446.41 Source: HUANG QI. Ref: 2.

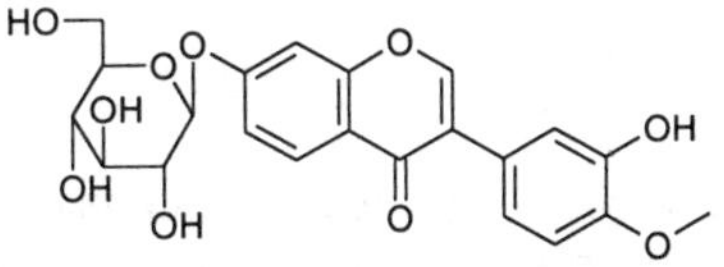

3236 7-Hydroxy-4-methoxy-5-methylcoumarin

$C_{11}H_{10}O_4$ MW: 206.20 Source: HU ZHANG. Ref: 2.

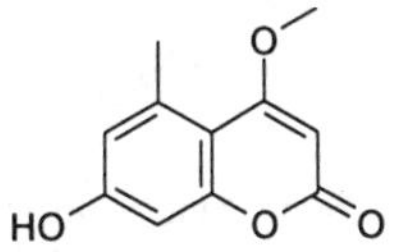

3237 5-Hydroxy-7-methoxy-3',4'-methylene-dioxy isoflavone

Property: colorless acicular crystal (MeOH), mp 232-4°C, slightly soluble in various organic solvents. Source: JIN QUE GEN. Ref: 489.

3238 7-Hydroxy-1-methoxy-2,3-methylenedioxy – xanthone

$C_{14}H_{10}O_6$ MW: 286.24 Property: light yellow acicular crystal (chloroform-methanol), mp 228-30°C. Source: HUANG HUA YUAN ZHI. Ref: 382.

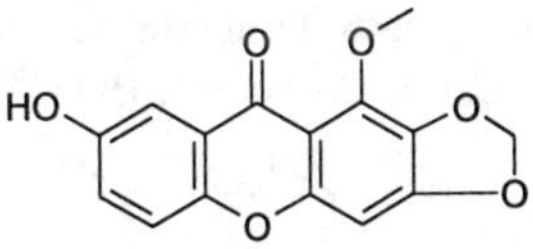

3239 2-Hydroxy-5-methoxy-3-pentadecenyl benzoquinone

$C_{22}H_{36}O_4$ MW: 362.51 Property: mp 67°C. Source: ZI JIN NIU. Ref: 6.

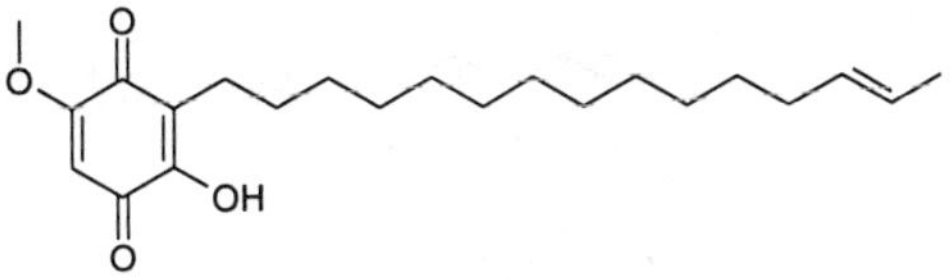

3240 1-(4-Hydroxy-3-methoxyphenyl)-3,5-diacetoxyoctane

$C_{19}H_{28}O_6$ MW: 352.43 Source: SHENG JIANG. Ref: 2.

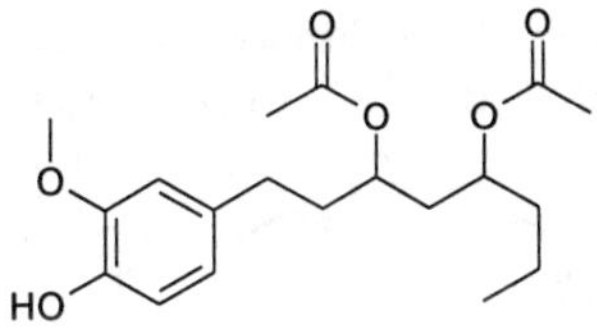

3241 6-Hydroxy-2-[2-(4'-methoxyphenyl)ethyl] chromone

$C_{18}H_{16}O_4$ MW: 296.33 Property: colorless lump crystal, mp 167-8°C. Source: BAI MU XIANG, GUO CHAN CHEN XIANG. Ref: 13, 140.

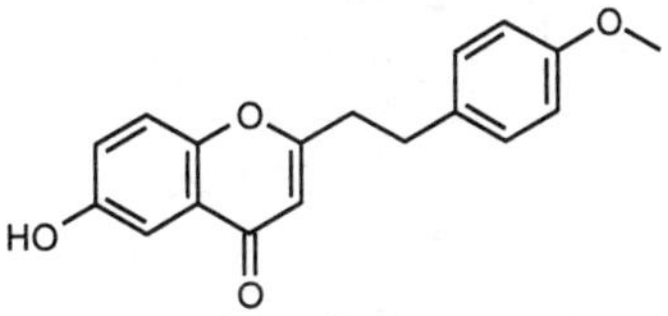

3243 2-(3-Hydroxy-4-methoxyphenyl)-ethyl-1-O-α-L-rhamnosyl-(1→3)-β-D-(4-feruloyl)-glucoside

$C_{31}H_{40}O_{15}$ MW: 652.66 Source: HUANG QIN. Ref: 2.

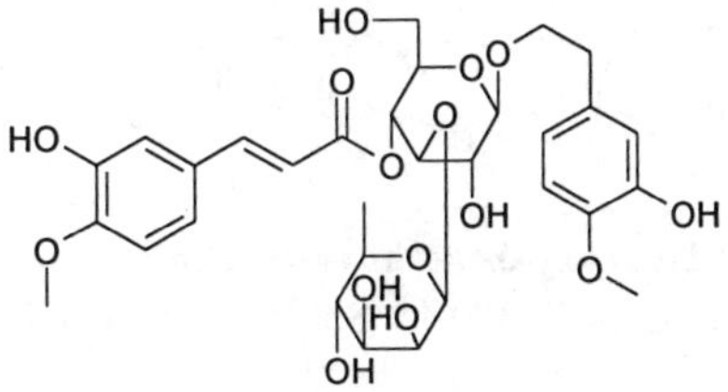

3244 1-(4-Hydroxy-3-methoxyphenyl-2-[4-(ω-hydroxypropyl)-2-methoxyphenoxy]propane, 3-diol

$C_{20}H_{26}O_7$ MW: 378.43 Source: HOU PO. Ref: 2.

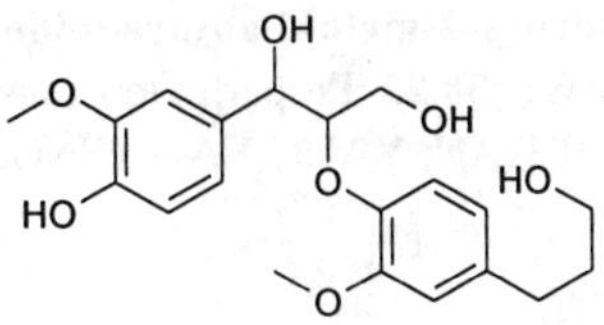

3245 1-(4-Hydroxy-3-methoxyphenyl)-3,5-octane-diol
$C_{15}H_{24}O_4$ MW: 268.36 Source: SHENG JIANG. Ref: 2.

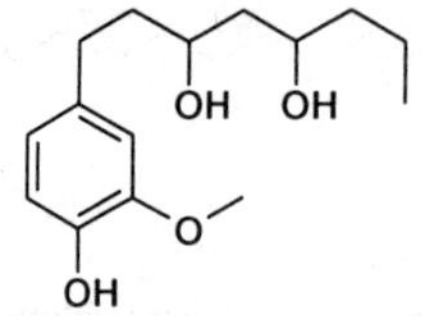

3246 7-(4''-Hydroxy-3''-methoxyphenyl)-1-phenyl-hept-4-en-3-one
$C_{20}H_{22}O_3$ MW: 310.40 Property: colorless oleaginous liquid. Source: GAO LIANG JIANG. Ref: 435.

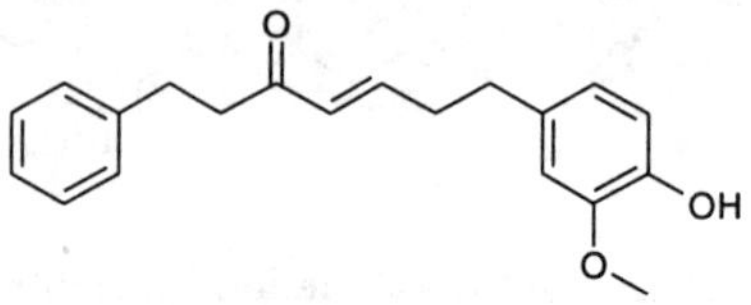

3247 L-3-Hydroxy-9-methoxypterocarpan
$C_{16}H_{16}O_4$ MW: 272.30 Source: HUANG QI. Ref: 2.

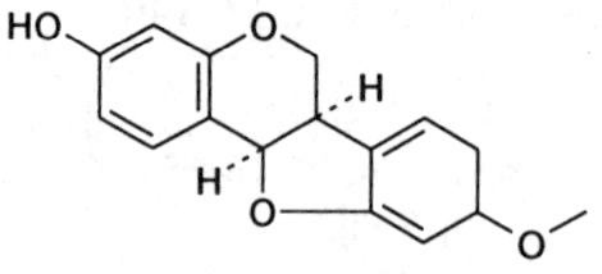

3248 2-Hydroxy-3-methoxystrychnine
$C_{22}H_{24}N_2O_4$ MW: 380.45 Source: MA QIAN ZI. Ref: 2.

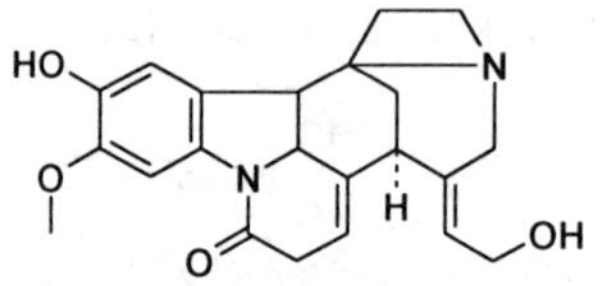

3249 4-Hydroxy-3-methoxystrychnine
$C_{22}H_{24}N_2O_4$ MW: 380.45 Source: MA QIAN ZI. Ref: 2.

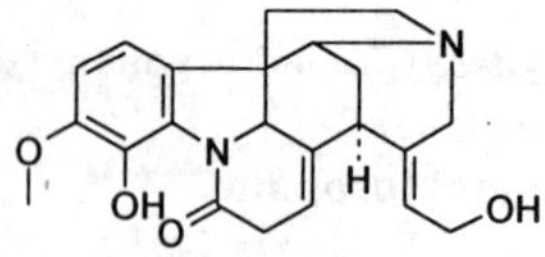

3250 1-Hydroxy-2-methyl-anthraquinone
$C_{15}H_{10}O_3$ MW: 238.25 Property: mp 184-5°C. Source: BA JI TIAN, YANG JIAO TENG. Ref: 6, 228.

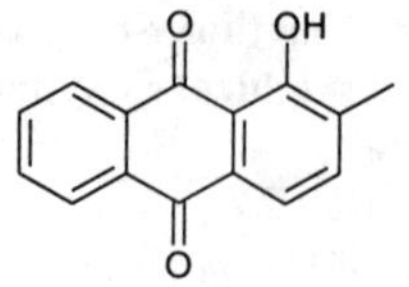

3251 1-Hydroxymethyl-β-carboline
$C_{12}H_{10}N_2O$ MW: 198.23 Source: KU SHU PI. Ref: 12.

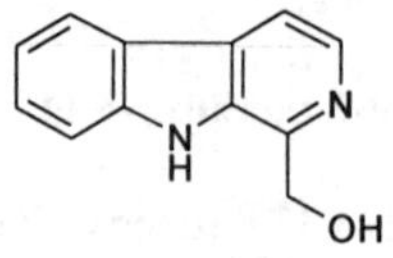

3252 5-Hydroxymethyl-6-endo-3'-methoxy-4'-hydroxyphenyl-8-oxa-bicyclo[3,2,1]-oct-3-en-2-one
$C_{16}H_{16}O_5$ MW: 288.30 Source: CHUAN XIONG. Ref: 2.

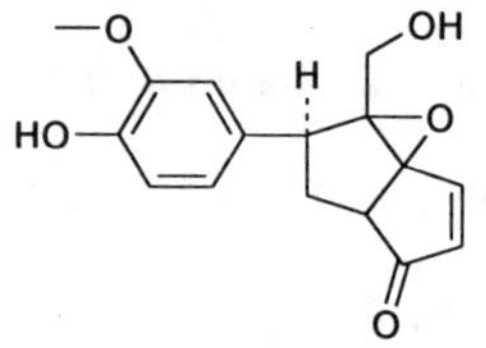

3253 β-Hydroxy-α-methylene-γ-butyllactone
$C_5H_6O_3$ MW: 114.10 Source: XIAO YE HUA. Ref: 6.

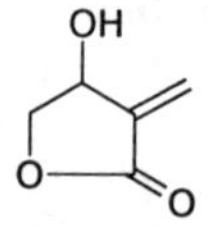

3254 6-Hydroxy-7-methylesculetin
$C_{10}H_8O_3$ MW: 176.17 Source: YIN CHEN HAO. Ref: 2.

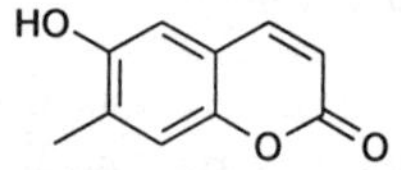

3255 5-Hydroxymethylfuraldehyde
$C_6H_6O_3$ MW: 126.11 Source: DANG SHEN, DU ZHONG. Ref: 2.

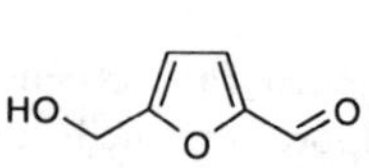

3256 6-Hydroxymethyllumazin
$C_7H_6N_4O_3$ MW: 194.15 Source: BO CAI. Ref: 6.

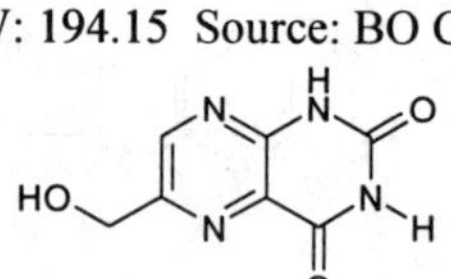

3257 cis-4-Hydroxymethylproline
$C_6H_{11}NO_3$ MW: 145.16 Property: mp 257-8°C (dec). Source: PI PA HE. Ref: 6.

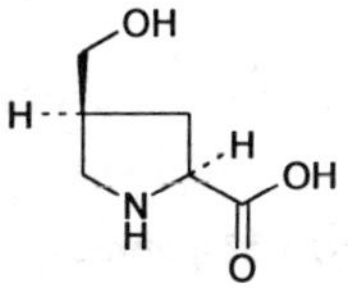

3258 trans-4-Hydroxymethyl-D-proline
$C_6H_{11}NO_3$ MW: 145.16 Property:mp 227.5-9.0°C. Source: PI PA HE. Ref: 6.

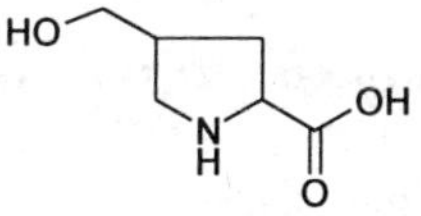

3259 α-Hydroxymethylserine
$C_4H_9NO_4$ MW: 135.12 Source: TIAN HUA FEN. Ref: 2.

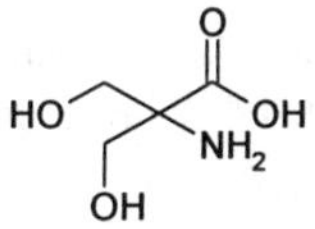

3260 Hydroxymuscopyridine A
$C_{16}H_{25}NO$ MW: 247.38 Source: SHE XIANG. Ref: 2.

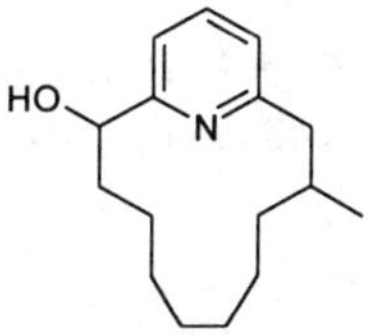

3261 Hydroxymuscopyridine B
$C_{16}H_{25}NO$ MW: 247.38 Source: SHE XIANG. Ref: 2.

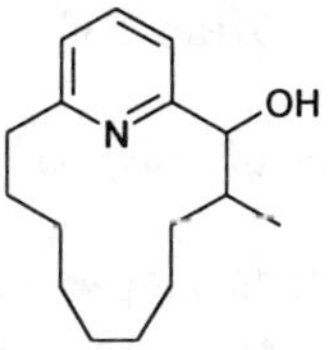

3262 6-Hydroxy-musizin-8-O-β-D-glucoside
$C_{19}H_{22}O_9$ MW: 394.38 Source: DA HUANG. Ref: 2.

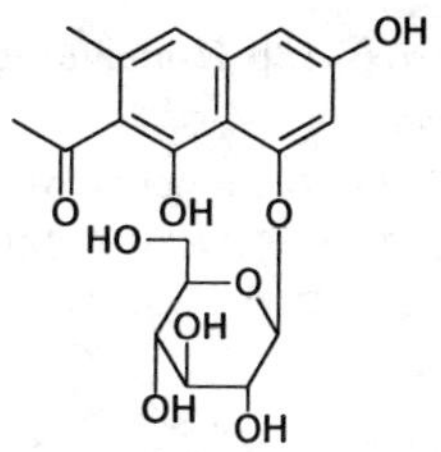

3263 3-Hydroxy-25-norfriedel-3,1(10)-dien-2-one-30-oic acid
$C_{29}H_{42}O_4$ MW: 454.66 Property: colorless acicular crystal, mp 286-7°C. Source: LEI GONG TENG. Ref: 190.

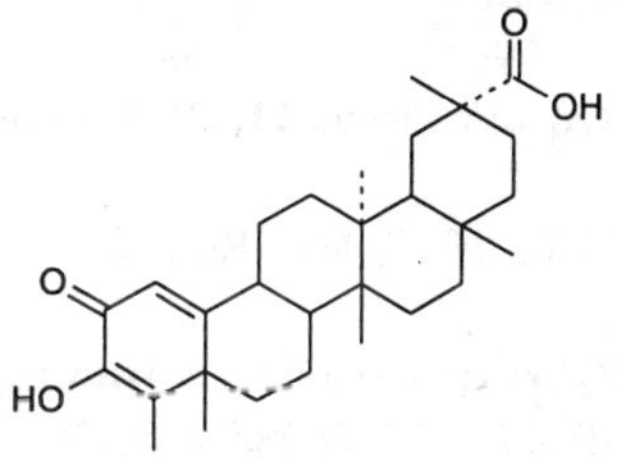

3264 21-Hydroxy-30-norhopan-22-one
$C_{29}H_{48}O_2$ MW: 428.70 Property: mp 281-4°C. Source: ZHU ZONG CAO. Ref: 6.

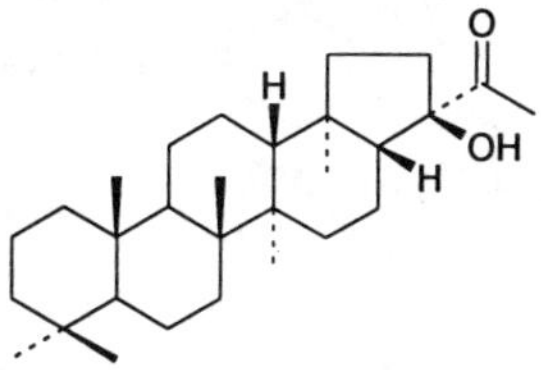

3265 9-D-Hydroxy-cis-12-octadecenoic acid
$C_{18}H_{34}O_3$ MW: 298.47 Property: mp (+): 30-2°C. Source: ZHI XIE MU PI. Ref: 6.

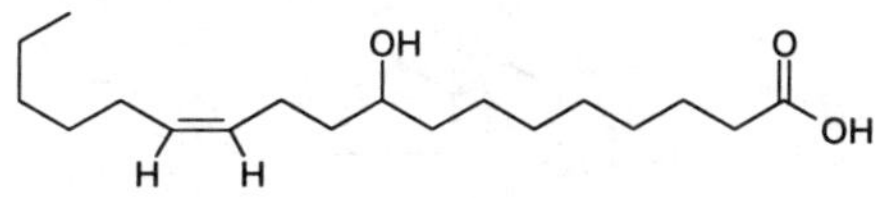

3266 Hydroxy oleanolic acid
2α,3α,19α-Trihydroxy-12-ursen-28-oic acid. Source: SHAN DI XIANG CHA CAI. Ref: 595.

3267 2β-Hydroxyoleanolic acid
$C_{30}H_{48}O_4$ MW: 472.71 Source: MI DIE XIANG. Ref: 6.

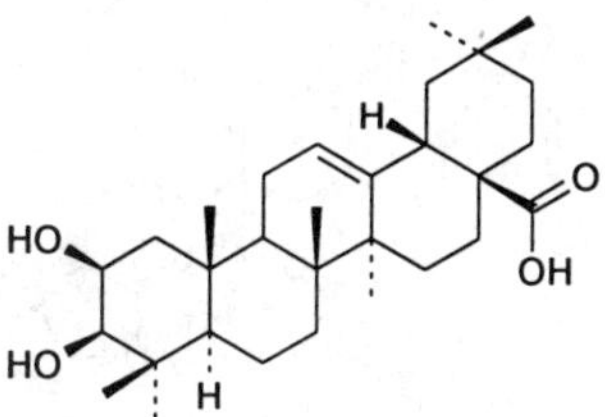

3268 16β-Hydroxy-18β-H-oleanolic acid-28-O-β-D-glucopyranoside
$C_{36}H_{58}O_9$ MW: 634.86 Property: white powder, mp 274-6°C. Source: TOU XU SONG MU. Ref: 398.

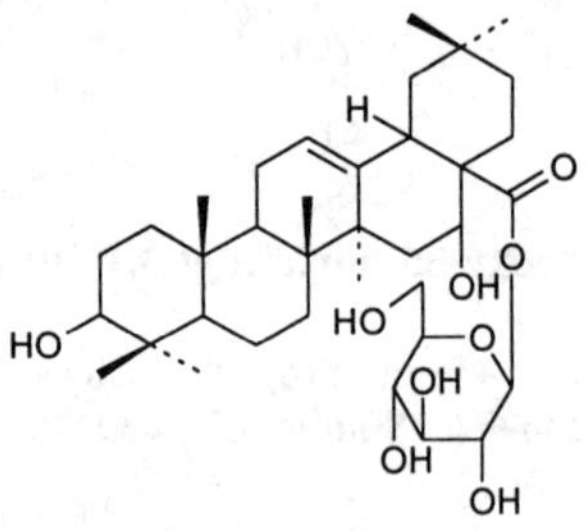

3269 3β-Hydroxy-oleans-11,13(18)-dien-28-oic acid
Source: AN HUI SONG MU. Ref: 622.

3270 3α-Hydroxy-6-oxo-5α-cholanic acid
$C_{24}H_{38}O_4$ MW: 390.57 Property: mp 194°C. Source: YE ZHU DA, ZHU DAN. Ref: 6.

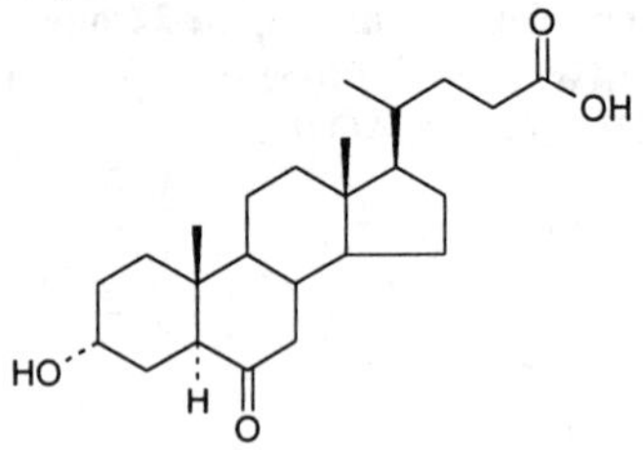

3271 (24Z)-27-Hydroxy-3-oxo-7,24-tirucalladien -21-al
$C_{30}H_{46}O_3$ MW: 454.70 Source: KU SHU PI. Ref: 12.

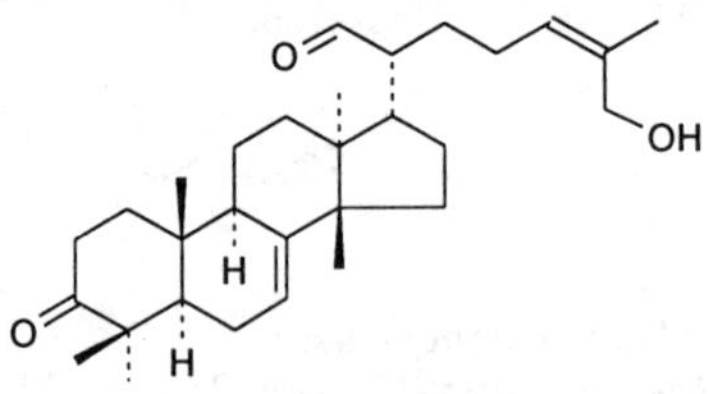

3272 12α-Hydroxypachyr(r)hizone
$C_{20}H_{14}O_8$ MW: 382.33 Property: mp 214°C. Source: DI GUA ZI. Ref: 6.

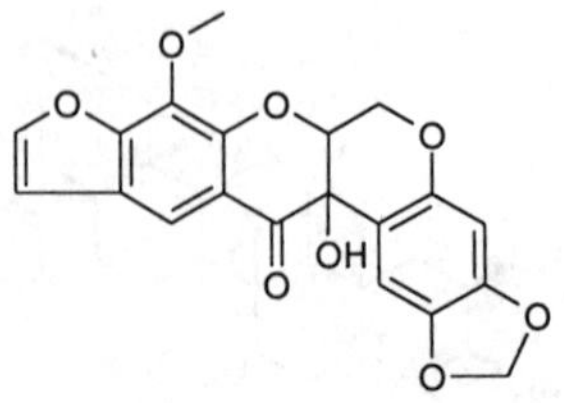

3273 γ-Hydroxypalmitic acid lactone
$C_{16}H_{30}O_2$ MW: 254.42 Property: mp 40.7-1. 3°C. Source: HONG MU JI CAO. Ref: 6.

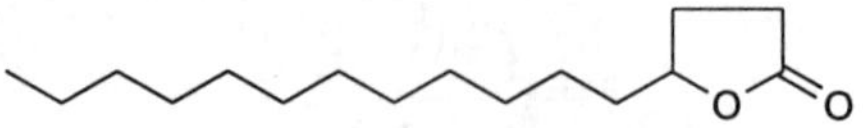

3274 9-Hydroxy-10,12-pentadecadienoic acid
$C_{15}H_{26}O_3$ MW: 254.37 Source: CU LIU GUO (SHA JI). Ref: 2.

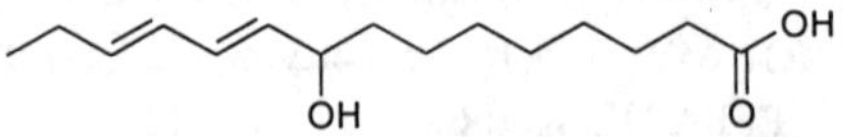

3274b 5-Hydroxy-6,7,3',4',5'-pentamethoxy flavone
Source: ZHI ZI. Ref: 626.

3274c 5-Hydroxy-3,4',5,6,7-pentamethoxy flavone
Source: ZHI ZI. Ref: 626.

3275 5-Hydroxy-3,6,7,3',4'-pentamethoxyflavone
$C_{20}H_{20}O_8$ MW: 388.38 Source: QING HAO. Ref: 2.

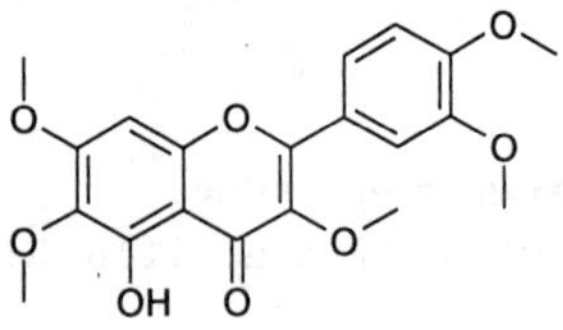

3276 5-Hydroxy-6,7,8,3',4'-pentamethoxyflavone
$C_{21}H_{22}O_9$ MW: 418.40 Source: JU PI. Ref: 2.

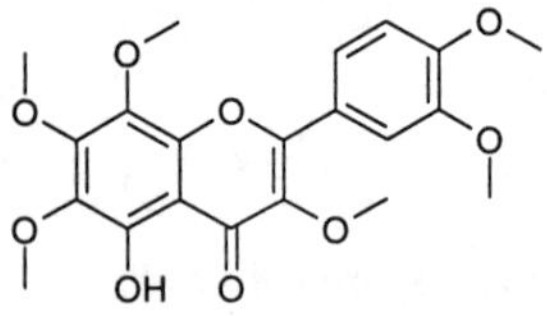

3277 p-Hydroxyphenethyl anisate
Source: QIANG HUO. Ref: 566.

3278 2-(p-Hydroxyphenoxy)-5,7dihydroxy-6-prenylchromone
$C_{20}H_{18}O_6$ MW: 354.36 Property: yellow-white powder. Source: CHAO XIAN YIN YANG HUO. Ref: 417.

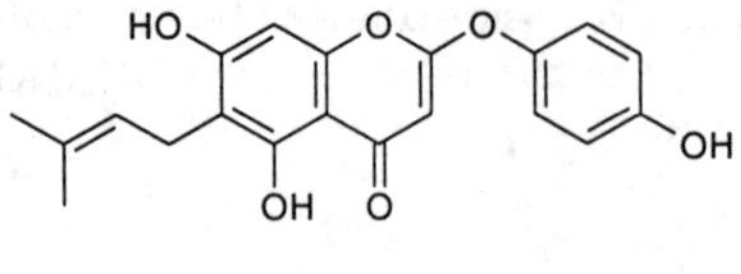

3279 2-Hydroxyphenyl acetic acid
$C_8H_8O_3$ MW: 152.15 Property: mp 147-9°C. Source: LUO XIN FU. Ref: 6.

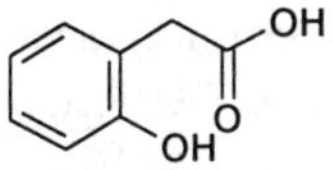

3280 p-Hydroxyphenyl acetic acid
$C_8H_8O_3$ MW: 152.15 Property: mp 148-50°C. Source: QIAN LI GUANG, NING MENG YE, NING MENG GEN. Ref: 6.

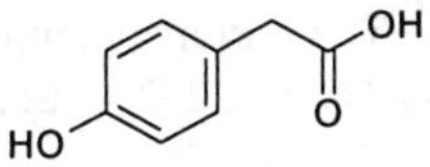

3281 6-Hydroxy-2-(2-phenylethyl) chromone
$C_{17}H_{14}O_3$ MW: 266.30 Property: colorless acicular crystal, mp 214-5°C. Source: BAI MU XIANG, CHEN XIANG. Ref: 13.

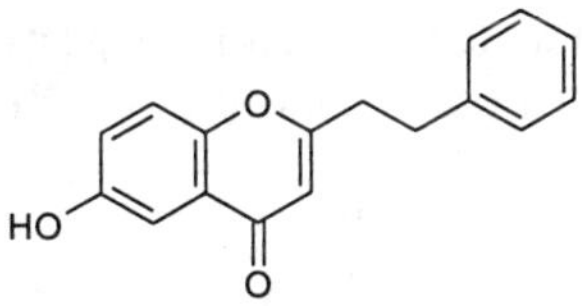

3282 4-Hydroxyphenyl-β-gentiobioside
$C_{18}H_{26}O_{12}$ MW: 434.40 Source: YUE JU YE. Ref: 6.

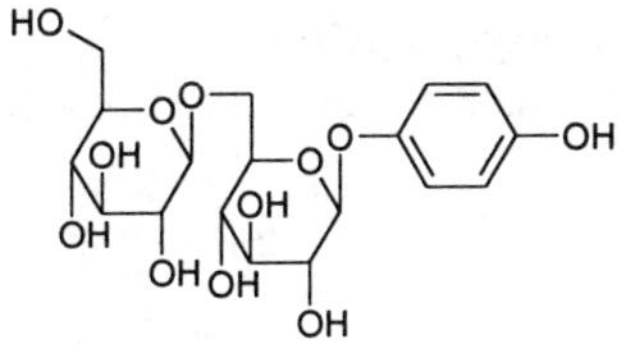

3283 m-Hydroxyphenylglycine
$C_8H_9NO_3$ MW: 167.17 Source: ZE QI. Ref: 6.

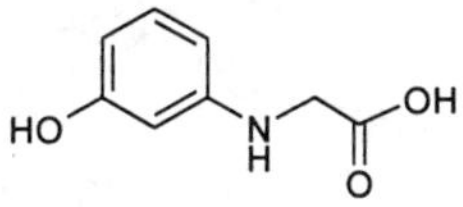

3284 3-(2-Hydroxyphenyl) propanoic acid
$C_9H_{10}O_3$ MW: 166.18 Source: GUI ZHI. Ref: 2.

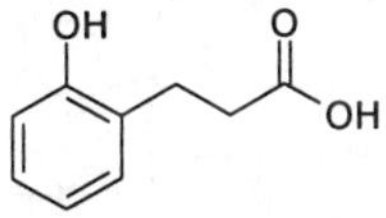

3285 3-(4-Hydroxyphenyl)-trans-propenoic acid-2,3-dihydroxypropyl ester
$C_{15}H_{16}O_7$ MW: 308.29 Source: PU HUANG. Ref: 2.

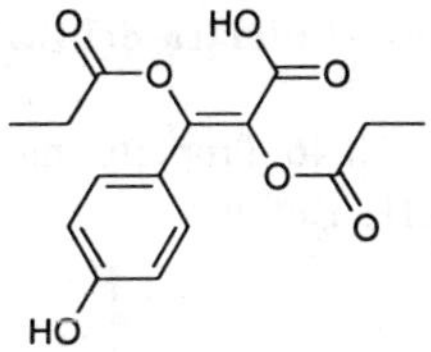

3286 o-Hydroxyphenylpyruvic acid
$C_9H_8O_4$ MW: 180.16 Source: NING MENG GEN. Ref: 6.

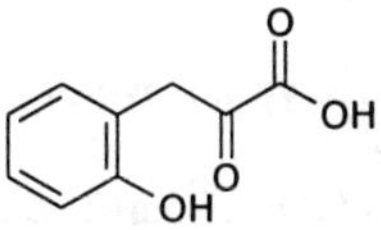

3287 m-Hydroxyphenylpyruvic acid
$C_9H_8O_4$ MW: 180.16 Source: NING MENG GEN. Ref: 6.

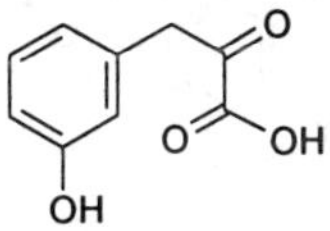

3288 p-Hydroxyphenylpyruvic acid
$C_9H_8O_4$ MW: 180.16 Property: mp 220°C. Source: NING MENG GEN. Ref: 6.

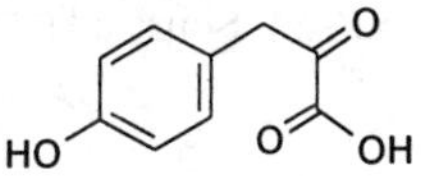

3289 Hydroxypiloselloidone
$C_{18}H_{24}O_4$ MW: 304.39 Source: MAO DA DING CAO. Ref: 6.

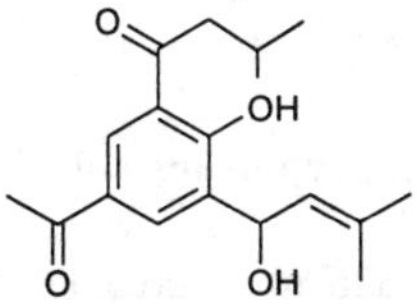

3290 7α-Hydroxy-l-pimara-8(14),15-dien-19-oic acid
$C_{20}H_{30}O_3$ MW: 318.46 Property: mp 292-4°C (dec). Source: TU DANG GUI (I). Ref: 6.

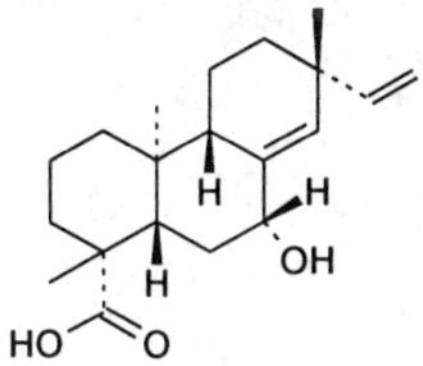

3291 7β-Hydroxy-l-pimara-8(14),15-dien-19-oic acid
$C_{20}H_{30}O_3$ MW: 318.46 Property: mp 218°C. Source: TU DANG GUI (I). Ref: 6.

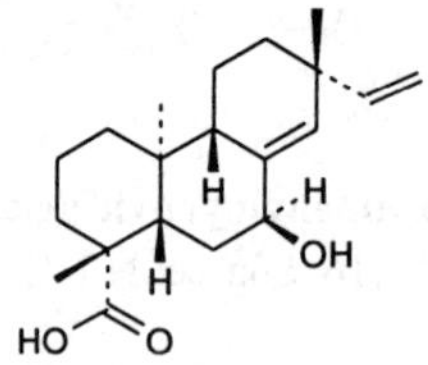

3292 (+)-1-Hydroxypinoresinol-4',4''-di-O-β-D-glucopyranoside
$C_{32}H_{42}O_{17}$ MW: 698.68 Source: DU ZHONG. Ref: 2.

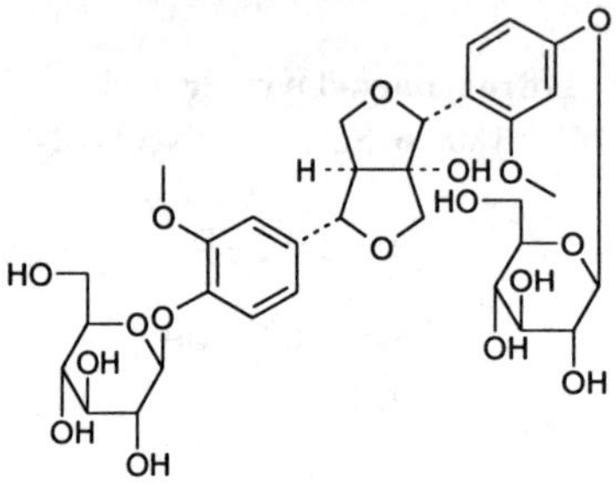

3293 (+)-1-Hydroxypinoresinol-4'-O-β-D-gluco-pyranoside
$C_{26}H_{32}O_{12}$ MW: 536.54 Source: DU ZHONG. Ref: 2.

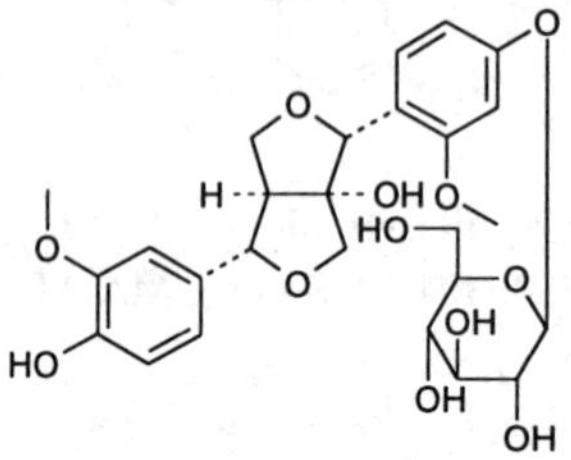

3294 (+)-1-Hydroxypinoresinol-4''-O-β-D-gluco - pyranoside
$C_{26}H_{32}O_{12}$ MW: 536.54 Source: DU ZHONG. Ref: 2.

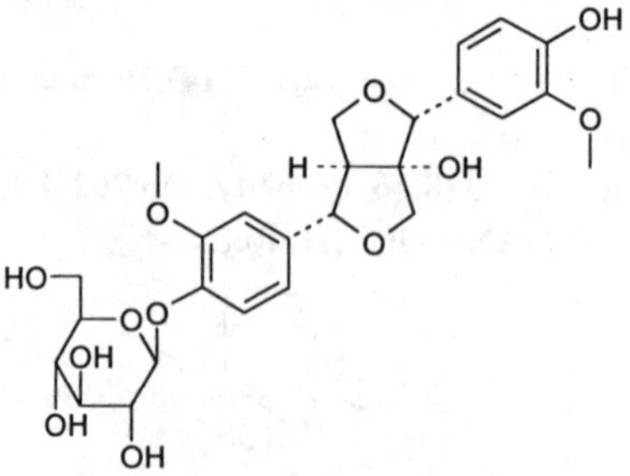

3295 Hydroxyproline
$C_5H_9NO_3$ MW: 131.13 Property: mp L-trans: 228-35°C (dec), DL-trans: 224-30°C, L-cis: 245-55°C (dec), DL-cis: 225-35°Cdec). Source: HUANG MING JIAO, WU LI, XIANG GU. Ref: 6.

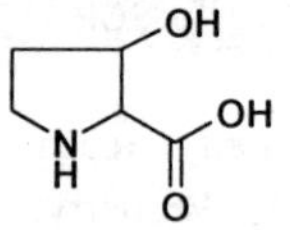

3296 cis-4-Hydroxyproline
$C_5H_9NO_3$ MW: 131.13 Property: mp D(+): 237-41°C, L(-): 238-41°C, DL: 250°C. Source: TAN XIANG. Ref: 6.

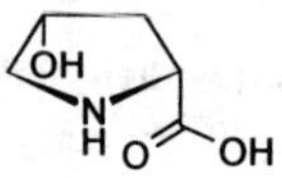

3297 trans-4-Hydroxyproline
$C_5H_9NO_3$ MW: 131.13 Property: mp D(+): 274°C, L(-): 274°C, DL: 261°C. Source: TAN XIANG. Ref: 6.

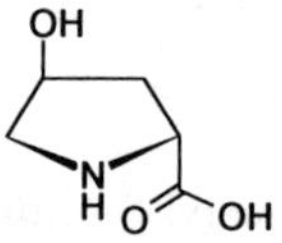

3298 2-Hydroxy-propylene
C_3H_6O MW: 58.08 Source: DA SUAN. Ref: 2.

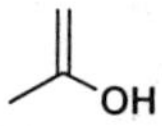

3299 5-Hydroxy-2-pyridinemethanol
$C_6H_7NO_2$ MW: 125.13 Source: DANG SHEN. Ref: 2.

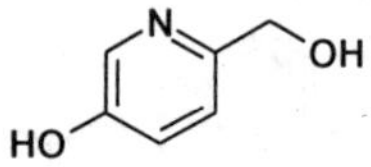

3300 11-Hydroxyrankinidine
$C_{20}H_{24}N_2O_4$ MW: 356.43 Property: mp 212-4°C, $[\alpha]_D$ -135°. Source: HU MAN TENG. Ref: 14.

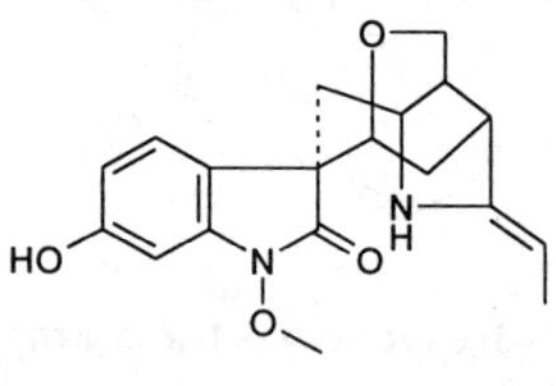

3301 4-Hydroxyrottlerin
$C_{30}H_{28}O_9$ MW: 532.55 Property: mp 208-10°C. Source: LU SONG QIU MAO. Ref: 6.

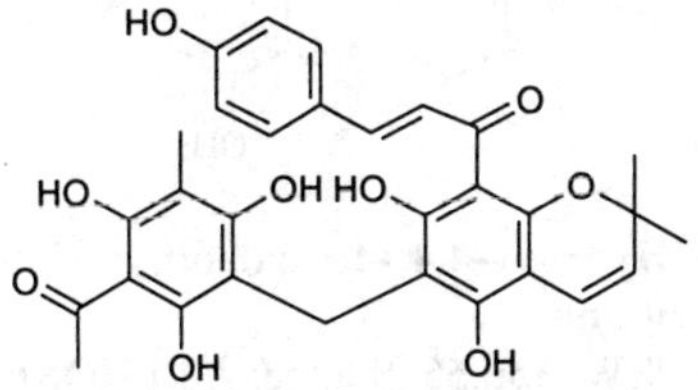

3302 3β-Hydroxysandara copimaric acid
$C_{20}H_{30}O_3$ MW: 318.46 Property: mp 261°C. Source: DU SONG SHI. Ref: 6.

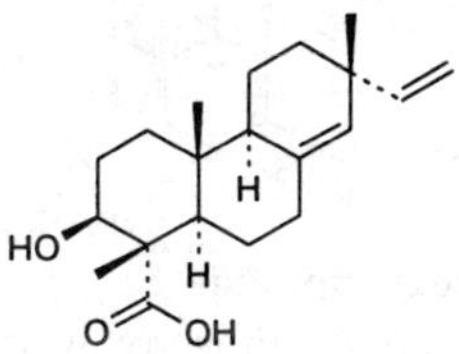

3303 15α-Hydroxysoladulcidine
$C_{27}H_{45}NO_3$ MW: 431. 66 Property: mp 156-9°C. Source: BAI MAO TENG. Ref: 6.

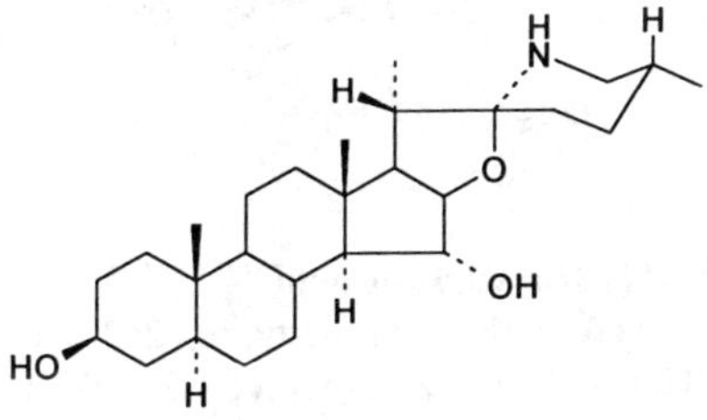

3304 15α-Hydroxysolasodine
$C_{27}H_{43}NO_3$ MW: 429.65 Source: BAI MAO TENG. Ref: 6.

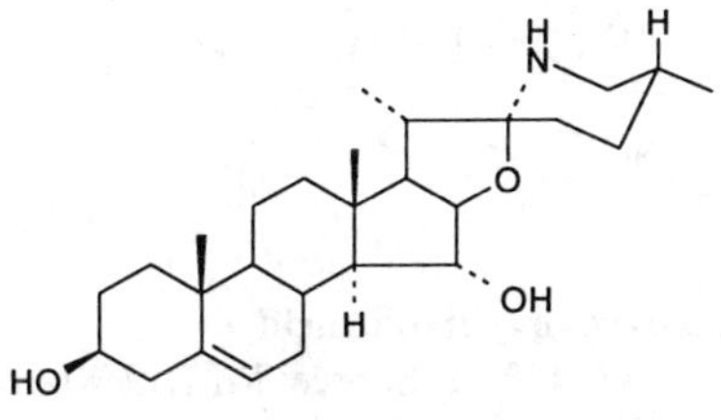

3305 9α-Hydroxysophoramine
$C_{15}H_{20}N_2O_2$ MW: 260.34 Source: KU SHEN. Ref: 2.

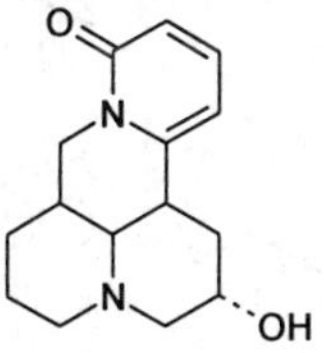

3306 4-Hydroxystrychnine
$C_{21}H_{22}N_2O_3$ MW: 364.45 Source: MA QIAN ZI. Ref: 2.

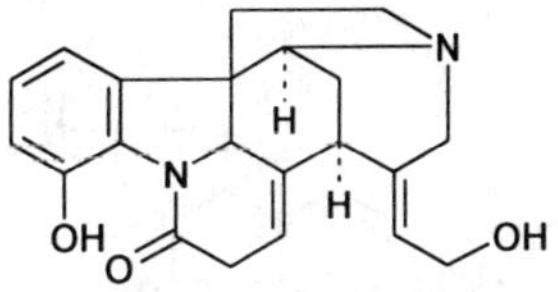

3307 Hydroxytanshinone IIA
3-α-Hydroxytanshinone II A. $C_{19}H_{18}O_4$ MW: 310.35 Property: mp 187°C. Source: DAN SHEN. Ref: 2, 6.

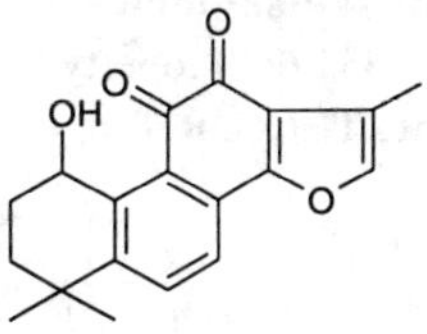

3308 5-Hydroxy-3,6,7,4'-tetramethoxyflavone
$C_{19}H_{18}O_7$ MW: 358.35 Source: QING HAO. Ref: 2.

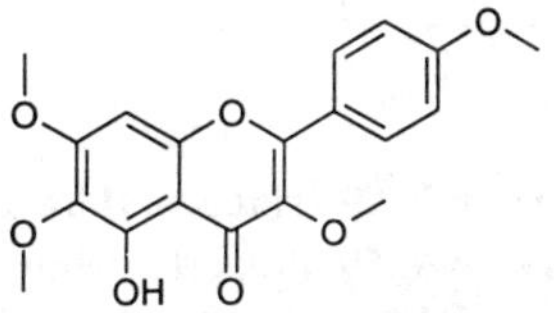

3309 1-Hydroxy-2,3,4,5-tetramethoxyxanthone
$C_{17}H_{16}O_7$ MW: 332.31 Source: HUA MAO. Ref: 6.

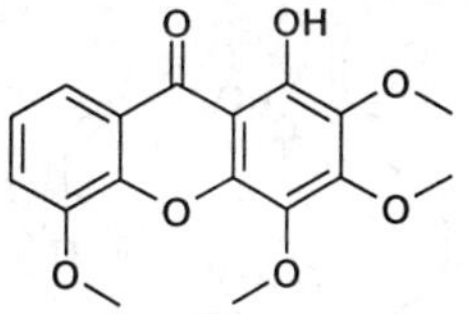

3310 1-Hydroxy-2,3,4,7-tetramethoxyxanthone
$C_{17}H_{16}O_7$ MW: 332.31 Property: mp 117.8-8.8°C. Source: HUA MAO. Ref: 6.

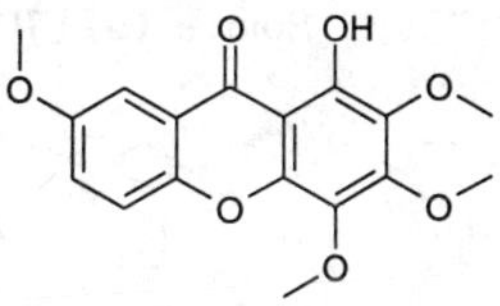

3311 (24Z)-27-Hydroxy-7, 24-tirucalladien-3-one
$C_{30}H_{48}O_2$ MW: 440.72 Source: KU SHU PI. Ref: 12.

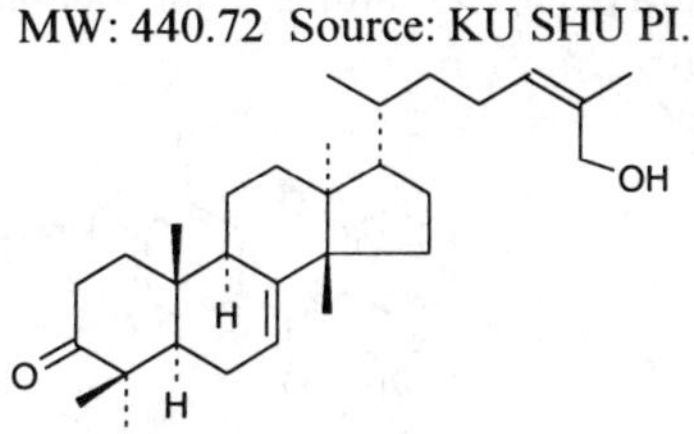

3312 15α-Hydroxytomatidenol
$C_{27}H_{43}NO_3$ MW: 429.65 Property: mp 237-40°C. Source: BAI MAO TENG. Ref: 6.

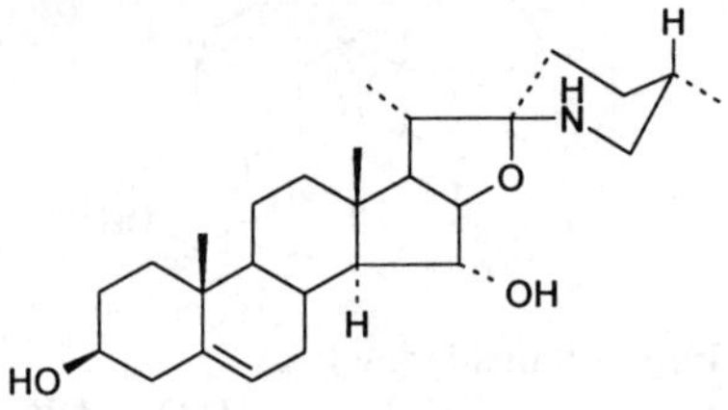

3313 15α-Hydroxytomatidine
$C_{27}H_{45}NO_3$ MW: 431.66 Property: mp 150-5°C. Source: BAI MAO TENG. Ref: 6.

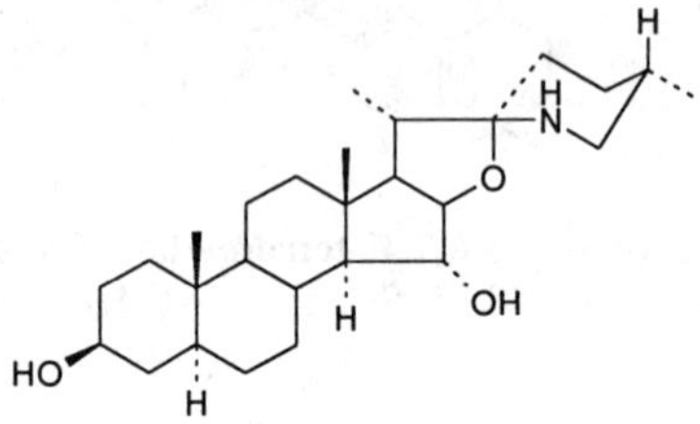

3314 1-Hydroxy-2,7,9-trideacetyl baccatin I
$C_{26}H_{38}O_{11}$ MW: 526.59 Property: white granular crystal, mp 232-5°C (methanol), $[\alpha]_D^{12}$ -52.94° (c=0.043, methanol). Source: YUN NAN HONG DOU SHAN. Ref: 296.

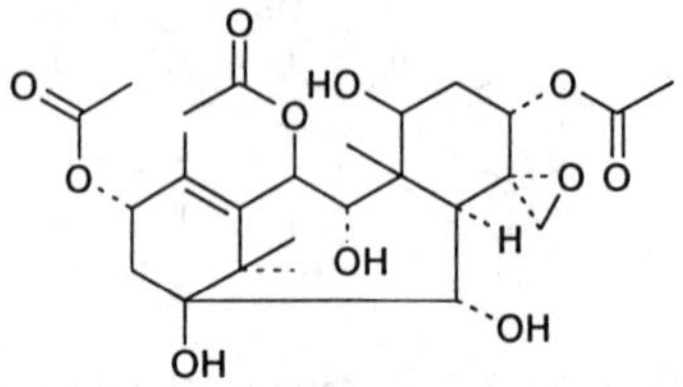

3315 11-Hydroxy-9-tridecenoicacid
$C_{13}H_{24}O_3$ MW: 228.33 Source: CU LIU GUO (SHA JI). Ref: 2.

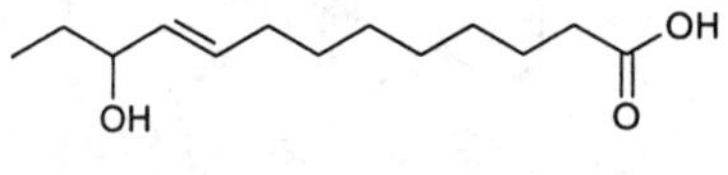

3316 1-Hydroxy-2,3,5-trimethoxyxanthone
$C_{16}H_{14}O_6$ MW: 302.29 Property: mp 189-90°C. Source: HUA MAO. Ref: 6.

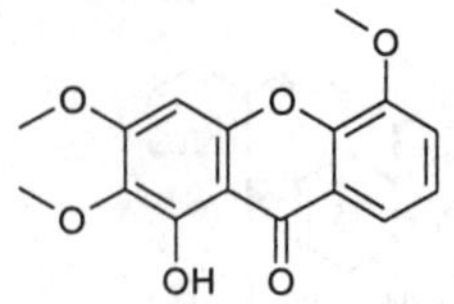

3317 1-Hydroxy-3,6,7-trimethoxy xanthone
$C_{16}H_{14}O_6$ MW: 302.29 Source: YUAN ZHI. Ref: 2.

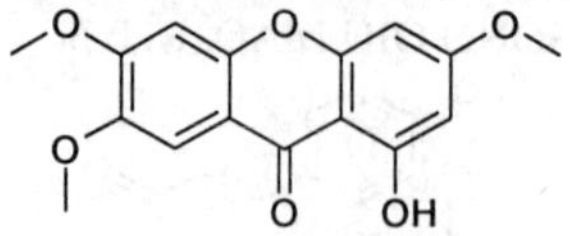

3318 3α-Hydroxy-4,4,14α-trimethyl-Δ2-5α-pregnen-20-one
$C_{24}H_{36}O_2$ MW: 356.55 Source: A LI HONG (LUO YE SONG XUN) . Ref: 6.

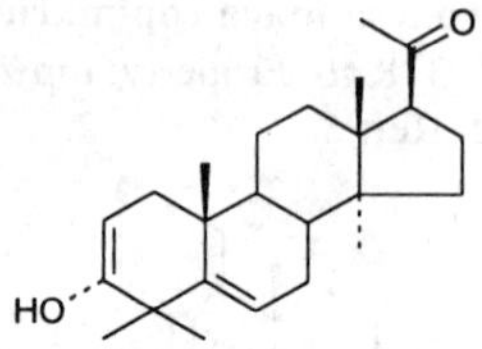

3319 16-Hydroxytriptolide
$C_{20}H_{24}O_7$ MW: 376.41 Property: white crystal, mp 232-3.5°C. Source: LEI GONG TENG. Ref: 204.

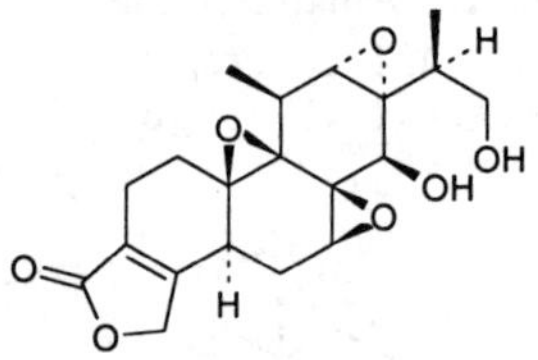

3320 2α-Hydroxyursolic acid
$C_{30}H_{48}O_4$ MW: 472.71 Property: mp 243-5°C. Source: HONG KUAI ZI, SAN YE SHU WEI CAO. Ref: 6, 570.

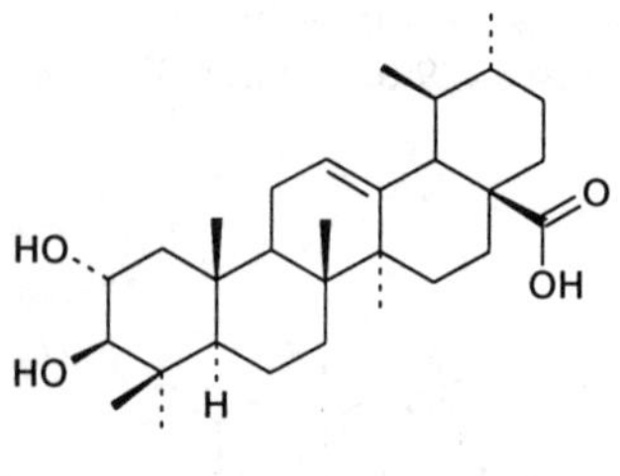

3321 19α-Hydroxyursolic acid
$C_{30}H_{48}O_4$ MW: 472.71 Source: MI DIE XIANG. Ref: 6.

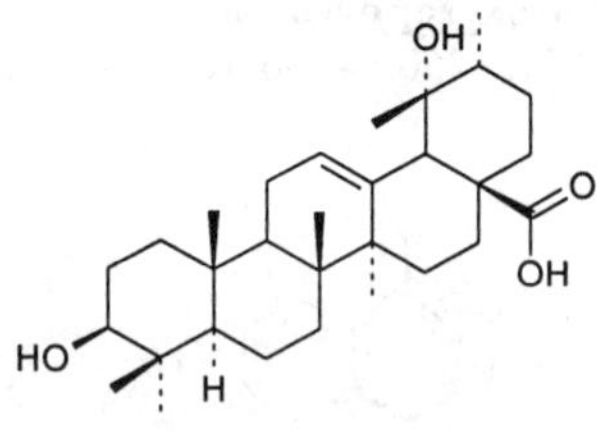

3322 Hygrine
$C_8H_{15}NO$ MW: 141.21 Property: bp (-): 193-5°C.
Source: JIA SUAN JIANG. Ref: 6.

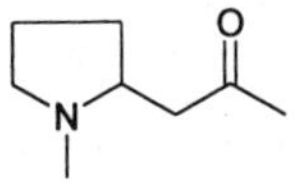

3323 Hyocholic acid
$C_{24}H_{40}O_5$ MW: 408.58 Property: mp 188-9°C.
Source: ZHU DAN. Ref: 6.

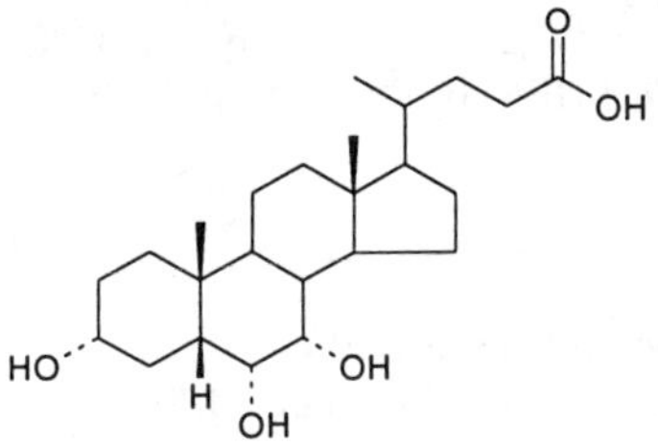

3324 α-Hyodeoxycholic acid
$C_{24}H_{40}O_4$ MW: 392.58 Property: mp 196-7°C.
Source: ZHU DAN. Ref: 6.

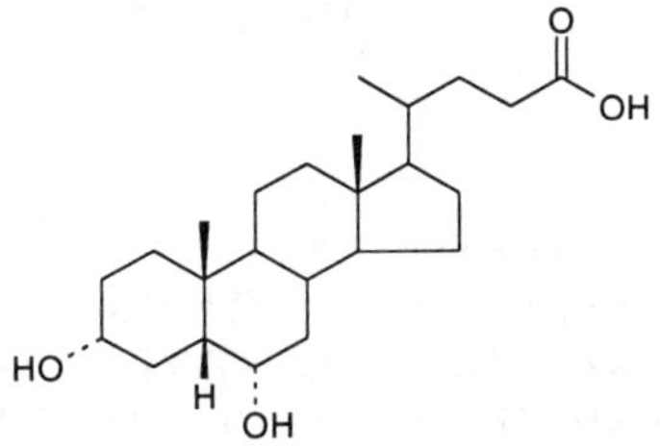

3325 β-Hyodeoxycholic acid
$C_{24}H_{40}O_4$ MW: 392.58 Property: mp 189-90°C.
Source: ZHU DAN. Ref: 6.

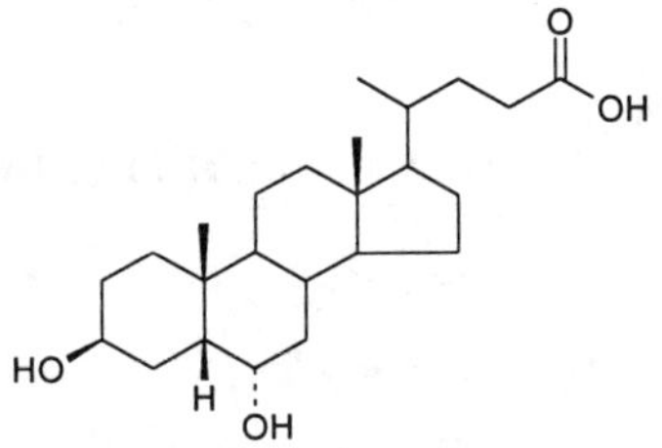

3326 Hyoerin
Source: CHUAN E YIN YANG HUO. Ref: 567.

3327 Hyoscine
$C_{17}H_{21}NO_4$ MW: 303.36 Source: YANG JIN HUA.
Ref: 2.

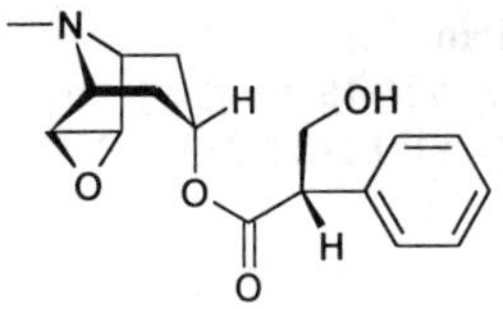

3328 Hyoscyamine
$C_{17}H_{23}NO_3$ MW: 289.38 Source: GOU QI ZI, YANG JIN HUA. Ref: 2.

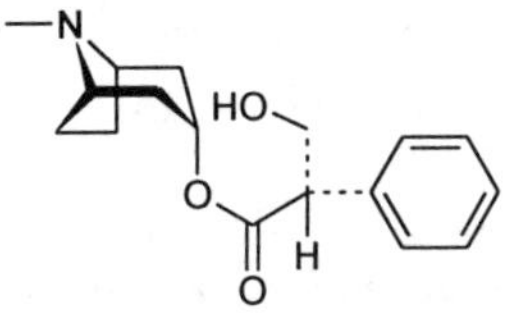

3329 Hypaconitine
$C_{33}H_{45}NO_{10}$ MW: 615.73 Property: white granular crystal, mp 197.5-8.5°C, $[\alpha]_D^{26}$ +21.6° (c=0.607, $CHCl_3$). Source: E ZHANG YE FU ZI, FU ZI.
Ref: 2, 6, 460.

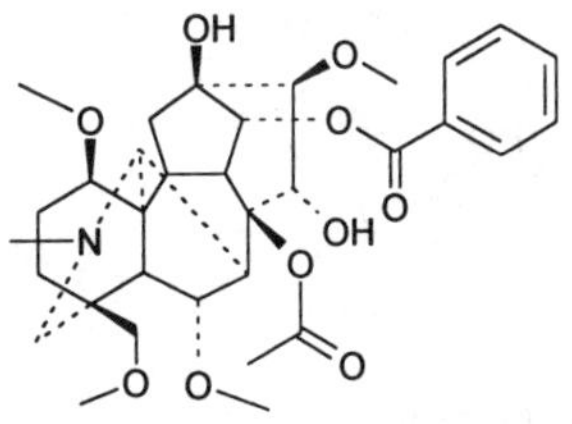

3330 Hypaphorine
$C_{14}H_{20}N_2O_2$ MW: 248.33 Property: mp 255°C (dec).
Source: HONG MU JI CAO, XIANG SI ZI. Ref: 6.

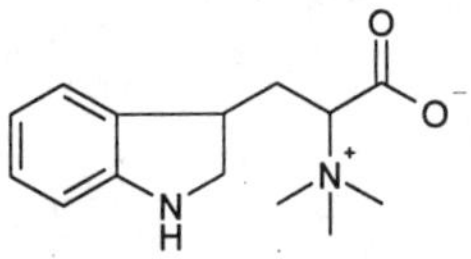

3330b Hypecoumine
$C_{19}H_{11}NO_6$ MW: 349.30 Property: colorless acicular crystal, mp 202-4°C, $[\alpha]_D^{32}$ +45.06° (c=0.07, $CHCl_3$)
Source: XI GUO JIAO HUI XIANG (Tibet drug).
Ref: 37.

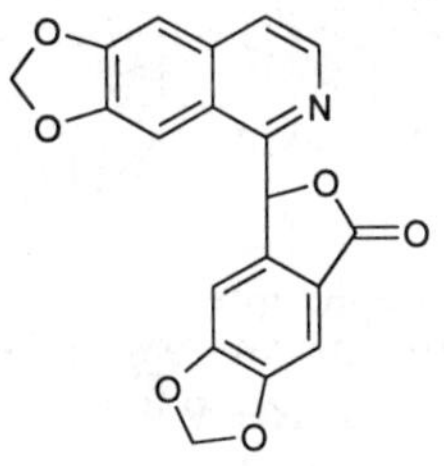

3331 Hypericin
$C_{30}H_{16}O_8$ MW: 504.46 Property: mp >330°C (dec). Source: GUAN YE LIAN QIAO, XIAO LIAN QIAO. Ref: 6.

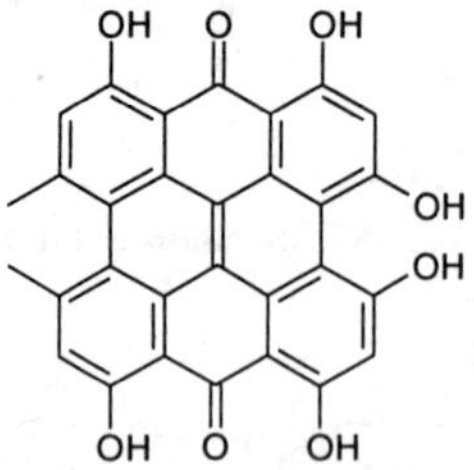

3332 Hyperin
Hyperoside; Quercetin-3-O-galactoside; 3',4',5,7-Tetrahydroxyflavonol-3-β-D-galactoside. CAS: 482-36-0 $C_{21}H_{20}O_{12}$ MW: 464.39 Source: GOU TENG, LING LAN, XIAN HE CAO, YIN CHEN HAO, YIN YANG HUO, YU XING CAO. Ref: 2, 4.

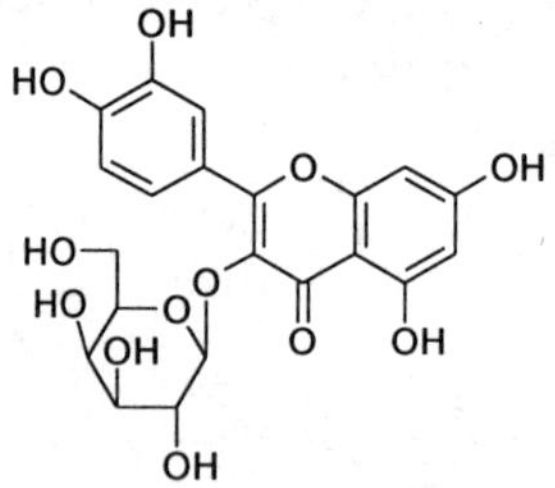

3333 Hypodematine
$C_{17}H_{13}NO$ MW: 247.30 Property: light yellow acicular crystal, mp 156-8°C. Source: SHAN DONG ZHONG ZU JUE. Ref: 180.

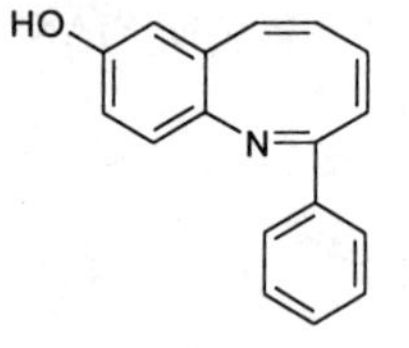

3334 Hypodiolide A
$C_{20}H_{30}O_3$ MW: 318.46 Property: white acicular crystal. mp 205-6°C. Source: KUN MING SHAN HAI TANG. Ref: 252.

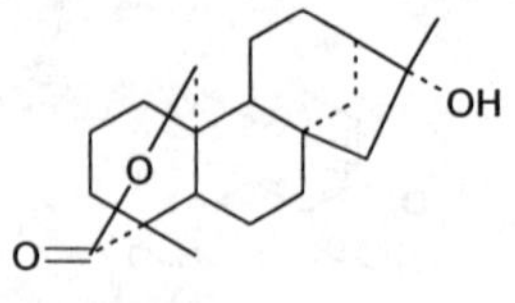

3335 Hypoepistephanine
$C_{36}H_{36}N_2O_6$ MW: 592.70 Property: mp 257°C. Source: QIAN JIN TENG. Ref: 6.

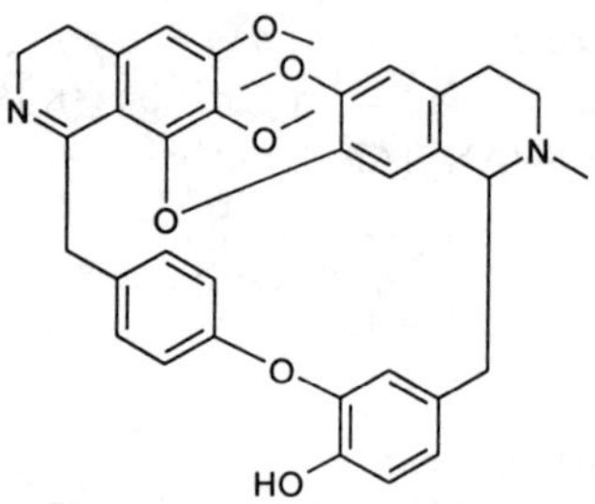

3336 Hypogaeic acid
$C_{14}H_{26}O_2$ MW: 226.36 Property: mp 33°C. Source: LUO HUA SHENG YOU, MI LA. Ref: 6.

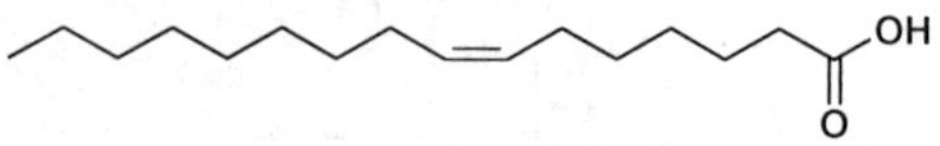

3337 Hypolide methyl ether
$C_{21}H_{26}O_3$ MW: 326.44 Source: LEI GONG TENG. Ref: 2.

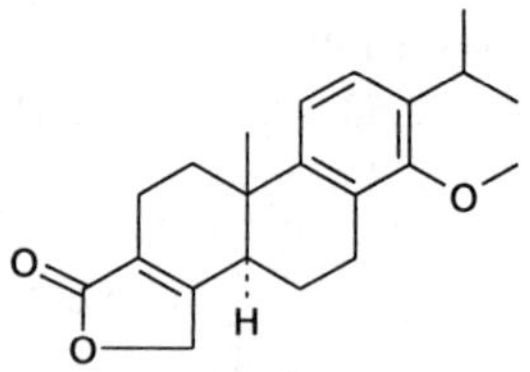

3338 Hypoxanthine
6-Hydroxypurine. $C_5H_4N_4O$ MW: 136.11 Property: mp 150°C (dec). Source: GOU QI YE, GUI GAI, GUI GAI, HAI XIA, QIU YIN, TIAN GAO, ZHANG YE BAN XIA. Ref: 2, 6, 586.

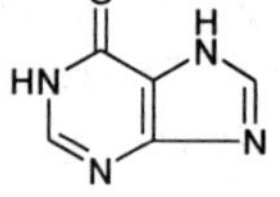

3339 I-23
$C_{20}H_{16}O_6$ MW: 352.35 Source: JIU LI XIANG. Ref: 11.

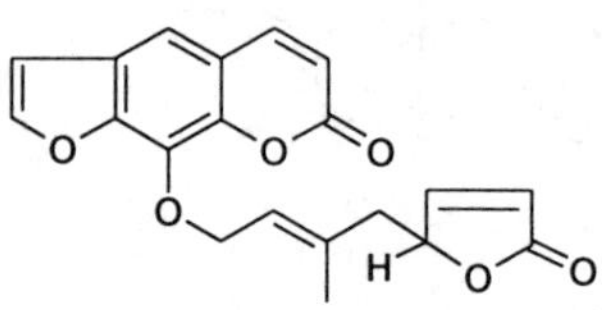

3340 Ibotenic acid
CAS: 2552-55-8 $C_5H_6N_2O_4$ MW: 158.11 Property: mp151-2°C (dec). Source: E GAO TAN. Ref: 5.

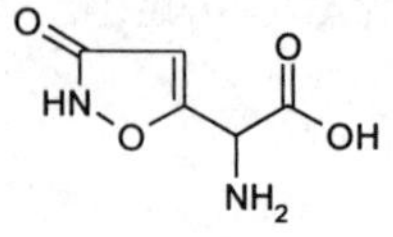

3341 Icajine

$C_{22}H_{24}N_2O_3$ MW: 364.45 Property: mp 271-2°C (dec). Source: MA QIAN ZI. Ref: 2, 542.

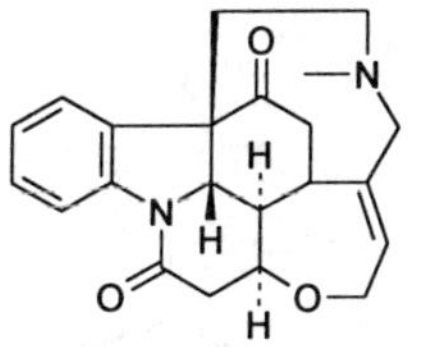

3342 Icaride A

$C_{22}H_{28}O_7$ MW: 404.46 Source: YIN YANG HUO. Ref: 2.

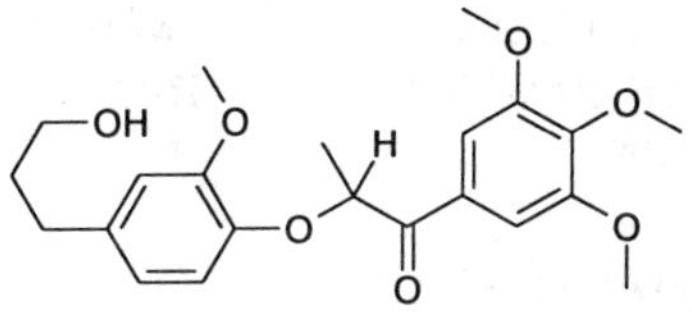

3343 Icaride A2

$C_{22}H_{28}O_9$ MW: 436.46 Source: YIN YANG HUO. Ref: 2.

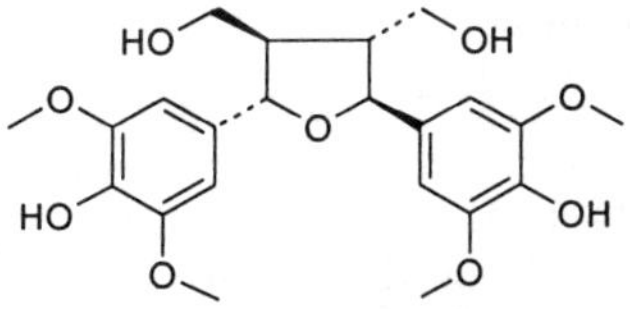

3344 Icariin

$C_{33}H_{40}O_{15}$ MW: 676.68 Source: CHUAN E YIN YANG HUO, CU MAO YIN YANG HUO, YIN YANG HUO. Ref: 2, 514, 568, 635.

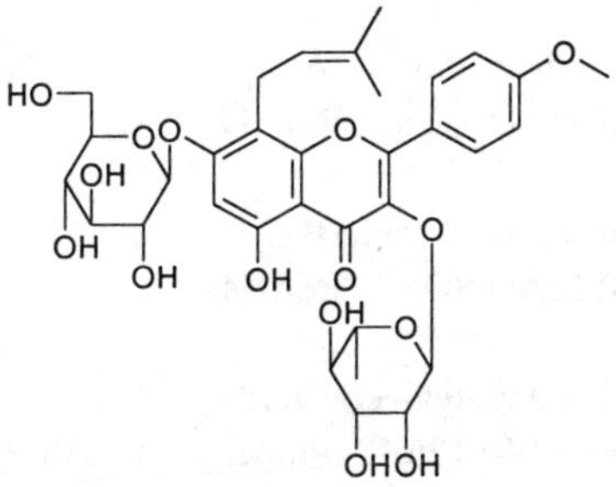

3345 Icariside

Property: mp 250-2°C. Source: CU MAO YIN YANG HUO. Ref: 539.

3346 Icariside A7

$C_{23}H_{26}O_{11}$ MW: 462.46 Property: white powder. Source: CHAO XIAN YIN YANG HUO. Ref: 417.

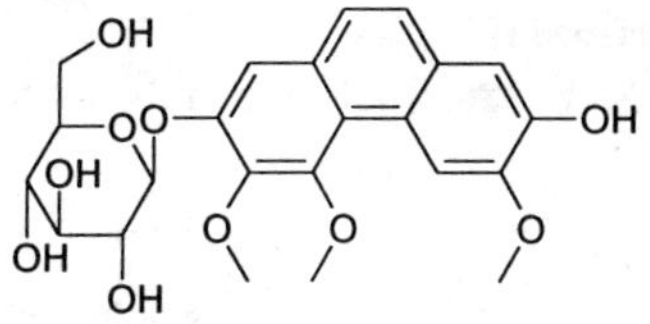

3347 Icariside B9

$C_{19}H_{32}O_7$ MW: 372.46 Source: YIN YANG HUO. Ref: 2.

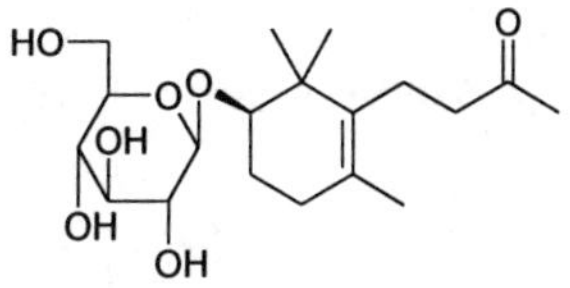

3348 Icariside D3

$C_{15}H_{20}O_7$ MW: 312.32 Source: YIN YANG HUO. Ref: 2.

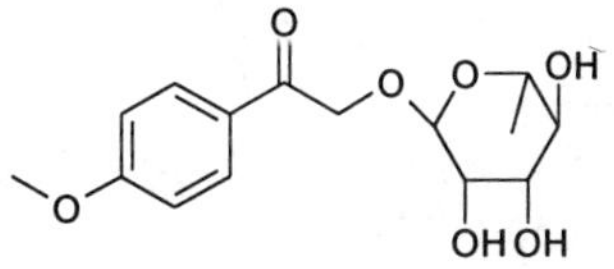

3349 Icariside E6

$C_{26}H_{36}O_{10}$ MW: 508.57 Source: YIN YANG HUO. Ref: 2.

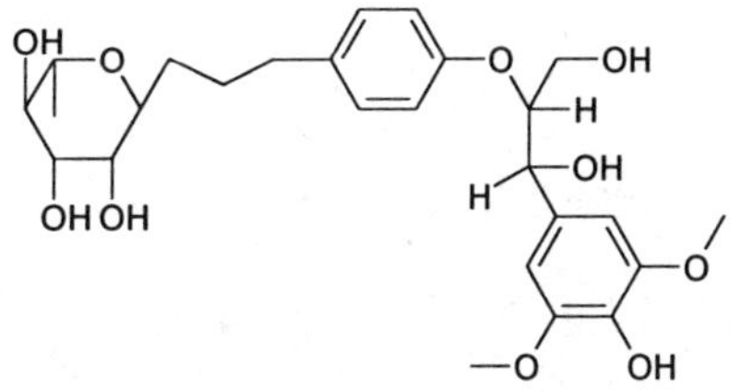

3350 Icariside E7

$C_{29}H_{38}O_{13}$ MW: 594.62 Source: YIN YANG HUO. Ref: 2.

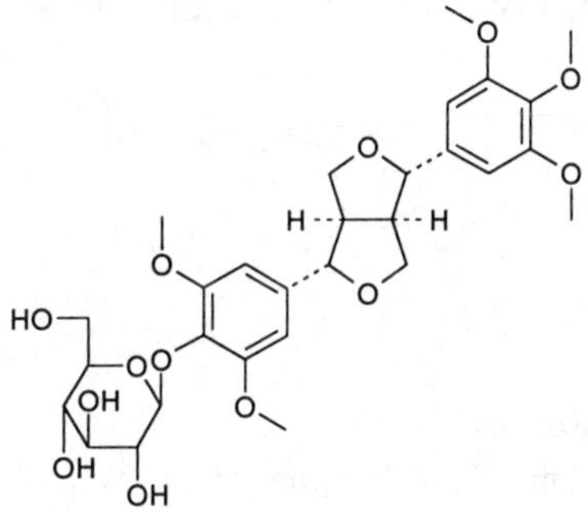

3351 Icariside H1
$C_{18}H_{26}O_9$ MW: 386.40 Source: YIN YANG HUO. Ref: 2.

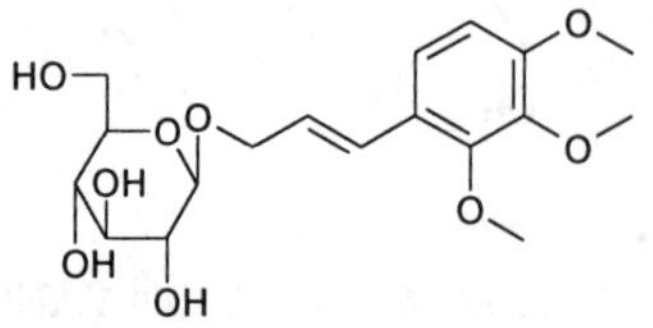

3352 Icariside I
$C_{27}H_{30}O_{11}$ MW: 530.53 Source: YIN YANG HUO. Ref: 2.

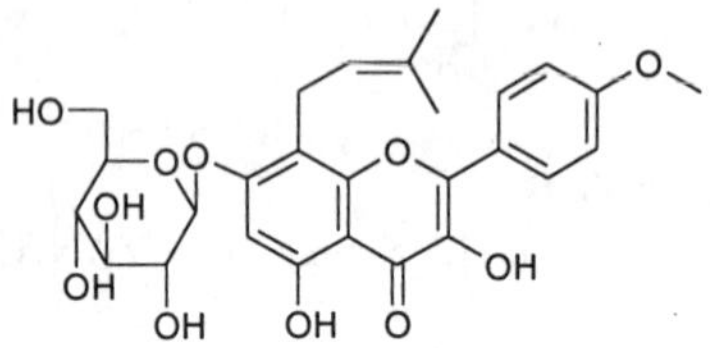

3353 Icaritin
Property: yellow powder, mp 230-1°C. Source: CHAO XIAN YIN YANG HUO, CU MAO YIN YANG HUO. Ref: 458, 539.

3354 Icaritin-3-O-α-rhamnoside
$C_{27}H_{32}O_{11}$ MW: 532.55 Source: YIN YANG HUO. Ref: 2.

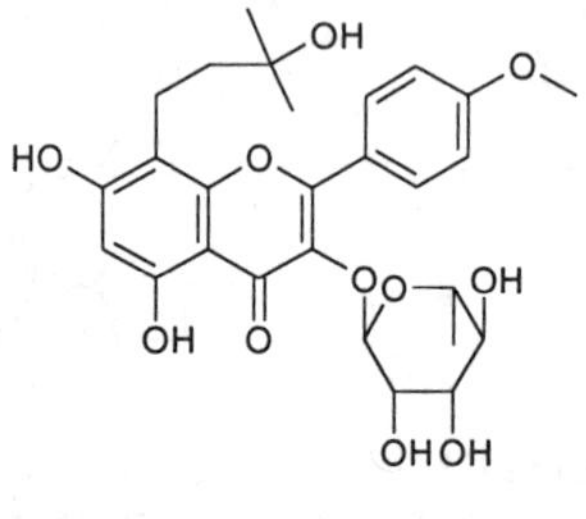

3355 Igagenin
$C_{27}H_{44}O_5$ MW: 448.65 Source: BEI XIE. Ref: 6.

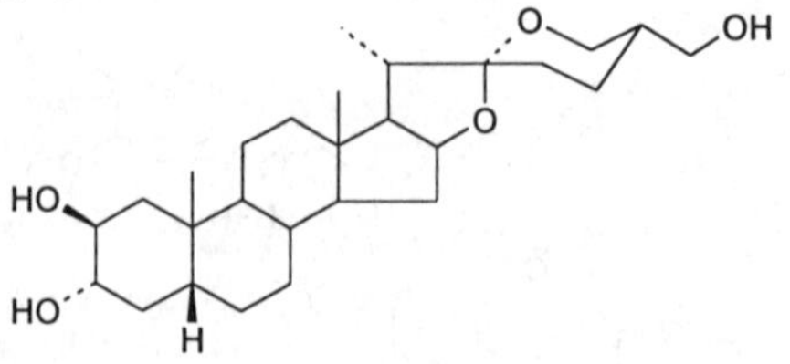

3356 Ignavine
Property: mp 226-8°C. Source: CAO WU TO. Ref: 6.

3357 Ikarisoside A
$C_{26}H_{28}O_{10}$ MW: 500.51 Property: mp 132-4°C. Source: CU MAO YIN YANG HUO, YIN YANG HUO. Ref: 2, 599.

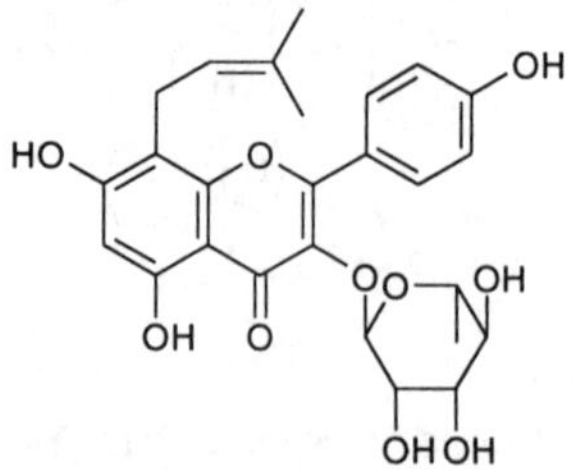

3358 Ikarisoside B
Property: mp 180-2°C. Source: CU MAO YIN YANG HUO, WAN SHAN YIN YANG HUO. Ref: 574, 599.

3359 Ikarisoside C
Source: CHUAN E YIN YANG HUO, CU MAO YIN YANG HUO, YIN YANG HUO. Ref: 565, 567, 624.

3360 Ikarisoside F
Source: YIN YANG HUO. Ref: 565.

3361 Ilexin A
$C_{19}H_{28}O_{10}$ MW: 436.43 Property: mp 194°C. Source: JIU BI YING. Ref: 6.

3362 Ilexin B
$C_{33}H_{34}O_{10}$ MW: 436.43 Property: mp 215-7°C. Source: JIU BI YING. Ref: 6.

3363 Imbricataflavone A
Source: JI MAO SONG. Ref: 544.

3364 Imbricataflavone B
Source: JI MAO SONG. Ref: 544.

3365 1-Imidazolylacetic acid
$C_5H_6N_2O_2$ MW: 126.12 Property: mp 268-9°C (dec). Source: GUI GAI. Ref: 6.

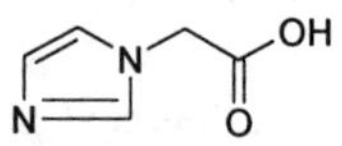

3366 2-4'-Imidazolylethanol
$C_5H_8N_2O$ MW: 112.13 Source: GUI GAI. Ref: 6.

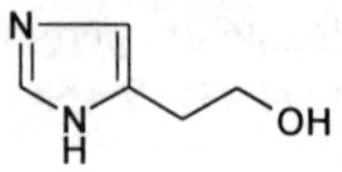

3367 Imidazolylethylamine

$C_5H_9N_3$ MW: 111.15 Property: mp 75-80°C; bp 167°/0.8 mm. Source: QIE YE. Ref: 6.

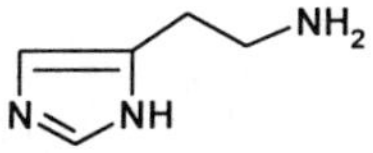

3368 Imidazolylpropionic acid

$C_6H_8N_2O_2$ MW: 140.14 Property: mp 206-8°C. Source: GUI GAI. Ref: 6.

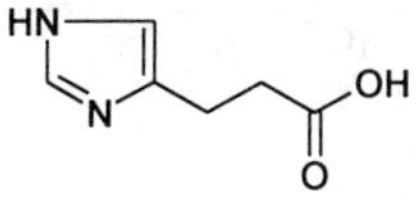

3369 Imperatorin

$C_{16}H_{14}O_4$ MW: 270.29 Property: mp 102-4°C. Source: BAI ZHI, FANG FENG, JIU LI XIANG, SONG YE FANG FENG, YUN NAN QIANG HUO, YUN QIAN HU. Ref: 2, 11, 177, 549, 551.

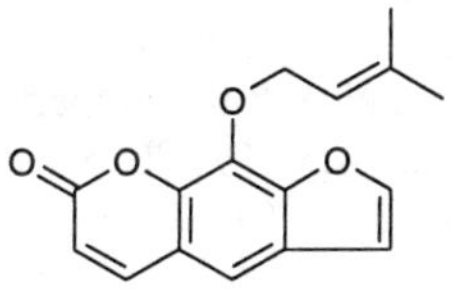

3370 Imperialine

Kashmirine; Sipeimine. CAS: 61825-98-7 $C_{27}H_{43}NO_3$ MW: 429.65 Property: mp 267-9°C. Source: CHUAN BEI MU, NING XIA BEI MU.
Ref: 4, 271.

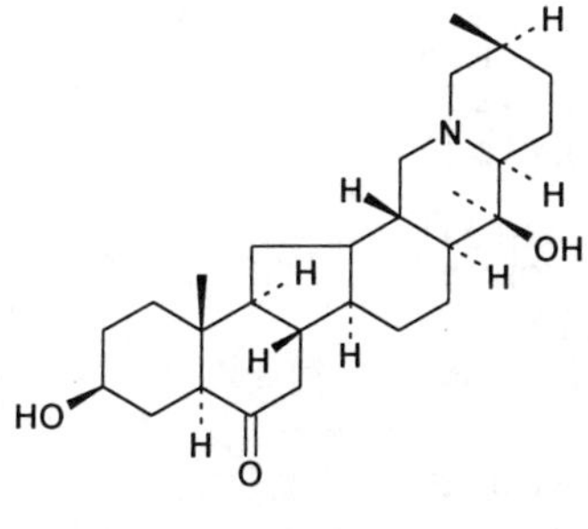

3371 1-Indanone

C_9H_8O MW: 132.16 Property: mp 42°C. Source: JUE. Ref: 6.

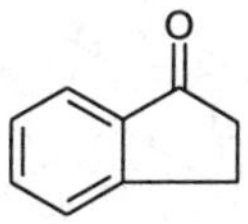

3372 Indican

$C_8H_9SO_4$ MW: 215.23 Source: REN NIAO. Ref: 6.

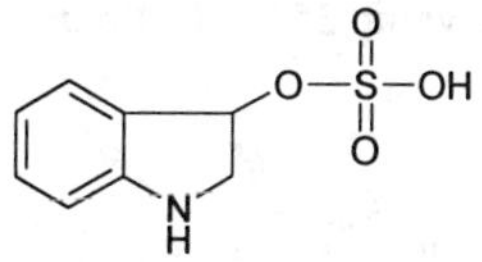

3373 Indican (glucoside)

$C_{14}H_{17}NO_6$ MW: 295.29 Property: mp 178-80°C (anhydride). Source: DA QING YE, GANG BAN GUI GEN, MU LAN. Ref: 6.

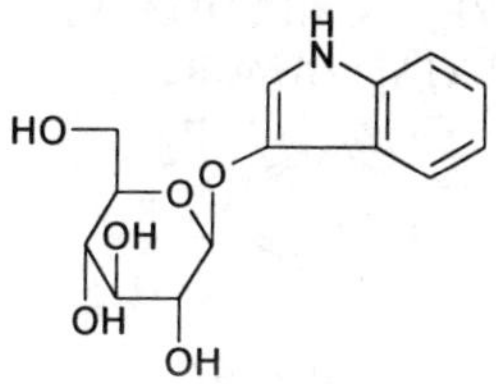

3374 Indicaxanthin

$C_{14}H_{16}N_2O_6$ MW: 308.29 Property: mp 160-2°C (dec). Source: ZI MO LI GEN. Ref: 6.

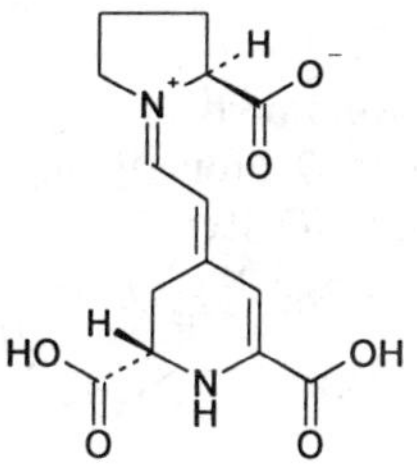

3375 Indicine

$C_{15}H_{25}NO_5$ MW: 299.37 Property: mp 97-8°C. Source: DA WEI YAO. Ref: 6.

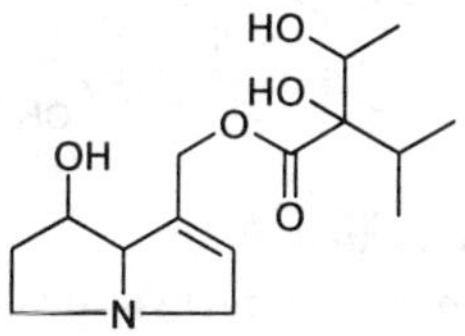

3376 Indigotin

$C_{16}H_{10}N_2O_2$ MW: 262.27 Source: DA QING YE. Ref: 2.

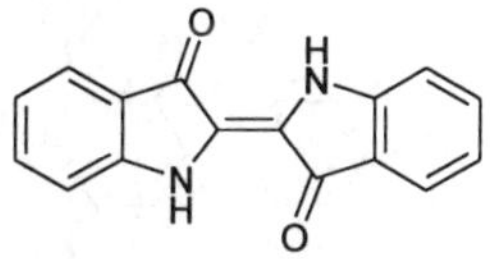

3377 Indirubin
Couroupitine B. CAS: 479-41-4 $C_{16}H_{10}N_2O_2$ MW: 262.27 Property: mp 356-8°C. Source: MU LAN. Ref: 4.

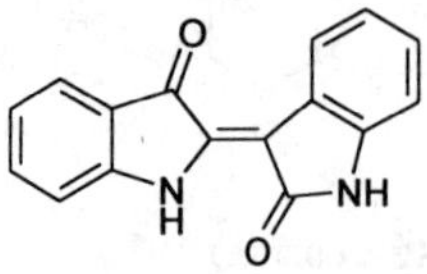

3378 Indole
C_8H_7N MW: 117.15 Property: mp 52°C, bp 253-4°C. Source: CHA YE, LA MEI HUA, LING MAO XIANG, SHUI XIAN HUA. Ref: 6.

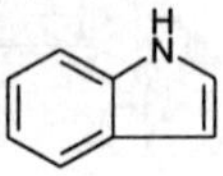

3379 Indole-3-acetaldehyde
$C_{10}H_9NO$ MW: 159.19 Source: GAN LAN. Ref: 6.

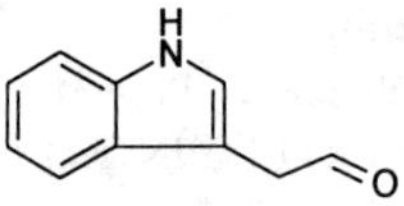

3380 Indole-3-acetonitrile
$C_{10}H_8N_2$ MW: 156.19 Property: mp 36-6.5°C. Source: TOU GU CAO. Ref: 6.

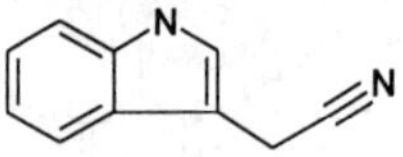

3381 3-Indolylacetic acid
$C_{10}H_9N_2O_2$ MW: 175.19 Property: mp 164-5°C. Source: LU SUN PIAN, WU HUA GUO. Ref: 6.

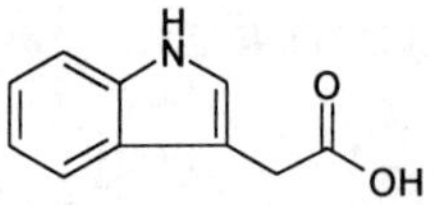

3382 Inflacoumarin A
4-(4'-Hydroxy-phenyl)-6-prenyl-7-hydroxy-coumarin. $C_{20}H_{18}O_4$ MW: 322.36 Property: colorless acicular crystal, mp 232-3°C. Source: ZHANG GUO GAN CAO. Ref: 302.

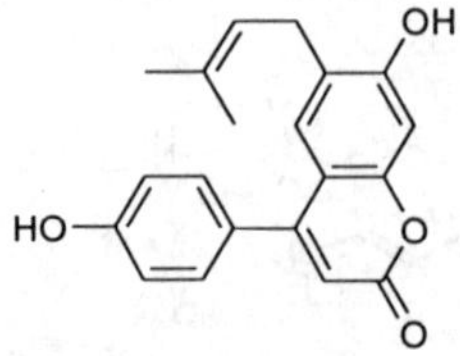

3383 Inflasaponin IV
Glycyrrhetic acid-3-O-β-D-6''-n-butyl-glucuronopyranosyl-(1→2)-β-D-6'-n-butyl-glucuronopyranoside. $C_{50}H_{78}O_{16}$ MW: 935.17 Property: colorless powder, mp 234-6°C. Source: ZHANG GUO GAN CAO. Ref: 301.

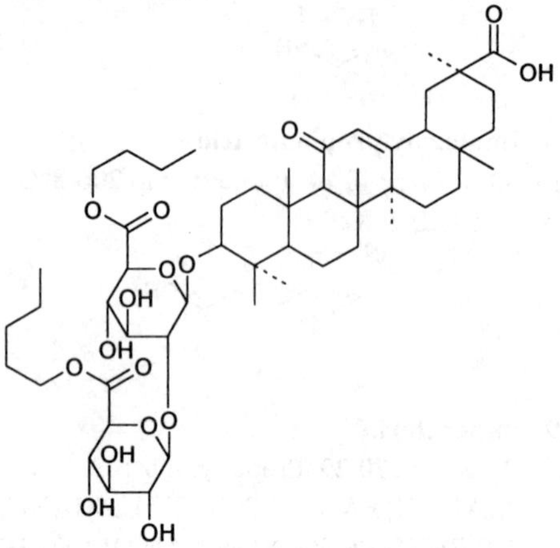

3384 Inflasaponin I
Glycyrrhetic acid-3-O-β-D-6''-n-methyl-glucuronopyranosyl-(1→2)-β-D-6'-n-butyl-glucuronopyranoside. $C_{47}H_{72}O_{16}$ MW: 893.03 Property: colorless amorphous powder, mp 256-8°C. Source: ZHANG GUO GAN CAO. Ref: 301.

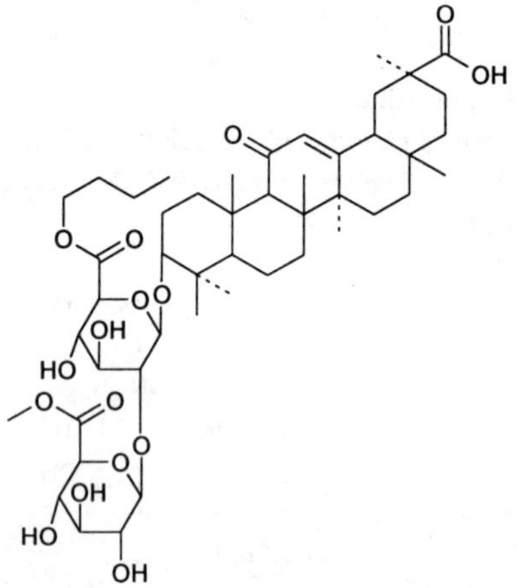

3385 Inflexusin B
$C_{20}H_{26}O_5$ MW: 346.43 Property: colorless rhomboid crystal (acetone), mp 221-3°C, $[\alpha]_D^{18}$ -187.6° (c=0.5, MeOH). Source: NEI ZHE XIANG CHA CAI. Ref: 491.

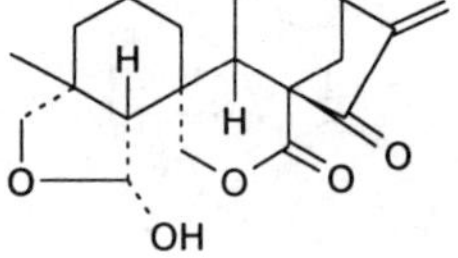

3386 Inokosterone
$C_{27}H_{44}O_7$ MW: 480.65 Source: NIU XI. Ref: 2.

3387 Inosine
$C_{10}H_{12}N_4O_5$ MW: 268.23 Property: mp 215°C. Source: GOU QI YE. Ref: 6.

3388 Inositol
$C_6H_{12}O_6$ MW: 180.16 Source: AI YE, CAO WU TOU, CHANG CHUN HUA, CHANG CHUN TENG, DI JIN CAO, FENG RU, FENG XIANG JI SHENG, JIN YIN HUA, LONG XU YAN ZI CAI, NIU RU, NIU SHE TOU, YANG YI, YU BAI FU, YU MI XU. Ref: 2, 6.

mp 247°C D(+) mp 238°C L(-) mp 218-9°C meso form

3389 Insularine
$C_{38}H_{40}N_2O_6$ MW: 620.75 Property: mp 160°C. Source: QIAN JIN TENG. Ref: 6.

3390 Integerrimine
Squalidine; Alkaloid S-D. $C_{18}H_{25}NO_5$ MW: 335.40 Property: mp 168-70°C, 172.5°C. Source: QUAN YUAN QIAN LI GUANG. Ref: 4.

3391 Inulicin
$C_{17}H_{24}O_5$ MW: 308.38 Property: mp 125.5-6.5°C. Source: JIN FO CAO, XUAN FU HUA. Ref: 6.

3392 Inulin
Property: mp 260°C. Source: DANG SHEN. Ref: 2.

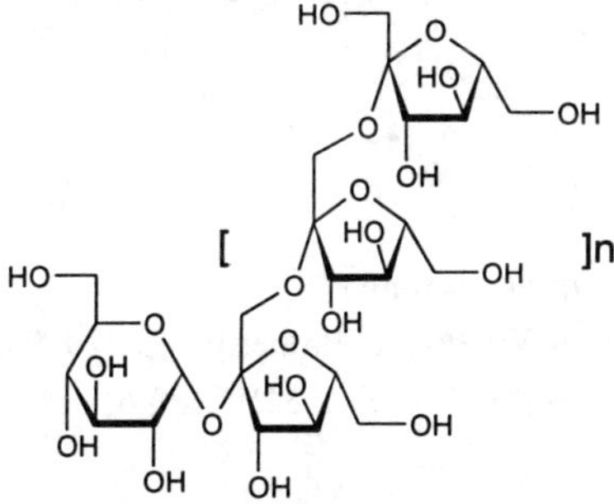

3393 Inumakilactone A
$C_{18}H_{20}O_8$ MW: 364.36 Property: mp 251-3°C (dec). Source: LUO HAN SONG SHI. Ref: 6.

3394 Inumakilactone A glucoside
$C_{24}H_{30}O_{13}$ MW: 526.50 Source: LUO HAN SONG SHI. Ref: 6.

3395 Inumakilactone B

$C_{18}H_{18}O_7$ MW: 346.34 Property: mp 295°C (dec). Source: LUO HAN SONG SHI. Ref: 6.

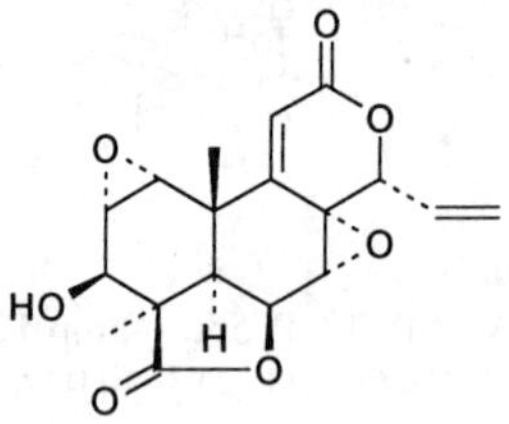

3396 Inumakilactone C

$C_{18}H_{22}O_9$ MW: 382.37 Property: mp 263-5°C (dec). Source: LUO HAN SONG SHI. Ref: 6.

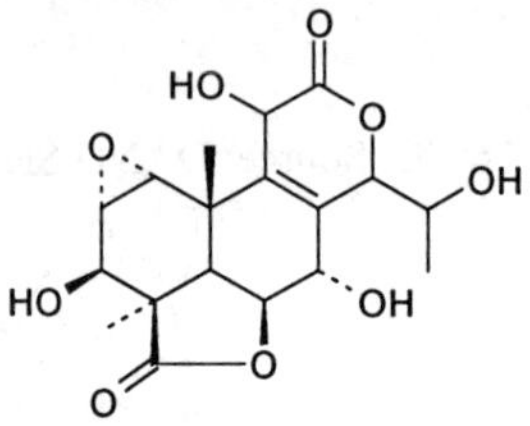

3397 Inumakilactone E

$C_{19}H_{24}O_7$ MW: 364.40 Property: mp 220-5°C. Source: LUO HAN SONG SHI. Ref: 6.

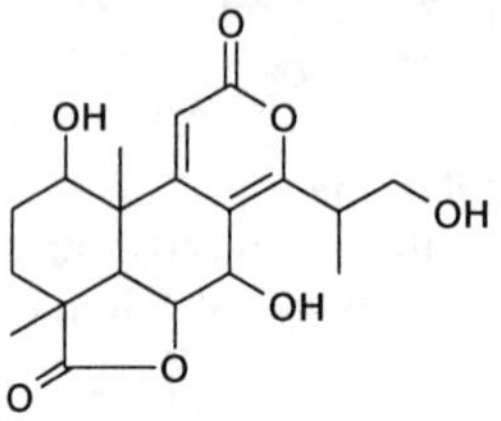

3398 Inunolide

$C_{15}H_{20}O_2$ MW: 232.31 Source: LUO HAN SONG SHI. Ref: 6.

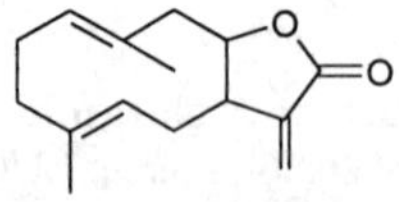

3399 α-Ionone

$C_{13}H_{20}O$ MW: 192.30 Property: bp (±): 146.5-7.5 °C/28mm. Source: MU XIANG. Ref: 2.

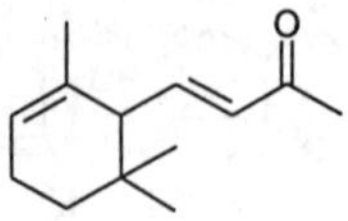

3400 β-Ionone

$C_{13}H_{20}O$ MW: 192.30 Property: bp 150-1.0°C/ 24mm. Source: XING REN. Ref: 2.

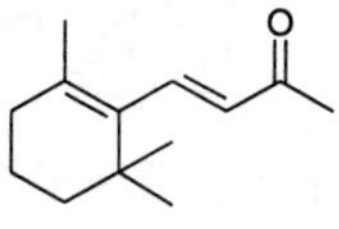

3401 Ipolamiide

$C_{17}H_{26}O_{11}$ MW: 406.39 Source: LUO HAN SONG SHI. Ref: 6.

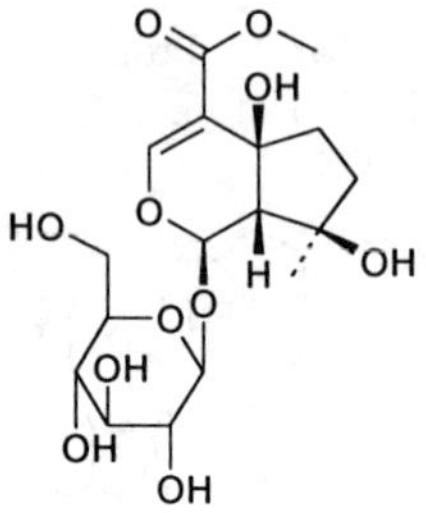

3402 Iridin

$C_{24}H_{26}O_{13}$ MW: 522.47 Property: mp 208°C. Source: BAI HUA SHE GAN, SHE GAN. Ref: 6.

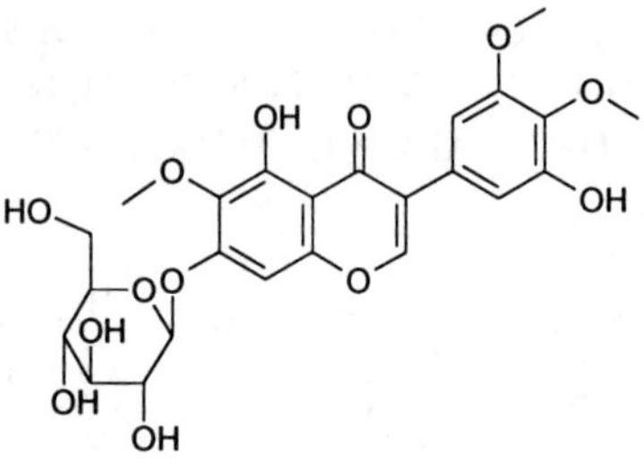

3403 Iridodiol

$C_{10}H_{20}O_2$ MW: 172.27 Source: MU TIAN LIAO. Ref: 6.

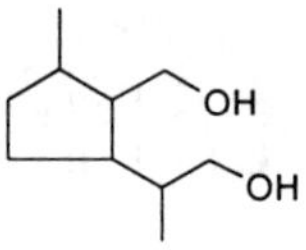

3404 Iridomyrmecin

$C_{10}H_{16}O_2$ MW: 168.24 Property: mp 60-1°C. Source: MU TIAN LIAO. Ref: 6.

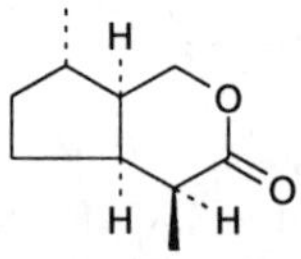

3405 Iristectorin A

$C_{23}H_{24}O_{12}$ MW: 492.44 Property: mp 212-4°C. Source: MU TIAN LIAO. Ref: 6.

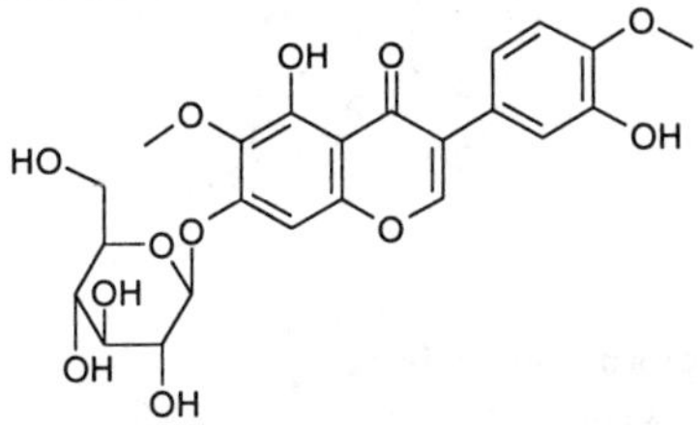

3406 Iristectorin B

$C_{23}H_{24}O_{12}$ MW: 492.44 Property: mp 153-5°C. Source: YUAN WEI. Ref: 6.

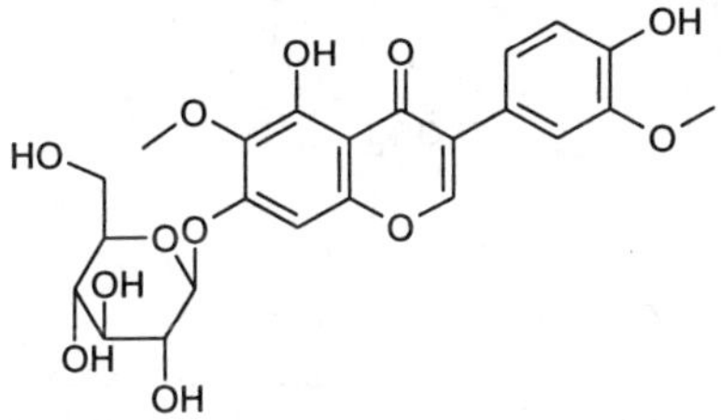

3407 Isatan B

$C_{14}H_{15}NO_7$ MW: 309.28 Source: DA QING YE. Ref: 2.

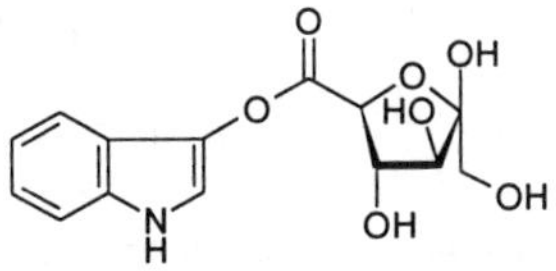

3408 Isatin

$C_8H_5NO_2$ MW: 147.13 Property: mp 203.5°C. Source: BAN LAN GEN. Ref: 6.

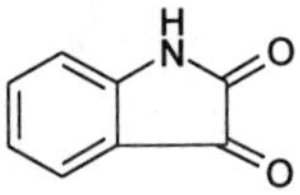

3409 Isoacolamone

$C_{15}H_{24}O$ MW: 220.36 Source: BAI CHANG. Ref: 6.

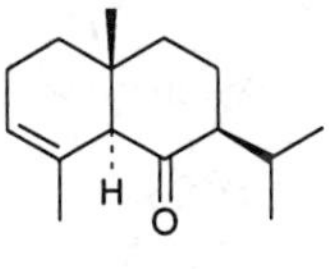

3410 Isoacteoside

$C_{29}H_{36}O_{15}$ MW: 624.60 Source: GAN DI HUANG. Ref: 2.

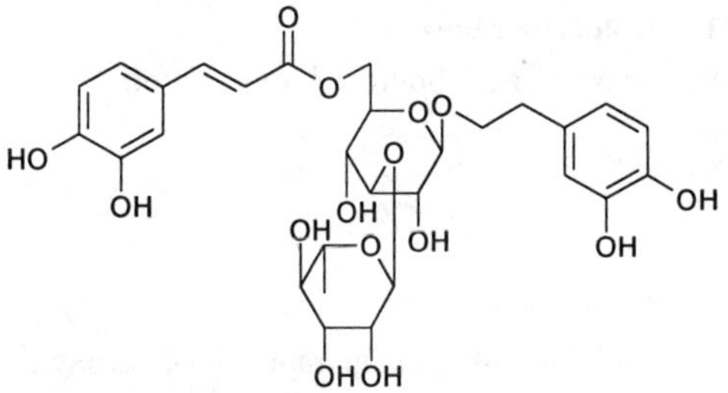

3411 Isoadiantone

$C_{29}H_{48}O$ MW: 412.71 Property: mp 232-3°C. Source: BIAN YE TIE XIAN JUE, TIE SI QI. Ref: 6.

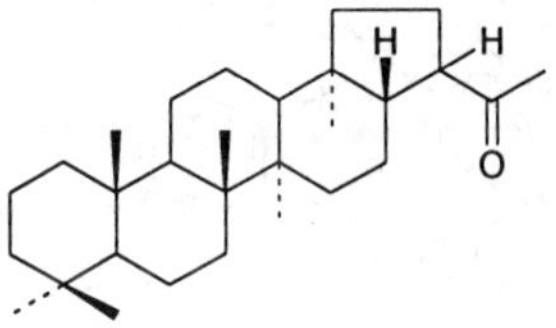

3412 Isoagarotetrol

AH2. $C_{17}H_{18}O_6$ MW: 318.33 Property: colorless lamellar crystal, mp 174-5°C (dec), $[\alpha]_D$ -58.6°. Source: CHEN XIANG. Ref: 13.

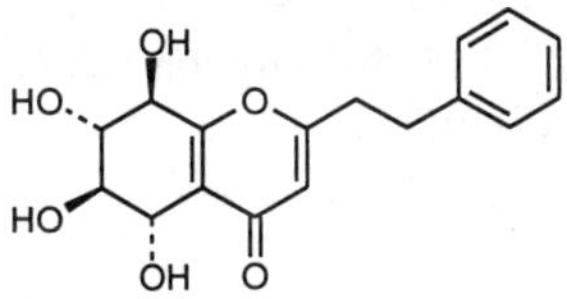

3413 Isoagastachoside

$C_{24}H_{24}O_{11}$ MW: 488.45 Source: HUO XIANG. Ref: 2.

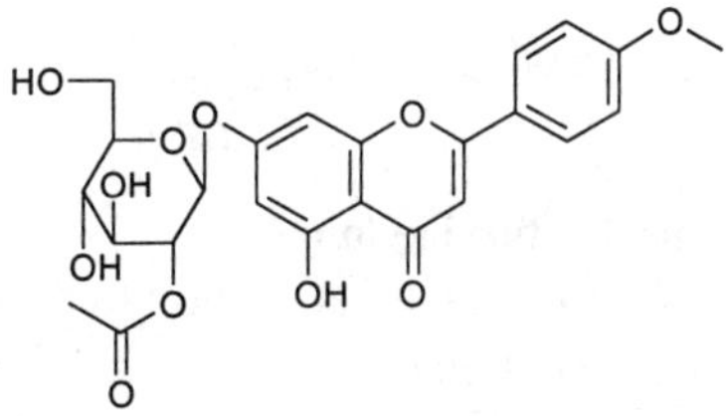

3414 Isoalantolactone

Isohenin. $C_{15}H_{20}O_2$ MW: 232.33 Property: mp 112-5°C. Source: MU XIANG. Ref: 4.

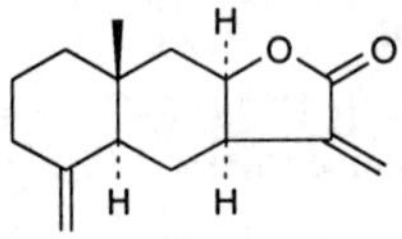

3415 Isoallylbenzene

C_9H_{10} MW: 118.18 Source: SAN QI. Ref: 2.

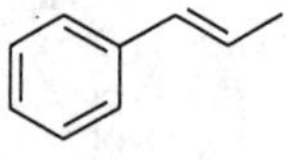

3416 Iso-aloesin

2-Acetonyl-6-C-β-D-glucopyranosyl-7-hydroxy-5-methyl-chromone. Source: LU HUI. Ref: 534.

3417 Isoamaranthin

$C_{30}H_{34}N_2O_{19}$ MW: 726.61 Source: QIAN RI HONG. Ref: 15.

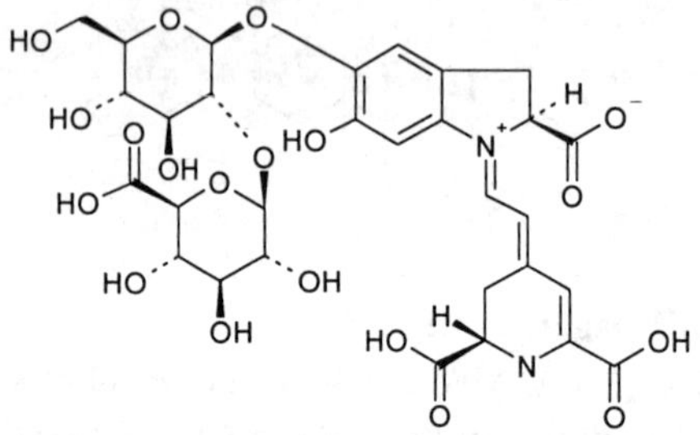

3418 Isoamyl alcohol

$C_5H_{12}O$ MW: 88.15 Property: bp 132°C. Source: SHAN ZHU YU. Ref: 2.

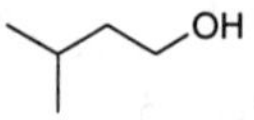

3419 Isoamylamine

$C_5H_{13}N$ MW: 87.17 Property: bp 95°C. Source: GUI GAI. Ref: 6.

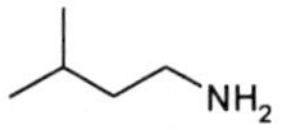

3420 Isoamyl-3-furyl ketone

$C_{10}H_{14}O_2$ MW: 166.22 Property: bp 130°C/30mm. Source: ZI SU YE. Ref: 6.

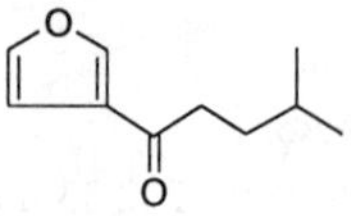

3421 Isoangelol

$C_{20}H_{24}O_7$ MW: 376.41 Property: colorless transparent substance, $[\alpha]_D^{20}$ -138.5° (c=0.33, chloroform). Source: ZHONG CHI MAO DANG GUI. Ref: 79.

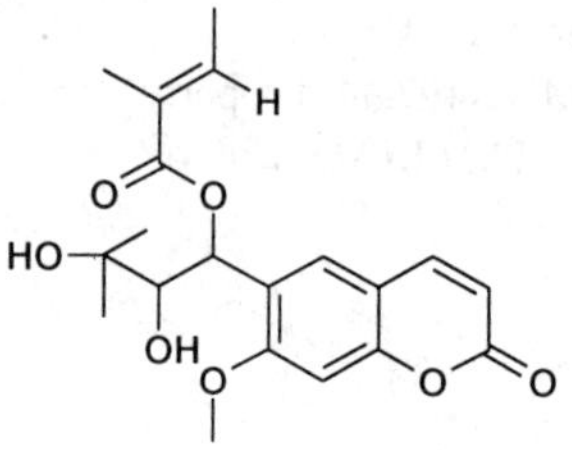

3422 Isoannonareticin (2)

$C_{37}H_{66}O_7$ MW: 622.93 Property: white crystal, mp 83-4°C. Source: NIU XIN FAN LI ZHI. Ref: 401.

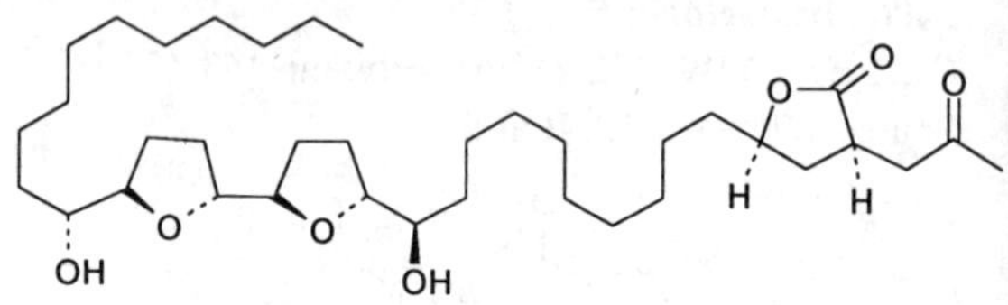

3423 2,4-cis-Isoannonareticin(2-1)

$C_{37}H_{66}O_7$ MW: 622.93 Property: white crystal, mp 83-4°C. Source: NIU XIN PAN LI ZHI. Ref: 432.

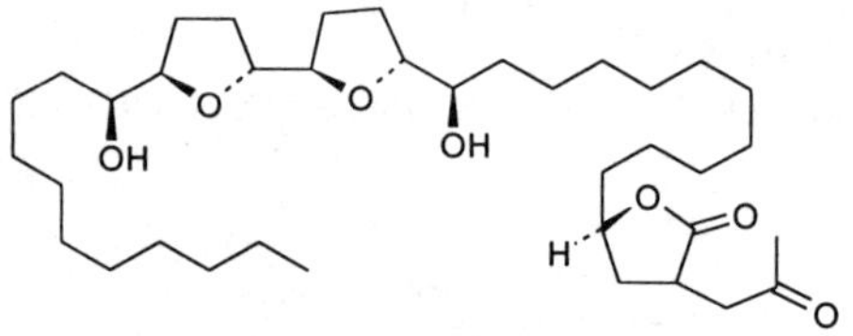

3424 2,4-trans-Isoannonareticin(2-2)

$C_{37}H_{66}O_7$ MW: 622.93 Property: white crystal, mp 83-4°C. Source: NIU XIN PAN LI ZHI. Ref: 432.

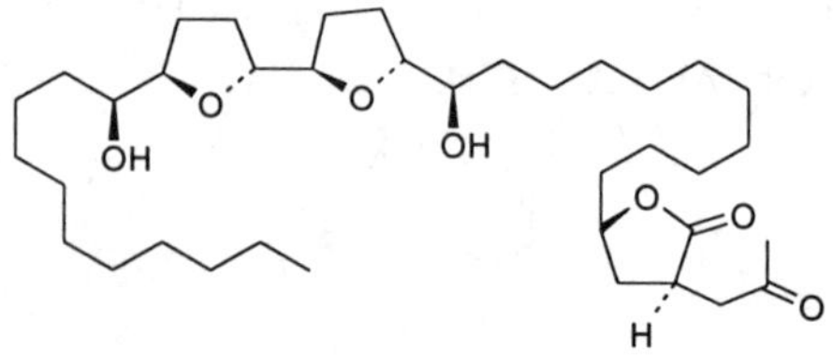

3425 Isoanthricin

$C_{22}H_{22}O_7$ MW: 398.24 Property: mp 170°C. Source: E SHEN. Ref: 6.

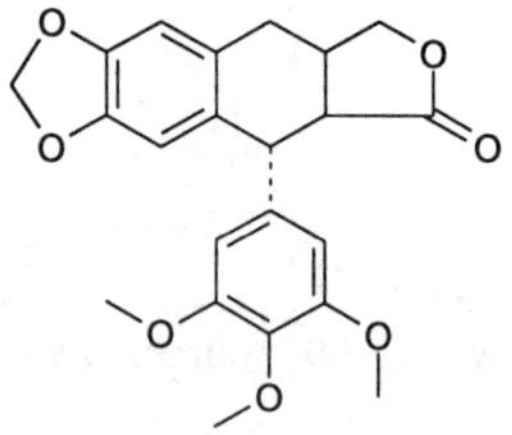

3426 Isoarborinol
$C_{30}H_{50}O$ MW: 426.73 Property: mp 294.0-4.5°C. Source: CHOU SHAN YANG. Ref: 6.

3427 Isoarcapillin
$C_{18}H_{16}O_8$ MW: 360.32 Source: YIN CHEN HAO. Ref: 2.

3428 Isoarctigenin
$C_{21}H_{24}O_6$ MW: 372.42 Property: mp cis-: (+): 92-3°C. Source: NIU BANG ZI. Ref: 6.

3429 Isoartemisia ketone
$C_{10}H_{16}O$ MW: 152.24 Source: QING HAO. Ref: 2.

3430 Isoastilbin
5,7,3',5'-tetrahydroxyl-flavanonol-3-O-α-L-rhamnopyranoside. $C_{21}H_{22}O_{11}$ MW: 450.40 Property: light yellow acicular crystal (methanol), mp 186-7°C. Source: TU FU LING. Ref: 366, 568.

3431 Isobaimuxinol
$C_{15}H_{26}O_2$ MW: 238.37 Source: BAI MU XIANG. Ref: 13.

3432 Isobavachin
$C_{20}H_{20}O_5$ MW: 340.38 Property: mp 187-8°C. Source: BU GU ZHI. Ref: 2, 630.

3433 Isobergapten
$C_{12}H_8O_4$ MW: 216.20 Property: mp 222-4°C. Source: DU HUO, LANG DU, YONG NING DU HUO. Ref: 6, 541.

3434 Isobetanidin-6-O-rhamnosyl sophoroside
$C_{30}H_{36}N_2O_{17}$ MW: 696.62 Source: YE ZI HUA. Ref: 6.

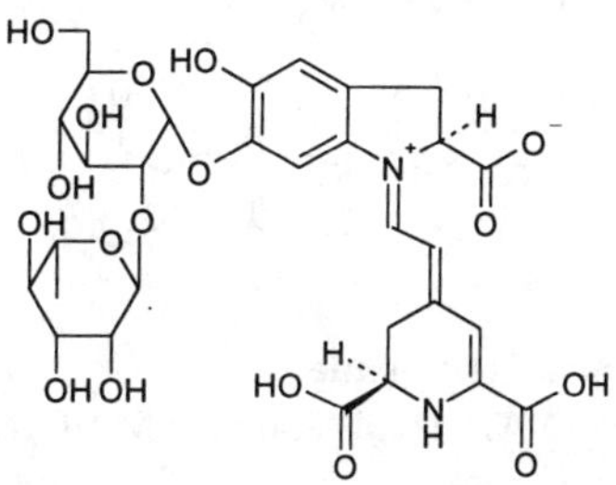

3435 Isobetanidin-6-O-β-sophoroside
$C_{30}H_{38}N_2O_{18}$ MW: 714.64 Source: YE ZI HUA. Ref: 6.

3436 β-Isobiotol
$C_{15}H_{24}O$ MW: 220.36 Source: BAI ZHI JIE. Ref: 6.

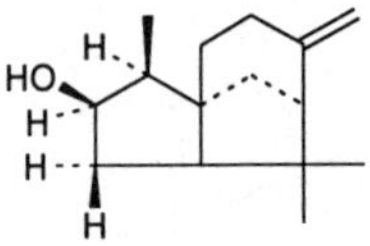

3437 Isoboldine
$C_{19}H_{21}NO_4$ MW: 327.38 Property: mp 178-80°C (dec). Source: BAI ZHI JIE. Ref: 6.

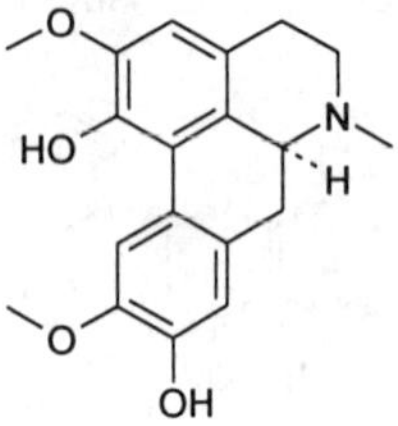

3438 Isoborneol
$C_{20}H_{36}O_2$ MW: 308.51 Source: BING PIAN, SHENG JIANG. Ref: 2.

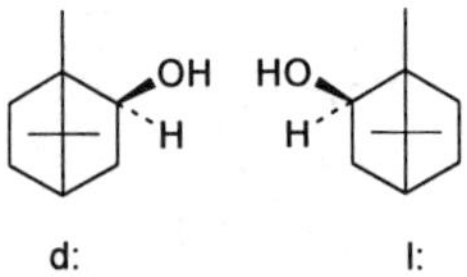

d: l:

3439 Isobrucine
$C_{23}H_{26}N_2O_4$ MW: 394.47 Property: mp 198-9°C Source: MA QIAN ZI. Ref: 2, 542.

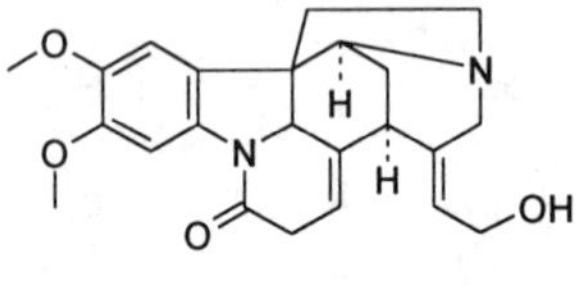

3440 Isobrucine N-oxide
$C_{23}H_{26}N_2O_5$ MW: 410.47 Source: MA QIAN ZI. Ref: 2, 542.

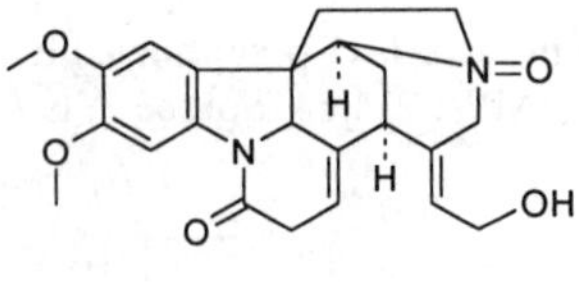

3441 Isobutanal
C_4H_8O MW: 72.11 Property: bp 63-4°C/757mm. Source: NIU BANG GEN. Ref: 6.

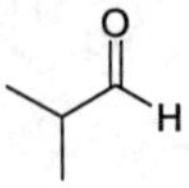

3442 Isobutyl alcohol
$C_4H_{10}O$ MW: 74.12 Source: SHAN ZHU YU. Ref: 2.

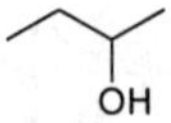

3443 N-Isobutyldeca-trans-2-trans-4-dienamide
$C_{14}H_{25}NO$ MW: 223.36 Property: mp 90°C. Source: BI BA. Ref: 6.

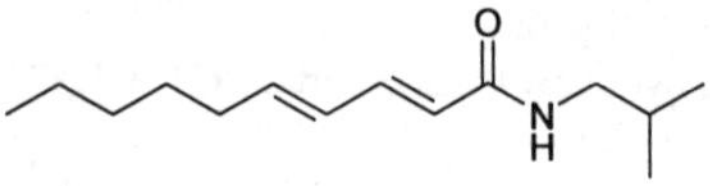

3444 Isobutylisovalerate
$C_9H_{18}O_2$ MW: 158.24 Property: bp 170-2°C/757.5mm. Source: BAN BIAN SU. Ref: 6.

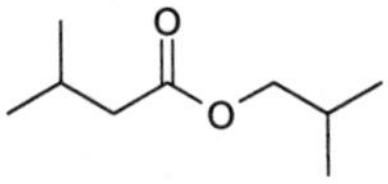

3445 Isobutyric acid
$C_4H_8O_2$ MW: 88.11 Property: mp -47°C, bp 154.3°C. Source: SANG YE. Ref: 6.

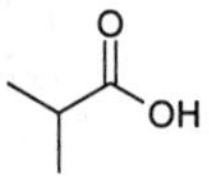

3446 3'-Isobutyryloxy-O-acetyl-2', 3'-dihydro-oroselol
$C_{20}H_{22}O_7$ MW: 374.39 Property: mp 153-4°C. Source: SHE CHUANG ZI. Ref: 6.

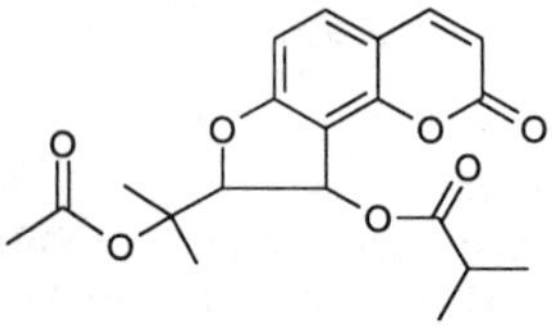

3447 Isobutyryl shikonin
$C_{20}H_{22}O_6$ MW: 358.39 Property: mp 89-90°C. Source: ZI CAO. Ref: 2, 6.

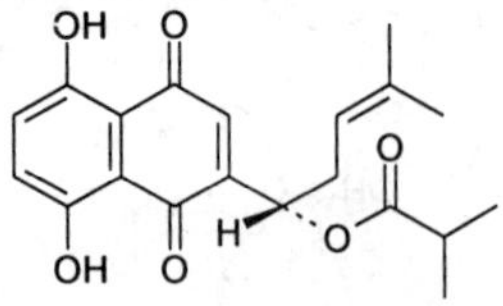

3448 Isobyakangelicol
Anhydrobyakangelicin. $C_{17}H_{16}O_6$ MW: 316.31 Property: mp 108-9°C. Source: BAI ZHI. Ref: 2.

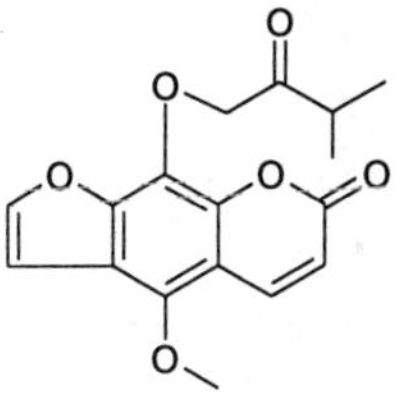

3449 Isocalamendiol
$C_{15}H_{26}O_2$ MW: 238.37 Property: mp 72.5-3.5°C. Source: BAI CHANG. Ref: 6.

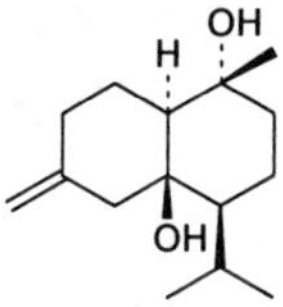

3450 Isocantlyine
5H-Pyridine-4-carboxylic acid, 6,7-dihydro-6-hydroxy-7-methyl-methyl ester. $C_{11}H_{13}NO_3$ MW: 207.23 Property: white feathery crystal, mp 124-5°C. Source: YIN XING CAO. Ref: 117.

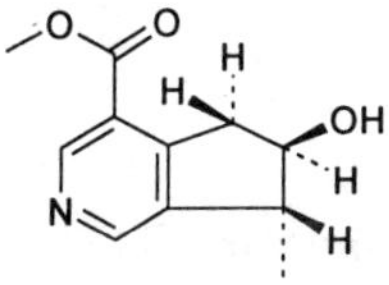

3451 Isocarneagenin
$C_{27}H_{44}O_5$ MW: 448.65 Property: mp 242-4°C. Source: JI XIANG CAO. Ref: 6.

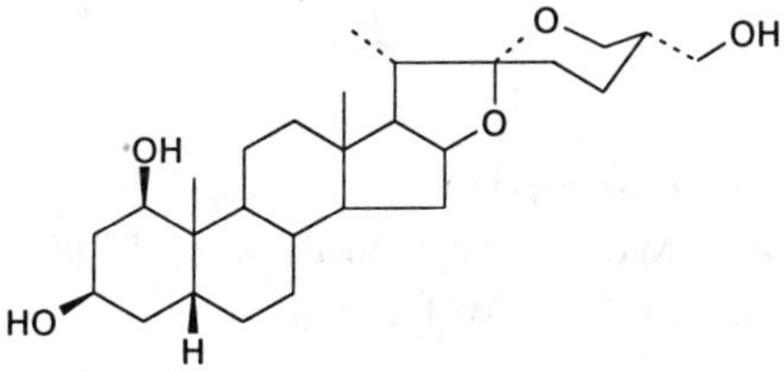

3452 Isocembrol
$C_{20}H_{34}O$ MW: 290.49 Source: HAI SONG ZI. Ref: 6.

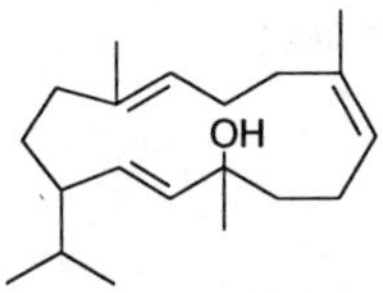

3453 Isocephalotaxinone
$C_{19}H_{19}NO_4$ MW: 325.37 Source: TU XIANG FEI. Ref: 2.

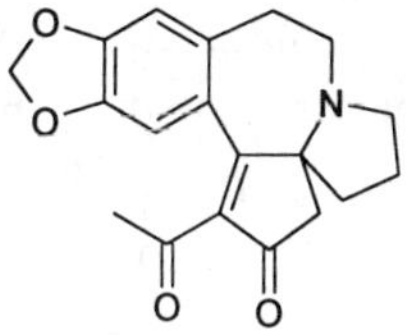

3454 Isochamanetin
CAS: 58777-17-6 $C_{22}H_{18}O_5$ MW: 362.39 Property: mp 215-7°C. Source: AI ZI YU PAN. Ref: 5.

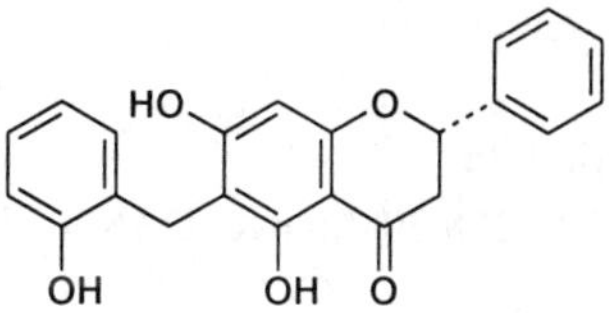

3455 Isochondrodendrin
$C_{36}H_{38}N_2O_6$ MW: 594.71 Property: mp 316°C (dec). Source: RU LAN, XI SHENG TENG, YIN BU HUAN. Ref: 6.

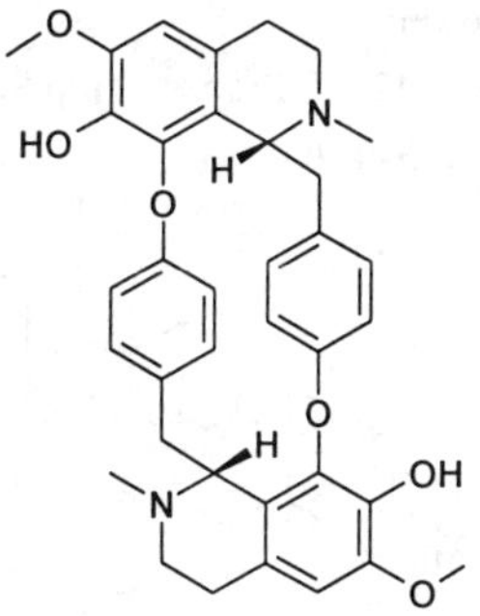

3456 Isocimicifugamide
N-(3'-methoxy-4'-hydroxyphenethyl)-4-O-β-D-galactopyranosyl-isoferulamide. $C_{25}H_{31}NO_{10}$ MW: 505.53 Property: white amorphous powder, mp 97-100°C, $[\alpha]_D^9$ -46.2° (c=0.13, methanol). Source: XING AN SHENG MA. Ref: 294.

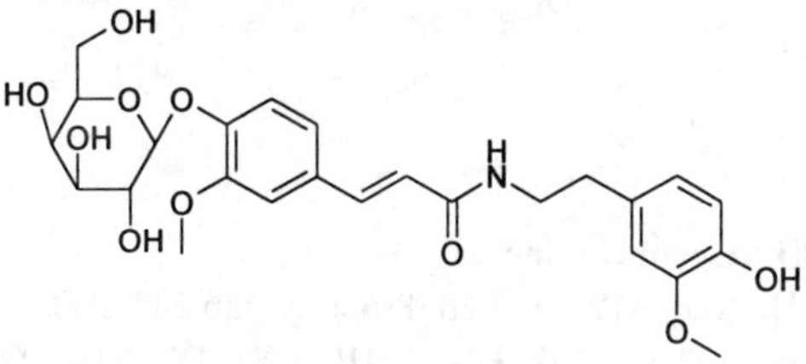

3457 Isocitric acid

$C_6H_8O_7$ MW: 192.13 Source: REN SHEN. Ref: 2.

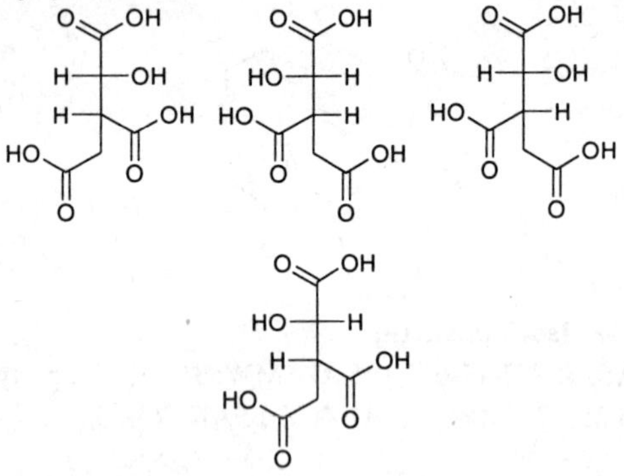

3458 Isocnidilide

$C_{13}H_{20}O_2$ MW: 208.30 Source: DANG GUI. Ref: 6.

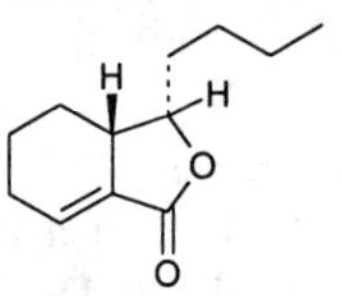

3459 Isoconessimine

$C_{23}H_{38}N_2$ MW: 342.57 Property: mp 92°C. Source: ZHI XIE MU PI. Ref: 6.

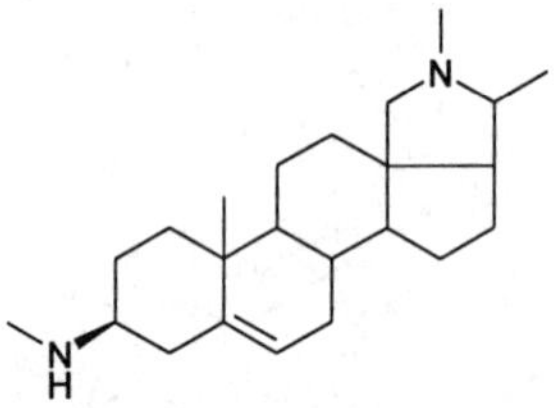

3460 Isocorydine

$C_{20}H_{23}NO_4$ MW: 341.41 Property: mp 185-6°C. Source: BI CHENG QIE, NAN TIAN ZHU ZI, YAN HU SUO. Ref: 6.

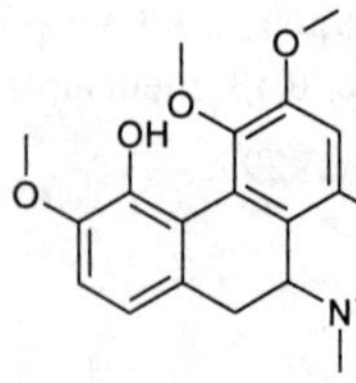

3461 Isocorynoline

$C_{20}H_{19}NO_5$ MW: 353.38 Property: mp 234-5°C. Source: YUN QIAN HU, ZI HUA YU DENG CAO (LIE BAO ZI JING). Ref: 6, 436.

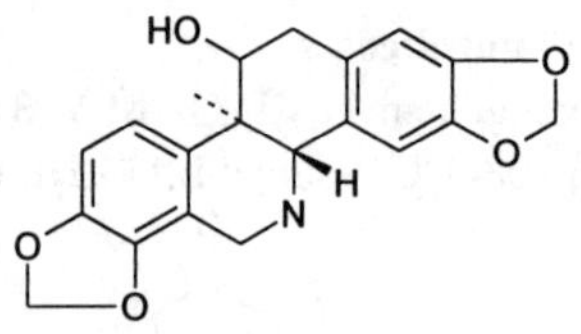

3462 Isocorynoxeine

$C_{22}H_{26}N_2O_4$ MW: 382.46 Source: GOU TENG. Ref: 2.

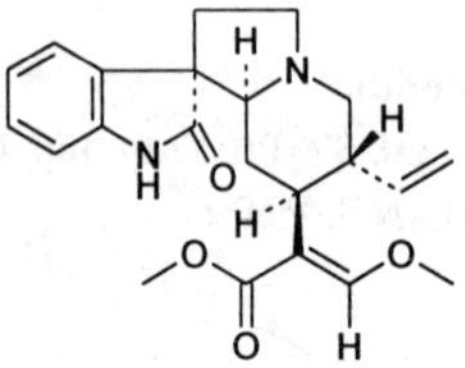

3463 Isocorypalmine

(-)-Tetrahydrocolumbamine. $C_{20}H_{23}NO_4$ MW: 341.41 Property: mp (+): 239-41°C, (-): 241-2°C, (±): 221-2°C. Source: YA PIAN, YAN HU SUO. Ref: 2, 6.

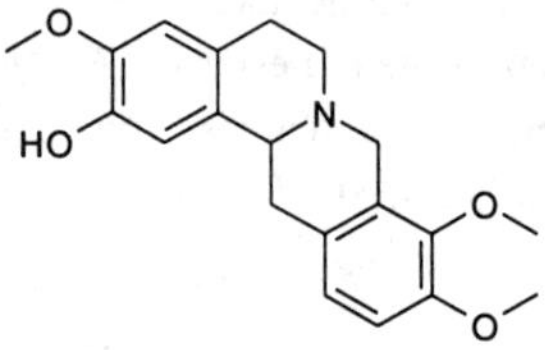

3464 Isocrotonylpterosin B

$C_{18}H_{22}O_3$ MW: 286.37 Source: JUE. Ref: 6.

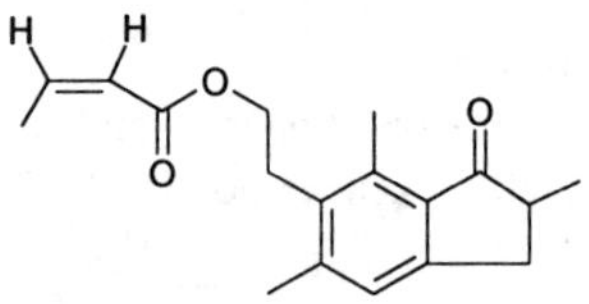

3465 Isocryptomerin

$C_{31}H_{20}O_{10}$ MW: 552.50 Property: mp 308-10°C (dec). Source: JUAN BAI. Ref: 6.

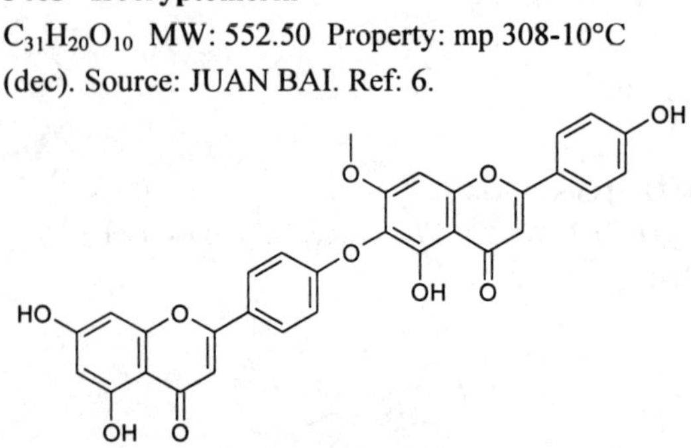

3466 Isocryptotanshinone
$C_{19}H_{20}O_3$ MW: 296.37 Property: mp 121°C. Source: DAN SHEN. Ref: 2, 6.

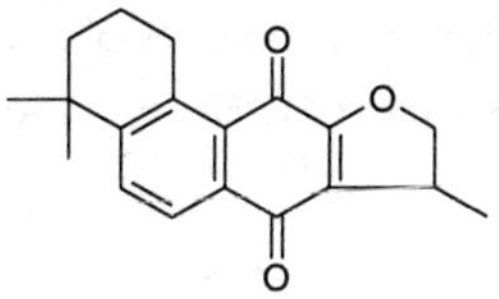

3467 Isocucurbitacin B
Property: mp 220-3°C. Source: HU BEI GUA LOU. Ref: 532.

3468 α-Isocuparenol
$C_{15}H_{22}O$ MW: 218.34 Property: mp 78.5°C. Source: BAI ZHI JIE. Ref: 6.

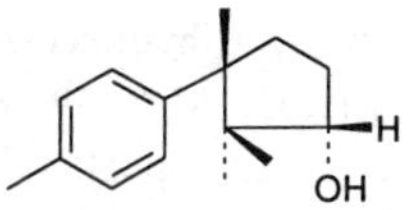

3469 Isocurcumenol
$C_{15}H_{22}O_2$ MW: 234.34 Property: mp 139-41°C. Source: PENG E SHU. Ref: 6.

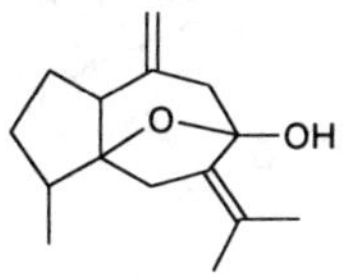

3470 Isocyasterone
$C_{29}H_{44}O_8$ MW: 520.67 Source: CHUAN NIU XI. Ref: 6.

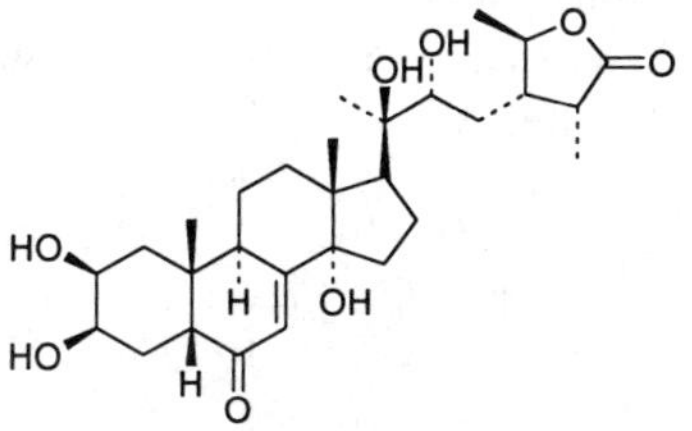

3471 Isocycleanine III
$C_{38}H_{42}N_2O_6$ MW: 622.77 Property: colorless powder, $[\alpha]_D^{25}$ 0°(c= 0.10, $CHCl_3$). Source: SI CHUAN LUN HUAN TENG. Ref: 274.

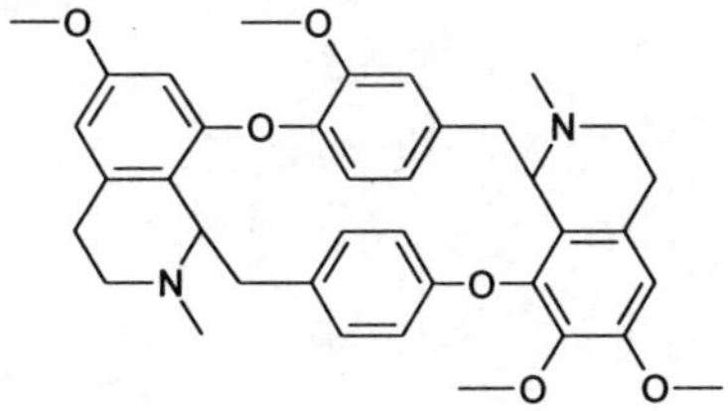

3472 Isocyperol
$C_{15}H_{24}O$ MW: 220.36 Source: XIANG FU. Ref: 6.

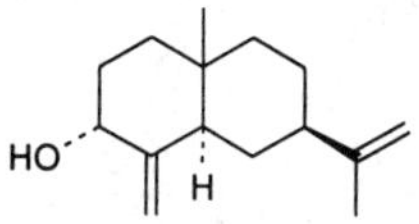

3473 Isodalbergin
$C_{16}H_{12}O_4$ MW: 268.27 Source: JIANG ZHEN XIANG. Ref: 6.

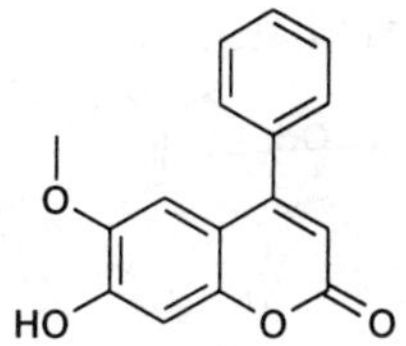

3474 Isodaphnoretin
7-Methoxydaphnoritin. $C_{20}H_{14}O_7$ MW: 366.33 Property: fine acicular crystal, mp 238-40°C, soluble in methanol, ethanol, insolublein chloroform, ether, acetone. Source: LANG DU. Ref: 488.

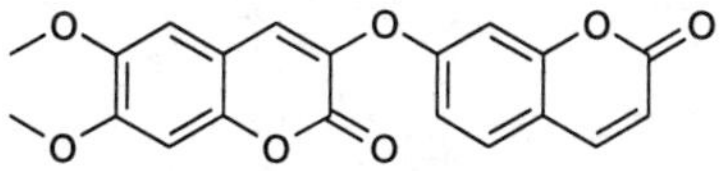

3475 Isodehydrocostus lactone
$C_{14}H_{17}NO_2$ MW: 231.30 Source: MU XIANG. Ref: 2.

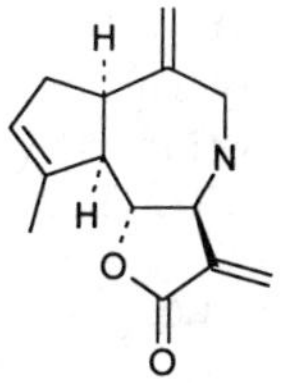

3476 3β-Isodihydrocadambine
$C_{27}H_{34}N_2O_{10}$ MW: 168.24 Source: GOU TENG. Ref: 2.

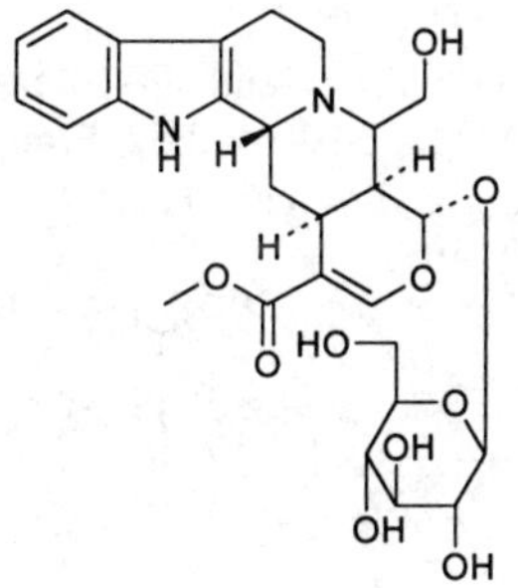

3478 Isodihydronepetalactone
$C_{10}H_{16}O_2$ MW: 168.24 Source: JIA JING JIE, MU TIAN LIAO. Ref: 6.

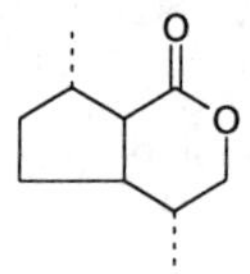

3479 Isodiospyrin
$C_{22}H_{14}O_6$ MW: 374.35 Property: mp 226-8°C. Source: JUN QIAN ZI. Ref: 6.

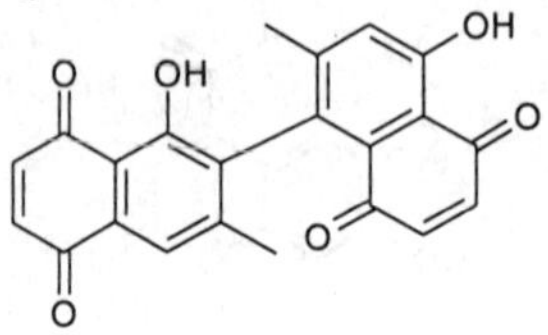

3480 Isodonal
CAS: 16964-56-0 $C_{22}H_{28}O_7$ MW: 404.46 Property: mp 245-7°C (dec). Source: DA YE XIANG CHA CAI. Ref: 5.

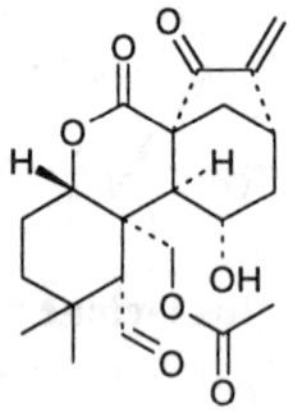

3481 Isodopharicin D
3α,11β,13α-Trihydroxy-entkaur-16-en-15-one. $C_{20}H_{30}O_4$ MW: 334.46 Property: white crystal, mp245-7°C. Source: CHUAN ZANG XIANGCHA CAI. Ref: 405.

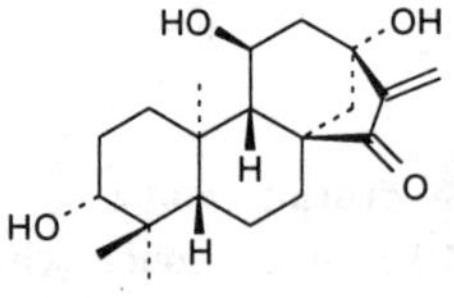

3482 Isodopharicin F
11β,13α,15α-Trihydroxy-entkaur-16-en-3α-β-D-glucoside. $C_{26}H_{42}O_9$ MW: 498.62 Property: white crystal, mp252-4°C. Source: CHUAN ZANG XIANG CHA CAI. Ref: 405.

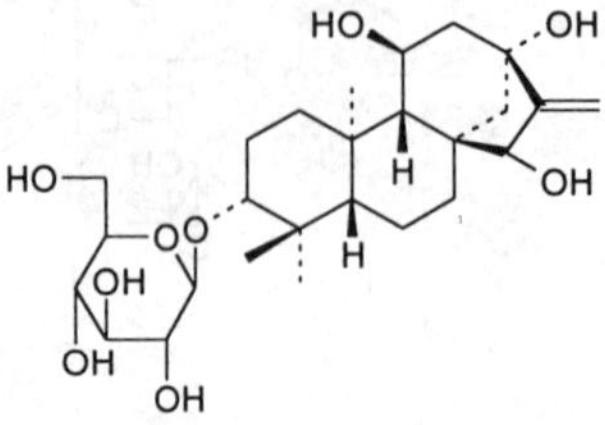

3483 Isodoternifolin A
β,11α,15β-Triacetoxy-7β-hydroxy-7α,20-epoxy-entkaur-16-ene. $C_{26}H_{36}O_8$ MW: 746.57 Property: colorless acicular crystal, mp 249-5°C, $[\alpha]_D^{20}$ -122.9° (chloroform). Source: CHONG YA YAO. Ref: 367.

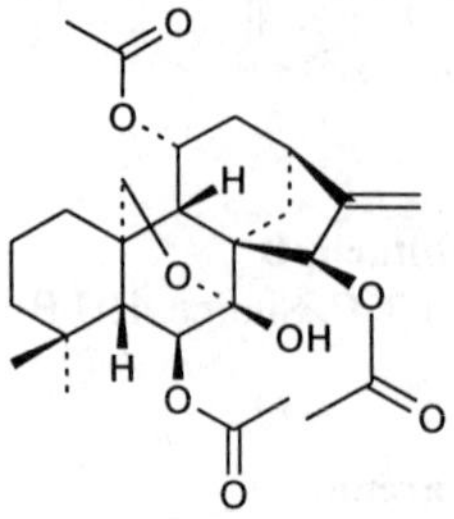

3484 Isodoternifolin B
11α-Acetoxy-6β,7β,15β-trihydroxy-7α,20-epoxy-entkaur-16-ene. $C_{22}H_{32}O_6$ MW: 392.50 Property: colorless prismatic crystal, mp 236-8°C (chloroform). Source: CHONG YA YAO. Ref: 367.

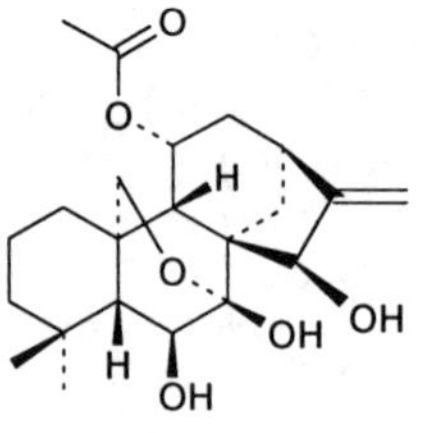

3485 Isodtrychnine N-oxide
Source: MA QIAN ZI. Ref: 542.

3486 Isoegomaketone
$C_{10}H_{12}O_2$ MW: 164.21 Property: mp 179-80°C. Source: ZI SU. Ref: 2.

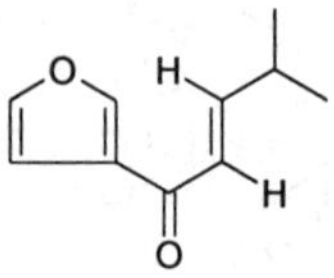

3487 Isoelemicine
$C_{12}H_{16}O_3$ MW: 208.26 Property: bp 153-6°C/10mm. Source: YE XIANG MAO. Ref: 6.

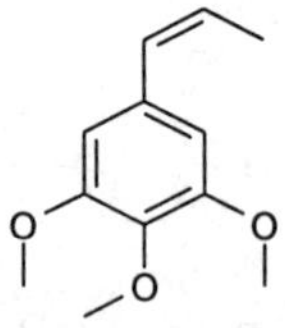

3488 Isoeleutherol glucoside

$C_{20}H_{22}O_9$ MW: 406.39 Source: LU HUI. Ref: 2.

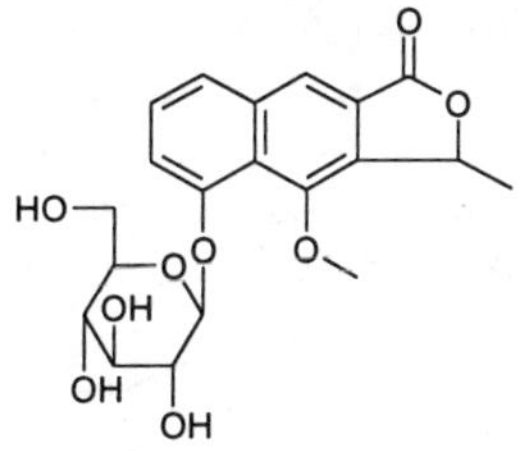

3489 Isoengelitin

$C_{21}H_{22}O_{10}$ MW: 434.40 Property: mp 295-6°C. Source: DING XIANG, TU FU LING. Ref: 6, 568.

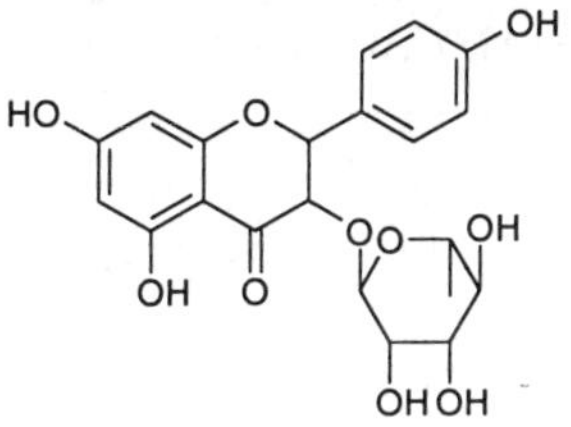

3490 Iso-eruboside B

$C_{51}H_{84}O_{24}$ MW: 1081.22 Property: white acicular crystal, mp 310-2°C, $[\alpha]_D^{20}$ -32.8° (c=1.0, C_5H_5N). Source: DASUAN. Ref: 362.

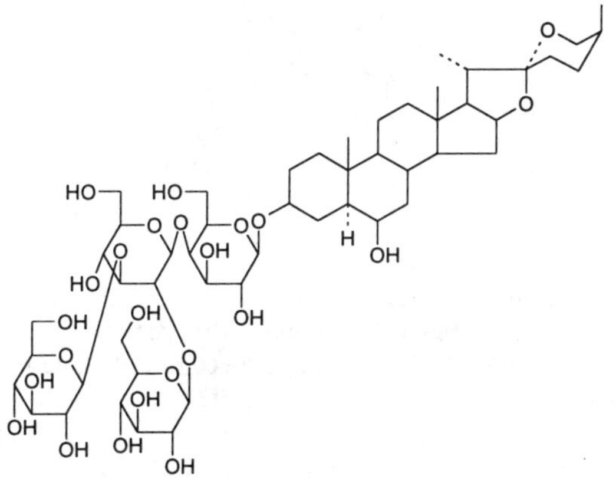

3491 Isoeugenitol

$C_{11}H_{10}O_4$ MW: 206.20 Property: mp 229-30°C. Source: DING XIANG. Ref: 6.

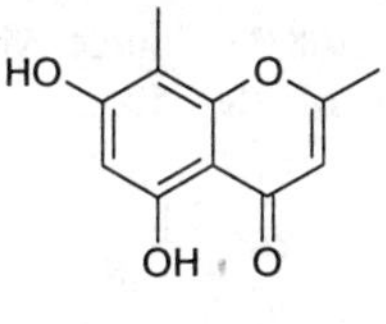

3492 Isoeugenol

$C_{10}H_{12}O_2$ MW: 164.21 Property: cis: bp 134: 5°C/13mm, trans: mp 33-4°C, bp 141-2°C/13mm. Source: DANG GUI. Ref: 2, 6.

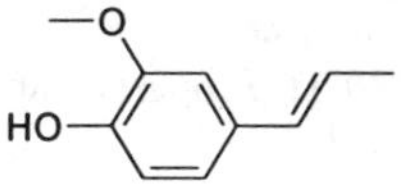

3493 Isofernene

$C_{30}H_{50}$ MW: 410.73 Property: mp 189-90°C. Source: TIE SI QI. Ref: 6.

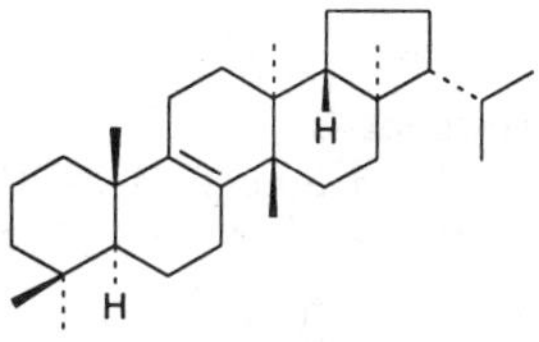

3494 Isoferulic acid

$C_{10}H_{10}O_4$ MW: 194.19 Property: colorless acicular crystal, mp 225-9°C. Source: DAN SHEN, MAO LIAN HAO. Ref: 2, 474.

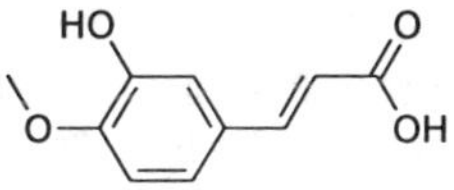

3495 Isofraxidin

CAS: 486-21-5 $C_{11}H_{10}O_5$ MW: 222.20 Property: mp 148-9°C. Source: CAO SHAN HU, CI WU JIA, DA JI (a). Ref: 5.

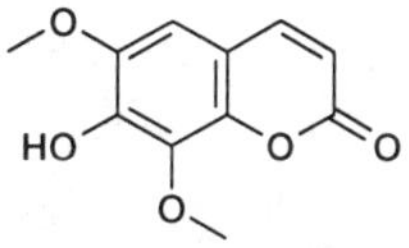

3496 Isofraxidin glucoside

$C_{17}H_{20}O_{10}$ MW: 384.34 Source: CI WU JIA. Ref: 2.

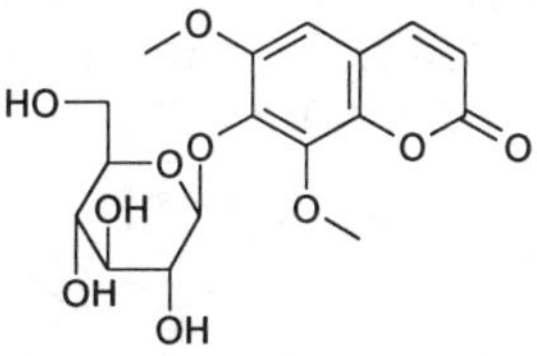

3497 28-Isofucosterol

$C_{29}H_{48}O$ MW: 412.71 Property: mp 133-5°C. Source: SHI CHUN. Ref: 6.

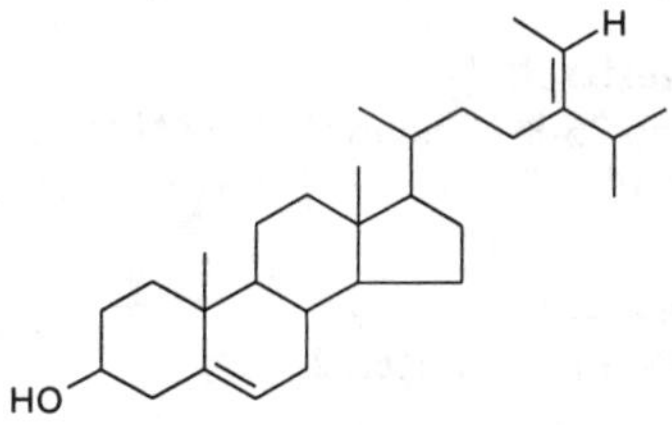

3498 Isofuranodienone
$C_{15}H_{18}O_2$ MW: 230.31 Property: mp 70-1°C. Source: PENG E SHU. Ref: 6.

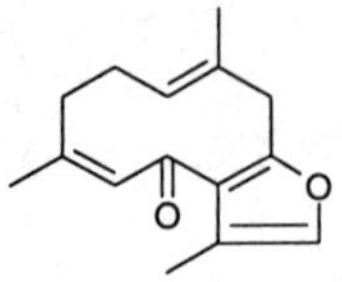

3499 Isogingerenone-B
$C_{22}H_{26}O_6$ MW: 386.45 Source: GAN JIANG, SHENG JIANG. Ref: 2.

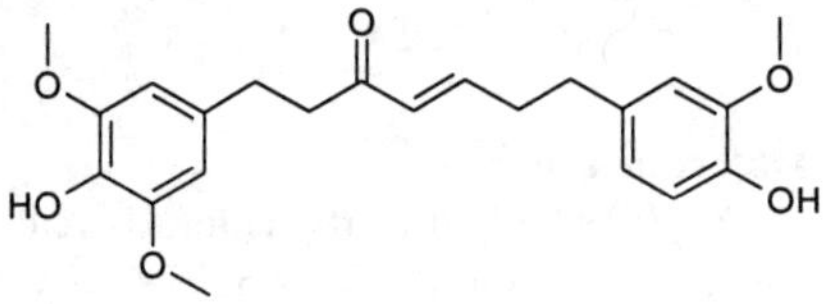

3500 Isoginkgetin
$C_{32}H_{22}O_{10}$ MW: 566.53 Property: yellow powder, mp 210°C. Source: BAI GUO YE, CHAO XIAN YIN YANG HUO. Ref: 6, 442.

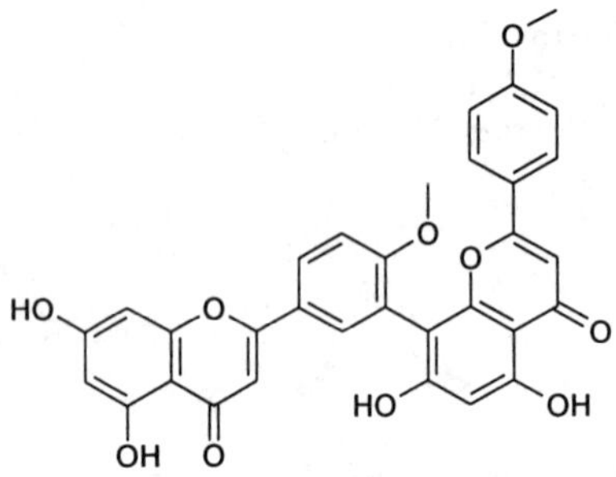

3501 Isoglycyrol
$C_{21}H_{18}O_6$ MW: 366.37 Property: mp 298-300°C (dec). Source: GAN CAO. Ref: 2.

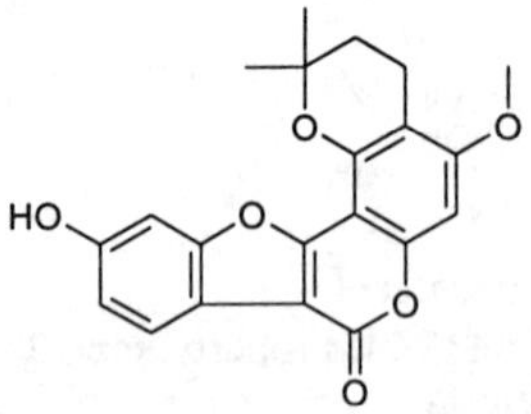

3502 Isogosferol
Property: mp 76-8°C. Source: YUN NAN QIANG HUO. Ref: 551.

3503 Isoguvacine
Source: BING LANG. Ref: 2.

3504 Isoharringtonine
CAS: 26833-86-3 $C_{28}H_{37}NO_9$ MW: 531.61 Source: SAN JIAN SHAN. Ref: 5.

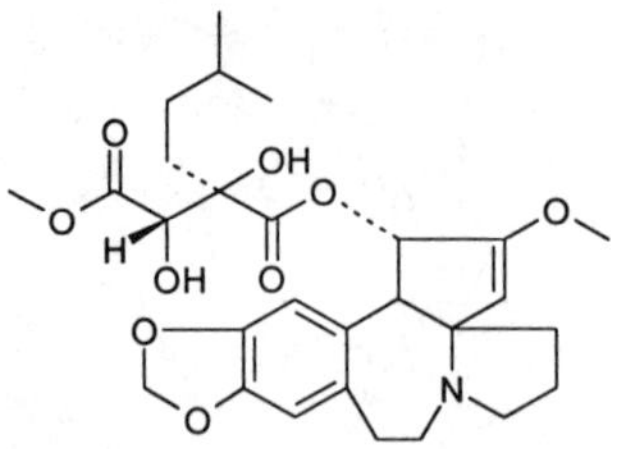

3505 Isohomoarbutin
$C_{13}H_{18}O_7$ MW: 286.28 Property: mp 175-6°C. Source: LU XIAN CAO. Ref: 6.

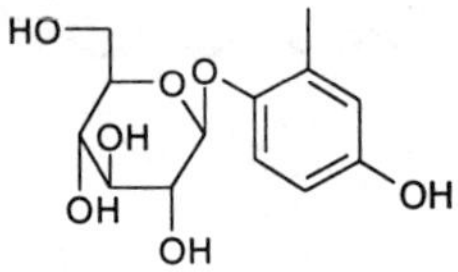

3506 Isohyperoside
$C_{21}H_{20}O_{12}$ MW: 464.39 Property: mp 242-5°C. Source: MAN SHAN HONG. Ref: 6.

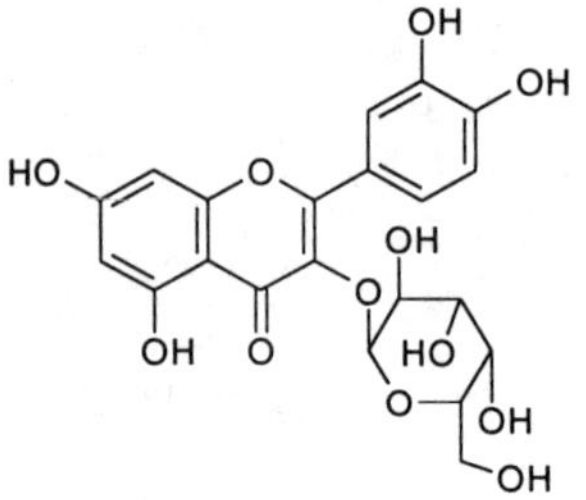

3507 Isoimperatorin
Ausraptin. CAS: 482-45-1 $C_{16}H_{14}O_4$ MW: 270.29 Property: mp 109-101°C. Source: BAI ZHI, QIANG HUO, ZHONG CHI MAO DANG GUI. Ref: 4, 325, 344, 507, 566.

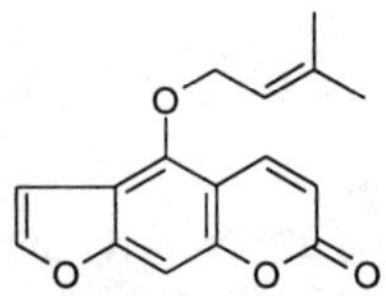

3508 6-Isoinosine
$C_{10}H_{12}N_4O_5$ MW: 268.23 Source: MAO GENG HONG MAO WU JIA. Ref: 525.

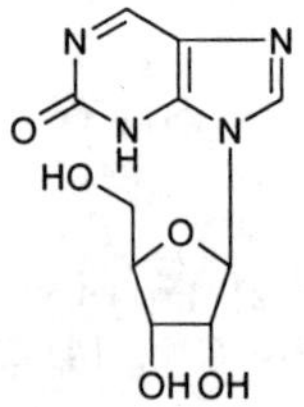

3509 Isoiridomyrmecin

$C_{10}H_{16}O_2$ MW: 168.24 Property: mp 58-9°C. Source: MU TIAN LIAO. Ref: 6.

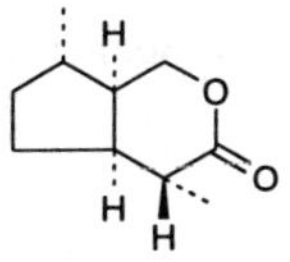

3510 Isokobusone

$C_{14}H_{22}O_2$ MW: 222.33 Source: XIANG FU. Ref: 6.

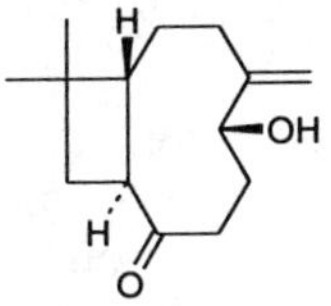

3511 Isokuraramine

$C_{12}H_{18}N_2O_2$ MW: 222.29 Source: KU SHEN. Ref: 2.

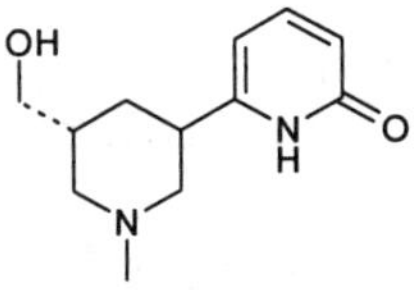

3512 Isokurarinone

$C_{26}H_{28}O_6$ MW: 436.51 Source: KU SHEN. Ref: 2.

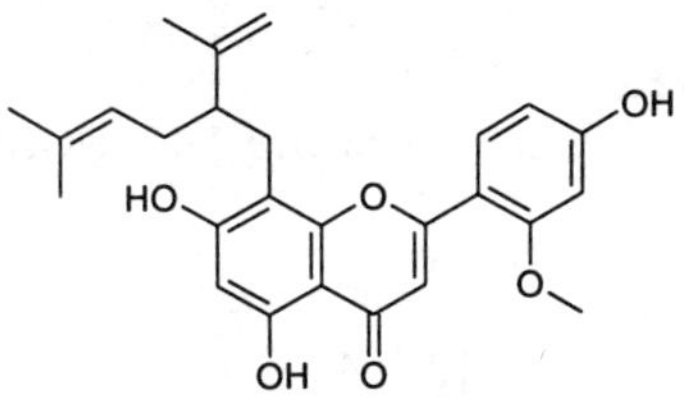

3513 Isoleurosine

$C_{46}H_{58}N_4O_8$ MW: 795.00 Property: mp 202-6.0°C. Source: CHANG CHUN HUA. Ref: 2.

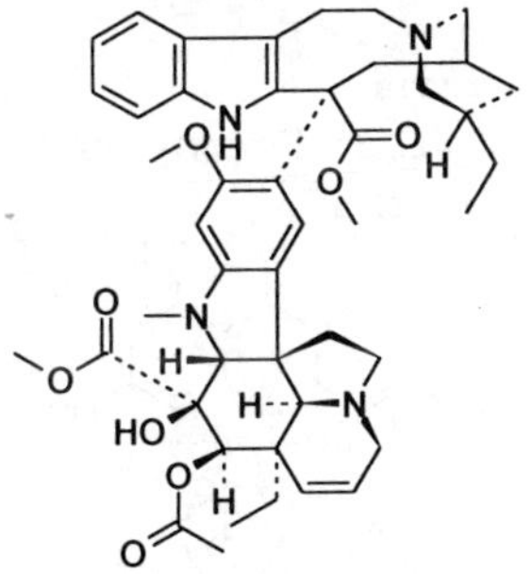

3514 Isolicoflavonol

$C_{20}H_{18}O_6$ MW: 354.36 Source: GAN CAO. Ref: 2.

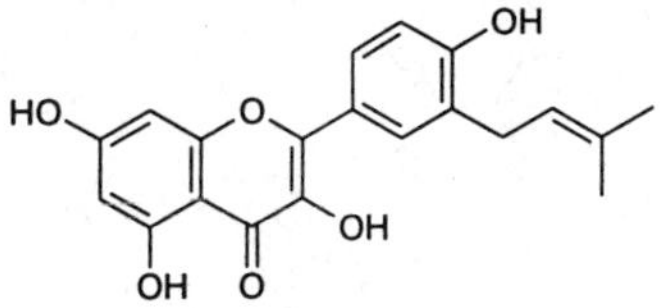

3515 Isoliensinine

$C_{37}H_{42}N_2O_6$ MW: 610.76 Source: LIAN ZI XIN. Ref: 6.

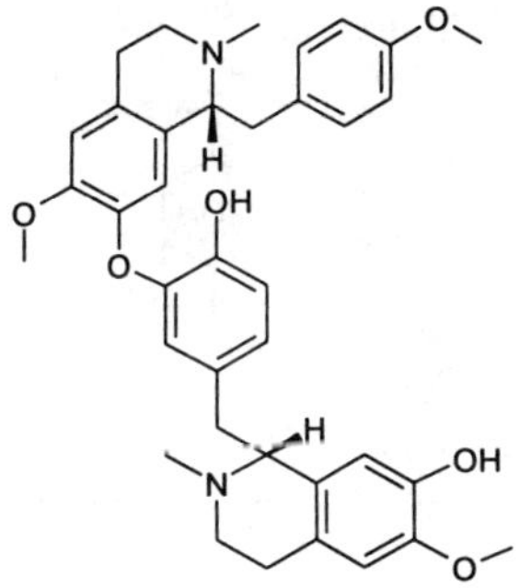

3516 Isolimocitrol-3-β-D-glucoside

$C_{24}H_{26}O_{14}$ MW: 538.47 Property: mp 220-5°C. Source: NING MENG. Ref: 6.

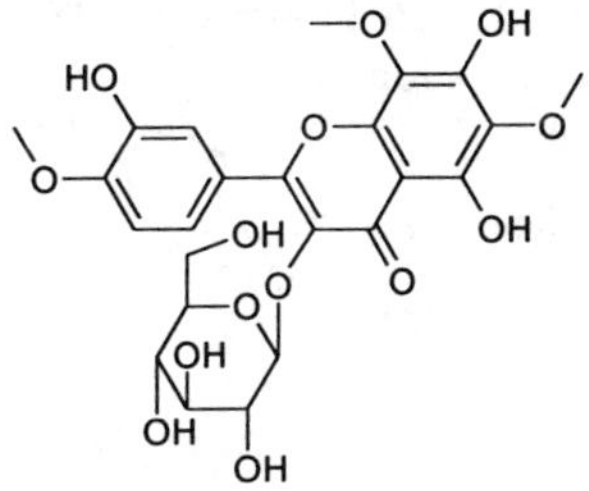

3517 Isolinderalactone

$C_{15}H_{16}O_3$ MW: 244.29 Property: mp 118-21°C. Source: WU YAO. Ref: 6.

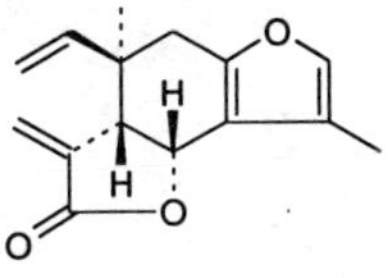

3518 Isolinderoxide

$C_{15}H_{18}O_2$ MW: 230.31 Property: bp 97-100°C /0.3 mm. Source: WU YAO. Ref: 6.

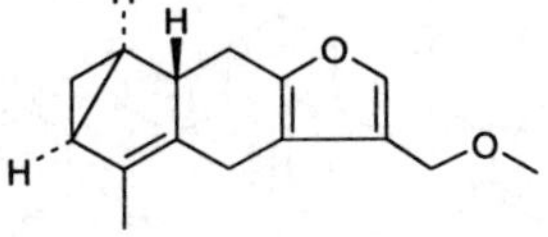

3519 Isolindleyin
$C_{23}H_{26}O_{11}$ MW: 478.46 Source: DA HUANG. Ref: 2.

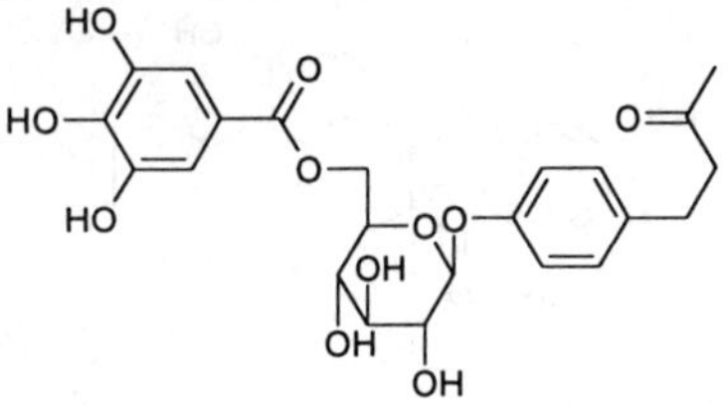

3520 Isolineolone
$C_{21}H_{32}O_5$ MW: 364.49 Property: mp 248-9°C. Source: XI SHUAI. Ref: 6.

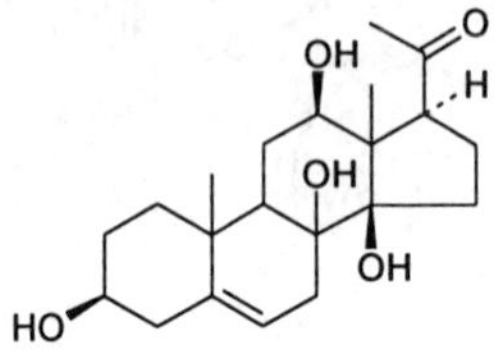

3521 Isolinolic acid
$C_{18}H_{32}O_2$ MW: 280.45 Property: mp 54°C. Source: SHU MI. Ref: 6.

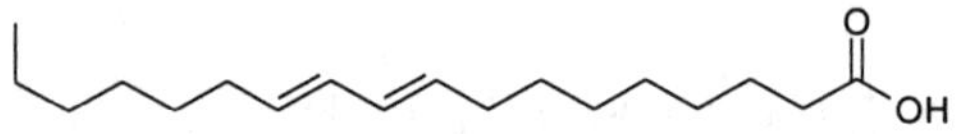

3522 Isoliquiritfigenin
$C_{15}H_{12}O_4$ MW: 256.26 Property: mp 185-6°C (dec). Source: GAN CAO. Ref: 2.

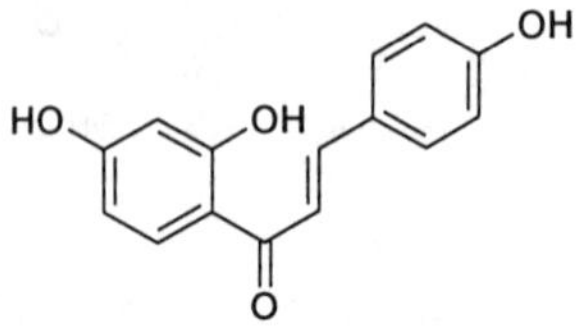

3523 Isoliquiritin
$C_{21}H_{22}O_9$ MW: 418.40 Property: mp 185-6°C. Source: GAN CAO. Ref: 2.

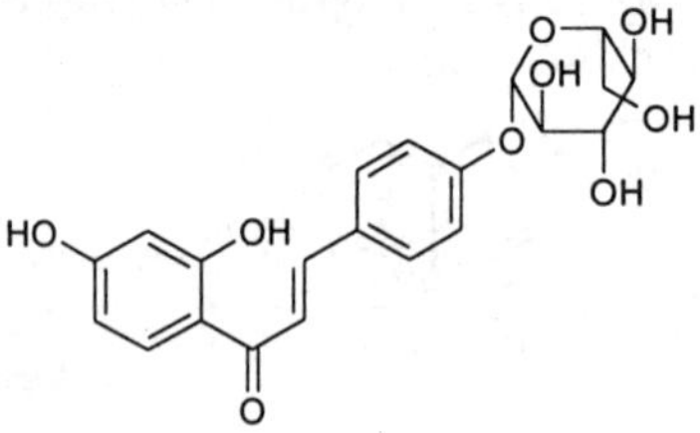

3524 Isolobelanine
$C_{21}H_{23}NO_2$ MW: 321.42 Property: mp 120-1°C. Source: BAN BIAN LIAN. Ref: 2.

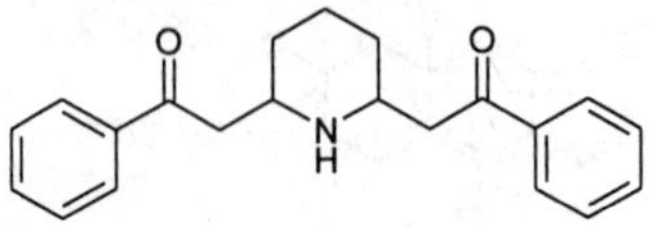

3525 Isolongifolene
$C_{15}H_{24}$ Source: WU WEI ZI. Ref: 2.

3526 Isolychnose
$C_{24}H_{42}O_{21}$ MW: 666.59 Source: BAI NIU XI. Ref: 6.

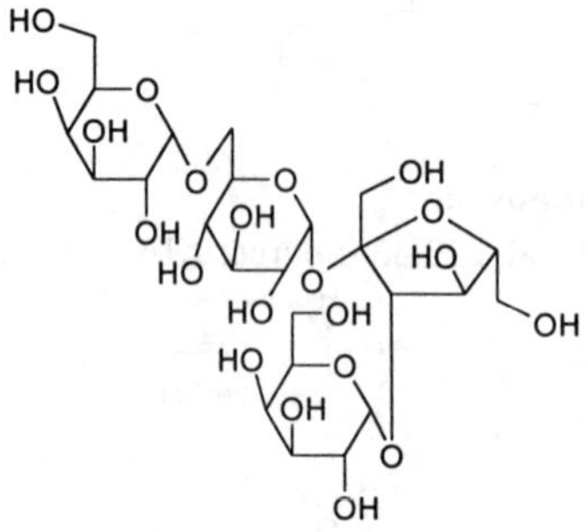

3527 Iso-magnolol
Hydromag-nolol. $C_{18}H_{18}O_2$ Property: mp 143.5°C. Source: HOU PO. Ref: 2.

3528 Isomahanimbine
$C_{23}H_{25}NO$ MW: 331.46 Source: YIN DU JIU LI XIANG. Ref: 11.

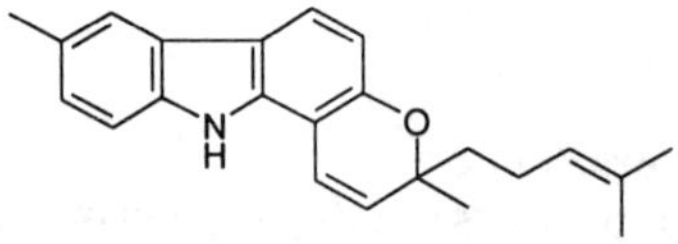

3529 Isomaltose
$C_{12}H_{22}O_{11}$ MW: 342.30 Source: DU ZHONG. Ref: 2.

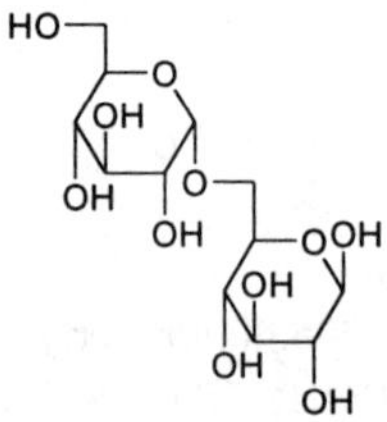

3530 Isomangiferin
$C_{19}H_{18}O_{11}$ MW: 422.35 Property: mp >260°C (dec). Source: ZHI MU. Ref: 2.

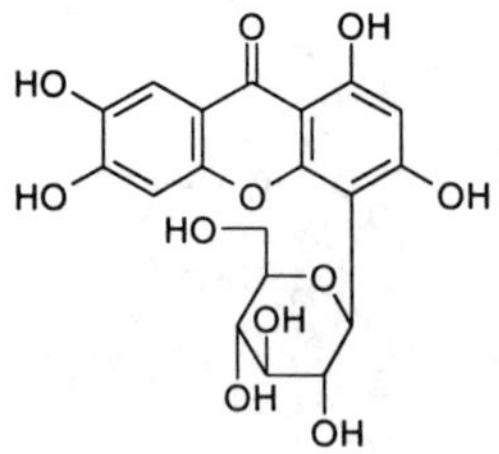

3531 Isomangiferolic acid

$C_{29}H_{46}O_3$ MW: 442.69 Property: mp 168-70°C. Source: MANG GUO, MANG GUO SHU PI. Ref: 6.

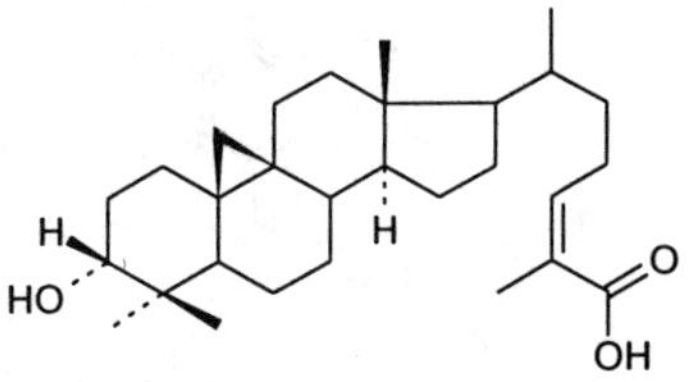

3532 Isomatrine

$C_{15}H_{24}N_2O$ MW: 248.37 Source: KU SHEN. Ref: 2.

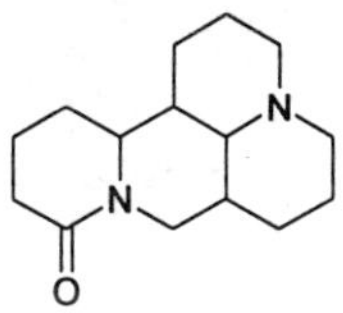

3533 Isomatsutakeol

$C_8H_{16}O$ MW: 128.22 Property: bp 87-9°C/11mm. Source: SONG XUN. Ref: 6.

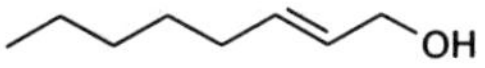

3534 Isomenthone

$C_{10}H_{18}O$ MW: 154.25 Property: mp (+): -35°C, bp (+): 212°C, (±): 210°C. Source: BO HE. Ref: 2.

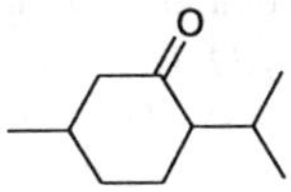

3535 Isomeramazin

$C_{15}H_{16}O_4$ MW: 260.29 Note: commonly in family Rutaceae, genus Murraya. Source: JIU LI XIANG. Ref: 11.

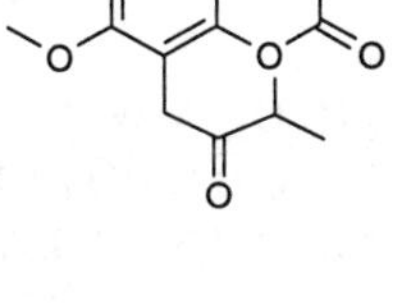

3536 Isomesityl oxide

$C_6H_{10}O$ MW: 98.15 Property: mp 135-45°C (dec). Source: YA ER QIN. Ref: 6.

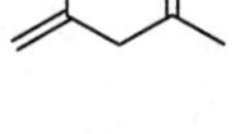

3537 L-Isomexoticin

$C_{16}H_{20}O_6$ MW: 308.33 Source: JIU LI XIANG. Ref: 11.

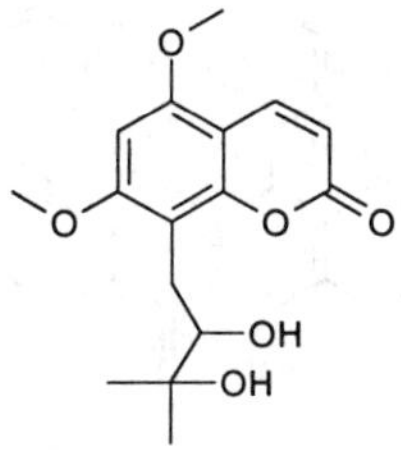

3538 Isomitraphyllic acid

$C_{20}H_{22}N_2O_4$ MW: 354.41 Property: white thin acicular crystal, mp 184-6°C. Source: HUA GOU TENG. Ref: 287.

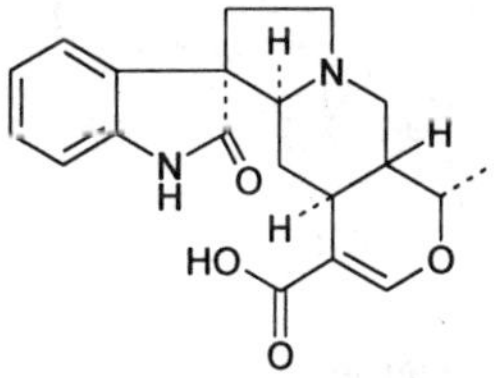

3539 Isomitraphyllic acid[16-1]-β-D-glucopyranosyl ester

$C_{26}H_{32}N_2O_9$ MW: 516.55 Property: white powder crystal, mp 206-9°C, $[\alpha]_D$ 0° (MeOH). Source: HUA GOU TENG. Ref: 287.

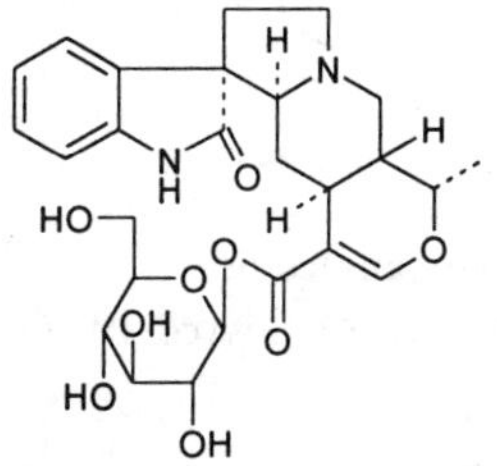

3540 Isomorellic acid

$C_{33}H_{36}O_8$ MW: 560.65 Source: TENG HUANG. Ref: 6.

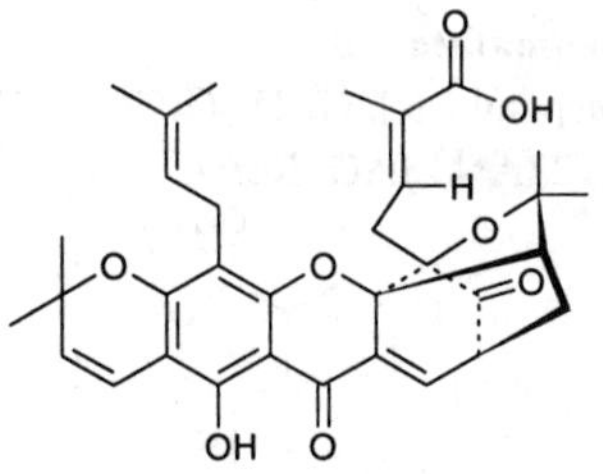

3541 Isomorellin

$C_{33}H_{36}O_7$ MW: 544.65 Property: mp 120-1°C. Source: TENG HUANG. Ref: 6.

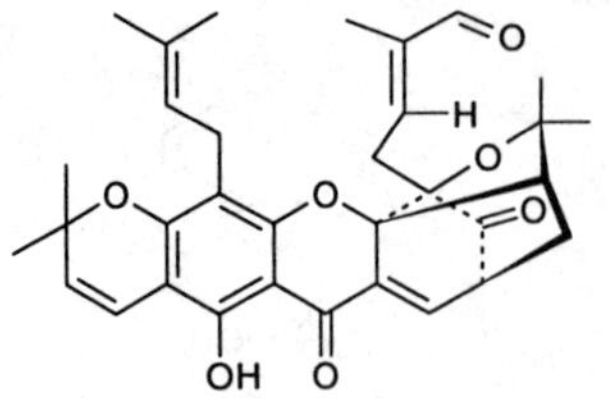

3542 Isomyricitrin

$C_{21}H_{20}O_{13}$ MW: 480.39 Source: FEI CAI. Ref: 6.

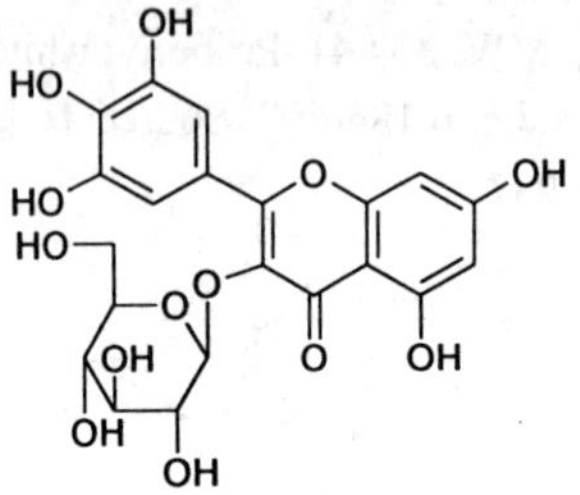

3543 Isonarthogenin

$C_{27}H_{42}O_4$ MW: 430.63 Source: CHA RUI SHU YU. Ref: 10.

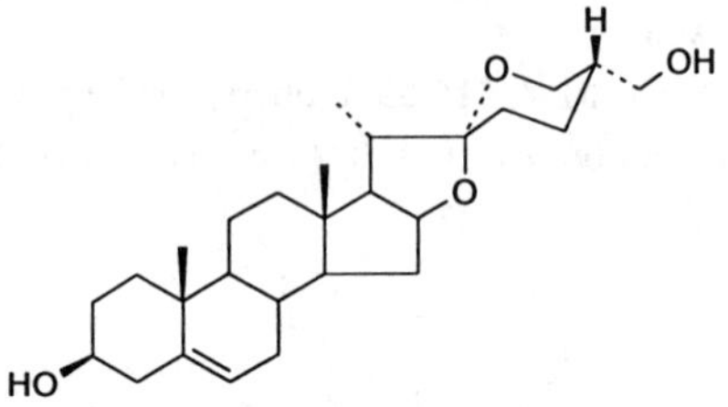

3544 Isoneobavachalcone

$C_{17}H_{14}O_5$ MW: 298.30 Source: BU GU ZHI. Ref: 2.

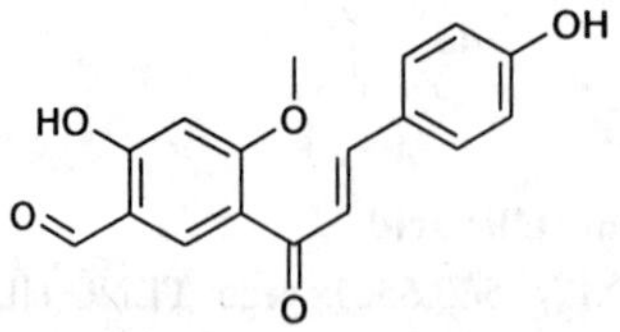

3545 Isoneomatatabiol

Isodihydronepetalactol. $C_{10}H_{18}O_2$ MW: 170.25 Source: MU TIAN LIAO. Ref: 6.

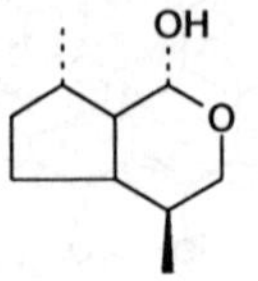

3546 Isoneotriptophenolide

$C_{21}H_{28}O_4$ MW: 344.45 Source: LEI GONG TENG. Ref: 2.

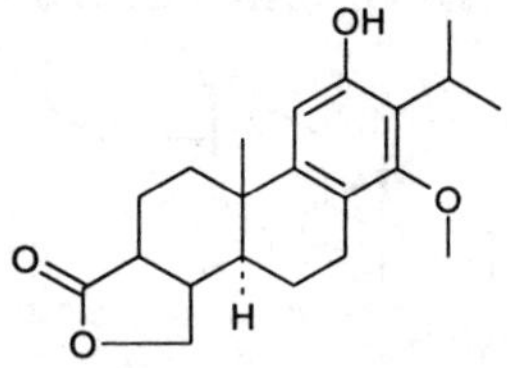

3547 Isonepetalactone

$C_{10}H_4O_2$ MW: 166.22 Property: mp 27.5-9.0°C. Source: JIA JING JIE. Ref: 6.

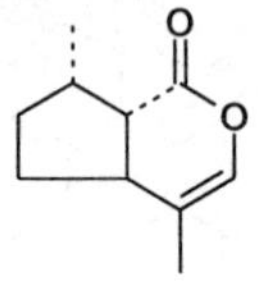

3548 Isooleic acid

$C_{16}H_{30}O_2$ MW: 254.42 Property: mp 52.5°C. Source: WEN PO. Ref: 6.

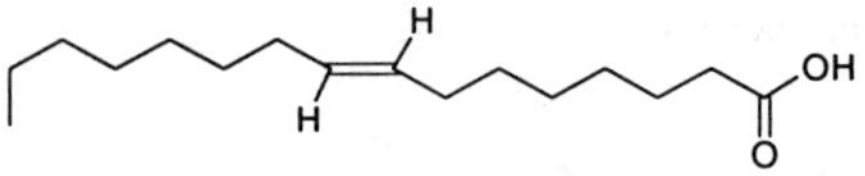

3549 Isoononin

Isoformononetin-4'-glucoside. $C_{22}H_{22}O_9$ MW: 430.42 Property: white acicular crystal, mp 216-8°C. Source: WU LA ER GAN CAO. Ref: 305.

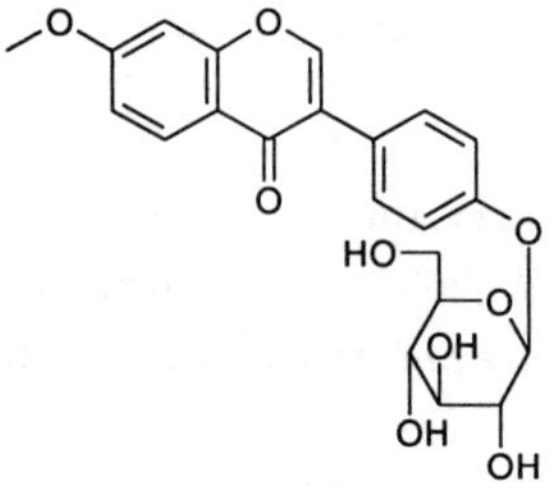

3550 Isoorientin

Homoorientin. $C_{21}H_{20}O_{11}$ MW: 448.39 Property: mp 235°C. Source: HU LU BA, HU ZHI ZI, NAN ZHU YE, QIAO MAI JIE, SUAN JIAO, YA MA, ZHANG YA CAI. Ref: 6.

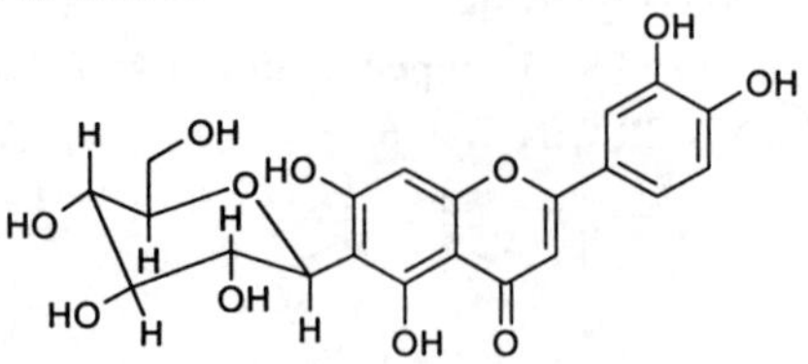

3551 Isooxypeucedanin
$C_{16}H_{14}O_5$ MW: 286.29 Source: BAI ZHI. Ref: 2.

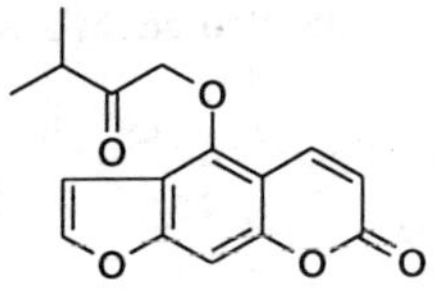

3552 Isopatrinene
$C_{15}H_{24}$ MW: 204.36 Source: BAI JIANG. Ref: 2.

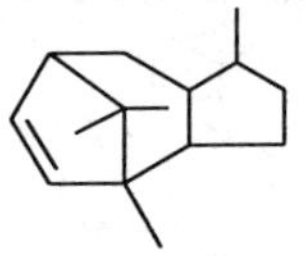

3553 Isopaulownin
$C_{20}H_{18}O_7$ MW: 370.36 Property: mp 132°C. Source: TONG MU. Ref: 6.

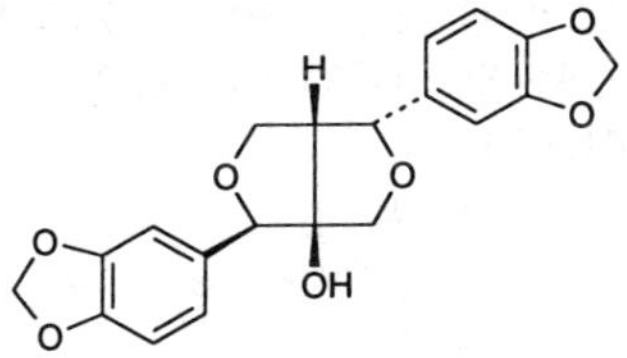

3554 Isopelletierine
$C_8H_{15}NO$ MW: 141.21 Property: bp (±): 91-2°C/14mm. Source: SHI LIU GEN. Ref: 6.

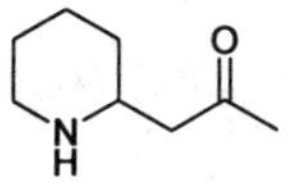

3555 Isopenniclavine
$C_{16}H_{18}N_2O_2$ MW: 270.33 Property: mp 163-5°C (dec). Source: QIAN NIU ZI. Ref: 6.

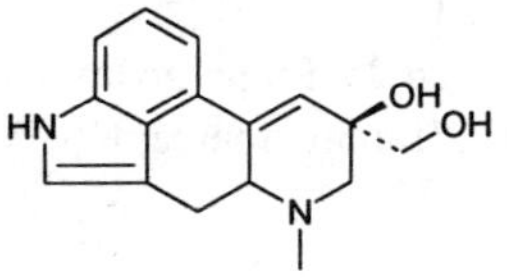

3556 8-Isopentenyl-kaempferol
$C_{20}H_{18}O_6$ MW: 354.36 Source: KU SHEN. Ref: 6.

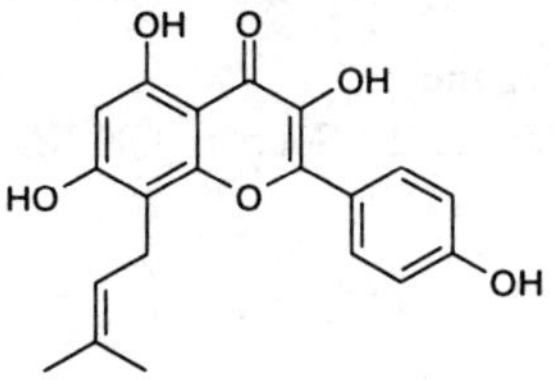

3557 8-Isopentenyllimettin
$C_{16}H_{18}O_4$ MW: 274.32 Note: commonly in family *Rutaceae*, genus *Murraya*. Source: JIU LI XIANG. Ref: 11.

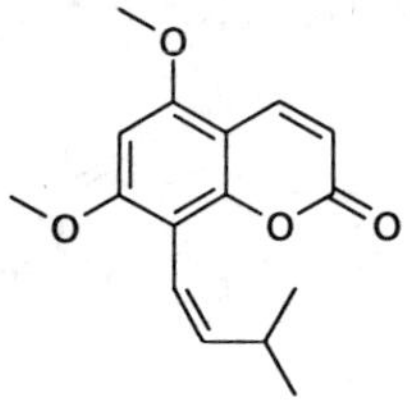

3558 6-Isopentenyloxyisobergapten
Property: mp 96-7°C. Source: YONG NING DU HUO. Ref: 541.

3559 8-(Δ3-Isopentenyl)-5,7,3',4',-tetrahydroxy-flavone
$C_{20}H_{18}O_6$ MW: 354.36 Property: mp 100°C. Source: CANG ER. Ref: 6.

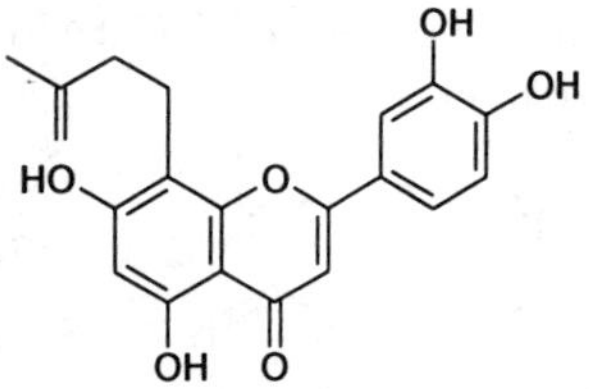

3560 Isopetasin
$C_{20}H_{28}O_3$ MW: 316.44 Property: mp 95-6°C. Source: FENG DOU CAI. Ref: 6.

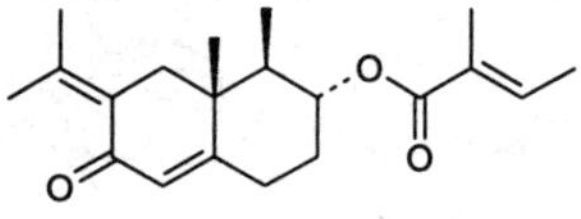

3561 Isopicropodophyllone
CAS: 55515-07-6 $C_{22}H_{20}O_8$ MW: 412.40 Property: mp 170-2°C. Source: BA JIAO LIAN. Ref: 5.

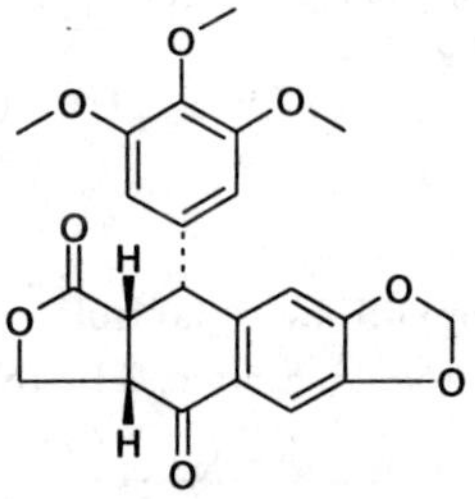

3562 Isopimpinellin

$C_{13}H_{10}O_5$ MW: 246.22 Property: mp 151°C. Source: CHOU CAO, DU HUO, FEI LONG ZHANG XUE, LANG DU, SHE CHUANG ZI, XIANG YUAN YE, YONG NING DU HUO. Ref: 6, 541.

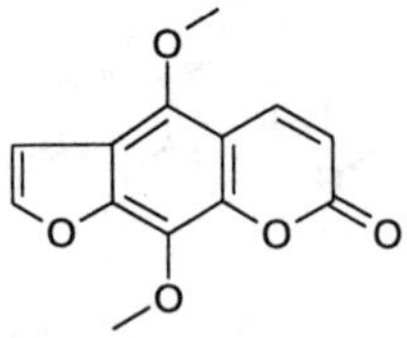

3563 Isopinocamphone

$C_{10}H_{16}O$ MW: 152.24 Property: bp (+): 213.4-5.0 °C; (-): 81°C/5mm. Source: JIN QIAN CAO. Ref: 6.

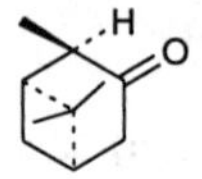

3564 Isopropenyl toluene

$C_{10}H_{12}$ MW: 132.21 Property: o: bp 172-3°C, m: bp 185-6°C, p: mp -20°C, bp 184-5°C. Source: JU PI (CHEN PI). Ref: 6.

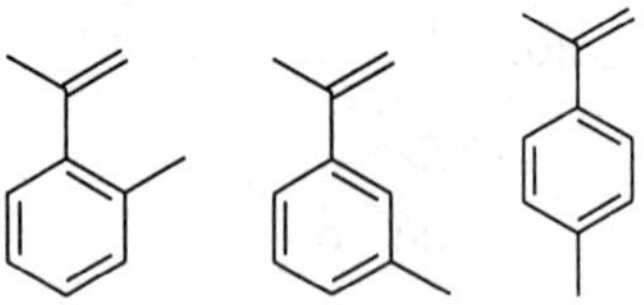

o m p

3565 Isopropyl idenekirenol

$C_{23}H_{38}O_4$ MW: 378.56 Source: XI XIAN. Ref: 2.

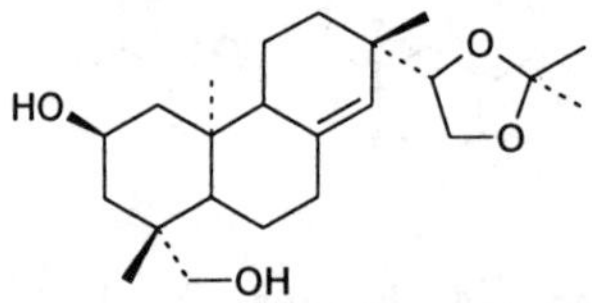

3566 Isopropyl isothiocyanate

C_4H_7NS MW: 101.17 Property: bp 137.0-7.5°C. Source: JIE ZI. Ref: 6.

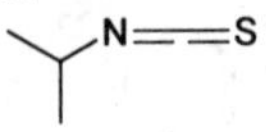

3567 2-Isopropyl-5-methylanisole

$C_{11}H_{16}O$ MW: 164.25 Source: XI XIN. Ref: 2.

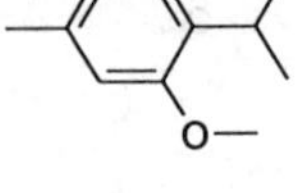

3568 (E)-9-Isopropyl-6-methyl-5,9-decadiene-2-one

$C_{14}H_{24}O$ MW: 208.35 Source: MU XIANG. Ref: 2.

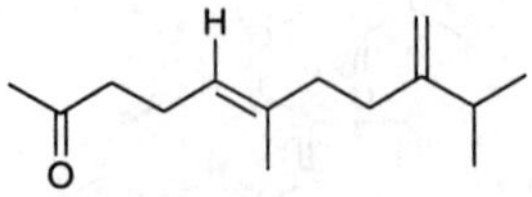

3569 1-Isopropyl-4-methylene-7-methyl-1,2,3,4,4a,5,6,8a-octahydronaphthalene

$C_{15}H_{24}$ MW: 204.36 Source: DU HUO. Ref: 2.

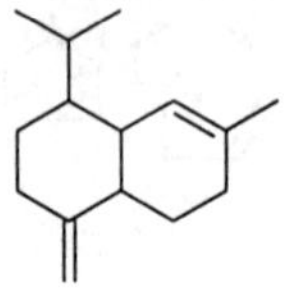

3570 Isopsoralen

Angelicin. $C_{11}H_6O_3$ MW: 186.17 Property: mp 135.0-9.5°C, 142°C. Source: BU GU ZHI, DU HUO, CHAI HU, GAN SONG, YONG NING DU HUO. Ref: 2, 6, 541, 630.

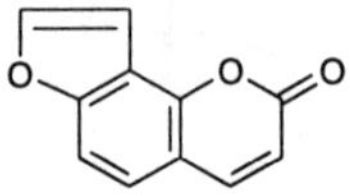

3571 Isopsoralidin

$C_{20}H_{16}O_5$ MW: 336.35 Source: BU GU ZHI. Ref: 2, 630.

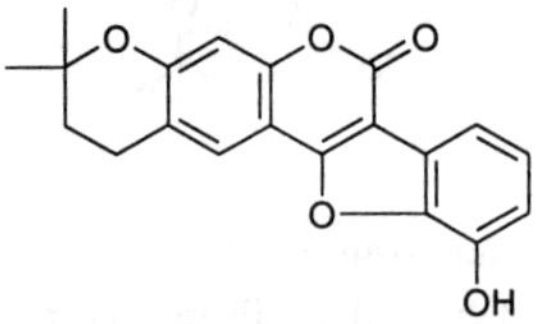

3572 Isopulegol

$C_{10}H_{18}O$ MW: 154.25 Property: bp (+): 93-4°C/14mm., (-): 94°C/14mm. Source: NING MENG AN YE. Ref: 6.

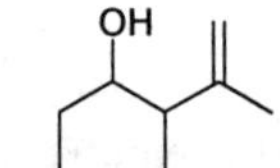

3573 Isopulegone

$C_{10}H_{16}O$ MW: 152.24 Source: JON JIE. Ref: 2.

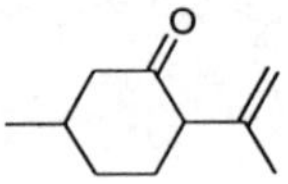

3574 Isoquercitrin
Isoquercetin. $C_{21}H_{20}O_{12}$ MW: 464.39 Property: mp 234-6°C. Source: GAN CAO, XIU MAO JI SHENG, YU XING CAO, etc. Ref: 2, 6, 231, 559.

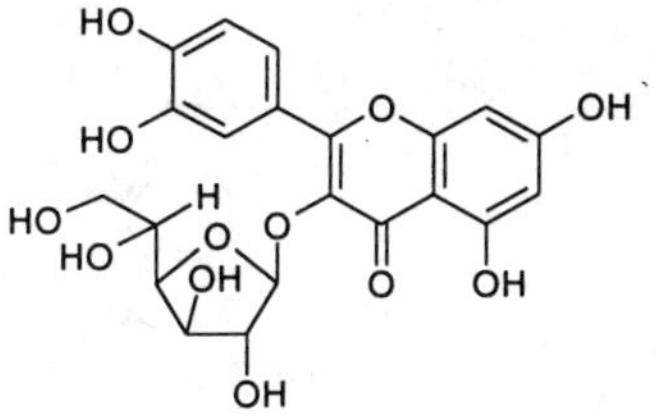

3575 Isoramanone
$C_{21}H_{32}O_4$ MW: 348.49 Property: mp 220-3.4°C. Source: FU SHOU CAO, LUO MO. Ref: 6.

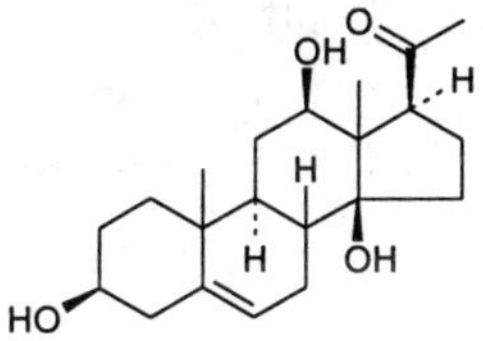

3576 Isoreineckiagenin
$C_{27}H_{44}O_5$ MW: 448.65 Property: mp 240-2°C. Source: JI XIANG CAO. Ref: 6.

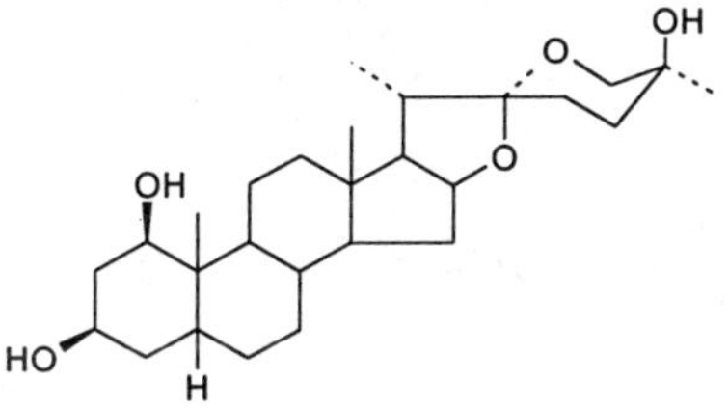

3577 Isorhamnetin
$C_{16}H_{12}O_7$ MW: 316.27 Property: mp 305°C (dec). Source: BAI GUO, CU LIU GUO (SHA JI), PU HUANG, YIN CHEN HAO. Ref: 2.

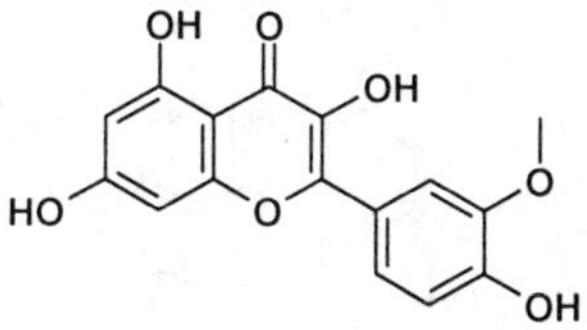

3578 Isorhamnetin-3-arabino-glucoside
$C_{27}H_{30}O_{16}$ MW:610.53 Source:NING MENG. Ref:6.

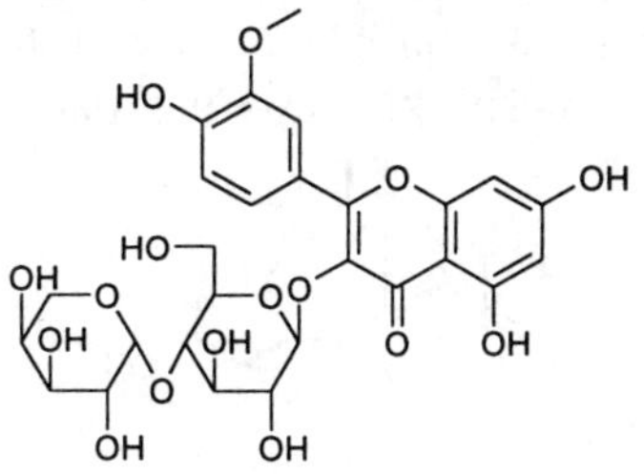

3579 Isorhamnetin-3-α-L-arabofuranoside
$C_{21}H_{20}O_{11}$ MW: 448.39 Source: GUI JIAN JIN JI ER. Ref: 6.

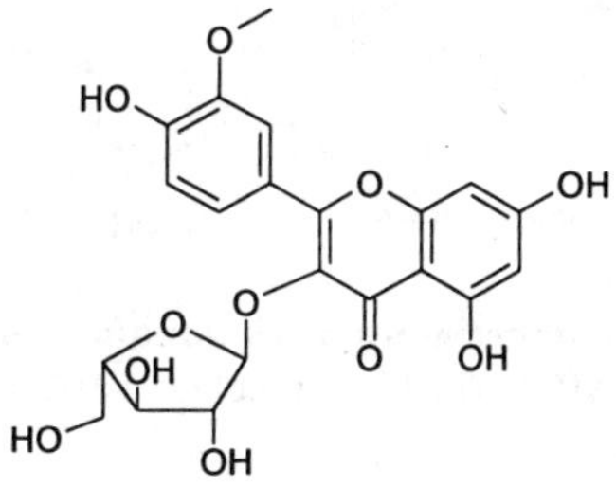

3580 Isorhamnetin-3-β-D-galactopyranoside
Isorhamnetin-3-O-galactoside. $C_{22}H_{22}O_{12}$ MW: 478.41 Property: mp 267-9°C. Source: GUI JIAN JIN JI ER, TIAN CONG. Ref: 6.

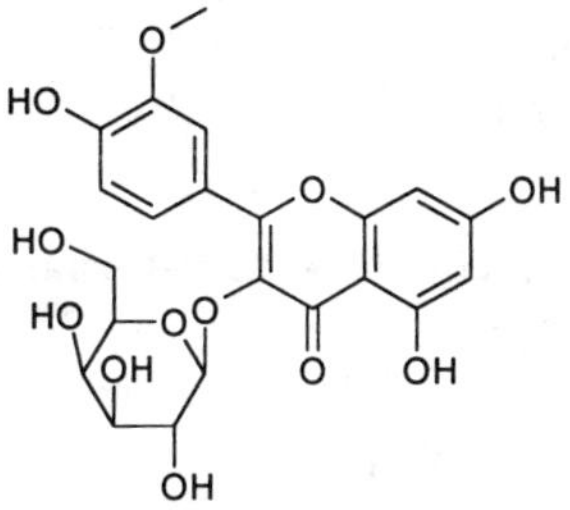

3581 Isorhamnetin-3-glucoside
$C_{22}H_{22}O_{12}$ MW: 478.41 Source: TIAN CONG, YIN CHEN HAO, ZHEN ZHU MEI. Ref: 2, 6.

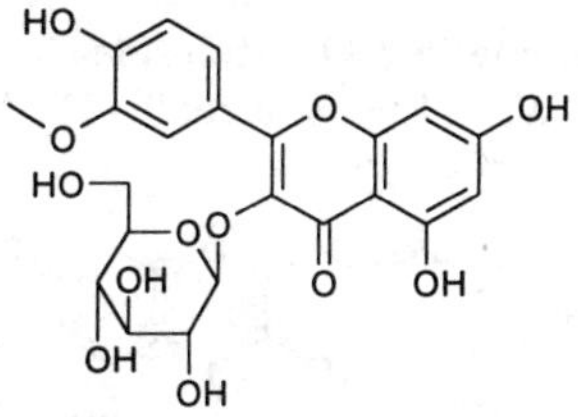

3582 Isorhamnetin-3-mono-β-D-glucoside
$C_{22}H_{22}O_{12}$ MW: 478.41 Property: mp 177-9°C. Source: TENG HUANG. Ref: 6.

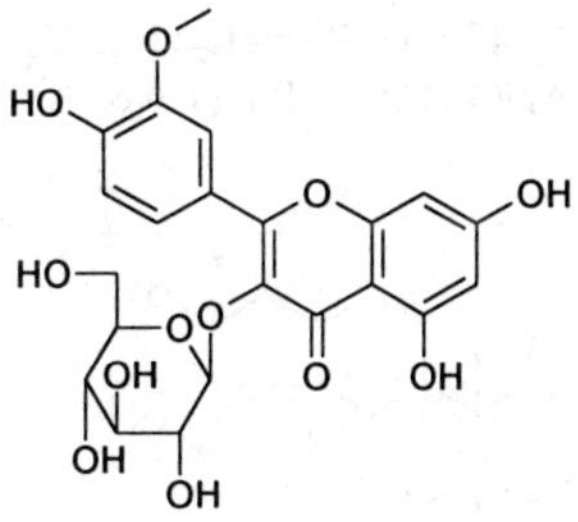

3583 Isorhamnetin-3-O-neohesperidoside
Source: PU HUANG. Ref: 2.

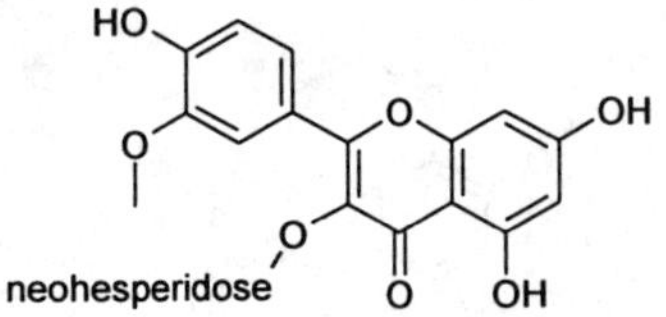

3584 Isorhamnetin-3-α-L-rhamnofuranoside
$C_{22}H_{22}O_{11}$ MW: 462.41 Source: GUI JIAN JIN JI ER. Ref: 6.

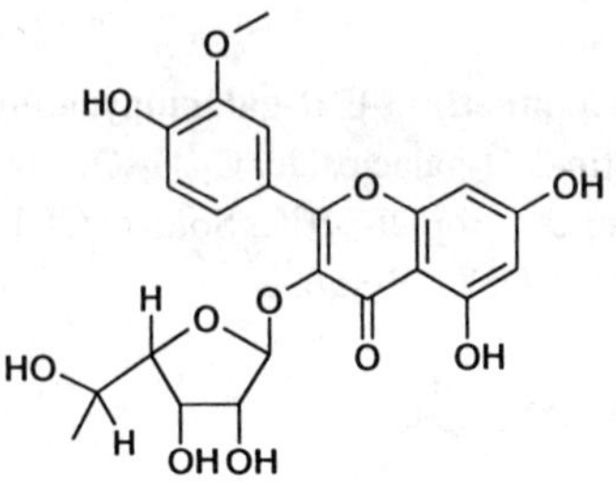

3585 Isorhamnetin-3-O-(2G-α-L-rhamnopyranosyl)-rutinoside
Source: PU HUANG. Ref: 2.

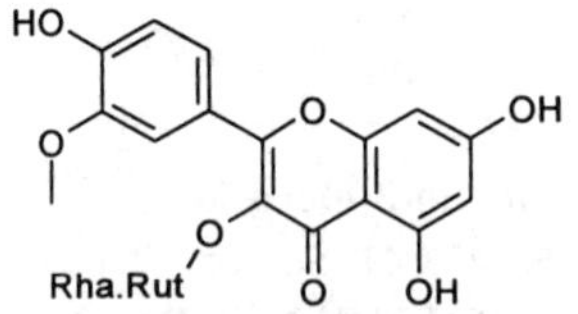

3586 Isorhamnetin-3-O-rutinoside
$C_{28}H_{32}O_{16}$ MW: 624.56 Source: PU HUANG. Ref: 2.

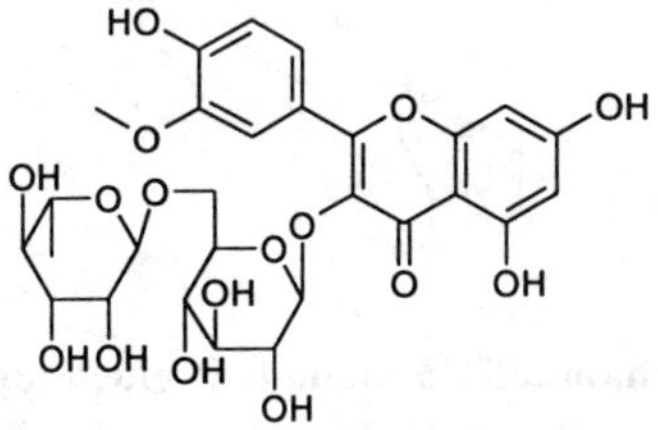

3587 Isorhodeasapogenin
$C_{27}H_{44}O_4$ MW: 432.65 Property: mp 239-40°C. Source: JI XIANG CAO, LING LAN. Ref: 6.

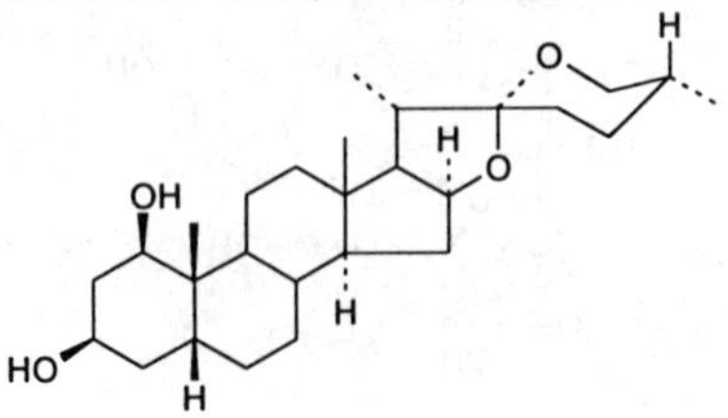

3588 Isorhoeadine
$C_{21}H_{21}NO_6$ MW: 383.40 Property: mp 165-7°C. Source: LI CHUN HUA. Ref: 6.

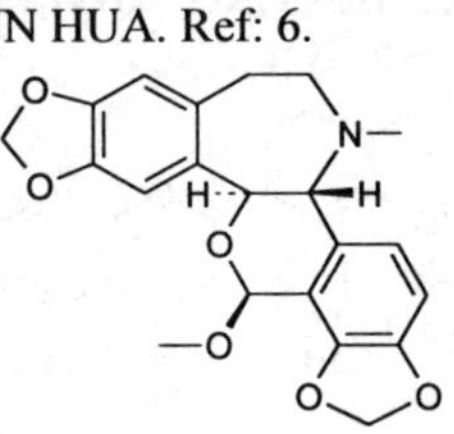

3589 Isorhynchophylline
$C_{22}H_{28}N_2O_4$ MW: 384.48 Property: mp 60-70°C. Source: GOU TENG. Ref: 2, 6.

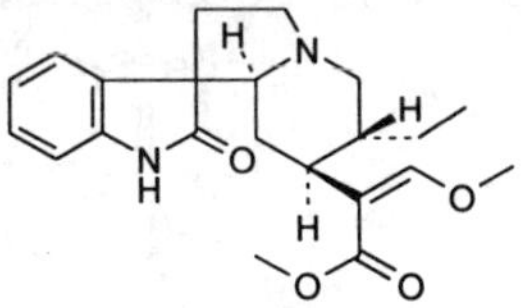

3590 Isorosmaricine
$C_{20}H_{27}NO_4$ MW: 345.44 Source: MI DIE XIANG. Ref: 6.

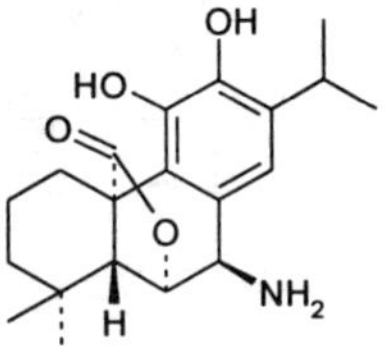

3591 Isorottlerin
$C_{30}H_{28}O_8$ MW: 516.55 Property: mp 180°C. Source: LU SONG QIU MAO. Ref: 6.

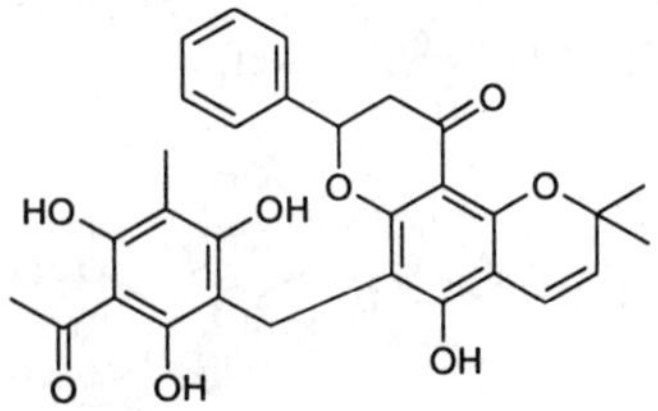

3592 Isorupestonic acid
$C_{15}H_{20}O_3$ MW: 248.32 Property: colorless bar crystal, mp 192-3°C, $[\alpha]_D^{14}$ 11° (c=0.62, methanol). Source: XI JIANGYI ZHI GAO. Ref: 196.

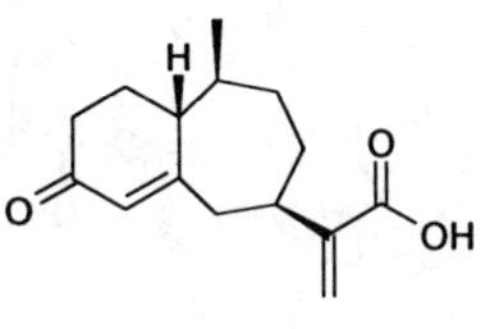

3593 Isosakuranetin-7-rutinoside
$C_{28}H_{34}O_{14}$ MW: 594.57 Property: mp 211-3°C. Source: TIAN CHEN. Ref: 6.

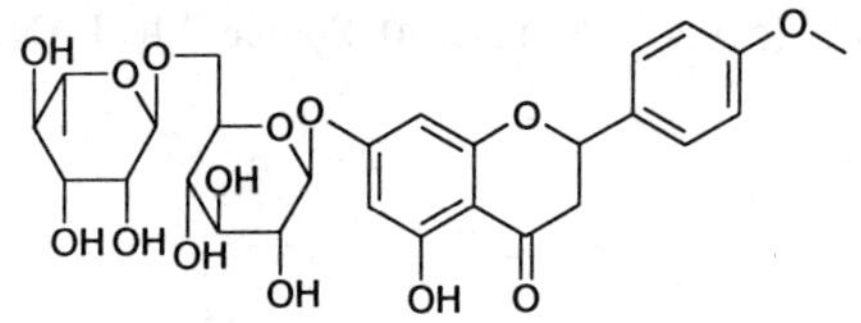

3594 Isosalipurposide
$C_{21}H_{22}O_{10}$ MW: 434.40 Property: mp 172-3°C. Source: SHUI YANG MU BAI PI. Ref: 6.

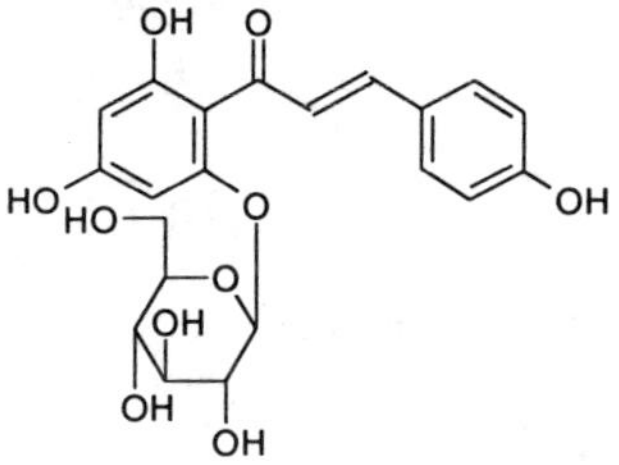

3595 Isosaponarin
$C_{27}H_{30}O_{16}$ MW: 610.53 Property: mp 236-7°C. Source: WANG BU LIU XING. Ref: 6.

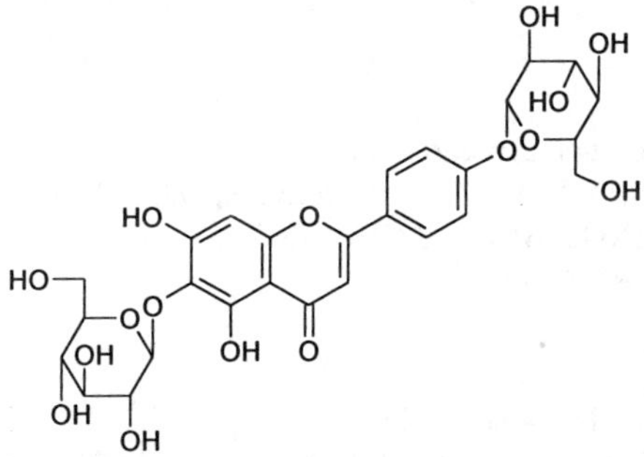

3596 Isoschisandrin
$C_{24}H_{32}O_7$ MW: 432.52 Source: WU WEI ZI. Ref: 2.

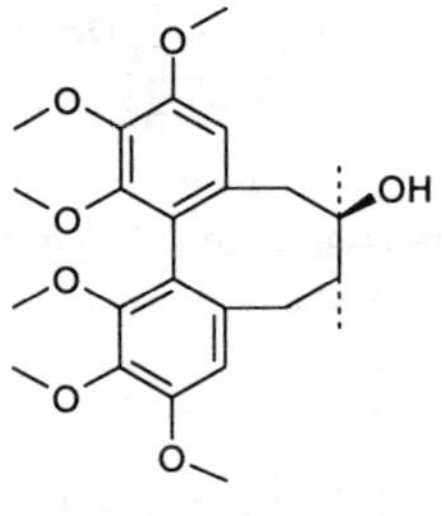

3597 Isoshyobunone
$C_{15}H_{24}O$ MW: 220.36 Source: BAI CHANG. Ref: 6.

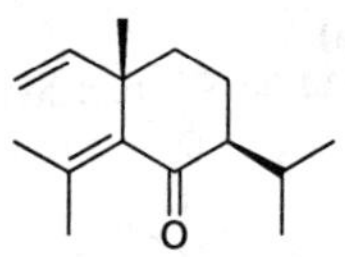

3598 Isosinomenine
$C_{19}H_{23}NO_4$ MW: 329.40 Property: mp (+): 198-202°C. Source: BAI CHANG. Ref: 6.

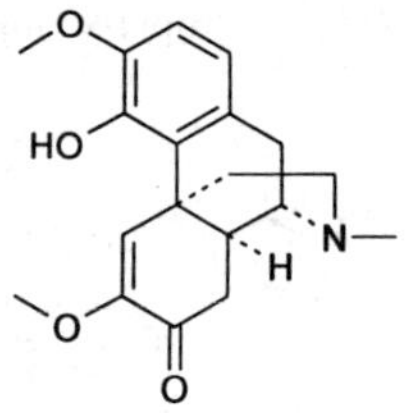

3599 Isositsivikine
$C_{21}H_{26}N_2O_3$ MW: 354.45 Source: CHANG CHUN HUA. Ref: 6.

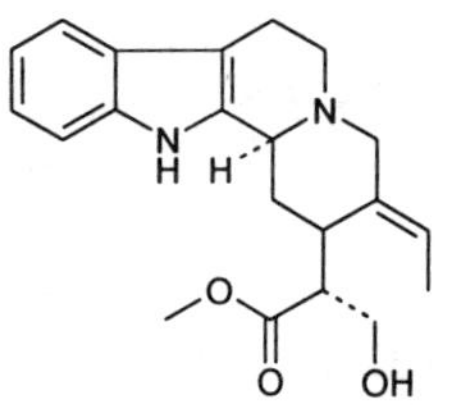

3600 Isosophocarpine
$C_{15}H_{22}N_2O$ MW: 246.36 Source: KU SHEN. Ref: 2.

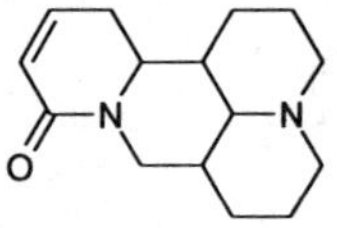

3601 Isostrychnine
$C_{21}H_{24}N_2O_2$ MW: 336.44 Source: MA QIAN ZI. Ref: 2, 542.

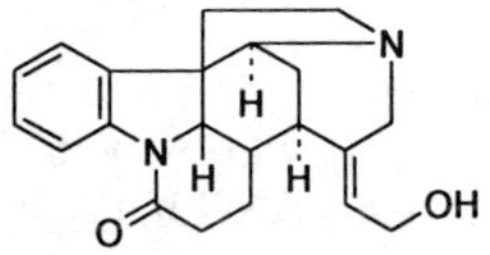

3602 Isostrychnine N-oxide
$C_{21}H_{24}N_2O_3$ MW: 352.44 Source: MA QIAN ZI. Ref: 2.

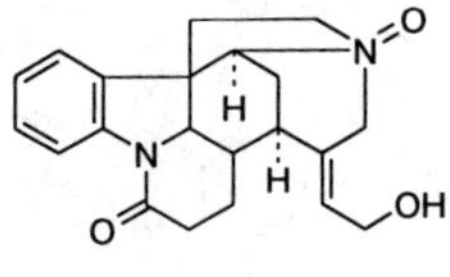

3603 Isotadeonal
$C_{15}H_{22}O_2$ MW: 234.34 Source: SHUI LIAO. Ref: 6.

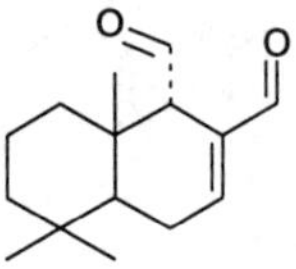

3604 Isotanshinone I
$C_{18}H_{12}O_3$ MW: 276.29 Property: mp 219°C. Source: DAN SHEN. Ref: 2.

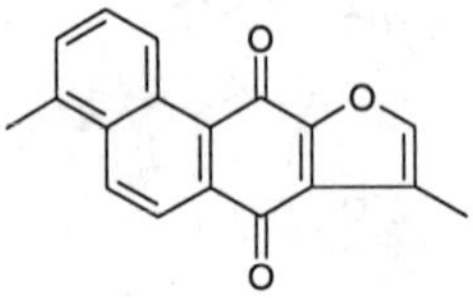

3605 Isotanshinone II
$C_{19}H_{18}O_3$ MW: 294.35 Property: mp 208°C. Source: DAN SHEN. Ref: 2.

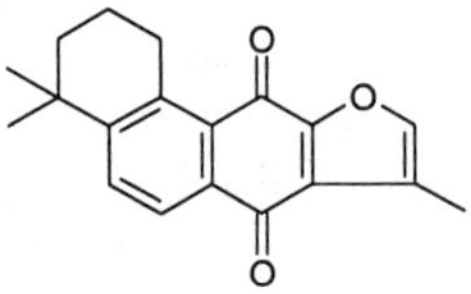

3606 Isotetrandrine
$C_{38}H_{42}N_2O_6$ MW: 622.77 Property: mp 182°C. Source: BAI YAO ZI, GONG LAO ZI, GONG LAO MU, SHI DA GONG LAO YE, YIN BU HUAN. Ref: 6.

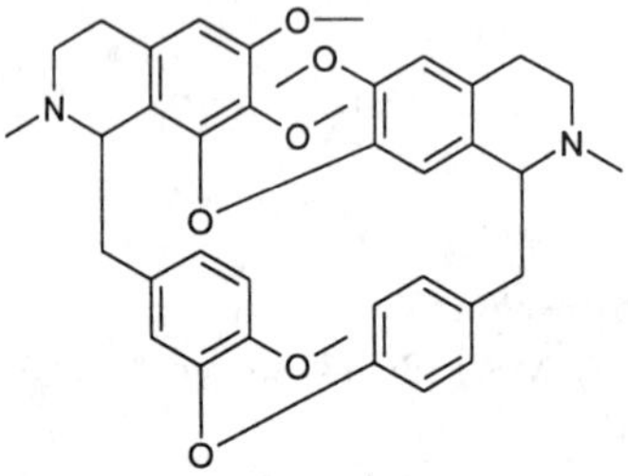

3607 Isotrilobine
Homotrilobine. $C_{36}H_{36}N_2O_5$ MW: 576.70 Property: mp 213-5°C. Source: FANG JI, FANG JI RU LAN. Ref: 6.

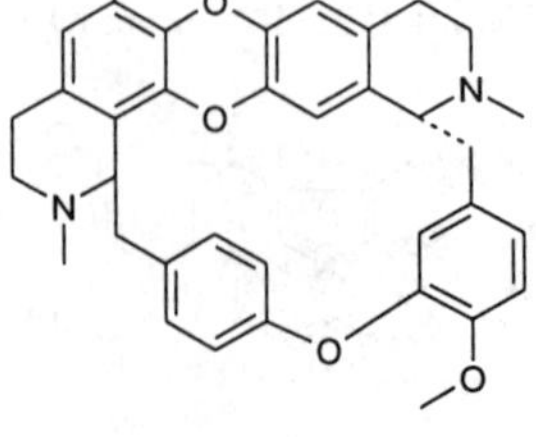

3608 Isotrilobine-N-2-oxide
$C_{36}H_{36}N_2O_6$ MW: 592.70 Property: light yellow crystalline powder, mp 178-9°C (methanol), $[\alpha]_D^{20.5}$ +150.9° (c=0.91, chloroform). Source: MU FANG JI. Ref: 203.

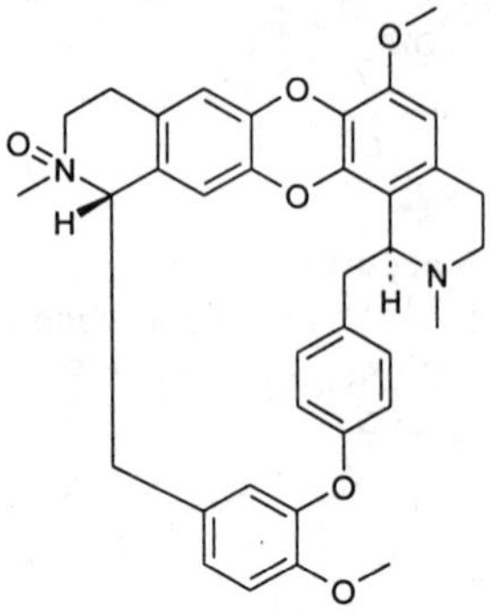

3609 Isotuberostemonine
$C_{22}H_{33}NO_4$ MW: 375.51 Property: mp 123-5°C. Source: BAI BU. Ref: 6.

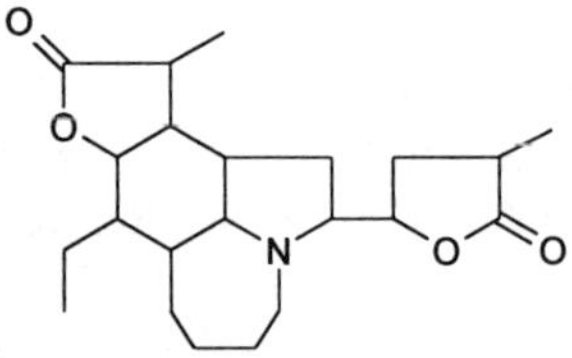

3610 Isovaleraldehyde
$C_5H_{10}O$ MW: 86.13 Property: mp 92.5°C. Source: SHENG JIANG, XI GUA. Ref: 2.

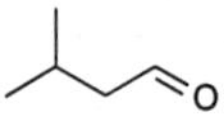

3611 Isovaleric acid
$C_5H_{10}O_2$ MW: 102.13 Property: mp -37.6°C, bp 176.7°C. Source: BAN BIAN SU, DIAO JING CAO, GAN SONG, HAI TUN YU, NIU BANG GEN, SANG YE, XIE CAO, YANG SHI CAO. Ref: 6.

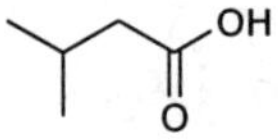

3612 Isovaleroxy-hydroxy dihydrovaltrate
$C_{27}H_{40}O_{11}$ MW: 540.61 Source: XIE CAO SHE CHUANG ZI. Ref: 6.

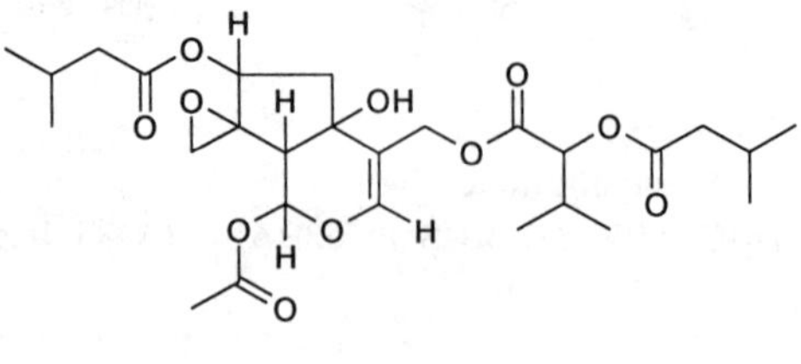

3613 o-Isovalerylcolum bianetin
$C_{19}H_{22}O_5$ MW: 330.38 Source: SHE CHUANG ZI. Ref: 6.

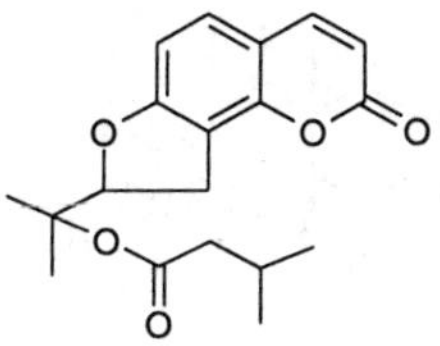

3614 Isovalerylshikonin
$C_{21}H_{24}O_6$ MW: 372.42 Source: ZI CAO. Ref: 2.

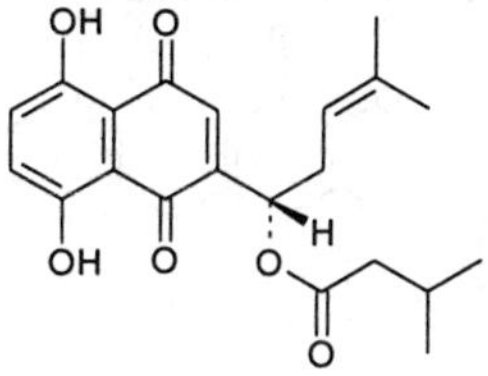

3615 Isovanillin
$C_8H_8O_3$ MW: 152.15 Property: mp 116-7°C, bp 179 °C/15mm. Source: SHI CHUN. Ref: 6.

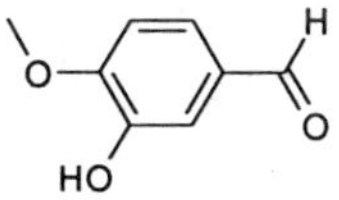

3616 Isovitexin
Homovitexin; Saponaretin. CAS: 38953-85-4
$C_{21}H_{20}O_{10}$ MW: 432.39 Property: mp 265°C, 239°C. Source: SUAN JIAO, YA MA, ZHANG YA CAI. Ref: 5, 6.

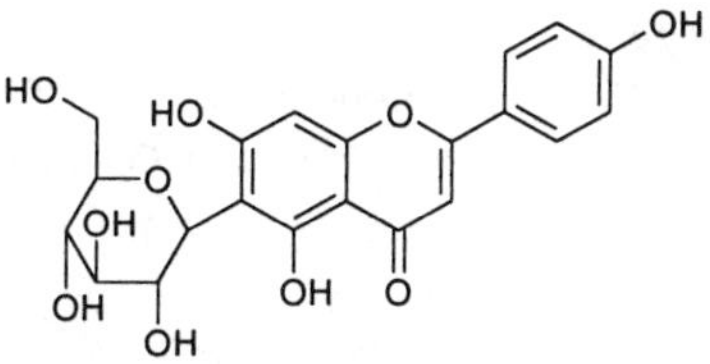

3617 Isowilfortrine
$C_{41}H_{47}NO_{20}$ MW: 873.83 Property: colorless lamellar crystal, mp 329-31°C. Source: LEI GONG TENG. Ref: 310.

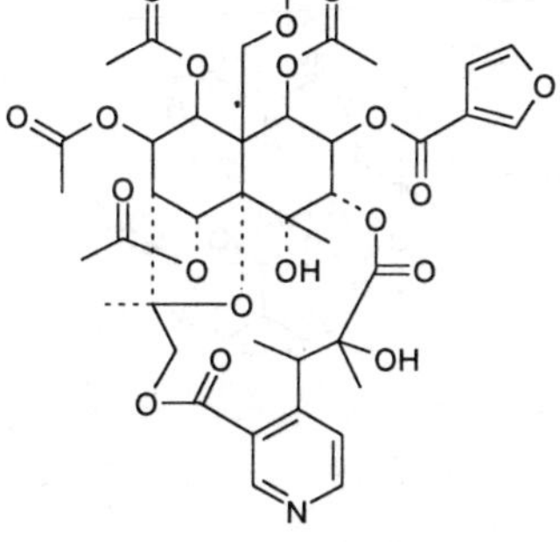

3618 Isoxanthohumol
$C_{21}H_{22}O_5$ MW: 354.41 Property: mp 198°C. Source: KU SHEN. Ref: 6.

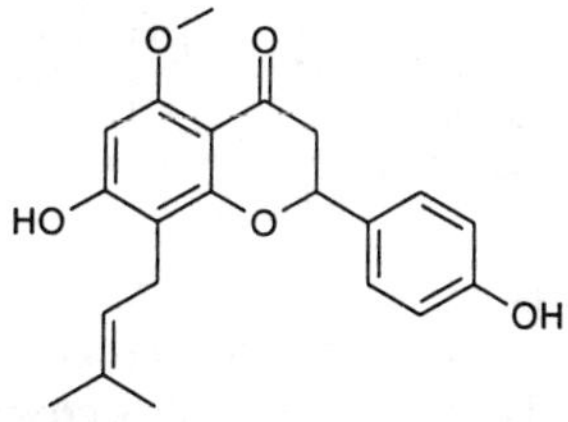

3619 Isoxanthopterin
$C_6H_5N_5O_2$ MW: 179.14 Property: mp >300°C (dec). Source: DIE DA LAO, JIN YU, QING WA. Ref: 6.

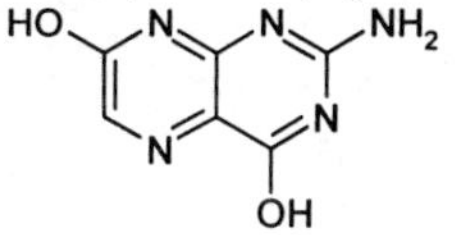

3620 Isoxanthopterin-6-carboxylic acid
$C_7H_5N_5O_4$ MW: 223.15 Source: JIN YU. Ref: 6.

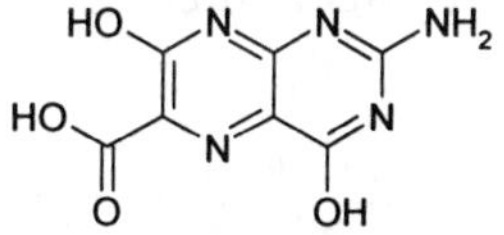

3621 Isozaluzanine
$C_{15}H_{18}O_3$ MW: 246.31 Source: MU XIANG. Ref: 2.

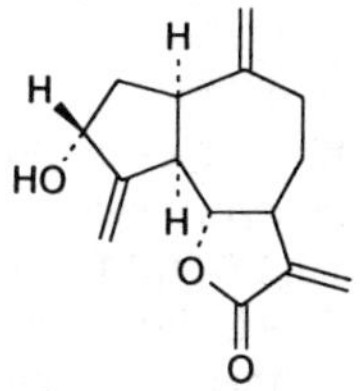

3622 (-)-Istanbulin A
$C_{15}H_{20}O_4$ MW: 264.32 Property: colorless granular crystal, mp 245°C, $[\alpha]_D^{17.5}$ -110° (c=0.6035, methanol). Source: CAO SHAN HU. Ref: 94.

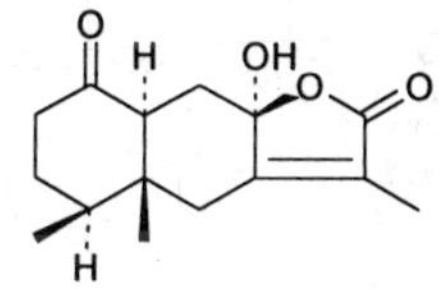

3623 Iupeol palmitate
Balanophorin B. $C_{46}H_{80}O_2$ MW: 665.15 Property: white amorphous powder (Me_2CO), mp 68-69°C. Source: YIN DU SHE GU. Ref: 633.

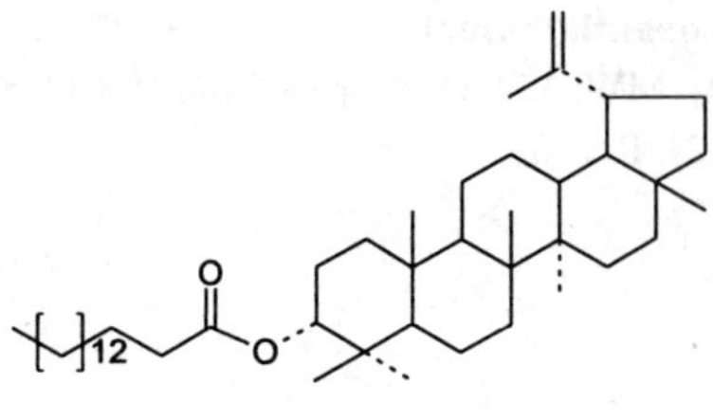

3624 Izalpinin
4H-1-Benzopyran-4-one,3,5,-dihydroxy-7-methoxy-2-phenyl. $C_{16}H_{12}O_5$ MW: 284.27 Property: yellow acicular crystal (CH_2Cl_2), mp 192-5°C. Source: FENG JIAO, JIN YU, LIAN JIANG. Ref: 6, 463.

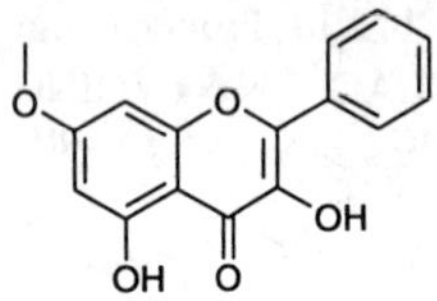

3626 Jacaranone
CAS: 60263-07-2 $C_9H_{10}O_4$ MW: 182.18 Property: mp 76-7°C, 80-1°C. Source: SONG YE QIAN LI GUANG, YI DIAN HONG. Ref: 5.

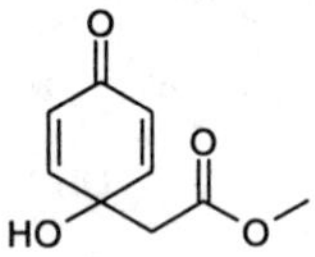

3627 Jacoumaric acid
Source: WU LING ZHI. Ref: 637.

3628 Japondipsaponin E1
3-O-α-L-rhamnopyranosyl(1→3)-β-D-glucopyranosyl(1→3)-α-L-rhamnopyranosyl(1→2)-α-L-arabinopyranosyl-hederagenin 28-O-β-D-glucopyranoside. $C_{59}H_{96}O_{26}$ MW: 1221.41 Property: white powder, mp 223-6°C, soluble in methanol, pyridine and water. Source: XU TUAN. Ref: 339.

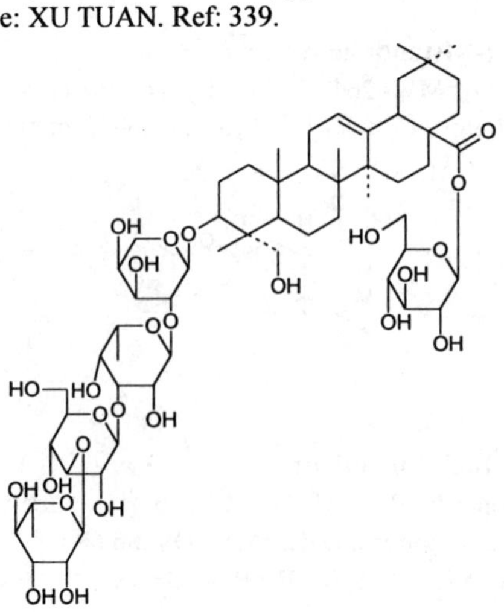

3629 S-Japonine
$C_{19}H_{28}O_3S$ MW: 336.52 Property: mp 116.5-7.0°C. Source: FENG DOU CAI. Ref: 6.

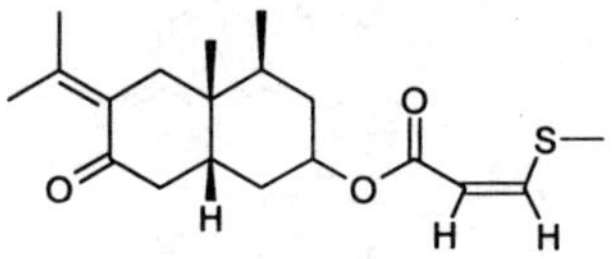

3630 Japonine
$C_{18}H_{17}NO_3$ MW: 295.34 Property: mp 143°C. Source: CHOU SHAN YANG. Ref: 6.

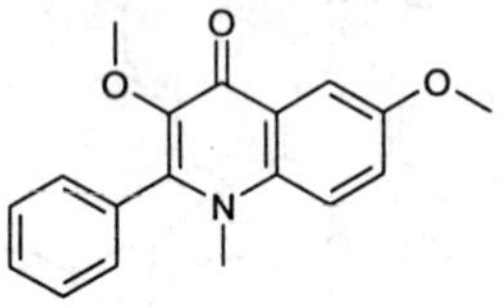

3631 Jasminoidin
$C_{17}H_{24}O_{10}$ MW: 388.37 Source: ZHI ZI. Ref: 2.

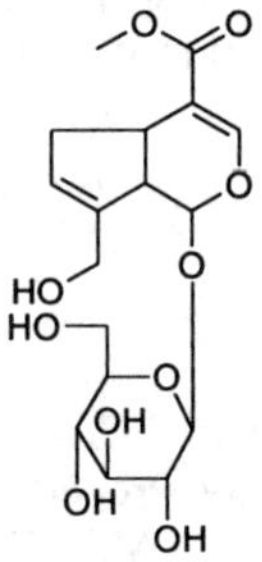

3632 Jasmone
$C_{11}H_{16}O$ MW: 164.25 Property: bp 134-5°C/12mm. Source: CHA YE, DAI DAI HUA, MO LI HUA. Ref: 6.

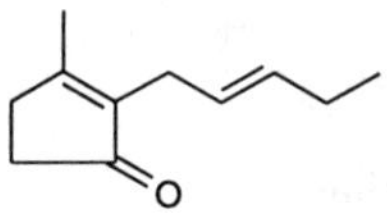

3633 Jatamansin
$C_{19}H_{20}O_5$ MW: 328.3 Property: mp 97-8°C. Source: GAN SONG. Ref: 6.

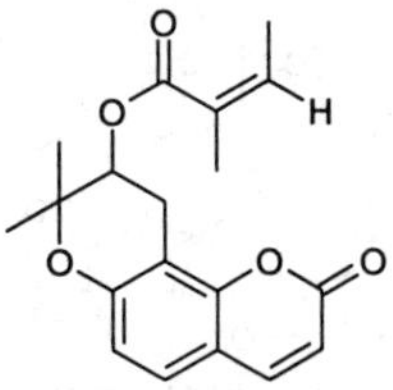

3634 Jatamansinol
$C_{15}H_{16}O_4$ MW: 260.29 Property: mp 182-3°C. Source: GAN SONG. Ref: 6.

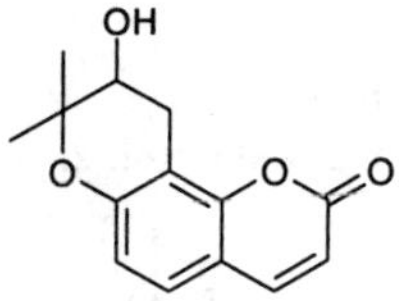

3635 Jatropham
Jatrophalactam. CAS: 656-76-3 $C_5H_7NO_2$ MW: 113.12 Property: mp 131-2°C. Source: *Jatropha macrorhiza* Benth. Ref: 5.

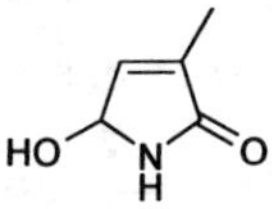

3636 Jatrophatrione
CAS: 58298-76-3 $C_{20}H_{26}O_3$ MW: 314.43 Property: mp 148-50°C. Source: *Jatropha macrorhiza* Benth. Ref: 5.

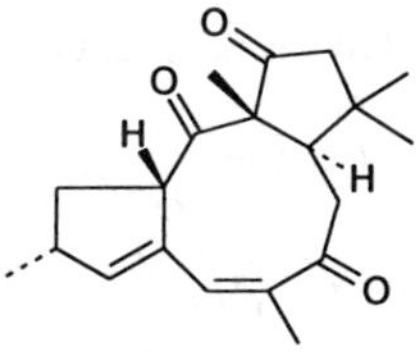

3637 Jatrophone
CAS: 29444-03-9 $C_{20}H_{24}O_3$ MW: 312.41 Property: mp 152-3°C. Source: *Jatropha gossypifolia* Benth. Ref: 5.

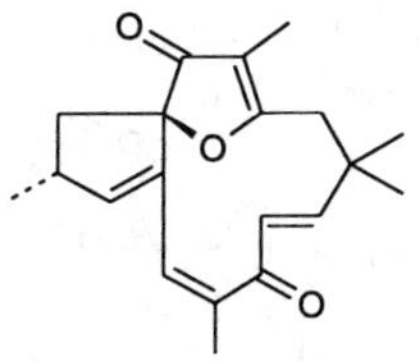

3638 Jatrorrhizine
Jateorrhizine; Neprotin; Yatrorizine. CAS: 3621-38-3 $C_{20}H_{20}NO_4$ MW: 338.39 Source: FANG JI, HE NAN TANG SONG CAO, HUANG BAI, HUANG LIAN. Ref: 2, 4, 537.

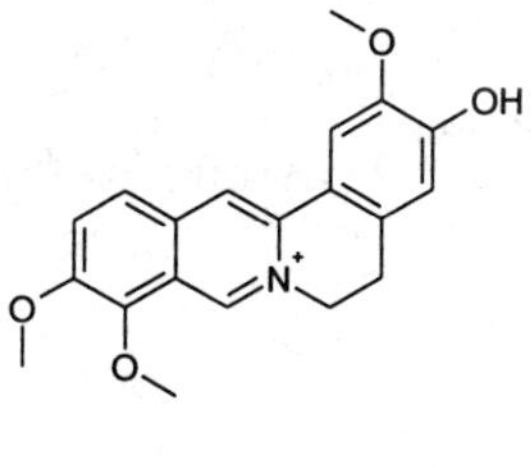

3639 Javanicin
$C_{23}H_{26}O_{12}$ MW: 494.46 Source: YA DAN ZI. Ref: 2.

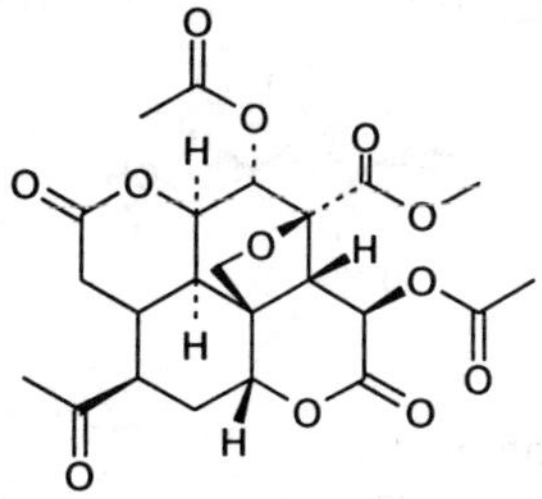

3640 Jervine
$C_{27}H_{39}NO_3$ MW: 425.62 Property: mp 237-8°C. Source: LI LU. Ref: 6.

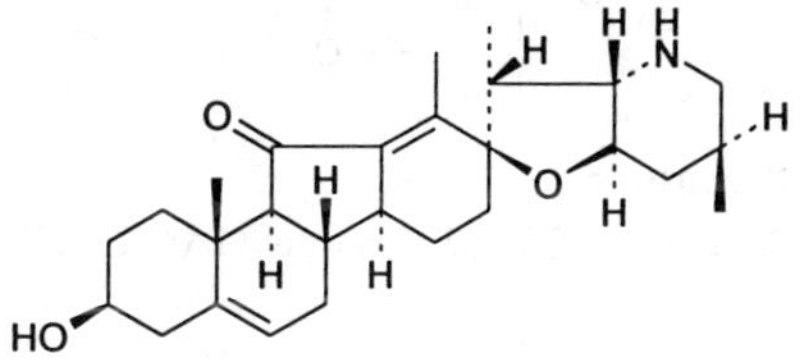

3641 Jinkoheremol
$C_{15}H_{26}O$ MW: 222.37 Source: BAI MU XIANG, CHEN XIANG. Ref: 13.

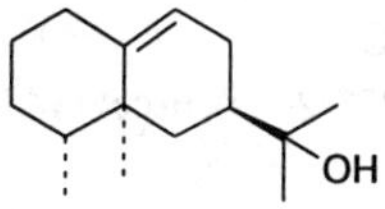

3642 Jinkohol
$C_{15}H_{26}O$ MW: 222.37 Source: CHEN XIANG. Ref: 13.

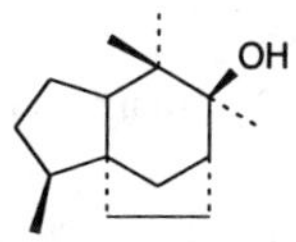

3643 Jinkohol II
$C_{15}H_{26}O$ MW: 222.37 Source: CHEN XIANG. Ref: 13.

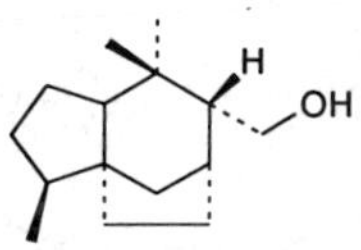

3644 Jiofuran
$C_9H_{12}O_4$ MW: 184.19 Source: GAN DI HUANG.
Ref: 2.

3645 Jioglutin A
$C_{10}H_{15}ClO_5$ MW: 250.68 Source: GAN DI HUANG.
Ref: 2.

3646 Jioglutin B
$C_{10}H_{15}ClO_5$ MW: 250.68 Source: GAN DI HUANG.
Ref: 2.

3647 Jioglutin C
$C_{10}H_{16}O_6$ MW: 232.24 Source: GAN DI HUANG.
Ref: 2.

3648 Jioglutin D
$C_{10}H_{16}O_5$ MW: 216.24 Source: GAN DI HUANG.
Ref: 2.

3649 Jioglutin E
$C_{11}H_{20}O_5$ MW: 232.28 Source: GAN DI HUANG.
Ref: 2.

3650 Jioglutolide
$C_9H_{14}O_4$ MW: 186.21 Source: GAN DI HUANG.
Ref: 2.

3651 Jioglutoside A
Source: GAN DI HUANG. Ref: 2.

3652 Jioglutoside B
Source: GAN DI HUANG. Ref: 2.

3653 Jionoside
$C_{22}H_{34}O_{12}$ MW: 490.51 Source: GAN DI HUANG.
Ref: 2.

3654 Jionoside A1
Source: GAN DI HUANG. Ref: 2.

3655 Jionoside A2
Source: GAN DI HUANG. Ref: 2.

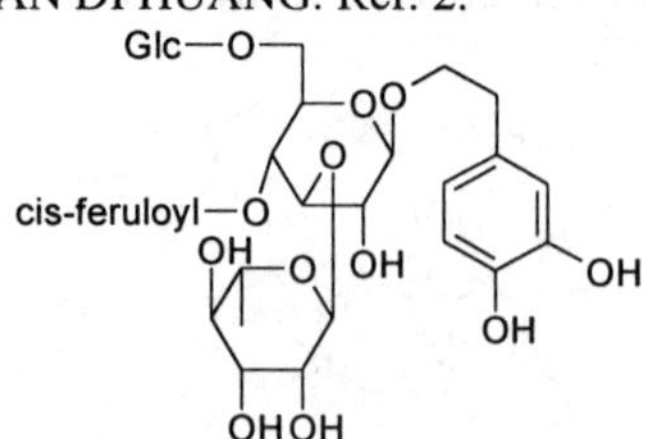

3656 Jionoside B1

Source: GAN DI HUANG. Ref: 2.

Glc—O trans-feruloyl—O O OH OH OH OH OH O

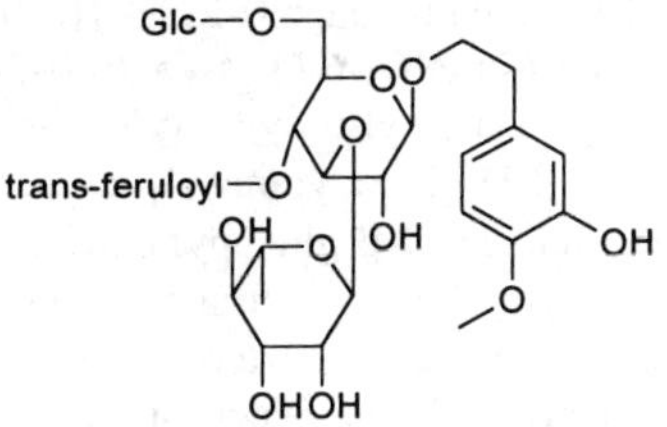

3657 Jionoside B2

Source: GAN DI HUANG. Ref: 2.

Glc—O cis-feruloyl—O O OH OH OH OH OH O

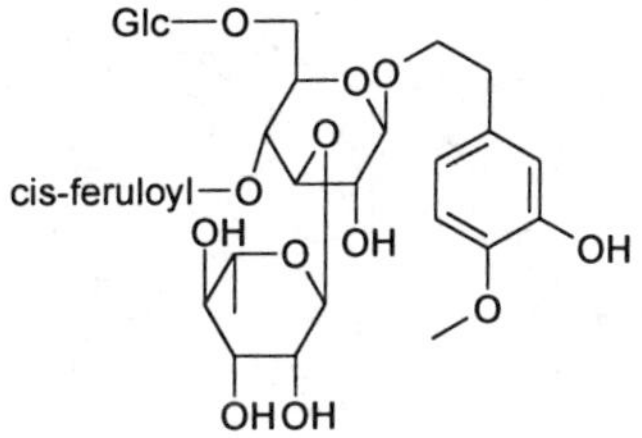

3658 Jionoside C

$C_{29}H_{36}O_{13}$ MW: 592.60 Source: GAN DI HUANG. Ref: 2.

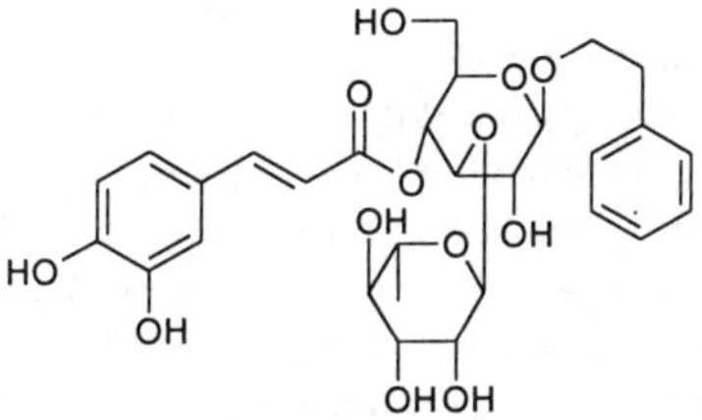

3659 Jionoside D

$C_{30}H_{38}O_{15}$ MW: 638.63 Source: GAN DI HUANG. Ref: 2.

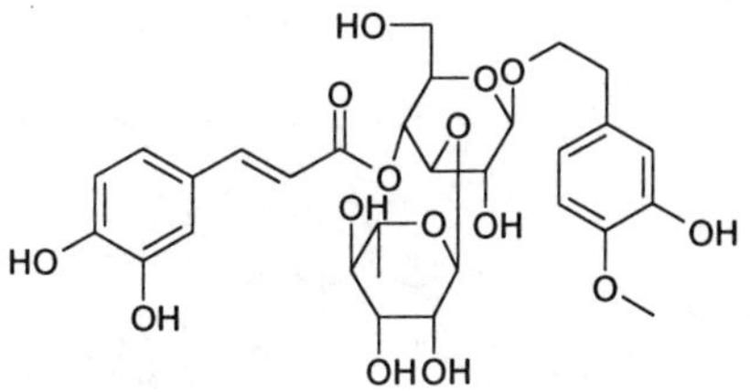

3660 Jolkinolide E

Property: mp 181-2°C. Source: DA LANG DU. Ref: 547.

3661 Juglanin

Kaempferol-arabinoside. $C_{20}H_{18}O_{10}$ MW: 418.36 Property: mp 224-5°C (containing1.5H_2O) Source: HU TAO YE, HUI XIANG JING YE, TOU GU CAO. Ref: 6.

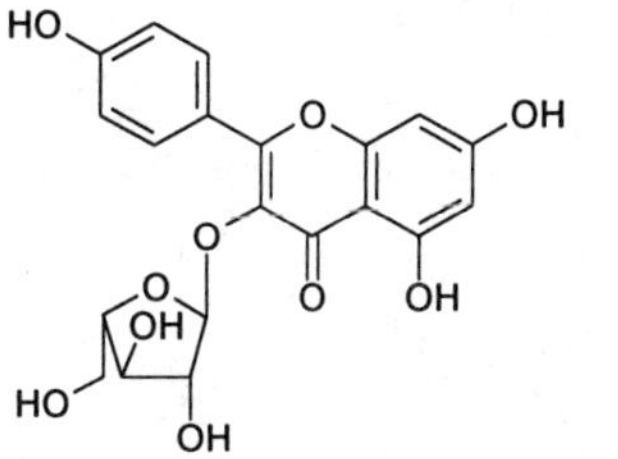

3662 Juglone

Yuglon. CAS: 481-39-0 $C_{10}H_6O_3$ MW: 174.16 Property: mp 153-5°C. Source: HU TAO REN. Ref: 5.

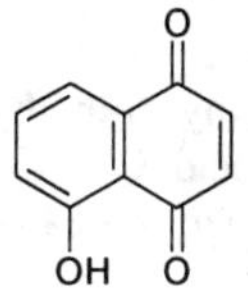

3663 Jujubogenin

$C_{30}H_{48}O_4$ MW: 472.71 Source: SUAN ZAO REN. Ref: 2.

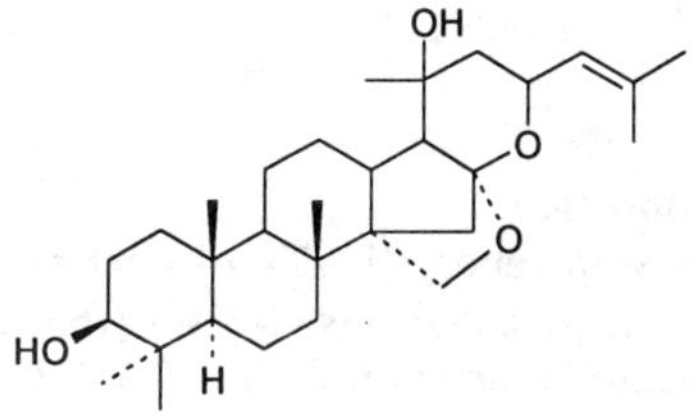

3664 Jujuboside A

$C_{58}H_{94}O_{26}$ MW: 1207.38 Source: DA ZAO, SUAN ZAO REN. Ref: 2.

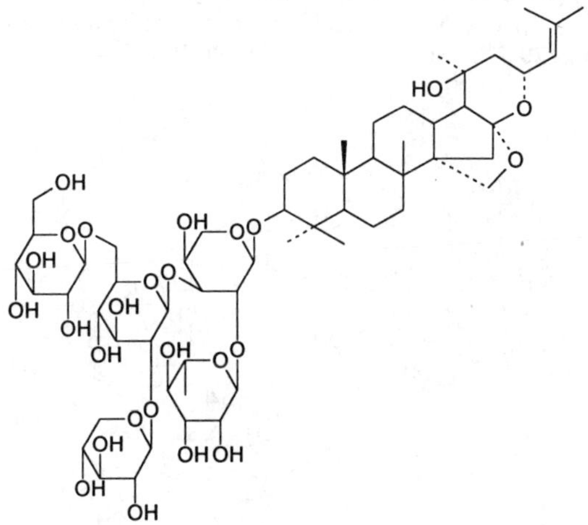

3665 Jujuboside B
$C_{52}H_{84}O_{21}$ MW: 1045.24 Source: DA ZAO, SUAN ZAO REN. Ref: 2.

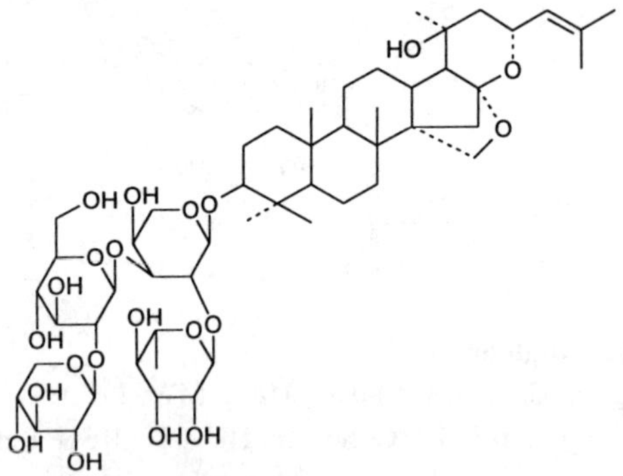

3666 Julibrogenin A
21-O-(2-Hydroxymethyl-6-methyl-6-methoxy-2,7-octadienoyl)-acacic acid. $C_{41}H_{64}O_8$ MW: 684.96 Property: white powder, mp 244-6 °C. Source: HE HUA PI. Ref: 375.

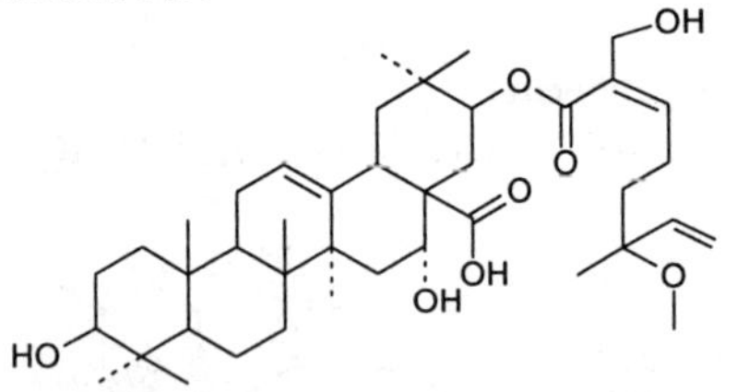

3667 Julibroside
3-O-[β-D-xylopyranosyl(1→2)-α-L-arabinopyranosyl(1→6)-β-D-glucopyranosyl]-21-O-{(6S)-2-trans-2-hydroxymethyl-6-methyl-6-O-[4-O-((6S)-2-trans-2,6-dimethyl-6-O-(6-deoxy-β-D-glucopyranosyl)-2,7-octadienoyl)-6-deoxy-β-D-glucopyranosyl]-2,7-octadienoyl}-acacic acid 28-O-β-glucopyransyl (1→3)-α-L-arabinofuranosyl(1→4)]-α-L- rhamnnopyranosyl(1→2)-β-D-glucopyranosyl ester. $C_{101}H_{160}O_{49}$ MW: 2158.37 Property: white powder, mp170-2 °C. Source: HE HUAN PI. Ref: 374.

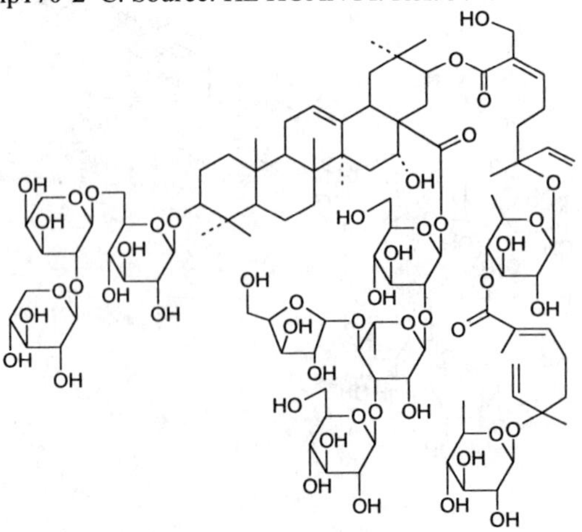

3668 Julibroside J2
3-O-[β-D-xylopyranosyl(1→2)-α-L-arabinopyranosyl(1→6)-β-D-glucopyranosyl]-21-O-{(6S)-2-trans-2-hydroxymethyl-6-methyl-6-O-[4-O-((6S)-2-trans-2-hydroxymethyl-6-methyl-6-hydroxyl-2,7-octadienoyl)-6-deoxy-β-D-glucopyranosyl]-2,-7-octadienoyl}-acacic acid 28-O-β-glucopyransyl(1→3)-α-L-arabinofuranosyl(1→4)]-α-L- rhamnnopyransyl (1→2)-β-D-glucopyranosyl ester. $C_{95}H_{150}O_{46}$ MW: 2028.23 Property: white powder, mp 202-4°C. Source: HE HUAN PI. Ref: 374.

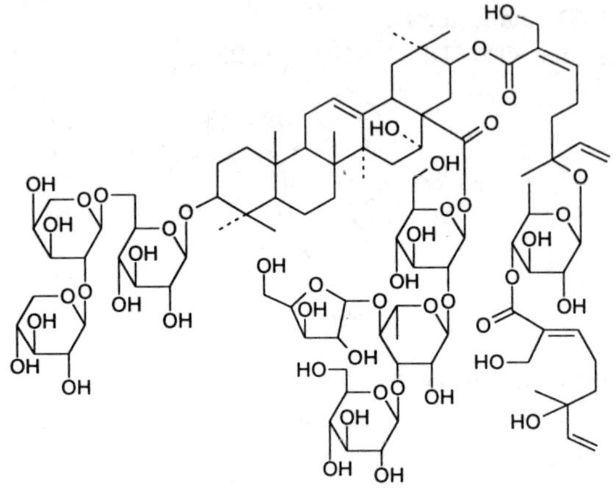

3669 Julibroside J3
3-O-[β-D-xylopyranosyl(1→2)-α-L-arabinopyranosyl(1→6)-2-acetamido-2-deoxy-β-D-glucopyranosyl] -21-O-{(6S)-2-trans-2-hydroxymethyl-6-methyl-6-O-[4-O-((6S)-2-trans-2,6-dimethyl-6-O-(6-deoxy-β-D-glucopyranosyl)-2,7-octadienoyl)-6-deoxy-β-D-glucopyranosyl]-2,-7-octadienoyl}-acacic acid 28-O-β-glucopyransyl(1→3)-α-L-arabinofuranosyl(1→4)]-α-L-rhamnnopyransyl(1→2)-β-D-glucopyranosyl ester. $C_{103}H_{163}O_{49}$ MW: 2199.42 Property: white powder, mp 204-6 °C. Source: HE HUAN PI. Ref: 374.

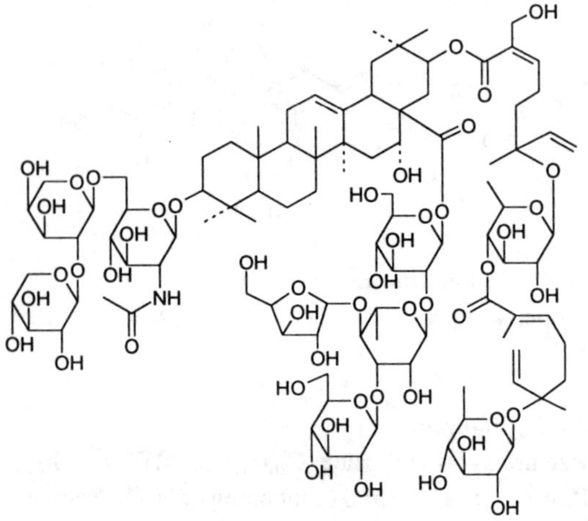

3670 Jurubine

$C_{33}H_{57}NO_8$ MW: 595.82 Source: SHUI QIE. Ref: 6.

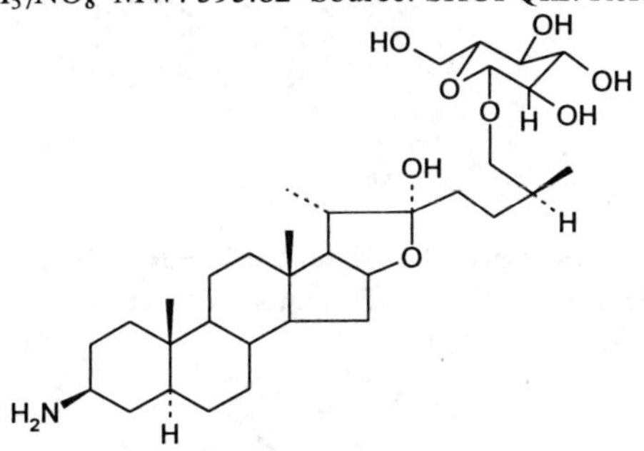

3671 Justicidin A

$C_{22}H_{18}O_7$ MW: 394.38 Property: mp 263°C. Source: JUE CHUANG. Ref: 6.

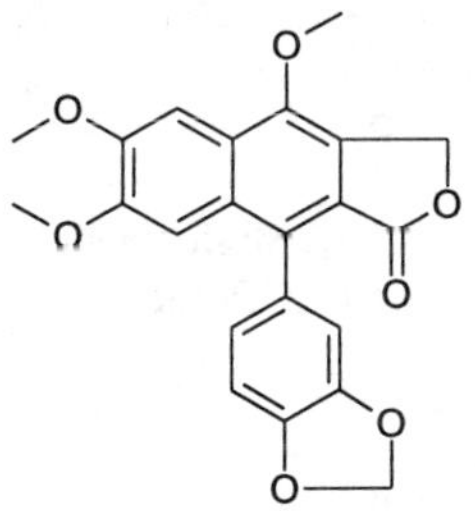

3672 Justicidin B

$C_{21}H_{16}O_6$ MW: 364.36 Property: mp 240°C. Source: JUE CHUANG. Ref: 6.

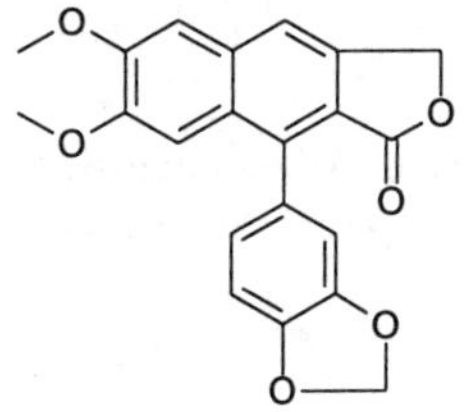

3673 Justicidin C

$C_{22}H_{18}O_7$ MW: 394.38 Property: mp 266°C. Source: JUE CHUANG. Ref: 6.

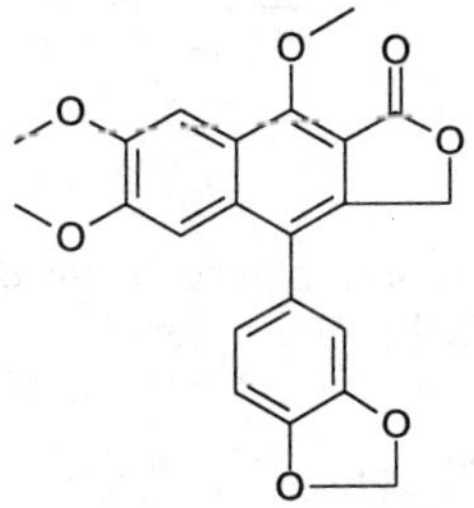

3674 Justicidin D

$C_{21}H_{14}O_7$ MW: 378.34 Property: mp 272°C. Source: JUE CHUANG. Ref: 6.

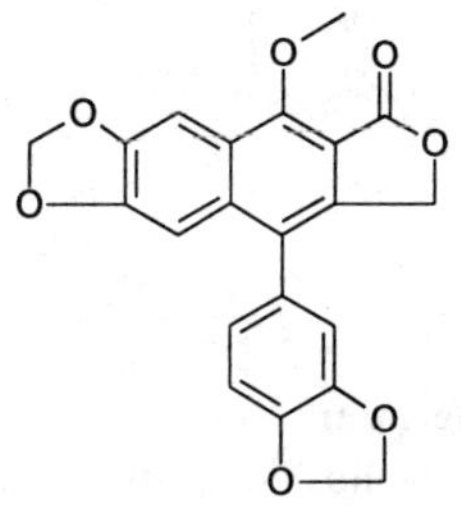

3675 Juzirine

Source: SUAN ZAO REN. Ref: 583.

3676 Juzunal

$C_{16}H_{10}O_6$ MW: 298.25 Property: mp 248°C. Source: HU CI. Ref: 6.

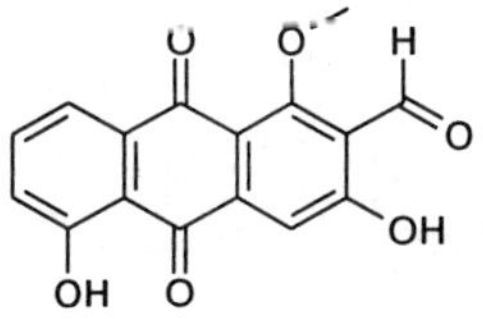

3677 Kadsulactone acid

$C_{30}H_{44}O_4$ MW: 468.68 Property: colorless massive crystal, mp 180-2°C. Source: CHANG GENG NAN WU WE IZI. Ref: 389.

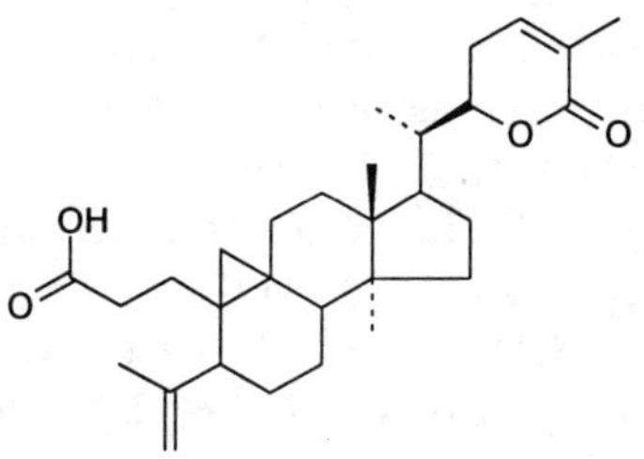

3678 Kadsurenin M

$C_{19}H_{20}O_5$ MW: 328.37 Property: colorless oleaginous substance, $[\alpha]_D^{15}$ -24.6° ($CHCl_3$). Source: HAN FENG TENG. Ref: 267.

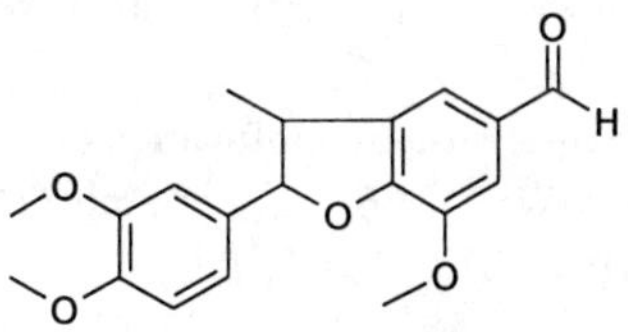

3679 Kaempferide
$C_{16}H_{12}O_6$ MW: 300.27 Property: mp 227-9°C.
Source: SHAN NAI, GAO LIANG JIANG. Ref: 6.

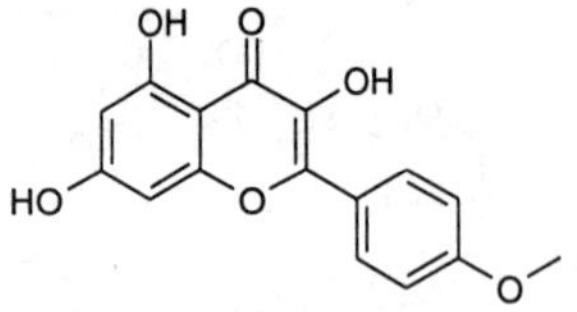

3680 Kaempferitrin
Kaempferol dirhamnoside; Lespenephryl; Lespidin.
CAS: 482-38-2 $C_{27}H_{30}O_{14}$ MW: 578.53 Property: mp 201-3°C. Source: CHAI HU, LAO GUAN CAO, MIAN TENG, SHAN MA HUANG, WAN SHOU JU YE, WANG GUA, YIN YANG HUO. Ref: 4, 6, 623.

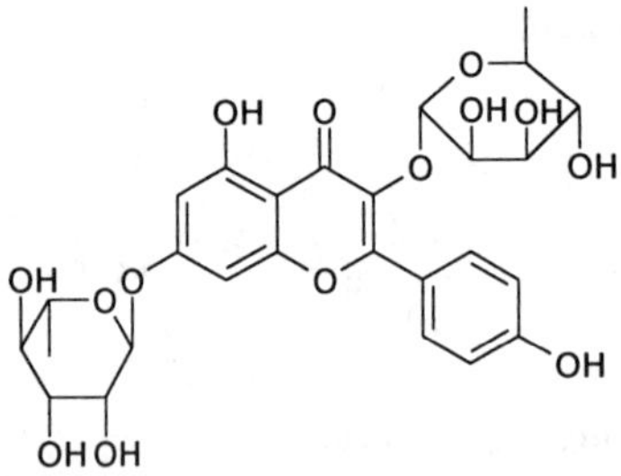

3681 Kaempferol
4H-1-Benzopyran-4-one,3,5,7-trihydroxy-2-(4-hydroxy-phenyl). $C_{15}H_{10}O_{16}$ MW: 286.24 Property: yellow acicular crystal (methanol), mp 274-8°C. Source: BAI GUO, CU LIU GUO (SHA JI), DA JIN QIAN CAO, DU ZHONG, FENG JIAO, MU ZEI, NAN FANG TU SI ZI, QING HAO, REN SHEN, SAN LING, SHAN HE YE, SHAN YE WAN DOU, SHE PU TAO, YE XIA ZHU. Ref: 2, 4, 279, 283, 397, 463, 468, 552, 573.

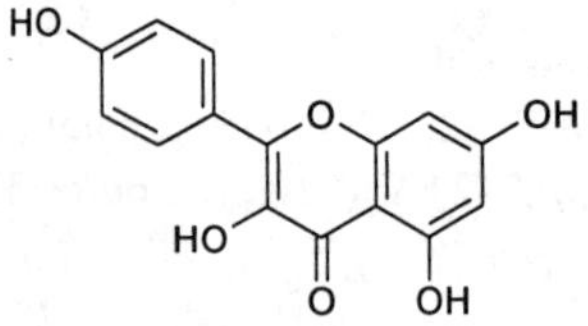

3682 Kaempferol-3-arabofuranoside
$C_{20}H_{18}O_{10}$ MW: 418.36 Property: mp 224-5°C.
Source: ZHEN ZHU MEI. Ref: 6.

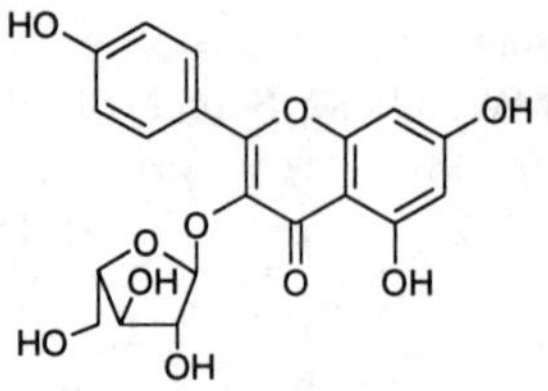

3683 Kaempferol-3-diglucose-7-glucoside
$C_{33}H_{40}O_{21}$ MW: 727.67 Source: MU ZEI.
Ref: 2.

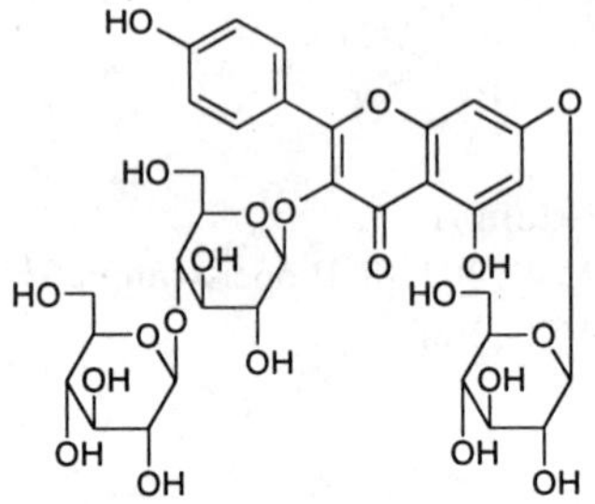

3684 Kaempferol-3,7-diglucoside
$C_{27}H_{30}O_{16}$ MW: 610.53 Property: mp 233°C. Source: MU ZEI. Ref: 2.

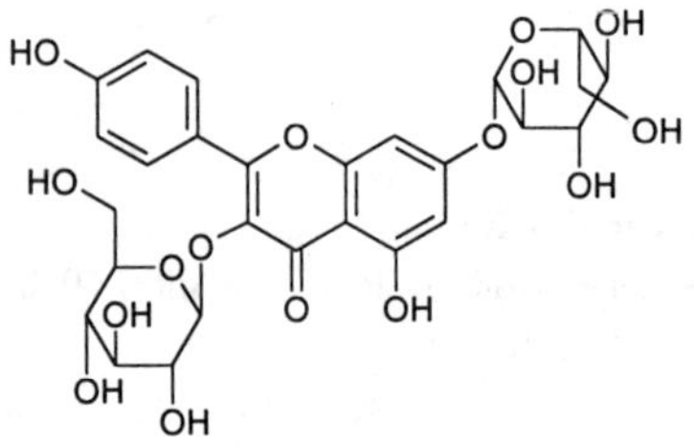

3685 Kaempferol-3-O-galactoside
$C_{21}H_{20}O_{11}$ MW: 448.39 Source: DA JIN QIAN CAO. Ref: 2.

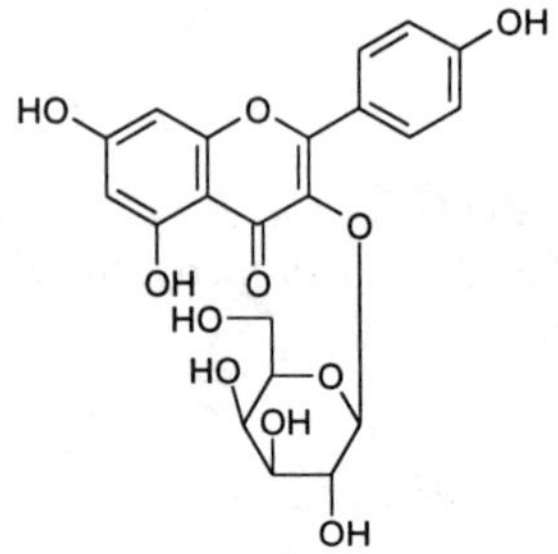

3686 Kaempferol-3-glucogalactoside
Source: YIN CHEN HAO. Ref: 2.

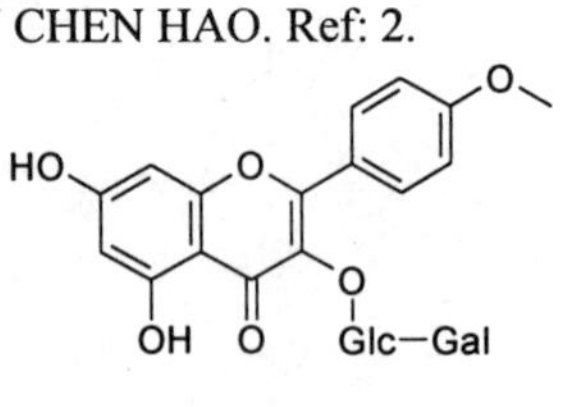

3687 Kaempferol-3-β-D-(2-O-β-D-glucopyranosidoglucopyranoside)-7-β-D-glucopyranoside
Source: MU ZEI. Ref: 2.

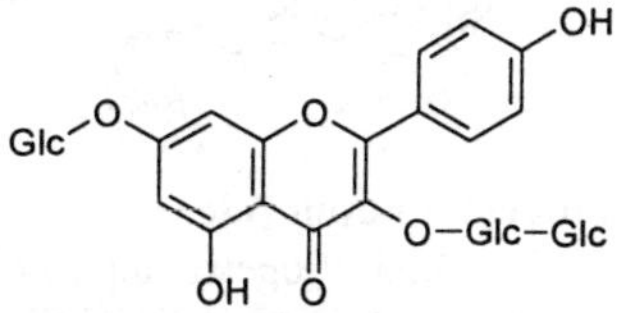

3688 Kaempferol-3-β-D-gluco-7-α-L-rhamnoside
$C_{27}H_{30}O_{15}$ MW: 594.53 Property: mp 249-51°C. Source: NAN SHE TENG YE. Ref: 6.

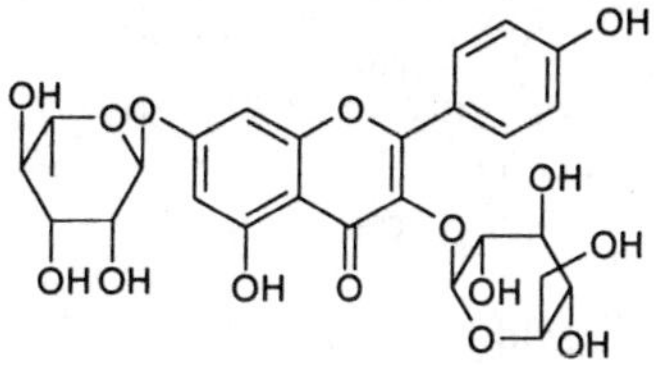

3689 Kaempferol-3-β-D-gluco-7-β-L-rhamnoside
$C_{27}H_{30}O_{15}$ MW: 594.53 Source: TIAO JING CAO. Ref: 6.

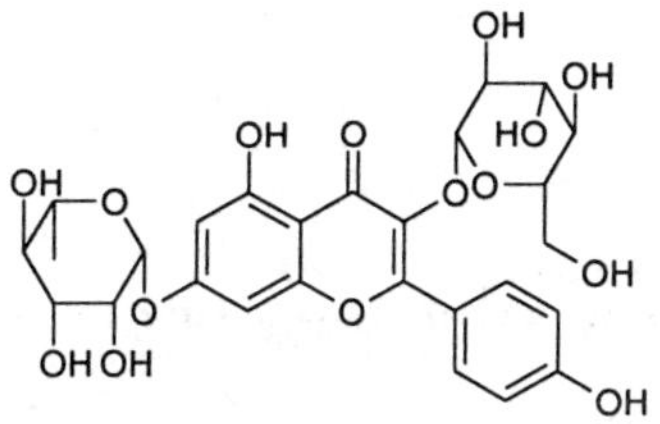

3690 Kaempferol-3-glucose-7-diglucoside
$C_{33}H_{40}O_{21}$ MW: 727.67 Source: MU ZEI. Ref: 2.

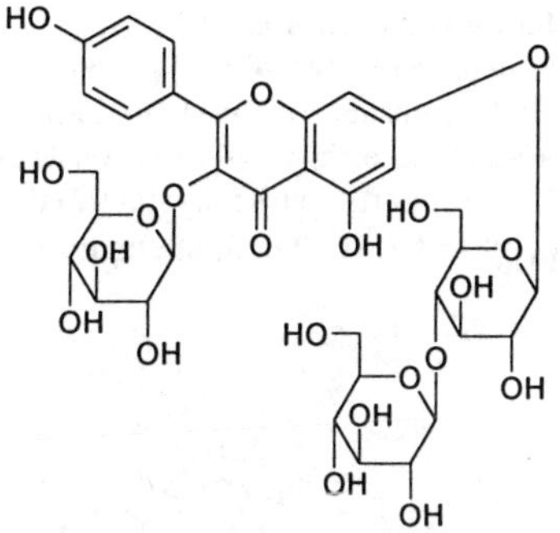

3691 Kaempferol-3-O-glucoside
Astragalin. $C_{21}H_{20}O_{11}$ MW: 448.39 Property: mp 178°C. Source: CU LIU GUO (SHA JI), GAN CAO, NAN FANG TU SI ZI, QING HAO. Ref: 2, 231, 468.

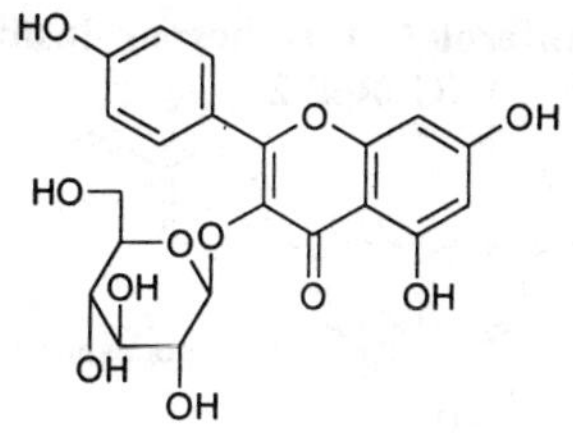

3692 Kaempferol-3-glucoside-7-rhamnoside
$C_{27}H_{30}O_{15}$ MW: 594.53 Property: mp 231-4°C. Source: CAN DOU YE. Ref: 6.

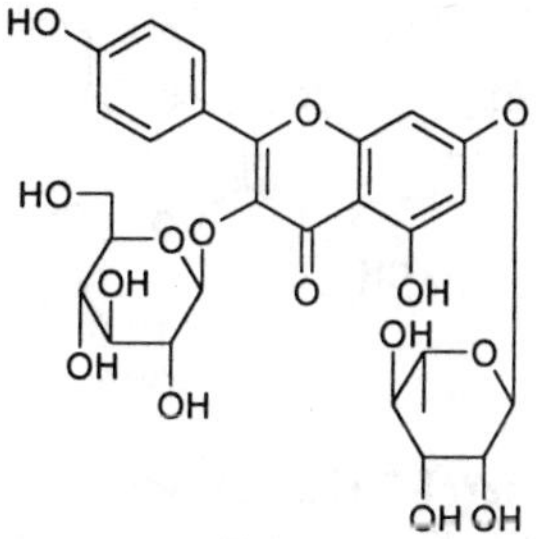

3693 Kaempferol-3-β-D-glucuronide
$C_{21}H_{18}O_{12}$ MW: 462.37 Property: mp 189-90.5°C. Source: JI CHANG LANG DU. Ref: 6.

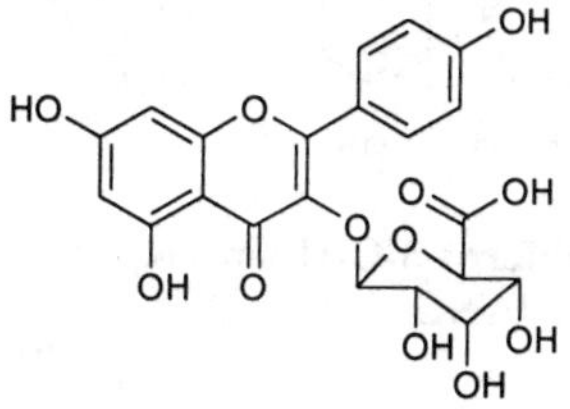

3694 Kaempferol-3-O-lysimachiatrioside
$C_{35}H_{40}O_{19}$ MW: 764.70 Source: DA JIN QIAN CAO. Ref: 2.

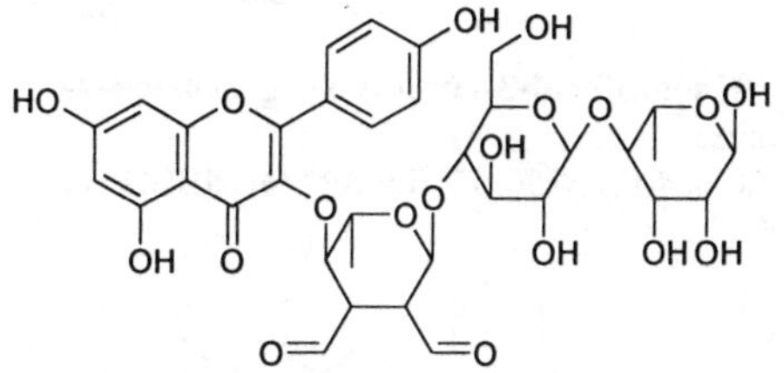

3695 Kaempferol-7-monomethyl ether
$C_{27}H_{12}O_6$ MW: 300.27 Source: NING MENG AN YE. Ref: 6.

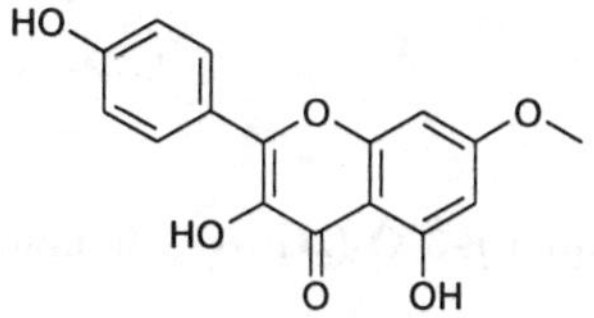

3696 Kaempferol-3-O-neohesperidoside
Source: PU HUANG. Ref: 2.

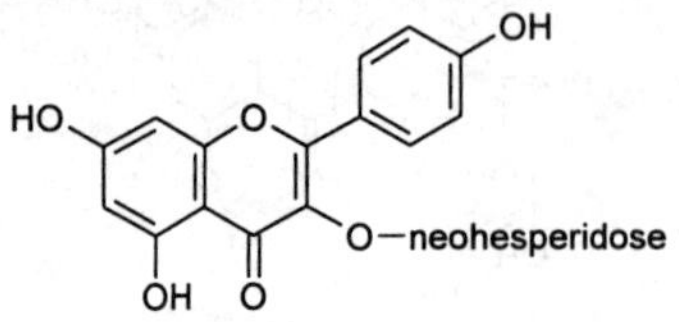

3697 Kaempferol rhamnoside
$C_{21}H_{20}O_{10}$ MW: 432.39 Source: BAI GUO YE, MA HUANG. Ref: 2, 603.

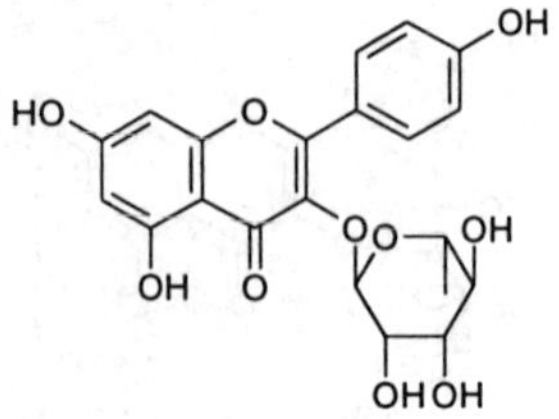

3698 Kaempferol-7-rhamnoside
$C_{21}H_{20}O_{10}$ MW: 432.39 Property: mp 239-42°C. Source: NAN SHE TENG YE, TU JING JIE. Ref: 6.

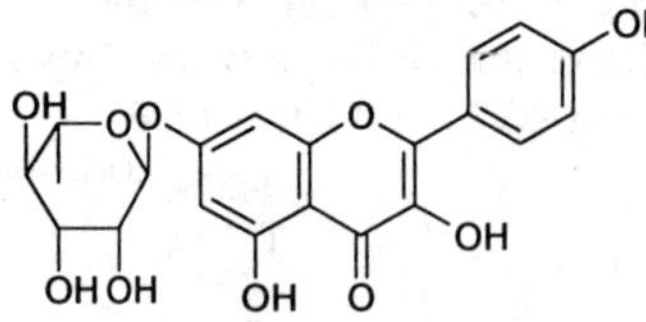

3699 Kaempferol-3-O-rhamnosylglucoside
Source: PU HUANG. Ref: 2.

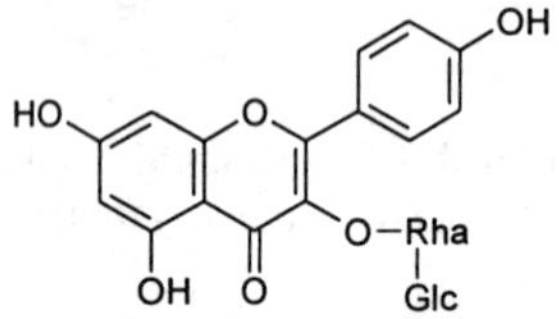

3700 Kaempferol-3-rhamnosyl glucoside-7-glucoside
$C_{33}H_{40}O_{20}$ MW: 756.67 Source: GU JIE CAO. Ref: 6.

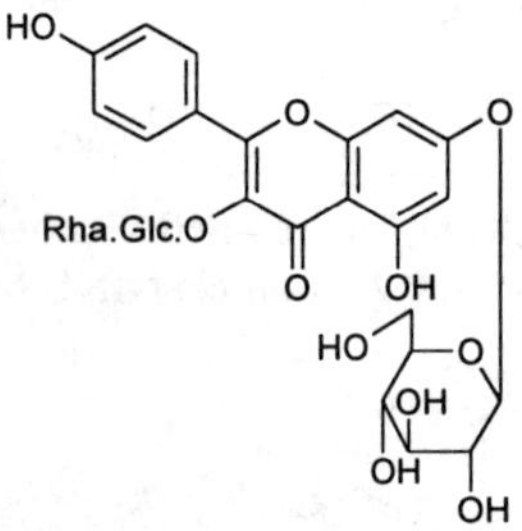

3701 Kaempferol-3-O-(2G-α-L-rhamnosyl)-rutinoside
Source: PU HUANG. Ref: 2.

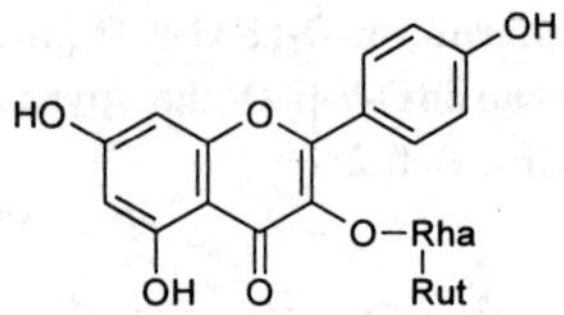

3702 Kaempferol-3-rutinoside
$C_{27}H_{30}O_{15}$ MW: 594.53 Property: mp 224°C. Source: BI MA YE, CI JI LI, JIN BIAN LONG SHE LAN. Ref: 6.

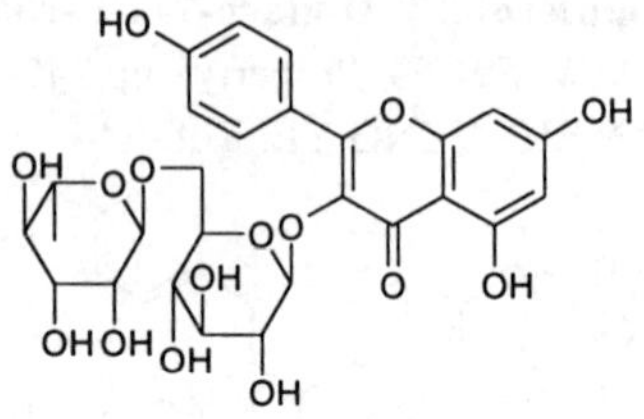

3703 Kainic acid
L-α-Kainic acid. $C_{10}H_{15}NO_4$ MW: 213.24 Property: mp 253-4°C (dec). Source: HAI REN CAO, ZHE GU CAI. Ref: 6.

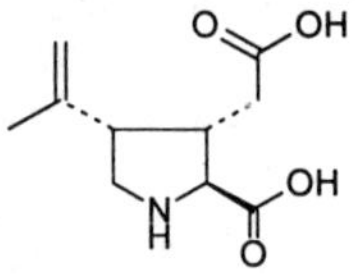

3704 Kakkonein
$C_{20}H_{18}O_5$ MW: 338.36 Source: GE GEN. Ref: 2.

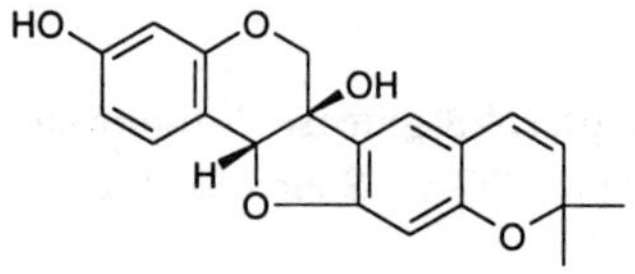

3705 Kalopanax saponin C
3-O-[α-L-rhamnopyranosyl-(1→2)-α-L-arabinopyra-nosyl]-hedragenin-28-[α-L-rhamnopyranosyl-(1→2)-β-D-glucopy-ranosyl(1→6)-β-D-glucopyranosyl] ester. $C_{59}H_{96}O_{26}$ MW: 1221.41 Property: white crystal (methanol), mp 226-8°C, $[\alpha]_D^{14}$ +14.2° (c=0.005, methanol). Source: CI QIU.
Ref: 148.

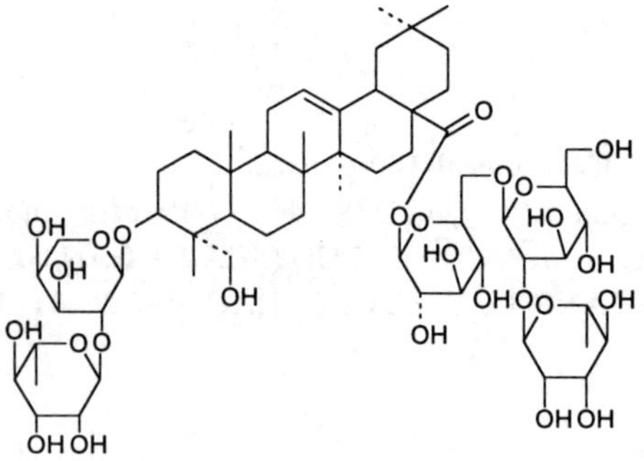

3706 Kalopanax saponin G
$C_{53}H_{84}O_{23}$ MW: 1089.25 Property: white powder, $[\alpha]_D^{20}$ +16.4° (c=0.67, H_2O). Source: CI QIU. Ref: 457.

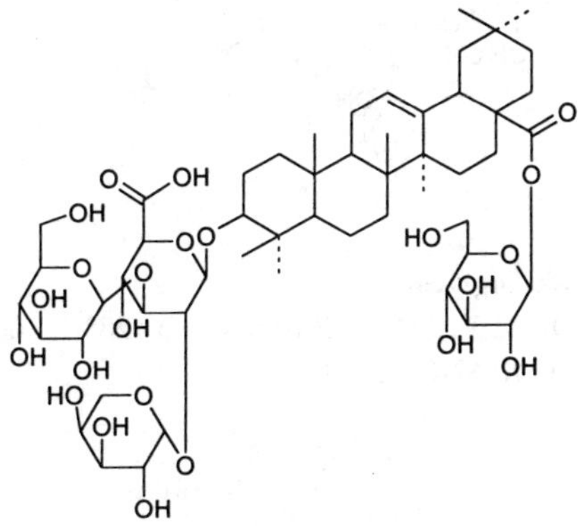

3707 Kalopanax saponin H
$C_{47}H_{76}O_{17}$ MW: 913.12 Property: white powdere, $[\alpha]_D^{20}$ +8.6° (c=0.5, methanol). Source: CI QIU. Ref: 457.

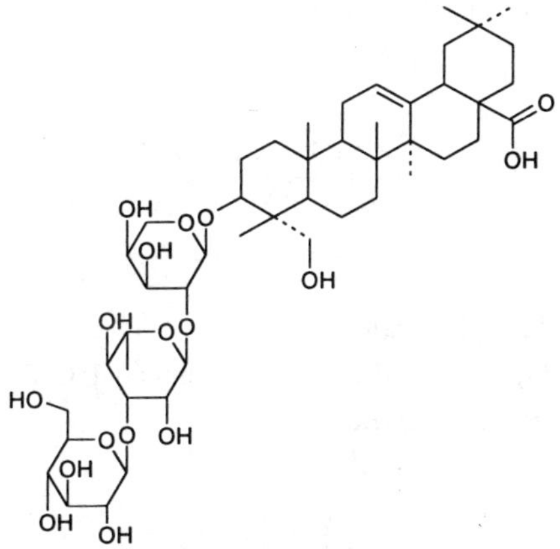

3708 Kalopanax septemlobus asponin A
$C_{41}H_{66}O_{12}$ MW: 750.98 Property: mp 228-30°C. Source: CI QIU SHU PI. Ref: 6.

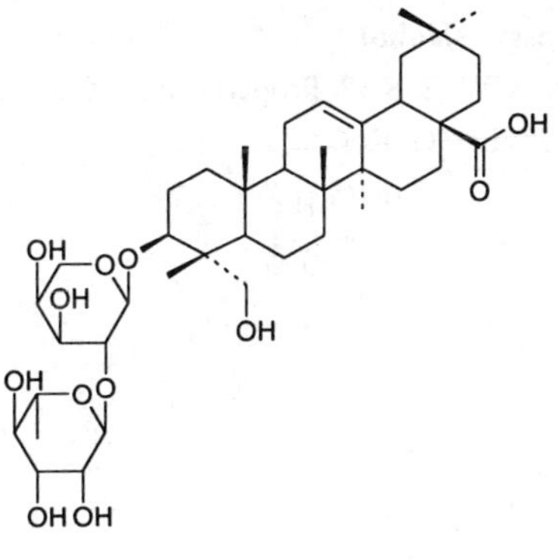

3709 Kamogenin
$C_{27}H_{40}O_5$ MW: 444.62 Property: mp 240-1°C. Source: JIN BIAN LONG SHE LAN. Ref: 6.

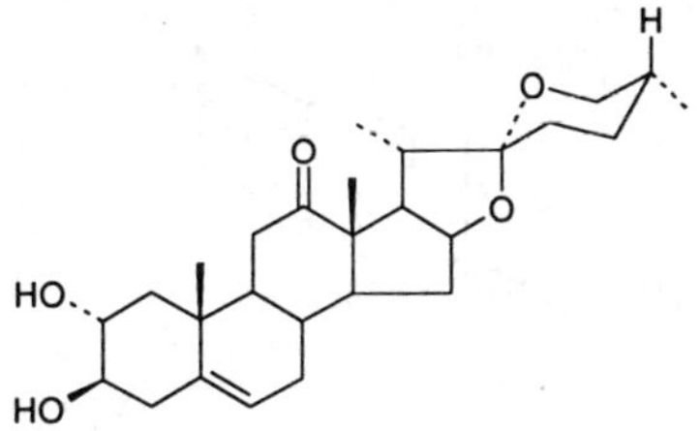

3710 Karacolidine
$C_{23}H_{39}NO_5$ MW: 409.57 Source: CAO WU TOU. Ref: 6.

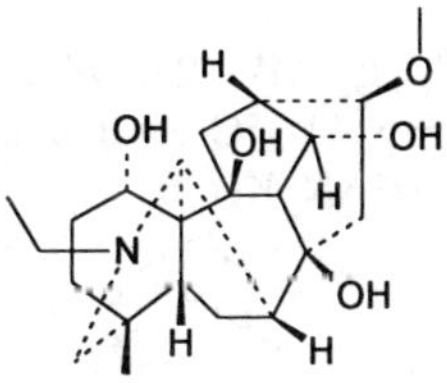

3711 Karacoline
$C_{22}H_{35}NO_4$ MW: 377.53 Source: CAO WU TOU, HUANG CAO WU TOU JIAN. Ref: 6, 239.

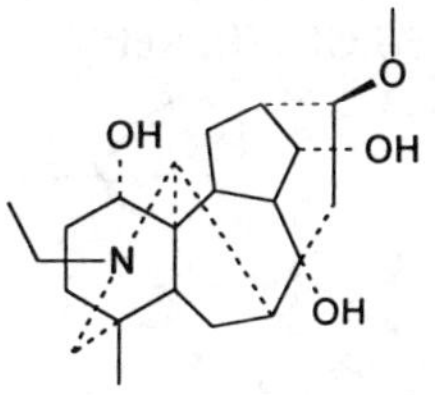

3712 Karajin
$C_{18}H_{12}O_4$ MW: 292.29 Property: mp 158.5°C. Source: SHUI LIU DOU. Ref: 6.

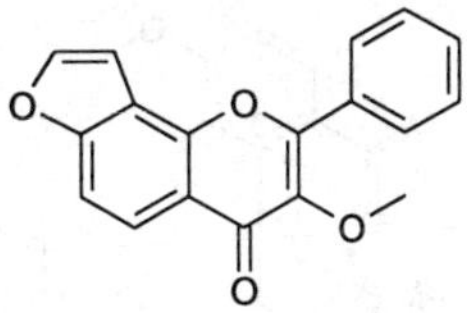

3713 (+)-Karanone
$C_{15}H_{20}O$ MW: 216.33 Source: CHEN XIANG. Ref: 13.

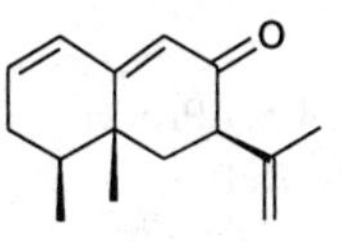

3714 Karounidiol

$C_{30}H_{48}O_2$ MW: 440.72 Source: GUA LOU. Ref: 2.

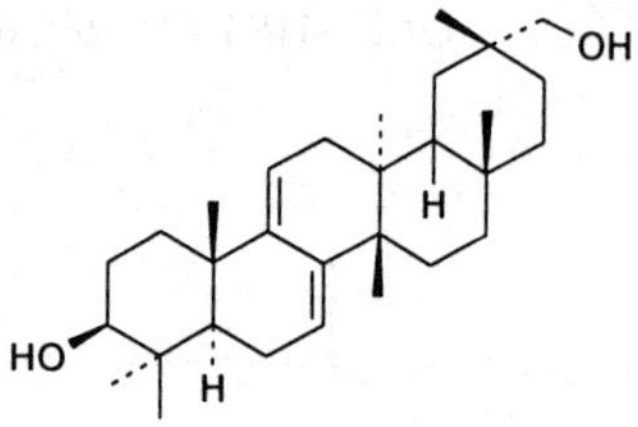

3715 ent-Kauran-16β,17-diol

Property: mp 188-90°C. Source: ZHE BEI MU. Ref: 528.

3716 Kaurene

Podocarprene. $C_{20}H_{32}$ MW: 272.48 Property: mp (+): 49°C, (-): 50°C, (±): 44-7°C. Source: LUO HAN SONG YE, LIU SHAN. Ref: 6.

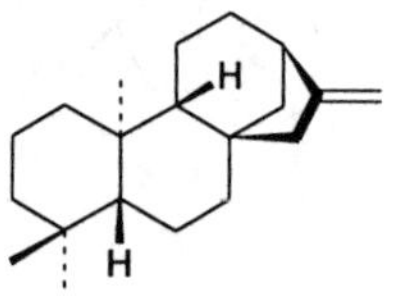

3717 l-Kaur-16-en-19-oic acid

$C_{20}H_{30}O_2$ MW: 302.46 Property: mp 179-81°C. Source: TU DANG GUI (I). Ref: 6.

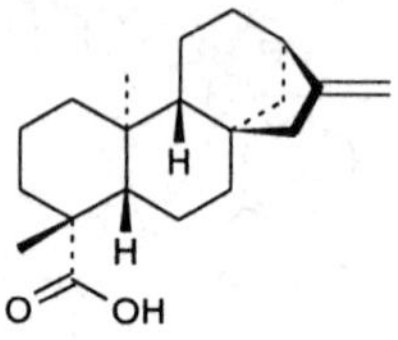

3718 Kayaflavone

$C_{33}H_{24}O_{10}$ MW: 580.55 Property: mp 335°C (dec). Source: LIU SHAN. Ref: 6.

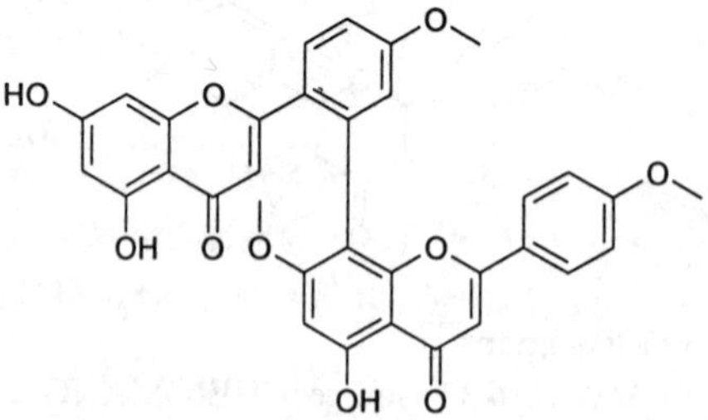

3719 Keioside

$C_{28}H_{32}O_{16}$ MW: 624.56 Property: mp 183-6°C. Source: LING LAN. Ref: 6.

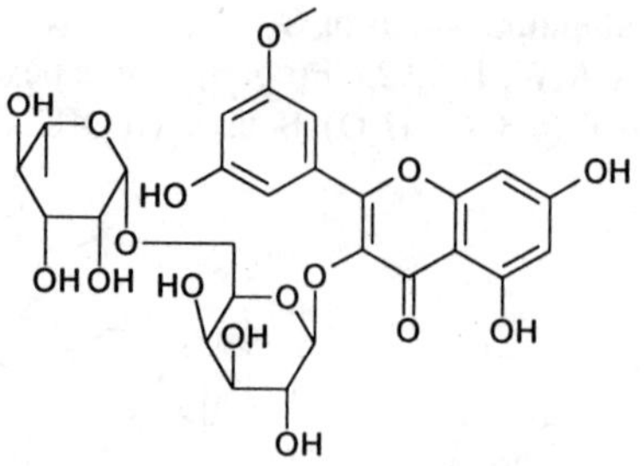

3720 Kessoglycol

$C_{15}H_{26}O_3$ MW: 254.37 Property: mp 128°C. Source: ZHI ZHU XIANG. Ref: 6.

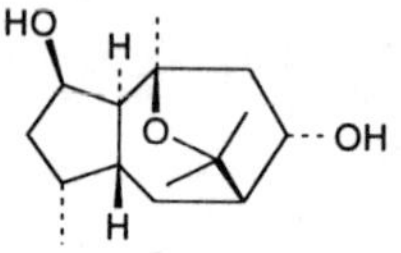

3721 Kessoglycol diacetate

$C_{19}H_{30}O_5$ MW: 338.45 Property: mp 117°C. Source: ZHI ZHU XIANG. Ref: 6.

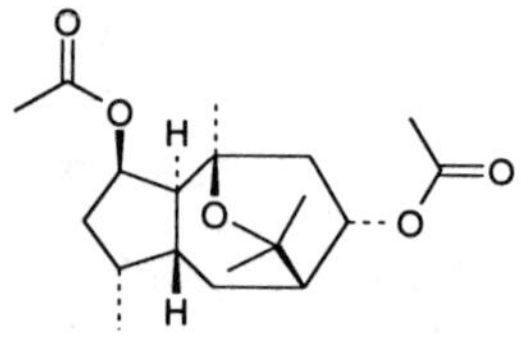

3722 Kessyl acetate

$C_{17}H_{28}O_3$ MW: 280.41 Property: mp 60-1°C. Source: ZHI ZHU XIANG. Ref: 6.

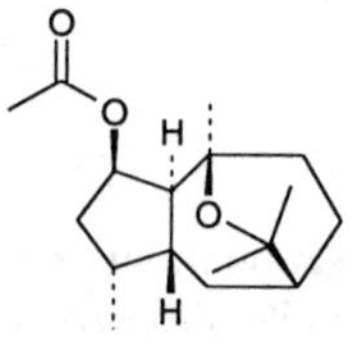

3723 Kessyl alcohol

$C_{15}H_{26}O_2$ MW: 238.37 Property: mp 85°C. Source: ZHI ZHU XIANG. Ref: 6.

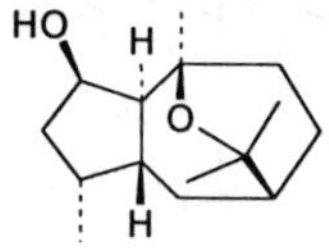

3724 1-Kestose
$C_{18}H_{32}O_{16}$ MW: 504.45 Source: GE CONG. Ref: 6.

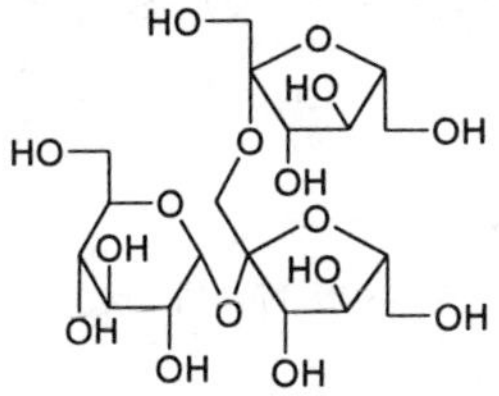

3725 α-Keto-δ-guanidino-valeric acid
$C_6H_{11}N_3O_3$ MW: 173.17 Source: XI SHUAI. Ref: 6.

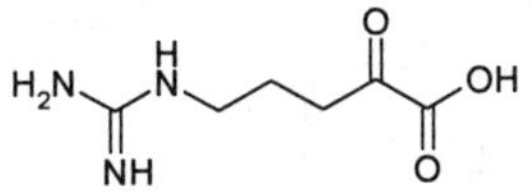

3726 4-Keto-4'-hydroxy-β-carotene
$C_{40}H_{54}O_2$ MW: 566.88 Source: JIN YU. Ref: 6.

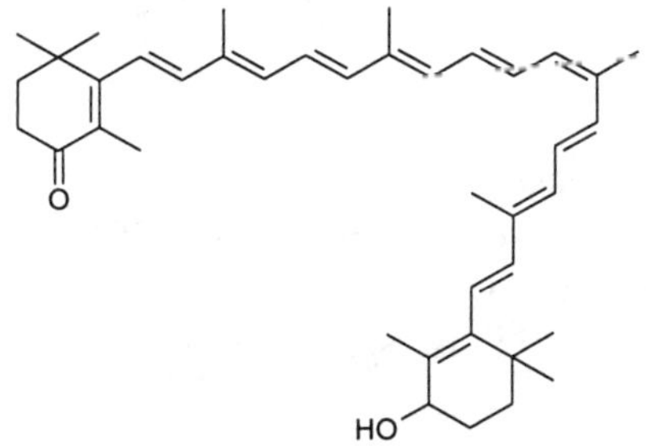

3727 7-Keto-l-pimara-8(14),15-dien-19-oic acid
$C_{20}H_{28}O_3$ MW: 316.44 Property: mp 241-5°C. Source: TU DANG GUI (I). Ref: 6.

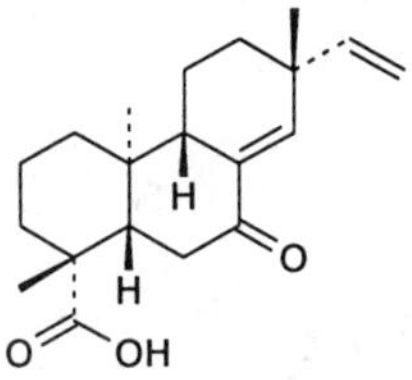

3728 Khellol
$C_{13}H_{10}O_5$ MW: 246.22 Property: mp 176-8°C. Source: YE SHENG MA. Ref: 6.

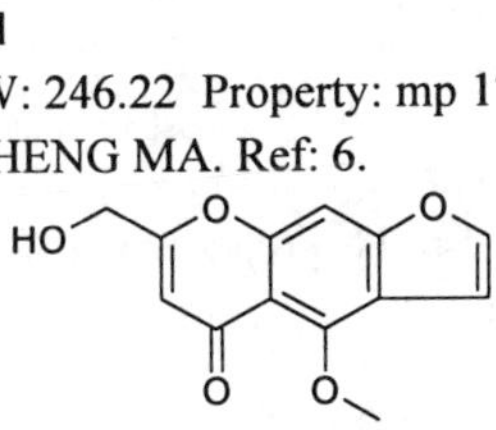

3729 Kidjolanin
$C_{30}H_{38}O_7$ MW: 510.63 Property: mp 148-9°C. Source: BAI SHOU WU. Ref: 6.

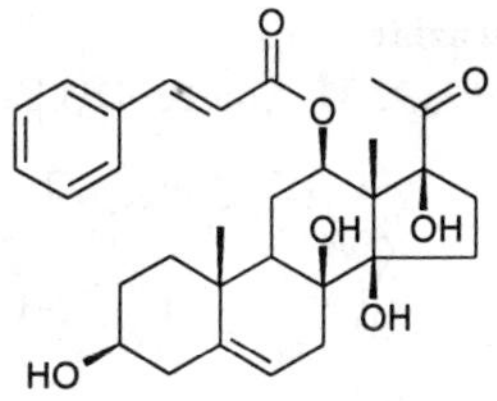

3730 Kikemanine
$C_{20}H_{23}NO_4$ MW: 341.41 Property: mp 177-8°C. Source: JU HUA HUANG LIAN. Ref: 6.

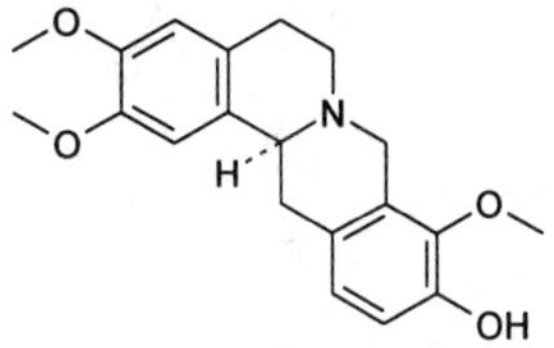

3731 Kinetin
$C_{10}H_9N_5O$ MW: 215.22 Property: mp 266-7°C. Source: BAN LAN GEN. Ref: 6.

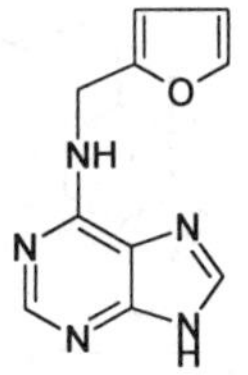

3732 Kirenol
$C_{20}H_{34}O_4$ MW: 338.49 Property: mp 190-2°C. Source: XI XIAN. Ref: 6, 377.

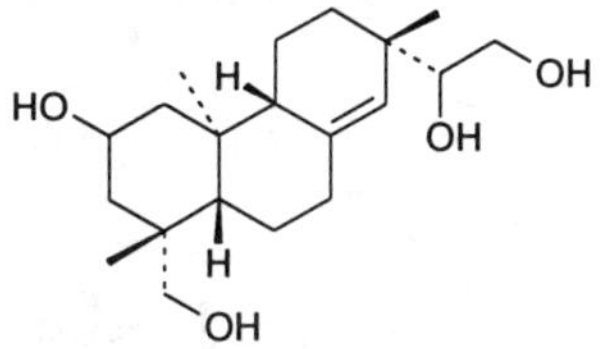

3733 Knoxiadin
1,3,5-Trihydroxy-2-methyl-6-methoxy-anthraquinone. $C_{16}H_{12}O_6$ MW: 300.27 Property: yellow acicular crystal, mp >310°C. Source: HONG YA DA JI. Ref: 35.

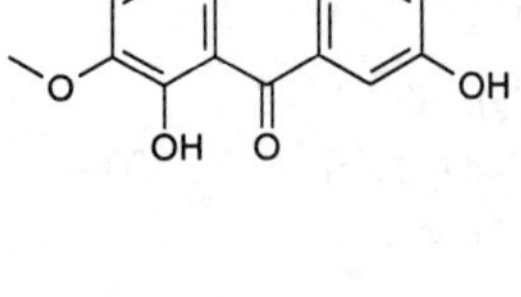

3734 Koaburaside

$C_{14}H_{20}O_9$ MW: 332.31 Source: DU ZHONG. Ref: 2.

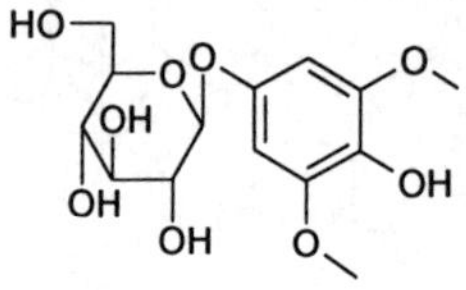

3735 Kobusone

$C_{14}H_{22}O_2$ MW: 222.33 Source: XIANG FU. Ref: 6.

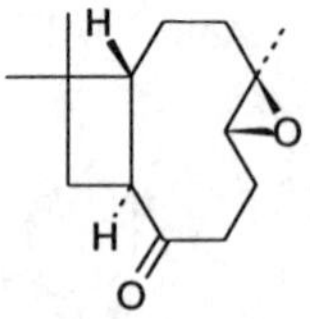

3736 Koelreuteria saponin A

$C_{35}H_{56}O_8$ MW: 604.83 Property: mp 224-6°C (dec). Source: LUAN HUA. Ref: 6.

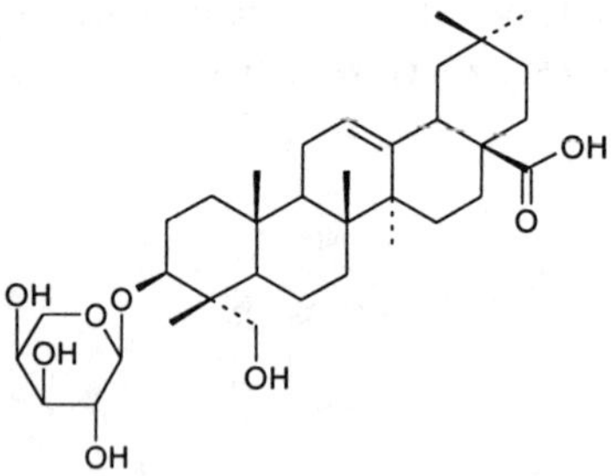

3737 Koelreuteria saponin B

$C_{53}H_{82}O_{23}$ MW: 1087.23 Source: LUAN HUA. Ref: 6.

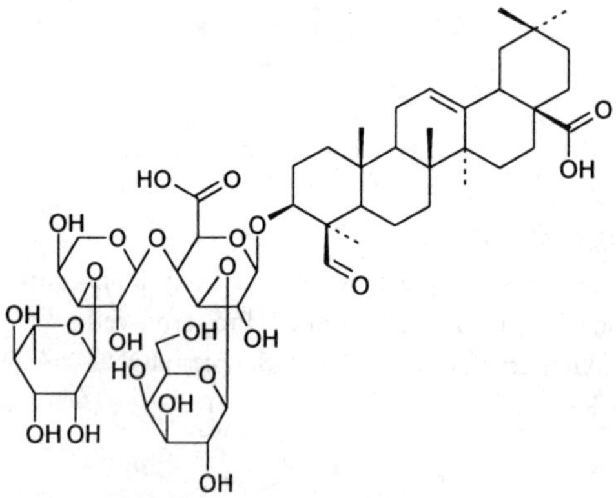

3738 Koenigicine

Koenidine. $C_{20}H_{21}NO_3$ MW: 323.4 Source: YIN DU JIU LI XIANG. Ref: 11.

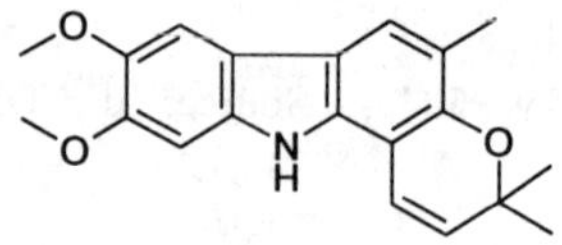

3739 Koenigine

$C_{19}H_{19}NO_3$ MW: 309.37 Source: YIN DU JIU LI XIANG. Ref: 11.

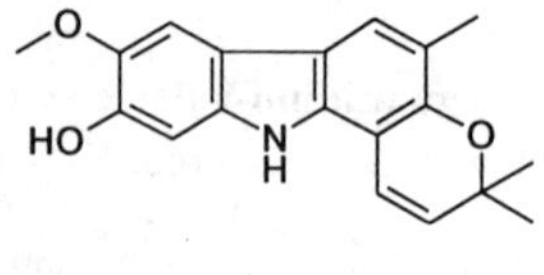

3740 Koenimbin

$C_{18}H_{17}NO_2$ MW: 279.34 Source: YIN DU JIU LI XIANG. Ref: 11.

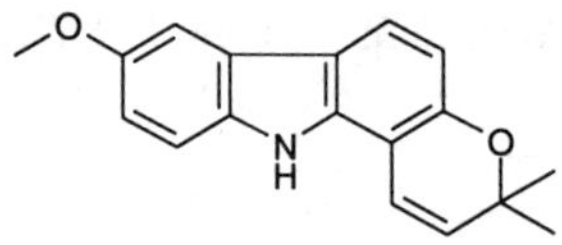

3741 Koenine

$C_{18}H_{17}NO_2$ MW: 279.34 Source: YIN DU JIU LI XIANG. Ref: 11.

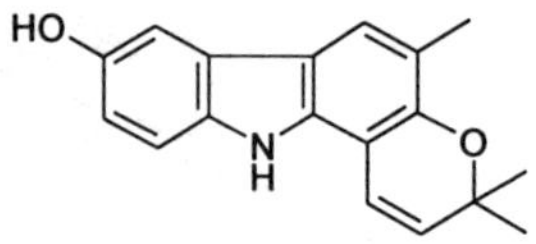

3742 Kogagenin

$C_{27}H_{44}O_6$ MW: 464.65 Property: mp 318-22°C (dec). Source: BEI XIE. Ref: 6.

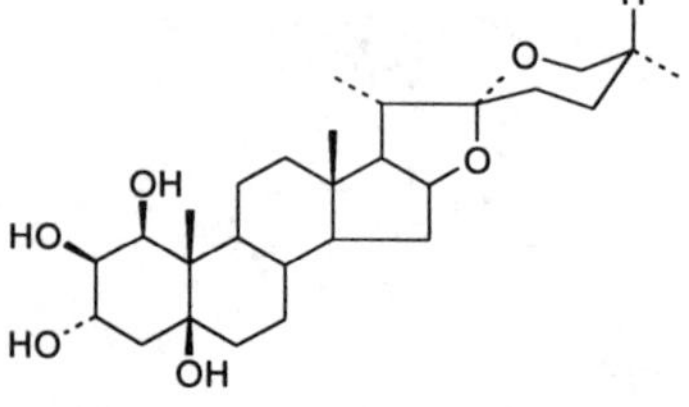

3743 Kojic acid

$C_6H_6O_4$ MW: 142.11 Property: mp 152°C. Source: JIANG. Ref: 6.

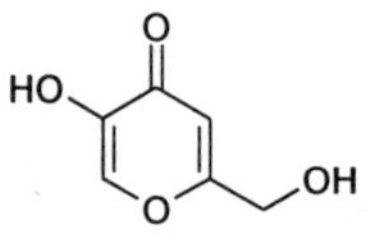

3744 Kokusagine
$C_{13}H_9NO_4$ MW: 243.22 Property: mp 195-7°C. Source: CHOU SHAN YANG. Ref: 6.

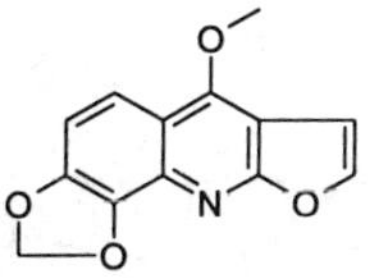

3745 Kokusaginine
$C_{14}H_{13}O_4$ MW: 259.26 Property: mp 171°C. Source: CHOU CAO, CHOU SHAN YANG. Ref: 6.

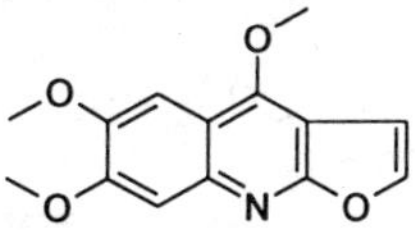

3746 Korepimedoside
$C_{41}H_{52}O_{21}$ MW: 880.86 Property: yellow powder. Source: CHAO XIAN YIN YANG HUO. Ref: 417.

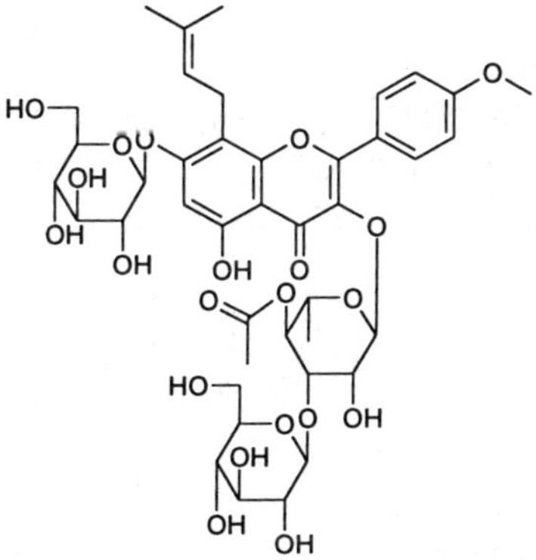

3747 Korepimedoside A
Anhydroicaritin 3-O-β-D-(6-acetyl) glucopyranosyl (1→3)-α-L-(4-acetyl)rhamnopyranoside. $C_{37}H_{44}O_{17}$ MW: 746.73 Property: yellow powder, mp 170-1°C. Source: CHAO XIAN YIN YANG HUO. Ref: 361.

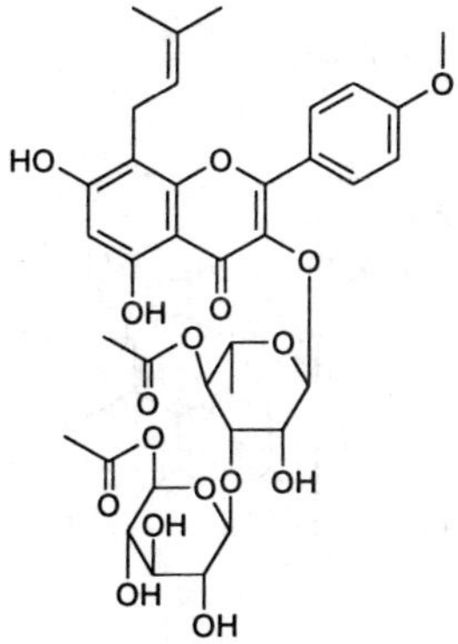

3748 Korepimedoside B
Anhydroicaritin 3-O-β-D-(2,6-diacetyl)gluco pyranosyl (1→3)-α-L-(4-acetyl) rhamnopyranoside-7-O-β-D-glucopyranosyl. $C_{45}H_{56}O_{23}$ MW: 964.93 Property: yellow powder, mp 170-1°C. Source: CHAO XIAN YIN YANG HUO. Ref: 361.

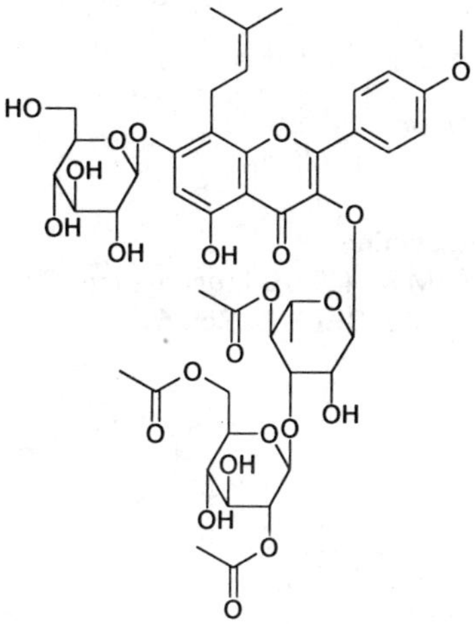

3749 Korseveramine
$C_{27}H_{45}NO_3$ MW: 431.66 Source: CHUAN BEI MU. Ref: 6.

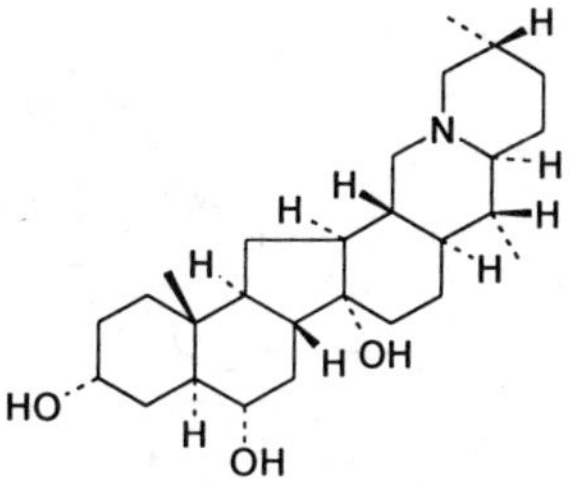

3750 Korseveriline
$C_{27}H_{45}NO_3$ MW: 431.66 Property: mp 240-2°C. Source: CHUAN BEI MU. Ref: 6.

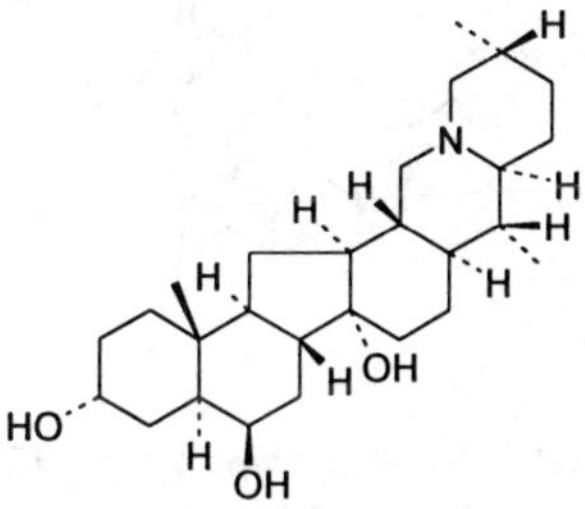

3751 Korseverinine
$C_{27}H_{43}NO_2$ MW: 413.65 Source: CHUAN BEI MU. Ref: 6.

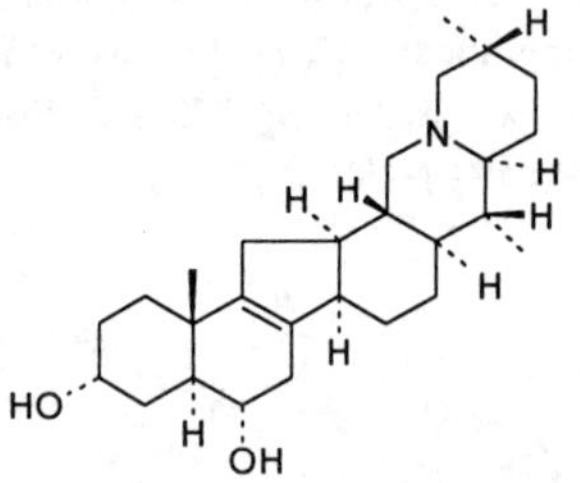

3752 Korsevinine
$C_{27}H_{41}NO_3$ MW: 427.63 Property: mp 224-5°C. Source: CHUAN BEI MU. Ref: 6.

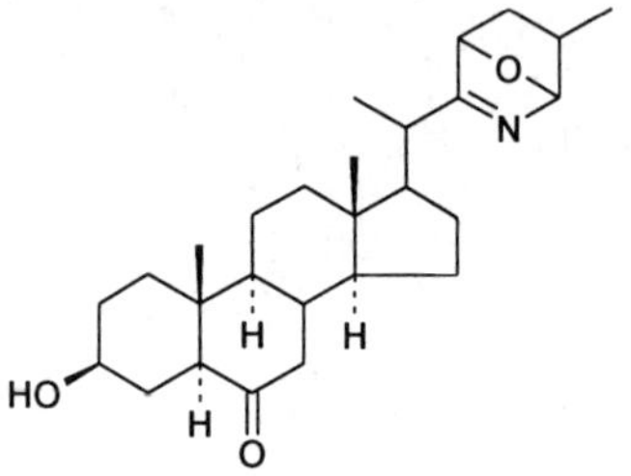

3753 Korsine
$C_{27}H_{43}NO_3$ MW: 429.65 Source: CHUAN BEI MU. Ref: 6.

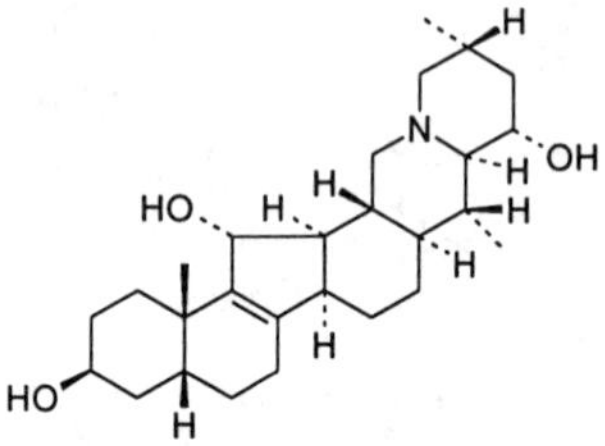

3754 Koumidine
$C_{19}H_{22}N_2O$ MW: 294.40 Property: mp 200-1°C. Source: HU MAN TENG. Ref: 14.

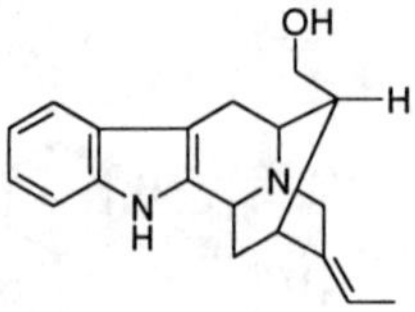

3755 Koumine
$C_{20}H_{22}N_2O$ MW: 306.41 Property: mp 170°C, $[\alpha]_D$ -254°. Source: HU MAN TENG. Ref: 14.

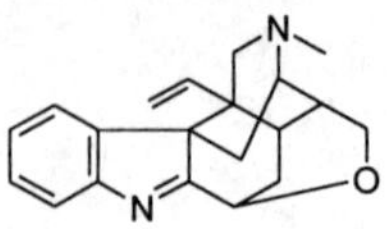

3756 Koumine N-oxide
$C_{20}H_{22}N_2O_2$ MW: 322.41 Property: mp 111-3°C. Source: HU MAN TENG. Ref: 14.

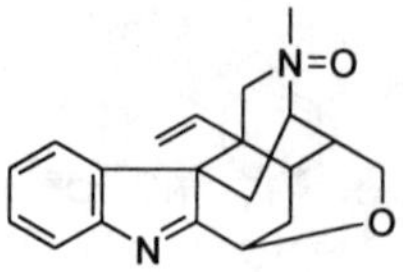

3757 Kukoamine A
$C_{28}H_{42}N_4O_6$ MW: 530.67 Source: DI GU PI. Ref: 2.

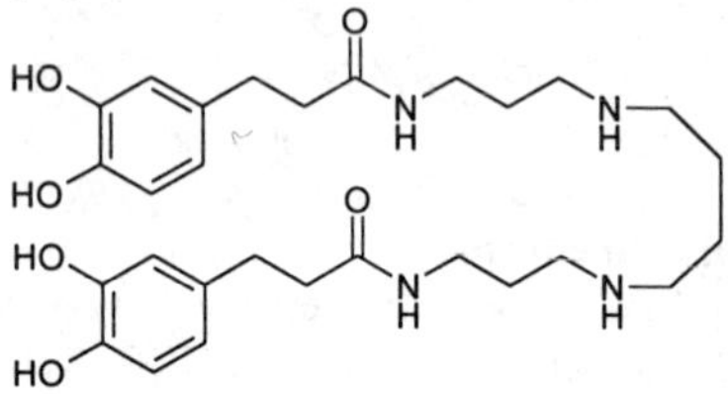

3758 Kulactone
$C_{30}H_{44}O_3$ MW: 452.68 Property: mp 163-4.5°C. Source: KU LIAN PI. Ref: 6.

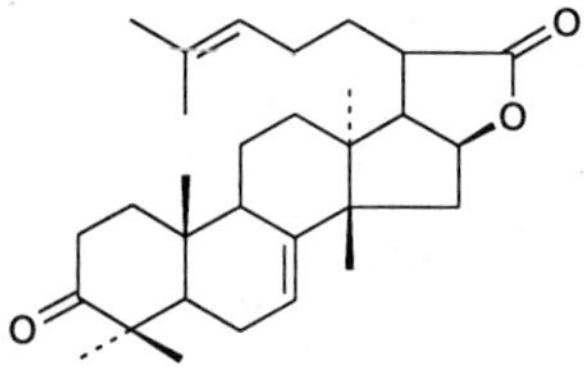

3759 Kulinone
$C_{30}H_{48}O_2$ MW: 440.72 Property: mp 138°C. Source: KU LIAN PI. Ref: 6.

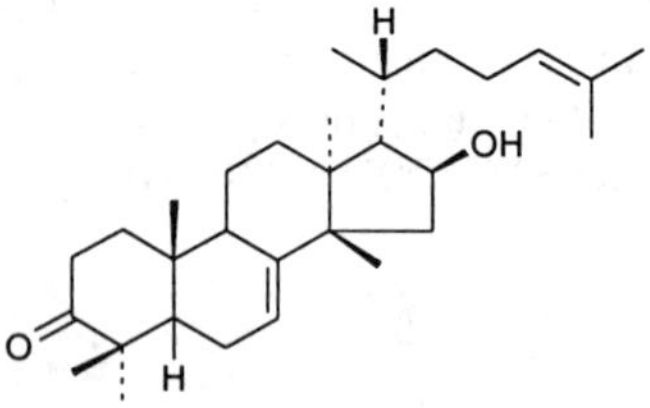

3760 Kulolactone
$C_{30}H_{46}O_3$ MW: 454.70 Source: KU LIAN PI. Ref: 6.

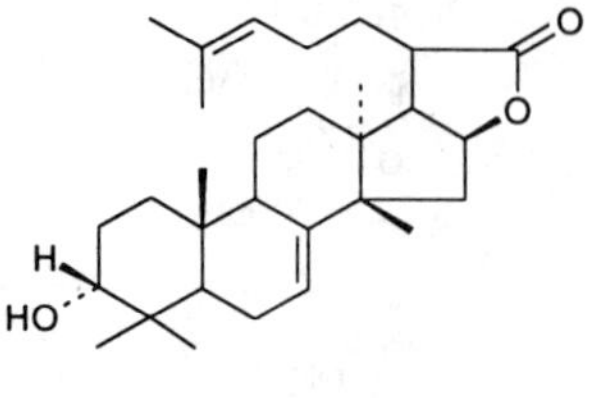

3761 Kumatakenin
$C_{17}H_{14}O_6$ MW: 314.30 Property: mp 246°C. Source: HUANG QI, TU SHA REN. Ref: 2, 6.

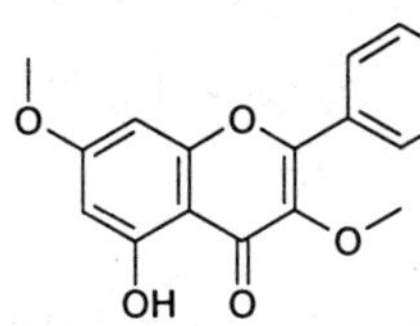

3762 Kumujansine A
$C_{28}H_{25}N_4O_2$•Cl MW: 449.54•35.45 Property: light yellow granular crystal, mp 249-50°C (dec). Source: KU SHU PI. Ref: 101.

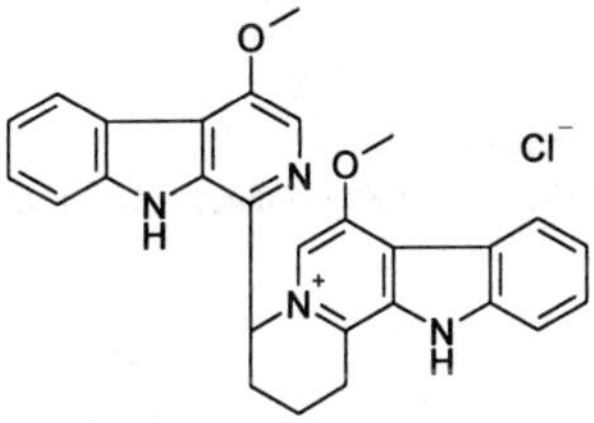

3763 Kumujansine B
$C_{30}H_{29}N_4O_4$•Cl MW:509.54•35.45 Property: light yellow granular crystal, mp 270°C (dec). Source: KU SHU PI. Ref: 101.

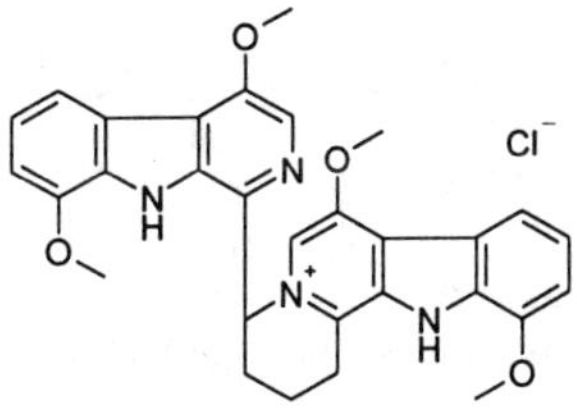

3764 Kuraramine
$C_{12}H_{18}N_2O_2$ MW: 222.29 Source: KU SHEN. Ref: 2.

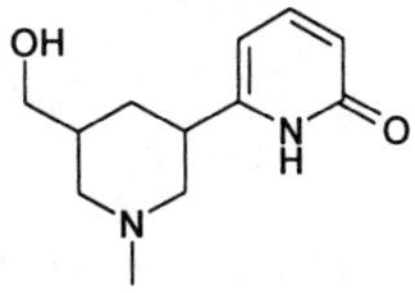

3765 Kuraridinol
$C_{26}H_{32}O_7$ MW: 456.54 Source: KU SHEN. Ref: 2.

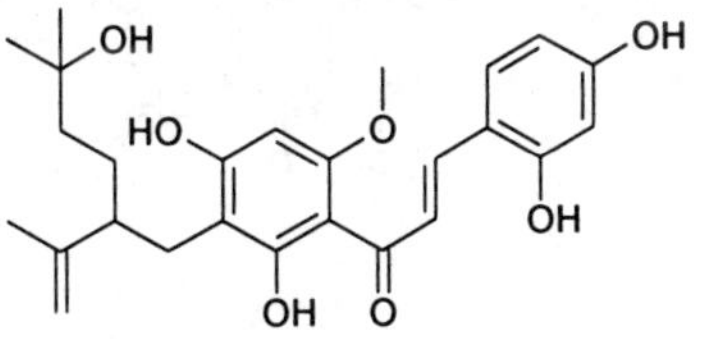

3766 Kurarinol
$C_{26}H_{30}O_7$ MW: 454.52 Source: KU SHEN. Ref: 2.

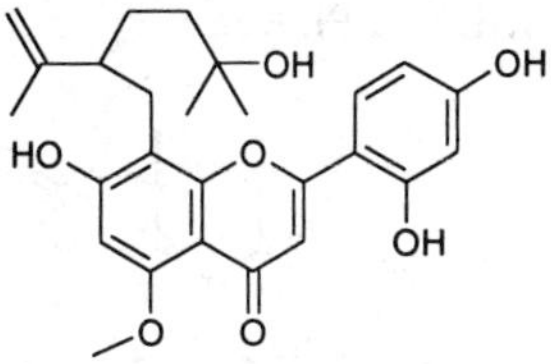

3767 Kurchaline
$C_{23}H_{37}O_2$ MW: 359.56 Property: mp 185°C. Source: ZHI XIE MU PI. Ref: 6.

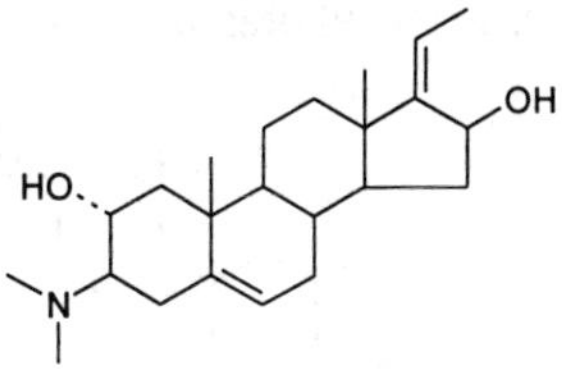

3768 Kurchamine
$C_{22}H_{36}N_2$ MW: 328.55 Property: mp 115-7°C. Source: ZHI XIE MU PI. Ref: 6.

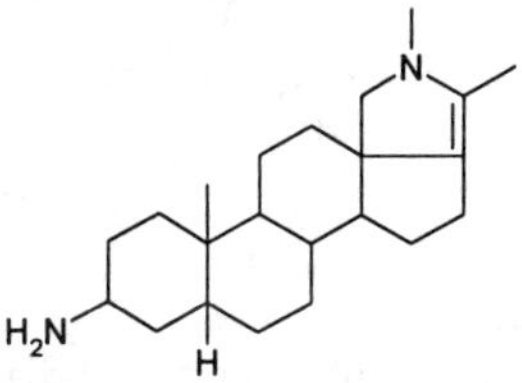

3769 Kurchessine
$C_{25}H_{44}N_2$ MW: 372.64 Property: mp 140-1°C. Source: ZHI XIE MU PI. Ref: 6.

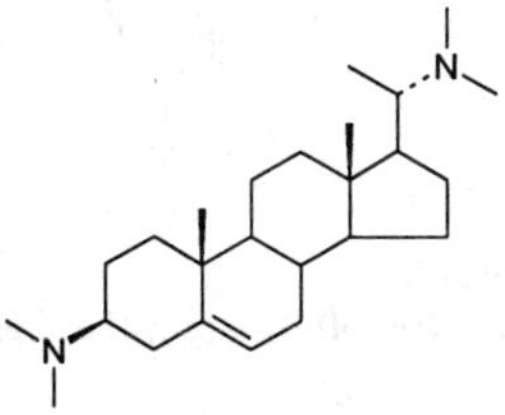

3770 Kurchiline
$C_{23}H_{37}NO_2$ MW: 359.56 Source: ZHI XIE MU PI. Ref: 6.

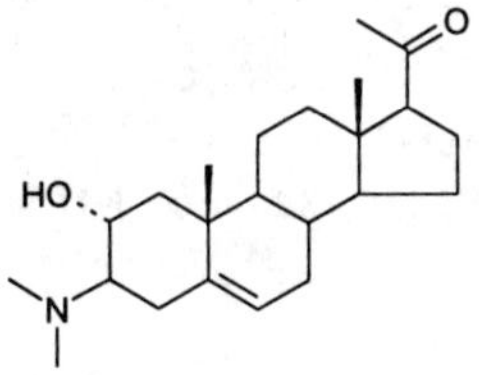

3771 Kurchiphyllamine
$C_{22}H_{35}NO_2$ MW: 345.53 Property: mp 161°C.
Source: ZHI XIE MU PI. Ref: 6.

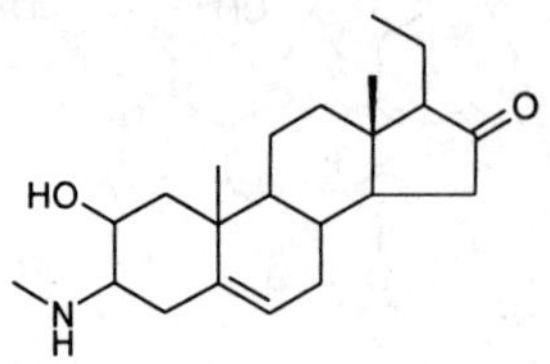

3772 Kurchiphylline
$C_{23}H_{37}NO_2$ MW: 359.56 Property: mp 184°C.
Source: ZHI XIE MU PI. Ref: 6.

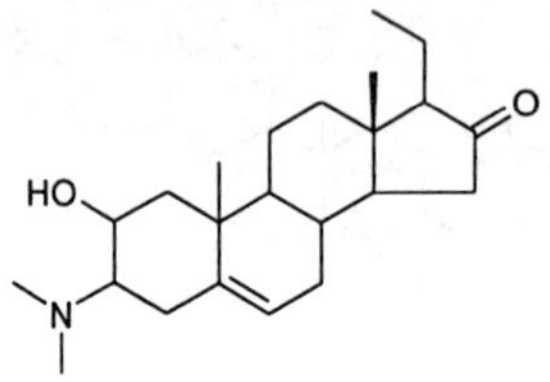

3773 Kushenin
$C_{16}H_{14}O_5$ MW: 286.29 Source: KU SHEN. Ref: 2.

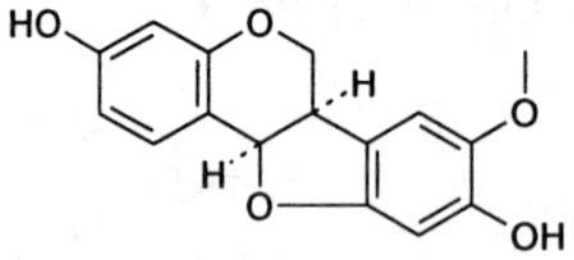

3774 Kushenol A
$C_{25}H_{26}O_5$ MW: 406.48 Source: KU SHEN. Ref: 2.

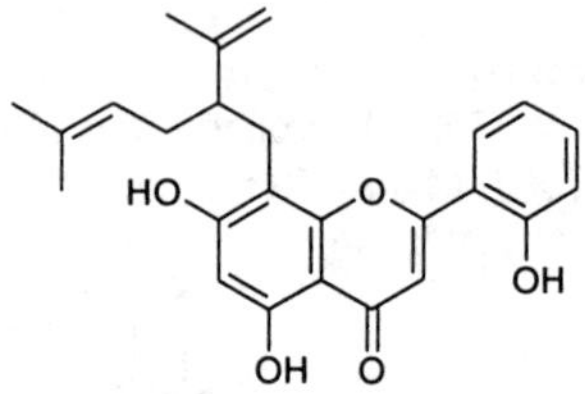

3775 Kushenol B
$C_{30}H_{34}O_6$ MW: 490.60 Source: KU SHEN. Ref: 2.

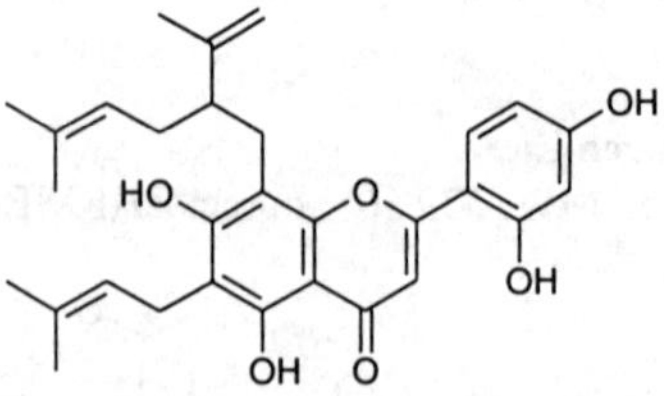

3776 Kushenol C
$C_{25}H_{26}O_7$ MW: 438.48 Source: KU SHEN. Ref: 2.

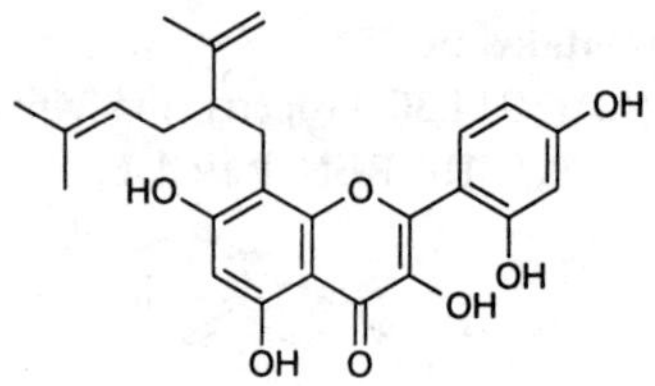

3777 Kushenol D
$C_{27}H_{32}O_6$ MW: 452.55 Source: KU SHEN. Ref: 2.

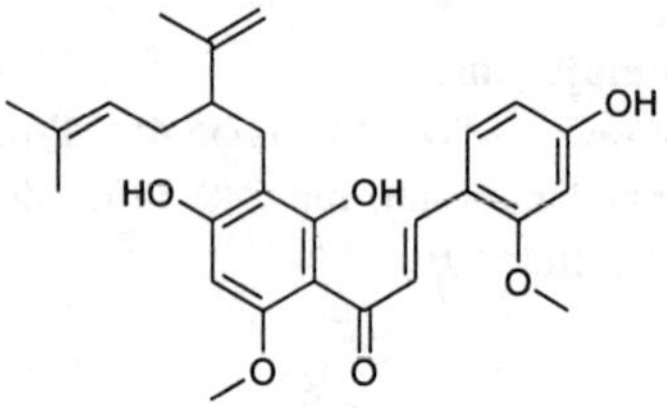

3778 Kushenol E
$C_{25}H_{26}O_6$ MW: 422.48 Source: KU SHEN. Ref: 2.

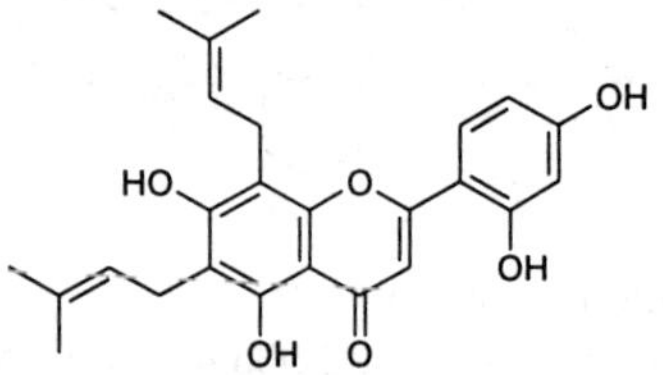

3779 Kushenol F
$C_{25}H_{26}O_6$ MW: 422.48 Source: KU SHEN. Ref: 2.

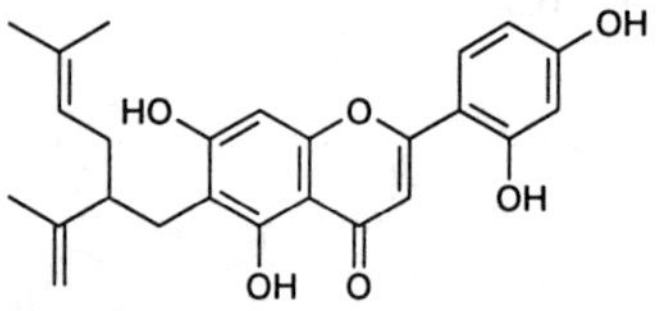

3780 Kushenol G
$C_{25}H_{28}O_8$ MW: 456.50 Source: KU SHEN. Ref: 2.

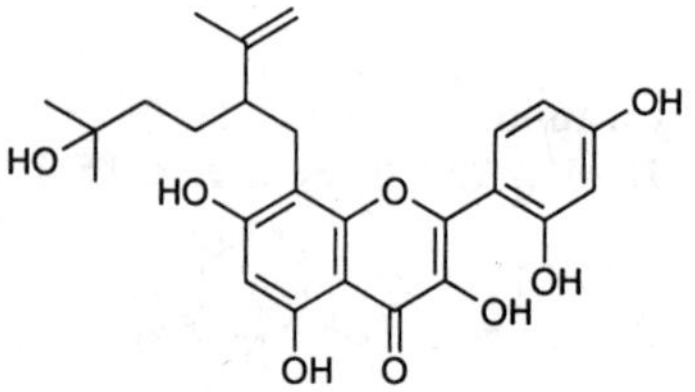

3781 Kushenol H
$C_{26}H_{30}O_8$ MW: 470.52 Source: KU SHEN. Ref: 2.

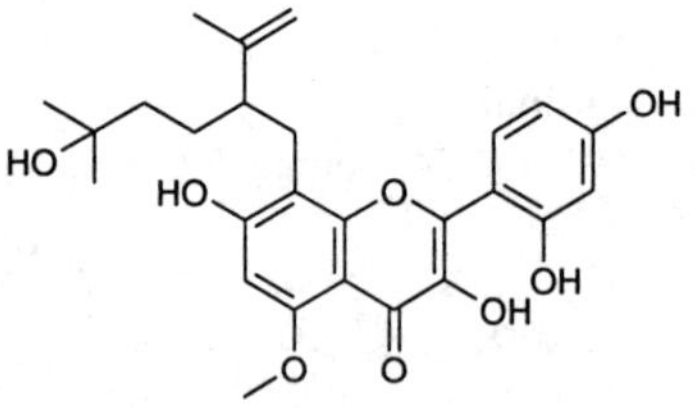

3782 Kushenol I
$C_{26}H_{28}O_7$ MW: 452.51 Source: KU SHEN. Ref: 2.

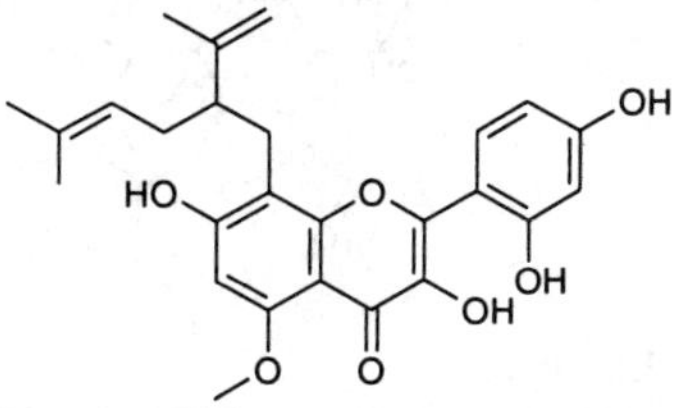

3783 Kushenol J
Source: KU SHEN. Ref: 2.

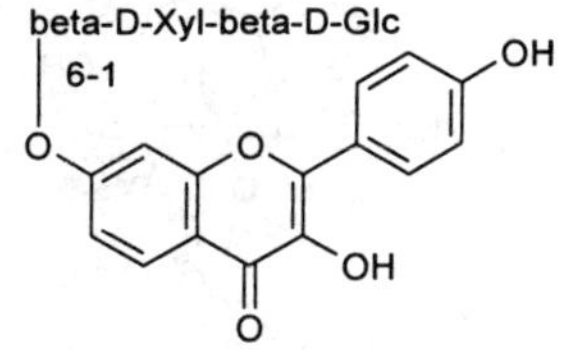

3784 Kushenol K
$C_{26}H_{32}O_8$ MW: 472.54 Source: KU SHEN. Ref: 2.

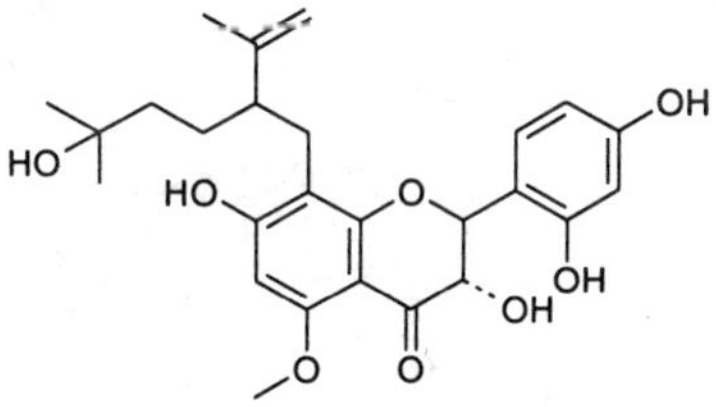

3785 Kushenol L
$C_{25}H_{26}O_7$ MW: 438.48 Source: KU SHEN. Ref: 2.

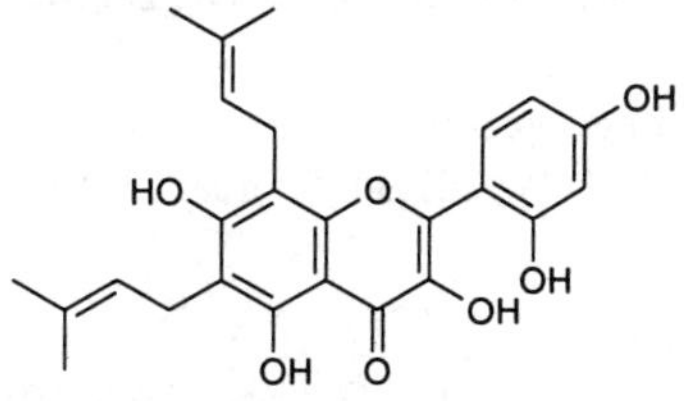

3786 Kushenol M
$C_{30}H_{34}O_7$ MW: 506.60 Source: KU SHEN. Ref: 2.

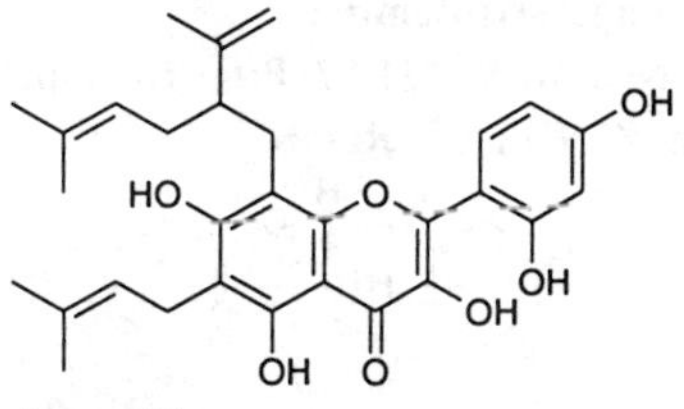

3787 Kushenol N
$C_{26}H_{30}O_7$ MW: 454.52 Source: KU SHEN. Ref: 2.

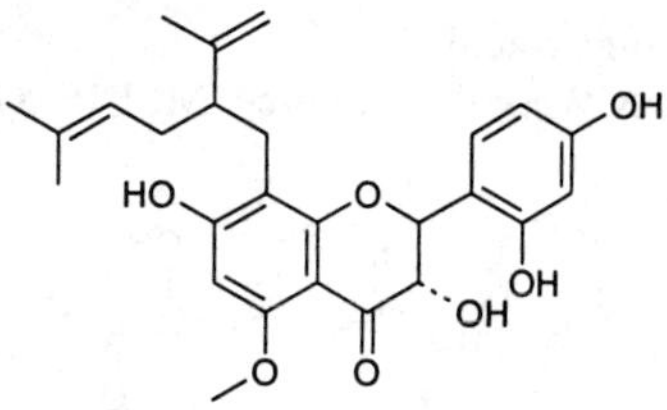

3788 Kushenol O
Source: KU SHEN. Ref: 2.

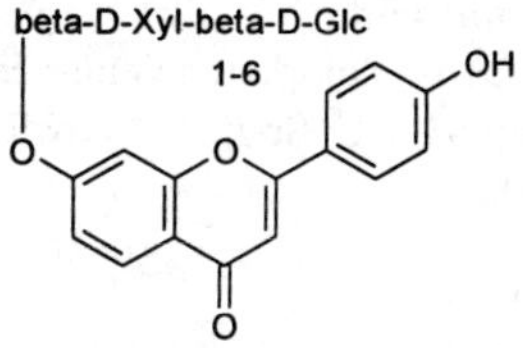

3789 Kushenquinone A
$C_{17}H_{22}O_4$ MW: 290.34 Source: KU SHEN. Ref: 2.

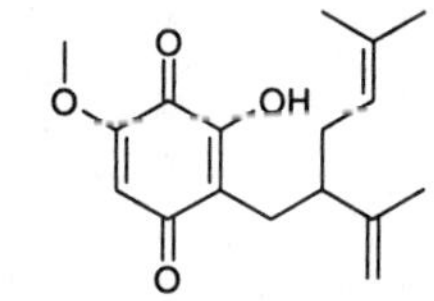

3790 Kusulactone
$C_{25}H_{34}O_9$ MW: 478.54 Source: KU SHU PI. Ref: 12.

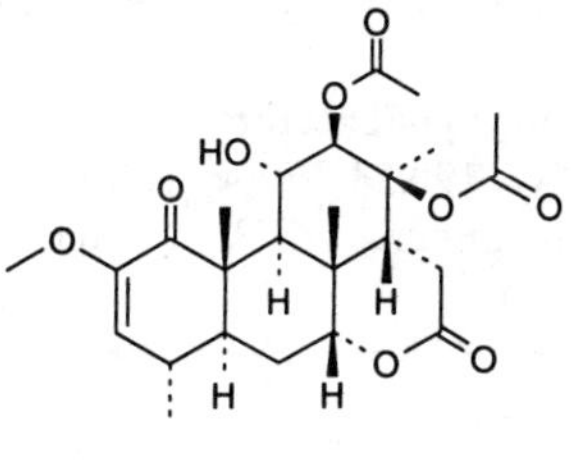

3791 Kusunol
$C_{15}H_{26}O$ MW: 222.37 Source: BAI MU XIANG, CHEN XIANG, ZHANG MU.
Ref: 6, 13.

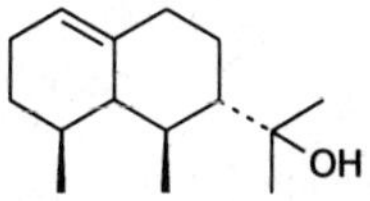

3792 Kynurenine
$C_{10}H_{12}N_2O_3$ MW: 208.22 Property: mp (+): 191°C, (-): 191°C, (±): 219°C (dec). Source: FENG RU, MO GU. Ref: 6.

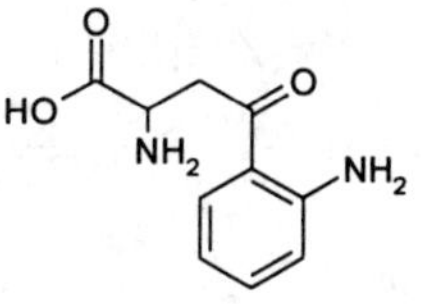

3793 Labiatic acid
$C_{18}H_{16}O_8$ MW: 360.32 Source: MI DIE XIANG. Ref: 6.

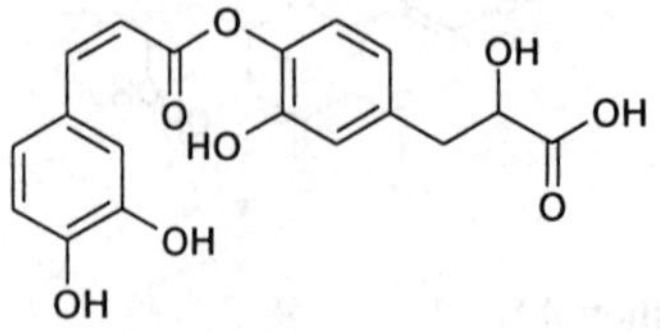

3794 Lacceroic acid
$C_{32}H_{64}O_2$ Property: colorless acicular crystal (methanol), mp 83-5°C. Source: NAN FANG TU SI ZI. Ref: 468.

3795 Laccol
$C_{23}H_{40}O_2$ MW: 348.57 Property: mp 23°C. Source: LIN BEI ZI. Ref: 6.

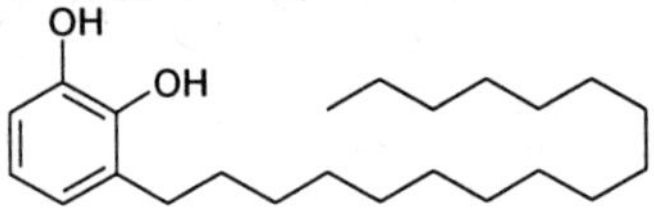

3796 Lachnophyllol
$C_{10}H_{12}O$ MW: 148.21 Property: mp trans-: 39-40°C. Source: ZI WAN. Ref: 6.

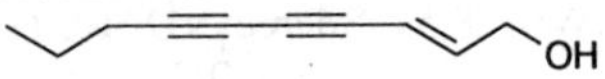

3797 Lachnophyllol acetate
$C_{12}H_{14}O_2$ MW: 190.24 Property: bp 90°C/0.001mm. Source: ZI WAN. Ref: 6.

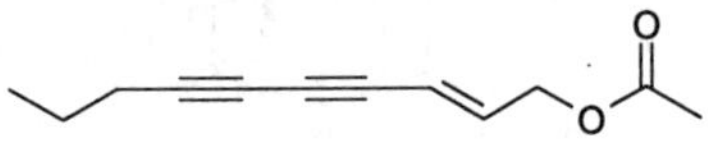

3798 Lactic acid
$C_3H_6O_3$ MW: 90.08 Source: PU HUANG, LU HUI. Ref: 2.

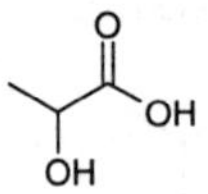

3799 Lactiflorasyne
$C_{19}H_{22}O_5$ MW: 330.38 Property: white granular crystal, mp 92.5-3.5°C, $[\alpha]_D^{29}$ +3° (c=0.37, chloroform). Source: BAI HUA HAO. Ref: 66.

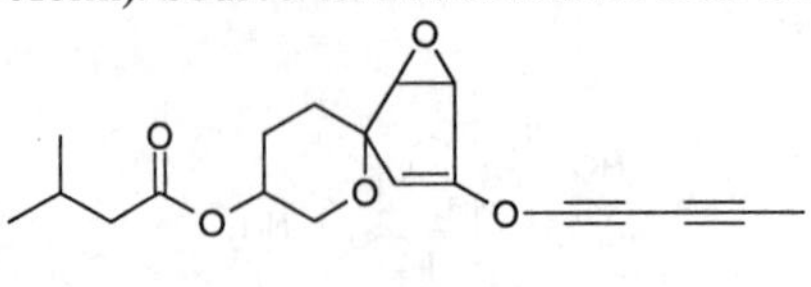

3800 Lactiflorin
$C_{23}H_{26}O_{10}$ MW: 462.46 Source: CHI SHAO YAO. Ref: 2.

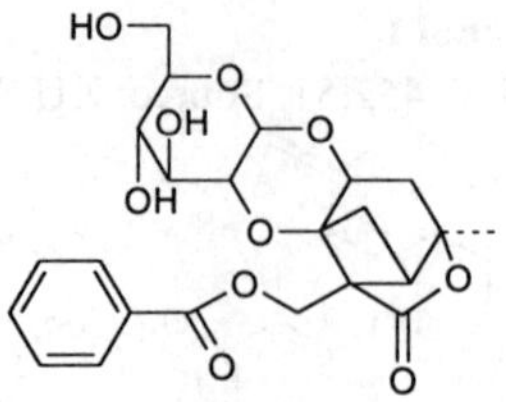

3801 Lactucin
CAS: 1891-29-8 $C_{15}H_{16}O_5$ MW: 276.29 Source: JU QU. Ref: 5.

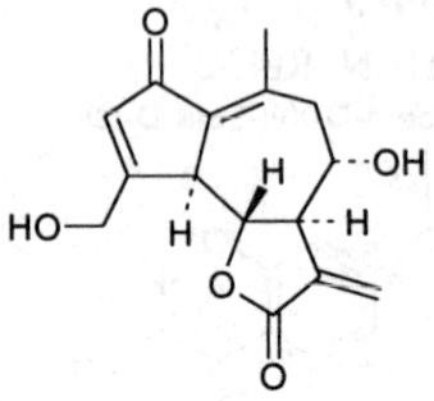

3802 Lactucopicrin
$C_{23}H_{22}O_7$ MW: 410.43 Source: JU QU. Ref: 6.

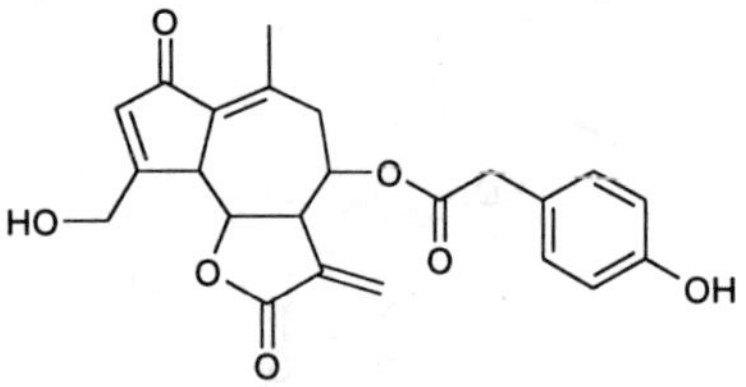

3803 Laevigatanoside A
2α,3β,19α,23-trihydroxy-12-ursorlic-28-glucopyester. Source: JIN YING ZI. Ref: 584.

3804 Lageracetal
$C_{12}H_{26}O_2$ MW: 202.34 Source: ZI WEI HUA. Ref: 6.

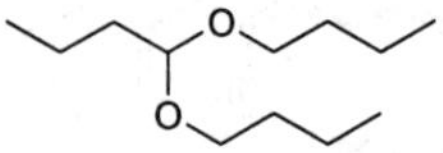

3805 Lagerstr(o)emine
$C_{27}H_{33}NO_5$ MW: 451.57 Property: mp 226-8°C. Source: ZI WEI YE. Ref: 6.

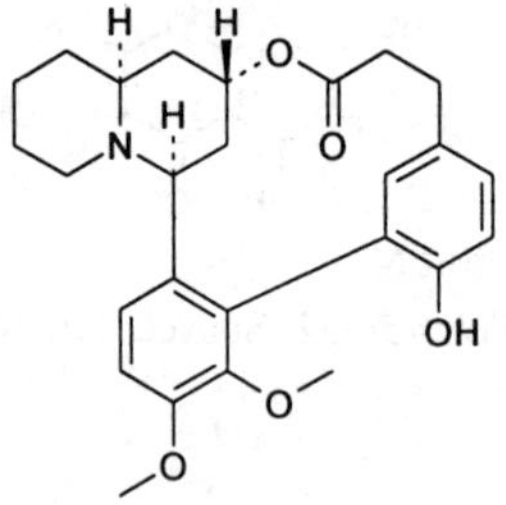

3806 Lambertianic acid
$C_{19}H_{26}O_3$ MW: 302.42 Property: mp 126.5-7.5 °C. Source: HAI SONG ZI. Ref: 6.

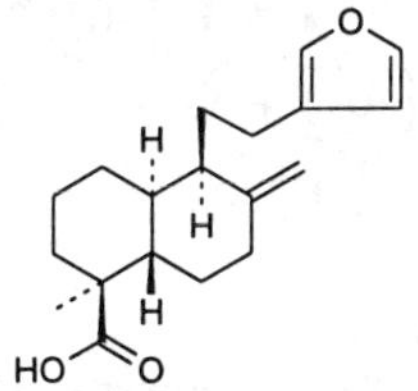

3807 Lamiide
$C_{17}H_{26}O_{12}$ MW: 422.39. Source: BAO GAI CAO. Ref: 6.

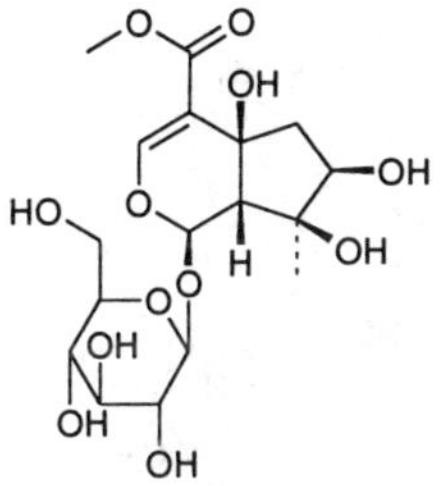

3808 Laminine
6-N-Trimethyl-L-lysine betaine. CAS: 2408-79-9 $C_9H_{20}N_2O_2$ MW: 188.27 Source: *Laminarin angustata* Kiellm, KUN BU, etc. Ref: 5, 6.

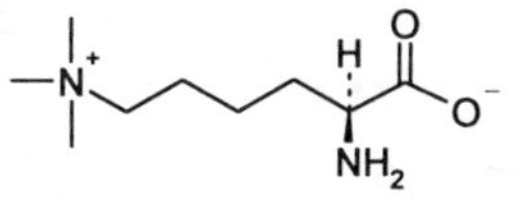

3809 Lamiol
$C_{16}H_{26}O_{10}$ MW: 378.38 Source: BAO GAI CAO. Ref: 6.

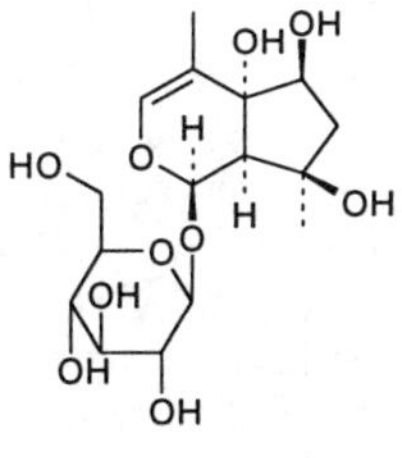

3810 Lamiophlomiol A
$C_{11}H_{14}O_6$ MW: 242.23 Property: colorless prismatic crystal (acetic ester-methanol), mp 159-63°C, $[\alpha]_D^{22}$ +43.2° (c=1.325, methanol). Source: DU YI WEI. Ref: 178.

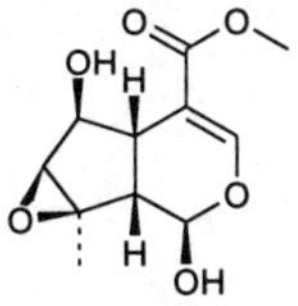

3811 Lamiophlomiol C
$C_{11}H_{14}O_7$ MW: 258.23 Property: colorless prismatic crystal, mp 155-7°C, $[\alpha]_D^{22}$ +66.7° (c=2.11, methanol). Source: DU YI WEI. Ref: 223.

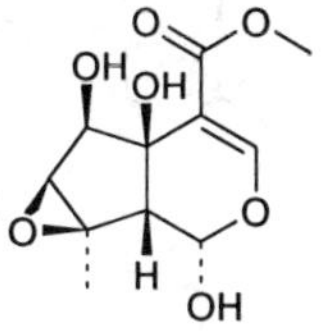

3812 Lamiophlomioside A
3-Methoxy-4-hydroxy-phenethyl-O-[α-L-rhamnopyranosyl (1→3)]-O-[β-D-apiofuranosyl (1→6)]-4-O-feruloyl-β-D-glucopyranoside. $C_{36}H_{48}O_{19}$ MW: 784.77 Property: light yellow powder, mp 107-8 °C. Source: ZANG YAO DU YI WEI. Ref: 323.

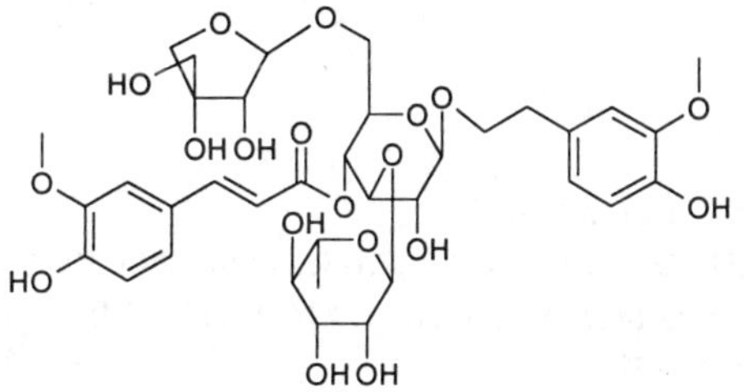

3813 Lamioside
$C_{18}H_{28}O_{11}$ MW: 420.42 Source: BAO GAI CAO. YE ZHI MA. Ref: 6.

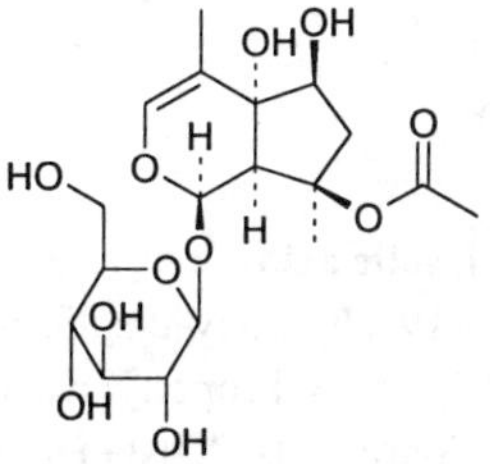

3814 Lanceolin
$C_{22}H_{24}O_{11}$ MW: 464.43 Property: mp 215-20°C. Source: XIAN YE JIN JI JU. Ref: 6.

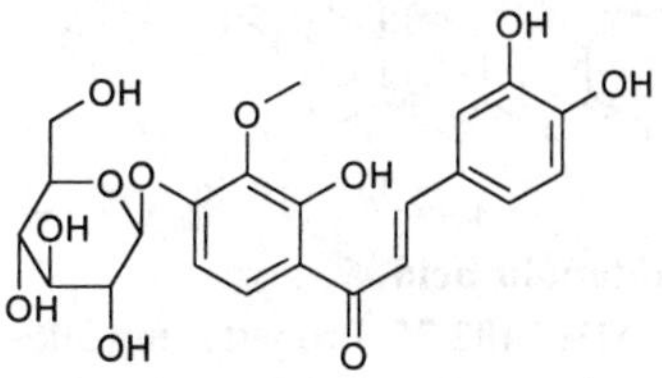

3815 Lanosterol
$C_{30}H_{50}O$ MW: 426.73 Property: mp 140-1°C. Source: HOU PI SHU. Ref: 6.

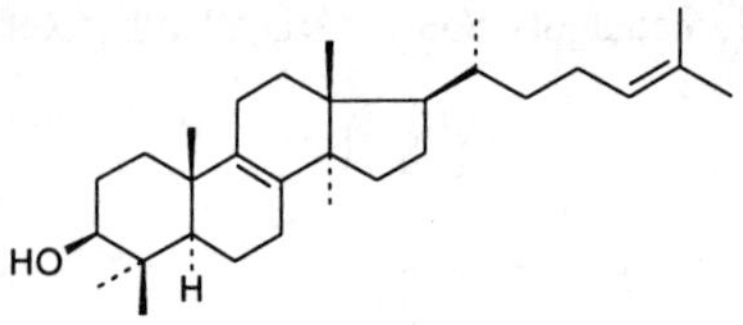

3816 Lantadene A
$C_{37}H_{56}O_4$ MW: 564.86 Property: mp 282-6°C. Source: MA YING DAN, WU SE MEI. Ref: 6, 253.

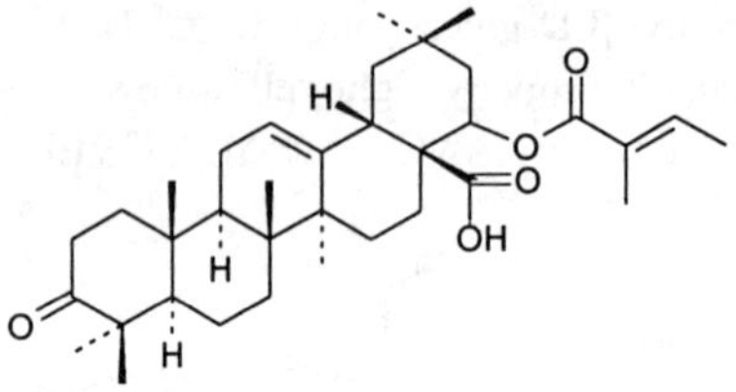

3817 Lantadene B
$C_{37}H_{56}O_4$ MW: 564.86 Property: mp 295-300°C (dec). Source: MA YING DAN, WU SE MEI. Ref: 6, 253.

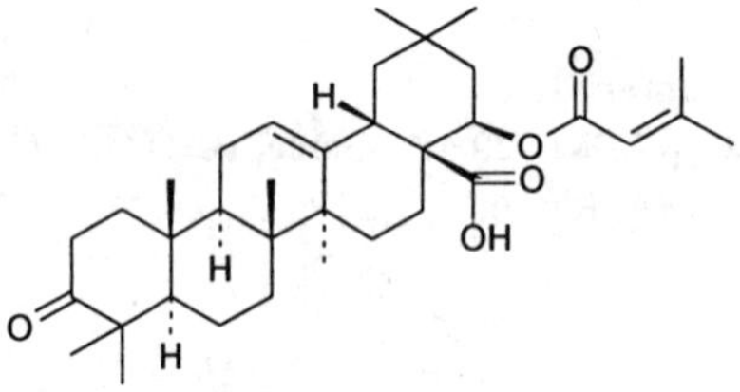

3818 Lantaiursolic acid
3β-isovalerroyl-19α-hydroxy-ursolic acid. $C_{35}H_{56}O_5$ MW: 556.83 Property: acicular crystal, mp 218-20°C. Source: MA YING DAN. Ref: 254.

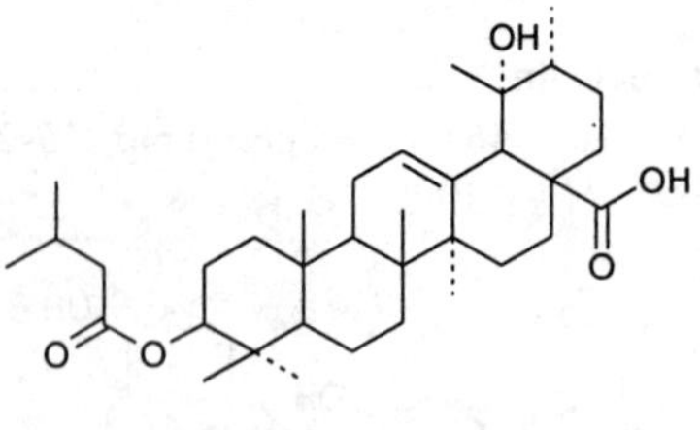

3819 Lantanolic acid
$C_{32}H_{50}O_3$ MW: 482.75 Property: mp 306-9°C. Source: MA YING DAN, WU SE MEI. Ref: 6, 254.

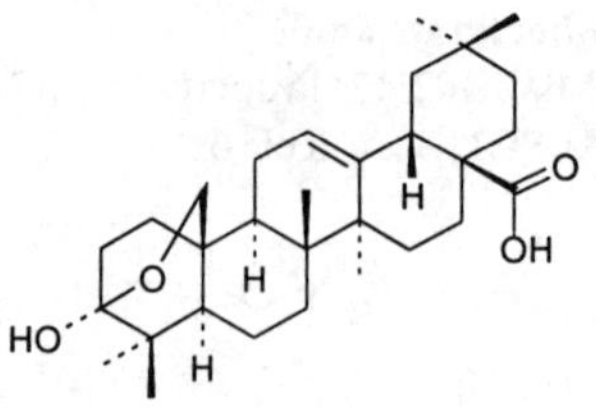

3820 Lantanose A
$C_{30}H_{52}O_{26}$ MW: 828.73 Property: white powder, $[\alpha]_D$ +166.0° (c=1.04, H_2O). Source: MA YING DAN. Ref: 234.

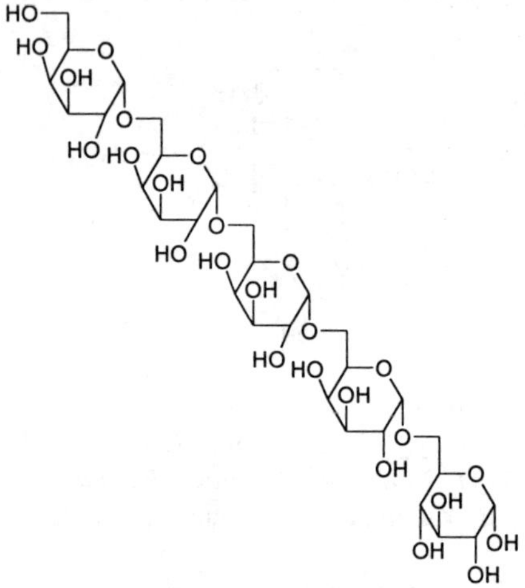

3821 Lantanose B
$C_{36}H_{62}O_{31}$ MW: 990.88 Property: white powder, $[\alpha]_D$ +114.2° (c=1.06, H_2O). Source: MA YING DAN. Ref: 234.

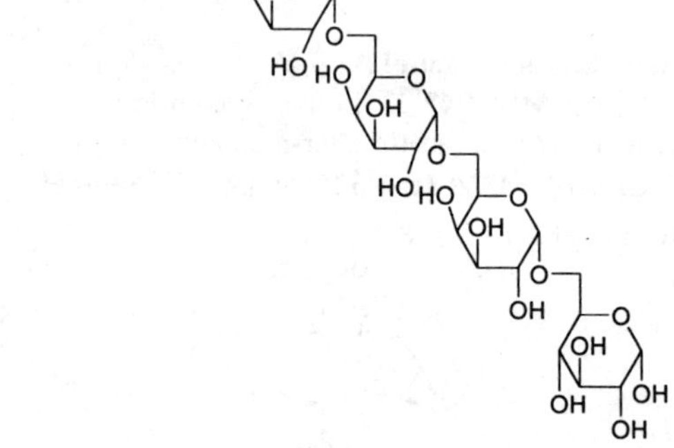

3822 Lanthopine
$C_{23}H_{25}NO_4$ MW: 379.46 Property: mp ≈200°C (dec). Source: YA PIAN. Ref: 6.

3823 Lantic acid
$C_{32}H_{50}O_3$ MW: 482.75 Property: mp 256-9°C. Source: WU SE MEI. Ref: 6.

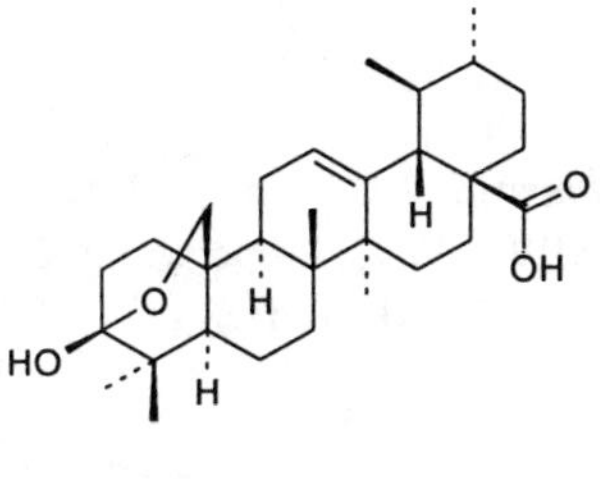

3824 Lanuginosine
$C_{18}H_{11}NO_4$ MW: 305.29 Property: mp 302-3°C (dec). Source: XIN YI. Ref: 6.

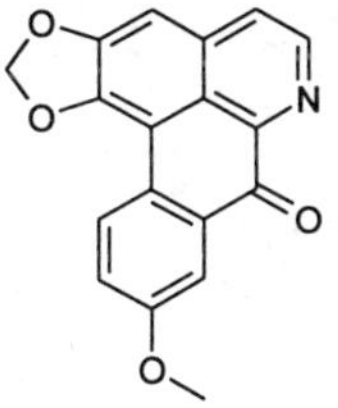

3825 Lapachol
Greenhartin; Lapachic acid; Tecomin. CAS: 84-79-7 $C_{15}H_{14}O_3$ MW: 242.28 Property: mp 140°C. Source: *Tabebula avellanedae, Markhamia stipulate* Wall.. Ref: 5.

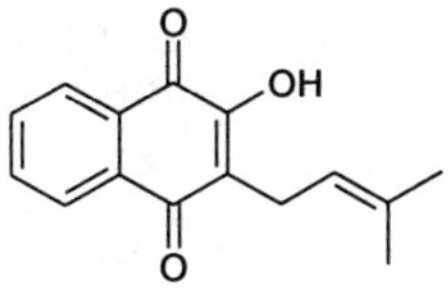

3826 α-Lapachone
$C_{15}H_{14}O_3$ MW: 242.28 Property: mp 117°C. Source: ZI MU. Ref: 6.

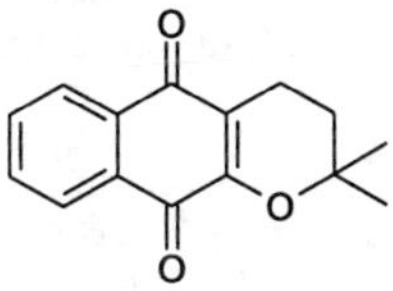

3827 Lasiocarpine
CAS: 303-34-4 $C_{21}H_{33}NO_7$ MW: 411.50 Property: mp 95°C. Source: DA BAI DING CAO, YAO YONG DAO TI HU. Ref: 5, 6.

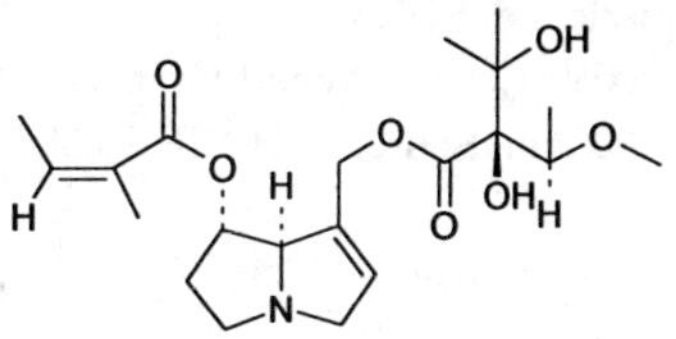

3828 Lasiokaurin
CAS: 28957-08-6 $C_{22}H_{30}O_7$ MW: 406.48 Property: mp 226-9°C. Source: MAO YE XIANG CHA CAI, XIAN MAI XIANG CHA CAI. Ref: 4, 504.

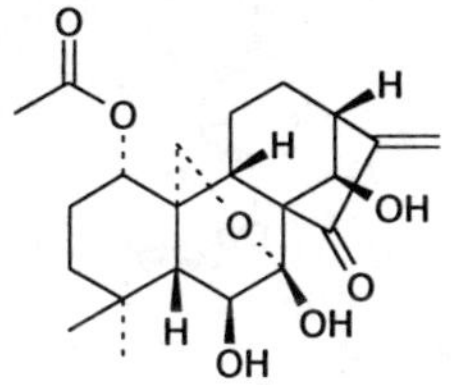

3829 Laudanidine
$C_{20}H_{25}NO_4$ MW: 343.43 Property: mp 181-2°C. Source: YA PIAN. Ref: 6.

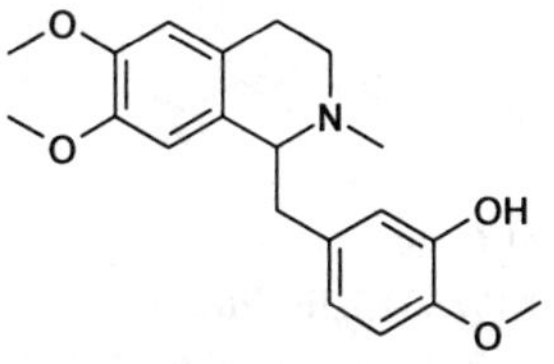

3830 Laudanosine
$C_{21}H_{27}NO_4$ MW: 357.45 Property: mp (+): 89°C. Source: YA PIAN. Ref: 6.

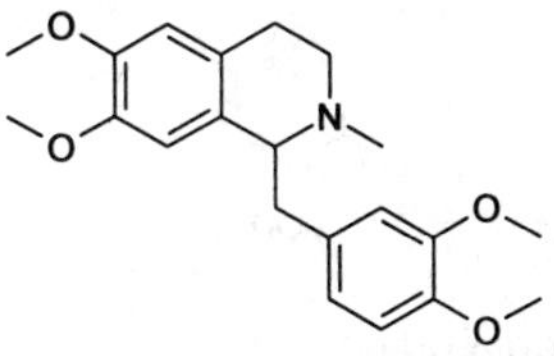

3831 Launobine
$C_{18}H_{17}NO_4$ MW: 311.34 Property: mp 214-5°C (dec). Source: DIAO ZHANG GEN PI, YUE GUI ZI, ZHEN CAI. Ref: 6.

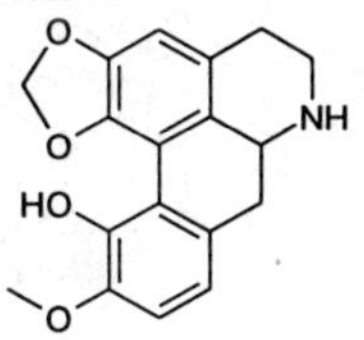

3832 Lauric aldehyde
$C_{12}H_{24}O$ MW: 184.32 Property: mp 44.5°C, bp 184-5°C/100 mm. Source: YU XING CAO. Ref: 6.

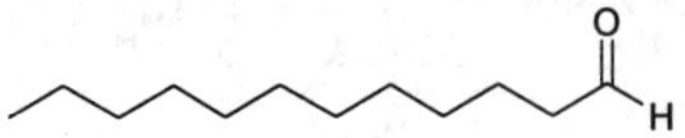

3833 Laurifoline
$C_{20}H_{24}NO_4$ MW: 342.42 Source: CHU YE HUA, HENG ZHOU WU YAO. Ref: 6.

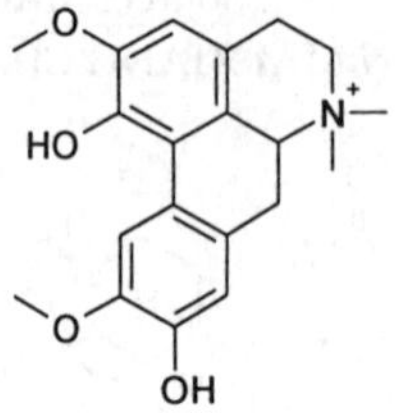

3834 Lauroic acid
$C_{12}H_{24}O_2$ MW: 220.32 Source: BA DOU, BING LANG, CU LIU GUO, DANG SHEN, FU LING, GAN DI HUANG, GUA LOU, HONG HUA, LU HUI. Ref: 2.

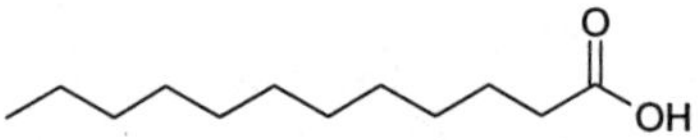

3835 Laurolitsine
$C_{18}H_{19}NO_4$ MW: 313.36 Property: mp 138-40°C. Source: DIAO ZHANG GEN PI, WU YAO, ZHANG MU. Ref: 6.

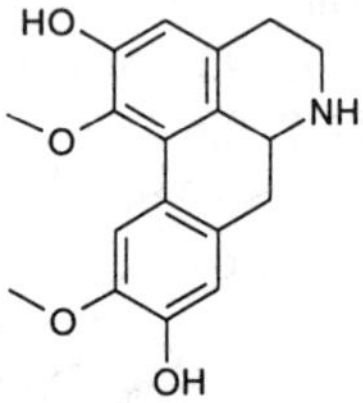

3836 Laurotetanine
$C_{19}H_{21}NO_4$ MW: 327.38 Property: mp 125°C. Source: BI BA, WU YE TENG, ZHEN CAI. Ref: 6.

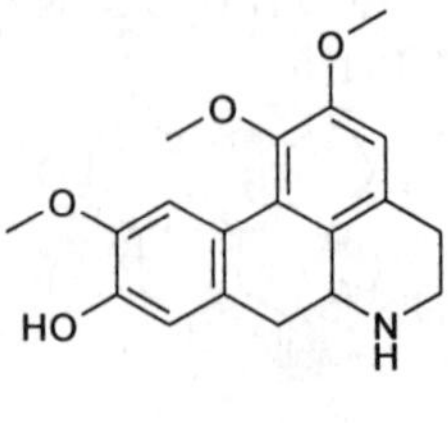

3837 Lawsone
$C_{10}H_6O_3$ MW: 174.16 Property: mp 192°C. Source: FENG XIAN HUA, ZHI JIA HUA YE. Ref: 6.

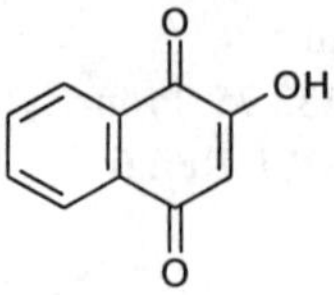

3838 Laxogenin
$C_{27}H_{42}O_4$ MW: 430.43 Property: mp 210°C. Source: NIAN YU XU. Ref: 6.

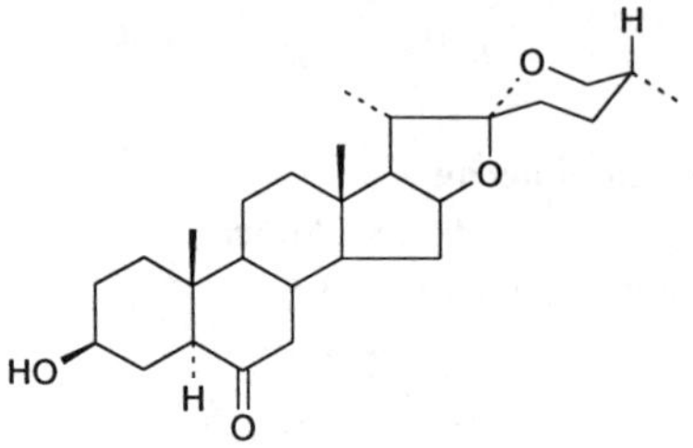

3839 Ledebouliellol
$C_{20}H_{22}O_7$ MW: 374.39 Source: FANG FENG. Ref: 2.

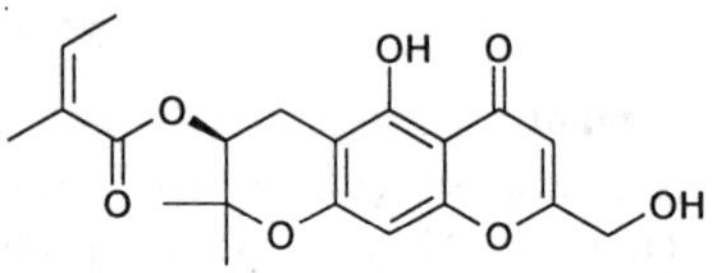

3840 Ledol
$C_{15}H_{26}O$ MW: 222.37 Source: CHAI HU. Ref: 2.

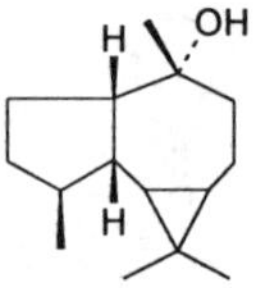

3841 Leiocarpaquinone
$C_{17}H_{12}O_6$ MW: 312.28 Property: orange yellow lamellar crystal, mp 175-8°C. Source: YI HE GUO. Ref: 97.

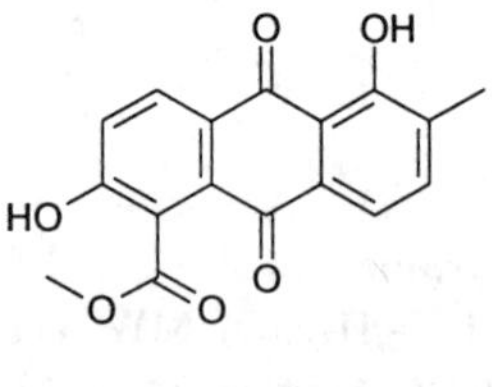

3842 Lemmasterone
$C_{29}H_{48}O_7$ MW: 508.70 Property: mp 263-5°C (dec). Source: LUO YAN CAO. Ref: 6.

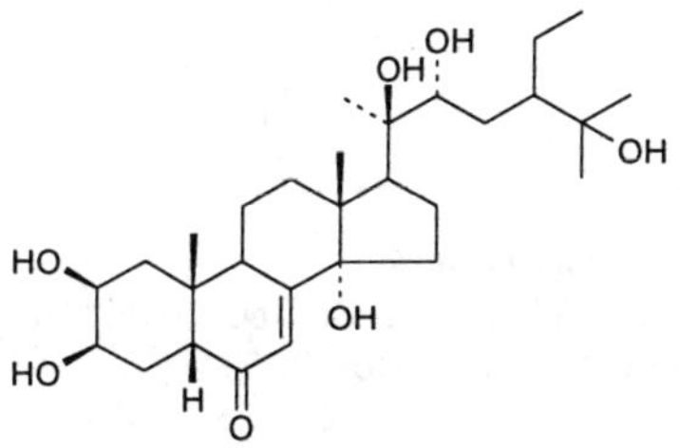

3843 Lentysine
$C_9H_{11}N_5O_4$ MW: 253.22 Property: mp 261-3°C (dec). Source: XIANG XUN. Ref: 6.

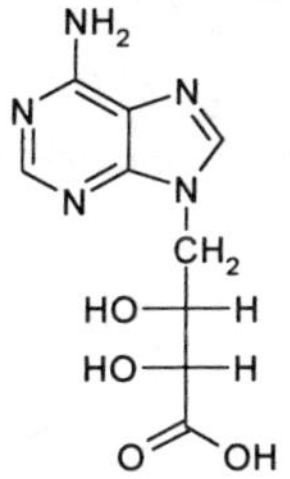

3844 Leonuride
$C_{15}H_{24}O_9$ MW: 348.35 Source: GAN DI HUANG, ROU CONG RONG. Ref: 2, 628.

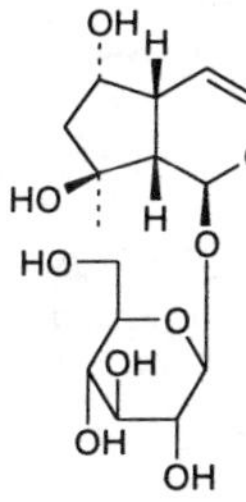

3845 Leonurine
$C_{14}H_{21}N_3O_5$ MW: 311.34 Property: mp 238°C (dec). Source: YI MU CAO. Ref: 4.

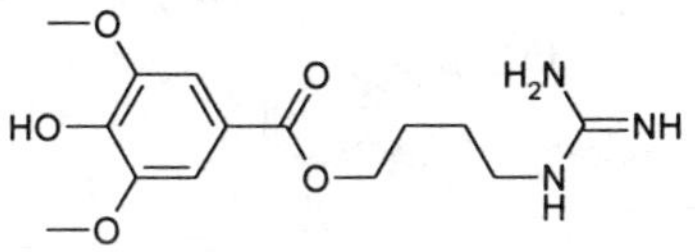

3846 Leptene B
$C_{15}H_{18}O_3$ MW: 246.31 Property: light yellow oleaginous substances. Source: SAN CHA KU. Ref: 393.

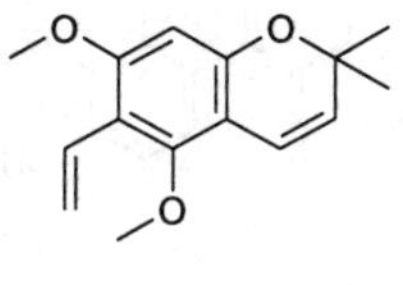

3847 Leptol B
$C_{15}H_{20}O_4$ MW: 264.32 Property: colorless oleaginous substances, $[\alpha]_D^{26}$ -0.6° (c=1.12, CH_3COCH_3). Source: SAN CHA KU. Ref: 393.

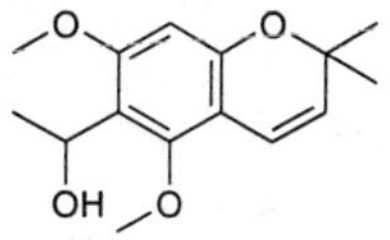

3848 Leptosin
$C_{22}H_{22}O_{11}$ MW: 462.41 Property: mp 229-31°C (dec). Source: XIAN YE JIN JI JU. Ref: 6.

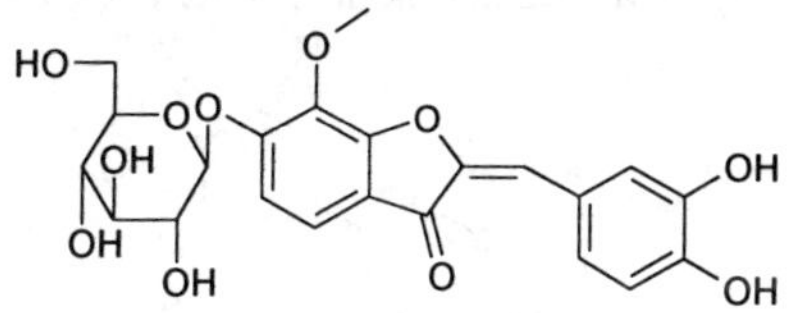

3849 Leptostachyol acetate
$C_{26}H_{28}O_{12}$ MW: 532.51 Source: LAO PO ZI ZHEN XIAN. Ref: 6.

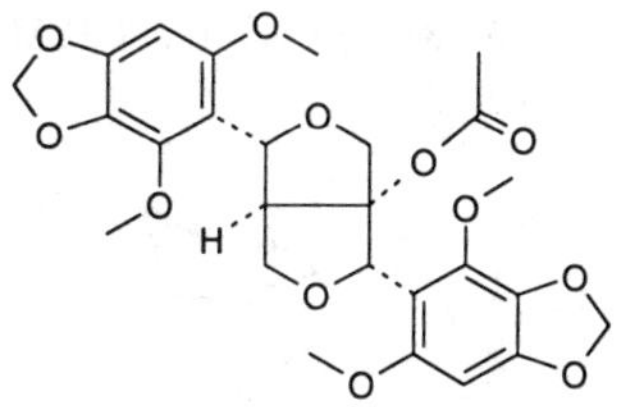

3850 Leucoanthocyanidin
$C_{15}H_{14}O_3$ MW: 242.28 Source: BING LANG. Ref: 2.

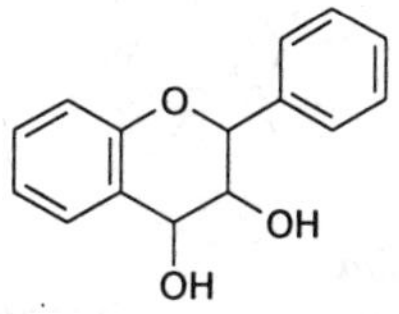

3851 Leucocyanidin
$C_{15}H_{14}O_7$ MW: 306.27 Property: mp (+): >355°C. Source: BAI FAN DOU, FAN SHI LIU GAN, FAN SHI LIU PI, FAN SHI LIU YE, HOU PI SHU, LUO HUA SHENG, OU, PI JIU HUA, SHAN ZHA YE. Ref: 6.

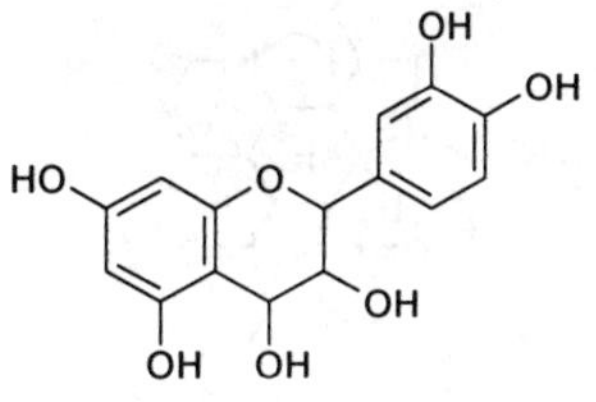

3852 Leucodelphinidin
$C_{15}H_{14}O_8$ MW: 322.27 Source: MA HUANG. Ref: 2.

3853 Leucopelargonidin
$C_{15}H_{14}O_6$ MW: 290.28 Source: BAI FAN DOU. Ref: 6.

3854 Leurocolombine
$C_{46}H_{58}N_4O_9$ MW: 811.00 Source: CHANG CHUN HUA. Ref: 2.

3855 Leurosidine
Inrosidine; Vinrosidine. CAS: 15228-71-4
$C_{46}H_{58}N_4O_9$ MW: 811.00 Property: mp 208-11°C (dec). Source: CHANG CHUN HUA. Ref: 2, 5.

3856 Levulinic acid
$C_5H_8O_2$ MW: 116.12 Property: mp 33-5°C, bp 245-6°C. Source: HEI DA DOU PI. Ref: 6

3857 Licochalcone A
$C_{21}H_{22}O_4$ MW: 338.41 Source: GAN CAO, HUANG GAN CAO. Ref: 2, 591.

3858 Licochalcone B
$C_{16}H_{14}O_5$ MW: 286.29 Source: GAN CAO. Ref: 2.

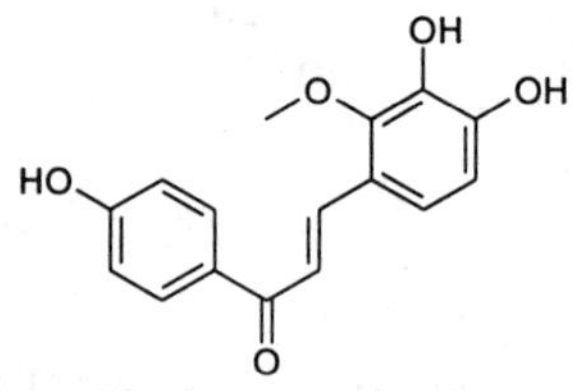

3859 Licocoumarone
$C_{20}H_{20}O_5$ MW: 340.38 Source: GAN CAO. Ref: 2.

3860 Licoflavone
$C_{20}H_{18}O_4$ MW: 322.36 Source: GAN CAO. Ref: 2.

3861 Licoisoflavone A
$C_{20}H_{18}O_6$ MW: 354.36 Source: GAN CAO. Ref: 2.

3862 Licopyranocoumarin
$C_{21}H_{20}O_7$ MW: 384.39 Source: GAN CAO.
Ref: 2.

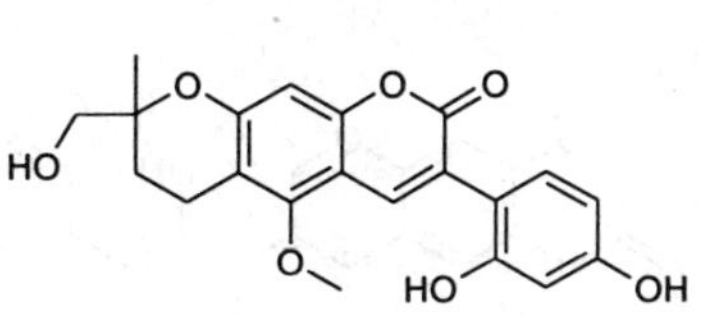

3863 Licoricesaponine A3
$C_{48}H_{72}O_{21}$ MW: 985.10 Source: GAN CAO.
Ref: 2.

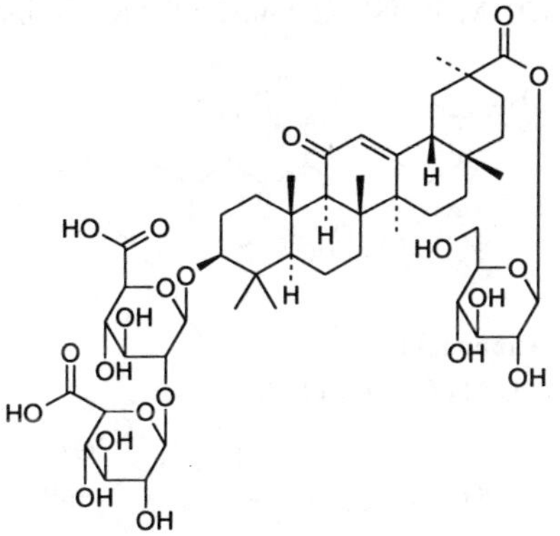

3864 Licoricesaponine B2
$C_{42}H_{64}O_{15}$ MW: 808.97 Source: GAN CAO.
Ref: 2.

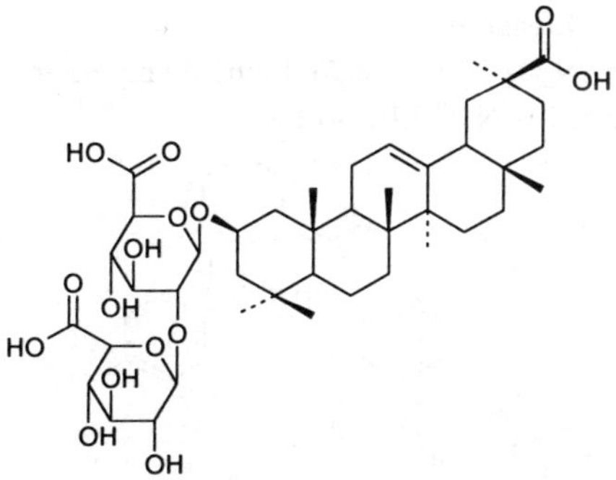

3865 Licoricesaponine C2
$C_{42}H_{62}O_{15}$ MW: 806.95 Source: GAN CAO.
Ref: 2.

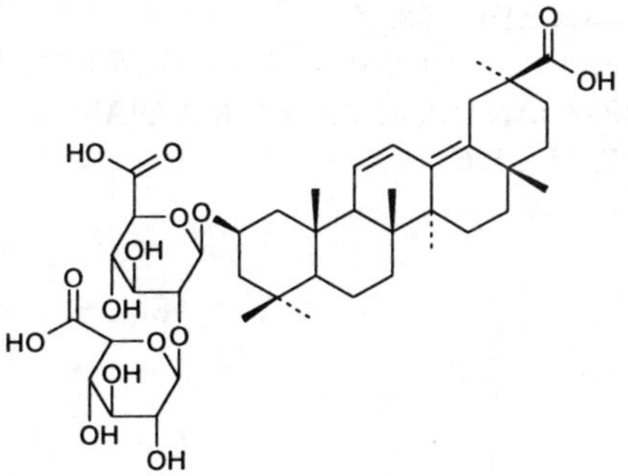

3866 Licoricesaponine D3
Source: GAN CAO. Ref: 2.

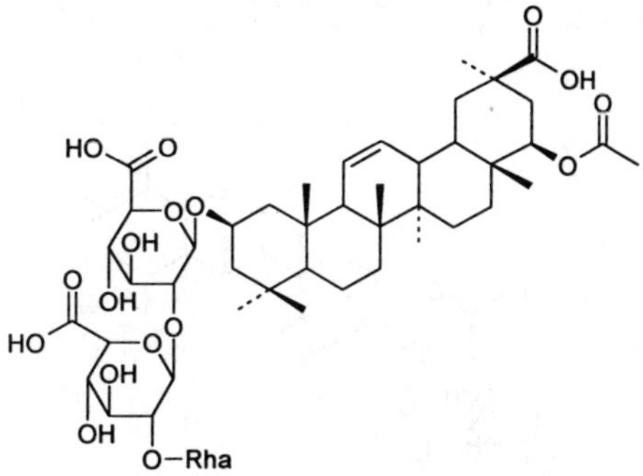

3867 Licoricesaponine F3
$C_{48}H_{72}O_{19}$ MW: 953.10 Source: GAN CAO.
Ref: 2.

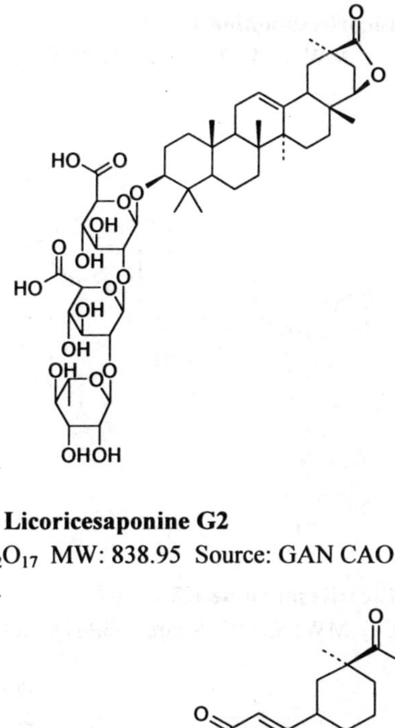

3868 Licoricesaponine G2
$C_{42}H_{62}O_{17}$ MW: 838.95 Source: GAN CAO.
Ref: 2.

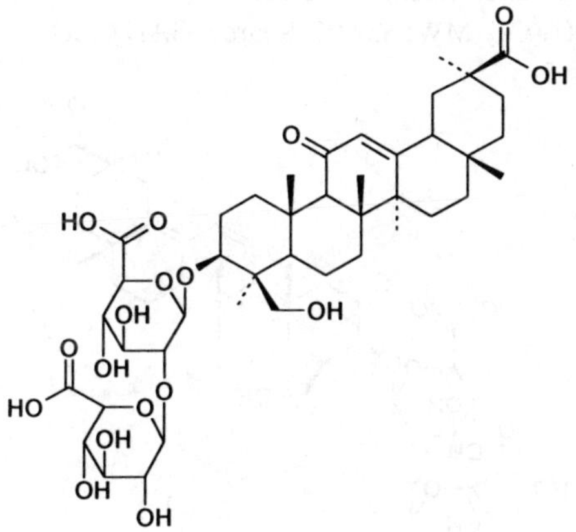

3869 Licoricesaponine H2
$C_{42}H_{62}O_{16}$ MW: 822.95 Source: GAN CAO.
Ref: 2.

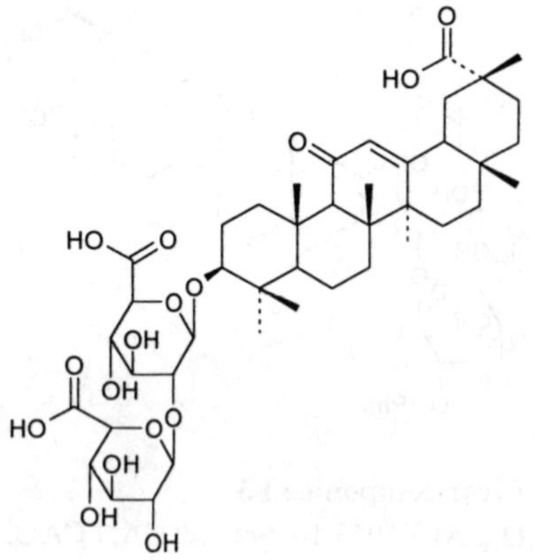

3870 Licoricesaponine J2
$C_{42}H_{64}O_{16}$ MW: 824.97 Source: GAN CAO.
Ref: 2.

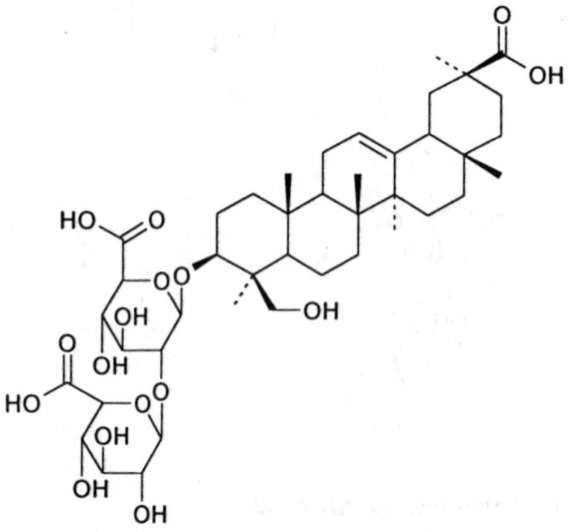

3871 Licoricesaponine K2
$C_{42}H_{62}O_{16}$ MW: 822.95 Source: GAN CAO.
Ref: 2.

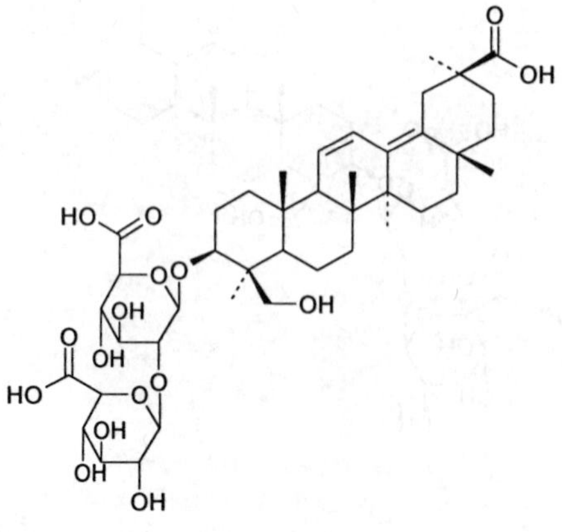

3872 Licoricidin
$C_{26}H_{32}O_5$ MW: 424.54 Source: GAN CAO.
Ref: 2.

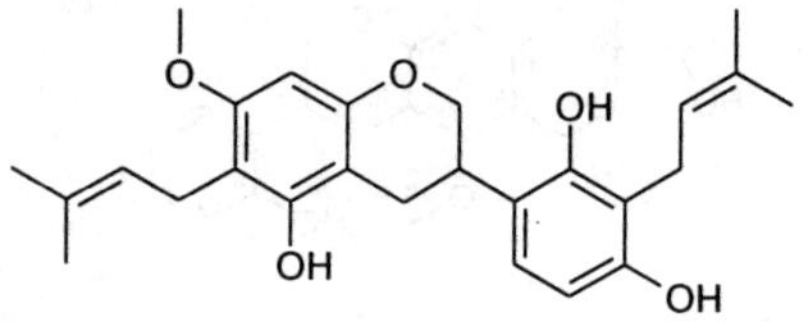

3873 Licoricone
$C_{22}H_{22}O_6$ MW: 382.42 Source: GAN CAO. Ref: 2.

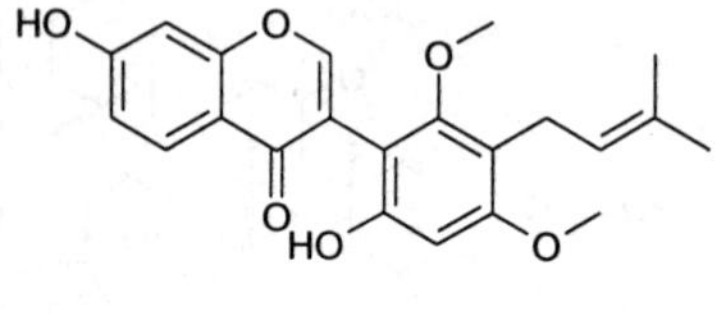

3874 Licuraside
Source: GAN CAO. Ref: 2.

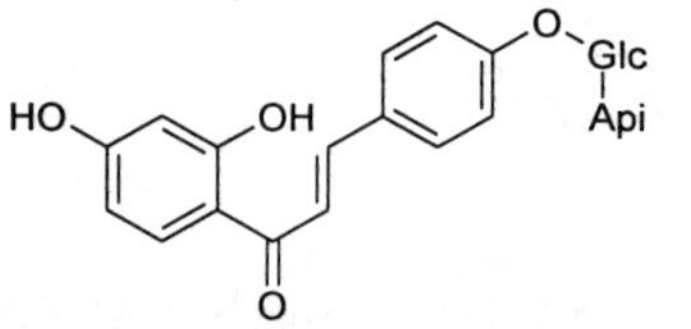

3875 Liensinine
$C_{37}H_{42}N_2O_6$ MW: 610.76 Property: mp 95-9°C.
Source: LIAN ZI XIN. Ref: 6.

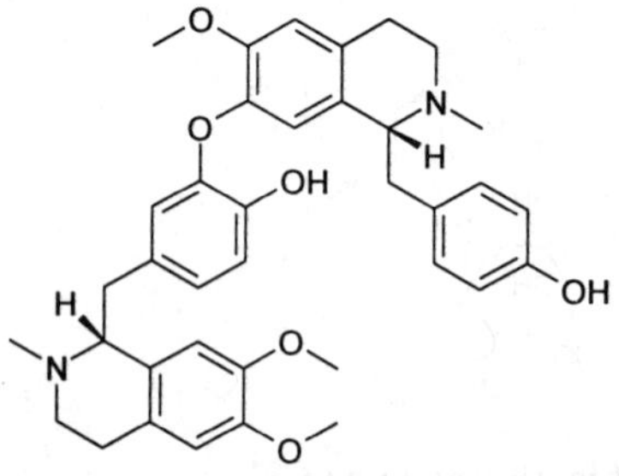

3876 Lignoceric acid
$C_{24}H_{48}O_2$ MW: 368.65 Property: mp 88°C.
Source: CHAI HU, FANG FENG, GUA LOU, LI JIANG QIAN HU, MAO ZHU MA QIAN.
Ref: 2, 557, 576.

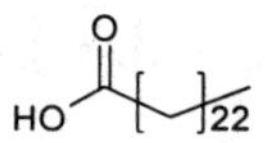

3877 N-Lignoceryl sphingosyl glucose
$C_{48}H_{93}NO_8$ MW: 812.28 Source: JING MI. Ref: 6.

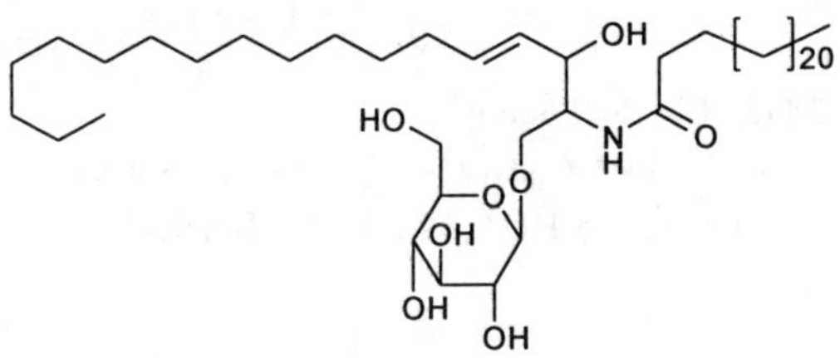

3878 Ligularine
$C_{23}H_{33}NO_9$ MW: 467.52 Source: HU LU QI. Ref: 6.

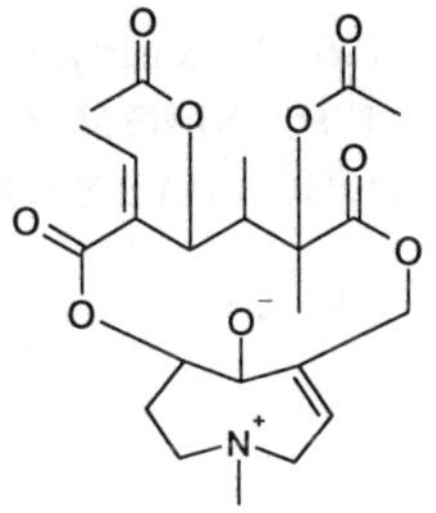

3879 Ligularone
$C_{14}H_{16}O_2$ MW: 216.28 Property: mp 64-5°C. Source: FENG DOU CAI, HU LU QI. Ref: 6.

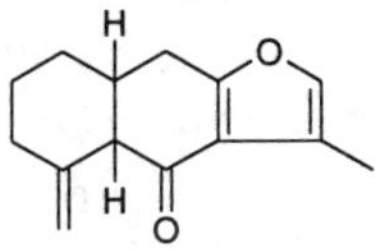

3880 Liguloxide
$C_{15}H_{26}O$ MW: 222.37 Property: mp 36°C. Source: HU LU QI. Ref: 6.

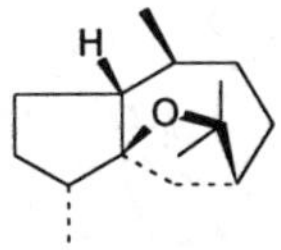

3881 Liguloxidol
$C_{15}H_{26}O_2$ MW: 238.37 Source: HU LU QI. Ref: 6.

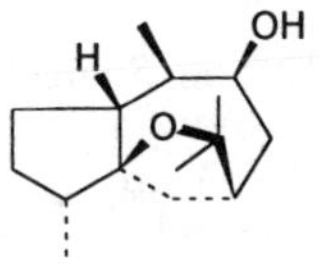

3882 Liguloxidol acetate
$C_{17}H_{28}O_3$ MW: 280.41 Property: mp 85°C. Source: HU LU QI. Ref: 6.

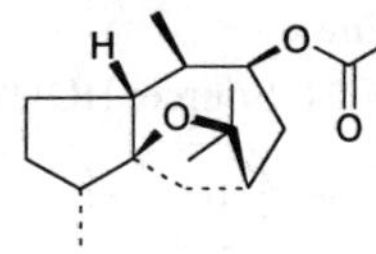

3883 Ligustilide
$C_{12}H_{14}O_2$ MW: 190.24 Source: CHUAN XIONG, DANG GUI, LIAO GAO BEN. Ref: 2, 343, 601.

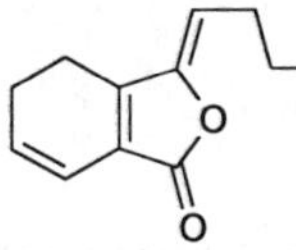

3884 Limocitrin-β-D-glucoside
$C_{23}H_{24}O_{13}$ MW: 508.44 Property: mp 150°C, 240-5°C. Source: NING MENG, TIAN CHEN. Ref: 6.

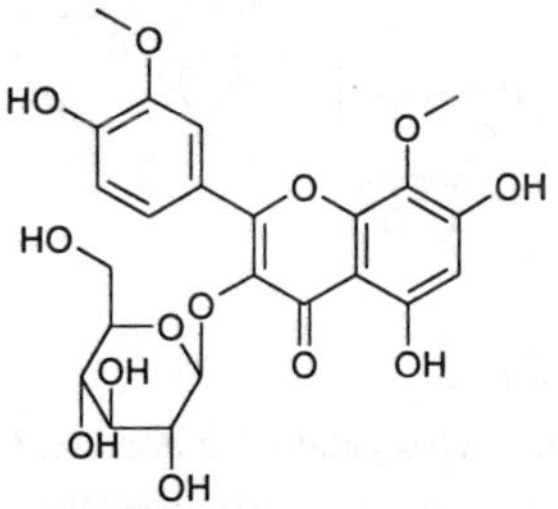

3885 Limocitrol-β-D-glucoside
$C_{24}H_{26}O_{14}$ MW: 538.47 Property: mp 163°C, 203-4°C. Source: NING MENG. Ref: 6.

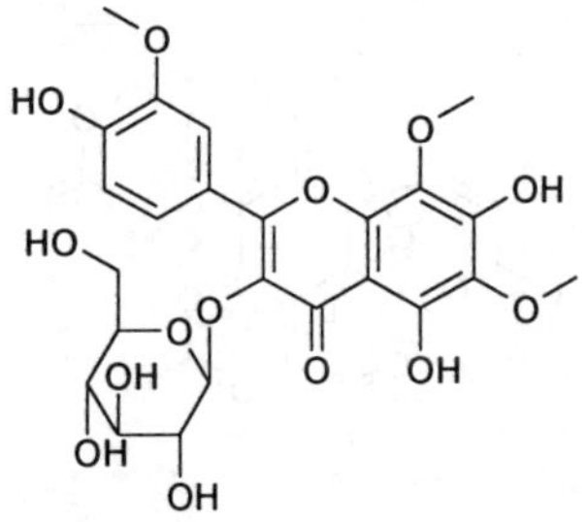

3886 Limonene
$C_{10}H_{16}$ MW: 136.24 Property: bp 178°C. Source: BO HE, CHAI HU, DONG LING CAO, GAN JIANG, JIU LI XIANG, JU PI, LIAN QIAO, QIANG HUO, QING HAO, SHENG JIANG, WU WEI ZI, WU ZHU YU, XI XIN. Ref: 2, 11.

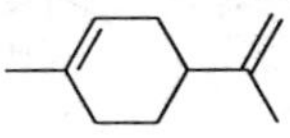

3887 α-Limonene

$C_{10}H_{16}$ MW: 136.24 Source: HOU PO. Ref: 2.

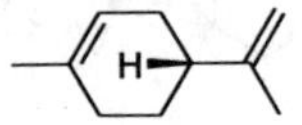

H

3888 d-Limonene

Source: HUO XIANG, JING JIE. Ref: 2.

3889 l-Limonene

Source: ZI SU. Ref: 2.

3891 Limonoic acid A-ring lactone

$C_{26}H_{32}O_9$ MW: 488.54 Source: TIAN CHEN. Ref: 6.

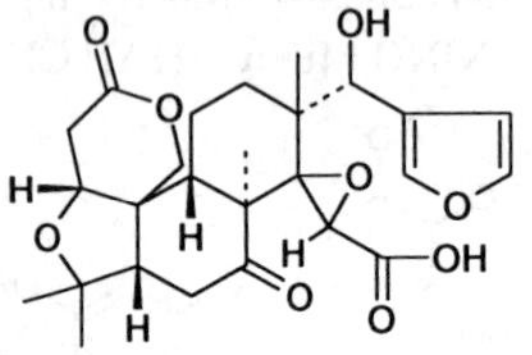

O OH O H H O H OH O O H

3892 Limonoid

6-Deoxy-6α-acetoxyatalantin acetate. $C_{31}H_{38}O_{11}$ MW: 586.64 Property: white lamellar prismatic crystal, mp 208-9°C. Source: DONG FENG JU. Ref: 402.

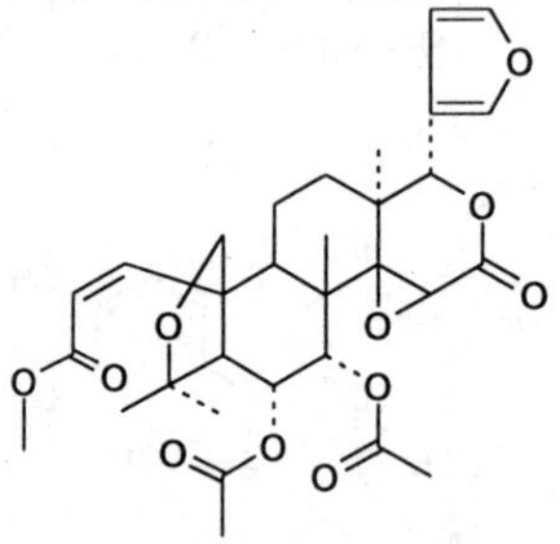

O O O O O O O O O O O

3893 Linalool

$C_{10}H_{18}O$ MW: 154.25 Source: CHAI HU, HOU PU, HUO XIANG, JIN YIN HUA, JU PI, LIAN QIAO, SHENG JIANG, WU WEI ZI, XING REN, YU XING CAO. Ref: 2, 638.

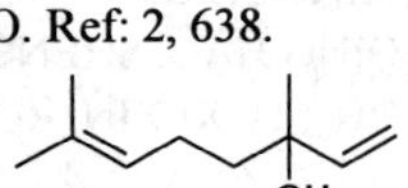

OH

3894 1-Linalool

$C_{10}H_{18}O$ MW: 154.25 Source: ZI SU. Ref: 2.

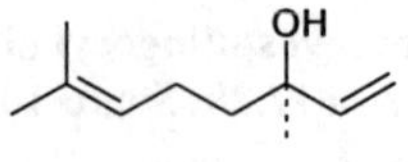

OH

3895 Linalool oxide

Epoxylinalool $C_{10}H_{18}O_2$ MW: 170.25 Source: GUI HUA, MA HUA, PI PA YE, XIANG YE. Ref: 6.

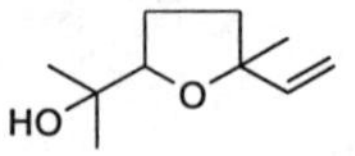

HO O

3896 Linalyl acetate

$C_{12}H_{20}O_2$ MW: 196.29 Property: bp 115-6°C/25 mm. Source: HOU PO, NING MENG, SHE XIANG CAO, YE HUA JIAO YE. Ref: 2, 6.

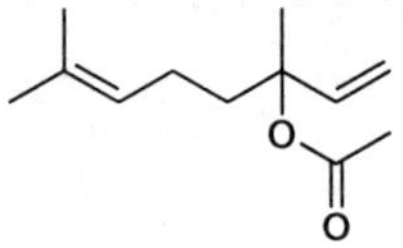

O O

3897 Linalyl benzoate

$C_{17}H_{22}O_2$ MW: 258.36 Source: MO LI HUA. Ref: 6.

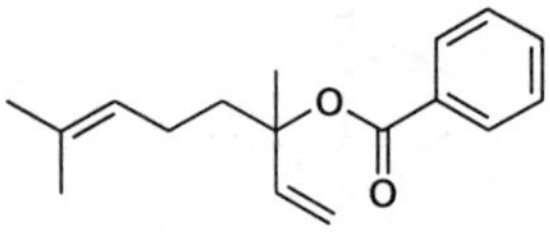

O O

3898 Linamarin

$C_{10}H_{18}NO_6$ MW: 247.25 Property: mp 142-3°C. Source: YA MA, YA MA ZI. Ref: 6.

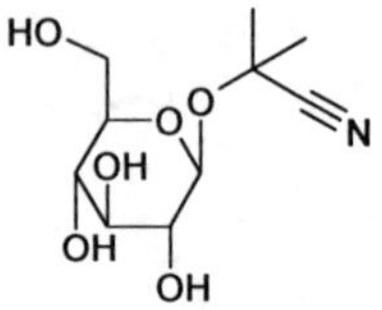

HO O O N OH OH OH

3899 Linarin

$C_{28}H_{32}O_{14}$ MW: 592.56 Source: HUO XIANG. Ref: 2.

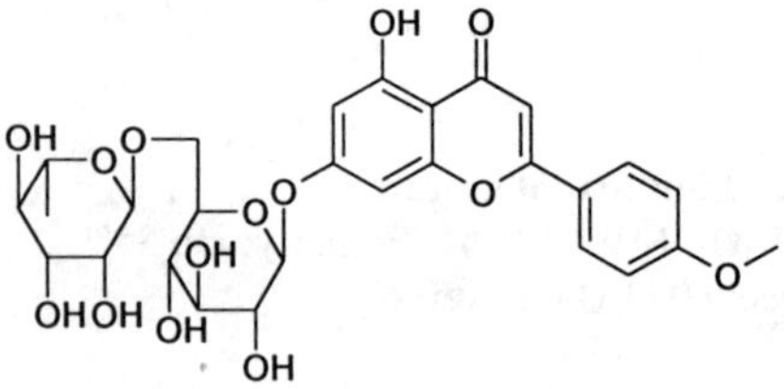

OH O OH O O O O O OH OH OH OH OH

3900 Linarin isovalerate
$C_{33}H_{40}O_{14}$ MW: 660.68 Property: mp 138-40°C. Source: ZHI ZHU XIANG. Ref: 6.

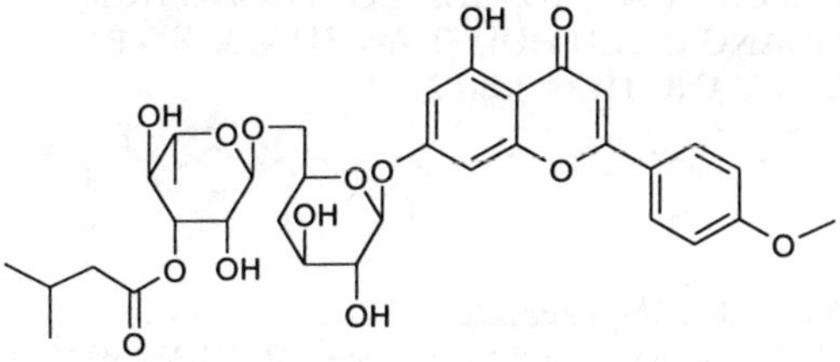

3901 Linarionoside A
$C_{19}H_{34}O_7$ MW: 374.48 Property: white powder, mp 108-10°C. Source: XI YANG SHEN. Ref: 445.

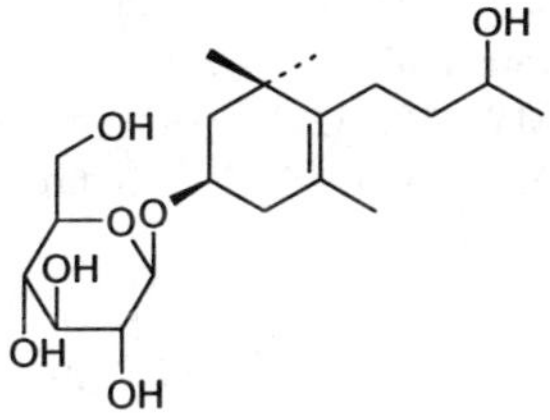

3902 Lindenene
$C_{15}H_{18}O$ MW: 214.31 Source: WU YAO. Ref: 6.

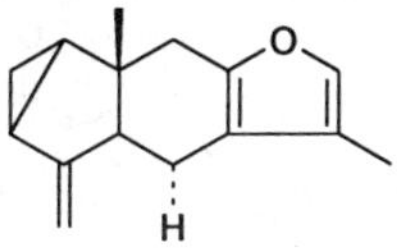

3903 Lindenenone
$C_{15}H_{16}O_2$ MW: 228.29 Property: mp 108°C. Source: WU YAO. Ref: 6.

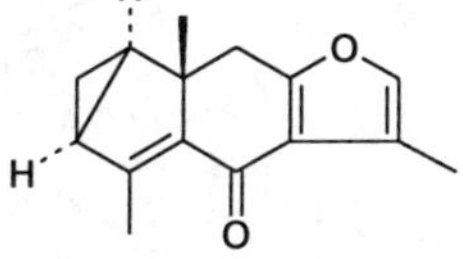

3904 Linderalactone
$C_{15}H_{16}O_3$ MW: 244.29 Property: mp 136-8°C. Source: WU YAO. Ref: 6.

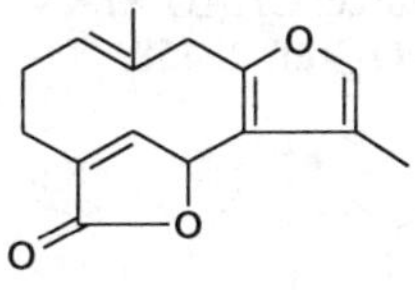

3905 Linderane
$C_{15}H_{16}O_4$ MW: 260.29 Property: mp 190-1°C (dec). Source: WU YAO. Ref: 6.

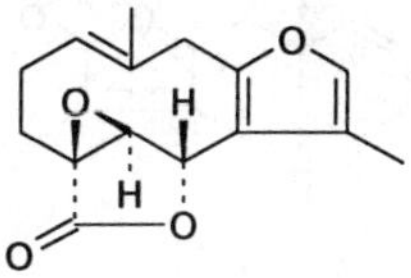

3906 Linderazulene
$C_{15}H_{14}O$ MW: 210.28 Property: mp 106-7°C. Source: WU YAO. Ref: 6.

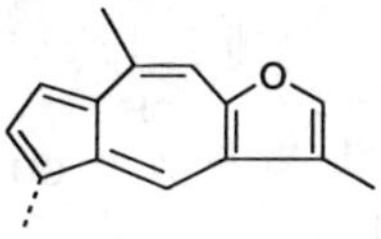

3907 Linderene
$C_{15}H_{18}O_2$ MW: 230.31 Property: mp 145°C. Source: WU YAO. Ref: 6.

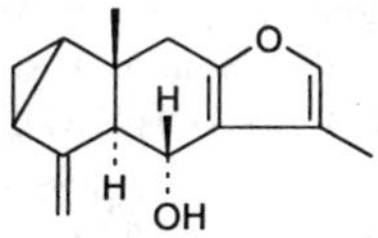

3908 linderene acetate
$C_{17}H_{20}O_3$ MW: 272.35 Property: mp 82°C. Source: WU YAO. Ref: 6.

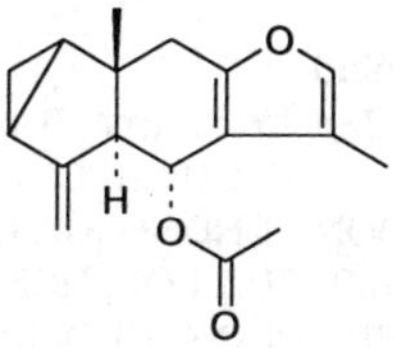

3909 Linderic acid
$C_{12}H_{22}O_2$ MW: 198.31 Source: MU XIANG. Ref: 2.

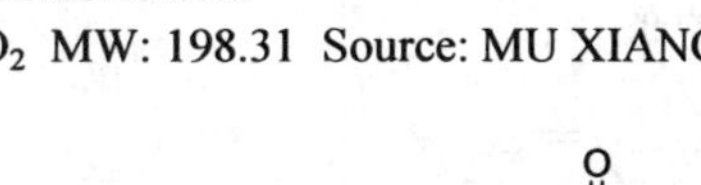

3910 Lindestrene
$C_{15}H_{18}O$ MW: 214.31 Property: bp 100-2°C/2 mm. Source: WU YAO. Ref: 6.

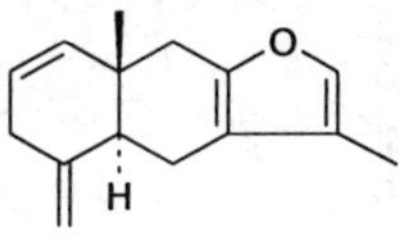

3911 Lindestrenolide
$C_{15}H_{18}O_2$ MW: 230.31 Property: bp 100-5°C/0.2°C. Source: WU YAO. Ref: 6.

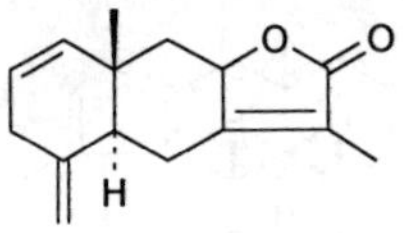

3912 Lindleyin
$C_{23}H_{26}O_{11}$ MW: 478.46 Source: DA HUANG. Ref: 2.

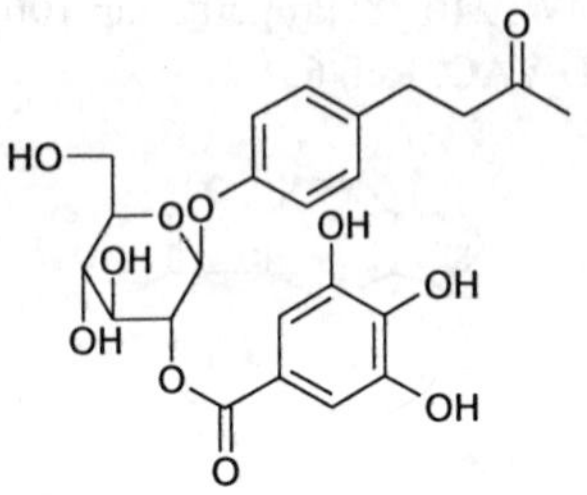

3913 Lineolone
Deacylcynanchogenin. $C_{21}H_{32}O_5$ MW: 364.49 Property: mp 240-4°C. Source: BAI SHOU WU, FU SHOU CAO, LUO MO, XU CHANG QING. Ref: 6.

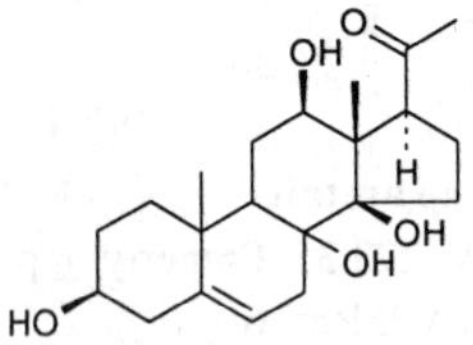

3914 Linoleic acid
$C_{18}H_{32}O_2$ MW: 280.45 Source: BAI GUO, BING LANG, CHUAN XIONG, CU LIU GUO (SHA JI), DA ZAO, DI GU PI, DONG CHONG XIA CAO, GAN DI HUANG, GOU QI ZI, GUA LOU, HONG HUA, HUANG QI, LU HUI, QIANG HUO, REN SHEN, SHAN ZHA, SHAN ZHU YU, XI YANG SHEN, XING REN, YA DAN ZI, YIN YANG HUO, YU XING. Ref: 2, 500.

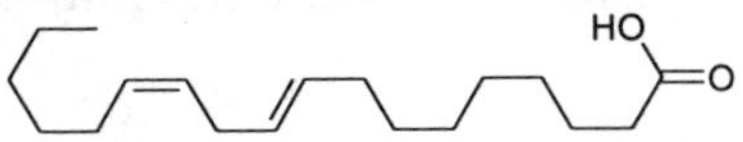

3915 Linolein
$C_{57}H_{98}O_6$ MW: 879.41 Property: mp -13°C. Source: BAI SU ZI. Ref: 6.

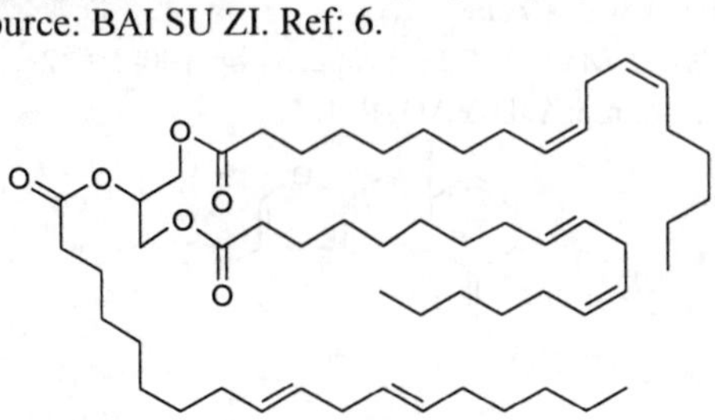

3916 Linolenic acid
$C_{18}H_{30}O_2$ MW: 278.44 Source: BA DOU, CHAI HU, CU LIU GUO (SHA JI), DI GU PI, DONG CHONG XIA CAO, GUA LOU, HONG HUA, HUANG QI, LU HUI, SHAN ZHA, XING REN, YIN YANG HUO. Ref: 2.

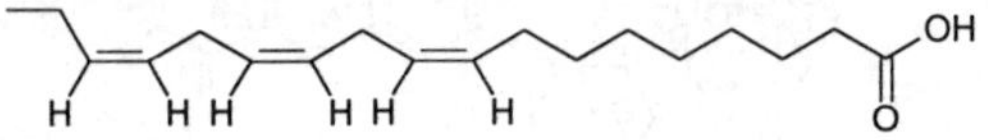

3917 Linoleyl acetate
$C_{20}H_{36}O_2$ MW: 308.51 Source: QI ZHOU YI ZHI HAO. Ref: 6.

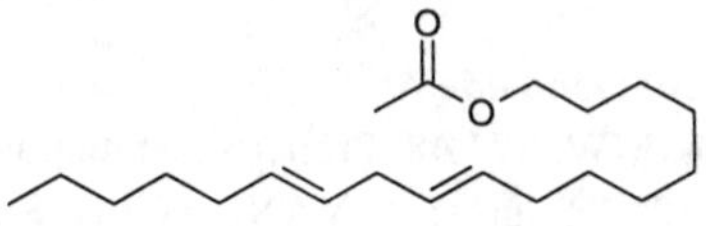

3918 α-Lipoic acid
$C_8H_{14}O_2S_2$ MW: 206.33 Property: mp (+): 46-8°C, (-): 45-7.5°C, (±): 59-61°C. Source: ZI CAI. Ref: 6.

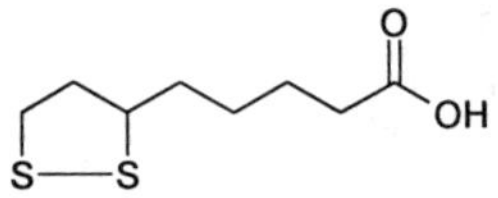

3919 β-Lipoic acid
$C_8H_{14}O_3S_2$ MW: 222.33 Source: ZI CAI. Ref: 6.

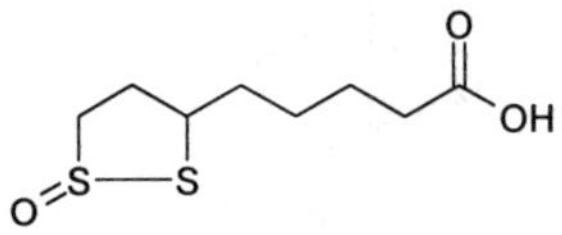

3920 Liquidambaric lactone
$C_{30}H_{44}O_4$ MW: 468.68 Property: white acicular crystal, mp >300 °C. Source: FENG XIANG SHU. Ref: 356.

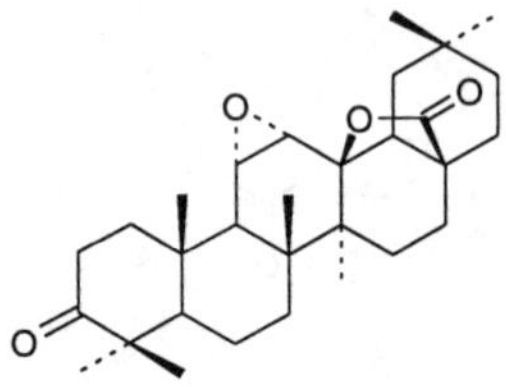

3921 Liquiritigenin
$C_{15}H_{12}O_4$ MW: 256.26 Property: white powder, mp 210-2°C. Source: CHAO XIAN YIN YANG HUO, GAN CAO. Ref: 2, 458.

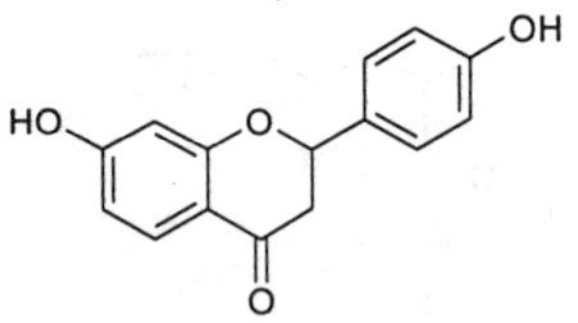

3922 Liquiritigenin-7-O-β-D-(3-O-acetyl)-apiofuranosyl-4'-O-β-D-glucopyranoside
$C_{28}H_{32}O_{14}$ MW: 592.56 Property: white powder, mp 201-2 °C. Source: ZHANG GUO GAN CAO. Ref: 376.

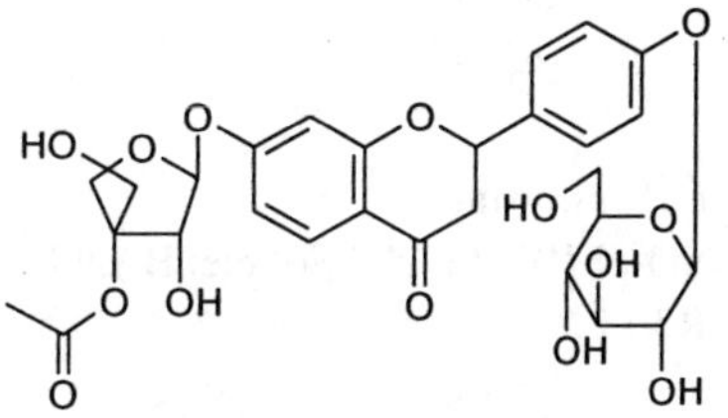

3923 Liquiritigenin-7-O-β-D-apiofuranosyl)-4'-O-β-D-glucopyranoside
$C_{26}H_{30}O_{13}$ MW: 550.52 Property: white powder, mp 214-5°C. Source: ZHANG GUO GAN CAO. Ref: 376.

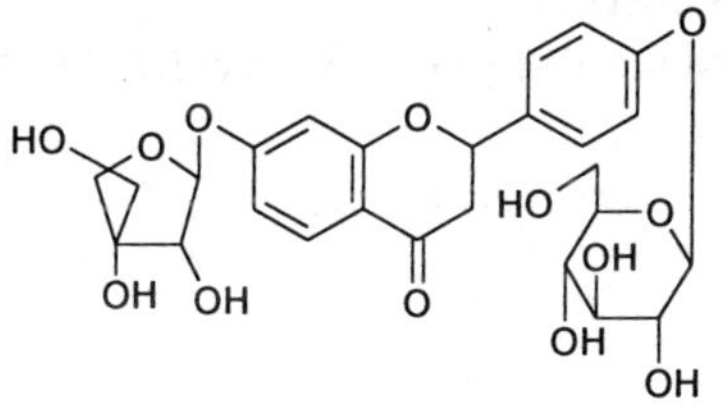

3924 Liquiritigenin-4'-apiosyl(1→2)glucoside
Source: GAN CAO. Ref: 2.

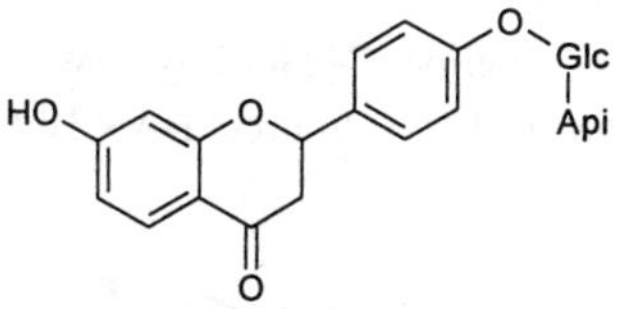

3925 Liquiritigenin-7,4'-diglucoside
$C_{27}H_{32}O_{14}$ MW: 580.55 Source: GAN CAO. Ref: 2.

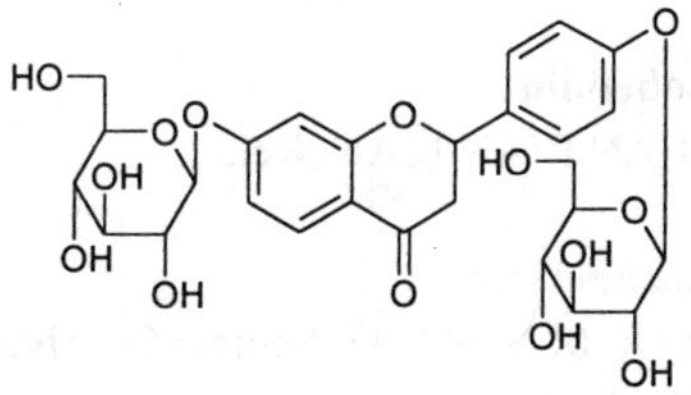

3926 Liquiritin
$C_{21}H_{22}O_9$ MW: 418.40 Source: GAN CAO. Ref: 2.

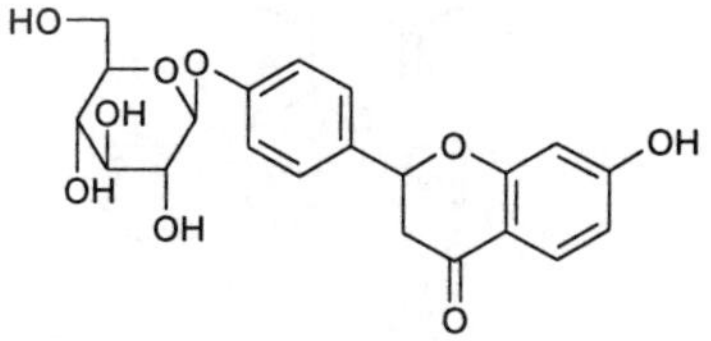

3927 Liquiritin-glucorhamnoside
Source: GAN CAO. Ref: 2.

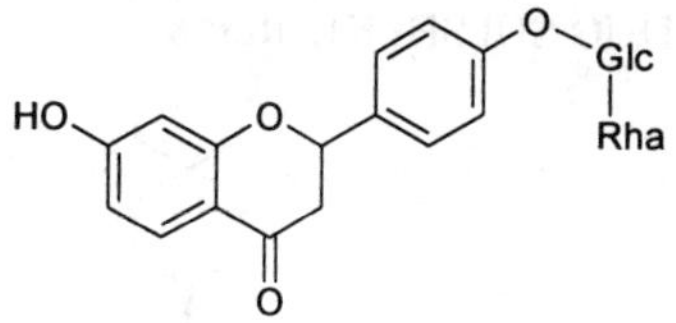

3928 Liquoric acid
$C_{30}H_{44}O_5$ MW: 484.68 Source: GAN CAO. Ref: 2.

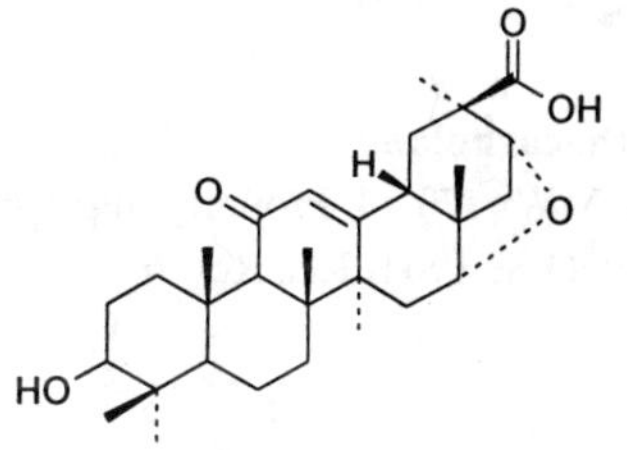

3929 Liriodendrin
$C_{34}H_{46}O_{18}$ MW: 742.73 Source: DU ZHONG. Ref: 2.

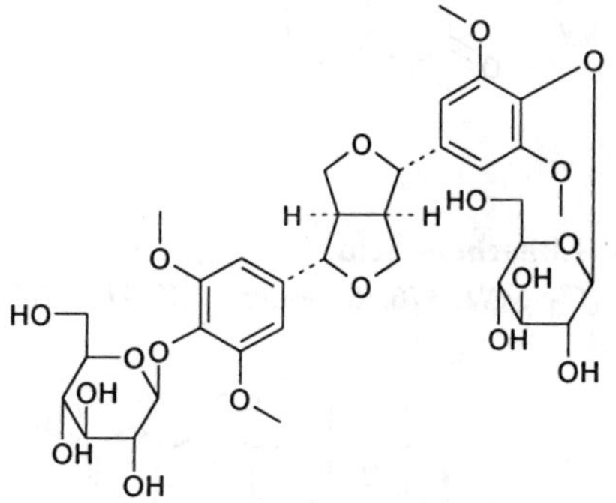

3930 Lirioresinol B dimethyl ether
$C_{24}H_{30}O_8$ MW: 446.50 Property: mp 122-3°C. Source: WANG CHUN MU LAN. Ref: 6, 543.

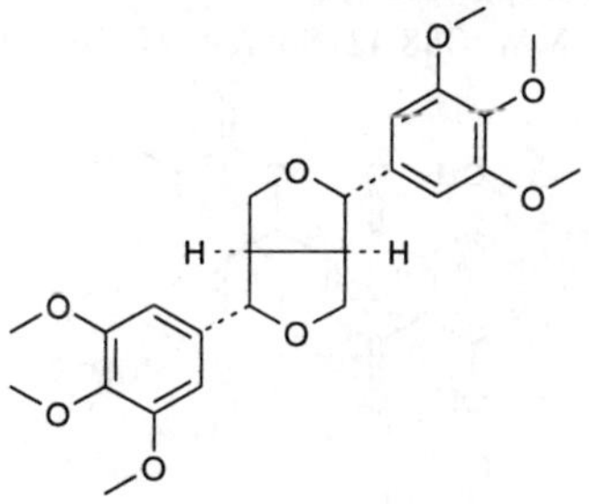

3931 Lithocarpdiol
$C_{31}H_{52}O_3$ MW: 472.76 Property: mp 179-80°C. Source: DUO SUI SHI KE. Ref: 6.

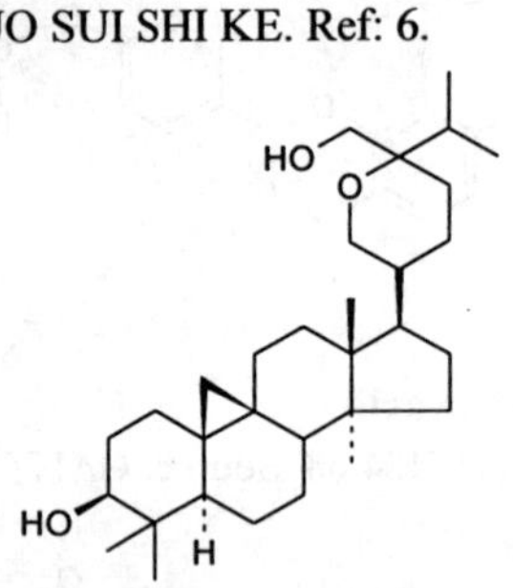

3932 Lithocarpolone
$C_{31}H_{50}O_3$ MW: 470.74 Property: mp 190-2°C. Source: DUO SUI SHI KE. Ref: 6.

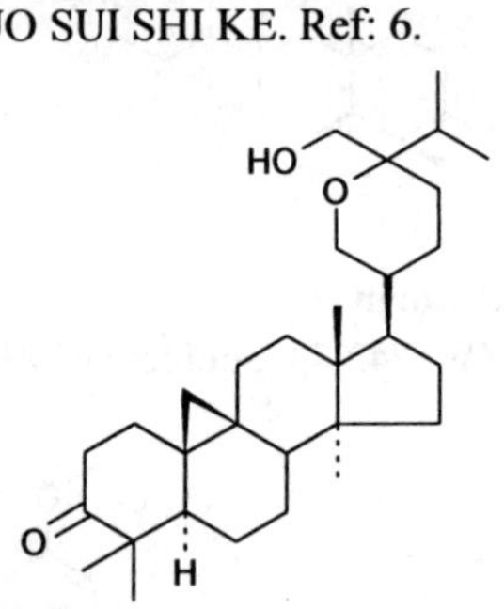

3933 Lithocholic acid
$C_{24}H_{40}O_3$ MW: 376.58 Source: NIU HUANG. Ref: 2.

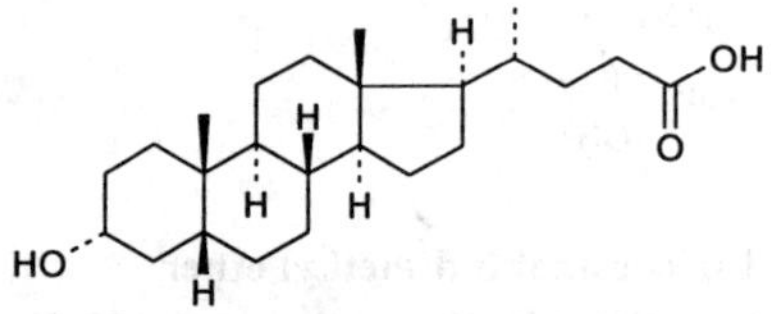

3934 Lithospermidin A
$C_{21}H_{24}O_7$ MW: 388.42 Source: ZI CAO. Ref: 2.

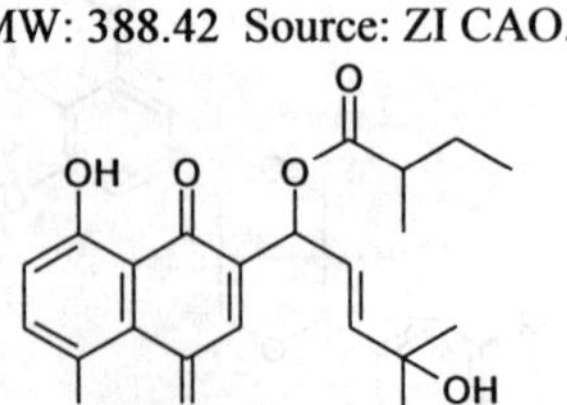

3935 Lithospermidin B
$C_{21}H_{24}O_7$ MW: 388.42 Source: ZI CAO. Ref: 2.

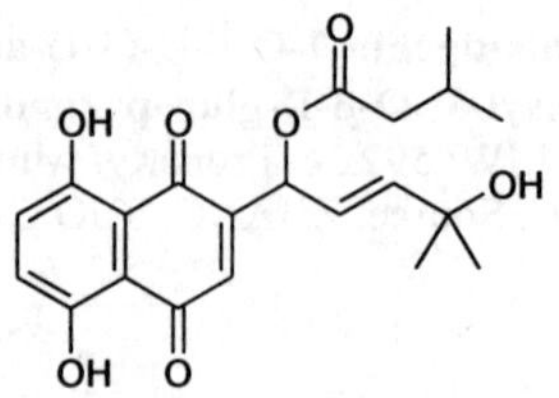

3936 Lobelanidine
$C_{22}H_{29}NO_2$ MW: 339.48 Source: BAN BIAN LIAN. Ref: 2.

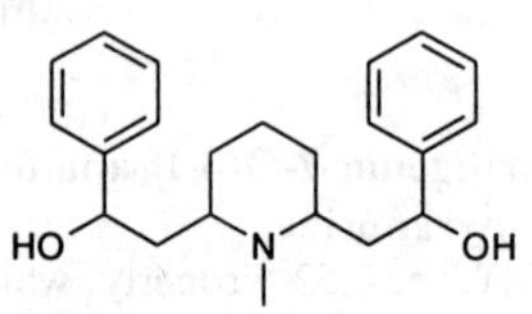

3937 Lobelanine
$C_{22}H_{25}NO_2$ MW: 335.45 Source: BAN BIAN LIAN. Ref: 2.

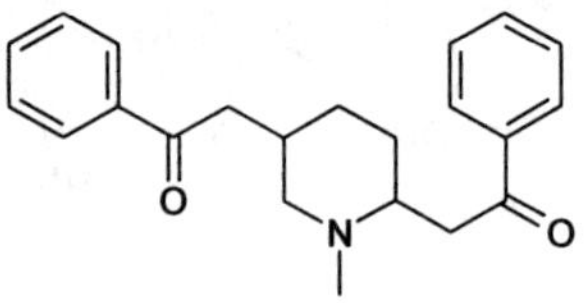

3938 Lobeline
Inflatine; α-Lobeline. $C_{22}H_{27}NO_2$ MW: 337.47 Property: mp 130-1°C. Source: BAN BIAN LIAN. Ref: 2, 4.

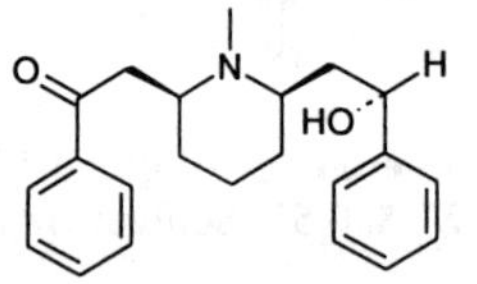

3939 Lobelinin
Source: BAN BIAN LIAN. Ref: 2.

3940 Lochnericine
$C_{21}H_{24}N_2O_3$ MW: 352.44 Source: CHANG CHUN HUA. Ref: 2.

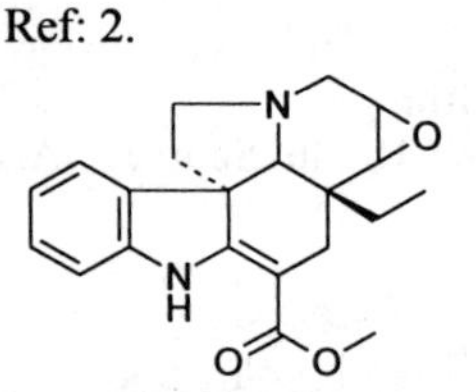

3941 Lochneridine
$C_{22}H_{28}N_2O_3$ MW: 368.48 Source: CHANG CHUN HUA. Ref: 2.

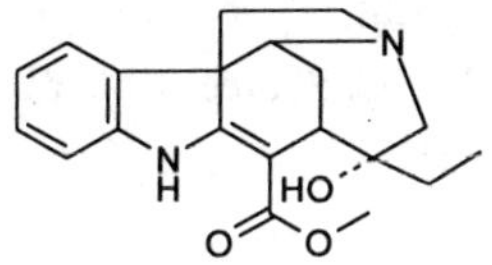

3942 Lochnerine
$C_{20}H_{24}N_2O_2$ MW: 324.43 Source: CHANG CHUN HUA. Ref: 2.

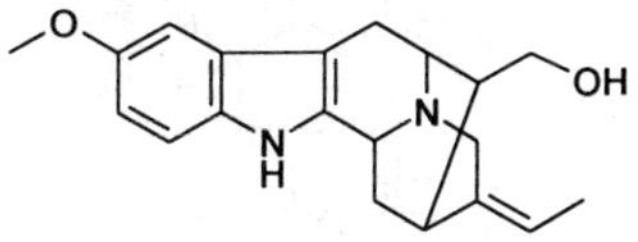

3943 Lochnerinine
$C_{22}H_{26}N_2O_4$ MW: 382.46 Source: CHANG CHUN HUA. Ref: 2.

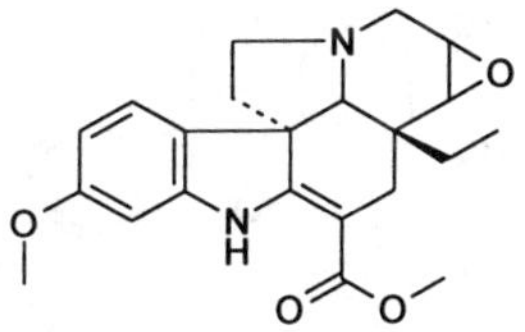

3944 Lochnerivine
$C_{24}H_{28}N_2O_5$ Source: CHANG CHUN HUA. Ref: 2.

3945 Lochrovicine
$C_{20}H_{22}N_2O_3$ Source: CHANG CHUN HUA. Ref: 2.

3946 Lochrovidine
$C_{22}H_{26}N_2O_4$ Source: CHANG CHUN HUA. Ref: 2.

3947 Lochrovine
$C_{23}H_{30}N_2O_3$ Source: CHANG CHUN HUA. Ref: 2.

3948 Loganic acid
$C_{15}H_{22}O_{11}$ MW: 378.34 Source: JIN YIN HUA, LONG DAN. Ref: 2, 638.

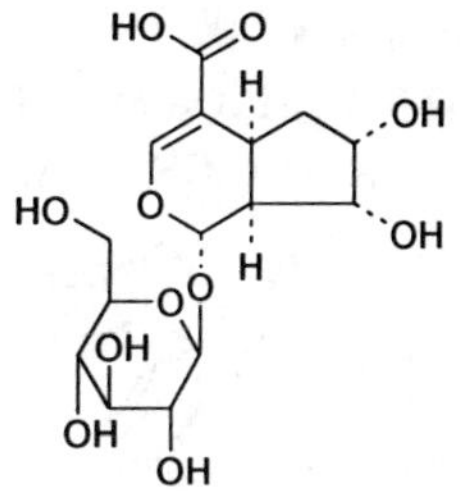

3949 Loganin
$C_{17}H_{26}O_{10}$ MW: 390.39 Source: BAI JIANG, CHANG CHUN HUA, JIN YIN HUA, SHAN ZHU YU. Ref: 2, 638.

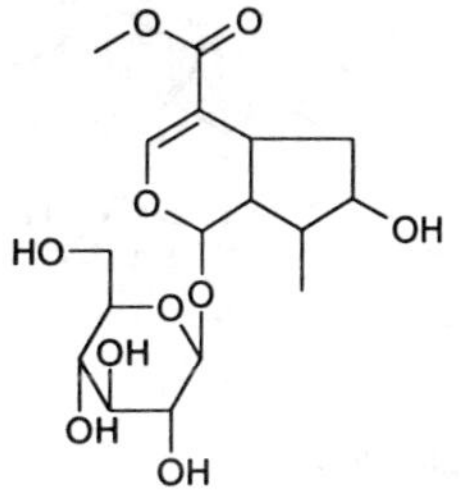

3950 Loganoside
$C_{16}H_{24}O_{11}$ MW: 392.36 Source: MA QIAN ZI. Ref: 2.

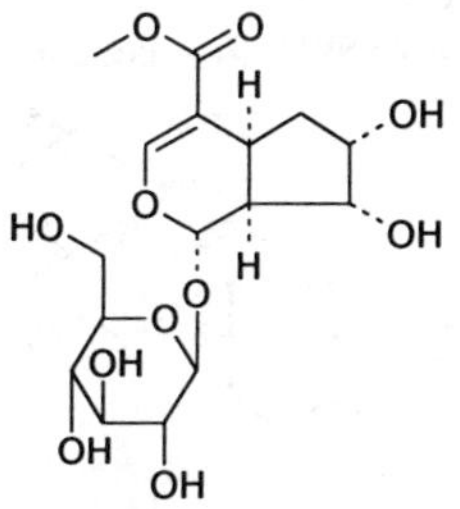

3952 Loliolide
$C_{11}H_{16}O_3$ MW: 196.25 Property: mp 149°C. Source: KUN BU. Ref: 6.

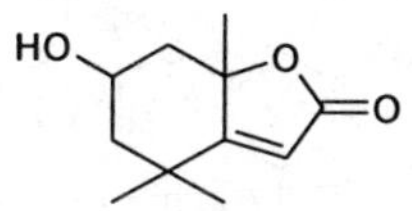

3953 Longifolene
$C_{15}H_{24}$ MW: 204.36 Source: CHAI HU, WU WEI ZI. Ref: 2.

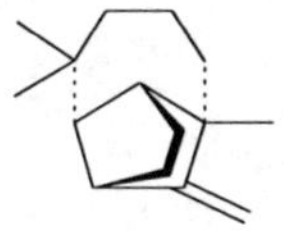

3954 Longikaurin A
CAS: 75207-67-9 $C_{20}H_{28}O_5$ MW: 348.44 Source: CHANG GUAN XIANG CHA CAI. Ref: 5.

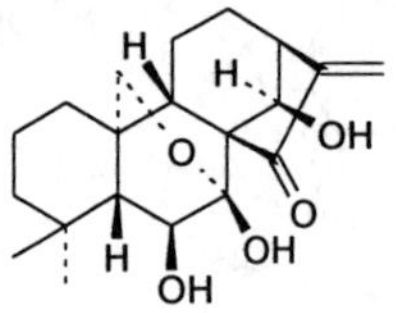

3955 Longikaurin B
CAS: 75207-66-8 $C_{22}H_{30}O_7$ MW: 406.48 Source: CHANG GUAN XIANG CHA CAI. Ref: 5.

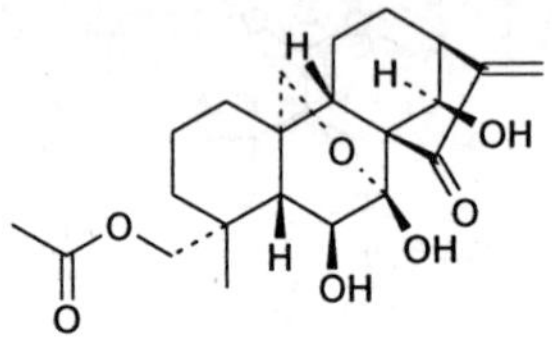

3956 α-Longipinene
$C_{15}H_{24}$ MW: 204.36 Source: CHAI HU, WU WEI ZI. Ref: 2.

3957 Longispinogenin
$C_{30}H_{50}O_3$ MW: 458.73 Source: CHAI HU. Ref: 2.

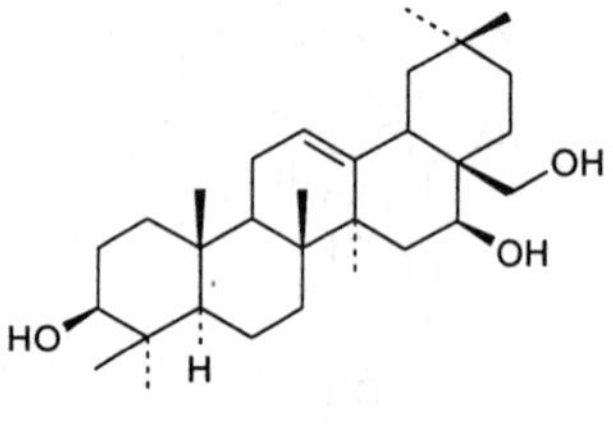

3958 Lonicerin
$C_{27}H_{30}O_{15}$ MW: 594.53 Source: ZHI SHI. Ref: 2.

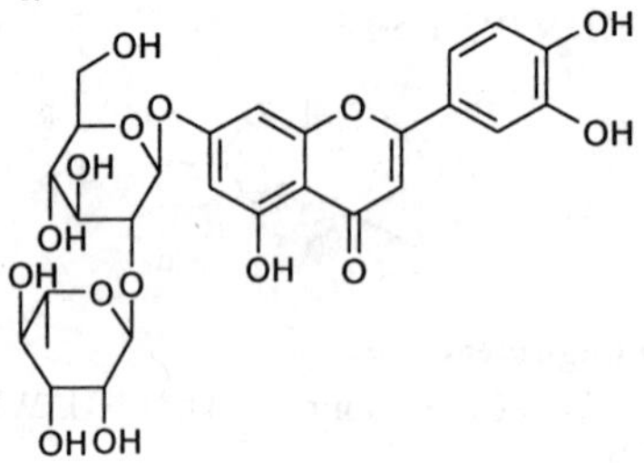

3959 Lophenol
Source: GUANG XI XUE JIE. Ref: 616.

3960 Lotaustralin
Property: mp 121°C. Source: XIA YE HONG JING TIAN. Ref: 516.

3961 Lotusine
$C_{19}H_{24}NO_3$ MW: 314.41 Source: LIAN ZI XIN. Ref: 6.

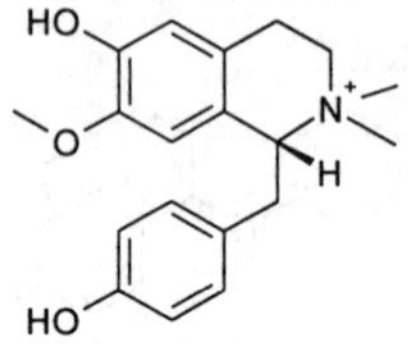

3962 Lucernol
$C_{15}H_8O_5$ MW: 268.23 Property: mp >350°C. Source: MU XU. Ref: 6.

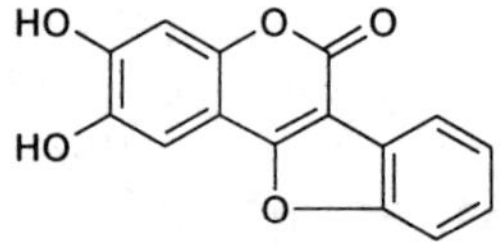

3963 Lucidin
$C_{15}H_{10}O_5$ MW: 270.24 Property: mp >330°C. Source: TU LIAN QIAO, YANG JIAO TENG. Ref: 6.

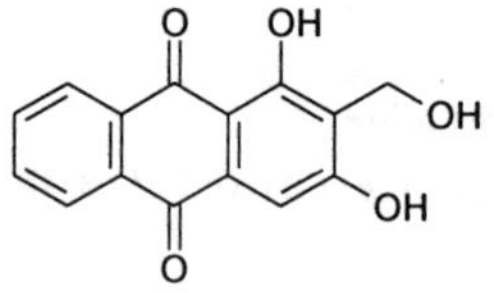

3964 Lucyin A
21β-Hydroxy-gypsogenin(L-2). $C_{30}H_{46}O_5$ MW: 486.70 Property: colorless claviform crystal, mp 240-2°C. Source: SI GUA. Ref: 284.

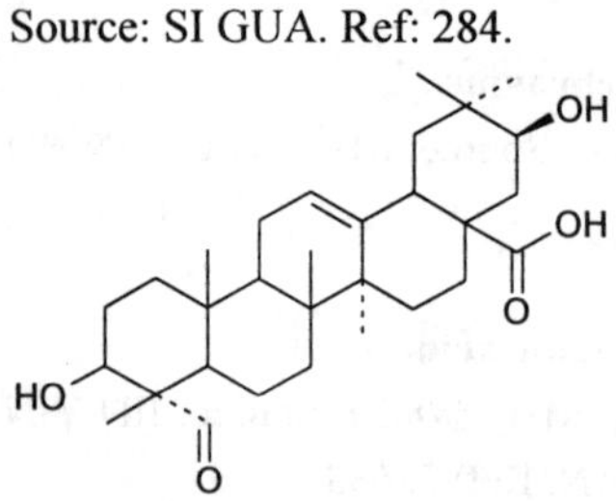

3965 Lucyoside N
3-O-β-D-glucopyranosyl-21-β-hydroxyhederangenin. $C_{36}H_{58}O_{10}$ MW: 650.86 Property: colorless granular crystal, mp 221-3°C. Source:SI GUA. Ref: 284.

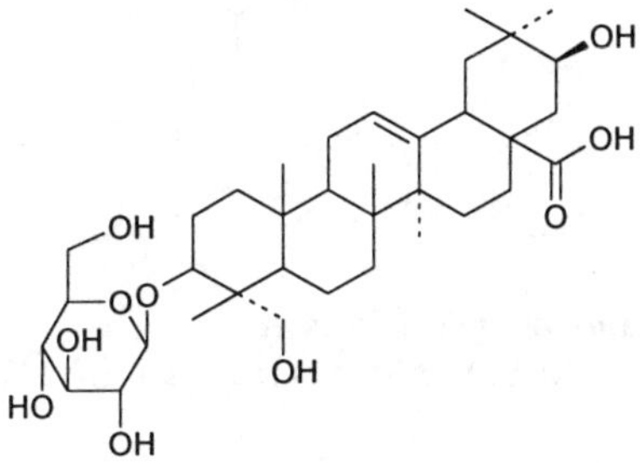

3966 Lucyoside Q
21β-Hydroxyloleanoic acid-28-O-β-D-glucopyranoside. $C_{36}H_{58}O_9$ MW: 634.86 Property: white powder, mp 238-40°C, $[\alpha]_D^{15}$ +23.5° (c=0.40, methanol). Source: SI GUA. Ref: 346.

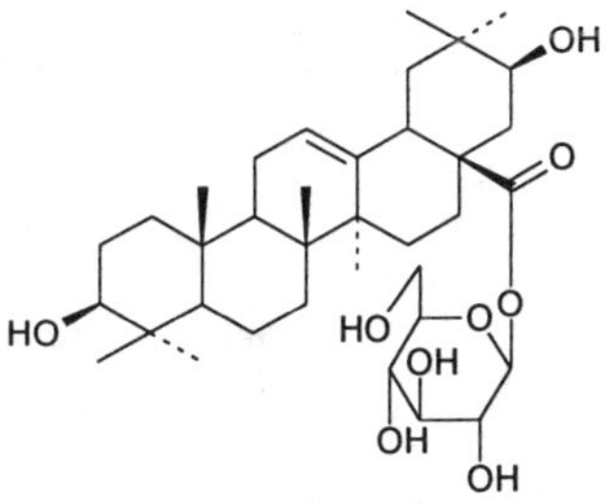

3967 Lucyoside R
2α,21β-Dihydroxyhederagenin-3-O-β-D-glucopyranoside. $C_{36}H_{58}O_{11}$ MW: 666.86 Property: colorless granular crystal, mp 234-6°C, $[\alpha]_D$ +35.7° (c=0.40, methanol). Source: SI GUA. Ref: 396.

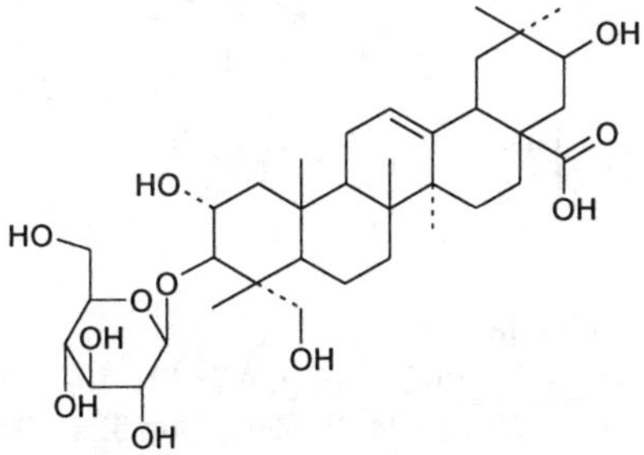

3968 Ludongnin
Property: mp 266-8°C. Source: DONG LING CAO. Ref: 501.

3969 Lumicaeruleic acid
Source: Huang Bai. Ref: 2.

3970 β-Lumicolchicine
$C_{22}H_{25}NO_6$ MW: 399.45 Property: mp 184-6°C. Source: CAO BEI MU. Ref: 6.

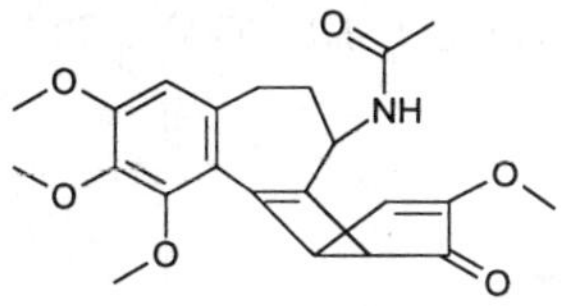

3971 Lunularic acid
$C_{15}H_{14}O_4$ MW: 258.28 Property: mp 192°C. Source: BA XIAN HUA. Ref: 6.

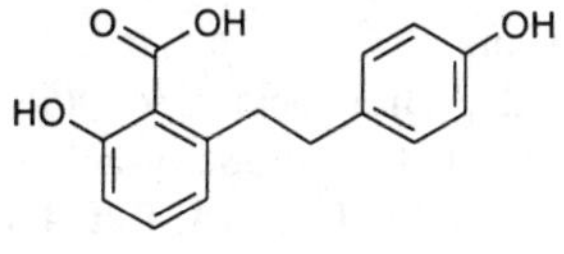

3972 Lupanine
$C_{15}H_{24}N_2O$ MW: 248.37 Property: mp (+): 44°C, (-): 44°C. Source: HONG MAO QI, KU SHEN, MU MA DOU. Ref: 2, 6.

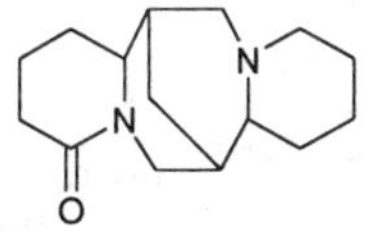

3973 Lupenone
$C_{30}H_{48}O_8$ MW: 424.72 Property: mp 170°C. Source: CHI YANG, WU TONG BAI PI. Ref: 6.

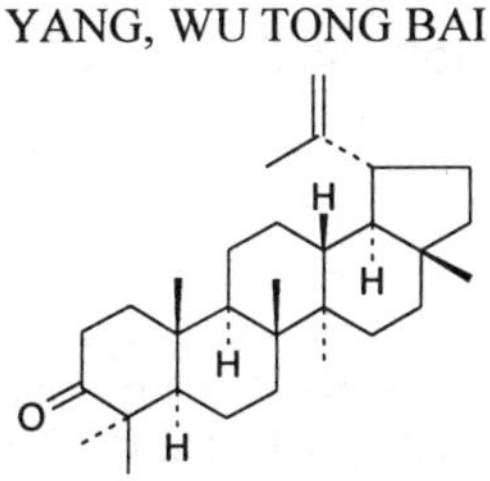

3974 Lupeol
$C_{30}H_{50}O$ MW: 426.73 Property: colorless acicular crystal, mp 214-6°C, $[\alpha]_D^{18}$ +20.0° (c= 0.101, $CHCl_3$). Source: BAI HUA, CAN JIAN, GUI GA, JUN QIAN ZI, KU DI DAN, KU DING CHA, SANG JI SHENG, SANG YE, SHAN DOU GEN, SHAN REN YE, WU HUA GUO YE, YANG MEI, YOU GAN GEN, YOU GAN MU PI, YOU GAN YE, YUAN CAN SHA. Ref: 6, 453.

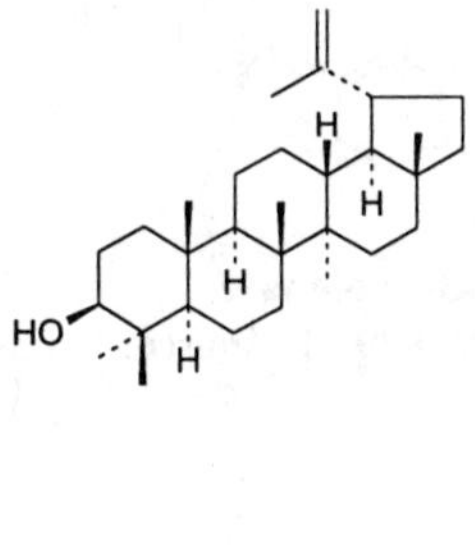

3975 Lupeol acetate
$C_{32}H_{52}O_2$ MW: 468.77 Property: mp 217-8°C. Source: HUANG HUA JIA ZHU TAO, KU DI DAN, MANG GUO SHU, XIANG PI MU. Ref: 6.

3976 Lupulone
β-Lupulic acid; β-Bitter acid. CAS: 468-28-0
$C_{26}H_{38}O_4$ MW: 414.59 Property: mp 92-4°C. Source: LU CAO, PI JIU HUA. Ref: 4, 6.

3977 Luteic acid
$C_{14}H_8O_9$ MW: 320.221 Property: mp 338-42°C (dec). Source: FAN SHI LIU PI. Ref: 6.

3978 Lutein
$C_{40}H_{56}O_2$ MW: 568.89 Property: mp 196°C. Source: DAO CAO, HAI XIA, HUO SUO MA, JI ZI BAI, JI ZI HUANG, JIA LIAN QIAO YE, JIN YU, LI YU PI, NING MENG YE, PU GONG YING, SU MI, SUAN SHUI CAO, TU SI ZI, ZI CAI. Ref: 6.

3979 Lutein-3-linolenate
$C_{58}H_{84}O_3$ MW: 829.31 Source: XIANG RI KUI YE. Ref: 6.

3980 Lutein oleic acid ester
$C_{58}H_{88}O_3$ MW: 833.35 Source: DI TANG HUA. Ref: 6.

3981 Lutein-3-palmitate
$C_{56}H_{86}O_3$ MW: 807.31 Source: XIANG RI KUI YE. Ref: 6.

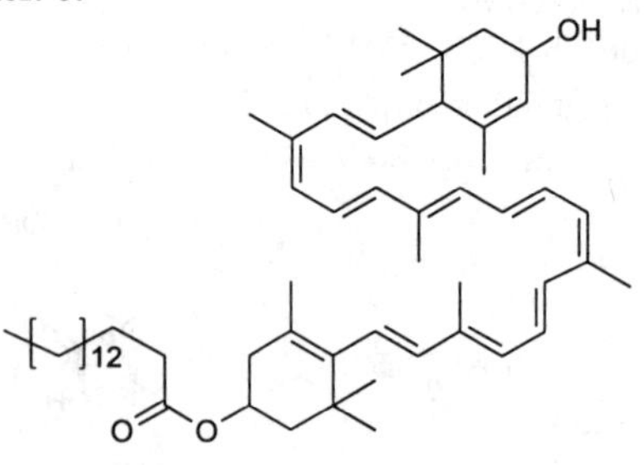

3982 Luteolin
Cyanidenon; Digitoflavone. CAS: 491-70-3
$C_{15}H_{10}O_6$ MW: 286.24 Property: mp 328-30°C (dec). Source: JIAN DI PU GONG YING, JIN YIN HUA, JING JIE, MI MENG HUA, QING HAO. Ref: 4, 369, 602.

3983 Luteolin 7-O-β-D-galactoside

$C_{21}H_{20}O_{11}$ MW: 448.39 Source: LIE YE JU MAI CAI, YA DAN ZI. Ref: 2, 521.

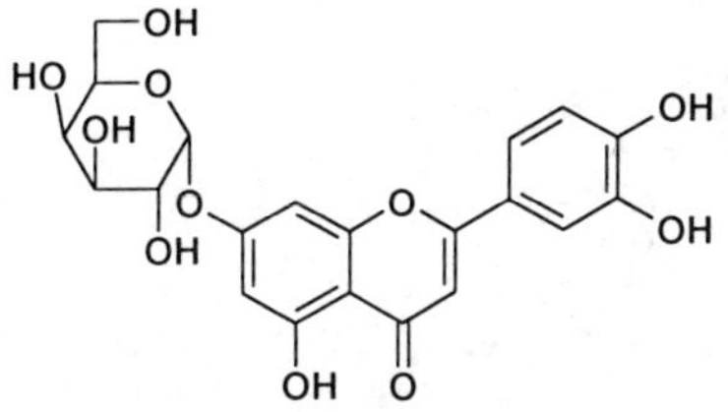

3984 Luteolin-7-O-glucoside

Cymaroside; Cynaroside; Gimaroside; Glucolutaolin; Luteoloside. CAS: 5373-11-5 $C_{21}H_{20}O_{11}$ MW: 448.39 Property: yellow granular crystal, mp 255-60°C. Source: HU ZHANGV, JIN JIE, PU GONG YING, PU GONG YING, QING HAO, XIAN HE CAO. Ref: 2, 4, 440, 475.

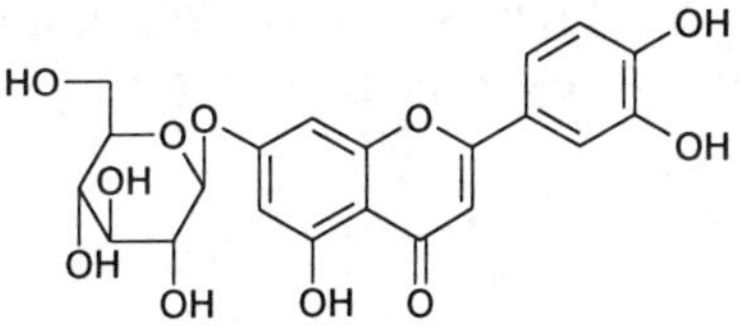

3985 Luteolin-4'-β-D-glucoside

$C_{15}H_{16}O_{10}$ MW: 356.29 Property: mp 168-78°C. Source: SHU QU CAO. Ref: 6.

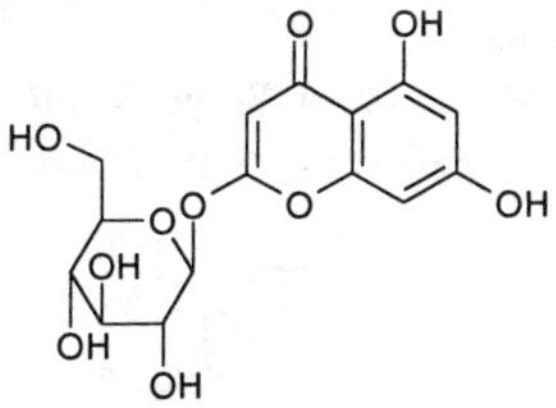

3986 Luteolin-7-β-D-glucuronide

$C_{21}H_{18}O_{12}$ MW: 462.37 Property: mp 182-2°C. Source: WO JU. Ref: 6.

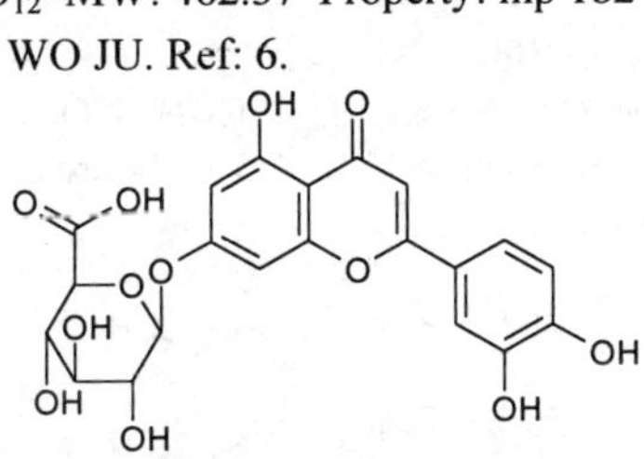

3987 Luteolin-7-rutinoside

$C_{27}H_{30}O_{15}$ MW: 594.53 Source: JI CAI. Ref: 6.

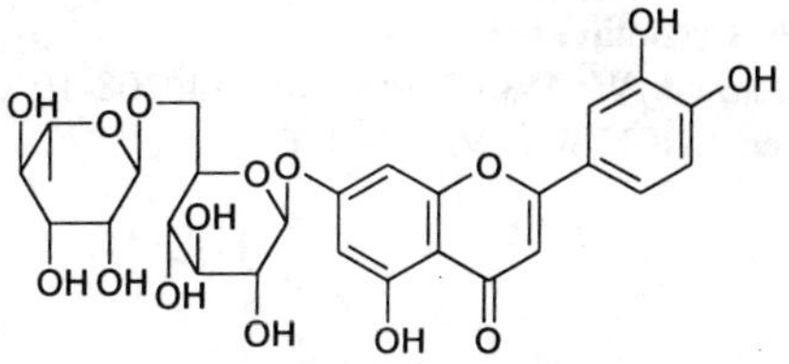

3988 Lychnose

$C_{24}H_{42}O_{21}$ MW: 666.59 Source: BAI NIU XI. Ref: 6.

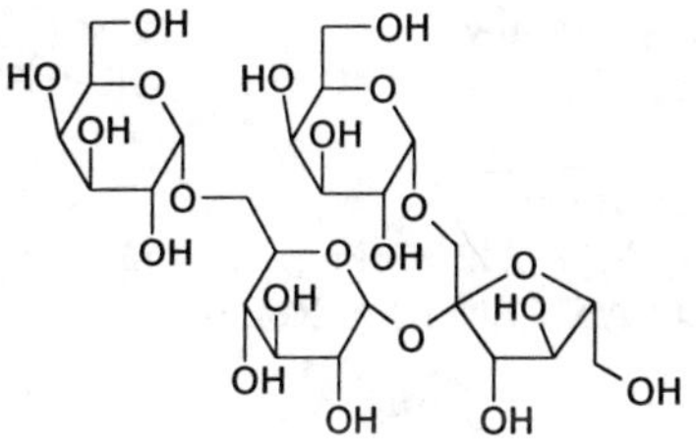

3989 Lyciumin A

$C_{15}H_{10}O_{6}$ MW: 286.24 Source: JIN YIN HUA, JIN JIE, QING HAO. Ref: 2.

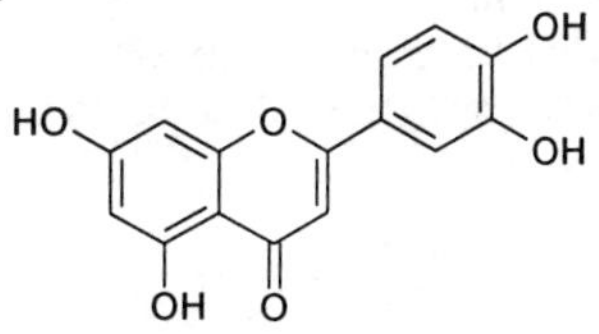

3990 Lycocernuine

$C_{16}H_{26}N_{2}O_{2}$ MW: 278.40 Property: mp 230°C. Source: PU DI WU GONG. Ref: 6.

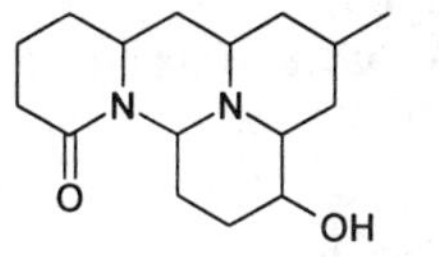

3991 Lycoclavanin

$C_{30}H_{48}O_{5}$ MW: 488.71 Property: mp 344-6°C. Source: SHEN JIN CAO. Ref: 6.

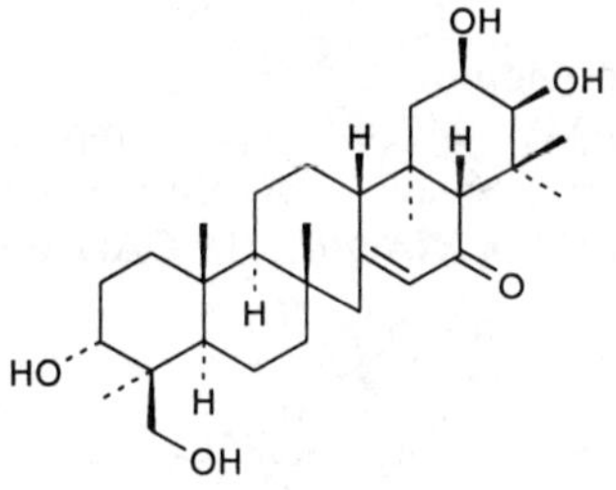

3992 Lycoclavanol
$C_{30}H_{50}O_3$ MW: 458.73 Property: mp 308-10°C. Source: SHEN JIN CAO. Ref: 6.

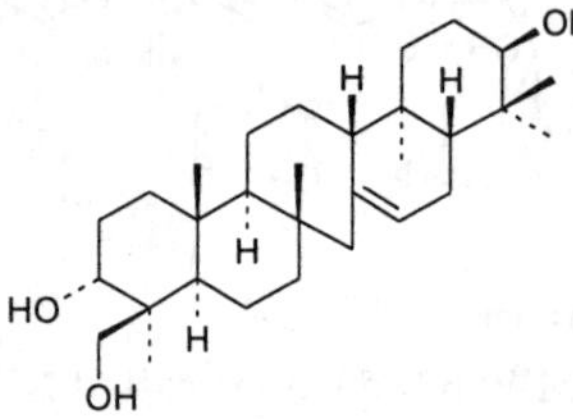

3993 Lycoctonine
Source: XUE SHANGYI ZHI HAO. Ref: 618.

3994 Lycodine
$C_{16}H_{22}N_2$ MW: 242.37 Property: mp 118°C. Source: QIAN CENG TA. Ref: 6.

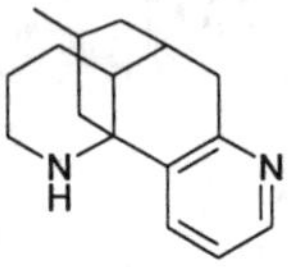

3995 Lycodoline
$C_{16}H_{25}NO_2$ MW: Property: mp 180°C. Source: QIAN CENG TA, SHEN JIN CAO, XIAO JIE JIN CAO. Ref: 6.

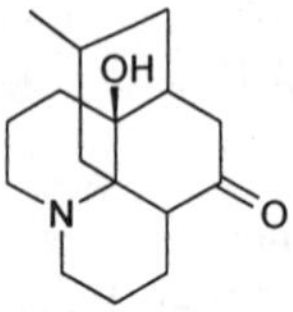

3996 Lycophyll
$C_{39}H_{54}O_2$ MW: 554.86 Property: mp 179°C. Source: KU QIE. Ref: 6.

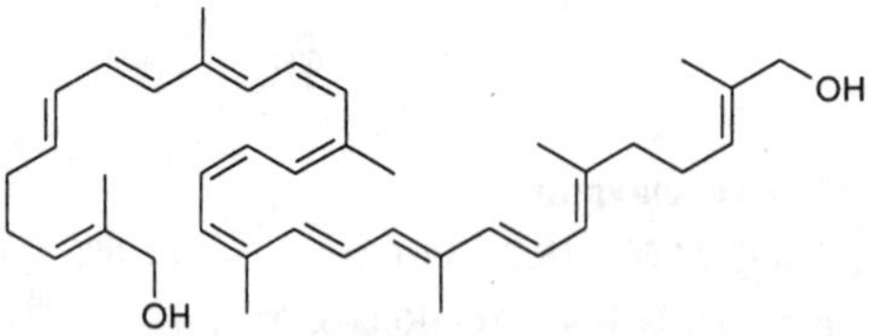

3997 Lycopodine
$C_{16}H_{25}NO$ MW: 247.38 Property: mp 116°C, bp 125°C/0.2 mm. Source: GUO JIANG LONG, SHEN JIN CAO, XIAO JIE JIN CAO. Ref: 6.

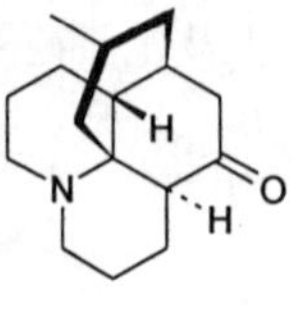

3998 Lycopose
$C_{36}H_{62}O_{31}$ MW: 990.88 Property: mp 270°C. Source: DI SUN, ZE LAN. Ref: 6.

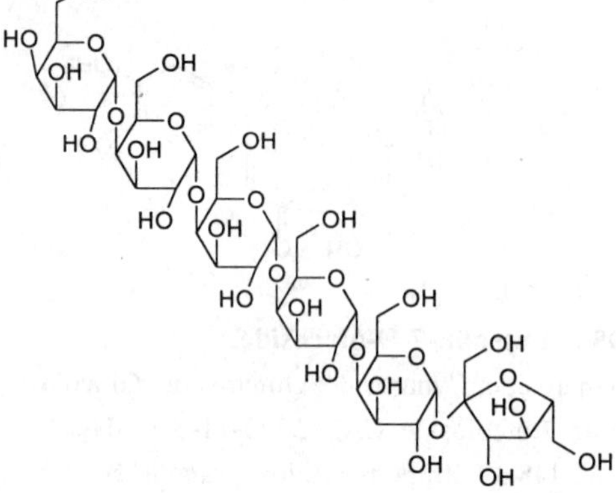

3999 Lycoramine
CAS: 21133-52-8 $C_{17}H_{23}NO_3$ MW: 289.38 Property: mp 121°C. Source: DA YI ZHI JIAN, SHUI XIAN GEN, SHI SUAN. Ref: 4.

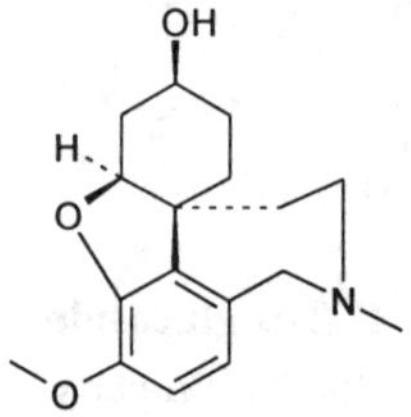

4000 Lycorenine
$C_{18}H_{23}NO_4$ MW: 317.39 Property: mp 198-200°C. Source: DA YI ZHI JIAN, SHI SUAN. Ref: 6.

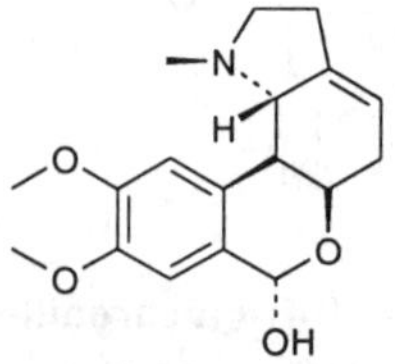

4001 Lycoricidine
Margetine. CAS: 19622-83-4 $C_{14}H_{13}NO_6$ MW: 291.26 Property: mp 214.5-5.5°C. Source: SHI SUAN. Ref: 5.

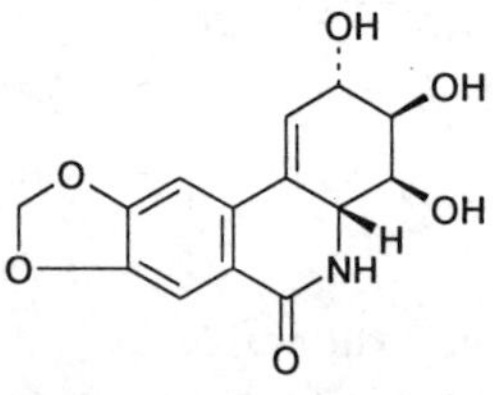

4002 Lycoricidinol
Narciclasine. CAS: 29477-83-6 $C_{14}H_{13}NO_7$ MW: 307.26 Property: mp 260°C (dec). Source: SHI SUAN. Ref: 5.

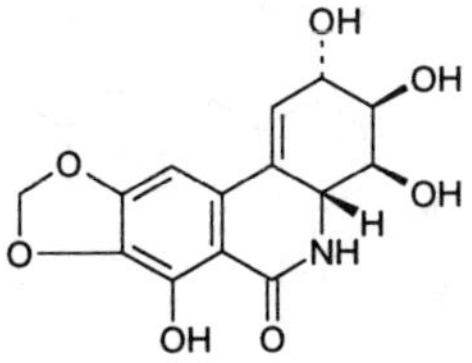

4003 Lycorine
Amarylline; Bellamlrine; Galanthidine. $C_{16}H_{17}NO_4$ MW: 287.32 Property: mp 275-80°C. Source: DA YI ZHI JIAN, GAN FENG CAO, LUO QUN DAI GEN, SHUI XIAN GEN, SHUI GUI JIAO YE, SHI SUAN. Ref: 4.

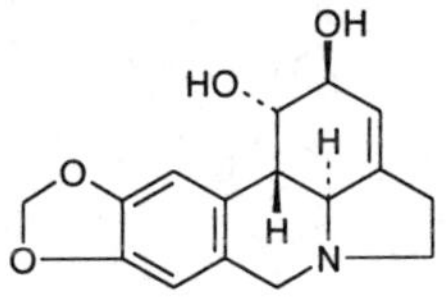

4004 Lycoxanthin
$C_{40}H_{56}O$ MW: 552.56 Property: mp 168°C. Source: KU QIE. Ref: 6.

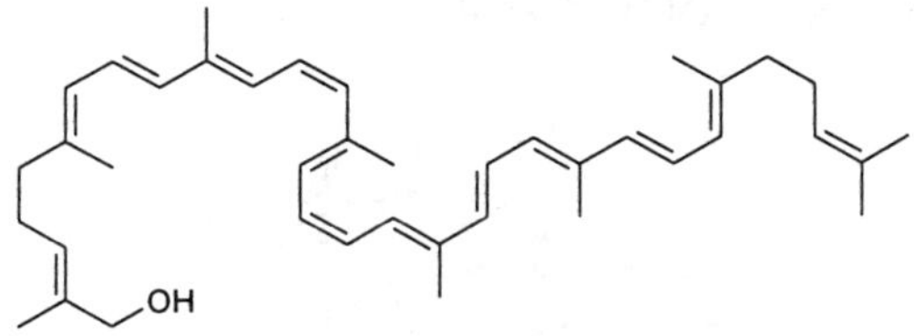

4005 Lyoniol A
$C_{22}H_{34}O_7$ MW: 410.51 Property: mp 250-3°C. Source: LI MU. Ref: 6.

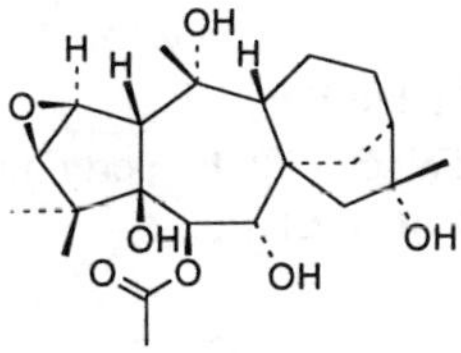

4006 Lyoniol B
$C_{20}H_{32}O_6$ MW: 368.47 Property: mp 280-3°C. Source: LI MU. Ref: 6.

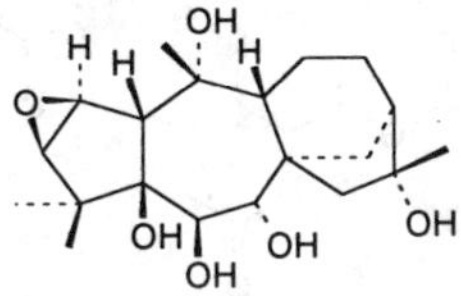

4007 Lyoniol C
$C_{18}H_{30}O_7$ MW: 358.44 Property: mp 255-9°C. Source: LI MU. Ref: 6.

4008 Lysergol
$C_{16}H_{18}N_2O$ MW: 254.33 Source: QIAN NIU ZI. Ref: 6.

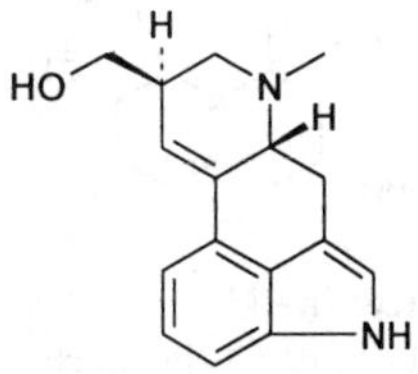

4009 Lysicamine
Source: SUAN ZAO REN. Ref: 583.

4010 Lysionotin
CAS: 10176-66-6 $C_{18}H_{16}O_7$ MW: 344.32 Property: mp 195-6°C. Source: SHI DIAO LAN, etc. Ref: 4.

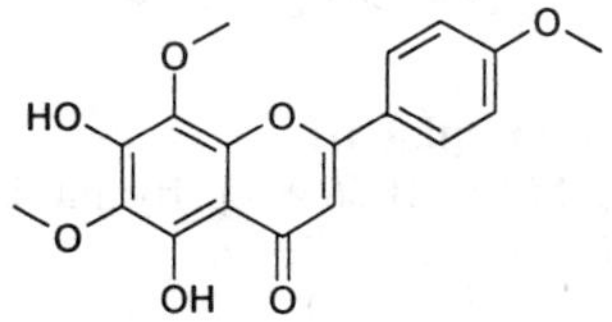

4011 Lysopine
$C_9H_{18}N_2O_4$ MW: 218.25 Source: DI JIN. Ref: 6.

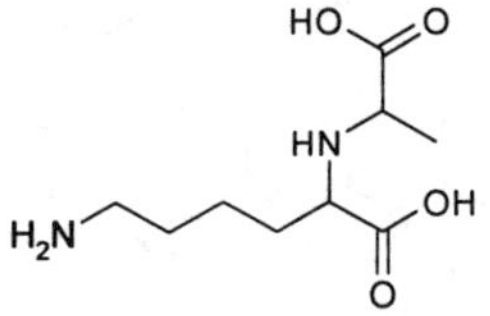

4012 Lythramine
$C_{29}H_{17}NO_5$ MW: 479.62 Source: QIAN QU CAI. Ref: 6.

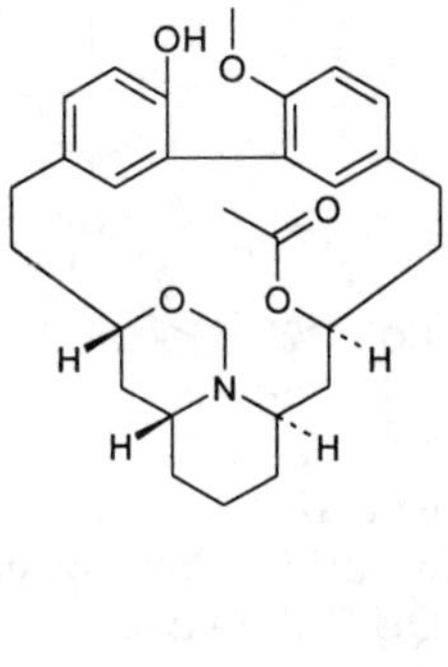

4013 Lythrancepine I
$C_{27}H_{35}NO_4$ MW: 437.58 Property: mp 149-51°C.
Source: QIAN QU CAI. Ref: 6.

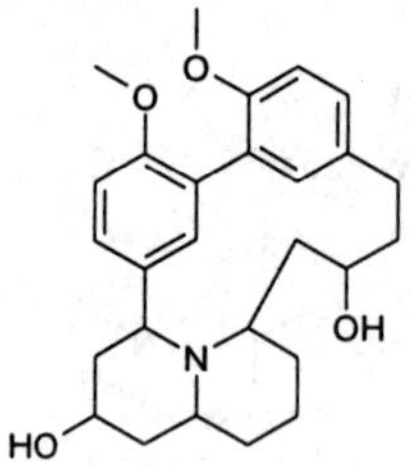

4014 Lythrancepine II
$C_{29}H_{37}NO_5$ MW: 479.62 Property: mp 187-9°C.
Source: QIAN QU CAI. Ref: 6.

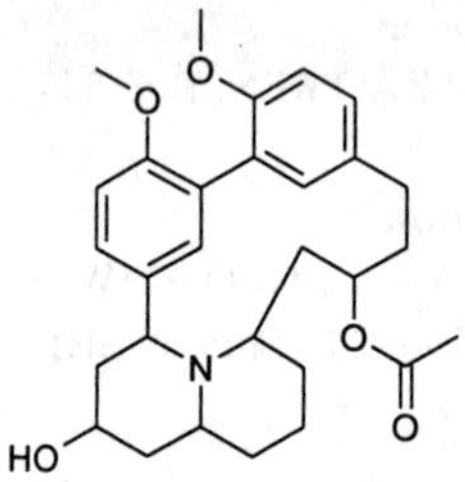

4015 Lythrancepine III
$C_{31}H_{39}NO_6$ MW: 521.66 Property: mp 174-8°C.
Source: QIAN QU CAI. Ref: 6.

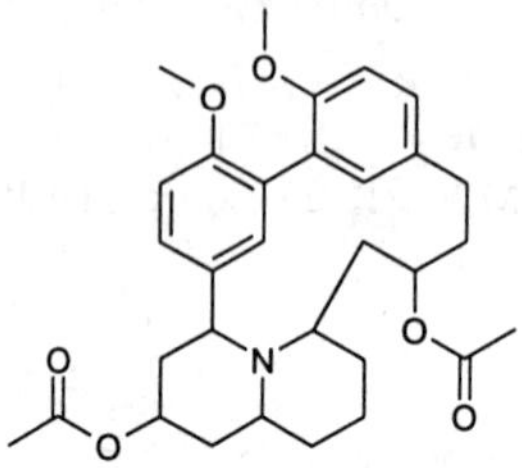

4016 Lythrancine I
$C_{27}H_{35}NO_5$ MW: 453.58 Source: QIAN QU CAI.
Ref: 6.

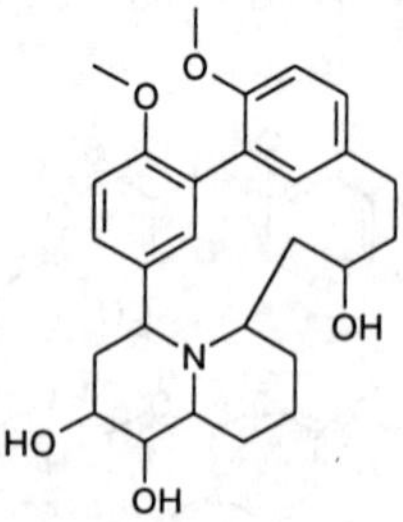

4017 Lythrancine II
$C_{29}H_{37}NO_6$ MW: 495.62 Property: mp 274-5°C.
Source: QIAN QU CAI. Ref: 6.

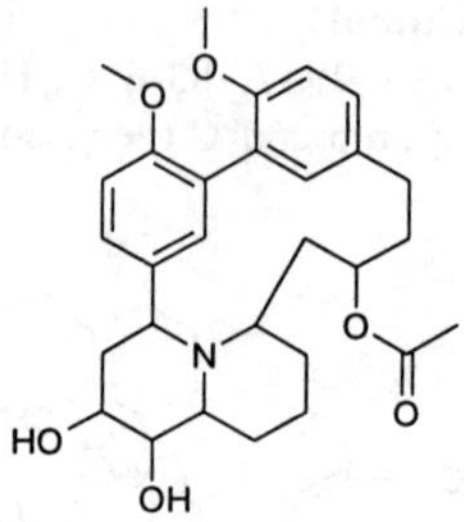

4018 Lythrancine III
$C_{31}H_{39}NO_7$ MW: 537.66 Property: mp 134-6°C.
Source: QIAN QU CAI. Ref: 6.

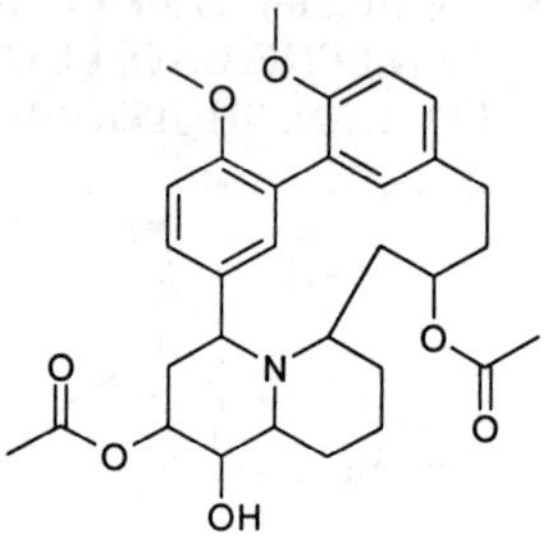

4019 Lythrancine IV
$C_{33}H_{41}NO_8$ MW: 579.70 Property: mp 237-8°C.
Source: QIAN QU CAI. Ref: 6.

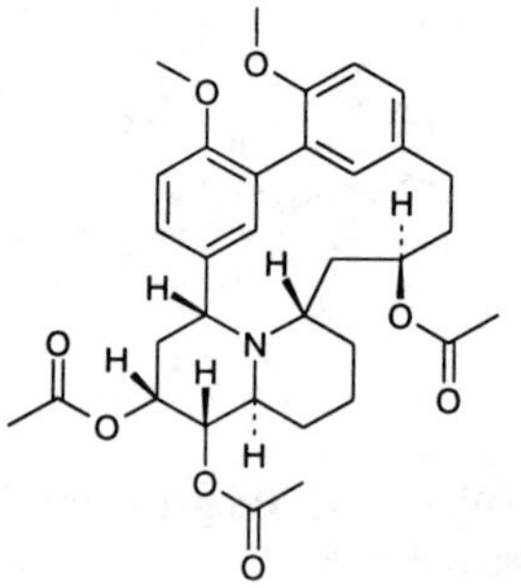

4020 Lythrancine V
$C_{33}H_{41}NO_8$ MW: 579.70 Property: mp 133-4°C.
Source: QIAN QU CAI. Ref: 6.

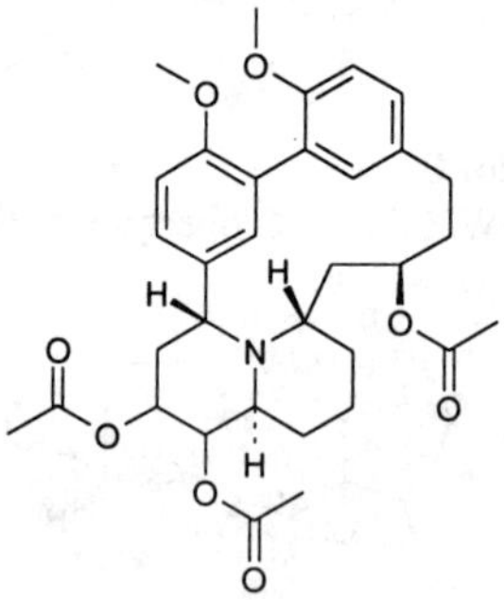

4021 Lythrancine VI
$C_{31}H_{38}NO_7$ MW: 537.66 Source: QIAN QU CAI. Ref: 6.

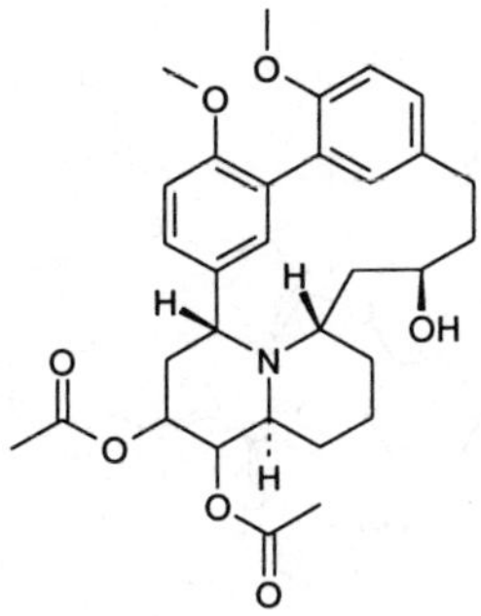

4022 Lythrancine VII
$C_{31}H_{39}NO_7$ MW: 537.66 Source: QIAN QU CAI. Ref: 6.

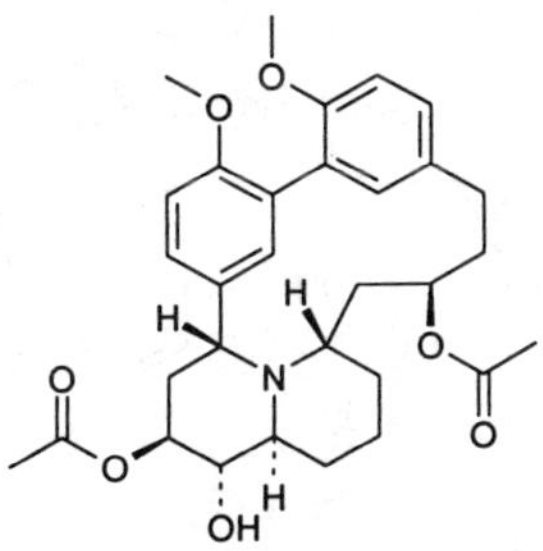

4023 Lythranidine
$C_{26}H_{35}NO_4$ MW: 425.57 Source: QIAN QU CAI. Ref: 6.

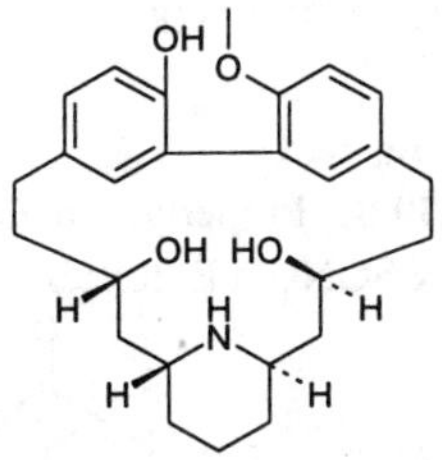

4024 Lythranine
$C_{28}H_{37}NO_5$ MW: 467.61 Source: QIAN QU CAI. Ref: 6.

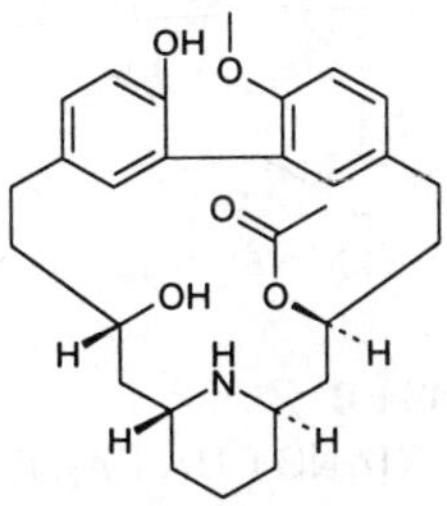

4025 Maackiain
$C_{16}H_{12}O_5$ MW: 284.27 Property: mp (-): 195-6 °C, (±): 199-200°C. Source: HUAI GEN, SHAN DOU GEN. Ref: 6.

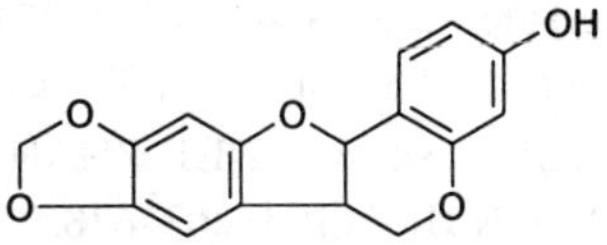

4026 α-Maackiain-mono-β-D-glucoside
$C_{22}H_{22}O_{10}$ MW: 446.41 Property: mp 202-4°C (dec). Source: HUAI GEN. Ref: 6.

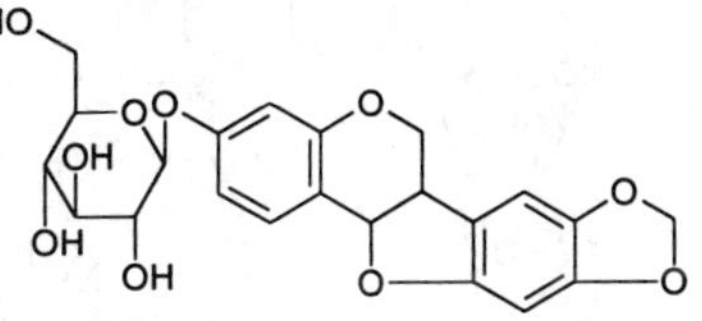

4027 Maali alcohol
$C_{15}H_{26}O$ MW: 222.37 Property: mp 103.5-5°C. Source: XIE CAO. Ref: 6.

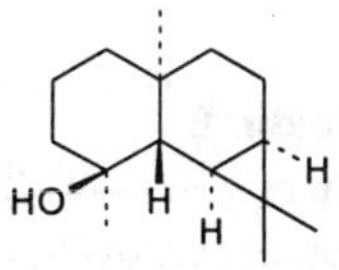

4028 β-Maaliene
$C_{15}H_{24}$ MW: 204.36 Source: QING HAO, REN SHEN. Ref: 2.

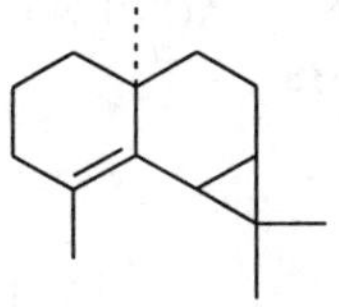

4029 Maclurin
$C_{13}H_{10}O_6$ MW: 262.22 Property: mp 220-2°C. Source: SANG ZHI. Ref: 6.

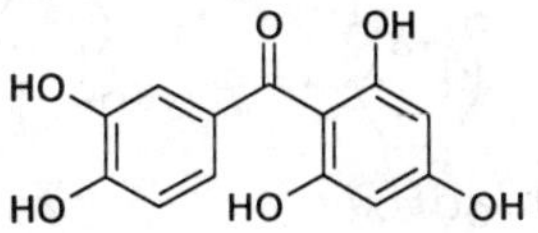

4030 Macranthoidin A
3-O-β-D-glucopyranosyl-(1→3)-α-L-rhamnopyanosyl(1→2)-α-L-arabinopyranosyl 3β, 23-dihydroxyl-olean-12-en-28-O-β-D-glucopyranosyl-(1→6)-β-D-glucopyranoside. $C_{59}H_{96}O_{27}$ MW:1237.41 Property: white cluster crystal, mp 229-232 °C, $[\alpha]_D^{16}$ -12.0° (c=3.2, MeOH). Source: HUI ZHAN MAO REN DONG, JIN YIN HUA. Ref: 263, 638.

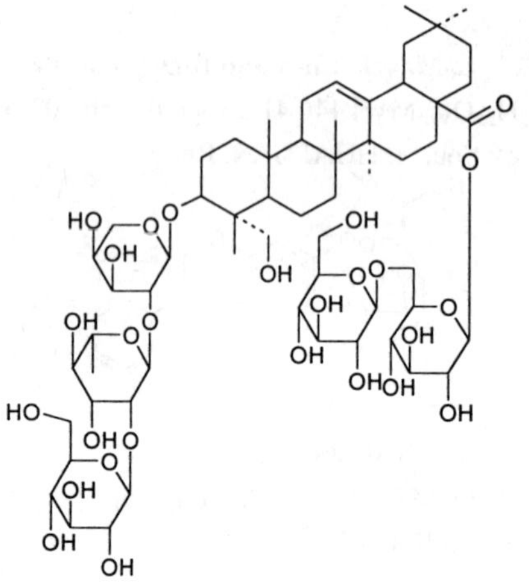

4031 Macranthoidin B
3-O-β-D-glucopyranosyl-(1→4)-β-D-glucopyranosyl(1→3)-α-L-rhamnopyanosyl-(1→2)-α-L-arabinopyranosyl 3β, 23-dihydroxyl-olean-12-en-28-O-β-D-glucopyranosyl-(1→6)-β-D-glucopyranoside. $C_{65}H_{106}O_{32}$ MW: 1399.55 Property: white acicular crystal, mp 230-233°C, $[\alpha]_D^{22}$ -13.4°(c=1.5, MeOH). Source: HUI ZHAN MAO REN DONG, JIN YIN HUA. Ref: 263, 638.

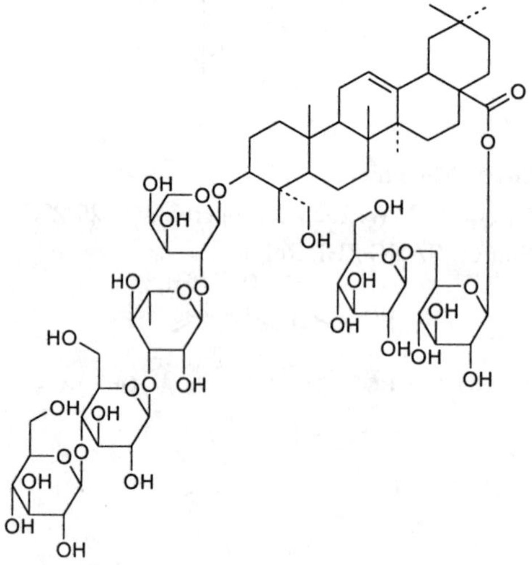

4032 Macranthoin F
$C_{26}H_{26}O_{12}$ MW: 530.49 Property: light yellow powder, mp 115-6°C. Source: HEI ZHAN MAO REN DONG. Ref: 311.

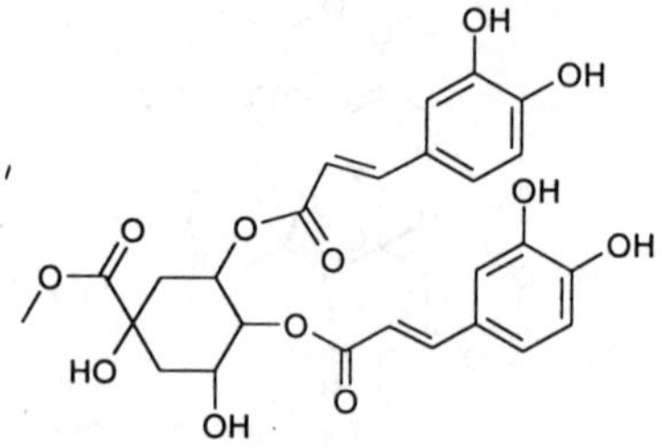

4033 Macranthoin G
$C_{26}H_{26}O_{12}$ MW: 530.49 Property: light yellow powder, mp 123-4°C. Source: HEI ZHAN MAO REN DONG. Ref: 311.

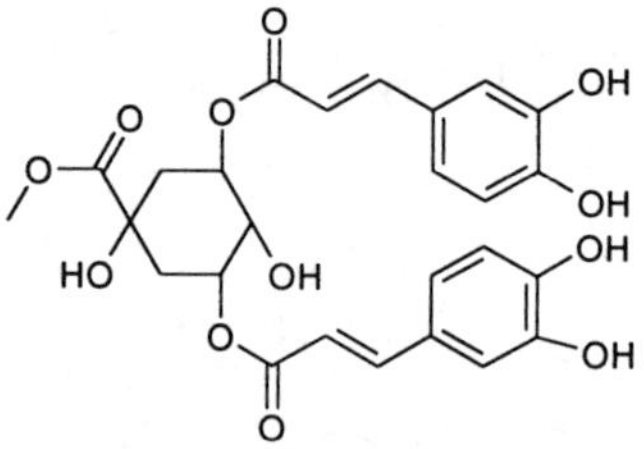

4034 Macranthoside A
Source: JIN YIN HUA. Ref: 638.

4035 Macranthoside B
Source: JIN YIN HUA. Ref: 638.

4036 Macrophyllic acid
$C_{40}H_{54}O_6$ MW: 630.87 Property: mp 237-8°C (dec). Source: LUO HAN SONG YE. Ref: 6.

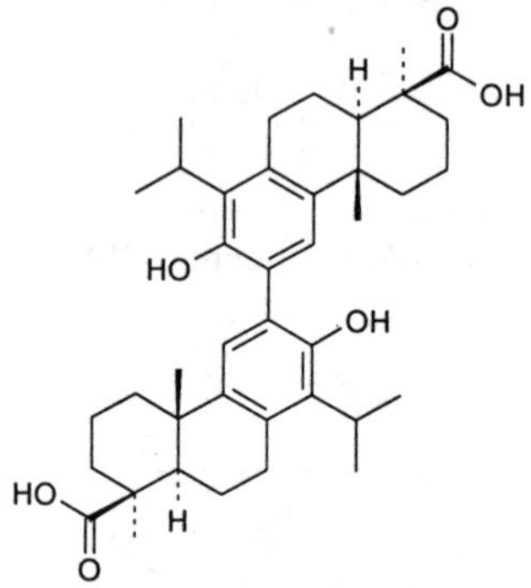

4037 Macrophyllin B
Source: MAO YE XIANG CHA CAI. Ref: 575.

4038 Macrophylline

$C_{13}H_{21}NO_3$ MW: 239.32 Property: mp 42-44°C, bp 100°C/0.2 mm. Source: HUANG WAN. Ref: 6.

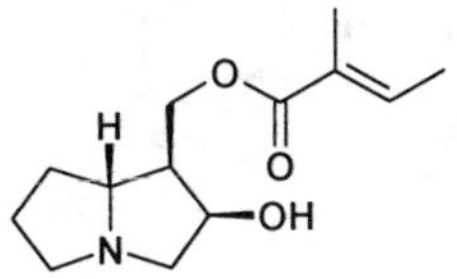

4039 Macrospegatrine

$C_{40}H_{46}N_4O_3{\bullet}Cl_2$ MW: 630.84•70.90 Property: colorless rhomboid crystal, mp 300°C (changing into black), $[\alpha]_D^{17}$ +215° (chloroform). Source: HAI NAN LUO FU MU. Ref: 89.

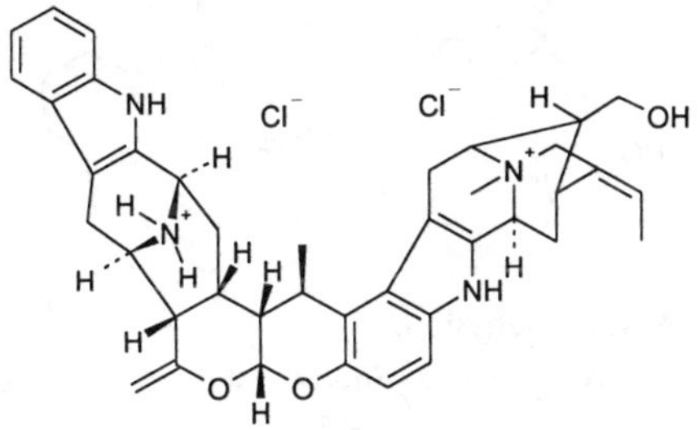

4040 Macrostemonoside A

Tigogenin-3-O-β-D-glucopyranosyl(1→2)[β-D-glucopyranosyl(1→3)]-β-D-glucopyranosyl(1→4)-β-D-galactopyranoside (1). $C_{51}H_{84}O_{23}$ MW: 1065.22 Property: white powder, mp 276-8°C, $[\alpha]_D^{20}$ 0° (c=0.1, pyridine). Source: XIE BAI. Ref: 250.

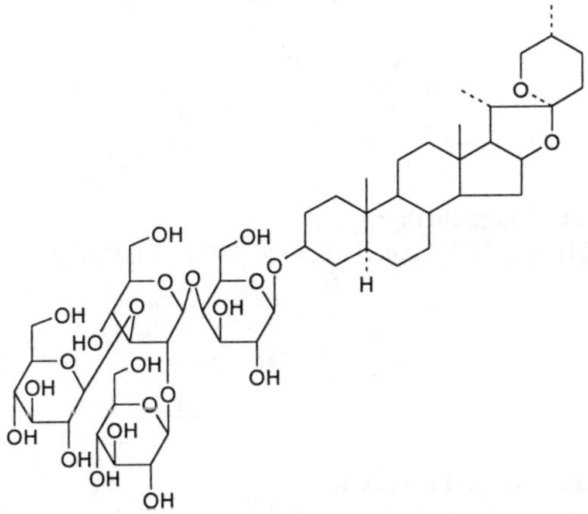

4041 Macrostemonoside D

Tigogenin-3-O-β-D-glucopyranosyl(1→2)[β-D-glucopyranosyl(1→3)(6-O-acetyl-β-D-glucopyranosyl)](1→4)-β-D-galactopyranoside. $C_{53}H_{86}O_{23}$ MW: 1107.26 Property: white powder, mp 270-3°C, $[\alpha]_D^{20}$ 0° (c=0.1, pyridine). Source: XIE BAI. Ref: 250.

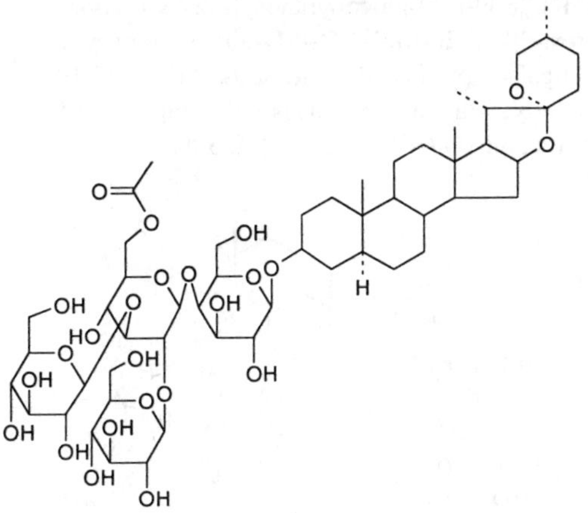

4042 Macrostemonoside E

$C_{57}H_{94}O_{28}$ MW: 1227.37 Property: white amorphous powder, mp 227.5-30°C. Source: XIE BAI. Ref: 273.

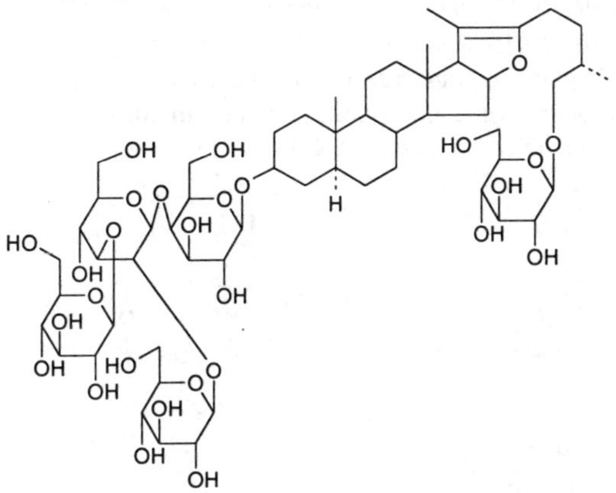

4043 Macrostemonoside F

$C_{45}H_{74}O_{18}$ MW: 903.38. Property: white amorphous powder, mp 196-198.5°C. Source: XIE BAI. Ref: 273.

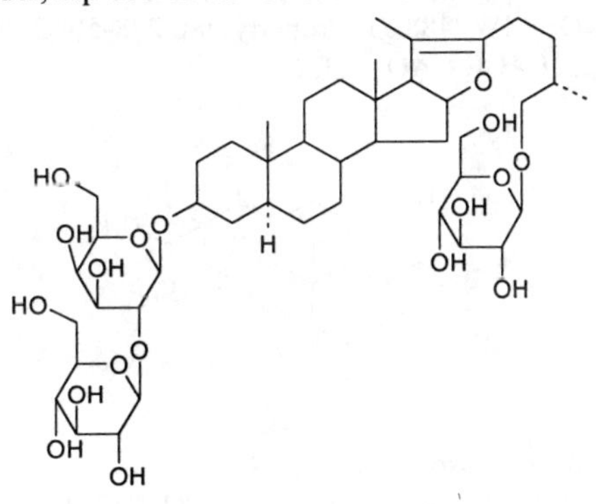

4044 Macrostemonoside J
(25R)-26-O-β-D-glucopyranosyl-22-hydroxy-5β-furost-2β,3β,26-triol-3-O-β-D-glucopyranosyl (1→2)-β-D-galactopyranoside. $C_{45}H_{76}O_{20}$ MW: 937.10 Property: white amorphous powder, mp 230-2°C. Source: XIAO GEN SUAN. Ref: 309.

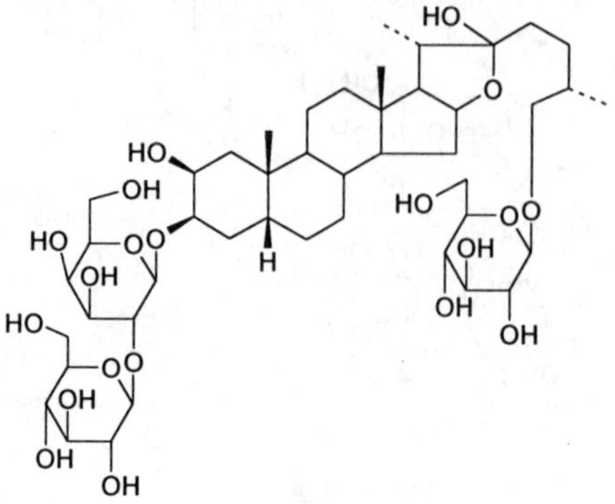

4045 Macrostemonoside L
(25R)-26-O-β-D-glucopyranosyl-22-methoxy-5β-furost-2β,3β,26-triol-3-O-β-D-glucopyranosyl (1→2)-β-D-galactopyranoside. $C_{45}H_{74}O_{19}$ MW: 919.08 Property: white amorphous powder, mp 206-8°C. Source: XIAO GEN SUAN. Ref: 309.

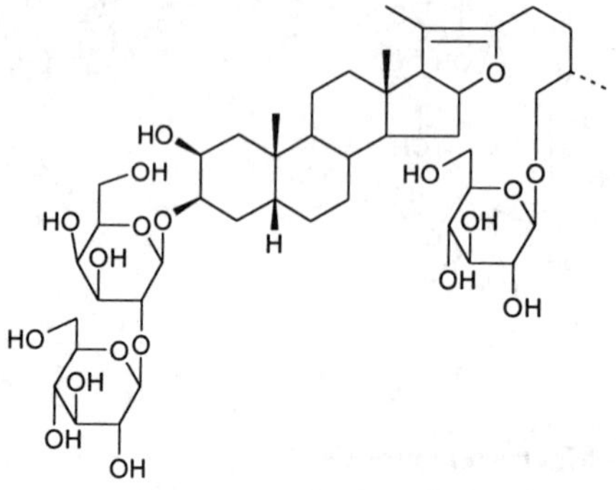

4046 Madasiatic acid
$C_{30}H_{48}O_5$ MW: 488.71 Property: mp 248-50°C (dec). Source: JI XUE CAO. Ref: 6.

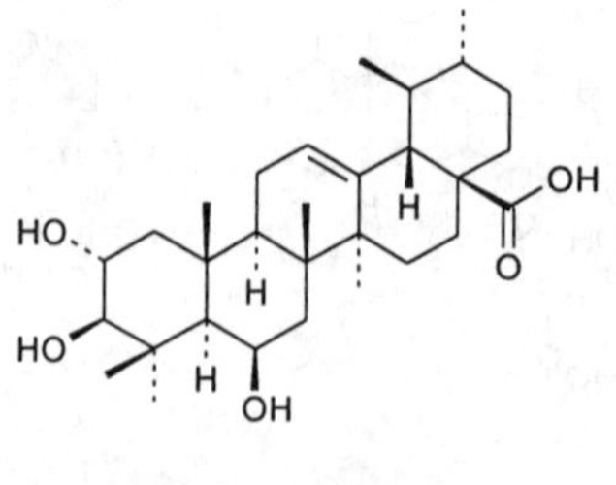

4047 Madecassoside
$C_{47}H_{76}O_{20}$ MW: 961.12 Source: JI XUE CAO. Ref: 6.

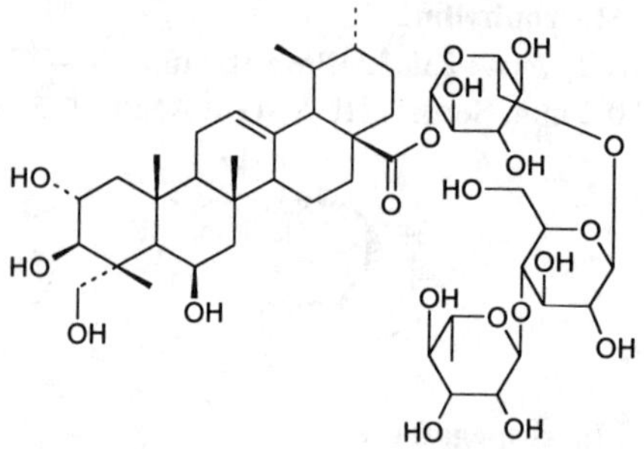

4048 Maesaquinone
$C_{26}H_{42}O_4$ MW: 418.62 Property: mp 122°C. Source: DU JING SHAN. Ref: 6.

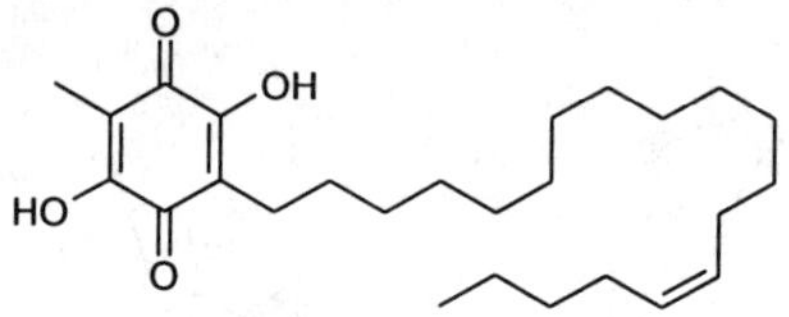

4049 Magnaldehyde B
$C_{18}H_{16}O_3$ MW: 280.33 Source: HOU PO. Ref: 2.

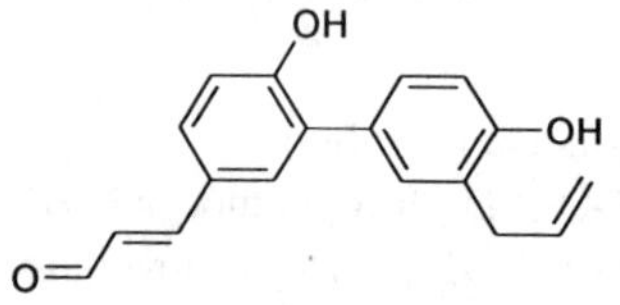

4050 Magnaldehyde C
$C_{18}H_{18}O_5$ MW: 314.34 Source: HOU PO. Ref: 2.

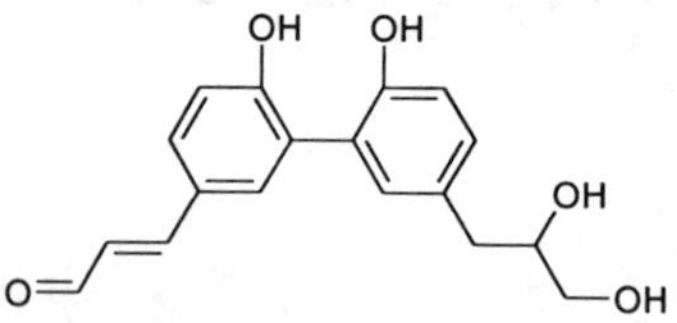

4051 Magnaldehyde D
$C_{16}H_{14}O_3$ MW: 254.29 Source: HOU PO. Ref: 2.

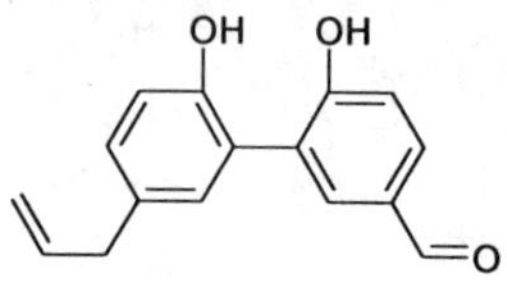

4052 Magnaldehyde E
$C_{16}H_{14}O_3$ MW: 254.29 Source: HOU PO. Ref: 2.

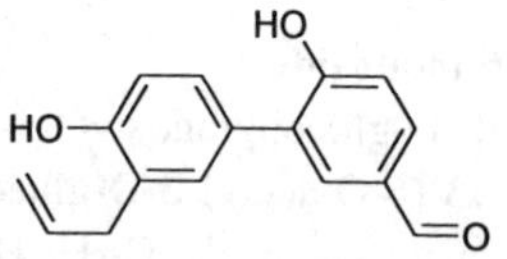

4053 Magnatriol B

$C_{15}H_{14}O_3$ MW: 242.28 Source: HOU PO. Ref: 2.

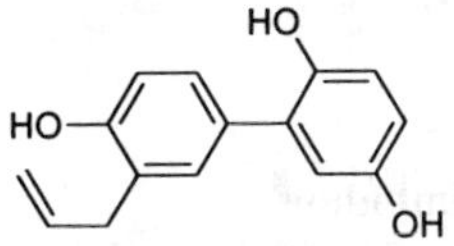

4054 Magnesium lactate

$C_3H_6M_gO_3$ MW: 114.39 Source: LU HUI. Ref: 2.

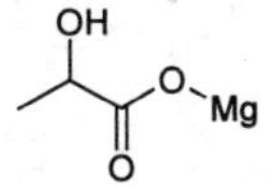

4055 Magnococline

$C_{18}H_{21}NO_3$ MW: 299.37 Source: YE HE HUA. Ref: 6.

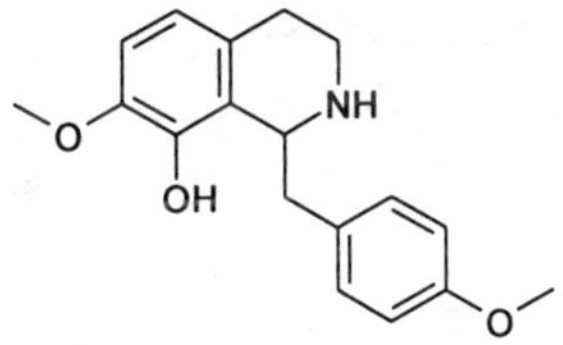

4056 Magnocurarine

$C_{19}H_{23}NO_3$ MW: 313.40 Property: mp (+) (s): 198-9°C (dec), (-) (r): 199-200°C. Source: DA YE MU LAN, HOU PO. Ref: 2, 4, 6, 625.

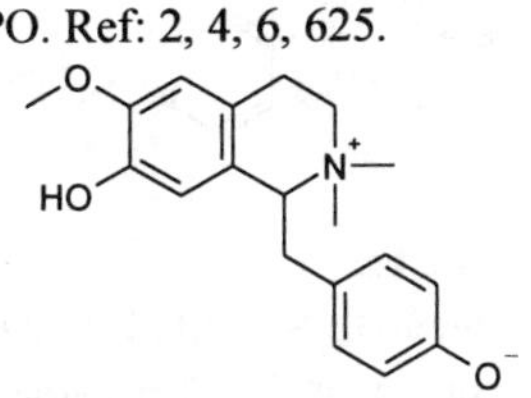

4057 Magnoflorine

Escholine; Thalictrine. CAS: 2141-09-5 $C_{20}H_{24}NO_4$ MW: 342.42 Property: mp 169-70°C. Source: HUANG BAI, HOU PU, HUANG LIAN, MA WEI LIAN, XIN YI, YAN GUO CAO, YIN YANG HUO. Ref: 2, 4, 6, 306, 625.

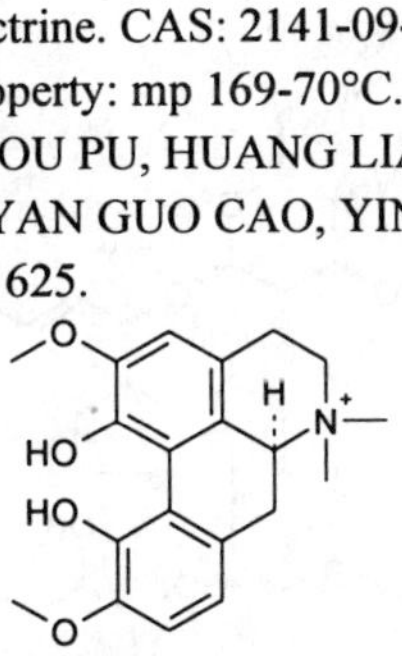

4058 Magnolignan A

$C_{18}H_{20}O_4$ MW: 300.36 Source: HOU PO. Ref: 2, 6.

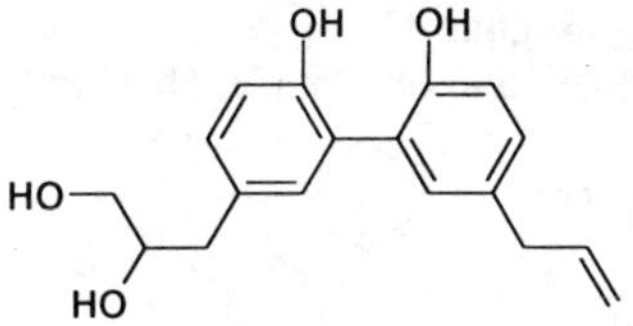

4059 Magnolignan B

$C_{18}H_{20}O_5$ MW: 316.36 Source: HOU PO. Ref: 2, 6

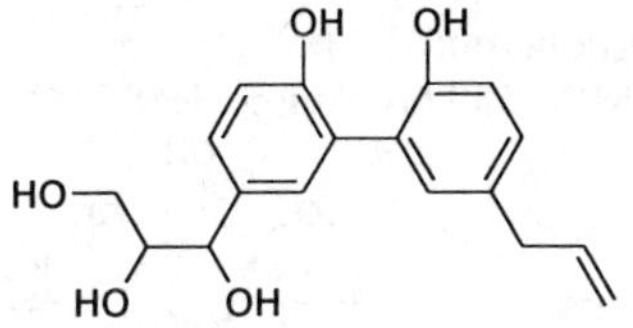

4060 Magnolignan C

$C_{18}H_{20}O_4$ MW: 300.36 Source: HOU PO. Ref: 2, 6

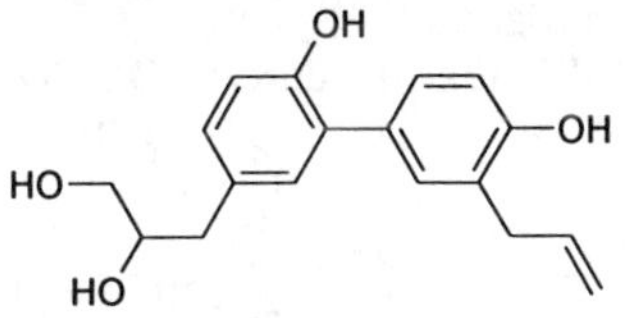

4061 Magnolignan D

$C_{19}H_{22}O_5$ MW: 330.38 Source: HOU PO. Ref: 2.

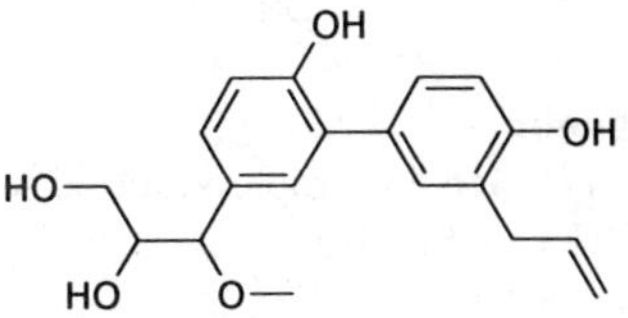

4062 Magnolignan E

$C_{18}H_{18}O_4$ MW: 298.34 Source: HOU PO. Ref: 2.

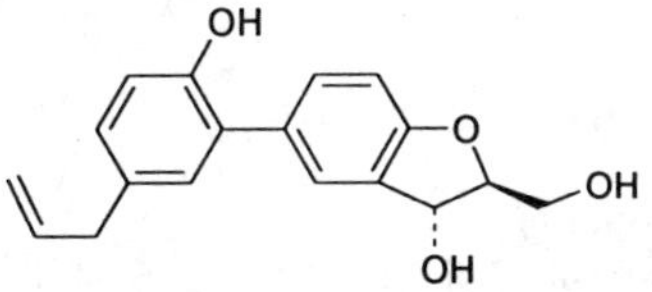

4063 Magnolignan F

$C_{36}H_{36}O_6$ MW: 564.68 Source: HOU PO. Ref: 2.

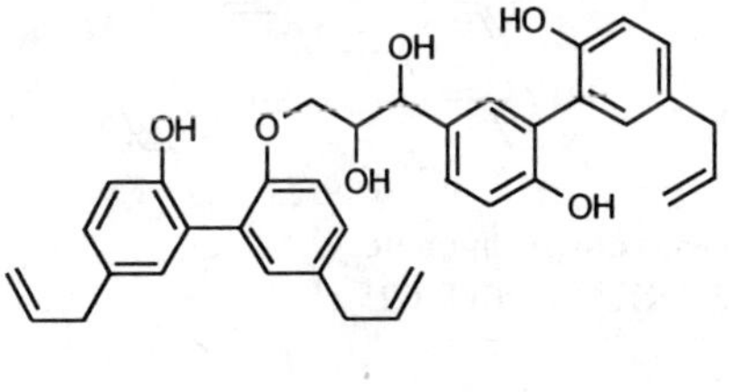

4064 Magnolignan G
$C_{36}H_{36}O_8$ MW: 596.68 Source: HOU PO. Ref: 2.

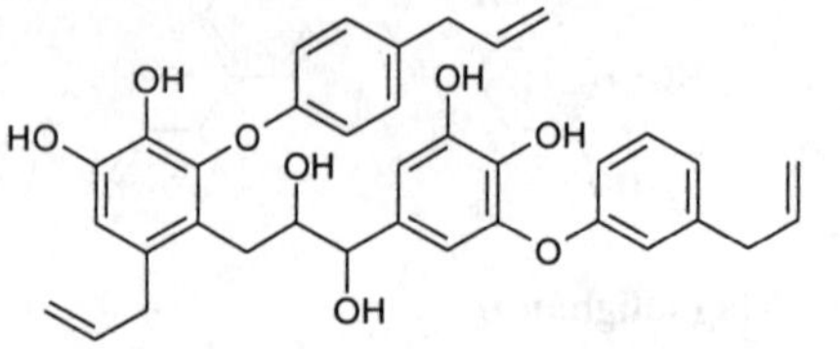

4065 Magnolignan H
$C_{35}H_{34}O_6$ MW: 550.66 Source: HOU PO. Ref: 2.

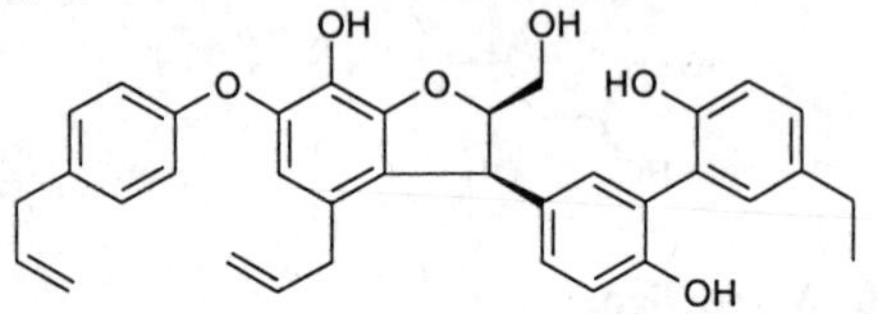

4066 Magnolignan I
$C_{33}H_{30}O_6$ MW: 522.60 Source: HOU PO. Ref: 2.

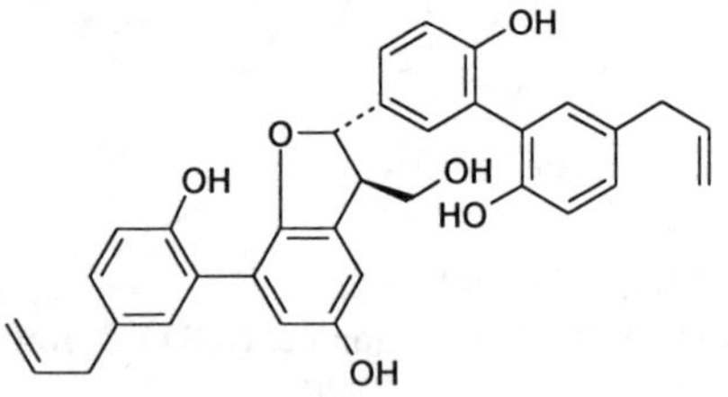

4067 Magnolin
$C_{23}H_{28}O_7$ MW: 416.48 Property: mp 97°C. Source: WANG CHUN MU LAN,
XIN YI. Ref: 6, 543.

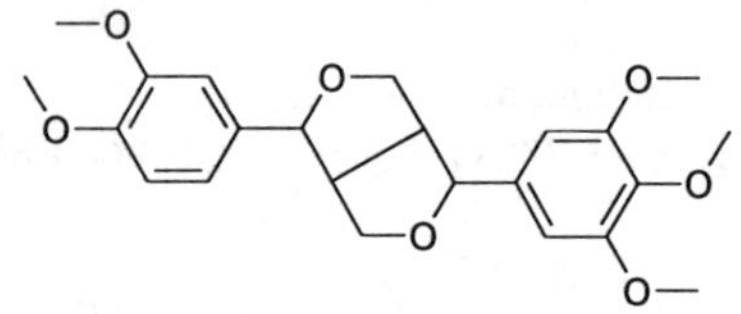

4068 Magnolol
CAS: 528-43-8 $C_{18}H_{18}O_2$ MW: 266.34 Property: mp 102°C. Source: DA YE MU LAN, HOU PO.
Ref: 4, 625.

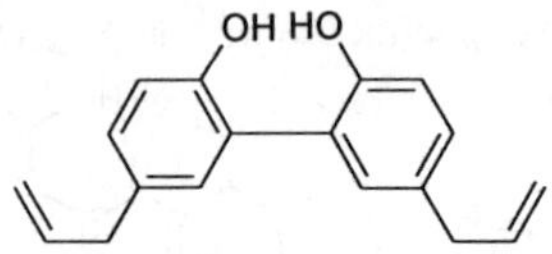

4069 Magnosprengerine
Source: HOU PO. Ref: 625.

4070 Mahanimbicine
$C_{23}H_{25}NO$ MW: 331.46 Source: YIN DU JIU LI XIANG. Ref: 11.

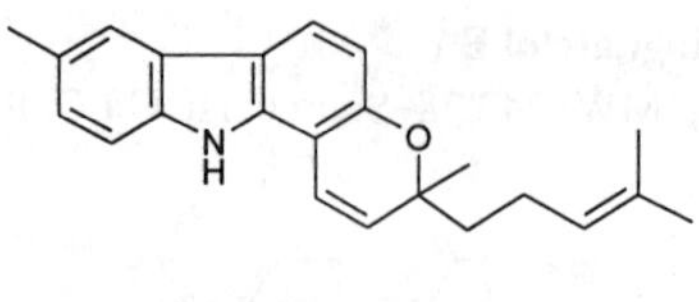

4071 Mahanimbidine
$C_{24}H_{29}NO$ MW: 347.50 Source: JIU LI XIANG. Ref: 11.

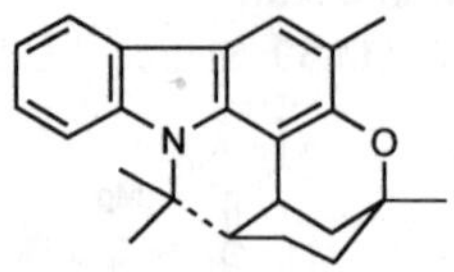

4072 (+) Mahanimbine
$C_{23}H_{25}NO$ MW: 331.46 Source: YIN DU JIU LI XIANG, ZHONG HUA JIU LI XIANG. Ref: 11.

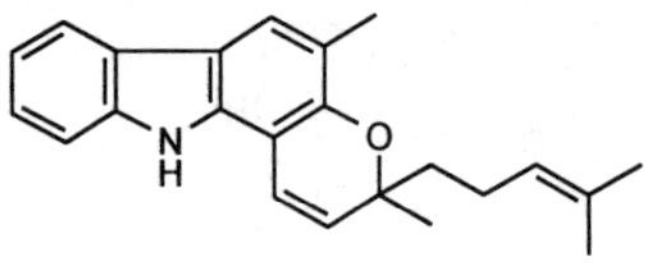

4073 Mahanimbinine
$C_{22}H_{25}NO_2$ MW: 335.45 Source: YIN DU JIU LI XIANG. Ref: 11.

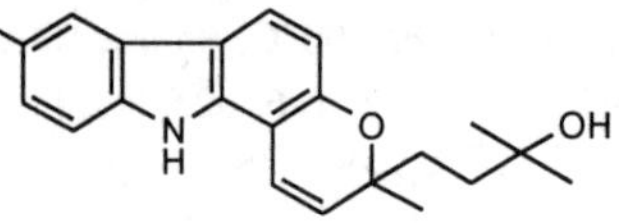

4074 Majoroside F5
Dammar-22(32)-ene-3β,6α,12β,20(S),24ξ-pentaol-(20-O-β-D-glucopyranosyl-6-O-α-L-rhamnopyranosyl(1-2)-β-D-glucopyranoside). $C_{48}H_{82}O_{19}$ MW: 963.18 Property: white powder, mp 192-4°C. Source: ZHU ZI SHEN. Ref: 137.

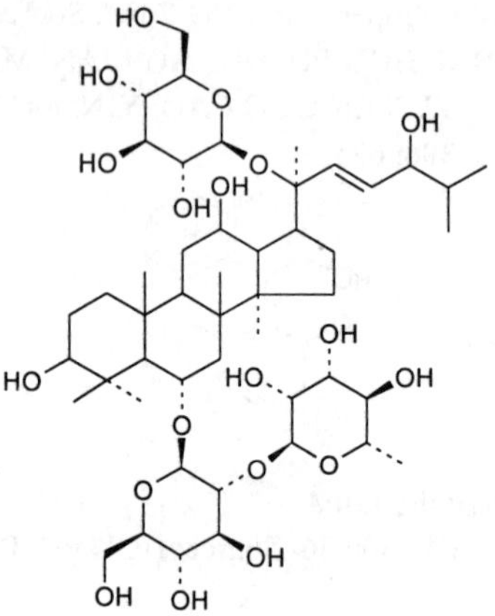

4075 Majoroside F6
Dammar-23(24)-ene-3β,6α,12β,20(S),25-pentaol-(20-O-β-D-glucopyranosyl-6-O-α-L-rhamnopyranosyl (1-2)-β-D-glucopyranoside). $C_{48}H_{82}O_{19}$ MW: 963.18 Property: white powder, mp 182.5-4°C. Source: ZHU ZI SHEN. Ref: 137.

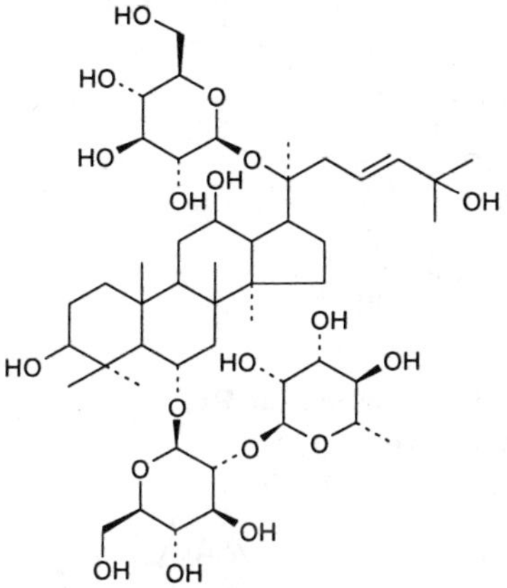

4076 Makisterone A
$C_{28}H_{46}O_7$ MW: 494.67 Property: mp 263-5°C (dec). Source: LUO HAN SONG YE. Ref: 6, 408.

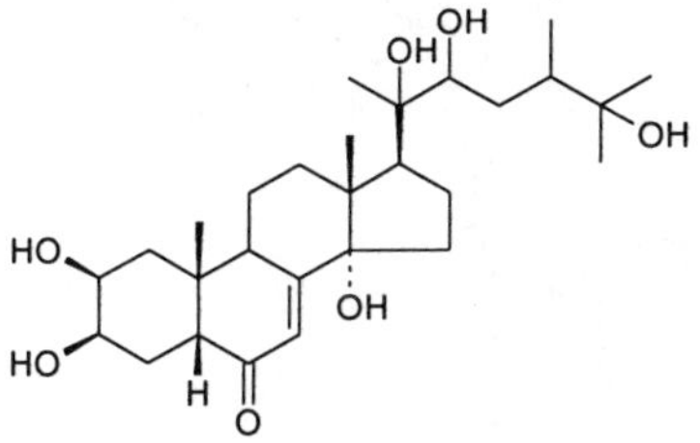

4077 Makisterone B
$C_{28}H_{46}O_7$ MW: 494.67 Property: mp 172-3°C (dec). Source: LUO HAN SONG YE. Ref: 6.

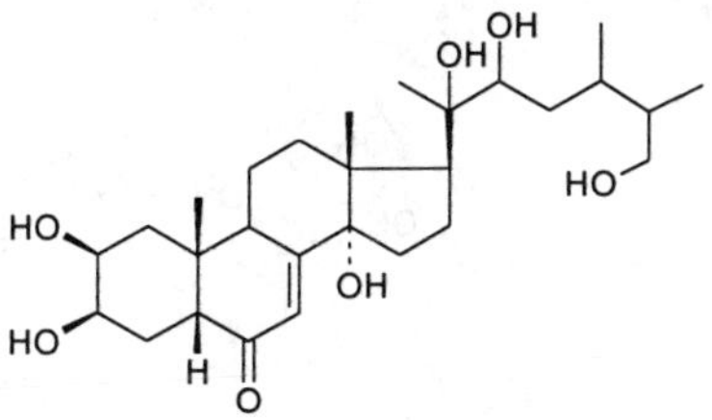

4078 Makisterone C
$C_{29}H_{48}O_7$ MW: 508.70 Property: mp 263-5°C (dec). Source: LUO HAN SONG YE. Ref: 6.

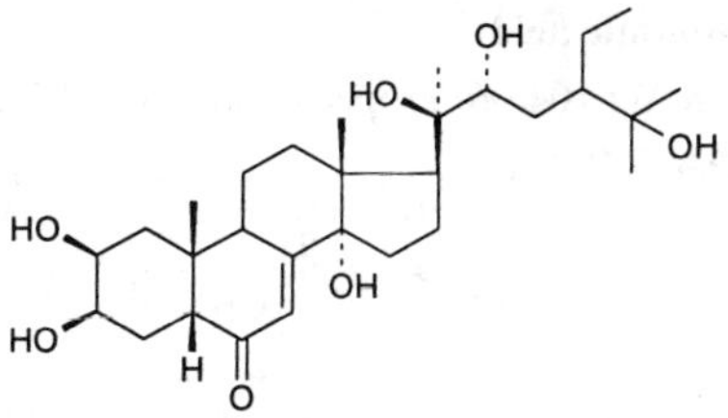

4079 Makisterone D
$C_{29}H_{48}O_7$ MW: 508.70 Source: LUO HAN SONG YE. Ref: 6.

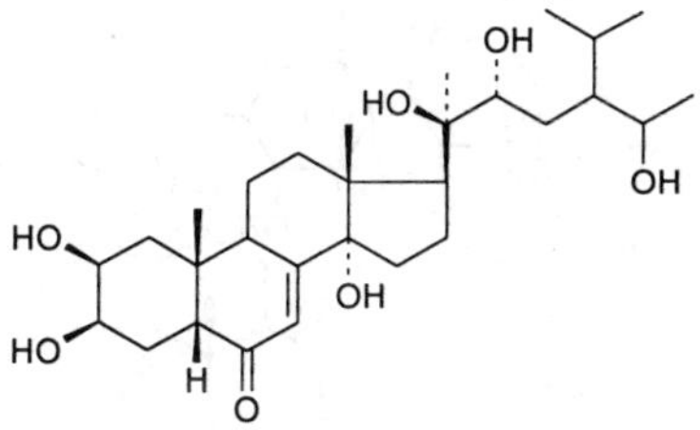

4080 Malic acid
$C_4H_6O_5$ MW: 134.09 Property: mp (+): 98-9°C, (-): 100°C, (±): 133°C, 125-6°C. Source: CU LIU GUO (SHA JI), DA ZAO, MA HUANG, PU HUANG, REN SHEN, SHAN ZHU YU, SHAN ZHA. Ref: 2.

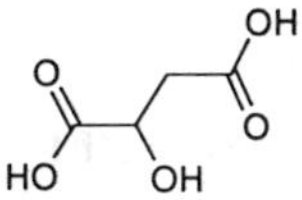

4081 Malloprenol
$C_{45}H_{74}O$ MW: 631.09 Source: YE WU TONG. Ref: 6.

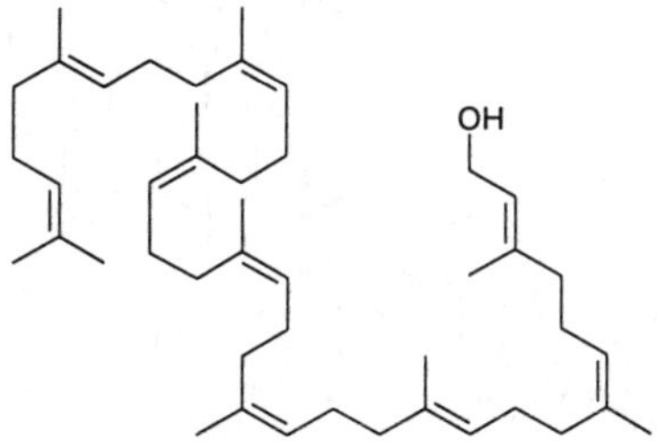

4082 Malloprenyl linolenate
$C_{63}H_{102}O_2$ MW: 891.51 Source: YE WU TONG. Ref: 6.

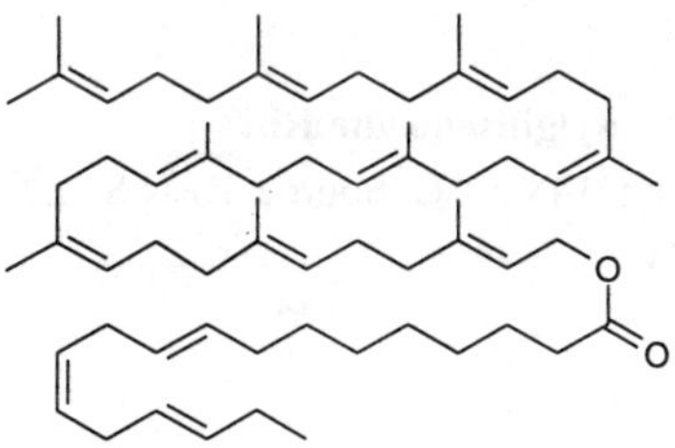

4083 Malonic acid

$C_3H_4O_4$ MW: 104.06 Property: mp 135.6°C. Source: QI YE DAN. Ref: 2.

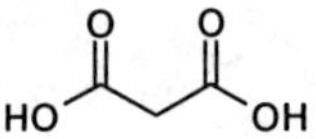

4084 6''-Malonylginsenoside Rb1

$C_{57}H_{94}O_{26}$ MW: 1195.37 Source: QI YE DAN. Ref: 2.

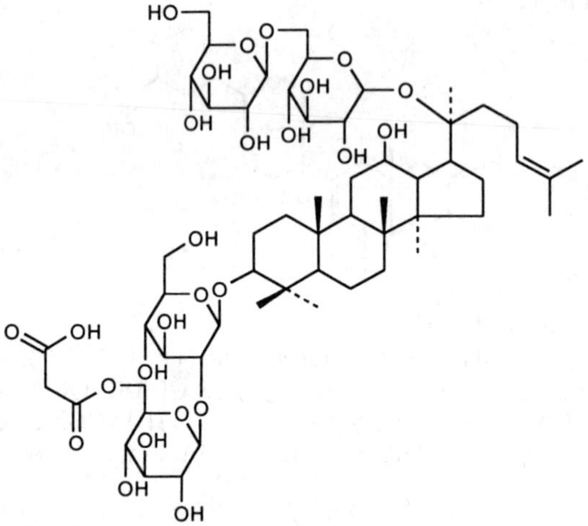

4085 Malonylginsenoside Rb1

Property: mp 150-2°C. Source: REN SHEN, XI REN SHEN. Ref: 2, 524, 613.

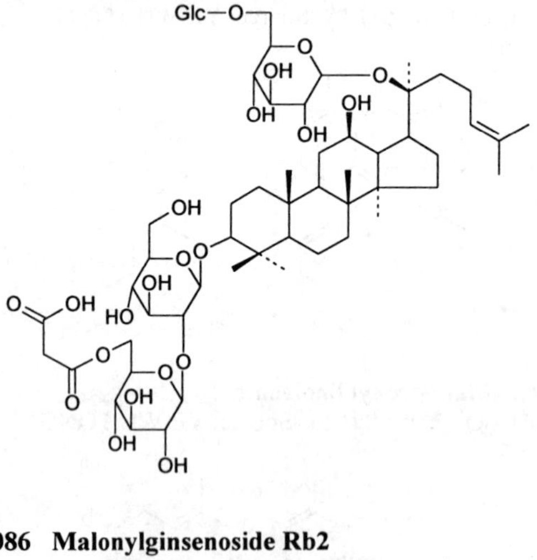

4086 Malonylginsenoside Rb2

Property: mp 148-50°C. Source: REN SHEN. Ref: 2, 524.

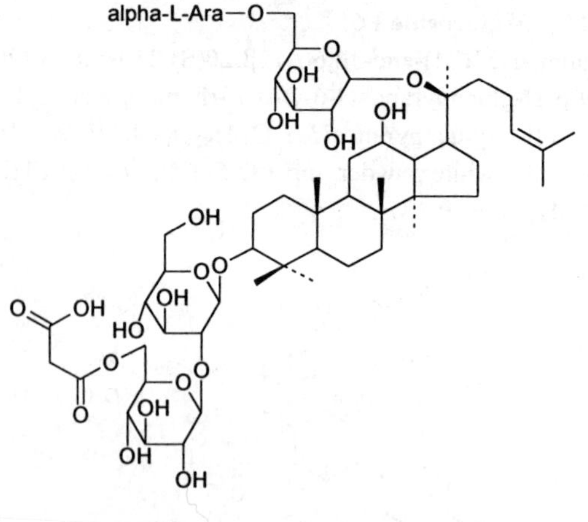

4087 Malonylginsenoside Rc

Source: REN SHEN. Ref: 2.

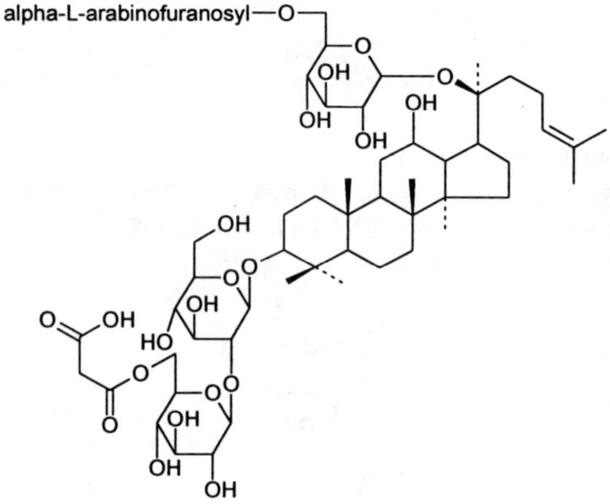

4088 Malonylginsenoside Rd

$C_{51}H_{84}O_{21}$ MW: 1033.23 Source: QI YE DAN. Ref: 2, 524.

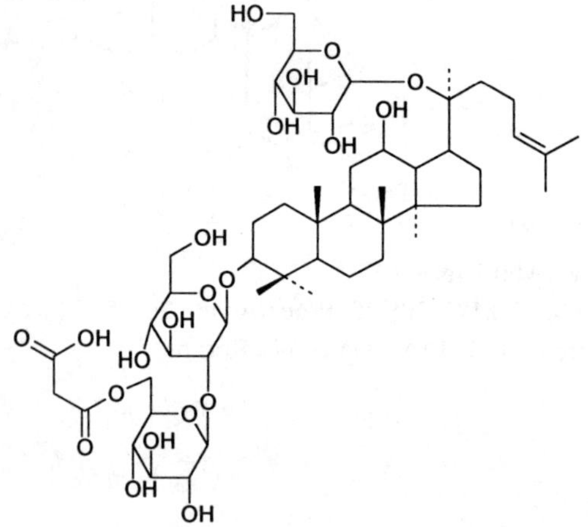

4089 6''-Malonylginsenoside Rd1
$C_{57}H_{94}O_{26}$ MW: 1195.37 Source: QI YE DAN. Ref: 2.

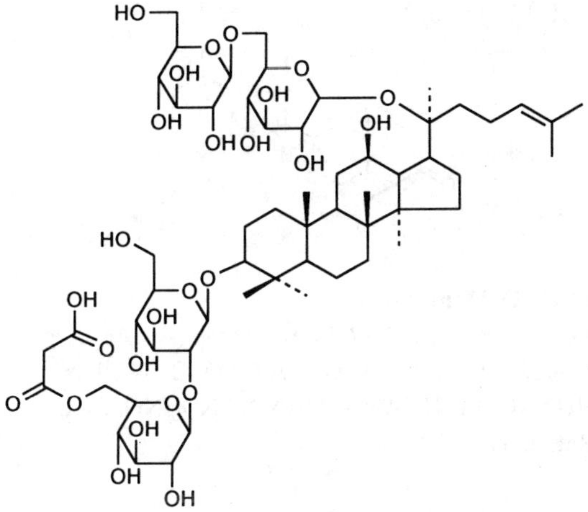

4090 7-(6-O-Malonyl-β-D-glucopyransyloxy)-3-(4-hydroxyphenyl)-4H-1-benzopyran-4-one
$C_{24}H_{24}O_{12}$ MW: 504.45 Source: GE GEN. Ref: 2.

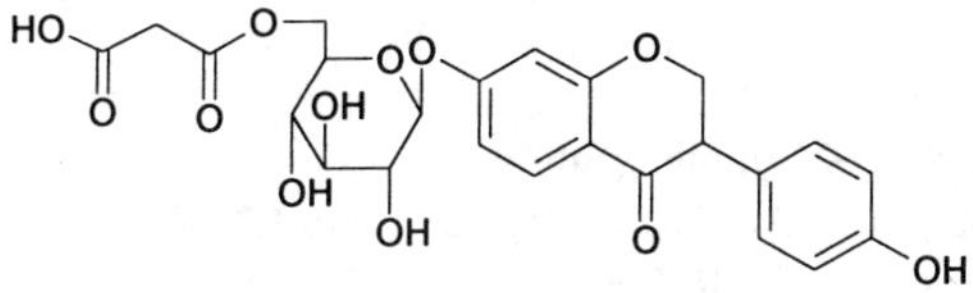

4091 6''-Malonylgypenoside V
$C_{57}H_{94}O_{25}$ MW: 1179.37 Source: QI YE DAN. Ref: 2.

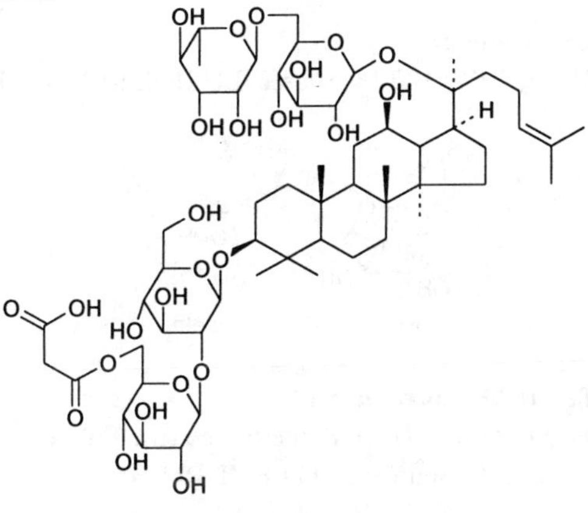

4092 Maltose
Source: REN SHEN. Ref: 2.

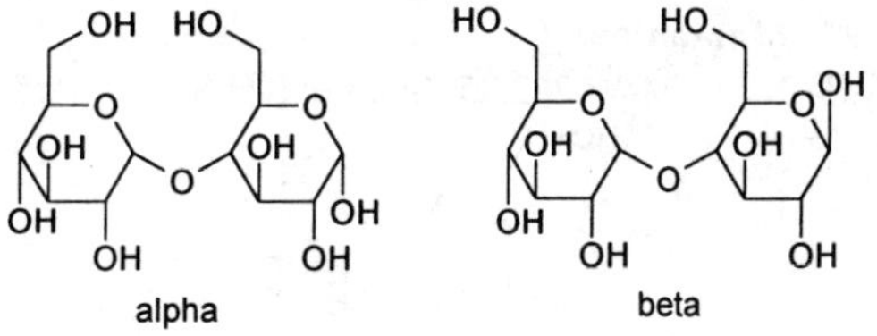

alpha

beta

4093 Malvic acid
$C_{18}H_{32}O_2$ MW: 200.45 Source: MU JIN ZI. Source: Ref: 6.

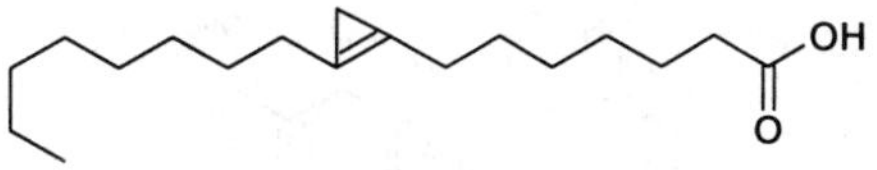

4094 Malvidin
$C_{17}H_{15}O_7$ MW: 331.30 Source: FENG XIAN HUA, JIU, MU XU, PU TAO. Ref: 6.

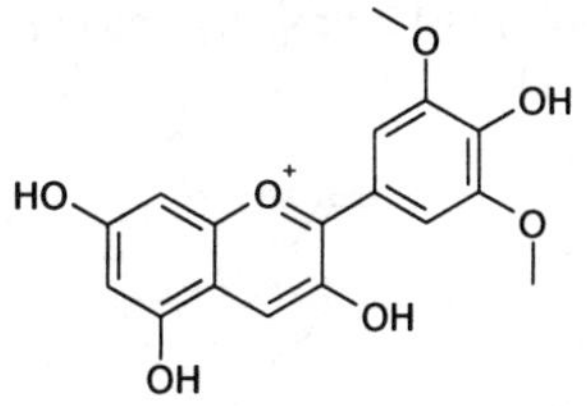

4095 Malvidin-3-arabinoside
$C_{22}H_{23}O_{11}$ MW: 463.42 Source: ZI BEI TIAN KUI CAO. Ref: 6.

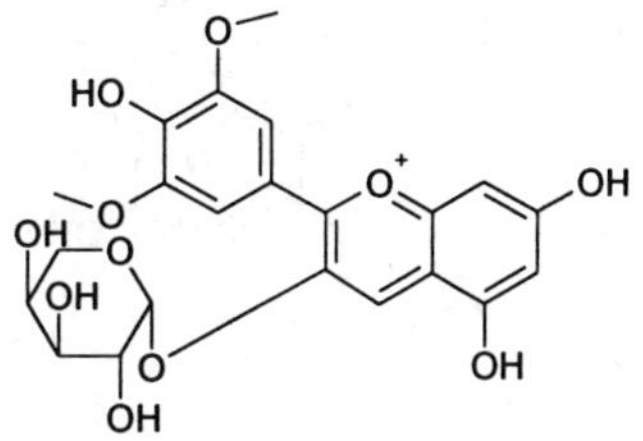

4096 Malvin
$C_{29}H_{35}O_{19}$ MW: 655.59 Property: mp 165°C. Source: QIAN QU CAI. Ref: 6.

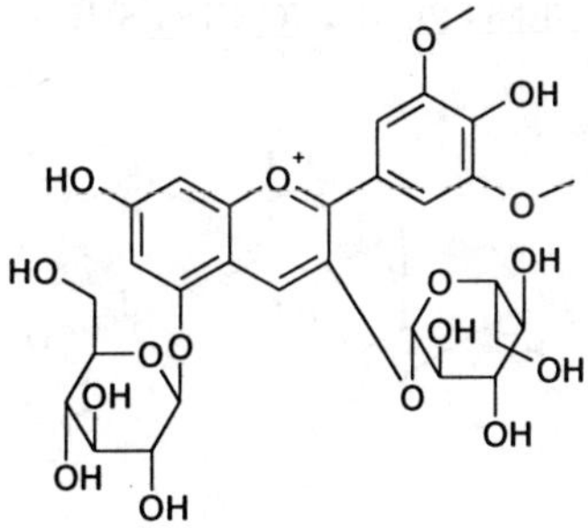

4097 Mamanine
$C_{15}H_{22}N_2O_2$ MW: 262.35 Source: KU SHEN. Ref: 2.

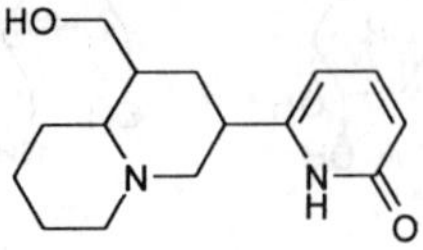

4098 Mamegakinone
$C_{20}H_{10}O_8$ MW: 374.35 Property: mp 253°C (dec). Source: JUN QIAN ZI. Ref: 6.

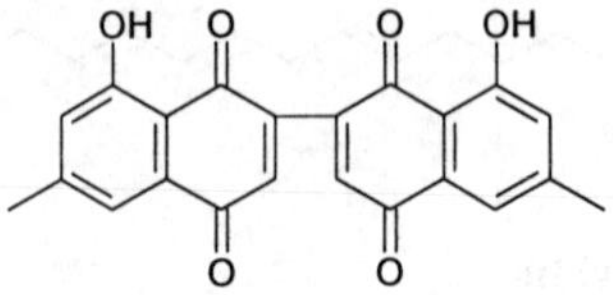

4099 Mandelonitrile
C_8H_7NO MW: 133.15 Property: mp (+): 28.5-9.5°C. Source: XING REN. Ref: 2.

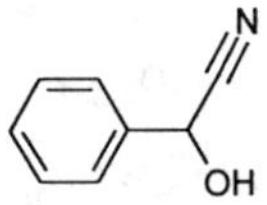

4100 Mangiferin
Chimonin; Euxanthogen. CAS: 4773-96-0 $C_{19}H_{18}O_{11}$ MW: 422.35 Property: mp 271-3°C. Source: BIAN TAO, ZHI MU, etc. Ref: 4, 6, 550.

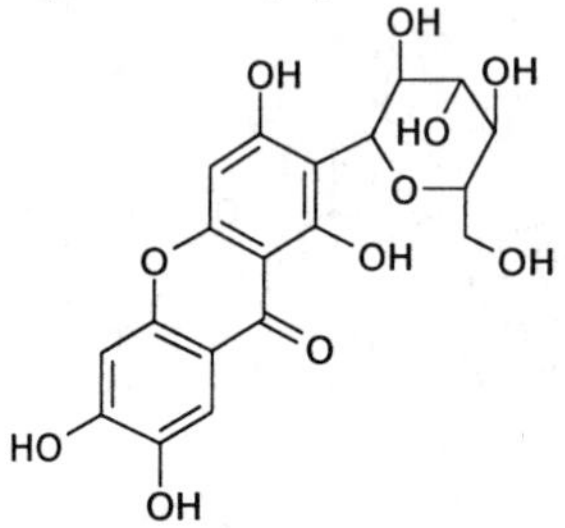

4101 Mangiferolic acid
$C_{29}H_{46}O_3$ MW: 442.69 Property: mp 181-3°C. Source: DI FENG PI, MANG GUO SHU PI. Ref: 6, 395.

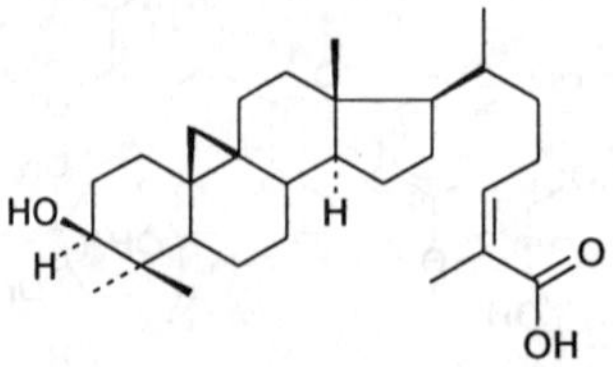

4102 Mangiferonic acid
$C_{29}H_{44}O_3$ MW: 440.67 Property: mp 184-7°C. Source: DI FENG PI, MANG GUO, MANG GUO SHU PI. Ref: 6, 395.

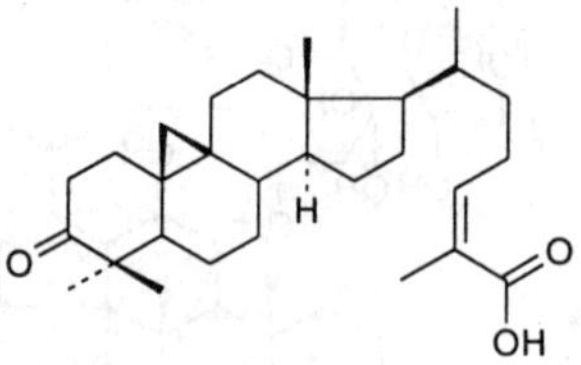

4103 D-Mannitol
$C_6H_{14}O_6$ MW: 182.17 Property: mp (-): 166°C. Source: DONG CHONG XIA CAO, GAN DI HUANG, PU HUANG, TIAN NAN XING, ZHI. Ref: 2, 373, 502.

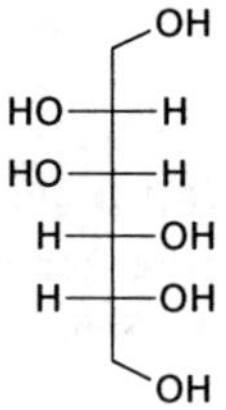

4104 D-Mannoheptulose
$C_7H_{14}O_7$ MW: 210.19 Property: mp 152°C. Source: YING SU KE. Ref: 6.

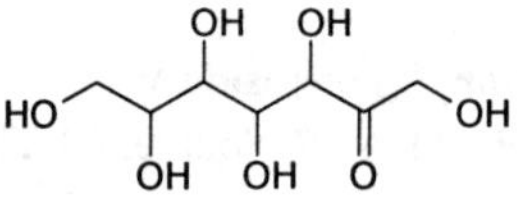

4105 Mannose
$C_6H_{12}O_6$ MW: 180.16 Source: LU HUI, REN SHEN. Ref: 2.

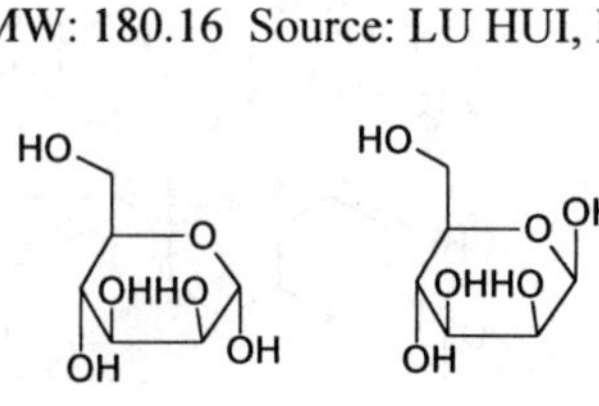

alpha beta

4106 D-Mannuronic acid
$C_6H_{10}O_7$ MW: 194.14 Property: mp (α): 120- 30°C, (β): 165-7°C. Source: LUO LE ZI. Ref: 6.

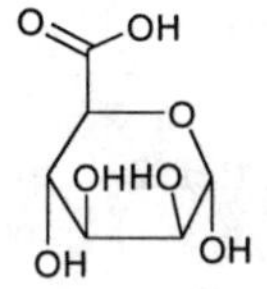

4107 Manogenin

$C_{27}H_{42}O_5$ MW: 446.63 Source: DONG YI HAO JIAN MA, DUAN YE LONG SHE LAN, FAN MA, WU CI FAN MA, XIA YE LONG SHE LAN.
Ref: 10.

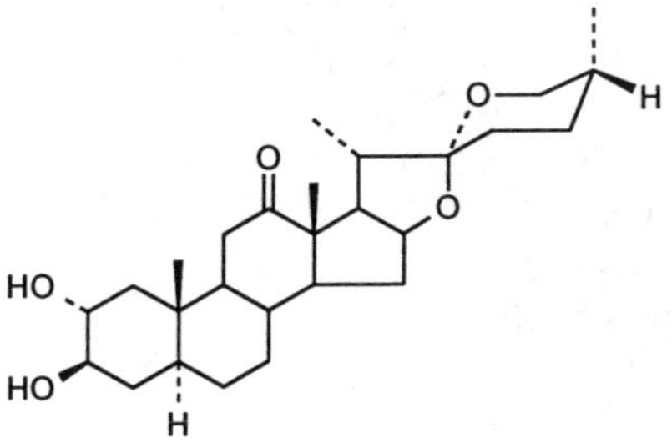

HO HO H H O O O

4108 Mansonone C

$C_{15}H_{16}O_2$ MW: 228.29 Property: mp 134-8°C.
Source: LANG YU PI. Ref: 6.

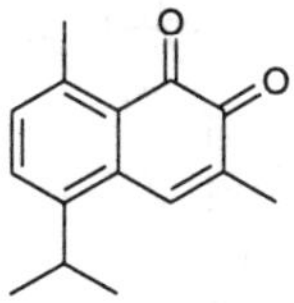

O O

4109 Mansonone G

$C_{15}H_{16}O_3$ MW: 244.29 Property: mp 210-3°C.
Source: LANG YU PI. Ref: 6.

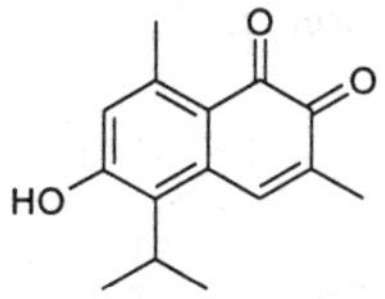

O O HO

4110 Margaric acid

$C_{17}H_{34}O_2$ MW: 270.46 Property: mp 256°C. Source: DANG SHEN[1], LU HUI. Ref: 2.

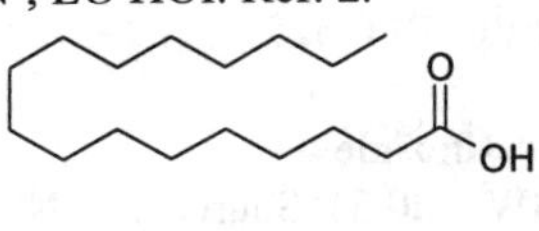

O OH

4111 Marinobufagin 3-suberoyl-L-glutamine ester

$C_{33}H_{46}O_7$ MW: 554.73 Source: CHAN SU. Ref: 2.

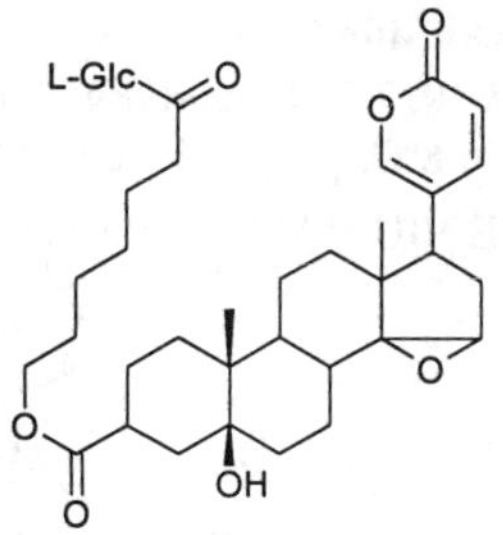

L-Glc O O O O O O OH

4112 Markogenin

$C_{27}H_{44}O_4$ MW: 432.65 Source: ZHI MU. Ref: 2.

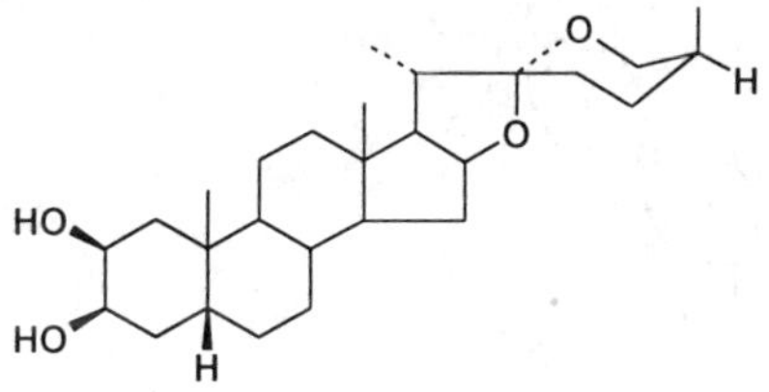

O H O HO HO H

4113 Markogenin3-O-β-D-glucopyranosyl-(1→2)-β-D-galactopyranoside

Source: ZHI MU. Ref: 2.

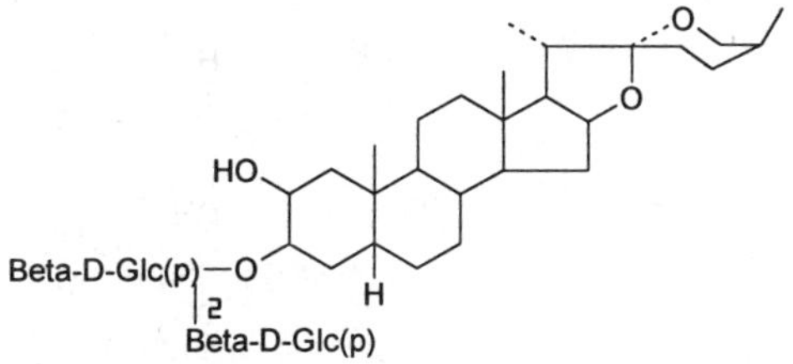

O O HO Beta-D-Glc(p)—O 2 Beta-D-Glc(p) H

4114 Marmesine

$C_{14}H_{14}O_4$ MW: 246.27 Property: mp (+): 188-90°C.
Source: BAI ZHI, QIANG HUO, YUN NAN QIANG HUO, YUN QIAN HU. Ref: 2, 177, 551.

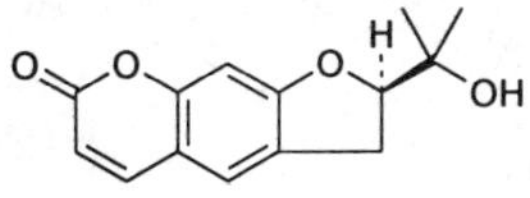

O O O H OH

4115 Marmesinin

$C_{20}H_{24}O_9$ MW: 408.41 Property: mp 129°C. Source: CHOU CAO, ZHONG CHI MAO DANG GUI.
Ref: 6, 344.

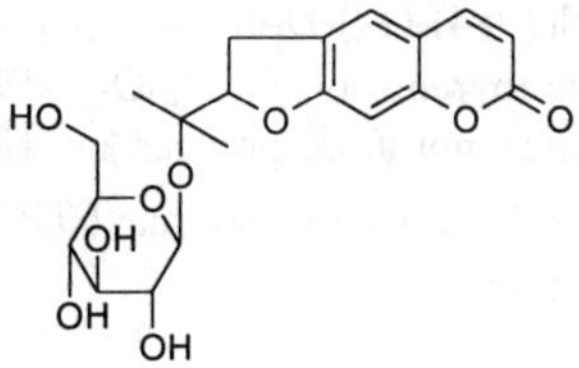

HO O O O O O OH OH OH

4116 Marsdekoiside C
$C_{46}H_{76}O_{18}$ MW: 917.11 Property: white amorphous powder, mp 156-8°C, $[\alpha]_D^{19}$ +25° (c=0.20, methanol). Source: DA YE NIU NAI CAI. Ref: 200.

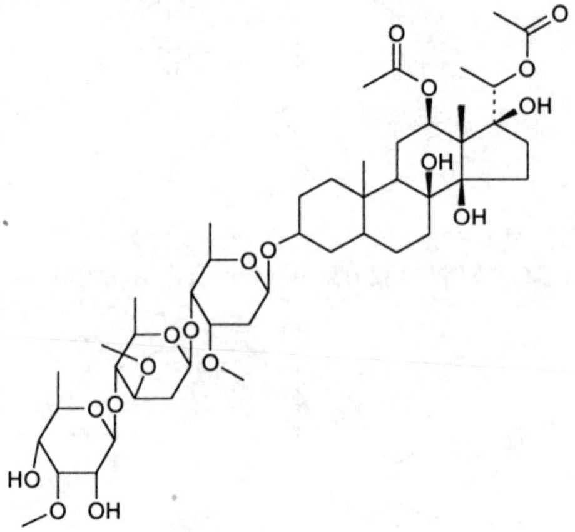

4117 Marsdekoiside E
$C_{51}H_{78}O_{17}$ MW: 963.18 Property: white amorphous powder, mp 154-60°C. Source: DA YE NIU NAI CAI. Ref: 449.

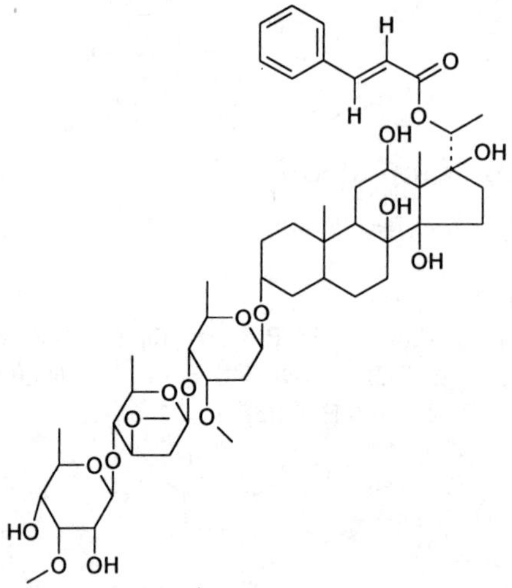

4118 Marsdeoreophiside B
12-O-Cinnamyldihydrosarcostin-3-O-β-D-glucopyranosyl(1→4)-O-3-O-methyl-6-deoxy-β-D-allopyranosyl(1→4)-O-β-D-oleandropyranosyl(1→4)-O-β-D-cymaropyranoside. $C_{57}H_{88}O_{22}$ MW: 1125.32 Property: white amorphous powder, mp 183-4°C, $[\alpha]_D^{19}$ +49.2° (c=0.065, methanol). Source: HUI ZHU NIU NAI CAI. Ref: 298.

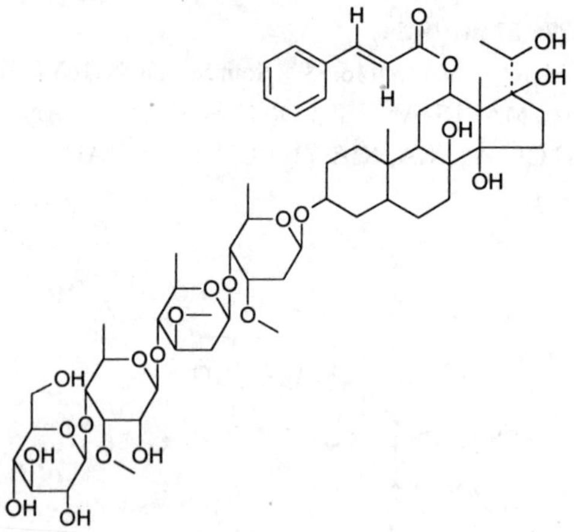

4119 Martynoside
$C_{31}H_{40}O_{15}$ MW: 652.66 Source: GAN DI HUANG. Ref: 2.

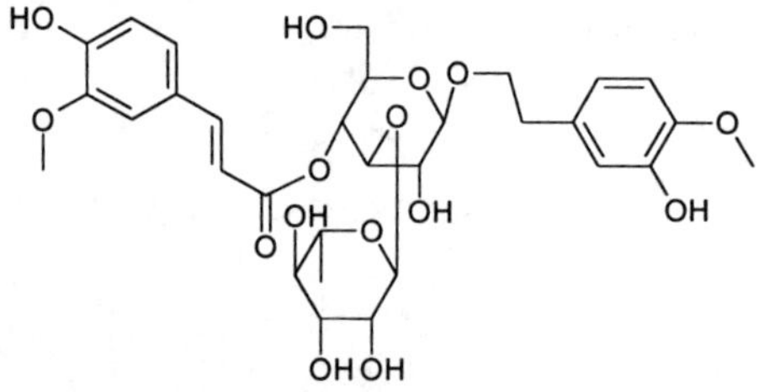

4120 Maslinic acid
$C_{30}H_{48}O_4$ MW: 472.71 Property: mp (-): 263-5°C. Source: DA ZAO. Ref: 2.

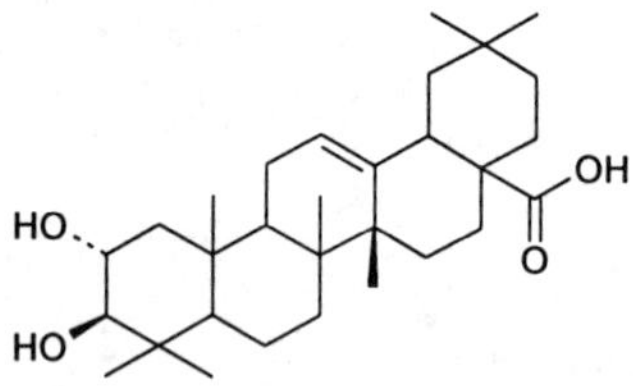

4121 Massaenosidic acid
Source: HOU PU. Ref: 625.

4122 Matairesinoside
$C_{26}H_{32}O_{11}$ MW: 520.54 Source: LIAN QIAO. Ref: 2.

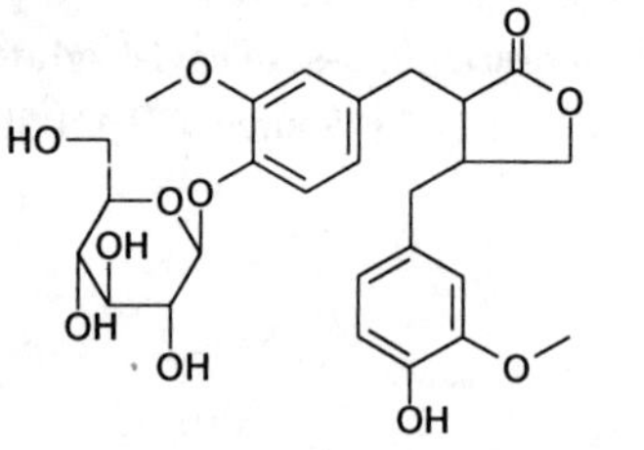

4123 Matricarin
$C_{17}H_{20}O_5$ MW: 304.35 Property: mp 193-5°C.
Source: MU JU. Ref: 6.

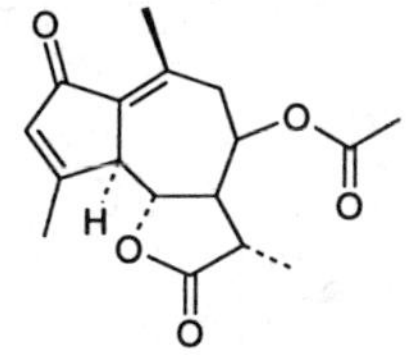

4124 Matricin
$C_{17}H_{22}O_5$ MW: 306.36 Property: mp 158-60°C.
Source: MU JU. Ref: 6.

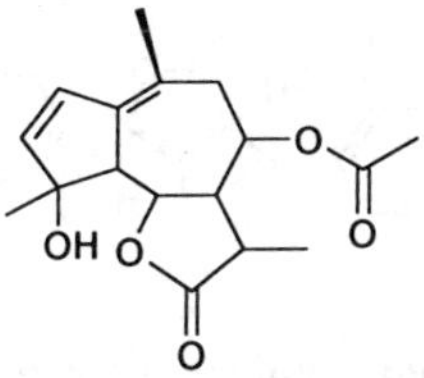

4125 Matrine
cis-Matrine. CAS: 519-02-8 $C_{15}H_{24}N_2O$ MW: 248.37
Property: mp α=76°C, β=87°C, δ=84°C,
γ=223°C/6mm. Source: BAI CI HUA, KU DOU ZI,
KU SHEN. Ref: 4, 546, 564, 593.

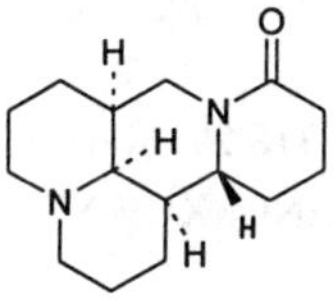

4126 Matsukaze lactone
$C_{20}H_{14}O_6$ MW: 350.33 Source: YAN JIAO CAO.
Ref: 6.

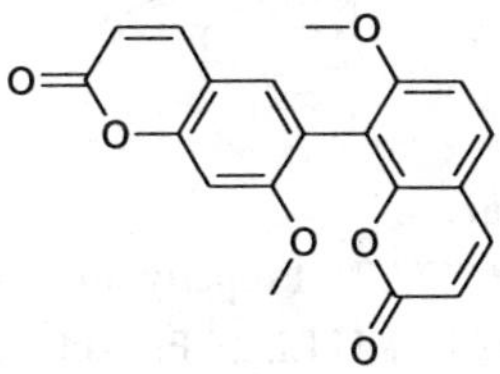

4127 Matsutake alcohol
$C_8H_{16}O$ MW: 128.22 Property: bp 165-75°C. Source:
BAI SU ZI, SONG XUN. Ref: 6.

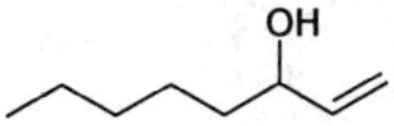

4128 Matteucinin
$C_{29}H_{36}O_{15}$ MW: 624.60 Property: mp 139-41°C.
Source: DU JUAN HUA YE. Ref: 6.

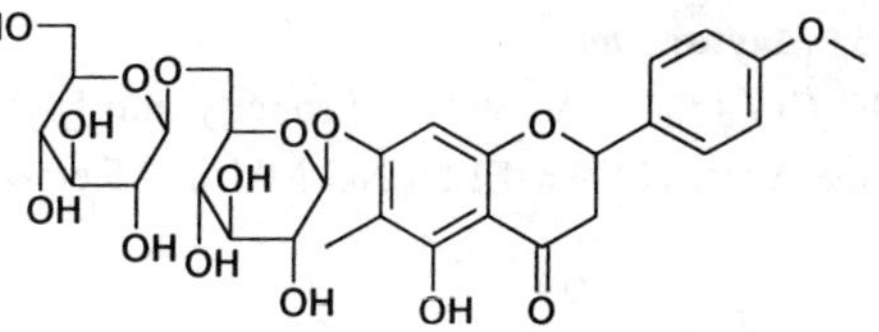

4129 Mauritine A
$C_{32}H_{41}N_5O_5$ MW: 575.71 Property: mp 104°C
Source: MIAN ZAO. Ref: 6.

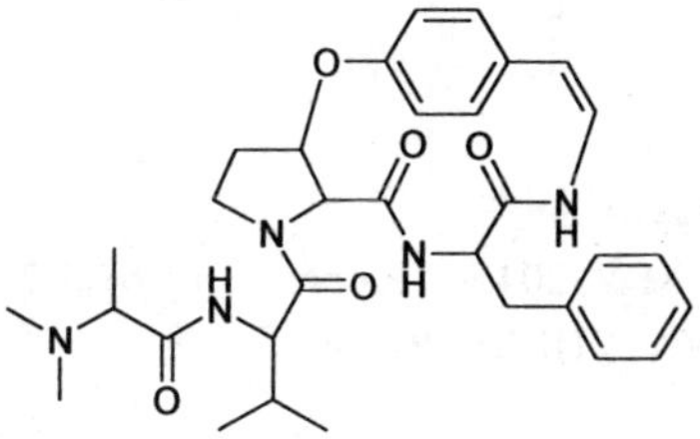

4130 Mauritine B
$C_{35}H_{47}N_5O_5$ MW: 617.81 Source: MIAN ZAO.
Ref: 6.

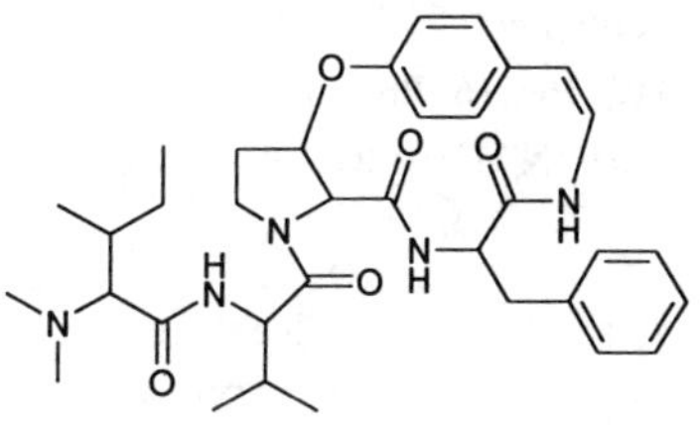

4131 Mavacurine
$C_{20}H_{25}N_2O$ MW: 309.44 Source: MA QIAN ZI.
Ref: 6.

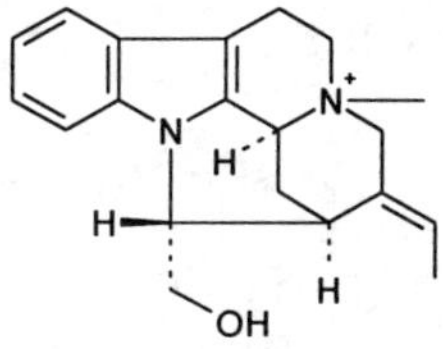

4132 Maytanprine
$C_{35}H_{48}ClN_3O_{10}$ MW: 706.24 Property: mp 178°C.
Source: YUN NAN MEI DENG MU, etc. Ref: 5.

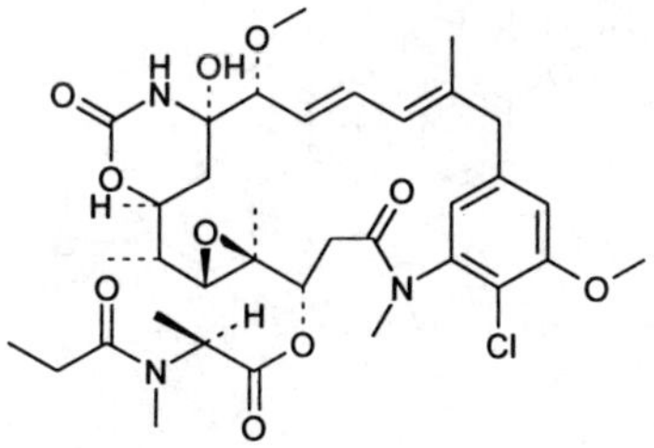

4133 Maytansine

$C_{34}H_{46}ClN_3O_{10}$ MW: 692.21 Property: mp 182°C.
Source: YUN NAN MEI DENG MU, etc. Ref: 4.

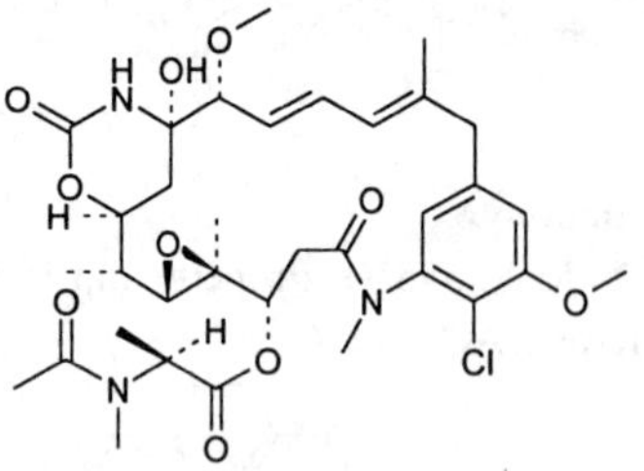

4134 Mayurone

$C_{14}H_{20}O$ MW: 204.31 Property: mp 69.5-70°C.
Source: BAI ZHI JIE. Ref: 6.

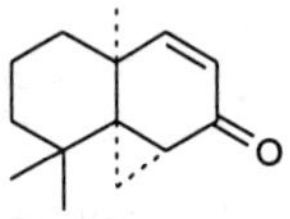

4135 Meconic acid

$C_9H_8O_5$ MW: 196.16 Property: mp 120°C (dec).
Source: LI CHUN HUA. Ref: 6.

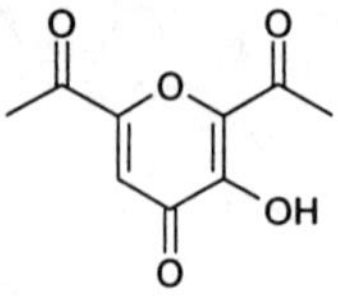

4136 Meconine

$C_{10}H_{10}O_4$ MW: 194.19 Property: mp 102.5°C.
Source: YA PIAN. Ref: 6.

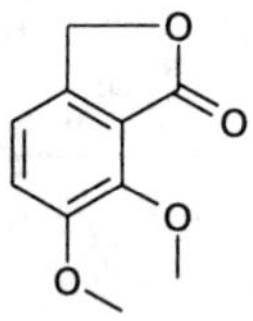

4137 Medicagol

$C_{16}H_8O_6$ MW: 296.24 Property: mp 324-5°C. Source: HUI HUI DOU. Ref: 6.

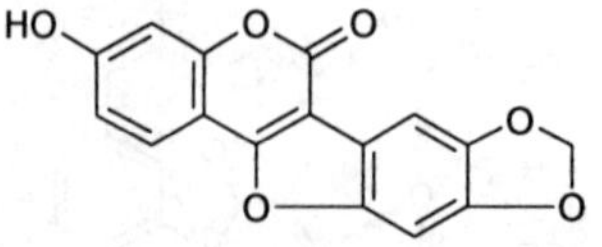

4138 (+)-Medioresinol di-O-β-D-glucopyranoside

Source: DU ZHONG. Ref: 2.

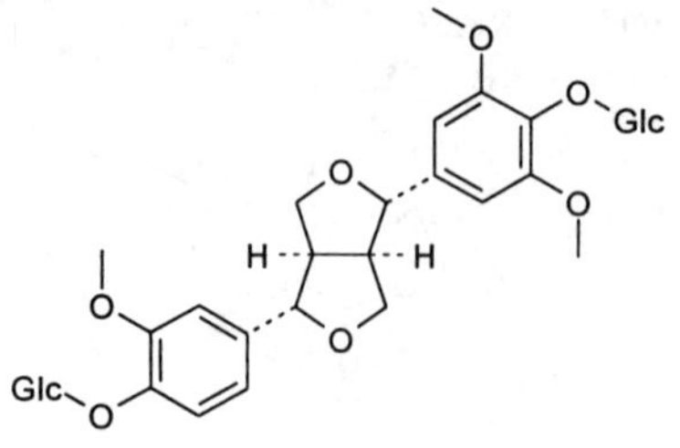

4139 (+)-Medioresinol-di-O-β-D-glucoside

Source: CI WU JIA. Ref: 2.

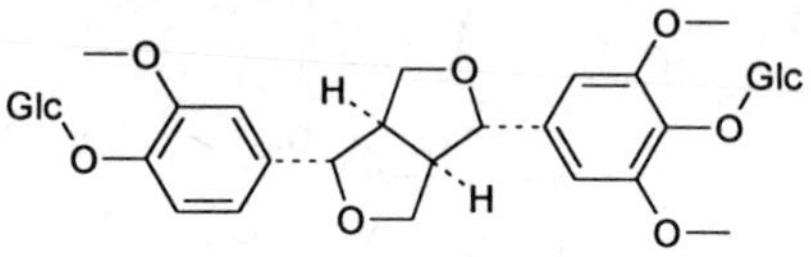

4140 (+)-Medioresinol monoglucoside

Source: DU ZHONG. Ref: 2.

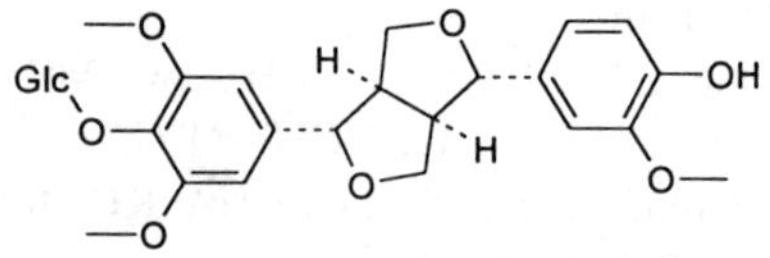

4141 Melanin

$C_{18}H_{10}N_2O_4$ MW: 318.29 Source: SI GUA ZI, WANG BU LIU XING, XUE YU, YANG PI. Ref: 6.

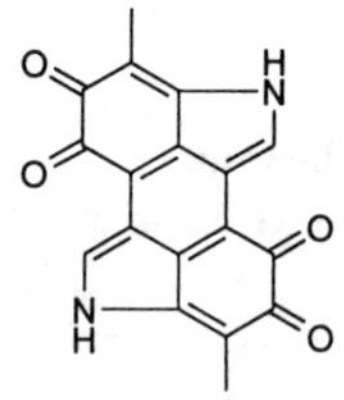

4142 Melianol

$C_{30}H_{48}O_4$ MW: 472.71 Property: mp 194-5°C.
Source: KU LIAN, KU LIAN PI. Ref: 6, 648.

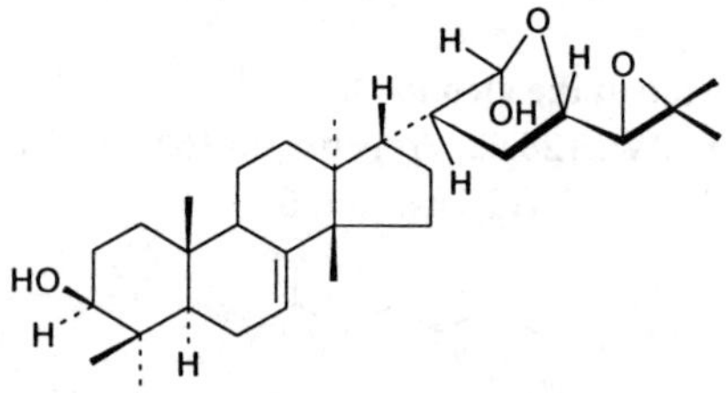

4143 Melianone

$C_{30}H_{46}O_4$ MW: 470.70 Property: mp 223-4°C (acetone and pentane), 232-3°C (chloroform and pentane). Source: KU LIAN, KU LIAN PI. Ref: 6, 648.

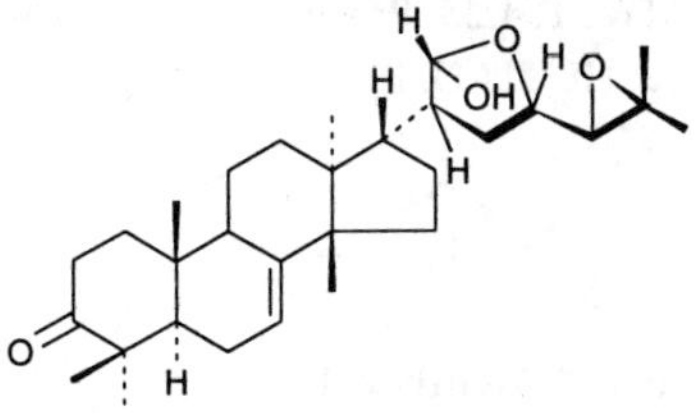

4144 Melianoninol

$C_{20}H_{20}O_6$ MW: 356.38 Property: light yellow prismatic crystal, mp 150-2°C, $[\alpha]_D^{18}$ -4.28° (c=0.46, methanol). Source: KU LIAN PI. Ref: 648.

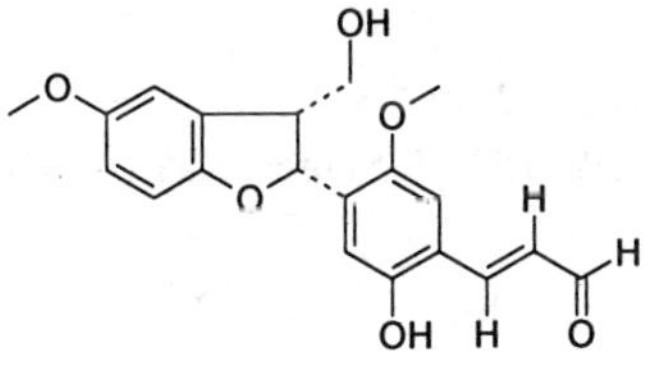

4145 Melianotriol

$C_{30}H_{50}O_5$ MW: 490.73 Property: mp 176-8°C. Source: KU LIAN PI. Ref: 6.

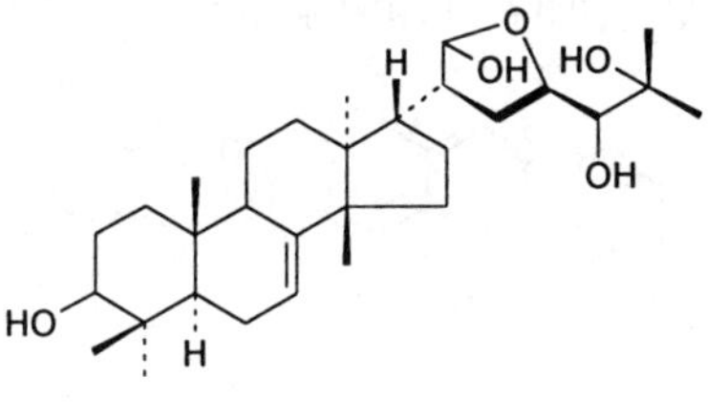

4146 Melicitrin

$C_{20}H_{18}O_{12}$ MW: 450.36 Source: LIAN HUA. Ref: 6.

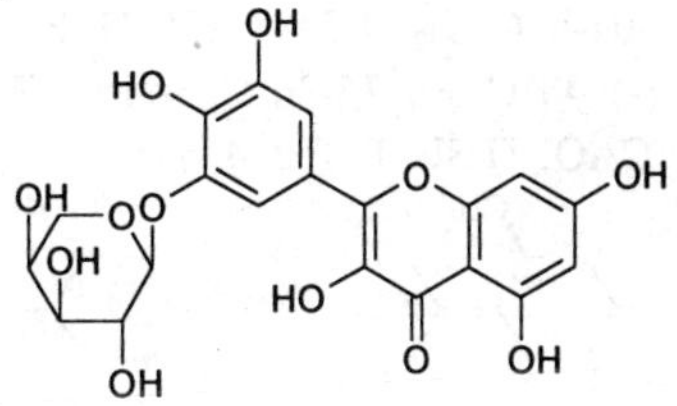

4148 Melissane

$C_{30}H_{62}$ MW: 422.83 Property: mp 73-4°C, bp 222°C/0.3 mm. Source: TU DING GUI. Ref: 6.

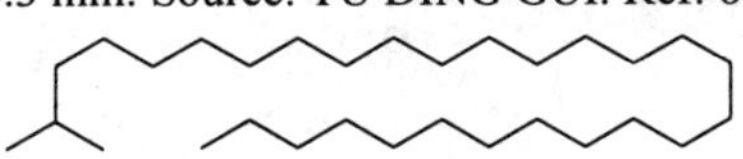

4149 Melissic acid A

$C_{30}H_{60}O_2$ MW: 452.81 Property: mp 93°C. Source: GUA LOU, YUN QIAN HU. Ref: 2, 177.

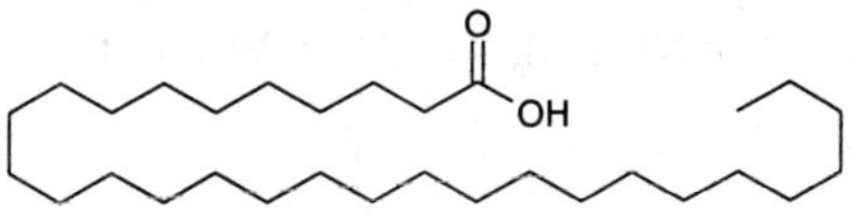

4150 Melissic acid B

$C_{31}H_{62}O_2$ MW: 466.84 Property: mp 93.5-4°C. Source: GUA LOU. Ref: 2.

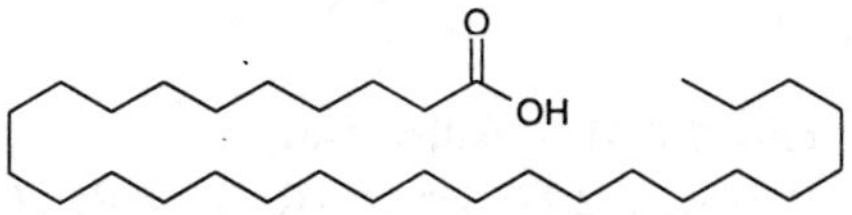

4151 Melissyl lignocerate

$C_{54}H_{108}O_2$ MW: 789.46 Source: CHONG BAI LA. Ref: 6.

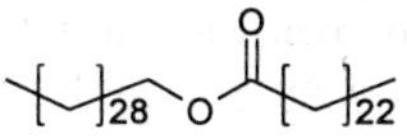

4152 Melittoside

Source: GAN DI HUANG. Ref: 2.

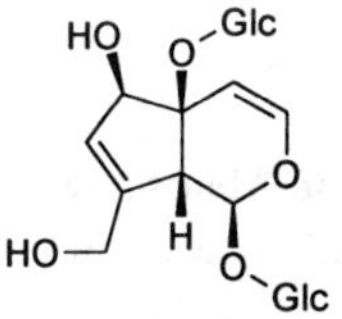

4153 Menisidine

$C_{37}H_{40}N_2O_6$ MW: 608.74 Source: FANG JI. Ref: 2.

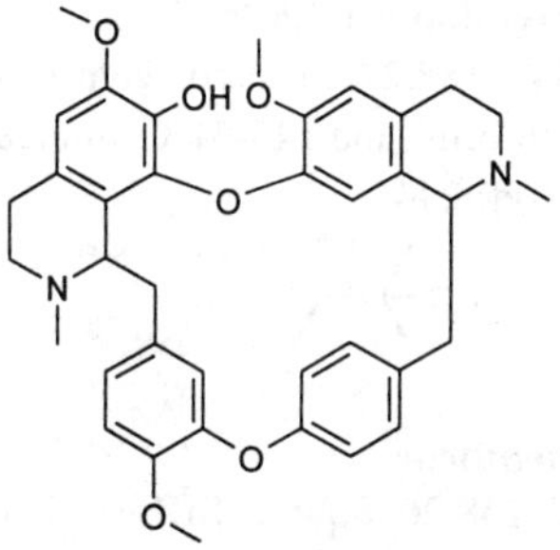

4154 Menisine

$C_{38}H_{42}N_2O_6$ MW: 622.77 Source: FANG JI. Ref: 2.

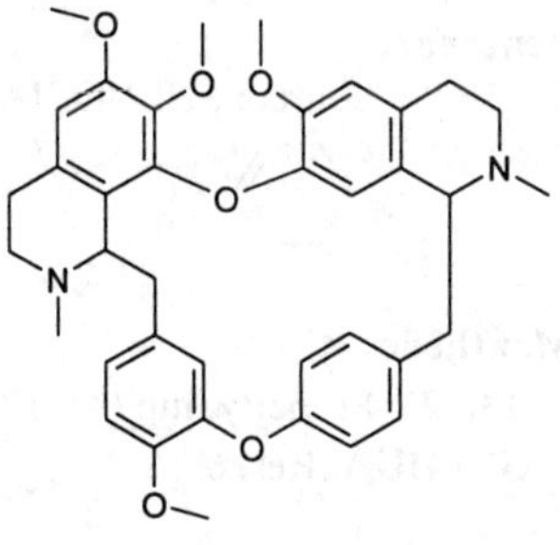

4155 Menisperine
$C_{21}H_{27}NO_4$ MW: 357.45 Property: mp 233°C. Source: HUANG BAI, XIA TIAN WU. Ref: 2, 512.

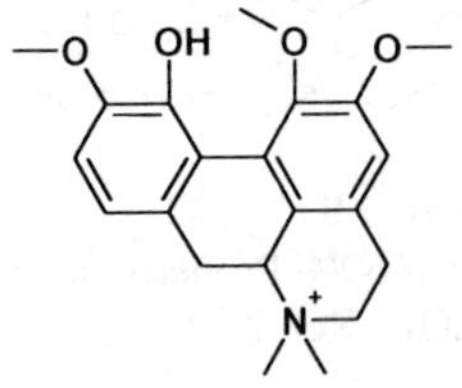

4156 cis-p-2,8-Menthadien-1-ol
$C_{10}H_{16}O$ MW: 152.24 Source: HU JIAO. Ref: 6.

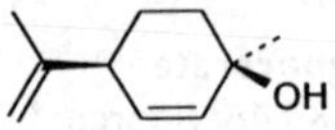

4157 1,8-Menthadien-10-ol acetate
$C_{12}H_{18}O_2$ MW: 194.28 Source: JU PI (CHEN PI). Ref: 6.

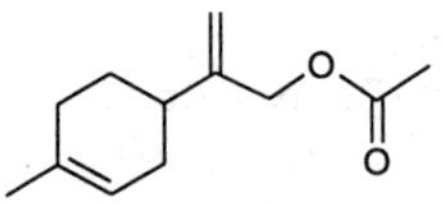

4158 (1s, 3s)-(+)-m-Menthane
$C_{10}H_{20}$ MW: 140.27 Source: SHAN ZHA. Ref: 2.

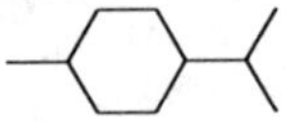

4159 4-p-Menthane-1,7,8-triol
$C_{10}H_{20}O_3$ MW: 188.27 Property: colorless prismatic crystal (chloroform), mp 149-51°C. Source: HUA BEI BAI QIAN. Ref: 244.

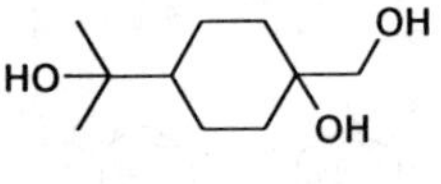

4160 Δ7-Menthene
$C_{10}H_{18}$ MW: 138.26 Source: SHENG JIANG. Ref: 2.

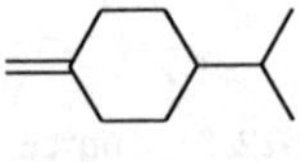

4161 Δ3-Menthene
$C_{10}H_{18}$ MW: 138.26 Source: SHENG JIANG. Ref: 2.

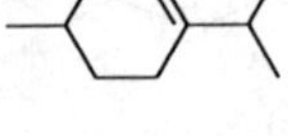

4162 p-1-Menthene
$C_{10}H_{18}$ MW: 138.25 Property: mp (+): 175-7°C. Source: MEI GUI HUA. Ref: 6.

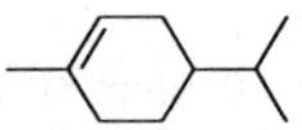

4163 cis-p-2-Menthen-1-ol
$C_{10}H_{18}O$ MW: 154.25 Property: bp (-): 110-5°C/25 mm. Source: HU JIAO. Ref: 6.

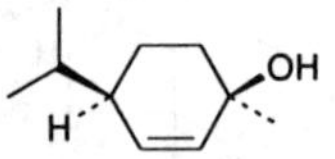

4164 trans-p-2-Menthen-1-ol
$C_{10}H_{18}O$ MW: 154.25 Source: BAI DOU KOU. Ref: 6.

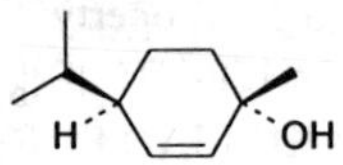

4165 p-Menth-2-en-7-ol
$C_{10}H_{18}O$ MW: 154.25 Source: MA HUANG. Ref: 2.

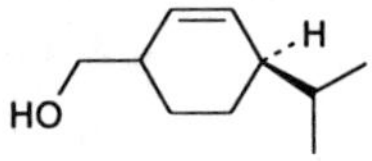

4166 Menthiafolin
$C_{28}H_{40}O_{12}$ MW: 568.62 Property: mp 186°C. Source: SHUI CAI, SHUI CAI GEN. Ref: 6.

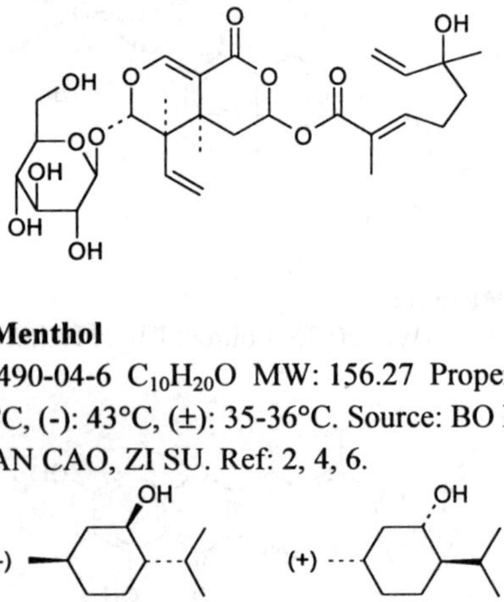

4167 Menthol
CAS: 1490-04-6 $C_{10}H_{20}O$ MW: 156.27 Property: mp (+): 42°C, (-): 43°C, (±): 35-36°C. Source: BO HE, JIN QIAN CAO, ZI SU. Ref: 2, 4, 6.

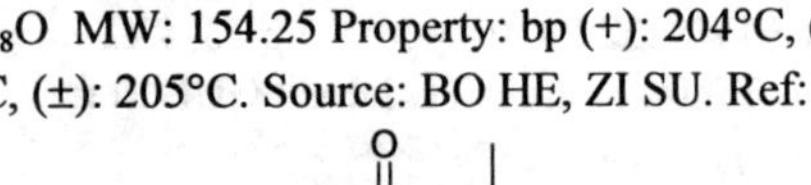

(-) (+)

4168 Menthone
$C_{10}H_{18}O$ MW: 154.25 Property: bp (+): 204°C, (-): 207°C, (±): 205°C. Source: BO HE, ZI SU. Ref: 2.

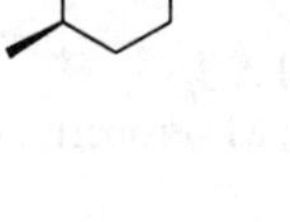

4169 Menthyl acetate
$C_{12}H_{22}O_2$ MW: 198.31 Property: bp 227°C. Source: BO HE. Ref: 2.

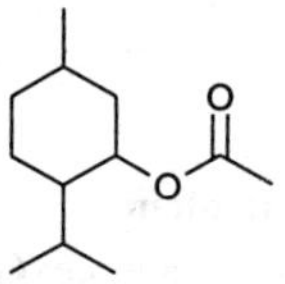

4170 Meranzin hydrate
$C_{15}H_{18}O_5$ MW: 278.31 Source: JIU LI XIANG, ZHONG CHI MAO DANG GUI. Ref: 11, 344.

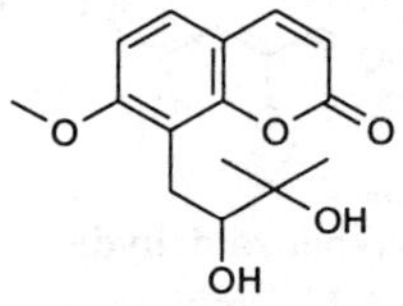

4171 Meratin
$C_{27}H_{30}O_{17}$ MW: 626.53 Property: mp 182-4°C. Source: DUO SUI LIAO, LA MEI HUA. Ref: 6.

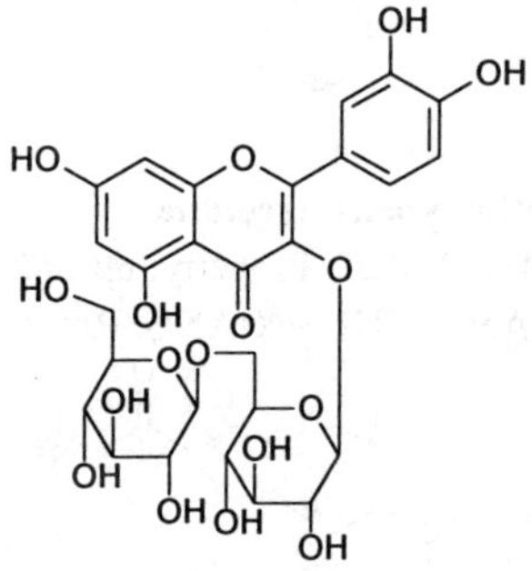

4172 Mesaconic acid
$C_5H_6O_4$ MW: 130.10 Property: mp 240.5°C. Source: GAN ZHE. Ref: 6.

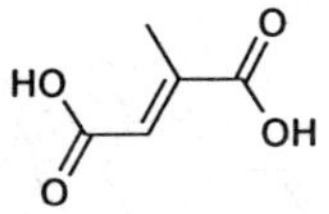

4173 Mesaconitine
$C_{33}H_{45}NO_{11}$ MW: 631.73 Property: white granular crystal, $[\alpha]_D^{26}$ +22.4° (c=1.511, $CHCl_3$). Source: E ZHANG YE FU ZI, FU ZI. Ref: 2, 460.

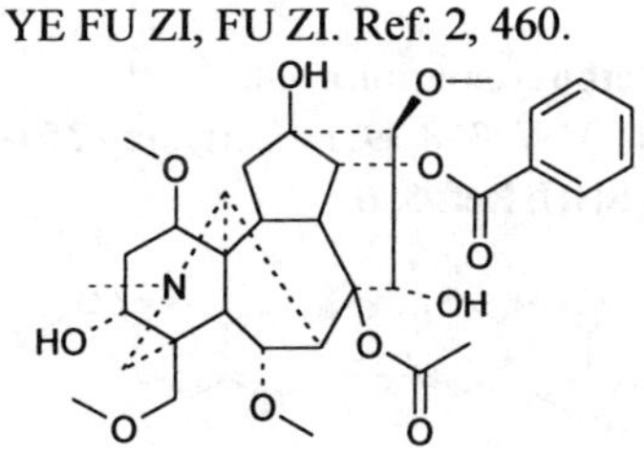

4174 Mesityl oxide
$C_6H_{10}O$ MW: 98.15 Property: bp 130-1°C. Source: YA ER QIN. Ref: 6.

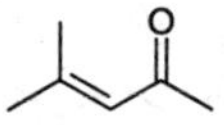

4175 Meso-3,5-diacetoxy-1,7-bis(4-hydroxy-3-methoxyphenyl) heptane
$C_{25}H_{32}O_8$ MW: 460.53 Source: GAN JIANG, SHENG JIANG. Ref: 2.

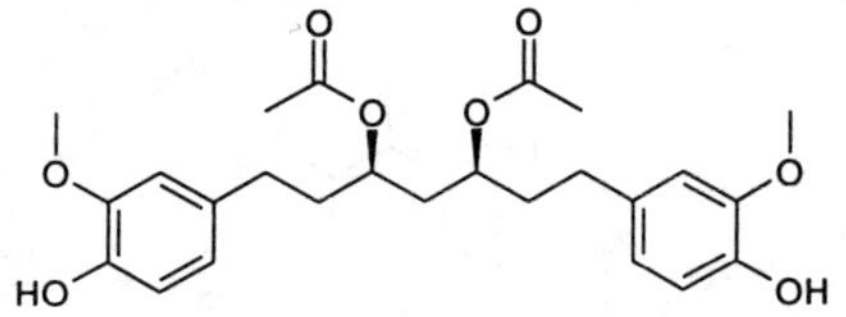

4176 Metaphanine
$C_{19}H_{23}NO_5$ MW: 345.40 Property: mp 233°C. Source: QIAN JIN TENG. Ref: 6.

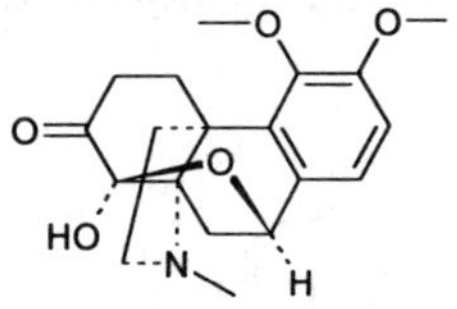

4177 Metaplexigenin
$C_{23}H_{34}O_7$ MW: 422.52 Property: mp 268-75°C. Source: LUO MO. Ref: 6.

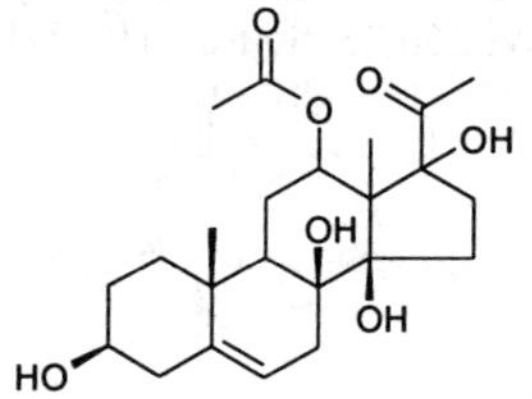

4178 Meteloidine
$C_{13}H_{21}NO_4$ MW: 255.32 Property: mp 141-2°C. Source: MAN TUO LUO YE, MAN TUO LUO GEN. Ref: 6.

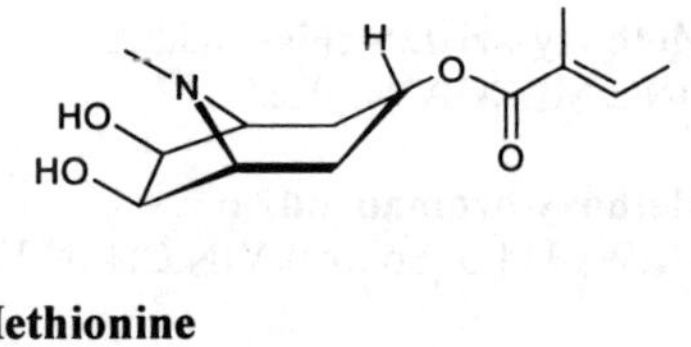

4179 Methionine
$C_5H_{11}NO_2S$ MW: 149.21 Source: BAI GUO. Ref: 2.

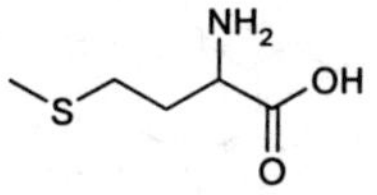

4180 Methionine sulfoxide
$C_5H_{11}NO_3S$ MW: 165.21 Property: mp 230-1°C (dec). Source: YUAN CAN ZI. Ref: 6.

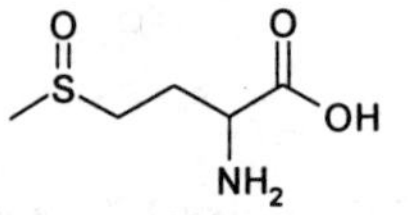

4181 12-Methoxy-6,8,11,13-abietatraen-11-ol
$C_{21}H_{30}O_2$ MW: 314.47 Source: DU SONG SHI. Ref: 6.

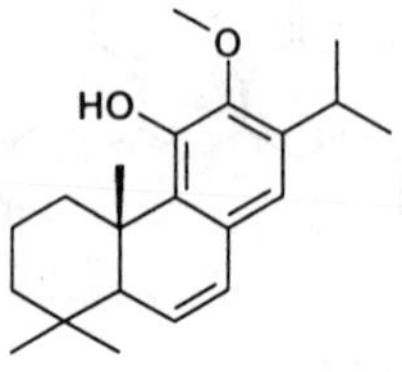

4182 12-Methoxy-8,11,13-abietatriene-7β,11-diol
$C_{21}H_{32}O_3$ MW: 332.49 Source: DU SONG SHI. Ref: 6.

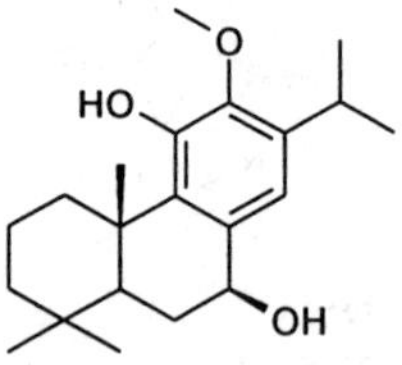

4183 2-Methoxy-6-acethyl-7-methyljuglone
$C_{14}H_{12}O_5$ MW: 260.25 Source: HU ZHANG. Ref: 2.

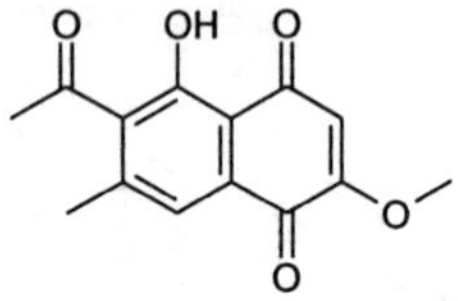

4184 4-Methoxy-acetophenone
$C_9H_{10}O_2$ MW: 150.18 Source: DU HUO. Ref: 2.

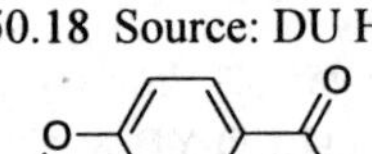

4185 7-Methoxy-aristolochiac acid A
Source: QING MU XIANG. Ref: 517.

4186 7-Methoxy-aromadendrin
$C_{17}H_{14}O_6$ MW: 314.0 Source: YIN CHEN HAO. Ref: 2.

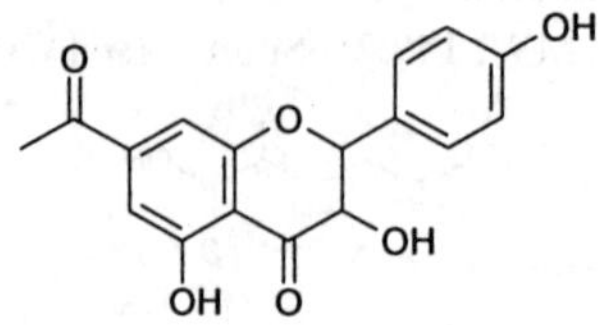

4187 6-Methoxy aurapten
$C_{20}H_{24}O_4$ MW: 328.41 Source: GOU JU HE. Ref: 6.

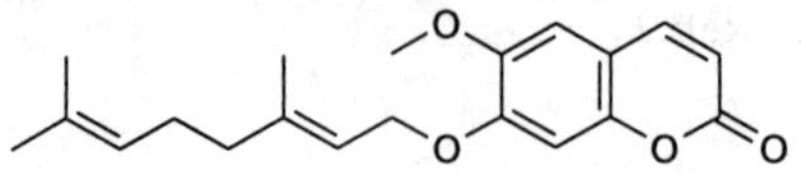

4188 7-Methoxybaicalein
$C_{16}H_{12}O_5$ MW: 284.27 Source: GUANG YE SHUI SU. Ref: 6.

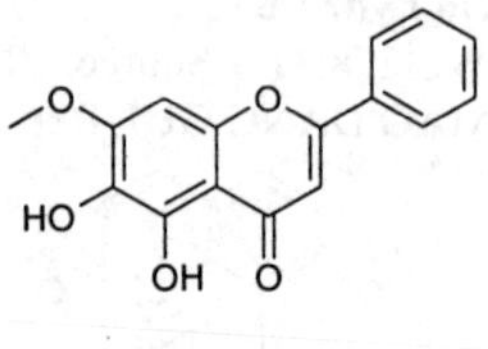

4189 m-Methoxybenzaldehyde
$C_8H_8O_2$ MW: 136.15 Property: bp 230°C. Source: DING XIANG. Ref: 6.

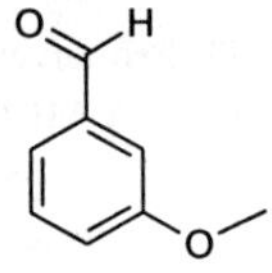

4190 p-Methoxybenzylacetone
$C_{11}H_{14}O_2$ MW: 178.23 Property: bp 277°C. Source: BAI MU XIANG, CHEN XIANG. Ref: 6, 13.

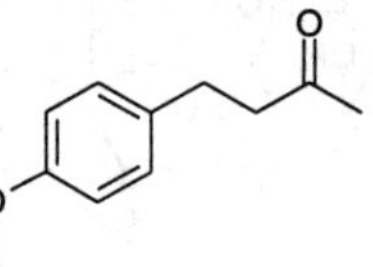

4191 5'-Methoxy-bilobetin
$C_{32}H_{22}O_{11}$ MW: 582.53 Source: BAI GUO. Ref: 2.

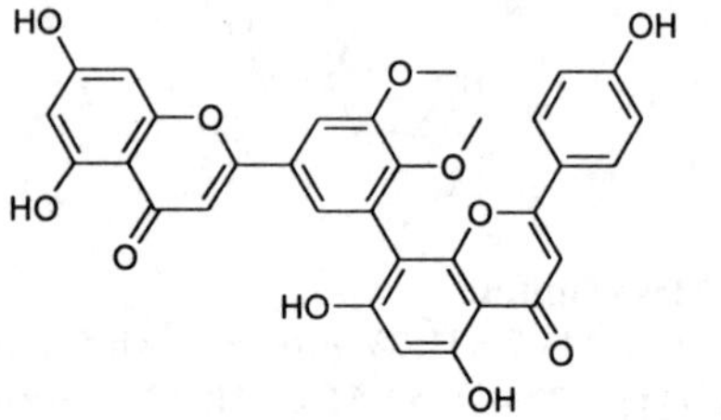

4192 9-Methoxycamptothecin
$C_{21}H_{18}N_2O_5$ MW: 378.39 Property: mp 254-5°C. Source: XI SHU. Ref: 5, 6.

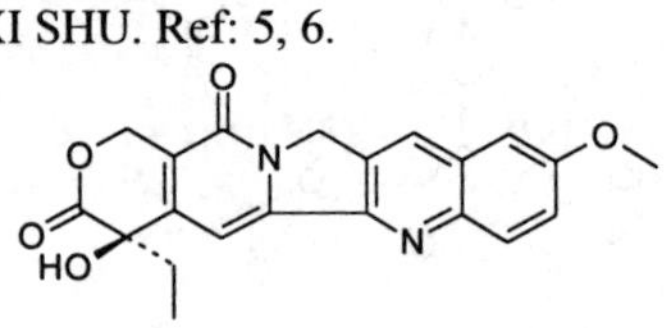

4193 10-Methoxycamptothecin
$C_{21}H_{18}N_2O_5$ MW: 378.39 Property: mp 255-6°C. Source: XI SHU. Ref: 6.

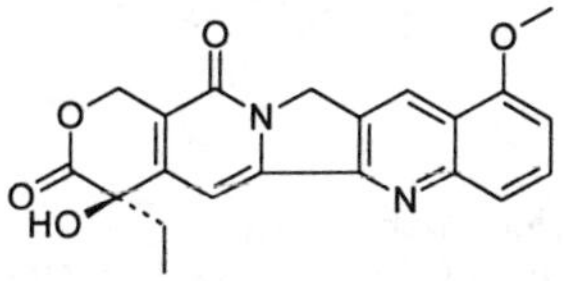

4194 o-Methoxycapillen
$C_{13}H_{12}O$ MW: 184.24 Source: YIN CHEN HAO. Ref: 2.

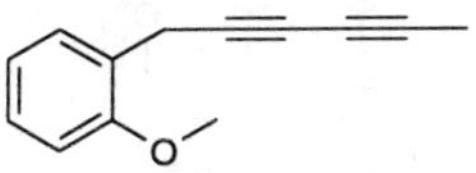

4195 Methoxychelidonine
$C_{21}H_{21}NO_6$ MW: 383.40 Property: mp 221°C. Source: BAI QU CAI. Ref: 6.

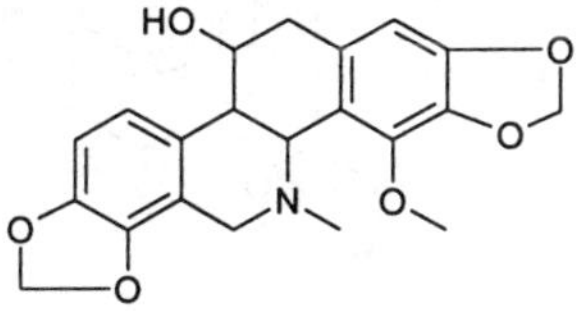

4196 p-Methoxy cinnamaldehyde
$C_{10}H_{10}O_2$ MW: 162.19 Property: mp 134°C. Source: HUO XIANG. Ref: 2.

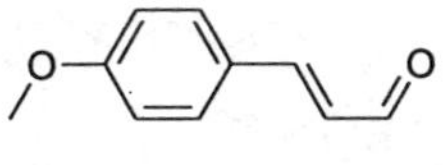

4197 p-Methoxycinnamic acid
$C_{10}H_{10}O_3$ MW: 178.19 Property: mp 170°C(174°C). Source: MU ZEI. Ref: 2.

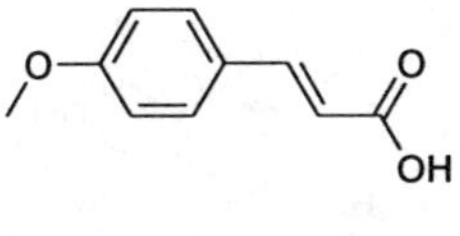

4198 m-Methoxycinnamic acid
$C_{10}H_{10}O_3$ MW: 178.19 Source: MU ZEI. Ref: 2.

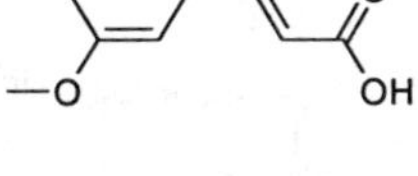

4199 6-Methoxy dictamnine
$C_{13}H_{11}NO_3$ MW: 229.24 Property: mp 134-5°C. Source: CHOU CAO. Ref: 6.

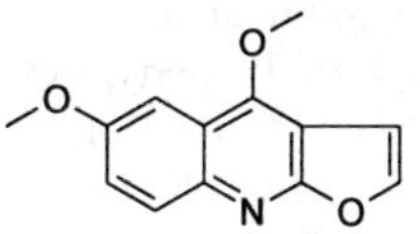

4200 12-Methoxydihydrodehydrocostus lactone
$C_{16}H_{22}O_3$ MW: 262.35 Source: MU XIANG. Ref: 2.

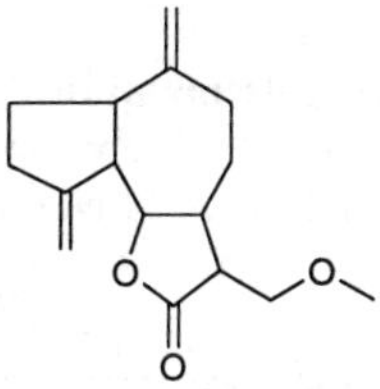

4201 4'-Methoxy-3',7-dihydroxy-flavone
Source: GUANG XI XUE JIE. Ref: 616.

4202 5-Methoxy-N,N-dimethyl-tryptamine
$C_{13}H_{18}N_2O$ MW: 218.30 Property: mp 47°C. Source: HONG MU JI CAO, PAI QIAN CAO. Ref: 6.

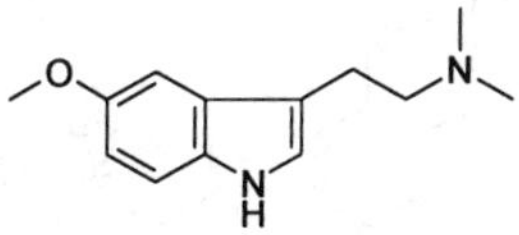

4203 5-Methoxy-N,N-dimethyl-tryptamine Nb-oxide
$C_{13}H_{18}N_2O_2$ MW: 234.30 Source: HONG MU JI CAO, PAI QIAN CAO. Ref: 6.

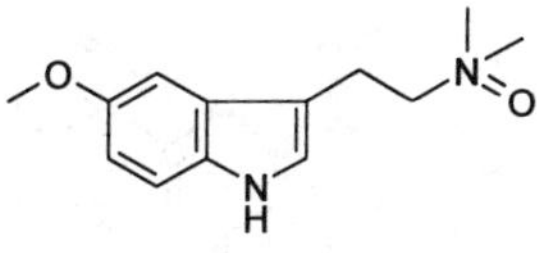

4204 7-Methoxy-8-(2'-formyl-2'-methylpropyl) coumarin
$C_{15}H_{16}O_4$ MW: 260.29 Source: JIU LI XIANG. Ref: 11.

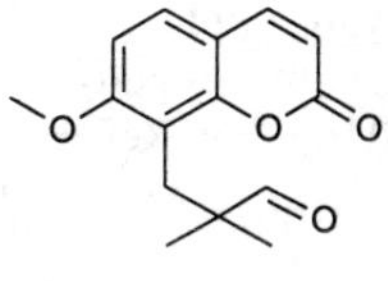

4205 5-Methoxyfuraldehyde
$C_6H_6O_3$ MW: 126.11 Source: DANG SHEN. Ref: 2.

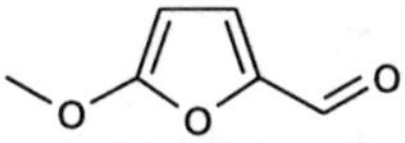

4206 3-Methoxygallic acid
$C_8H_8O_5$ MW: 184.15 Property: mp 220°C(131-2°C). Source: SHUI JIE GU DAN. Ref: 6.

4207 11–Methoxygelsemamide
$C_{20}H_{24}N_2O_4$ MW: 356.43 Property: mp 140°C, $[\alpha]_D$ +215.5°. Source: HU MAN TENG. Ref: 14.

4208 3'-Methoxyglabridin
$C_{21}H_{22}O_5$ MW: 354.41 Source: GAN CAO. Ref: 2.

4209 8-Methoxy-5-O-glucoside flavone
$C_{22}H_{22}O_9$ MW: 430.42 Source: HUANG QIN. Ref: 2.

4210 6-Methoxygossypol
$C_{31}H_{34}O_8$ MW: 534.61 Property: mp 146-9°C. Source: MIAN HUA GEN. Ref: 6.

4211 6-Methoxyhemigossypol
$C_{16}H_{18}O_4$ MW: 274.32 Source: MIAN HUA GEN. Ref: 6.

4212 3-Methoxyherbacetin
$C_{16}H_{12}O_7$ MW: 316.27 Source: MA HUANG. Ref: 2.

4213 11-Methoxyhumantenine
$C_{22}H_{28}N_2O_4$ MW: 384.48 Property: powder, $[\alpha]_D$ -146.5°. Source: HU MAN TENG. Ref: 14.

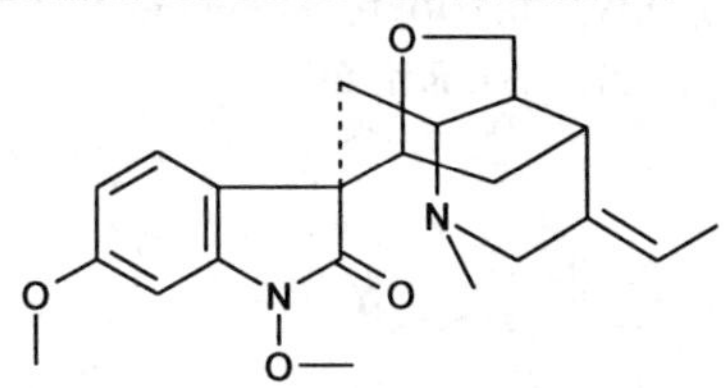

4214 p-Methoxyhydrocinnamic acid
$C_{10}H_{12}O_3$ MW: 180.21 Property: mp 104-5°C Source: CHEN XIANG. Ref: 6.

4215 3-Methoxy-4-hydroxybenzoic acid
$C_8H_8O_4$ MW: 168.15 Source: GAN DI HUANG. Ref: 2.

4216 3-Methoxy-7-hydroxycadalenal
$C_{16}H_{18}O_3$ MW: 258.32 Property: mp 137-9°C. Source: LANG YU PI. Ref: 6.

4217 4-Methoxy-5-hydroxycanthin-6-one
$C_{15}H_{10}N_2O_3$ MW: 266.26 Source: KU SHU PI. Ref: 12.

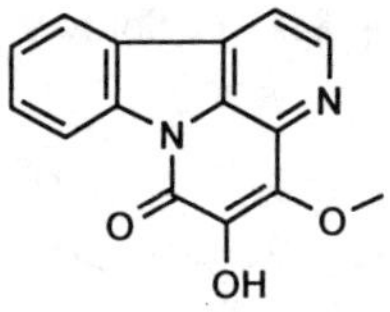

4218 6-Methoxy-7-hydroxycoumarin
$C_{10}H_8O_4$ MW: 192.17 Source: DANG GUI, QING HAO. Ref: 2.

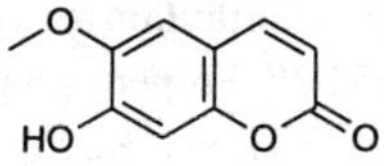

4219 4'-Methoxy-5-hydroxy-8-3,3-dimethylallyl-flavone-3-glucosyl(1→2)rhamnoside-7-glucoside
$C_{40}H_{52}O_{19}$ MW: 836.85 Source: YIN YANG HUO. Ref: 2.

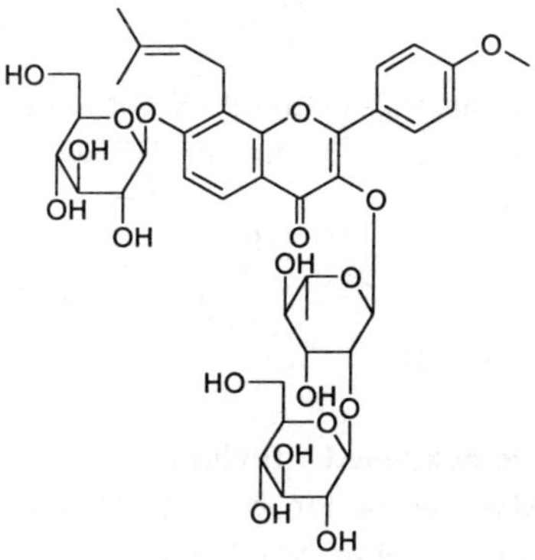

4220 4'-Methoxy-5-hydroxy-8-3,3-dimethyl allylflavone-3-rhamnosyl(1→2)rhamnoside-7-glucoside
$C_{39}H_{50}O_{18}$ MW: 806.82 Source: YIN YANG HUO. Ref: 2.

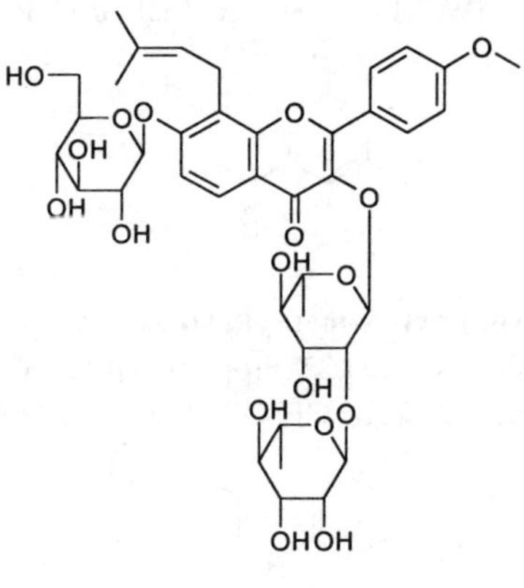

4221 4'-Methoxy-5-hydroxy-8-3,3-dimethyl allylflavone-3-xyloxyl(1→2)rhamnoside-7-glucoside
$C_{38}H_{48}O_{18}$ MW: 792.80 Source: YIN YANG HUO. Ref: 2.

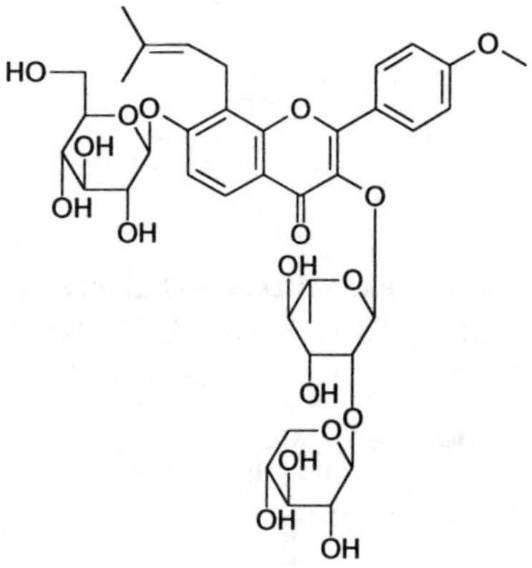

4222 11-Methoxy-19-(R)-Hydroxygelselegine
$C_{21}H_{28}N_2O_6$ MW: 404.47 Property: mp 234-6°C, $[\alpha]_D$ -110°. Source: HU MAN TENG. Ref: 14.

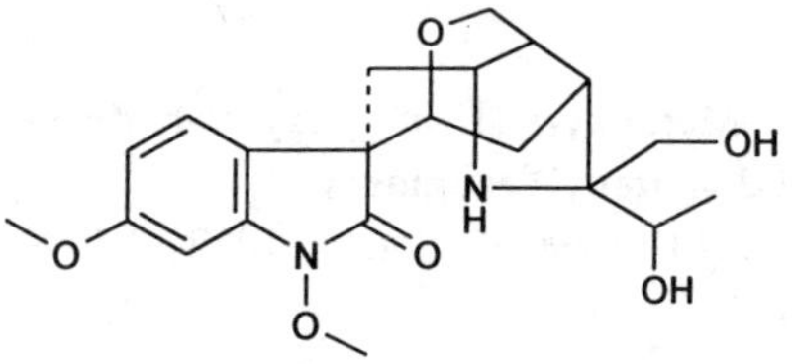

4223 5-methoxy-7-(4''-hydroxy-3''-methoxy phenyl)-1-phenyl-3-heptanone
$C_{20}H_{24}O_4$ MW: 328.41 Property: colorless oleaginous liquid, $[\alpha]_D^{20}$ -11.6° (c=0.43, $CHCl_3$). Source: GAO LIANG JIANG. Ref: 435.

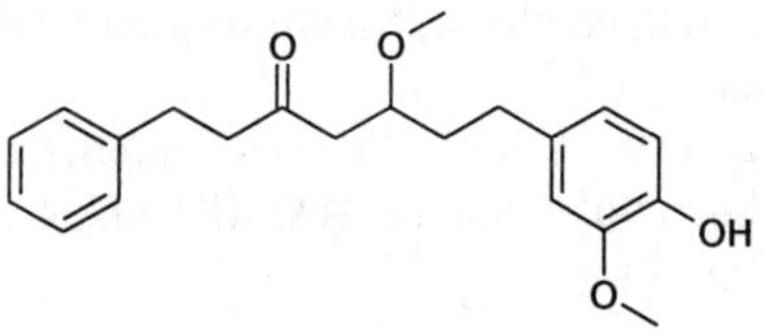

4224 5-Methoxy-8-hydroxy-psoralen
$C_{12}H_8O_5$ MW: 232.19 Source: BAI ZHI. Ref: 2.

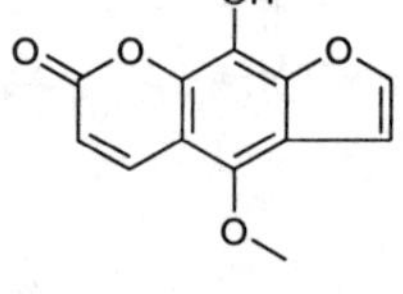

4225 3-Methoxyicajine
$C_{23}H_{26}N_2O_4$ MW: 394.47 Source: MA QIAN ZI. Ref: 2.

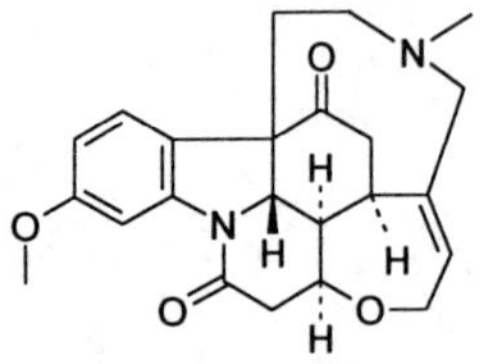

4226 6-Methoxykaempferol 3-O-glycoside
$C_{22}H_{22}O_{12}$ MW: 478.41 Source: QING HAO. Ref: 2.

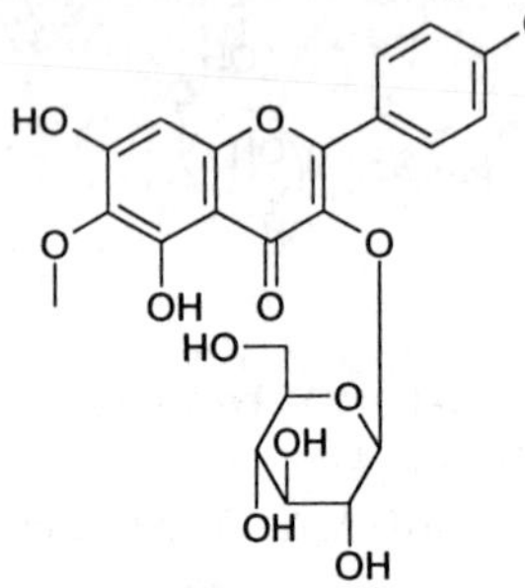

4227 7-Methoxy-8-(1'-methoxy-2'-hydroxy-3'-methyl-3'-butenyl) coumarin
$C_{16}H_{18}O_5$ MW: 290.32 Source: JIU LI XIANG. Ref: 11.

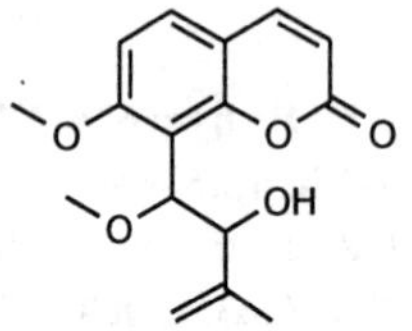

4228 6-Methoxy-2-[2-(3'-methoxyphenyl) ethyl] chromone
$C_{19}H_{18}O_4$ MW: 310.35 Property: colorless acicular crystal, mp 97-9°C. Source: BAI MU XIANG, CHEN XIANG. Ref: 13.

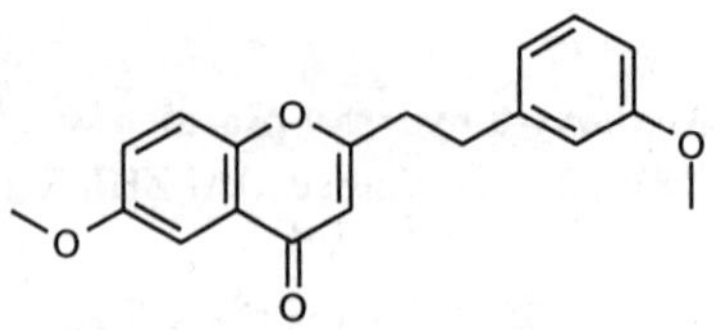

4229 6-Methoxy-2-[2-(4'methoxyphenyl) ethyl] chromone
$C_{19}H_{18}O_4$ MW: 310.35 Property: colorless fine acicular crystal, mp 84-5°C. Source: CHEN XIANG. Ref: 13.

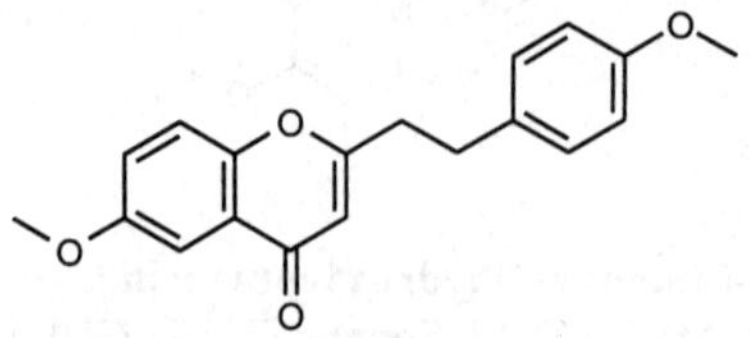

4230 1-Methoxy-2-methylan-thraquinone
$C_{16}H_{12}O_3$ MW: 252.27 Property: mp 150-7°C. Source: YANG JIAO TENG. Ref: 6.

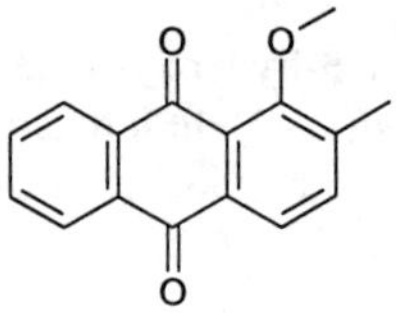

4231 6-Methoxy-2-methyl-β-carbolinium
$C_{13}H_{13}N_2O$ MW: 213.26 Source: HONG MU JI CAO. Ref: 6.

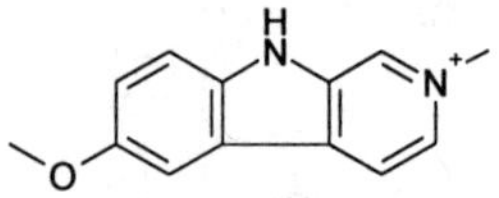

4232 5-Methoxy-methylfurfural
$C_7H_8O_3$ MW: 140.14 Property: bp 98°C/7mm. Source: TIAN MEN DONG. Ref: 6.

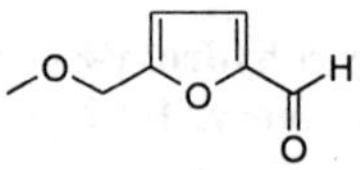

4233 3-Methoxy-7-methyljuglone
$C_{12}H_{10}O_4$ MW: 218.21 Source: SHI GEN. Ref: 6.

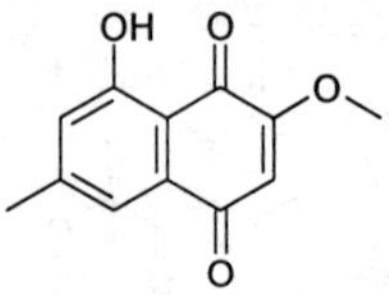

4234 5-Methoxy-N-methyltryptamine
$C_{12}H_{16}N_2O$ MW: 204.27 Property: bp 150°C/0.05 mm. Source: LU ZHU GEN, PAI QIAN CAO. Ref: 6.

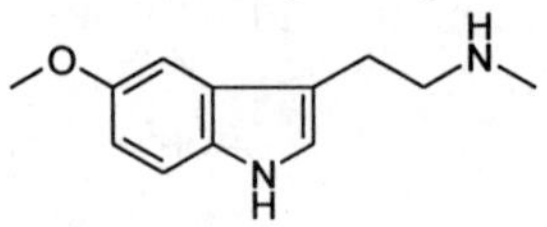

4235 11-Methoxy-nor-yangonin
$C_{15}H_{14}O_5$ MW: 274.28 Source: GUA LOU. Ref: 2.

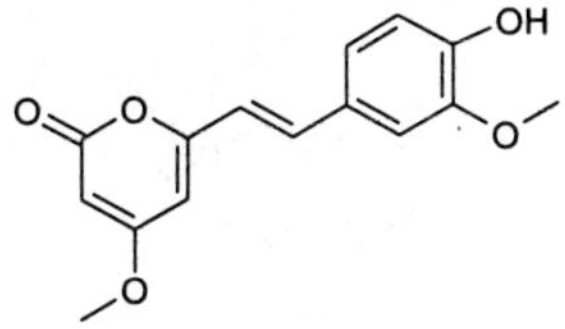

4236 2-Methoxy-obtusifolin
$C_{17}H_{14}O_5$ MW: 298.30 Source: XUAN CAO GEN. Ref: 6.

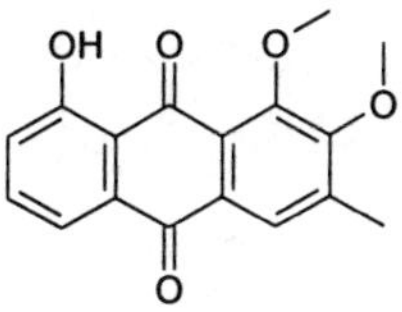

4237 o-Methoxy phenol
$C_7H_8O_2$ MW: 124.14 Source: CHAI HU. Ref: 2.

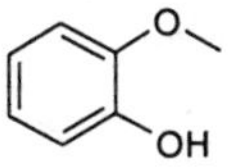

4238 5-Methoxy-3-(2-phenyl-E-E-ethenyl)-2,4-bis(4-hydroxybenzyl) phenol
$C_{29}H_{26}O_4$ MW: 438.53 Property: white acicular crystal, mp 193-6°C. Source: SHAN HU LAN. Ref: 280.

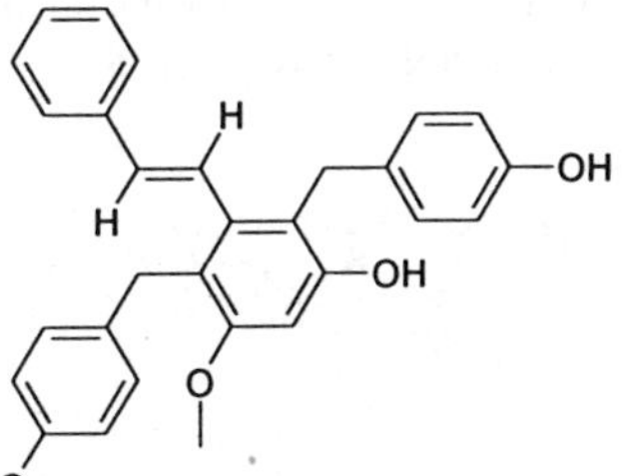

4239 2-[2-(4'-Methoxyphenyl) ethyl] chromone
$C_{18}H_{16}O_3$ MW: 280.33 Property: yellowish lamellar crystal, mp 60-1°C. Source: CHEN XIANG. Ref: 13.

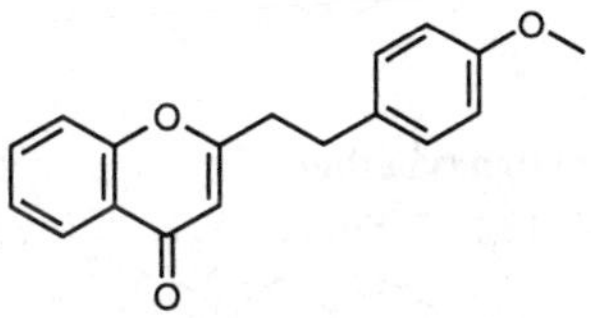

4240 6-Methoxy-2-(2-phenylethyl) chromone
$C_{18}H_{16}O_3$ MW: 280.33 Property: colorless acicular crystal, mp 68-70°C. Source: BAI MU XIANG, CHEN XIANG. Ref: 13.

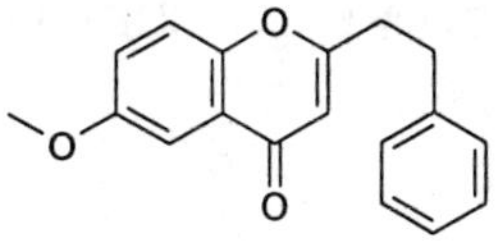

4241 2-Methoxy-4-(1-propenyl)-phenol
$C_{10}H_{12}O_2$ MW: 164.21 Source: XI YANG SHEN. Ref: 2.

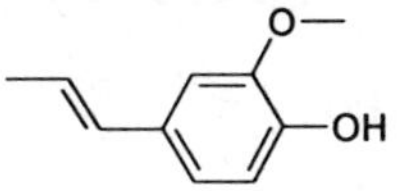

4242 4'-Methoxypuerarin
Source: GE GEN. Ref: 2.

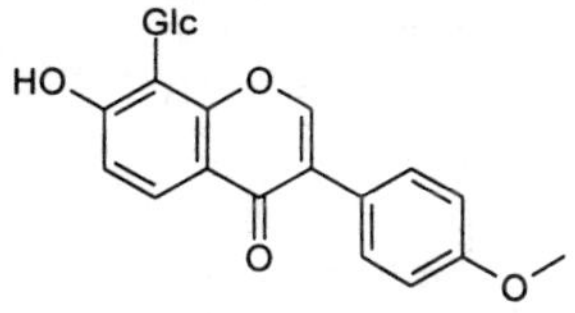

4243 3-Methoxy pyridine
C_6H_7NO MW: 109.13 Source: WEN JING. Ref: 6.

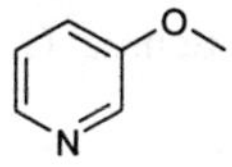

4244 4-Methoxysalicylaldehyde
$C_8H_8O_3$ MW: 152.15 Property: mp 40-2°C Source: SHENG TENG, XIANG JIA PI. Ref: 6.

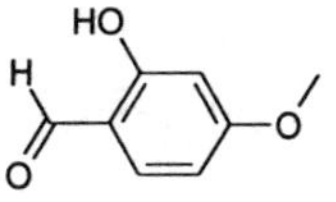

4245 16-Methoxystrychnine
$C_{22}H_{24}N_2O_3$ MW: 364.45 Property: mp 214-8°C. Source: LU SONG GUO. Ref: 6.

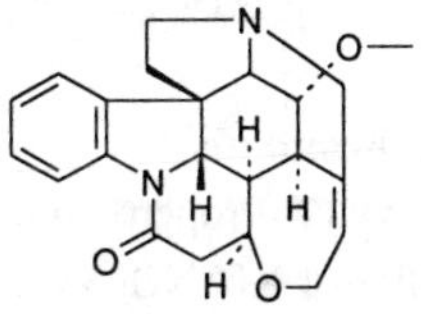

4246 p-Methoxystyrene
$C_9H_{10}O$ MW: 134.18 Property: bp 204-5°C/756 mm Source: SHAN NAI. Ref: 6.

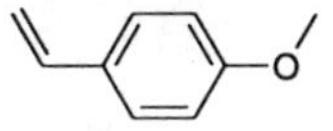

4247 Methyl acetate
$C_3H_6O_2$ MW: 74.08 Source: SHENG JIANG. Ref: 2.

4248 β-Methylaesculetin
$C_{10}H_8O_4$ MW: 192.17 Property: mp 272-4°C. Source: TIAN XUAN HUA. Ref: 6.

4249 6-Methylalizarin
$C_{15}H_{10}O_4$ MW: 254.24 Property: mp 220°C. Source: TU LIAN QIAO. Ref: 6.

4250 Methyl allyl disulfide
$C_4H_8S_2$ MW: 120.24 Source: GE CONG, JIU CAI. Ref: 6.

4251 Methyl allyl sulfide
C_4H_8S MW: 88.17 Source: DA SUAN, SHENG JIANGV. Ref: 2, 6.

4252 Methylamine
CH_5N MW: 31.06 Property: mp -92.5°C, bp -6.5°C. Source: BAI QU CAI, HAI XIA, MAI JIAO. Ref: 6.

4253 Methyl anthranilate
$C_8H_9NO_2$ MW: 151.17 Property: mp 24-5°C. Source: DAI DAI HUA, JIU LI XIANG, YOU. Ref: 6, 11.

4254 N-Methylanthranylamide
$C_8H_{10}N_2O$ MW: 150.18 Source: WU ZHU YU. Ref: 2, 347.

4255 2-Methylanthraquinone
$C_{15}H_{10}O_2$ MW: 222.25 Property: mp 177-9°C. Source: YANG JIAO TENG. Ref: 6.

4256 Methyl arteannuate
$C_{16}H_{24}O_2$ MW: 248.37 Source: QING HAO. Ref: 2.

4257 o-Methylbalfourodinium salt
$C_{17}H_{22}NO_4$ MW: 304.37 Property: mp x=ClO_4^-, 124.5°C, x=I^-, (±): 152-3°C, x= ClO_4^-, (±): 203-4°C. Source CHOU SHAN YANG. Ref: 6.

4258 Methylbenzene
C_7H_8 MW: 92.14 Source: SHAN ZHA. Ref: 2.

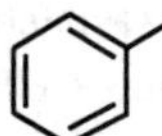

4259 Methyl benzyl ether
$C_8H_{10}O$ MW: 122.17 Source: WU WEI ZI. Ref: 2.

4260 Methylbetulinate
$C_{31}H_{50}O_3$ MW: 470.74 Property: mp 223-4°C.
Source: QIAO MU ZI ZHU, QIU FENG MU. Ref: 6.

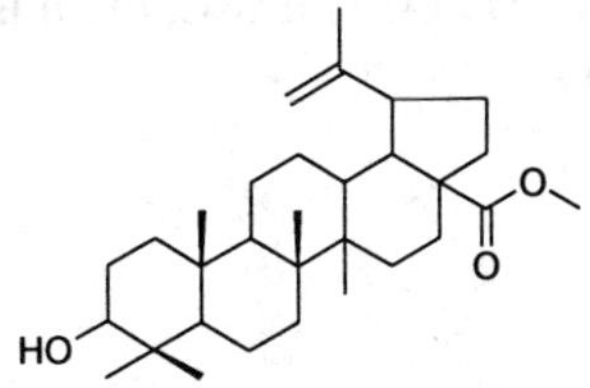

4261 Methyl brevifolin carboxylate
$C_{14}H_{10}O_8$ MW: 306.23 Property: light yellow acicular crystal, mp 200°C. Source:YE XIA ZHU. Ref: 283, 607.

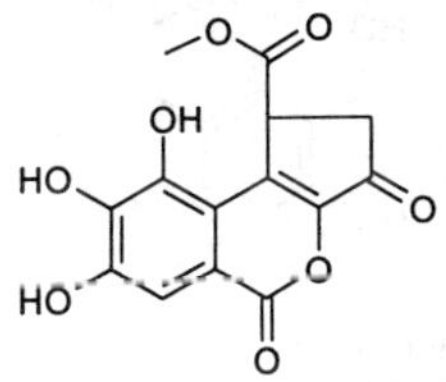

4262 2-Methyl-3-buten-2-ol
$C_5H_{10}O$ MW: 86.13 Source: FANG FENG. Ref: 2.

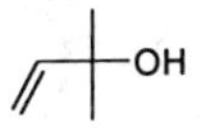

4263 N-3-methyl-2-butenyl urea
$C_6H_{12}N_2O$ MW: 128.18 Property: colorless acicular crystal, mp 104-5°C. Source: XUN DAO NIU. Ref: 324.

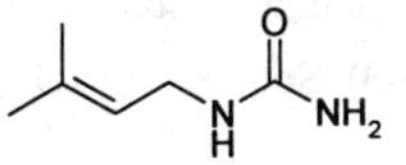

4264 4-(3'-Methyl-but-2'-one)oxy,N-benzoyl phenethyl amine
$C_{20}H_{23}NO_2$ MW: 309.41 Property: yellow acicular crystal, mp 103.5-4.5°C. Source: DONG FENG JU. Ref: 67.

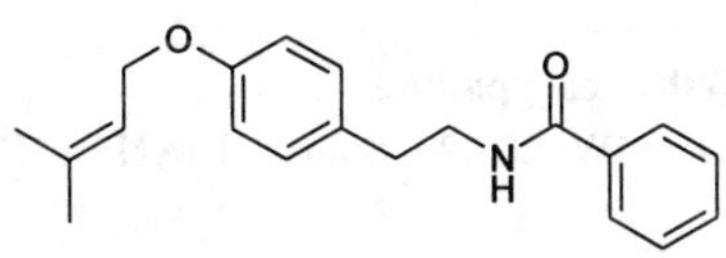

4265 2-Methyl butyric acid
$C_5H_{10}O_2$ MW: 102.13 Property: bp 177°C. Source: XING ZI. Ref: 6.

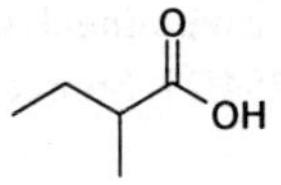

4266 α-Methyl-n-butyrylshikonin
$C_{20}H_{22}O_6$ MW: 358.39 Source: ZI CAO. Ref: 2.

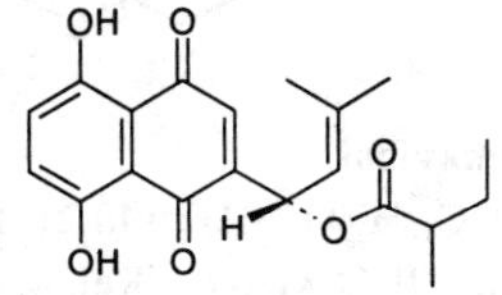

4267 3-Methyl-canthin-2,6-dione
$C_{15}H_{10}N_2O_2$ MW: 250.26 Source: KU SHU PI. Ref: 12.

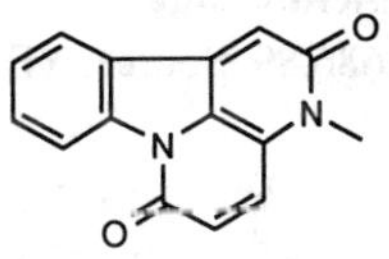

4268 4'-Methylcapillarisin
$C_{17}H_{14}O_7$ MW: 330.30 Source: YIN CHEN HAO. Ref: 2.

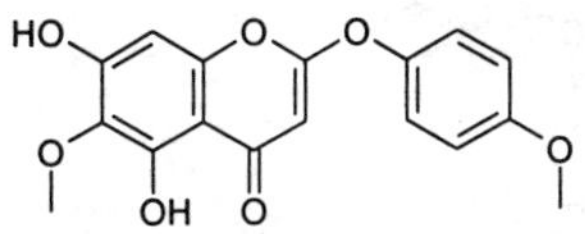

4269 7-Methylcapillarisin
$C_{17}H_{14}O_7$ MW: 330.30 Source: YIN CHEN HAO. Ref: 2.

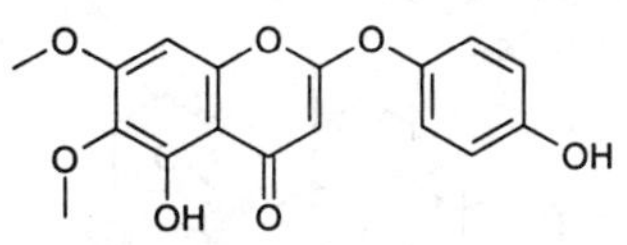

4270 8-Methyl capric acid
$C_{11}H_{22}O_2$ MW: 186.30 Source: XI YANG SHEN. Ref: 2.

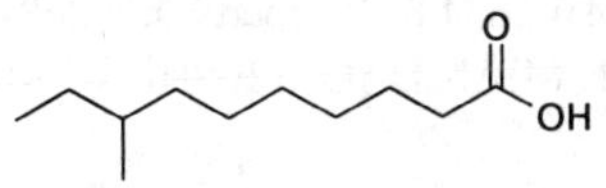

4271 Methyl caprylate
$C_9H_{18}O_2$ MW: 158.24 Source: DANG SHEN. Ref: 2.

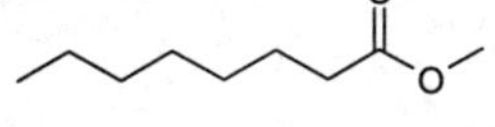

4272 Methyl-3-(β-carboline-1-yl) propionate
$C_{15}H_{14}N_2O_2$ MW: 254.29 Source: KU SHU PI. Ref: 12.

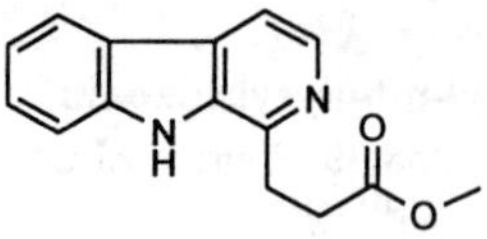

4273 Methylchavicol
CAS: 140-67-0 $C_{10}H_{12}O$ MW: 148.21 Property: bp 215-6°C. Source: HUO XIANG. Ref: 4.

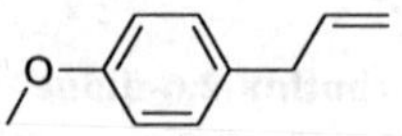

4274 Methylcimicifugoside
$C_{39}H_{58}O_{10}$ MW: 686.89 Source: YE SHENG MA. Ref: 6.

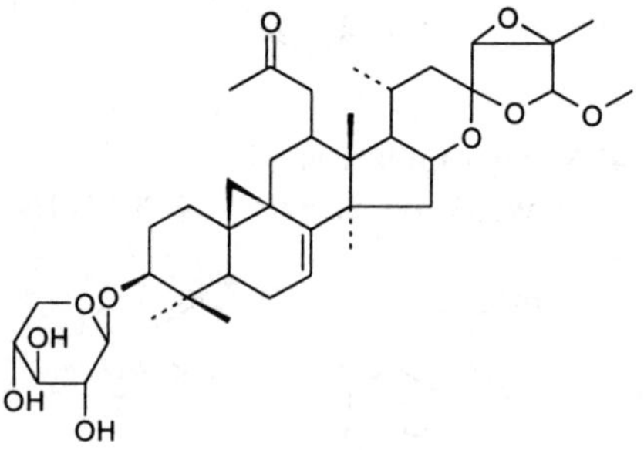

4275 15-O-Methylcimigenol
$C_{31}H_{50}O_5$ MW: 502.74 Property: mp 199.5-200.5°C. Source: SAN MIAN DAO. Ref: 6.

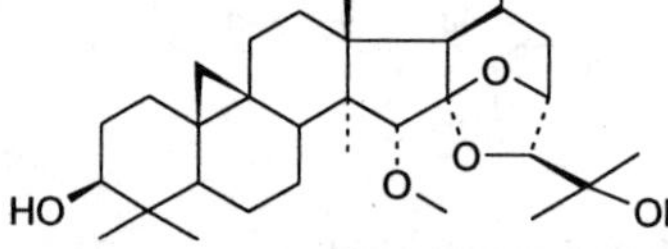

4276 25-O-Methylcimigenoside
$C_{36}H_{58}O_9$ MW: 634.89 Property: mp 268-70°C. Source: SAN MIAN DAO, YE SHENG MA. Ref: 6.

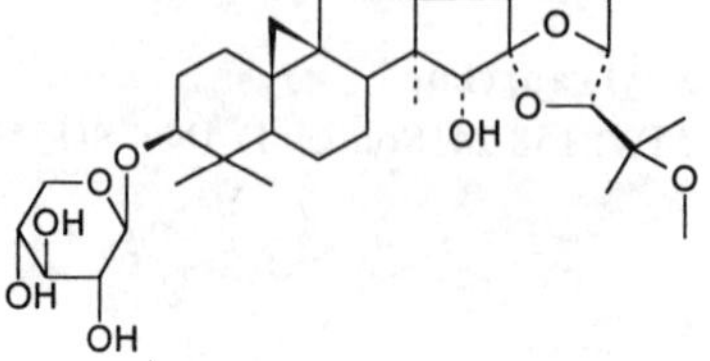

4277 Methylcinnamate
$C_{10}H_{10}O_2$ MW: 162.19 Property: mp 36.5°C, bp 261°C/750 mm. Source: DA LIANG JIANG, DA CAO KOU, GAO LIANG JIANG, LUOLE, SONG XUN. Ref: 6.

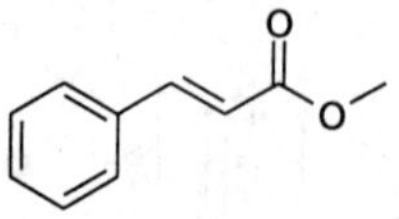

4278 D-N-Methyl coclaurine
$C_{18}H_{21}NO$ MW: 299.37 Property: mp 94.5-5°C. Source: HE YE, HENG ZHOU WU YAO. Ref: 6.

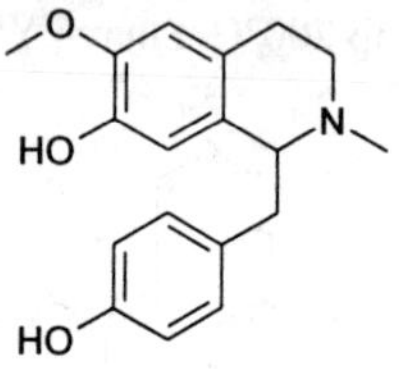

4279 6-Methylcodeine
$C_{19}H_{23}NO_3$ MW: 313.40 Source: YA PIAN. Ref: 6.

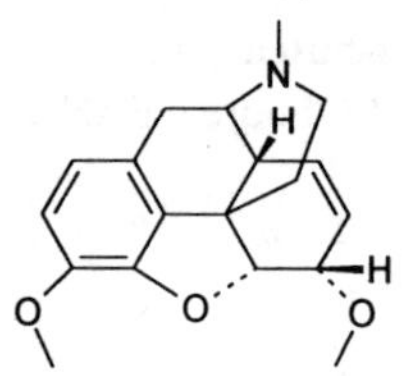

4280 Methylconiferin
3'-O-Methylconiferin. $C_{17}H_{24}O_8$ MW: 356.38 Property: white acicular crystal, mp 167-9°C, $[\alpha]_D^{21}$ -69.5° (c=0.1, H2O). Source: TONG QIAO SHE GU. Ref: 490.

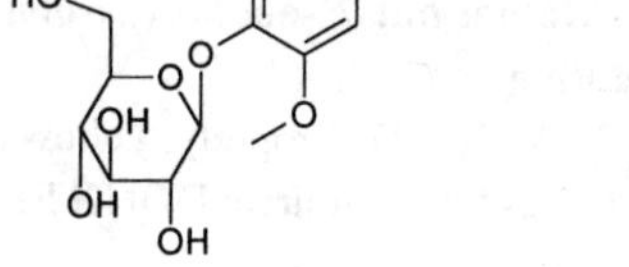

4281 Methyl-corypalline
$C_{12}H_{17}NO_2$ MW: 207.27 Source: LIAN ZI XIN. Ref: 6.

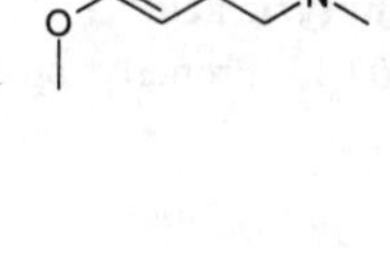

4282 5-Methylcoumarin-4-cellobioside

$C_{22}H_{28}O_{13}$ MW: 500.46 Property: acicular crystal, mp 217-9°C, $[\alpha]_D^{21}$ -94° (c=0.515, methanol). Source: DA DING CAO. Ref: 77.

4283 5-Methylcoumarin-4-gentiobioside

$C_{22}H_{28}O_{13}$ MW: 500.46 Property: acicular crystal, mp 155-7°C, $[\alpha]_D^{21}$ -80° (c=0.902, methanol). Source: DA DING CAO. Ref: 77.

4284 12-O-Methylcoumestrol

$C_{16}H_{10}O_5$ MW: 282.2 Source: HUI HUI DOU. Ref: 6.

4285 (+)-4''-O-Methylcurine

$C_{37}H_{40}N_2O_6$ MW: Property: mp 164°C. Source: XI SHENG TENG. Ref: 6.

4286 24-Methylcycloartanol ferulate

$C_{41}H_{62}O_4$ MW: 618.95 Source: MI PI KANG. Ref: 6.

4287 Methyl cyclodecane

C_9H_{18} MW: 126.24 Source: BAI ZHI. Ref: 2.

4288 Methylcyclohexane

C_7H_{14} MW: 98.19 Source: SHAN ZHA. Ref: 2.

4289 3-Methylcyclohexanone

$C_7H_{12}O$ MW: 112.17 Source: JIN JIE. Ref: 2.

4290 4-Methyl cyclohexanone

$C_7H_{12}O$ MW: 112.17 Source: DU HUO. Ref: 2.

4291 3-Methyl-1,2-cyclopentanediol

$C_6H_{12}O_2$ MW: 116.16 Source: SHAN ZHA. Ref: 2.

4292 2-Methyl cyclopentanone

$C_6H_{10}O$ MW: 98.15 Source: CHAI HU. Ref: 2.

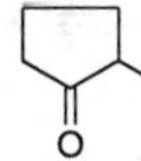

4293 3-Methylcyclotridecan-1-one

$C_{14}H_{26}O$ MW: 210.36 Source: SHE XIANG. Ref: 2.

4294 S-Methyl-L-cysteine sulfoxide
$C_4H_9NO_3S$ MW: 151.19 Property: mp (+): 164°C (dec). Source: DA SUAN. Ref: 6.

4295 N-Methylcytisine
$C_{12}H_{16}N_2O$ MW: 204.27 Property: mp (-):137°C. Source: KU SHEN. Ref: 2.

4296 o-Methyldalbergin
$C_{17}H_{14}O_4$ MW: 282.30 Property: mp 145-6°C. Source: JIANG ZHEN XIANG. Ref: 6.

4297 Methyldeacetylasperulosidate
$C_{17}H_{24}O_{11}$ MW: 402.40 Source: SHUI ZHI. Ref: 6.

4298 Methyl 2-decen-4,6,8-triynate
$C_{11}H_8O_2$ MW: 172.19 Property: mp cis-, 114-5°C. Source: AI YE. Ref: 6.

4299 Methyl-trans-2-decene-4,6,8-triynoate
$C_{11}H_8O_2$ MW: 172.19 Property: mp 105°C. Source: BI MA GEN. Ref: 6.

4300 Methyl dehydro-15-hydroxy-abietan-18-oate
$C_{21}H_{30}O_3$ MW: 330.47 Source: HAI SONG ZI. Ref: 6.

4301 N-Methyldendrobium
$C_{17}H_{28}NO_2$ MW: 278.42 Source: SHI SUAN. Ref: 6.

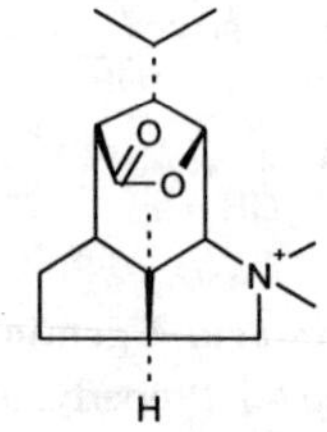

4302 N-Methyl-14-O-desmethyl-epiporphyroxine
$C_{20}H_{21}NO_6$ MW: 371.39 Source: YA PIAN. Ref: 6.

4303 Methyl β,γ-dihydroxy-α-methylene butylate
$C_7H_{12}O_3$ MW: 144.17 Source: XIAO YE HUA. Ref: 6.

4304 6-Methyl-2,5-dihydroxymethyl-γ-pyranone (III)
$C_8H_{10}O_4$ MW: 170.17 Property: colorless columnar crystal, mp 122-3°C. Source: HOU GU JUN. Ref: 161.

4305 2-Methyl-4-(1,1-dimethylethyl) phenol
$C_{11}H_{16}O$ MW: 164.25 Source: DU HUO. Ref: 2.

4306 2-Methyl-5-(1,5-dimethyl-4-hexenyl)-1,3-cyclo-hexadiene
$C_{15}H_{24}$ MW: 204.36 Source: DU HUO. Ref: 2.

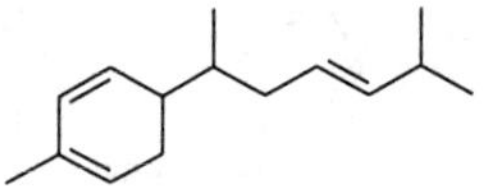

4307 Methyl disulfide
$C_2H_6S_2$ MW: 94.20 Property: bp 116-8°C. Source: YANG CONG. Ref: 6.

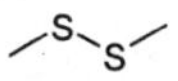

4308 4-Methyl-1,2-dithio-3-cyclopentene
$C_4H_6S_2$ MW: 118.22 Source: DA SUAN. Ref: 2.

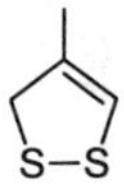

4309 5-Methyl-1,2-dithio-3-cyclopentene
$C_4H_6S_2$ MW: 118.22 Source: DA SUAN. Ref: 2.

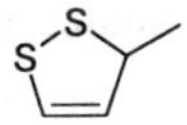

4310 2-Methyl-dodecane-5-one
$C_{13}H_{26}O$ MW: 198.35 Source: DANG GUI. Ref: 2.

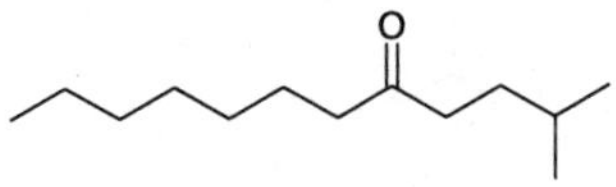

4311 O-Methyl domesticine
$C_{20}H_{21}NO_4$ MW: 339.39 Property: mp (+): 138-9°C. Source: NAN TIAN ZHU ZI, NAN TIAN ZHU GEN, NAN TIAN ZHU GENG. Ref: 6.

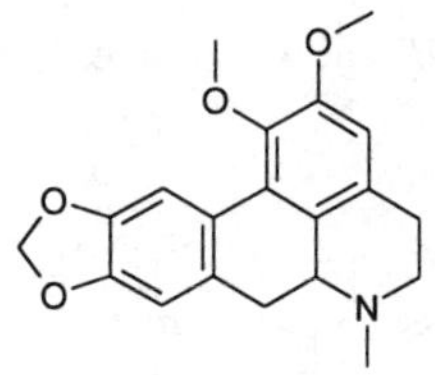

4312 4,4'-Methylene bis[2,3,5,6-tetramethyl phenol]
$C_{22}H_{30}O_2$ MW: 326.48 Source: DU HUO. Ref: 2.

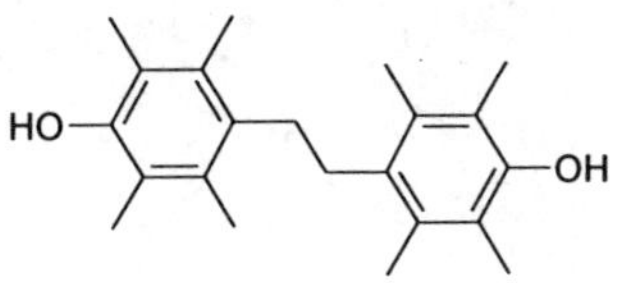

4313 24-Methylene cholesterol
$C_{28}H_{46}O$ MW: 398.68 Property: mp 142°C. Source: LUO HUA SHENG, ZHI XIE MU PI. Ref: 6.

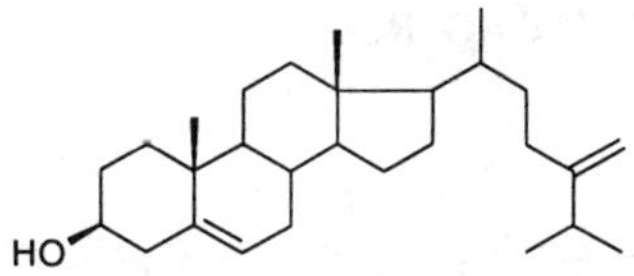

4314 24-Methylene cycloartan-3β,21-diol
$C_{31}H_{52}O_2$ MW: 456.76 Property: mp 105-8°C. Source: DUO SUI SHI KE YE. Ref: 6.

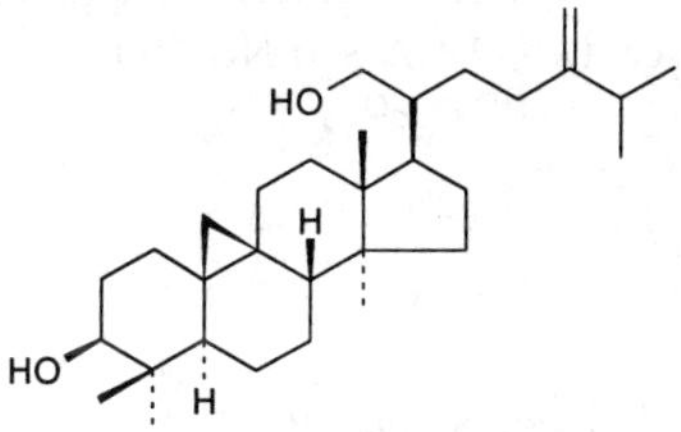

4315 24-Methylene cycloartanol
$C_{31}H_{52}O$ MW: 440.76 Property: mp 122-2.5°C. Source: JI CHANG LANG DU, SHI CHUN, XI YE DA JI. Ref: 6.

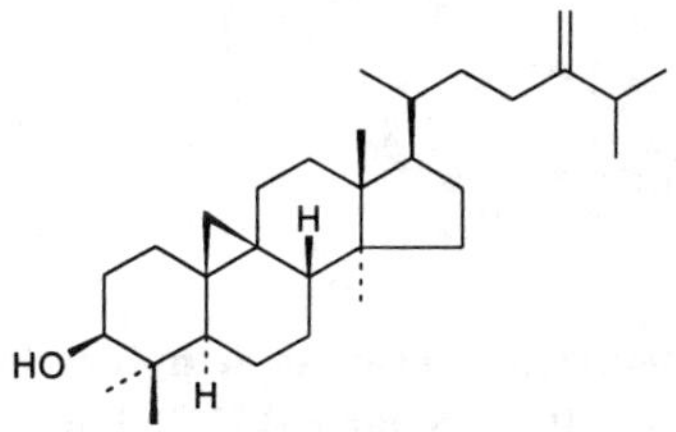

4316 24-Methylene cycloartanol ferulate
$C_{41}H_{60}O_4$ MW: 616.93 Property: mp 162-4°C/193-4°C. Source: MI PI KANG. Ref: 6.

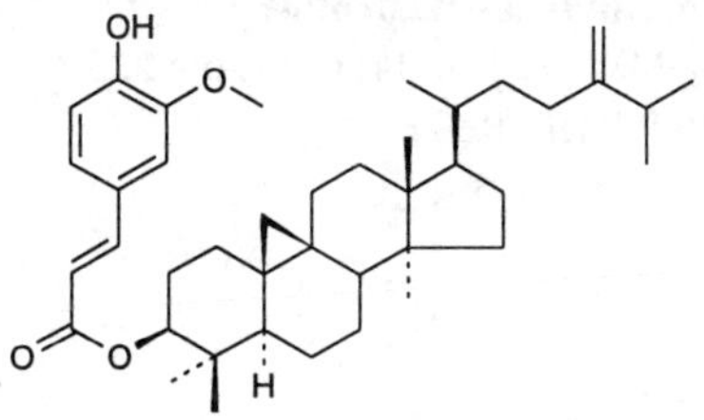

4317 α-(Methylenecyclopropyl) glycine
$C_6H_9NO_2$ MW: 127.14 Property: 202°C(dec). Source: LI ZHI HE. Ref: 6.

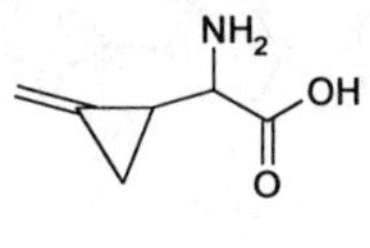

4318 2-[4(3,4-Methylenedioxyphenyl) butyl]-4-quinolone
$C_{20}H_{19}NO_3$ MW: 321.38 Property: mp 224°C. Source: CHOU CAO. Ref: 6.

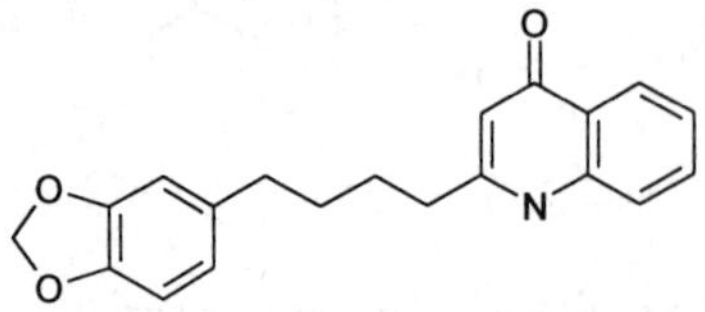

4319 γ-Methylene glutamic acid
$C_6H_9NO_4$ MW: 159.14 Property: mp (DL): 203-10°C (dec). Source: LUO HUA SHENG. Ref: 6.

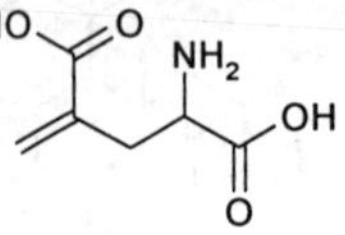

4320 24-Methylenelophenol
$C_{29}H_{48}O$ MW: 412.71 Property: mp 172-3°C. Source: GAN ZHE. Ref: 6.

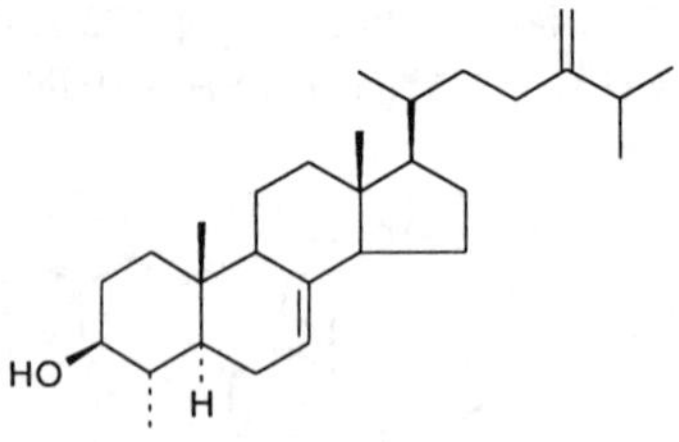

4321 3-Methylene-6-(1-methylethyl) cyclohexene
$C_{10}H_{16}$ MW: 136.24 Source: BAI ZHI. Ref: 2.

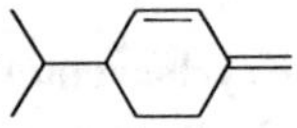

4322 4-Methylene-DL-proline
$C_6H_9NO_2$ MW: 127.14 Property: mp 225°C (dec). Source: PI PA HE. Ref: 6.

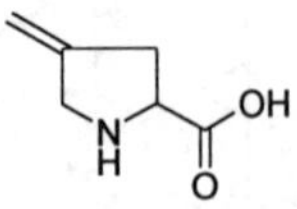

4323 Methylene tanshinquinone
$C_{18}H_{14}O_3$ MW: 278.31 Source: BAI ZHI. Ref: 2.

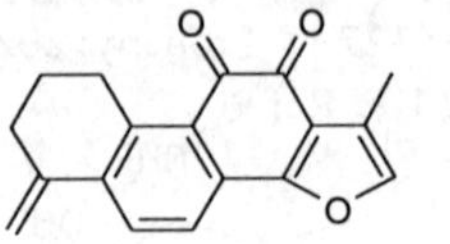

4324 l-N-Methylephedrine
$C_{11}H_{17}NO$ MW: 179.26 Property: mp (-): 87-8°C. Source: MA HUANG. Ref: 2.

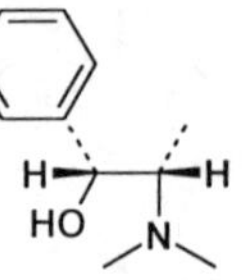

4325 14α-Methyl-5α-ergosta-9(11),24(28)-dien-3β-ol
$C_{29}H_{48}O$ MW: 412.71 Source: QI YE DAN. Ref: 2.

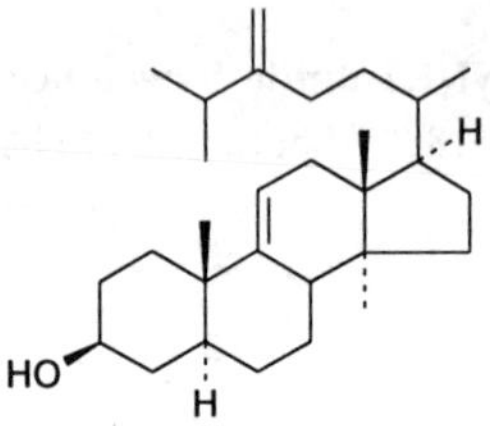

4326 14α-Methyl-5α-ergosta-9(11)-en-3β-ol
$C_{29}H_{50}O$ MW: 414.72 Source: QI YE DAN. Ref: 2.

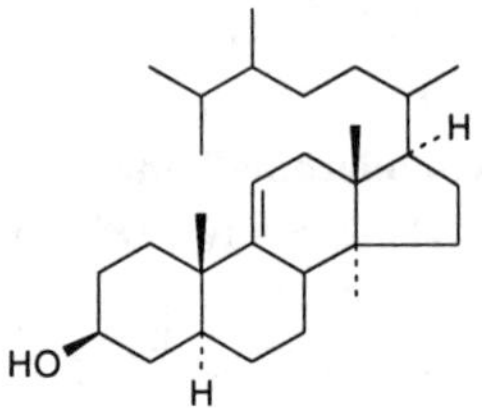

4327 Methyl ester dehydrochebulic acid
Source:YE XIA ZHU. Ref: 607.

4328 Methyl ester of N,N-dimethyl-tryptophan methocation
$C_{15}H_{21}N_2O_2$ MW: 261.35 Source: XIANG SI ZI. Ref: 6.

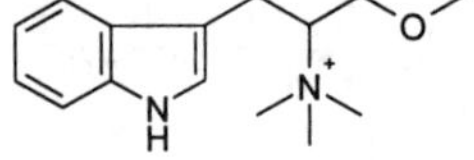

4329 3-Methyl-3-ethylhexane
C_9H_{20} MW: 128.26 Source: ROU CONG RONG. Ref: 2.

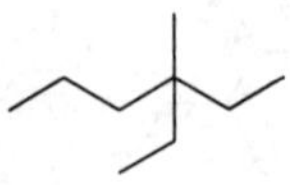

4330 Methyl eugenol
Eugenol methyl ether. CAS: 93-15-2 $C_{11}H_{14}O_2$ MW: 178.23 Property: bp 248-9°C. Source: LUO LE, JU JIANG YE, SHAN ZHU YU, SHENG JIANG, XI XIN, YIN CHEN HAO. Ref: 2, 4.

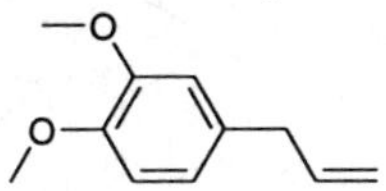

4331 (+)-2-N-Methylfangchinoline
$C_{38}H_{44}N_2O_6$ MW: 624.78 Source: FANG JI. Ref: 2.

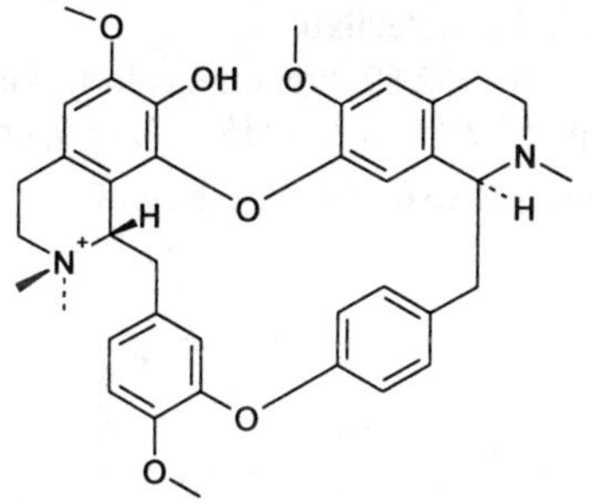

4332 α-Methylfurfural
$C_6H_6O_2$ MW: 110.11 Property: bp 187°C. Source: SHUI SONG. Ref: 6.

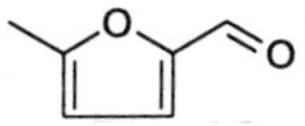

4333 Methyl D-galactoside
$C_7H_{14}O_6$ MW: 194.19 Property: mp α: 125.5°C, β: 178-80°C. Source: LU JIAO CAI. Ref: 6.

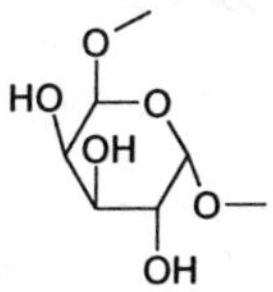

4334 Methyl gallate
Gallicin. CAS: 99-24-1 $C_8H_8O_5$ MW: 184.15 Property: mp 197-8°C. Source: LUAN HUA, YAN FU YE, ZI WEI HUA. Ref: 4, 6.

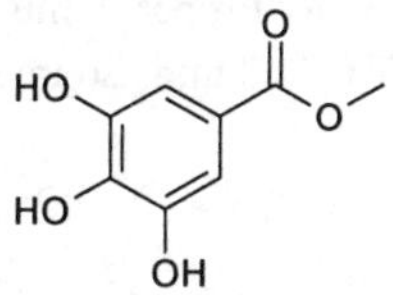

4335 6-Methylgingediacetate
$C_{22}H_{34}O_6$ MW: 394.51 Source: SHENG JIANG. Ref: 2.

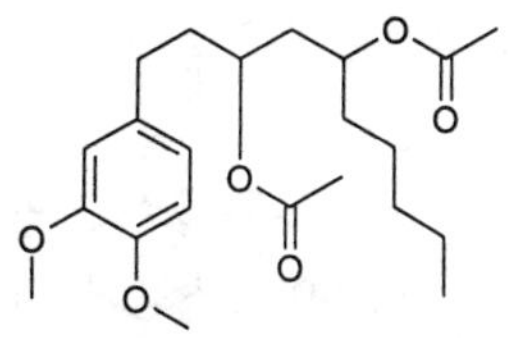

4336 6-Methylgingediol
$C_{18}H_{30}O_4$ MW: 310.44 Source: SHENG JIANG. Ref: 2.

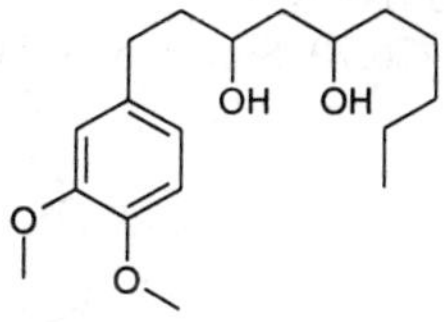

4337 4'-O-Methylglabridin
$C_{21}H_{22}O_4$ MW: 338.41 Source: GAN CAO. Ref: 2.

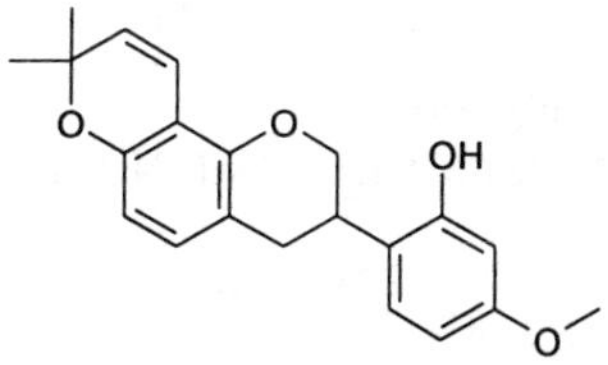

4338 β-Methyl-D-glucoside
$C_7H_{14}O_6$ MW: 194.19 Source: MU XU. Ref: 6.

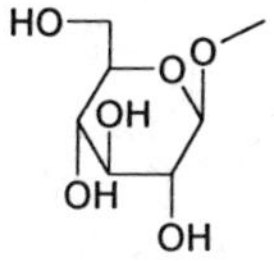

4339 Methyl glutarate
$C_6H_{10}O_4$ MW: 146.14 Source: MU ZEI. Ref: 2.

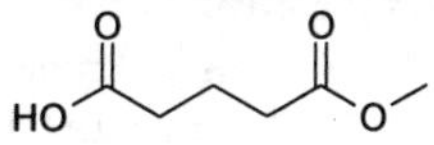

4340 Methylglutathione (S)
$C_{11}H_{19}N_3O_6S$ MW: 321.35 Source: NIU FEI. Ref: 6.

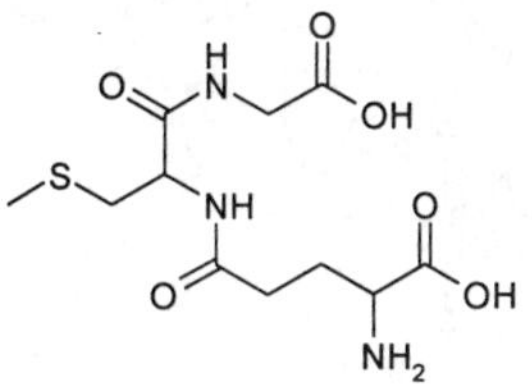

4341 5-O-Methyl glycyrol
$C_{22}H_{20}O_6$ MW: 380.40 Property: mp 259-60°C. Source: GAN CAO. Ref: 6.

4342 Methylglycyrrhetate
$C_{30}H_{46}O_4$ MW: 470.70 Source: GAN CAO. Ref: 2.

4343 Methylglyoxal
$C_3H_4O_2$ MW: 72.06 Source: SHENG JIANG. Ref: 2.

4344 Methyl guaia-1(10),11-dien-15-carboxylate
$C_{16}H_{24}O_2$ MW: 248.37 Source: CHEN XIANG. Ref: 13.

4345 Methyl gymnaconitine
$C_{35}H_{49}NO_8$ MW: 611.78 Property: amorphous powder, $[\alpha]_D^{20.5}$ +33.2°. Source: LU RUI WU TOU. Ref: 52.

4346 Methyl helicterate
$C_{40}H_{56}O_6$ MW: 632.89 Property: colorless lamellar crystal, mp 196-7°C, $[\alpha]_D^{20}$ -12.3° (c=8.0, chloroform). Source: SHAN ZHI MA. Ref: 40.

4347 Methyl helicterilate
$C_{40}H_{56}O_6$ MW: 632.89 Property: colorless acicular crystal, mp 152-3°C, $[\alpha]_D^{20}$ +118.8° (c=5.9, chloroform). Source: SHAN ZHI MA. Ref: 40.

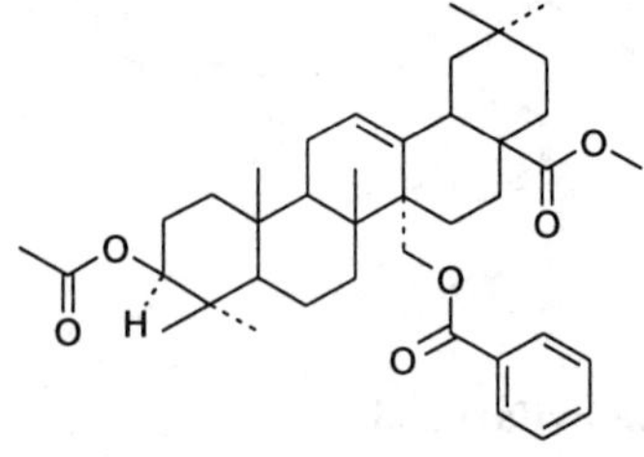

4348 2-Methylheptane
C_8H_{18} MW: 114.23 Source: SHAN ZHA. Ref: 2.

4349 Methylheptenone
$C_8H_{14}O$ MW: 126.20 Source: GAN JIANG. Ref: 2.

4350 Methylheptyl-ketone
$C_9H_{18}O$ MW: 142.24 Source: YIN CHEN HAO. Ref: 2.

4351 Methyl hexadecanate
$C_{17}H_{34}O_2$ MW: 270.46 Property: mp 30.5°C (29.5°C), bp 415-8°C/747 mm. Source: QING FENG TENG. Ref: 6.

4352 14-Methyl hexadecanoic acid
$C_{17}H_{34}O_2$ MW: 270.46 Source: QIANG HUO. Ref: 2.

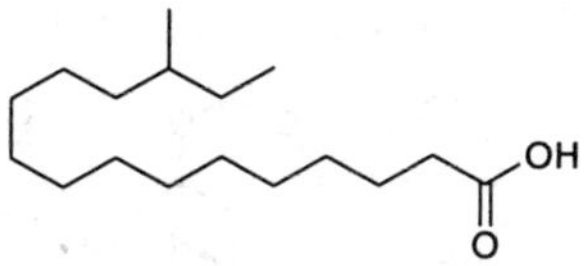

4353 3-Methylhexane
C_7H_{16} MW: 100.21 Source: SHAN ZHA. Ref: 2.

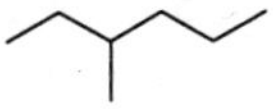

4354 3-Methylhistidin(e)
$C_8H_{12}N_2O_2$ MW: 168.20 Property: mp (L-): 248-50°C (dec). Source: JI ROU, WU LI. Ref: 6.

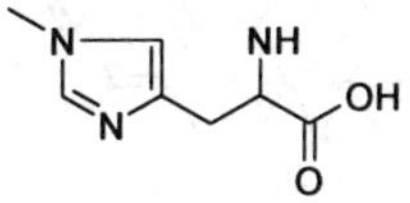

4355 6'-O-Methylhonokiol
$C_{19}H_{20}O_2$ MW: 280.37 Source: HOU PO. Ref: 2.

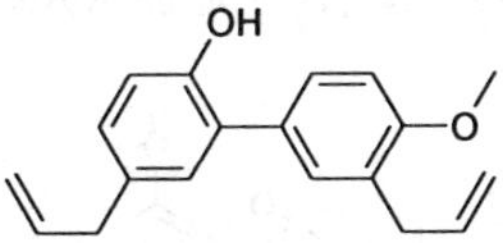

4356 Methyl-24-hydroxy-11-deoxoglycyrrhetate
$C_{31}H_{52}O_4$ MW: 488.76 Property: mp 263-4°C. Source: GAN CAO. Ref: 6.

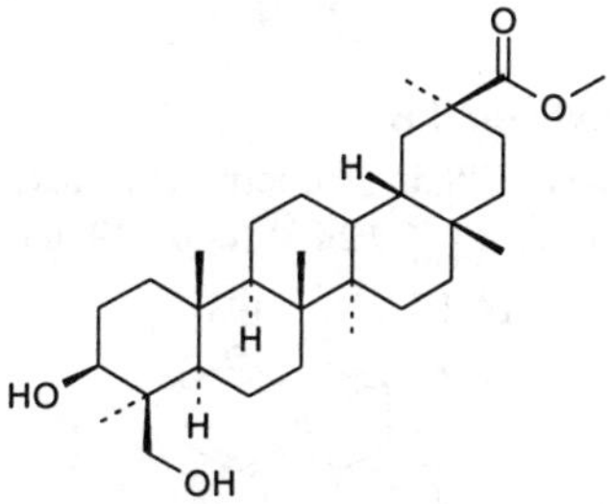

4358 Methyl 18 α-hydroxyglycyrrhetate
$C_{31}H_{48}O_5$ MW: 500.73 Property: white acicular crystal (95% ethanol), 302-3°C, 284-90°C. Source: GAN CAO, WU LA ER GAN CAO. Ref: 6, 82.

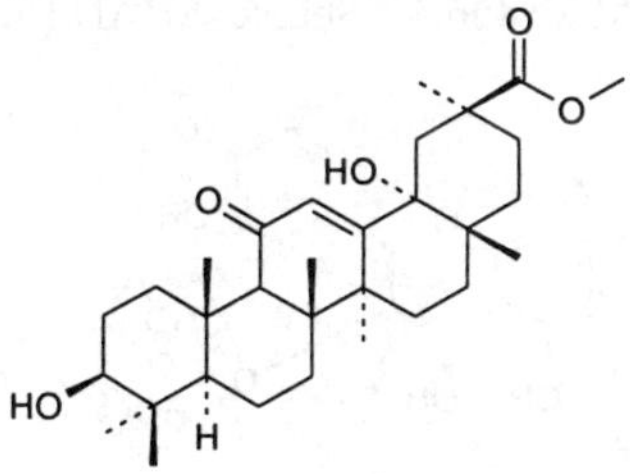

4359 Methyl-24-hydroxyglycyrrhetate
$C_{31}H_{48}O_5$ MW: 500.73 Property: mp 247-8°C. Source: GAN CAO. Ref: 6.

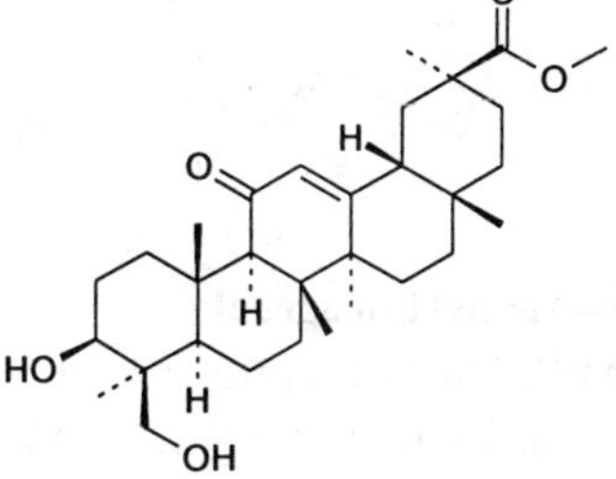

4360 Methyl(24Z)-27-hydroxy-3-oxo-7,24-titucalla-dienoate
$C_{31}H_{48}O_4$ MW: 484.73 Source: KU SHU PI. Ref: 12.

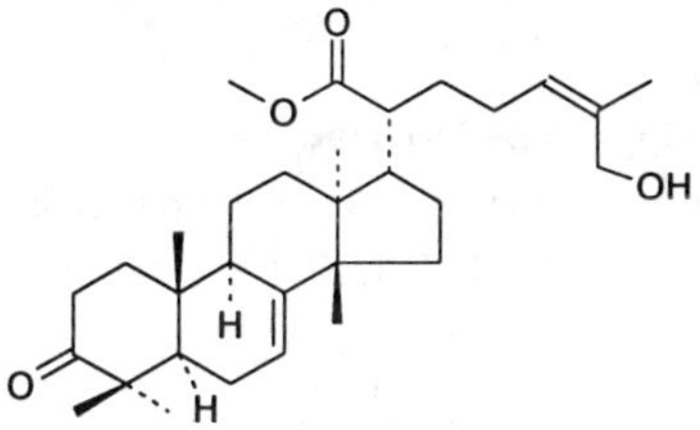

4361 Methyl 9-hydroxyselina-4,11-dien-14-oate
$C_{15}H_{24}O$ MW: 240.36 Source: CHEN XIANG. Ref: 13.

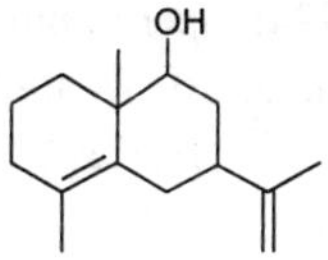

4362 6-Methyl indole
C_9H_9N MW: 131.18 Source: ROU CONG RONG. Ref: 2.

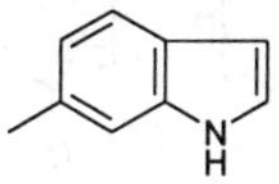

4363 1-Methyl-4-isoallyl-cyclohexane
$C_{10}H_{18}$ MW: 138.25 Source: SAN QI. Ref: 2.

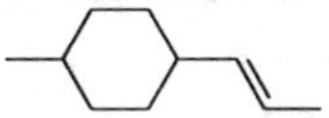

4364 Methyl isobutyl ketone
$C_6H_{12}O$ MW: 100.16 Source: SHENG JIANG. Ref: 2.

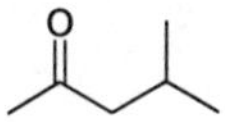

4365 cis-Methyl isoeugenol
$C_{11}H_{14}O_2$ MW: 178.23 Property: bp 138-40°C/12 mm. Source: BAI CHANG. Ref: 6.

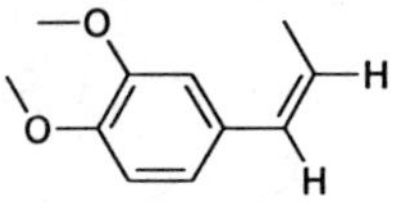

4366 trans-Methyl isoeugenol
$C_{11}H_{14}O_2$ MW: 178.23 Property: mp 16-7°C, bp 143-4°C/11 mm. Source: BAI CHANG, YE XIANG MAO. Ref: 6.

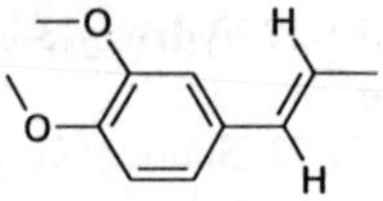

4367 Methyl isopelletierine
$C_9H_{17}NO$ MW: 155.24 Property: bp (±): 96-8°C/13 mm. Source: SHI ZHI JIA, SHI LIU GEN. Ref: 6.

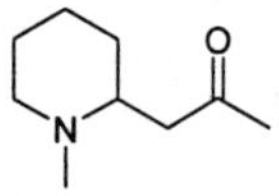

4368 Methyl isothiocyanate
C_2H_3NS MW: 73.12 Property: mp 35.93°C, bp 119°C/758 mm. Source: JIE ZI. Ref: 6.

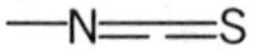

4369 7-Methyl juglone
$C_{11}H_8O_3$ MW: 188.18 Source: JUN QIAN ZI. Ref: 6.

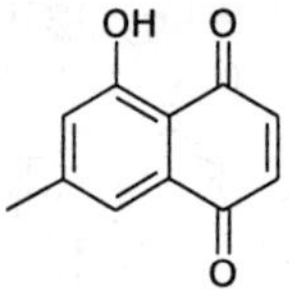

4370 5-Methyl kaempferol
$C_{16}H_{12}O_6$ MW: 300.27 Source: YING SHAN HONG. Ref: 6.

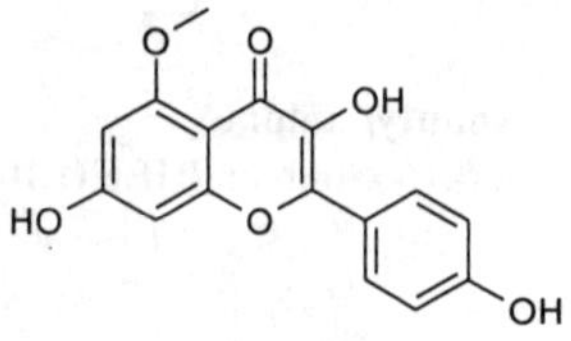

4371 Methyl lagerine
$C_{26}H_{31}NO_5$ MW: 437.54 Source: ZI WEI HUA. Ref: 6.

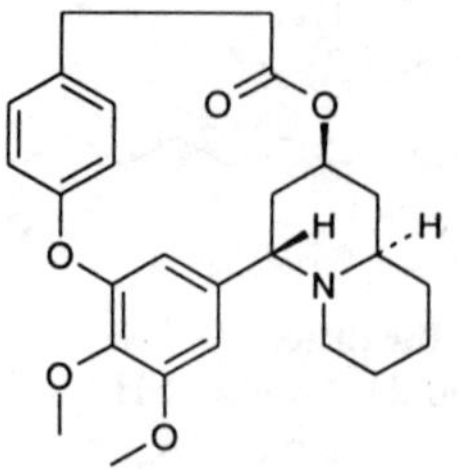

4372 Methyl lambertianate
$C_{21}H_{30}O_3$ MW: 330.47 Source: HAI SONG ZI. Ref: 6.

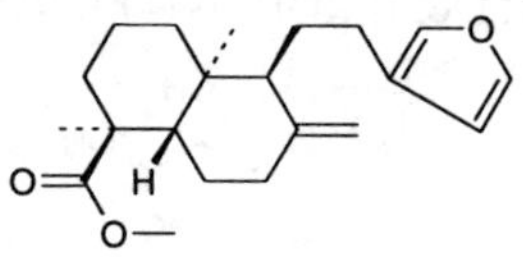

4373 (+)-N-Methyl laurotetanine
$C_{20}H_{23}NO_4$ MW: 341.41 Source: YAN HU SUO. Ref: 2.

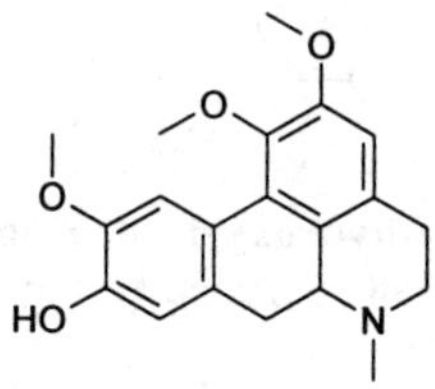

4374 Methyl leptol B
$C_{16}H_{22}O_4$ MW: 278.35 Property: colorless columnar crystal (acetone), $[\alpha]_D^{18}$ +24.3° (c=0.339, CH_3COCH_3). Source: SAN CHA KU. Ref: 393.

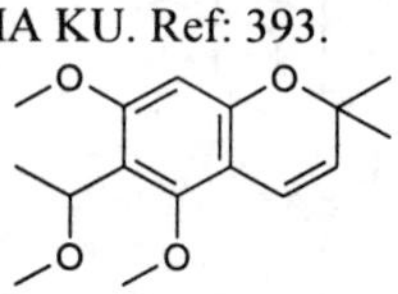

4375 4'-O-Methyl leucopelargonidin-3-monogluco furanoside
$C_{22}H_{26}O_{11}$ MW: 466.45 Source: SHAN FAN YE. Ref: 6.

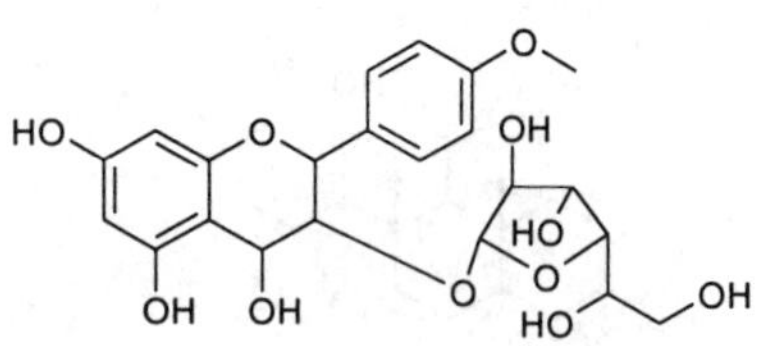

4376 7-O-Methyl leucopelargonidin-3-mono-gluco furanoside
$C_{22}H_{26}O_{11}$ MW: 466.45 Source: SHAN FAN YE Ref: 6.

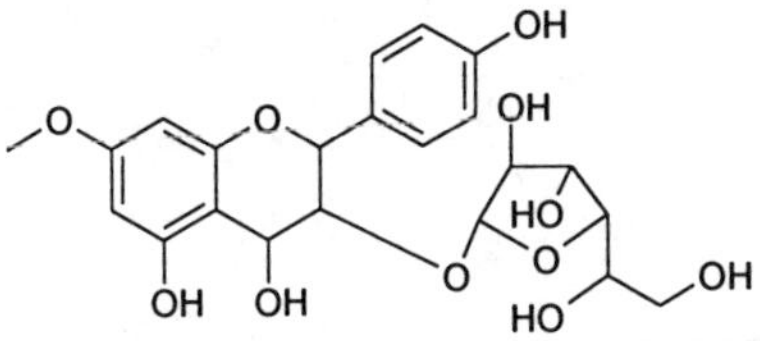

4377 Methyl leugenol
$C_{11}H_{14}O_2$ MW: 178.23 Source: XI XIN. Ref: 2.

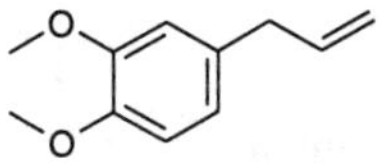

4378 5-O-Methyl licoricidin
$C_{27}H_{34}O_5$ MW: 438.57 Source: GAN CAO. Ref: 2.

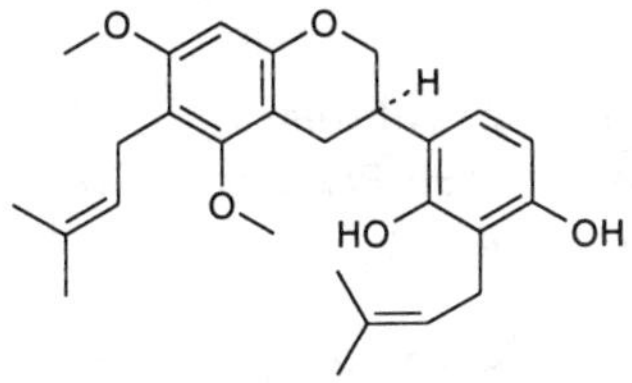

4379 Methyl linoleate
$C_{19}H_{34}O_2$ MW: 294.48 Source: CHUAN XIONG. Ref: 2.

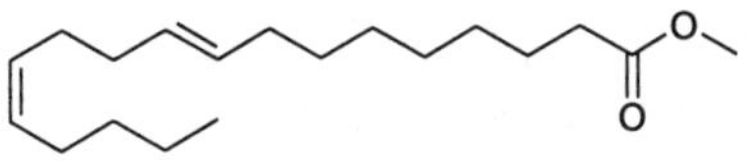

4380 Methyllinolenate
$C_{19}H_{32}O_2$ MW: 292.47 Property: bp 177-80°C/3.5 mm. Source: KUN BU. Ref: 6.

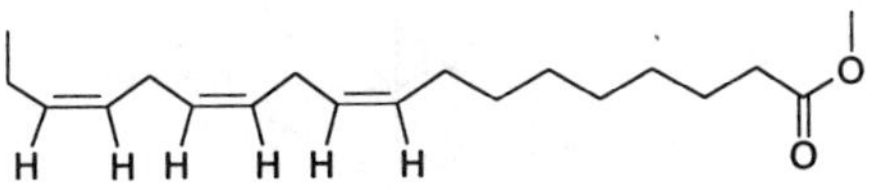

4381 Methyllycaconitine
$C_{37}H_{50}N_2O_{10}$ MW: 682.82 Property: mp 128°C. Source: CUI QUE HUA. Ref: 6.

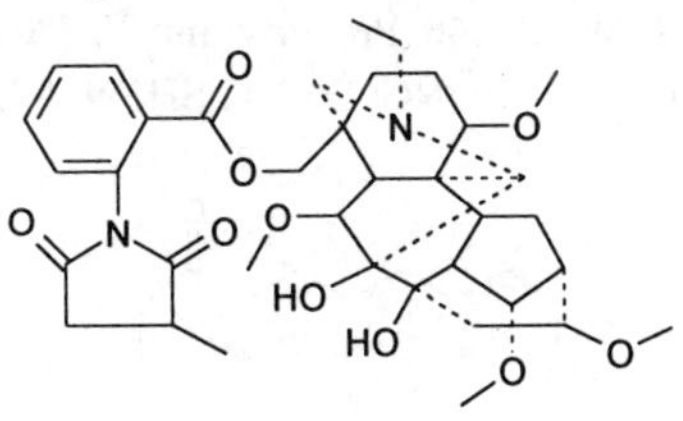

4382 14-Methylmangiferolic aldehyde
$C_{30}H_{48}O_2$ MW: 440.72 Property: mp 66-70°C. Source: MANG GUO SHU PI. Ref: 6.

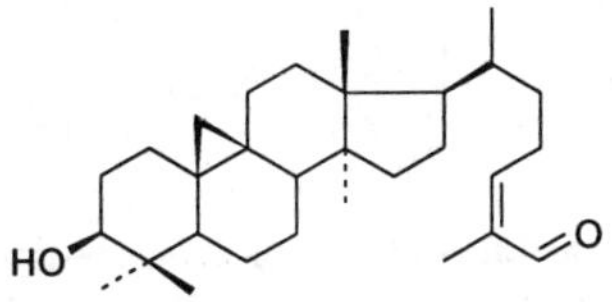

4383 Methyl mercaptan
CH_4S MW: 48.11 Property: mp -123°C, bp 5.8-6.2°C. Source: XIANG YE, LAI FU, LAI FU ZI. Ref: 6.

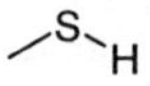

4384 3-Methyl-6-methoxy-8-hydroxy-3,4-dihydroisocoumarin
$C_{11}H_{12}O_4$ MW: 208.22 Property: mp 75-76°C. Source: HU LUO BO. Ref: 6.

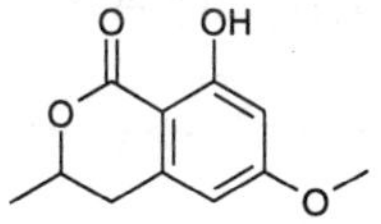

4385 14-Methyl-24-methylene-dihydromangiferodiol
$C_{31}H_{52}O_2$ MW: 456.76 Source: MANG GUO SHU PI. Ref: 6.

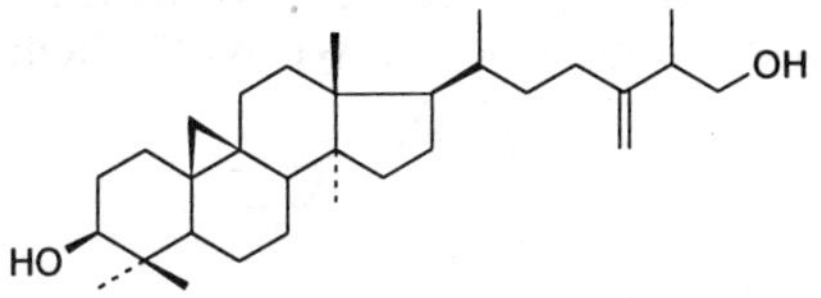

4386 (14-Methyl-24-methylene-dihydroman-giferodiol)-14-methyl -24-methylene dihydroman-giferonate
$C_{62}H_{98}O_4$ MW: 907.47 Source: MANG GUO SHU PI. Ref: 6.

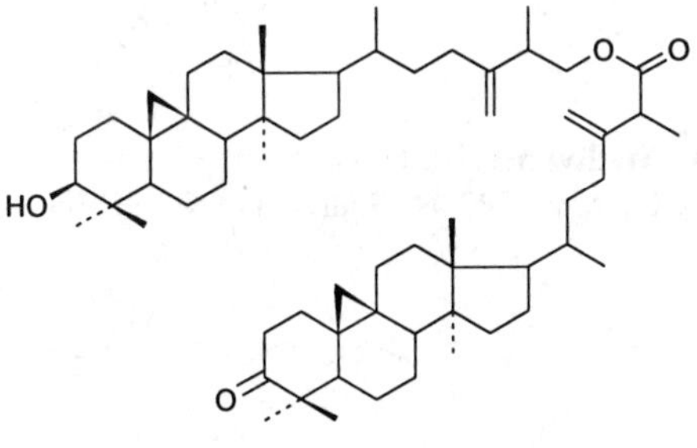

4387 2-Methyl-3-methylene-2-(4-methyl-3-pentenyl)-bicyclo[2,2,1] heptane
$C_{15}H_{24}$ MW: 204.36 Source: WU WEI ZI. Ref: 2.

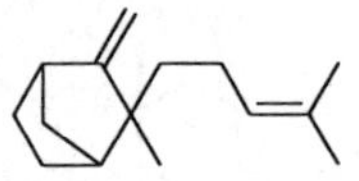

4388 2-Methyl-6-methylene-2,7-octadienol
$C_{10}H_{16}O$ MW: 152.24 Source: HUO XIANG CAO. Ref: 6.

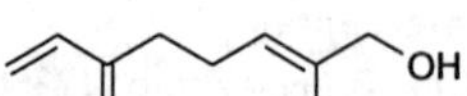

OH

4389 2-Methyl-6-methylene-2,7-octadienol acetate
$C_{12}H_{18}O_2$ MW: 194.28 Source: SHE XIANG CAO. Ref: 6.

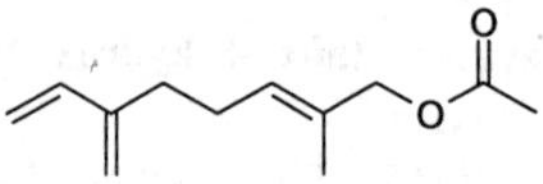

4390 4-Methyl-1-(1-methylethyl)-3-cyclohexen-1-ol -acetate
$C_{12}H_{20}O_2$ MW: 196.29 Source: SHENG JIANG. Ref: 2.

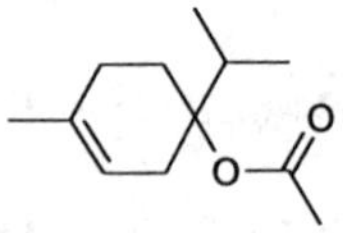

4391 1-Methyl-4-methylethenylcyclohexene
$C_{10}H_{16}$ MW: 136.24 Source: WU WEI ZI. Ref: 2.

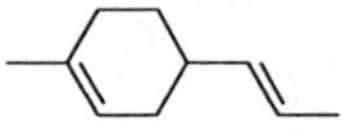

4392 5-Methylmyricetin
$C_{16}H_{12}O_8$ MW: 332.27 Source: YING SHAN HONG. Ref: 6.

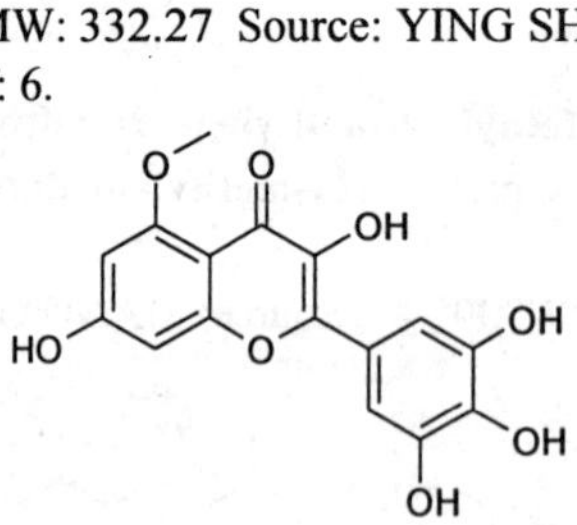

OH
HO
OH
OH
OH

4393 Methyl myristate
$C_{15}H_{30}O_2$ MW: 242.41 Source: DANG SHEN. Ref: 2.

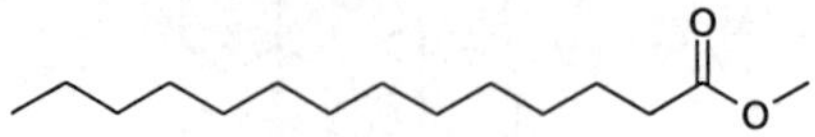

4394 Methyl nigakinone
$C_{16}H_{12}N_2O_3$ MW: 280.29 Property: mp 145-6°C. Source: KU SHU PI. Ref: 6.

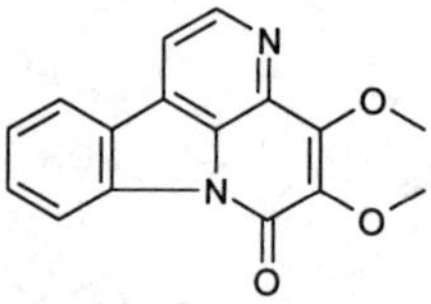

N
N

4395 3-Methylnonane
$C_{10}H_{22}$ MW: 142.29 Source: DU HUO. Ref: 2.

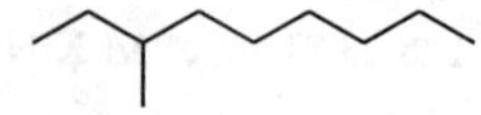

4396 4-Methyl-nonane
$C_{10}H_{22}$ MW: 142.29 Source: SHAN ZHA. Ref: 2.

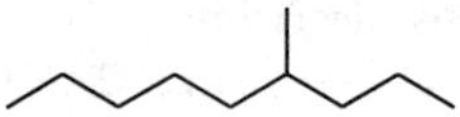

4397 Methyl-n-nonylketone
$C_{11}H_{22}O$ MW: 170.30 Property: bp 228°C. Source: YU XING CAO. Ref: 2.

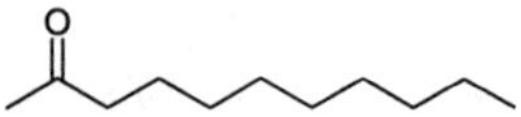

4398 2-Methyl octane
C_9H_{20} MW: 128.26 Source: DU HUO, SHAN ZHA. Ref: 2.

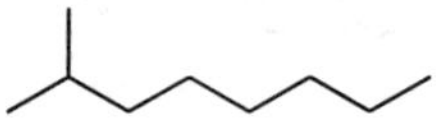

4399 N-Methyl pachysamine A
$C_{25}H_{46}N_2$ MW: 374.66 Property: mp 165.5-7°C. Source: XUE SHAN LIN. Ref: 6.

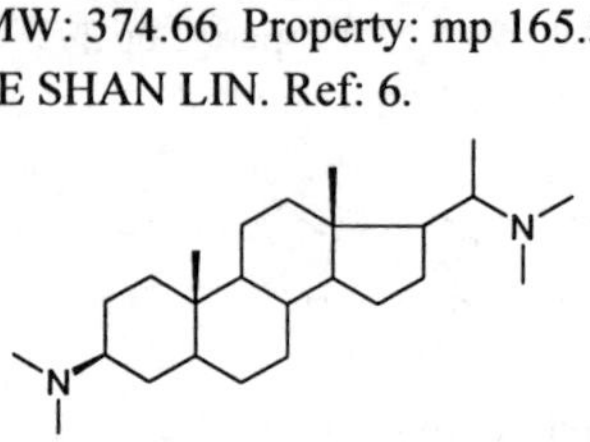

N
N

4400 Methyl palmitate
$C_{17}H_{34}O_2$ MW: 270.46 Property: mp 30.5°C(29.5°C). Source: CHUAN XIONG, DANG SHEN, SAN QI. Ref: 2.

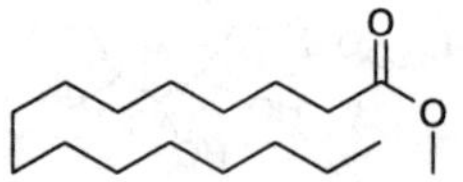

4401 1-Methyl-2-[(6Z,9Z)-6, 9-pentadecadienyl]-4(1H)-quinolone
$C_{25}H_{35}NO$ MW: 365.56 Source: WU ZHU YU. Ref: 2.

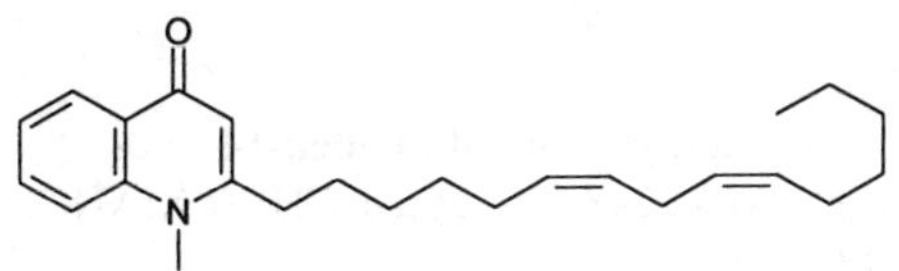

4402 Methyl pentadecanoate
$C_{16}H_{32}O_2$ MW: 256.43 Source: CHUAN XIONG, DANG SHEN. Ref: 2.

4403 13-Methyl pentadecanoic acid
$C_{17}H_{34}O_2$ MW: 270.46 Source: BAI ZHI. Ref: 2.

4404 1-Methyl-2-[(Z)-6-pentadecenyl]-4(1H)-quinolone
$C_{25}H_{37}NO$ MW: 367.58 Source: WU ZHU YU. Ref: 2.

4405 1-Methyl-2-[(Z)-10-pentadecenyl]-4(1H)-quinolone
$C_{25}H_{37}NO$ MW: 367.58 Source: WU ZHU YU. Ref: 2.

4406 1-Methyl-2-pentadecyl-4(1H)-quinolone
$C_{25}H_{39}NO$ MW: 369.60 Source: WU ZHU YU. Ref: 2.

4407 2-Methyl-2-pentenal
$C_6H_{10}O$ MW: 98.15 Source: XI XIANG CONG. Ref: 6.

4408 Methyl-n-pentyl ketone
$C_7H_{14}O$ MW: 114.19 Property: bp 151.45°C. Source: DING XIANG. Ref: 6.

4409 Methyl phenylacetate
$C_9H_{10}O_2$ MW: 150.18 Source: CHUAN XIONG. Ref: 2.

4410 Methyl phenyl carbinol
$C_8H_{10}O$ MW: 122.17 Property: bp (+): 98-9°C/20 mm, (-):93°C/14 mm, (±): 100°C /18 mm. Source: CHA YE. Ref: 6.

4411 Methyl phenyl ethyl ether
$C_9H_{12}O$ MW: 136.20 Source: LU DOU LE HUA. Ref: 6.

4412 N-Methylplatydesmin
$C_{16}H_{20}NO$ MW: 274.34 Source: CHOU CAO. Ref: 6.

4413 Methyl propyl disulfide
$C_4H_{10}S_2$ MW: 122.25 Source: DA SUAN, XI YANG CONG, ZHI ZI. Ref: 6.

4414 2-Methyl-5-propyl nonane
$C_{13}H_{28}$ MW: 184.37 Source: ROU CONG RONG. Ref: 2.

4415 Methyl propyl trisulfide
$C_4H_{10}S_3$ MW: 154.32 Source: DA SUAN. Ref: 2.

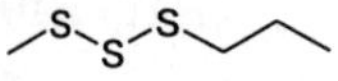

4416 d-N-Methyl-pseudoephedrine
$C_{11}H_{17}NO$ MW: 179.26 Source: MA HUANG. Ref: 2.

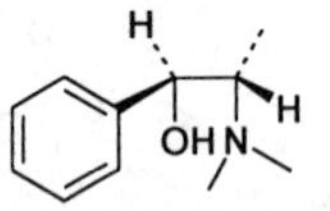

4417 3-O-Methylquercetin-7-O-diglucoside-4'-O-glucoside
$C_{34}H_{42}O_{22}$ MW: 802.70 Source: PING ER XIAO CAO. Ref: 6.

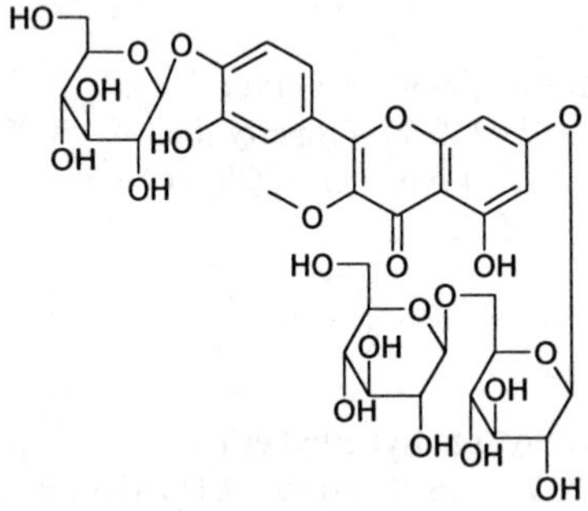

4418 Methyl-β-resorcylate
$C_8H_8O_4$ MW: 168.15 Property: mp 118-9°C. Source: CI HUAI HUA. Ref: 6.

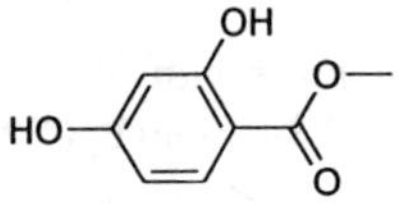

4419 4-Methyl salicylaldehyde
$C_8H_8O_2$ MW: 136.15 Property: mp 60-1°C. Source: WU JIA PI. Ref: 6.

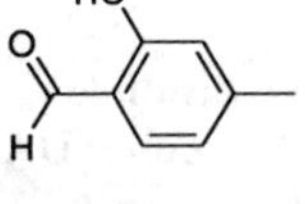

4420 Methyl salicylate
$C_8H_8O_3$ MW: 152.15 Property: bp 223°C. Source: DING XIANG, JIU LI XIANG, PAO DAN GUO, QU MAI, SANG YE, TOU GU XIANG. Ref: 6, 11.

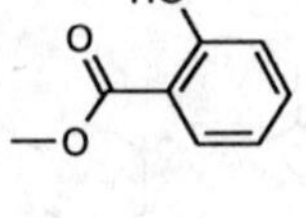

4421 (-)-Methyl selina-3,11-dien-14-oate
$C_{16}H_{24}O_2$ MW: 248.37 Source: CHEN XIANG. Ref: 13.

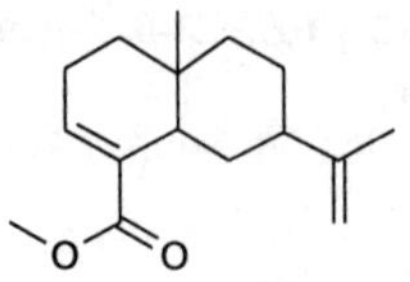

4422 (+)-Methyl selina-4,11-dien-14-oate
$C_{16}H_{24}O_2$ MW: 248.37 Source: CHEN XIANG. Ref: 13.

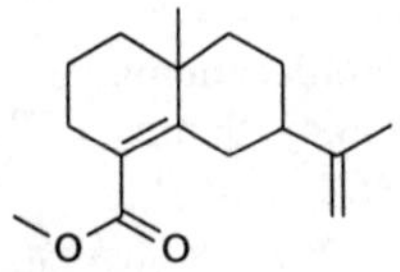

4423 Methyl stearate
$C_{19}H_{38}O_2$ MW: 298.51 Source: DANG SHEN. Ref: 2.

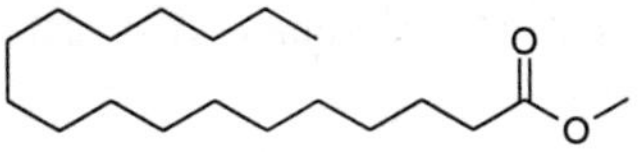

4424 Methyl syramuraldehydate
$C_{11}H_{14}O_6$ MW: 242.23 Property: colorless oleaginous, $[\alpha]_D^{22}$ -87.4° (c=2, chloroform). Source: BAO MA ZI. Ref: 70.

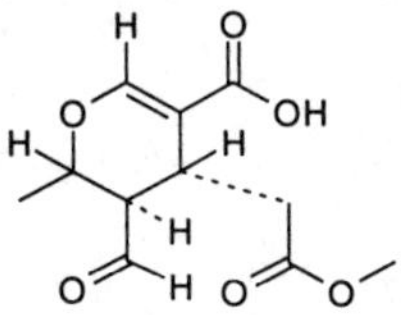

4425 Methyl tanshinonate
$C_{20}H_{18}O_5$ MW: 338.36 Property: 175-6°C. Source: DAN SHEN. Ref: 2.

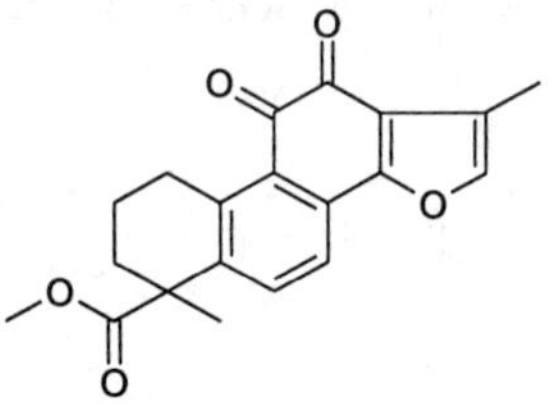

4426 O-Methyltaxodine
$C_{20}H_{29}NO_3$ MW: 331.46 Source: SAN JIAN SHAN. Ref: 2.

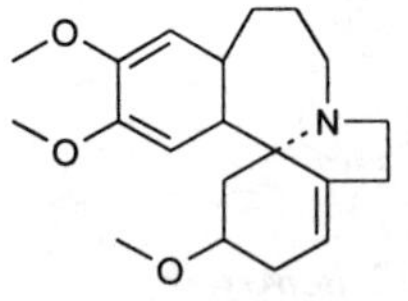

4427 12-Methyl tetradecanoic acid

$C_{15}H_{30}O_2$ MW: 242.41 Source: QIANG HUO. Ref: 2.

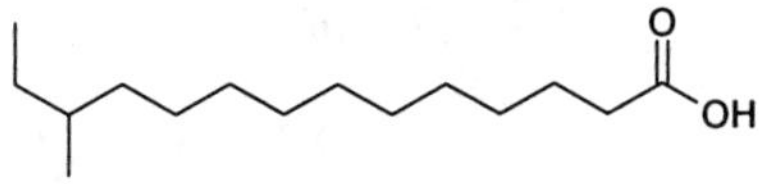

4428 13-Methyl tetradecanoic acid

$C_{15}H_{30}O_2$ MW: 242.41 Source: BAI SHAO YAO. Ref: 6.

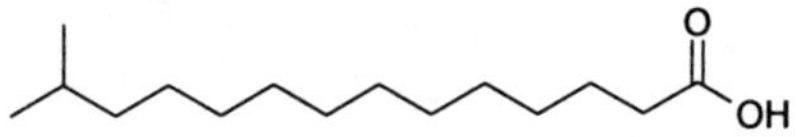

4429 2-Methyl-1,2,3,4-tetrahydro-β-carboline

$C_{12}H_{16}NO_2$ MW: 188.27 Property: mp 216-8°C. Source: SHA ZAO SHU PI. Ref: 6.

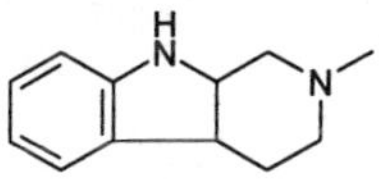

4430 N-Methyltetrahydrocytisine

$C_{12}H_{20}N_2O$ MW: 208.31 Source: HONG DOU. Ref: 6.

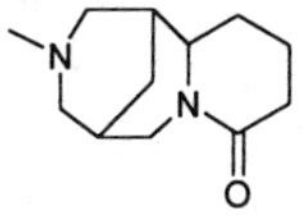

4431 Nb-Methyltetrahydroharman

$C_{13}H_{16}N_2$ MW: 200.29 Property: mp 112°C. Source: HONG MU JI CAO. Ref: 6.

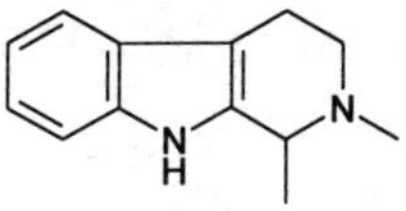

4432 N-Methyltetrahydroharmol

$C_{14}H_{18}N_2$ MW: 214.31 Property: mp 268-70°C. Source: SHA ZAO SHU PI. Ref: 6.

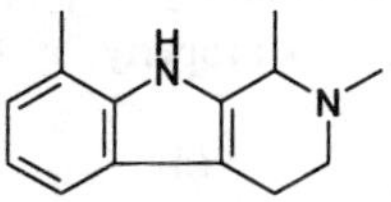

4433 (+)-2-N-Methyltetrandrine

$C_{39}H_{45}N_2O_6$ MW: 637.80 Source: FANG JI. Ref: 2.

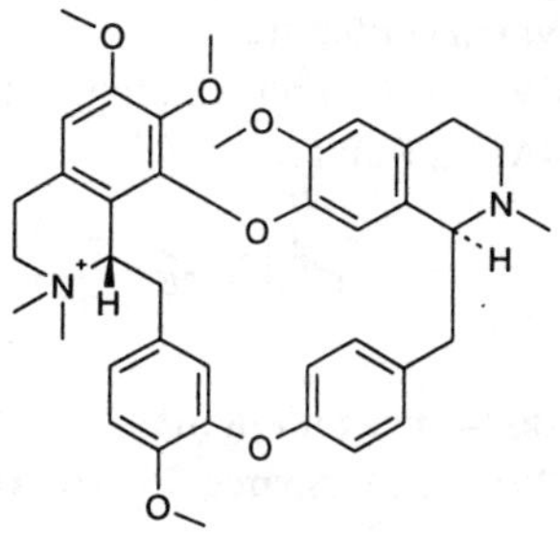

4434 O-Methyl thalicberine

$C_{38}H_{42}N_2O_6$ MW: 622.77 Property: mp 186-7°C. Source: YAN GUO CAO. Ref: 6.

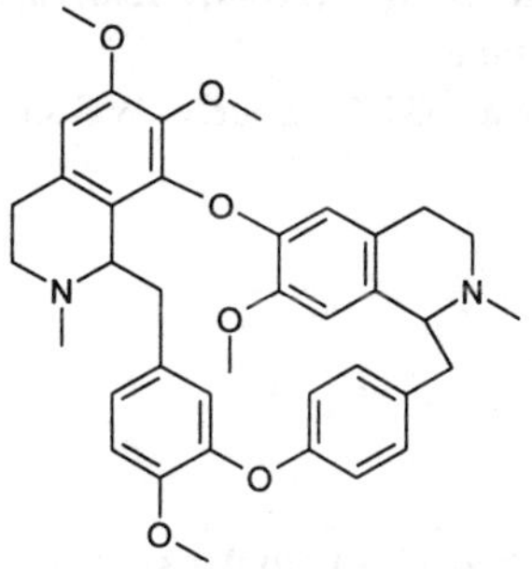

4435 Methyl trans-5-(2-thienyl)-2-penten-4-yn-1-oate

$C_{10}H_8O_2S$ MW: 192.24 Property: mp 67°C. Source: YANG SHI CAO. Ref: 6.

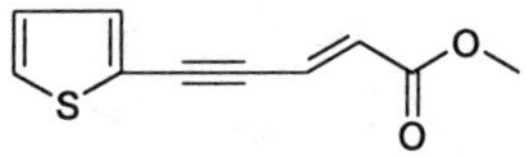

4436 6-Methyl-1-thio-2,4-cyclohexadiene

C_6H_8S MW: 112.19 Source: DA SUAN. Ref: 2.

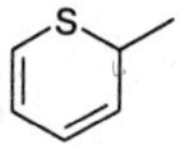

4437 3-Methylthiopropyl

$C_5H_9NS_2$ MW: 147.26 Property: bp 120.5-2°C/12 mm. Source: JIE ZI. Ref: 6.

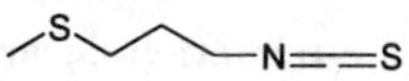

4438 5-Methyl thymol ether

$C_{11}H_{16}O$ MW: 164.25 Property: bp 216°C. Source: PEI LAN. Ref: 6.

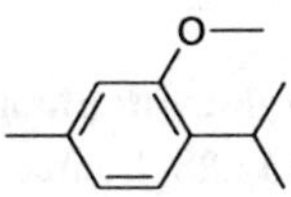

4439 Methyl triacontanate
$C_{31}H_{62}O_2$ MW: 466.84 Property: mp 71.5°C. Source: TAO JING BAI PI. Ref: 6.

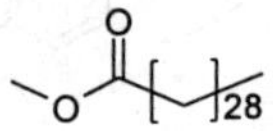

4440 7-Methyl-4-triacontanone
$C_{51}H_{102}O$ MW: 731.38 Source: PU HUANG. Ref: 2.

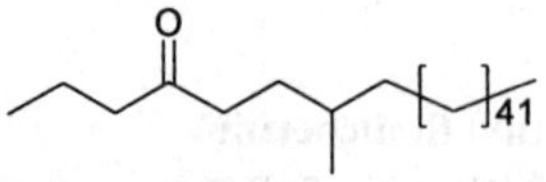

4441 1-Methyl-2-[(4Z,7Z)-4,7-tridecadienyl]-4(1H)-quinolone
$C_{23}H_{31}NO$ MW: 337.51 Source: WU ZHU YU. Ref: 2.

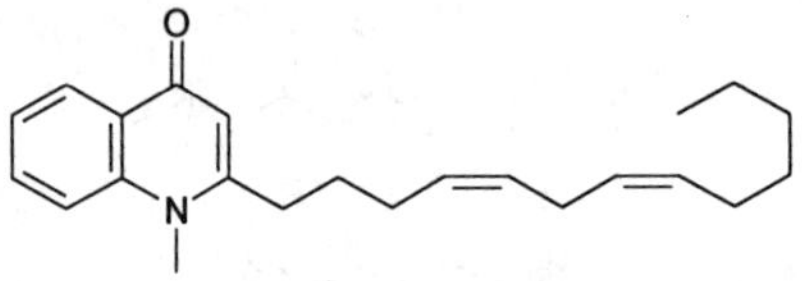

4442 2-Methyl-1,3,6-trihydroxy-9,10-anthraquinone-3-O-β-D-xylosyl(1→2)-β-D-(6'-O-acetyl) glucoside
$C_{28}H_{30}O_{15}$ MW: 606.54 Property: yellow acicular crystal, mp 284-6°C. Source: QIAN CAO. Ref: 242.

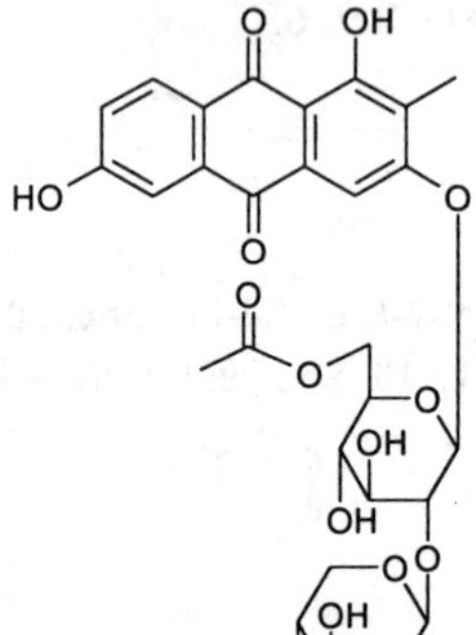

4443 Methyl-2,4,6-trimethyl-decanoate
$C_{14}H_{28}O_2$ MW: 228.38 Source: DU HUO. Ref: 2.

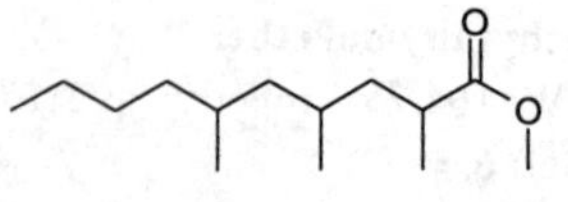

4444 (+)-Nb-Methyl tryptophan methyl ester (S)
$C_{13}H_{16}N_2O_2$ MW: 232.28 Source: HUANG HUA ZI. Ref: 6.

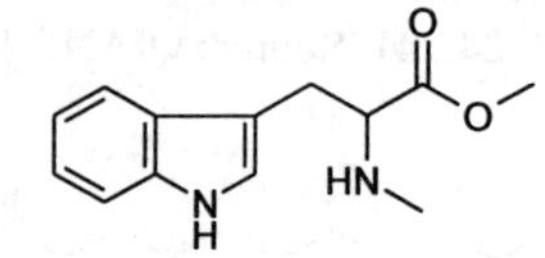

4445 N-Methyltyramine
CAS: 370-89-9 $C_9H_{13}NO$ MW: 151.21 Property: mp 130-1°C, bp 183-5°C/9mm. Source: ZHI SHI. Ref: 4.

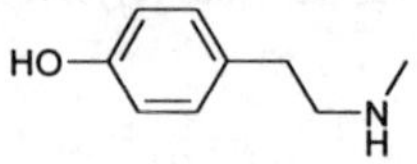

4446 1-Methyl-2-[(Z)-6-undecenyl]-4(1H)-quinolone
$C_{21}H_{29}NO$ MW: 311.47 Source: WU ZHU YU. Ref: 2.

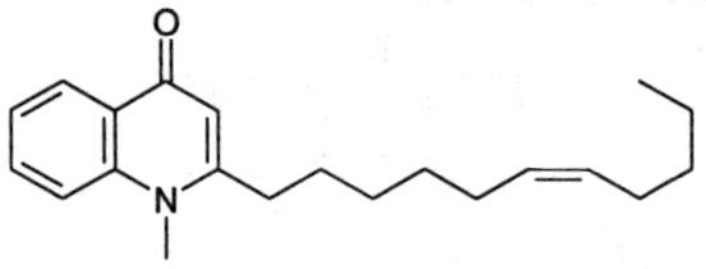

4447 1-Methyl-2-undecyl-4(1H)-quinolone
$C_{21}H_{31}NO$ MW: 313.49 Source: WU ZHU YU. Ref: 2.

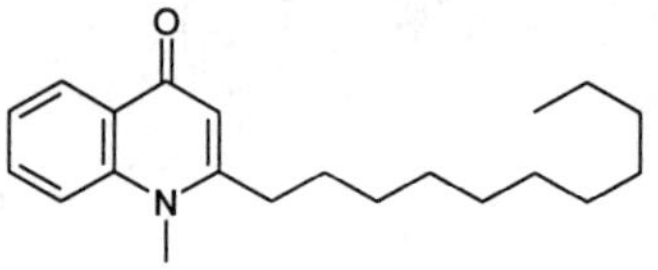

4448 Methylvanillin
$C_9H_{10}O_3$ MW: 166.18 Property: mp 44°C, 58°C. Source: PENG ZI CAI, SHOU ZHANG SHEN. Ref: 6.

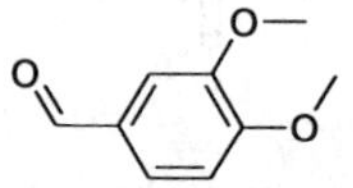

4449 2-Methyl-2-vinyl-3-isopropenyl-5-isopropylidene cyclohexanol
$C_{15}H_{24}O$ MW: 220.36 Property: bp 46-7°C. Source: XI XIN. Ref: 6.

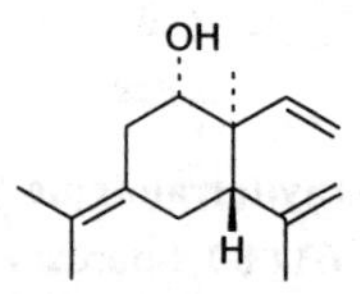

4450 5-O-Methylvisamminol

$C_{16}H_{18}O_5$ MW: 290.32 Source: FANG FENG. Ref: 2.

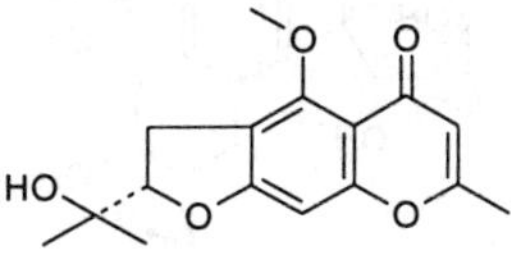

4451 2-O-Methyl-D-xylose

$C_6H_{12}O_5$ MW: 164.16 Property: mp β-D (+): 137-8°C. Source: HAI DAI (DA YE ZAO). Ref: 6.

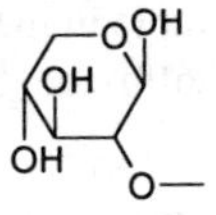

4452 Methyl-D-xyloside

$C_6H_{12}O_5$ MW: 164.16 Property: mp α: 90-2°C, β: 157°C. Source: LU JIAO CAI. Ref: 6.

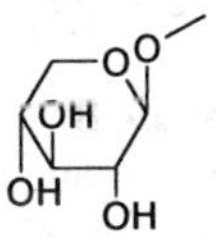

4453 Mexoticin

5,7-Dimethoxy-8-(2,3-dihydroxyisopentyl) coumarin. $C_{16}H_{20}O_6$ MW: 308.33 Property: mp 185°C. Source: JIU LI XIANG, YUN QIAN HU. Ref: 6, 11, 177.

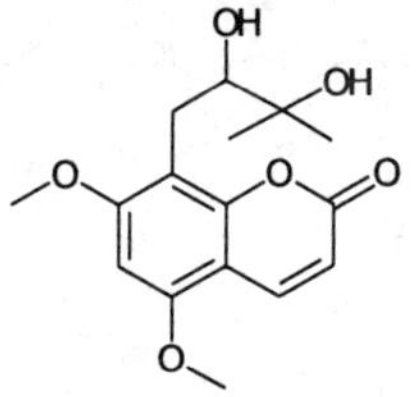

4454 Michelalbine

$C_{17}H_{15}NO_3$ MW: 281.31 Property: mp 205-7°C. Source: BAI LAN HUA, HOU PU, QING FENG TENG. Ref: 6, 625.

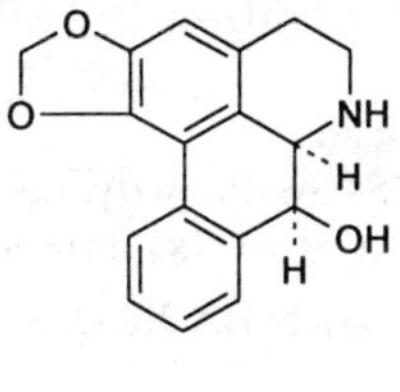

4455 Microhelenin A

$C_{15}H_{18}O_4$ MW: 262.31 Property: mp 140-1°C. Source: XIAO TOU DUI XIN JU. Ref: 5.

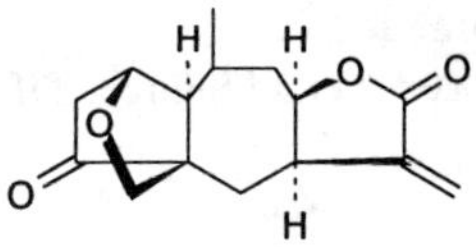

4456 Microlenin

$C_{29}H_{34}O_7$ MW: 494.59 Property: mp 280°C (dec). Source: XIAO TOU DUI XIN JU. Ref: 5.

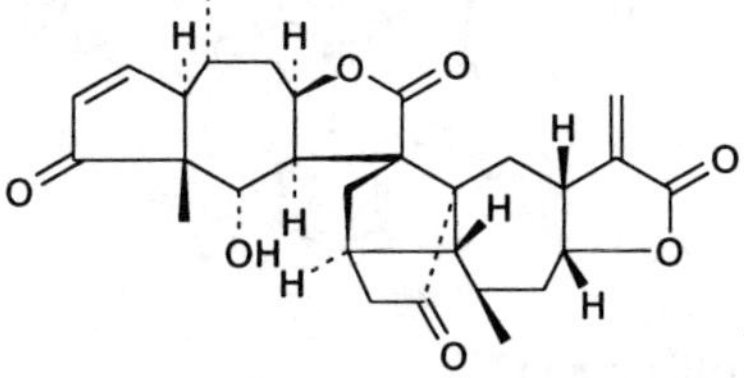

4457 Miliacin

$C_{31}H_{52}O$ MW: 440.76 Property: mp 282-3°C. Source: SHU MI. Ref: 6.

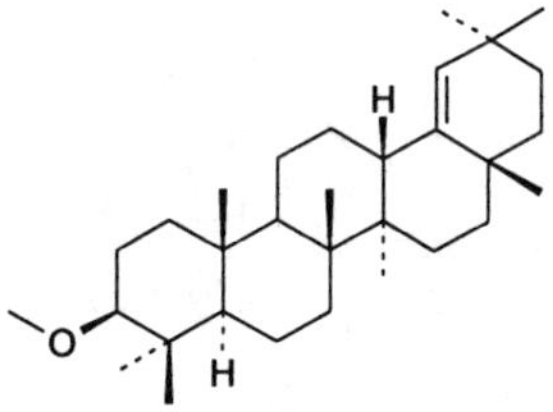

4458 Millefin

$C_{19}H_{26}O_6$ MW: 350.42 Property: mp 209-10°C. Source: YANG SHI CAO. Ref: 6.

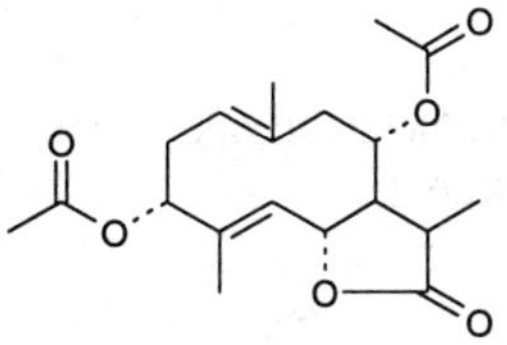

4459 Milliamine A

$C_{45}H_{49}N_3O_{10}$ MW: 791.91 Source: TIE HAI TANG. Ref: 6.

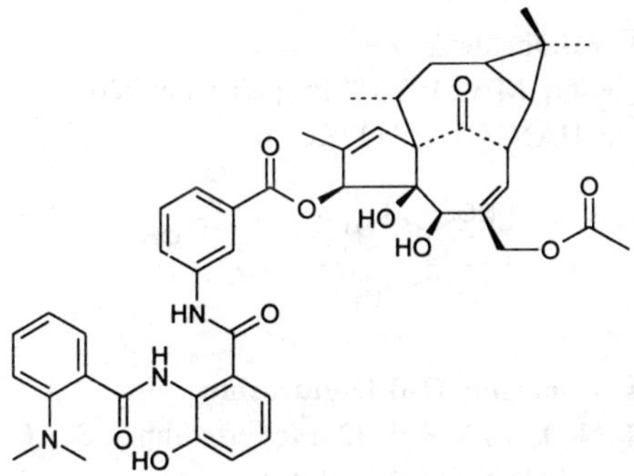

4460 Milliamine B
$C_{43}H_{47}N_3O_{10}$ MW: 749.87 Source: TIE HAI TANG. Ref: 6.

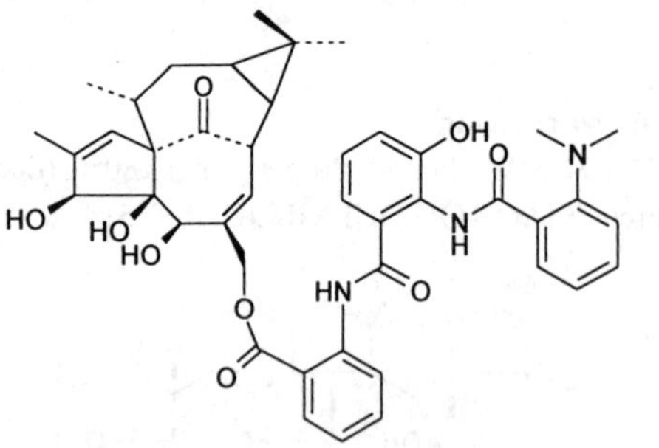

4461 Milliamine C
$C_{43}H_{47}N_3O_8$ MW: 733.89 Source: TIE HAI TANG. Ref: 6.

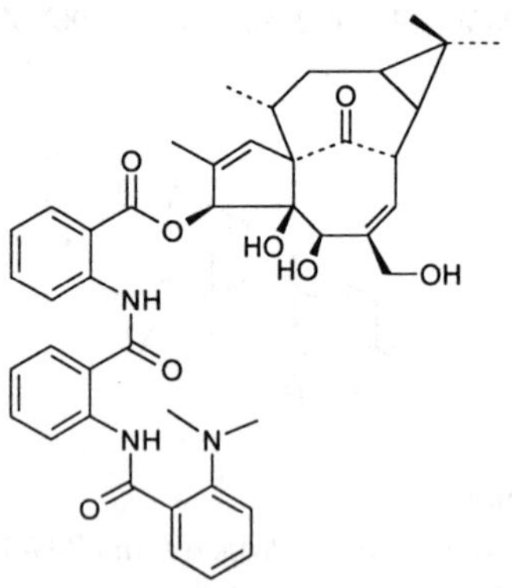

4462 Miltirone
$C_{19}H_{22}O_2$ MW: 282.39 Property: mp 100°C. Source: DAN SHEN. Ref: 2.

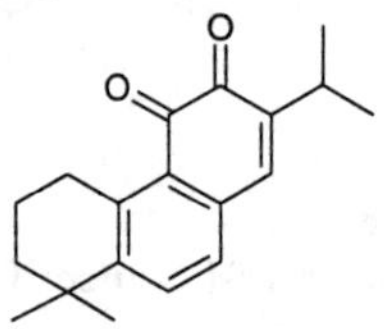

4463 Mimosine
$C_8H_{10}N_2O_4$ MW: 198.18 Property: mp 226-7°C. Source: HAN XIU CAO. Ref: 6.

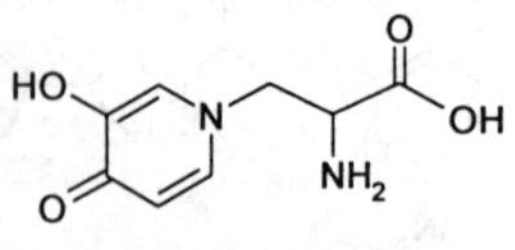

4464 Mimosine-O-β-D-glucoside
$C_{14}H_{20}N_2O_9$ MW: 360.32 Property: mp 178-9°C. Source: HAN XIU CAO. Ref: 6.

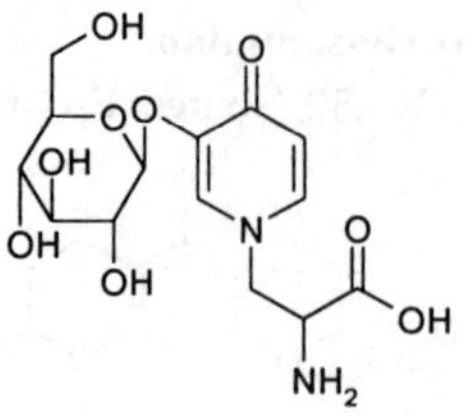

4465 Mingjinianuronide A
3,5,7,8,4'-pentahydroxyflavone-7-O-β-D-glucuronide. $C_{21}H_{18}O_{13}$ MW: 478.37 Property: yellow powder, mp 230°C, soluble in methanol, ethanol acetone and dimethyl sulfoxide. Source: ZI HUA BA BAO. Ref: 308.

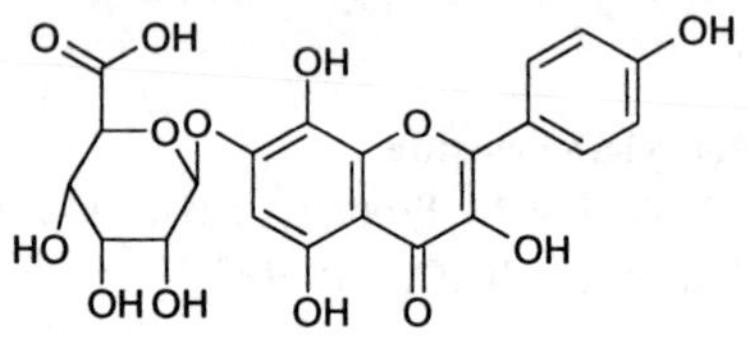

4466 Mingjinianuronide B
3,5,7,8,4'-pentahydroxyflavone-8-O-β-D-2''-O-(2-methylbutanoyl) glucuronide. $C_{26}H_{26}O_{14}$ MW: 562.49 Property: yellow powder, mp 206-7°C, soluble in methanol, ethanol acetone and dimethyl sulfoxide; unsoluble in chloroform and water. Source: ZI HUA BA BAO. Ref: 308.

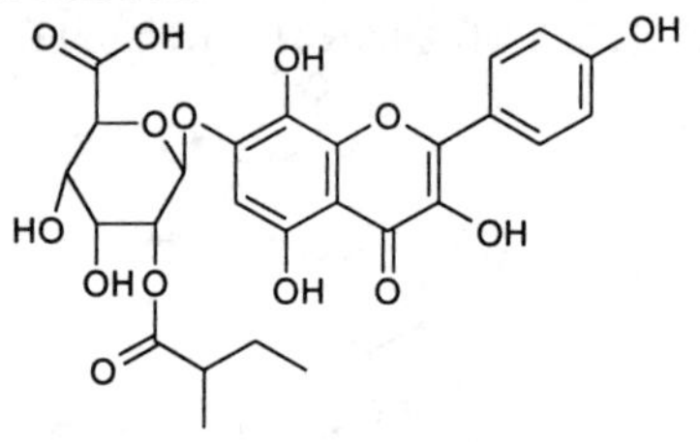

4467 Minpeimine
$C_{27}H_{43}NO_2$ Source: CHUAN BEI MU. Ref: 2.

4468 Minpeiminine
$C_{27}H_{41}NO_3$ Source: CHUAN BEI MU. Ref: 2.

4469 Minwanensin
$C_{15}H_{24}O_5$ MW: 284.36 Property: colorless acicular crystal, mp 171-3°C, $[\alpha]_D^{14}$ -87.4° (c=0.1075, methanol). Source: MIN WAN BA JIAO. Ref: 315.

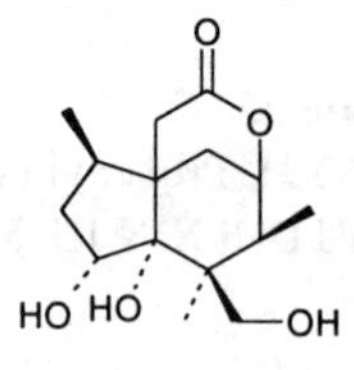

4470 Miraxanthin I
$C_{14}H_{18}N_2O_7S$ MW: 358.37 Source: ZI JIN NIU GEN. Ref: 6.

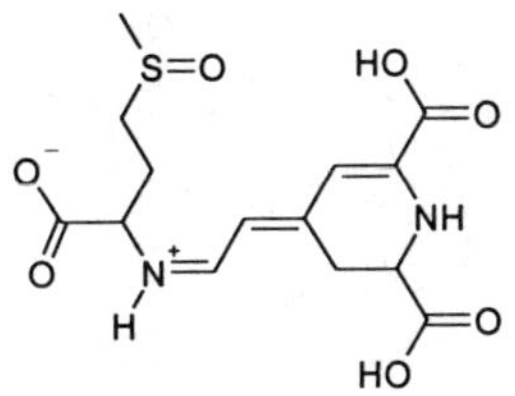

4471 Miraxanthin II
$C_{13}H_{14}N_2O_8$ MW: 326.27 Source: ZI JIN NIU GEN. Ref: 6.

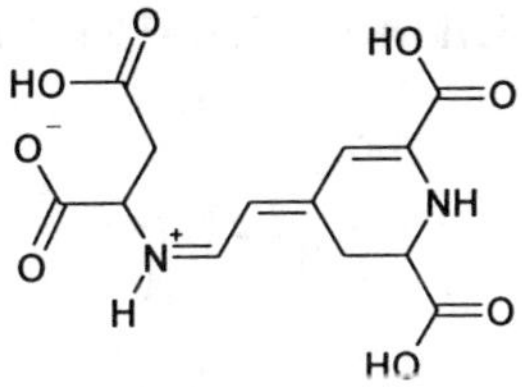

4472 Miraxanthin III
$C_{17}H_{16}N_2O_5$ MW: 328.33 Source: ZI JIN NIU GEN. Ref: 6.

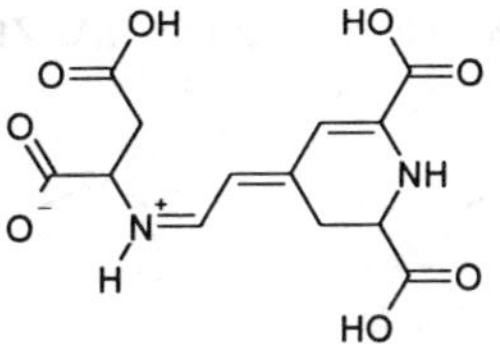

4473 Miraxanthin V
$C_{17}H_{16}N_2O_6$ MW: 344.33 Source: ZI JIN NIU GEN. Ref: 6.

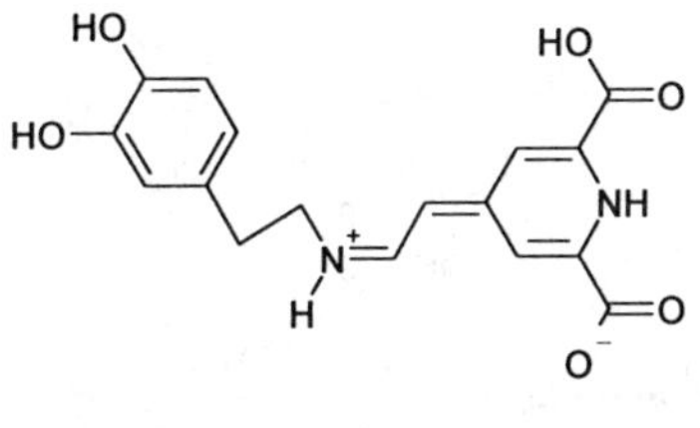

4474 Miroestrol
$C_{20}H_{22}O_6$ MW: 358.39 Property: mp 268-70°C (dec). Source: GUO YE GE. Ref: 4.

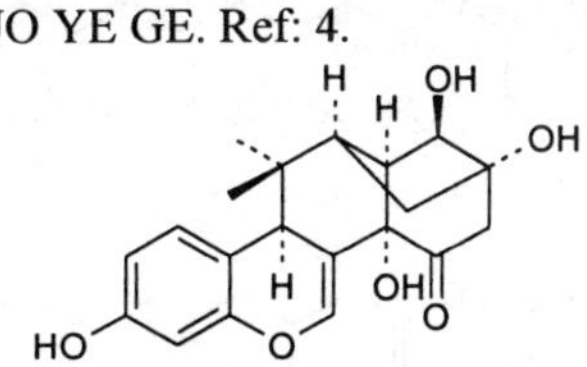

4475 Miscanthoside
$C_{21}H_{22}O_{11}$ MW: 450.40 Property: mp 158-63°C. Source: MANG JING. Ref: 6.

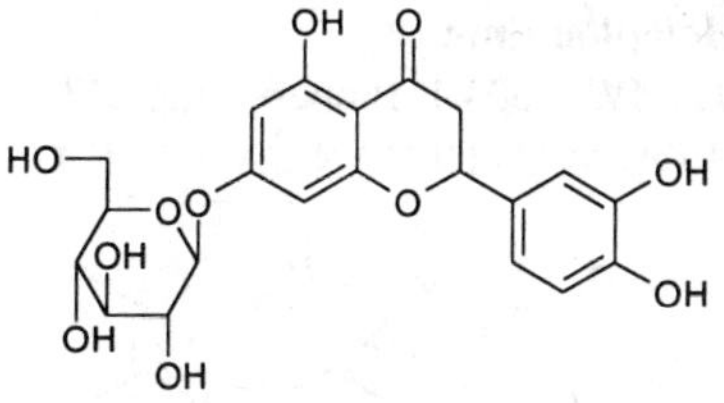

4476 Mitraphyllic acid [16-1]-β-D-gluco-pyranosyl ester
$C_{26}H_{32}N_2O_9$ MW: 516.55 Property: white amorphous powder crystal, $[\alpha]_D$ -48.8° (MeOH). Source: HUA GOU TENG. Ref: 287.

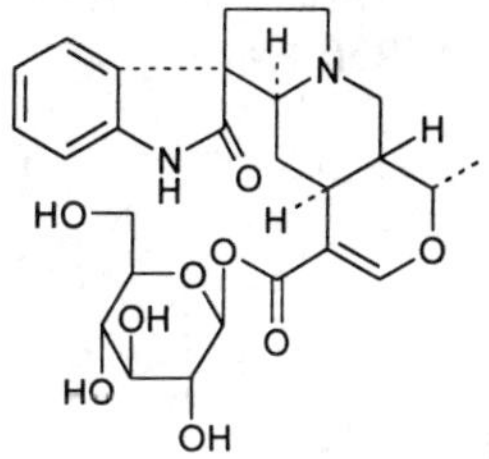

4477 Mitraphylline
$C_{21}H_{24}O_2O_4$ MW: 368.44 Source: CHANG CHUN HUA. Ref: 2.

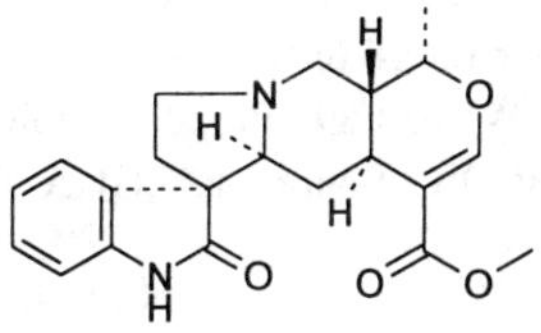

4478 Moellendorffiline
$C_{26}H_{20}O_{10}$ MW: 492.44 Property: light yellow column crystal, mp 244-6°C. Source: LI JIANG QIAN HU, ZOU MA QIN. Ref: 61, 557.

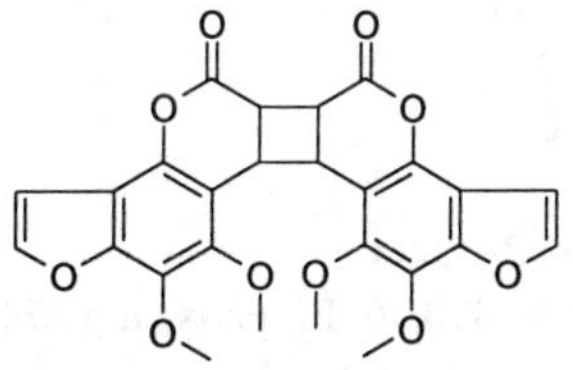

4479 Molephantin
$C_{19}H_{22}O_6$ MW: 346.38 Property: mp 214-6°C. Source: ROU MAO DI DAN CAO. Ref: 4.

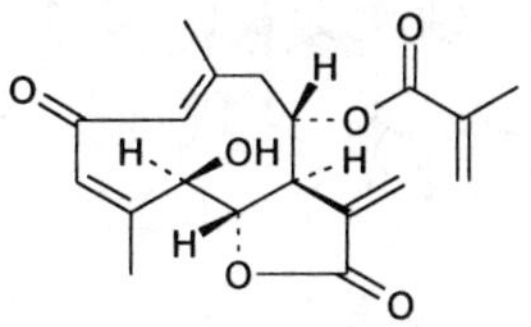

4480 Molephantinin
$C_{20}H_{24}O_6$ MW: 360.41 Property: mp 223-5°C. Source: ROU MAO DI DAN CAO. Ref: 4.

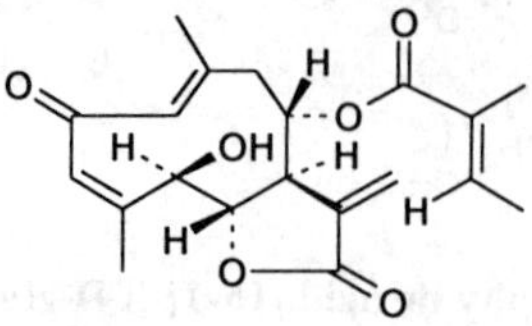

4481 Momorcharaside A
$C_{42}H_{72}O_{15}$ MW: 817.03 Property: colorless prismatic crystal, mp 170-2°C, $[\alpha]_D^{19}$ +0.80° (c=1.80, methanol). Source: KU GUA. Ref: 176.

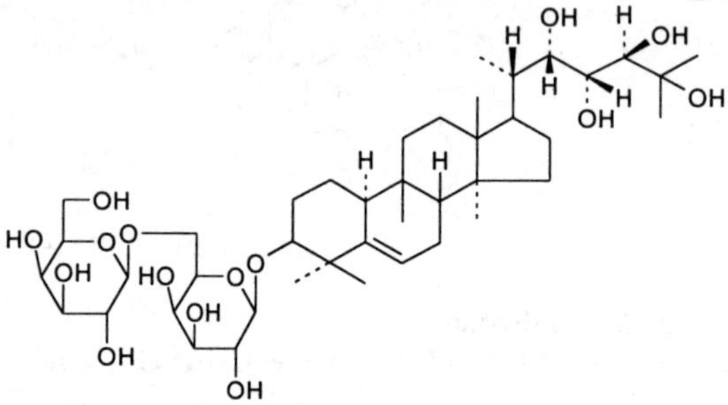

4482 Momorcharaside B
$C_{36}H_{62}O_{10}$ MW: 654.89 Property: colorless acicular crystal, mp 186-9°C. Source: KU GUA. Ref: 176.

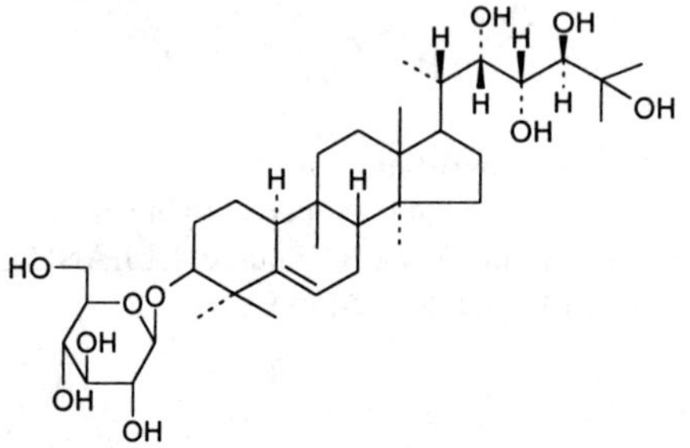

4483 Momordic acid
$C_{30}H_{46}O_4$ MW: 470.70 Property: mp 274-6°C. Source: MU BIE ZI. Ref: 6.

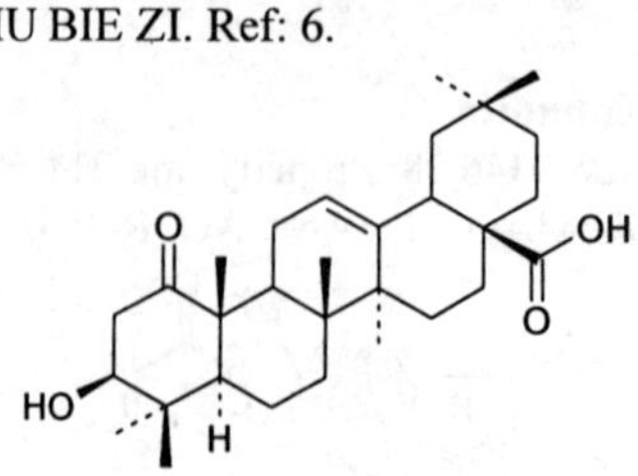

4484 Monocaffeyltartaric acid
$C_{13}H_{12}O_9$ MW: 312.24 Property: mp 146-7°C. Source: JU QU. Ref: 6.

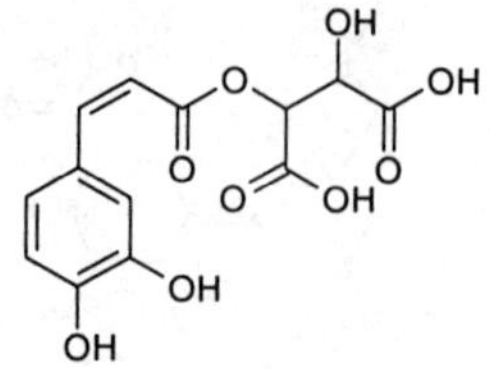

4485 Monocrotaline
Crotaline; Retronecine. CAS: 315-22-0 $C_{16}H_{23}NO_6$ MW: 325.36 Property: mp 197-8°C (dec). Source: MEI LI ZHU SHI DOU, YE BAI HE, ZI XIAO RONG. Ref: 4.

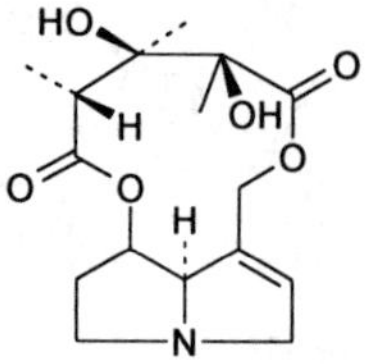

4486 1-Monolinolein
$C_{20}H_{36}O_4$ MW: 340.51 Source: BAI ZHI. Ref: 2.

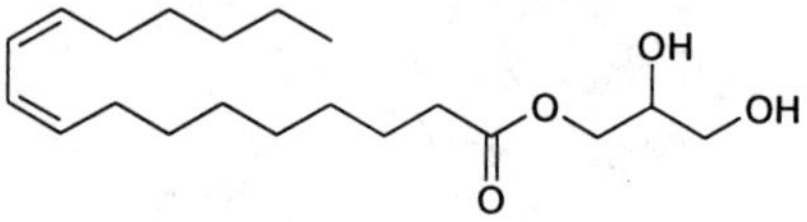

4487 Mono-O-methylwightin
$C_{19}H_{18}O_7$ MW: 358.35 Property: mp 150°C. Source: CHUAN XIN LIAN. Ref: 2.

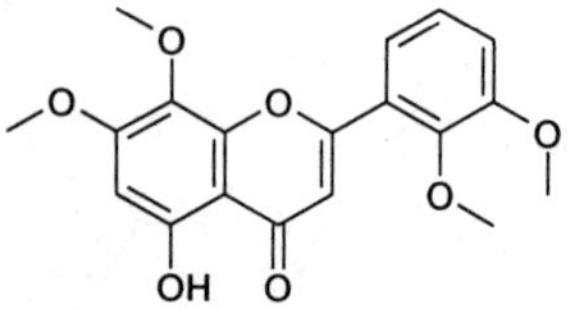

4488 Monoolein
$C_{21}H_{40}O_4$ MW: 356.55 Property: mp α: 35°C, β: 26°C. Source: MANG GUO HE. Ref: 6.

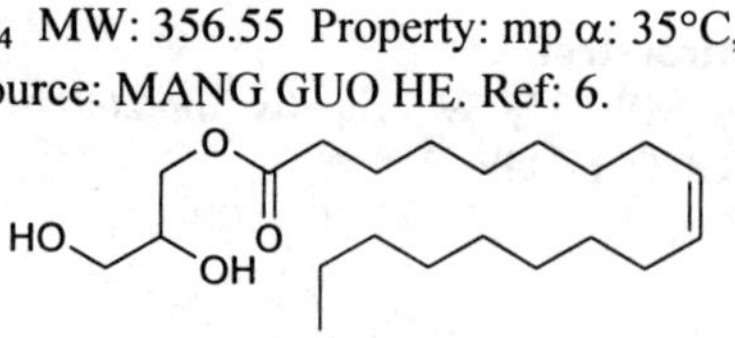

α–:

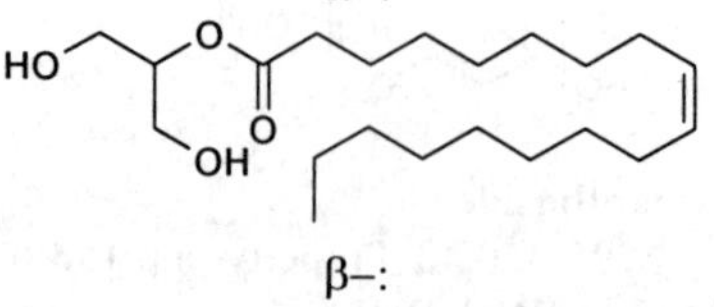

β–:

4489 L-(-)-α-Monopalmitin
$C_{19}H_{38}O_4$ MW: 330.51 Source: GUA LOU. Ref: 2.

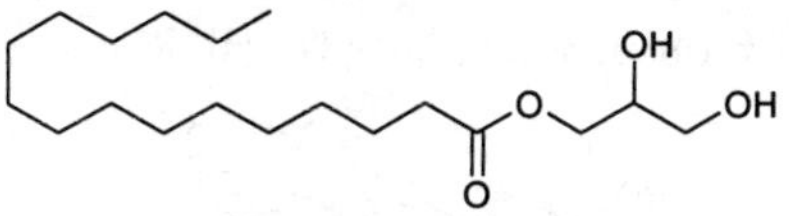

OH OH O

4490 Monoricinolein
$C_{21}H_{40}O_5$ MW: 372.55 Source: BI MA YOU. Ref: 6.

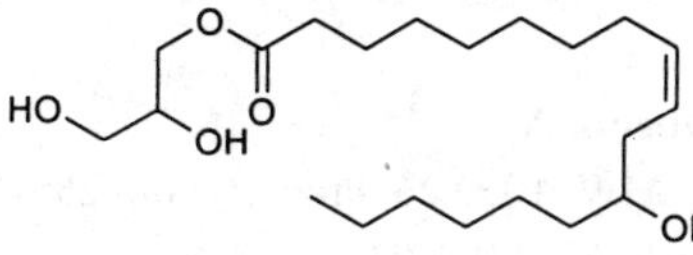

HO O O OH OH

4491 Monotropein
$C_{16}H_{22}O_{11}$ MW: 290.35 Property: mp 175°C (dec). Source: LU SHOU CAO, SHUI JINGLAN. Ref: 6.

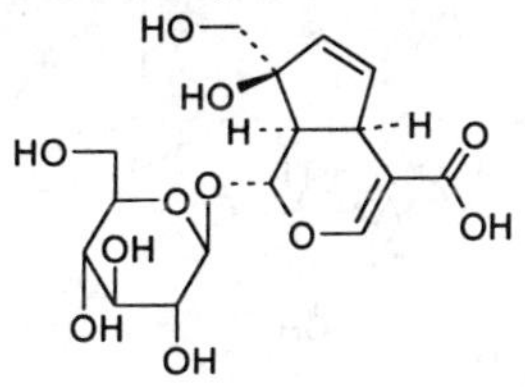

HO HO H H HO O O O OH OH OH OH O

4492 Montanic acid
$C_{28}H_{56}O_2$ MW: 424.76 Source: GUA LOU. Ref: 2.

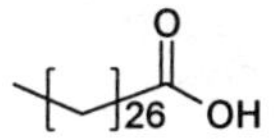

O 26 OH

4493 Moracetin
$C_{33}H_{40}O_{22}$ MW: 788.67 Property: mp 211-4°C. Source: SANG YE. Ref: 6.

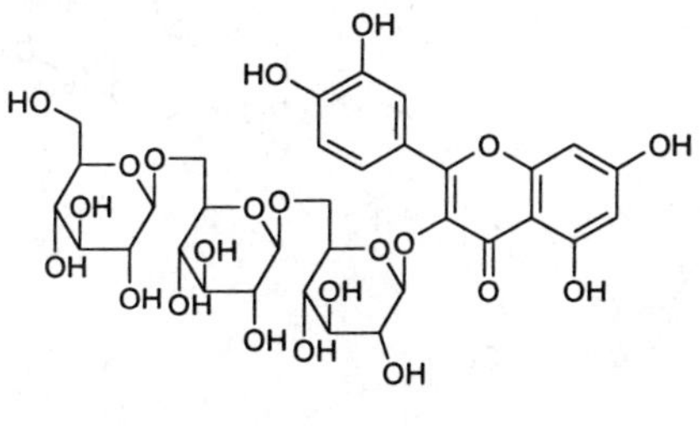

OH HO HO O O OH OH OH OH OH OH O O OH OH OH O O OH OH

4494 Morellic acid
$C_{33}H_{36}O_8$ MW: 560.65 Source: TENG HUANG. Ref: 6.

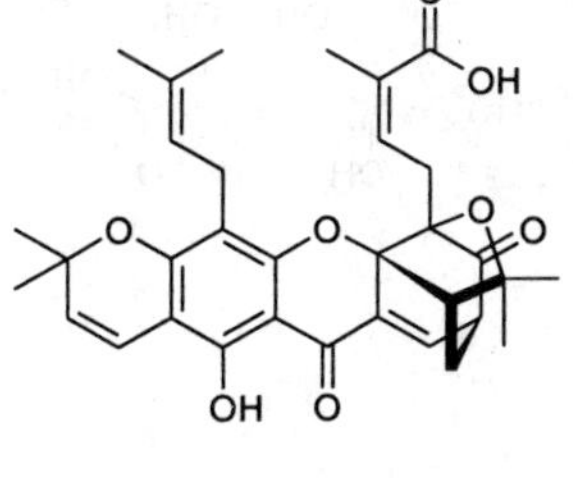

O OH O O O O OH O

4495 Morellin
$C_{33}H_{36}O_7$ MW: 544.65 Property: mp 157-9°C. Source: TENG HUANG. Ref: 6.

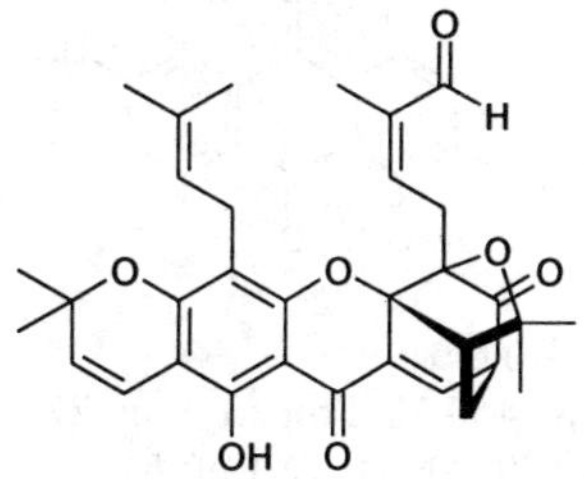

O H O O O O OH O

4496 Morelloflavone
$C_{30}H_{20}O_{11}$ MW: 556.49 Property: mp (+): 244-5°C (dec), (±): 298°C (dec). Source: SHAN ZHU ZI, TENG HUANG. Ref: 6.

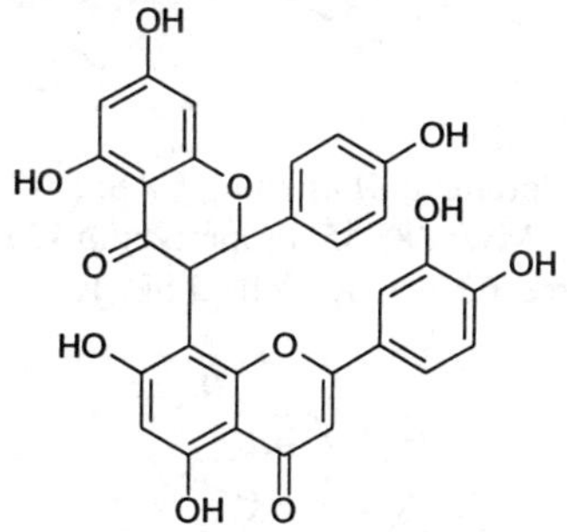

OH OH HO O OH O OH HO O OH O

4497 Morin
$C_{15}H_{10}O_7$ MW: 302.24 Property: mp 303-4°C. Source: SANG ZHI. Ref: 6.

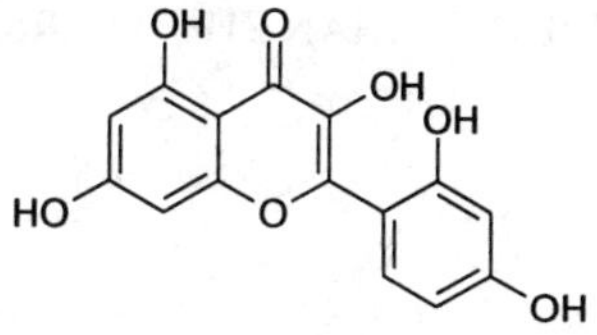

OH O OH OH HO O OH

4498 Morindin
$C_{27}H_{30}O_{14}$ MW: 578.53 Property: mp 264.5°C (dec). Source: BA JI TIAN. Ref: 6.

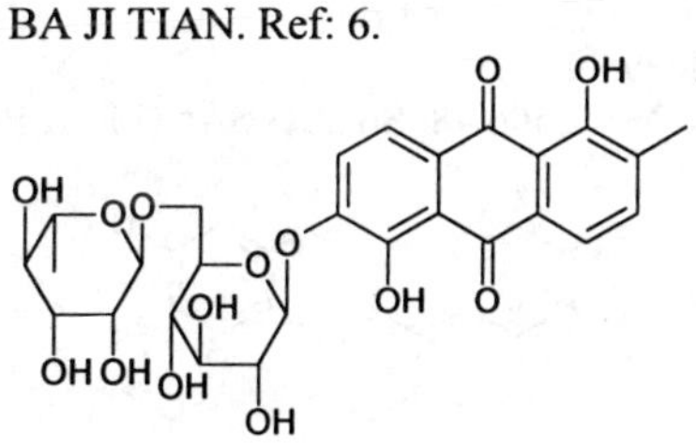

O OH OH O O O OH OH OH OH OH OH O

4499 Morindon
$C_{14}H_8O_6$ MW: 272.22 Property: mp 282°C. Source: TU LIAN QIAO. Ref: 6.

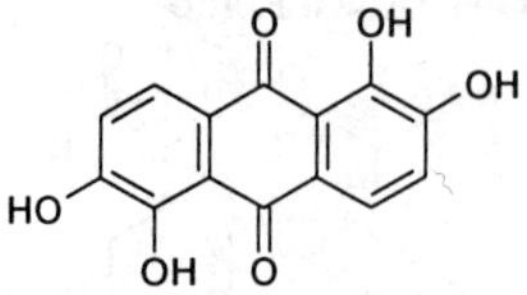

4500 Morolic acid
$C_{30}H_{48}O$ MW: 456.72 Property: mp 273°C (dec). Source: SHUI TUAN HUA. Ref: 6.

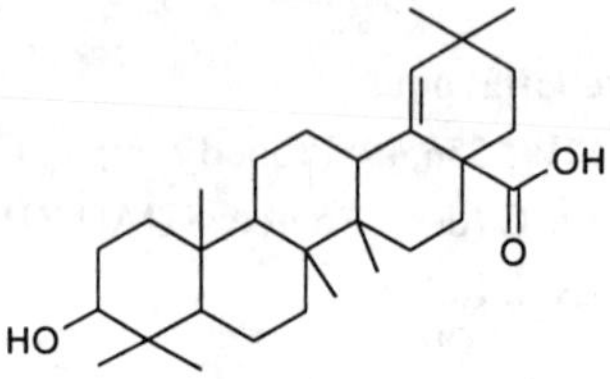

4501 Morphine
Morphia; Morphina; Morphium. CAS: 57-27-2
$C_{17}H_{19}NO_3$ MW: 285.35 Property: mp 154-6°C (dec). Source: CHAN SU, YING SU. Ref: 2, 4.

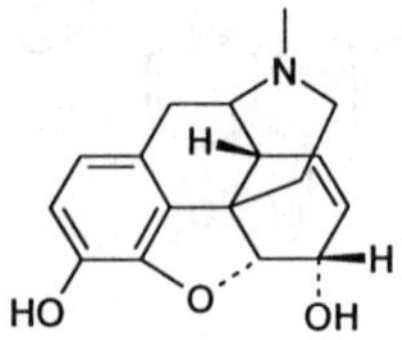

4502 Morroniside
$C_{17}H_{26}O_{11}$ MW: 406.39 Property: mp 103-5°C. Source: BAI JIANG, SHAN ZHU YU. Ref: 2.

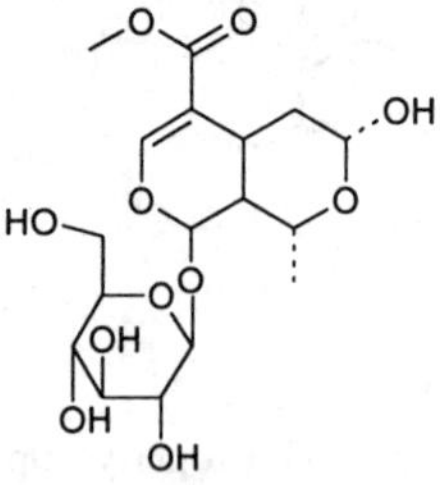

4503 Morusin
$C_{25}H_{26}O_5$ MW: 406.48 Source: SANG BAI PI. Ref: 6.

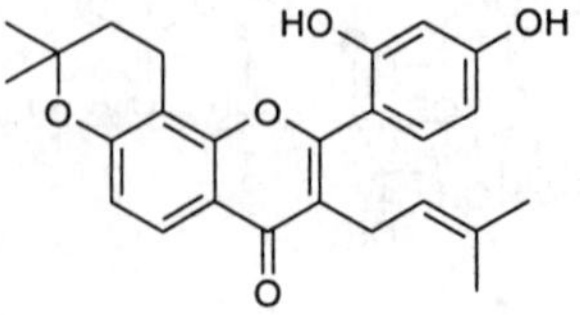

4504 Motin
CAS: 480-16-0 $C_{15}H_{10}O_7$ MW: 302.24 Property: mp 285-90°C (dec). Source: SANG ZHI. Ref: 4.

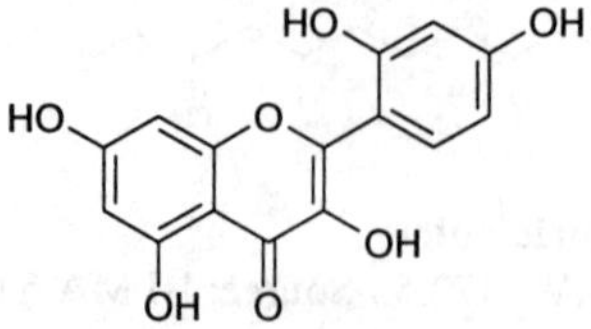

4505 Mubenin A
$C_{53}H_{86}O_{21}$ MW: 1059.26 Property: mp 255-9°C (dec). Source: YE MU GUA. Ref: 6.

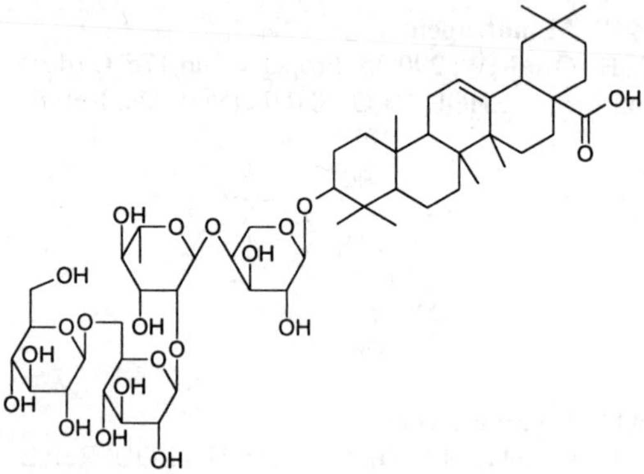

4506 Mubenin B
$C_{41}H_{66}O_{11}$ MW: 734.98 Property: mp 234-235°C (dec). Source: YE MU GUA. Ref: 6.

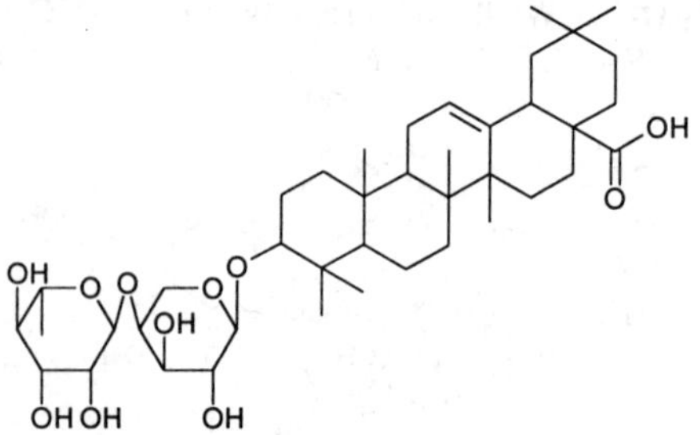

4507 Mucic acid
$C_6H_{10}O_8$ MW: 210.14 Property: mp 255°C. Source: AN MO LE. Ref: 6.

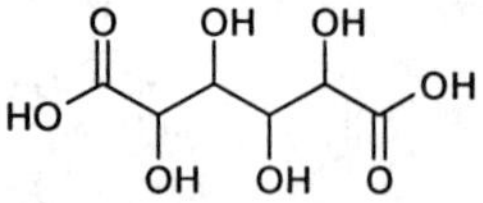

4508 Mucronatinine
$C_{18}H_{25}NO_6$ MW: 351.40 Property: mp 161-3°C. Source: XIANG LING CAO. Ref: 6.

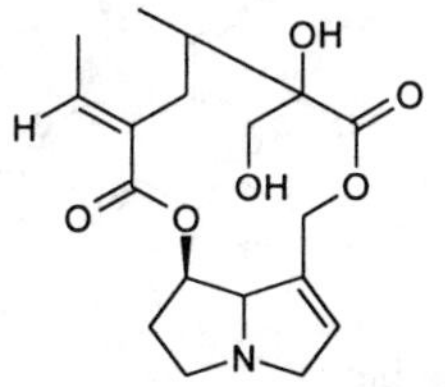

4509 3S-(-)Mucronulatol-7-D-glucopyranoside
$C_{23}H_{28}O_{10}$ MW: 464.47 Property: white acicular crystal, mp 167-9°C. Source: MENG GU HUANG QI. Ref: 167.

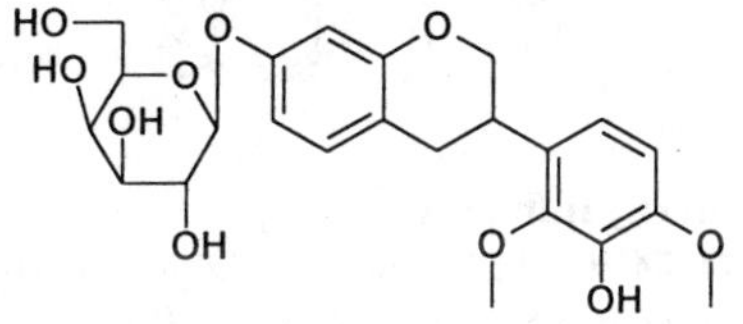

4510 Mulberrin
$C_{25}H_{26}O_6$ MW: 422.48 Property: mp 153-6°C. Source: SANG ZHI, SANG BAI PI. Ref: 6.

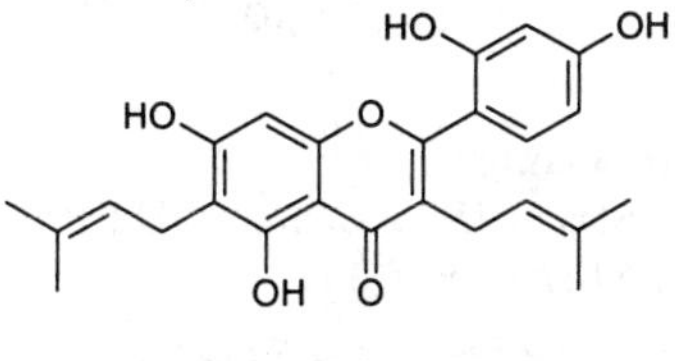

4511 Mulberrochromene
$C_{25}H_{24}O_6$ MW: 420.47 Property: mp 232-5°C. Source: SANG ZHI, SANG BAI PI. Ref: 6.

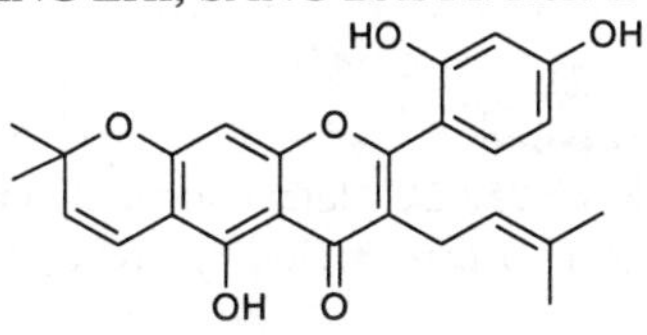

4512 Multiflorin A
Source: FENG WEI PA SHAN HU. Ref: 533.

4513 Multigilin
CAS: 64937-25-3 $C_{20}H_{24}O_6$ MW: 360.41 Source: BAI LAI SHI JU. Ref: 5.

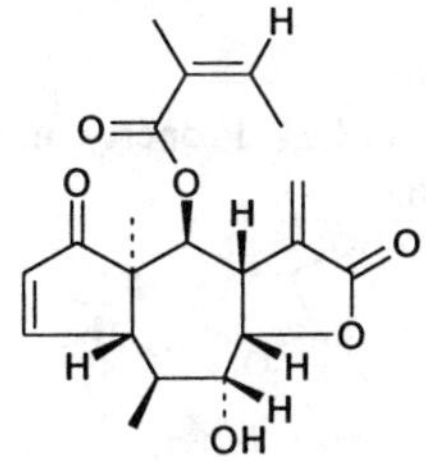

4514 Multiradiatin
CAS: 58262-52-5 $C_{20}H_{22}O_6$ MW: 358.39 Property: mp 226-30°C (dec). Source: BAI LAI SHI JU. Ref: 5.

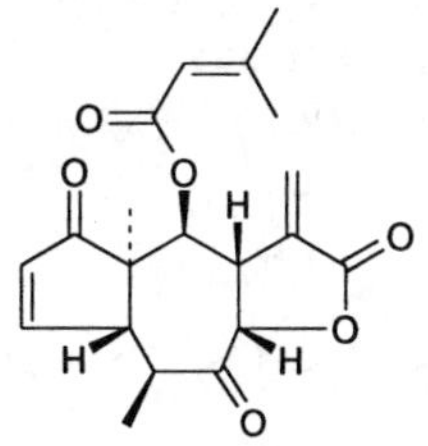

4515 Multistatin
CAS: 64937-26-4 $C_{20}H_{22}O_6$ MW: 358.39 Property: mp 257-60°C. Source: BAI LAI SHI JU. Ref: 5.

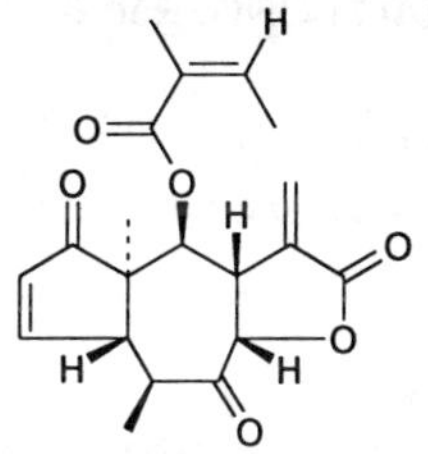

4516 Munjistin
$C_{15}H_8O_6$ MW: 284.23 Property: mp 229-30°C. Source: QIAN CAO GEN, YANG JIAO TENG. Ref: 6.

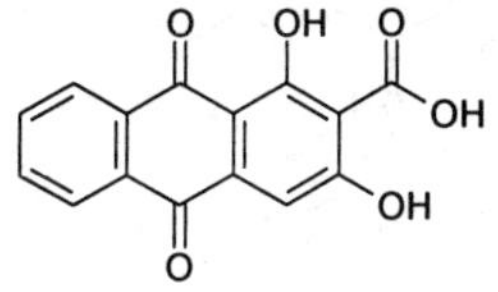

4517 Mupinensisone
$C_{30}H_{48}O_2$ MW: 440.72 Property: colorless acicular crystal (methanol), mp 230-231°C. Source: BAO XING WEI MAO. Ref: 278.

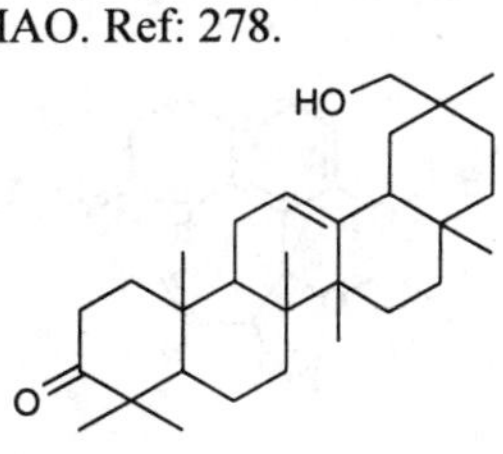

4518 Muricatalicin(I)
$C_{35}H_{64}O_8$ MW: 612.50 Property: white crystal, mp 105-6°C, $[\alpha]_D^{20}$ +17.7 (c=0.4, methanol). Source: CI GUO FAN LI ZHI. Ref: 385.

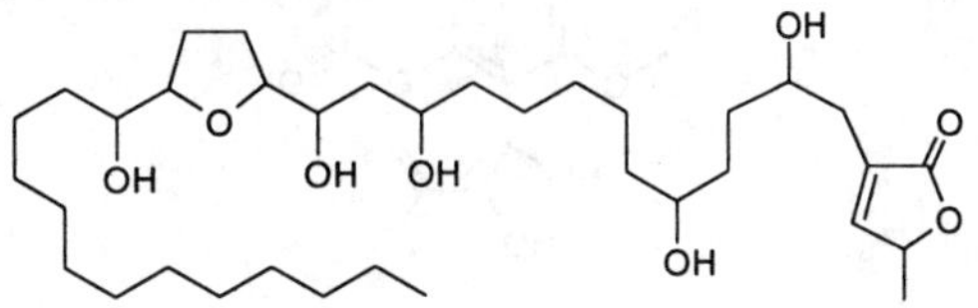

4519 Muricatalicin(VI)
$C_{35}H_{64}O_8$ MW: 612.90 Property: white crystal, mp 143-4°C, $[\alpha]_D^{16}$ +8.8 (c=0.06, methanol). Source: CI GUO FAN LI ZHI. Ref: 385.

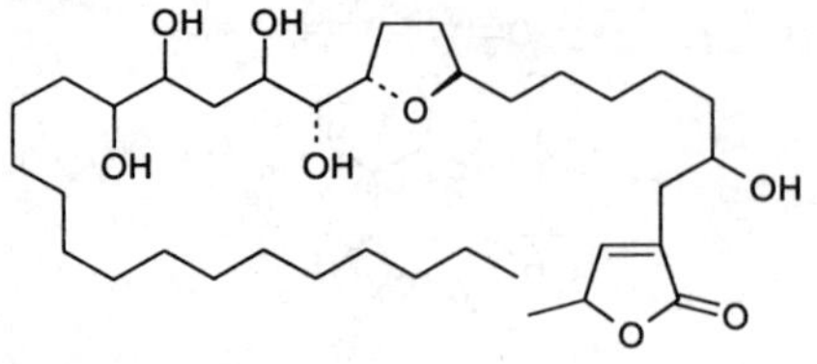

4520 Muricatin A
$C_{32}H_{60}O_{14}$ MW: 668.83 Property: mp 115-8°C. Source: WU ZHAO LONG. Ref: 6.

4521 Muricatin B
$C_{30}H_{54}O_{13}$ MW: 622.76 Source: WU ZHAO LONG. Ref: 6.

4522 Murisolin
$C_{35}H_{64}O_6$ MW: 580.90 Property: mp 62-4°C. Source: JIN PING GE NA XIANG, NIU XIN PAN LI ZHI. Ref: 420, 432.

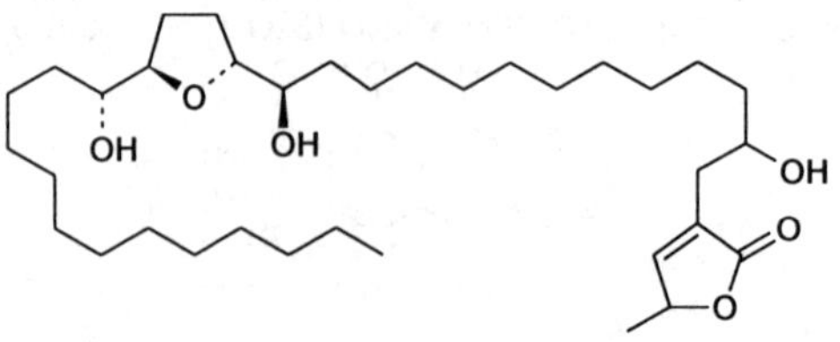

4524 Murpanicin
$C_{17}H_{20}O_5$ MW: 304.35 Source: JIU LI XIANG. Ref: 11.

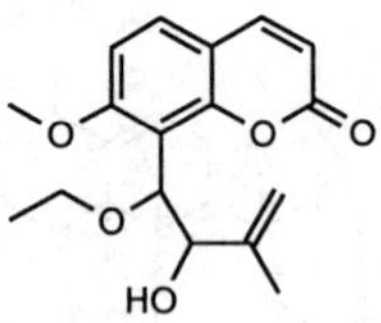

4525 Murpanidin (S)
$C_{15}H_{16}O_5$ MW: 276.29 Source: JIU LI XIANG. Ref: 11.

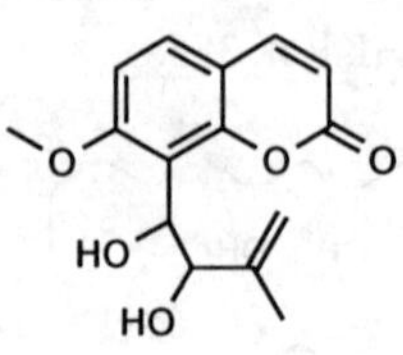

4526 Murralogin
$C_{15}H_{14}O_4$ MW: 258.28 Source: JIU LI XIANG. Ref: 11.

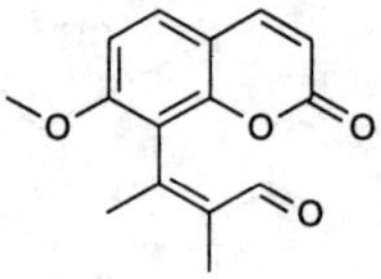

4527 Murrayacine
$C_{18}H_{15}NO_2$ MW: 277.33 Source: YIN DU JIU LI XIANG. Ref: 11.

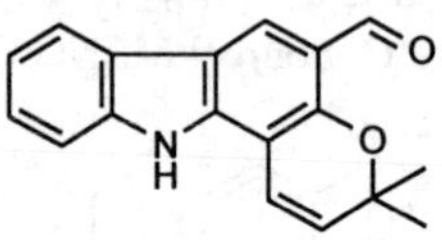

4528 Murrayafoline A
$C_{14}H_{13}NO$ MW: 211.27 Source: DOU YE JIU LI XIANG, TAI WAN JIU LI XIANG. Ref: 11.

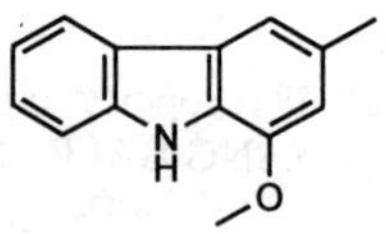

4529 Murrayanine
$C_{14}H_{11}NO$ MW: 225.25 Source: JIU LI XIANG, YIN DU JIU LI XIANG. Ref: 11.

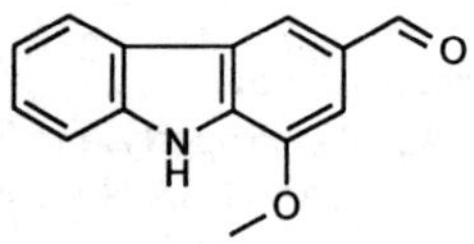

4530 Murrayone
$C_{15}H_{14}O_4$ MW: 258.28 Note: commonly in family *Rutaceae*, genus *Murraya*. Source: JIU LI XIANG. Ref: 11.

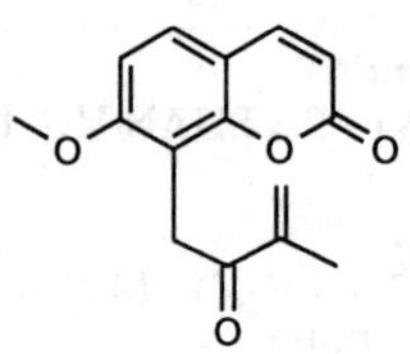

4531 Muscarine
$C_9H_{20}NO_2$ MW: 174.24 Property: mp 182°C. Source: MA HUA. Ref: 6.

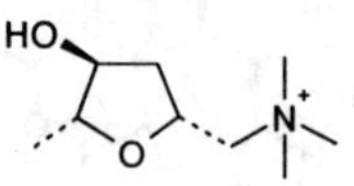

4532 Muscol

$C_{16}H_{32}O$ MW: 240.43 Source: SHE XIANG. Ref: 2.

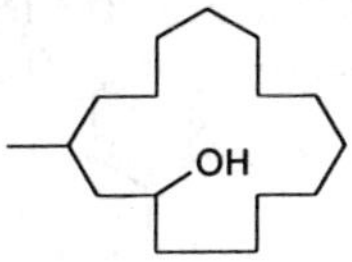

OH

4533 Muscone

$C_{16}H_{30}O$ MW: 238.42 Property: bp (-): 130°C/0.5 mm. Source: SHE XIANG. Ref: 2, 4, 6.

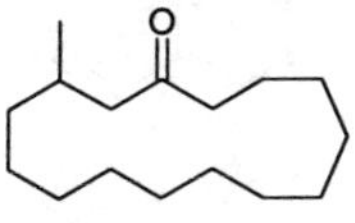

O

4534 Muscopyridine

$C_{16}H_{25}N$ MW: 231.38 Source: SHE XIANG. Ref: 2.

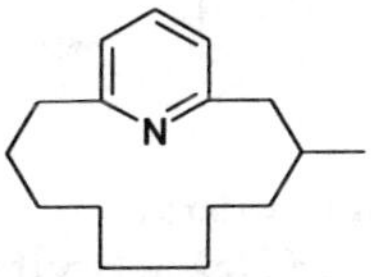

N

4535 Musizin-8-O-β-D-glucoside

$C_{19}H_{22}O_8$ MW: 378.38 Source: DA HUANG. Ref: 2.

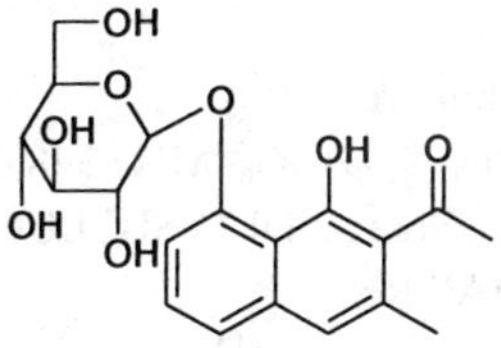

OH O OH OH O OH OH

4536 α-Muurolene

$C_{15}H_{24}$ MW: 204.36 Source: REN SHEN, SAN QI. Ref: 2.

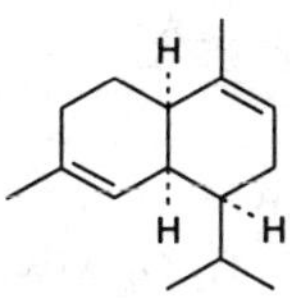

H H H

4537 Myoinositol

$C_6H_{12}O_6$ MW: 180.16 Property: mp 218-9°C. Source: DI JIN, DI JIN CAO, LI MU, MAO XU CAO, NAN ZHU YE, SANG YE, YANG MEI, YING SU KE. Ref: 6.

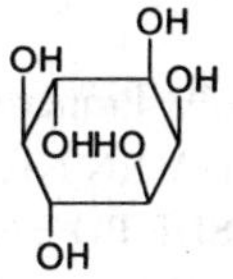

OH OH OH OHHO OH

4538 Myrcene

$C_{10}H_{16}$ MW: 136.24 Source: CHAI HU, DU HUO, JU PI, LIAN QIAO, MA HUANG, QIANG HUO, QING HAO, WU WEI ZI, XI XIN, YU XING CAO. Ref: 2.

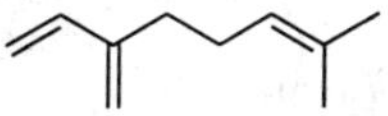

4539 Myricetin

Cannabiscetin; Myricetol. CAS: 529-44-2 $C_{15}H_{10}O_8$ MW: 318.24 Property: mp >330°C. Source: CU LIU GUO (SHA JI), XIAN CHI SHE PU TAO. Ref: 2, 4, 605.

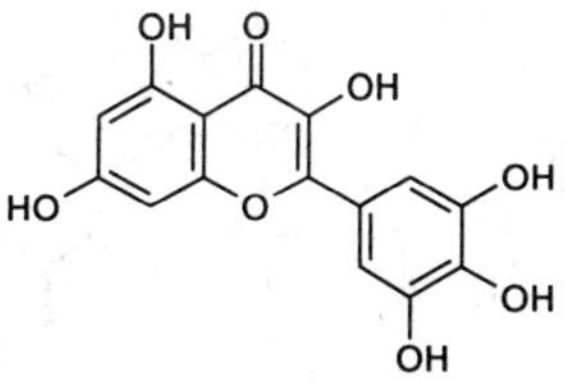

OH O OH HO O OH OH OH

4540 Myricetin-3-glucoside

$C_{21}H_{20}O_{13}$ MW: 480.39 Source: BAI FAN DOU. Ref: 6.

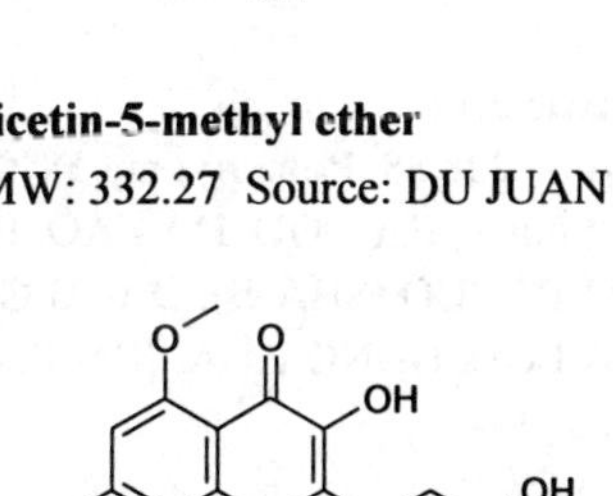

OH O O HO O OH HO O OH OH OH OH OH

4541 Myricetin-5-methyl ether

$C_{16}H_{12}O_8$ MW: 332.27 Source: DU JUAN HUA. Ref: 6.

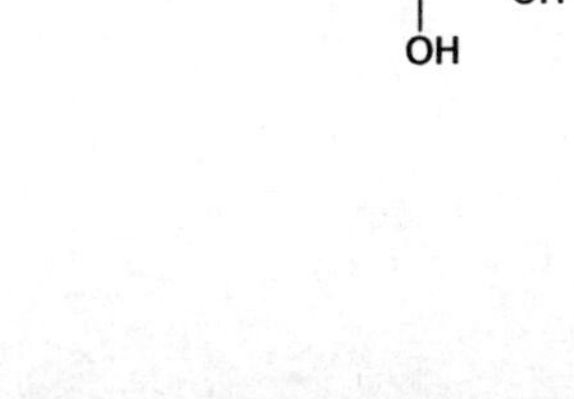

O O OH HO O OH OH OH

4542 Myricitrin

$C_{21}H_{20}O_{12}$ MW: 464.39 Property: mp 197-9°C (anhydrate). Source: DA JIN NIU CAO, FEI CAI, SHI YE, XIAN CHI SHE PU TAO, YANG MEI, YANG MEI SHU PI, ZI JIN NIU. Ref: 6, 605.

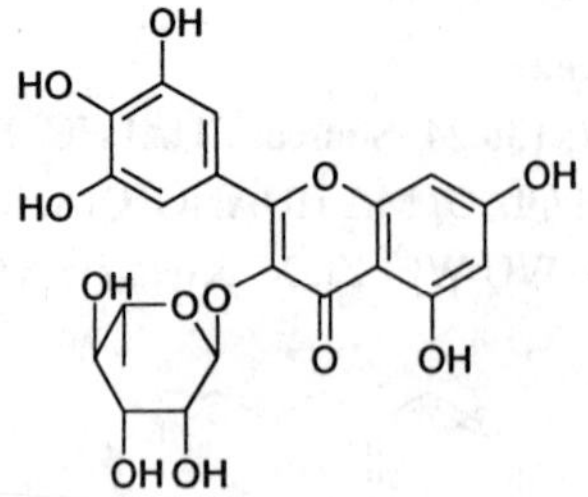

4543 Myricomplanoside

$C_{22}H_{22}O_{13}$ MW: 494.41 Property: yellow acicular crystal, mp 255-7°C. Source: BIAN JIN HUANG QI. Ref: 123.

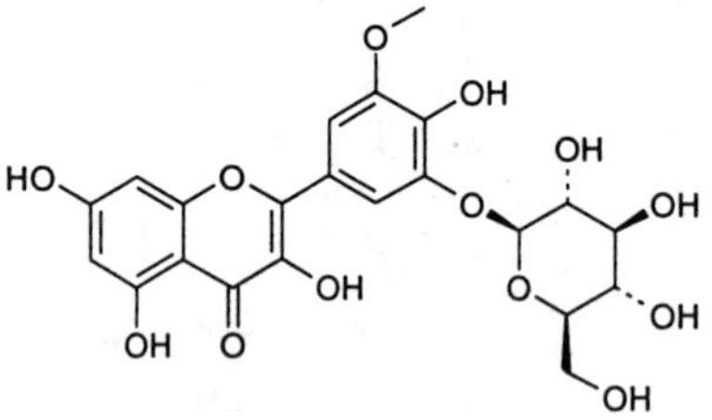

4544 Myricyl hypogaeate

$C_{46}H_{90}O_2$ MW: 675.23 Source: MI LA. Ref: 6.

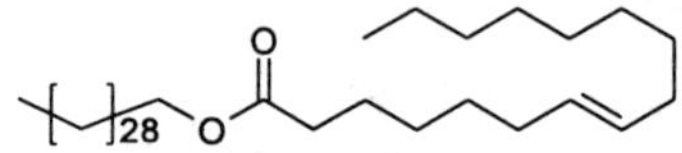

4545 Myricyl palmitate

$C_{46}H_{92}O_2$ MW: 677.24 Source: MI LA. Ref: 6.

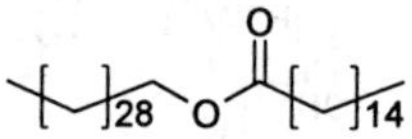

4546 Myristic acid

$C_{14}H_{28}O_2$ MW: 228.38 Property: mp 58°C, bp 250.5 °C/100mm. Source: BA DOU, DA ZAO, BING LANG, CU LIU GUO (SHA JI), DANG GUI, DANG SHEN, GUA LOU, HONG HUA, XIN JIANG GAO MU. Ref: 2, 333.

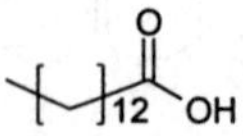

4547 Myristicin

$C_{11}H_{12}O_3$ MW: 192.22 Property: bp (+): 99-100°C/ 15mm, (-): 220-1°C. Source: XI XIN. Ref: 2.

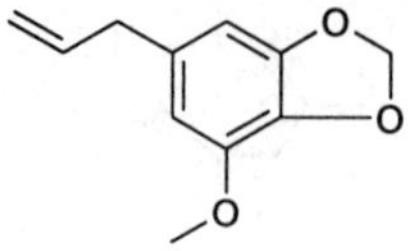

4548 Myrtenal

$C_{10}H_{14}O$ MW: 150.22 Source: DU HUO. Ref: 2.

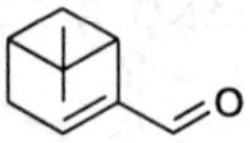

4549 Myrtenol

$C_{10}H_{16}O$ MW: 152.24 Property: bp (-): 221-2°C. Source: CHAI HU. Ref: 2.

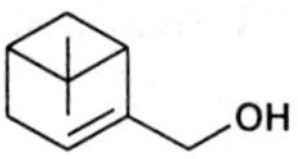

4550 l–Myrtenyl isovalerate

$C_{15}H_{24}O_2$ MW: 236.36 Source: XIE CAO. Ref: 6.

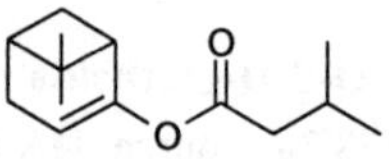

4551 Nagilactone A

CAS: 19891-50-0 $C_{19}H_{24}O_6$ MW: 348.40 Property: mp 305°C (sub). Source: DUO SUI LUO HAN SONG, ZHU BAI. Ref: 5.

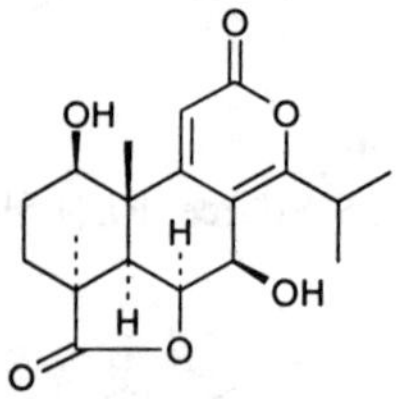

4552 Nagilactone B

CAS: 19891-51-1 $C_{19}H_{24}O_7$ MW: 364.40 Property: mp 258-61°C (dec). Source: ZHU BAI. Ref: 5.

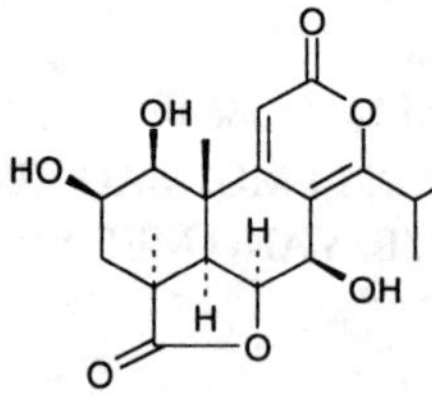

4553 Nagilactone C
CAS: 19891-53-2 $C_{19}H_{22}O_7$ MW: 362.38 Property: mp 325°C, 290°C (dec). Source: LUO HAN SONG SHI, ZHU BAI. Ref: 5, 6.

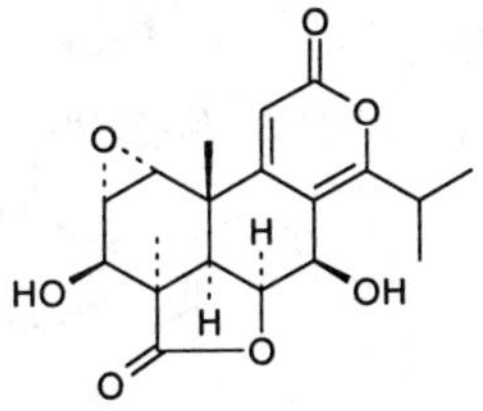

4554 Nagilactone D
CAS: 19891-53-3 $C_{18}H_{20}O_6$ MW: 332.36 Property: mp 265-6°C (dec). Source: ZHU BAI. Ref: 5.

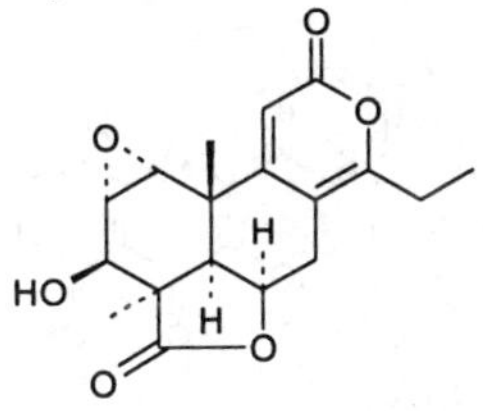

4555 Nagilactone E
CAS: 368.95-12-2 $C_{19}H_{24}O_6$ MW: 348.40 Source: *Podocarpus* sp. Ref: 5.

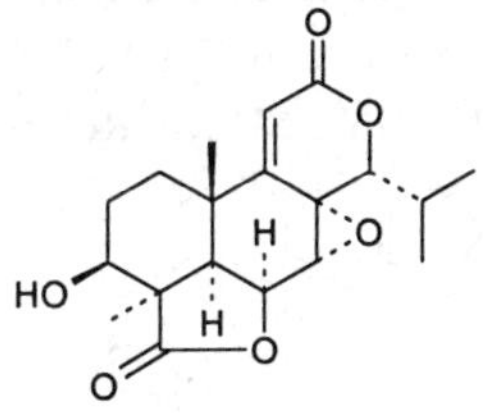

4556 Nagilactone F
CAS: 36912-00-2 $C_{19}H_{24}O_4$ MW: 316.40 Source: LUO HAN SONG SHI. Ref: 5, 6.

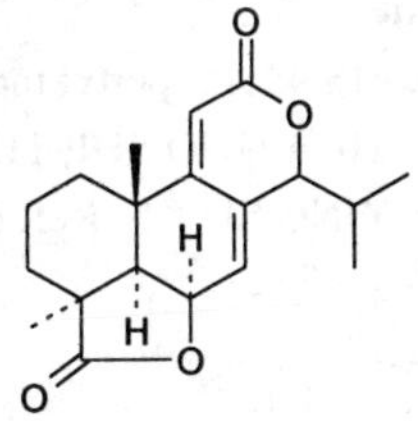

4557 Naginataketone
$C_{10}H_{12}O_2$ MW: 164.21 Property: bp 116-9°C/20mm. Source: BAN BIAN SU. Ref: 6.

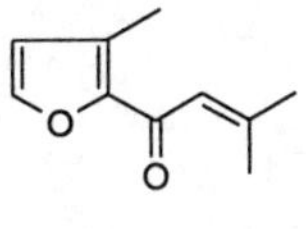

4558 α-Naginatene
$C_{10}H_{14}O$ MW: 150.22 Source: BAN BIAN SU. Ref: 6.

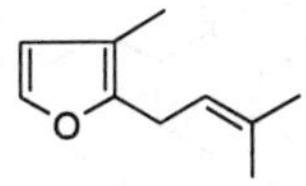

4559 β-Naginatene
$C_{10}H_{14}O$ MW: 150.22 Source: BAN BIAN SU. Ref: 6.

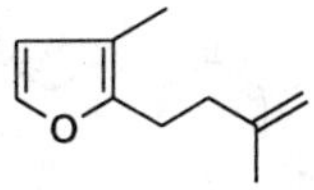

4560 Nandazurine
$C_{19}H_{13}NO_5$ MW: 335.32 Property: mp 250-1°C. Source: NAN TIAN ZHU GEN, NAN TIAN ZHU GENG. Ref: 6.

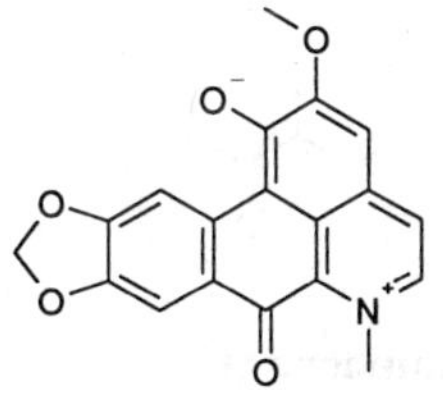

4561 Nandinine
$C_{19}H_{19}NO_4$ MW: 325.37 Property: mp 146°C. Source: NAN TIAN ZHU Z, NAN TIAN ZHU GEN. Ref: 6.

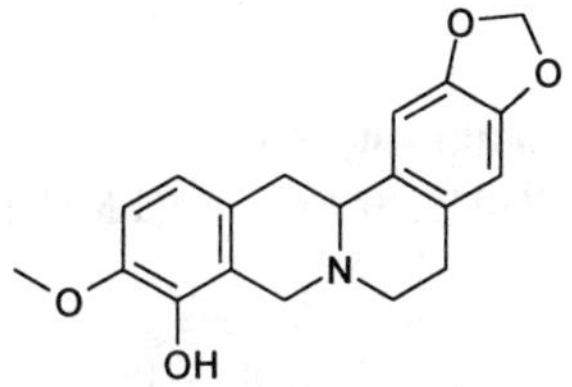

4562 β-Naphthaldehyde
$C_{11}H_8O$ MW: 156.19 Property: mp 59°C. Source: WU MU XIE. Ref: 6.

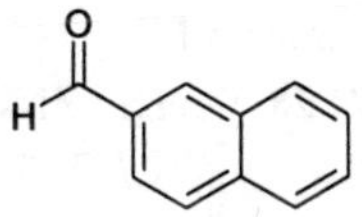

4563 Naphthalene
$C_{10}H_8$ MW: 128.18 Source: FANG FENG, XI XIN. Ref: 2.

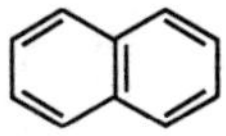

4564 Naphthoquinone I
$C_{15}H_{18}O_2$ MW: 230.31 Source: ZI MU. Ref: 6.

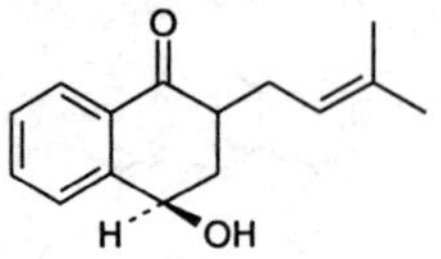

4565 Naphthoquinone II
$C_{15}H_{16}O_2$ MW: 228.29 Source: ZI MU. Ref: 6.

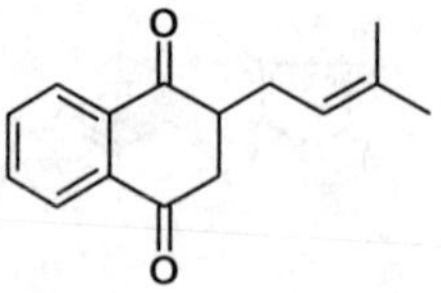

4566 Naphthoquinone III
$C_{15}H_{16}O_3$ MW: 244.29 Source: ZI MU. Ref: 6.

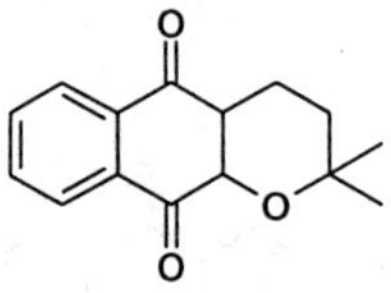

4567 Naphthoquinone IV
$C_{15}H_{14}O_4$ MW: 258.28 Source: ZI MU. Ref: 6.

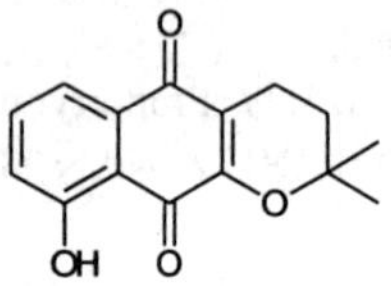

4568 Naphthoquinone V
$C_{16}H_{16}O_4$ MW: 272.30 Source: ZI MU. Ref: 6.

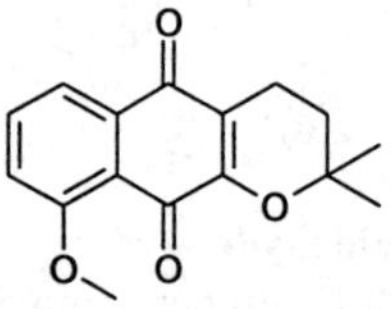

4569 Naphthoquinone VI
$C_{15}H_{14}O_5$ MW: 274.28 Source: ZI MU. Ref: 6.

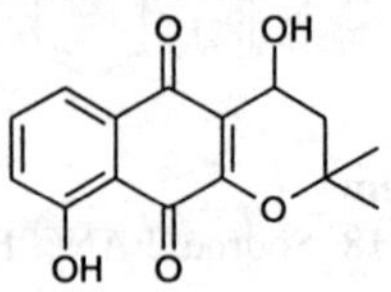

4570 Narceine
$C_{23}H_{27}NO_8$ MW: 445.47 Property: mp 145.2°C. Source: YA PIAN. Ref: 6.

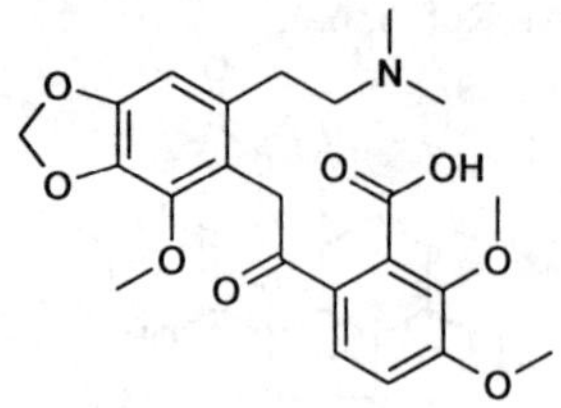

4571 Narcissin
$C_{28}H_{32}O_{16}$ MW: 624.56 Property: mp 174°C. Source: SHUI XIAN HUA, WU LA ER GAN CAO. Ref: 6, 231.

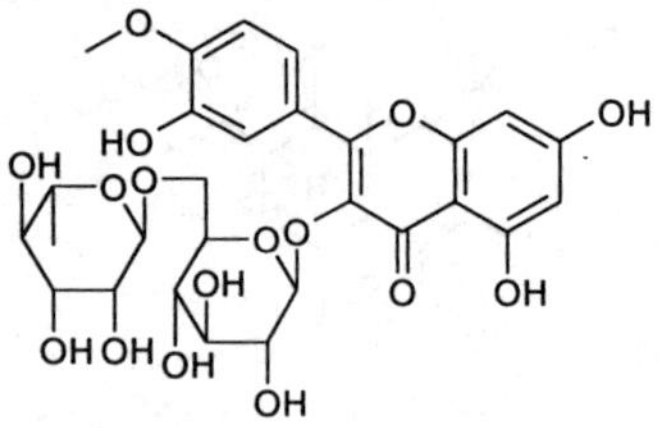

4572 α-Narcotine
$C_{22}H_{23}NO_7$ MW: 441.49 Property: mp 176°C. Source: LI CHUN HUA GUO SHI, TIAN CHEN, YA PIAN, YING SU, YING SU KE. Ref: 6.

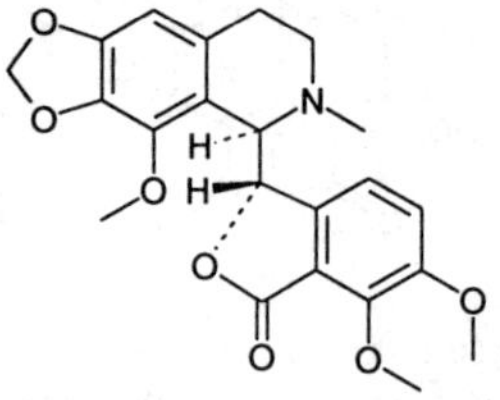

4573 β-Narcotine
$C_{22}H_{23}NO_7$ MW: 413.42 Property: mp 176°C. Source: LI CHUN HUA GUO SHI, TIAN CHEN, YA PIAN, YING SU, YING SU KE. Ref: 6.

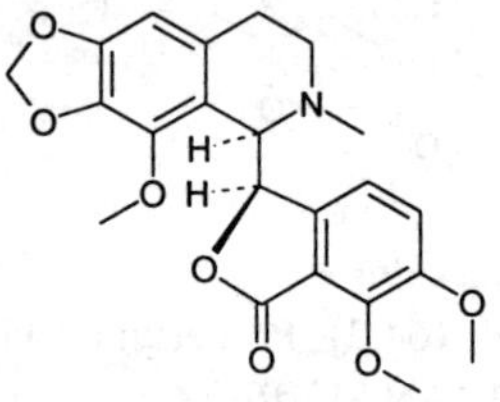

4574 Narcotoline
$C_{21}H_{21}NO_7$ MW: 399.40 Property: mp 202°C. Source: YA PIAN, YING SU KE. Ref: 6.

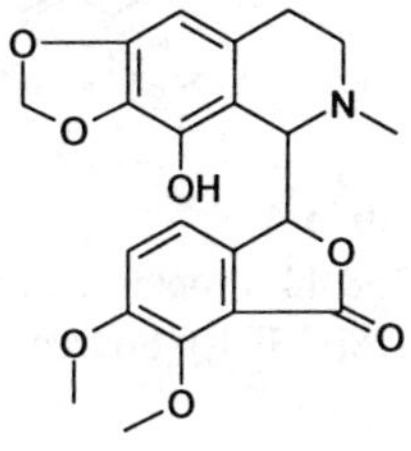

4575 Nardol
$C_{15}H_{26}O$ MW: 222.37 Property: bp 120-5°C/0.5 mm. Source: GAN SONG. Ref: 6.

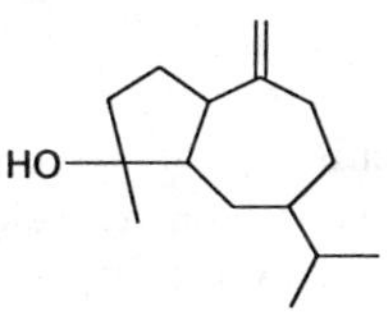

4576 Nardosinone
$C_{15}H_{22}O_3$ MW: 250.34 Property: mp 108-10°C. Source: GAN SONG. Ref: 6.

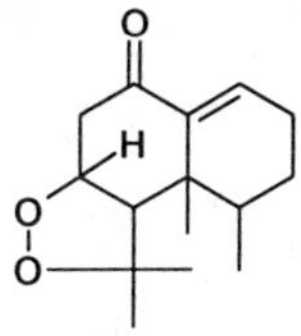

4577 Nardostachone
$C_{15}H_{20}O$ MW: 216.33 Property: bp 130-5°C/0.09 mm. Source: GAN SONG. Ref: 6.

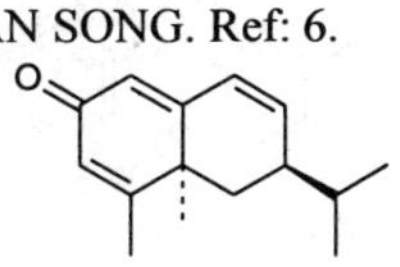

4578 Naringenin
5,7,4'-Trihydroxyflavanone. CAS: 480-41-1 $C_{15}H_{12}O_5$ MW: 272.26 Property: mp 251°C. Source: HU LU BA. PU ER CHA, PU HUANG, TAO YE, TAO HUA, TAO ZHI, TAO JING BAI PI. Ref: 4, 6, 581, 615.

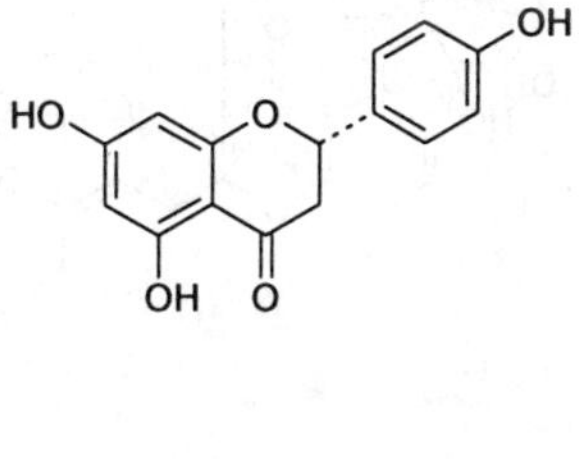

4579 Naringenin-4'-glucoside-7-neohesperidoside
$C_{33}H_{42}O_{19}$ MW: 742.69 Source: YOU. Ref: 6.

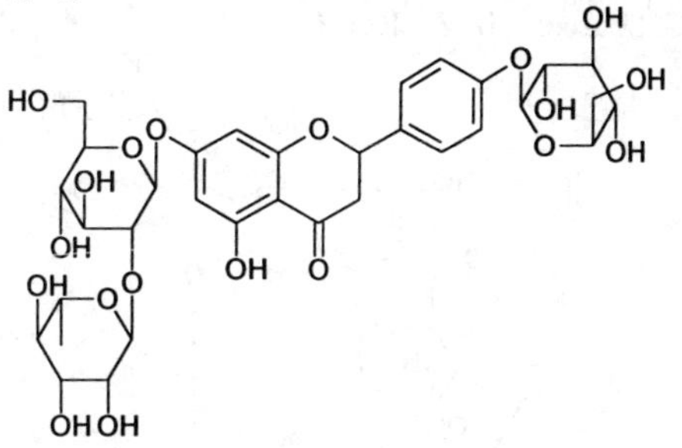

4580 Naringenin-4'-glucoside-7-rutinoside
$C_{33}H_{42}O_{21}$ MW: 774.69 Source: TIAN CHEN. Ref: 6.

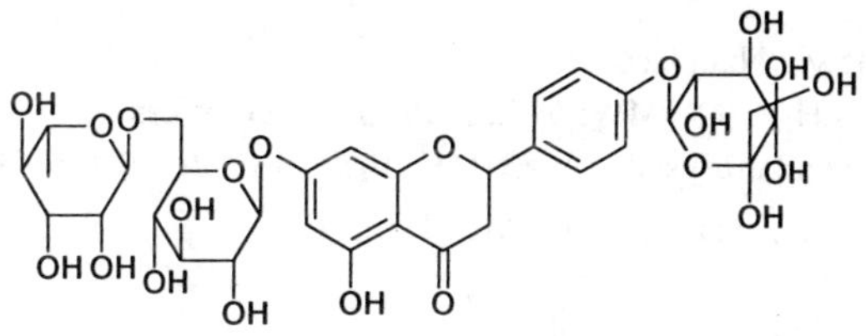

4581 Naringin
Aurantiin. CAS: 10236-47-2 $C_{27}H_{32}O_{14}$ MW: 580.55 Property: mp 82°C, 171°C. Source: GUAN ZHONG, GOU JU, GU SUI BU, NING MENG, TIAN JU, YOU, ZHI KE, ZHI SHI. Ref: 2, 4.

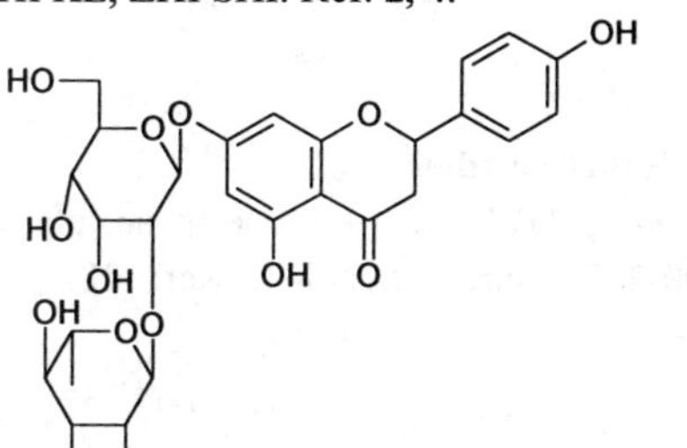

4582 Narirutin
$C_{27}H_{32}O_{14}$ MW: 580.55 Property: mp 160-5°C. Source: TIAN CHEN. Ref: 6.

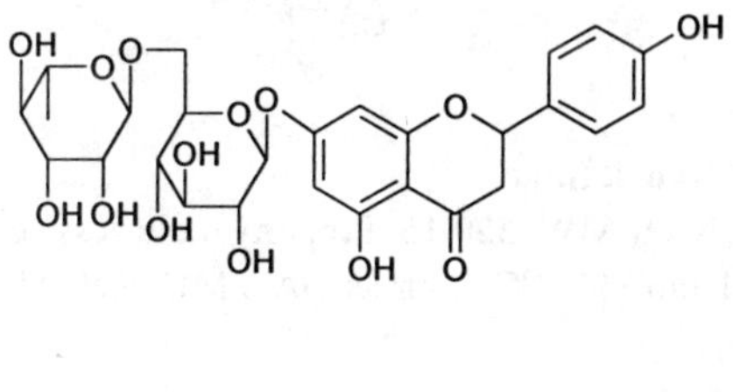

4583 Nasunin
$C_{42}H_{47}O_{23}$•Cl MW: 919.83•35.45 Property: mp 179-80°C. Source: QIE ZI. Ref: 6.

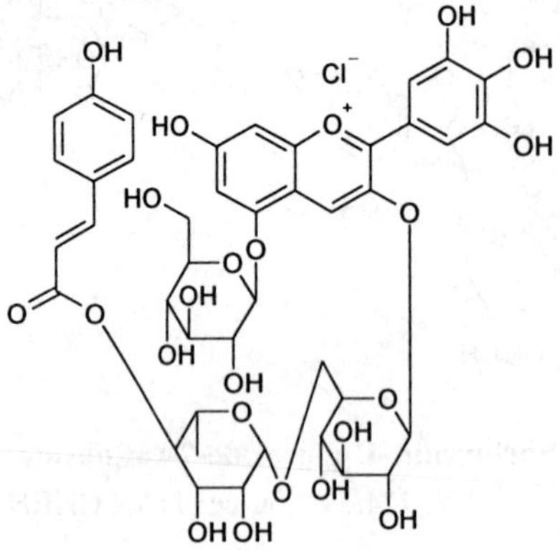

4584 Nauclecoside
$C_{26}H_{28}N_2O_9$ MW: 512.52 Property: colorless granular crystal, mp >310°C, $[\alpha]_D^{25}$ -149° (c= 0.1, 50% EtOH). Source: DAN MU. Ref: 118.

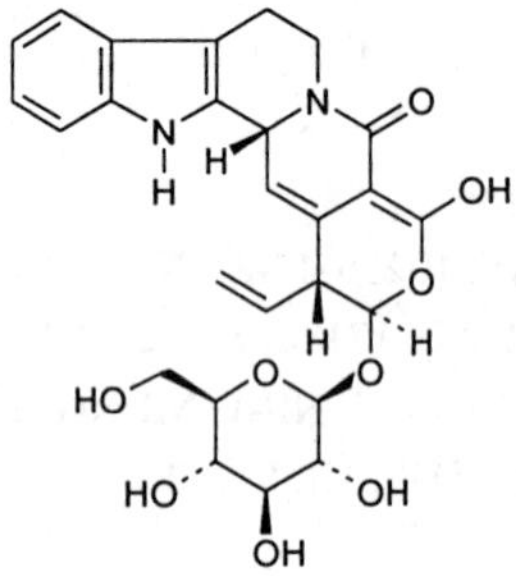

4585 Nauclecosidine
$C_{25}H_{26}N_2O_9$ MW: 498.49 Property: acicular crystal, mp 200-2°C. Source: DAN MU. Ref: 118.

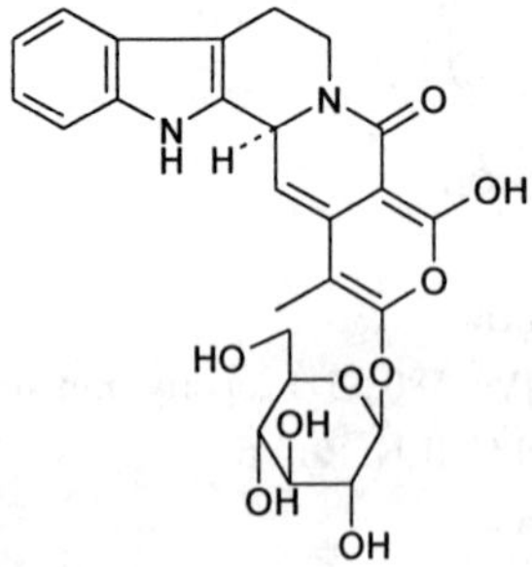

4586 Nauclefiline
$C_{20}H_{20}N_2O_2$ MW: 320.15 Property: colorless acicular crystal, mp 315-7°C. Source: DAN MU. Ref: 41.

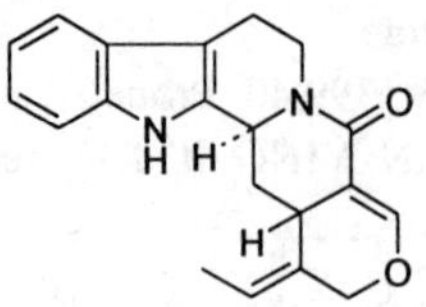

4587 (-)-Nectandrin A
$C_{21}H_{26}O_5$ MW: 358.44 Property: colorless oleaginous substance, $[\alpha]_D^{25}$ -28($CHCl_3$). Source: DUAN JU. Ref: 424.

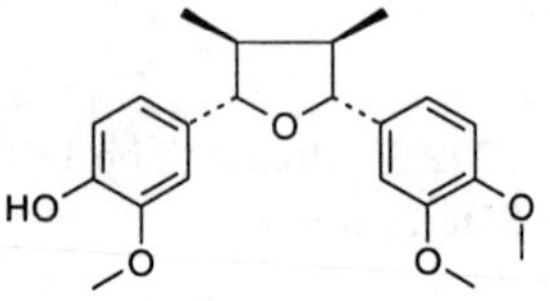

4588 Nectandrin B
$C_{20}H_{24}O_5$ MW: 344.41 Property: colorless oleaginous substance. Source: DUAN JU. Ref: 424.

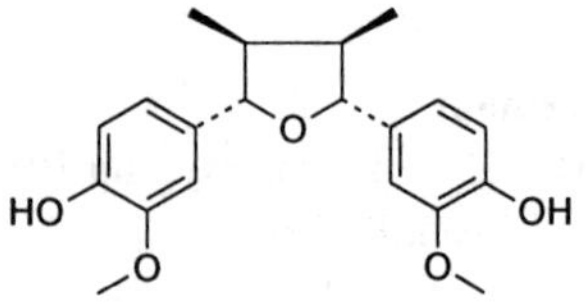

4589 Neferine
$C_{38}H_{44}N_2O_6$ MW: 624.78 Source: LIAN ZI XIN. Ref: 6.

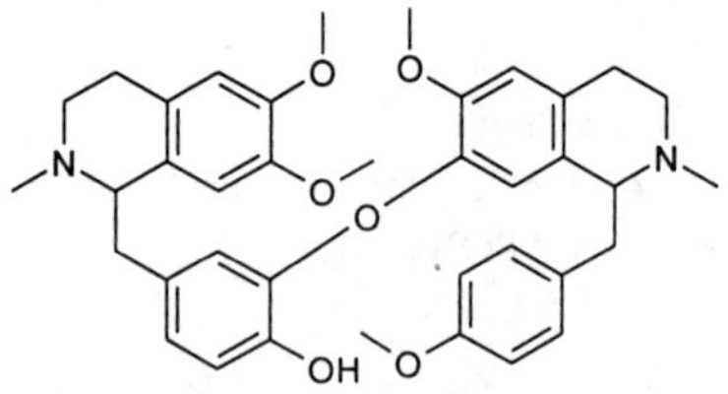

4590 Nelumboside
$C_{27}H_{28}O_{18}$ MW: 640.51 Property: mp 174-5°C. Source: HUI XIANG JING YE, HE YE. Ref: 6.

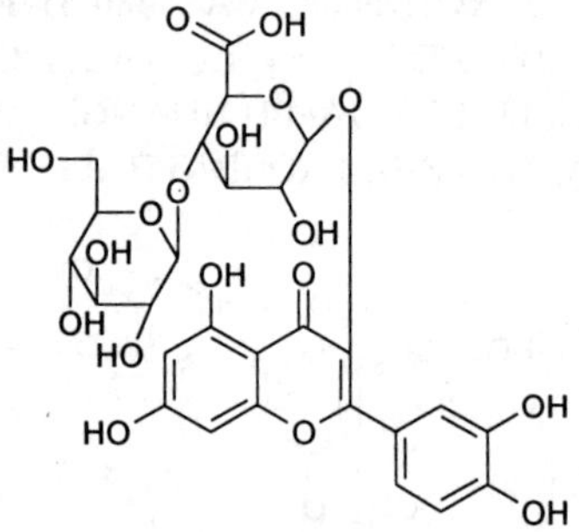

4591 Nematocyphol acetate IV
$C_{32}H_{52}O_2$ MW: 468.77 Property: white lamellar crystal, mp 264-5°C, $[\alpha]_D^{21}$ 0° (c=0.049, chloroform). Source: DA LANG DU. Ref: 232.

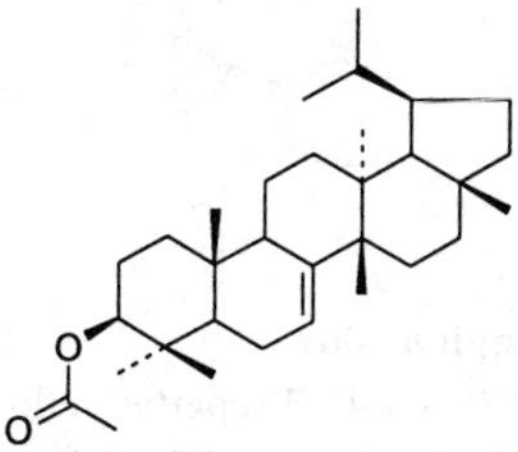

4592 cis-Neoabienol
$C_{20}H_{34}O$ MW: 290.49 Source: HAI SONG ZI. Ref: 6.

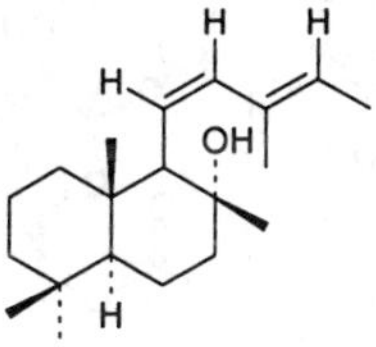

4593 Neoandrographolide
$C_{26}H_{40}O_8$ MW: 480.60 Property: mp 168-9°C. Source: CHUAN XIN LIAN. Ref: 2.

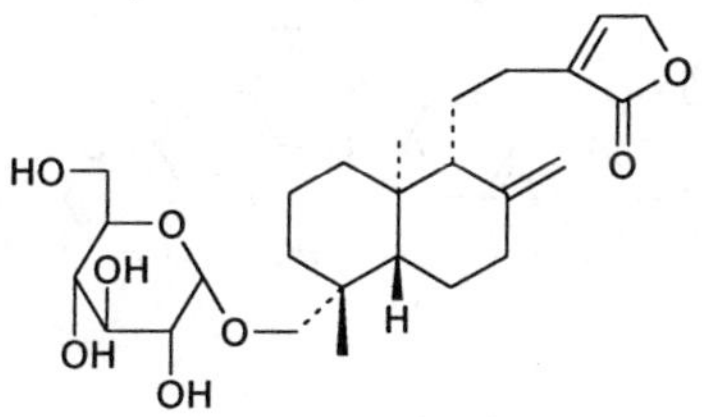

4594 Neoarctin B
$C_{42}H_{46}O_{12}$ MW: 742.83 Property: light yellow amorphous powder, mp 102-3.5°C, $[\alpha]_D^{15}$ -46.86° (c=0.083, $CHCl_3$). Source: NIU BANG ZI. Ref: 288.

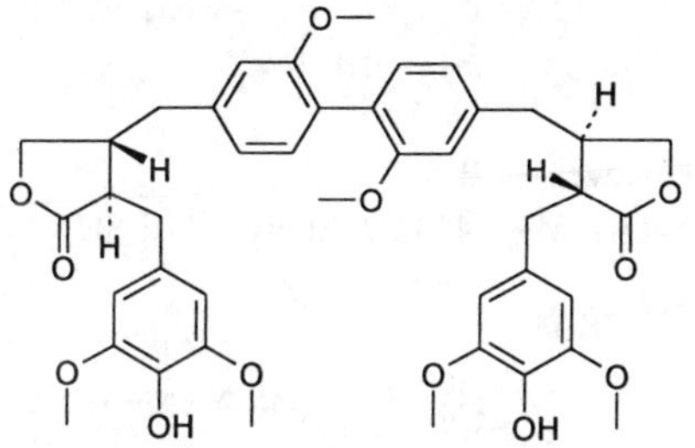

4595 Neoaristolacton
$C_{15}H_{20}O_2$ MW: 232.33 Property: white acicular crystal, mp 138-40°C, $[\alpha]_D^{15}$ +38° (c=1.0, ethanol). Source: MIAN MAO MA DOU LING. Ref: 215.

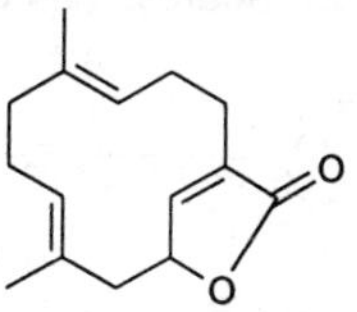

4596 Neobavachalcone
$C_{17}H_{14}O_5$ MW: 298.30 Source: BU GU ZHI. Ref: 2, 630.

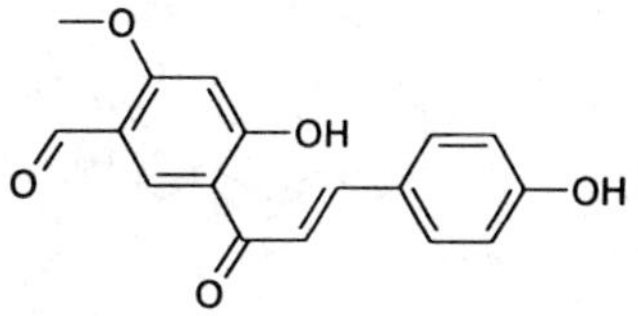

4597 Neobavaisoflavone
$C_{20}H_{18}O_4$ MW: 322.36 Source: BU GU ZHI. Ref: 2, 630.

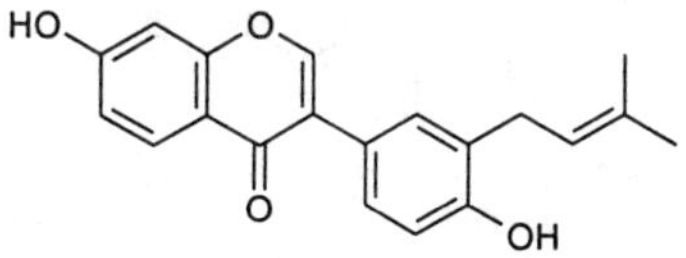

4598 Neobudofficide
5,7-Dihydroxy-4'-methoxyflavone-7-O-α-L-rhamnopyranosyl-(1→2)-[α-L-rhamnopyranosyl-(1→6)]-β-D-glucopyranoside. $C_{34}H_{42}O_{18}$ MW: 738.70 Property: light yellow powder, mp 180-2 °C. Source: MI MENG HUA. Ref: 369.

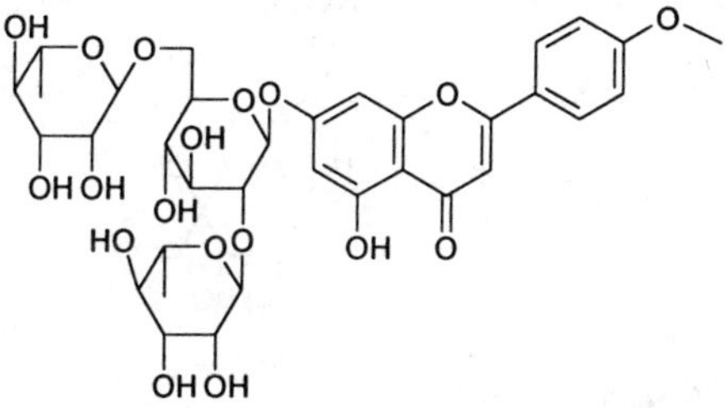

4599 Neobyakangelicol
$C_{17}H_{16}O_6$ MW: 316.31 Property: mp 106-7°C. Source: BAI ZHI. Ref: 2.

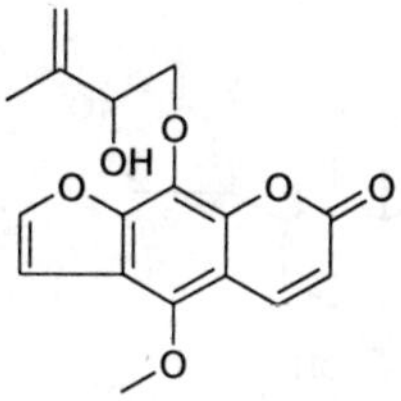

4600 Neocapillene
$C_{12}H_{10}$ MW: 154.21 Source: YIN CHEN HAO. Ref: 2.

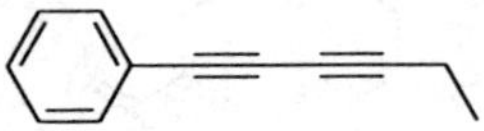

4601 Neo-β-carotene B
$C_{40}H_{56}$ MW: 536.89 Source: BO CAI. Ref: 6.

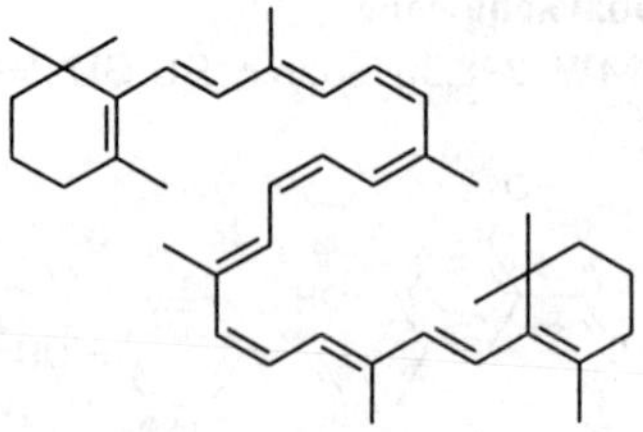

4602 Neocarthamin
$C_{21}H_{22}O_{11}$ MW: 450.40 Source: HONG HUA. Ref: 2.

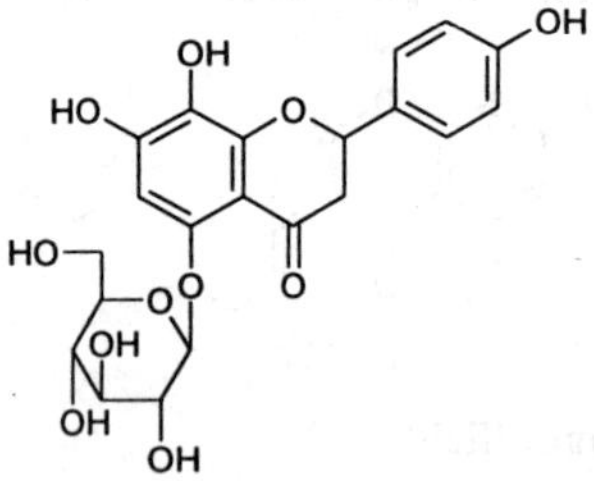

4603 Neochlorogenic acid
$C_{16}H_{18}O_{9}$ MW: 354.32 Property: mp 218-9°C. Source: BIAN YE TIE XIAN JUE, MENG GU SHAN LUO BO, SHA ZAO, TANG LI, XIANG RI KUI YE, XIANG RI KUI JING SUI. Ref: 6.

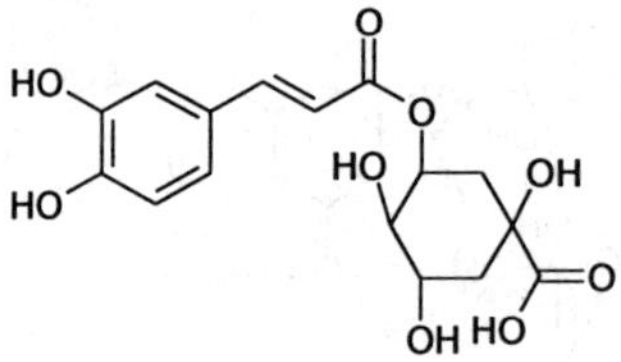

4604 Neochlorogenin
$C_{27}H_{44}O_{4}$ MW: 432.65 Property: mp 269-70°C. Source: XIA YE LONG SHE LAN. Ref: 10.

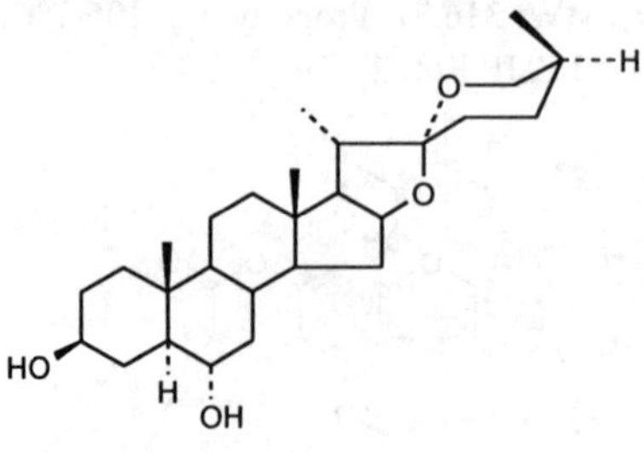

4605 Neocnidilide
$C_{12}H_{18}O_{2}$ MW: 194.27 Property: mp 24-7°C, bp 147-8°C/4mm. Source: CHA XIONG, CHUAN XIONG. Ref: 2, 531.

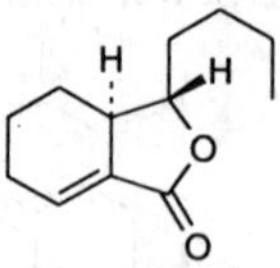

4606 Neocomplanoside
$C_{24}H_{24}O_{12}$ MW: 504.45 Property: yellow acicular crystal, mp 217-9°C. Source: BIAN JIN HUANG QI. Ref: 123.

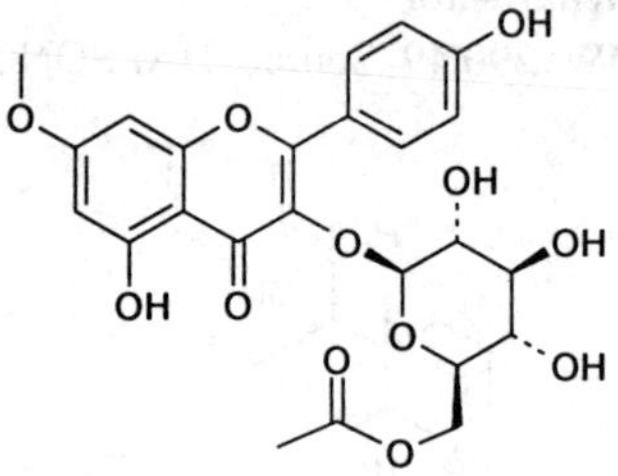

4607 Neocryptomerin
$C_{31}H_{20}O_{10}$ MW: 552.50 Source: LUO HAN SONG YE. Ref: 6.

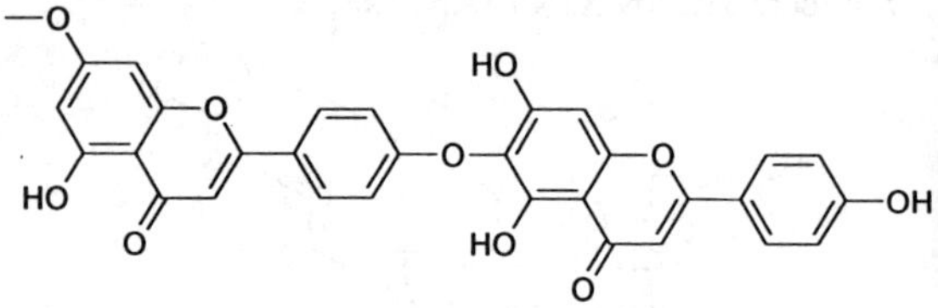

4608 Neocycasin A
$C_{14}H_{26}N_{2}O_{12}$ MW: 414.37 Source: TIE SHU GUO. Ref: 6.

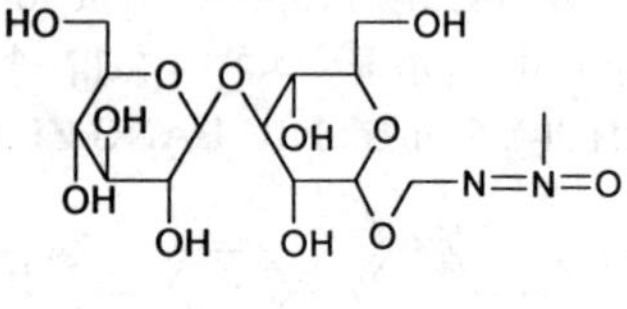

4609 Neocycasin B
$C_{14}H_{26}N_{2}O_{12}$ MW: 414.37 Source: TIE SHU GUO. Ref: 6.

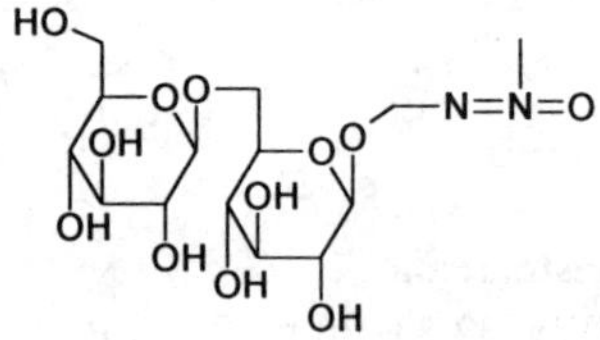

4610 Neocycasin C
$C_{20}H_{36}N_2O_{17}$ MW: 576.51 Source: TIE SHU GUO. Ref: 6.

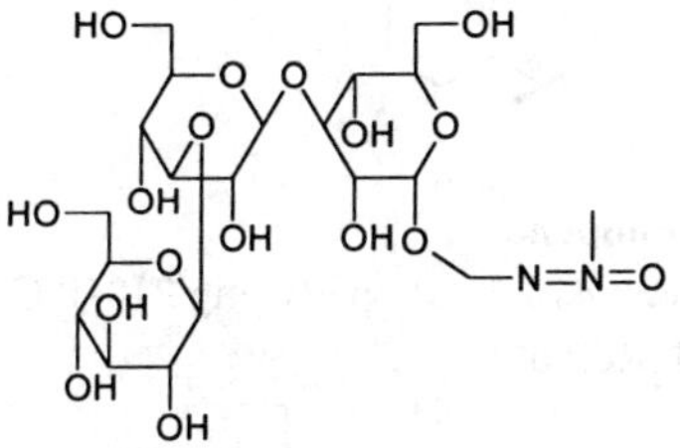

4611 Neocycasin D
$C_{26}H_{46}N_2O_{22}$ MW: 738.66 Source: TIE SHU GUO. Ref: 6.

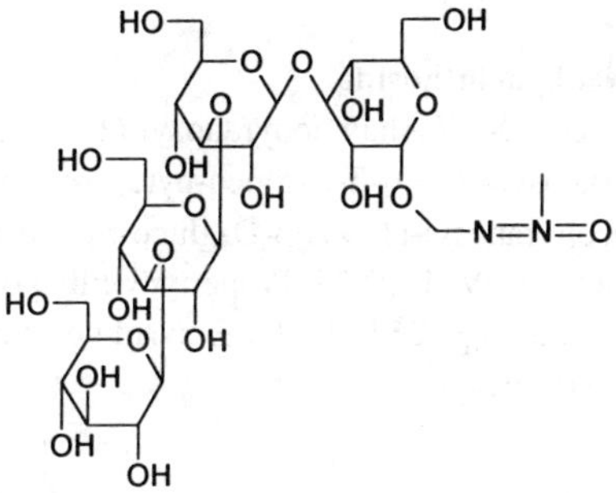

4612 Neocycasin E
$C_{14}H_{28}N_2O_{12}$ MW: 416.39 Source: TIE SHU GUO. Ref: 6.

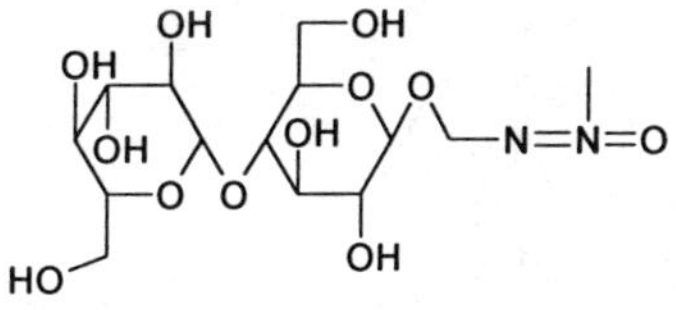

4613 Neocycasin F
$C_{20}H_{36}N_2O_{17}$ MW: 576.51 Source: TIE SHU GUO. Ref: 6.

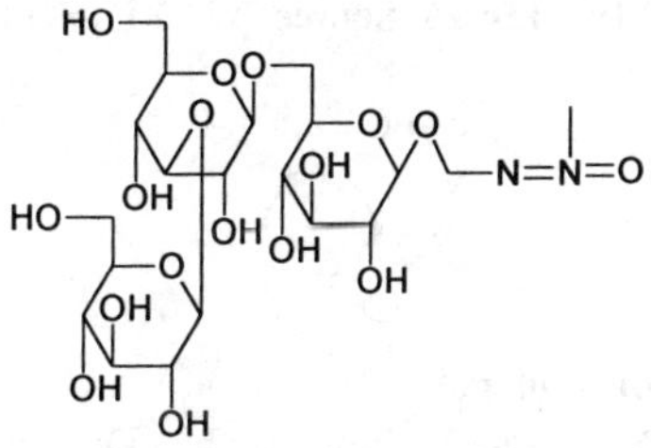

4614 Neocycasin G
$C_{20}H_{36}N_2O_{17}$ MW: 576.51 Source: TIE SHU GUO. Ref: 6.

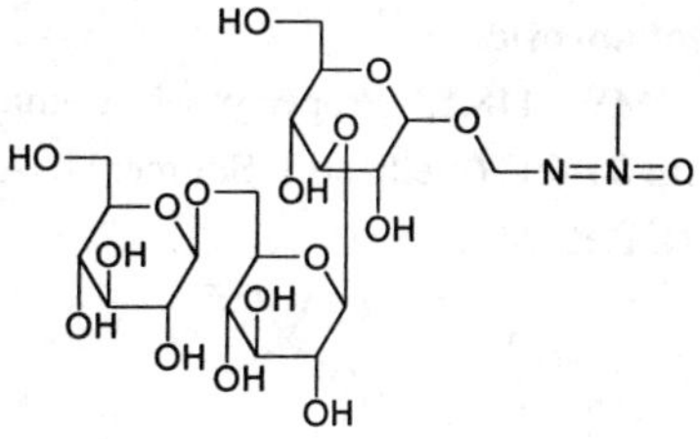

4615 Neodiospyrin
$C_{22}H_{14}O_6$ MW: 374.35 Property: mp 253-4°C. Source: SHI GEN. Ref: 6.

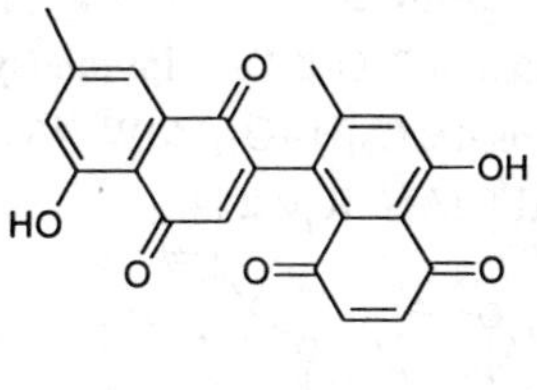

4616 A'-Neogammacer-22(29)-en-3β-ol(18β,21α)
Property: mp 209-11°C. Source: DA LANG DU. Ref: 547.

4617 Neogitogenin
$C_{27}H_{44}O_4$ MW: 432.65 Source: ZHI MU. Ref: 2.

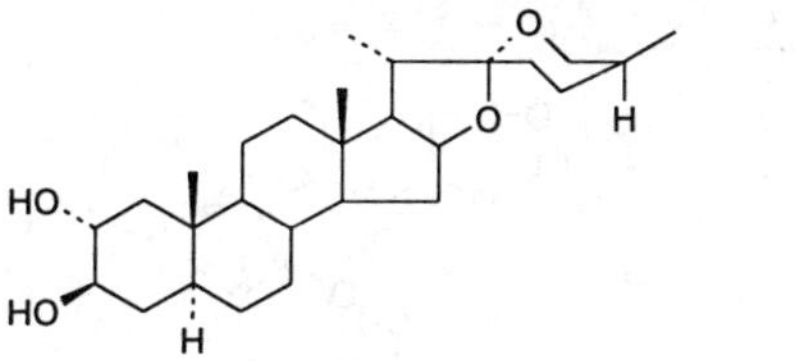

4618 Neoglucobrassicin
$C_1H_{21}N_2O_{10}S_2$ MW: 477.49 Source: DA QING YE. Ref: 2.

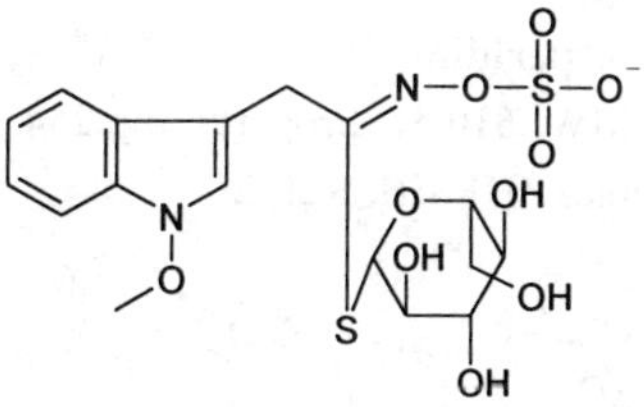

4619 Neoglycyrol
$C_{21}H_{18}O_6$ MW: 366.37 Property: light yellow acicular crystal, mp 263-5°C. Source: WU LA ER GAN CAO. Ref: 181.

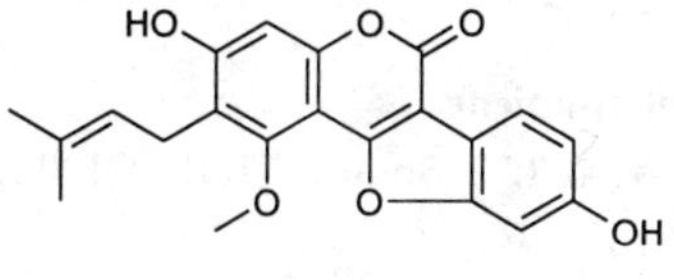

4620 Neohancoside A
$C_{21}H_{36}O_{10}$ MW: 448.52 Property: white amorphous powder, mp 84-6°C (methanol). Source: HUA BEI BAI QIAN. Ref: 244.

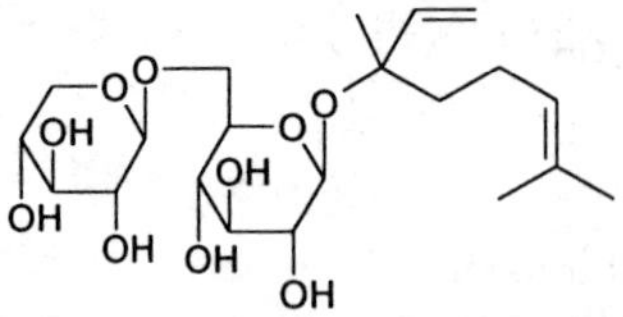

4621 Neohancoside B
8-Hydroxy-linalool-3-O-β-D-xylpyranosyl(1→6)-β-D-glucopyranoside. $C_{21}H_{36}O_{11}$ MW: 464.51 Source: HUA BEI BAI QIAN. Ref: 244.

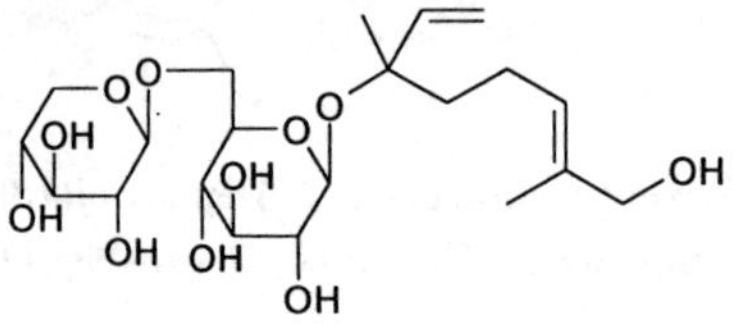

4622 Neoharringtonine
$C_{30}H_{31}NO_8$ MW: 533.58 Source: SAN JIAN SHAN. Ref: 2.

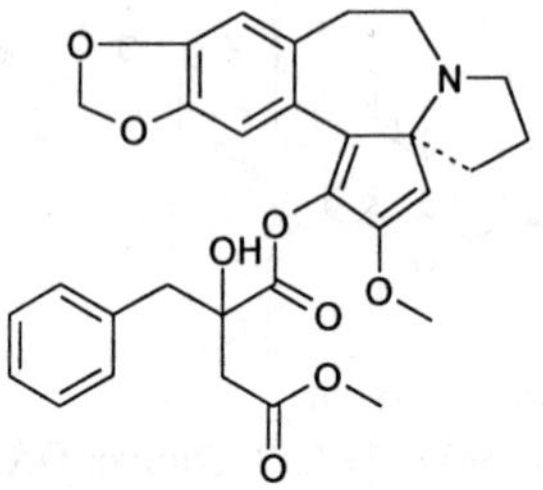

4623 Neohesperidin
$C_{28}H_{34}O_{15}$ MW: 610.57 Property: mp 234-5°C, 244°C. Source: ZHI SHI. Ref: 2.

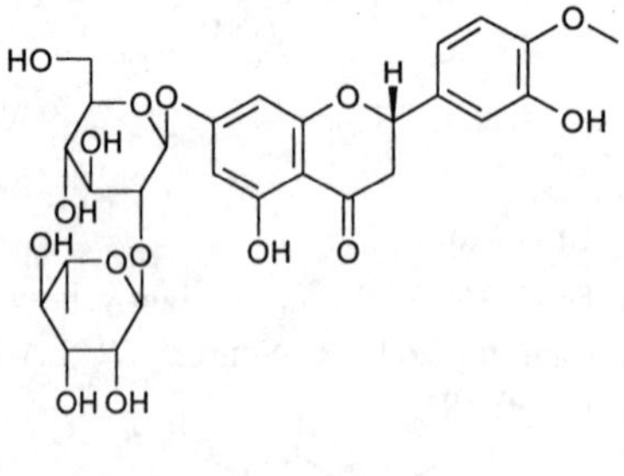

4624 Neohopadiene
$C_{30}H_{48}$ MW: 408.72 Source: TIE SI QI. Ref: 6.

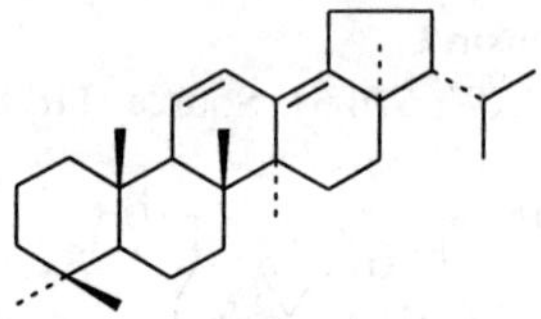

4625 Neohopene
$C_{30}H_{50}$ MW: 410.73 Property: mp 210-1°C. Source: TIE SI QI. Ref: 6.

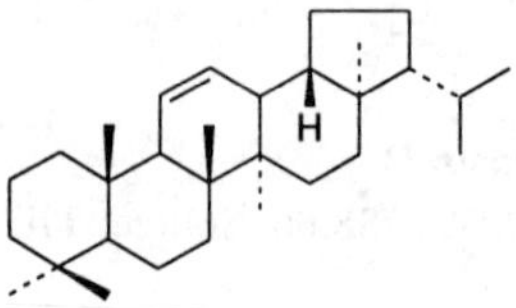

4626 Neohyacinthoside
Solanidine-3-O-α-L-rhamnopyranosyl-(1→2)-[β-D-glucopyranosyl-(1→6)-β-D-gluco-pyranosyl-(1→3)-β-D-glucopyranosyl-(1→4)]β-D-gluco-pyranoside. $C_{57}H_{92}NO_{25}$ MW: 1192.37 Property: white powder, mp 262-5°C, $[\alpha]_D^{20}$ -25.9° (c=0.29, pyridine). Source: JIA BAI HE. Ref: 93.

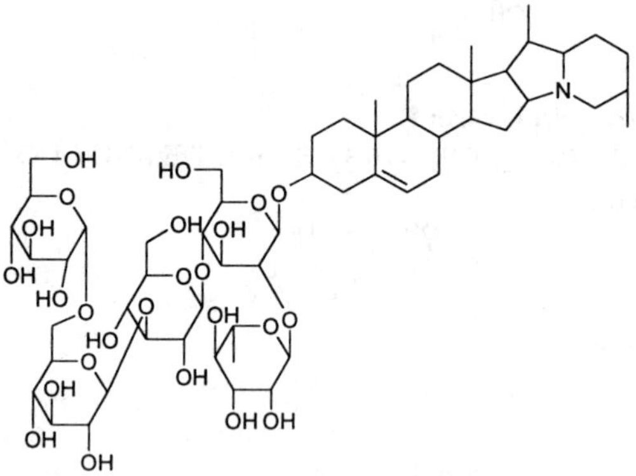

4627 Neoisoisopulegol
$C_{10}H_{18}O$ MW: 154.25 Source: YU XIANG CAO. Ref: 6.

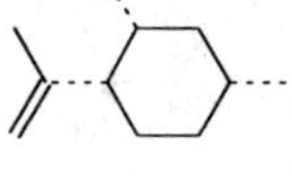

4628 Neoisopulegol
$C_{10}H_{18}O$ MW: 154.25 Property: bp (+): 95°C/17 mm. Source: YU XIANG CAO. Ref: 6.

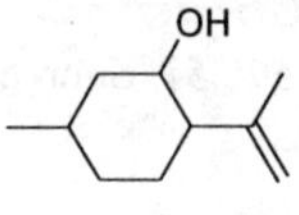

4629 Neoisoliquiritin

Isoliquiritigenin-4-β-glucoside. $C_{21}H_{22}O_9$ MW: 418.40 Property: mp 228-30°C. Source: GAN CAO. Ref: 2.

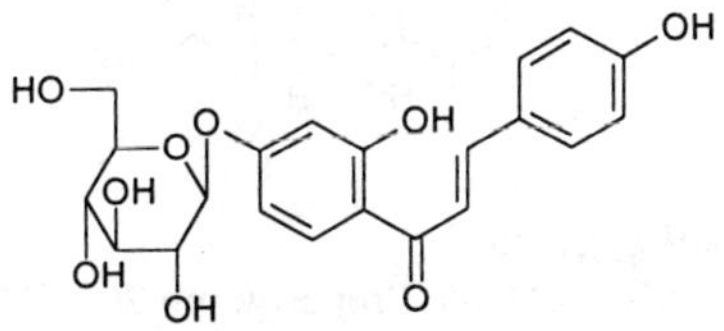

4630 Neoisorutin

$C_{27}H_{30}O_{16}$ MW: 610.53 Source: LUO BU MA, PAO NANG CAO. Ref: 6.

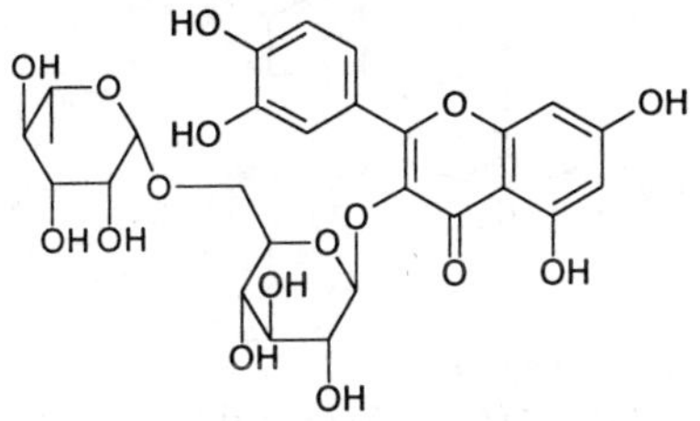

4631 Neojiangyouaconitine

Aconitane-13,14,15-trihydroxyl,20-ethyl-1,6,8,16-tetramethoxy-4-(methoxymethyl)-14-benzoate (1α,6α,14α,15α,16β). $C_{33}H_{47}NO_9$ MW: 601.74 Property: white lamellar crystal, mp 201-4°C, $[\alpha]_D^{14.4}$ -9.46° (c=0.22, methanol). Source: JIANG YOU FU ZI. Ref: 239.

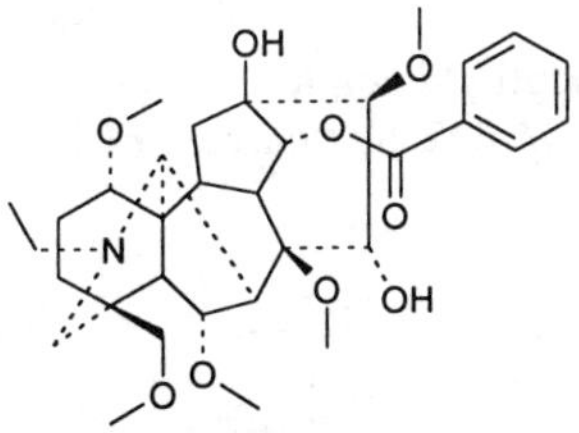

4632 Neojusticin A

$C_{21}H_{14}O_7$ MW: 378.34 Property: mp 273-5°C. Source: JUE CHUANG. Ref: 6.

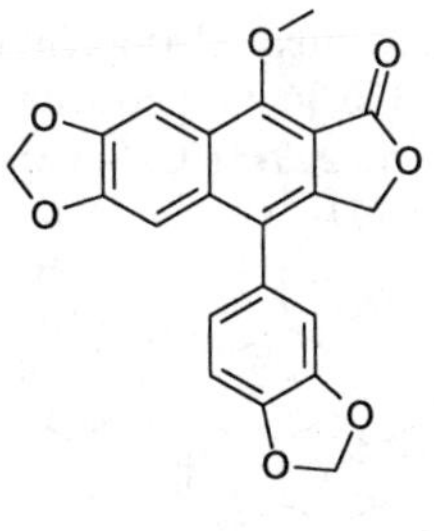

4633 Neojusticin B

$C_{22}H_{18}O_7$ MW: 394.38 Property: mp 262-5°C. Source: JUE CHUANG. Ref: 6.

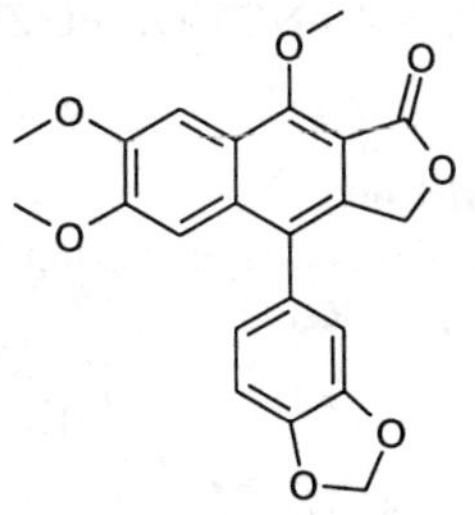

4634 Neokestose

$C_{18}H_{32}O_{16}$ MW: 504.45 Source: GE CONG. Ref: 6.

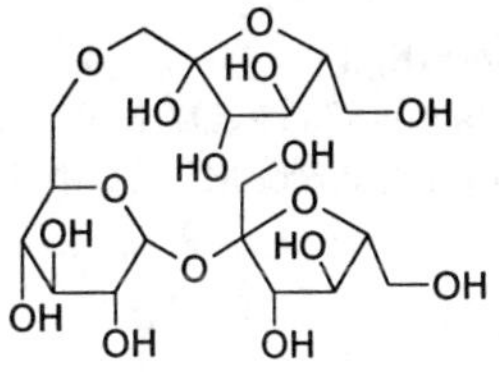

4635 Neokurarinol

$C_{27}H_{32}O_7$ MW: 468.55 Source: KU SHEN. Ref: 2.

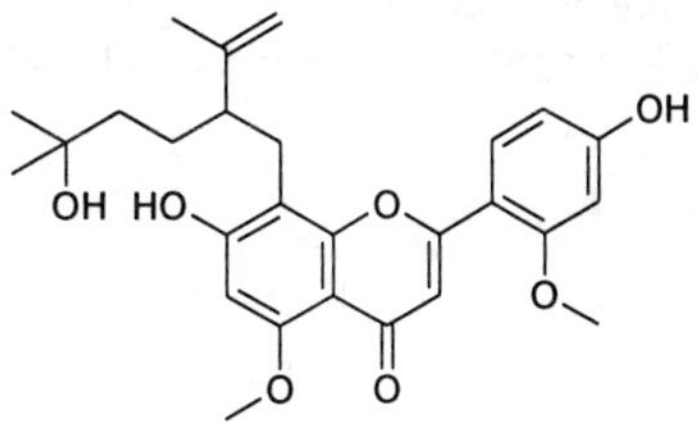

4636 Neoligustilide

$C_{12}H_{14}O_2$ MW: 190.24 Property: colorless massive crystal, mp 58-60°C. Source: LIAO GAO BEN. Ref: 343.

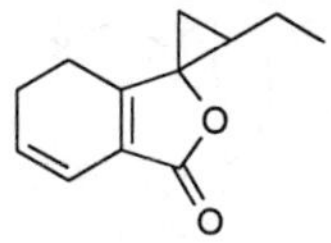

4637 Neolinderalactone

$C_{15}H_{16}O_3$ MW: 244.29 Property: mp 116-8°C. Source: WU YAO. Ref: 6.

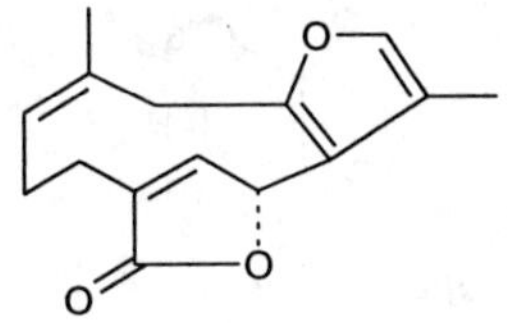

4638 Neoline
$C_{24}H_{39}NO_6$ MW: 437.27 Property: colorless powder, $[\alpha]_D^{26}$ +19.2° (c=0.826, EtOH). Source: E ZHANG YE FU ZI, SI CHUAN JIANG YOU FU ZI.
Ref: 239, 461.

4639 Neoliquiritin
$C_{21}H_{22}O_9$ MW: 418.40 Property: mp 164-6°C.
Source: GAN CAO. Ref: 2.

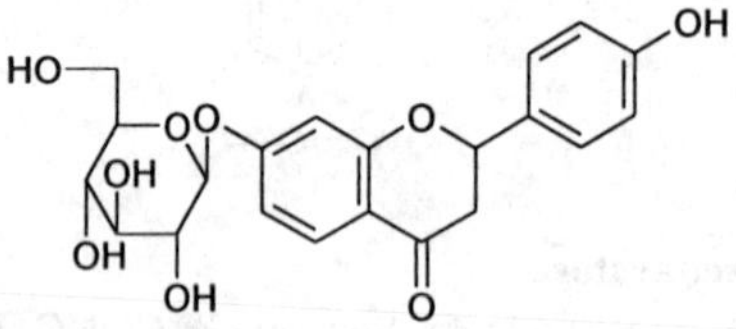

4640 Neomatatabiol
Dihydronepetalactol. $C_{10}H_{18}O_2$ MW: 170.25 Property: bp 95°C/5 mm. Source: MU TIAN LIAO. Ref: 6.

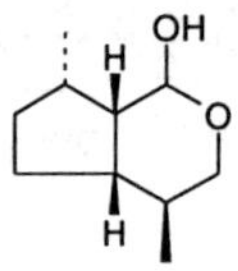

4641 Neonepetalactone
$C_{10}H_{14}O_2$ MW: 166.22 Source: MU TIAN LIAO.
Ref: 6.

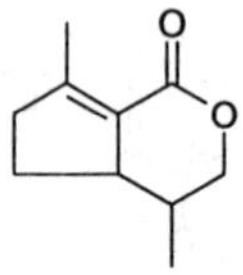

4642 Neopetasone
$C_{15}H_{22}O$ MW: 218.34 Source: CHEN XIANG.
Ref: 13.

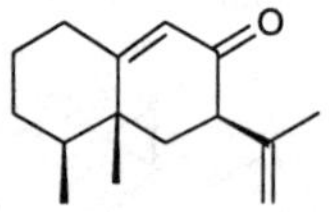

4643 Neopine
$C_{18}H_{21}NO_3$ MW: 299.37 Property: mp 127-7.5°C.
Source: YA PIAN. Ref: 6.

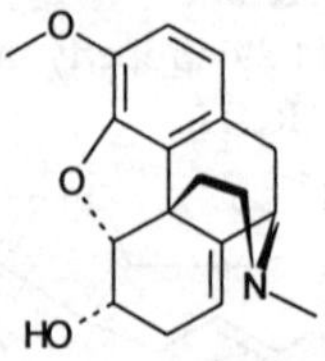

4644 Neoquassin
$C_{22}H_{30}O_6$ MW: 390.48 Source: KU SHU PI. Ref: 12.

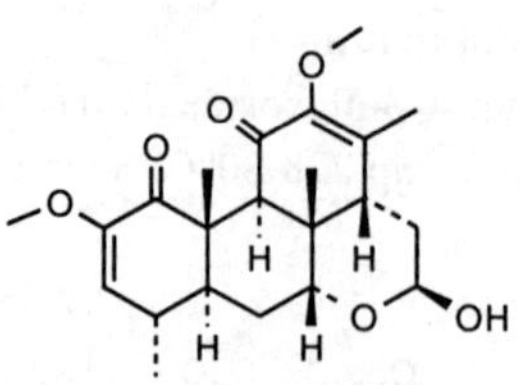

4645 Neotigogenin
$C_{27}H_{44}O_3$ MW: 416.65 Property: mp 202-3°C.
Source: JIN BIAN LONG SHE LAN, JIAN MA, NIAN YU XU, XIA YE LONG SHE LAN. Ref: 6, 10.

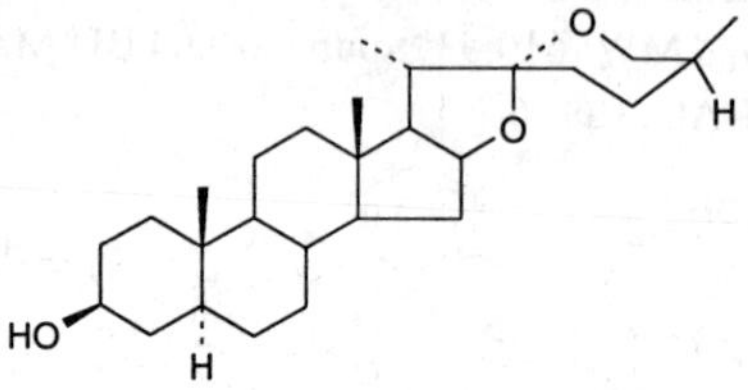

4646 Neotigogenone
$C_{27}H_{42}O_3$ MW: 414.63 Source: JIAN MA. Ref: 10.

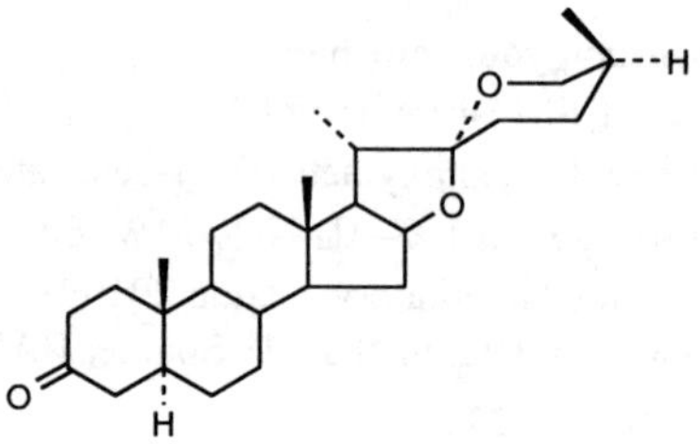

4647 Neotriptophenolide
$C_{21}H_{26}O_4$ MW: 342.44 Source: LEI GONG TENG.
Ref: 2.

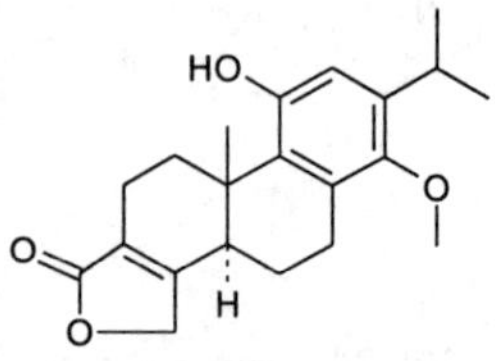

4648 Neouralenol
3,6,7,3',4'-Pentahydroxy-2'-isoprenylflavone.
$C_{20}H_{18}O_7$ MW: 370.36 Property: dark yellow acicular crystal, mp 229-31°C. Source: WU LA ER GAN CAO. Ref: 171.

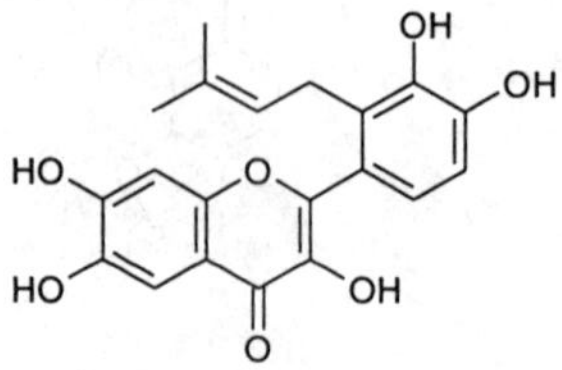

4649 Neowilforine
$C_{44}H_{51}NO_{16}$ MW: 849.89 Source: LEI GONG TENG. Ref: 2.

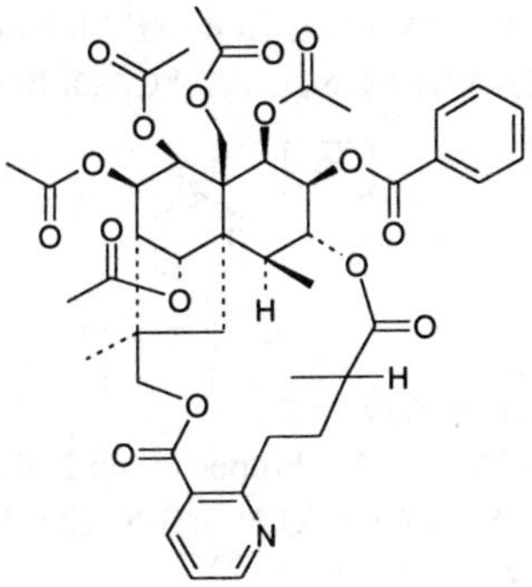

4650 Neoxanthin
$C_{40}H_{56}O_4$ MW: 600.89 Property: mp ≈134°C. Source: DAO CAO, SUAN SHUI CAO. Ref: 6.

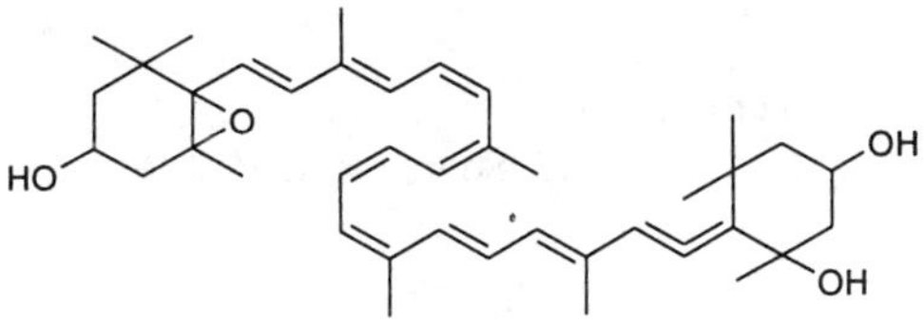

4651 Nepetalic acid
$C_{10}H_{16}O_3$ MW: 184.24 Property: mp 75-6°C. Source: JIA JING JIE. Ref: 6.

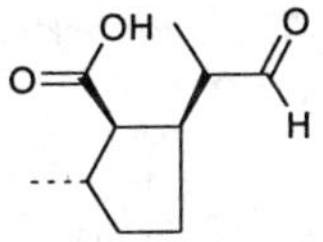

4652 Nepetalic anhydride
$C_{21}H_{32}O_5$ MW: 364.49 Property: mp 139-40°C. Source: JIA JING JIE. Ref: 6.

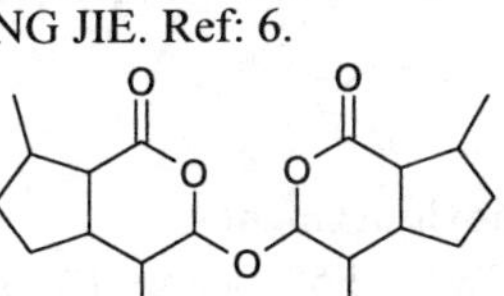

4653 Nepodin
2-Acetyl-1,8-dihydroxy-3-methyl naphthalene. $C_{13}H_{12}O_3$ MW: 216.24 Property: mp 162-3°C. Source: YANG TI . Ref: 6.

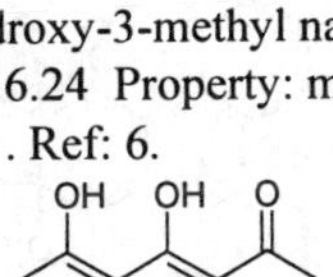

4654 Neral
$C_{10}H_{16}O$ MW: 152.24 Property: bp 103°C/12mm. Source: GAN JIANG, JU PI , SHENG JIANG. Ref: 2.

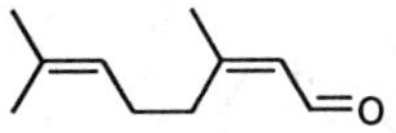

4655 Neriantin
$C_{29}H_{42}O_9$ MW: 534.65 Property: mp 206-8°C. Source: JIA ZHU TAO. Ref: 6.

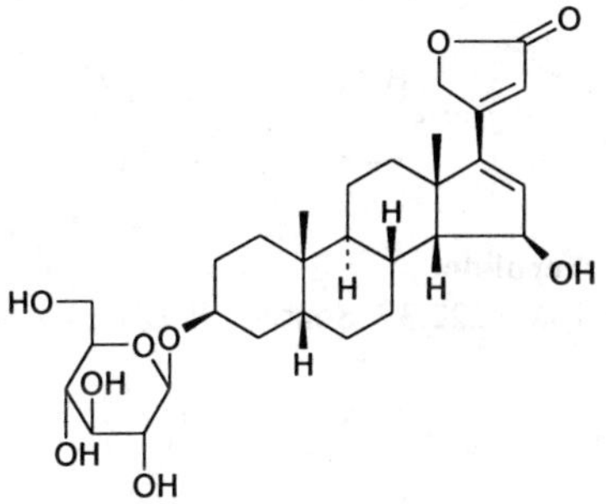

4656 Neriifolin
CAS: 466-07-9 $C_{30}H_{46}O_8$ MW: 534.70 Property: mp 218-25°C. Source: HUANG HUA JIA ZHU TAO. Ref: 4, 5.

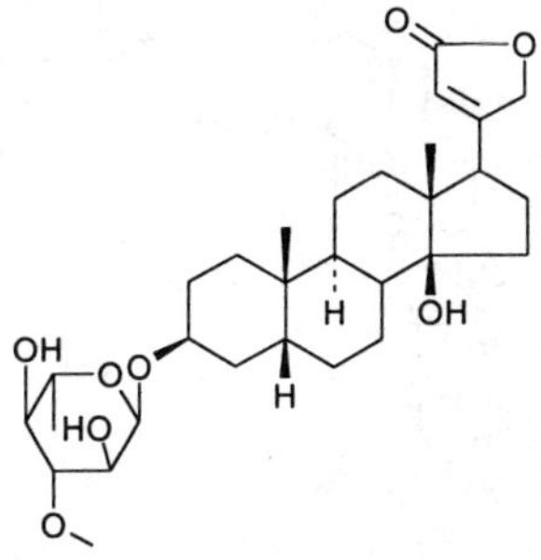

4657 Nerinine
$C_{19}H_{25}NO_5$ MW: 347.41 Property: mp 209-10°C. Source: GAN FENG CAO. Ref: 6.

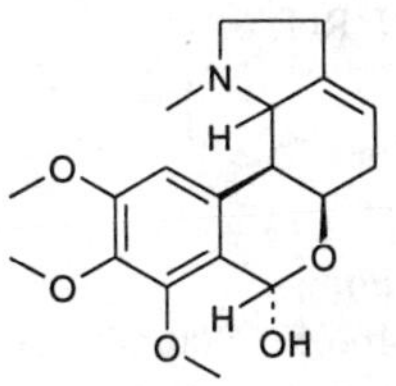

4658 Nerol
$C_{10}H_{18}O$ MW: 154.25 Property: bp 224-7°C. Source: DAI DAI HUA, GUI HUA, JU PI , MEI GUI HUA, PI BA YE, SHAN BUO HE, SHENG JIANG. Ref: 2.

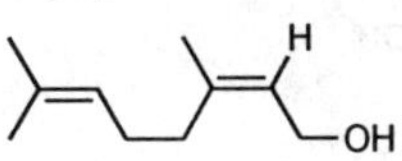

4659 Nerolidol
$C_{15}H_{26}O$ MW: 222.37 Property: bp (+): 276°C. Source: DA DA HUA, DU HUO, MI LU XIANG JIAO, PI BA YE, SHA RE, SHENG JIANG, ZHANG MU. Ref: 2.

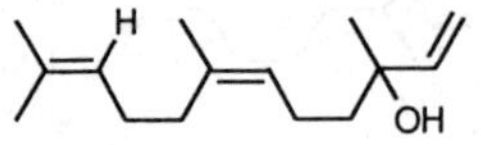

4660 Z-Nerolidol
$C_{15}H_{26}O$ MW: 222.37 Source: SHENG JIANG. Ref: 2.

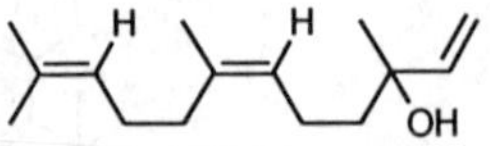

4661 E-Nerolidol
$C_{15}H_{26}O$ MW: 222.37 Source: SHENG JIANG. Ref: 2.

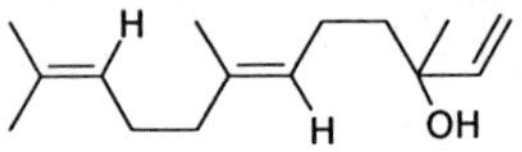

4662 Nervosine
$C_{36}H_{53}NO_{12}$ MW: 691.82 Property: mp 130-1°C. Source: JIAN XUE QING. Ref: 6.

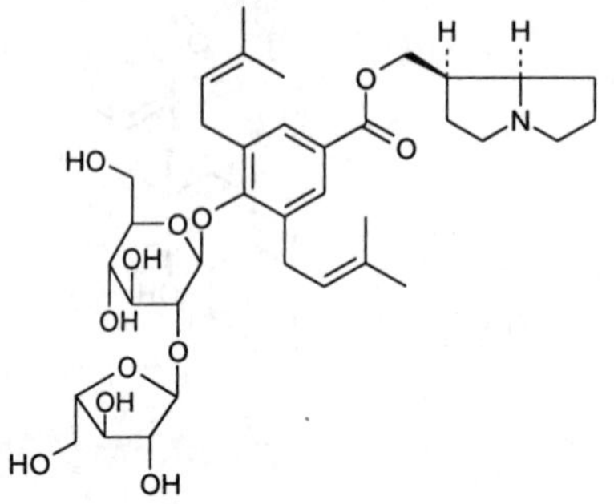

4663 Neryl acetate
$C_{12}H_{20}O_2$ MW: 196.29 Property: bp 134°C/25 mm. Source: PEI LAN. Ref: 6.

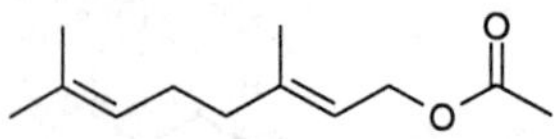

4664 Nicandrenone
$C_{28}H_{34}O_6$ MW: 466.58 Source: JIA SUAN JIANG. Ref: 6.

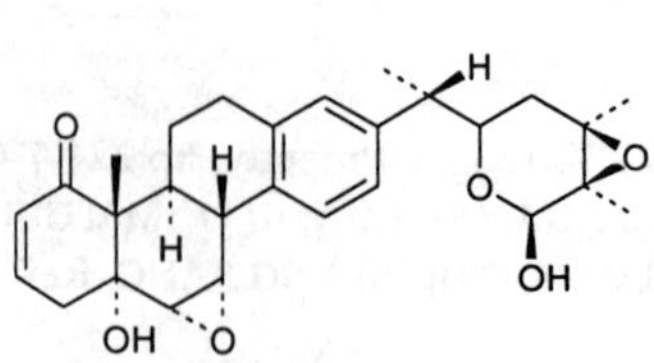

4665 Nicotine
$C_{10}H_{14}N_2$ MW: 162.24 Property: bp (+): 245.5-6.5°C/729mm, (-): 246.1°C/730.5mm. Source: DANG SHEN, GU JIE CAO, KU DOU ZI, MOU HAN LIAN, PU DI WU GONG, YAN CAO. Ref: 2, 593.

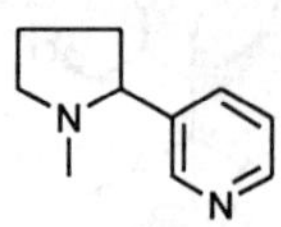

4666 Nicotinic acid
$C_6H_5NO_2$ MW: 123.11 Property: mp 236°C. Source: DA ZAO, DANG GUI, REN SHEN, ZHI MU, GOU QI ZI. Ref: 2.

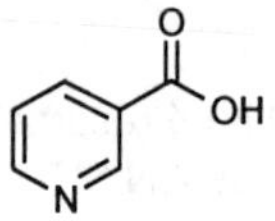

4667 Nicotinamide
$C_6H_6N_2O$ MW: 122.13 Source: ZHI MU. Ref: 2.

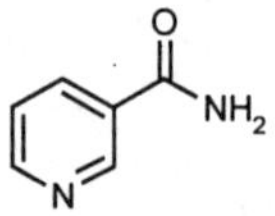

4668 12-O-Nicotinoylisolineolone
$C_{27}H_{35}NO_6$ MW: 469.58 Property: mp 250-4°C. Source: FU SHOU CAO. Ref: 6.

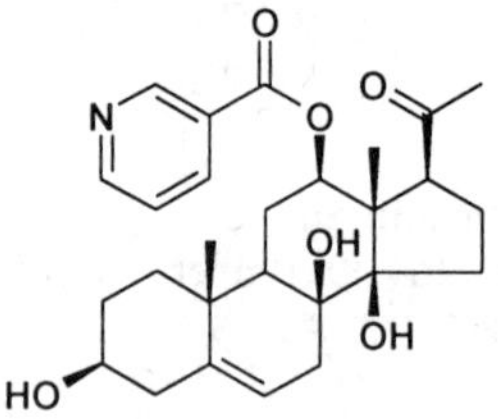

4669 Nicotinoylisoramanon
$C_{27}H_{35}NO_5$ MW: 453.58 Source: FU SHOU CAO. Ref: 6.

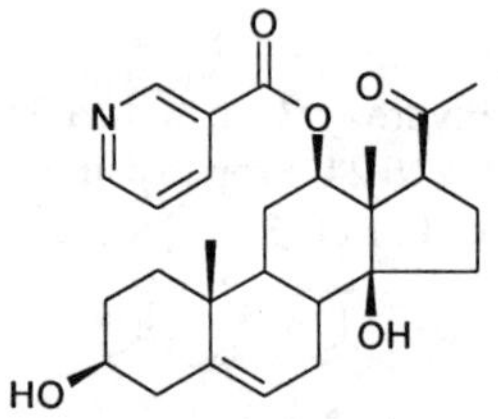

4670 Nigainchigoside F1
Property: mp 229-33°C. Source: CU YE XUAN GOU ZI, MAO MEI. Ref: 509, 606.

4671 Nigakihemiacetal A
$C_{22}H_{34}O_7$ MW: 410.51 Property: mp 262-3°C. Source: KU SHU PI. Ref: 6.

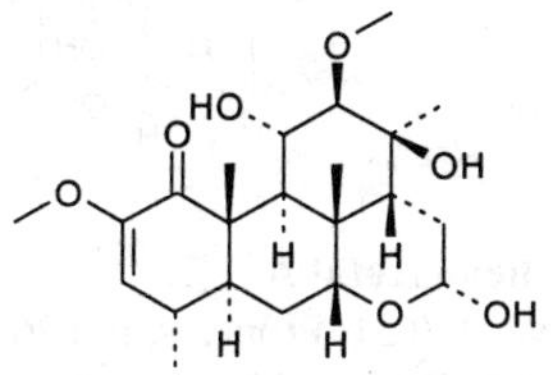

4672 Nigakilactone
$C_{24}H_{34}O_7$ MW: 434.53 Property: mp 252.5-253°C. Source: KU SHU PI. Ref: 12.

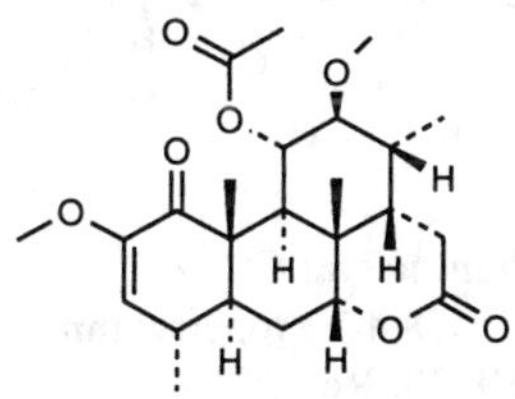

4673 Nigakilactone A
$C_{21}H_{30}O_6$ MW: 378.47 Property: mp 237.5-238°C. Source: KU SHU PI. Ref: 12.

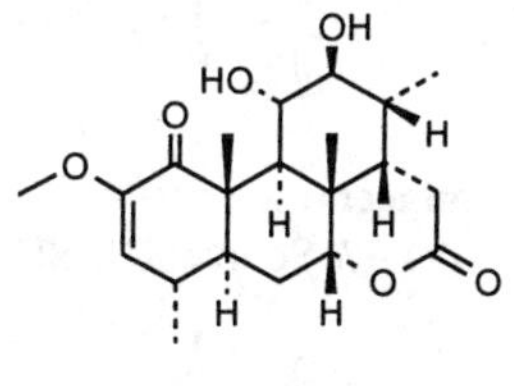

4674 Nigakilactone B
$C_{22}H_{32}O_6$ MW: 392.50 Property: mp 278.5°C. Source: KU SHU PI. Ref: 12.

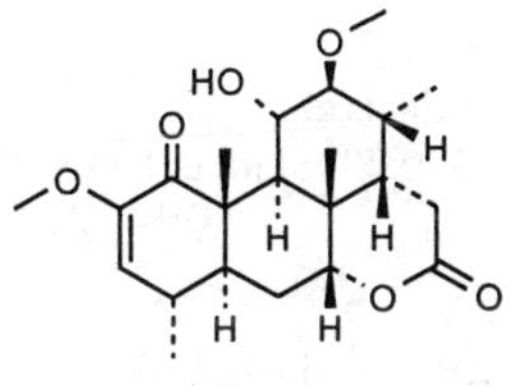

4675 Nigakilactone E
$C_{24}H_{34}O_8$ MW: 450.53 Property: mp 280°C. Source: KU SHU PI. Ref: 12.

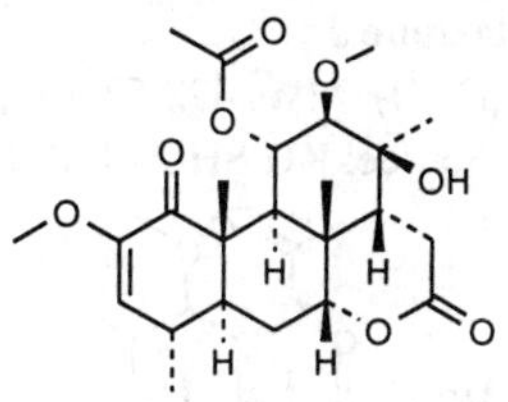

4676 Nigakilactone F
$C_{22}H_{32}O_7$ MW: 408.50 Property: mp 265-265.5°C. Source: KU SHU PI. Ref: 12.

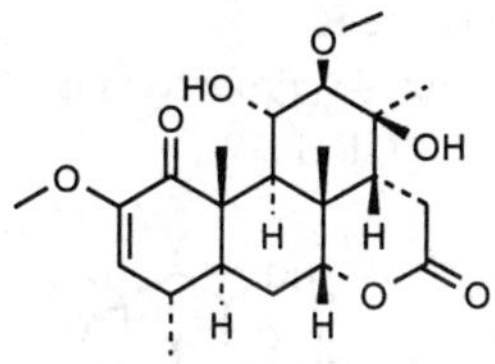

4677 Nigakilactone G
Picrasin A. $C_{26}H_{34}O_8$ MW: 474.56 Property: mp 297-9°C. Source: KU SHU PI. Ref: 12.

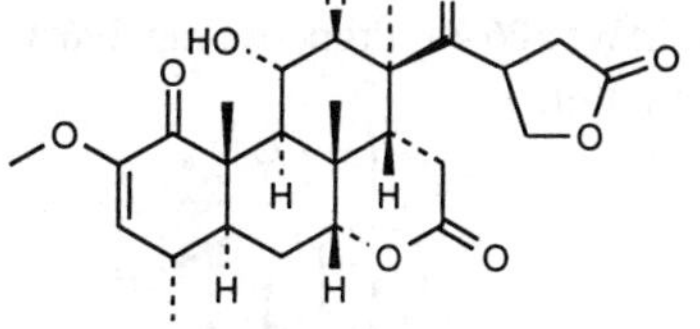

4678 Nigakilactone H
$C_{22}H_{32}O_8$ MW: 424.50 Property: mp 274-275.5°C. Source: KU SHU PI. Ref: 12.

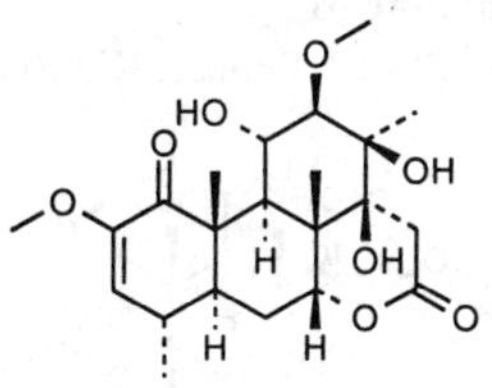

4679 Nigakilactone I
Picrasin B. $C_{21}H_{28}O_6$ MW: 376.45 Property: mp 255-7°C. Source: KU SHU PI. Ref: 12.

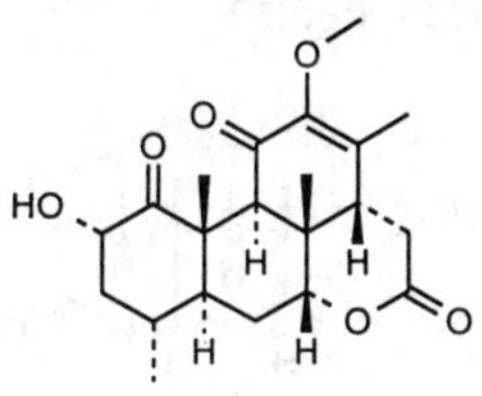

4680 Nigakilactone J
Picrasin C. $C_{23}H_{34}O_7$ MW: 422.52 Property: mp 240-1°C, 250-2°C. Source: KU SHU PI. Ref: 6, 12.

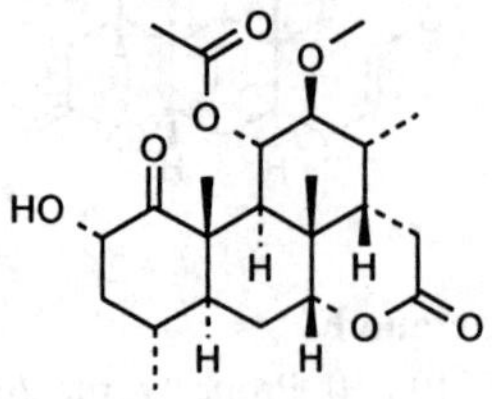

4681 Nigakilactone K
$C_{22}H_{30}O_7$ MW: 406.48 Property: mp 226-7°C. Source: KU SHU PI. Ref: 12.

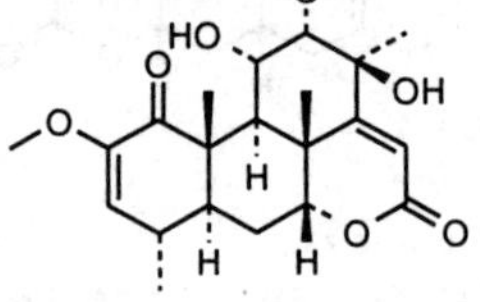

4682 Nigakilactone L
$C_{22}H_{30}O_7$ MW: 406.48 Property: mp 296°C. Source: KU SHU PI. Ref: 12.

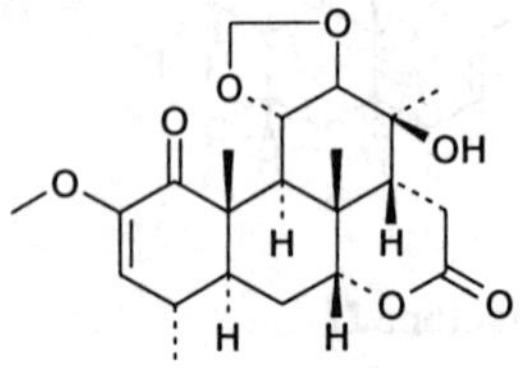

4683 Nigakilactone M
$C_{21}H_{30}O_7$ MW: 394.47 Source: KU SHU PI. Ref: 12.

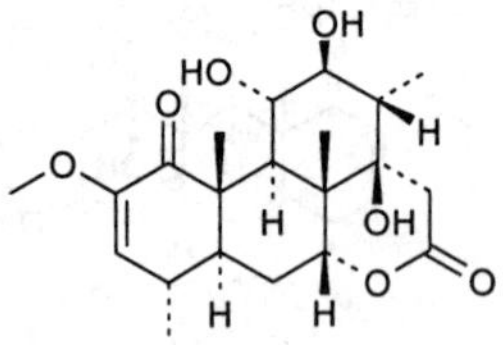

4684 Nigakilactone N
$C_{21}H_{30}O_7$ MW: 394.47 Property: mp 207-11°C. Source: KU SHU PI. Ref: 12.

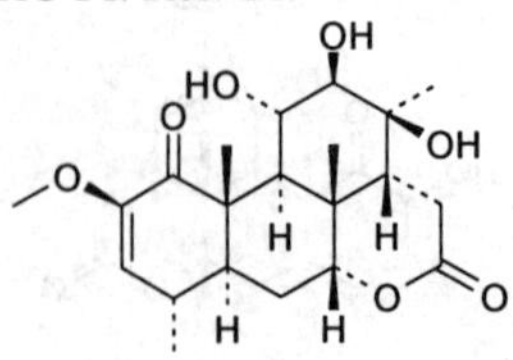

4685 Nigakilactone O
$C_{30}H_{36}O_{11}$ MW: 572.61 Source: KU SHU PI. Ref: 12.

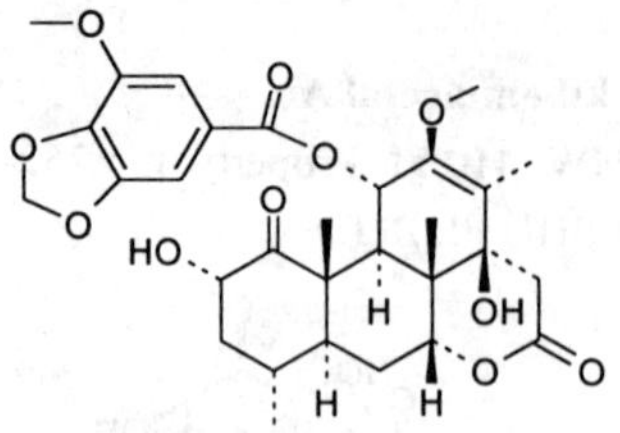

4686 Nigakihemiacetal A
$C_{22}H_{34}O_7$ MW: 410.51 Property: mp 262-3°C. Source: KU SHU PI. Ref: 12.

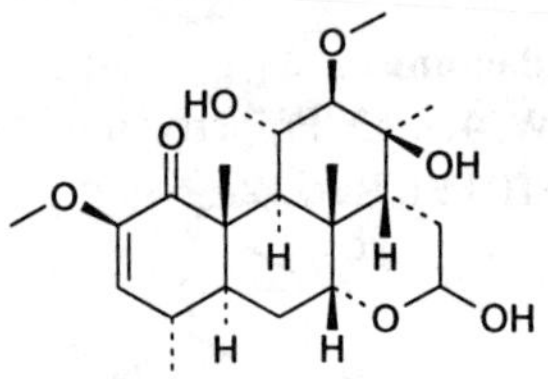

4687 Nigakihemiacetal C
$C_{21}H_{30}O_6$ MW: 378.47 Property: mp 265-5.5°C. Source: KU SHU PI. Ref: 12.

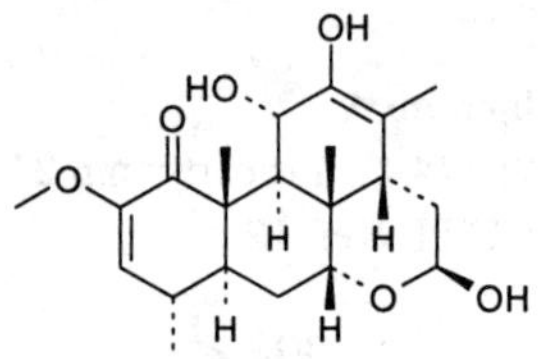

4688 Nigakihemiacetal E
$C_{21}H_{30}O_7$ MW: 394.47 Source: KU SHU PI. Ref: 12.

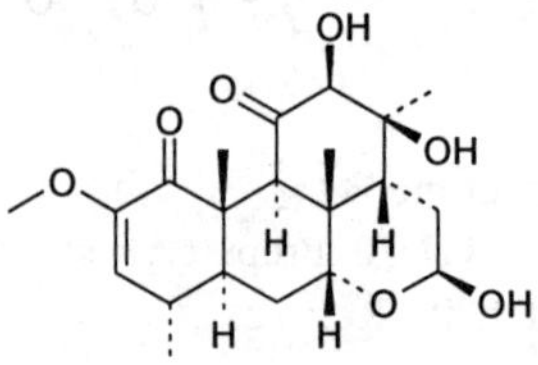

4689 Nigakihemiacetal F
$C_{21}H_{32}O_6$ MW: 380.49 Source: KU SHU PI. Ref: 12.

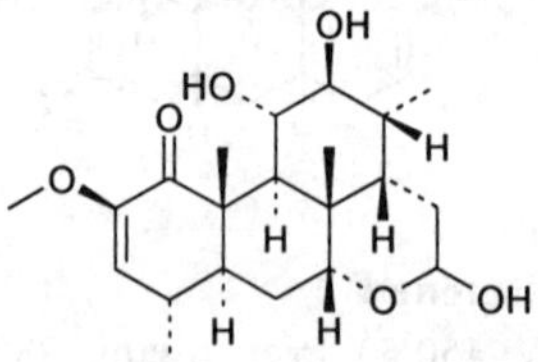

4690 Nigakinone
$C_{15}H_{10}N_2O_3$ MW: 266.26 Source: KU SHU PI. Ref: 6.

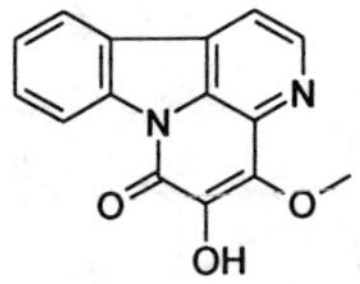

4691 Nilgirine
$C_{17}H_{23}NO_5$ MW: 321.38 Property: mp 127-8°C. Source: XIANG LING CAO. Ref: 6.

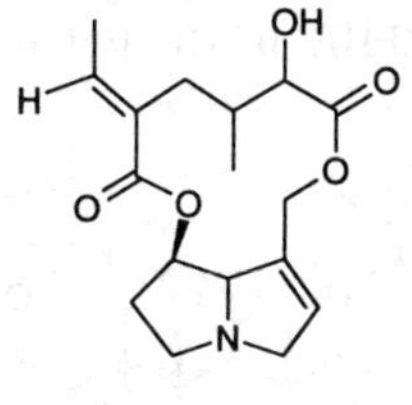

4692 Nilic acid
$C_5H_{11}O_3$ MW: 118.13 Source: QIAN NIU ZI. Ref: 6.

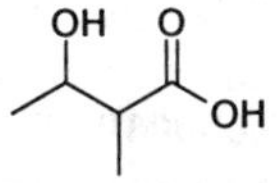

4693 Nimbolin A
$C_{39}H_{46}O_8$ MW: 642.80 Property: mp 180-3°C. Source: KU LIAN PI. Ref: 6.

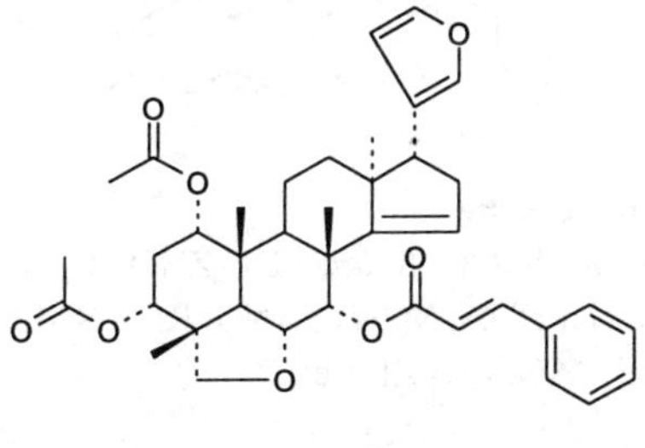

4694 Nimbolin B
$C_{39}H_{46}O_{10}$ MW: 674.80 Property: mp 243-5°C. Source: KU LIAN PI. Ref: 6.

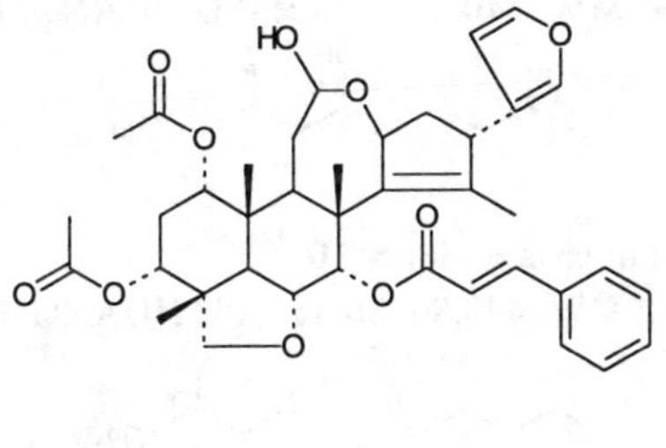

4695 Ningpeisine
N-methyl-3β-hydroxy-5α-veratranine-6-one. $C_{28}H_{47}NO_2$ MW: 429.69 Property: colorless acicular clustered crystal, mp 228-30°C, $[\alpha]_D^{20}$ +20° (c=0.5, anhydrous ethanol). Source: NING GUO BEI MU. Ref: 105.

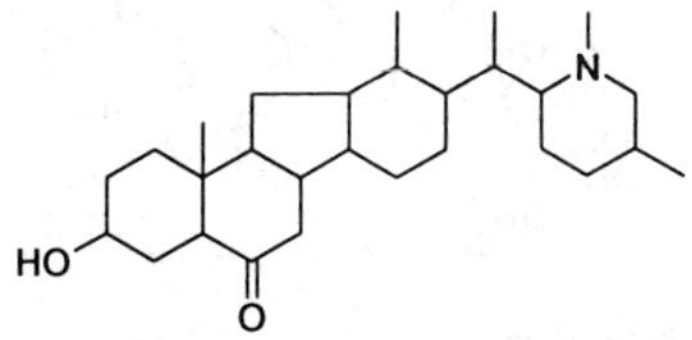

4696 Ningpeisinoside
N-methyl-5α-veratranine-6-oxo-3β-O-β-D-glucoside. $C_{34}H_{57}NO_7$ MW: 575.84 Property: thin acicular crystal, mp 284-6°C, $[\alpha]_D^{20}$ +24° (c=0.24, chloroform-methanol). Source: NING GUO BEI MU. Ref: 205.

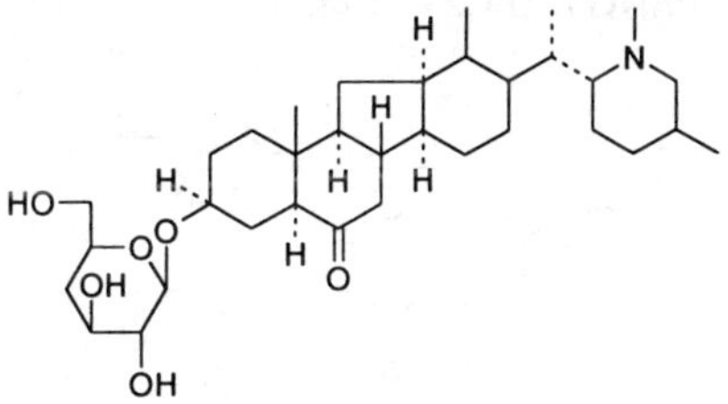

4697 Nitidine
CAS: 6872-57-7 $C_{21}H_{18}NO_4$ MW: 348.38 Property: mp 215-8°C. Source: CHU YE HUA JIAO PI, HUA JIAO, RU DI JIN NIU. Ref: 4, 5, 6.

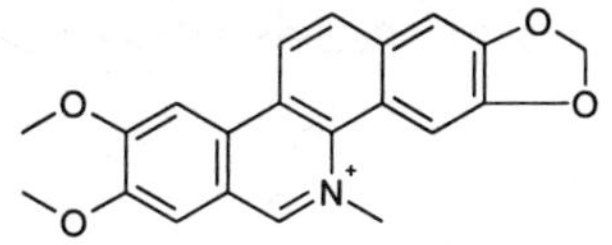

4698 Nobiletin
CAS: 10236-47-2 $C_{21}H_{22}O_8$ MW: 402.40 Property: mp 137-8°C. Source: GAN, GAN PI, JIN JU YE. Ref: 4, 5.

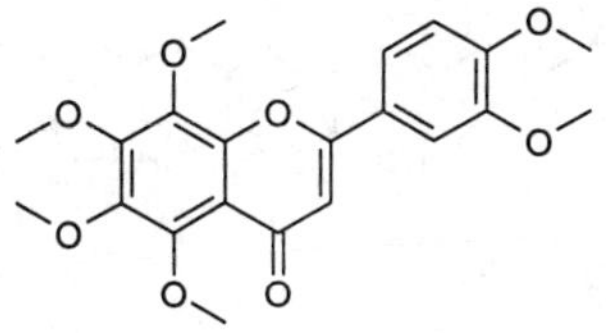

4699 Nobilonine
$C_{17}H_{27}NO_3$ MW: 293.41 Property: mp 86°C. Source: SHI HU. Ref: 6.

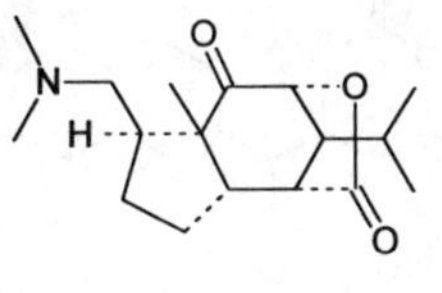

4700 Nodakenin
$C_{20}H_{24}O_9$ MW: 408.41 Source: QIANG HUO. Ref: 2, 566.

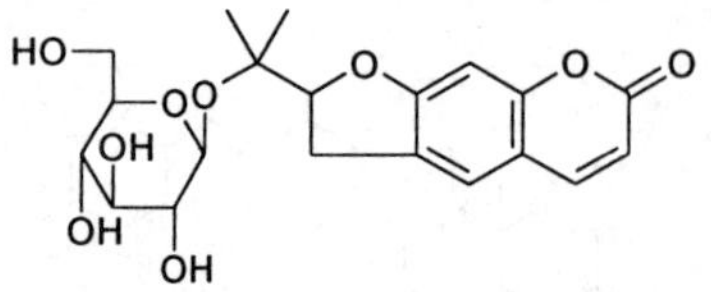

4701 Nodakenitin
Source: BAI HUA QIAN HU, QIANG HUO. Ref: 297, 566.

4702 Nodifloretin
$C_{16}H_{12}O_7$ MW: 316.27 Property: mp 250-3°C. Source: PENG LAI CAO. Ref: 6.

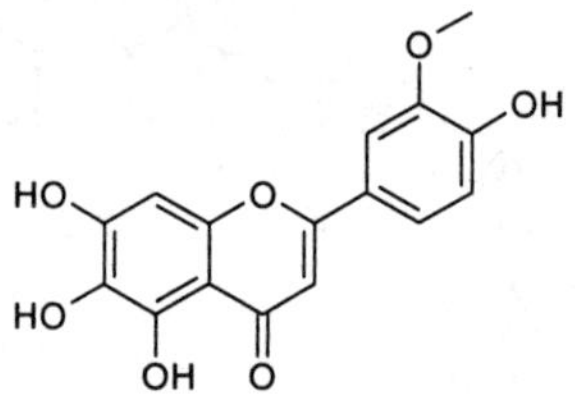

4703 Nodifloridin A
$C_{22}H_{24}O_7$ MW: 400.43 Source: PENG LAI CAO. Ref: 6.

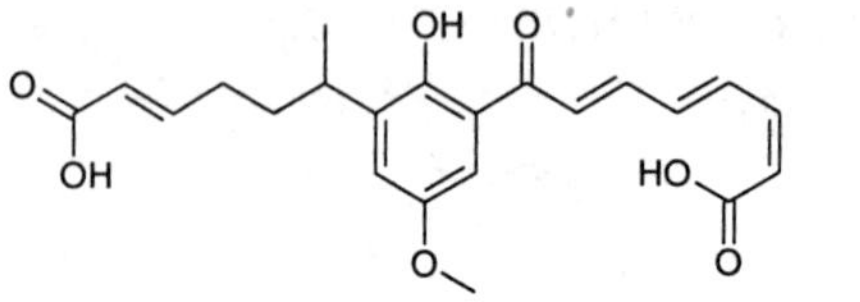

4704 Nodifloridin B
$C_{21}H_{24}O_9$ MW: 420.42 Source: PENG LAI CAO. Ref: 6.

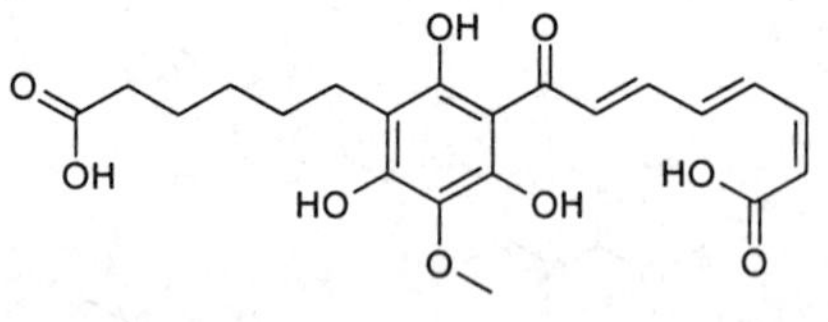

4705 Nodolidate
$C_{32}H_{60}O_4$ MW: 508.83 Property: mp 69-70°C. Source: HUANG DOU. Ref: 6.

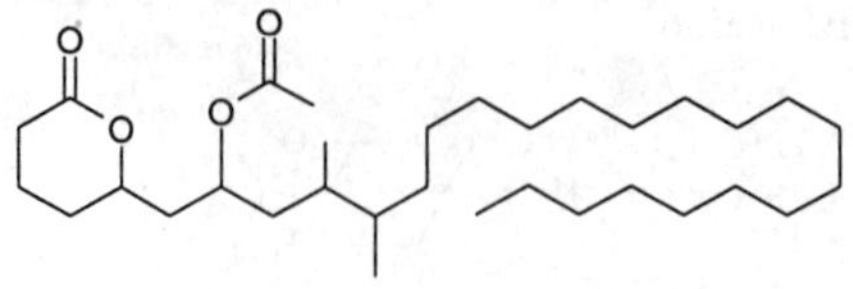

4706 Nodososide
$C_{22}H_{22}O_{11}$ MW: 462.41 Source: SHEN HUANG DOU. Ref: 6.

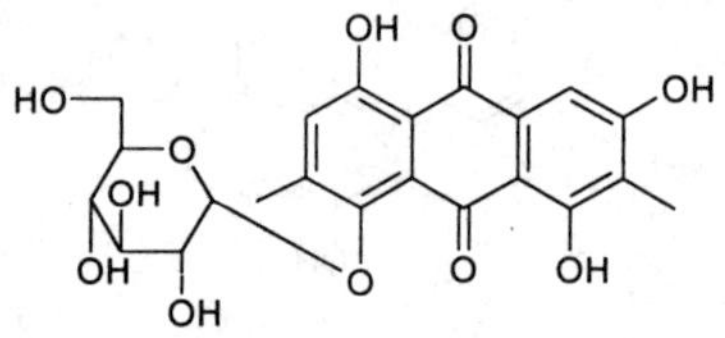

4707 Nomilin
$C_{28}H_{34}O_9$ MW: 514.58 Property: mp 278-9°C. Source: CHEN ZI HE, JU HE. Ref: 6.

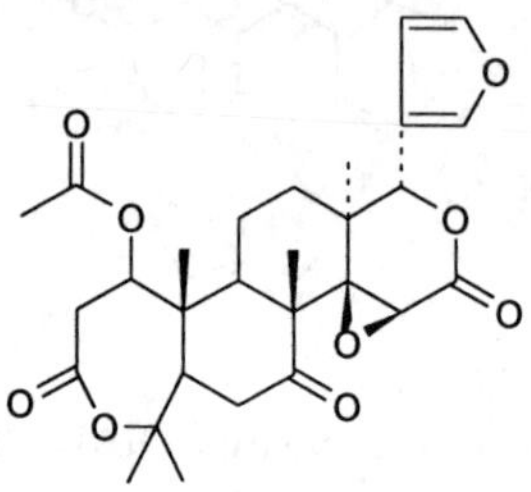

4709 Nonacasyl alcohol-10
Celidoniol; Ginnol; 10-Nonacosanol. $C_{19}H_{40}O$ MW: 284.53 Property: mp 82.5°C. Source: BAI GUO, BAI GUO YE, BAI QU CAI, JU HUA HUANG LIAN. Ref: 2, 6.

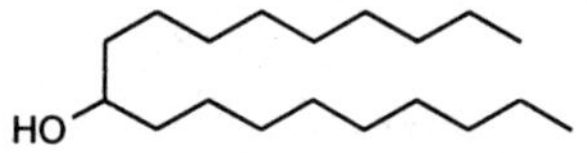

4710 Nonacosane
$C_{29}H_{60}$ MW: 408.80 Source: DU ZHONG, GUA LOU, HONG HUA, MA HUANG, REN SHEN, XIAN HE CAO, ZHI ZI. Ref: 2.

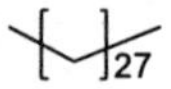

4711 Nonacosanediol-6, 8
$C_{29}H_{60}O_2$ MW: 440.80 Source: PU HUANG. Ref: 2.

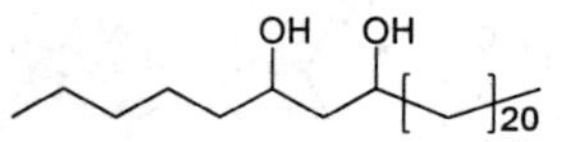

4712 Nonacosanediol-6, 10
$C_{29}H_{60}O_2$ MW: 440.80 Source: PU HUANG. Ref: 2.

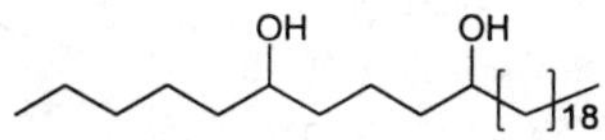

4713 Nonacosanediol-6, 21
$C_{29}H_{60}O_2$ MW: 440.80 Source: PU HUANG. Ref: 2.

4714 Nonacosanol
$C_{29}H_{60}O$ MW: 424.80 Source: MA HUANG. Ref: 2.

4715 2-Nonacosanone
$C_{29}H_{58}O$ MW: 422.79 Source: ROU CONG RONG. Ref: 2.

4716 10-Nonacosanone
$C_{29}H_{58}O$ MW: 422.79 Property: mp 74-5°C. Source: BAI GUO YE, JI MAO SONG. Ref: 6, 544.

4717 n-Nonadecane
$C_{19}H_{40}$ MW: 268.53 Source: DANG SHEN, ROU CONG RONG, SAN QI. Ref: 2.

4718 Nonadecanoic acid
$C_{19}H_{38}O_2$ MW: 298.51 Source: GAN DI HUANG. Ref: 2.

4719 2,6-Nonadienal
$C_9H_{14}O$ MW: 138.21 Property: bp 85-7°C/11 mm. Source: HUANG GUA. Ref: 6.

4720 2,4-Nonadienic
$C_9H_{14}O_2$ MW: 154.21 Source: DANG SHEN. Ref: 2.

4721 2,6-Nonadienol
$C_9H_{16}O$ MW: 140.23 Property: bp 95.5-100°C/11 mm. Source: HUANG GUA. Ref: 6.

4722 Nonaldehyde
$C_9H_{18}O$ MW: 142.24 Source: DONG LING CAO. Ref: 2.

4723 2,6-Nonamethylene dihydropyran
Source: SHE XIANG. Ref: 2.

4724 2,6-Nonamethylene pyridine
$C_{14}H_{21}N$ MW: 203.33 Source: SHE XIANG. Ref: 2.

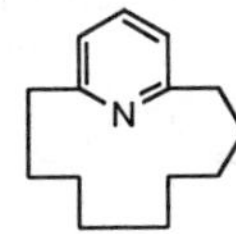

4725 n-Nonane
C_9H_{20} MW: 128.26 Source: SHENG JIANG, DU HUO. Ref: 2.

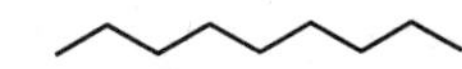

4726 Nonanedioic acid
Source: MU JIN PI. Ref: 519.

4727 Nonanoic acid
$C_9H_{18}O_2$ MW: 158.24 Source: GAN DI HUANG, GUA LOU, SAN QI, XI YANG SHEN. Ref: 2.

4728 2-Nonanol
$C_9H_{20}O$ MW: 144.26 Source: GAN JIANG. Ref: 2.

4729 n-Nonanol
$C_9H_{20}O$ MW: 144.26 Source: SHENG JIANG. Ref: 2.

4730 2-Nonanone
$C_9H_{18}O$ MW: 142.24 Source: SHENG JIANG. Ref: 2.

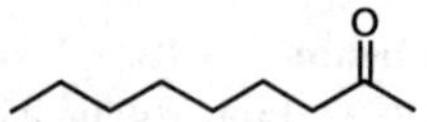

4731 (E)-2-Nonenal
$C_9H_{16}O$ MW: 140.23 Source: XING REN. Ref: 2.

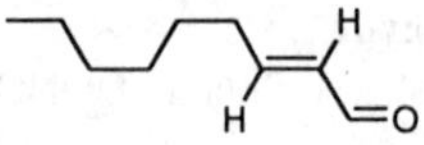

4732 1-Nonene
C_9H_{18} MW: 126.24 Property: bp 146°C. Source: FENG DOU CAI. Ref: 6.

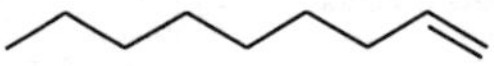

4733 2-Nonenic acid
$C_9H_{16}O_2$ MW: 156.23 Source: CHAI HU. Ref: 2.

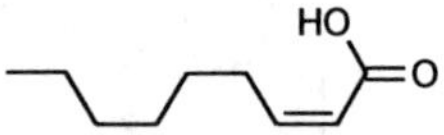

4734 8-Nonenoic acid
$C_9H_{16}O_2$ MW: 156.23 Source: BAI ZHI. Ref: 2.

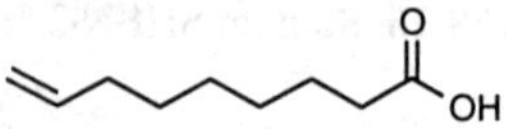

4735 1-Nonen-3-ol
$C_9H_{18}O$ MW: 142.24 Property: bp 193-4°C. Source: FENG DOU CAI. Ref: 6.

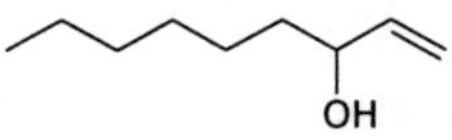

4736 Nonoyl vanillylamide
$C_{17}H_{17}NO_3$ MW: 293.41 Source: LA JIAO. Ref: 6.

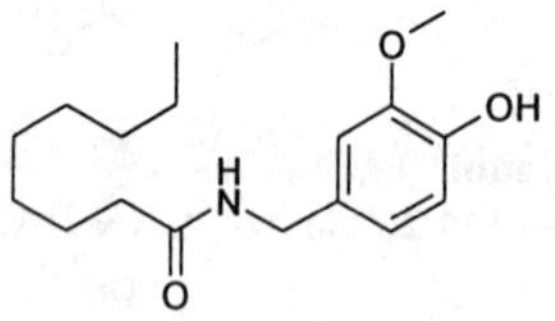

4737 2-Nonyl acetate
$C_{11}H_{22}O_2$ MW: 186.30 Source: CHOU CAO. Ref: 6.

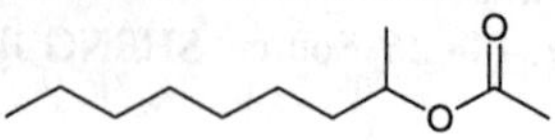

4738 Nonyl alcohol
$C_9H_{20}O$ MW: 144.26 Property: bp 215°C. Source: SHENG JIANG. Ref: 2.

4739 Nonylaldehyde
$C_9H_{18}O$ MW: 142.24 Source: GAN JIANG. Ref: 2.

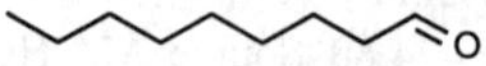

4740 Nonyl cyclopropane
$C_{11}H_{22}$ MW: 154.30 Source: BAI ZHI. Ref: 2.

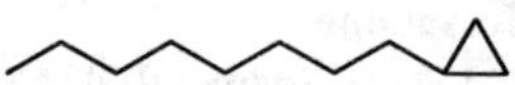

4741 Nonyl ethyl ether
$C_{11}H_{24}O$ MW: 172.31 Property: bp 88°C/21 mm. Source: WEN PO. Ref: 6.

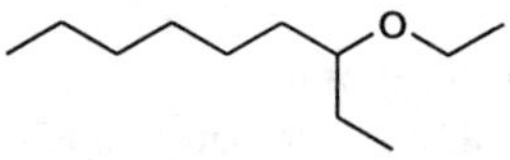

4742 Nonylphenol
$C_{15}H_{24}O$ MW: 220.36 Source: WU WEI ZI. Ref: 2.

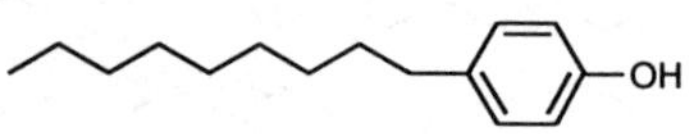

4743 Nootkatin
$C_{15}H_{20}O_2$ MW: 232.33 Property: mp 95°C. Source: SHAN CI BAI. Ref: 6.

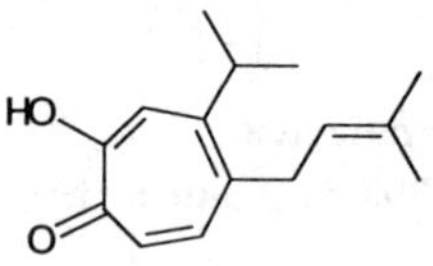

4744 Nootkatinol
$C_{15}H_{22}O_3$ MW: 250.34 Property: mp 102-3°C. Source: DU SONG SHI. Ref: 6.

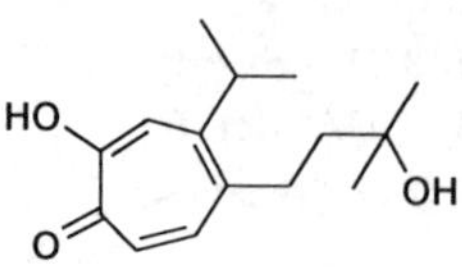

4745 Nootkatone
Source: CHAI HU. Ref: 2.

4746 Noracronycine
$C_{19}H_{17}NO_3$ MW: 307.35 Source: JIU LI XIANG. Ref: 11.

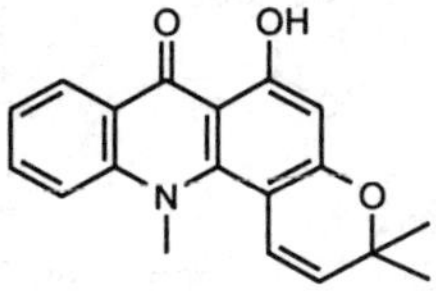

4747 Noradrenaline
$C_8H_{11}NO_3$ MW: 169.18 Property: mp (+): 215-7°C (dec), (-): 216.5-8°C, (±): 191°C (dec). Source: JIN YU, MA CHI XIAN, NIU SHEN, WEI NAO, WEI XIN GAN, XIANG JIAO. Ref: 6.

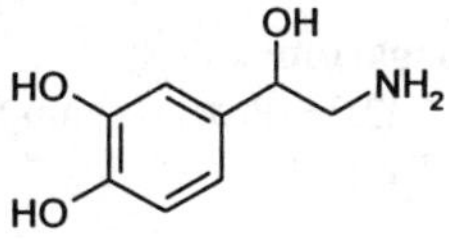

4748 Norarmepavine
$C_{18}H_{21}NO_3$ MW: 299.37 Property: mp D(+): 157-8°C, L(-): 157-8°C. Source: HONG NAN PI, LIAN ZI. Ref: 6.

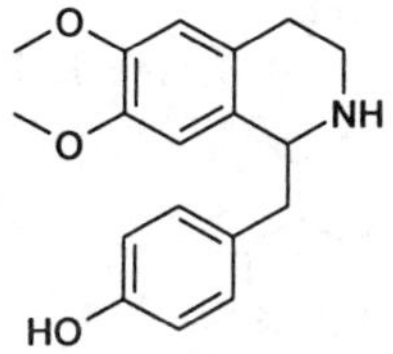

4749 Norbellidifodin
$C_{13}H_8O_6$ MW: 260.21 Property: yellow powder, mp 276-8°C. Source: BAO E ZHANG YA CAI. Ref: 634.

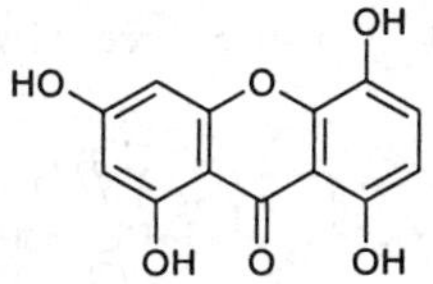

4750 Norcapillene
$C_{11}H_8$ MW: 140.19 Source: YIN CHEN HAO. Ref: 2.

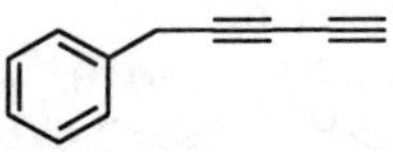

4751 24-nor-cholesta-5,22E-dien-3β-ol
Property: colorless lamellar crystal, mp 135-8°C (methanol-chloroform). Source: TOU JIE HAI MIAN. Ref: 459.

4752 31-Norcycloartanol
$C_{29}H_{50}O$ MW: 414.72 Property: mp 128-32°C. Source: SHUI LONG GU. Ref: 6.

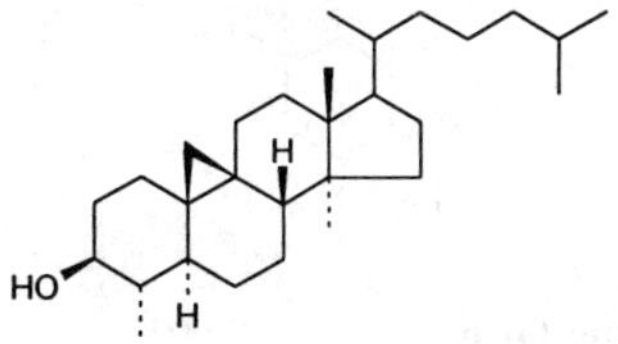

4753 31-Norcyclolaudenol
$C_{31}H_{52}O$ MW: 440.76 Source: SHUI LONG GU. Ref: 6.

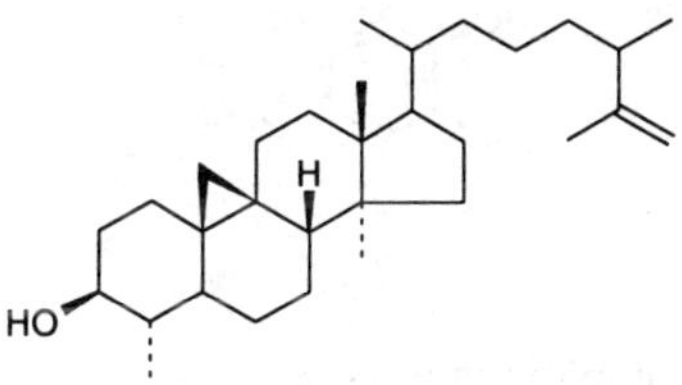

4754 Nordalbergin
$C_{15}H_{10}O_4$ MW: 254.24 Property: mp 274-6°C. Source: JIANG ZHEN. Ref: 6.

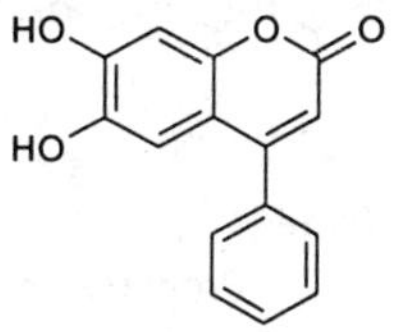

4755 Nordamnacanthal
$C_{15}H_8O_5$ MW: 268.23 Source: HU CI, TU LIAN QIAO. Ref: 6.

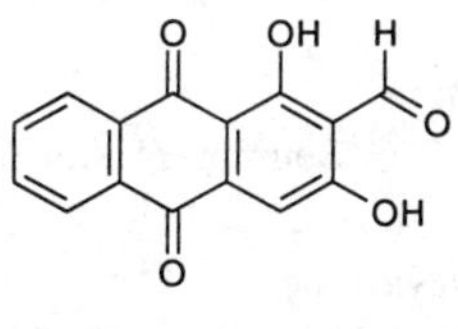

4756 18-Nordehydroabietan-4α-ol
$C_{19}H_{28}O$ MW: 272.43 Source: HAI SONG ZI. Ref: 6.

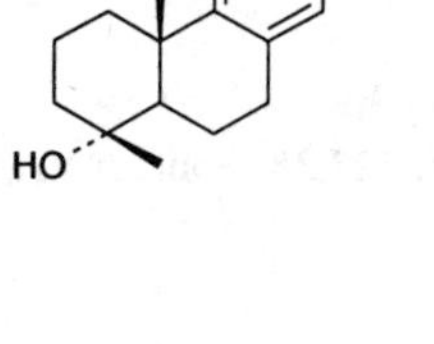

4757 19-Nordehydroabiet-4(8)-ene
$C_{19}H_{26}$ MW: 254.42 Source: HAI SONG ZI. Ref: 6.

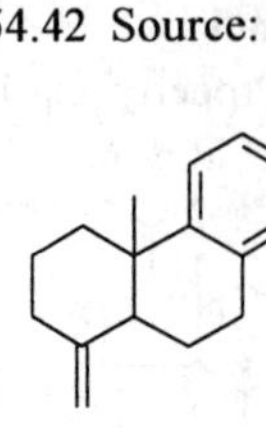

4758 Nordentatin
$C_{19}H_{20}O_4$ MW: 312.37 Property: mp 182°C. Source: YE HUANG PI. Ref: 6.

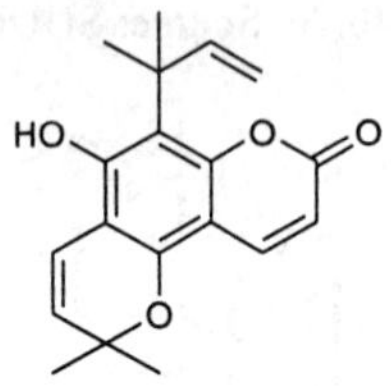

4759 Nordihydrocapsacine
$C_{17}H_{27}NO_3$ MW: 293.41 Source: LA JIAO. Ref: 15.

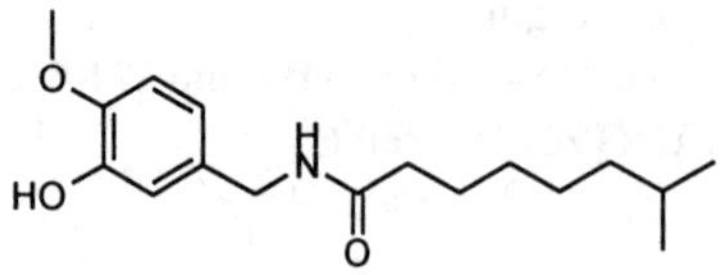

4760 l-Norephedrine
$C_9H_{13}NO$ MW: 151.21 Property: mp (-): 50°C. Source: MA HUANG. Ref: 2.

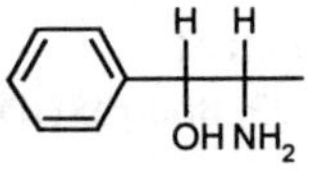

4761 Norharman
Property: mp 197°C. Source: YUAN ZHI. Ref: 538.

4762 Norhyoscyamine
$C_{16}H_{21}NO_3$ MW: 275.35 Property: mp (-): 140.5°C. Source: DONG LANG DANG. Ref: 6.

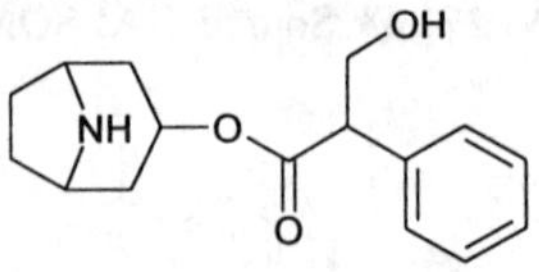

4763 Norisocorydine
$C_{19}H_{21}NO_4$ MW: 327.38 Source: YAN HU SUO. Ref: 6.

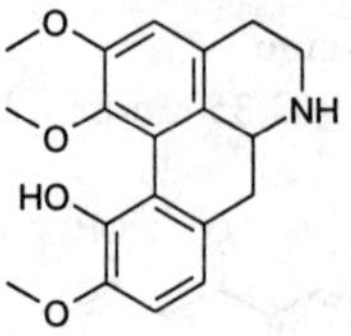

4764 Norjuzunal
$C_{15}H_8O_6$ MW: 284.23 Property: mp 265°C. Source: HU CI. Ref: 6.

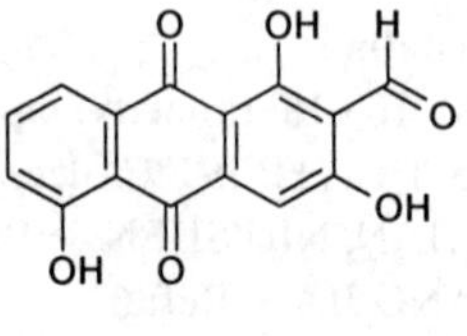

4765 Nor-ketoagarofuran
$C_{14}H_{22}O_2$ MW: 222.33 Property: mp 56-7°C. Source: CHEN XIANG. Ref: 13.

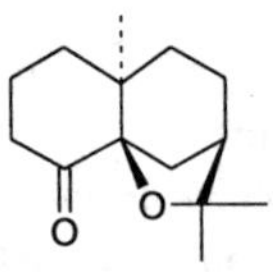

4766 Norkurarinol
$C_{25}H_{28}O_7$ MW: 440.50 Source: KU SHEN. Ref: 2.

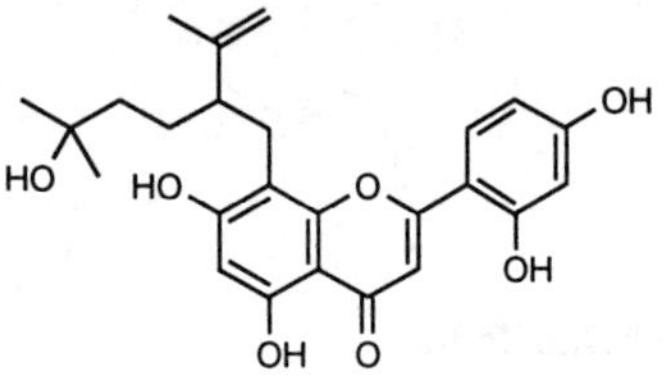

4767 Normacusine B
$C_{19}H_{22}N_2O$ MW: 294.40 Source: MA QIAN ZI. Ref: 2.

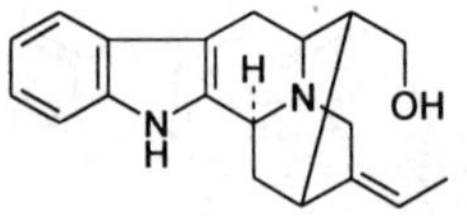

4768 Normenisarine
$C_{35}H_{32}N_2O_6$ MW: 576.66 Property: mp 223°C. Source: FANG JI. Ref: 6.

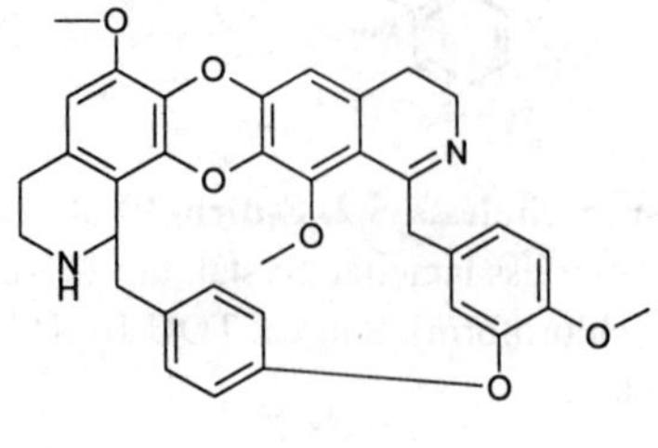

4769 Normuscone
$C_{15}H_{28}O$ MW: 224.39 Source: SHE XIANG. Ref: 2.

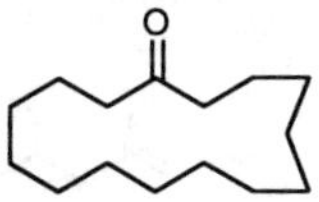

4770 Nornuciferine
$C_{18}H_{19}NO_2$ MW: 281.36 Property: mp 195-6°C. Source: HE YE, HE GENG, HE YE DI. Ref: 6.

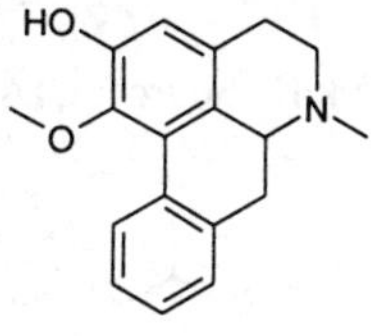

4771 N-Nornuciferine
$C_{18}H_{19}NO_2$ MW: 281.36 Property: mp (-): 128-9°C. Source: HE YE, LIAN ZI. Ref: 6.

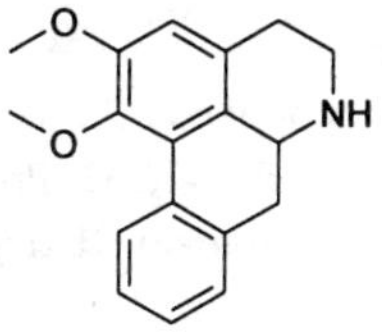

4772 Nor-orixine
$C_{16}H_{19}NO_6$ MW: 321.33 Property: mp 199-200°C. Source: CHOU SHAN YANG. Ref: 6.

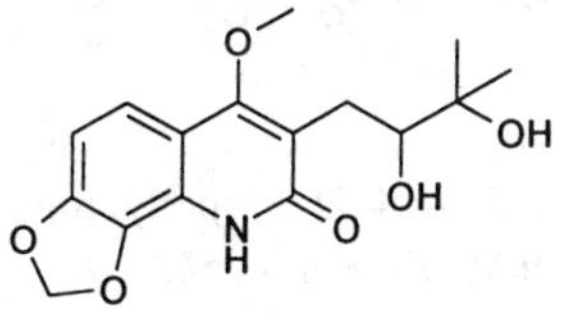

4773 Norpluviine
$C_{16}H_{19}NO_3$ MW: 273.33 Property: mp 239-41°C (dec), 274-5°C. Source: SHI SUAN. Ref: 6.

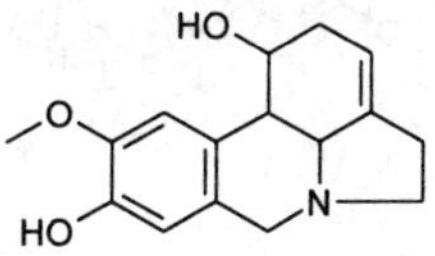

4774 d-Nor-pseudoephedrine
$C_9H_{13}NO$ MW: 151.21 Source: MA HUANG. Ref: 2.

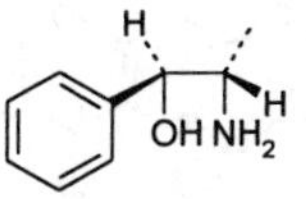

4775 Nor-rubrofusarin
$C_{14}H_{10}O_5$ MW: 258.23 Source: JUE MING ZI. Ref: 2.

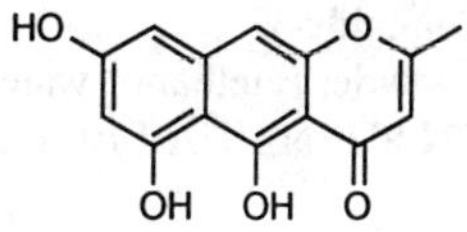

4776 Norsanguinarine
$C_{19}H_{11}NO_4$ MW: 317.30 Source: YING SU KE. Ref: 6.

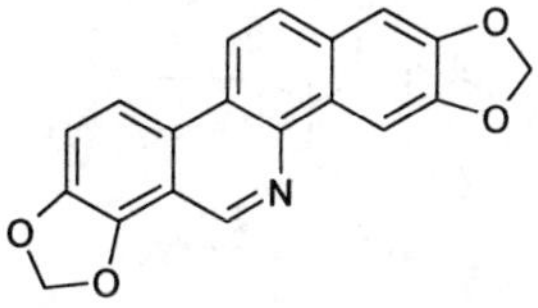

4777 Nortanshinone
$C_{17}H_{14}O_5$ MW: 298.30 Source: DAN SHEN. Ref: 2.

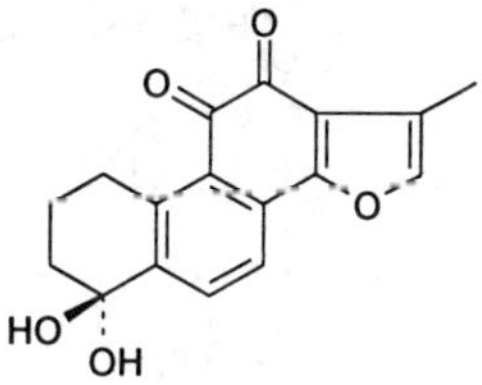

4778 Nortracheloside
$C_{26}H_{32}O_{12}$ MW: 536.54 Property: mp 95-100°C. Source: LUO SHI TENG. Ref: 6.

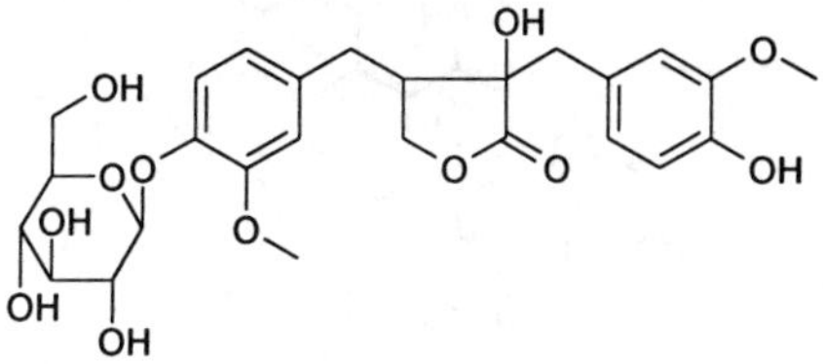

4779 Nor-wogonin
$C_{15}H_{10}O_5$ MW: 270.24 Source: HUANG QIN. Ref: 2.

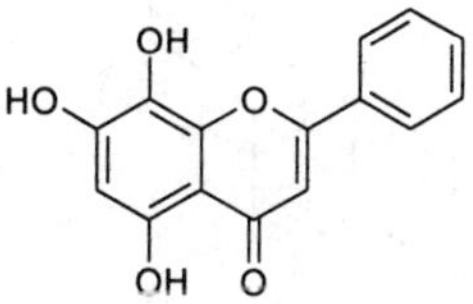

4780 Nothosmyrnol
$C_{11}H_{14}O_2$ MW: 178.22 Source: XIANG GEN QIN. Ref: 6.

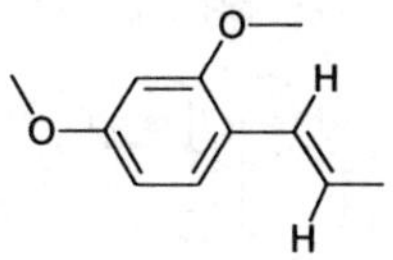

4781 Notoginsenoside-E
Property: white powder (methanol-water), mp 204-6°C. Source: REN SHEN HUA LEI. Ref: 446.

4782 Notoginsenoside R1
Source: REN SHEN, SAN QI. Ref: 2.

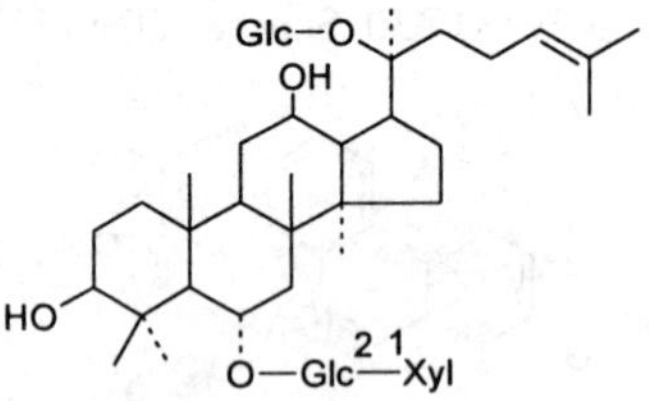

4783 Notoginsenoside R2
Source: SAN QI. Ref: 2.

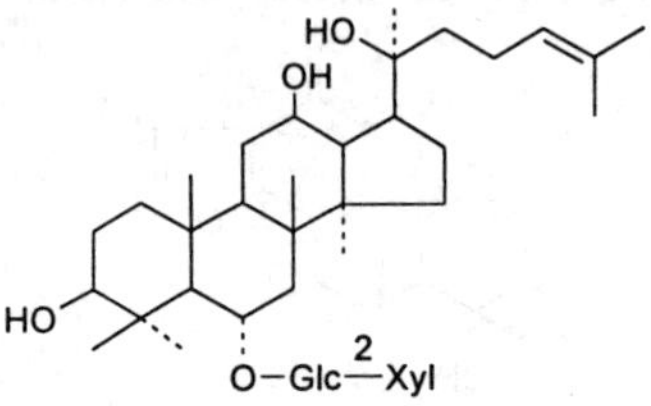

4784 Notoginsenoside R3
Source: SAN QI. Ref: 2.

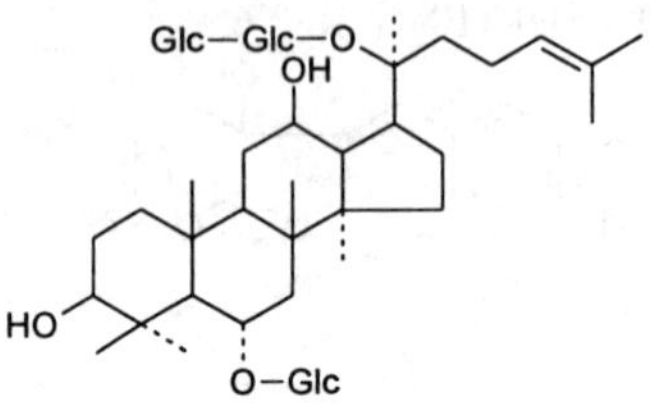

4785 Notoginsenoside R4
Source: REN SHEN, SAN QI. Ref: 2.

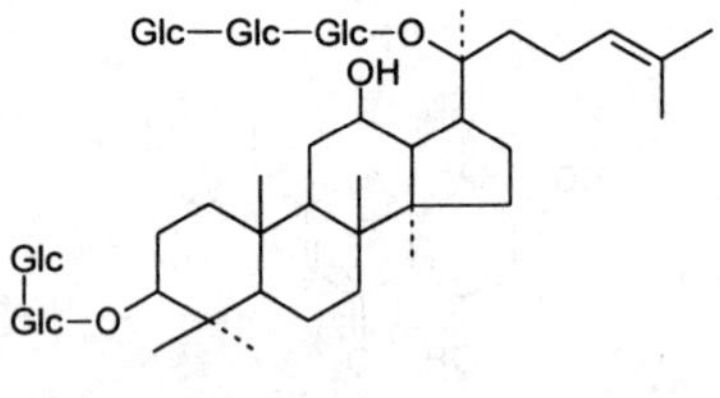

4786 Notoginsenoside R6
Source: SAN QI. Ref: 2.

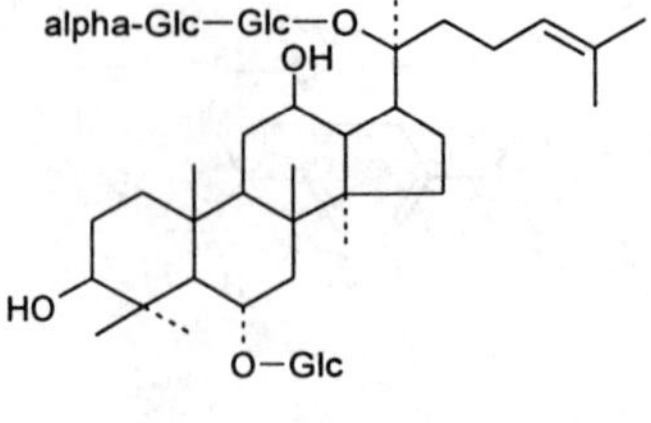

4787 Notopterol
$C_{21}H_{22}O_5$ MW: 354.41 Source: QIANG HUO. Ref: 2, 325, 507, 566.

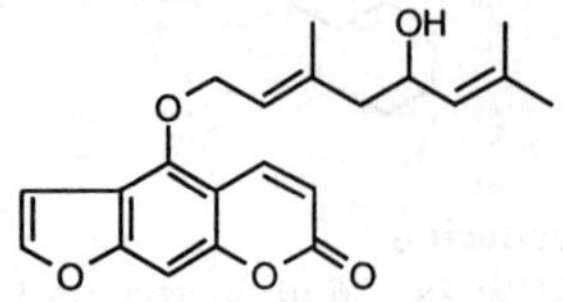

4788 Notoptol
$C_{21}H_{22}O_5$ MW: 354.41 Source: QIANG HUO. Ref: 2, 507.

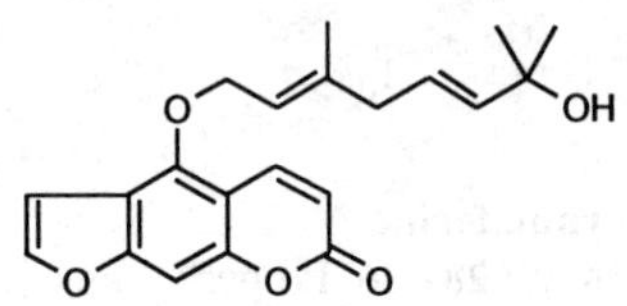

4789 Notoptolide
5-(2E)-3,7-dimethyl-5-ethoxy-2,6-octadienyloxy psoralen. $C_{25}H_{30}O_6$ MW: 426.51 Property: colorless oleaginous substance. Source: QIANG HUO. Ref: 325.

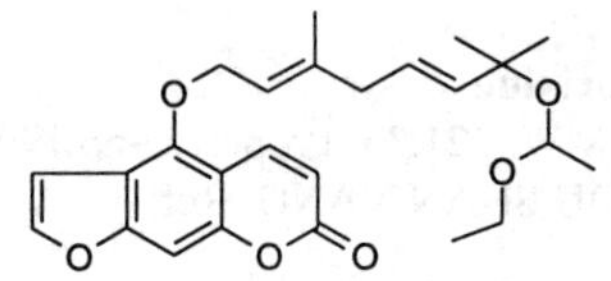

4790 Novacine
$C_{24}H_{28}N_2O_5$ MW: 424.50 Property: mp 231-2°C. Source: MA QIAN ZI. Ref: 6, 542.

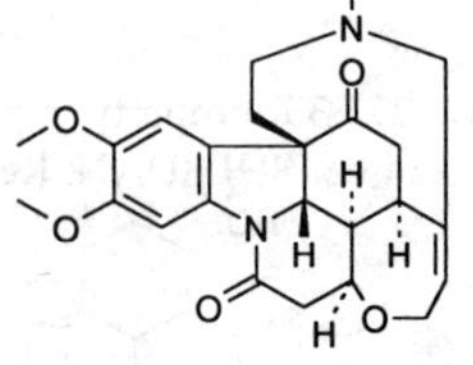

4791 Nuciferine
$C_{19}H_{21}NO_2$ MW: 295.38 Property: mp (-): 165.5°C, (±): 136-7°C. Source: HE YE, HE YE DI, LIAN ZI, LIAN ZI XIN. Ref: 6.

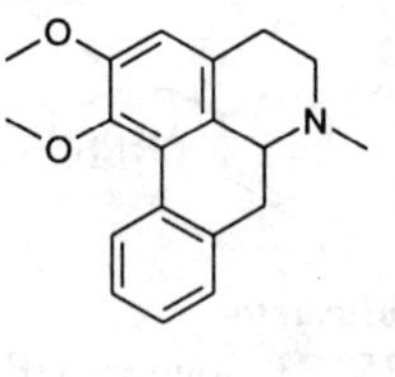

4792 Nuezhengalaside

$C_{18}H_{28}O_9$ MW: 388.42 Property: colorless powder, mp 144-7°C. Source: NU ZHEN ZI. Ref: 386.

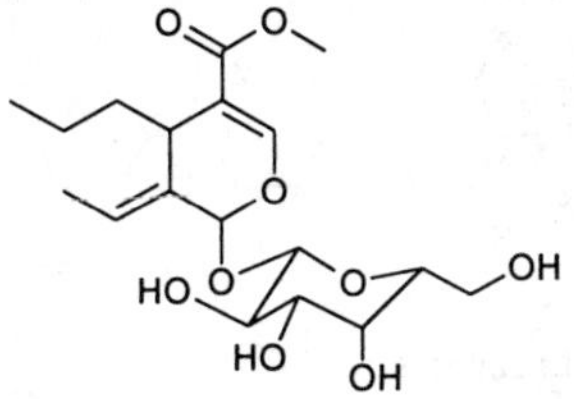

4793 Nyssoside

3'-O-Methyl-3,4-O,O-methylideneellagic acid-4'-O-β-D-glucopyranoside. $C_{22}H_{18}O_{13}$ MW: 490.38 Property: white acicular crystal (MeOH), mp 273-5°C, soluble in pyridine, slightly soluble in methanol, water. Source: ZI SHU. Ref: 492.

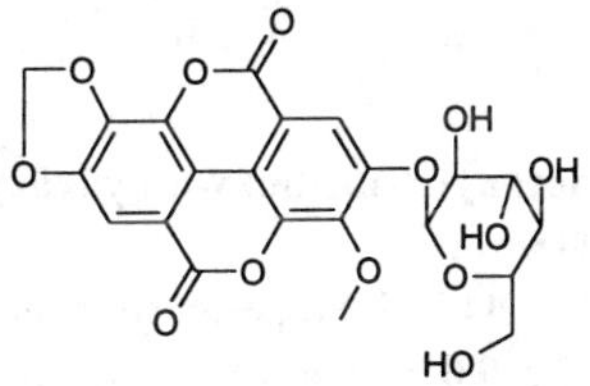

4794 Obaberine

$C_{38}H_{42}N_2O_6$ MW: 622.77 Property: mp 139-40°C. Source: HUANG XIAO BO, XIA YE TANG SONG CAO, XIAO TANG SONG CAO. Ref: 4.

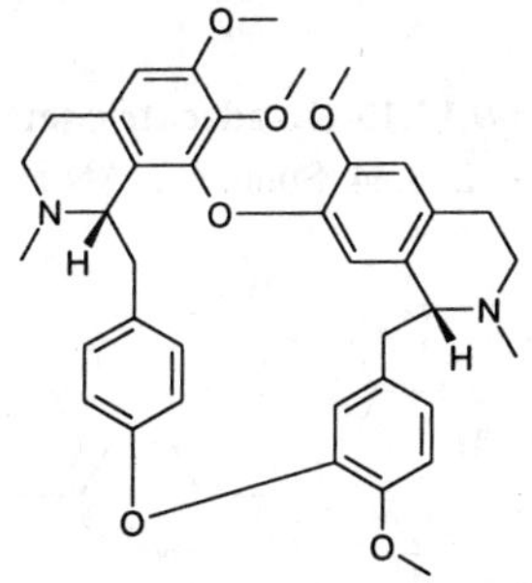

4795 Obaculactone

Dictamnolactone; Evodin; Limonin. $C_{26}H_{30}O_8$ MW: 470.52 Property: mp 297-8°C (dec). Source: BAI XIAN PI, CHENG ZI HE, HUANG BAI, HUANG LIAN, JU HE, TIAN CHENG, WU ZHU YU, XIANG YUAN, YOU HE. Ref: 2, 6.

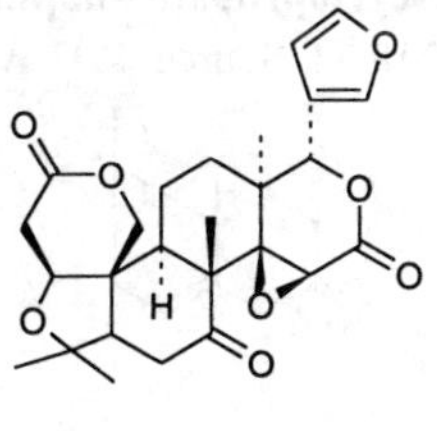

4796 Obacunoic acid

$C_{26}H_{32}O_8$ MW: 472.54 Property: mp 205-6°C. Source: BAI XIAN PI, HUANG BAI. Ref: 2.

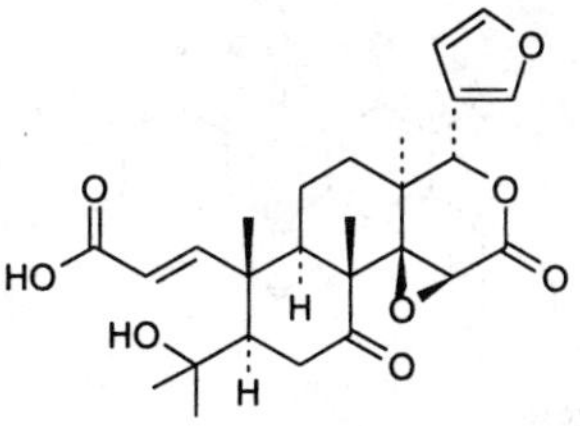

4797 Obacunone

$C_{26}H_{30}O_7$ MW: 454.52 Source: HUANG LIAN, WU ZHU YU. Ref: 2.

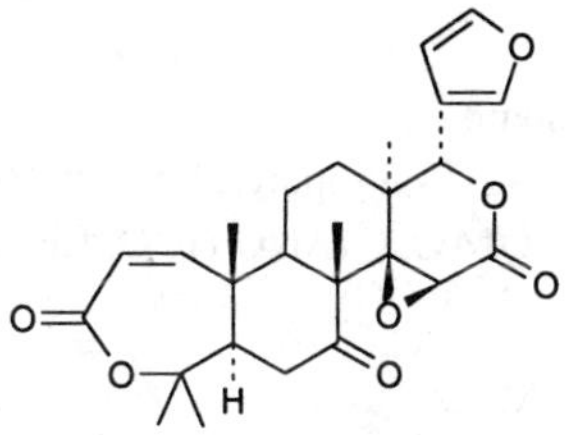

4798 α-Obscurine

$C_{17}H_{26}N_2O$ MW: 274.41 Property: mp 322-3°C. Source: GUO JIANG LONG, XIAO JIE JIN CAO. Ref: 6.

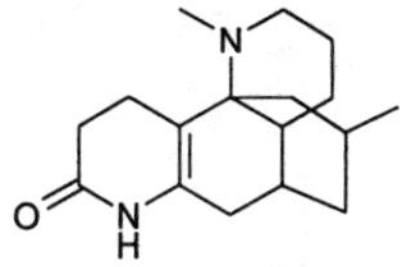

4799 β-Obscurine

$C_{17}H_{24}N_2O$ MW: 272.39 Property: mp 322-3°C(dec). Source: XIAO JIE JIN CAO. Ref: 6.

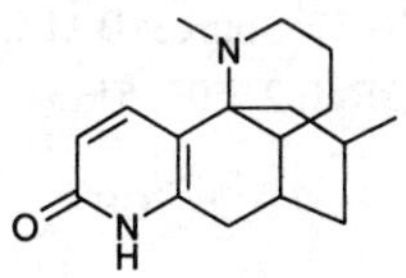

4800 Obtusifolin

$C_{16}H_{12}O_5$ MW: 284.27 Property: mp 237-8°C. Source: JUE MING ZI. Ref: 2.

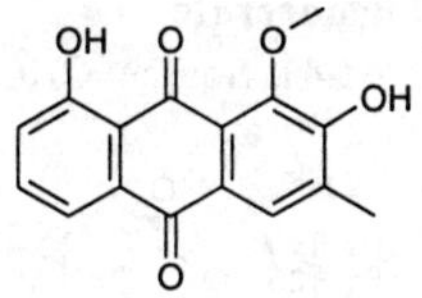

4801 Obtusin

$C_{18}H_{16}O_7$ MW: 344.32 Property: mp 242-3°C. Source: JUE MING ZI. Ref: 2.

4802 Ocimene

α-Ocimene $C_{10}H_{16}$ MW: 136.24 Source: JU PI , WU ZHU YU. Ref: 2.

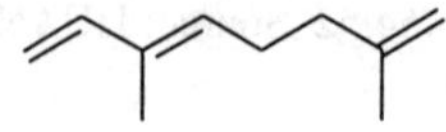

4803 β-Ocimene

$C_{20}H_{32}$ MW: 272.48 Property: bp 81°C/30mm. Source: LIAN QIAO, QIANG HUO. Ref: 2.

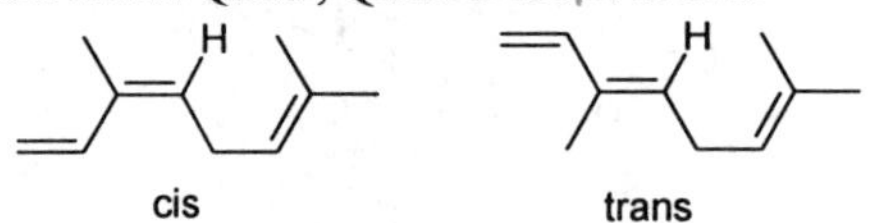

4804 Octacosanedioic acid

$C_{28}H_{54}O_4$ MW: 454.74 Source: WEN JING. Ref: 6.

4805 Octacosanic acid

Source: HUI BAO HAO. Ref: 503.

4806 Octacosanol-1

$C_{28}H_{58}O$ MW: 410.77 Source: BAI GUO, HUI BAO HAO, MU JIN PI. Ref: 2, 503, 519.

4807 Octacosanyl ferulate

Source: GUANG XI XUE JIE. Ref: 616.

4808 Octacosyl lignocerate

$C_{52}H_{104}O_2$ MW: 761.41 Source: CHONG BAI LA. Ref: 6.

4809 (Z,Z)-9,12-Octadecadienoic acid

$C_{18}H_{32}O_2$ MW: 280.45 Source: TIAN HUA FEN. Ref: 2.

4810 n-Octadecane

$C_{18}H_{38}$ MW: 254.50 Source: DANG SHEN. Ref: 2.

4811 Octadecanol

$C_{18}H_{38}O$ MW: 270.50 Source: BAI ZHI. Ref: 2.

4812 Octadecanyl-3-methoxy-4-hydroxy benzeneacrylate

$C_{28}H_{46}O_4$ MW: 446.68 Property: white acicular crystal, mp 67.5-9.0 °C. Source: DA JI (a). Ref: 360.

4813 (Z,Z,Z)-9,12,15-Octadecatrienoic acid

$C_{18}H_{30}O_2$ MW: 278.44 Source: TIAN HUA FEN. Ref: 2.

4814 9(Z)-Octadecen-1-ol

$C_{18}H_{36}O$ MW: 268.49 Source: BAI ZHI. Ref: 2.

4815 1,1a,2,4,6,7,7a,7b-Octahydro-1,1,7,7a-tetramethyl-5H-cyclopropa(α)-naphthalen-5-one

$C_{15}H_{22}O$ MW: 218.34 Source: WU WEI ZI. Ref: 2.

4816 1,1a,4,5,6,7,7a,7b-Octahydro-1,1,7,7a-tetramethyl-2H-cyclopropa(α)-naphthalen-2-one
$C_{15}H_{22}O$ MW: 218.34 Source: WU WEI ZI. Ref: 2.

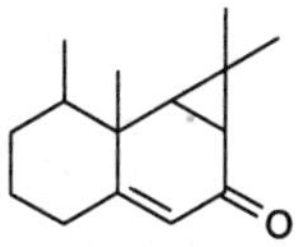

4817 γ-Octalactone
$C_8H_{14}O_2$ MW: 142.20 Property: bp 132-3°C/20 mm. Source: XING ZI. Ref: 6.

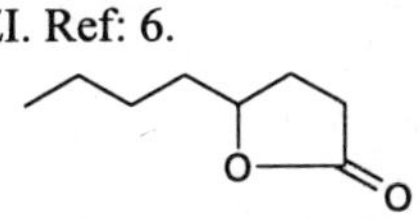

4818 Octanal
$C_8H_{16}O$ MW: 128.22 Source: FANG FENG, JU PI, QIANG HUO, REN SHEN, SHENG JIANG. Ref: 2.

4819 n-Octane
C_8H_{18} MW: 114.23 Source: DU HUO, SHENG JIANG. Ref: 2.

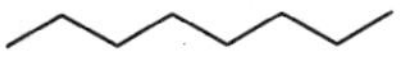

4820 Octanoic acid
$C_8H_{16}O_2$ MW: 144.22 Source: SAN QI, XI YANG SHEN. Ref: 2.

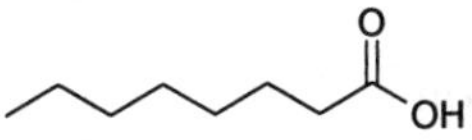

4821 Octanol
$C_8H_{18}O$ MW: 130.23 Source: FANG FENG, JU PI, XI YANG SHEN. Ref: 2.

4822 3-Octanol
$C_8H_{18}O$ MW: 130.23 Source: HUO XIANG, JIN JIE. Ref: 2.

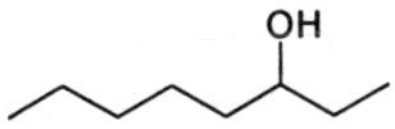

4823 3-Octanone
$C_8H_{16}O$ MW: 128.22 Property: bp (+): 178-9.5°C, (-): 82°C/24mm. Source: HUO XIANG, JIN JIE. Ref: 2.

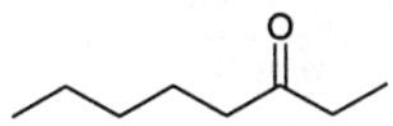

4824 Octasulpher
Property: mp 113-4°C. Source: SONG YE FANG FENG. Ref: 549.

4825 1-Octen-3-ol
$C_8H_{16}O$ MW: 128.22 Source: JIN JIE. Ref: 2.

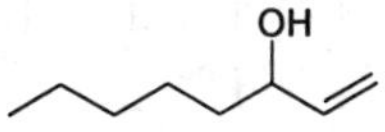

4826 7-Octen-4-ol
$C_8H_{16}O$ MW: 128.22 Source: FANG FENG. Ref: 2.

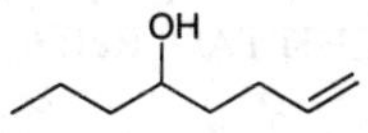

4827 2-Octenic acid
$C_8H_{14}O_2$ MW: 142.20 Source: CHAI HU. Ref: 2.

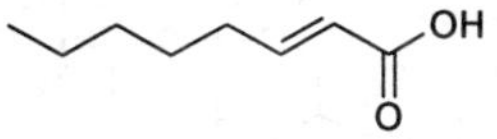

4828 Octopinic acid
$C_8H_{16}N_2O_4$ MW: 204.23 Source: DI JIN. Ref: 6.

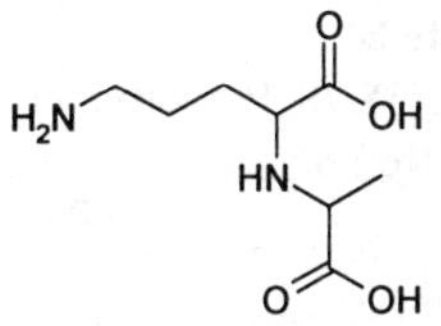

4829 Odoroside D
$C_{36}H_{56}O_{12}$ MW: 680.84 Property: mp 254-6°C. Source: JIA ZHU TAO. Ref: 6.

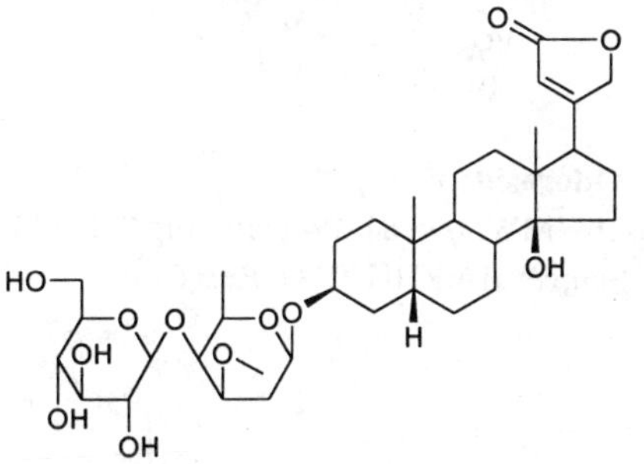

4830 Odontoside
$C_{23}H_{26}O_{11}$ MW: 478.46 Source: CHI YE CAO. Ref: 6.

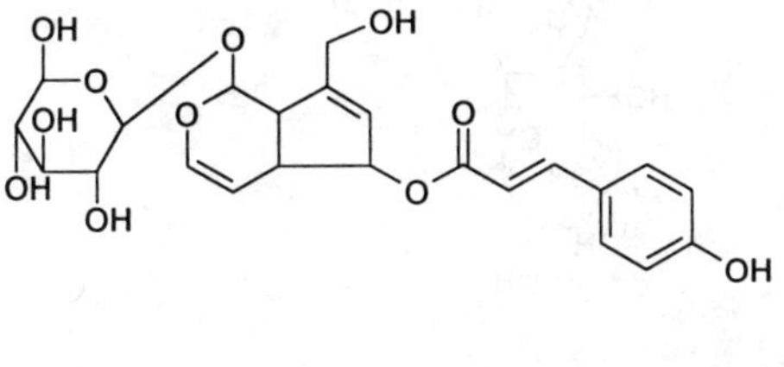

4831 Odoratin
CAS: 19908-77-1 $C_{15}H_{22}O_4$ MW: 266.34 Property: mp 165-7°C. Source: BAI LAI SHI JU, MO ZHI JU. Ref: 5.

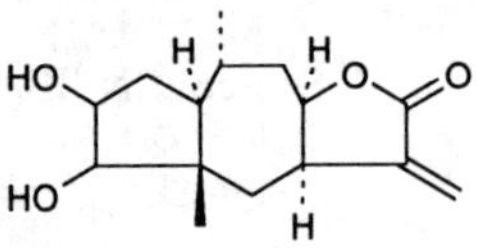

4832 Odoroside A
$C_{30}H_{46}O_7$ MW: 518.70 Property: mp 180-5°C/200-6°C. Source: JIA ZHU TAO. Ref: 6.

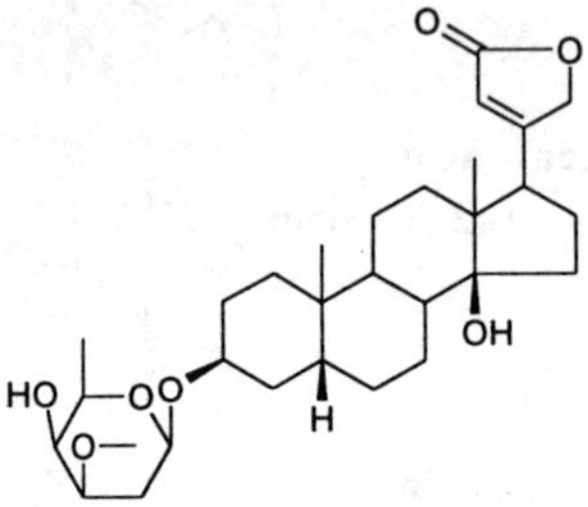

4833 Odoroside B
$C_{30}H_{46}O_7$ MW: 518.70 Property: mp 220°C. Source: JIA ZHU TAO. Ref: 6.

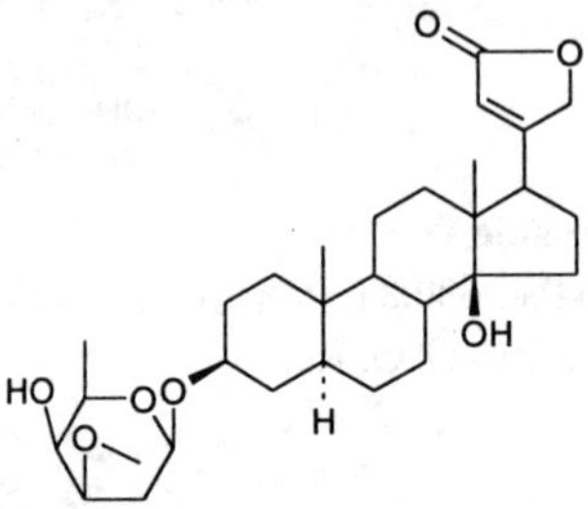

4834 Odoroside F
$C_{36}H_{56}O_{13}$ MW: 696.84 Property: mp 298-302°C (dec). Source: JIA ZHU TAO. Ref: 6.

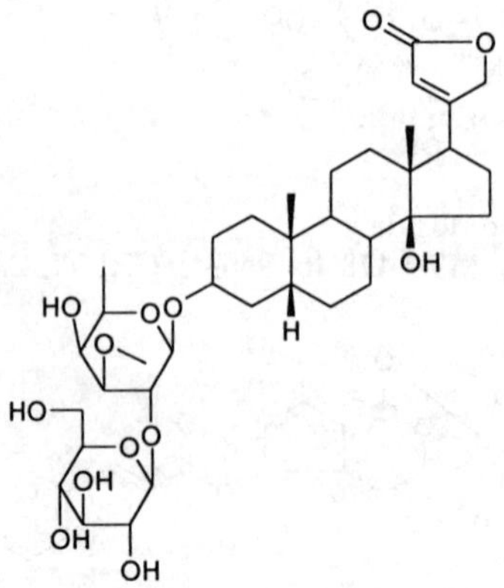

4835 Odoroside H
$C_{30}H_{46}O_8$ MW: 534.70 Property: mp 228-32°C. Source: JIA ZHU TAO. Ref: 6.

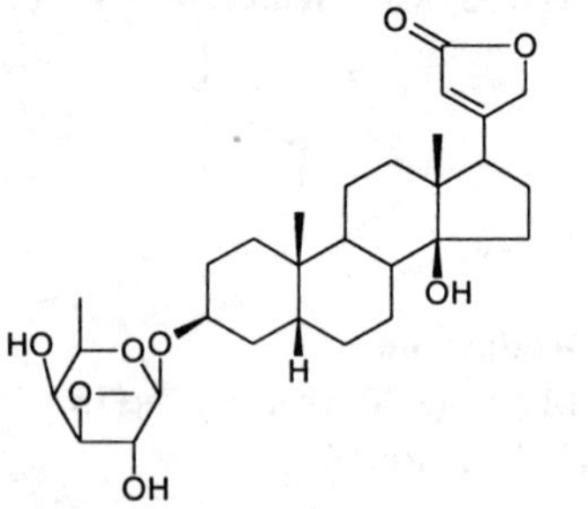

4836 Oenin
$C_{23}H_{25}O_{12}$ MW: 493.45 Source: JIU, PU TAO. Ref: 6.

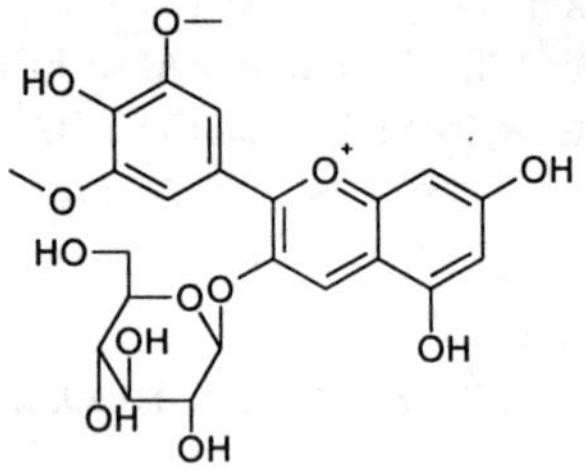

4837 Okinalein
$C_4H_6O_2$ Source: BAI TOU WENG. Ref: 2.

4838 Okinalin
$C_{32}H_{64}O_2$ Source: BAI TOU WENG. Ref: 2.

4839 Oleandrin
$C_{32}H_{48}O_9$ MW: 576.73 Property: mp 250°C (dec). Source: JIA ZHU TAO, PAO DAN GUO. Ref: 6.

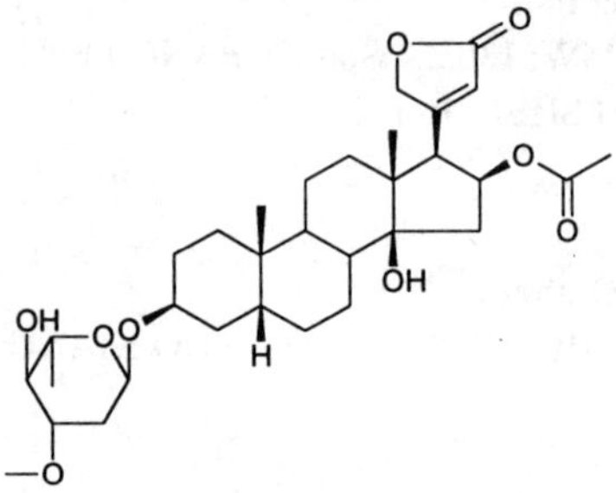

4840 Oleandrose
$C_7H_{14}O_4$ MW: 162.19 Property: mp 68-70°C. Source: FU SHOU CAO, LUO MO ZI. Ref: 6.

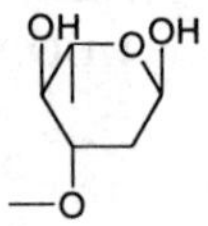

4841 Olean-12-en-3,28-diol
$C_{30}H_{50}O_2$ MW: 442.73 Source: MANG GUO SHU PI. Ref: 6.

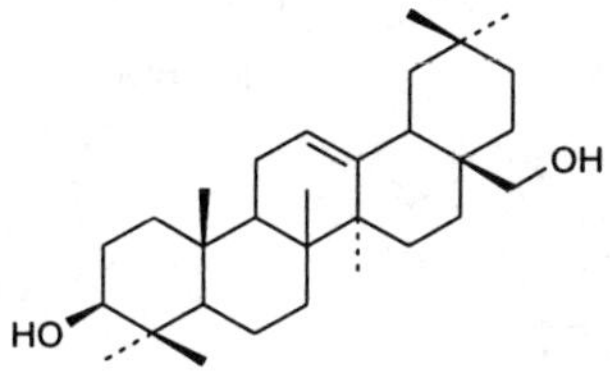

4842 Oleanolic acid
Astrantiagenin C; Caryophyltin; Giganteumgenin C; Oleand; Virhaureqgenin B. CAS: 508-02-1 $C_{30}H_{48}O_3$ MW: 456.72 Property: mp 306-10°C. Source: BAI HUA SHE SHE CAO, BAI JIANG, BING PIAN, DI YANG XI, DING XIANG, FENG XIANG JI SHENG, GUAN MU TONG, HONG KUI ZI, JI SHI TENG GUO, LIAN CHI, MEI SHANG LU, NU ZHEN ZI, PI BA YE, SHI YE, SHI DI, SANG JI SHENG, SHAN ZHA, XIA KU YE, etc. Ref: 4, 6, 439, 453, 455, 462, 471, 472, 592, 600, 622.

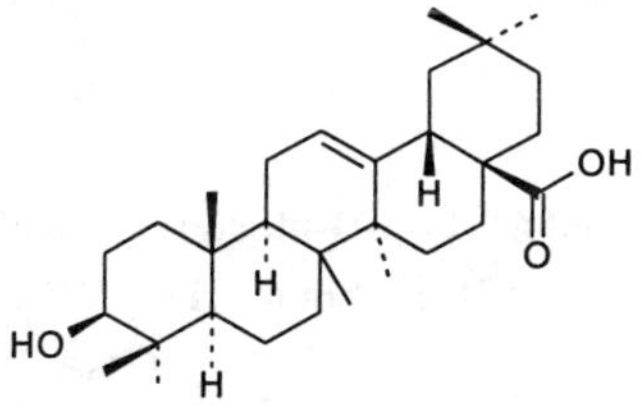

4843 Oleanolic aldehyde
$C_{30}H_{48}O_2$ MW: 440.72 Property: mp 230-1°C (168-72°C). Source: MANG GUO SHU PI. Ref: 6.

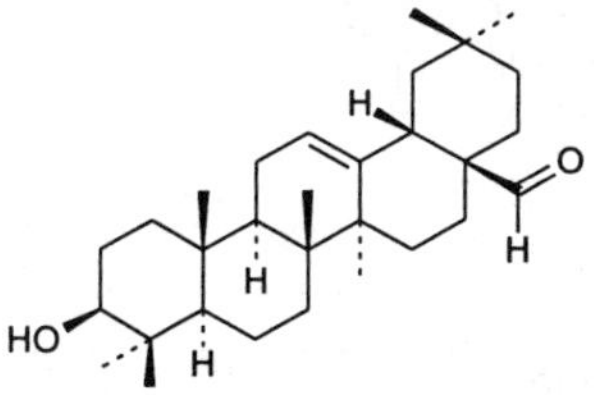

4844 Oleanonic acid
$C_{30}H_{46}O_3$ MW: 454.70 Property: white acicular crystal (ethanol), mp>300°C. Source: BAI HUA, CAO CONG RONG, JIN QUE GEN, SU HE XIANG, TAI BAI HU MU, XI NAN REN DONG, YI YE BAI JIANG, etc. Ref: 6.

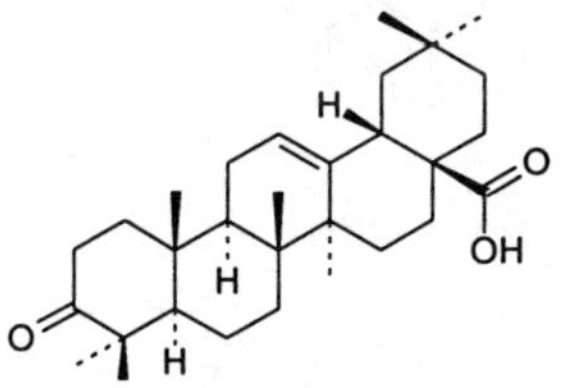

4845 Oleanolic acid-28O-β-D-glucopyranoside
$C_{36}H_{58}O_8$ MW: 618.86 Property: white crystalline powder, mp 218-20°C, $[\alpha]_D^{20}$ +25.59° (c=0.104, MeOH). Source: TAI BAI HU MU. Ref: 470.

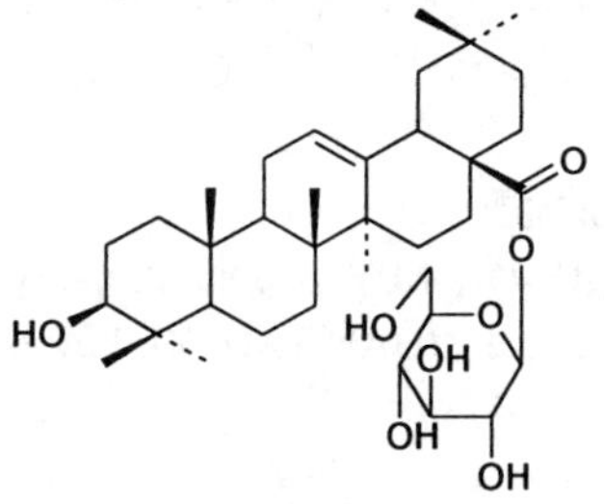

4846 Oleanolic acid-3-O-β-D-glucopyranosyl (1→4)-α-L-arabinopyranoside
MW: 750 Property: white amorphous powder, mp 257-9°C. Source: YI YE BAI JIANG. Ref: 472.

4847 Oleanolic acid-3-O-β-D-glucopyranosyl (1→3)-α-L-rhamnopyranosyl (1→2)-α-L-arabinopyranoside
MW: 896 Property: white amorphous powder, mp 245-7°C. Source: YI YE BAI JIANG. Ref: 472.

4848 Oleic acid
$C_{18}H_{34}O$ MW: 282.47 Property: mp 16°C, bp 285.5-6°C/100mm. Source: QIANG HUO, many.
Ref: 2, 500.

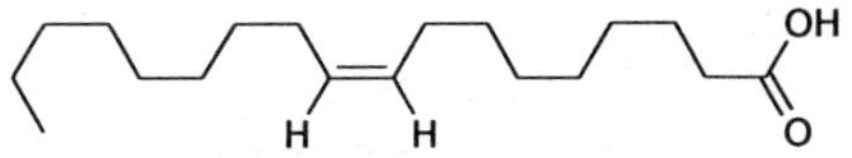

4849 Oleovitamin A
$C_{20}H_{30}O$ MW: 286.46 Source: LU RONG. Ref: 2.

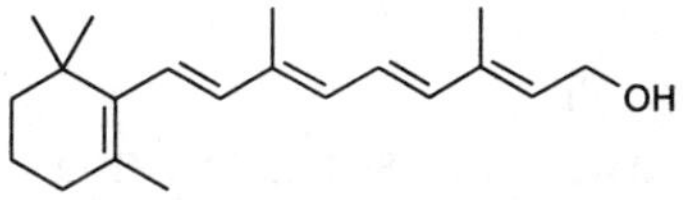

4850 Oleuropein
CAS: 32619-42-4 $C_{25}H_{32}O_{13}$ MW: 540.53 Property: mp 87-9°C. Source: NU ZHEN ZI, YOU GAN LAN. Ref: 4.

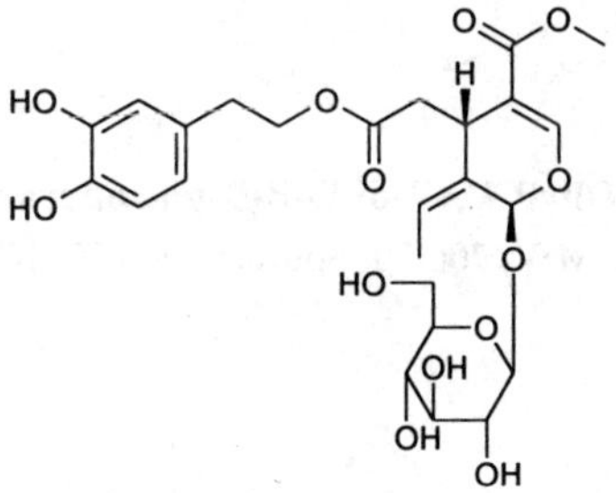

4851 Oleyl alcohol
$C_{18}H_{36}O$ MW: 268.49 Property: bp 205-10°C/15 mm. Source: LI. Ref: 6.

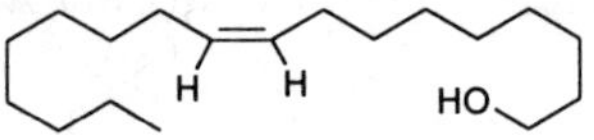

4852 Olitoriside
Olitorin. $C_{35}H_{52}O_{14}$ MW: 696.80 Property: mp 204-6°C (dec). Source: HUANG MA ZI. Ref: 4, 6.

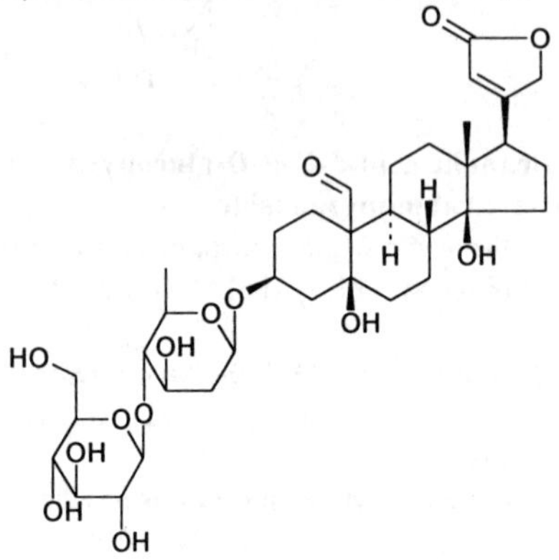

4853 Olivacine
Guatambuinine. CAS: 484-49-1 $C_{17}H_{14}N_2$ MW: 246.31 Property: mp 317-25°C. Source: BAI JIAN MU, etc. Ref: 5.

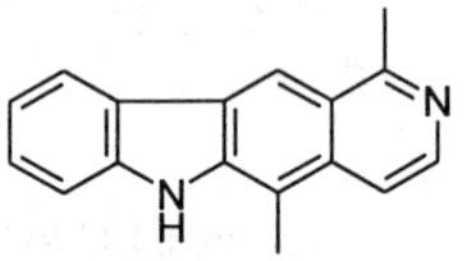

4854 (-)-Olivil
$C_{20}H_{24}O_7$ MW: 376.41 Source: DU ZHONG. Ref: 2.

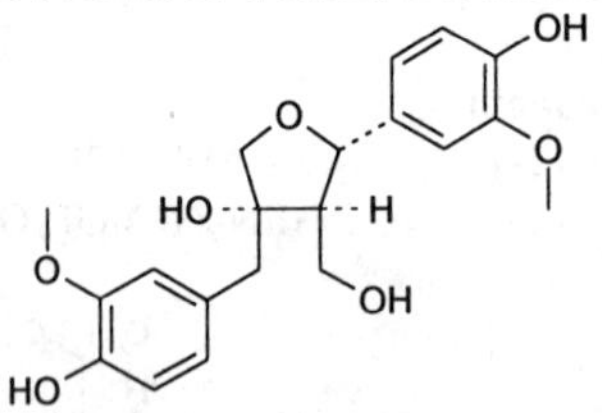

4855 (-)-Olivil 4',4''-di-O-β-D-glucopyranoside
$C_{32}H_{44}O_{17}$ MW: 700.70 Source: DU ZHONG. Ref: 2.

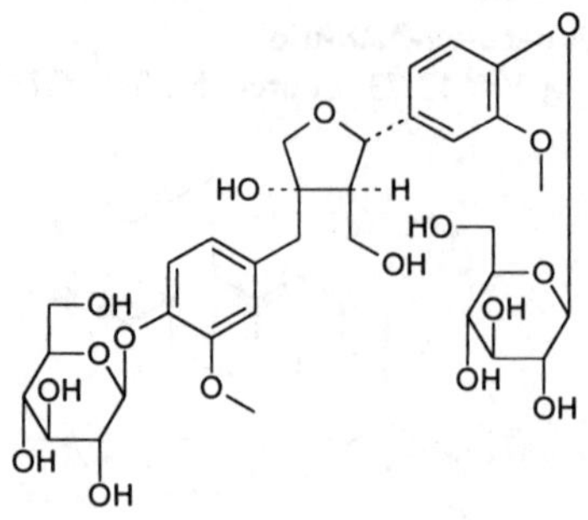

4856 (-)-Olivil 4'-O-β-D-glucopyranoside
$C_{26}H_{34}O_{12}$ MW: 538.55 Source: DU ZHONG. Ref: 2.

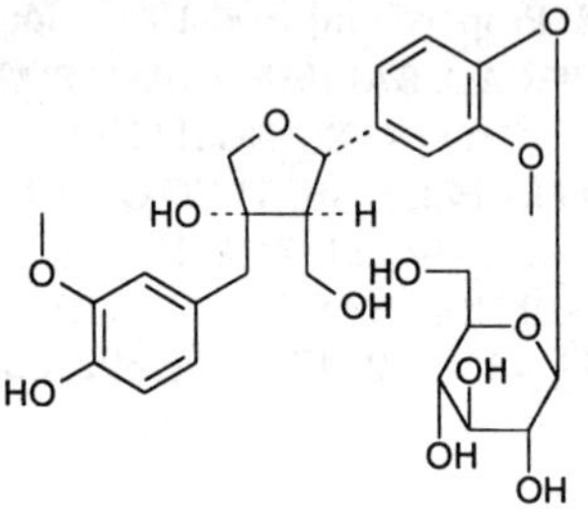

4857 (-)-Olivil 4''-O-β-D-glucopyranoside
$C_{26}H_{34}O_{12}$ MW: 538.55 Source: DU ZHONG. Ref: 2.

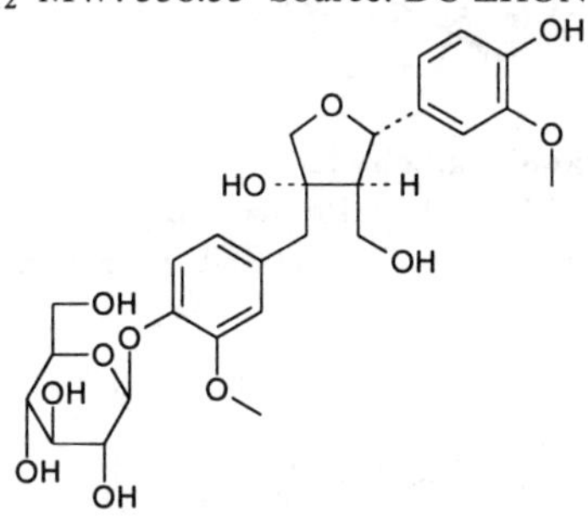

4858 Ombuin
$C_{17}H_{14}O_7$ MW: 330.39 Source: HUO XIANG, QI YE DAN (JIAO GU LAN). Ref: 2.

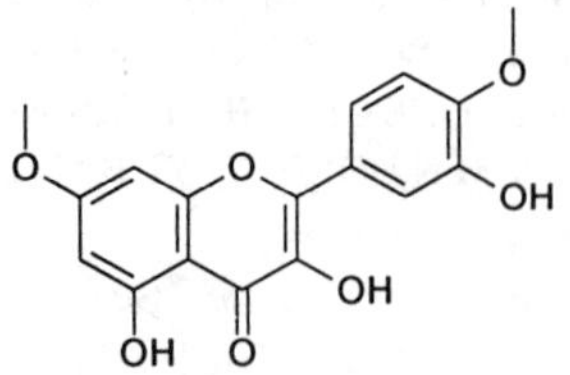

4859 Onjisaponin F

$C_{74}H_{110}O_{36}$ MW: 1575.68 Source: LIAN QIAO. Ref: 2.

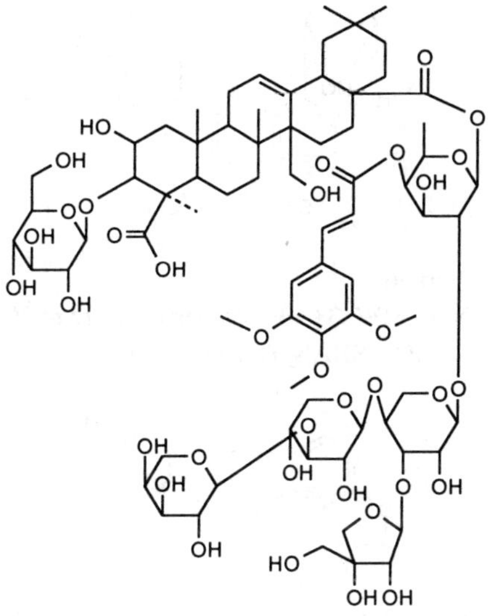

4860 Onjisaponin G

$C_{69}H_{102}O_{32}$ MW: 1443.56 Source: LIAN QIAO. Ref: 2.

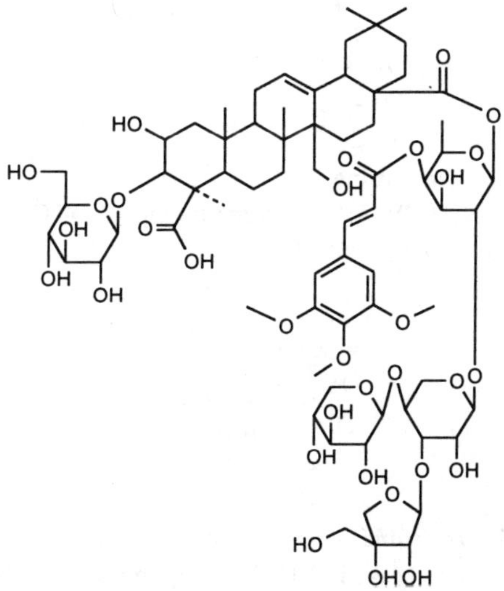

4861 Onjixanthone I

$C_{16}H_{14}O_6$ MW: 302.29 Source: HONG HUA. Ref: 2.

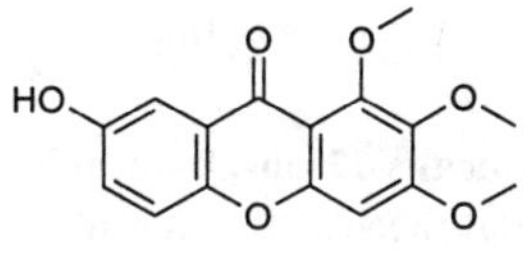

4862 Onjixanthone II

$C_{15}H_{12}O_7$ MW: 304.26 Source: HONG HUA. Ref: 2.

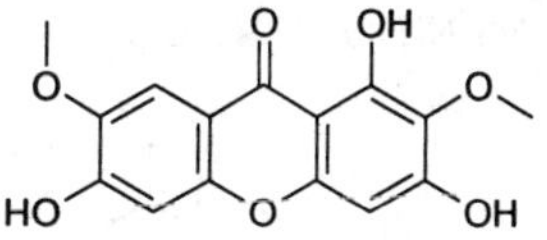

4863 α-Onocerin

$C_{30}H_{50}O_2$ MW: 442.73 Property: mp 232°C (202-3°C). Source: PU DI WU GONG, SHEN JIN CAO. Ref: 6.

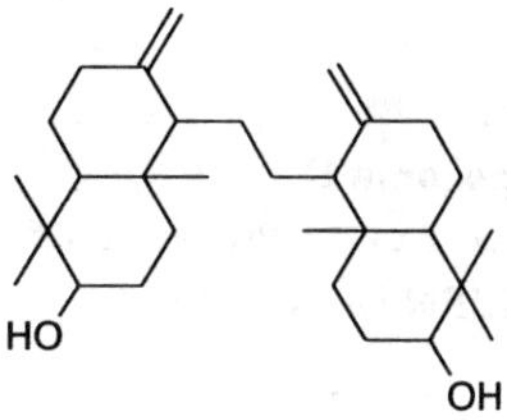

4864 Ononin

$C_{22}H_{22}O_9$ MW: 430.42 Source: GAN CAO. Ref: 2.

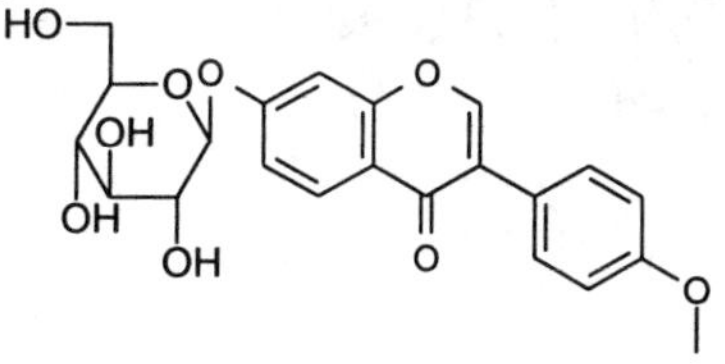

4865 Ononitol

$C_7H_{14}O_6$ MW: 194.19 Property: mp 173°C. Source: MU XU. Ref: 6.

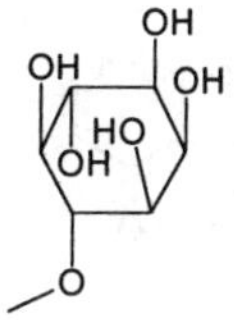

4866 Onopordopicrin

CAS: 19889-00-0 $C_{19}H_{24}O_6$ MW: 348.40 Property: mp 55-6°C. Source: DA CHI JI. Ref: 5.

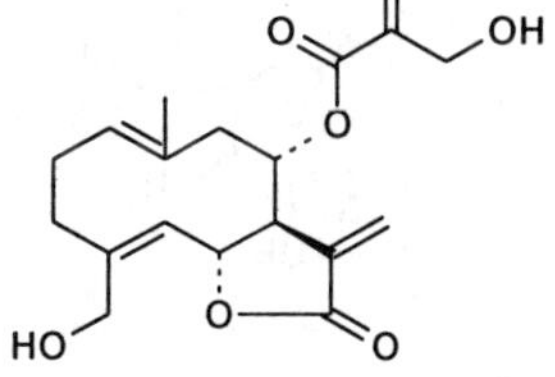

4867 Ophiopogonin B
$C_{40}H_{64}O_{12}$ MW: 736.95 Property: mp 269-71°C. Source: MAI MEN DONG. Ref: 6.

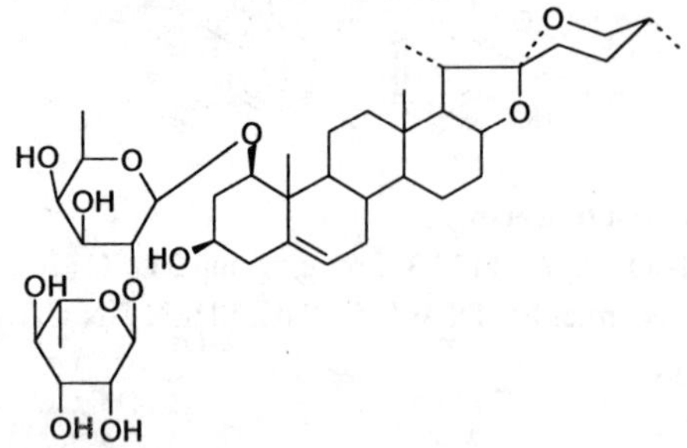

4868 Ophiopogonin D
$C_{46}H_{74}O_{16}$ MW: 883.09 Property: mp 263-5°C. Source: MAI MEN DONG. Ref: 6.

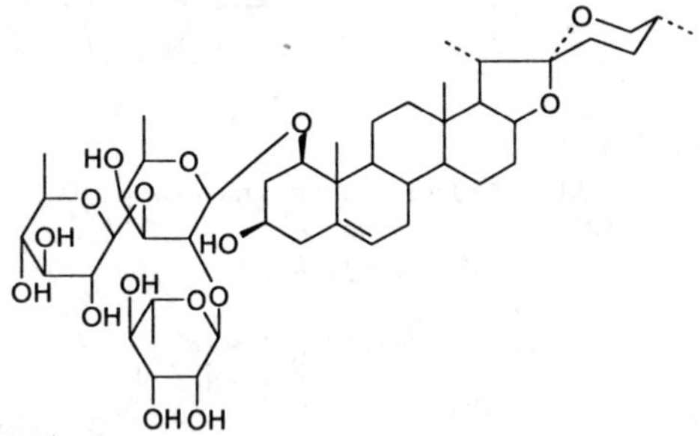

4869 Ophioside
$C_{27}H_{30}O_{16}$ MW: 610.53 Property: mp 227-8°C. Source: MAI MEN DONG. Ref: 6.

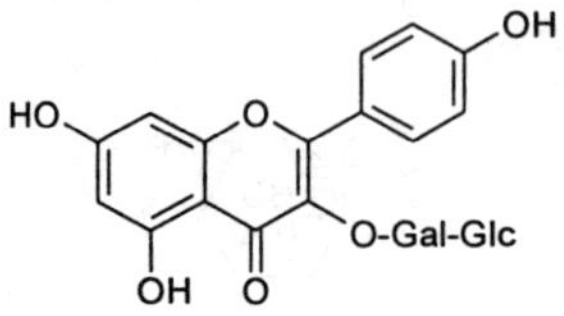

4870 Oridonin
Rubescensine A. CAS: 28957-04-2 $C_{20}H_{28}O_6$ MW: 364.44 Property: mp 247-50°C. Source: DONG LING CAO, XIAN MAI XIANG CHA CAI. Ref: 2, 4, 504.

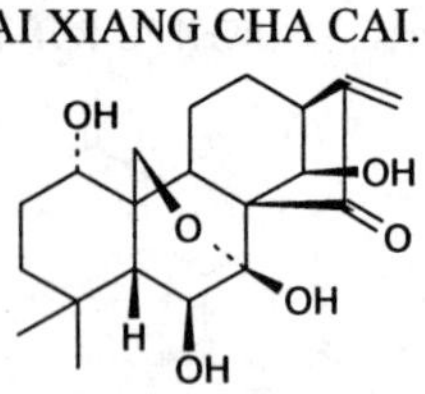

4871 Orientin
$C_{21}H_{20}O_{11}$ MW: 448.39 Property: mp 265-70°C (dec). Source: CHANG BAN JIN LIAN HUA, HONG CAO, HU ZHI ZI, QIAO MAI JIE, QUAN QU CAI, SUAN JIAO, XI XIAN, YA MA. Ref: 2, 6, 245.

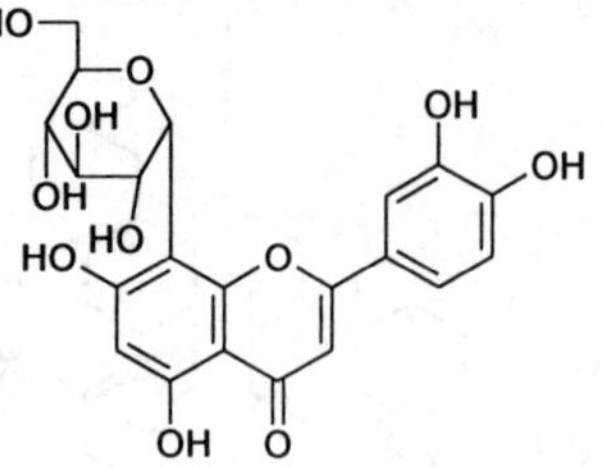

4872 Orixine
$C_{17}H_{21}NO_6$ MW: 335.36 Property: mp 152.5°C. Source: CHOU SHAN YANG. Ref: 6.

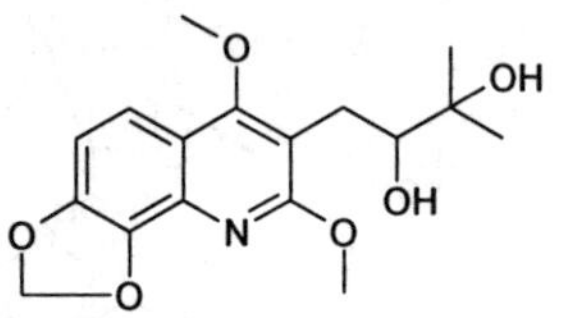

4873 Orixinone
$C_{17}H_{19}NO_5$ MW: 317.34 Property: mp 102-3°C. Source: CHOU SHAN YANG. Ref: 6.

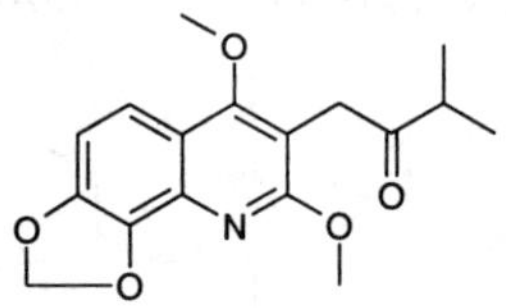

4874 Ormosanine
$C_{20}H_{35}N_3$ MW: 317.52 Property: mp 183-4°C. Source: HONG DOU. Ref: 6.

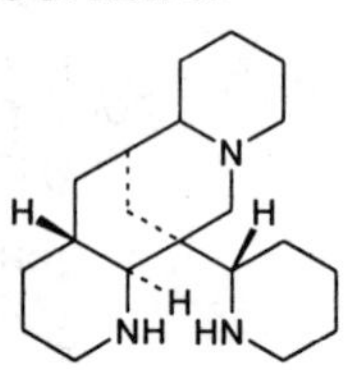

4875 Ornithine
$C_5H_{12}N_2O_2$ MW: 132.16 Property: mp L (+): 140°C. Source: LIE DANG. Ref: 6.

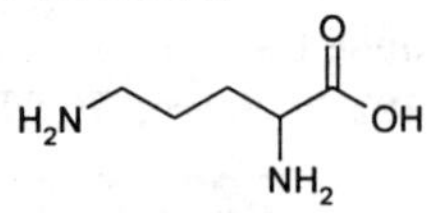

4876 3-Oxo-oleans-12-en-28-oic acid
Source: AN HUI SONG MU. Ref: 622.

4877 Oroselol
$C_{14}H_{12}O_4$ MW: 244.25 Property: mp 148-51°C. Source: GAN SONG. Ref: 6.

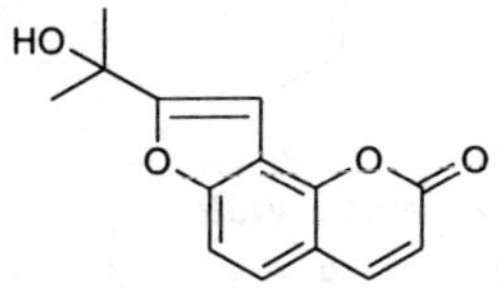

4878 Orotic acid
$C_5H_4N_2O_4$ MW: 156.10 Property: mp 345-6°C (322-5°C). Source: NIU RU. Ref: 6.

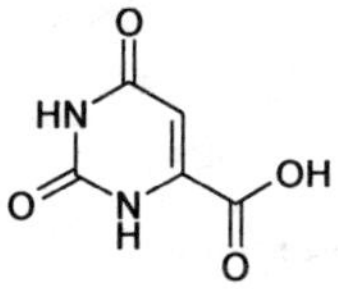

4879 Oroxin A
$C_{21}H_{20}O_{10}$ MW: 432.39 Property: mp 178-80°C. Source: MU HU DIE. Ref: 6.

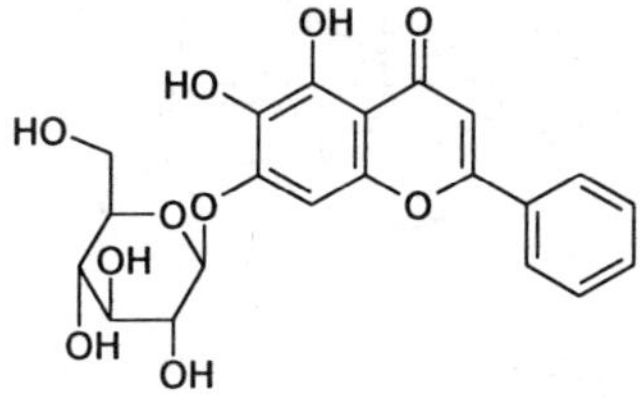

4880 Oroxin B
$C_{27}H_{30}O_{15}$ MW: 594.53 Property: mp 155-7°C. Source: MU HU DIE. Ref: 6.

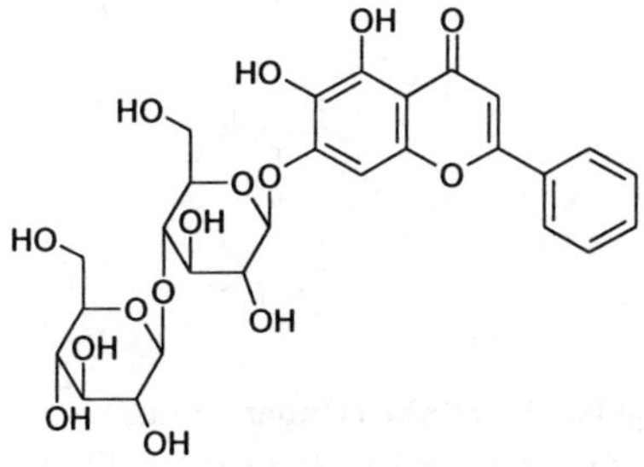

4881 Oroxylin
$C_{16}H_{12}O_5$ MW: 284.27 Property: mp 231-2°C. Source: MU HU DIE SHU PI. Ref: 6.

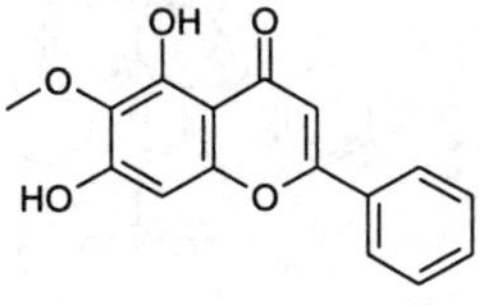

4882 Osladin
$C_{45}H_{74}O_{17}$ MW: 887.08 Property: mp 198-9°C. Source: SHUI LONG GU. Ref: 6.

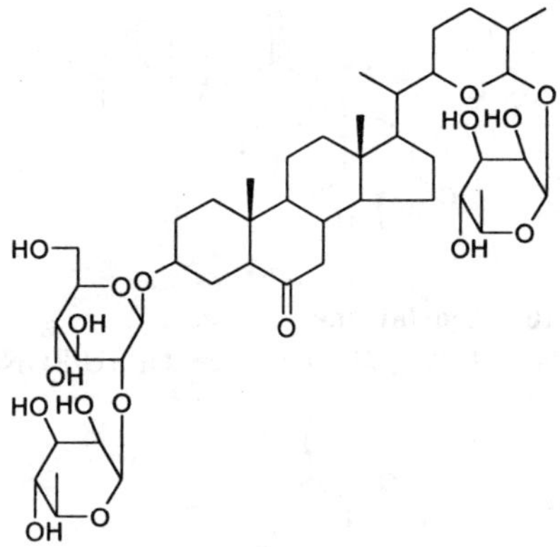

4883 Osthenol
$C_{14}H_{14}O_3$ MW: 230.27 Source: QIANG HUO. Ref: 2.

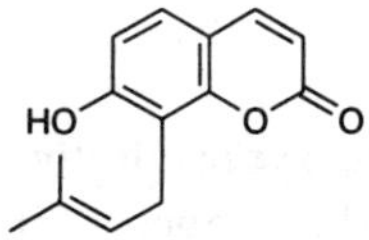

4884 Osthole
CAS: 484-12-8 $C_{15}H_{16}O_3$ MW: 244.29 Property: mp 83-4°C, bp 145-50°C. Source: DU HUO, JIU LI XIANG, SHE CHUANG ZI, XIAN HE CAO, YUN QIAN HU, ZHONG CHI MAO DANG GUI. Ref: 4, 6, 11, 177, 344.

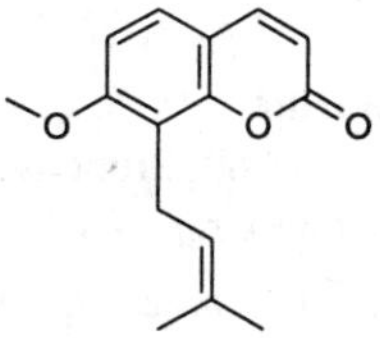

4885 Oxalacetic acid
$C_4H_4O_5$ MW: 132.07 Property: mp 189.5°C. Source: GUI JIAN YU. Ref: 6.

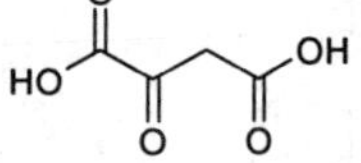

4886 Oxalic acid
$C_2H_2O_4$ MW: 90.04 Property: mp 189.5°C. Source: CU LIU GUO (SHA JI), MA HUANG, SHAN ZHA, YIN CHEN HAO. Ref: 2, 6.

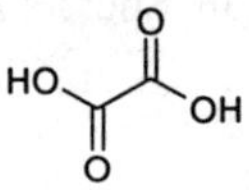

4887 12-Oxoarundoin
$C_{31}H_{50}O_2$ MW: 454.74 Source: MAO CAO YE. Ref: 6.

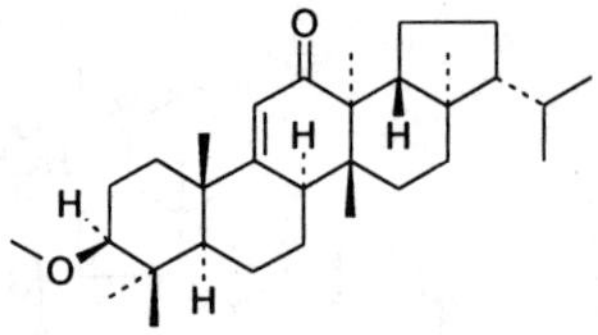

4888 16-Oxodelavaine
$C_{20}H_{21}NO_6$ MW: 371.39 Source: DI BU RONG. Ref: 6.

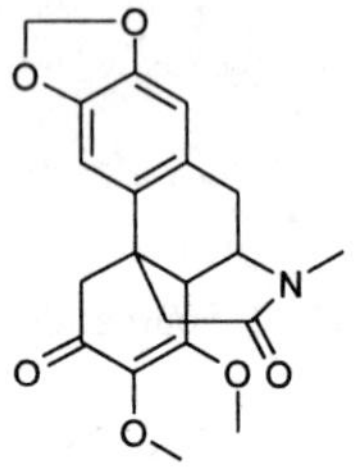

4889 2-Oxo-6-deoxyneoanisatin
$C_{15}H_{18}O_7$ MW: 310.31 Source: YE BA JIAO. Ref: 649.

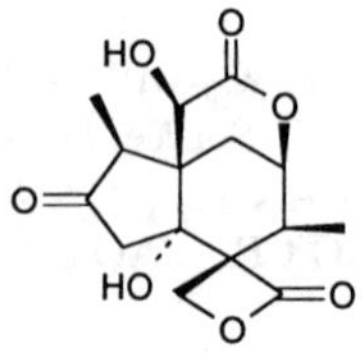

4890 Oxofangchirine
$C_{37}H_{34}N_2O_7$ MW: 618.69 Property: light yellow square crystal (acetone), mp 184-6°C, $[\alpha]_D^{20}$ +47° (c=0.42, chloroform). Source: FEN FANG JI. Ref: 44.

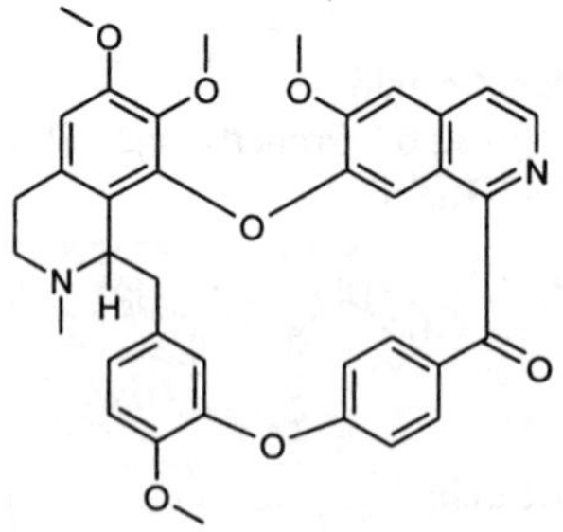

4891 9-Oxofarnesol
$C_{15}H_{24}O_2$ MW: 236.36 Source: ZHANG SHU YE. Ref: 6.

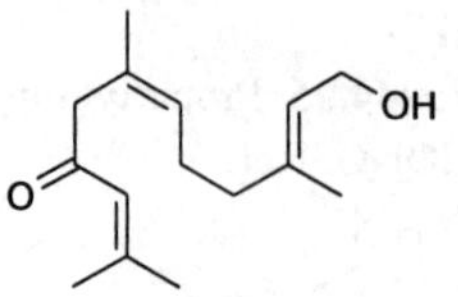

4892 9-Oxofarnesyl acetate
$C_{17}H_{24}O_3$ MW: 276.38 Source: ZHANG SHU YE. Ref: 6.

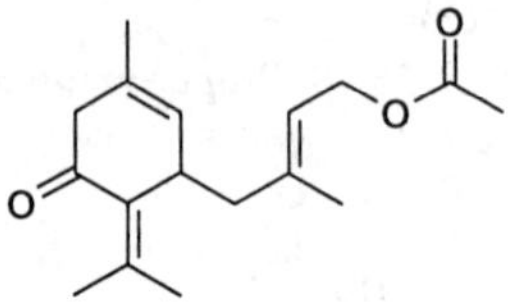

4893 19-Oxo-gelsenicine
$C_{19}H_{20}N_2O_4$ MW: 340.38 Property: mp 226-7°C. Source: HU MAN TENG. Ref: 14.

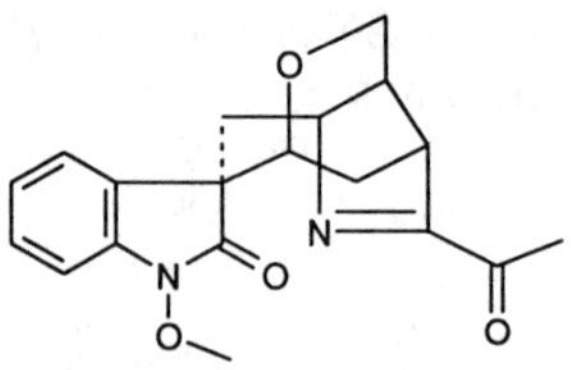

4894 Oxoglaucine
O-Methylatheroline; Noraporphine. $C_{20}H_{17}NO_5$ MW: 351.34 Property: mp 225-7°C. Source: JIAN LIE HAI YING SU. Ref: 5.

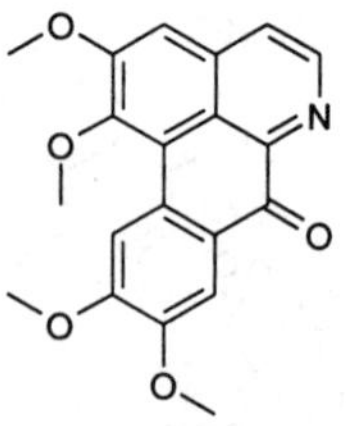

4895 3-Oxo-11-methoxytabersonine
$C_{22}H_{24}N_2O_4$ MW: 380.45 Property: light yellow transparent things, $[\alpha]_D^{30}$ -67.4° (chloroform). Source: JI GU CHANG SHAN. Ref: 49.

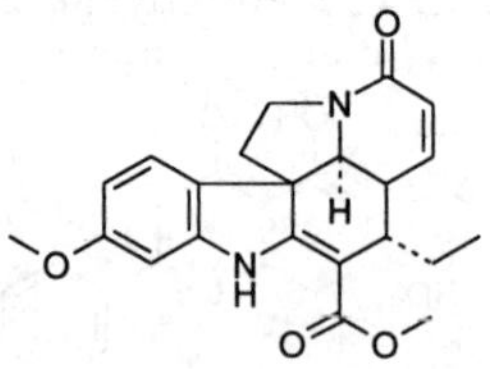

4896 9-Oxonerolidol
$C_{15}H_{24}O_2$ MW: 236.36 Source: NAN MU. Ref: 6.

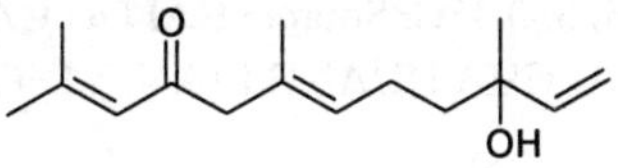

4897 16-Oxoseratenediol
$C_{30}H_{48}O_3$ MW: 456.72 Property: mp 294-7°C. Source: SHEN JIN CAO. Ref: 6.

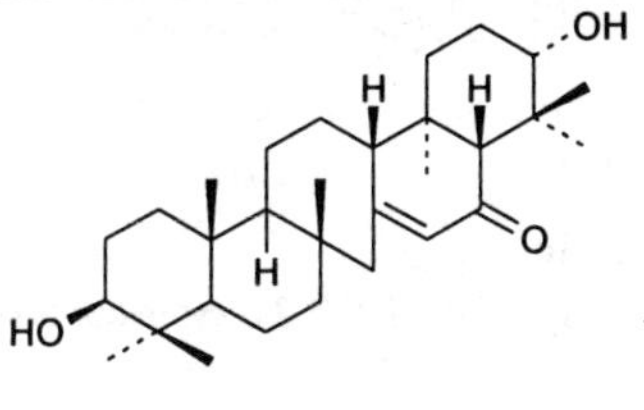

4898 11-Oxotriacontanoic acid
$C_{30}H_{58}O_3$ MW: 466.79 Property: mp 99-101°C. Source: YING SU. Ref: 6.

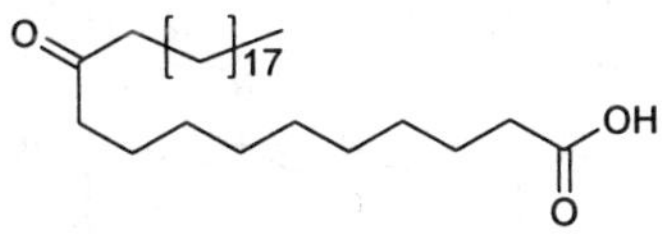

4899 Oxotuberostemonine
$C_{22}H_{31}NO_5$ MW: 389.50 Property: mp 217°C. Source: BAI BU. Ref: 6.

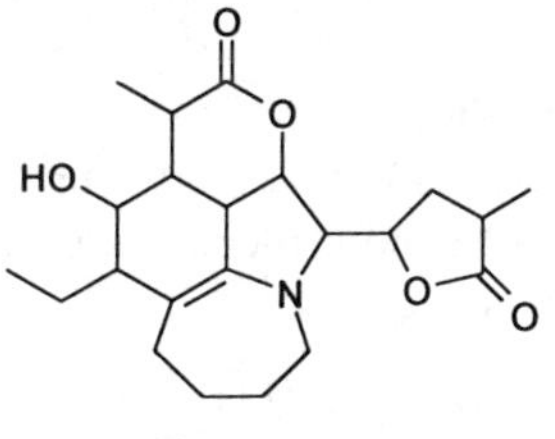

4900 Oxoushinsunine
$C_{17}H_9NO_3$ MW: 275.27 Property: mp 289°C (dec). Source: BAI LAN HUA, HUANG MIAN GUI, LIAN ZI, YE HE HUA. Ref: 6.

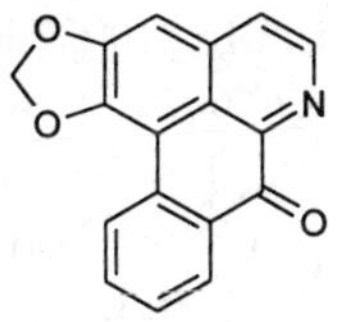

4901 Oxyacanthine
Oxycanthine. CAS: 548-40-3 $C_{37}H_{40}N_2O_6$ MW: 608.74 Property: mp 208-14°C, 216-7°C. Source: GONG LAO MU, XIAO BO. Ref: 4, 6.

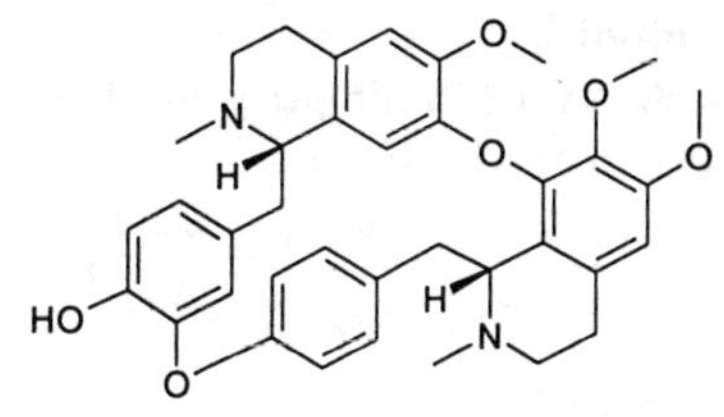

4902 Oxyberberine
$C_{20}H_{17}NO_5$ MW: 351.36 Property: mp 198-200°C. Source: XIAO BO. Ref: 6.

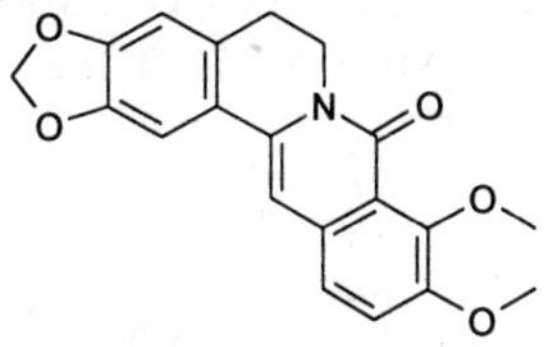

4903 17-Oxycorticosterone
$C_{21}H_{30}O_5$ MW: 362.47 Property: mp 220°C. Source: REN NIAO. Ref: 6.

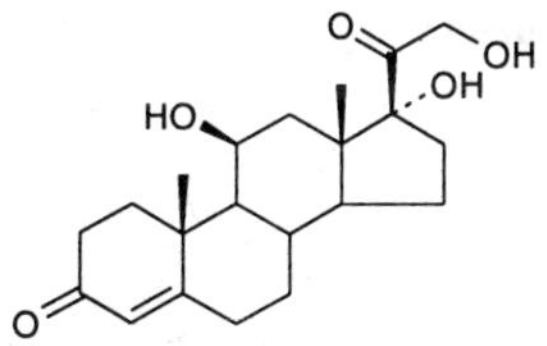

4904 Oxymatrine
Matrine N-oxide. $C_{15}H_{24}N_2O_2$ MW: 264.37 Property: mp 206-8°C. Source: BAI CI HUA, KU DOU ZI, KU SHEN, SHAN DOU GEN. Ref: 4, 546, 564, 593.

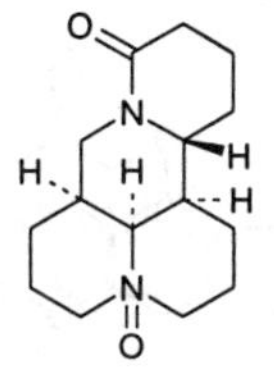

4905 Oxynarcotine
$C_{22}H_{25}NO_8$ MW: 431.45 Property: mp 229°C (dec). Source: YA PIAN. Ref: 6.

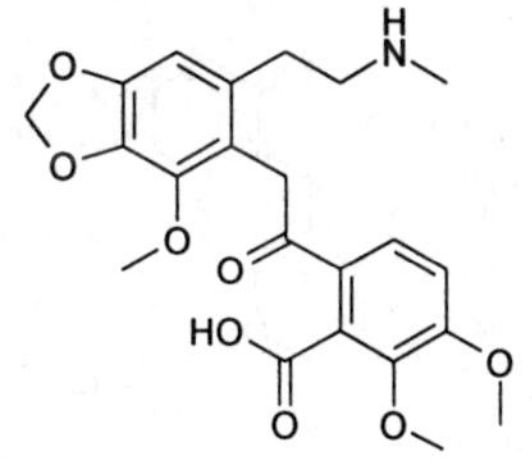

4906 Oxynitidine
$C_{21}H_{17}NO_5$ MW: 363.37 Property: mp 284-5°C. Source: RU DI JIN NIU. Ref: 6.

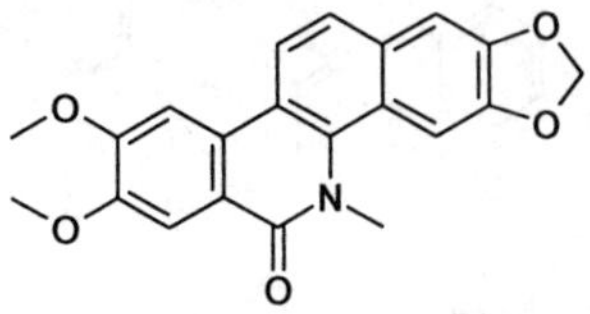

4907 Oxypaeoniflorin
$C_{16}H_{14}O_5$ MW: 286.29 Source:BAI SHAO YAO, CHI SHAO YAO, MU DAN PI. Ref: 2.

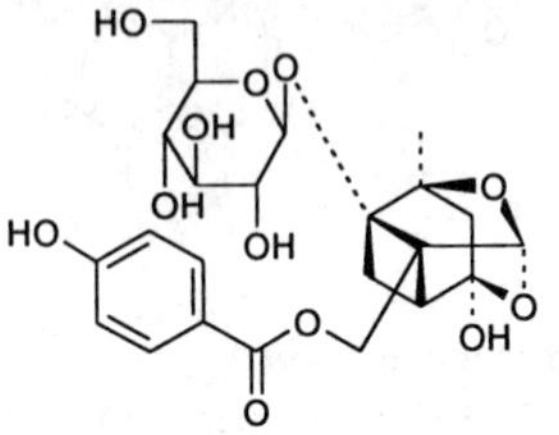

4908 Oxypeucedanin
$C_{16}H_{14}O_5$ MW: 286.27 Property: mp 142-3°C. Source: BAI ZHI. Ref: 4.

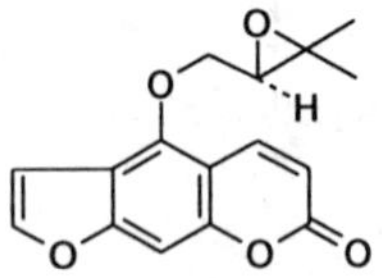

4909 Oxypeucedanin hydrate
$C_{16}H_{16}O_6$ MW: 304.30 Property: mp 134°C. Source: BAI ZHI. Ref: 2.

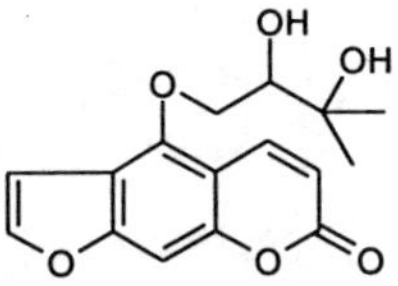

4910 Oxysophocarpine
$C_{15}H_{22}N_2O_2$ MW: 262.35 Property: mp 198-9°C, 206-8°C. Source: BAI CI HUA, KU DOU ZI. Ref: 2, 546. 564, 593.

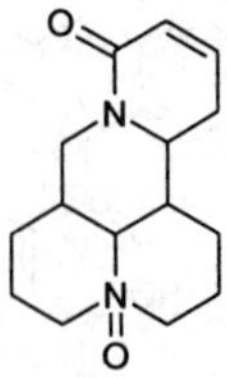

4911 Oxysanguinarine
Hydroxysanguiarine. $C_{20}H_{13}NO_5$ MW: 347.33 Property: mp 360-1°C. Source: BAI QU CAI, BO LUO HUI, JU HUA HUANG LIAN, YING SU KE. Ref: 6.

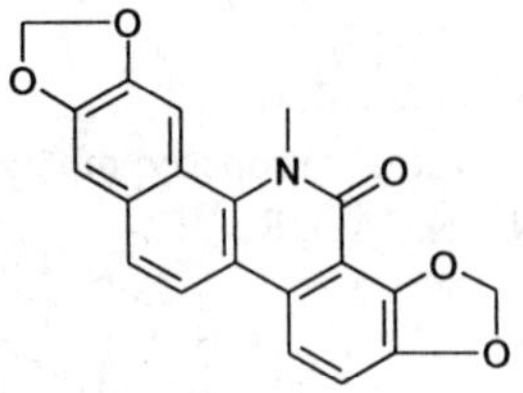

4912 Oxytocin
$C_{43}H_{66}N_{12}O_{12}S_2$ MW: 1007.21 Source: NIU NAO. Ref: 6.

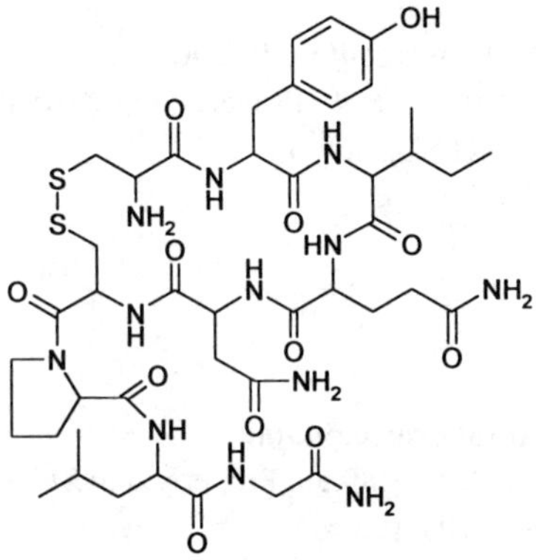

4913 α-Oxyvaline
$C_5H_{11}NO_3$ MW: 133.15 Property: mp L (+): 205°C, D (-): 205°C, DL: 240°C (dec). Source: XIONG ZHANG. Ref: 6.

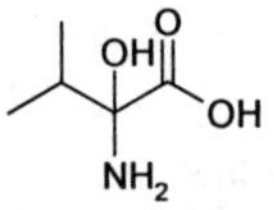

4914 β-Oxyvaline
$C_5H_{11}NO_3$ MW: 133.15 Property: mp mp L (+): 205°C, D (-): 205°C, DL: 240°C (dec). Source: XIONG ZHANG. Ref: 6.

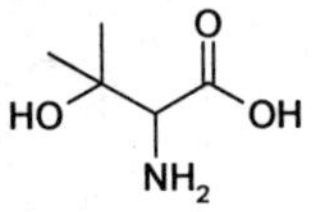

4915 Pabularinone
Property: mp 144-6°C. Source: YUN NAN QIANG HUO. Ref: 551.

4916 Pabulenol
$C_{16}H_{16}O_5$ MW: 288.30 Source: BAI ZHI. Ref: 2.

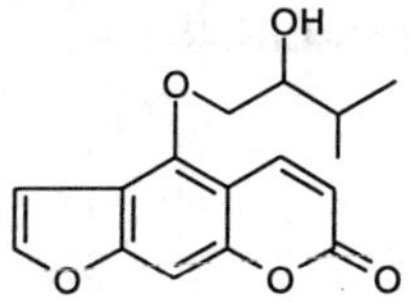

4917 Pachycarpine
$C_{15}H_{26}N_2$ MW: 234.39 Property: bp 173-4°C/8mm. Source: YE JUE MING. Ref: 6.

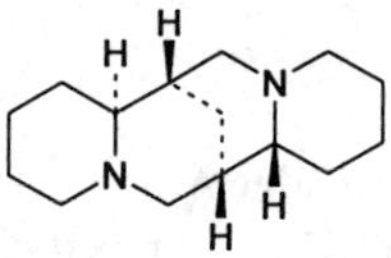

4918 Pachymaic acid
$C_{31}H_{46}O_4$ MW: 528 Property: white acicular crystal, mp 295-6°C. Source: FU LING. Ref: 403.

4919 β-Pachyman
Source: FU LING. Ref: 2.

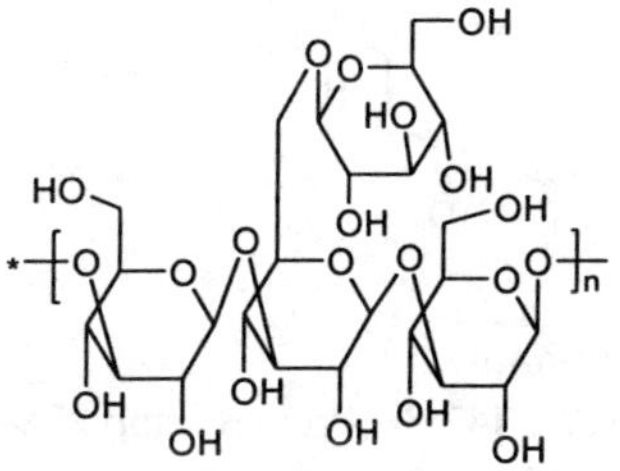

4920 Pachymic acid
$C_{33}H_{52}O_5$ MW: 528.78 Source: FU LING. Ref: 2.

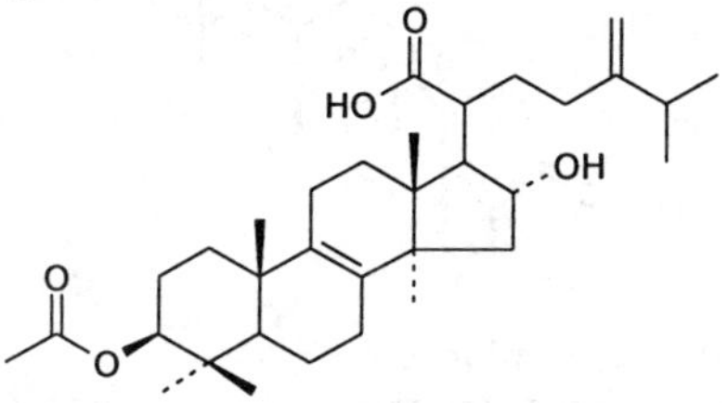

4921 Pachypodol
$C_{18}H_{16}O_7$ MW: 344.32 Property: mp 164-6°C. Source: HUO XIANG. Ref: 2, 505.

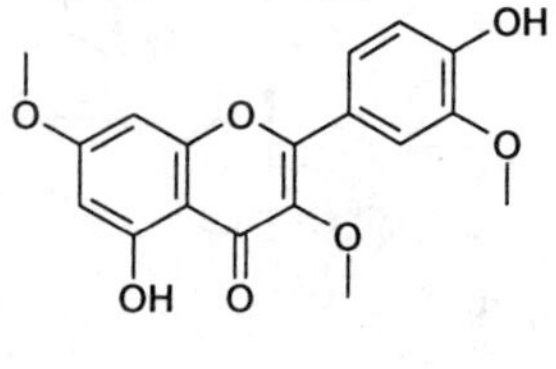

4922 Pachyrhizin
$C_{19}H_{12}O_6$ MW: 336.30 Property: mp 207-9°C. Source: DI GUA ZI. Ref: 6.

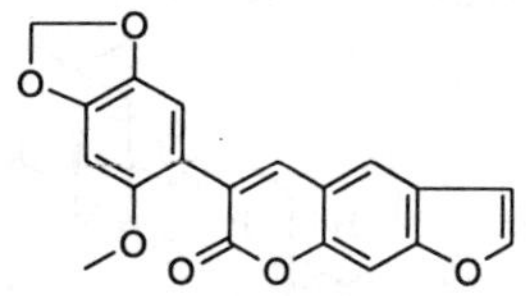

4923 Pachyrhizone
$C_{20}H_{14}O_7$ MW: 366.33 Property: mp 232-40°C (dec). Source: DI GUA ZI. Ref: 6.

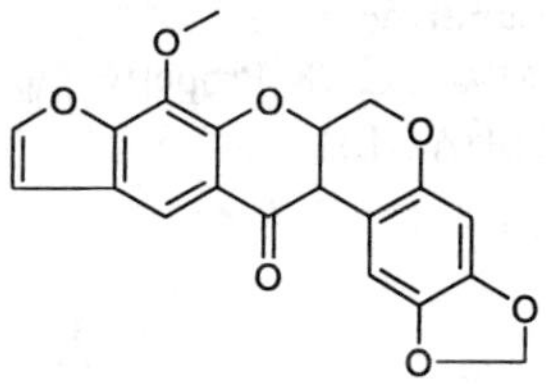

4924 Pachysamine A
$C_{24}H_{44}N_2$ MW: 360.63 Property: mp 167-8 °C. Source: HAI NAN YE SHAN HUA, JIN GANG DA, XUE SHAN LIN. Ref: 6, 261, 399.

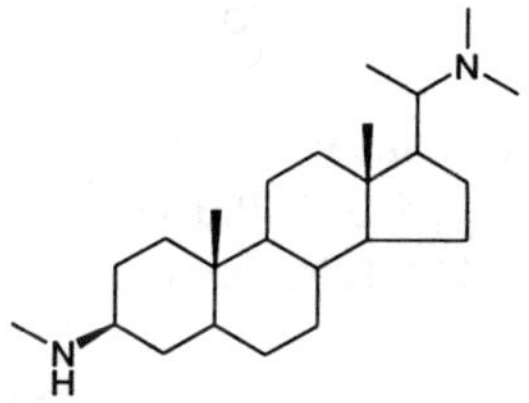

4925 Pachysamine B
$C_{29}H_{50}N_2O$ MW: 442.73 Property: mp 171-3°C. Source: XUE SHAN LIN. Ref: 6.

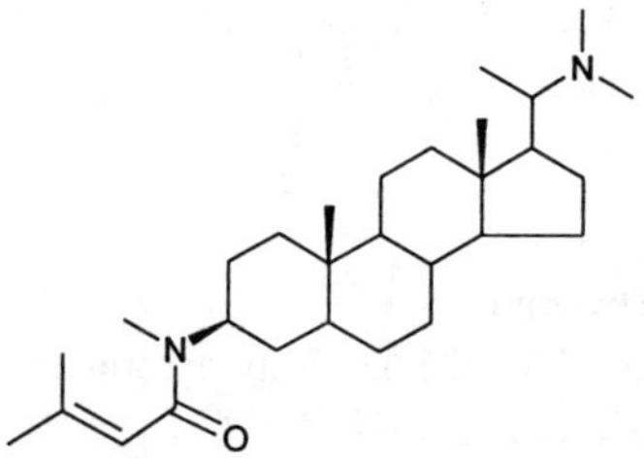

4926 Pachysandiol A
$C_{30}H_{52}O_2$ MW: 444.75 Property: mp 278-80°C. Source: XUE SHAN LIN. Ref: 6.

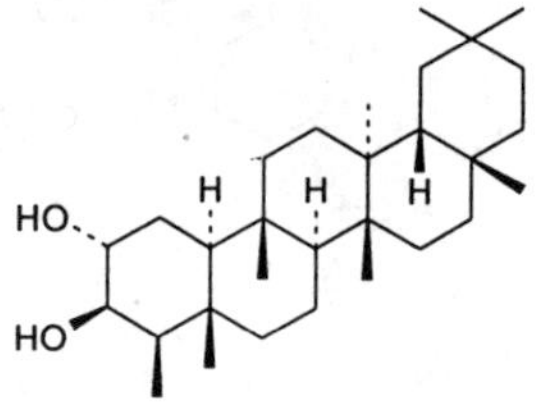

4927 Pachysandiol B
$C_{30}H_{52}O_2$ MW: 444.75 Property: mp 280-2°C.
Source: XUE SHAN LIN. Ref: 6.

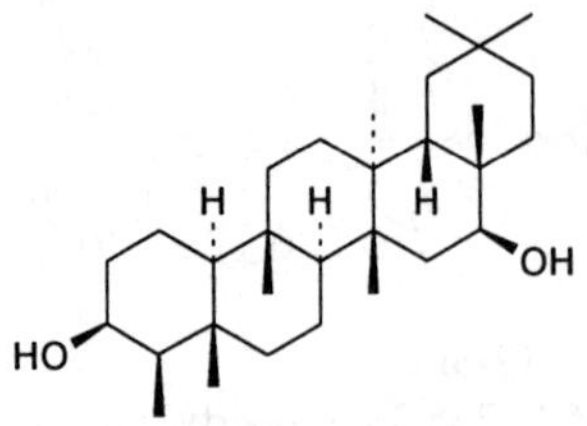

4928 Pachysandrine A
$C_{33}H_{50}N_2O_3$ MW: 522.78 Property: mp 235-6°C.
Source: XUE SHAN LIN. Ref: 6.

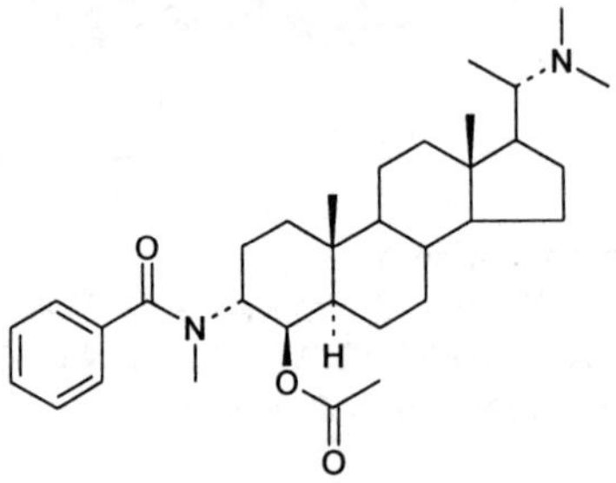

4929 Pachysandrine B
$C_{31}H_{52}N_2O_3$ MW: 500.77 Property: mp 187-9°C.
Source: XUE SHAN LIN. Ref: 6.

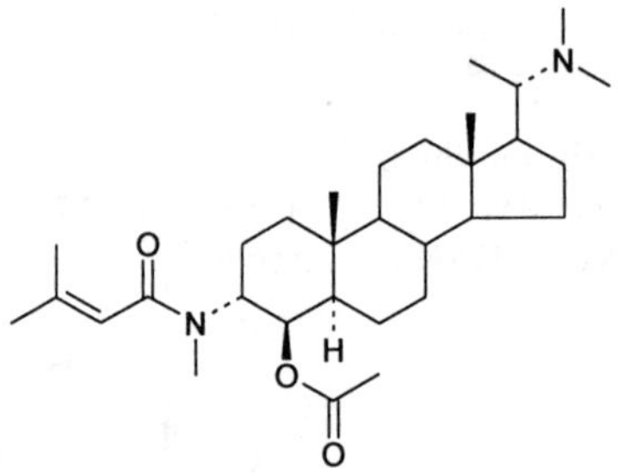

4930 Pachysandrine C
$C_{24}H_{44}N_2O$ MW: 376.63 Property: mp 212-4°C.
Source: XUE SHAN LIN. Ref: 6.

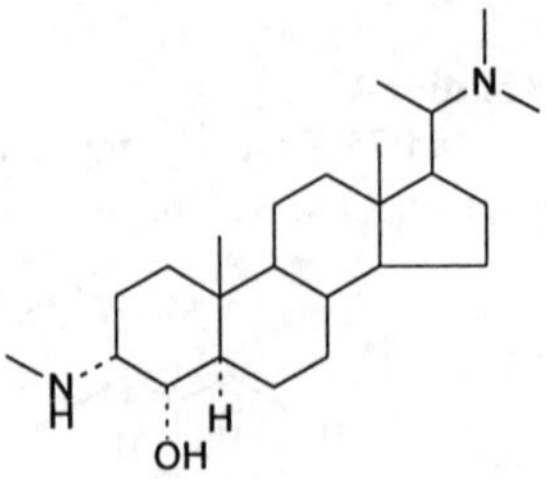

4931 Pachysandrine D
$C_{29}H_{50}N_2O_2$ MW: 458.73 Property: mp 184-5°C.
Source: XUE SHAN LIN. Ref: 6.

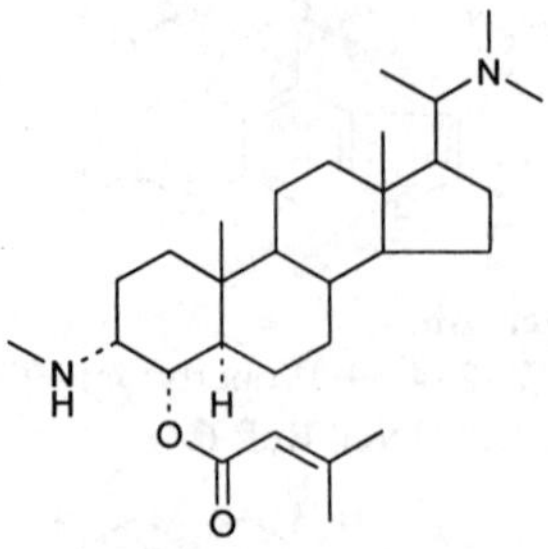

4932 Pachysantermine A
$C_{29}H_{48}N_2O_2$ MW: 456.72 Property: mp 260-3°C.
Source: XUE SHAN LIN. Ref: 6.

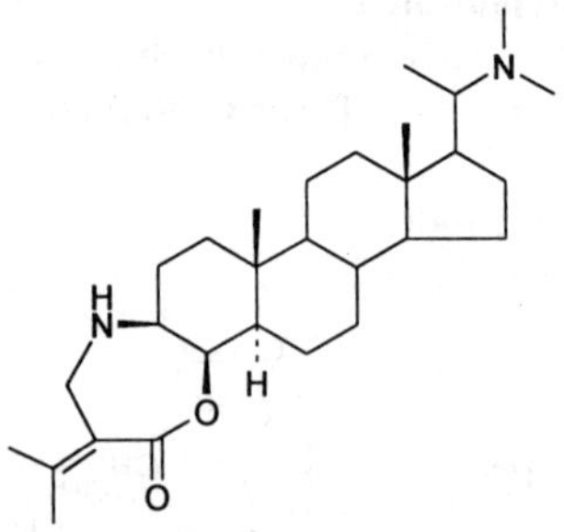

4933 Pachysonol
$C_{30}H_{50}O_2$ MW: 442.73 Property: mp 278-80°C.
Source: XUE SHAN LIN. Ref: 6.

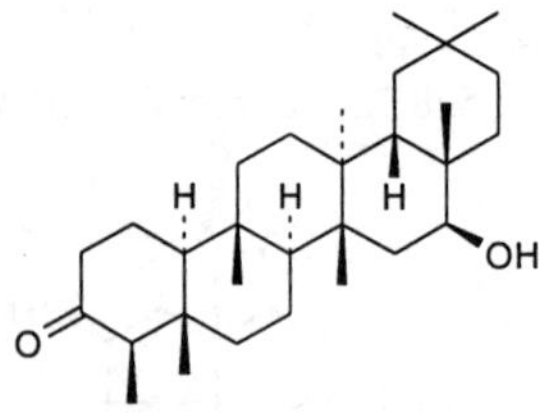

4934 Pachystermine A
$C_{29}H_{48}N_2O_2$ MW: 456.72 Property: mp 220-4°C.
Source: XUE SHAN LIN. Ref: 6.

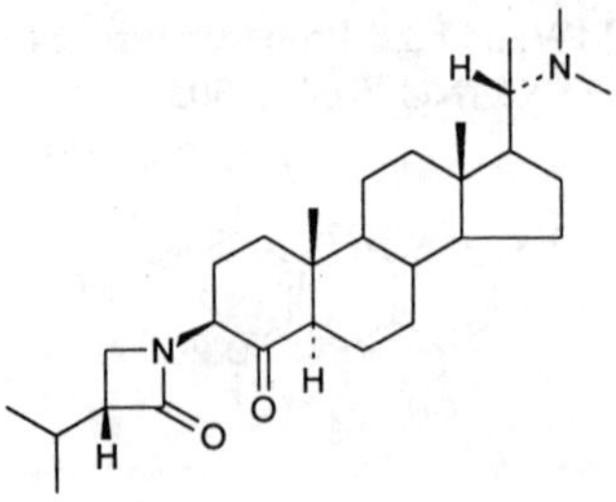

4935 Pachystermine B

$C_{29}H_{50}N_2O_2$ MW: 458.73 Property: mp 256-8°C. Source: XUE SHAN LIN. Ref: 6.

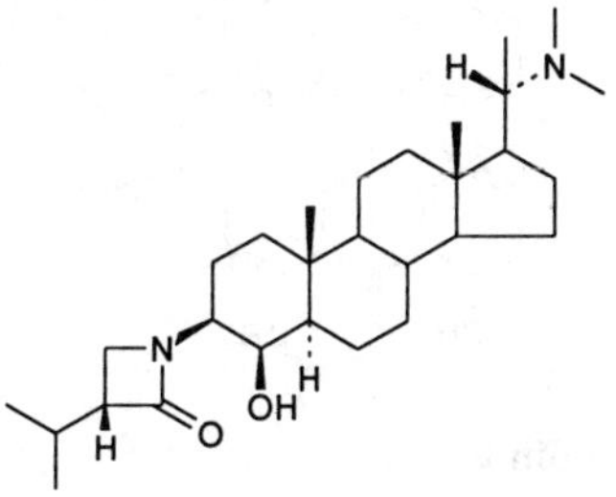

4936 Paederoside

$C_{18}H_{22}O_{10}S$ MW: 430.43 Property: mp 122-3°C. Source: JI SHI TENG. Ref: 6.

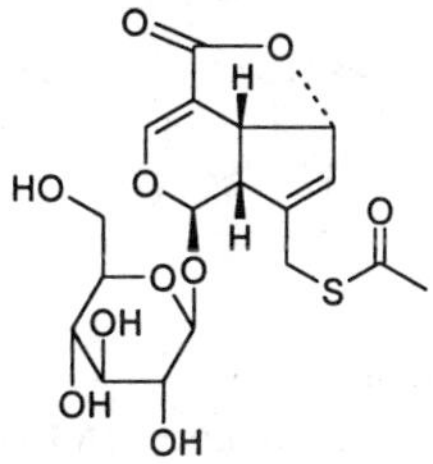

4937 Paeonidin

$C_{16}H_{13}O_6 \cdot Cl$ MW: 301.28•35.45 Source: MU LAN HUA. Ref: 6.

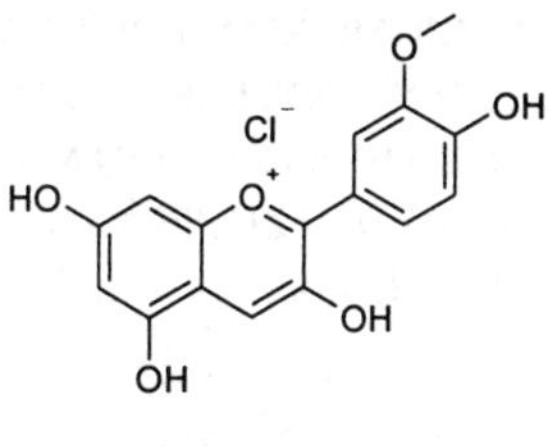

4938 Paeoniflorigenone

$C_{17}H_{18}O_6$ MW: 318.33 Source: BAI SHAO YAO, CHI SHAO YAO. Ref: 2.

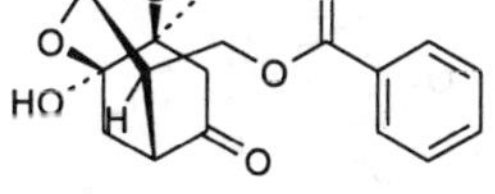

4939 Paeoniflorin

CAS: 23180-57-6 $C_{23}H_{28}O_{11}$ MW: 480.47 Property: white hygroscopic powder, mp 196°C. Source: BAI SHAO YAO, CHI SHAO YAO, CHUAN CHI SHAO, MU DAN PI. Ref: 2, 4, 448.

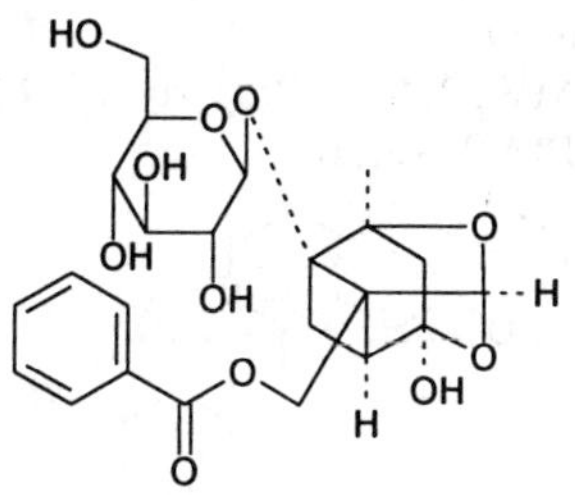

4940 Paeonin

$C_{28}H_{33}O_{16} \cdot Cl$ MW: 625.57•35.45 Source: BAI SHAO YAO. Ref: 2.

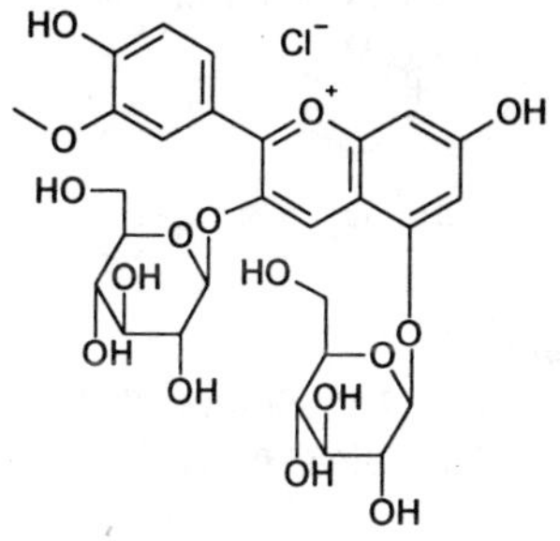

4941 Paeonol

Paeonal; Peonol. CAS: 552-41-0 $C_9H_{10}O_3$ MW: 166.18 Property: mp 50°C. Source: BAI SHAO YAO, MU DAN PI. Ref: 2, 4.

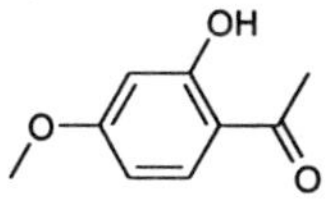

4942 Paeonolide

$C_{20}H_{28}O_{12}$ MW: 460.44 Source: MU DAN PI. Ref: 2.

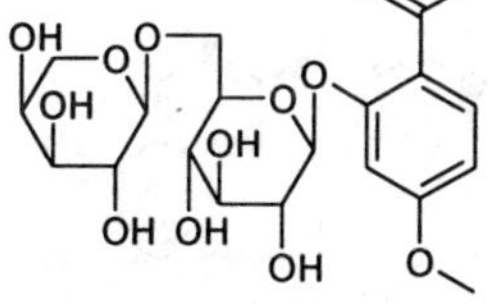

4943 Paeonoside

$C_{15}H_{20}O_8$ MW: 328.32 Source: MU DAN PI. Ref: 2.

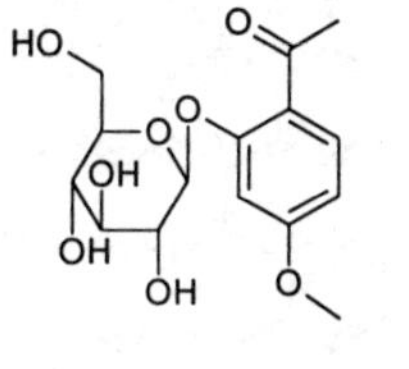

4944 Palaudine
$C_{19}H_{19}NO_4$ MW: 325.37 Property: mp 175-6°C. Source: YA PIAN. Ref: 6.

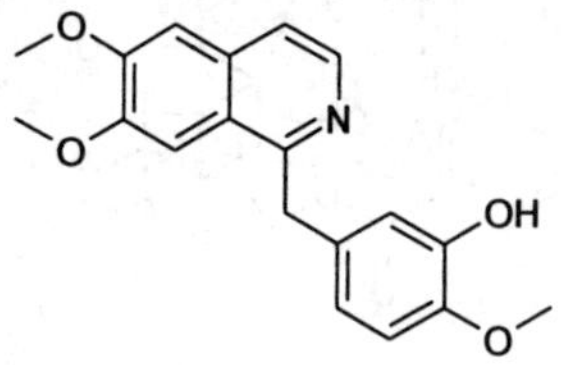

4945 Pallidiflorin
5-Hydroxy-4'-methoxy isoflavone. $C_{16}H_{12}O_4$ MW: 268.27 Property: white lamellar crystal, mp 265-8°C. Source: CI GUO GAN CAO. Ref: 166.

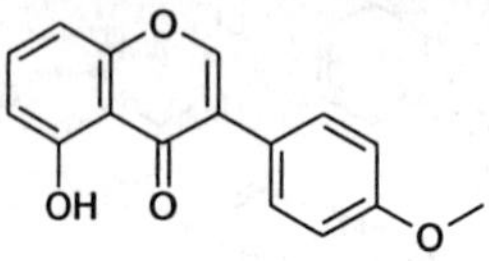

4946 Pallidine
$C_{19}H_{21}NO_4$ MW: 327.38 Source: JU HUA HUANG LIAN, ZI HUA YU DENG CAO (LIE BAO ZI JING). Ref: 6.

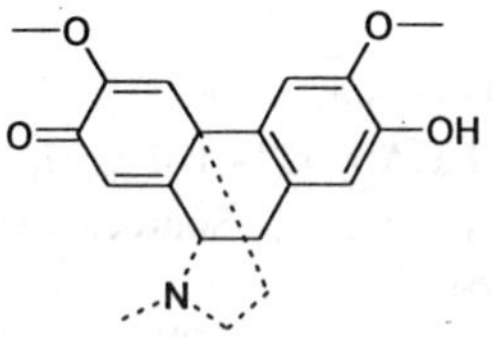

4947 Palmatine
Berbericinine. CAS: 3486-67-7 $C_{21}H_{22}NO_4$ MW: 352.41 Property: mp 198-201°C. Source: HUANG LIAN, HUANG BAI, YAN HU SUO. Ref: 2, 4, 408.

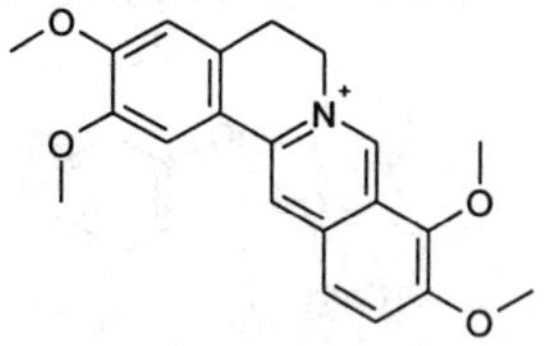

4948 Palmidin A
$C_{30}H_{22}O_8$ MW: 510.51 Source: DA HUANG. Ref: 2.

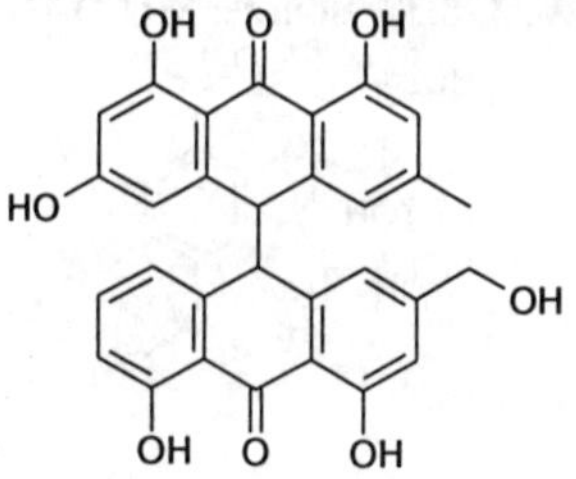

4949 Palmidin B
$C_{30}H_{22}O_7$ MW: 494.51 Source: DA HUANG. Ref: 2.

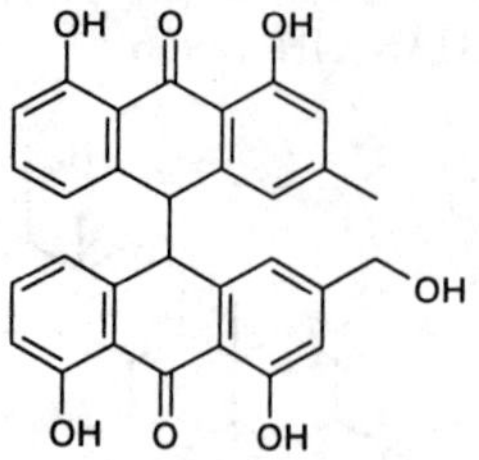

4950 Palmidin C
$C_{30}H_{22}O_7$ MW: 494.51 Source: DA HUANG. Ref: 2.

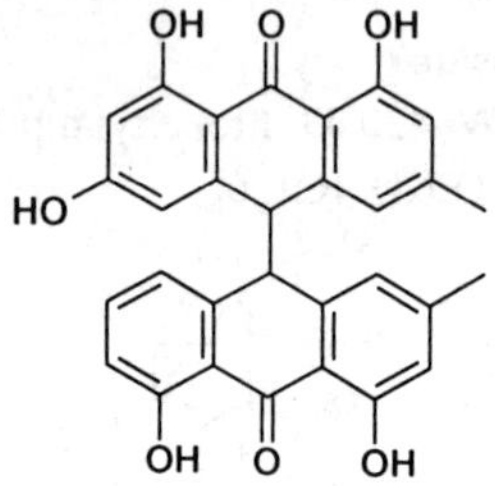

4951 Palmitic acid
$C_{16}H_{32}O_2$ MW: 256.43 Source: BA DOU, BING LANG, CHAI HU, CHUAN XIONG, CU LIU GUO (SHA JI), DA QING YE, DA ZAO, DANG GUI, DANG SHEN, DONG CHONG XIA CAO, DONG LING CAO, FU LING, GAN DI HUANG, GUA LOU, HONG HUA, HUANG QI, HUANG QIN, LU HUI, MU XIANG, PU HUANG, QING HAO, QUAN XIE, REN SHEN, SAN QI, SHAN ZHA, SHAN ZHU YU, TIAN HUA FEN, TIAN MA, XI YANG SHEN, XING REN, YA DAN ZI, YIN YANG HUO, YU XING CAO, etc. Ref: 2, 531, 549, 551, 557, 576, 582, 596, 601.

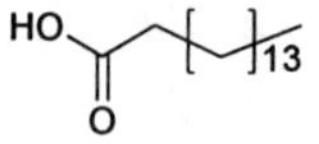

4952 Palmitin
$C_{51}H_{98}O_6$ MW: 807.35 Source: REN SHEN. Ref: 2.

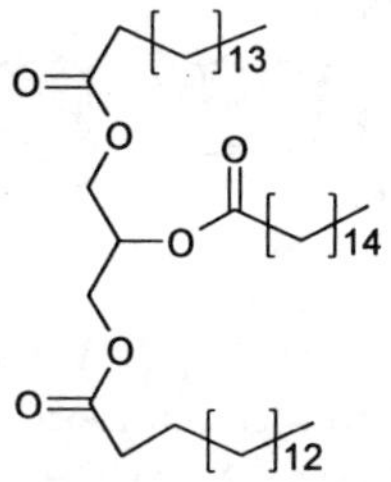

4953 Palmitoleic acid

$C_{16}H_{30}O_2$ MW: 254.42 Source: CU LIU GUO (SHA JI), LU HUI, GUA LOU, XING REN. Ref: 2.

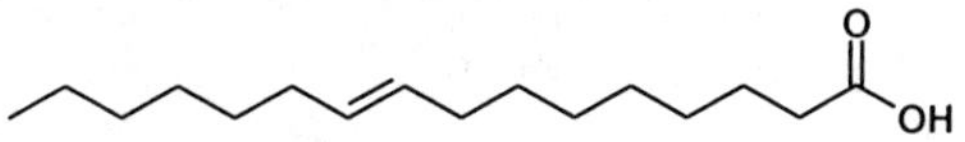

4954 Palmitone

$C_{31}H_{62}O$ MW: 450.84 Property: mp 82.8°C. Source: ZHEN CAI. Ref: 6.

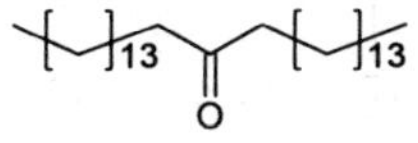

4955 Palmitylpterosin A

$C_{31}H_{50}O_4$ MW: 486.74 Property: mp 50-1°C. Source: JUE. Ref: 6.

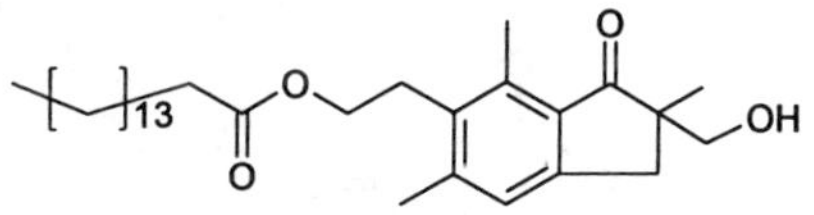

4956 Palmitylpterosin B

$C_{30}H_{48}O_3$ MW: 456.72 Property: mp 51-2°C. Source: JUE. Ref: 6.

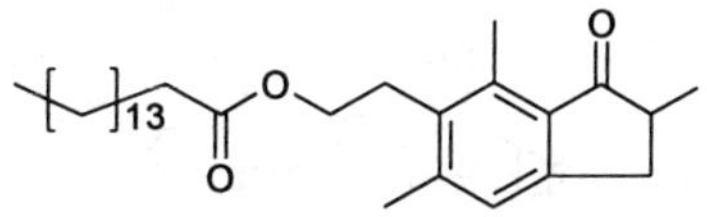

4957 Palmitylpterosin C

$C_{30}H_{48}O_4$ MW: 472.71 Property: mp 95-7°C. Source: JUE. Ref: 6.

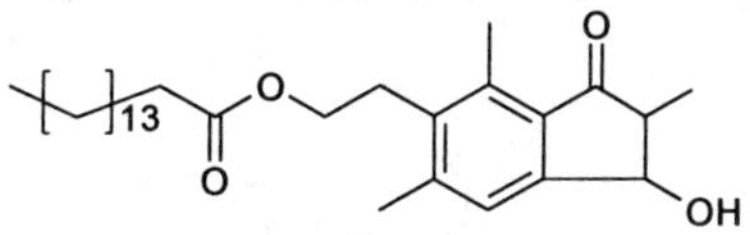

4958 Palustridine

$C_{18}H_{31}N_3O_3$ MW: 337.47 Source: GU JIE CAO. Ref: 6.

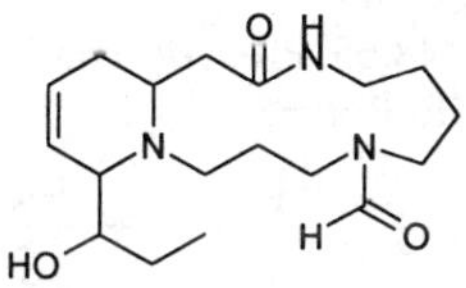

4959 Palustrine

$C_{17}H_{31}N_3O_2$ MW: 309.46 Source: MU ZEI. Ref: 2.

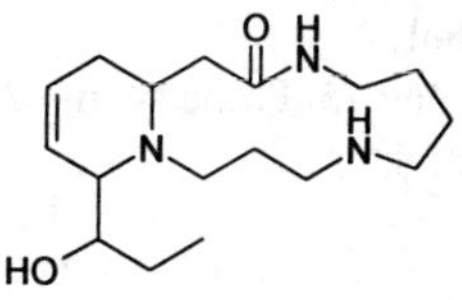

4960 Palustrinoside

$C_{22}H_{20}O_{11}$ MW: 460.40 Source: GUANG YE SHUI SU. Ref: 6.

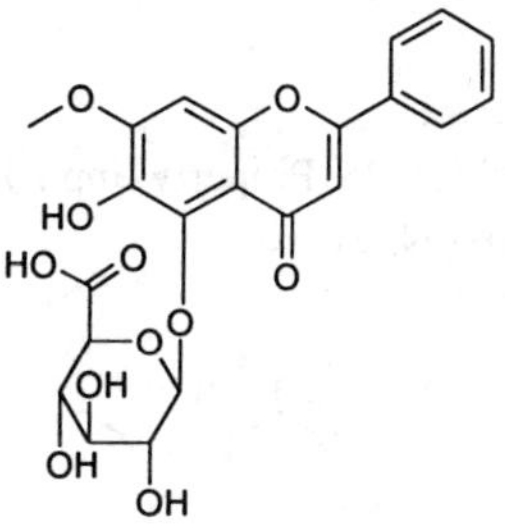

4961 Palustroside

$C_{27}H_{30}O_{15}$ MW: 594.53 Property: mp 178-80°C. Source: PENG ZI CAI. Ref: 6.

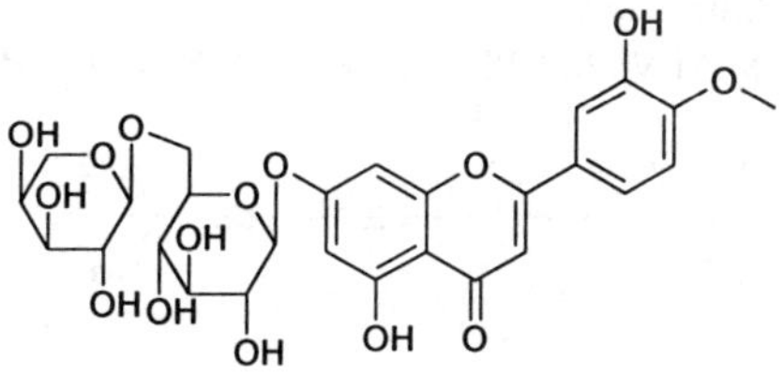

4962 Panacon

$C_{36}H_{62}O_8$ MW: 622.89 Source: REN SHEN. Ref: 6.

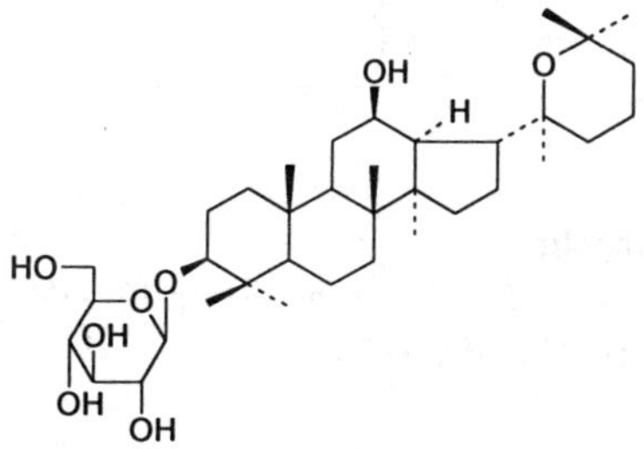

4963 Panasenoside

Source: REN SHEN. Ref: 2.

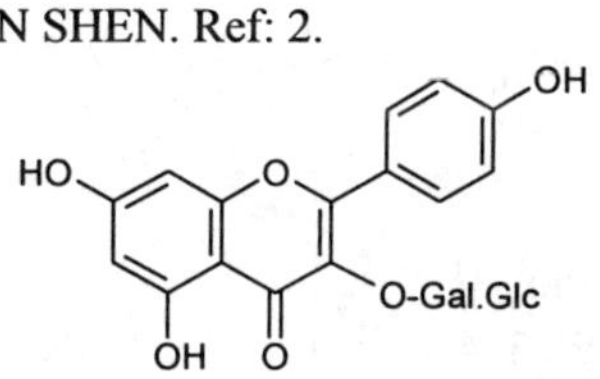

4964 Panaxadiol
$C_{30}H_{52}O_3$ MW: 460.75 Property: mp 250°C. Source: REN SHEN. Ref: 6.

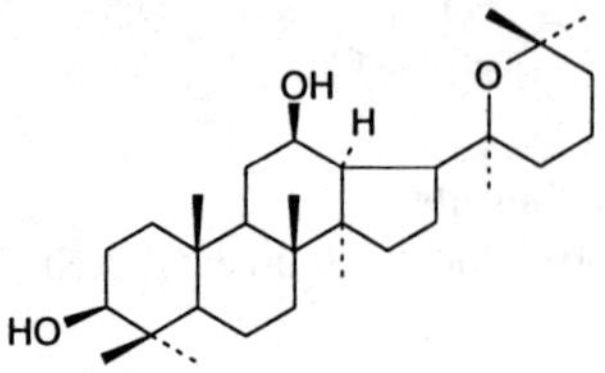

4965 Panaxatriol
$C_{30}H_{52}O_4$ MW: 476.75 Property: mp 238-9°C. Source: REN SHEN. Ref: 6.

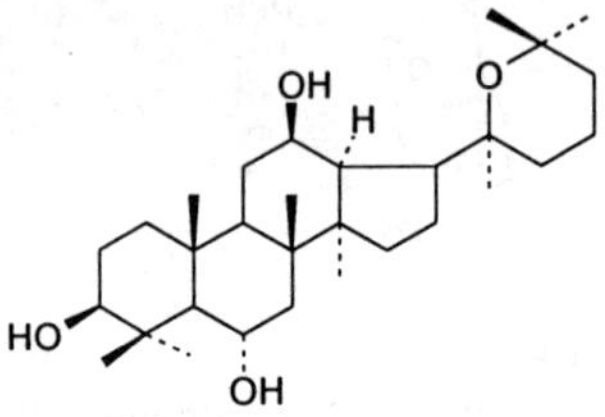

4966 Panaxynol
$C_{17}H_{24}O_2$ MW: 260.38 Source: REN SHEN. Ref: 2.

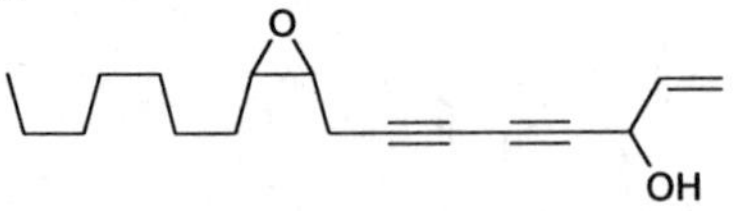

4967 Panaxytriol
$C_{17}H_{26}O_3$ MW: 278.40 Source: REN SHEN. Ref: 2.

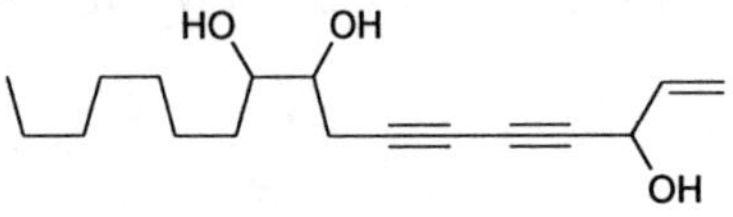

4968 Pangeline
$C_{16}H_{14}O_5$ MW: 286.29 Property: mp 122-3°C. Source: CHOU CAO. Ref: 6.

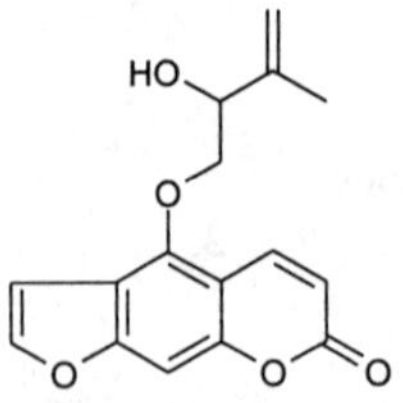

4969 Panicolin
$C_{17}H_{14}O_6$ MW: 314.30 Source: CHUAN XIN LIAN. Ref: 2.

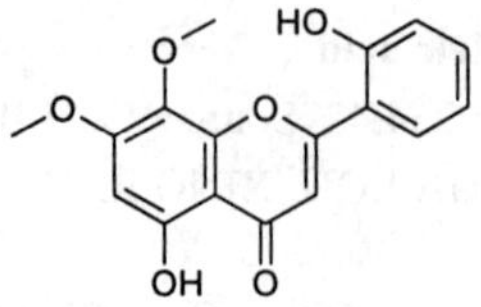

4970 Paniculatin
$C_{20}H_{24}O_6$ MW: 360.41 Property: mp 263°C. Source: JIU LI XIANG. Ref: 6.

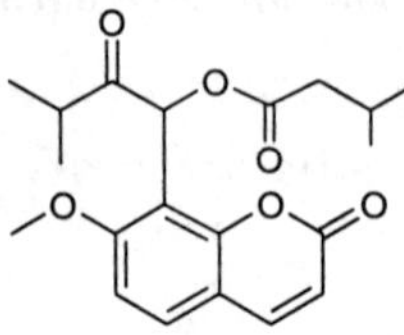

4971 Paniculide A
$C_{15}H_{20}O_4$ MW: 264.32 Source: CHUAN XIN LIAN. Ref: 2.

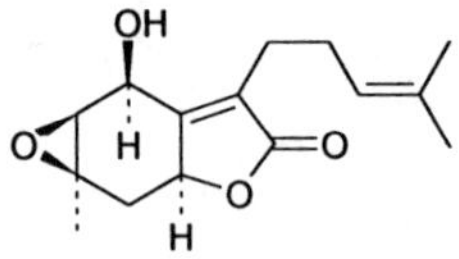

4972 Paniculide B
$C_{15}H_{20}O_5$ MW: 280.32 Source: CHUAN XIN LIAN. Ref: 2.

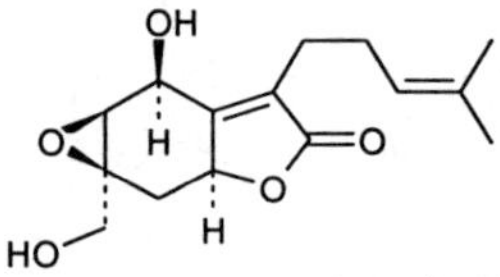

4973 Paniculide C
$C_{15}H_{18}O_5$ MW: 278.31 Source: CHUAN XIN LIAN. Ref: 2.

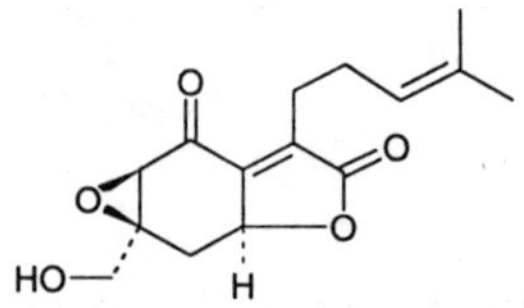

4974 Paniculogenin
$C_{27}H_{44}O_5$ MW: 448.65 Property: mp 214-6°C. Source: SHUI QIE. Ref: 6.

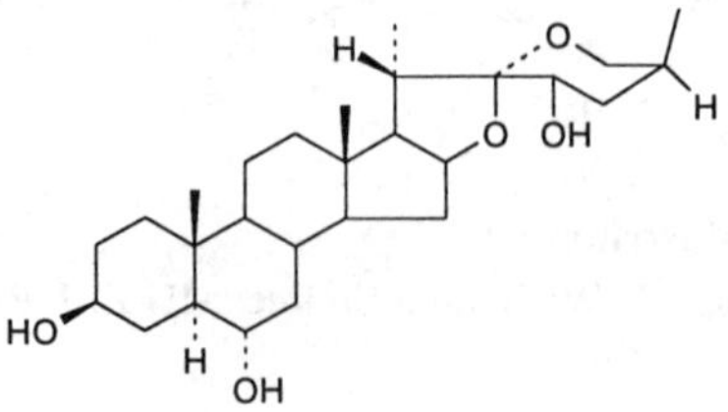

4975 Panose

$C_{18}H_{32}O_{16}$ MW: 504.45 Source: XI YANG SHEN. Ref: 2.

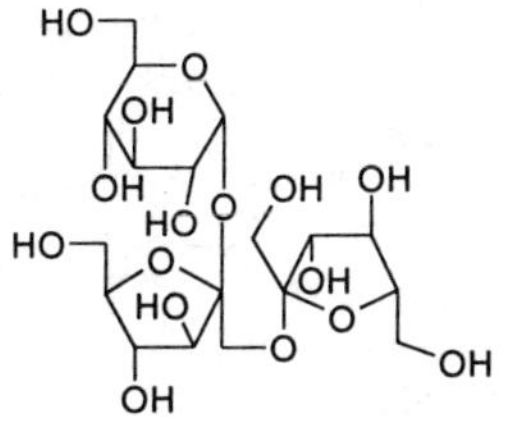

4976 Panose B

$C_{18}H_{32}O_{16}$ MW: 504.45 Source: XI YANG SHEN. Ref: 2.

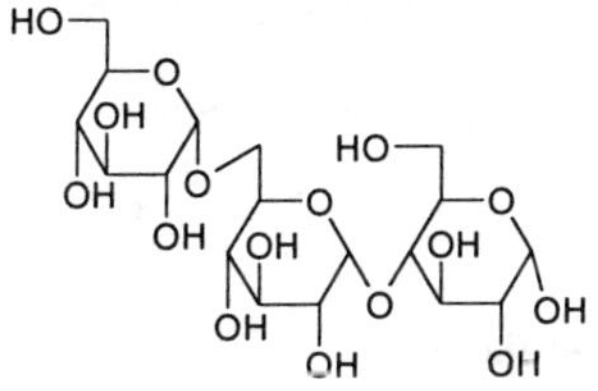

4977 Panose C

$C_{18}H_{32}O_{16}$ MW: 504.45 Source: XI YANG SHEN. Ref: 2.

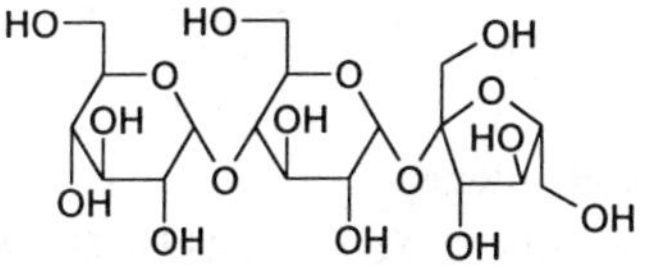

4978 Papaverine

CAS: 58-74-2 $C_{20}H_{21}NO_4$ MW: 339.39 Property: mp 147°C. Source: BAI YAO ZI, YA PIAN, YING SU, YING SU KE. Ref: 4, 5, 6.

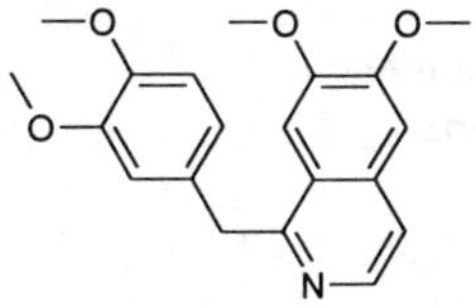

4979 Papaverrubine B

$C_{21}H_{23}NO_6$ MW: 385.42 Property: mp 202-4°C. Source: YA PIAN. Ref: 6.

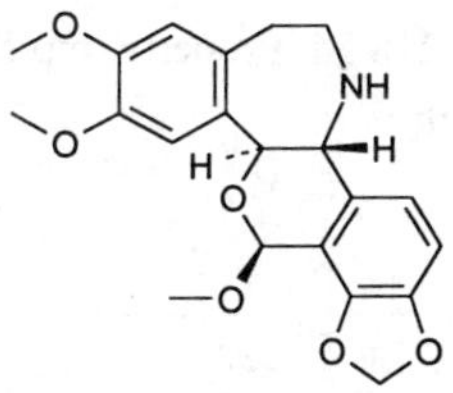

4980 Papaverrubine C

$C_{20}H_{21}NO_6$ MW: 371.39 Property: mp 190-1.5°C. Source: YA PIAN. Ref: 6.

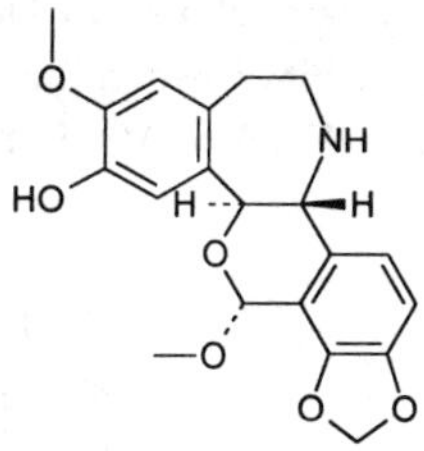

4981 Papyramine

$C_{18}H_{23}NO_4$ MW: 317.39 Property: mp 137-8°C. Source: SHUI XIAN GEN. Ref: 6.

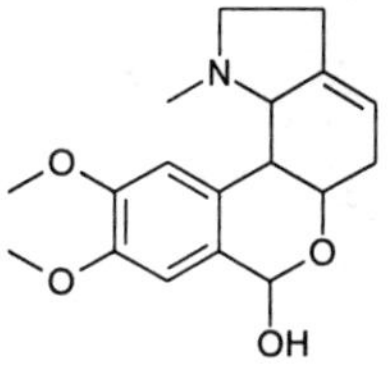

4982 Para-aspidin

$C_{25}H_{32}O_8$ MW: 460.53 Property: mp 123-5°C. Source: GUAN ZHONG. Ref: 6.

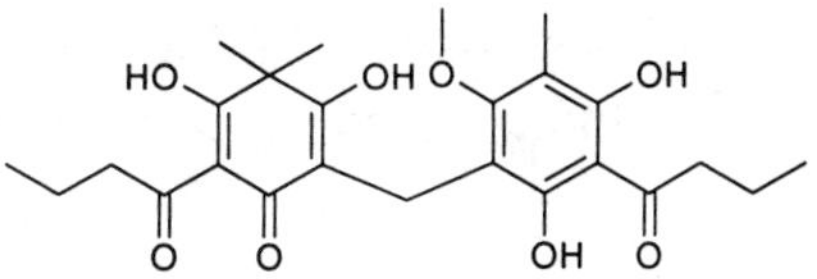

4983 Parasorbic acid

$C_6H_8O_2$ MW: 112.13 Property: bp (+): 105°C/14 mm. Source: TIAN SHAN HUA QIU. Ref: 6.

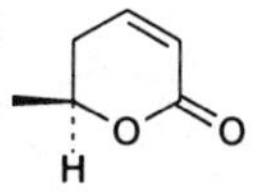

4984 Pareirine

$C_{19}H_{26}N_2O$ MW: 298.43 Property: mp 142.5-3°C. Source: XI SHENG TENG. Ref: 6.

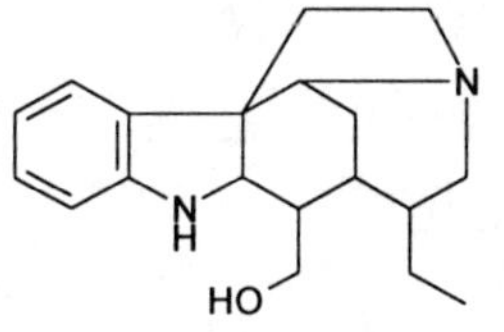

4985 Paridiformoside

3-O-(β-D-Glucopyranosyl-(1→3)-O-[-α-L-rhamnopyransyl-(1→2)-β-D-glucopyranosyl(1→2)] β-D-glucopyranosyl) cyclamiretin A. $C_{54}H_{88}O_{23}$ MW: 1105.29 Property: white powder, mp 163-5°C. Source: CHONG LOU PAI CAO. Ref: 86.

4986 Parinaric acid

$C_{18}H_{28}O_2$ MW: 276.42 Property: mp 85-6°C. Source: JI XING ZI. Ref: 6.

4987 Pariphyllin

$C_{44}H_{70}O_{16}$ MW: 855.04 Property: mp 294-8°C. Source: ZAO XIU. Ref: 6.

4988 Parmatic acid

$C_{18}H_{12}O_{10}$ MW: 388.29 Property: mp 260°C (dec). Source: SHI HUA. Ref: 6.

4989 Parthenolide

$C_{15}H_{20}O_3$ MW: 248.32 Property: colorless massive crystal, mp 114-5°C. Source: YU NAN HAN XIAO. Ref: 426.

4990 Patchoulane

$C_{15}H_{26}$ MW: 206.37 Source: CHAI HU. Ref: 2.

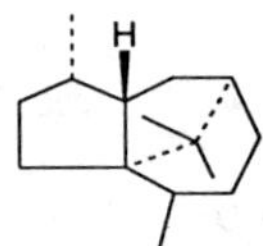

4991 γ-Patchoulene

$C_{15}H_{26}$ MW: 206.37 Source: DU HUO. Ref: 2.

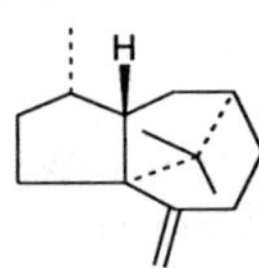

4992 α-Patchoulene

$C_{15}H_{24}$ MW: 204.36 Source: HUO XIANG. Ref: 2.

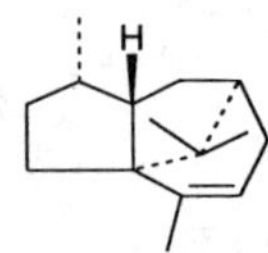

4993 Patchoulenone

$C_{15}H_{22}O$ MW: 218.34 Property: mp 52.5°C. Source: XIANG FU. Ref: 6.

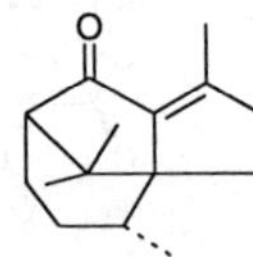

4994 Patchouli alcohol
$C_{15}H_{26}O$ MW: 222.37 Source: HUO XIANG. Ref: 2, 505.

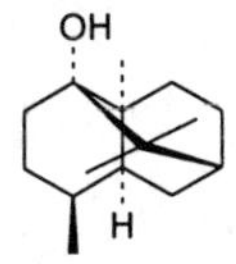

4995 Patchoulipyridine
$C_{15}H_{21}N$ MW: 215.34 Source: HUO XIANG. Ref: 2.

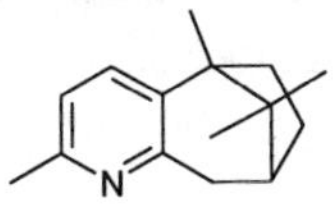

4996 Patrinene
$C_{15}H_{24}$ MW: 204.36 Source: BAI JIANG. Ref: 2.

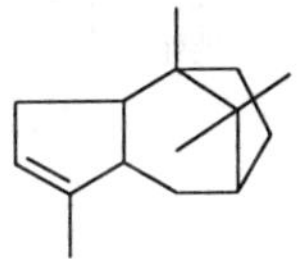

4997 Patrinoside C
$C_{65}H_{106}O_{31}$ MW: 1383.55 Source: BAI JIANG. Ref: 6.

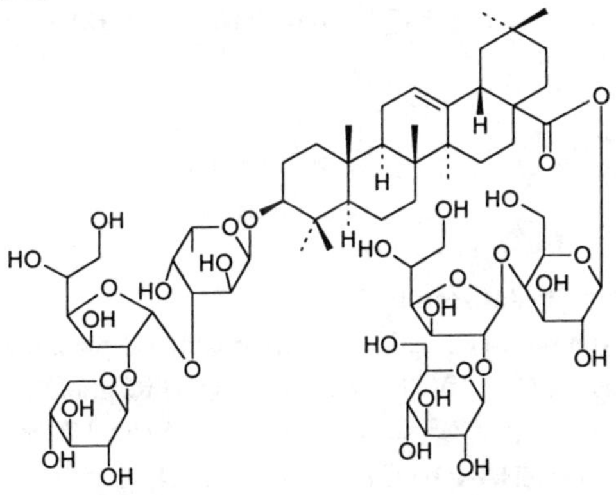

4998 Patrinoside C1
$C_{47}H_{76}O_{16}$ MW: 897.12 Source: BAI JIANG. Ref: 6.

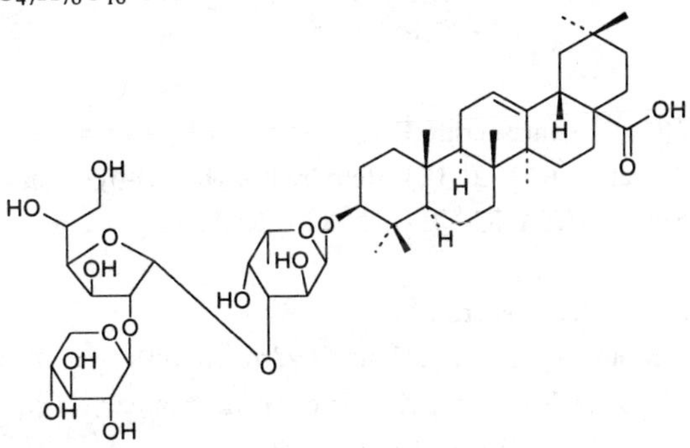

4999 Patrinoside D
$C_{70}H_{114}O_{36}$ MW: 1531.67 Source: BAI JIANG. Ref: 2.

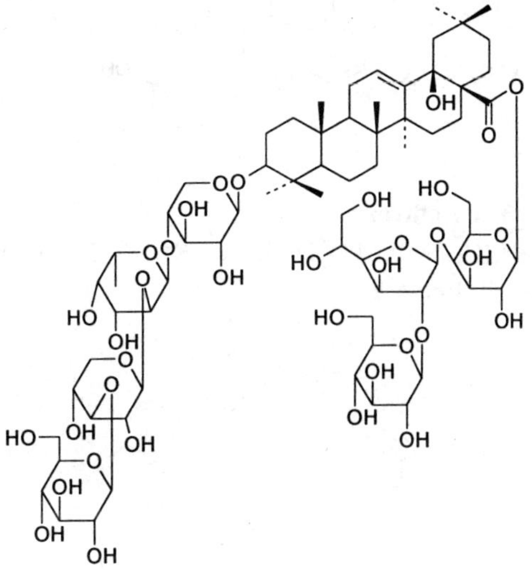

5000 Patrinoside D1
$C_{52}H_{84}O_{22}$ MW: 1061.24 Source: BAI JIANG. Ref: 2.

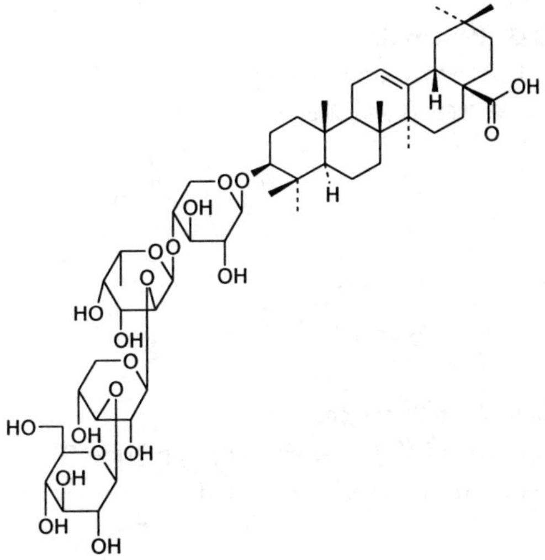

5001 Patuletin
$C_{16}H_{12}O_8$ MW: 332.27 Source: QING HAO. Ref: 2.

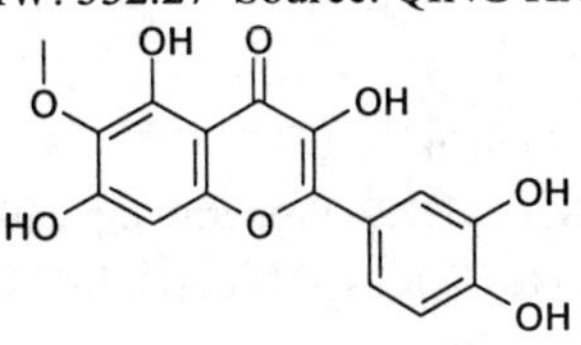

5002 Patuletin 3-O-glycoside
Source: QING HAO. Ref: 2.

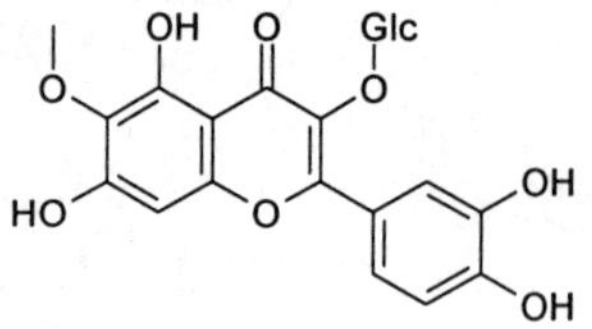

5003 Patulitrin
$C_{22}H_{22}O_{13}$ MW: 494.41 Source: KONG QUE CAO, MU JU. Ref: 6.

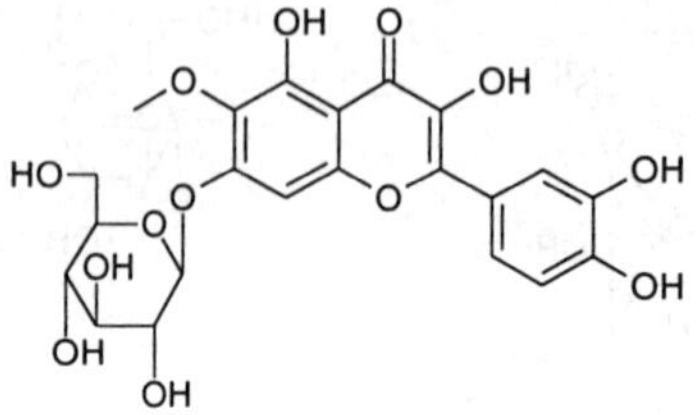

5004 Paucin
CAS: 26836-43-1 Property: mp 178-9°C. Source: BAI LAI SHI JU, MO ZHI JU. Ref: 5.

5005 Paulownin
$C_{20}H_{18}O_7$ MW: 370.36 Property: mp 84°C, 104-5°C. Source: TONG MU. Ref: 6.

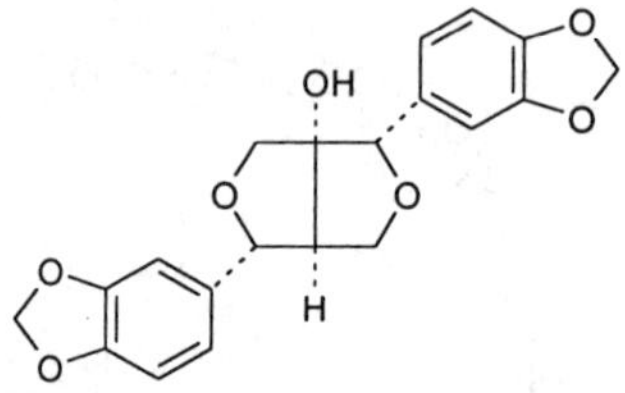

5006 Pectolinarigenin
$C_{17}H_{14}O_6$ MW: 314.30 Property: mp 215-6°C. Source: JIA LIAN QIAO YE. Ref: 6.

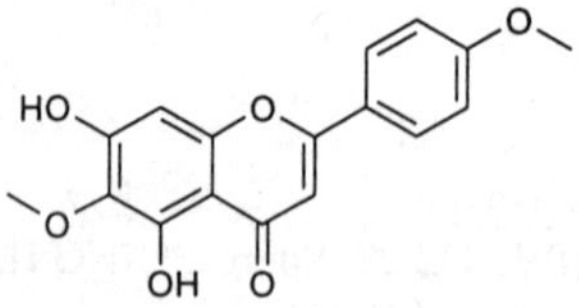

5007 Pectolinarin
$C_{29}H_{34}O_{15}$ MW: 622.9 Property: mp 240-50°C (dec). Source: HONG CHE ZHOU CAO, LIU CHUAN YU. Ref: 6.

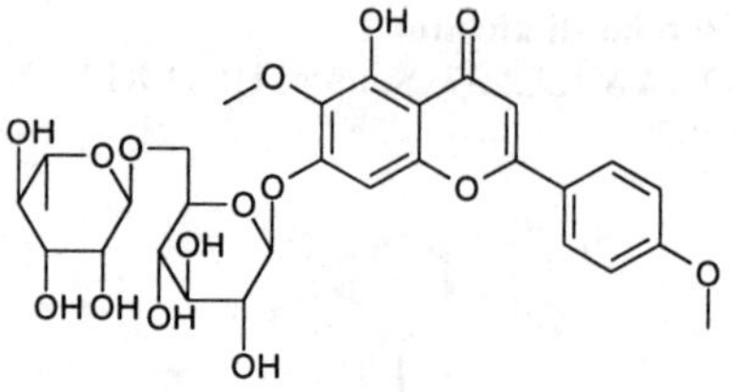

5008 Pedaliin
$C_{22}H_{22}O_{12}$ MW: 478.41 Property: mp 254°C (dec). Source: HU MA YE. Ref: 6.

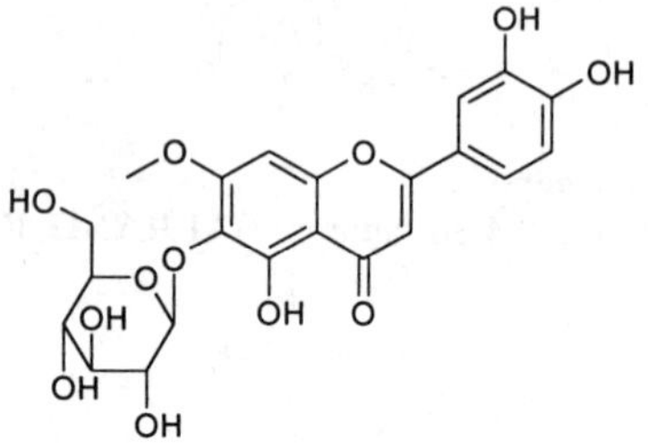

5009 Pedatisectine D
2-Methyl-3-(2',3',4'-trihydroxybutyl)-pyrazine. $C_9H_{14}N_2O_3$ MW: 198.22 Property: white granular crystal, mp 110-2°C. Source: ZHANG YE BAN XIA. Ref: 477.

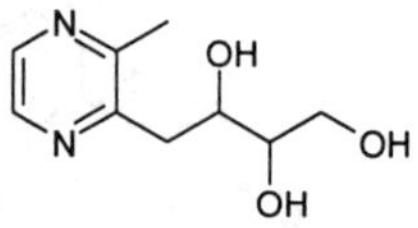

5010 Pedatisectine E
2-Methyl-5-(1',2',3',4'-tetrahydroxybutyl)pyrazine. $C_9H_{14}N_2O_4$ MW: 214.22 Property: white granular crystal, mp 202-3°C, $[\alpha]_D^{17}$ -87.8° (c=0.165, DMSO). Source: ZHANG YE BAN XIA. Ref: 477.

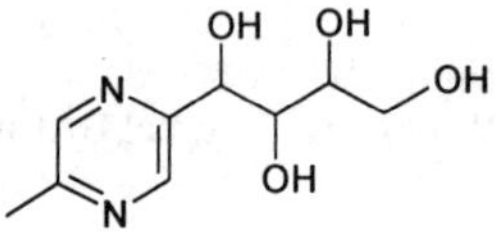

5011 Pedatisectine F
2-Methyl-6-(1',2',3',4',-tetrahydroxybutyl)-pyrazine. Source: ZHANG YE BAN XIA. Ref: 586.

5012 Pedatisectine G
2-Methyl-6-(1',2',3',4',-tetrahydroxybutyl)-5-(2'',3'',4''-trihydroxybutyl)-pyrazine. Source: ZHANG YE BAN XIA. Ref: 586.

5013 Pedunculagin

$C_{34}H_{24}O_{22}$ MW: 784.56 Property: earthy yellow amorphous powder, easy soluble in MeOH and Me_2CO. Source: TAO JIN NIANG. Ref: 429.

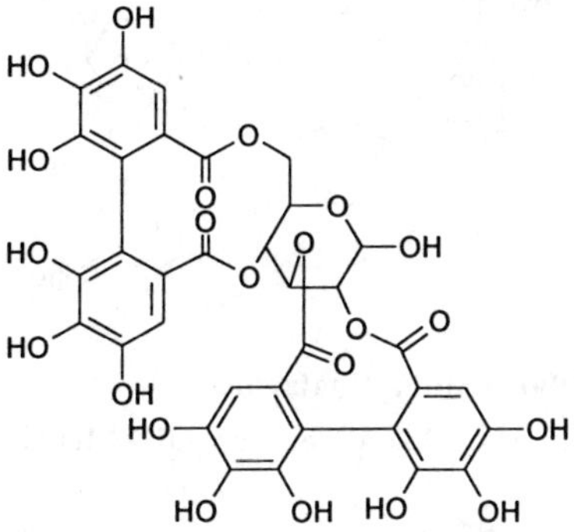

5014 Peduneuloside

$C_{36}H_{58}O_{10}$ MW: 650.86 Source: SI JI QING. Ref: 527.

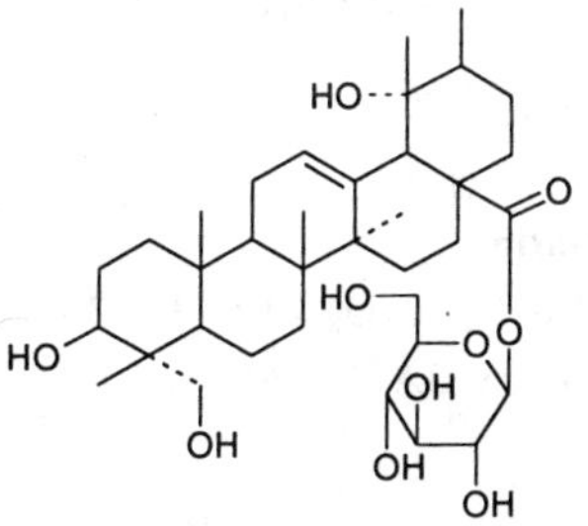

5015 Pegaline

$C_6H_{11}NO_3$ MW: 145.16 Property: mp 294°C. Source: LUO TUO PENG. Ref: 6.

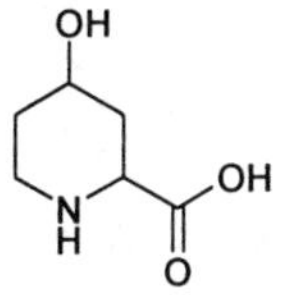

5016 Pegamine

$C_{11}H_{12}N_2O_2$ MW: 204.23 Source: LUO TUO PENG. Ref: 6.

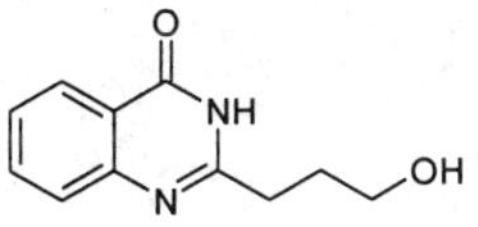

5017 Peganidin

$C_{14}H_{16}N_2O_2$ MW: 244.30 Property: mp 189-90°C. Source: LUO TUO PENG. Ref: 6.

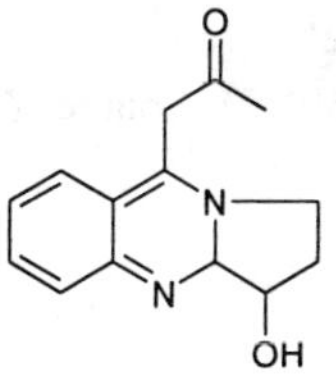

5018 Peganine

$C_{11}H_{12}N_2O$ MW: 188.23 Property: mp (-): 211-2°C, (±): 209-10°C. Source: LIU CHUAN YU, LUO TUO PENG, LUO TUO PENG ZI. Ref: 6.

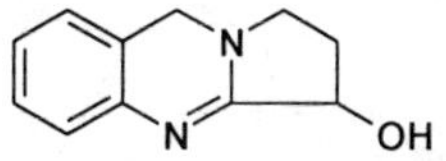

5019 Peganol

$C_{11}H_{12}N_2O$ MW: 188.23 Property: mp 178-80°C. Source: LUO TUO PENG. Ref: 6.

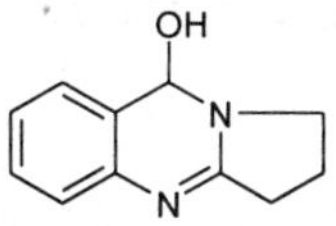

5020 Peimine

Verticine. CAS: 23496-41-5 $C_{27}H_{45}NO_3$ MW: 431.66 Property: mp 223-4°C, 268-70°C. Source: ZHE BEI MU. Ref: 4, 528.

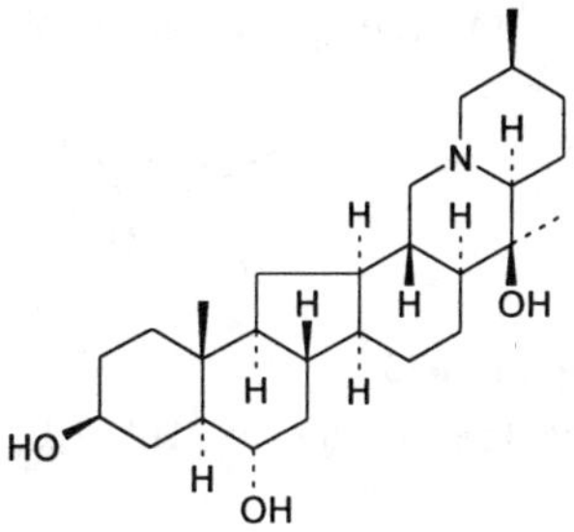

5021 Peiminine

$C_{27}H_{43}NO_3$ MW: 429.65 Property: mp 212-3°C. Source: ZHE BEI MU. Ref: 6.

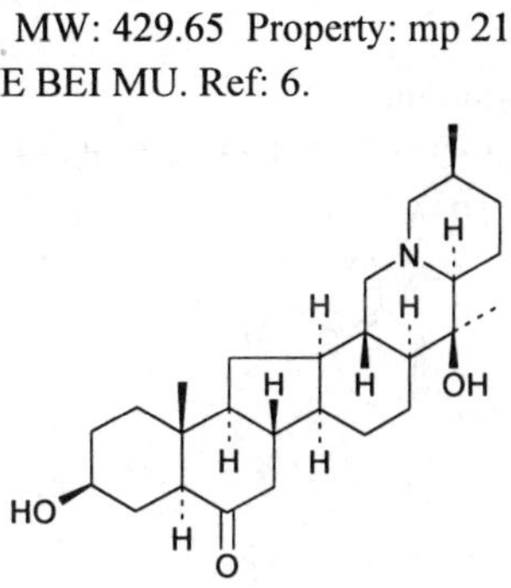

5022 Peiminoside

$C_{33}H_{55}NO_8$ MW: 593.81 Source: ZHE BEI MU. Ref: 6.

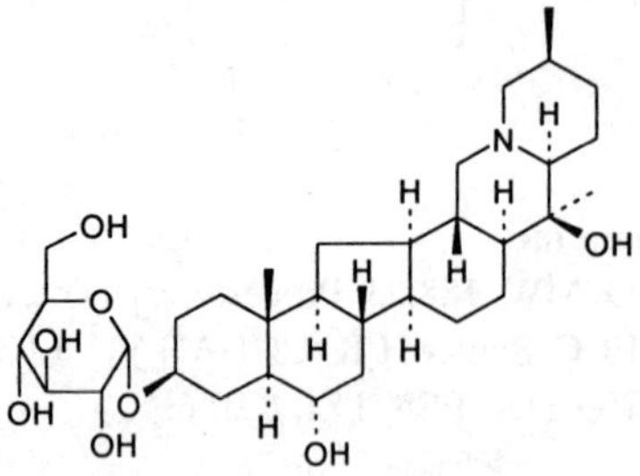

5023 Peimisine

$C_{27}H_{41}NO_3$ MW: 427.63 Property: colorless acicular crystal, mp 268-70°C (acetic ester-methanol), $[\alpha]_D^{20}$ -34.8° (c=0.24, methanol). Source: HUA XI BEI MU, NING XIA BEI MU. Ref: 225, 271.

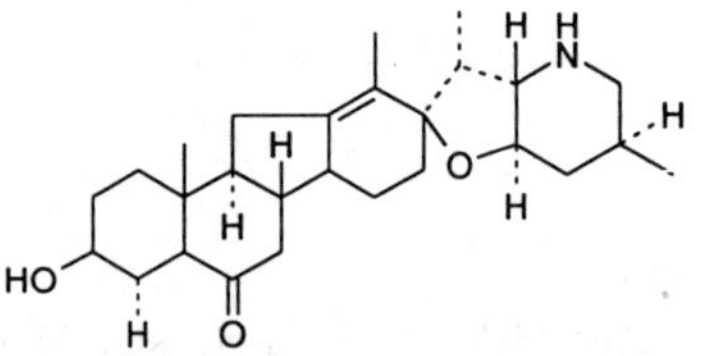

5024 Pelargonaldehyde

$C_9H_{18}O$ MW: 142.24 Property: bp 190-2°C. Source: GUI HUA. Ref: 6.

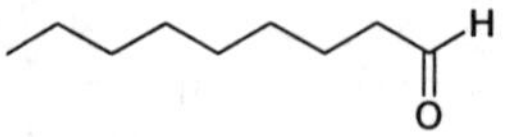

5025 Pelargonic acid

$C_9H_{18}O_2$ MW: 158.24 Source: CHAI HU, DANG SHEN. Ref: 2.

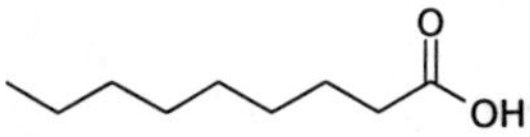

5026 Pelargonidin

$C_{15}H_{11}O_5$ MW: 271.25 Source: CHOU MO LI, FENG XIAN HUA. Ref: 6.

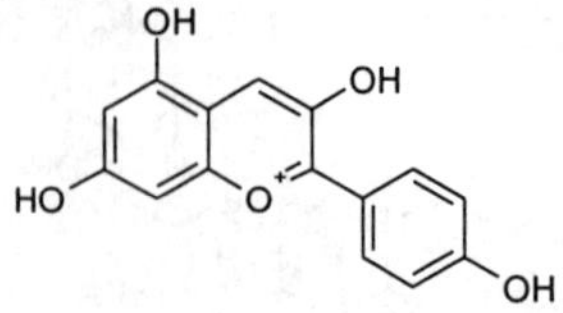

5027 Pelargonidin-3,5-diglucoside

$C_{27}H_{31}O_{15}$ MW: 595.54 Source: BAI FAN DOU. Ref: 6.

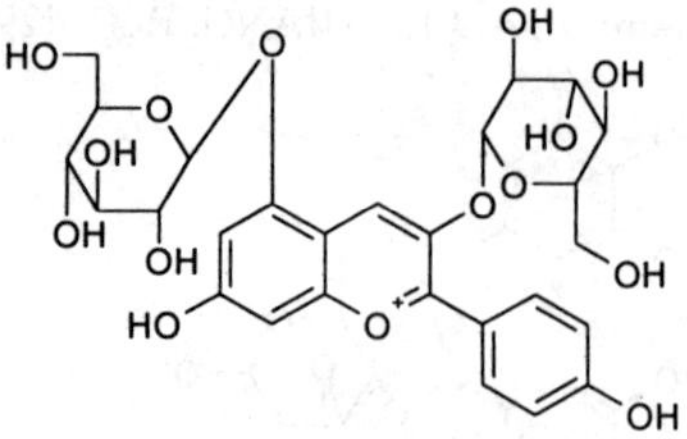

5028 Pelargonidin-3-galactoside

$C_{21}H_{21}O_{10}$ MW: 433.40 Source: QIU MU GUA. Ref: 6.

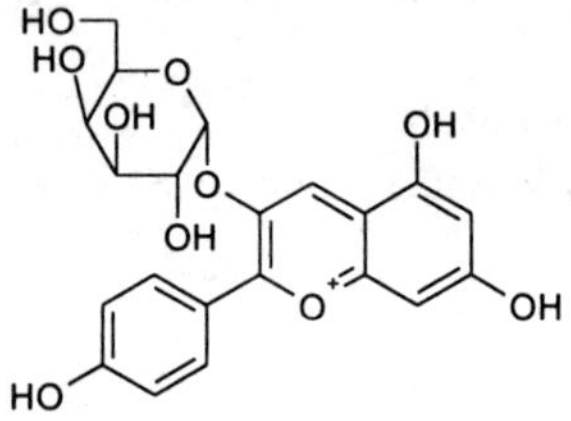

5029 α-Peltatin

CAS: 568-53-6 $C_{21}H_{20}O_8$ MW: 400.39 Property: mp 236-46°C. Source: BAI YA MA, DUN YE GUI JIU. Ref: 4, 5.

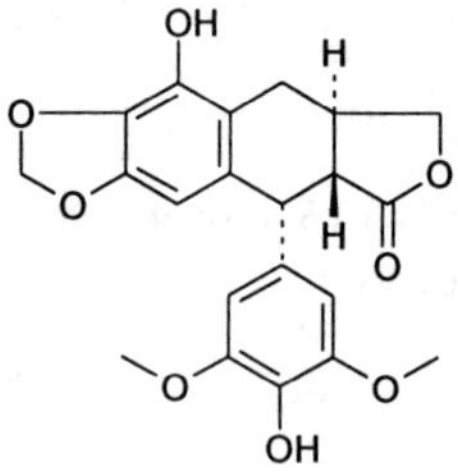

5030 β-Peltatin

$C_{22}H_{22}O_8$ MW: 414.42 Property: mp 238-41°C (dec). Source: BAI YA MA, DUN YE GUI JIU. Ref: 4, 5.

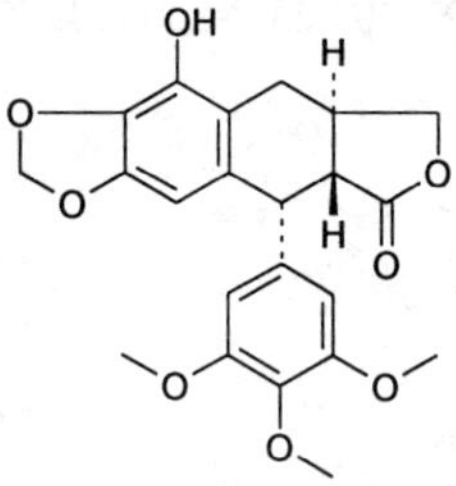

5031 α-Peltatin glucoside
Property: mp 168-71°C. Source: DUN YE GUI JIU. Ref: 5.

5032 β-Peltatin glucoside
Property: mp 156-9°C. Source: DUN YE GUI JIU. Ref: 5.

5033 Penduletin
$C_{18}H_{16}O_7$ MW: 344.32 Source: QING HAO. Ref: 2.

5034 Penniclavine
$C_{16}H_{18}N_2O_2$ MW: 270.33 Property: mp 222-5°C (dec). Source: MAI JIAO, QIAN NIU ZI. Ref: 6.

5035 Pennogenin
$C_{27}H_{42}O_4$ MW: 430.63 Source: YU ER QI. Ref: 6.

5036 Pennogenin rhamnosyl chacotrioside
$C_{51}H_{82}O_{21}$ MW: 1031.21 Property: mp 223-7°C (dec). Source: WANG SUN. Ref: 6.

5037 Pentacosane
$C_{25}H_{52}$ MW: 352.69 Source: PU HUANG. Ref: 2.

5038 n-Pentacosanoic acid
$C_{25}H_{50}O_2$ MW: 382.68 Source: QIANG HUO, ETC. Ref: 2.

5039 7,10-Pentadecadiynoic acid
$C_{15}H_{24}$ MW: 204.36 Source: DU HUO. Ref: 2.

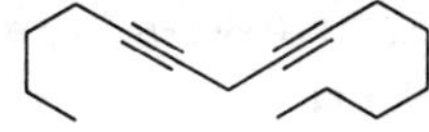

5040 n-Pentadecane
$C_{15}H_{32}$ MW: 212.42 Source: DANG SHEN, REN SHEN, SAN QI, XI XIN. Ref: 2.

5041 Pentadecanoic acid
$C_{15}H_{30}O_2$ MW: 242.41 Source: DANG SHEN, GAN DI HUANG, GUA LOU, LU HUI. Ref: 2.

5042 1-Pentadecene
$C_{15}H_{30}$ MW: 210.41 Source: BAI ZHI. Ref: 2.

5043 1,2,3,4,6-Pentagalloylglucose
$C_{41}H_{32}O_{26}$ MW: 940.70 Source: MU DAN PI. Ref: 2.

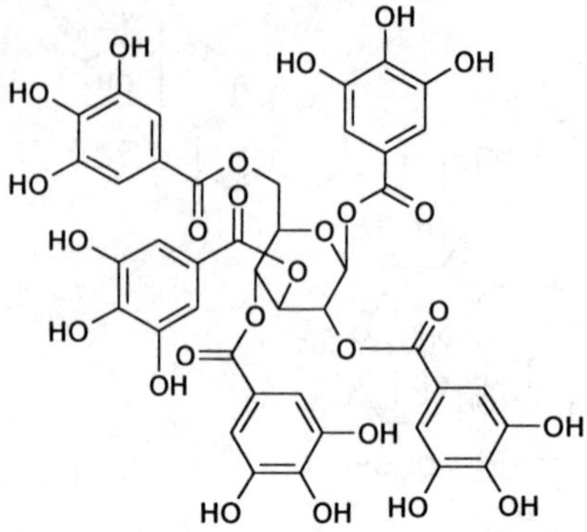

5044 (+)-3,3',5',5,7-Pentahydroflavanone
$C_{15}H_{12}O_7$ MW: 304.26 Property: light yellow acicular crystal, mp 218-20 °C, $[\alpha]_D^{15}$ +23.7° (c=0.11, methanol). Source: ZHI YU ZI. Ref: 391.

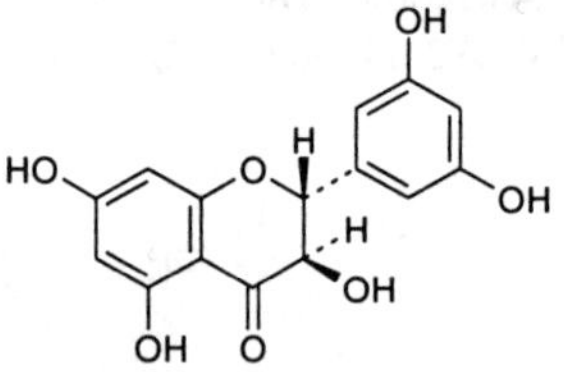

5045 Pentahydroxybufostane
$C_{28}H_{50}O_5$ MW: 466.71 Property: mp 172°C. Source: CHAN CHU DAN. Ref: 6.

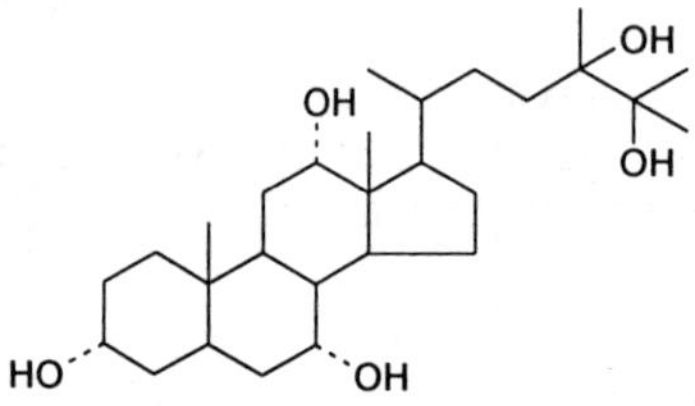

5046 3,4,5,2',4'-Pentahydroxychalcone
$C_{15}H_{12}O_6$ MW: 288.26 Source: CI HUAI HUA. Ref: 6.

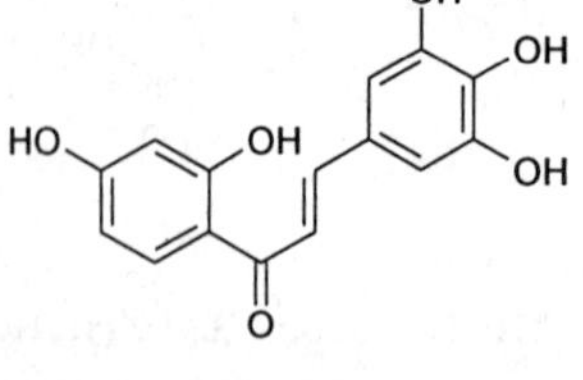

5047 3,5,7,2'6'-Pentahydroxy flavanonol
$C_{15}H_{12}O_7$ MW: 304.26 Source: HUANG QIN. Ref: 2.

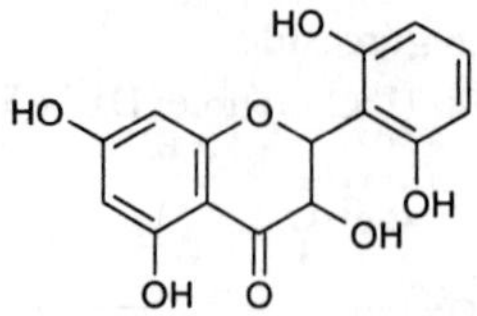

5048 3,5,7,2',6'-Pentahydroxy flavonol
$C_{15}H_{10}O_7$ MW: 302.24 Source: HUANG QIN. Ref: 2.

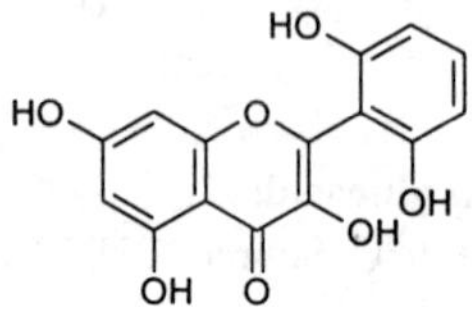

5049 3,3'4',5,7-Pentahydroxyvone-3-L-rhamnoside
$C_{21}H_{20}O_{11}$ MW: 448.39 Property: mp 178-82°C. Source: MAO YAN CAO. Ref: 6.

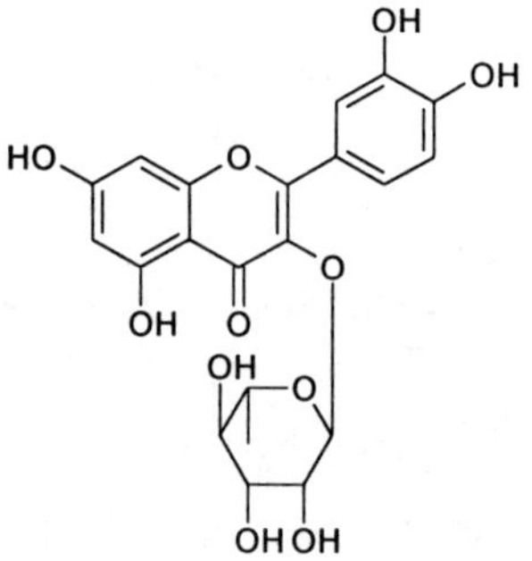

5050 3',3',5,7,8-Pentamethoxyflavone
$C_{20}H_{20}O_7$ MW: 372.38 Property: mp 197-200°C. Source: JIN JU. Ref: 6.

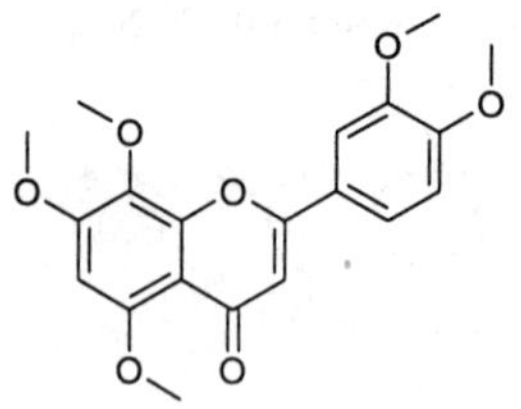

5051 5,6,7,8,4'-Pentamethoxyflavone3
$C_{20}H_{20}O_7$ MW: 372.38 Source: JU PI. Ref: 2.

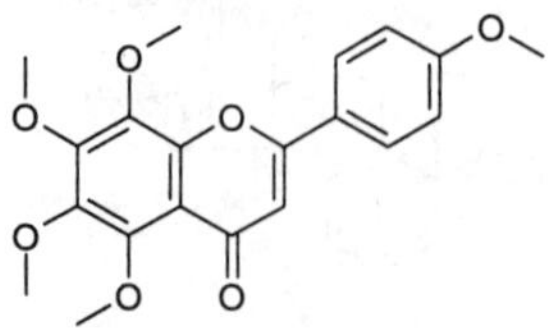

5052 Pentanal
$C_5H_{10}O$ MW: 86.13 Source: FANG FENG. Ref: 2.

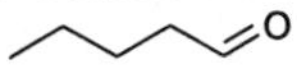

5053 Pentanic acid
$C_5H_{10}O_2$ MW: 102.13 Source: CHAI HU. Ref: 2.

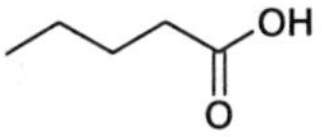

5054 Pentanol
$C_5H_{12}O$ MW: 88.15 Source: FANG FENG. Ref: 2.

5055 1-Penter-3-ol
$C_5H_{10}O$ MW: 86.13 Property: bp 114-6°C. Source: LUO HUA SHENG ZHI YE. Ref: 6.

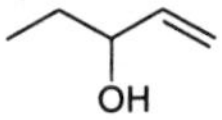

5056 4-Pentenyl isothiocyanate
C_6H_9NS MW: 127.21 Property: bp 75°C/12mm. Source: JIE ZI. Ref: 6.

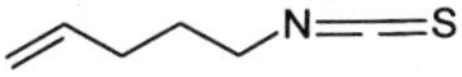

5057 Penupogenin
$C_{30}H_{40}O_7$ MW: 512.65 Property: mp 145-50°C. Source: BAI SHOU WU. Ref: 6.

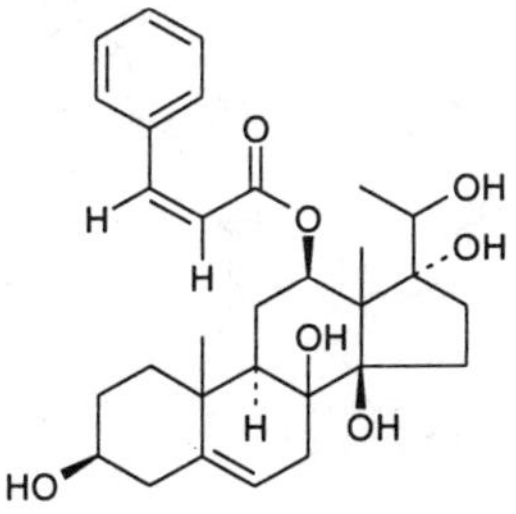

5058 Peraksine
$C_{19}H_{20}N_2O_2$ MW: 308.38 Property: mp 196-8°C. Source: LUO FU MU. Ref: 6.

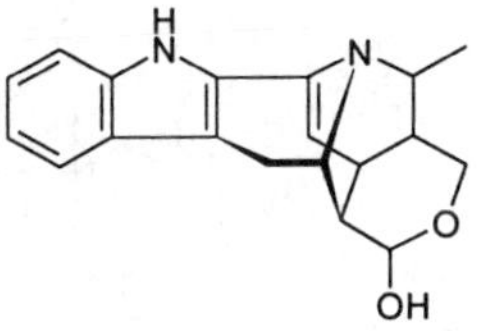

5059 Pergularin
$C_{21}H_{32}O_5$ MW: 364.49 Property: mp 220-30°C. Source: FU SHOU CAO, LUO MO. Ref: 6.

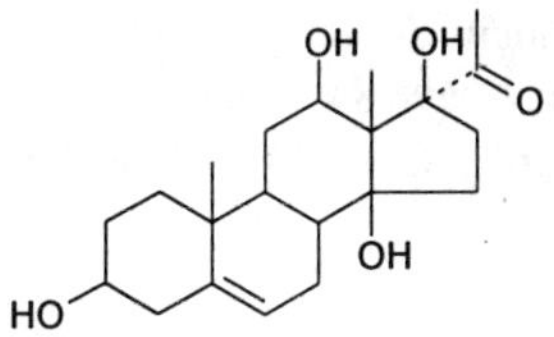

5060 Pericalline
$C_{18}H_{20}N_2$ MW: 264.37 Property: mp 198-9°C. Source: CHANG CHUN HUA. Ref: 6.

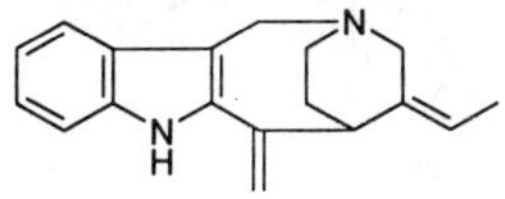

5061 Pericyclivine
$C_{20}H_{22}N_2O_2$ MW: 322.41 Source: CHANG CHUN HUA. Ref: 2.

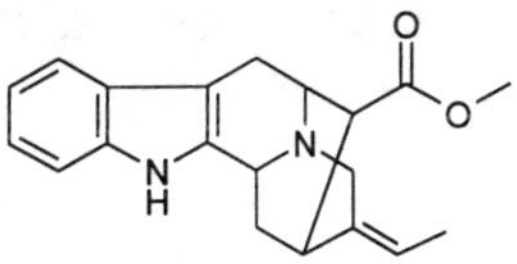

5062 Perilla ketone
$C_{10}H_{14}O_2$ MW: 166.22 Source: ZI SU. Ref: 2.

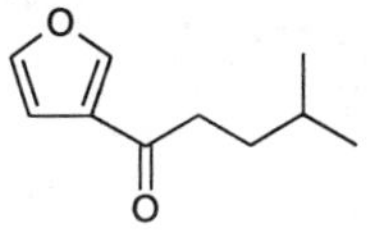

5063 Perilal
$C_{10}H_{16}O$ MW: 152.24 Source: SHENG JIANG. Ref: 2.

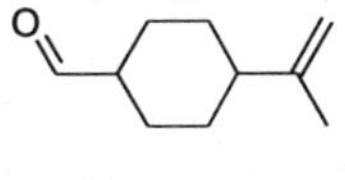

5064 Perillyl alcohol
Perilla alcohol. $C_{10}H_{16}O$ MW: 152.24 Property: bp (+): 228-9°C/755mm, (-): 244.5°C. Source: JIU LI XIANG, ZI SU. Ref: 6, 11.

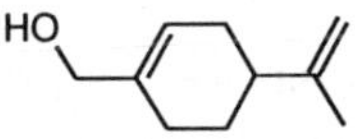

5065 Perillylaldehyde
Perillaldehyde. $C_{10}H_{14}O$ MW: 150.22 Property: bp (+): 234-6°C/743mm, (-): 235-7°C/750mm. Source: JIU LI XIANG, JU PI, ZI SU. Ref: 6, 11.

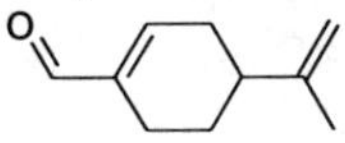

5066 Periplocin
$C_{36}H_{56}O_{13}$ MW: 696.84 Property: mp 209°C (dec), 232-3°C. Source: XIANG JIA PI. Ref: 6.

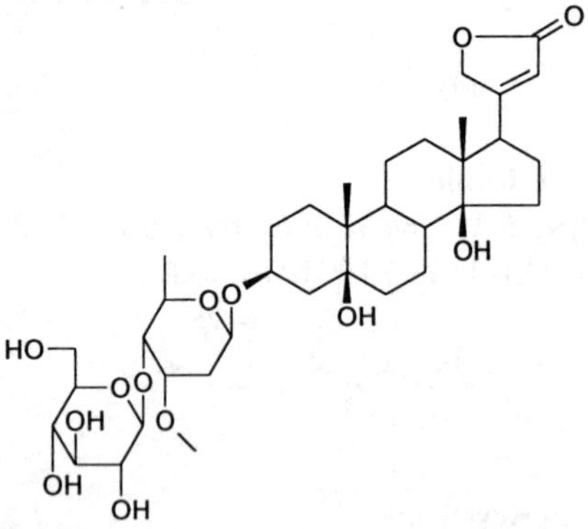

5067 Periplogenin-3-O-α-L-rhamnopyranoside
$C_{29}H_{44}O_{9}$ MW: 536.67 Property: mp 170-4°C, 219-26°C. Source: LING LAN. Ref: 6.

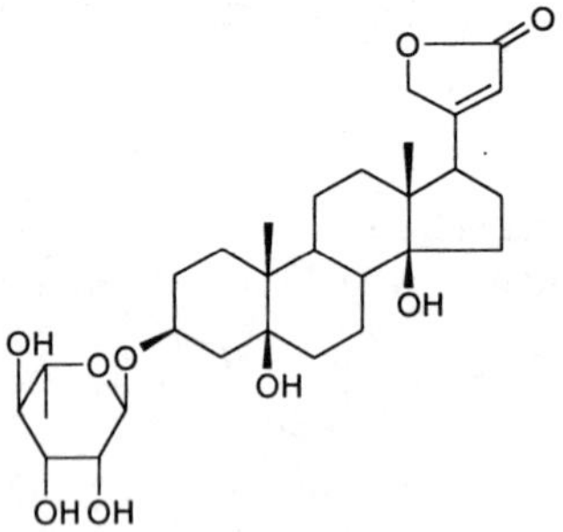

5068 Perivine
CAS: 2673-40-7 $C_{20}H_{22}N_{2}O_{3}$ MW: 338.41 Property: mp 218-21°C (dec). Source: CHANG CHUN HUA. Ref: 4, 5.

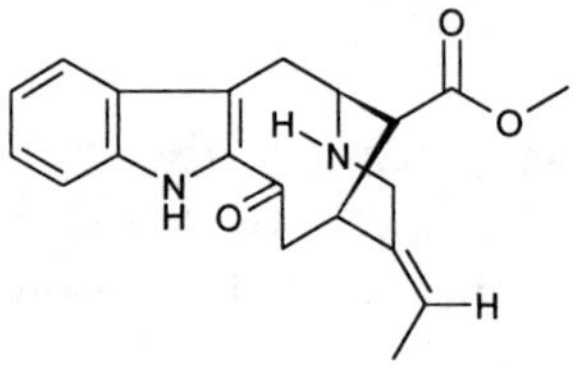

5069 Perlatolic acid
$C_{25}H_{32}O_{7}$ MW: 444.53 Property: mp 108°C. Source: TAI BAI HUA. Ref: 6.

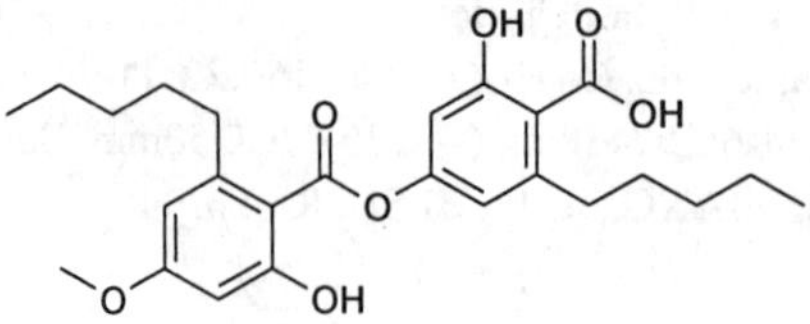

5070 Perlolyrine
Property: mp 165°C. Source: YUAN ZHI. Ref: 538.

5071 Persicarin
$C_{16}H_{11}KO_{9}S$ MW: 418.43 Property: mp 280°C. Source: QIN HUA, SHUI LIAO, SHUI MA TIAO. Ref: 6.

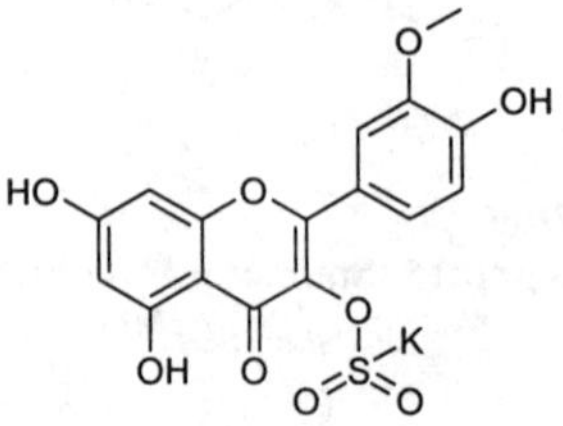

5072 Persicogenin
$C_{17}H_{14}O_{6}$ MW: 314.30 Source: TAO ZHI, TAO JING BAI PI. Ref: 6.

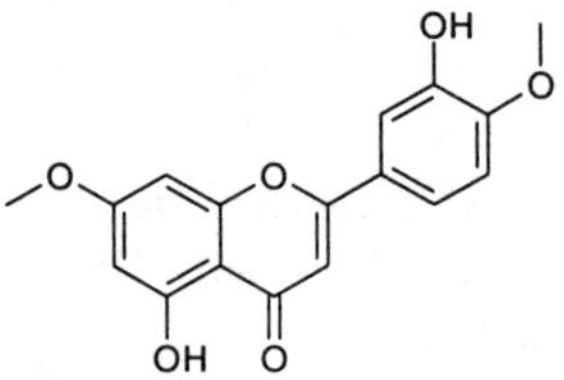

5073 Persicoside
$C_{23}H_{24}O_{11}$ MW: 476.44 Property: mp 250-60°C. Source: TAO ZHI, TAO JING BAI PI. Ref: 6.

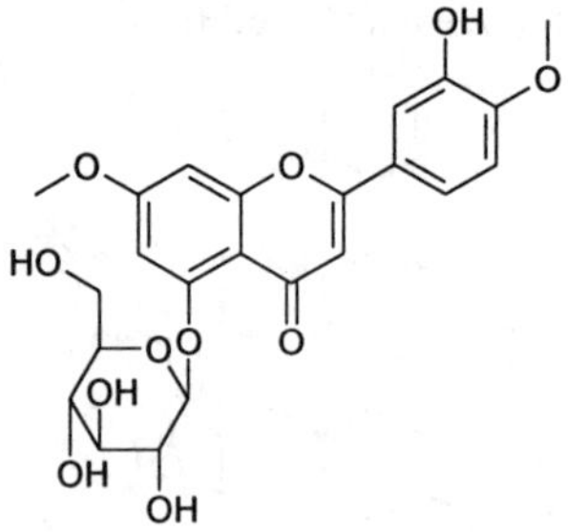

5074 Perusitin
$C_{30}H_{44}O_{10}$ MW: 564.68 Property: mp 168-70°C. Source: HUANG HUA JIA ZHU TAO. Ref: 6.

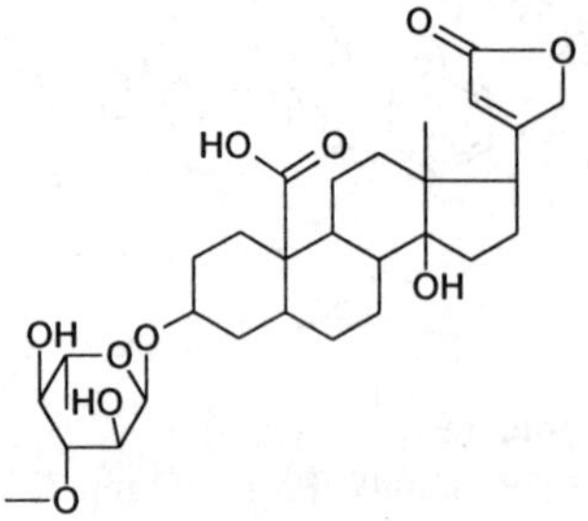

5075 Peruvoside
Encordin. CAS: 1182-87-2 $C_{30}H_{44}O_9$ MW: 548.68 Property: mp 161-4°C. Source: HUANG HUA JIA ZHU TAO. Ref: 4.

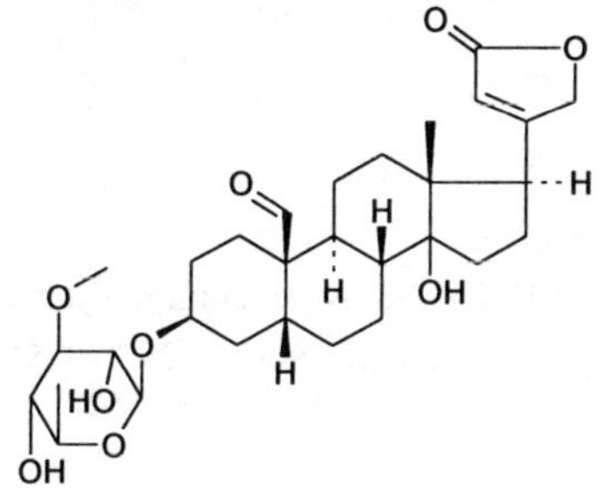

5076 Peruvoside-2'-monoacetate
$C_{32}H_{46}O_{10}$ MW: 590.72 Property: mp 212-7°C. Source: HUANG HUA JIA ZHU TAO. Ref: 6.

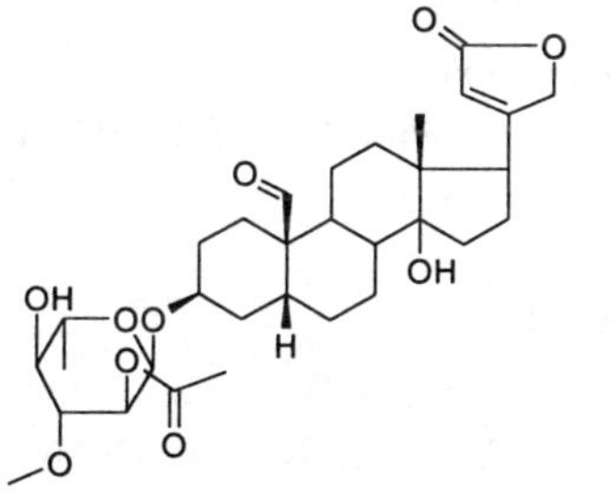

5077 Petasalbin
$C_{15}H_{22}O_2$ MW: 234.34 Property: mp 81-2°C. Source: FENG DOU CAI. Ref: 6.

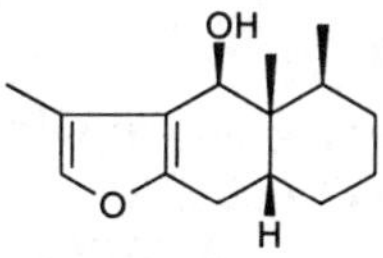

5078 Petasalbin methyl ether
$C_{16}H_{24}O_2$ MW: 248.37 Property: bp 90-100°C/ 4×10^{-4} mm. Source: ENG DOU CAI. Ref: 6.

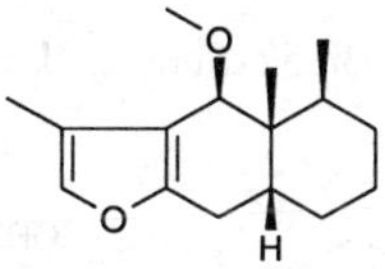

5079 Petasin
$C_{20}H_{28}O_3$ MW: 316.44 Property: mp 65-8°C. Source: FENG DOU CAI. Ref: 6.

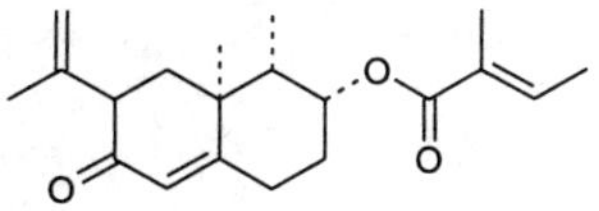

5080 Petasitin
$C_{20}H_{28}O_4$ MW: 332.44 Source: FENG DOU CAI. Ref: 6.

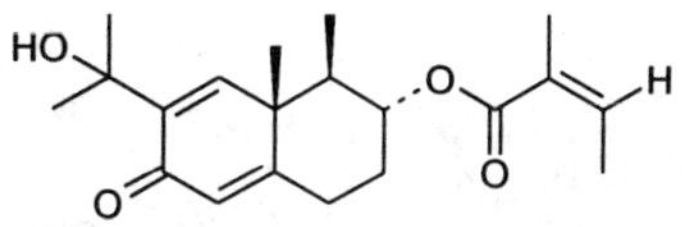

5081 Petasitolone
$C_{15}H_{24}O_2$ MW: 236.36 Property: bp 92°C/0.15 mm. Source: FENG DOU CAI. Ref: 6.

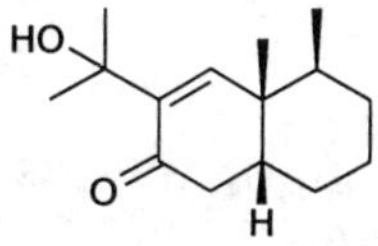

5082 Petroselic acid
$C_{18}H_{34}O_2$ MW: 282.47 Property: mp 33°C. Source: CHAI HU. Ref: 6.

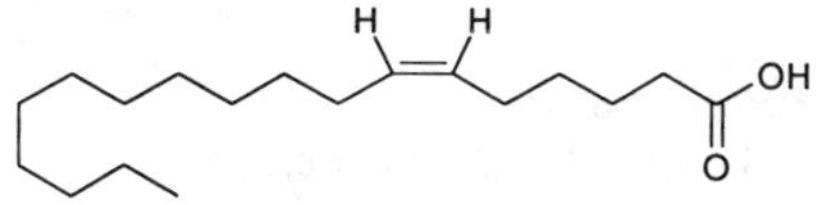

5083 Petroselidic acid
$C_{18}H_{34}O_2$ MW: 282.47 Property: mp 54-9°C. Source: CHAI HU, HAN QIN. Ref: 6.

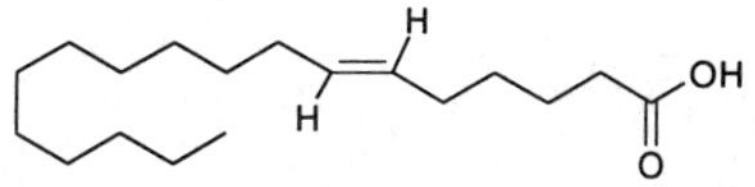

5084 Petunidin
$C_{16}H_{13}O_7$ MW: 317.28 Source: MU XU, PU TAO. Ref: 6.

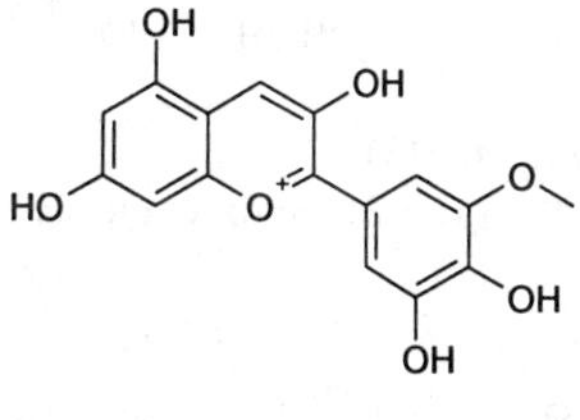

5085 Petunidin-3-arabinoside
$C_{21}H_{21}O_{11}$ MW: 449.39 Source: ZI WEI HUA. Ref: 6.

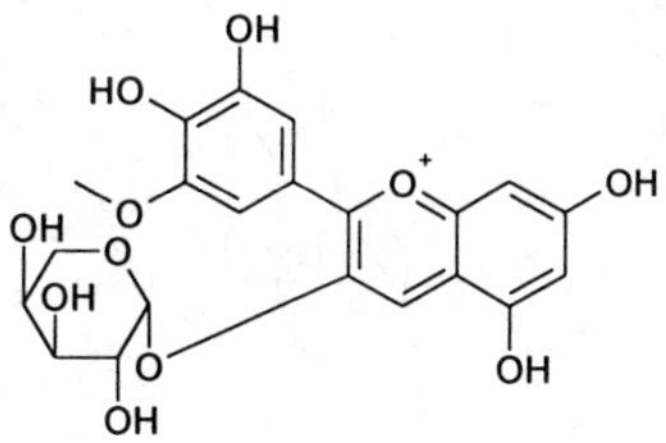

5086 Petunidin-3-glucoside
$C_{22}H_{23}O_{12}$ MW: 479.42 Source: BAI FAN DOU, HUANG LU ZHI YE. Ref: 6.

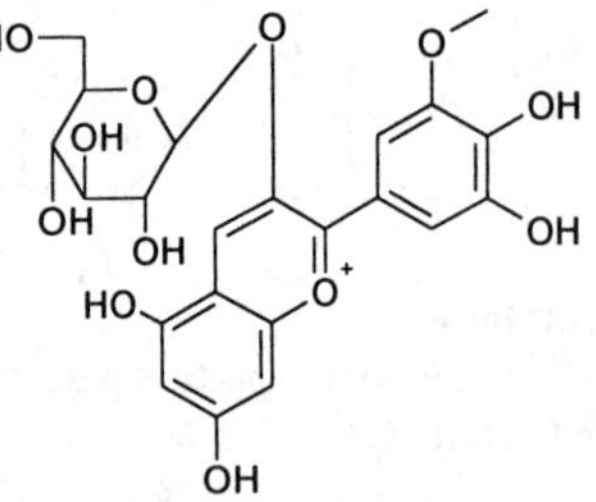

5087 Peucedanin
CAS: 133-26-6 $C_{15}H_{14}O_4$ MW: 258.26 Property: mp 97-9°C. Source: QIAN HU. Ref: 5.

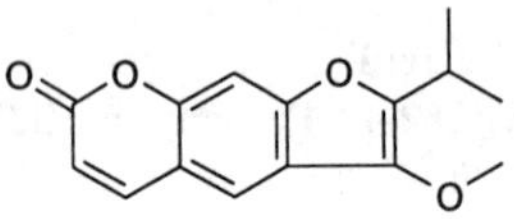

5088 Peucedanocomarin
Source: LI JIANG QIAN HU. Ref: 557.

5089 Pharbitic acid C
$C_{38}H_{68}O_{21}$ MW: 860.95 Source: QIAN NIU ZI. Ref: 6.

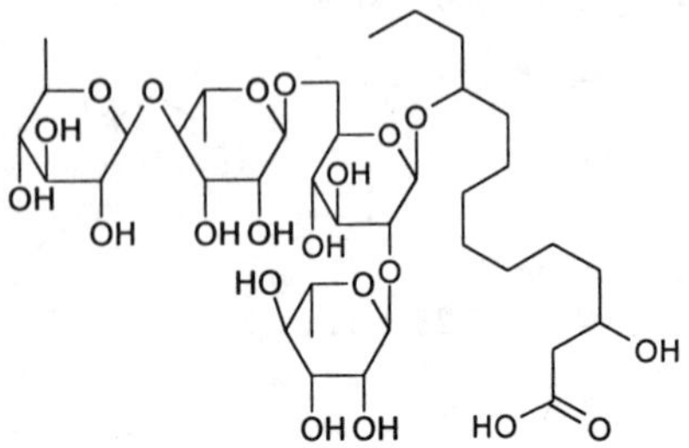

5090 Pharbitic acid D
$C_{49}H_{86}O_{30}$ MW: 1155.21 Source: QIAN NIU ZI. Ref: 6.

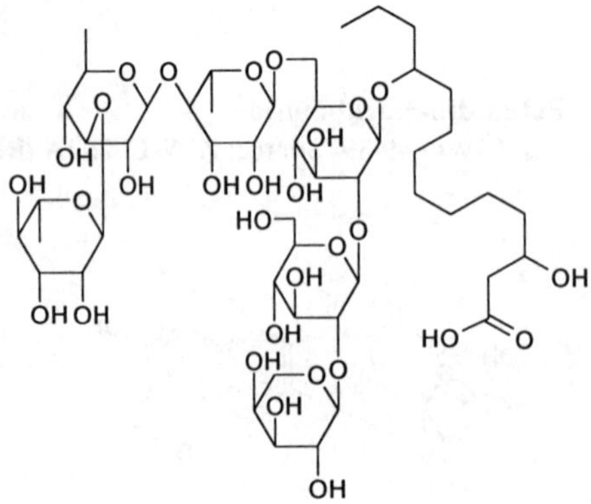

5091 Phaseollinisoflavan
$C_{20}H_{20}O_4$ MW: 324.38 Source: GAN CAO. Ref: 2.

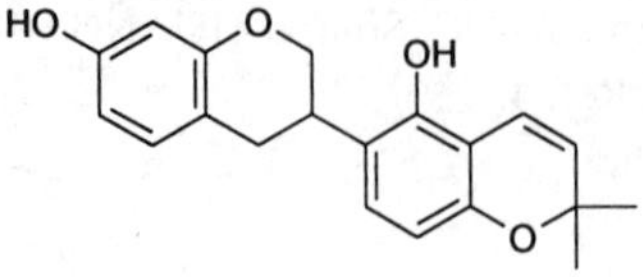

5092 Phebalosin
$C_{15}H_{14}O_4$ MW: 258.28 Note: commonly in family *Rutaceae*, genus *Murraya*. Source: JIU LI XIANG, etc. Ref: 11.

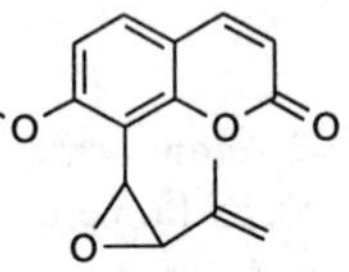

5093 Phellamurin
CAS: 52589-11-4 Property: mp 205°C. Source: HUANG BAI. Ref: 5.

5094 α-Phellandrene
Phellandrene. $C_{10}H_{16}$ MW: 136.24 Source: DU HUO, GAN JIANG, JU PI, MU XIANG, QIANG HUO. Ref: 2.

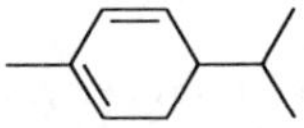

5095 β-Phellandrene
$C_{10}H_{16}$ MW: 136.24 Source: DANG GUI, LIAN QIAO, SHENG JIANG. Ref: 2.

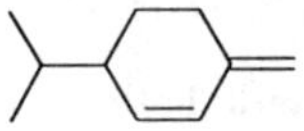

5096 Phellatin
$C_{26}H_{30}O_{12}$ MW: 534.52 Source: HUANG BAI. Ref: 6.

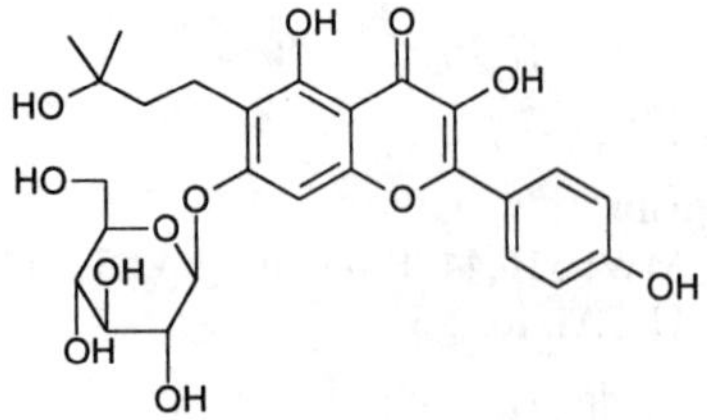

5097 Phellavin
$C_{26}H_{32}O_{12}$ MW: 536.54 Source: HUANG BAI. Ref: 6.

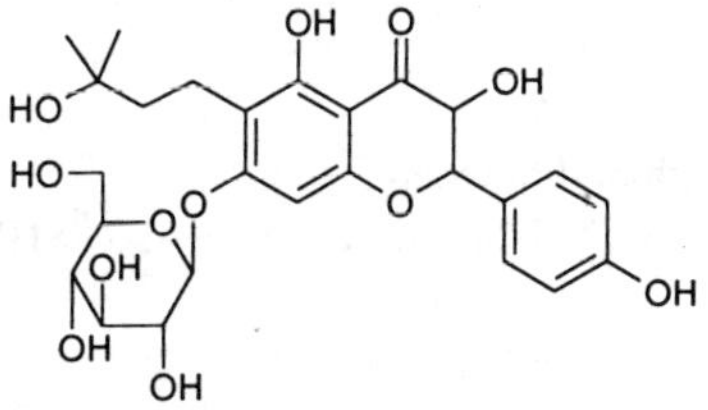

5098 Phellodendrine
CAS: 6873-13-8 $C_{20}H_{24}NO_4$ MW: 342.42 Property: mp 258°C. Source: HUANG BAI. Ref: 4.

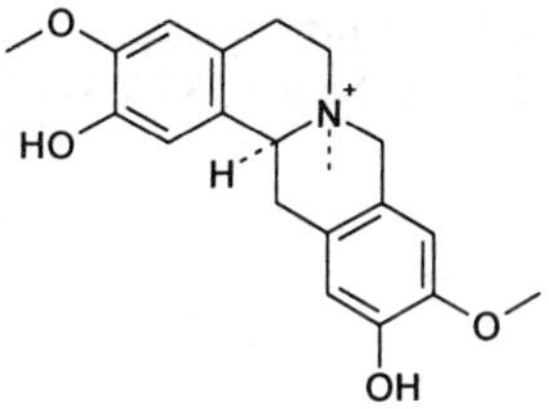

5099 Phellopterin
$C_{17}H_{16}O_5$ MW: 300.31 Source: BAI ZHI, FANG FENG, QIANG HUO. Ref: 2, 566.

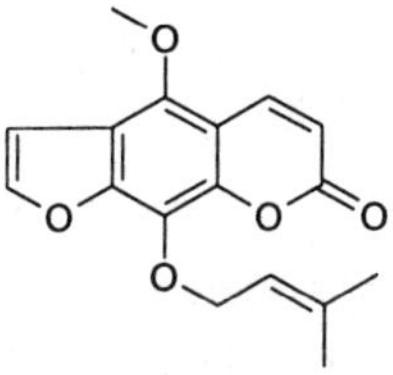

5100 Phenethyl ferulate
Source: QIANG HUO. Ref: 507.

5101 3-Phenglundecane
$C_{17}H_{28}$ MW: 232.41 Source: XI YANG SHEN. Ref: 2.

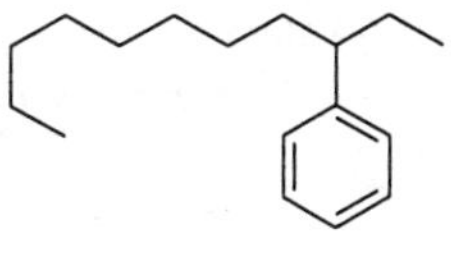

5102 Phenol
C_6H_6O MW: 94.11 Source: CHAI HU, DANG GUI. Ref: 2.

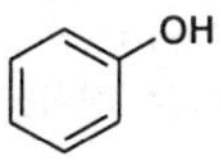

5103 Phenylacetic acid
$C_8H_8O_2$ MW: 136.15 Source: GAN DI HUANG. Ref: 2.

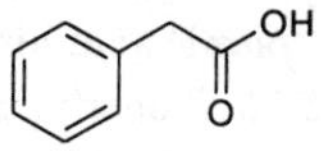

5104 Phenylalanine
$C_9H_{11}NO_2$ MW: 165.19 Source: BING LANG. Ref: 2.

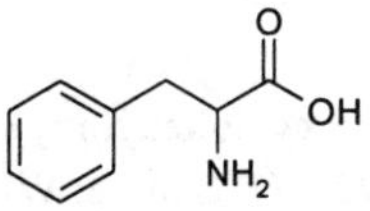

5105 4-Phenylbicyclo[2,2,2]octan-1-ol
$C_{14}H_{18}O$ MW: 202.30 Source: WU WEI ZI. Ref: 2.

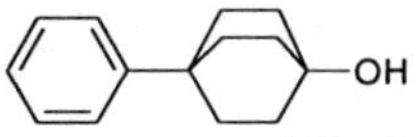

5106 1-Phenyl-1,3-butanedion
$C_{10}H_{10}O_2$ MW: 182.19 Source: HUANG QIN. Ref: 2.

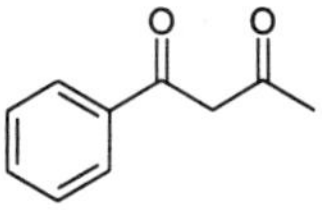

5107 4-Phenylbutan-2-one
$C_{10}H_{12}O$ MW: 148.21 Property: mp 235°C. Source: XIAO YE PI PA. Ref: 6.

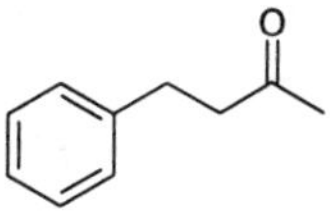

5108 Phenylbutanone-glucoside
$C_{16}H_{22}O_7$ MW: 326.35 Source: DA HUANG. Ref: 2.

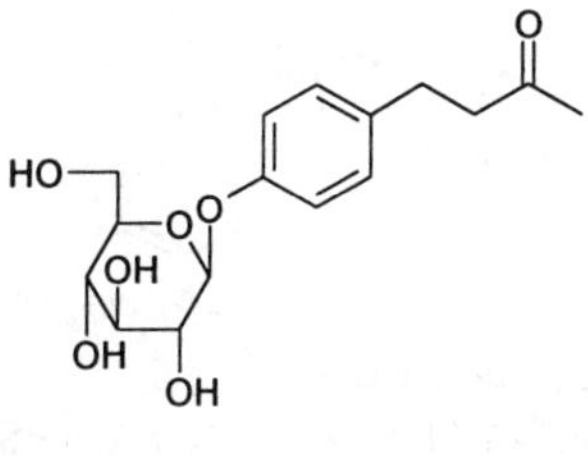

5109 (E)-4-phenyl-3-buten-2-one
$C_{10}H_{10}O$ MW: 146.19 Source: HUANG QIN. Ref: 2.

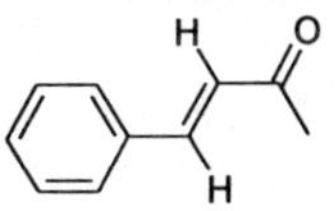

5110 α-Phenylcinnamic acid nitrile
$C_{15}H_{11}N$ MW: 205.26 Property: mp 49-51°C, bp 213-4°C/23 mm. Source: HAN LIAN HUA. Ref: 6.

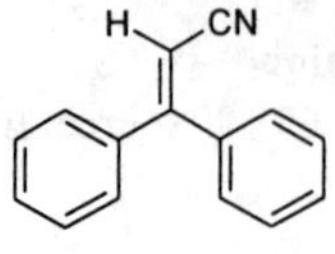

5111 2-(2-Phenyl cyclohexyloxy) ethanol
$C_{14}H_{20}O_2$ MW: 220.31 Source: WU WEI ZI. Ref: 2.

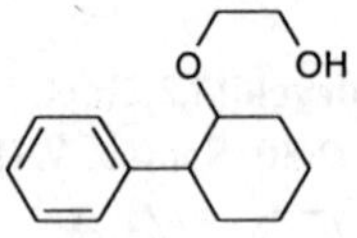

5112 2-Phenyldodecane
$C_{18}H_{30}$ MW: 246.44 Source: XI YANG SHEN. Ref: 2.

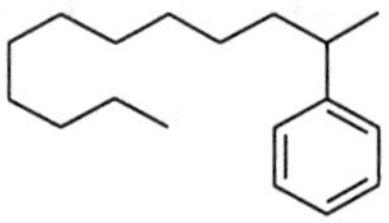

5113 3-Phenyldecane
$C_{16}H_{26}$ MW: 218.39 Source: XI YANG SHEN. Ref: 2.

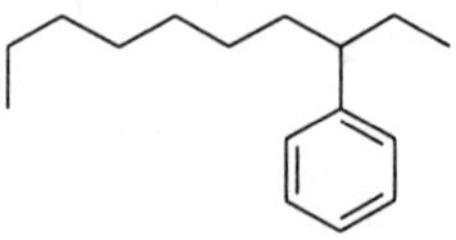

5114 3-Phenyldodecane
$C_{18}H_{30}$ MW: 246.44 Source: XI YANG SHEN. Ref: 2.

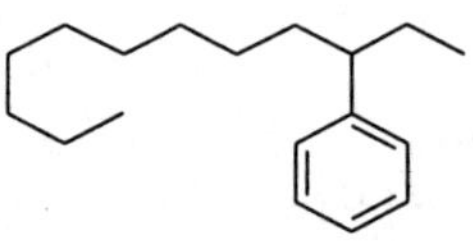

5115 4-Phenyldodecane
$C_{18}H_{30}$ MW: 246.44 Source: XI YANG SHEN. Ref: 2.

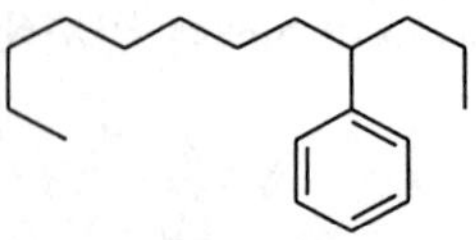

5116 5-Phenyldodecane
$C_{18}H_{30}$ MW: 246.44 Source: XI YANG SHEN. Ref: 2.

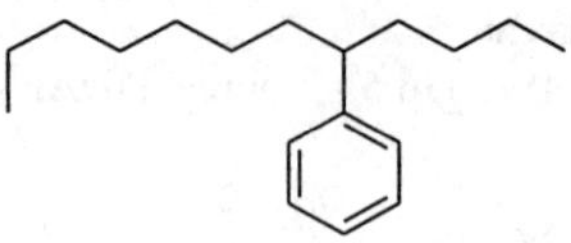

5117 6-Phenyldodecane
$C_{18}H_{30}$ MW: 246.44 Source: XI YANG SHEN. Ref: 2.

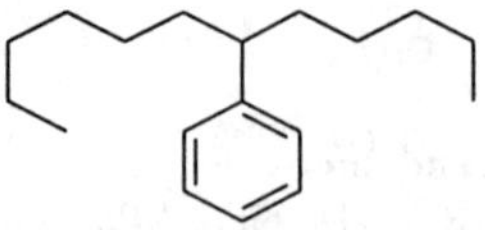

5118 5-Phenyldolecane
$C_{19}H_{32}$ MW: 260.47 Source: XI YANG SHEN. Ref: 2.

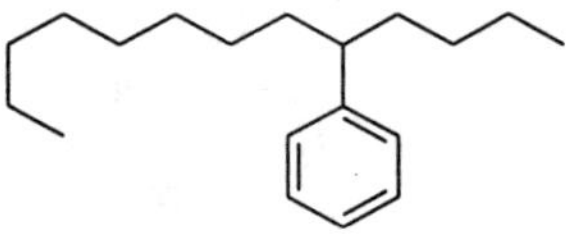

5119 Phenylethanone
C_8H_8O MW: 120.15 Source: SAN QI. Ref: 2.

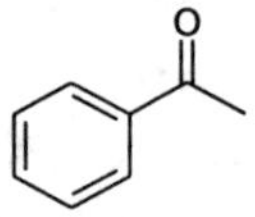

5120 Phenylethyl acetate
$C_{10}H_{12}O_2$ MW: 164.21 Property: bp 224°C. Source: LU DOU LE HUA, MEI GUI HUA, SHUI XIAN HUA. Ref: 6.

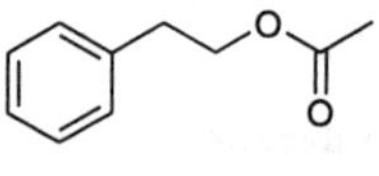

5121 β-Phenylethyl alcohol
$C_8H_{10}O$ MW: 122.17 Source: SHAN ZHU YU. Ref: 2.

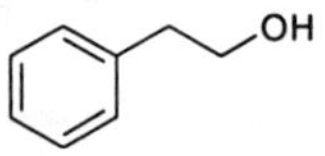

5122 Phenylethylamine
$C_8H_{11}N$ MW: 121.18 Property: bp 197-8°C. Source: GUI GAI, HUANG HUA ZI, HONG MU JI CAO. Ref: 6.

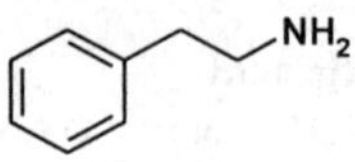

5123 2-(2-Phenylethyl) chromone
$C_{17}H_{14}O_2$ MW: 250.30 Property: white acicular crystal, mp 65°C. Source: BAI MU XIANG, CHEN XIANG. Ref: 13.

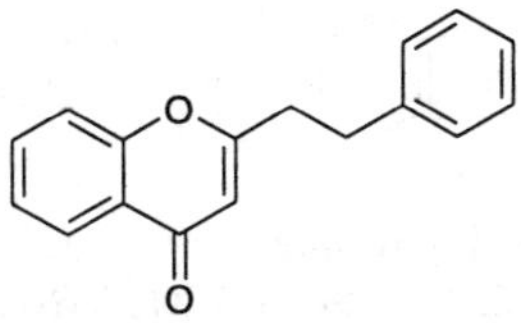

5124 Phenyl ethyl formate
$C_9H_{10}O_2$ MW: 150.18 Property: bp 94°C/9 mm. Source: CHA YE. Ref: 6.

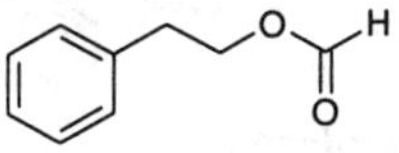

5125 β-Phenylethyl isothiocyanate
C_9H_9NS MW: 163.24 Property: bp 142°C/13 mm. Source: JIE ZI. Ref: 6.

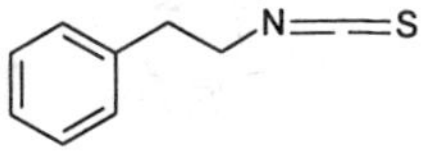

5126 **(5R,6R,7S,8R)-2-(2-Phenylethyl)-5e',6a, 7e,8e'-tetrahydroxy-5,6,7,8-tetrahydro-chromone (AH16)**
$C_{17}H_{18}O_6$ MW: 318.33 Property: white powder, mp 100-5°C, $[\alpha]_D$ +4.76°. Source: CHEN XIANG. Ref: 13.

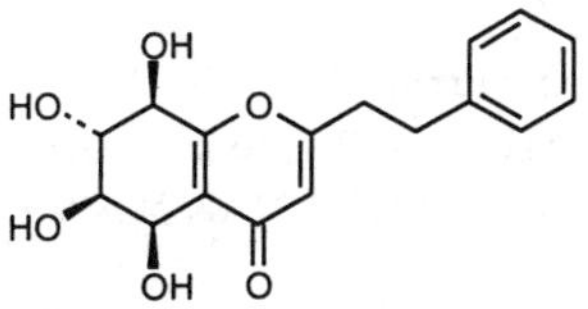

5127 (5S,6R,7R,8S)-2-(2-Phenylethyl)-5,6,7-trihydroxy-5,6,7,8-tetrahydro-8-[2-(2-phenylethyl)-7-methoxy-chromonyl-6-oxy] chromone (AH12)
$C_{35}H_{32}O_9$ MW: 596.64 Property: colorless acicular crystal, mp 227°C, $[\alpha]_D$ +0.7°. Source: CHEN XIANG. Ref: 13.

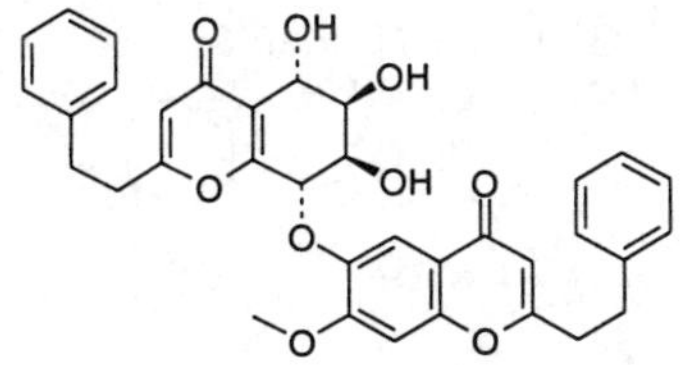

5128 (5S,6R,7R,8S)-2-(2-Phenylethyl)-5,6,7-trihydroxy-5,6,7,8-tetrahydro-8-[2-(2-phenylethyl) chromonyl-6-oxy] chromone (AH13)
$C_{34}H_{30}O_8$ MW: 566.61 Property: colorless acicular crystal, mp 193-4°C, $[\alpha]_D$ +2°. Source: CHEN XIANG. Ref: 13.

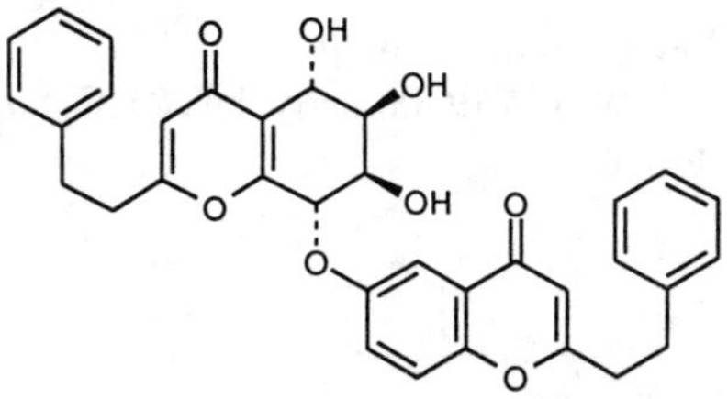

5129 (5S,6S,7S,8R)-2-(2-Phenylethyl)-6,7,8-trihydroxy-5,6,7,8-tetrahydro-5-[2-(2-phenylethyl) chromonyl-6-oxy] chromone (AH14)
$C_{34}H_{30}O_8$ MW: 566.61 Property: white powder, mp 86-8°C, $[\alpha]_D$ +64.4°. Source: CHEN XIANG. Ref: 13.

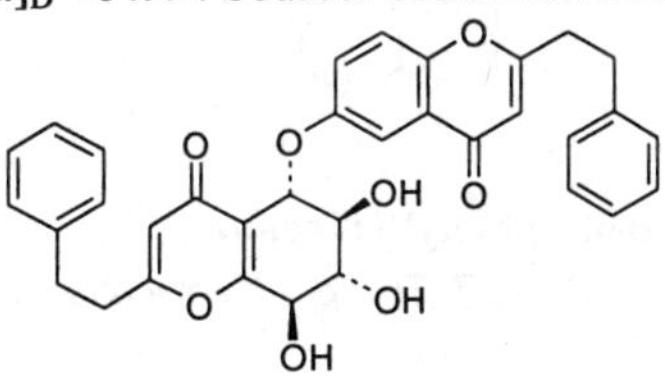

5130 (5S,6S,7R,8S)-2-(2-Phenylethyl)-6,7,8-trihydroxy-5,6,7,8-tetrahydro-5-[2-(2-phenylethyl)-7-hydroxy-chromonyl-6-oxy]-chromone (AH15)
$C_{34}H_{30}O_9$ MW: 582.61 Property: colorless acicular crystal, mp 244-5°C, $[\alpha]_D$ +5.8°. Source: CHEN XIANG. Ref: 13.

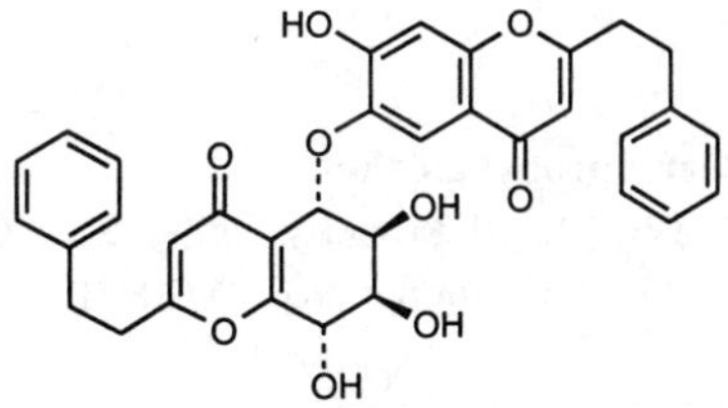

5131 1-Phenyl-2,4-hexadiyne-1-ol
$C_{12}H_{10}O$ MW: 170.21 Source: YIN CHEN HAO. Ref: 2.

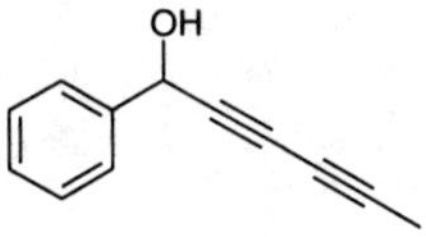

5132 1-Phenylhexane
$C_{12}H_{18}$ MW: 162.28 Source: XI YANG SHEN. Ref: 2.

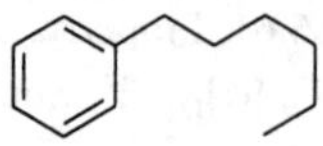

5133 Phenyl isothiocyanate
C_7H_5NS MW: 135.19 Property: bp 221°C. Source: JIE ZI. Ref: 6.

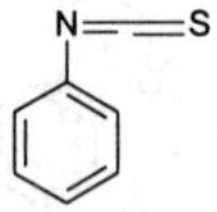

N=S

5134 N-Phenyl-2-naphthalene amine
$C_{15}H_{13}N$ MW: 207.28 Property: mp 107-8°C. Source: QIN PI. Ref: 2, 548.

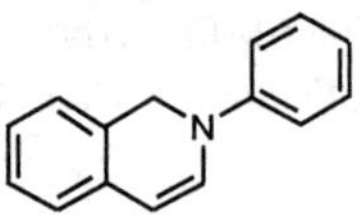

N

5135 4-Phenylphenyltridecane
$C_{19}H_{32}$ MW: 260.47 Source: XI YANG SHEN. Ref: 2.

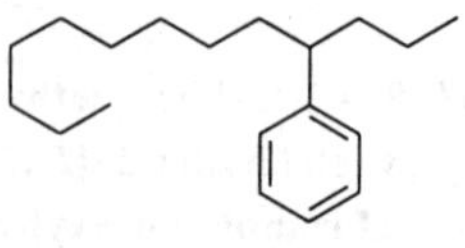

5136 Phenyl-2-propanone
$C_9H_{10}O$ MW: 134.18 Source: WU WEI ZI. Ref: 2.

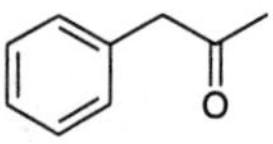

O

5137 Phenylpropyl alcohol
$C_9H_{12}O$ MW: 136.20 Property: bp (-): 94-5°C/10 mm, (±): 217-21°C. Source: SHUI XIAN HUA. Ref: 6.

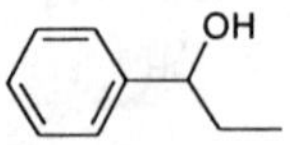

OH

5138 Phenylpropyl cinnamate
$C_{18}H_{18}O_2$ MW: 266.34 Source: AN XI XIANG. Ref: 6.

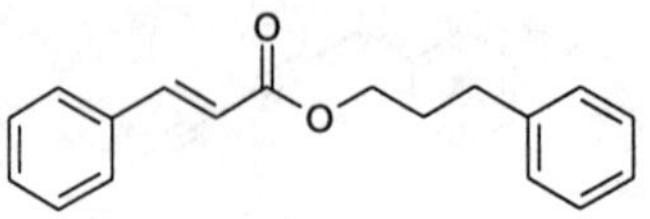

O
O

5139 Phenyl pyruvic acid
$C_9H_8O_3$ MW: 164.16 Property: mp 157°C (dec). Source: LAI FU. Ref: 6.

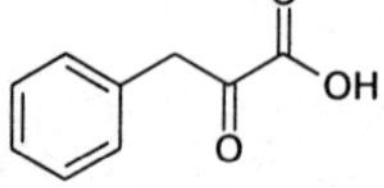

O
OH
O

5140 4-Phenylundecane
$C_{17}H_{28}$ MW: 232.41 Source: XI YANG SHEN. Ref: 2.

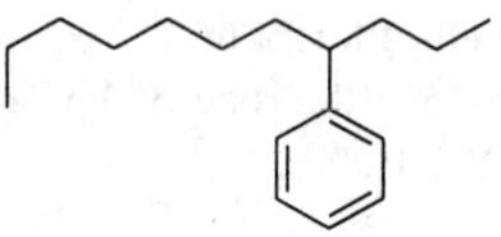

5141 6-Phenylundecane
$C_{17}H_{28}$ MW: 232.41 Source: XI YANG SHEN. Ref: 2.

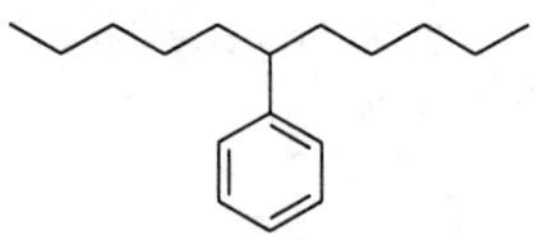

5142 Phlegmariuine-N
$C_{11}H_{11}NO$ MW: 173.22 Property: white acicular crystal, 179-81°C. Source: MA WEI SHAN. Ref: 122.

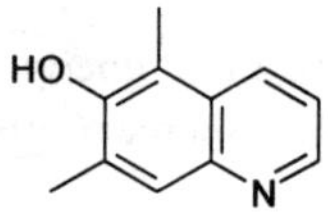

HO
N

5143 Phlegmariurine C
$C_{32}H_{44}N_2O_4$ MW: 520.72 property: acicular crystal, mp 151-2°C. Source: HUA NAN MA WEI SHAN. Ref: 95.

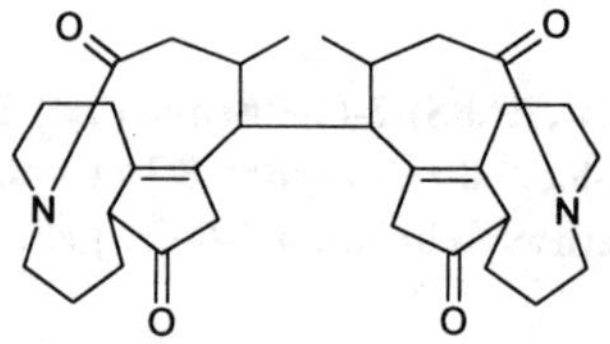

O O
N N
O O

5144 Phloretin
$C_{15}H_{14}O_5$ MW: 274.28 Property: mp 262-4°C (dec). Source: NING MENG YE. Ref: 6.

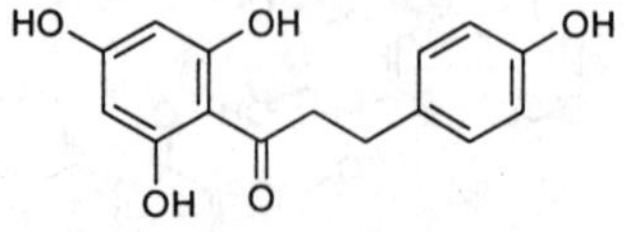

HO OH OH
OH O

5145 Phlorin

$C_{12}H_{16}O_8$ MW: 288.26 Property: mp 231-3°C. Source: JI SU ZI, TIAN CHEN. Ref: 6.

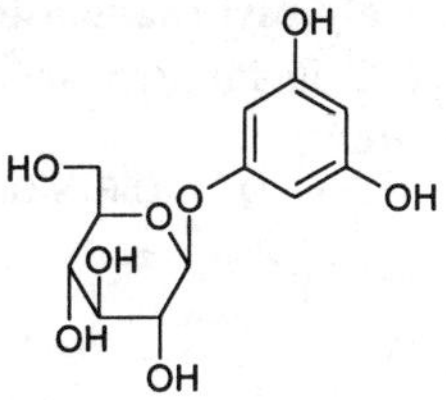

5146 Phloroacetophenone

$C_{10}H_{12}O_4$ MW: 196.20 Property: mp 85-8°C. Source: AI NA XIANG. Ref: 6.

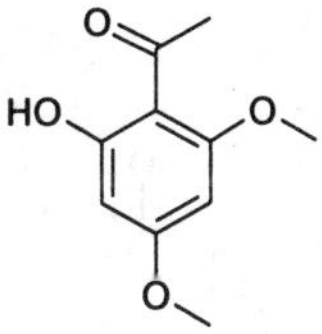

5147 Phloroglucinol

$C_6H_6O_3$ MW: 126.11 Property: mp 217-9°C. Source: LU SONG QIU MAO. Ref: 6.

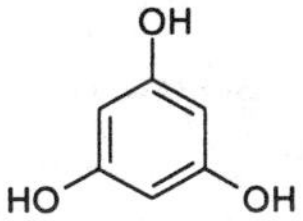

5148 Phloyoside II

Source: XIAN SHENG MA XIAN HAO. Ref: 579.

5149 Pholidotanin

25-Methylenecycloartanyl-p-hydroxy-trans-cinnamate. $C_{39}H_{56}O_3$ MW: 572.88 Property: white acicular crystal, mp 202-4°C, $[\alpha]_D^{14}$ +45.6° (c=0.19, chloroform). Source: YUN NAN SHI XIAN TAO. Ref: 478.

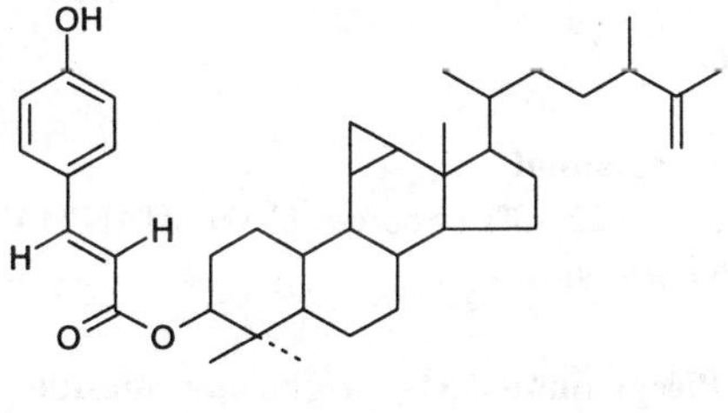

5150 Phorbol

$C_{20}H_{28}O_6$ MW: 364.44 Source: BA DOU. Ref: 2.

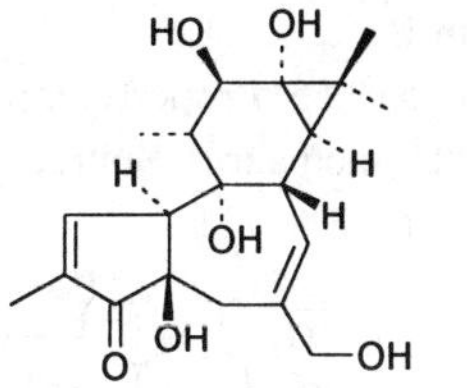

5151 Phrymarolin-II

$C_{23}H_{22}O_{10}$ MW: 458.43 Property: mp 160-1°C. Source: LAO PO ZI ZHEN XIAN. Ref: 6.

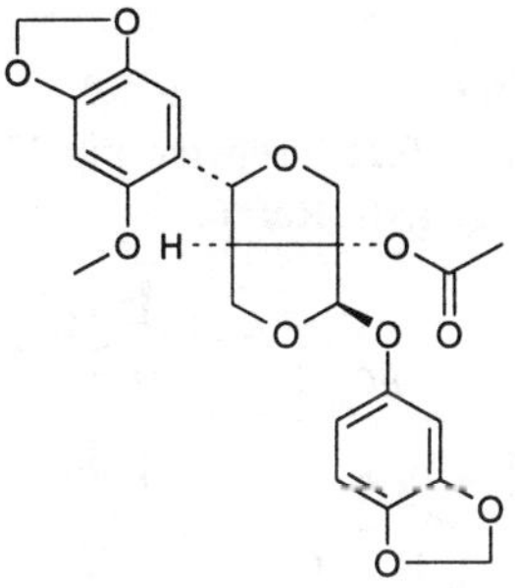

5152 Phthalic anhydride

$C_8H_4O_3$ MW: 148.12 Source: DANG GUI. Ref: 2.

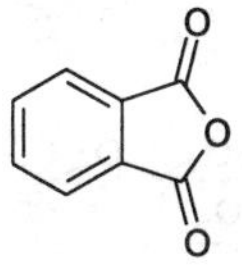

5153 Physalien

Zeaxanthin dipalmitate. $C_{72}H_{116}O_4$ MW: 1045.72 Source: GOU QI ZI. Ref: 2.

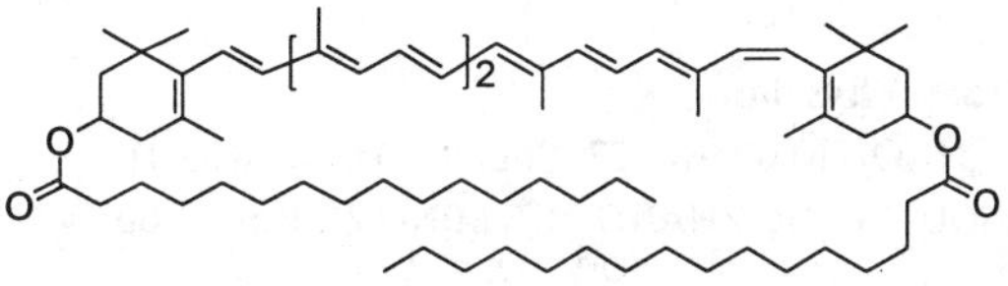

5154 Physalin A

$C_{28}H_{30}O_{10}$ MW: 526.55 Property: mp 266°C. Source: SUAN JIANG. Ref: 6.

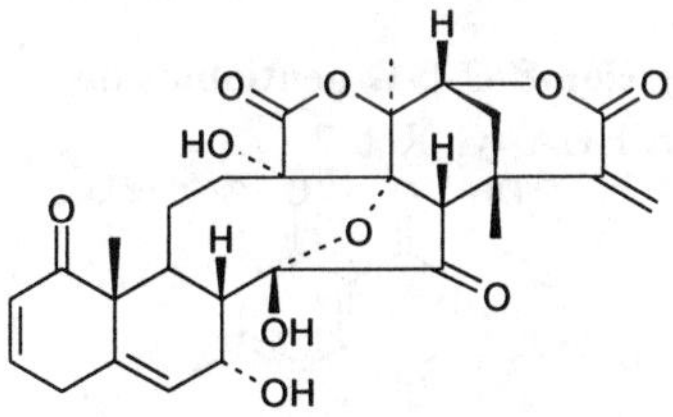

5155 Physalin B
$C_{28}H_{30}O_9$ MW: 510.55 Property: mp 250°C (acetone), 271°C (methanol). Source: SUAN JIANG. Ref: 6.

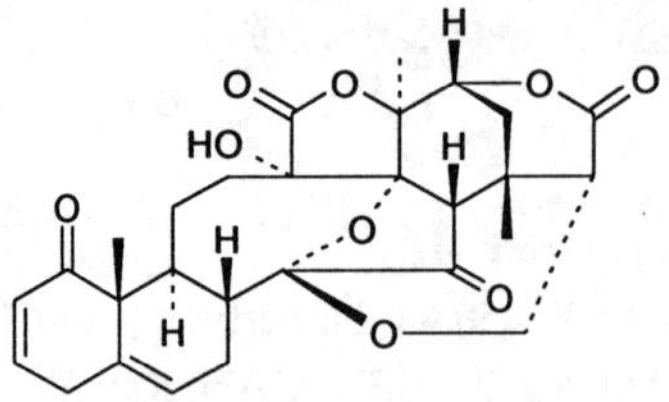

5156 Physalin C
$C_{28}H_{30}O_9$ MW: 510.55 Property: mp 274-7°C. Source: SUAN JIANG. Ref: 6.

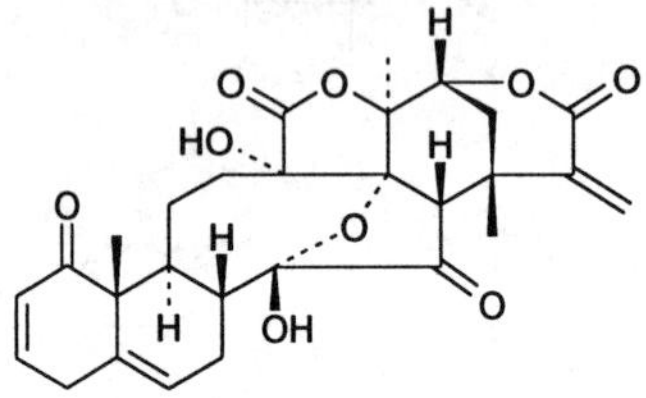

5157 Physalin D
$C_{28}H_{32}O_{11}$ MW: 544.56 Source: SUAN JIANG. Ref: 6.

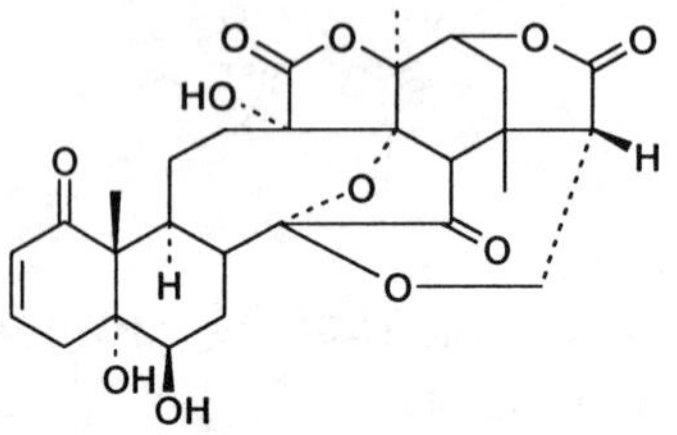

5158 Physcion
$C_{16}H_{12}O_5$ MW: 284.27 Source: DA HUANG, HE SHOU WU, HU ZHANG, JUE MING ZI. Ref: 2, 608.

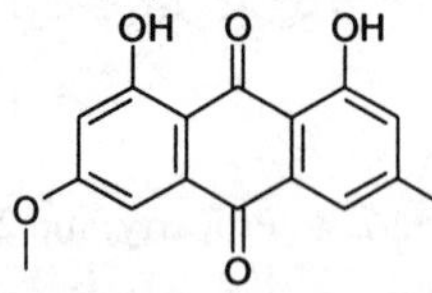

5159 Physcion-8-O-β-D-gentiobioside
Source: DA HUANG. Ref: 2.

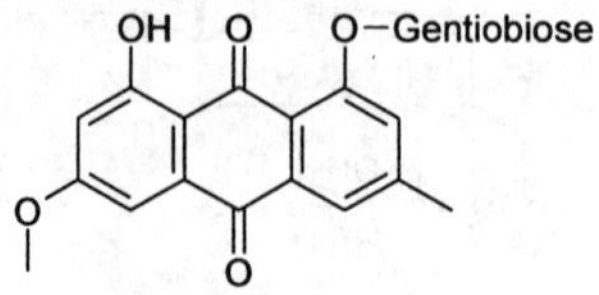

5160 Physcion-8-O-β-D-glucopyranoside
Source: TIAN SHAN DA HUANG. Ref: 608.

5161 Physcion-1-glycosyl rhamnoside
$C_{28}H_{32}O_{14}$ MW: 592.56 Property: mp 220°C. Source: PAI QIAN CAO. Ref: 6.

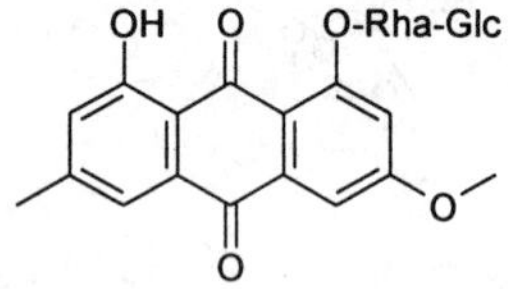

5162 Phytic acid
$C_6H_{18}O_{24}P_6$ MW: 660.04 Source: SHAN YAO. Ref: 2.

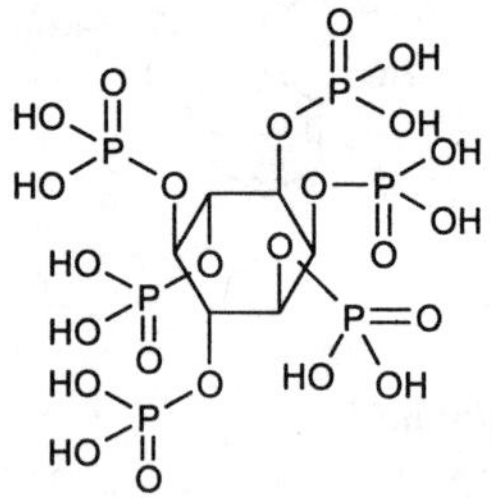

5163 Phytofluene
$C_{40}H_{62}$ MW: 542.94 Source: HU LUO BO, SAN SE JIN, XI GUA. Ref: 6.

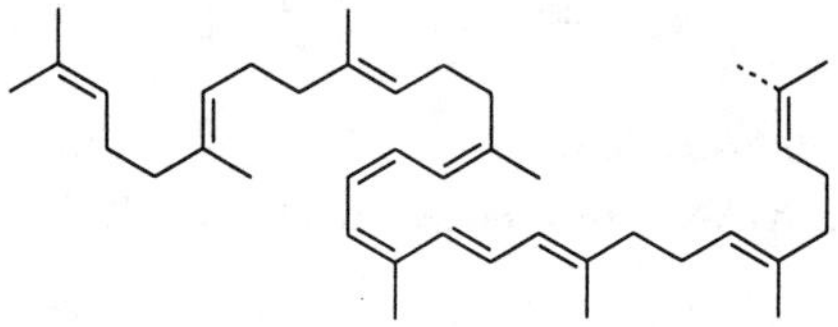

5164 Phytol
$C_{20}H_{40}O$ MW: 296.54 Property: bp 145°C/0.03 mm. Source: KUN BU, YUAN CAN SHA. Ref: 6.

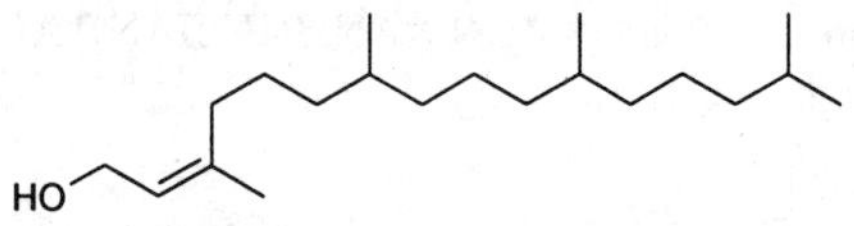

5165 Piceatannol
Property: mp 222-3°C. Source: TIAN SHAN DA HUANG. Ref: 609.

5166 Piceatannol-4'-O-β-D-glucopyranoside
Property: mp 206-8°C. Source: TIAN SHAN DA HUANG. Ref: 609.

5167 Piceid

$C_{20}H_{22}O_8$ MW: 390.39 Source: DA HUANG, HU ZHANG. Ref: 2.

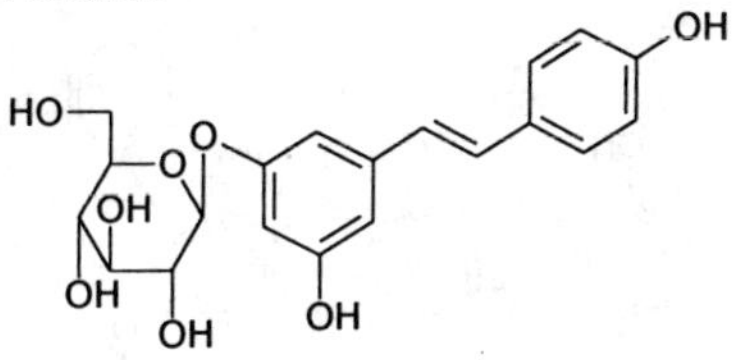

5168 Picralinal

$C_{21}H_{22}N_2O_4$ MW: 366.42 Property: mp 179-80°C. Source: XIANG PI MU. Ref: 6.

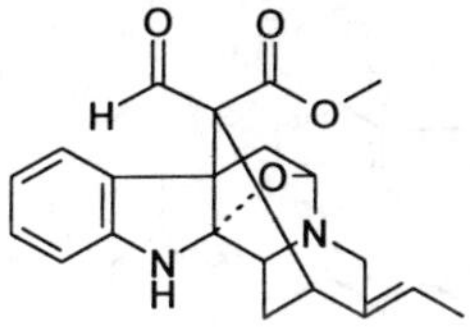

5169 Picrasidine E

$C_{18}H_{16}N_2O_5$ MW: 340.34 Source: KU SHU PI. Ref: 12.

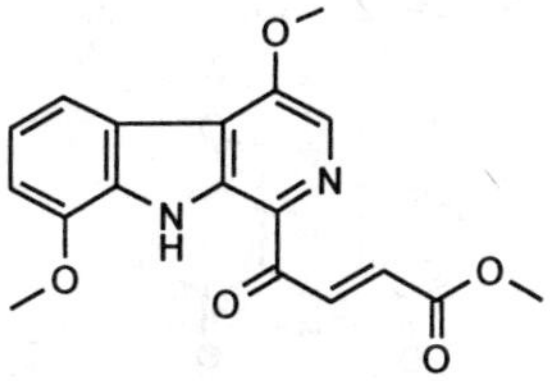

5170 Picrasidine F

$C_{28}H_{26}N_5O_3$•Cl MW: 480.55•35.45 Source: KU SHU PI. Ref: 12.

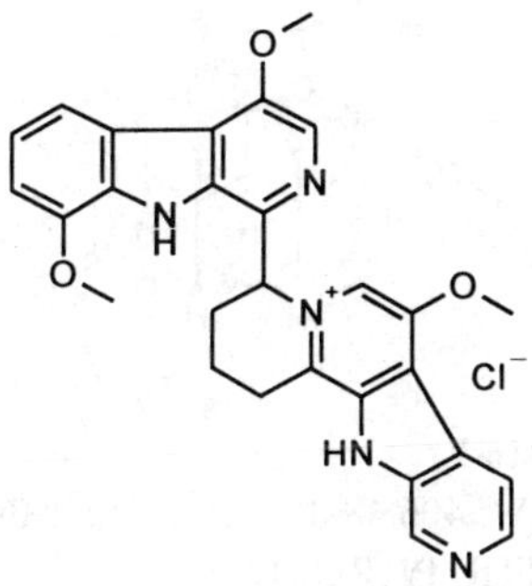

5171 Picrasidine H

$C_{28}H_{24}N_4O_4$ MW: 480.55 Source: KU SHU PI. Ref: 12.

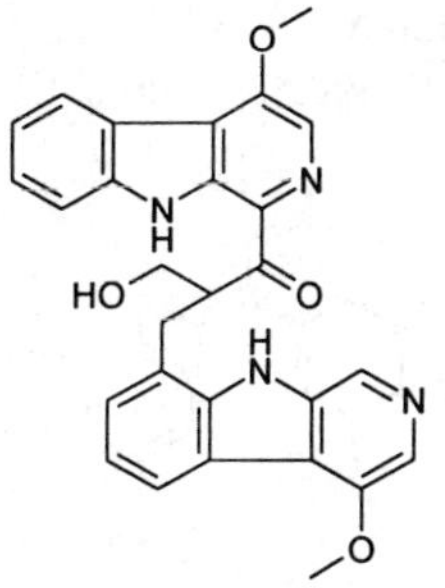

5172 Picrasidine I

$C_{14}H_{12}N_2O_2$ MW: 240.26 Source: KU SHU PI. Ref: 12.

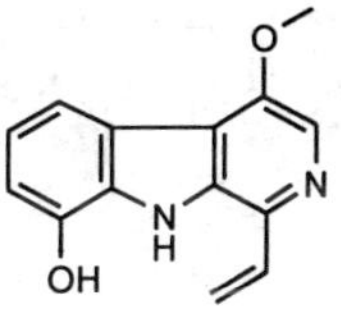

5173 Picrasidine J

$C_{14}H_{14}N_2O_2$ MW: 242.28 Source: KU SHU PI. Ref: 12.

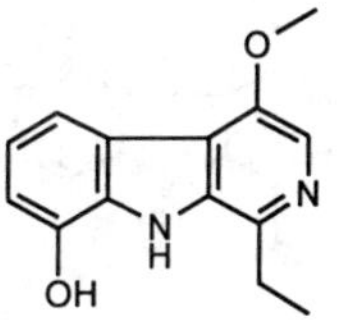

5174 Picrasidine K

$C_{18}H_{23}N_3O_2$ MW: 313.40 Source: KU SHU PI. Ref: 12.

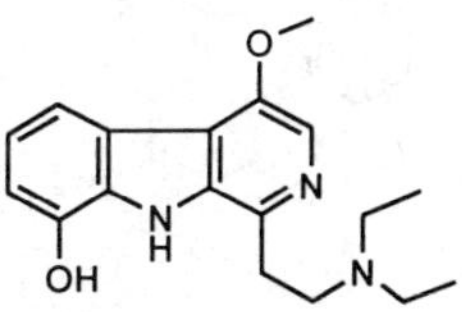

5175 Picrasidine M

$C_{31}H_{22}N_4O_4$ MW: 514.55 Source: KU SHU PI. Ref: 12.

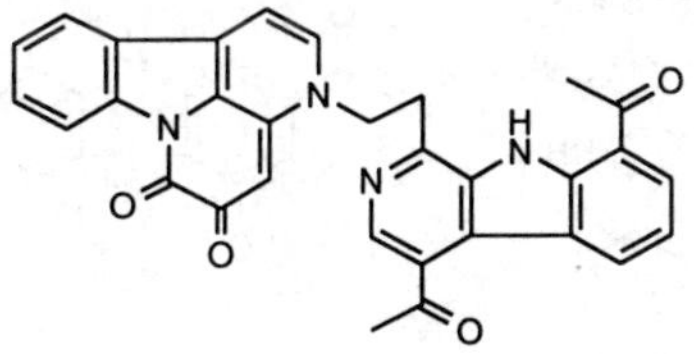

5176 Picrasidine N
$C_{29}H_{22}N_4O_4$ MW: 490.52 Source: KU SHU PI. Ref: 12.

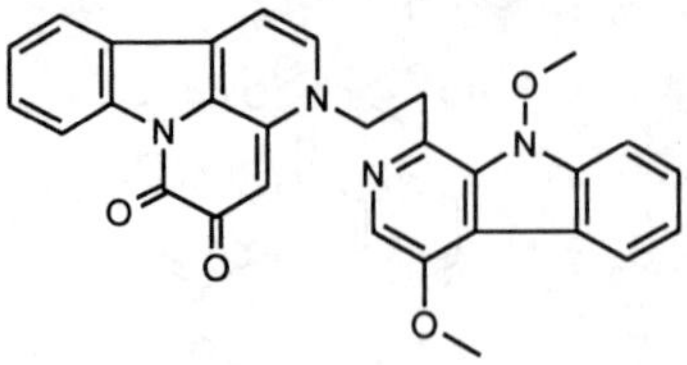

5177 Picrasidine O
$C_{16}H_{12}N_2O_3$ MW: 280.29 Source: KU SHU PI. Ref: 12.

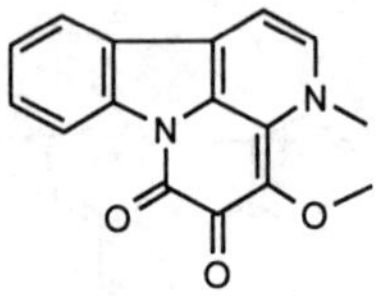

5178 Picrasidine P
$C_{15}H_{12}N_2O_2$ MW: 252.28 Source: KU SHU PI. Ref: 12.

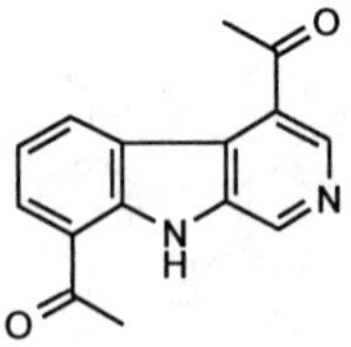

5179 Picrasidine Q
$C_{15}H_{10}N_2O_3$ MW: 266.26 Source: KU SHU PI. Ref: 12.

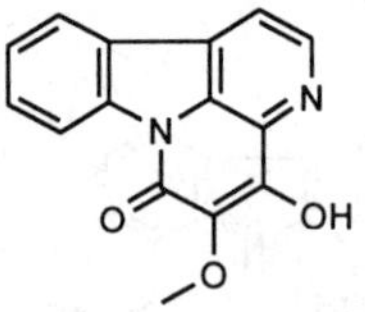

5180 Picrasidine R
$C_{30}H_{28}N_4O_6$ MW: 540.58 Source: KU SHU PI. Ref: 12.

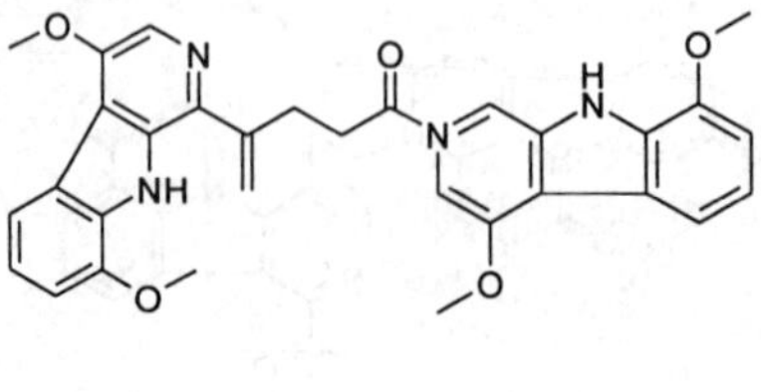

5181 Picrasidine T
$C_{27}H_{24}N_5O_4 \cdot Cl$ MW: 482.54 • 35.45 Source: KU SHU PI. Ref: 12.

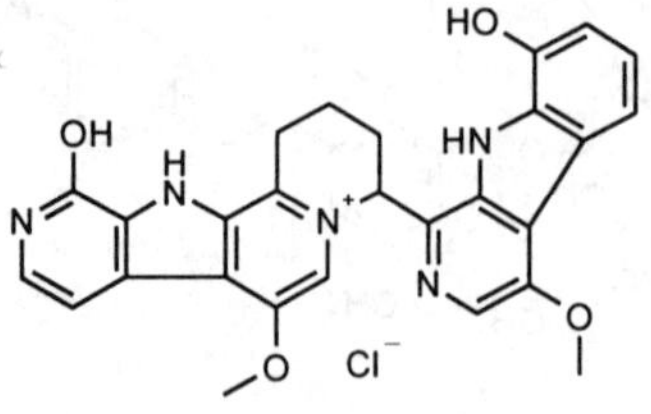

5182 Picrasidine U
$C_{30}H_{24}N_4O_5$ MW: 520.55 Source: KU SHU PI. Ref: 12.

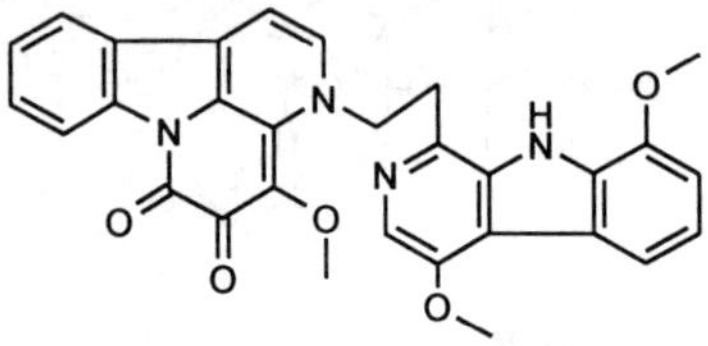

5183 Picrasidine V
$C_{14}H_8N_2O_4$ MW: 244.21 Source: KU SHU PI. Ref: 12.

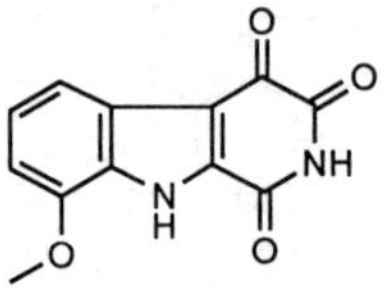

5184 Picrasin D
$C_{22}H_{30}O_6$ MW: 390.48 Property: mp 283.5-5°C. Source: KU SHU PI. Ref: 12.

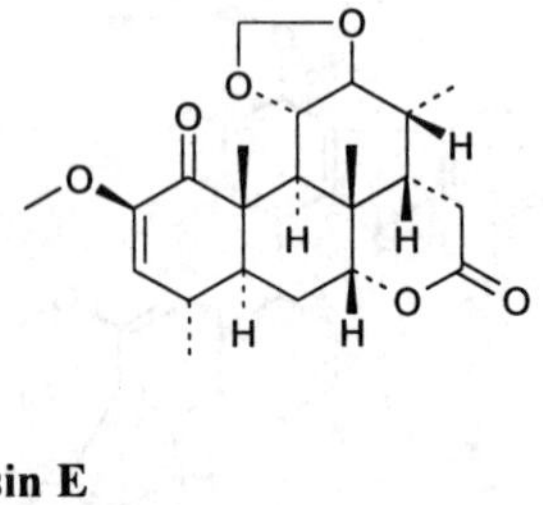

5185 Picrasin E
$C_{22}H_{30}O_7$ MW: 406.48 Property: mp 293-5°C. Source: KU SHU PI. Ref: 12.

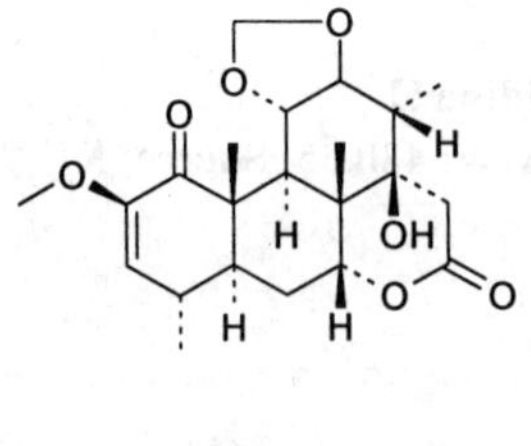

5186 Picrasin F
$C_{22}H_{30}O_8$ MW: 422.48 Property: mp 282-3°C.
Source: KU SHU PI. Ref: 12.

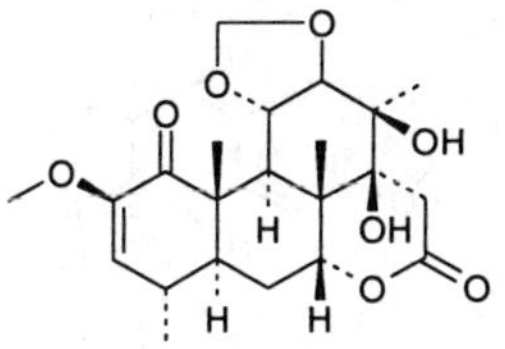

5187 Picrasin G
$C_{21}H_{28}O_7$ MW: 392.45 Source: KU SHU PI. Ref: 12.

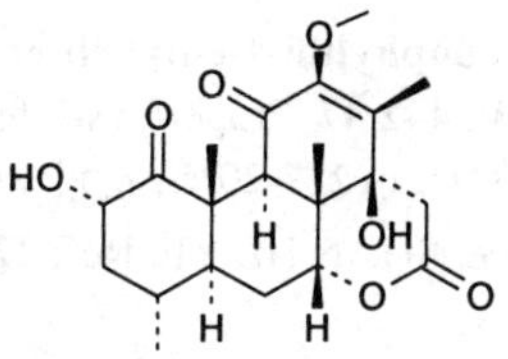

5188 Picrasinol A
$C_{24}H_{36}O_7$ MW: 436.55 Source: KU SHU PI. Ref: 12.

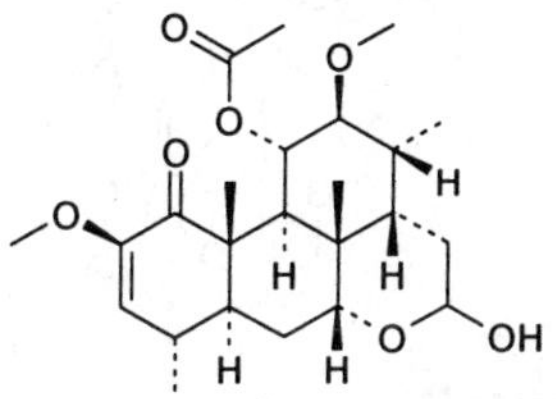

5189 Picrasinol B
$C_{22}H_{32}O_6$ MW: 392.50 Source: KU SHU PI. Ref: 12.

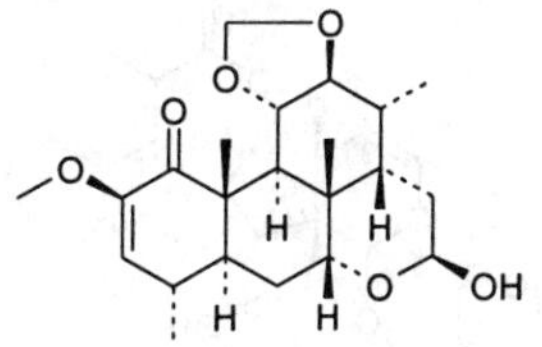

5190 Picrasinoside A
$C_{27}H_{38}O_{11}$ MW: 538.60 Source: KU SHU PI.
Ref: 12.

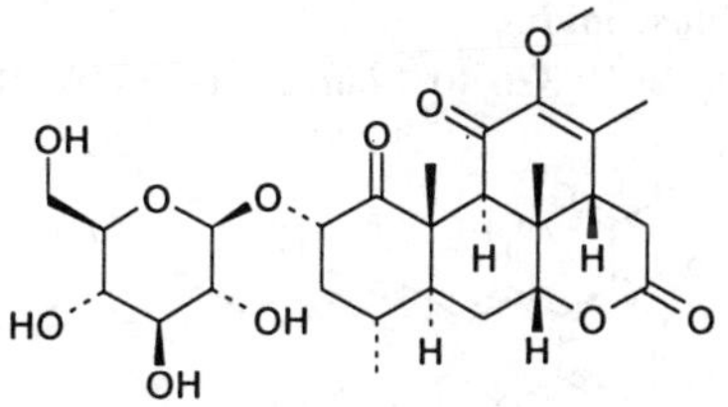

5191 Picrasinoside B
$C_{28}H_{40}O_{11}$ MW: 552.62 Source: KU SHU PI.
Ref: 12.

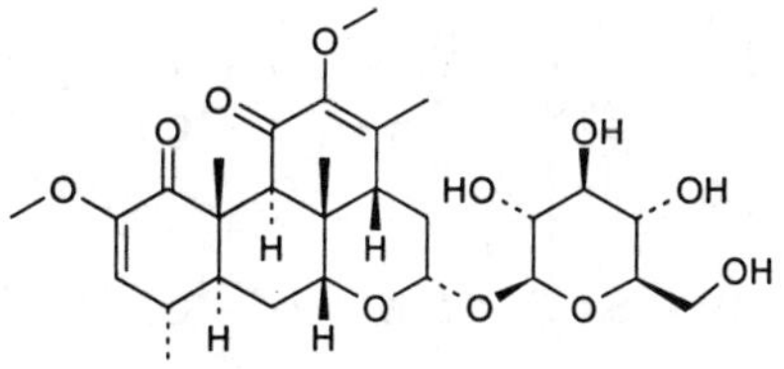

5192 Picrasinoside C
$C_{28}H_{42}O_{11}$ MW: 554.64 Source: KU SHU PI.
Ref: 12.

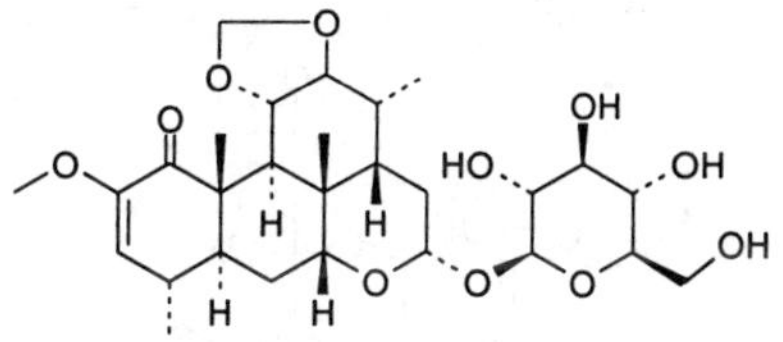

5193 Picrasinoside D
$C_{28}H_{44}O_{11}$ MW: 556.66 Source: KU SHU PI.
Ref: 12.

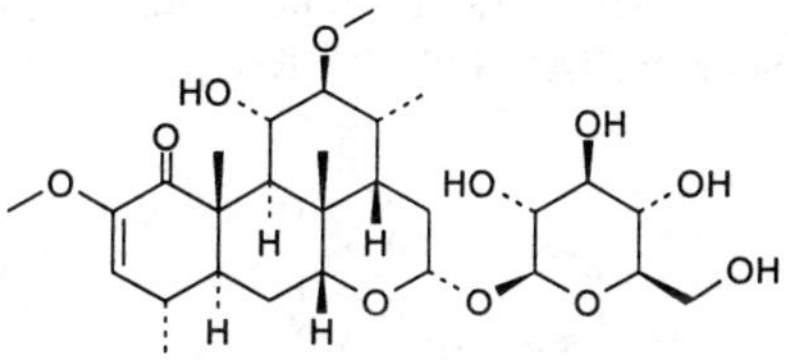

5194 Picrasinoside E
$C_{30}H_{46}O_{13}$ MW: 614.69 Source: KU SHU PI.
Ref: 12.

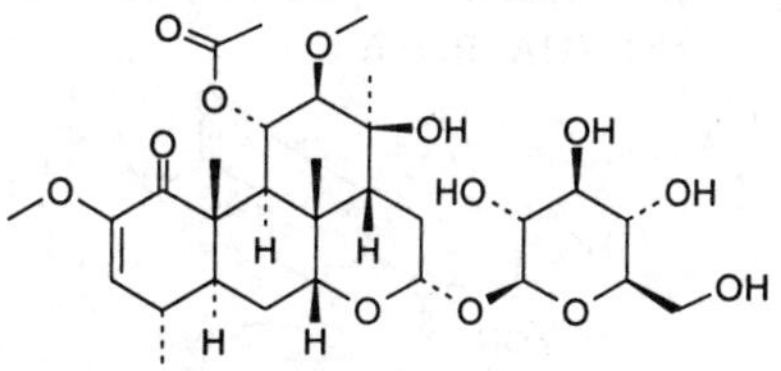

5195 Picrasinoside G
$C_{28}H_{44}O_{12}$ MW: 572.66 Source: KU SHU PI.
Ref: 12.

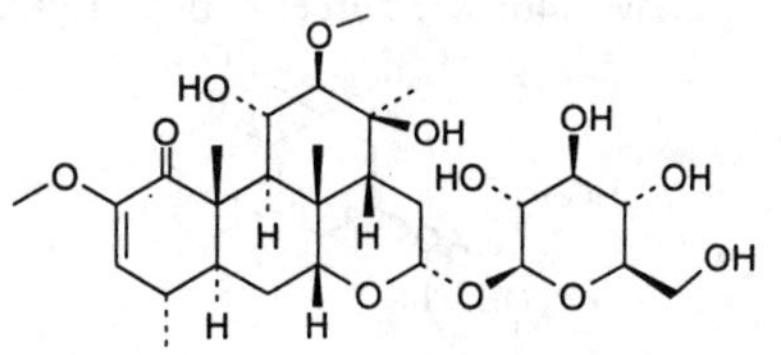

5196 Picrasinoside H
$C_{30}H_{44}O_{13}$ MW: 612.68 Source: KU SHU PI. Ref: 12.

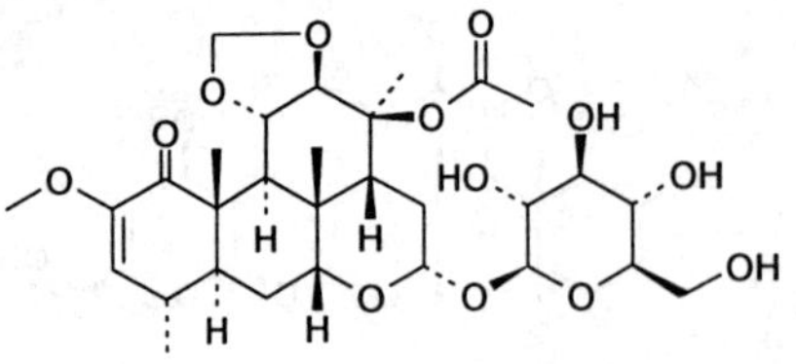

5197 Picrasmin
$C_{22}H_{28}O_6$ MW: 388.46 Property: mp 291°C. Source: KU SHU PI. Ref: 6.

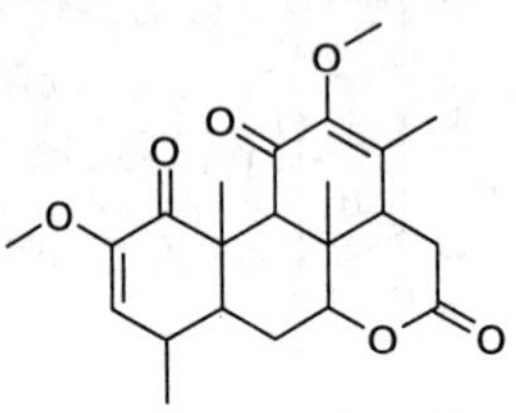

5198 Picrinine
$C_{20}H_{22}N_2O_3$ MW: 338.41 Property: mp 223-5°C (dec). Source: XIANG PI MU. Ref: 6.

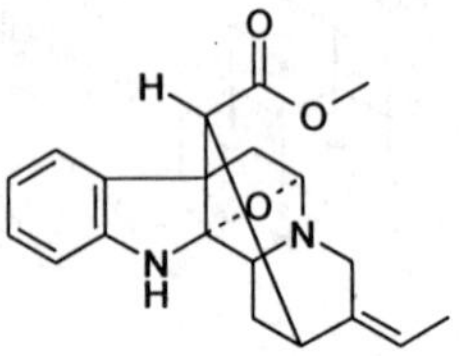

5199 Picrocrocin
$C_{16}H_{26}O_7$ MW: 330.38 Property: mp 156°C. Source: ZANG HONG HUA. Ref: 6.

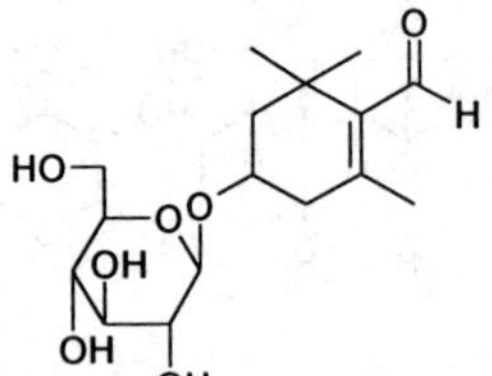

5200 Picrocrocinic acid
$C_{16}H_{26}O_8$ MW: 346.38 Source: ZHI ZI. Ref: 2, 626.

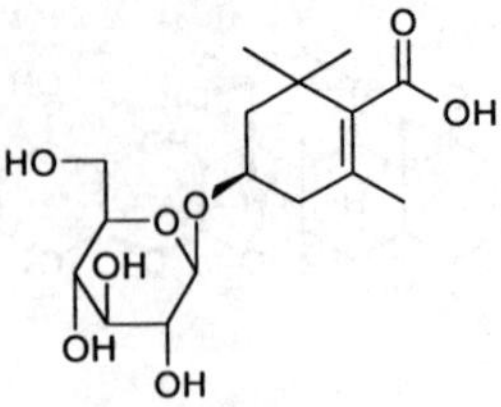

5201 Picropodophyllin
$C_{22}H_{22}O_8$ MW: 414.42 Property: mp 228°C. Source: SHAN HE YE, WO ER QI. Ref: 6, 279.

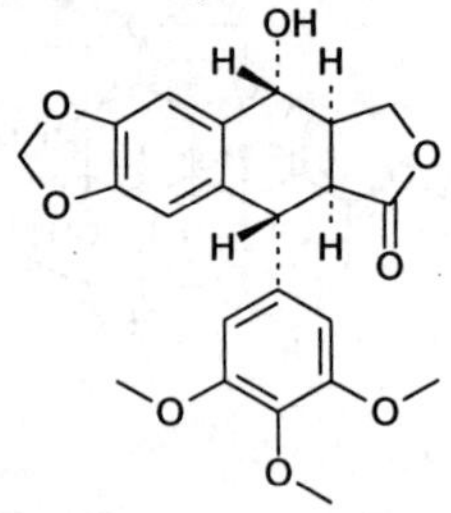

5202 Picropodophyllin-1-ethyl ether
$C_{24}H_{26}O_8$ MW: 442.47 Property: white thin acicular crystal (Me_2CO), mp 217-20°C, $[\alpha]_D^{17}$ +69° (c=0.01, $CHCl_3$). Source: SHAN HE YE. Ref: 279.

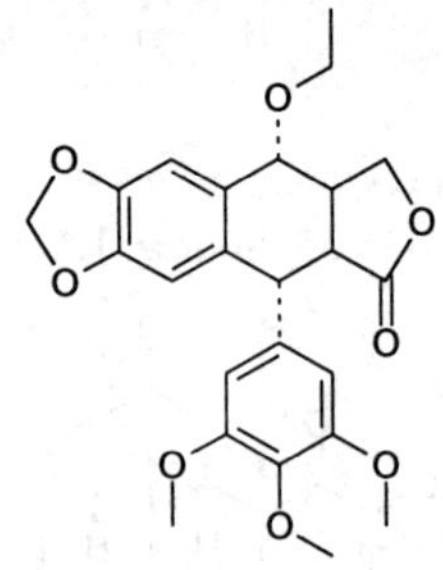

5203 Picroside II
$C_{23}H_{28}O_{13}$ MW: 512.47 Source: HU HUANG LIAN. Ref: 6.

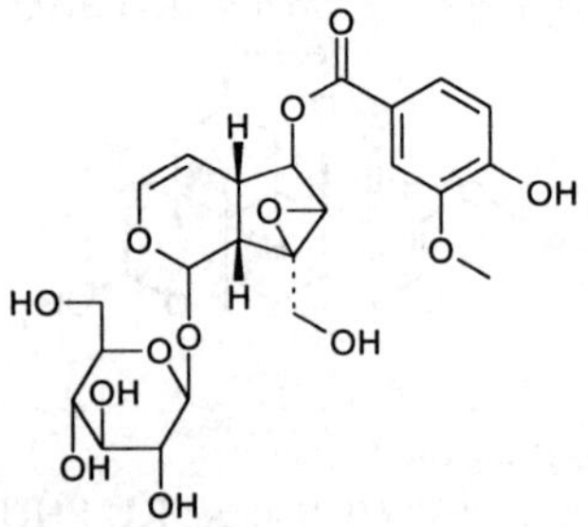

5204 Piloselloidal
$C_{20}H_{22}O_4$ MW: 326.40 Source: MAO DA DING CAO. Ref: 6.

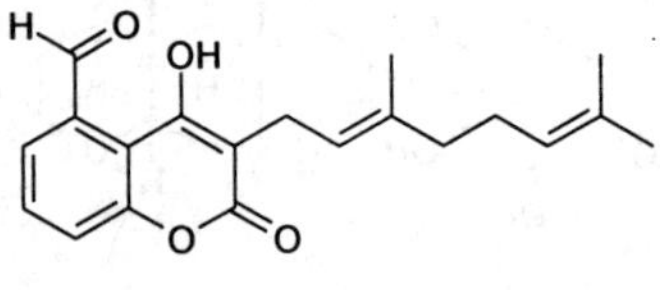

5205 Piloselloidone
$C_{18}H_{24}O_3$ MW: 288.39 Source: MAO DA DING CAO. Ref: 6.

5206 l-Pimara-8-(14),15-dien-19-oic acid
$C_{20}H_{30}O_2$ MW: 302.46 Property: mp (-): 163-4°C. Source: TU DANG GUI (I). Ref: 6.

5207 l-Pimara-8-(14),15-dien-19-ol
$C_{20}H_{32}O$ MW: 288.48 Property: mp (-): 109-10°C. Source: TU DANG GUI (I). Ref: 6.

5208 Pimpinellin
$C_{13}H_{10}O_5$ MW: 246.22 Property: mp 119°C. Source: FEI LONG ZHANG XUE, LI JIANG QIAN HU, YONG NING DU HUO. Ref: 6, 541, 557.

5209 Pinene
$C_{10}H_{16}$ MW: 136.24 Source: BO HE, DANG SHEN, DONG LING CAO, DU HUO, FANG FENG, HOU PO, HUO XIANG, JIN JIE, JIN YIN HUA, JU PI, LIAN QIAO, QIANG HUO, QING HAO, SHENG JIANG, WU WEI ZI, XI XIN, YIN CHEN HAO, YU XING CAO, ZI SU. Ref: 2.

5210 α-Pinene
$C_{10}H_{16}$ MW: 136.24 Property: bp (+): 155-6°C/755 mm, (-): 155-6°C/746mm, (±): 156.2°C/741mm. Source: JIU LI XIANG. Ref: 11.

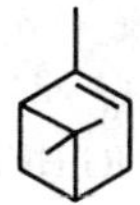

5211 β-Pinene
$C_{10}H_{16}$ MW: 136.24 Property: bp (+): 162-6°C, (-): 163.5-164°C/746mm. Source: JIU LI XIANG, many. Ref: 2, 11.

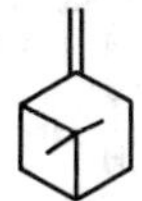

5212 (Z)-(IS,5R)-β-Pinen-10-yl-β-vicianoside
$C_{21}H_{34}O_{10}$ MW: 446.50 Source: CHI SHAO YAO. Ref: 2.

5213 Pingbeidinoside
$C_{34}H_{57}NO_9$ MW: 623.83 Property: colorless acicular crystal, mp 242-3.2°C, $[\alpha]_D^{25}$ +6.9°(c=0.145 MeOH). Source: PING BEI MU. Ref: 138.

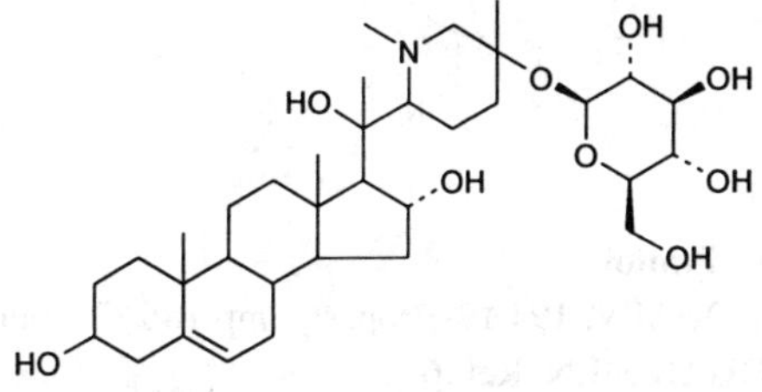

5214 Pingbeimin C
C-nor-D-homosteroid alkaloid. $C_{27}H_{48}NO_6$ MW: 477.65 Property: colorless prismatic crystal, mp 171.53°C, $[\alpha]_D^{25}$ -24.6° (c=1.1, methanol). Source: DONG BEI PING BEI MU. Ref: 150.

5215 Pingpeimine B
5α,17β,22α-cevanine-3β,6α,12α,14α,16β,20β-hexol. $C_{27}H_{45}NO_6$ MW: 479.66 Property: colorless acicular crystal, mp 242-4°C, $[\alpha]_D$ +24.9° (c=0.08, methanol). Source: DONG BEI PING BEI MU. Ref: 117.

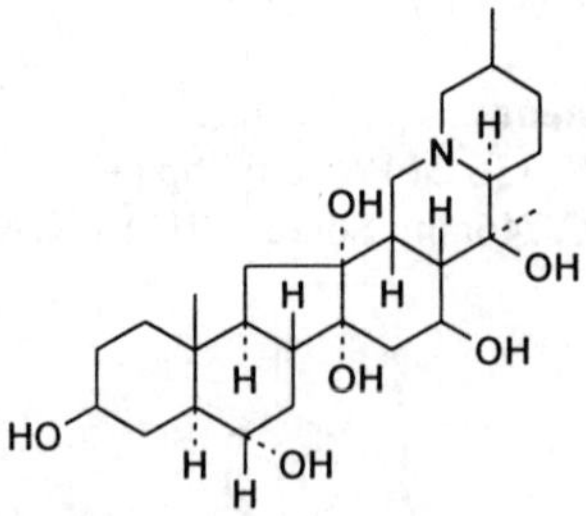

5216 Pinicolic acid
$C_{30}H_{46}O_3$ MW: 454.70 Source: FU LING. Ref: 2.

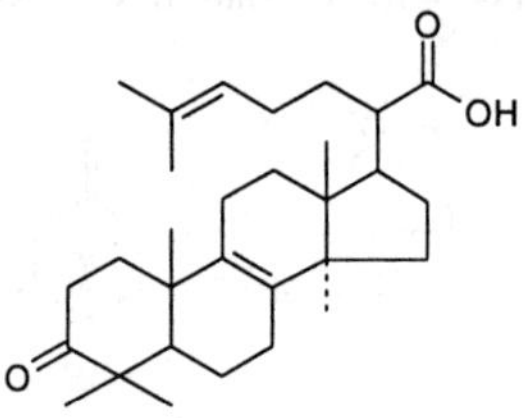

5217 Pinidine
$C_9H_{17}O$ MW: 139.24 Property: bp 176-7°C/751mm. Source: HAI SONG ZI. Ref: 6.

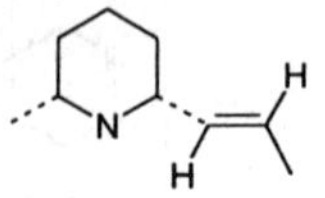

5218 Pinitol
$C_7H_{14}O_6$ MW: 194.19 Property: mp 186°C. Source: YE GUAN MEN. Ref: 6.

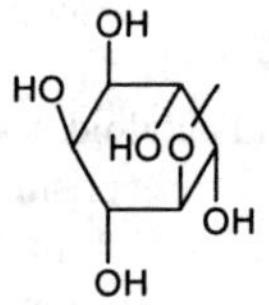

5219 Pinnatin
$C_{18}H_{12}O_4$ MW: 292.29 Property: mp 176-7°C. Source: SHUI LIU DOU. Ref: 6.

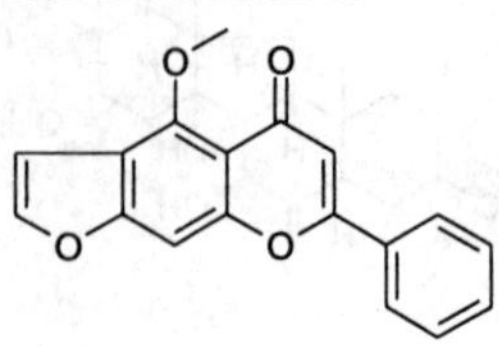

5220 l-Pinocamphone
$C_{10}H_{16}O$ MW: 152.24 Property: mp (-): 212°C. Source: JIN QIAN CAO. Ref: 6.

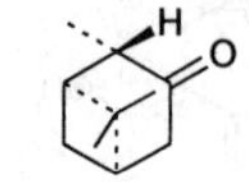

5221 trans-Pinocarveol
$C_{10}H_{16}O$ MW: 152.24 Property: mp (+):7°C, (-): 5°C, (±): 14°C. Source: HU JIAO. Ref: 6.

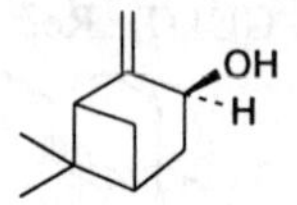

5222 (+)-Pinoresinol di-O-β-D-glucopyranoside
Source: DU ZHONG. Ref: 2.

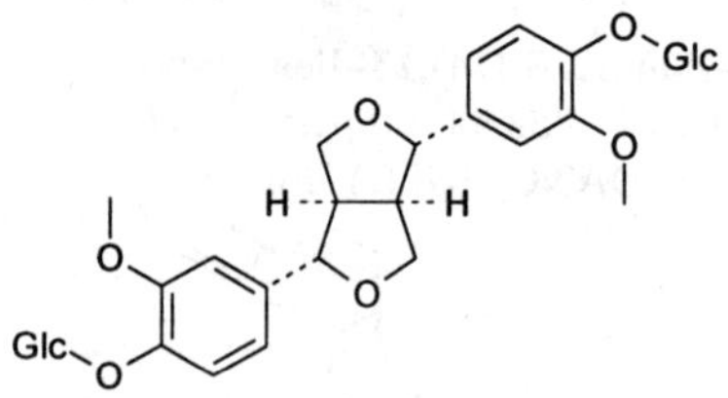

5223 (+)-Pinoresinol-di-O-β-D-glucoside
Source: CI WU JIA. Ref: 2.

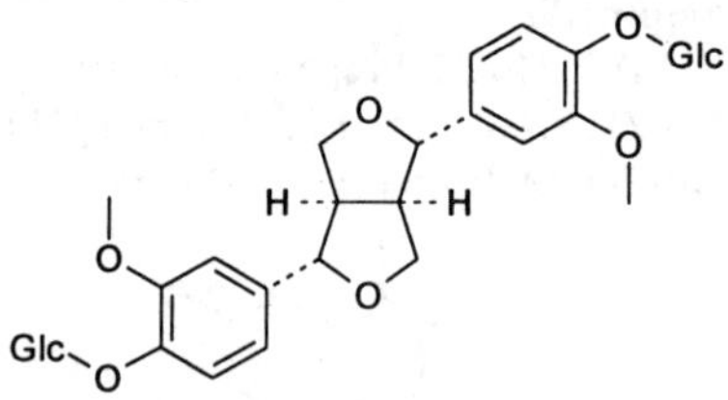

5224 Pinoresinol dimethyl ether
Source: WANG CHUN MU LAN. Ref: 543.

5225 (+)-Pinoresinol-O-β-D-glucopyranoside
Source: DU ZHONG. Ref: 2.

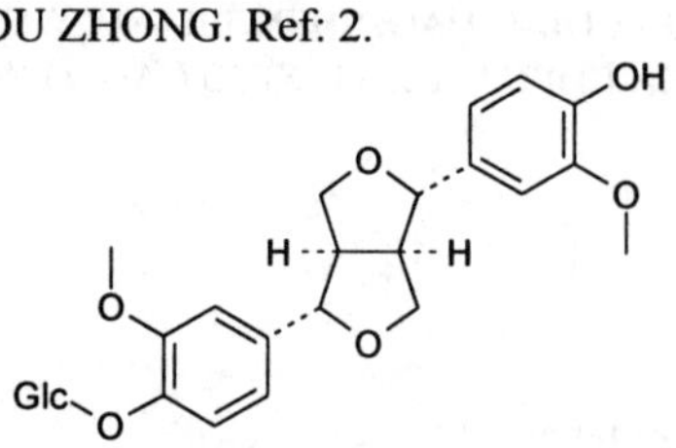

5226 Pipecolic acid
$C_6H_{11}NO_2$ MW: 129.16 Property: mp (+):270°C, (-): 270°C, (±): 264°C. Source: BIAN DOU, CAN DOU, HAI JIU CAI, SHENG JIANG, SUAN JIAO, WANG GUA ZI. Ref: 6.

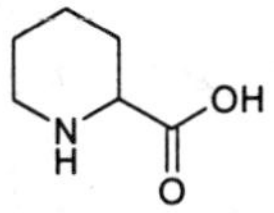

5227 d-α-Pipecoline
$C_6H_{13}N$ MW: 99.18 Property: bp (+): 117-7.5°C. Source: HAI SONG ZI. Ref: 6.

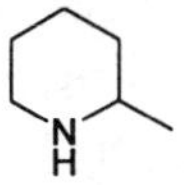

5228 Piperanine
$C_{17}H_{21N}O_3$ MW: 287.36 Source: HU JIAO. Ref: 6.

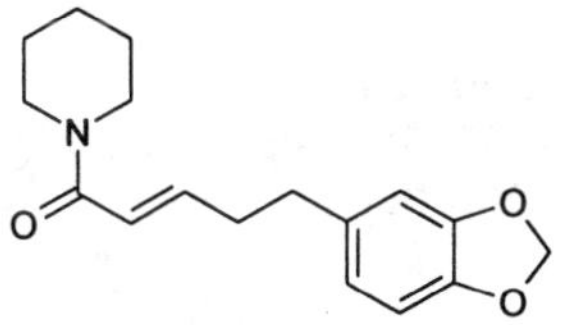

5229 Piperidine
$C_5H_{11}N$ MW: 85.15 Property: mp -9°C, bp 106°C. Source: BI BA, MA HUA. Ref: 6.

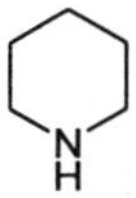

5230 Piperine
$C_{17}H_{19}NO_3$ MW: 285.35 Property: mp 129.5°C. Source: BI BA, BI BA GEN, HU JIAO. Ref: 6.

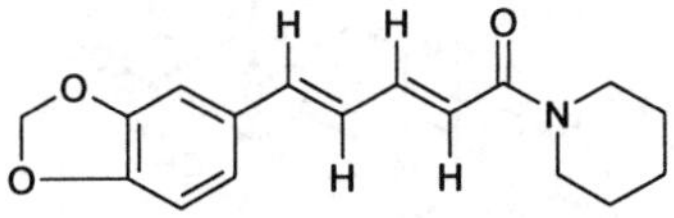

5231 Piperitenone
$C_{10}H_{14}O$ MW: 150.22 Source: JIN JIE. Ref: 2.

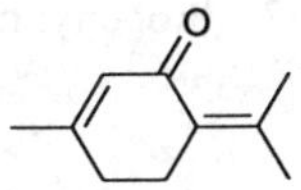

5232 Piperitone
3-Carvomenthenone. CAS: 89-81-6 $C_{10}H_{16}O$ MW: 152.24 Property: bp (+): 116-8.5°C/20mm, (-): 109.5-10.5°C/15mm, (±): 232-3°C/769mm. Source: JIN JIE, HU JIAO. Ref: 2, 4, 6.

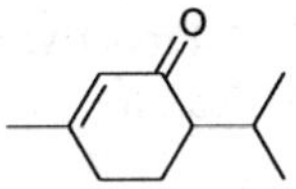

5233 Piperitylmagnolol
$C_{28}H_{34}O_2$ MW: 402.58 Source: HOU PO. Ref: 2.

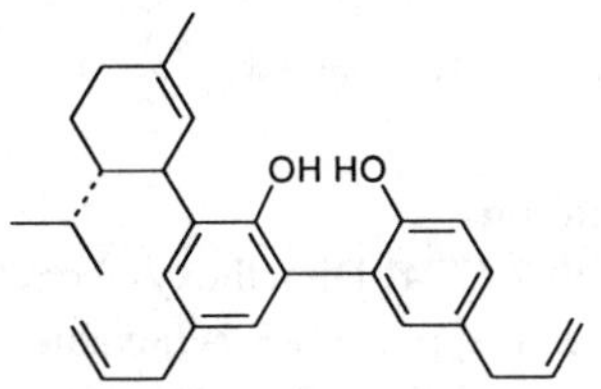

5234 Piperitylhonokiol
$C_{28}H_{34}O_2$ MW: 402.58 Source: HOU PO. Ref: 2.

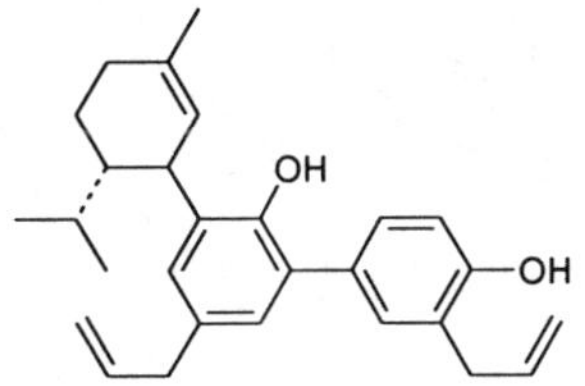

5235 Piperlonguminine
$C_{16}H_{19}NO_3$ MW: 273.33 Property: mp 166-8°C. Source: BI BA GEN. Ref: 6.

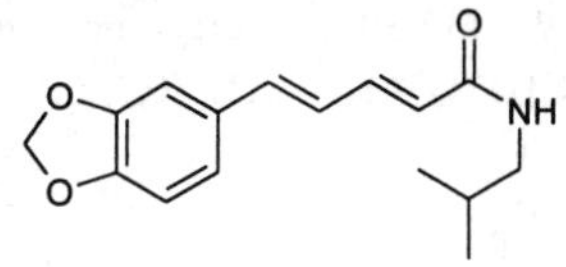

5236 Piperonal
$C_8H_6O_3$ MW: 150.11 Property: mp 37°C. Source: HU JIAO, PENG ZI CAI, SHOU ZHANG SHEN. Ref: 6.

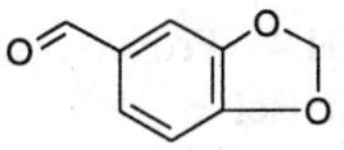

5237 Piplartine
$C_{17}H_{19}NO_5$ MW: 317.34 Property: mp 124°C. Source: BI BA GEN. Ref: 6.

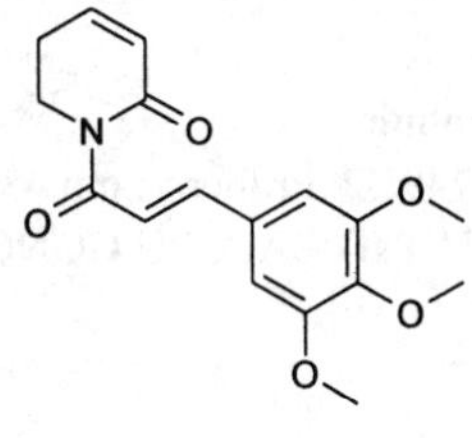

5238 Piptanthine
$C_{20}H_{35}N_3$ MW: 317.52 Property: mp 142-3°C.
Source: HONG DOU. Ref: 6.

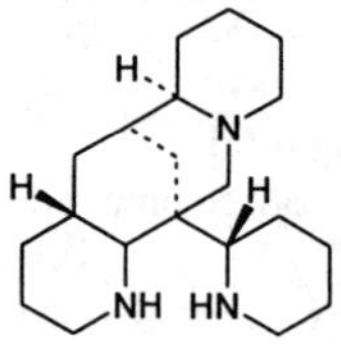

5239 L-Planinin
(1R,2R,5R,6S)-2-(3',4'-Dimethoxy-phenyl)-6-(3'', 4''-methylene dioxyphenyl)-3,7-dioxabicyclo(3,3,0) octane. $C_{21}H_{22}O_6$ MW: 370.41 Property: colorless columnar crystal, mp 133-3.5°C. Source: ZHU YE JIAO. Ref: 106.

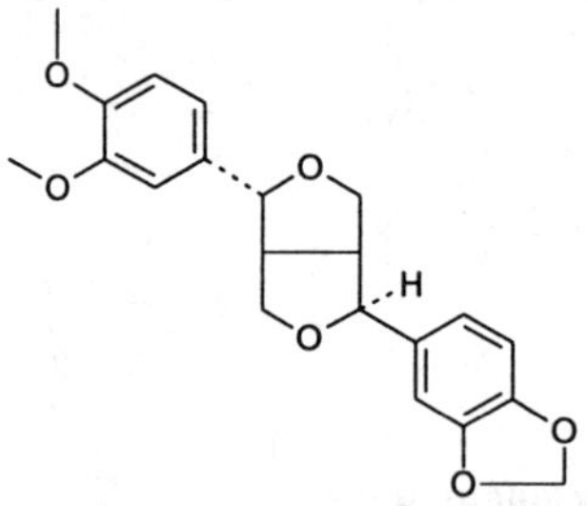

5240 Plantaginin
$C_{21}H_{20}O_{10}$ MW: 432.39 Property: mp 214°C. Source: CHE QIAN (CHE QIAN CAO). Ref: 6.

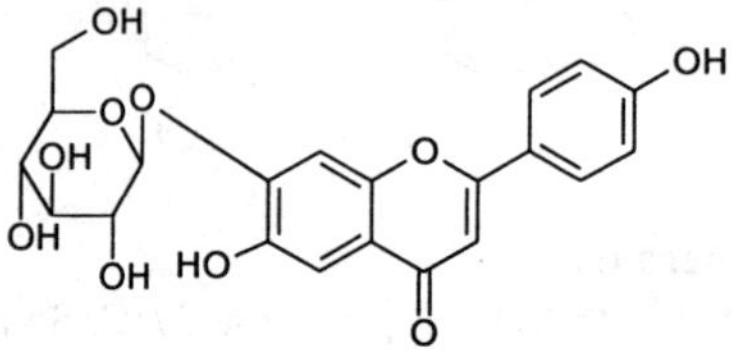

5241 Planteose
$C_{18}H_{32}O_{16}$ MW: 504.45 Property: mp 123-4°C.
Source: LUO LE ZI. Ref: 6.

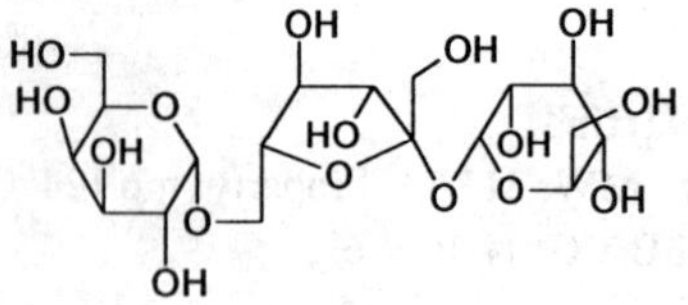

5242 Plastoquinone
$C_{53}H_{80}O_2$ MW: 749.32 Property: mp 48-9°C. Source: CAN DOU YE, HONG CAO, PU GONG YING.
Ref: 6.

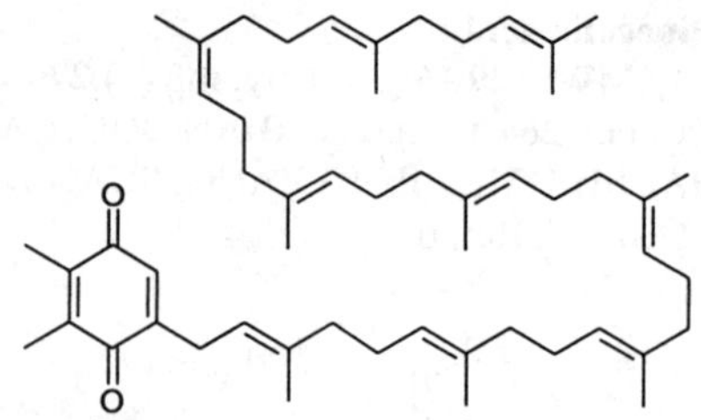

5243 Platycodigenin
$C_{30}H_{48}O_7$ MW: 520.71 Property: mp 241-2°C.
Source: JIE GENG. Ref: 6.

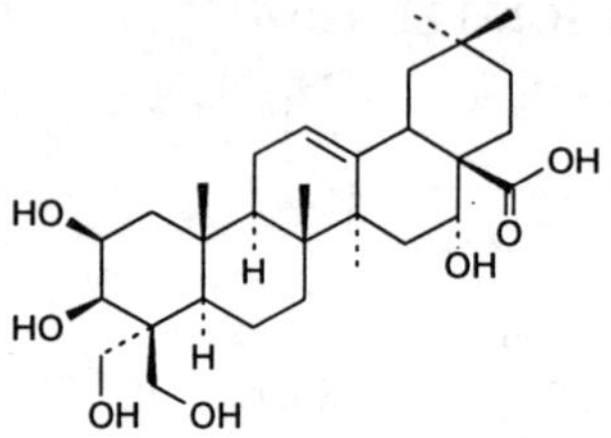

5244 Platycogenic acid A
$C_{30}H_{46}O_8$ MW: 534.70 Property: mp 243-9°C.
Source: JIE GENG. Ref: 6.

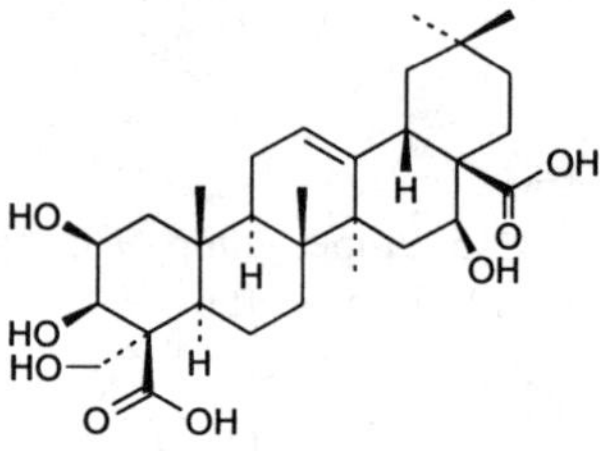

5245 Platycogenic acid B
$C_{30}H_{46}O_8$ MW: 534.70 Property: mp 274-7°C (dec).
Source: JIE GENG. Ref: 6.

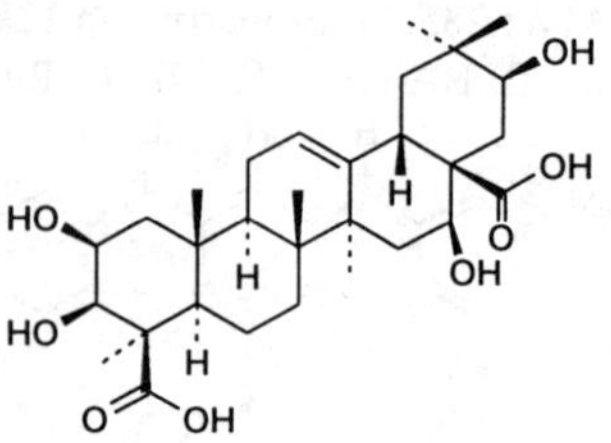

5246 Platycogenic acid C
$C_{30}H_{48}O_6$ MW: 504.71 Property: mp 282-8°C (dec).
Source: JIE GENG. Ref: 6.

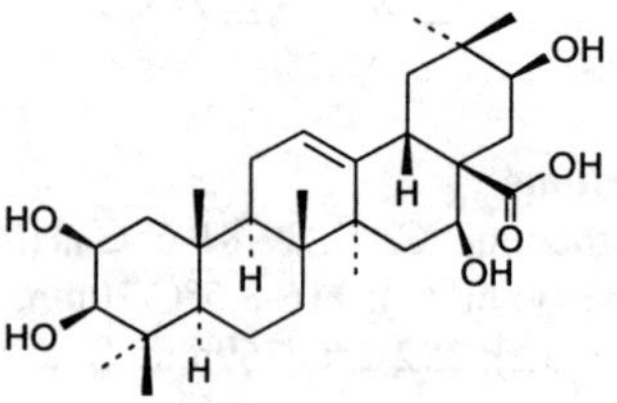

5247 Platyphylline
$C_{18}H_{27}NO_5$ MW: 337.42 Property: mp 124-5°C. Source: DA BAI DING CAO, GOU SHE CAO, YAO YONG DAO TI HU. Ref: 6.

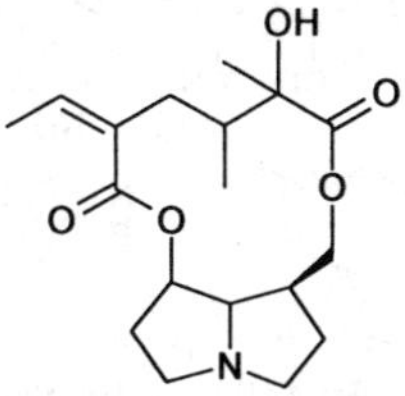

5248 Pleicarpamine
$C_{20}H_{24}N_2O_2$ MW: 324.43 Source: CHANG CHUN HUA. Ref: 2.

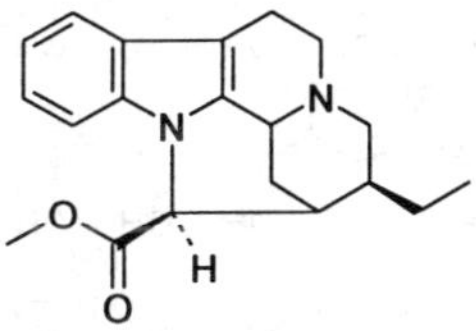

5249 Pleniradin
CAS: 25941-24-6 $C_{15}H_{20}O_4$ MW: 264.32 Source: BAI LAI SHI JU. Ref: 5.

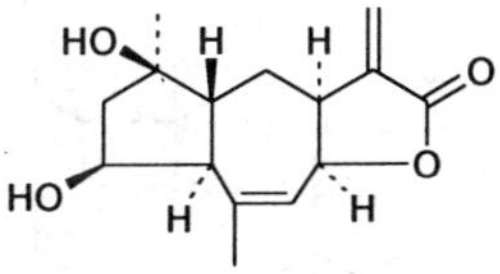

5250 Plumbagin
CAS: 481-42-5 $C_{11}H_8O_3$ MW: 188.18 Property: mp 78-9°C. Source: BAI HUA DAN, JI WA CAO, MAO GAO CAI, ZI JIN LIAN, ZI XUE HUA. Ref: 4, 621.

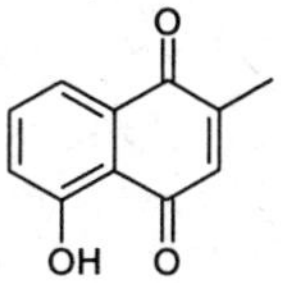

5251 Pluviine
$C_{17}H_{21}NO_3$ MW: 287.36 Property: mp 225-7°C. Source: SHI SUAN. Ref: 6.

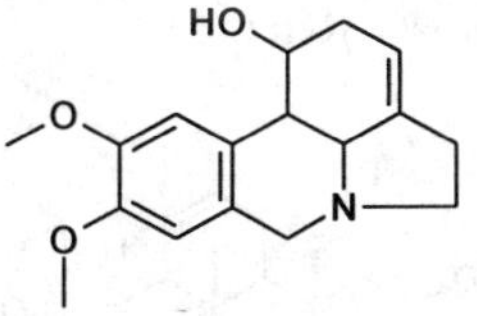

5252 Podocarpamide
$C_{20}H_{21}NO_4$ MW: 339.39 Property: acicular clustered crystal, mp 85-6°C. Source: BING GUO HUA JIAO. Ref: 119.

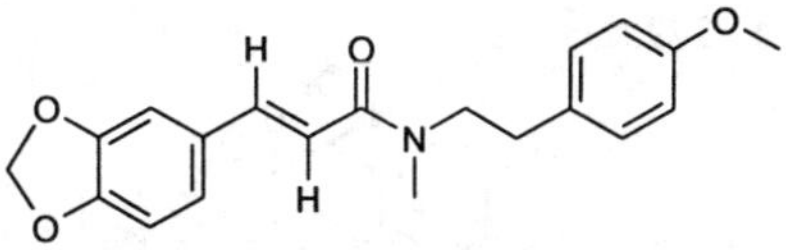

5254 Podocarpusflavone A
$C_{31}H_{20}O_{10}$ MW: 552.50 Source: DU SONG SHI, JI MAO SONG, LUO HAN SONG YE. Ref: 6, 544.

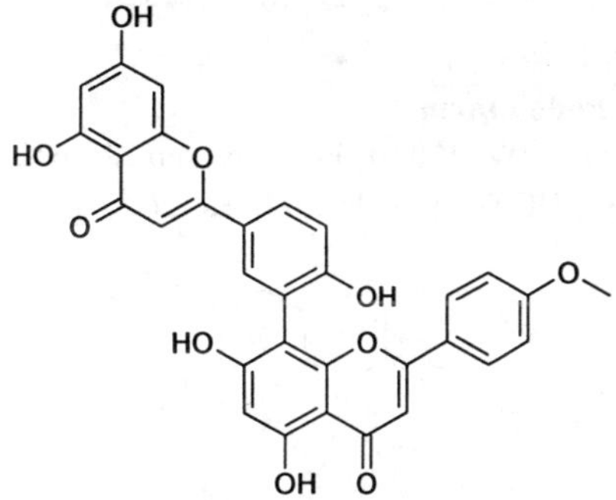

5255 Podocarpusflavone B
$C_{32}H_{22}O_{10}$ MW: 566.53 Source: LUO HAN SONG YE. Ref: 6.

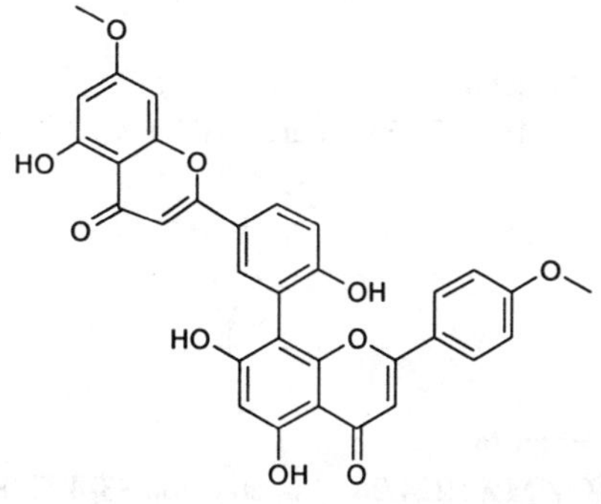

5256 Podolide
CAS: 55786-36-2 $C_{15}H_{22}O_5$ MW: 330.38 Property: mp 296-8°C. Source: XI LUO HAN SONG. Ref: 5.

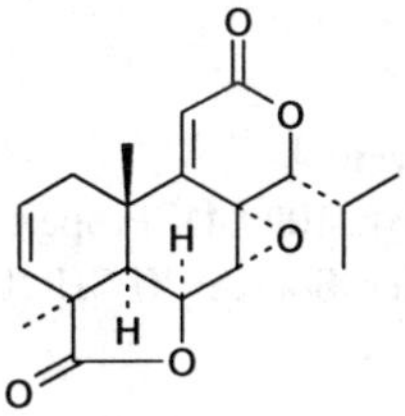

5257 Podophyllotoxin
CAS: 477-47-4 $C_{22}H_{22}O_8$ MW: 414.42 Property: mp 114-8°C. Source: BA JIAO LIAN, CHOU BAI, GUI JIU, SHAN HE YE, TAO ER QI, WO ER QI. Ref: 4, 6, 279.

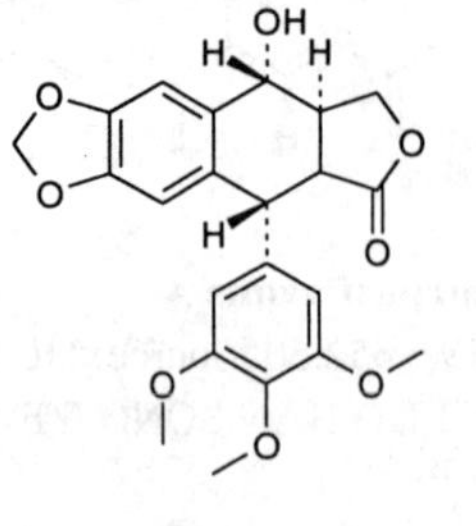

5258 Podototarin
$C_{40}H_{58}O_2$ MW: 570.91 Property: mp 225-6°C. Source: LUO HAN SONG YE. Ref: 6.

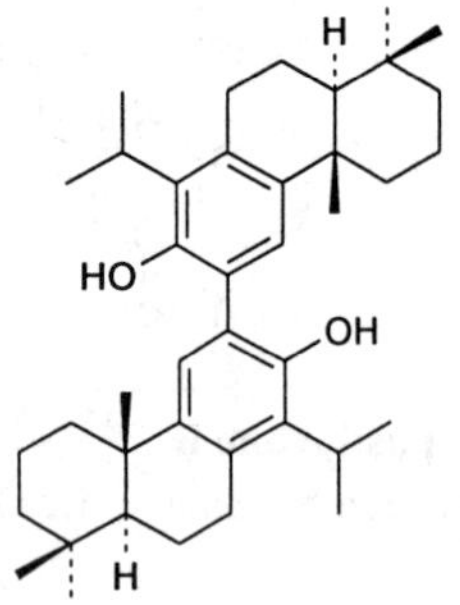

5259 Pogostol
$C_{15}H_{26}O$ MW: 222.37 Source: HUO XIANG. Ref: 2.

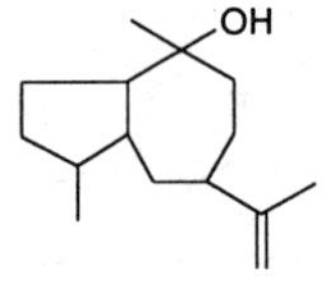

5260 Pogostone
$C_{12}H_{16}O_4$ MW: 224.26 Property: mp 33-4°C. Source: HUO XIANG. Ref: 2, 505.

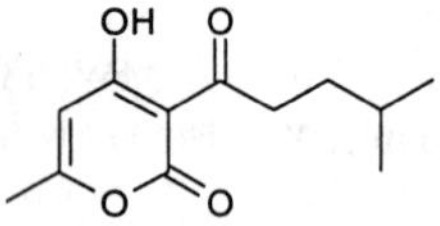

5261 Polaramycin A
$C_{55}H_{99}N_3O_{18}$ MW: 1090.41 Property: white crystalline powder. Source: XI SHUI LIAN MEI JUN. Ref: 380.

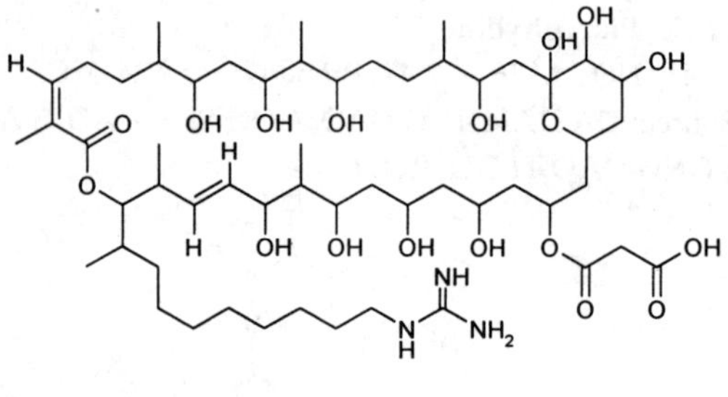

5262 Polaramycin B
$C_{56}H_{101}N_3O_{18}$ MW: 1104.44 Property: white crystalline powder. Source: XI SHUI LIAN MEI JUN. Ref: 380.

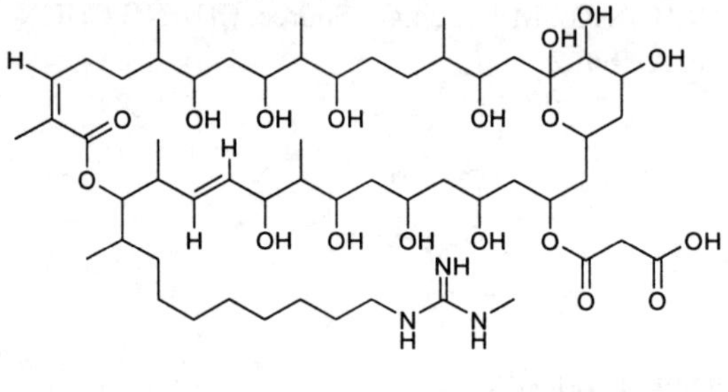

5263 Pollinastanol
$C_{28}H_{48}O$ MW: 400.69 Property: mp 95°C. Source: SHUI LONG GU. Ref: 6.

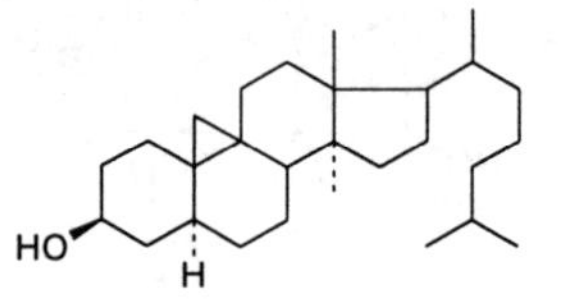

5264 Polydatin
$C_{20}H_{22}O_8$ MW: 390.39 Property: mp 225-6°C. Source: HU ZHANG. Ref: 2.

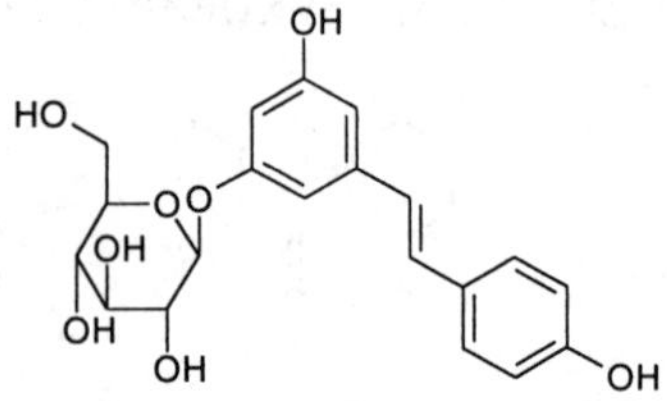

5265 Polygalacic acid
$C_{30}H_{48}O_6$ MW: 504.71 Property: mp 300-5°C. Source: JIE GENG. Ref: 6.

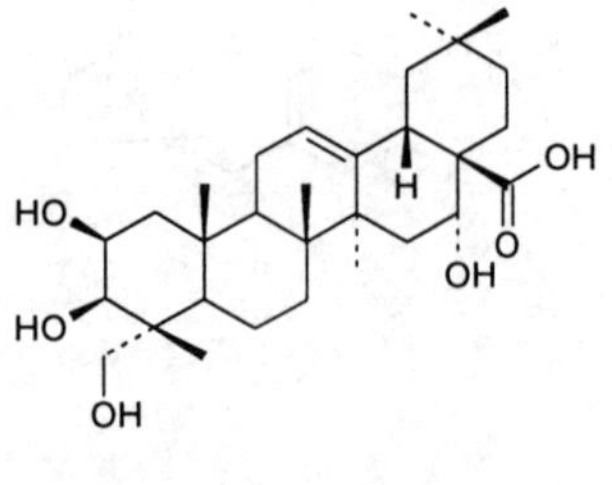

5266 Polygalytol
$C_6H_{12}O_5$ MW: 164.16 Property: mp 142-3°C. Source: HUAN HUA YUAN ZHI, YUAN ZHI. Ref: 2.

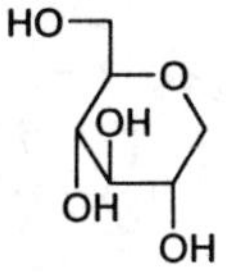

5267 Polygoacetophenoside
$C_{14}H_{18}O_{10}$ MW: 346.29 Source: HE SHOU WU. Ref: 2.

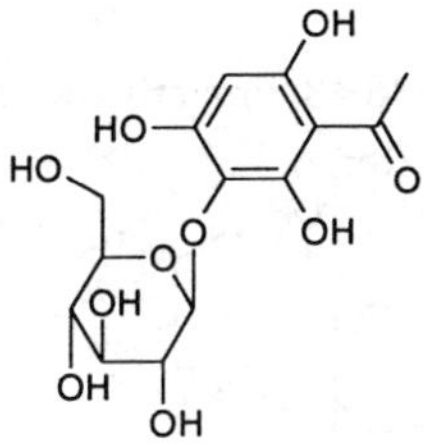

5268 Polygodial
$C_{15}H_{22}O_2$ MW: 234.34 Property: mp 57°C. Source: SHUI LIAO. Ref: 6.

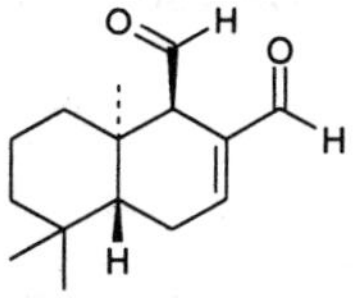

5269 Polyporenic acid C
$C_{31}H_{46}O_4$ MW: 482 Property: white columnar crystal, mp 258-60°C. Source: FU LING. Ref: 473.

5270 Polystachoside
$C_{20}H_{18}O_{11}$ MW: 434.36 Property: mp 246-7°C. Source: DUO SUI LIAO. Ref: 6.

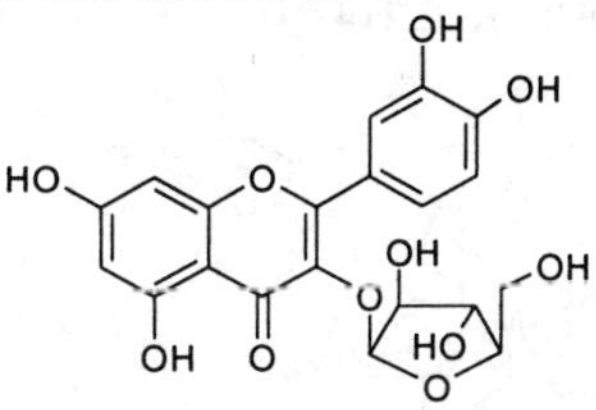

5271 Polysyphorin
Threo-$\Delta^{7'}$-7-hydroxy-3,4,5,3',5'-pentamethoxy-8-O-4'-neolignan. $C_{23}H_{30}O_7$ MW: 418.49 Property: colorless prismatic crystal, mp 147-8°C, $[\alpha]_D^{25}$ 0° (c= 0.40, chloroform). Source: ZHANG YE HU JIAO. Ref: 191.

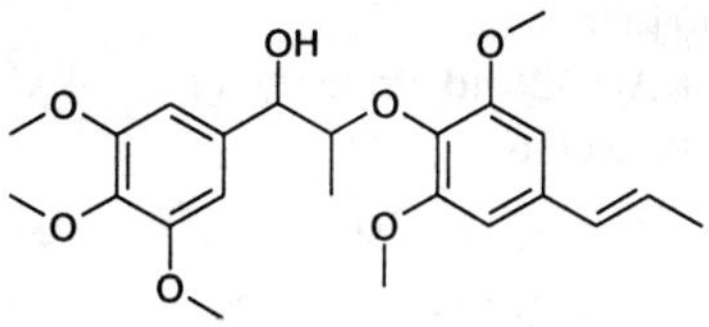

5272 Pomolic acid
Source: CHI NAN, WU LING ZHI. Ref: 600, 638.

5273 Ponasterone A
$C_{27}H_{44}O_6$ MW: 464.65 Property: mp 259-60°C (dec). Source: DONG FANG GOU JI, GUAN ZHONG, JUE, LUO HAN SONG YE, ZI SHAN. Ref: 6.

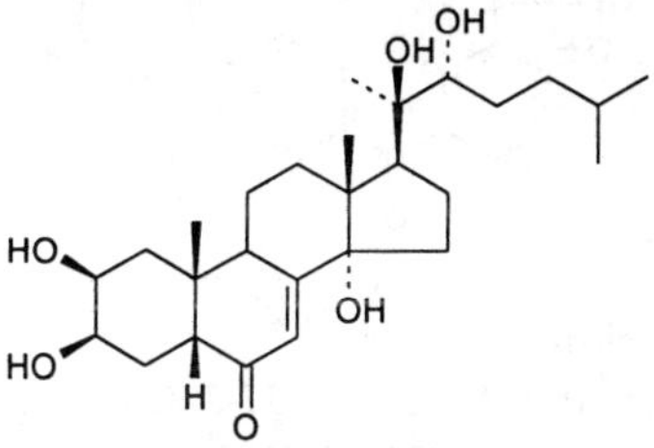

5274 Ponasteroside A
Warabisterone. $C_{33}H_{54}O_{11}$ MW: 626.79 Property: mp 278-9.5°C. Source: JUE. Ref: 6.

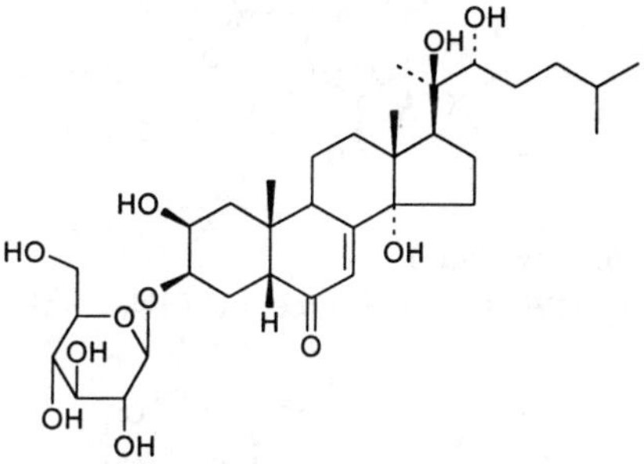

5275 Poncirin
$C_{28}H_{34}O_{14}$ MW: 594.57 Property: mp 211-2°C. Source: GOU JU, GOU JU YE, YOU. Ref: 6.

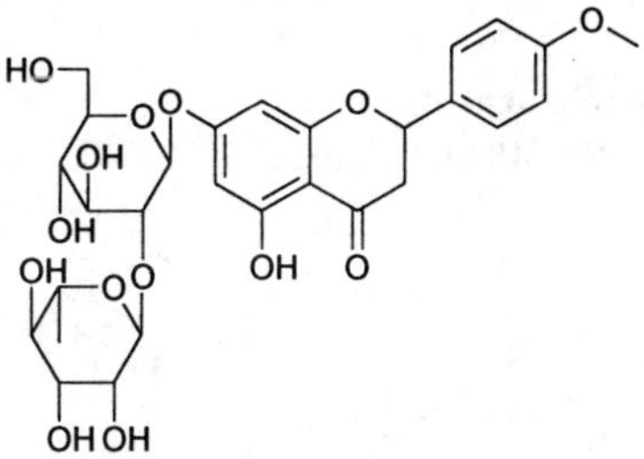

5276 Poncitrin
$C_{20}H_{22}O_4$ MW: 326.40 Property: mp 93-4°C. Source: ZHI GEN PI. Ref: 6.

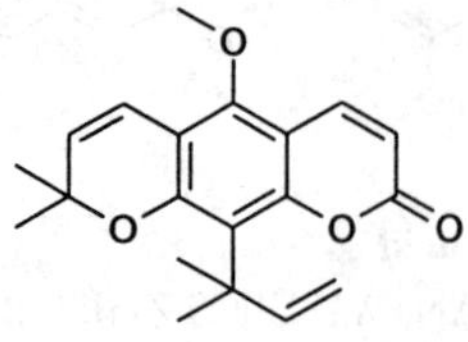

5277 Pongapin
$C_{19}H_{12}O_6$ MW: 336.30 Property: mp 190-1°C. Source: SHUI LIU DOU. Ref: 6.

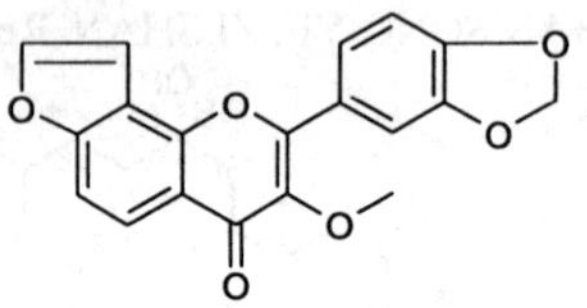

5278 Ponicidin
Rubescensine B. CAS: 52617-37-5 $C_{20}H_{26}O_6$ MW: 362.43 Property: mp 236-41°C. Source: DONG LING CAO, XIAN MAI XIANG CHA CAI. Ref: 5, 504.

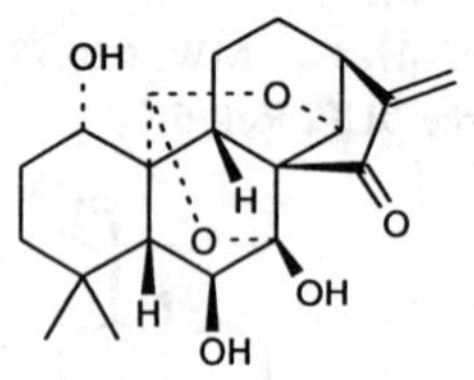

5279 Poricoic acid A
$C_{31}H_{46}O_5$ MW: 498.71 Source: FU LING. Ref: 2.

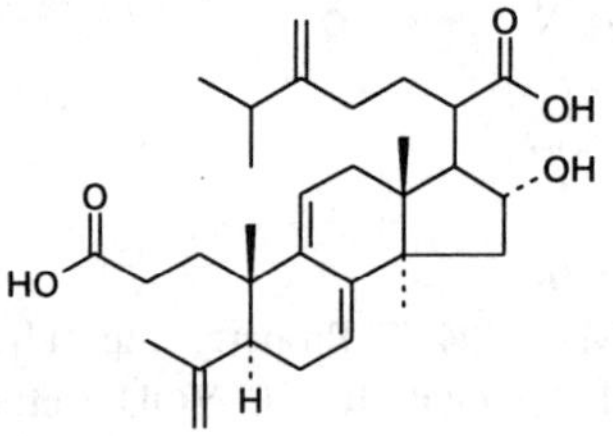

5280 Poricoic acid B
$C_{30}H_{44}O_5$ MW: 484.68 Source: FU LING. Ref: 2.

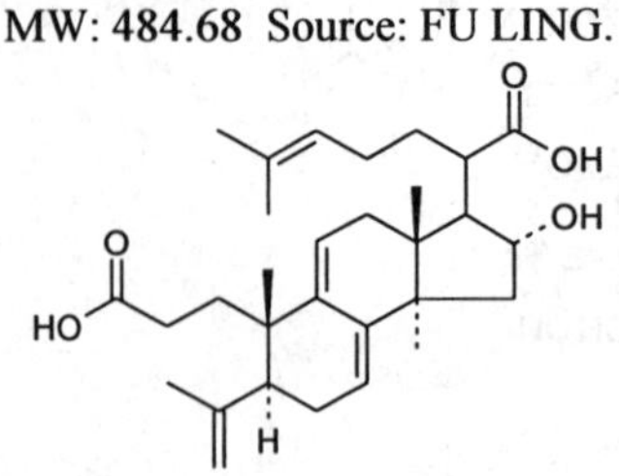

5281 Porphyroxine
$C_{20}H_{21}NO_6$ MW: 371.39 Property: mp 234-6°C (dec). Source: YA PIAN. Ref: 6.

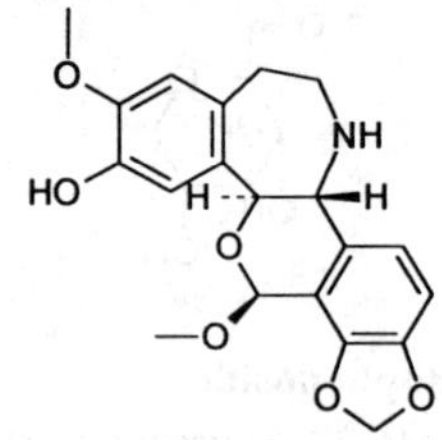

5282 Portulal
$C_{20}H_{32}O_4$ MW: 336.48 Property: mp 113°C. Source: BAN ZHI LIAN. Ref: 6.

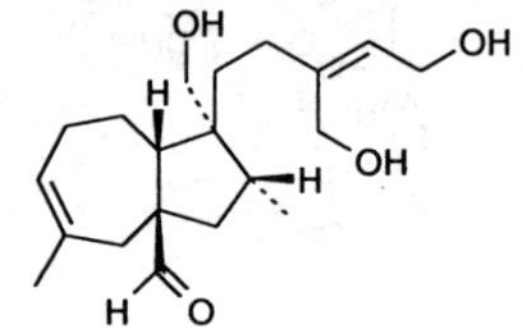

5283 Poststerone
$C_{21}H_{30}O_5$ MW: 362.47 Source: CHUAN NIU XI. Ref: 6.

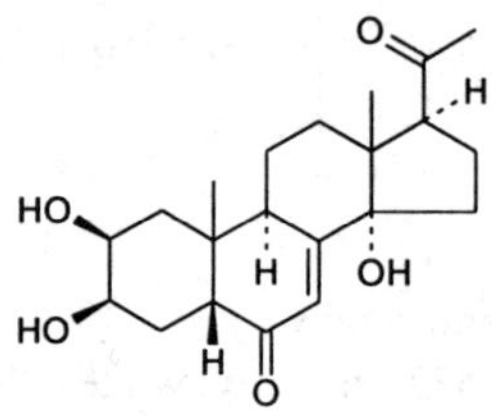

5284 potanidine A
$C_{41}H_{60}O_{11}$ MW: 756.94 Property: white amorphous powder, $[\alpha]_D^{10}$ +15.5° (c=1.0, methanol). Source: HEI SHUI CUI QUE. Ref: 314.

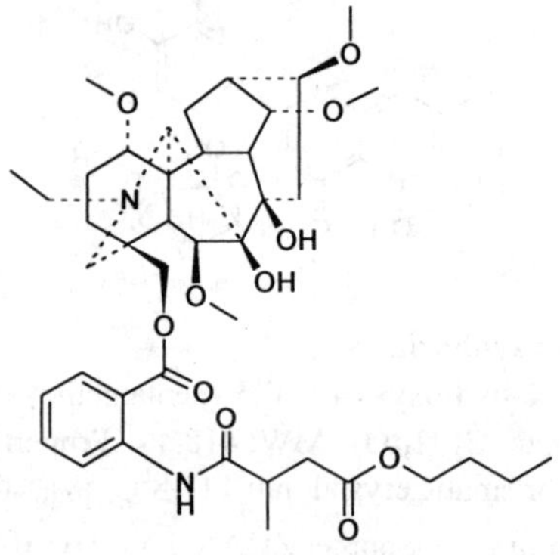

5285 Potanidine B
$C_{37}H_{48}N_2O_{11}$ MW: 696.80 Property: white amorphous powder, $[\alpha]_D^{24}$ +28.6° (c=0.07, chloroform). Source: HEI SHUI CUI QUE. Ref: 314.

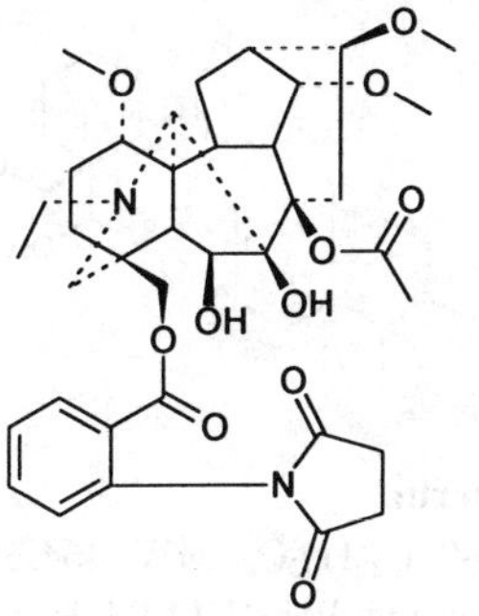

5286 PQ-1
$C_{18}H_{28}O_3$ MW: 292.42 Source: XI YANG SHEN. Ref: 2.

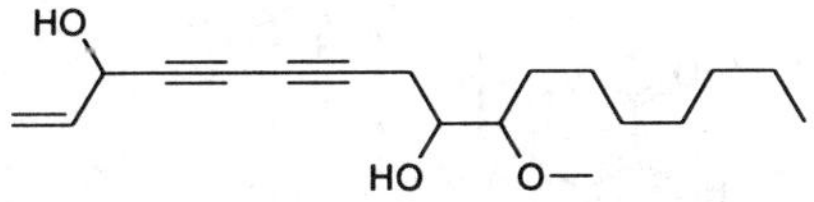

5287 PQ-2
$C_{18}H_{26}O_4$ MW: 306.41 Source: XI YANG SHEN. Ref: 2.

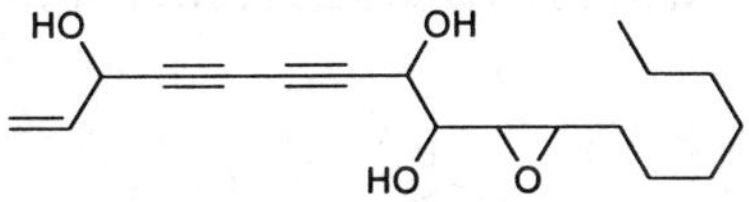

5288 PQ-3
$C_{17}H_{22}O_2$ MW: 258.36 Source: XI YANG SHEN. Ref: 2.

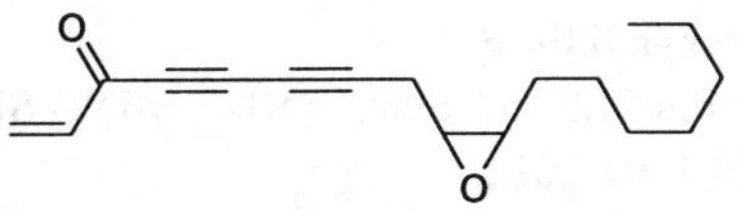

5289 (+)-Praeruptorin
Source: LI JIANG QIAN HU. Ref: 557.

5290 Pratensein
$C_{16}H_{12}O_6$ MW: 300.27 Property: mp 272-3°C. Source: HONG CHE ZHOU CAO. Ref: 6.

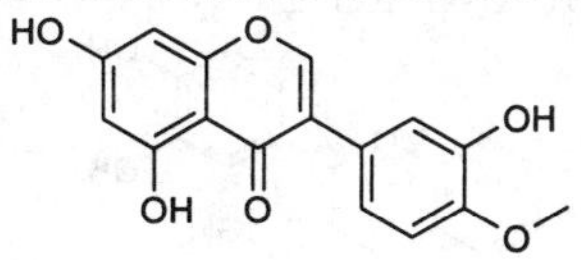

5291 Pratol
$C_{16}H_{12}O_4$ MW: 268.27 Property: mp 263-4°C. Source: HONG CHE ZHOU CAO. Ref: 6.

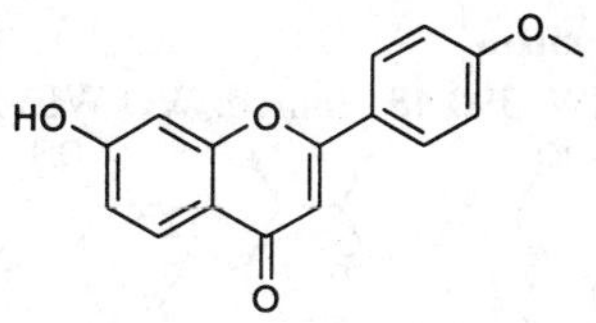

5292 Precatorine
$C_{14}H_{11}NO_6$ MW: 289.25 Property: mp 218-20°C. Source: XIANG SI ZI. Ref: 6.

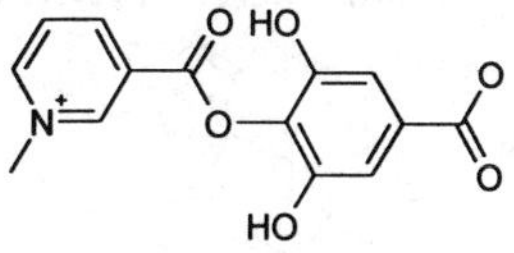

5293 Precyasterone
$C_{29}H_{44}O_8$ MW: 520.67 Source: CHUAN NIU XI. Ref: 6.

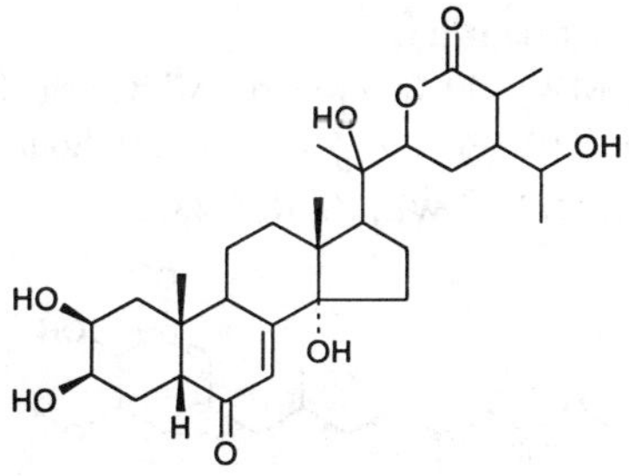

5294 5α-Pregnane-3β,20β-diol
$C_{21}H_{36}O_2$ MW: 320.52 Source: JIAN MA. Ref: 6.

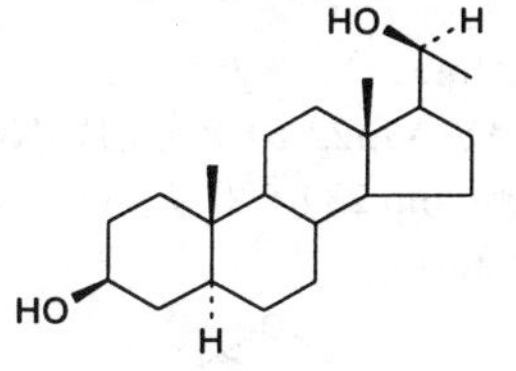

5295 Pregna-5,16-dien-3β-ol-20-one 3-O-β-chacotrioside
$C_{39}H_{60}O_{15}$ MW: 768.90 Property: mp 260-2°C (dec). Source: ZAO XIU. Ref: 6.

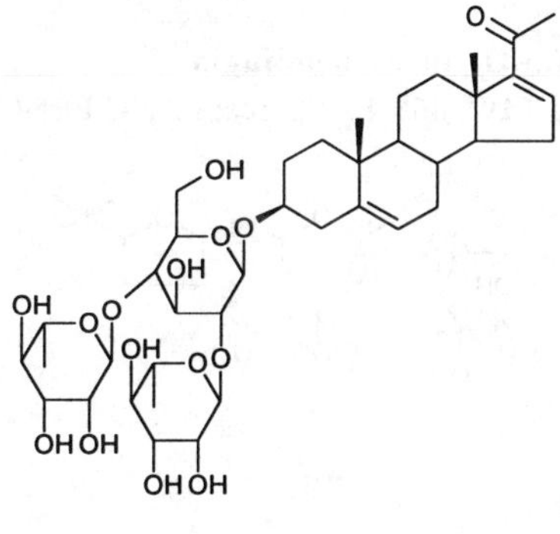

5296 Pregomisin
$C_{22}H_{30}O_6$ MW: 390.48 Source: WU WEI ZI. Ref: 2.

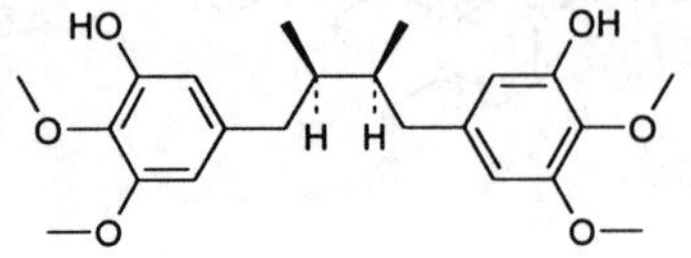

5297 Prehispanolone
$C_{20}H_{30}O_3$ MW: 318.46 Source: YI MU CAO. Ref: 2.

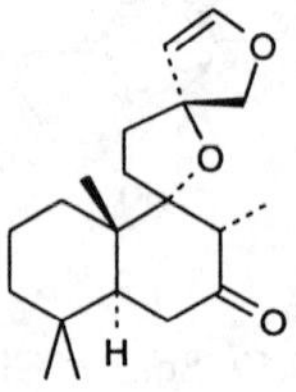

5298 Preschisanthrin
$C_{22}H_{30}O_6$ MW: 390.48 Property: white acicular crystal, mp 119-20°C, $[\alpha]_D^{19}$ 0° (MeOH). Source: ZHONG JIAN WU WEI ZI. Ref: 486.

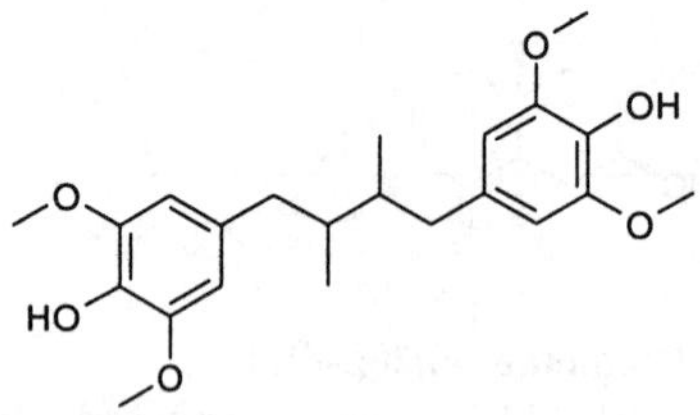

5299 Pretazettine
Isotazettine. CAS: 17322-84-8 $C_{18}H_{21}NO_5$ MW: 331.37 Property: mp 234-6°C. Source: SHUI XIAN GEN, etc. Ref: 5.

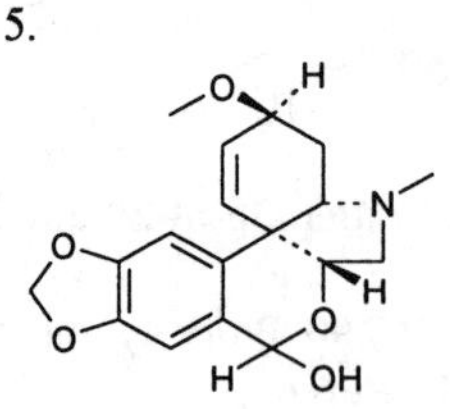

5300 Prim-O-glucosylcimifugin
$C_{11}H_{28}O_{11}$ MW: 468.42 Source: FANG FENG. Ref: 2.

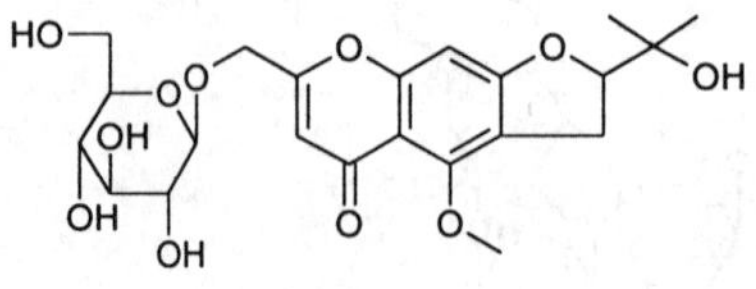

5301 Primulagenin A
$C_{30}H_{50}O_3$ MW: 458.73 Property: mp 249.5-50°C. Source: DA HONG PAO, ZHEN ZHU CAI (ZHEN ZHU YE). Ref: 6.

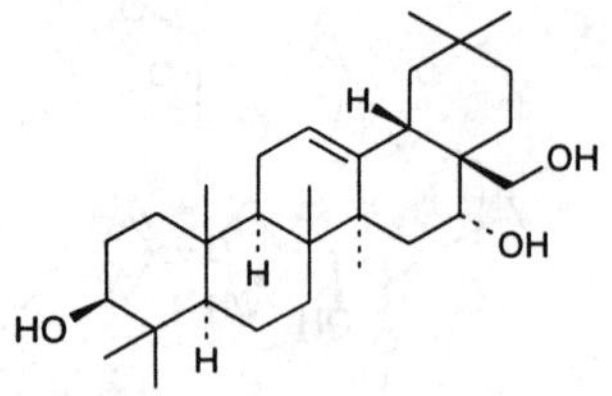

5302 Pristimerin
CAS: 1258-84-0 $C_{30}H_{40}O_4$ MW: 464.65 Property: mp 214-7°C. Source: PU RUI MU. Ref: 5.

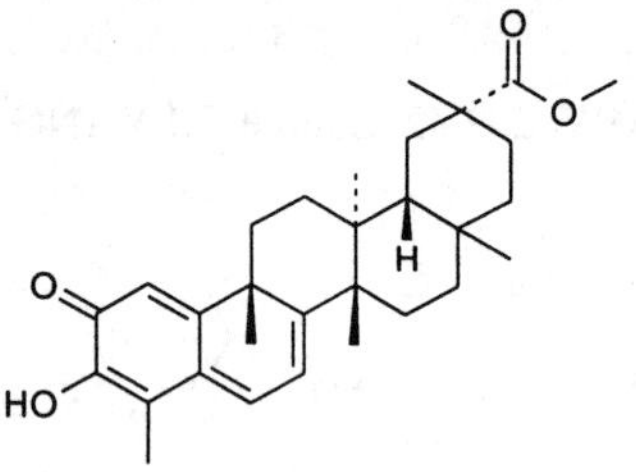

5303 Procurcumenol
$C_{15}H_{22}O_2$ MW: 234.34 Source: PENG E SHU. Ref: 6.

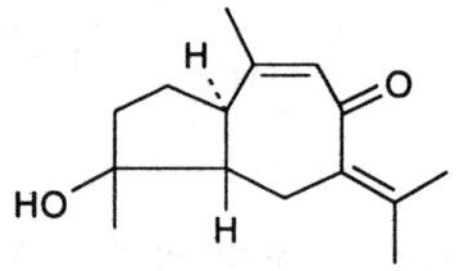

5304 Procyanidin B-3
Property: mp 212-5°C. Source: KUN MING SHAN HAI TANG. Ref: 612.

5305 Procyanidin B-4
Property: mp 207-10°C. Source: KUN MING SHAN HAI TANG. Ref: 612.

5306 Procyanidin B-13'-O-gallate
Source: DA HUANG. Ref: 2.

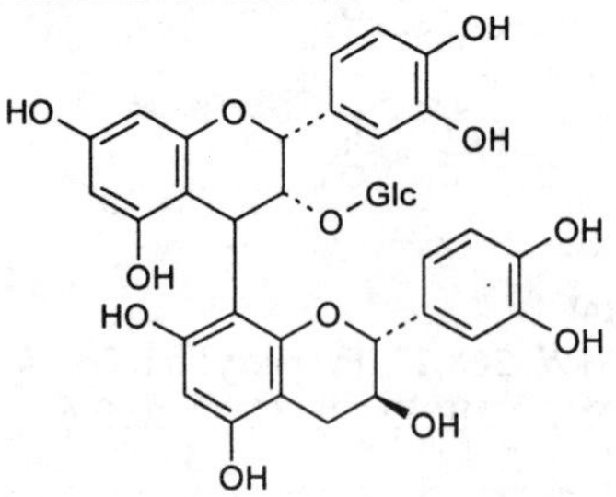

5307 Procyanidin B-23,3'-di-O-gallate
Source: DA HUANG. Ref: 2.

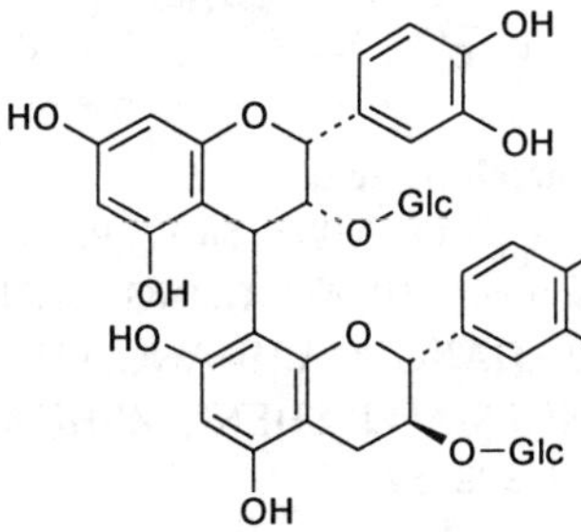

5308 Progesterone
$C_{21}H_{30}O_2$ MW: 314.47 Property: mp (α): 128.5°C, (β): 121-2°C. Source: ZI HE CHE. Ref: 6.

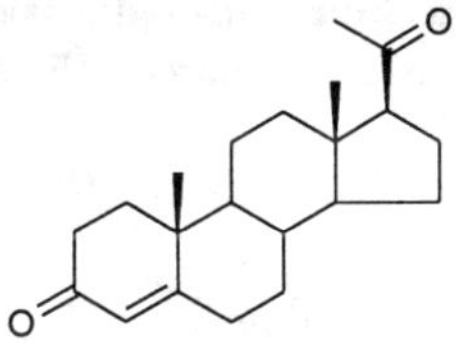

5309 Proglobeflowery acid
3-methoxy-4-hydroxyl-5-(3'-methyl-2'-) butylenyl benzoic acid. $C_{13}H_{16}O_4$ MW: 236.27 Property: white acicular crystal (ethanol-water), mp 141-2°C, hardly soluble in water, easy soluble in 5MNaHCO$_3$. Source: CHANG BAN JIN LIAN HUA. Ref: 245.

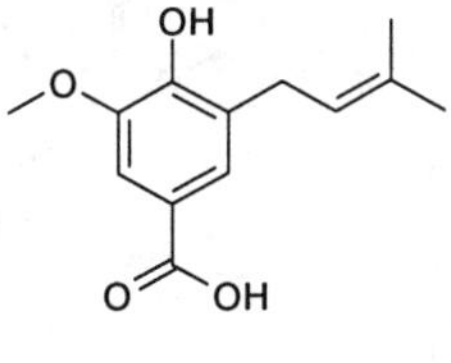

5310 Prometaphanine
$C_{20}H_{25}NO_5$ MW: 359.43 Source: QIAN JIN TENG. Ref: 6.

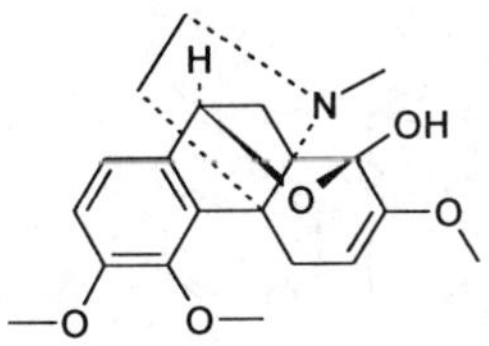

5311 Pronuciferine
$C_{19}H_{21}NO_3$ MW: 311.38 Property: mp (+): 127- 9°C, (±): 148-51°C. Source: HE YE, LIAN ZI XIN. Ref: 6.

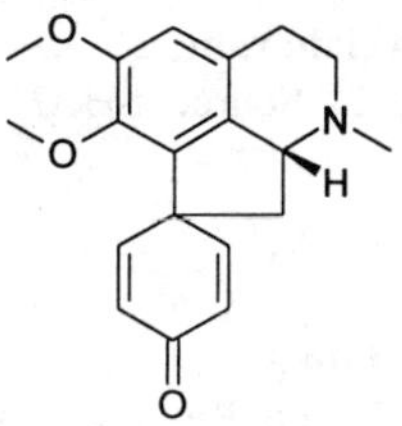

5312 n-Propanol
C_3H_8O MW: 60.10 Source: SHENG JIANG. Ref: 2.

5313 1-Propenyl-cyclohexane
C_9H_{16} MW: 124.23 Source: SHAN ZHA. Ref: 2.

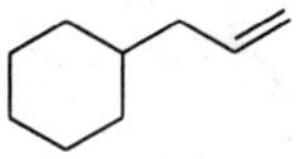

5314 Propenyl propyl disulfide
$C_6H_{12}S_2$ MW: 148.29 Source: XI XIANG CONG. Ref: 6.

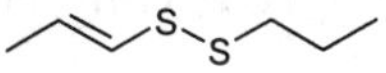

5315 Propionaldehyde
C_3H_6O MW: 58.08 Source: SHENG JIANG. Ref: 2.

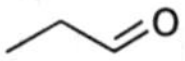

5316 Propionic acid
$C_3H_6O_2$ MW: 74.08 Property: bp 141.35°C. Source: BAI GUO. Ref: 2.

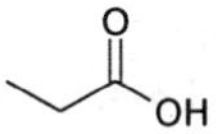

5317 16-Propoxystrychnine
$C_{24}H_{28}N_2O_3$ MW: 32.50 Property: mp 174-5°C. Source: LU SONG GUO. Ref: 6.

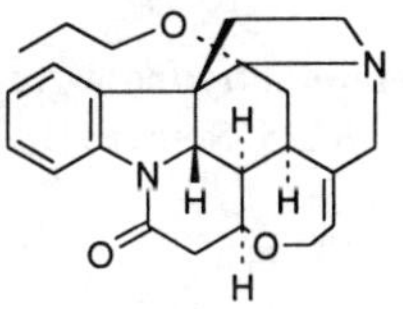

5318 Propylamine
C_3H_9N MW: 59.11 Property: bp 49°C. Source: LING MAO XIANG. Ref: 6.

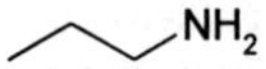

5319 Propyl-cyclohexane
C_9H_{18} MW: 126.24 Source: SHAN ZHA. Ref: 2.

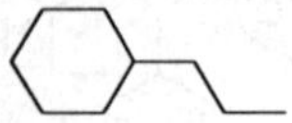

5320 Proscillaridin A
$C_{30}H_{42}O_8$ MW: 530.66 Property: mp 215-8°C. Source: MIAN ZAO ER. Ref: 6.

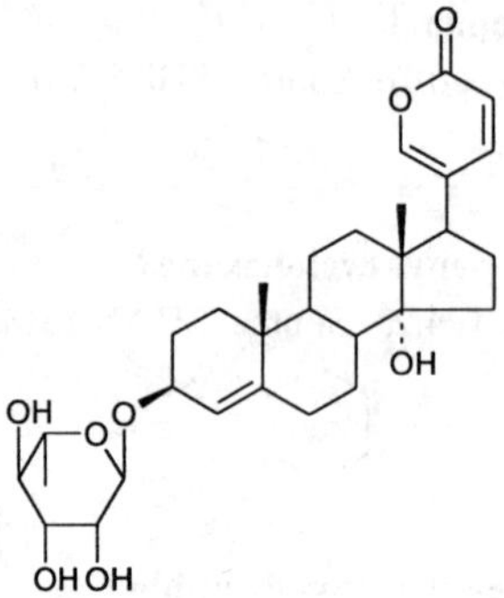

5321 Protoaescigenin
$C_{30}H_{50}O_6$ MW: 506.73 Property: mp 310°C. Source: SUO LUO ZI. Ref: 6.

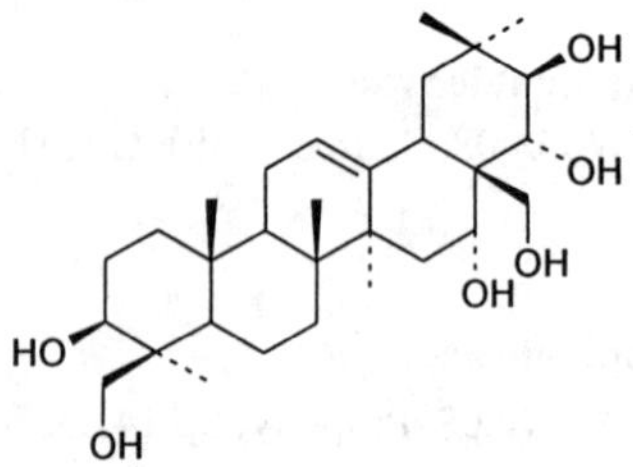

5322 Protoanemonin
$C_5H_4O_2$ MW: 96.09 Property: bp 45°C/1.5 mm. Source: MA TI YE, MAO GEN, SHI LONG RUI, ZI KOU CAO. Ref: 6.

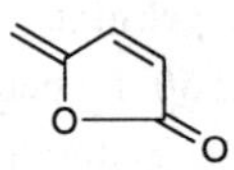

5323 Protoanemonin hydrate glucoside
$C_{11}H_{16}O_8$ MW: 276.25 Source: BAI HUA TENG. Ref: 6.

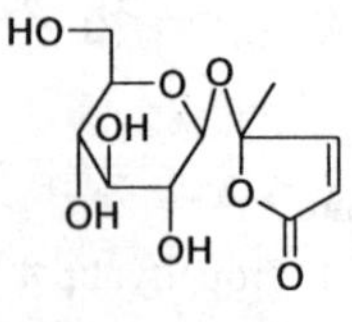

5324 Protocatechualdehyde
Protocatechuic aldehyde; Rancinamycin IV. CAS: 139-85-5 $C_7H_6O_3$ MW: 138.12 Property: mp 153-4°C. Source: SI JI QING. Ref: 4, 6.

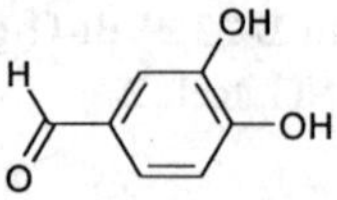

5325 Protocatechuic acid
CAS: 99-50-3 $C_7H_6O_4$ MW: 154.12 Property: mp 199-200°C. Source: CHUAN XIONG, DAN SHEN, GUI ZHI, HU ZHANG, MA HUANG, PU HUANG, SI JI QING, XIU MAO JI SHENG, ZI HUA BA BAO. Ref: 2, 4, 308, 527, 559.

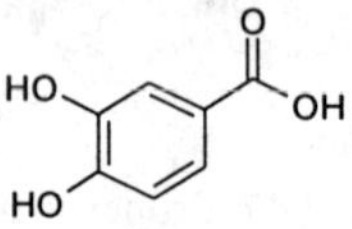

5326 Protocatechuic acid-3-glucoside
$C_{13}H_{16}O_9$ MW: 316.27 Source: YE LI ZHI YE. Ref: 6.

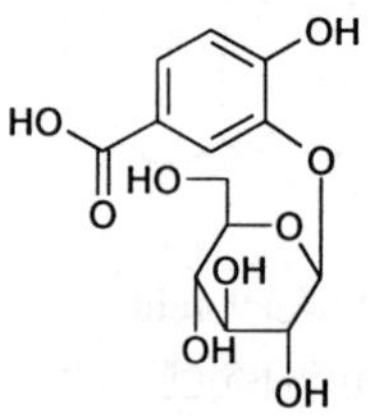

5327 Protocatechuoyl calleryanin
$C_{20}H_{022}O_{11}$ MW: 438.39 Source: YE LI ZHI YE. Ref: 6.

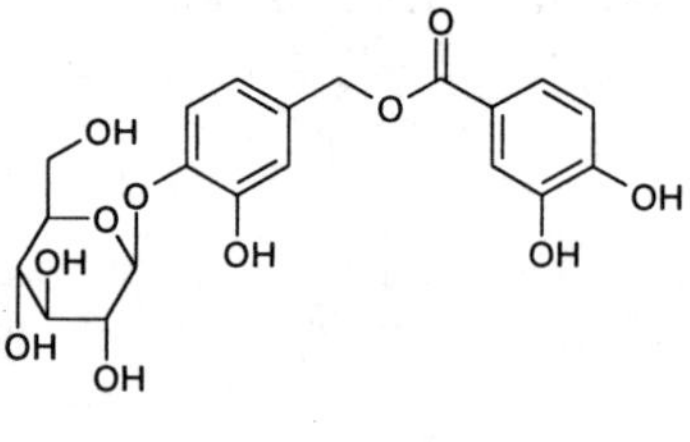

5328 Protocrocin
$C_{76}H_{116}O_{34}$ MW: 1573.75 Source: ZANG HONG HUA. Ref: 6.

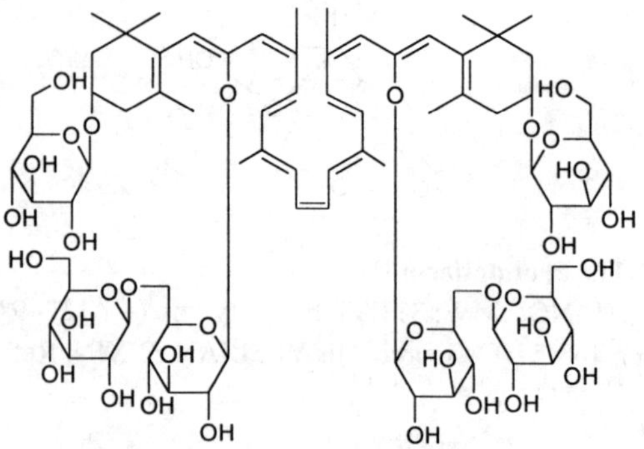

5329 Protoeruboside B
Source: DA SUAN. Ref: 2.

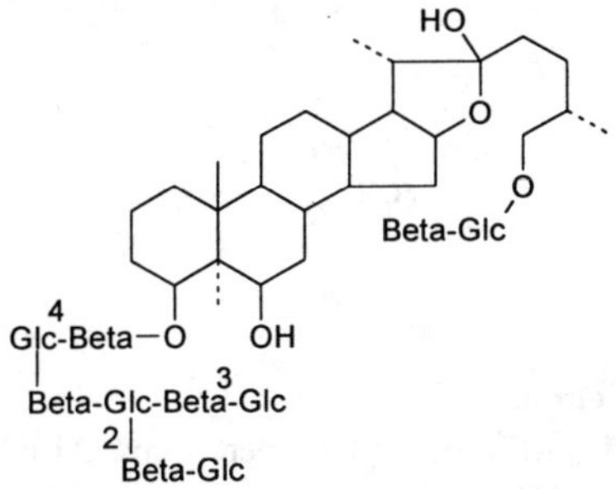

5330 Protogracillin
$C_{51}H_{82}O_{23}$ MW: 1063.21 Source: DUN YE SHU YU, fresh rhizome, XIAO HUA DUN YE SHU YU, fresh rhizome, XIAN XI SHU YU. Ref: 10, 15.

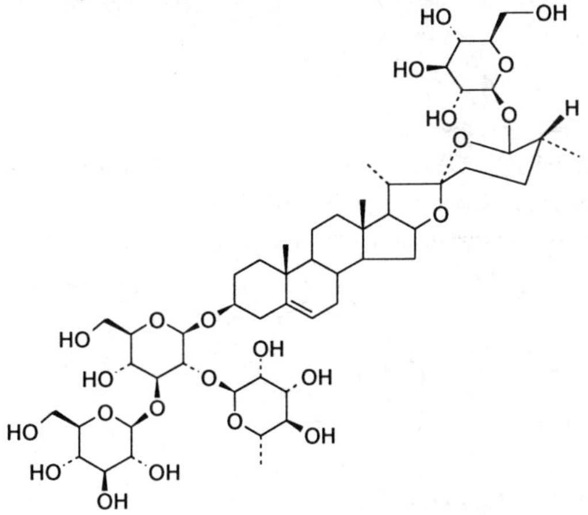

5331 Proto-iso-eruboside B
$C_{57}H_{96}O_{30}$ MW: 1261.38 Property: white powder, mp 218-20 °C, $[\alpha]_D^{20}$ -26° (c=0.1, C_5H_5N). Source: DA SUAN. Ref: 362.

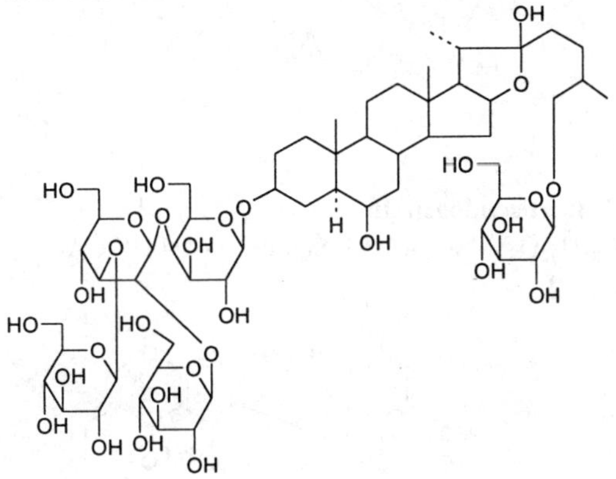

5332 Protopanaxadiol
$C_{30}H_{56}O_3$ MW: 460.75 Property: mp 236-8°C. Source: REN SHEN. Ref: 6.

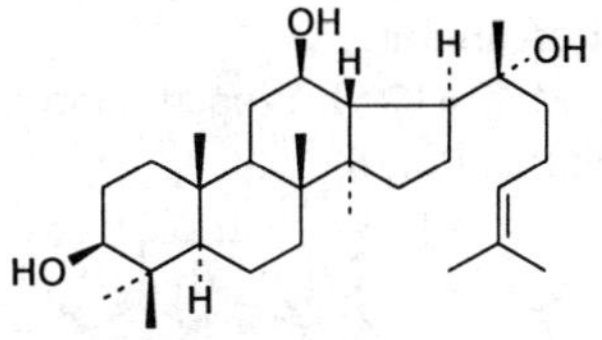

5333 Protopanaxatriol
$C_{30}H_{52}O_4$ MW: 476.75 Property: mp 233-5°C. Source: REN SHEN. Ref: 6.

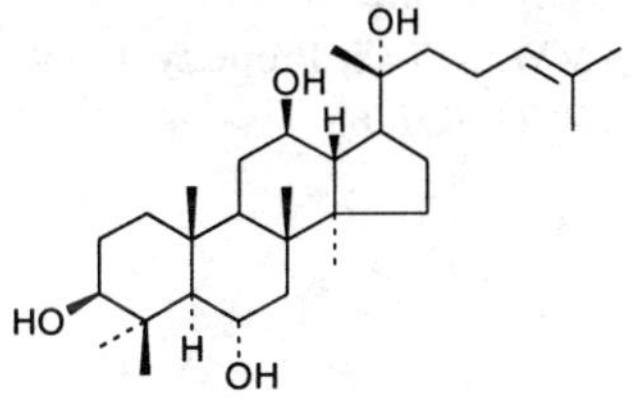

5334 20(R)-Protopanaxatriol
Property: colorless acicular crystal (chloroform-ether), mp 248-50°C. Source: REN SHEN HUA LEI. Ref: 446.

5335 Protopine
$C_{20}H_{19}NO_5$ MW: 353.38 Source: YAN HU SUO. Ref: 2.

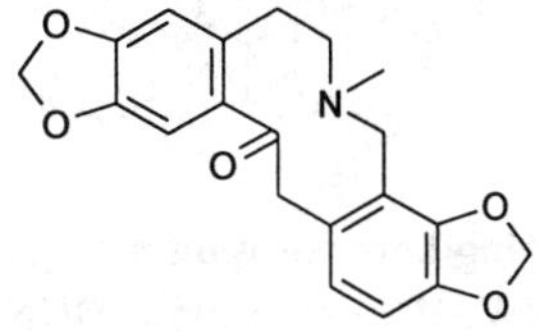

5336 Protoporphyrin
$C_{34}H_{34}N_4O_4$ MW: 562.67 Property: mp 225-30°C. Source: NIU XUE. Ref: 6.

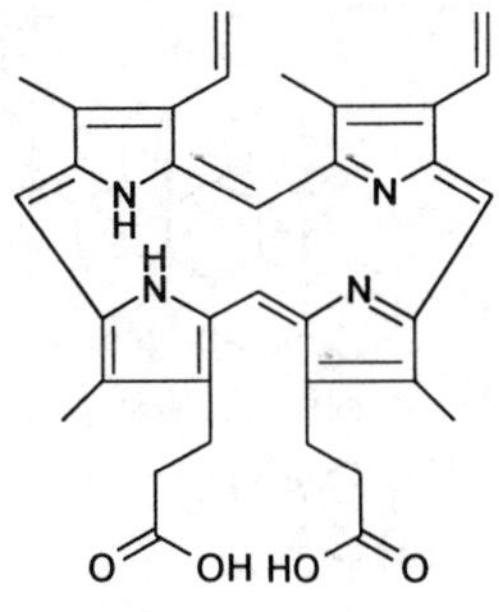

5337 Protosappanin A
Property: mp 250-2°C. Source: SU MU. Ref: 508.

5338 Protostemonine
$C_{23}H_{31}NO_6$ MW: 417.51 Property: mp 172°C. Source: BAI BU. Ref: 6.

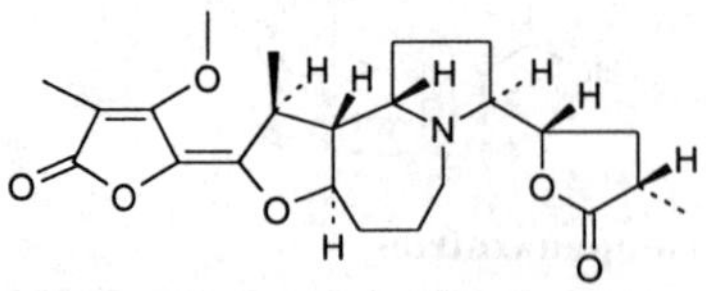

5339 Protostephanine
$C_{21}H_{27}NO_4$ MW: 357.45 Property: mp 91°C. Source: QIAN JIN TENG. Ref: 6.

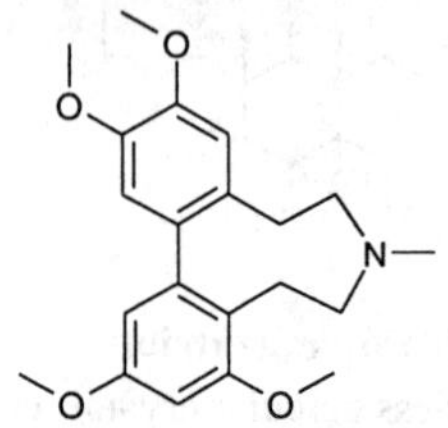

5340 Protostrychnine
$C_{21}H_{26}N_2O_3$ MW: 354.45 Source: MA QIAN ZI. Ref: 2.

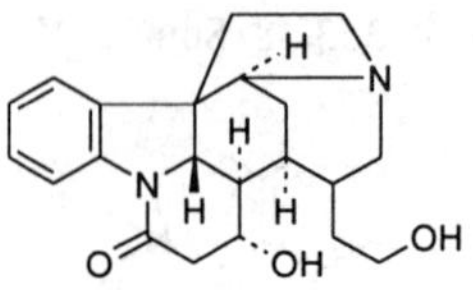

5341 Protozingiberensisaponin
$C_{51}H_{82}O_{24}$ MW: 1079.21 Source: DUN YE SHU YU. Ref: 10.

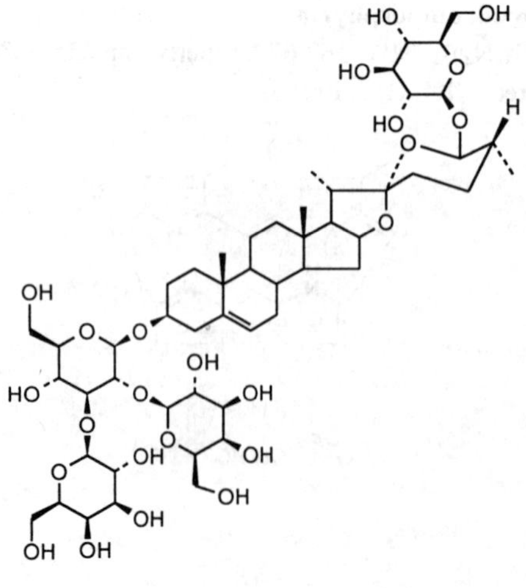

5342 Prunasine
$C_{14}H_{17}NO_6$ MW: 295.29 Source: XING REN. Ref: 2.

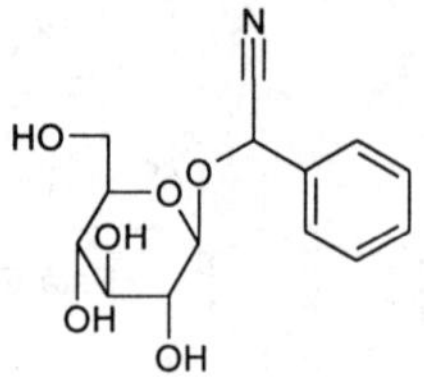

5343 Prunin
$C_{21}H_{22}O_{10}$ MW: 434.40 Property: mp 224-6°C. Source: MANG JING. Ref: 6.

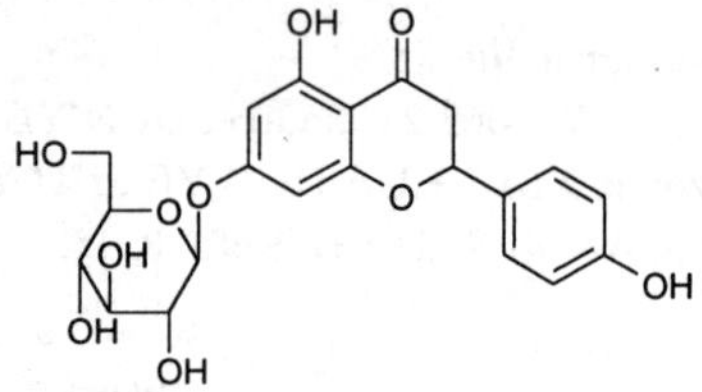

5344 Przewaquinone A
$C_{19}H_{18}O_4$ MW: 310.35 Property: mp 173-5°C (dec). Source: *Salvia przewalskii* Maxim. var. *mandarinorum*. Stib (root). Ref: 5.

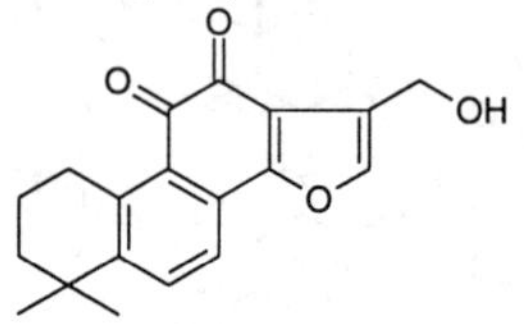

5345 Pseudaconitine
$C_{36}H_{51}NO_{12}$ MW: 689.81 Property: mp 214°C (dec). Source: CAO WU TOU. Ref: 6.

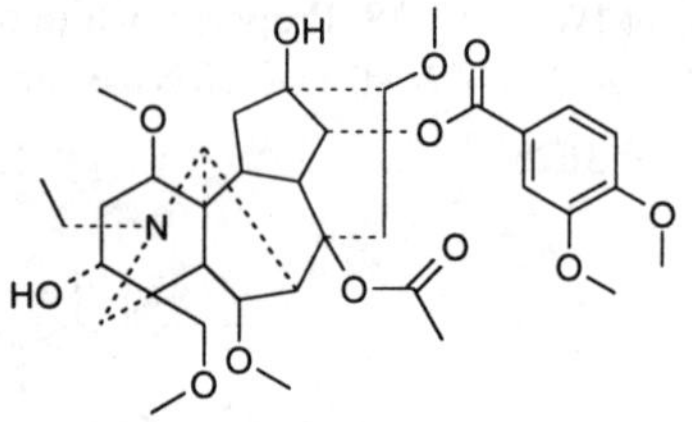

5346 Pseudoaspidin
$C_{25}H_{32}O_8$ MW: 460.53 Source: XIAN HE CAO. Ref: 2.

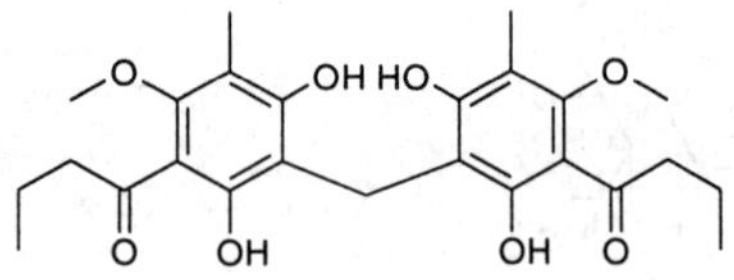

5347 Pseudobrucine
$C_{23}H_{26}N_2O_5$ MW: 410.47 Property: mp 258°C. Source: MA QIAN ZI. Ref: 2.

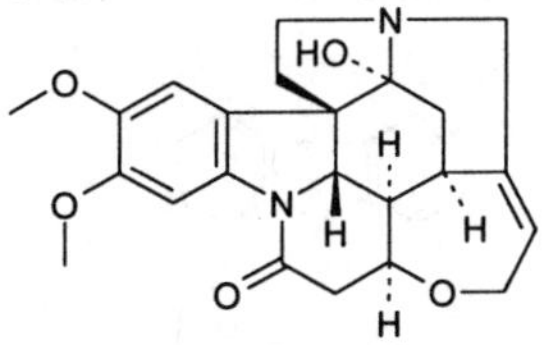

5348 Pseudocarpaine
ψ-Carpaine. $C_{28}H_{50}N_2O_4$ MW: 478.72 Property: mp 65-8°C. Source: FAN MU GUA YE. Ref: 6.

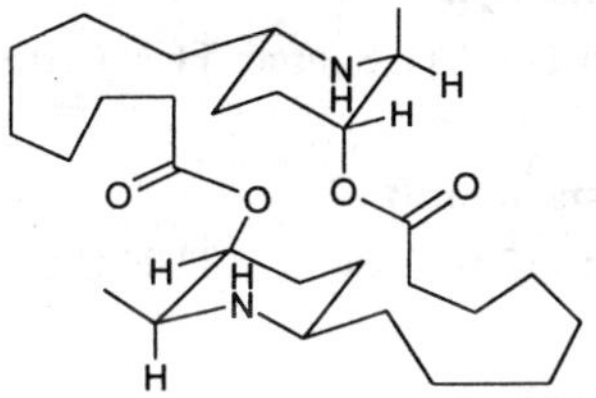

5349 d-Pseudoephedrine
$C_{10}H_{15}NO$ MW: 165.24 Property: mp (+): 117-8°C. Source: HUANG HUA ZI, MA HUANG. Ref: 2, 6.

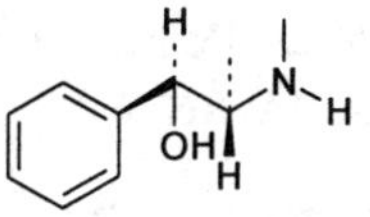

5350 Pseudoginsenoside F11
Ginsenoside A. Source: REN SHEN. Ref: 2.

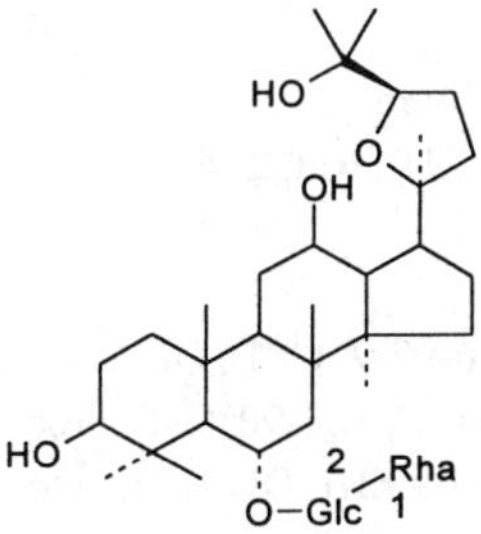

5351 Pseudojervine
$C_{33}H_{49}NO_8$ MW: 587.76 Property: mp 300-1°C (dec). Source: LI LU. Ref: 6.

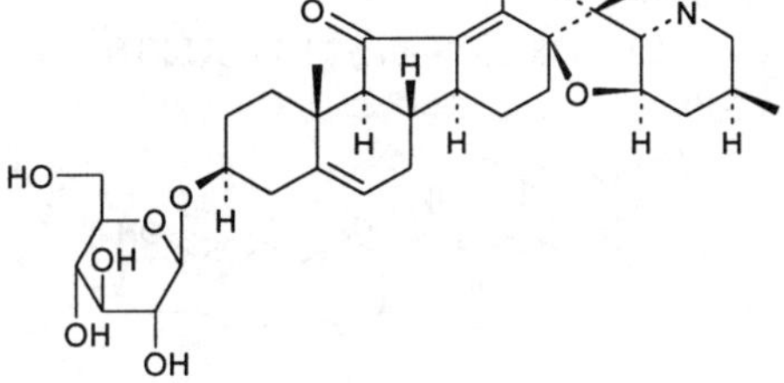

5352 Pseudolycorine
CAS: 29429-03-6 $C_{16}H_{19}NO_4$ MW: 289.33 Property: mp 247-8°C. Source: DA YI ZHI JIAN, SHUI XIAN GEN, SHI SUAN. Ref: 4, 5.

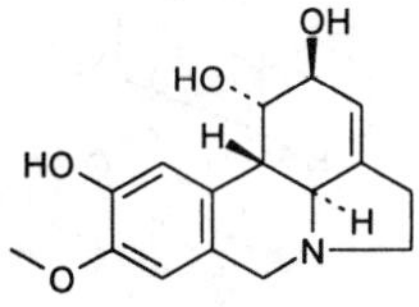

5353 d-N-Pseudomethylephedrine
$C_{11}H_{17}NO$ MW: 179.26 Property: mp (+): 30°C. Source: MA HUANG. Ref: 6.

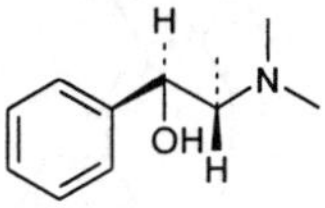

5354 Pseudomorphine
$C_{34}H_{36}N_2O_6$ MW: 568.68 Property: mp 327°C (dec). Source: YA PIAN. Ref: 6.

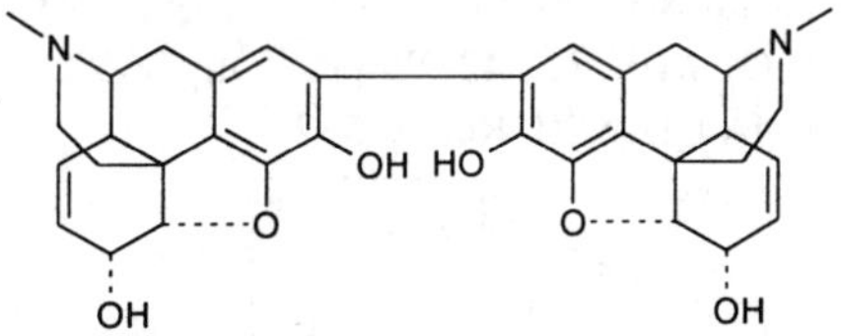

5355 Pseudopelletierine
$C_9H_{15}NO$ MW: 153.23 Property: mp 54°C. Source: SHI LIU GEN. Ref: 6.

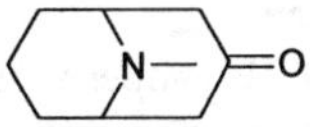

5356 Pseudopurpurin
$C_{15}H_8O_7$ MW: 300.23 Property: mp 222-4°C (dec). Source: QIAN CAO GEN. Ref: 6.

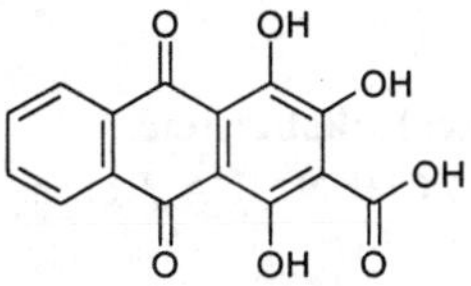

5357 Pseudosantonin
$C_{15}H_{20}O_4$ MW: 264.32 Property: mp 183-4°C. Source: HUANG HUA HAO. Ref: 6.

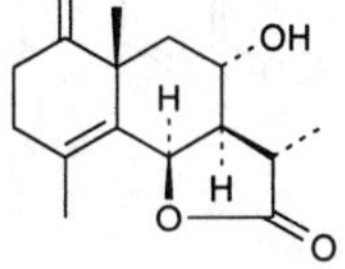

5358 Pseudoselagine
$C_{16}H_{25}NO_2$ MW: 263.38 Property: mp 163°C. Source: XIAO JIE JIN CAO. Ref: 6.

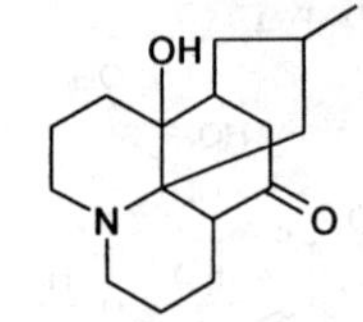

OH
N
O

5359 Pseudo-γ-schisandrin
$C_{23}H_{28}O_6$ MW: 400.48 Property: mp 92-3°C. Source: WU WEI ZI. Ref: 2.

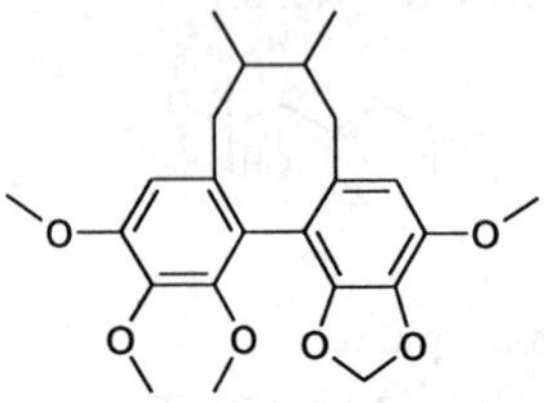

O O O O O O

5360 Pseudostrychnine
$C_{21}H_{22}N_2O_3$ MW: 350.42 Property: mp 266°C. Source: MA QIAN ZI. Ref: 2, 542.

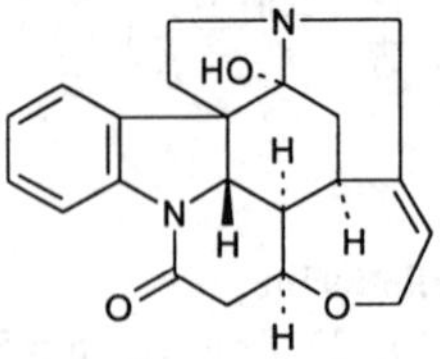

N HO H N H H O H O

5361 Pseudotropine
$C_8H_{15}NO$ MW: 141.21 Property: mp 108-9°C, bp 240-1°C. Source: MAN TUO LUO GEN. Ref: 6.

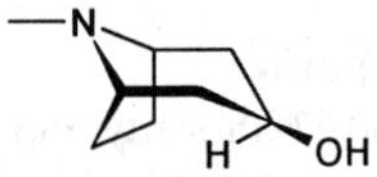

N H OH

5362 Psedovincaleukoblastine
Source: CHANG CHUN HUA. Ref: 2.

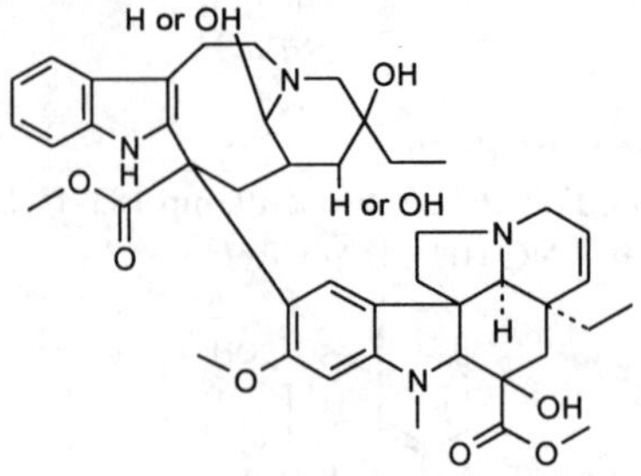

H or OH N OH N H O O H or OH N H O N OH O O

5363 Pseudoyohimbine
$C_{21}H_{26}N_2O_3$ MW: 354.45 Property: white powder, $[\alpha]_D^{25.4}$ +24.3° (c=0.8, pyridine). Source: YANG JIAO MIAN. Ref: 633.

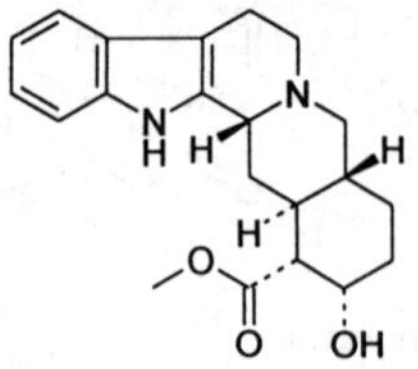

N N H H H H O O OH

5364 Psilostachyin
Property: mp 212-4°C. Source: TUN CAO. Ref: 526.

5365 Psilostachyin B
Property: mp 117-9°C. Source: TUN CAO. Ref: 526.

5366 Psilostachyin C
Property: mp 225-6°C. Source: TUN CAO. Ref: 526.

5367 Psilotin
$C_{17}H_{20}O_8$ MW: 352.34 Property: mp 130-1°C. Source: SHI SHUA BA. Ref: 6.

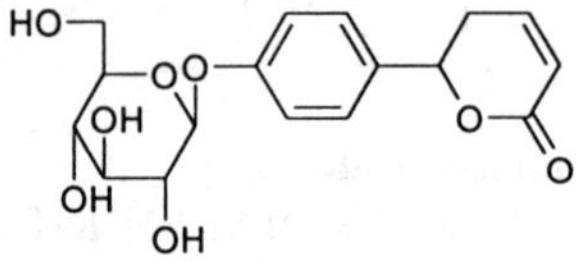

HO O O OH OH OH O O

5368 Psoraldehyde
Source: BU GU ZHI. Ref: 2, 630.

5369 Psoralen
Ficusin. CAS: 66-97-7 $C_{11}H_6O_3$ MW: 186.17 Property: mp 171°C, 189-90°C. Source: BAI HUA QIAN HU, BU GU ZHI, DU HUO, etc. Ref: 2, 4, 5, 268.

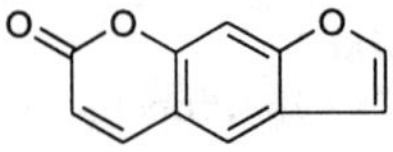

O O O

5370 Psoralenol
$C_{20}H_{18}O_5$ MW: 338.36 Source: BU GU ZHI. Ref: 2, 630.

HO O O OH O

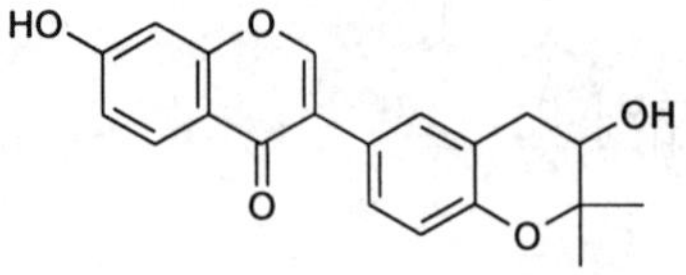

5371 Psoralidin
$C_{20}H_{16}O_5$ MW: 336.35 Source: BU GU ZHI. Ref: 2, 630.

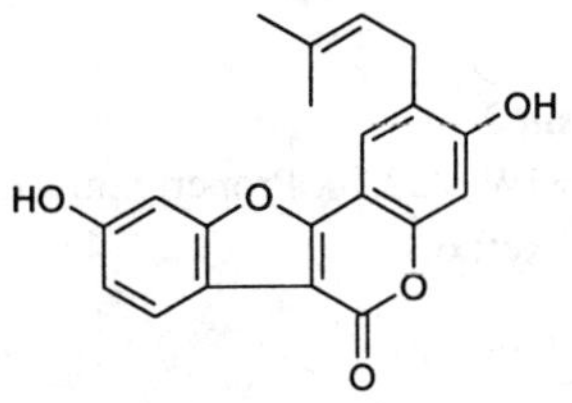

5372 Psoromic acid
$C_{18}H_{14}O_8$ MW: 358.31 Property: mp 265°C. Source: TAI BAI HUA. Ref: 6.

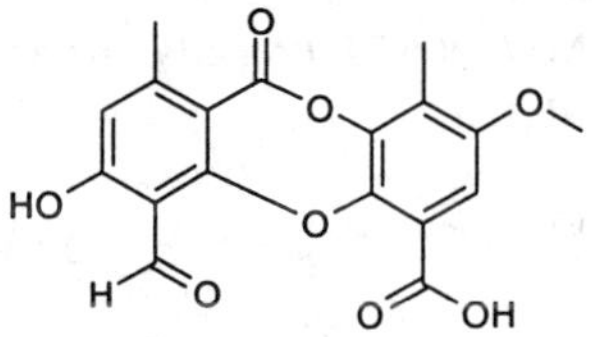

5373 Psorospermin
CAS: 74045-97-9 $C_{19}H_{16}O_6$ MW: 340.34 Property: mp 227-8°C. Source: PU SUO CAO. Ref: 5.

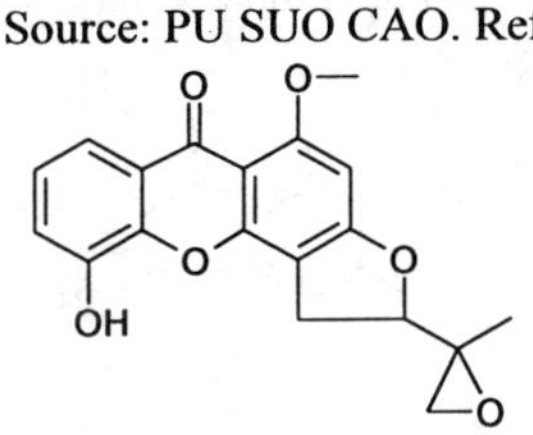

5374 Psyllic acid
$C_{33}H_{66}O_2$ MW: 494.89 Property: mp 94-5°C. Source: MI LA. Ref: 6.

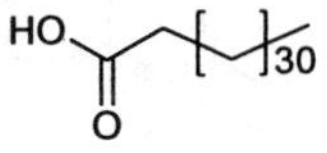

5375 Pterocarpine
CAS: 524-97-0 $C_{17}H_{14}O_5$ MW: 298.30 Property: mp (+): 159- 60°C, (-): 164-5°C, (±): 185-6°C. Source: SHAN DOU GEN, ZI TAN, etc. Ref: 5, 6.

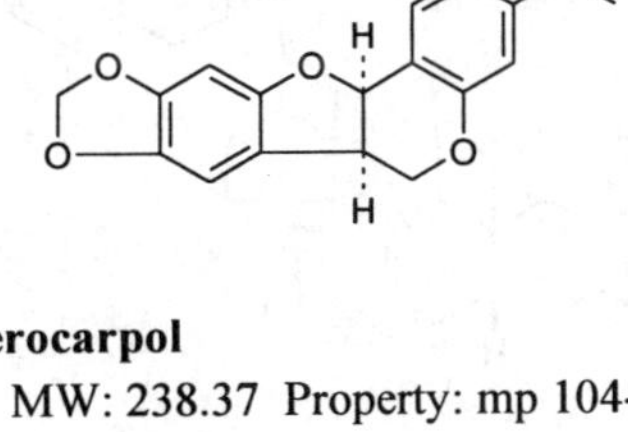

5376 Pterocarpol
$C_{15}H_{26}O_2$ MW: 238.37 Property: mp 104-5°C. Source: ZI TAN. Ref: 6.

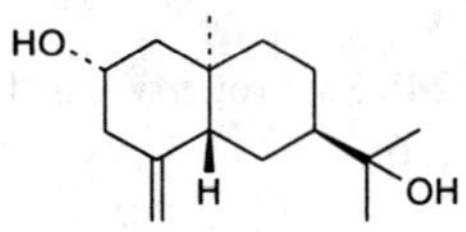

5377 Pterolactam
$C_5H_9NO_2$ MW: 115.13 Property: mp 56-7°C. Source: JUE. Ref: 6.

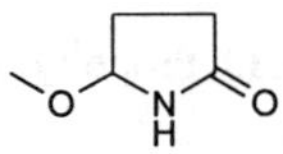

5378 Pteroside A
$C_{21}H_{30}O_8$ MW: 410.47 Source: JUE. Ref: 6.

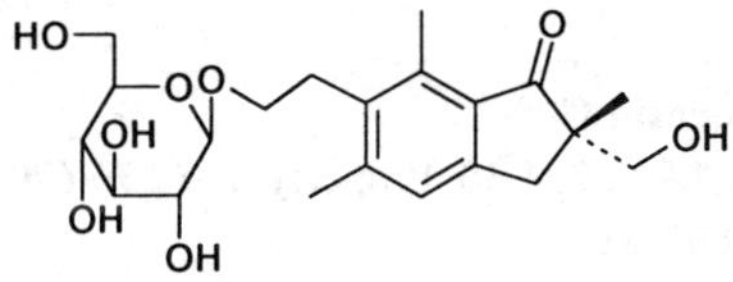

5379 Pteroside B
$C_{20}H_{28}O_7$ MW: 380.44 Property: mp 119-21°C. Source: JUE. Ref: 6.

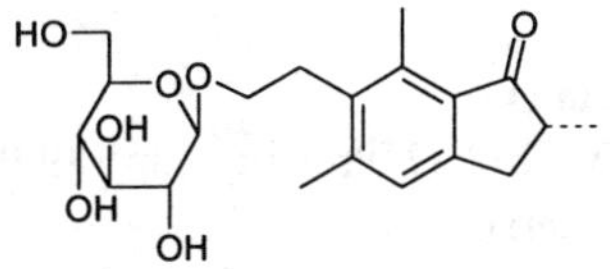

5380 Pteroside C
$C_{20}H_{28}O_8$ MW: 396.44 Source: JUE. Ref: 6.

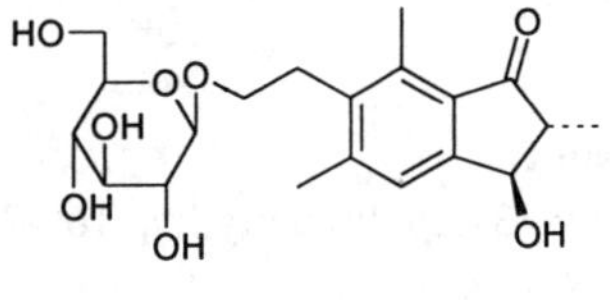

5381 Pteroside D
$C_{21}H_{30}O_8$ MW: 410.47 Source: JUE. Ref: 6.

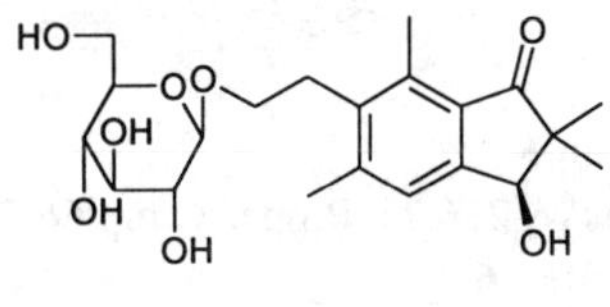

5382 Pteroside Z
$C_{21}H_{30}O_7$ MW: 394.47 Source: JUE. Ref: 6.

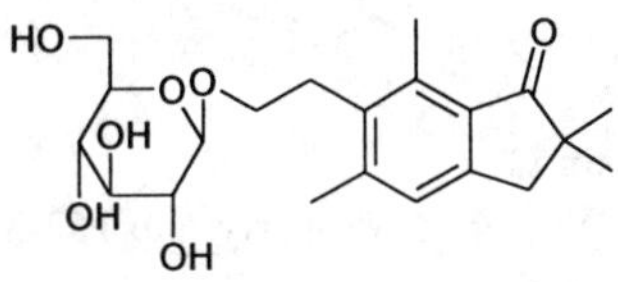

5383 Pterosin A
$C_{15}H_{20}O_3$ MW: 248.32 Property: mp 125-7°C.
Source: JUE. Ref: 6.

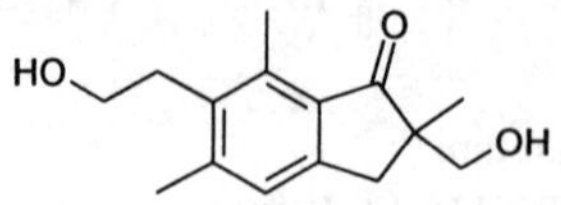

5384 Pterosin B
$C_{14}H_{18}O_2$ MW: 218.30 Property: mp 109-10°C.
Source: JUE. Ref: 6.

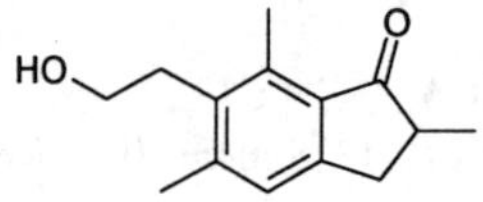

5385 Pterosin C
$C_{14}H_{18}O_3$ MW: 234.30 Property: mp 153-6°C.
Source: JUE. Ref: 6.

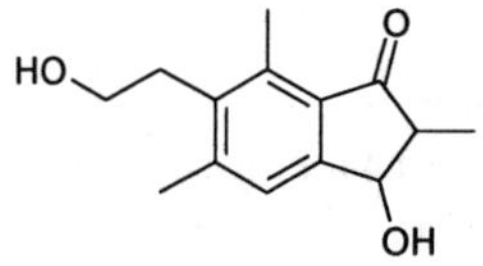

5386 Pterosin D
$C_{15}H_{20}O_3$ MW: 248.32 Property: mp 189-90°C.
Source: JUE. Ref: 6.

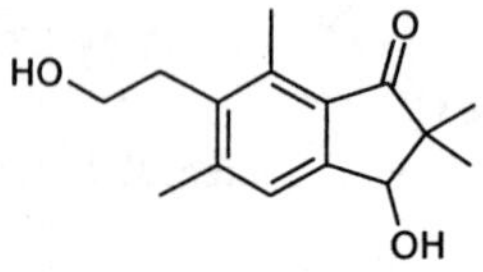

5387 Pterosin E
$C_{14}H_{16}O_3$ MW: 232.28 Property: mp 160-2°C.
Source: JUE. Ref: 6.

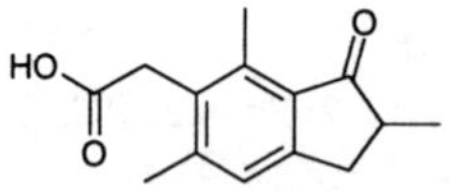

5388 Pterosin F
$C_{14}H_{17}ClO$ MW: 236.74 Property: mp 66-7°C.
Source: JUE. Ref: 6.

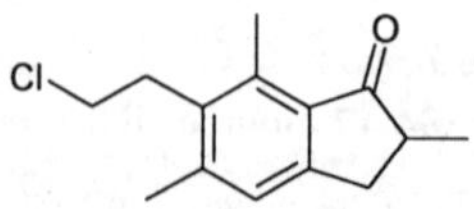

5389 Pterosin G
$C_{14}H_{18}O_3$ MW: 234.30 Property: mp 152-3°C.
Source: JUE. Ref: 6.

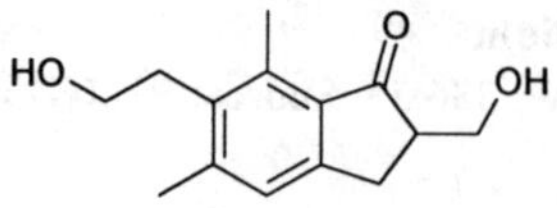

5390 Pterosin J
$C_{14}H_{17}ClO_2$ MW: 252.74 Property: mp 136-7°C.
Source: JUE. Ref: 6.

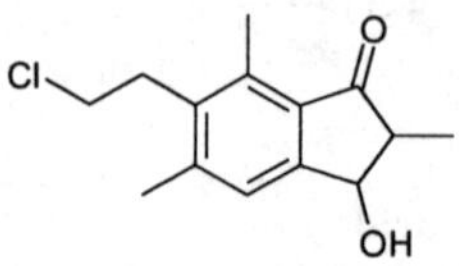

5391 Pterosin K
$C_{15}H_{19}ClO_2$ MW: 266.77 Property: mp 85-7°C.
Source: JUE. Ref: 6.

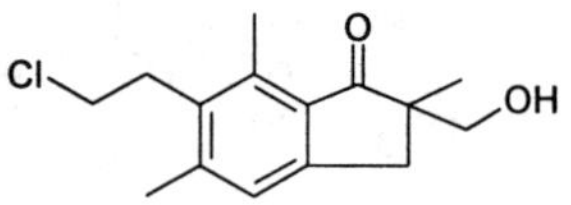

5392 Pterosin L
$C_{15}H_{20}O_4$ MW: 264.32 Property: mp 139-41°C.
Source: JUE. Ref: 6.

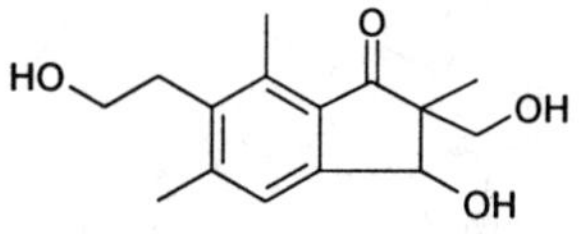

5393 Pterosin Z
$C_{15}H_{20}O_2$ MW: 232.33 Property: mp 86-88°C.
Source: JUE. Ref: 6.

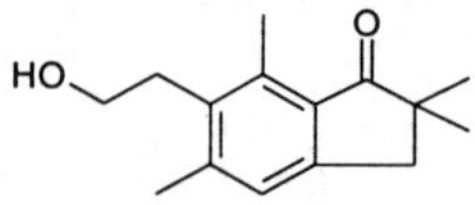

5394 Pterosterone
$C_{27}H_{44}O_7$ MW: 480.65 Property: mp 229-30°C.
Source: GUAN ZHONG, JUE, LUO YAN CAO.
Ref: 6.

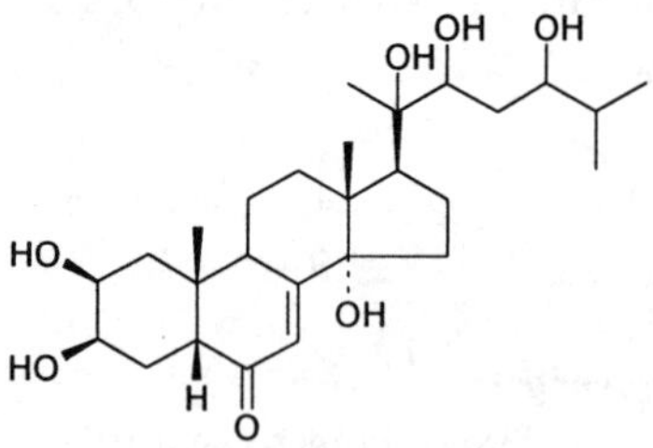

5395 Pterostilbene
$C_{16}H_{16}O_3$ MW: 256.30 Property: mp 86°C. Source: GUANG XI XUE JIE, ZI TAN. Ref: 6, 616.

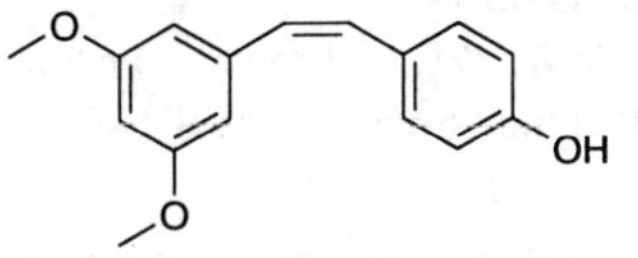

5396 Pteryxin
$C_{21}H_{22}O_7$ MW: 386.41 Property: mp 82°C, 87-8°C. Source: LI JIANG QIAN HU, *Pteryxia terebinthina* (Hook.) Coulter. Ref: 4, 557.

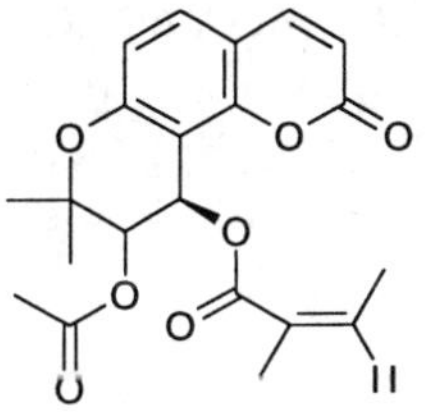

5397 Puerarin
CAS: 3681-99-0 $C_{21}H_{20}O_9$ MW: 416.39 Property: mp 187°C (dec). Source: GE GEN. Ref: 4.

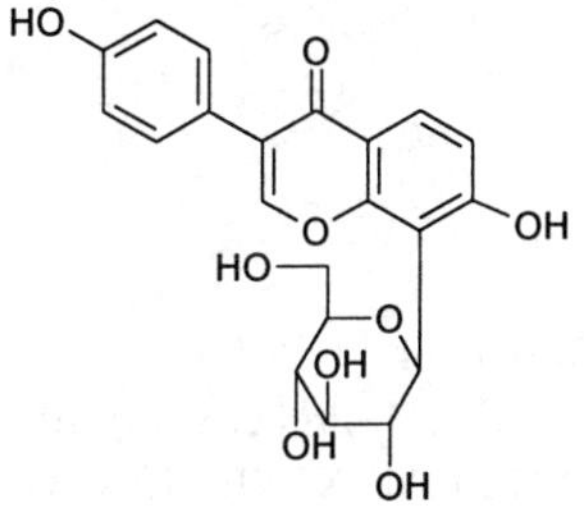

5398 Puerarin-xyloside
Source: GE GEN. Ref: 2.

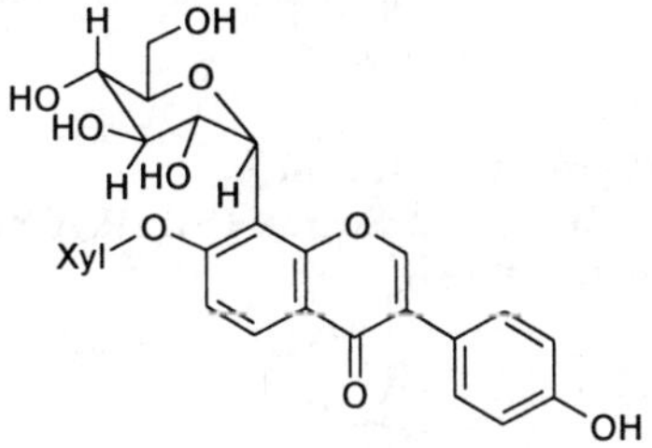

5399 Puerarol
$C_{26}H_{26}O_5$ MW: 418.49 Source: GE GEN. Ref: 2.

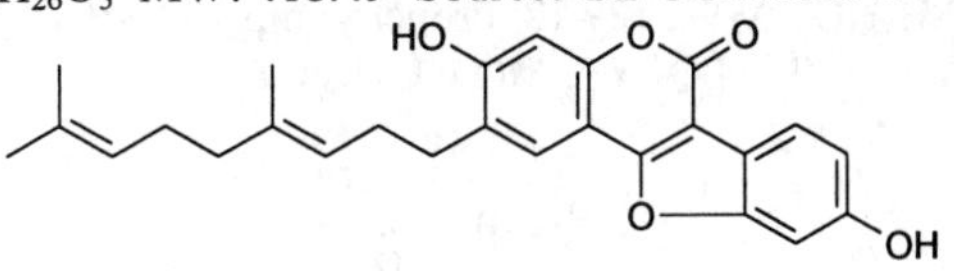

5400 Pukeensine
$C_{44}H_{64}N_2O_3$ MW: 669.01 Property: amorphous powder. Source: PU GE WU TOU. Ref: 229.

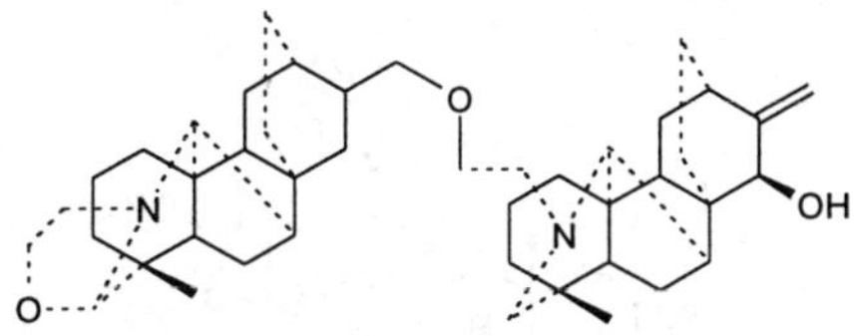

5401 Pulchinenoside A
Source: BAI TOU WENG. Ref: 2.

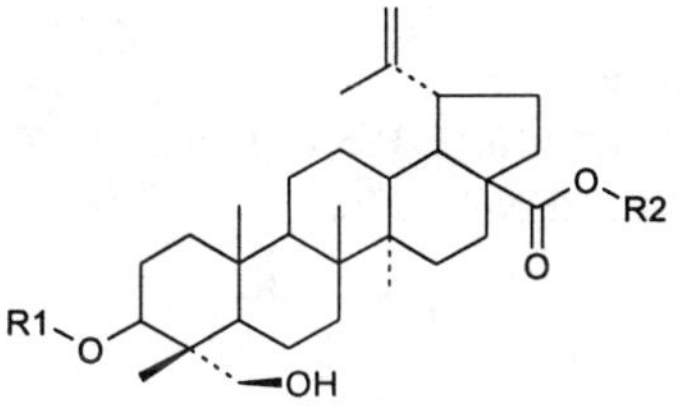

R1=α-L-Rha-(1→2)-α-L-Ara- R2=H

5402 Pulchinenoside B
Source: BAI TOU WENG. Ref: 2.

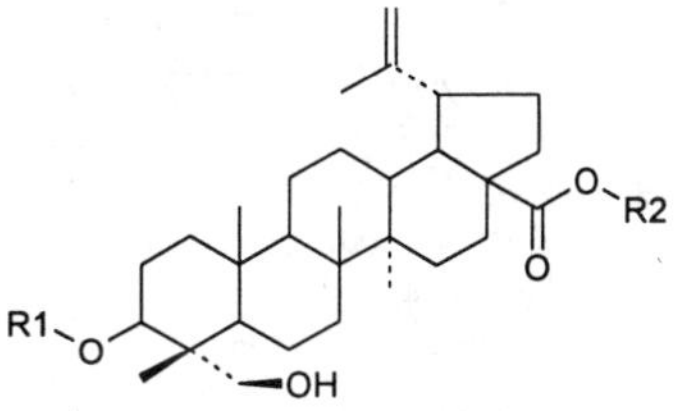

R1=α-L-Ara
R2=α-L-Rha-(1→4)-β-D-Glc-(1→6)-β-Glc-

5403 Pulchinenoside C
Source: BAI TOU WENG. Ref: 2.

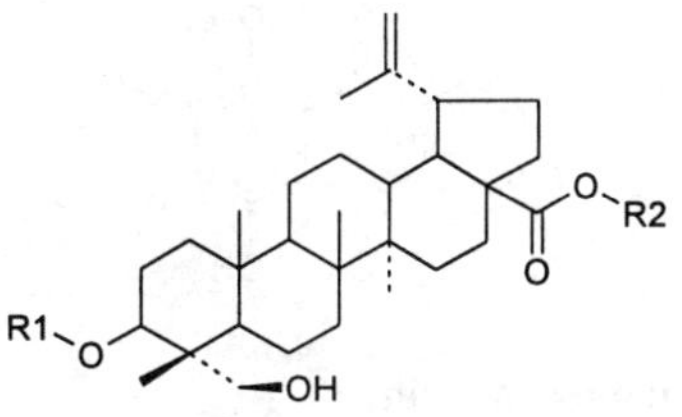

R1=α-L-Rha-(1→2)-α-L-Ara-
R2=α-L-Rha-(1→4)-β-D-Glc-(1→6)-β-Glc-

5404 Pulegone
$C_{10}H_{16}O$ MW: 152.24 Property: bp (+): 224°C, (-): 109°C/20mm. Source: CHAI HU, JIU LI XIANG, XI YANG SHEN. Ref: 2, 11.

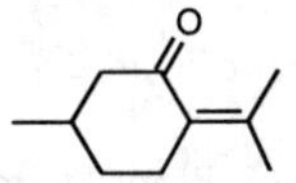

5405 Pulsatillic acid
$C_{30}H_{46}O_4$ MW: 470.70 Source: Ref: BAI TOU WONG. Ref: 2.

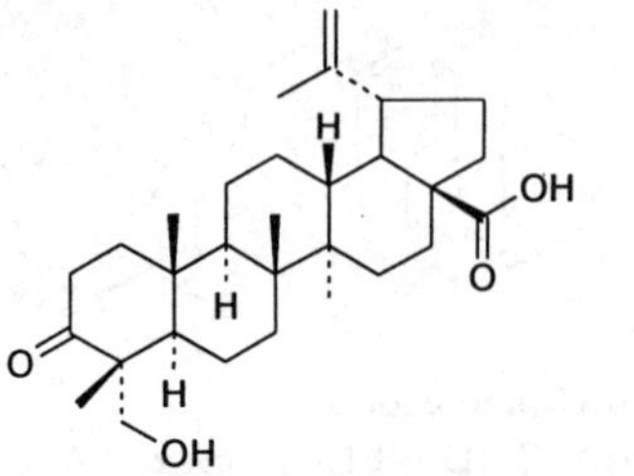

5406 Purine
$C_5H_4N_4$ MW: 120.11 Property: mp 216-7°C. Source: LUO HUA SHENG. Ref: 6.

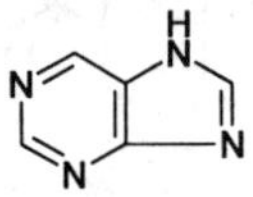

5407 Purpureaside C
Source: GAN DI HUANG. Ref: 2.

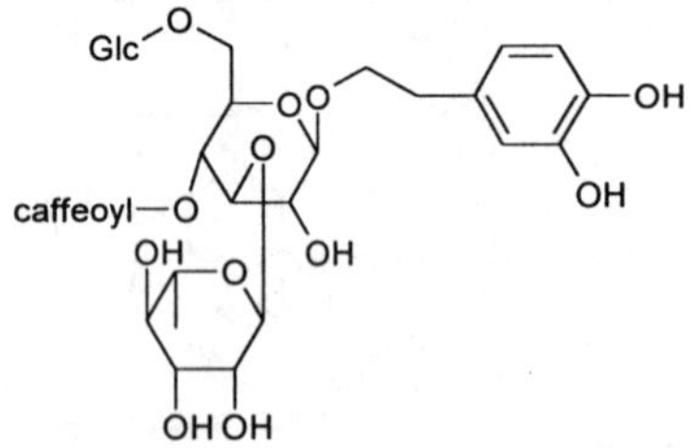

5408 Purpurin
$C_{14}H_8O_5$ MW: 256.22 Property: mp 263°C. Source: QIAN CAO GEN. Ref: 6.

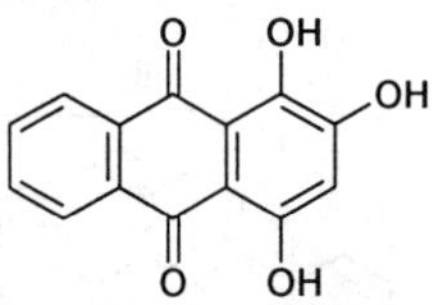

5409 Purpuroxanthin
$C_{14}H_8O_4$ MW: 240.22 Property: mp 268-70°C. Source: YANG JIAO TENG. Ref: 6.

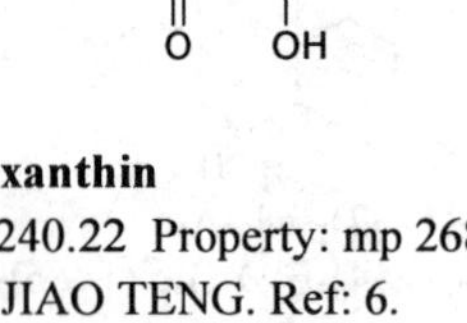

5410 Putrescine
$C_4H_{12}N_2$ MW: 88.15 Property: mp 27-8°C, bp 158-9°C. Source: JIANG. Ref: 6.

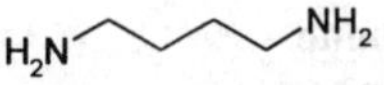

5411 Pyrethrin I
$C_{21}H_{28}O_3$ MW: 328.46 Property: bp 146-50°C/0.0005 mm. Source: BAI SHAO YAO. Ref: 6.

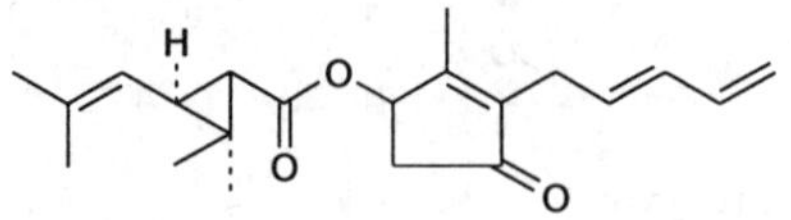

5412 Pyrethrin II
$C_{22}H_{28}O_5$ MW: 372.47 Property: bp 192-3°C/0.007 mm. Source: BAI SHAO YAO. Ref: 6.

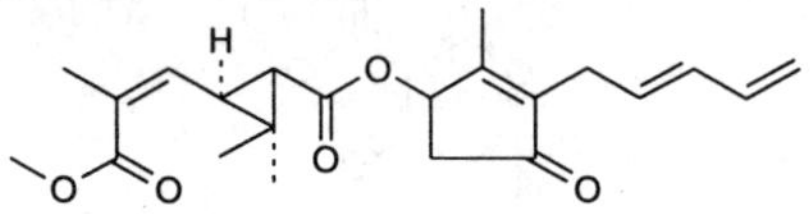

5413 Pyridoxine
Vitamin B_6. $C_8H_{11}NO_3$ MW: 169.18 Property: mp 160°C (sub). Source: BA JIAO HUI XIANG, GAN ZHE, FENG MI, MO GU, NIU RU, YU SHU SHU. Ref: 6.

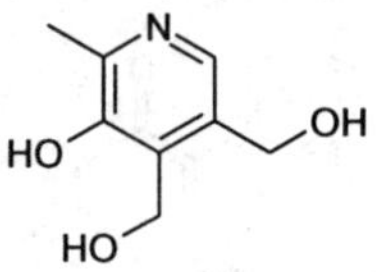

5414 Pyrocatechol
$C_6H_6O_2$ MW: 110.11 Property: mp 105°C, bp 240°C. Source: DENG ZHAN XI XIN, LIANG YE HUA PI, SI GUA ZI, XI FAN LIAN. Ref: 6.

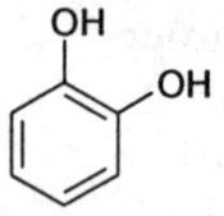

5415 o-Pyrocatechuic acid
$C_7H_6O_4$ MW: 154.12 Source: BAI HUA YING SHAN HONG. Ref: 6.

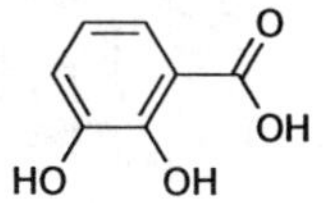

5416 Pyroglutamic acid
$C_5H_7NO_3$ MW: 129.12 Property: mp 182-3°C. Source: GOU QI YE, MO GU. Ref: 6.

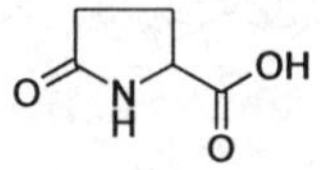

5417 Pyroglutamyl glucosamine
$C_{11}H_{18}N_2O_7$ MW: 290.28 Source: MO GU. Ref: 6.

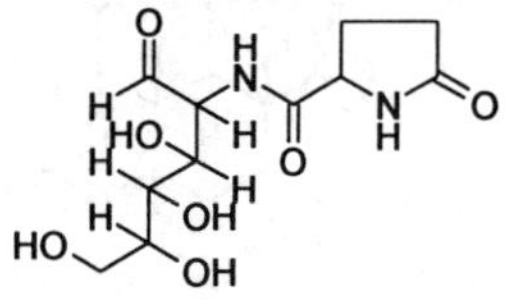

5418 Pyromeconic acid
$C_5H_4O_3$ MW: 112.09 Property: mp 117°C, bp 227-8°C. Source: YI NIAN PENG. Ref: 6, 415.

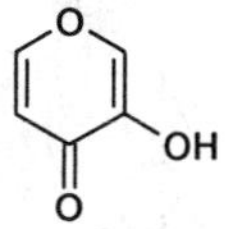

5419 Pyroracemic acid
$C_3H_4O_3$ MW: 88.06 Source: PU HUANG, REN SHEN. Ref: 2.

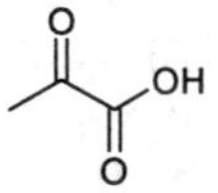

5420 Pyrrole-2-aldehyde
C_5H_5NO MW: 95.10 Property: mp 46-7°C. Source: CHA YE. Ref: 6.

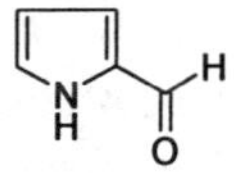

5421 Pyrrolidine
C_4H_9N MW: 71.12 Property: mp 88.5-9°C. Source: HU LUO BO, HE SHI FENG. Ref: 6.

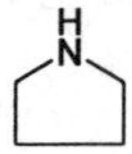

5422 Pyrrolidine carboxylic acd
$C_5H_9NO_2$ MW: 115.13 Property: mp (+): 215-20°C (dec), (-): 220-2°C (dec), (±): 213°C. Source: WU HUA GUO. Ref: 6.

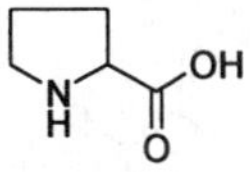

5423 Pyrryl-α-methyl ketone
C_6H_7NO MW: 109.13 Source: XIE CAO. Ref: 6.

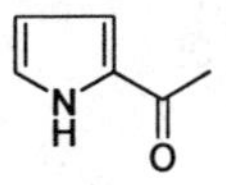

5424 Qianhucoumarin A
3'(R)-Hydroxy-4'(R)-tigloyloxy-3',4'-dihydroseslin. $C_{19}H_{20}O_6$ MW: 344.37 Property: white prismatic crystal, mp 123-6°C, $[\alpha]_D^{20}$ +209.6° (c=0.5, $CHCl_3$). Source: BAI HUA QIAN HU. Ref: 268.

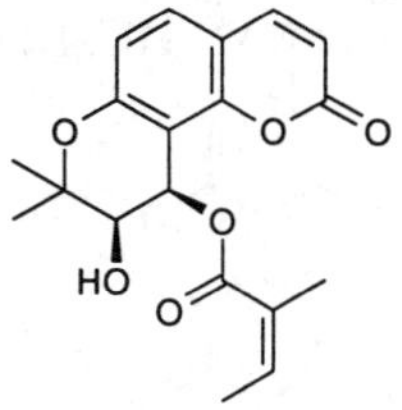

5425 Qianhucoumarin B
3'(S)-Acetoxy-4'(S)-hydroxy-3',4'-dihydroseselin. $C_{16}H_{16}O_6$ MW: 304.30 Property: color-less crystal (petroleum spirit-acetic ester), mp 159-61°C, $[\alpha]_D^{20}$ +3.9° (c=1.0, $CHCl_3$). Source: BAI HUA QIAN HU. Ref: 281.

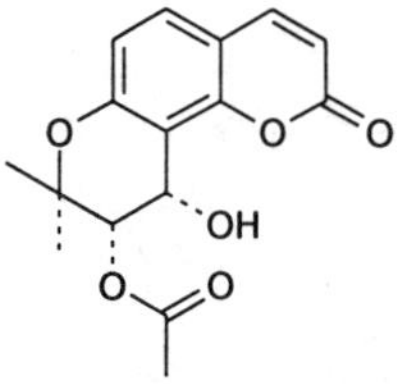

5426 Qianhucoumarin C
3'(S)-Hydroxy-4'(S)-acetoxy-3',4'-dihydroseselin. $C_{16}H_{16}O_6$ MW: 304.30 Property: color-less crystal (petroleum spirit-acetic ester), mp 186-8°C, $[\alpha]_D^{20}$ +7.6° (c=1.0, $CHCl_3$). Source: BAI HUA QIAN HU. Ref: 281.

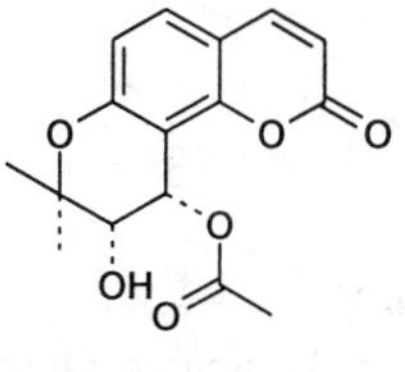

5427 Qianhucoumarin D
3'(S),4'(S)-Diacetoxy-3',4'-dihydroseselin. $C_{18}H_{18}O_7$ MW: 346.34 Property: colorless prismatic crystal, mp 160.5-2.5°C, $[\alpha]_D^{20}$ +4.0° (c=1.0, chloroform). Source: BAI HUA QIAN HU. Ref: 289.

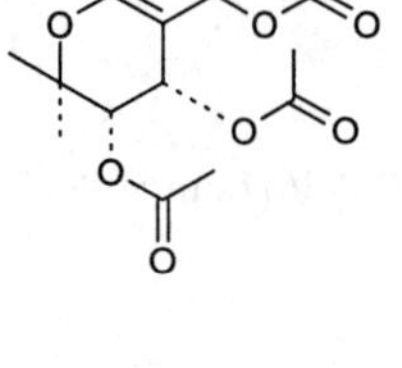

5428 Qianhucoumarin E
3'(R)-Tigloyloxy-4'-keto-3',4'-dihydroseselin. $C_{19}H_{18}O_6$ MW: 342.35 Property: colorless prismatic crystal, mp 103.5-5.5°C, $[\alpha]_D^{20}$ +19.6° (c=1.0, chloroform). Source: BAI HUA QIAN HU. Ref: 289.

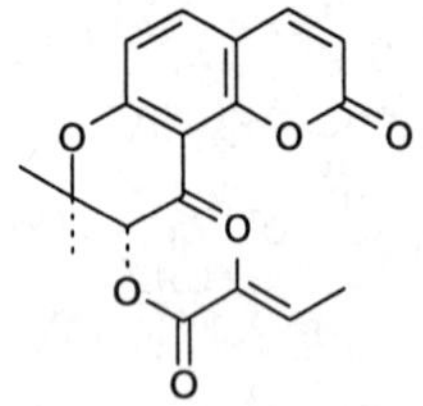

5429 Qingdainone
Indolo[2,1b]-quinazoline-6,12-dione. $C_{23}H_{13}N_3O_2$ MW: 363.39 Property: dark purple acicular crystal, mp 273-80°C. Source: LIAO LAN. Ref: 21.

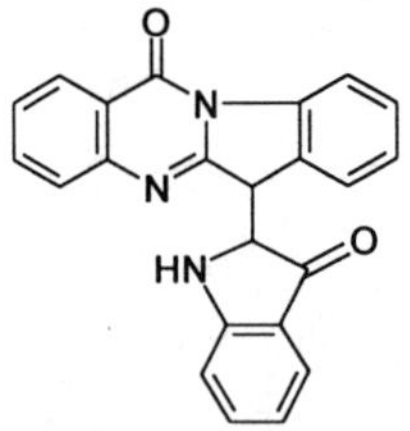

5430 Qinghaosu IV
$C_{15}H_{22}O_5$ MW: 282.34 Source: QING HAO. Ref: 2.

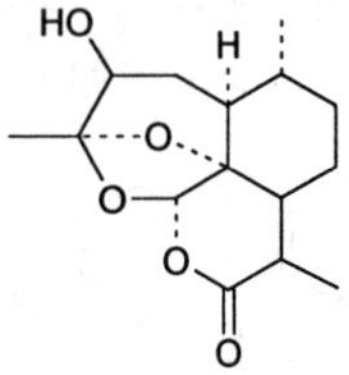

5431 Qinghaosu V
$C_{15}H_{22}O_3$ MW: 250.34 Source: QING HAO. Ref: 2.

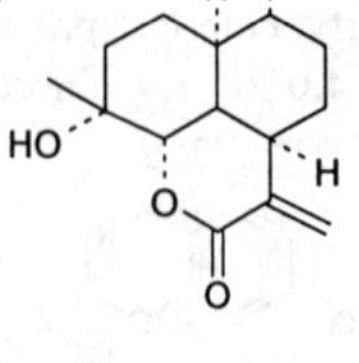

5432 Quassin
$C_{22}H_{28}O_6$ MW: 388.46 Source: KU SHU PI. Ref: 12.

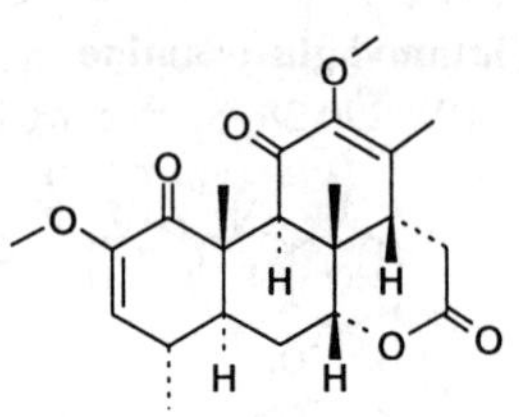

5433 L-Quebrachitol
$C_7H_{14}O_6$ MW: 194.19 Property: mp (-): 191°C. Source: AI YE. Ref: 6.

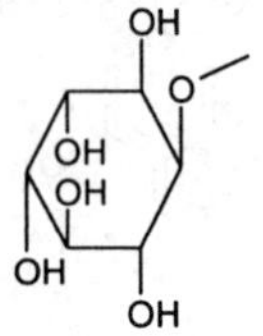

5434 Quercetagetin
$C_{15}H_{10}O_8$ MW: 318.28 Property: mp 318-20°C. Source: DA BAI DING CAO, HAI ER CHA, KONG QUE CAO. Ref: 6.

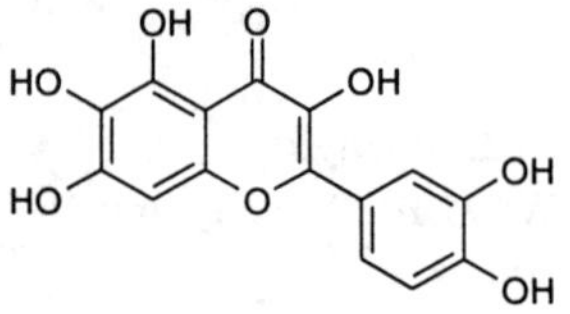

5435 Quercetagetin-3,4'-dimethyl ether
$C_{17}H_{14}O_8$ MW: 346.30 Source: QING HAO. Ref: 2.

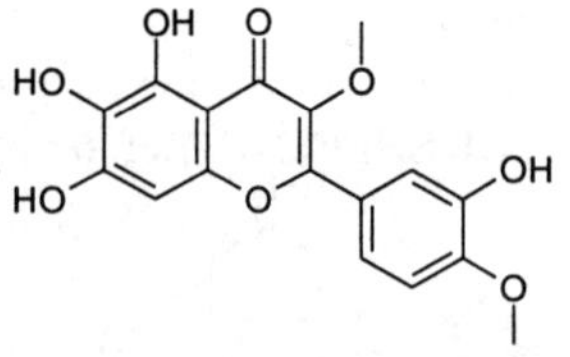

5436 Quercetagetin-3-galactoside
$C_{21}H_{20}O_{13}$ MW: 480.39 Property: mp 200°C. Source: DI YANG QUE. Ref: 6.

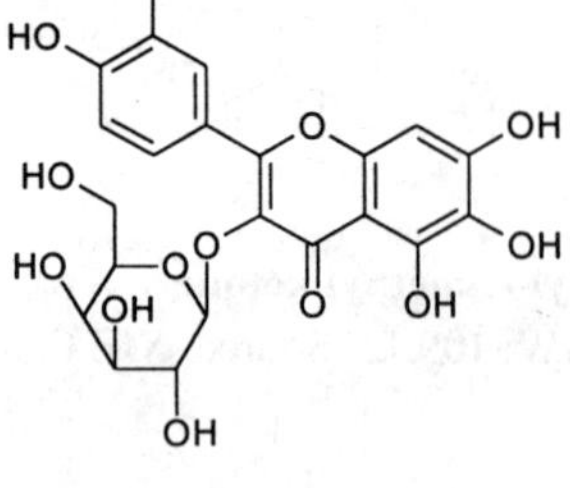

5437 Quercetagetin-6,7,3',4'-tetramethyl ether
$C_{19}H_{18}O_9$ MW: 390.35 Source: Ref: 2.

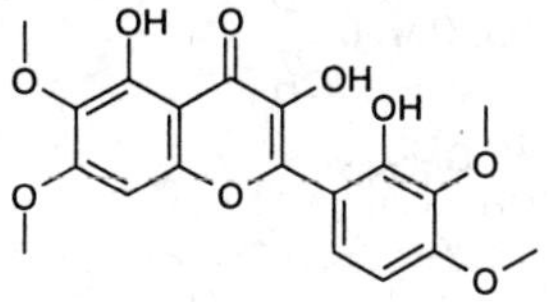

5438 Quercetagitrin
$C_{21}H_{20}O_{13}$ MW: 480.39 Property: mp 236-238°C (dec). Source: DA BAI DING CAO, KONG QUE CAO. Ref: 6.

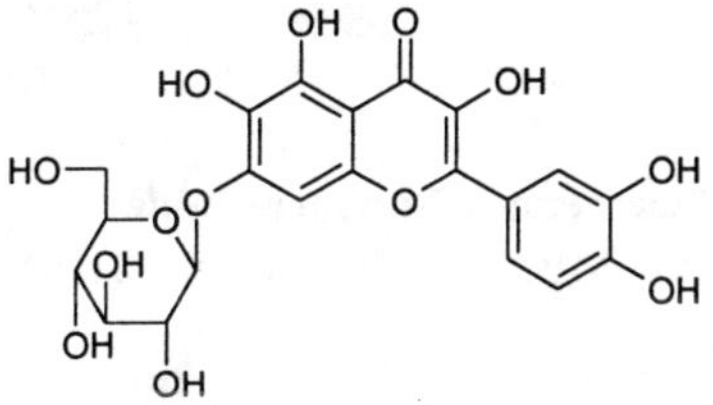

5439 Quercetin
Meletin; Sophoretin. CAS: 117-39-5 $C_{15}H_{10}O_7$ MW: 302.24 Property: yellow acicular crystal (methanol), mp 313-4°C. Source: BAI GUO, CU LIU GUO (SHA JI), BIAN TAO, DA JIN QIAN CAO, HU ZHANG, JIN LONG DAN CAO, JIN QIAO MAI, LI JIANG QIAN HU, MU ZEI, NAN FANG TU SI ZI, PU GONG YING, PU HUANG, QING HAO, SAN QI, XIAN HE CAO, YIN CHEN HAO, YIN YANG HUO, YU XING CAO. Ref: 2, 4, 468, 475, 550, 557, 594, 604, 615.

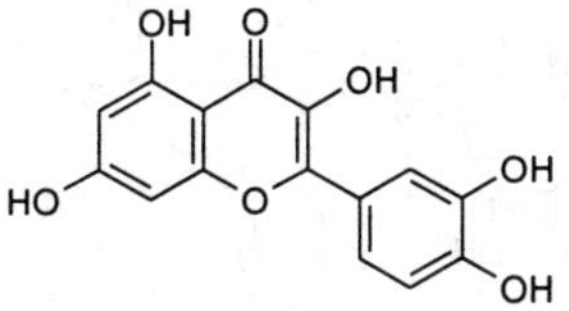

5440 Quercetin-3-L-arabino-7-D-glucoside
$C_{26}H_{28}O_{17}$ MW: 612.50 Source: MEI SHANG LU. Ref: 6.

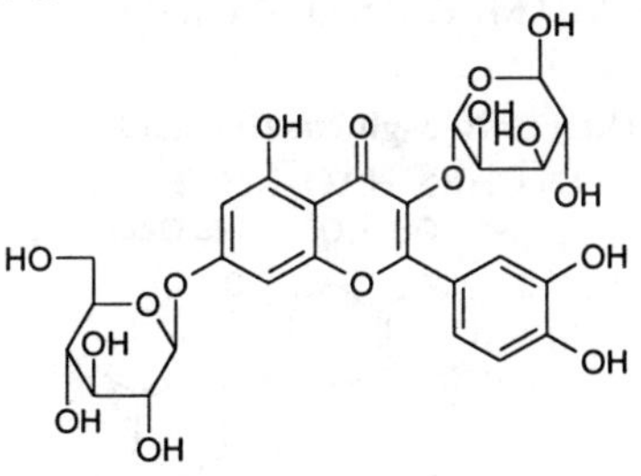

5441 Quercetin-3-O-α-L-arabinopyranoside
$C_{21}H_{20}O_{11}$ MW: 448.39 Property: yellow crystal, mp 166-8°C. Source: CHI ZI SHU. Ref: 433.

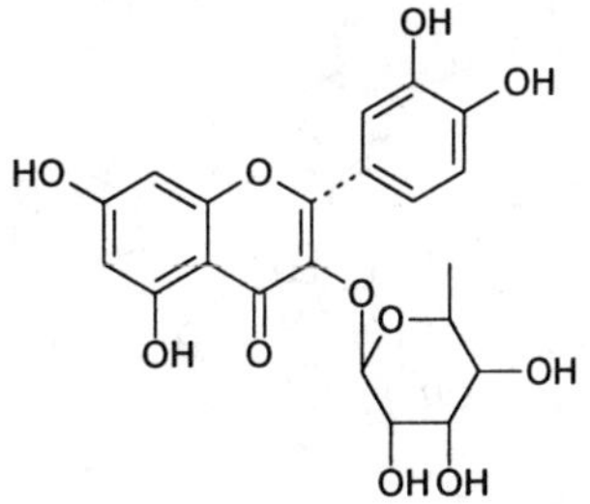

5442 Quercetin-3-O-arabinoside
$C_{20}H_{18}O_{11}$ MW: 434.36 Source: HE SHOU WU, HU ZHANG. Ref: 2.

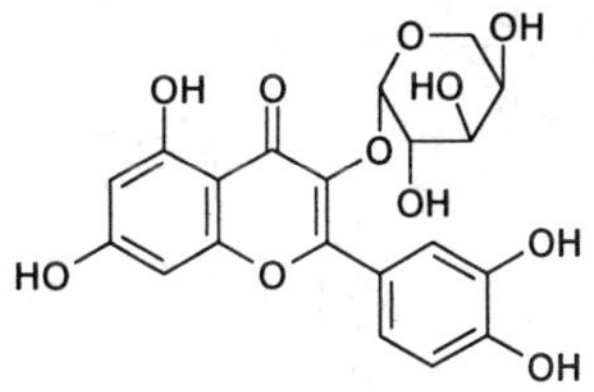

5443 Quercetin-3-diarabinoside
$C_{25}H_{26}O_{15}$ MW: 566.48 Source: LUO DI SHENG GEN. Ref: 6.

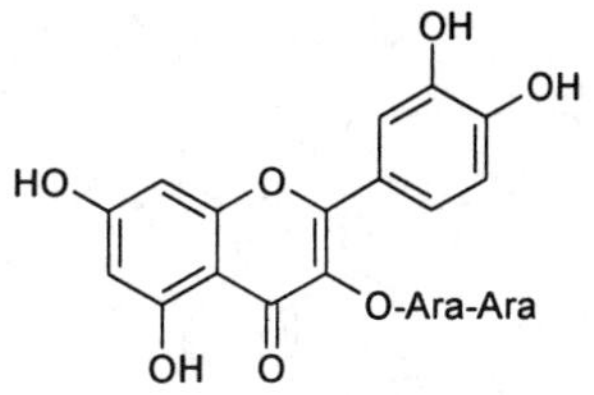

5444 Quercetin-5,3-di-D-galactoside
$C_{27}H_{30}O_{17}$ MW: 626.53 Property: mp 196-7°C, 219-20°C (solidifing), 270°C. Source: ZE QI. Ref: 6.

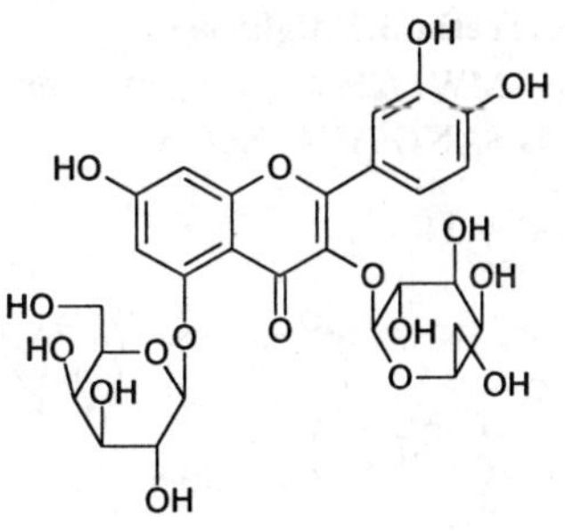

5445 Quercetin-3-diglucoside
$C_{27}H_{30}O_{17}$ MW: 626.53 Property: mp 182-4°C. Source: FU SANG HUA. Ref: 6.

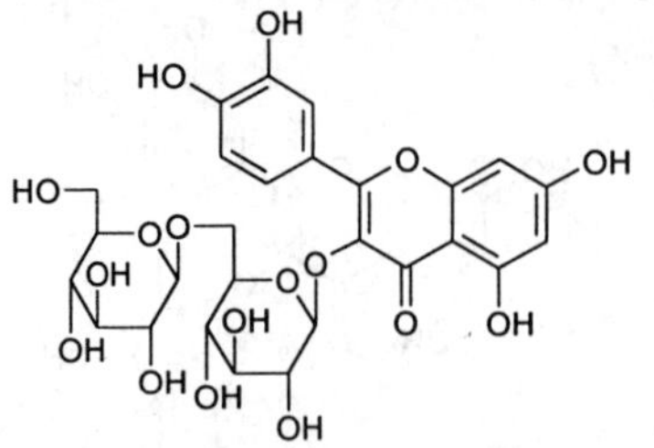

5446 Quercetin-3,4'-diglucoside
$C_{27}H_{30}O_{17}$ MW: 626.53 Source: HU CONG, YANG CONG. Ref: 6.

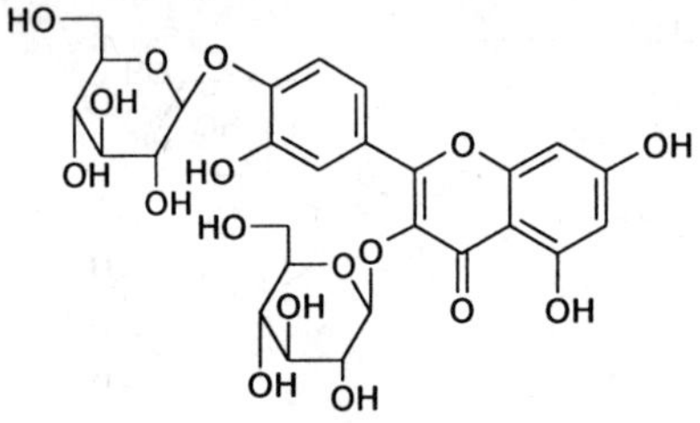

5447 Quercetin-3,5-diglucoside
$C_{27}H_{30}O_{17}$ MW: 626.53 Source: NING MENG. Ref: 6.

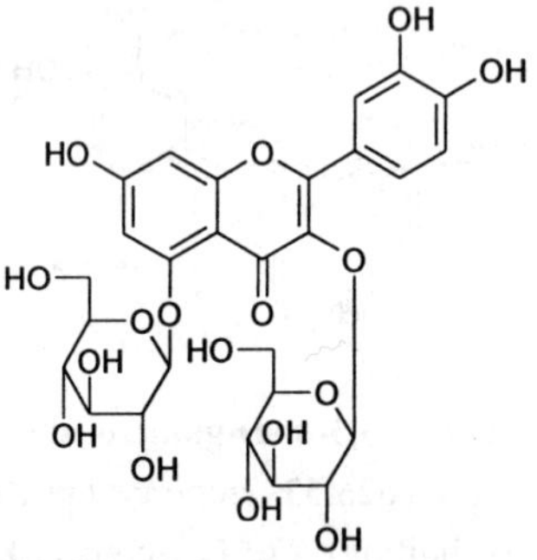

5448 Quercetin-3,7-diglucoside
$C_{27}H_{30}O_{17}$ MW: 626.53 Property: mp 218-20°C. Source: FU SANG HUA. Ref: 6.

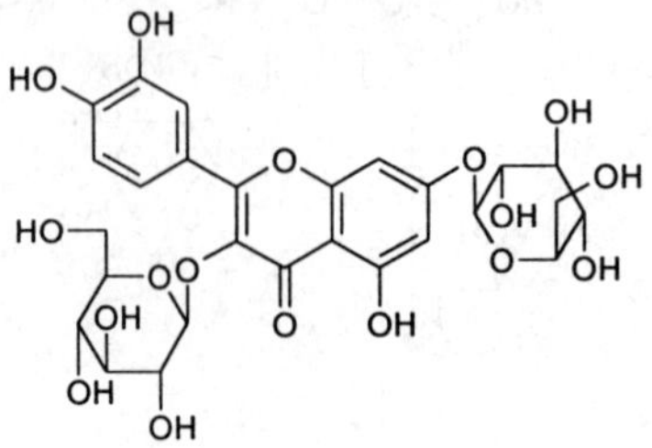

5449 Quercetin-7,4'-diglucoside
$C_{27}H_{30}O_{17}$ MW: 626.53 Source: HU CONG, YANG CONG. Ref: 6.

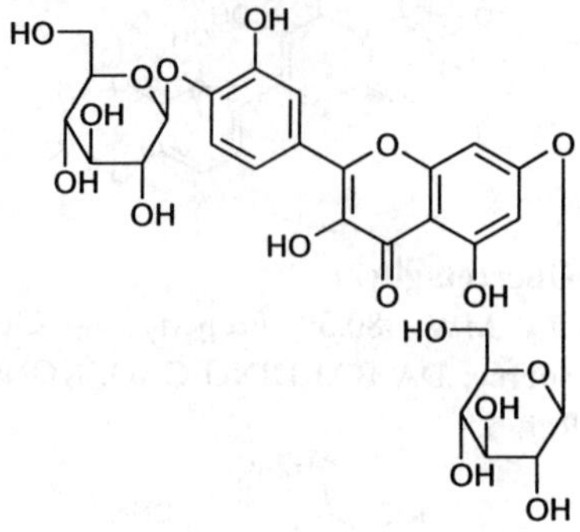

5450 Quercetin-3,7-diglucuronide
$C_{27}H_{26}O_{19}$ MW: 654.50 Source: JIN JIN BANG. Ref: 6.

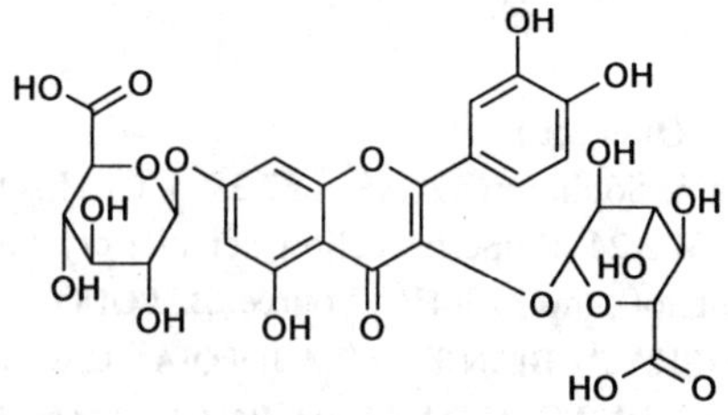

5451 Quercetin-3,7-α-L-dirhamnoside
$C_{27}H_{30}O_{15}$ MW: 594.53 Property: mp 185-6°C. Source: NAN SHE TENG YE. Ref: 6.

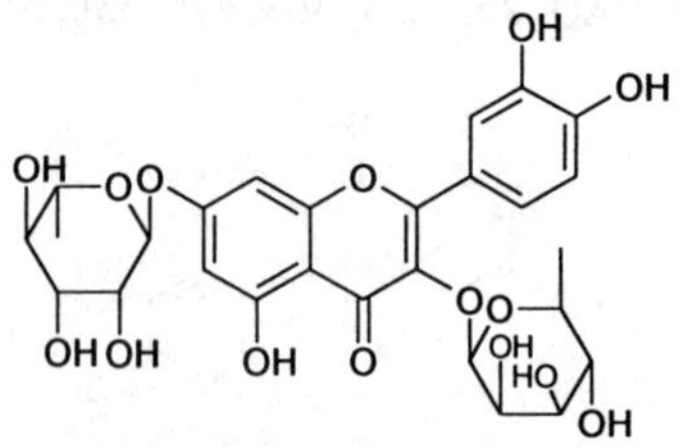

5452 Quercetin-3-O-(6''-galloyl)-β-D-glucoside
Source: XIU MAO JI SHENG. Ref: 559.

5453 Quercetin-3-glucogalactoside
Source: YIN CHEN HAO. Ref: 2.

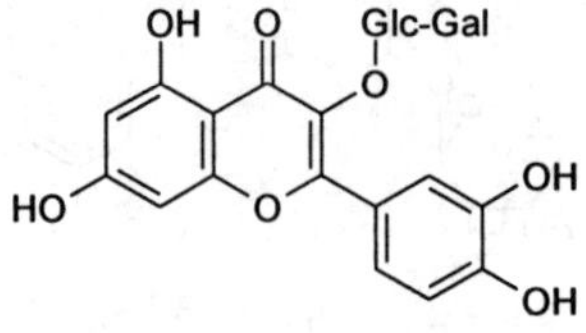

5454 Quercetin-3-β-D-gluco-7-α-L-rhamnoside
$C_{27}H_{30}O_{16}$ MW: 610.53 Property: mp 186-188°C. Source: DIAO JING CAO, NAN SHE TENG YE. Ref: 6.

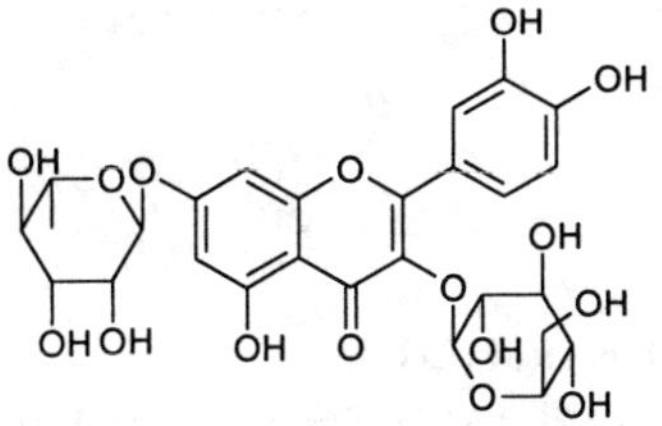

5455 Quercetin-4'-glucoside
$C_{21}H_{20}O_{12}$ MW: 464.39 Property: mp 211°C. Source: MU FU RONG HUA. Ref: 6.

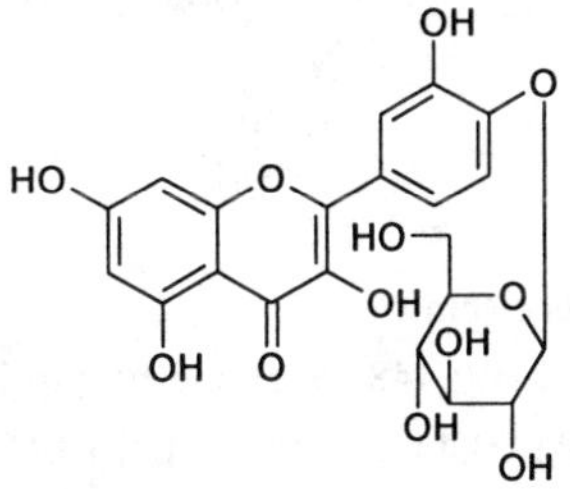

5456 Quercetin-3-O-glycoside
$C_{21}H_{20}O_{12}$ MW: 464.39 Source: DA JIN QIAN CAO, QING HAO. Ref: 2.

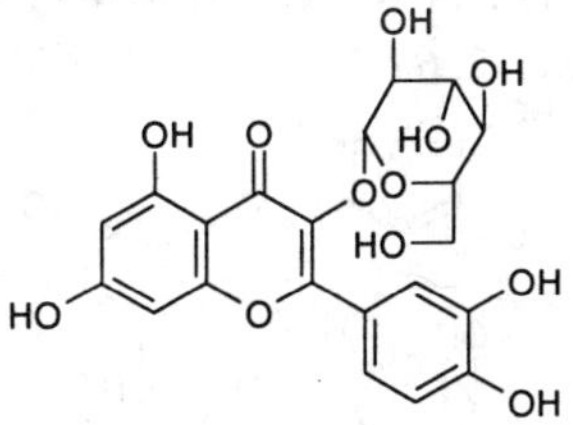

5457 Quercetin-3-O-malonyl-β-D-glucoside
$C_{24}H_{22}O_{15}$ MW: 550.43 Source: WO JU. Ref: 6.

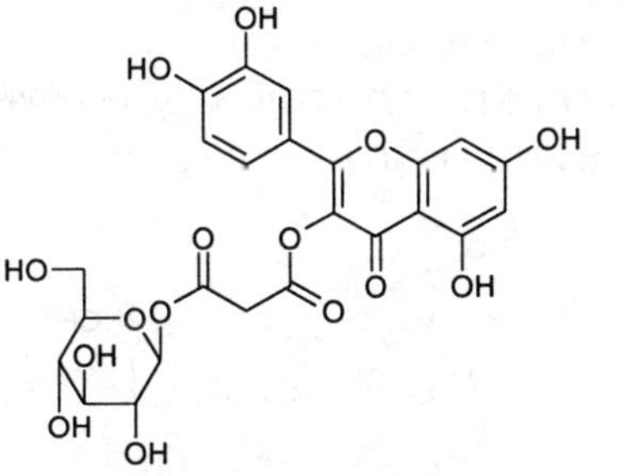

5458 Quercetin-3-methyl ether
$C_{16}H_{12}O_7$ MW: 316.27 Source: QING HAO. Ref: 2, 6.

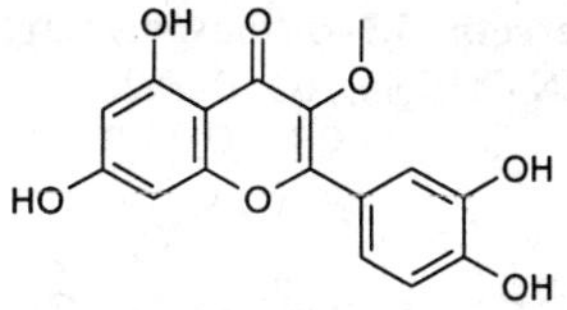

5459 Quercetin-3-O-neohesperidoside
Source: PU HUANG. Ref: 2.

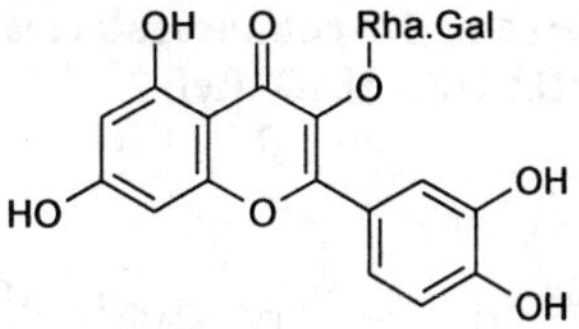

5460 Quercetin-3-α-L-rhamnofurancside
$C_{21}H_{20}O_{11}$ MW: 448.39 Source: GUI JIAN JIN JI ER. Ref: 6.

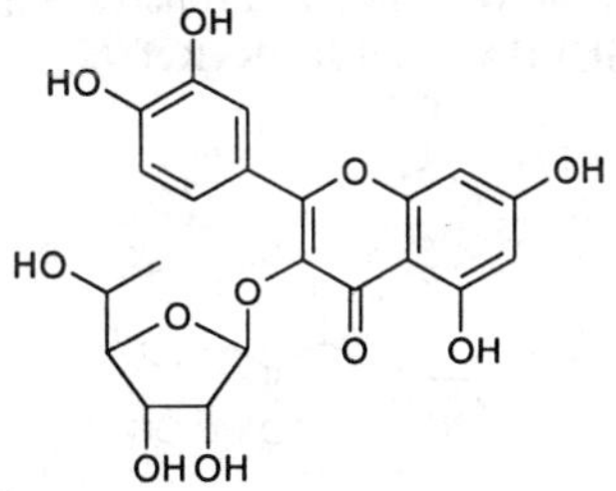

5461 Quercetin-3-rhamnoside
$C_{21}H_{20}O_{11}$ MW: 448.39 Source: HU ZHANG. Ref: 2.

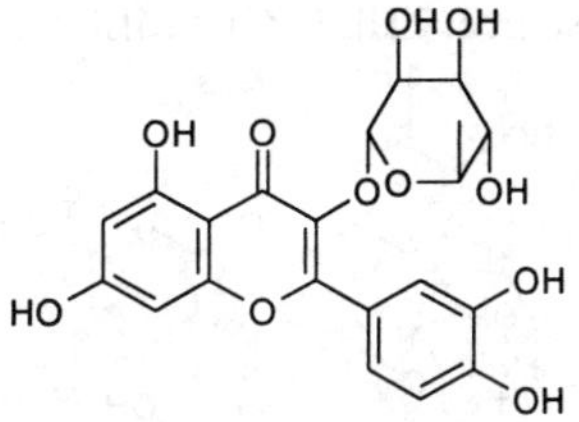

5462 Quercetin-3-rhamnoside-7-glucoside
$C_{27}H_{30}O_{16}$ MW: 610.53 Source: MIAN TENG. Ref: 6.

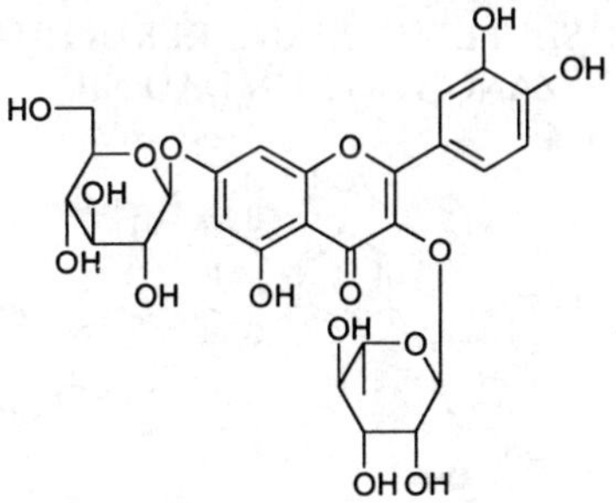

5463 Quercetin-3,7-rutinosodigalactoside
Source: YIN CHEN HAO. Ref: 2.

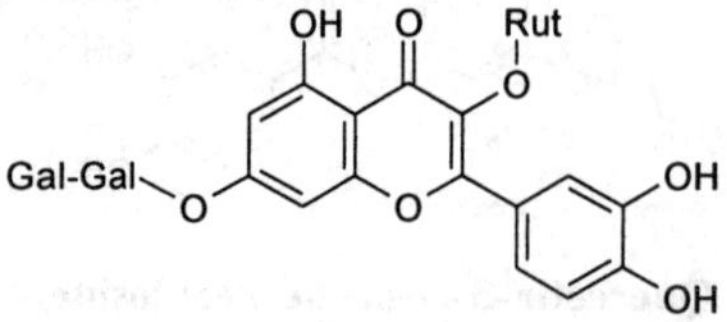

5464 Quercetin-3,7-rutinosogalactoside
Source: YIN CHEN HAO. Ref: 2.

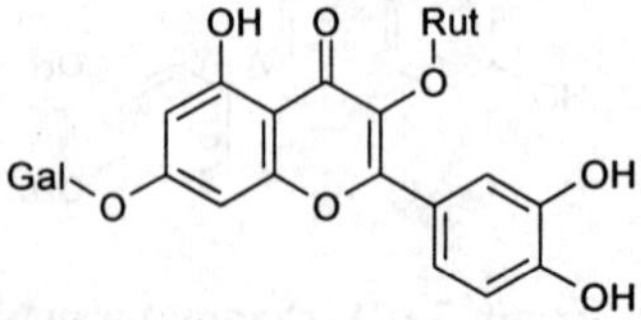

5465 Quercetin-3-β-D-xylopyranoside
$C_{20}H_{18}O_{11}$ MW: 434.36 Property: mp 210-1°C. Source: GUI JIAN JIN JI ER. Ref: 6.

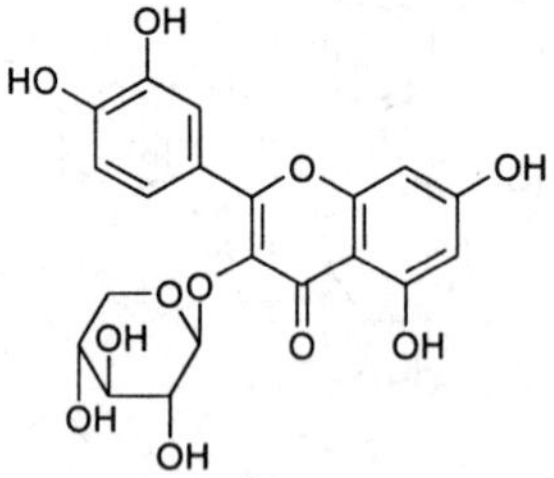

5466 Quercetin-3-xyloside
Reynoutrin. $C_{20}H_{18}O_{11}$ MW: 434.36 Property: mp 203-4°C. Source: ZHEN ZHU MEI. Ref: 6.

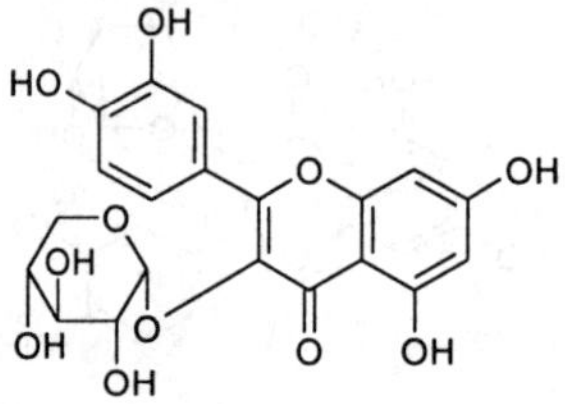

5467 Quercimeritrin
$C_{21}H_{20}O_{12}$ MW: 464.39 Property: mp 247-9°C. Source: LIANG QI LIAO, MU FU RONG HUA, MU JU, SHUI LIAO, XIANG RI KUI HUA, YE ZHI MA, ZANG YAO XUN DAO NIU. Ref: 6, 324.

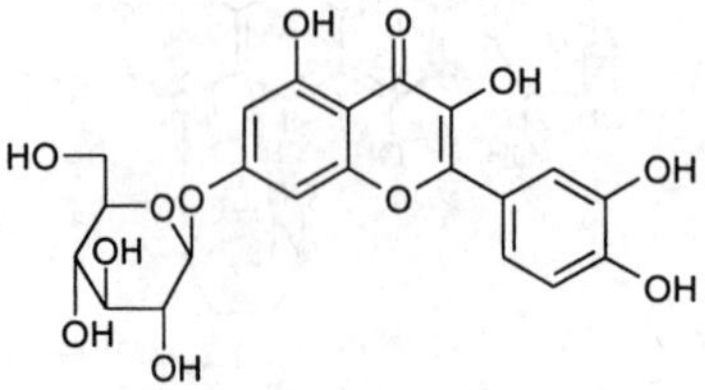

5468 Quercitol (D-)
$C_6H_{12}O_5$ MW: 164.16 Property: mp 235-7°C. Source: DA HONG PAO, HU CONG, RU LAN, XI SHENG TENG. Ref: 6.

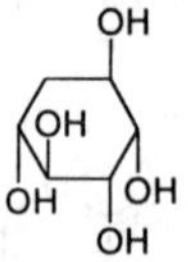

5469 Quercitol (L-)
$C_6H_{12}O_5$ MW: 164.16 Property: mp 180-1°C. Source: DA HONG PAO, HU CONG, RU LAN, XI SHENG TENG. Ref: 6.

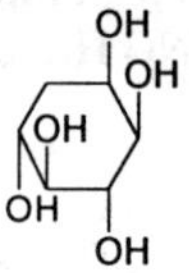

5470 Quercitrin
$C_{21}H_{20}O_{11}$ MW: 448.39 Property: mp 182-5°C. Source: BAI GUO YE, DUO HUI LIAO, LONG YAN YE, PIAN XU, SAN BAI CAO, SHAN YING TAO, SHUI LIAO, SHUI MA DIAO, TIAN QIAO MAI GENG, YI ZHI HUANG HUA, YANG TI YE, YUN TAI, YU XING CAO, ZI JIN NIU, etc. Ref: 2, 6.

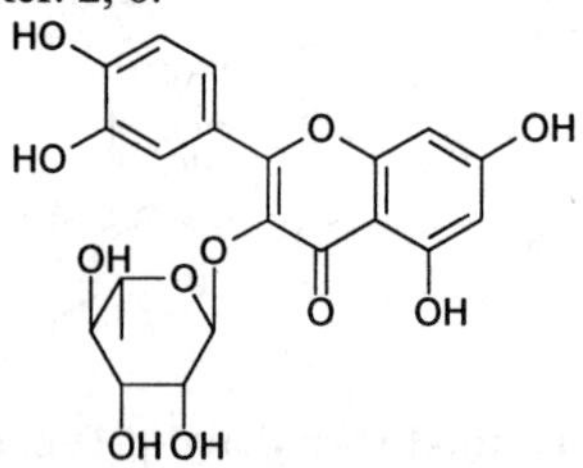

5471 Querciturone
$C_{21}H_{18}O_{13}$ MW: 478.37 Property: mp 190°C. Source: ZHU ZONG CAO. Ref: 6.

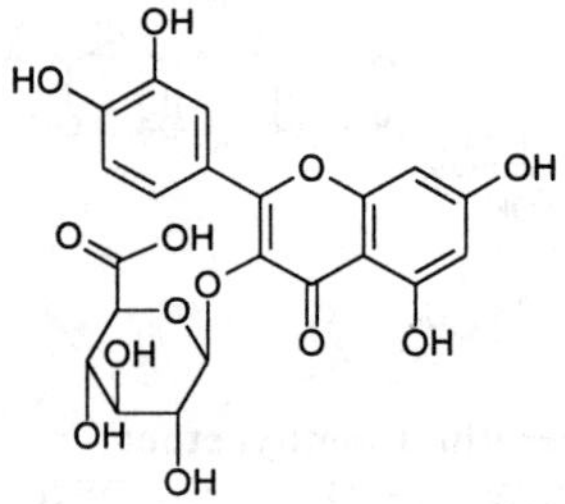

5472 Queretaroic avid
$C_{30}H_{48}O_4$ MW: 472.71 Property: mp 318-23°C. Source: SAN TAI HONG HUA. Ref: 6.

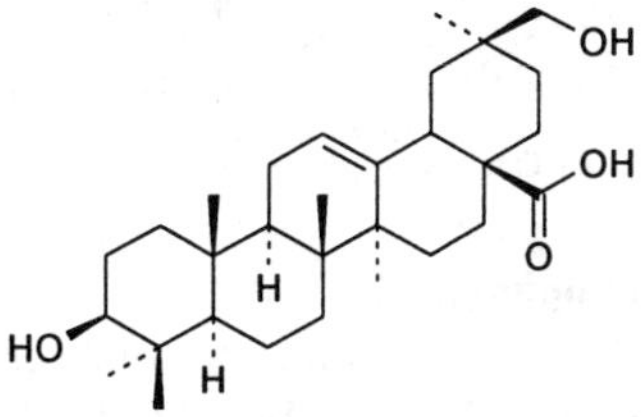

5473 Questin
$C_{16}H_{12}O_5$ MW: 284.27 Source: HU ZHANG. Ref: 2.

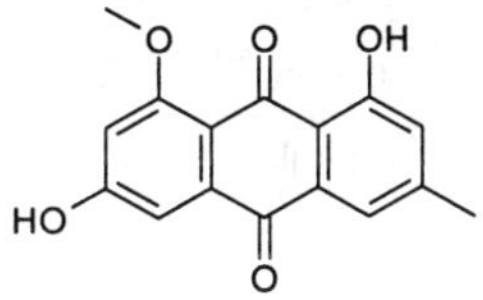

5474 Questinol
$C_{16}H_{12}O_6$ MW: 300.27 Source: HU ZHANG. Ref: 2.

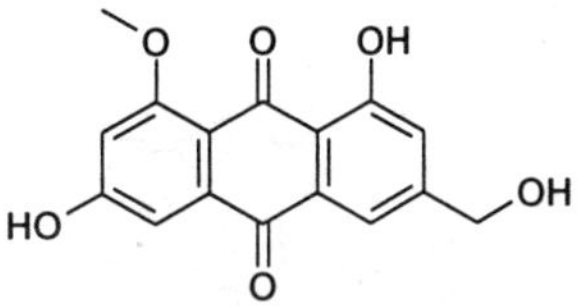

5475 Quinamine
$C_{19}H_{24}N_2O_2$ MW: 312.42 Property: mp 185-6°C. Source: JIN JI LE. Ref: 6.

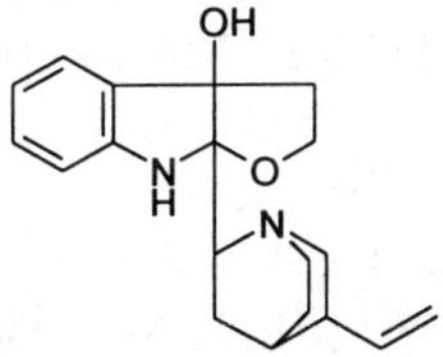

5476 4-Quinazolone
$C_8H_6N_2O$ MW: 146.15 Property: mp 211-2°C. Source: CHANG SHAN. Ref: 6.

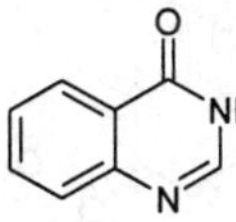

5477 Quinic acid
$C_7H_{12}O_6$ MW: 192.17 Property: mp (-): 172°C. Source: BAI GUO, HE ZI, HE ZI YE, HUI XIANG JING YE, JIN JI LE, MEI GUI HUA, NING MENG, NING MENG AN YE, PING GUO, PU TAO TENG YE, TAO YE, WU HUA GUO, XIANG RI KUI ZI, Ref: 2, 6.

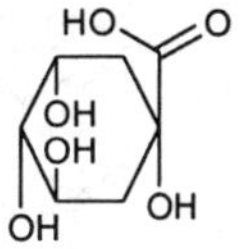

5478 Quinicine
$C_{20}H_{24}N_2O_2$ MW: 324.43 Property: mp (+): ≈60°C. Source: JIN JI LE. Ref: 6.

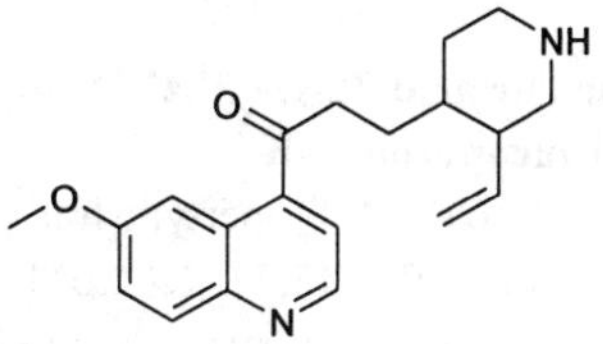

5479 Quinidine
β-Quinine; Pitayine. CAS: 56-54-2 $C_{20}H_{24}N_2O_2$ MW: 324.43 Property: mp (+): 174-5°C (anhydrate). Source: *Cinchona suceirubra* Pav. Ref: 4.

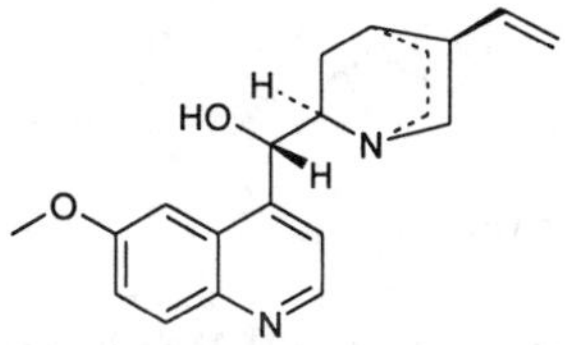

5480 Quinine
CAS: 56-54-2 $C_{20}H_{24}N_2O_2$ MW: 324.43 Property: mp 177°C (dec). Source: *Cinchona suceirubra* Pav. Ref: 4.

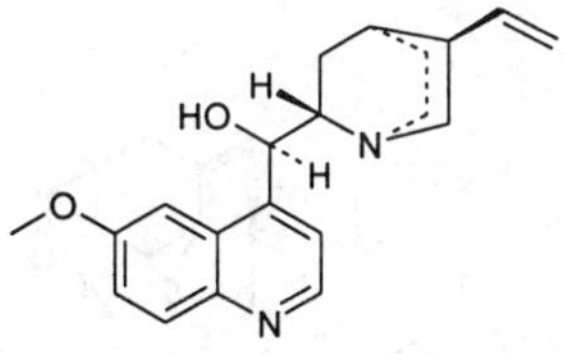

5481 Quininone
$C_{20}H_{22}N_2O_2$ MW: 322.41 Property: mp 108°C. Source: JIN JI LE. Ref: 6.

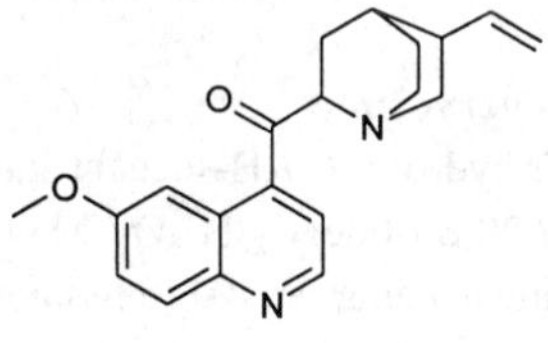

5482 Quinovic acid
$C_{30}H_{46}O_5$ MW: 486.70 Property: mp 298°C. Source: SHUI TUAN HUA. Ref: 6.

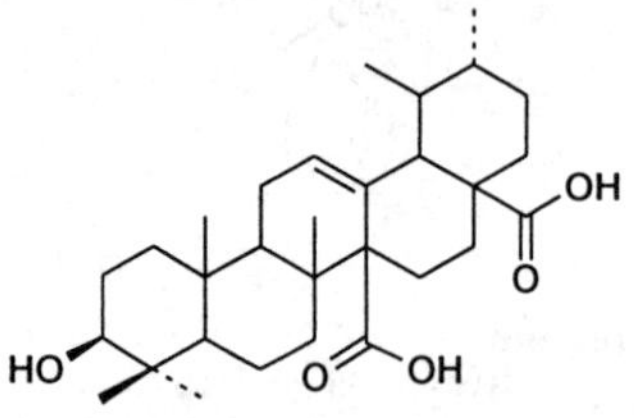

5483 Quinovic acid-3β-O-(3',4'-O-isopropylidene)-β-D-fucopyranoside
$C_{39}H_{60}O_9$ MW: 672.91 Property: white powder, mp 220°C (dec), $[\alpha]_D^{30}$ +48.77° (c=0.611, MeOH). Source: SHUI YANG MEI (II). Ref: 651.

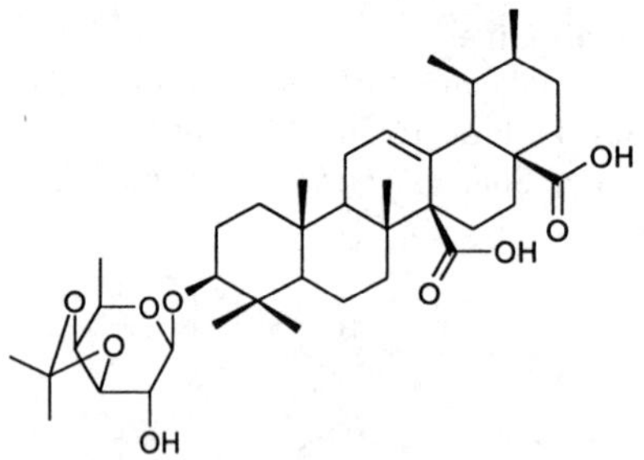

5484 Quinovic acid-3β-(2',3'-O-isopropylidene)-α-L-rhamnopyranoside
$C_{39}H_{60}O_9$ MW: 672.91 Property: white powder, mp 268-72°C (dec), $[\alpha]_D^{22}$ +47.29° (c=0.317, MeOH). Source: SHUI YANG MEI (II). Ref: 651.

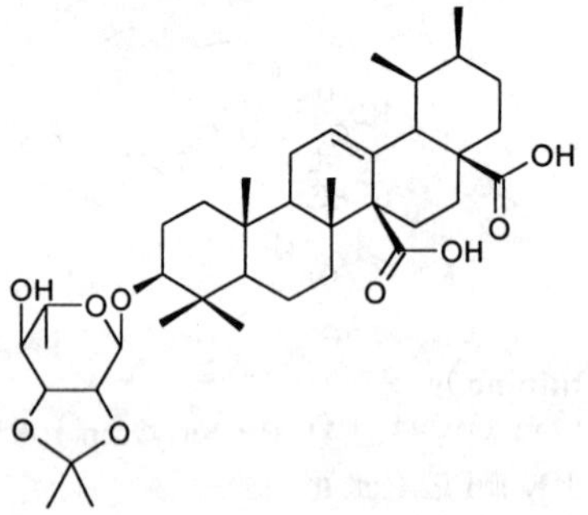

5485 Rabdonervosin A
1α,6β,15β-Trihydroxy-6,7-B-secoent-kaur-16-en-6,20-epoxy-7,20-δ-olide. $C_{20}H_{28}O_6$ MW: 364.44 Property: white acicular crystal (ethyl acetate), mp 312-4°C. Source: XIAN MAI XIANG CHA CAI. Ref: 496.

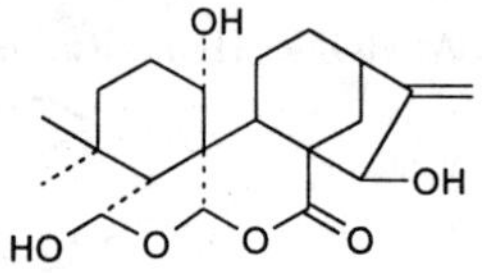

5486 Rabdophyllin H
$C_{24}H_{36}O_9$ MW: 468.55 Property: white crystal, mp 234-6°C. Source: DA YE XIANG CHA CAI. Ref: 45.

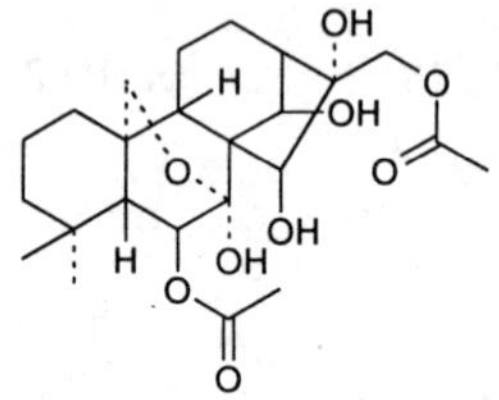

5487 Rabdoserrin A
$C_{20}H_{26}O_5$ MW: 346.43 Property: colorless lamellar crystal (chloroform-ethanol), mp 312-4°C, $[\alpha]_D^{20}$ -98.2° (c=1.4, DMF). Source: XI HUANG CAO. Ref: 29.

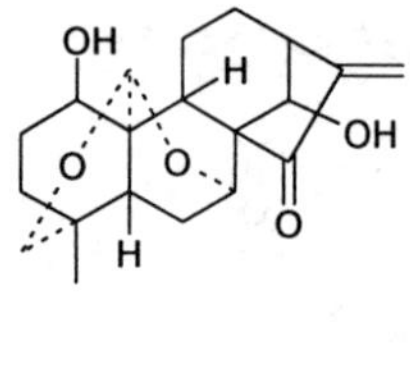

5488 Rabdosin A
CAS: 84304-91-6 $C_{21}H_{28}O_6$ Property: mp 200-202°C. Source: MAO YE XIANG CHA CAI. Ref: 5.

5489 Rabdosin B
CAS: 84304-91-7 $C_{24}H_{32}O_8$ MW: 448.52 Property: mp 182-4°C. Source: MAO YE XIANG CHA CAI. Ref: 5.

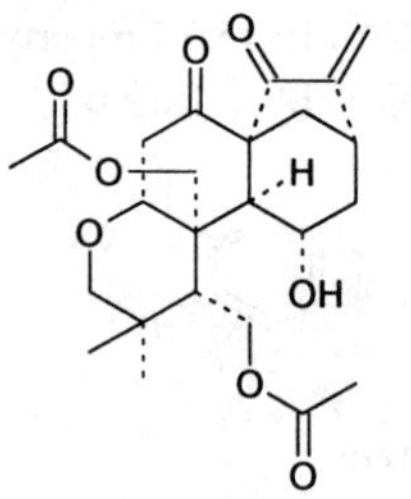

5490 Rabdosin C
CAS: 82460-75-1 $C_{22}H_{30}O_7$ MW: 406.48
Property: mp 266-8°C. Source: MAO YE XIANG CHA CAI. Ref: 5.

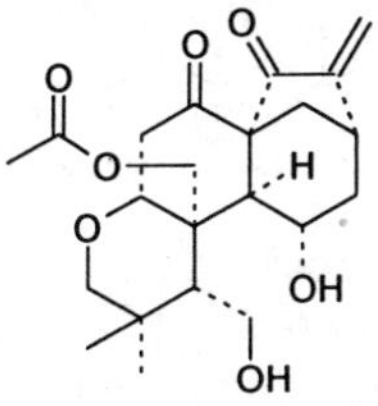

5491 Raddeanine
$C_{27}H_{43}NO_3$ MW: 429.65 Property: mp 265-7°C. Source: CHUAN BEI MU. Ref: 6.

5492 Radiatin
CAS: 25873-31-8 $C_{19}H_{24}O_6$ MW: 348.40
Property: mp 184-8°C, 202-4°C. Source: BAI LAI SHI JU. Ref: 5.

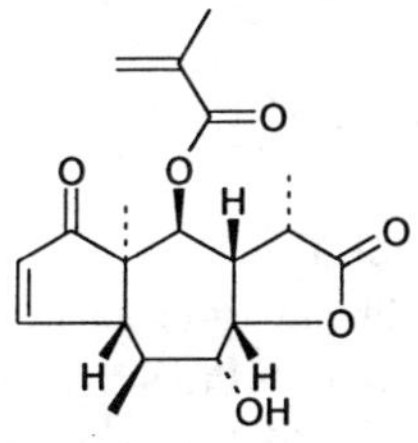

5493 Raffinose
$C_{18}H_{32}O_{16}$ MW: 504.45 Property: mp 118-9°C. Source: GAN DI HUANG, REN SHEN. Ref: 2.

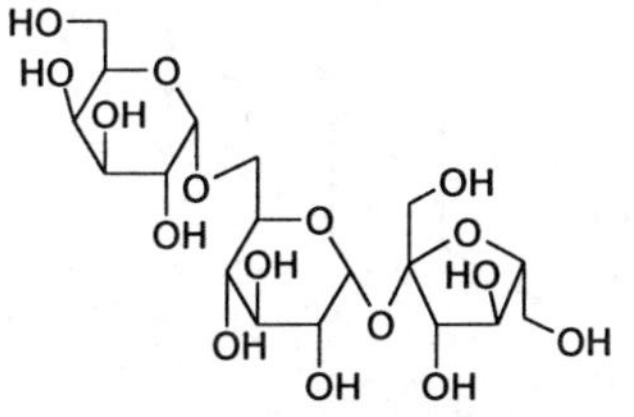

5494 Ramalic acid
$C_{18}H_{18}O_7$ MW: 346.34 Property: mp 203°C (dec). Source: SONG LUO. Ref: 6.

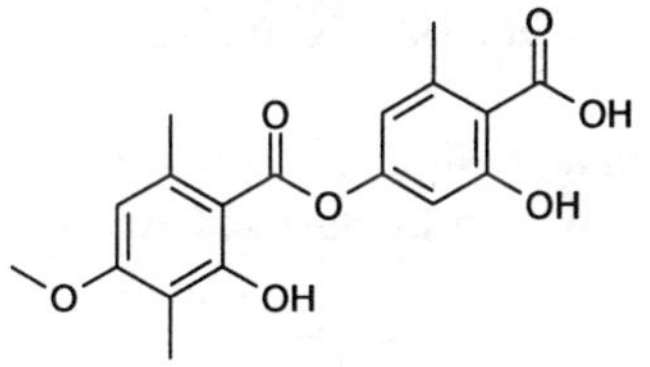

5495 Ranachrome 1
$C_9H_{11}N_5O_3$ MW: 237.22 Property: 243-80°C (carbonization). Source: QING WA. Ref: 6.

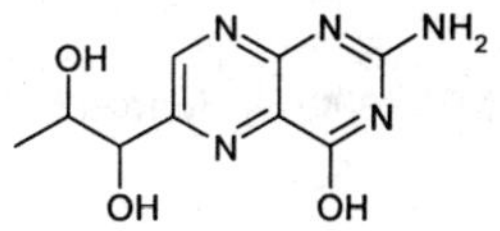

5496 Ranachrome 3
$C_7H_7N_5O_2$ MW: 193.17 Source: QING WA. Ref: 6.

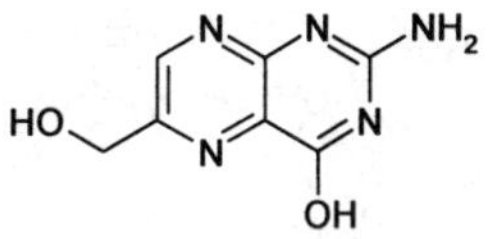

5497 Ranachrome 4
$C_6H_5N_5O_2$ MW: 179.14 Property: mp >300°C (dec). Source: QING WA. Ref: 6.

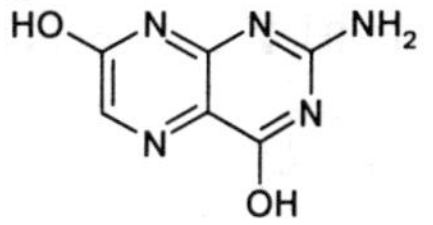

5498 Ranachrome 5
$C_7H_5N_5O_3$ MW: 207.15 Source: QING WA. Ref: 6.

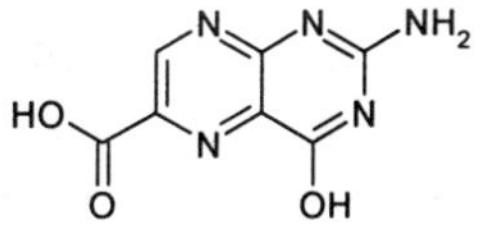

5499 Randainal
$C_{18}H_{16}O_3$ MW: 280.33 Source: HOU PO. Ref: 2.

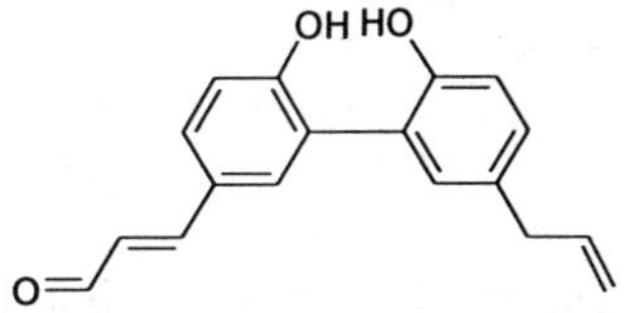

5500 Randaiol
$C_{15}H_{14}O_3$ MW: 242.28 Source: HOU PO. Ref: 2.

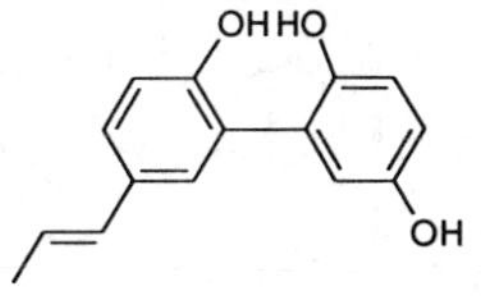

5501 Rankinidine
$C_{20}H_{24}N_2O_3$ MW: 340.43 Property: mp 175-8°C, $[\alpha]_D$ -126°. Source: HU MAN TENG. Ref: 14.

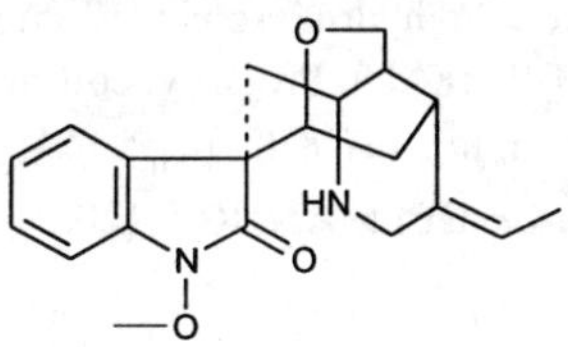

5502 Ranol
$C_{32}H_{44}N_2O_9$ MW: 600.72 Source: HA SHI MA. Ref: 6.

5503 Ranunculin
$C_{11}H_{16}O_2$ MW: 276.25 Property: mp 141-2°C. Source: SHI LONG RUI. Ref: 6.

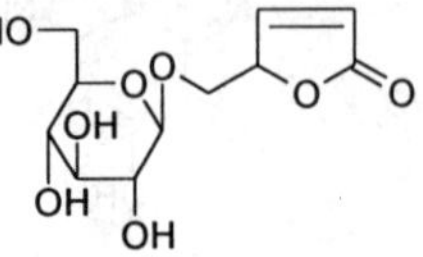

5504 Raunescine
$C_{31}H_{36}N_2O_8$ MW: 564.64 Property: mp 160-70°C. Source: LUO FU MU. Ref: 6.

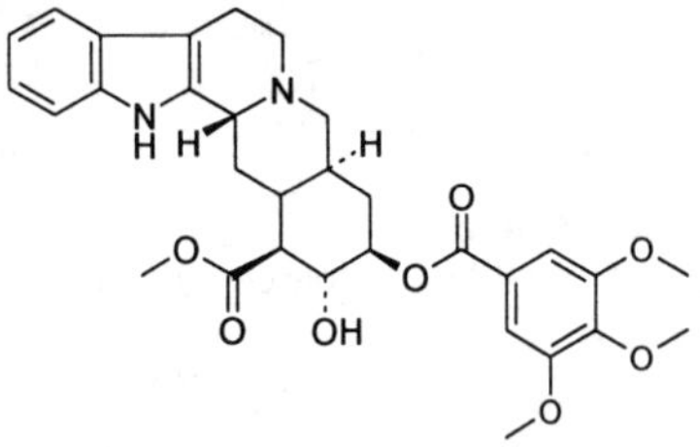

5505 Rauwolfia A
$C_{25}H_{28}N_2O_2$ MW: 388.51 Property: mp 274°C. Source: LUO FU MU. Ref: 6.

5506 Regelin C
Methyl 3-oxo-22α-acetoxy-23-hydroxy-urs-12-ene-30-oate. $C_{33}H_{50}O_6$ MW: 542.76 Property: colorless massive crystal, mp 161-3°C, $[\alpha]_D^{20}$ +60° (c= 0.5, $CHCl_3$). Source: HEI MAN. Ref: 120.

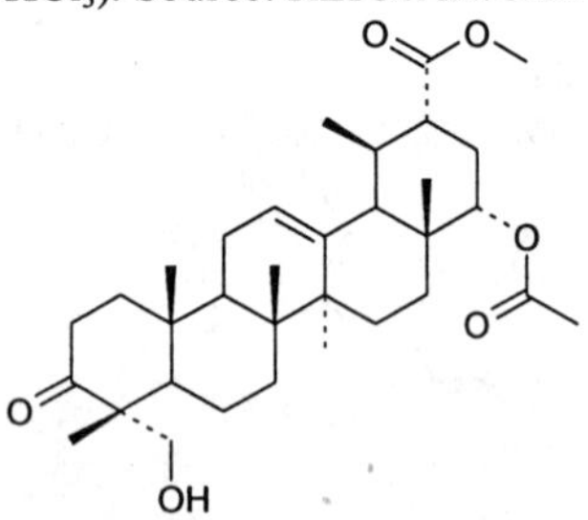

5507 Regelin D
Methyl 3-oxo-22α-hydroxy-olean-12-ene-29-oate. $C_{31}H_{48}O_4$ MW: 484.73 Property: colorless acicular crystal, mp 197-8°C, $[\alpha]_D^{20}$ +54° (c=0.3, $CHCl_3$). Source: HEI MAN. Ref: 120.

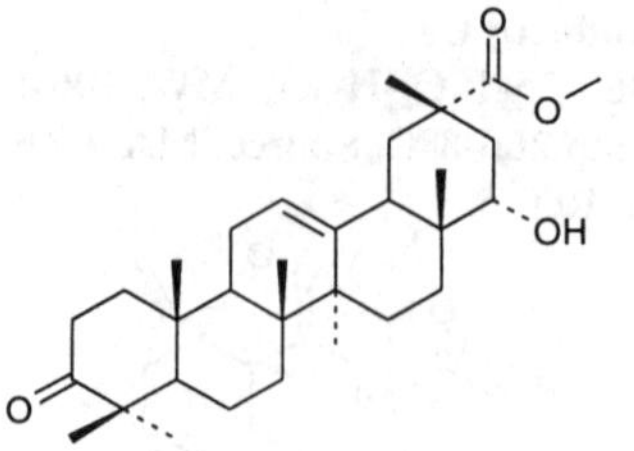

5508 Regelindiol A
Methyl-3β,22α-dihydroxy-urs-12-ene-30-oate. $C_{31}H_{50}O_4$ MW: 486.74 Property: colorless acicular crystal, mp 241-2°C, $[\alpha]_D^{20}$ +57° (c=0.2, $CHCl_3$). Source: HEI MAN. Ref: 120.

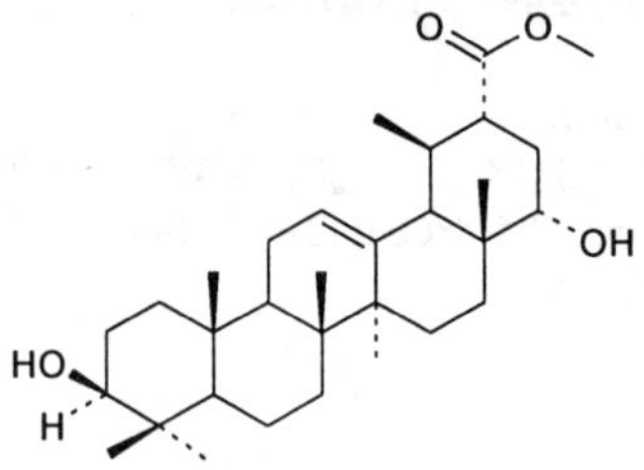

5509 Regelindiol B
Methyl 3β,22α-dihydroxy-olean-12-ene-29-oate. $C_{31}H_{50}O_4$ MW: 486.74 Property: colorless acicular crystal, mp 198-9°C, $[\alpha]_D^{20}$ +44° (c=0.2, $CHCl_3$). Source: HEI MAN. Ref: 120.

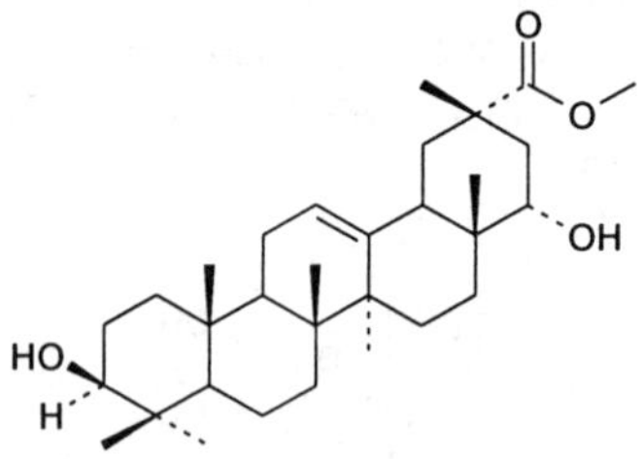

5510 Rehmaglutin A
Source: GAN DI HUANG. Ref: 2.

5511 Rehmaglutin B
Source: GAN DI HUANG. Ref: 2.

5512 Rehmaglutin C
$C_9H_{12}O_5$ MW: 200.19 Source: GAN DI HUANG. Ref: 2.

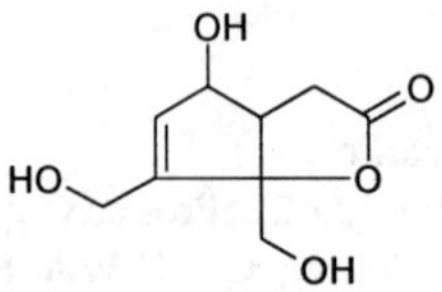

5513 Rehmaglutin D
Source: GAN DI HUANG. Ref: 2.

5514 Rehmaionoside A
$C_{19}H_{34}O_8$ MW: 390.48 Source: GAN DI HUANG. Ref: 2.

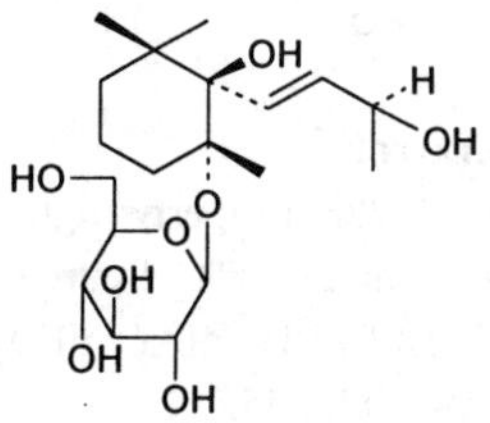

5515 Rehmaionoside B
$C_{19}H_{34}O_8$ MW: 390.48 Source: GAN DI HUANG. Ref: 2.

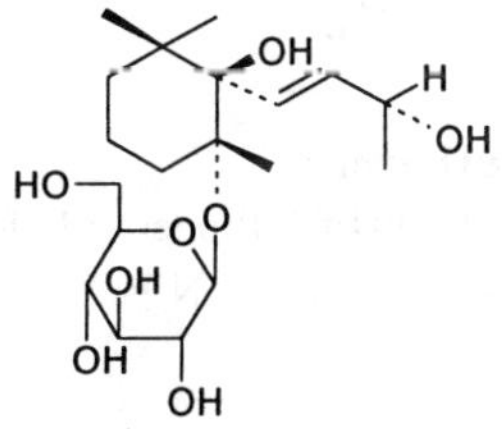

5516 Rehmaionoside C
$C_{19}H_{32}O_8$ MW: 388.46 Source: GAN DI HUANG. Ref: 2.

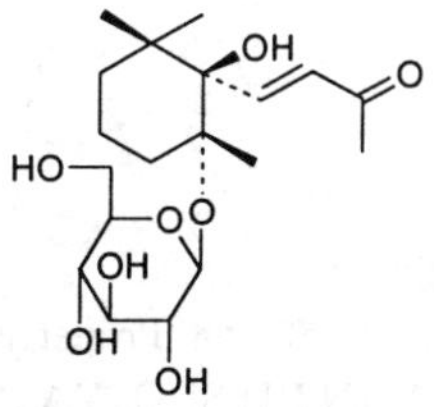

5517 Rehmannioside A
Source: GAN DI HUANG. Ref: 2.

5518 Rehmannioside B
Source: GAN DI HUANG. Ref: 2.

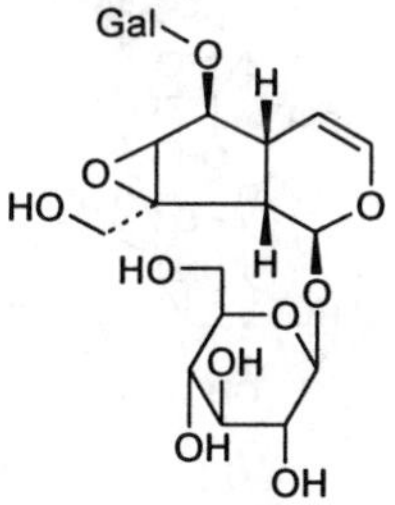

5519 Rehmannioside C
$C_{21}H_{34}O_{14}$ MW: 510.50 Source: GAN DI HUANG. Ref: 2.

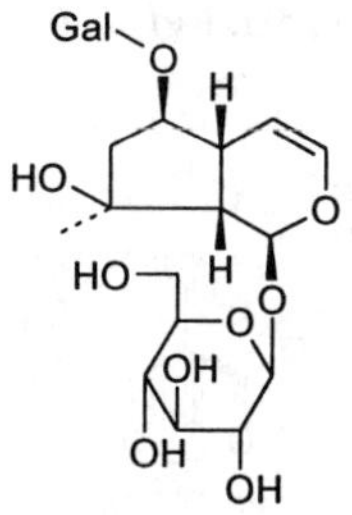

5520 Rehmannioside D
Source: GAN DI HUANG. Ref: 2.

5521 Rehmapicroside
$C_{16}H_{26}O_8$ MW: 346.38 Source: GAN DI HUANG. Ref: 2.

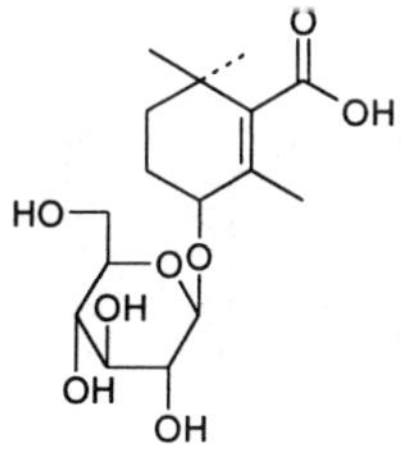

5522 Reineckiagenin
$C_{27}H_{44}O_5$ MW: 448.65 Property: mp 278-80°C. Source: JI XIANG CAO. Ref: 6.

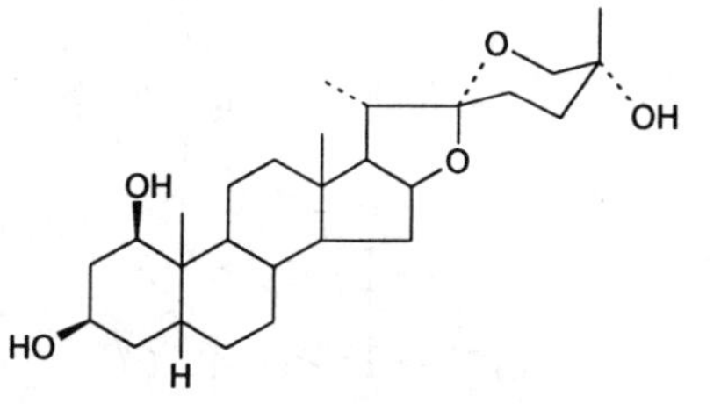

5523 Renifolin
$C_{18}H_{24}O_7$ MW: 352.39 Property: mp 236-8°C (dec). Source: LU XIAN CAO. Ref: 6.

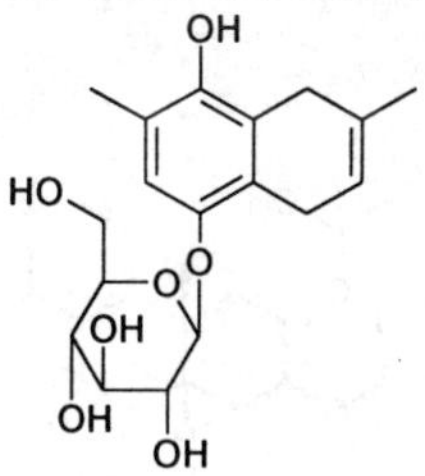

5524 Reserpine
CAS: 50-55-5 $C_{33}H_{40}N_2O_9$ MW: 608.69 Property: mp 262-3°C. Source: DIAN JI GU CHANG SHAN, LUO FU MU. Ref: 5, 6.

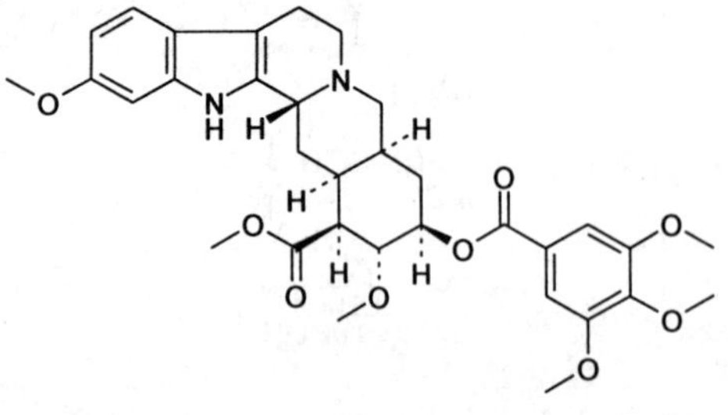

5525 Resibufagin
$C_2H_{30}O_5$ MW: 398.50 Property: mp 210-2°C. Source: CHAN SU. Ref: 2, 6.

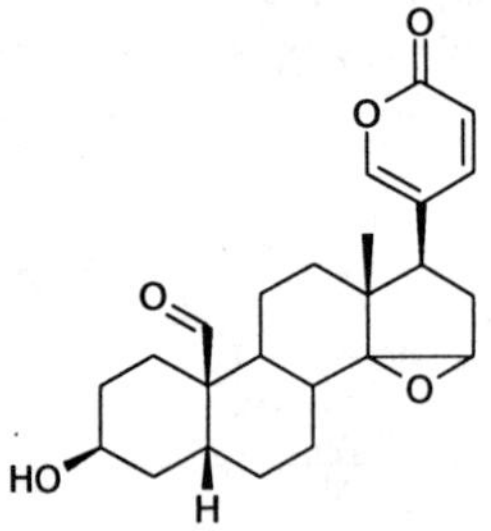

5526 Resibufogenin
$C_{24}H_{32}O_4$ MW: 384.52 Property: mp 113-40°C, 155-68°C. Source: CHAN SU, CHAN PI. Ref: 2, 6, 617.

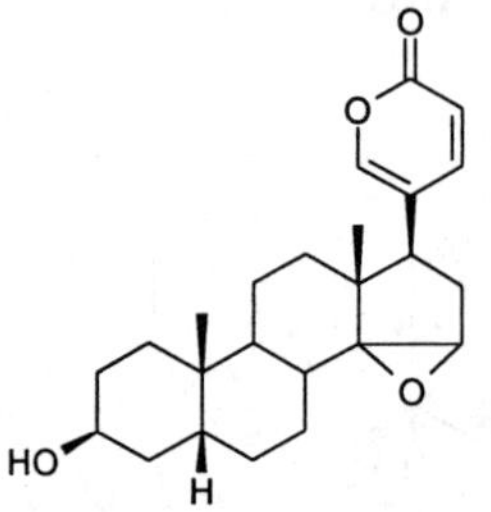

5527 Resibufogenin 3-hydrogen suberate
$C_{32}H_{44}O_7$ MW: 540.70 Source: CHAN SU. Ref: 2.

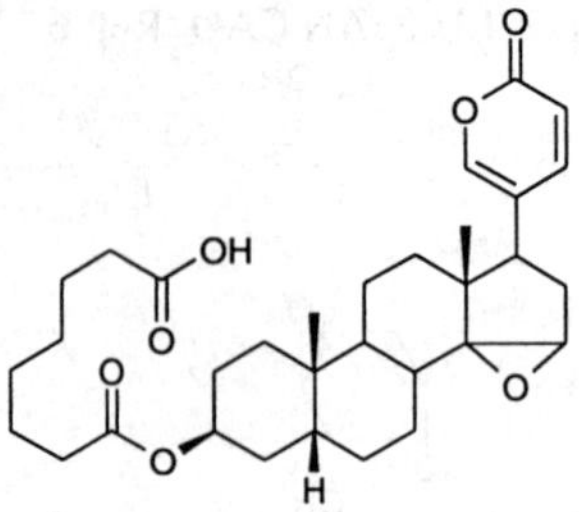

5528 β-Resorcylic acid
$C_7H_6O_4$ MW: 154.12 Property: mp 218-9°C. Source: CI HUAI HUA. Ref: 6.

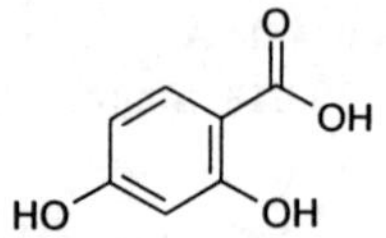

5529 Resveratrol
$C_{27}H_{38}O_{15}$ MW: 228 Property: light yellow acicular crystal, mp 264-5°C. Source: SHE PU TAO, WU SU LI LI LU, XIAO YE MAIMA TENG. Ref: 193, 438, 552.

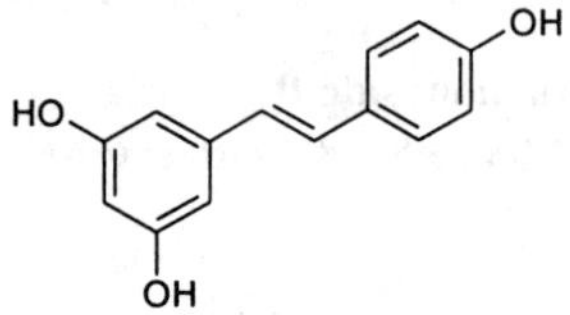

5530 Reticulacinone
$C_{35}H_{62}O_7$ MW: 594.88 Property: light yellow wax solid, mp 68-70°C. Source: NIU XIN PAN LI ZHI. Ref: 432.

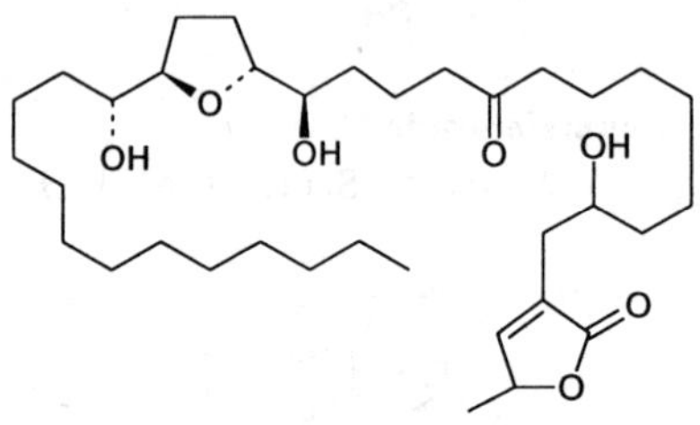

5531 Reticulin
$C_{21}H_{39}N_7O_{12}$ MW: 581.58 Property: mp 200°C (dec). Source: YAN HU SUO, YA PIAN. Ref: 6.

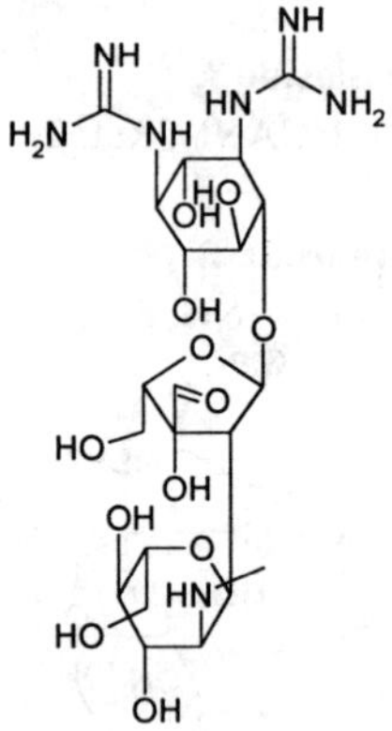

5532 Reticuline
CAS: 485-19-8 $C_{19}H_{23}NO_4$ MW: 329.40
Property: mp 146°C. Source: HE BAO MU DAN GEN, HENG ZHOU WU YAO, HONG NAN PI, ZHANG MU, ZI HUA YU DENG CAO. Ref: 6.

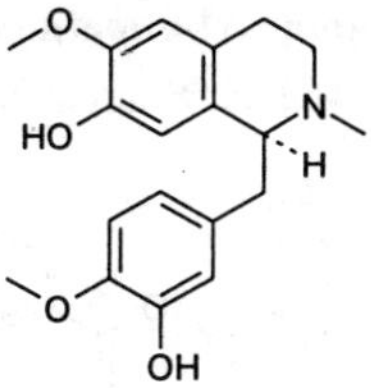

5533 Retrorsine
$C_{18}H_{25}NO_6$ MW: 351.40 Property: mp 207-8°C, 216-6.5°C. Source: DA BAI DING CAO. Ref: 6.

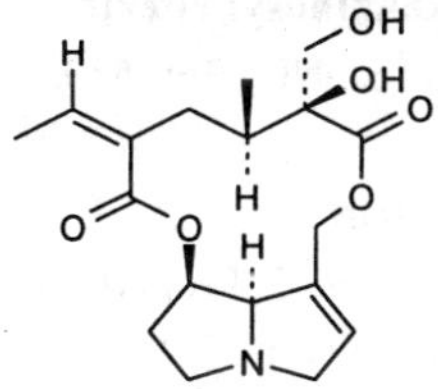

5534 Retusine
Property: mp 163-4°C. Source: HUO XIANG. Ref: 505.

5535 Reynosin
$C_{15}H_{20}O_3$ MW: 248.32 Property: colorless acicular crystal, mp 145-6°C. Source: YU NAN HAN XIAO. Ref: 426.

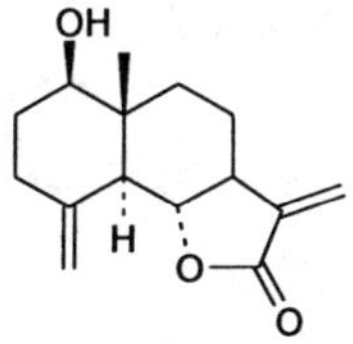

5536 Rhamnazin
$C_{17}H_{14}O_7$ MW: 330.30 Property: mp 216-8°C. Source: DUO SUI LIAO. Ref: 6.

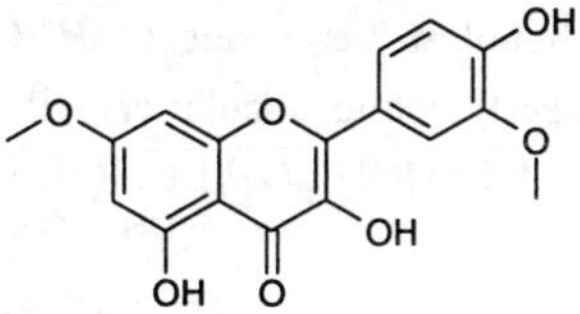

5537 Rhamnetin
4H-1-benzopyran-4-one,2-(3,4-dihydroxy-phenyl) -3,5-dihydroxy-7-methoxy. $C_{16}H_{12}O_7$ MW: 316.27 Property: yellow powder crystal (MeOH), mp 288-90°C. Source: DING XIANG, FENG JIAO, HUO XIANG, QING HAO, XI YE TENG.
Ref: 2, 6, 463.

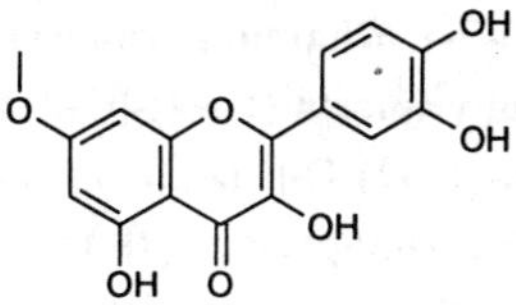

5538 Rhamnocitrin
$C_{16}H_{12}O_6$ MW: 300.27 Property: mp 221-2°C. Source: QING HAO, TU SHA REN, XI YE TENG, YIN CHEN HAO. Ref: 2, 372.

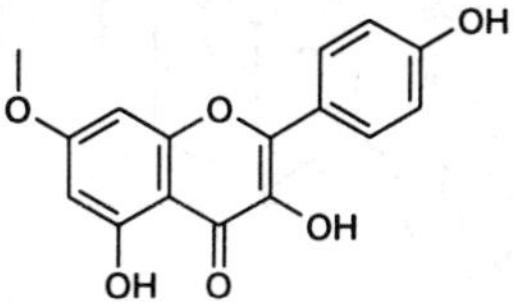

5539 Rhamno-isoliquiritin
Property: mp 127°C. Source: GAN CAO. Ref: 2.

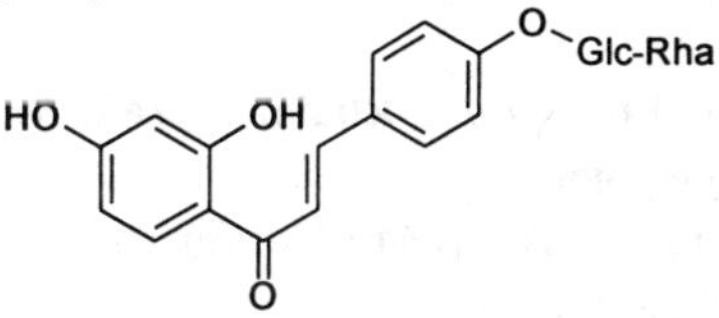

5540 28-O-α-L-rhamnopyranosyl(1→4)-β-D-glucopyranosyl(1→6)-β-D-glucopyranoside
$C_{48}H_{78}O_{18}$ MW: 942 Property: white powder, mp 214-6°C, $[\alpha]_D^{20}$ -3.0° (c=0.5, MeOH). Source: CI REN SHEN. Ref: 467.

5541 3-O-2-L-Rhamnopyranosyl(1→3)-β-D-glucopyranosyl(1→3)-α-L-rhamnopyranosyl (1→2)-α-L-arabinopyranosyl hederagenin 28-O-β-D-gluco-pyra-nosyl(1→6)-β-D-glucopyra-nosyl ester (VIII)
$C_{65}H_{106}O_{31}$ MW: 1385.55 Property: white powder, mp 220-4°C, $[\alpha]_D^{19}$ -27.6° (c=0.2, metha-nol). Source: CHUAN XU DUAN. Ref: 211.

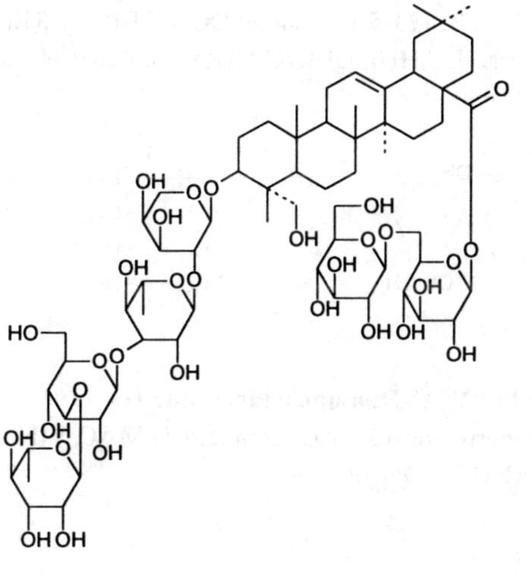

5542 3β-{O-α-L-Rhamnopyranosyl-(1→4)-O-α-L-rhamnopyranosyl-(1→4)-[O-α-L-rhamnopyranosyl-(1→2)-O-β-D-glucopyranosyl(1→x)-O-β-D-glucuronopyranosyl}-16α-hydroxy-13β, 28-epoxyoleahane

Source: CI WU JIA. Ref: 2.

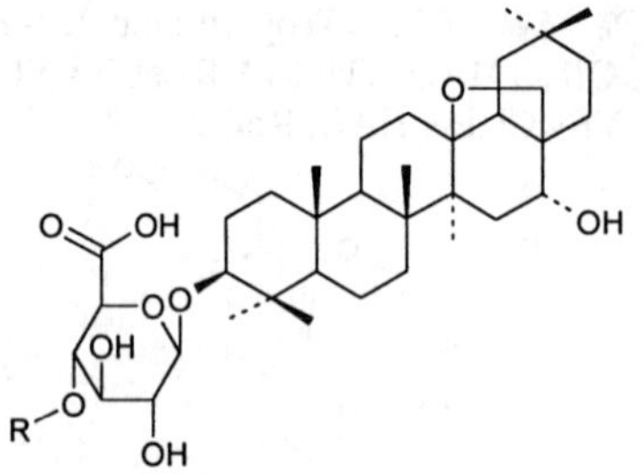

R=O-α-L-Rha-(1→4)-O-α-L-Rha-(1→4)-[O-α-L-Rha-(1→2)-β-D-Glc-

5543 6-O-(4''-O-α-L-Rhamnopyranosyl) vanilloylajugol

$C_{29}H_{40}O_{16}$ MW: 644.63 Source: GAN DI HUANG. Ref: 2.

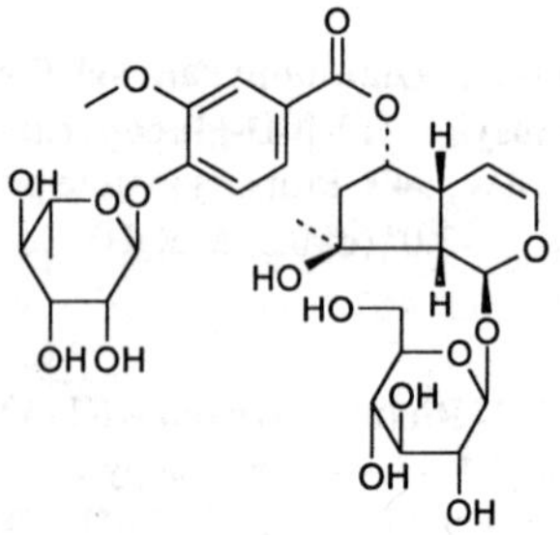

5544 Rhamnose

$C_6H_{12}O_5$ MW: 164.16 Property: (L): white powder crystal, mp 289-90°C (MeOH), mp (L) α: 105°C, β: 123-5°C. Source: DONG BEI CI REN SHEN, LU HUI, QIANG HUO, REN SHEN. Ref: 2, 6, 450.

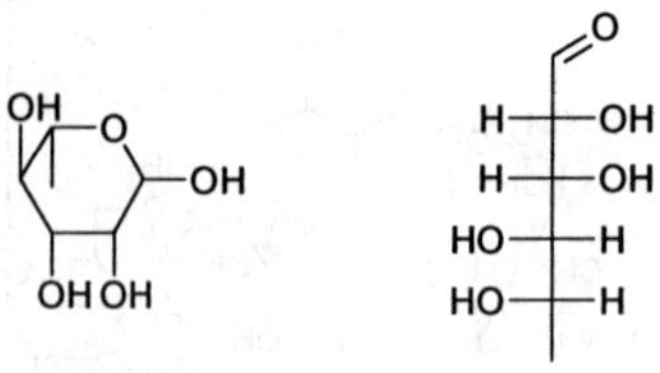

L

5545 2''-O-Rhamnosyl icariside II

Property: mp 151-3°C. Source: CU MAO YIN YANG HUO. Ref: 599.

5546 2''-O-Rhamnosyl ikarisoside A

Property: mp 170.5-172°C. Source: CU MAO YIN YANG HUO. Ref: 599.

5547 7α-L-Rhamnosyl-6-methoxylutcolin

$C_{22}H_{22}O_{11}$ MW: 462.41 Source: KONG XIN XIAN. Ref: 6.

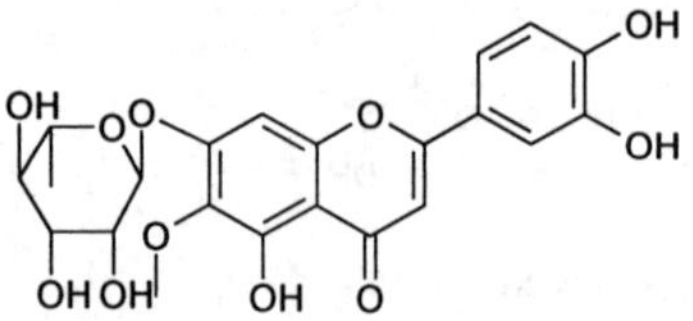

5548 2''-O-Rhamnosyl vitexin

Source: JI MAO SONG. Ref: 580.

5549 Rhaponticin

$C_{21}H_{24}O_9$ MW: 420.42 Property: mp 231°C. Source: DA HUANG. Ref: 2.

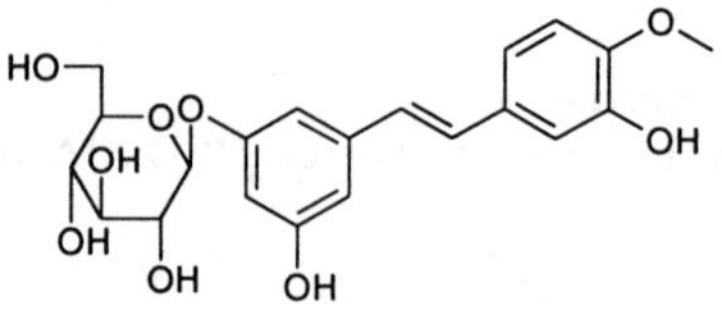

5550 Rhapontigenin

$C_{15}H_{14}O_4$ MW: 258.28 Property: mp 186-7°C. Source: DA HUANG. Ref: 6.

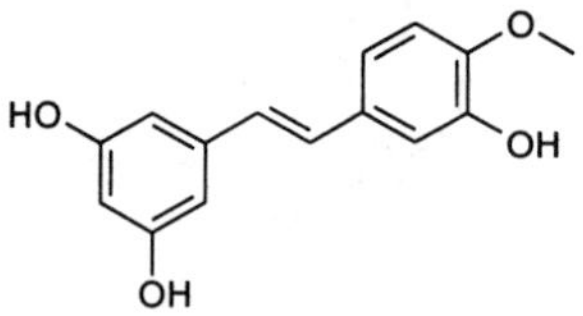

5551 Rhapontisterone

(20R,22R,24S)-2β,3β,11α,14α20,22,24-Heptahydroxy-5β-cholest-7-en-6-one. $C_{27}H_{44}O_8$ MW: 496.65 Property: white acicular crystal, mp 234-6°C. Source: QI ZHOU LOU LU. Ref: 194.

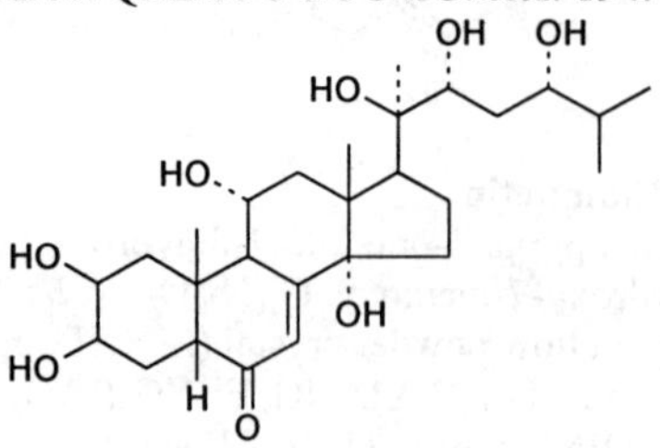

5552 Rhazine
$C_{21}H_{26}N_2O_3$ MW: 354.45 Property: mp 245-7.5°C (ethanol), 243-6°C (benzene). Source: XIANG PI MU. Ref: 6.

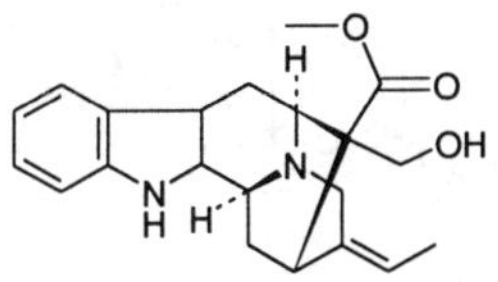

5553 Rheidin A
$C_{30}H_{20}O_9$ MW: 524.49 Source: DA HUANG. Ref: 2.

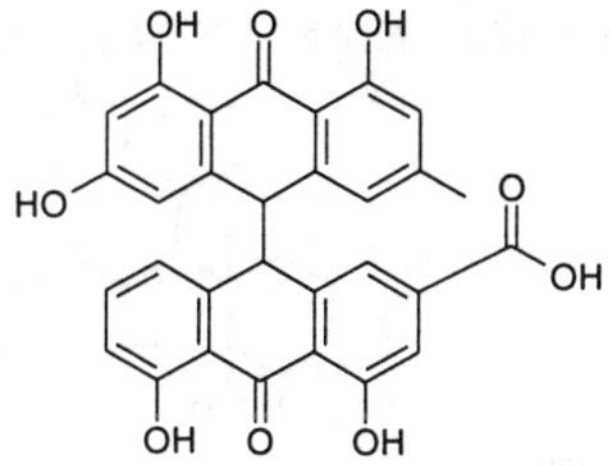

5554 Rheidin B
$C_{30}H_{20}O_8$ MW: 508.49 Source: DA HUANG. Ref: 2.

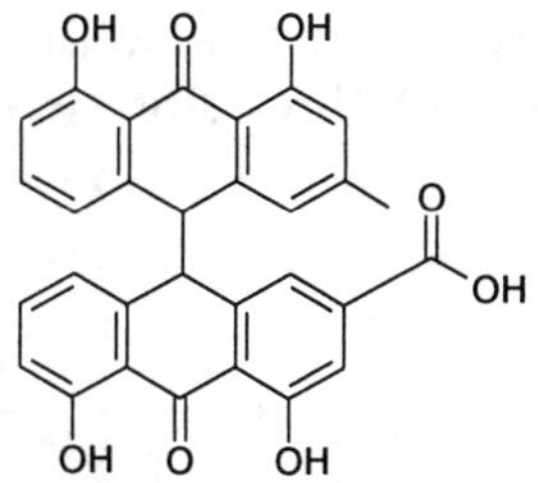

5555 Rheidin C
$C_{31}H_{22}O_9$ MW: 538.52 Source: DA HUANG. Ref: 2.

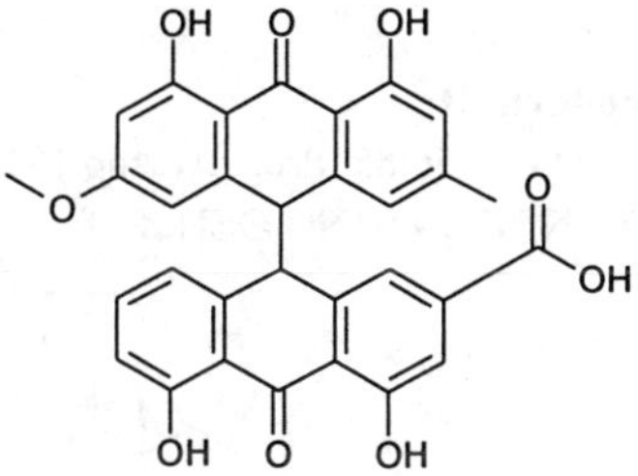

5556 Rhein
Cassic acid; Monorhein; Parietic acid; Rheic acid; Rhubarb yel-low, CAS: 478-43-3 $C_{15}H_8O_6$ MW: 284.23 Property: mp 321-2°C. Source: DA HUANG, HE SHOU WU, HU ZHANG, JUE MING ZI. Ref: 2, 4, 627.

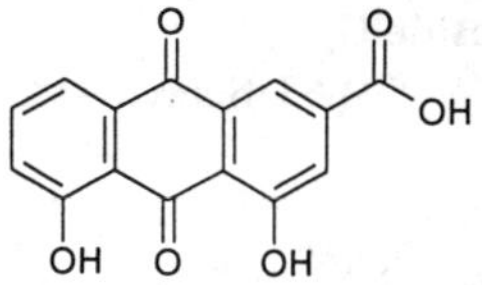

5557 Rhein diglucoside
$C_{27}H_{28}O_{16}$ MW: 608.51 Source: DA HUANG. Ref: 6.

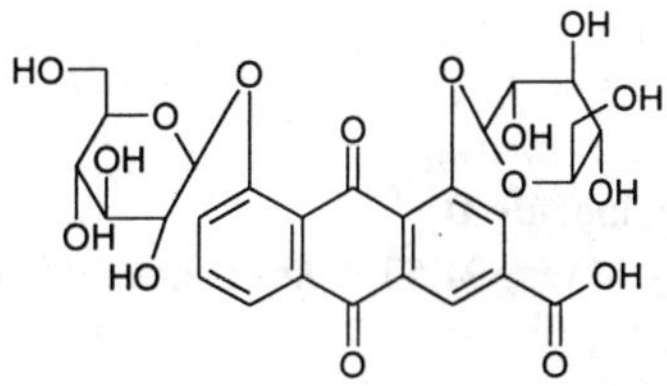

5558 Rhein-8-O-β-D-glucopyranoside
Rhein-8-monoglucoside. $C_{21}H_{18}O_{11}$ MW: 446.37 Property: mp 260-6°C. Source: DA HUANG. Ref: 2, 6.

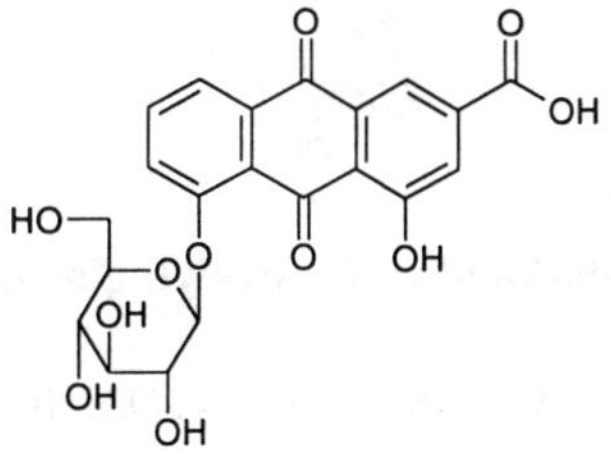

5559 Rheinoside A
$C_{27}H_{30}O_{16}$ MW: 610.53 Source: DA HUANG. Ref: 2.

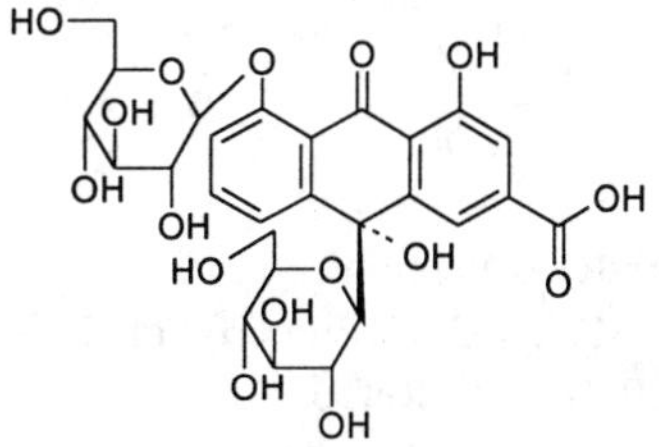

5560 Rheinoside B
$C_{27}H_{30}O_{16}$ MW: 610.53 Source: DA HUANG. Ref: 2.

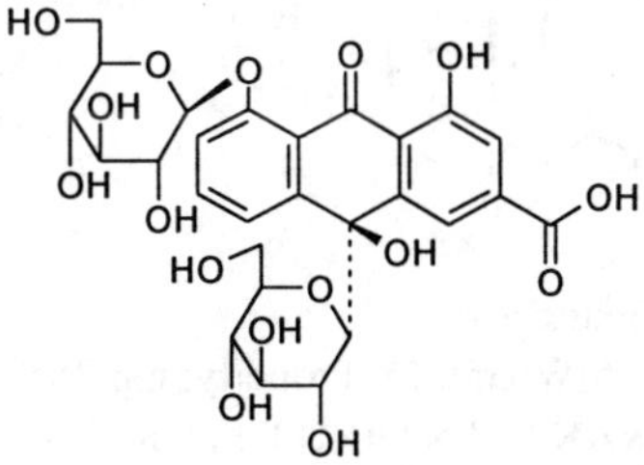

5561 Rheinoside C
$C_{27}H_{30}O_{15}$ MW: 594.53 Source: DA HUANG. Ref: 2.

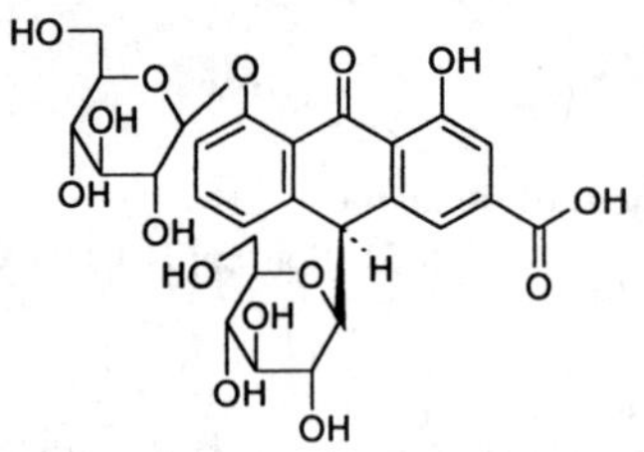

5562 Rheinoside D
$C_{27}H_{30}O_{15}$ MW: 594.53 Source: DA HUANG. Ref: 2.

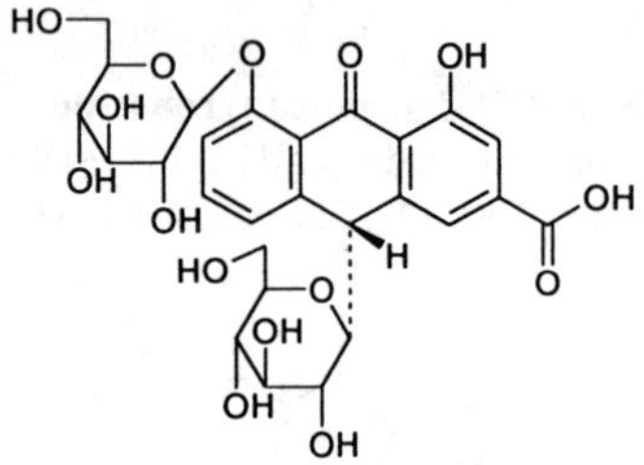

5563 Rhein-8-O-β-D-(6'-oxalyl)-glucopyranoside
$C_{23}H_{18}O_{14}$ MW: 518.39 Source: DA HUANG. Ref: 2.

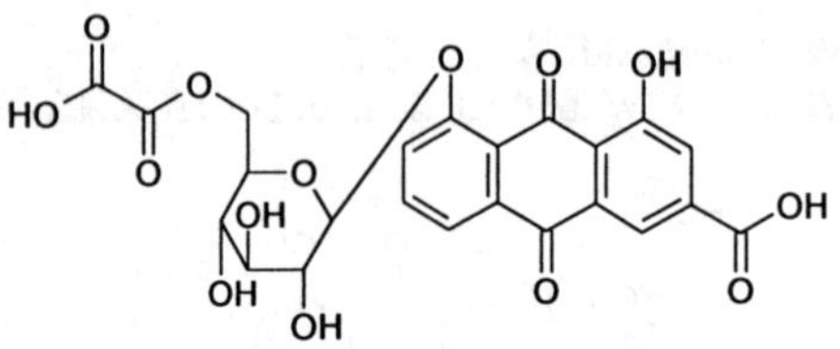

5564 Rhodeasapogenin
$C_{27}H_{44}O_4$ MW: 432.65 Property: mp 293-5°C. Source: LING LAN. Ref: 6.

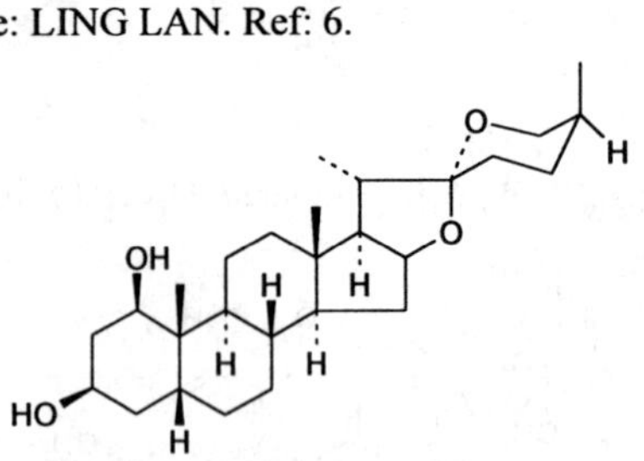

5565 Rhodexin A
$C_{29}H_{44}O_9$ MW: 356.67 Property: mp 265°C (dec). Source: WAN NIAN QING GEN. Ref: 6.

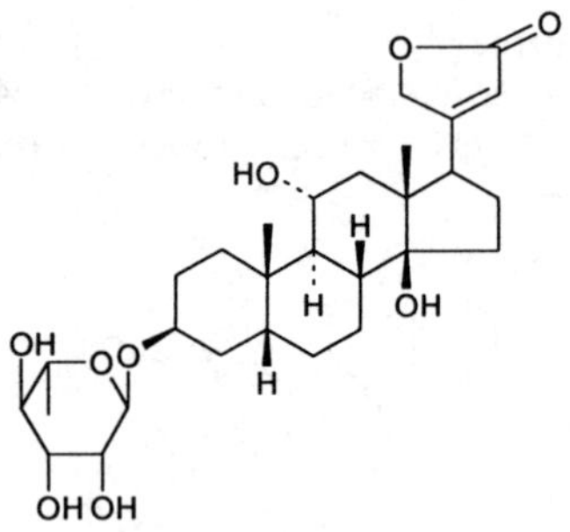

5566 Rhodexin B
$C_{31}H_{46}O_{10}$ MW: 578.71 Property: mp 262°C (dec). Source: WAN NIAN QING GEN. Ref: 6.

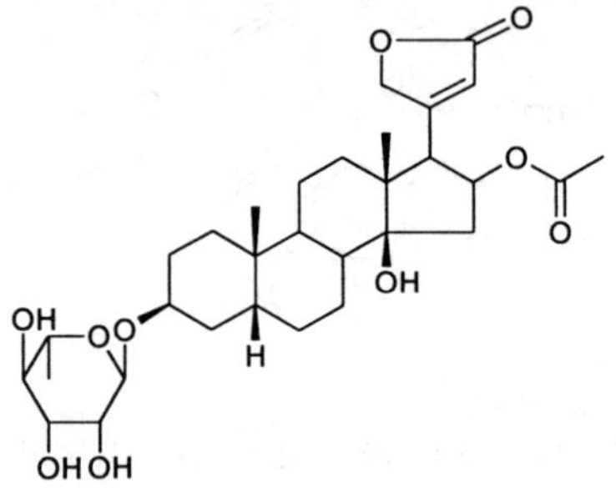

5567 Rhodexin C
$C_{37}H_{56}O_{15}$ MW: 746.85 Property: mp 275°C (dec). Source: WAN NIAN QING GEN. Ref: 6.

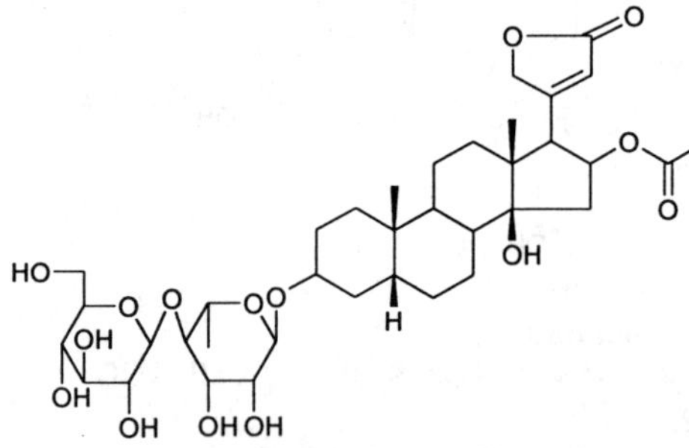

5568 Rhodexin D
$C_{37}H_{56}O_{16}$ MW: 756.85 Property: mp 181-184°C. Source: WAN NIAN QING GEN. Ref: 6.

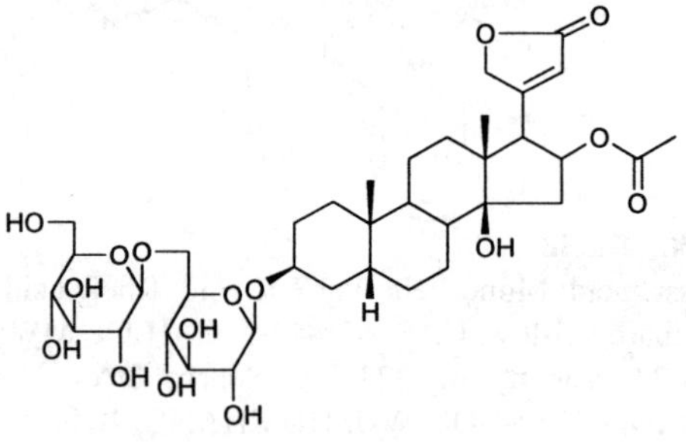

5569 Rhododendrol

$C_{10}H_{14}O_2$ MW: 166.22 Property: mp (-): 82°C. Source: BAI HUA YING SHAN HONG, MAN SHAN HONG. Ref: 6.

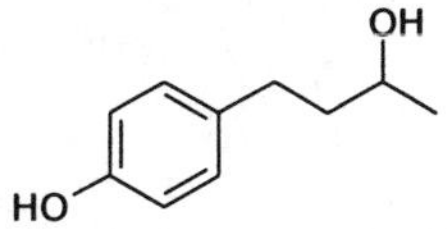

5570 Rhodomollein III

$C_{22}H_{36}O_8$ MW: 428.53 Property: white acicular crystal, mp 228-30°C, $[\alpha]_D^{20}$ -23.4° (c=0.1, methanol). Source: YANG ZHI ZHU. Ref: 173.

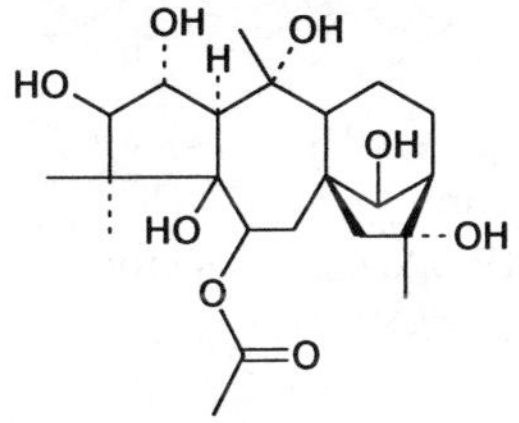

5571 Rhoeadine

$C_{21}H_{21}NO_6$ MW: 383.40 Property: mp 256-7°C. Source: LI CHUN HUA, YA PIAN. Ref: 6.

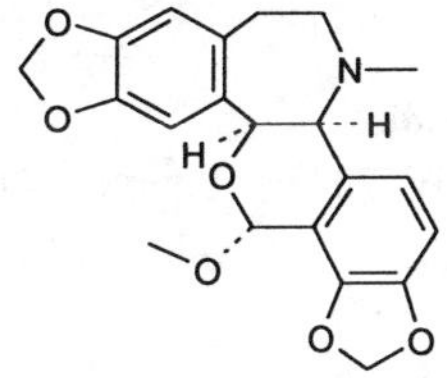

5572 Rhoeagenine

$C_{20}H_{19}NO_6$ MW: 369.38 Property: mp 236-8°C. Source: LI CHUN HUA. Ref: 6.

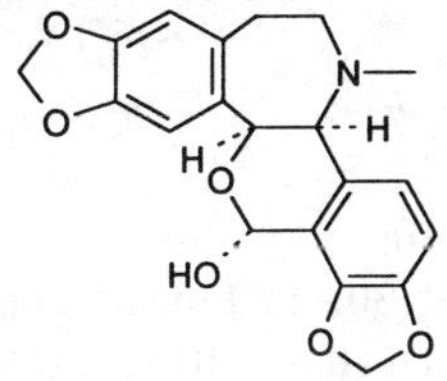

5573 Rhoifolin

$C_{27}H_{30}O_{14}$ MW: 578.53 Property: mp 205-8°C, 245°C. Source: GOU JU, GOU JU YE, LIN BEI ZI, YE QI SHU YE, ZHI SHI. Ref: 6.

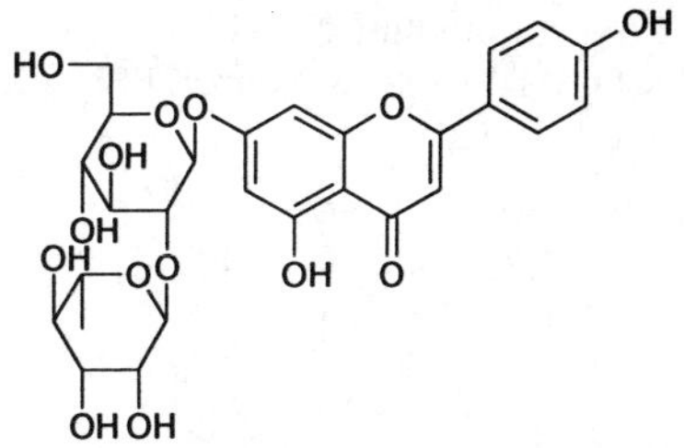

5574 Rhombifoline

$C_{15}H_{20}N_2O$ MW: 244.34 Property: bp 120°C/0.2 mm. Source: MU MA DOU. Ref: 6.

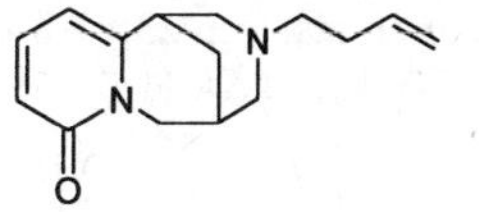

5575 Rhusone

1-(2',3'-Dihydroxylphenyl)-2-n-heptyl-1-nonene-3-one. $C_{22}H_{34}O_3$ MW: 346.51 Property: light grey amorphous powder, mp 60-2°C, soluble in liposoluble organic solvents, insoluble in water. Source: TAI SHAN YAN FU MU. Ref: 494.

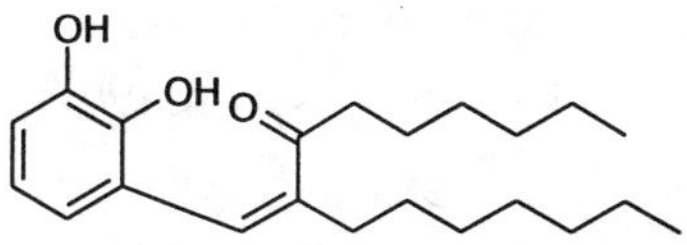

5576 Rhynchonhine

$C_{36}H_{38}N_2O_{11}$ MW: 674.71 Source: GOU TENG. Ref: 2.

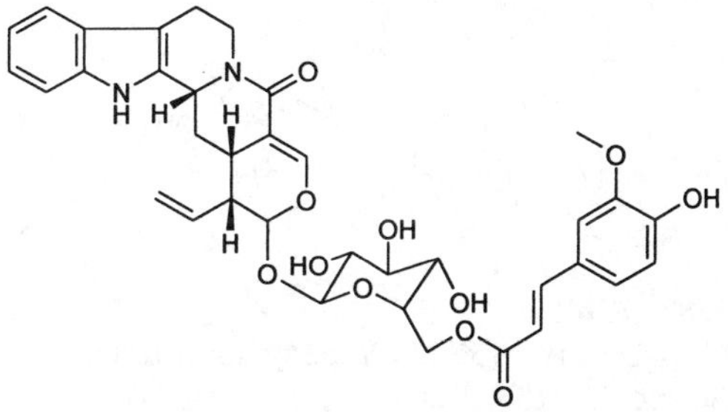

5577 Rhynchophylline

Mitrinermine. CAS: 77-66-4 $C_{22}H_{28}N_2O_4$ MW: 384.48 Property: mp 208-9°C, 216°C. Source: GOU TENG. Ref: 4.

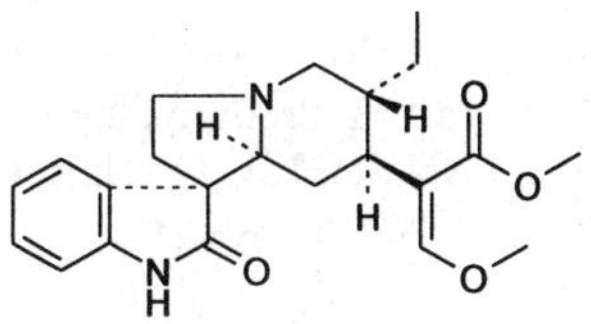

5578 Rhynchophylline N-oxide
$C_{22}H_{28}N_2O_5$ MW: 400.48 Source: FENG XIANG SHU YE (a) . Ref: 6.

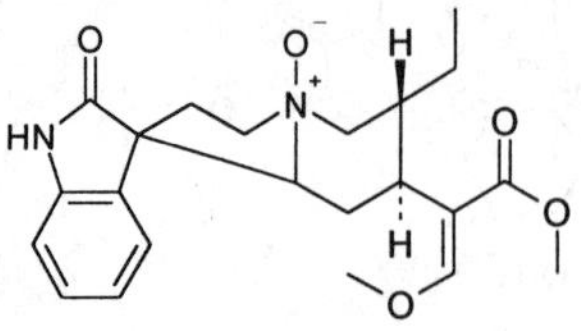

5579 Rhynchotechol V
1,6-Dihydroxy-7,8-dimethoxy-2-methyl-9,10-anthraquinone. $C_{17}H_{14}O_6$ MW: 314.30 Property: orange acicular crystal, mp 236.5-8°C. Source: MAO XIAN ZHU JU TAI. Ref: 168.

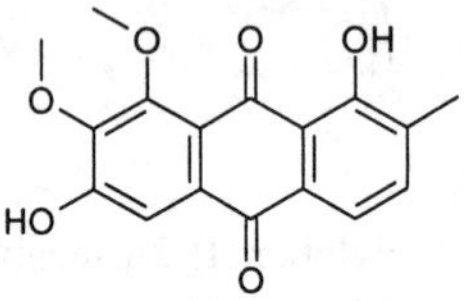

5580 Ribalinidine
$C_{15}H_{17}NO_4$ MW: 275.31 Property: mp 257-8°C (dec). Source: CHOU CAO. Ref: 6.

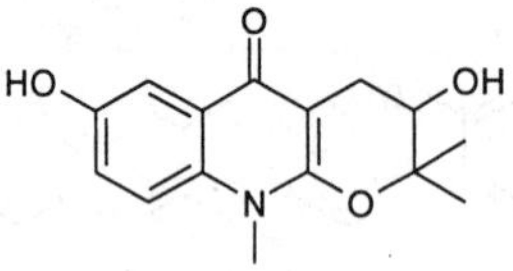

5581 Ribalinium
$C_{16}H_{20}NO_4$ MW: 290.34 Source: CHOU CAO. Ref: 6.

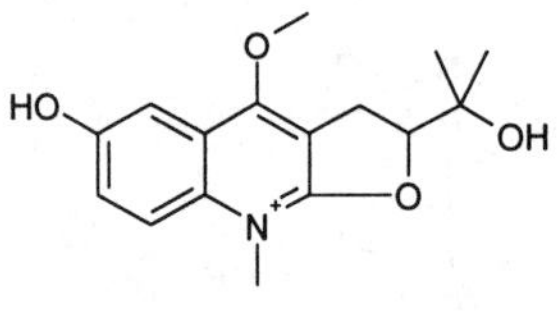

5582 Ribitol
$C_5H_{12}O_5$ MW: 152.15 Property: mp 102°C. Source: E SHEN. Ref: 6.

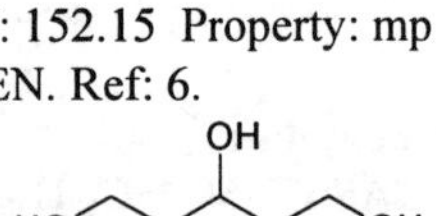

5583 Ribose
$C_5H_{10}O_5$ MW: 150.13 Property: mp D: 86-7°C, 95°C. Source: FAN SHI LIU GAN. Ref: 6.

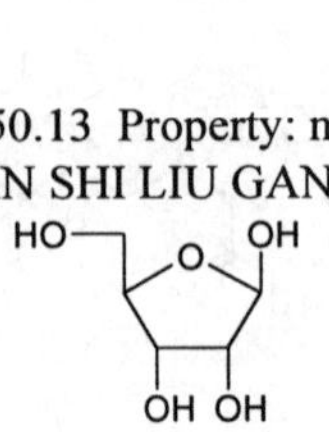

5584 Ricinine
$C_8H_8N_2O_2$ MW: 164.17 Property: mp 201.5°C. Source: BI MA ZI, BI MA YE. Ref: 6.

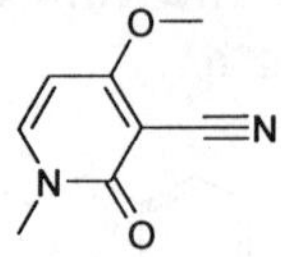

5585 Ricinoleic acid
Ricinolic acid. CAS: 141-22-0 $C_{18}H_{34}O_3$ MW: 298.47 Property: mp 5.5°C, bp 245°C/10 mm. Source: BI MA YOU, LING ZHI CAO. Ref: 4.

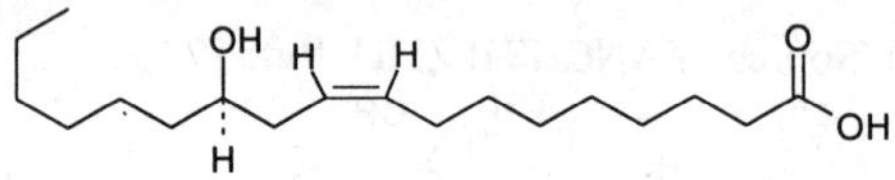

5586 Ridentin
$C_{15}H_{20}O_4$ MW: 264.32 Property: mp 215-8°C (dec). Source: AI YE. Ref: 6.

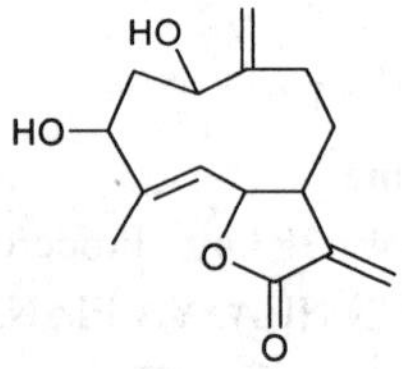

5587 Rindoside
$C_{34}H_{40}O_{21}$ MW: 784.69 Source: LONG DAN. Ref: 2.

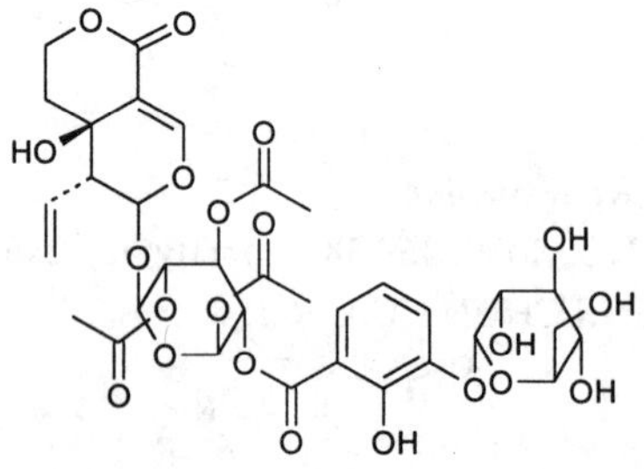

5588 Robinetin
$C_{15}H_{10}O_7$ MW: 302.24 Property: mp 325-30°C (dec). Source: CI HUAI HUA, JI CAI. Ref: 6.

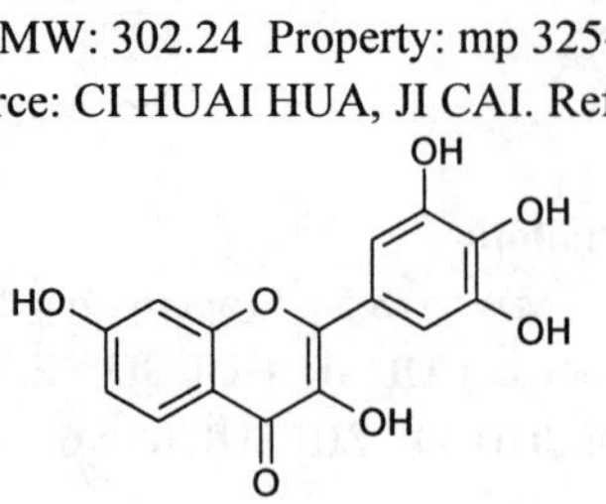

5589 Robinin
$C_{33}H_{40}O_{19}$ MW: 740.68 Property: mp (α): 195-7°C (water), (β): 249-50°C (ethanol). Source: GE YE , LUO FU MU JING YE. Ref: 5, 6.

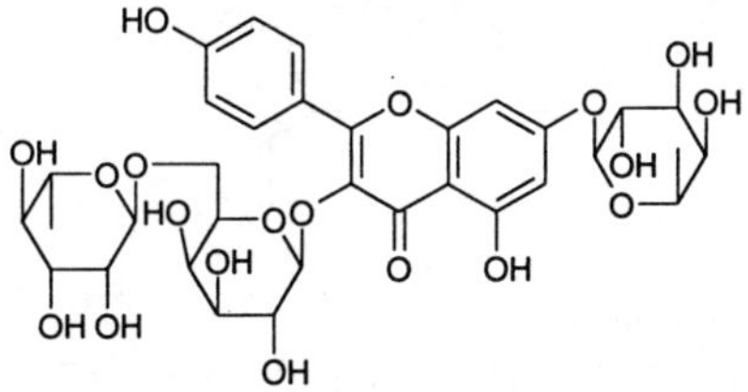

5590 Robustaflavone
Source: JI MAO SONG. Ref: 544.

5591 Robustaflavone-7''-methyl ether
Source: JI MAO SONG. Ref: 544.

5592 Rockogenin
$C_{27}H_{44}O_4$ MW: 432.65 Property: mp 208-10°C (methanol), 217-20°C (ether). Source: DONG YI HAO JIAN MA, FAN MA, JIAN MA. Ref: 10.

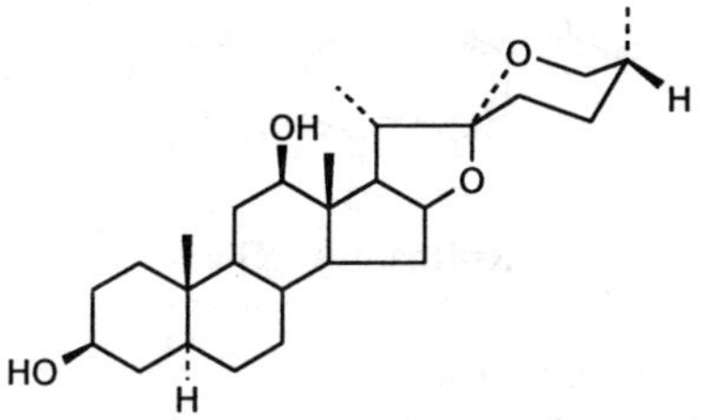

5593 Roemerine
$C_{18}H_{17}NO_2$ MW: 279.34 Property: mp 102-3°C. Source: HE YE, HE GENG, HE YE DI. Ref: 6.

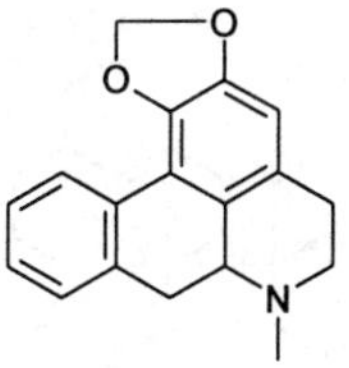

5594 Rorifone
$C_{11}H_{21}NO_2S$ MW: 231.36 Property: mp 40-6°C, bp 188-92°C /1mm. Source: HAN CAI. Ref: 4.

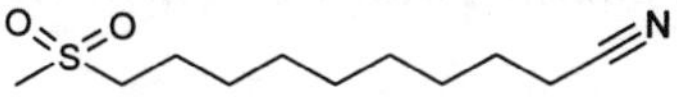

5595 Rosacea acid A
$C_{30}H_{48}O_4$ MW: 472.71 Property: white powder, mp 266-7°C (methanol), $[\alpha]_D^{18}$ +16.8° (c=0.05, pyridine). Source: KU HONG GU. Ref: 289.

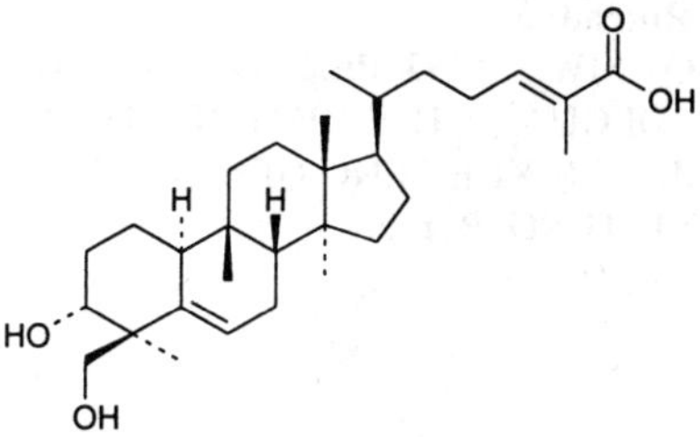

5596 Rosacea acid B
$C_{30}H_{48}O_3$ MW: 456.72 Property: white powder, mp 198-201°C (methanol), $[\alpha]_D^{18}$ +16.6° (c=0.10, pyridine). Source: KU HONG GU. Ref: 289.

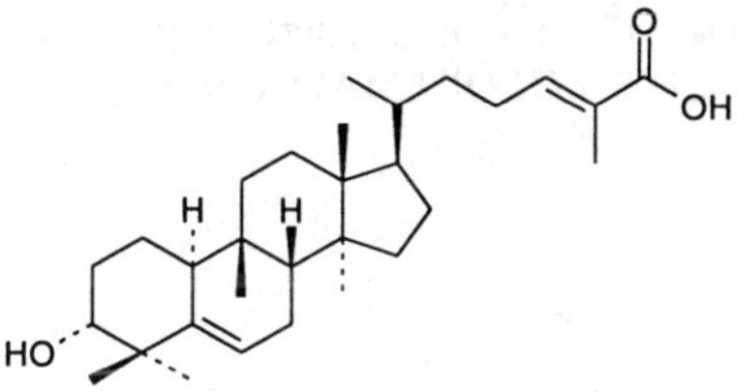

5597 Rosamultin
Source: DA HONG PAO. Ref: 592.

5598 Roseoside
Source: CHANG CHUN HUA, DA ZAO. Ref: 2.

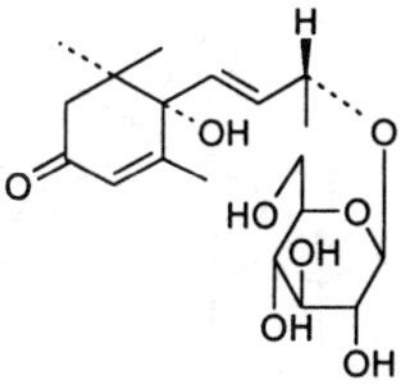

5599 Rosmaricine
$C_{20}H_{27}NO_4$ MW: 345.44 Property: mp 199-200°C. Source: MI DIE XIANG. Ref: 6.

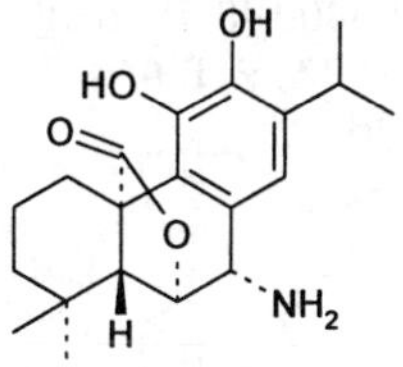

5600 Rosmarinic acid
$C_{18}H_{16}O_8$ MW: 360.32 Property: mp 204°C (dec). Source: BO HE. Ref: 2.

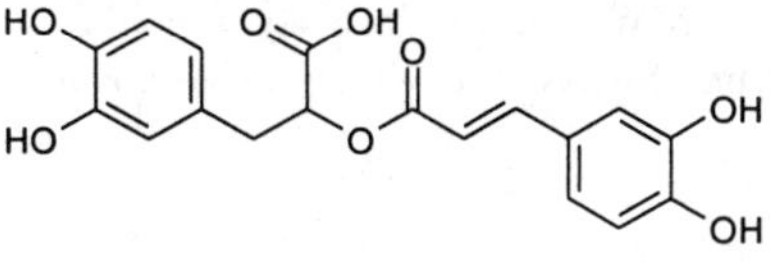

5601 Rotenone
$C_{23}H_{22}O_6$ MW: 394.43 Property: mp (-): 163°C. Source: DI GUA ZI, HUI YE GEN, KU TAN ZI, KUN MING JI XUE TENG GEN, MAO RUI HUA, YU TENG. Ref: 6.

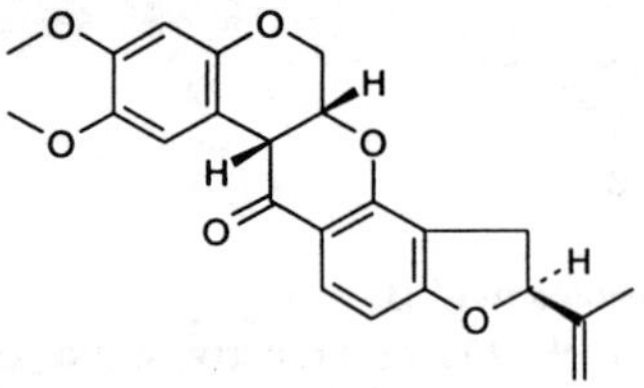

5602 Rottlerin
$C_{30}H_{28}O_8$ MW: 516.55 Property: mp 212°C. Source: LU SONG QIU MAO. Ref: 6.

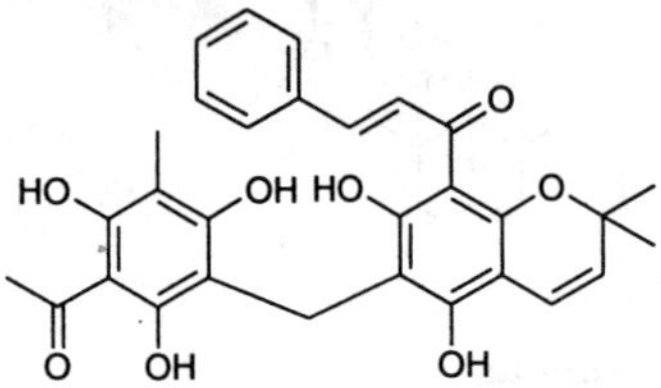

5603 Rotundic acid
$C_{30}H_{48}O_5$ MW: 488.71 Source: JIU BI YING, SI JI QING. Ref: 6, 527.

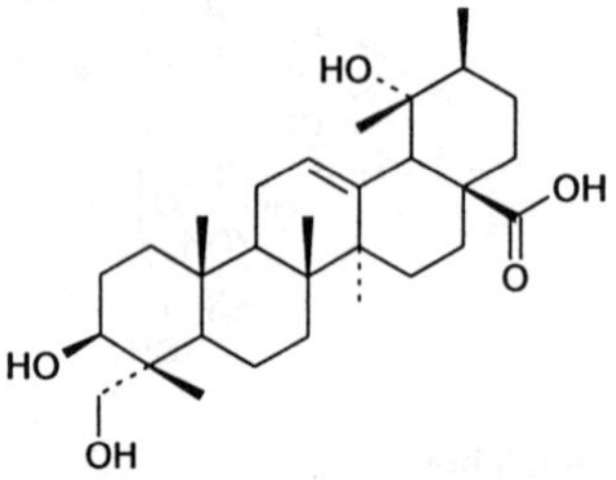

5604 Rotundifoline
$C_{22}H_{28}N_2O_5$ MW: 400.48 Property: mp 238-40°C. Source: HAI ER CHA. Ref: 6.

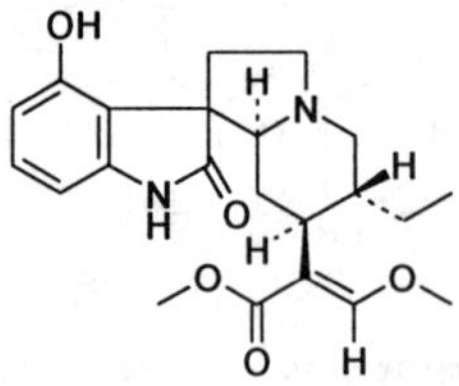

5605 Rotundifolone
$C_{10}H_{14}O_2$ MW: 166.22 Property: mp 27.5°C, bp 86°C/1mm. Source: YU XIANG CAO. Ref: 6.

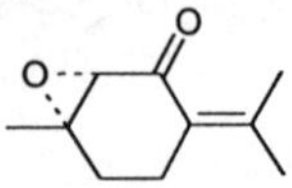

5606 Rotundone
$C_{15}H_{22}O$ MW: 218.34 Property: bp 128-9°C/1mm. Source: XIANG FU. Ref: 6.

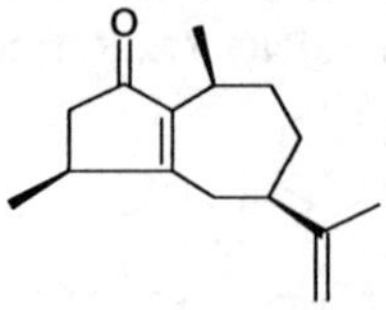

5607 Rotunol
$C_{15}H_{22}O_2$ MW: 234.34 Property: mp α: 87.5-8.5°C, β: 118-9°C. Source: XIANG FU. Ref: 6.

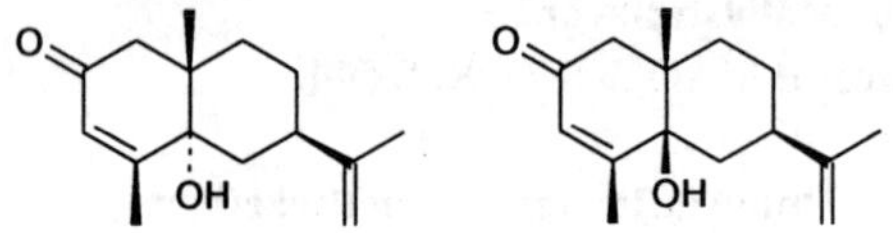

α: β:

5608 Rouhuoside
Source: YIN YANG HUO. Ref: 2.

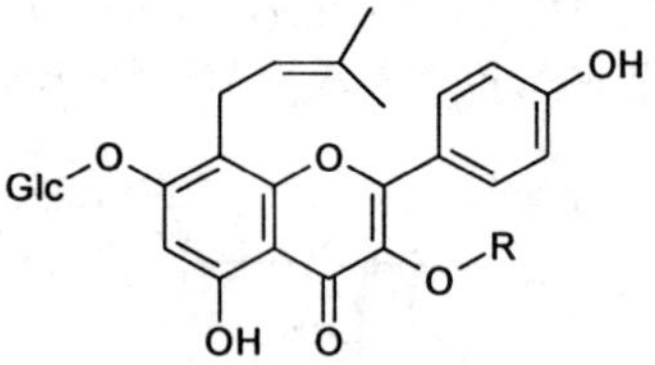

R=Rha(4→1)Glc

5609 Roxburic acid
2β,3β,7β,19α-Tetrahydroxyurs-12-en-28-oic acid. $C_{30}H_{48}O_6$ MW: 504.71 Property: white amorphous powder, mp 292°C (decomposition), $[\alpha]_D^{18}$ 0° (c=0.1550, pyridine). Source: CI LI. Ref: 74.

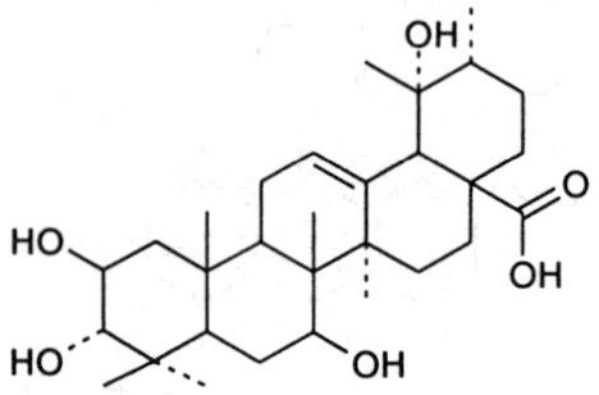

5610 Rubiadin
$C_{15}H_{10}O_4$ MW: 254.24 Property: mp 270-1°C. Source: TU LIAN QIAO, YANG JIAO TENG. Ref: 6.

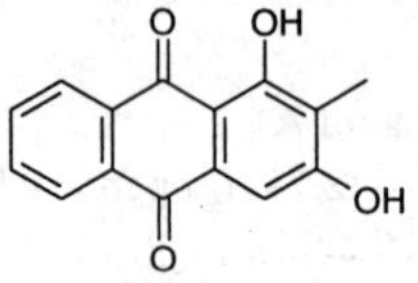

5611 Rubiadin-1-methyl ether
$C_{16}H_{12}O_4$ MW: 268.27 Property: mp 291°C. Source: TU LIAN QIAO, YANG JIAO TENG. Ref: 6.

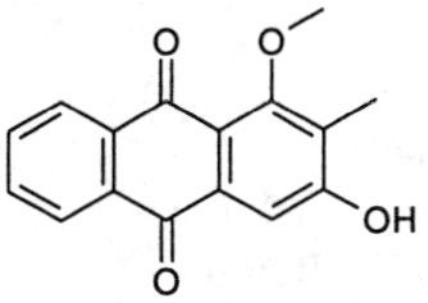

5612 Rubiadin primeveroside
$C_{26}H_{28}O_{13}$ MW: 548.51 Property: mp 248-50°C. Source: PENG ZI CAI. Ref: 6.

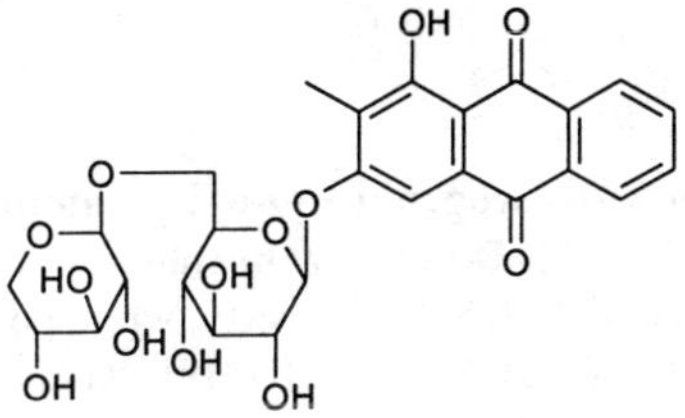

5613 Rubichrome
$C_{50}H_{68}O_2$ MW: 701.10 Property: mp 154°C (vaccum). Source: KONG QUE CAO. Ref: 6.

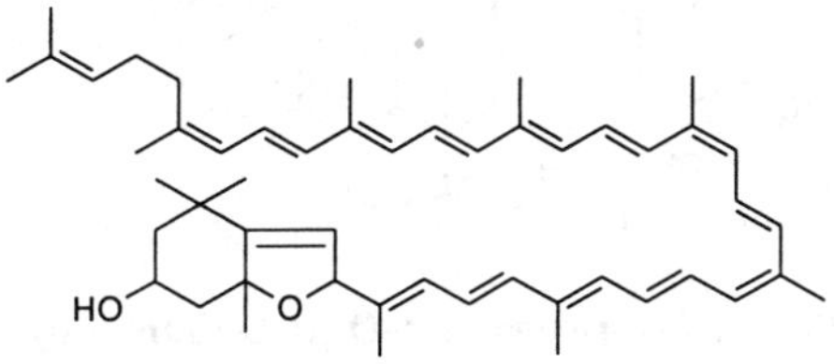

5614 Rubijervine
$C_{27}H_{43}NO_2$ MW: 413.65 Property: mp 242°C. Source: LI LU. Ref: 6.

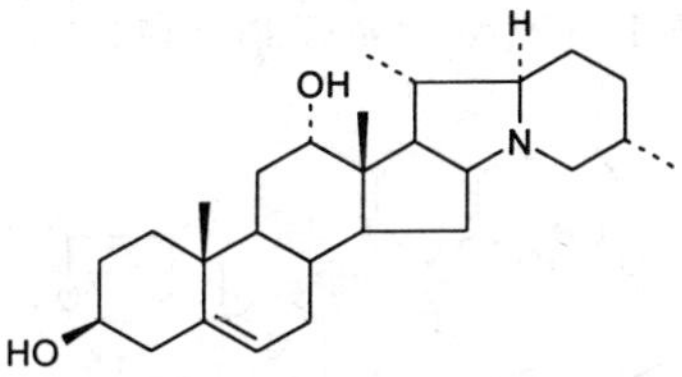

5615 Rubilactone
$C_{15}H_{10}O_5$ MW: 270.24 Property: light yellow crystal, mp 216-8°C. Source: QIAN CAO. Ref: 226.

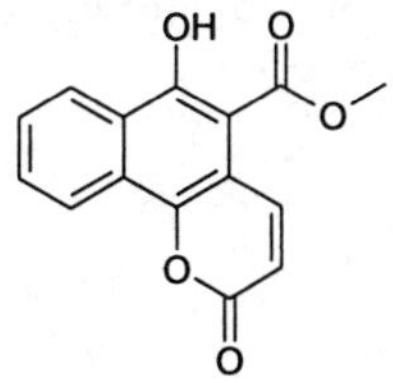

5616 Rubimaillin
3'-Carbomethoxy-4'-hydroxy-6,6-dimethylnaphtho(1',2'-2,3)pyran. $C_{17}H_{16}O_4$ MW: 284.31 Property: light yellow lamellar crystal, mp 128-30°C (recrystallization in alcohol), easily soluble in chloroform, benzene and acetic acid, soluble in ether, methanol and acetone, slightly soluble in ethanol, insoluble in water, but soluble in the water solution of sodium hydroxide or potassium hydroxide. Source: DA YE QIAN CAO. Ref: 22.

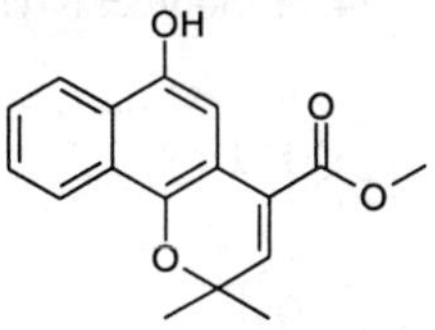

5617 Rubixanthin
$C_{40}H_{56}O$ MW: 552.89 Property: mp 160°C. Source: JIN ZHAN JU, MEI GUI HUA. Ref: 6.

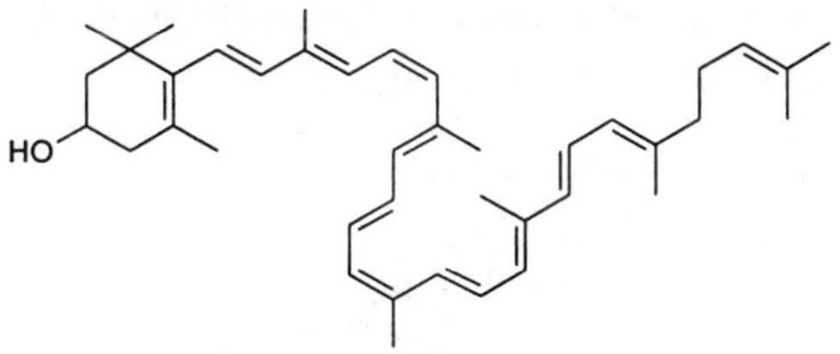

5618 Rubricauloside
5,7-Dimethoxy-8-[2'-hydroxy-3'-methyl, 3'-O-β-D-apiofuranosyl(1→6)-β-D-glucopyranosylbutyl]-coumaring. $C_{27}H_{38}O_{15}$ MW: 602.59 Property: white amorphous, mp 123-7°C, $[\alpha]_D^{16}$ -38.5° (c=0.31, DMSO). Source: YUN QIAN HU. Ref: 177, 476.

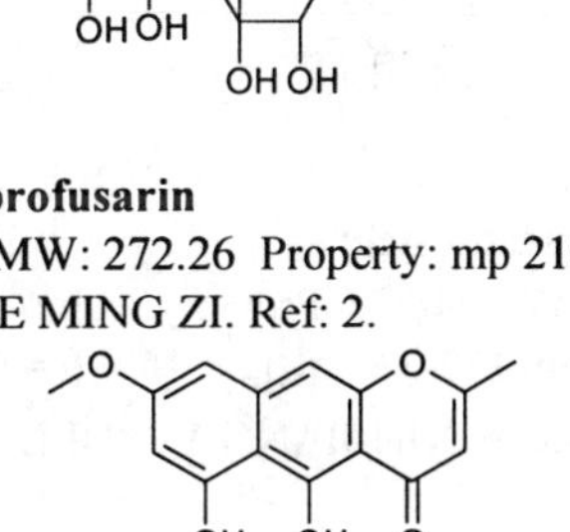

5619 Rubrofusarin
$C_{15}H_{12}O_5$ MW: 272.26 Property: mp 210-1°C. Source: JUE MING ZI. Ref: 2.

5620 Rubrofusarin-6-β-gentiobioside
$C_{27}H_{32}O_{15}$ MW: 596.55 Source: Ref: 2.

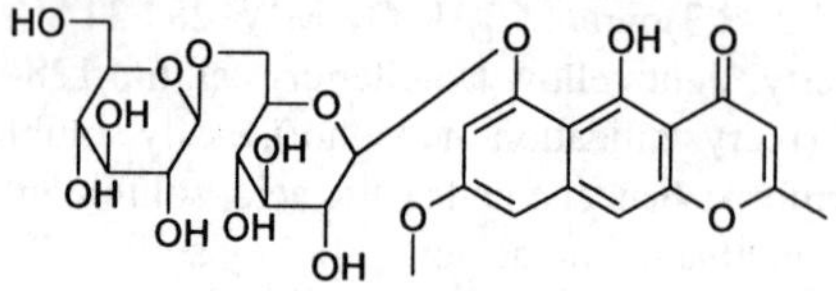

5621 Rubrosterone
$C_{19}H_{26}O_5$ MW: 334.42 Source: NIU XI. Ref: 2.

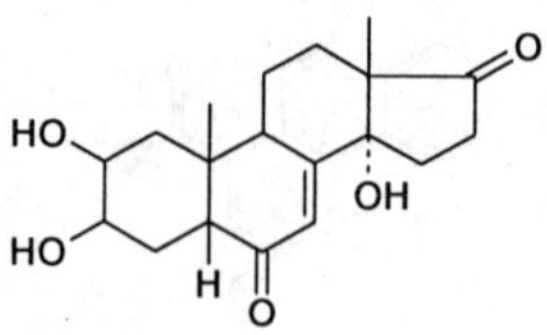

5622 Rubschisantherin
$C_{25}H_{30}O_8$ MW: 458.51 Property: amorphism powder, $[\alpha]_D^{18}$ -69° (ethanol). Source: HONG HUA WU WEI ZI, WU WEI ZI. Ref: 39.

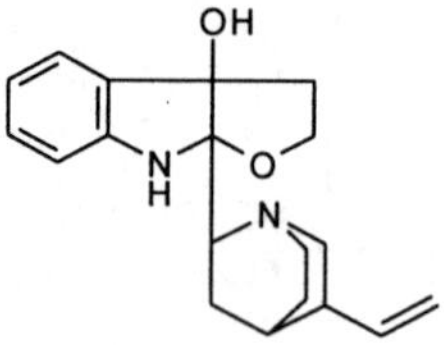

5623 γ-Rudecalactone
$C_{11}H_{20}O_2$ MW: 184.28 Source: CHAI HU. Ref: 2.

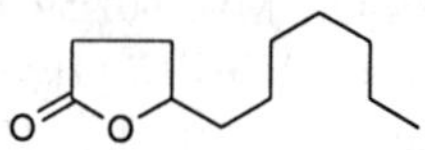

5624 Ruine
$C_{19}H_{22}N_2O_7$ MW: 390.40 Property: mp 227-9°C. Source: LUO TUO PENG. Ref: 6.

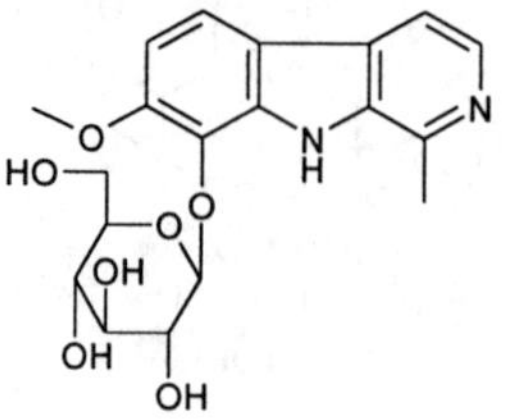

5625 Rupestonic acid
$C_{15}H_{20}O_3$ MW: 248.32 Property: colorless acicular crystal, mp 132-3°C, $[\alpha]_D^{25}$ +150° (c= 0.176 ethanol). Source: XIN JIANG YI ZHI HAO. Ref: 96.

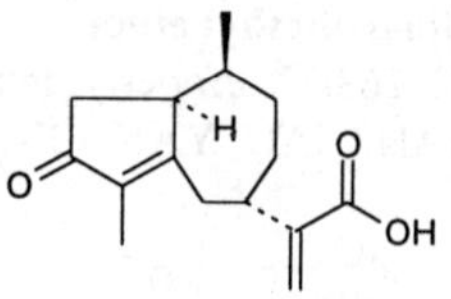

5626 Ruscogenin
$C_{27}H_{42}O_4$ MW: 430.63 Property: mp 205-11°C. Source: JI LI GEN. Ref: 6.

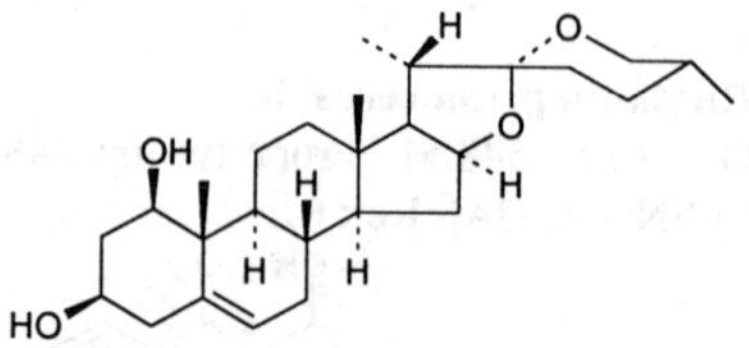

5627 25(S)-Ruscogenin 1-O-α-L-rhamnopyranosyl(1→2)-β-D-xylopyranoside
$C_{38}H_{62}O_{12}$ MW:708.89 Property: white powder, mp 232-4°C (dec). Source: HU BEI SHAN MAI DONG. Ref: 142.

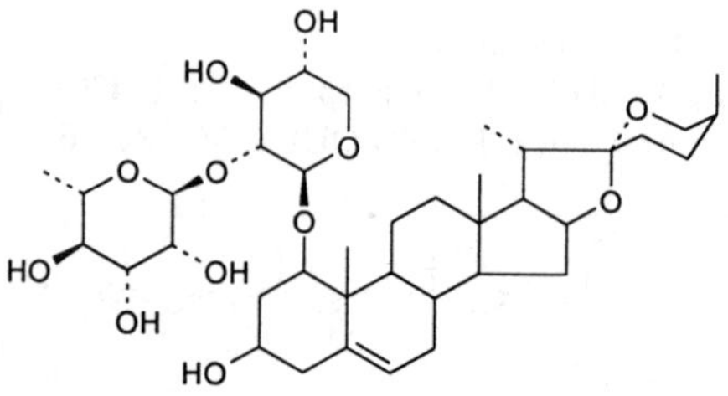

5628 25(S)-Ruscogenin 1-O-[α-L-rhamnopyranosyl(1→2)][β-D-xylopyra-nosyl(1→3)]-β-D-fucopyranoside
$C_{44}H_{70}O_{16}$ MW: 855.04 Property: colorless acicular crystal, mp 240-2°C, $[\alpha]_D^{24}$ -100.9°. Source: HU BEI SHAN MAI DONG. Ref: 142.

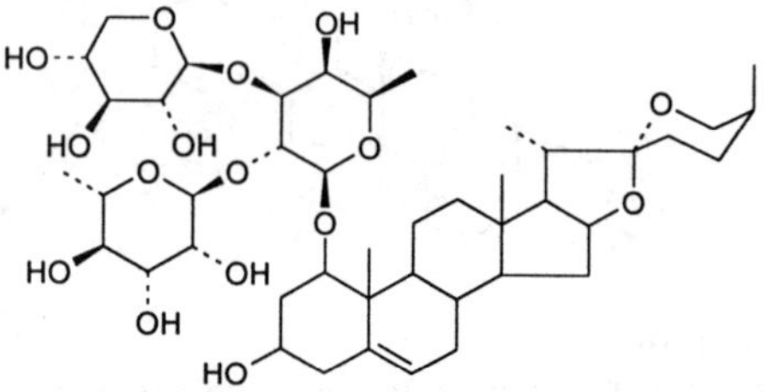

5629 Rutacridone
$C_{19}H_{17}NO_3$ MW: 307.35 Property: mp 161-2°C. Source: CHOU CAO. Ref: 6.

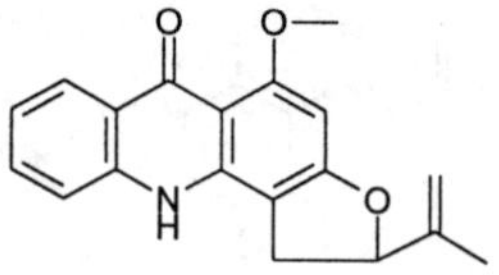

5630 Rutacultin
$C_{16}H_{18}O_4$ MW: 274.32 Property: mp 100-2°C. Source: CHOU CAO. Ref: 6.

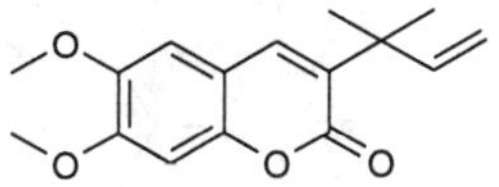

5631 Rutaecarpine
$C_{18}H_{15}N_3O$ MW: 289.34 Property: mp 256°C. Source: WU ZHU YU. Ref: 2, 347.

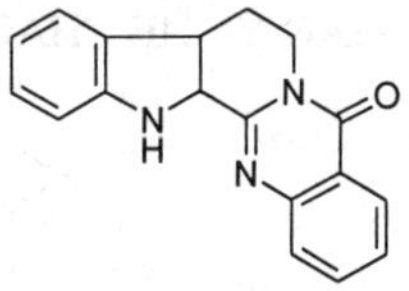

5632 Rutaevine
$C_{26}H_{30}O_9$ MW: 486.52 Source: WU ZHU YU. Ref: 2.

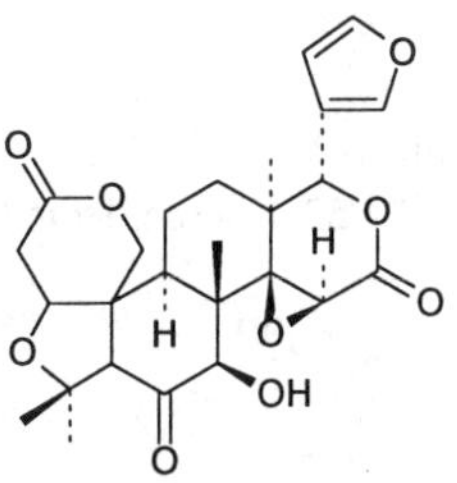

5633 Rutaevine acetate
$C_{28}H_{32}O_{10}$ MW: 528.56 Source: WU ZHU YU. Ref: 2.

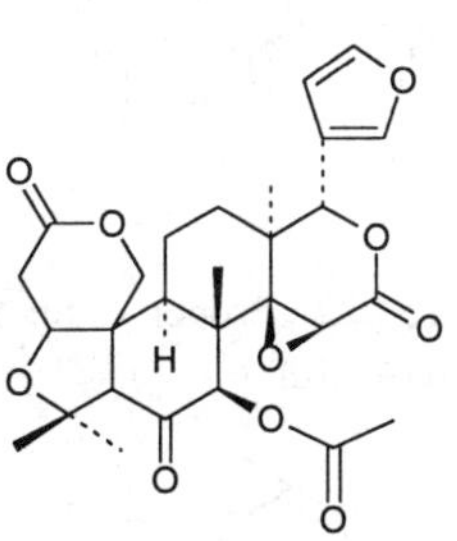

5634 Rutalinidine
$C_{15}H_{17}NO_4$ MW: 275.31 Source: CHOU CAO. Ref: 6.

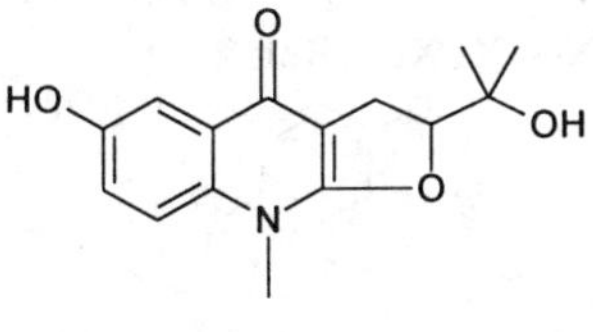

5635 Rutalinium
$C_{16}H_{23}NO_4$ MW: 293.37 Source: CHOU CAO. Ref: 6.

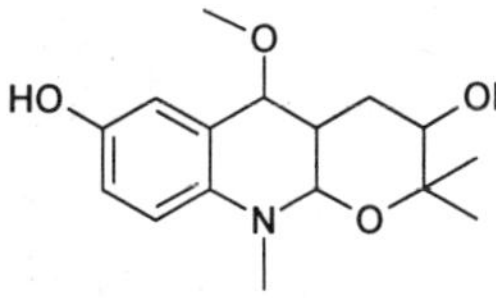

5636 Rutamarin
Chalepin acetate. CAS: 14882-94-1 $C_{21}H_{24}O_5$ MW: 356.42 Property: mp 107-8°C. Source: CHOU CAO, YAN JIAO CAO. Ref: 5.

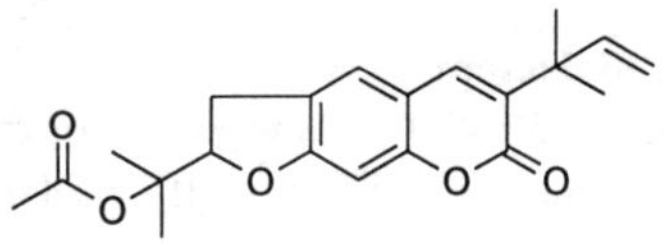

5637 Rutamarin alcohol
$C_{19}H_{22}O_4$ MW: 314.38 Property: mp 165°C. Source: CHOU CAO. Ref: 6.

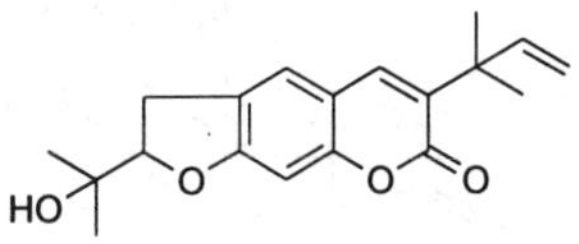

5638 Rutin
Quercetin 3-rutinoside; Violaquercitrin. CAS: 153-18-4 $C_{27}H_{30}O_{16}$ MW: 610.53 Source: BAI GUO, CU LIU GUO (SHA JI), DA ZAO, HUI HUA, JIN QIAO MAI, LU HUI, NING MA YE, QIAO MAI JIE, QI YE DAN, QING HAO, PU HUANG, SHAN ZHA, WU LA ER GAN CAO, XIAN HE CAO, YE WU TONG, YE XIA ZHU, YI MU CAO, YIN CHEN HAO, YU XING CAO. Ref: 2, 4, 6, 231, 283, 594.

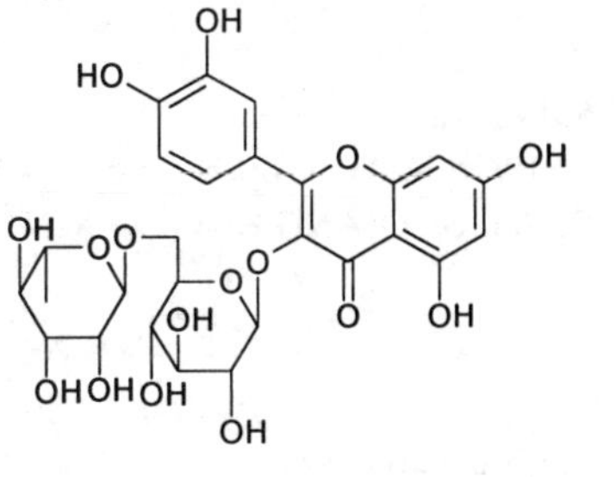

5639 Rutinoside
Property: light yellow acicular crystal, mp 174-6°C. Source: PU GONG YING. Ref: 440.

5640 Ruvoside

$C_{30}H_{46}O_9$ MW: 550.70 Property: mp 232-4°C. Source: HUANG HUA JIA ZHU TAO. Ref: 6.

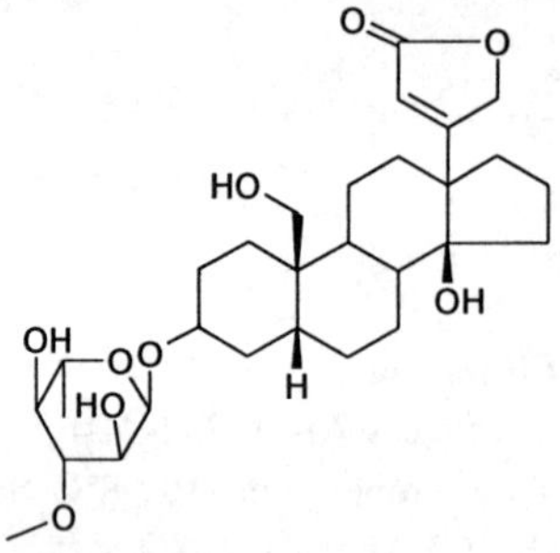

5642 Sabialactone

$C_{30}H_{46}O_4$ MW: 470.70 Property: colorless granular crystal , mp 273-5°C, $[\alpha]_D^{13}$ +78.65° (c=0.09, chloroform). Source: JIAN YE QING FENG TENG . Ref: 326, 403, 407, 377.

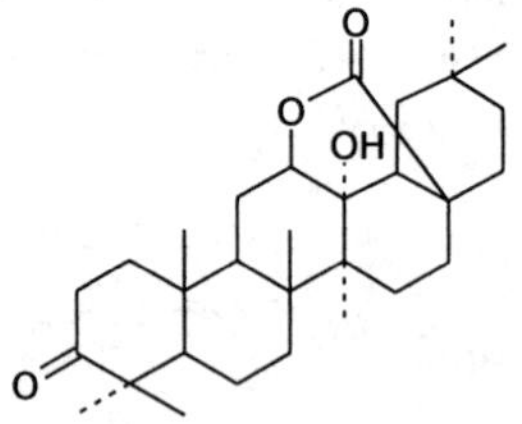

5643 Sabianone

$C_{30}H_{48}O_2$ MW: 440.72 Property: white amorphous powder, mp 185°C. Source: JIAN YE QING FENG TENG . Ref: 326.

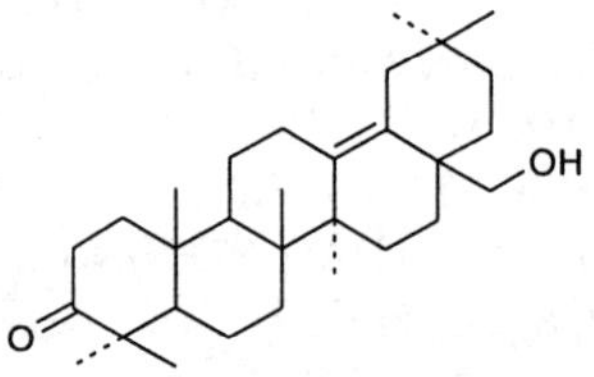

5644 Sabinene

$C_{10}H_{16}$ MW: 136.24 Property: bp (+): 163-5°C, (-): 162-6°C. Source: QIANG HUO, XI XIN. Ref: 2.

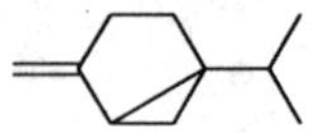

5645 Sabinene hydrate

$C_{11}H_{20}$ MW: 152.28 Property: mp (+): 36.5-7.2°C. Source: Ref: 2.

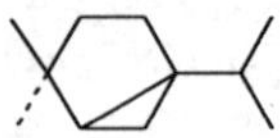

5646 Sabinol

$C_{10}H_{16}O$ MW: 152.24 Property: bp 208°C. Source: CHOU BAI. Ref: 6.

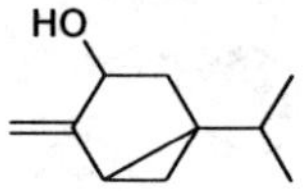

5647 Sackogenin Q

oleana-11,13,(18)-diene-3β,16β,28,30-pentol.

$C_{30}H_{48}O_5$ MW: 488.71 Property: white powder, mp 302-4°C. Source: XIAO YE HE CHAI HU. Ref: 327.

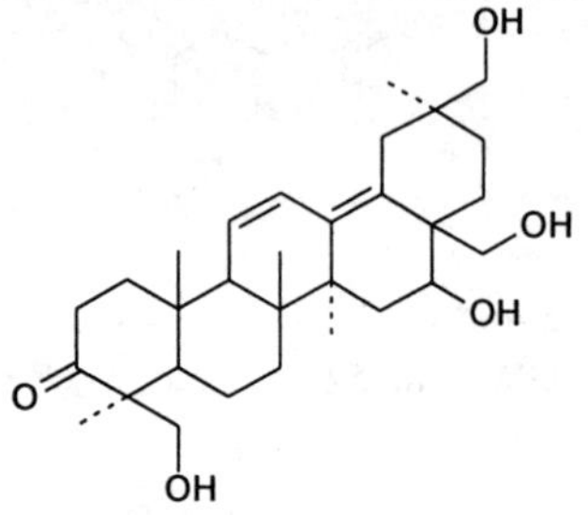

5648 Safflor yellow-A

$C_{27}H_{30}O_{15}$ MW: 594.53 Source: HONG HUA. Ref: 2.

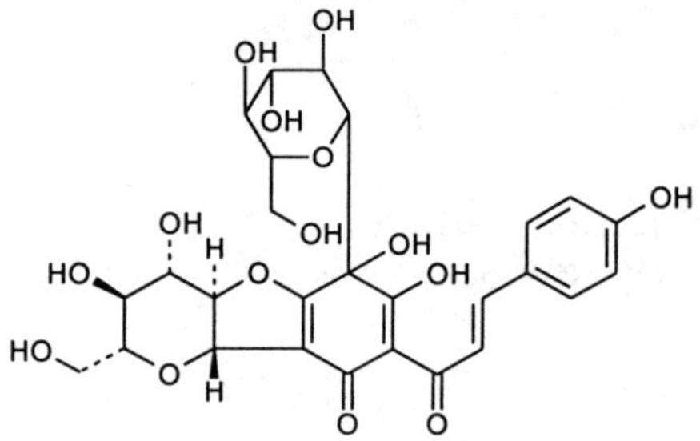

5649 Safranal

$C_{10}H_{14}O$ MW: 150.22 Property: bp 172°C. Source: ZANG HONG HUA. Ref: 6.

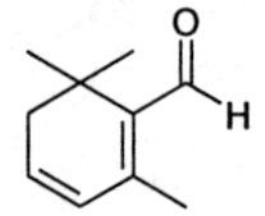

5650 Safrole

$C_{10}H_{10}O_2$ MW: 162.19 Source: LIAN QIAO, SHENG JIANG, XI XIN. Ref: 2.

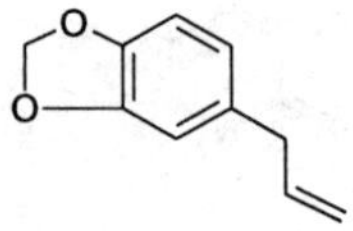

5651 Sagittariol
$C_{19}H_{32}O_2$ MW: 292.47 Property: mp 109-10°C. Source: CI GU. Ref: 6.

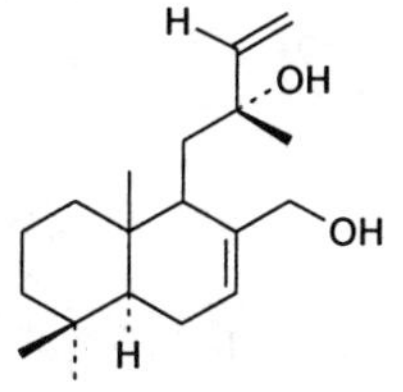

5652 Sagittatin A
Source: YIN YANG HUO. Ref: 2.

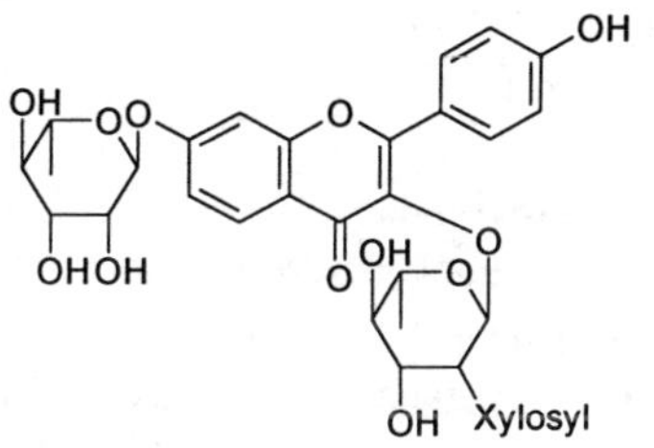

5653 Sagittatin B
Source: YIN YANG HUO. Ref: 2.

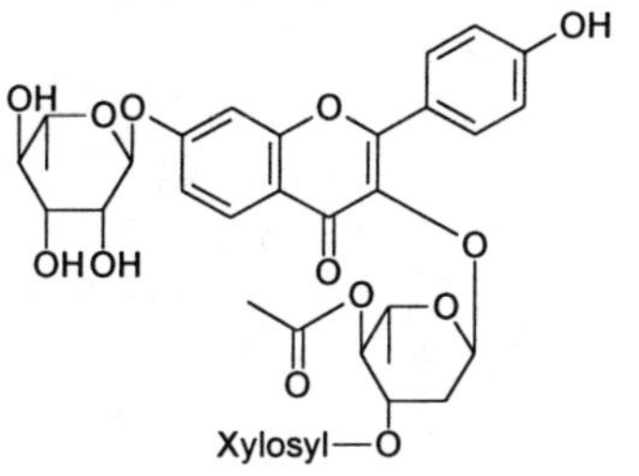

5654 Sagittatoside A
Source: WAN SHAN YIN YANG HUO, YIN YANG HUO. Ref: 2, 574.

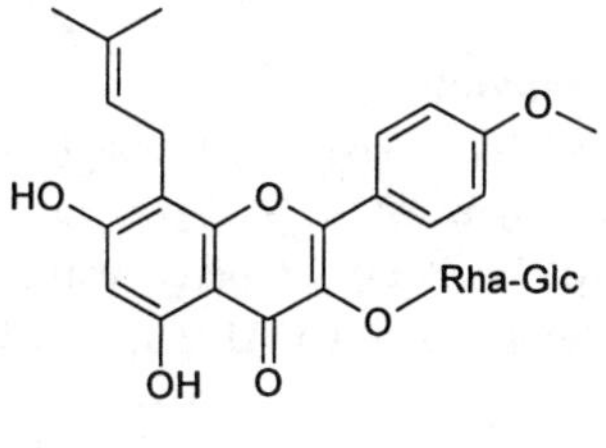

5655 Sagittatoside B
Source: WAN SHAN YIN YANG HUO, YIN YANG HUO. Ref: 2, 565, 574.

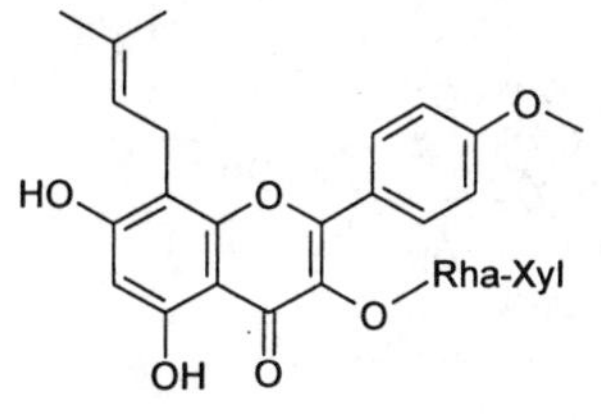

5656 Sagittatoside C
Source: YIN YANG HUO. Ref: 2.

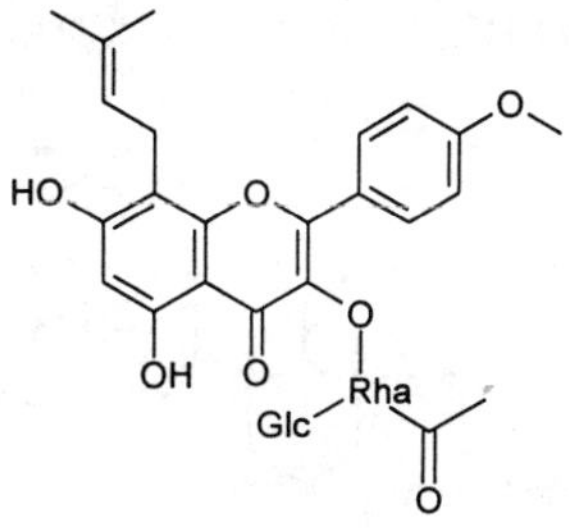

5657 Sagittin
5-Hydroxy-6,7-dimethoxy-3',4'-methylene-dioxy-flavone. $C_{18}H_{14}O_7$ MW: 342.31 Property: yellow acicular crystal, mp 254-257°C (230°C, sub). Source: YIN YANG HUO. Ref: 485.

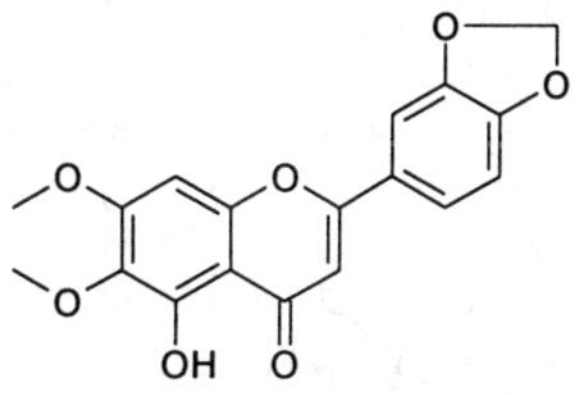

5658 Saikogenin E
$C_{30}H_{48}O_3$ MW: 456.72 Property: mp 289°C (dec). Source: CHAI HU. Ref: 2.

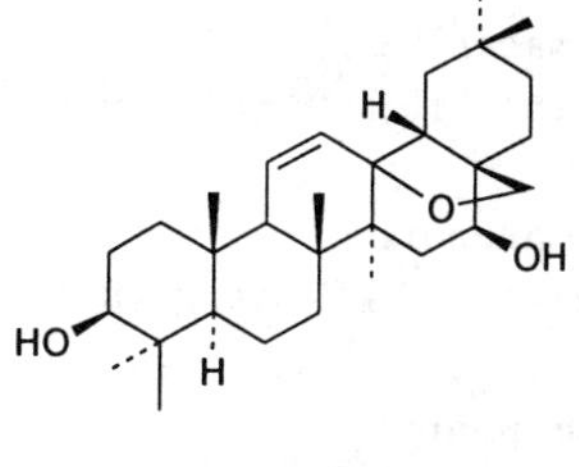

5659 Saikogenin F
$C_{30}H_{48}O_4$ MW: 472.71 Property: mp 265-73°C. Source: CHAI HU, XIAO YE HEI CHAI HU. Ref: 2, 598.

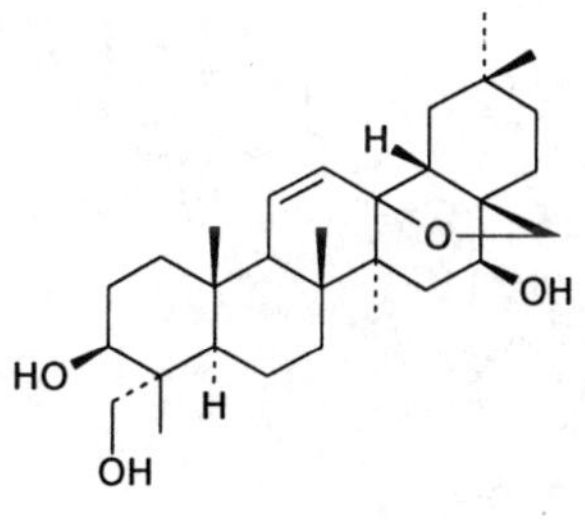

5660 Saikogenin G

$C_{30}H_{48}O_4$ MW: 472.71 Property: mp 238-45°C. Source: CHAI HU, XIAO YE HEI CHAI HU. Ref: 2, 598.

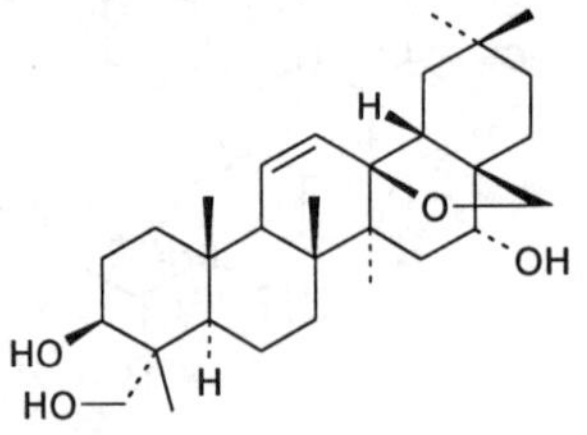

5661 Saikosaponin a

CAS: 20736-09-8 $C_{42}H_{68}O_{13}$ MW: 781.00 Property: mp 225-32°C. Source: CHAI HU, XIAO YE HEI CHAI HU. Ref: 5, 403, 598.

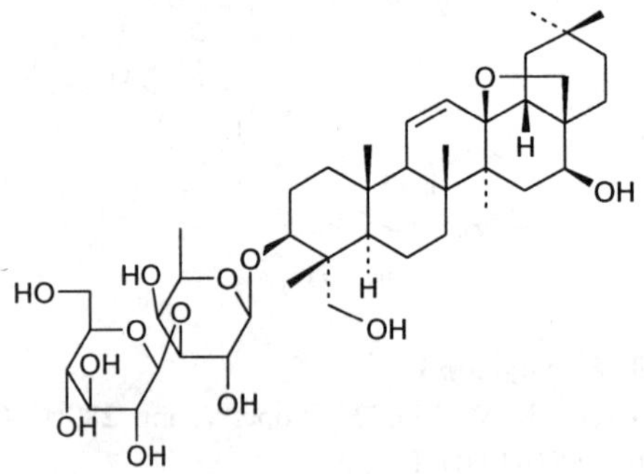

5662 Saikosaponin b2

Source: XIAO YE HEI CHAI HU. Ref: 598.

5663 Saikosaponin b4

Source: XIAO YE HEI CHAI HU. Ref: 598.

5664 Saikosaponin c

$C_{48}H_{78}O_{17}$ MW: 927.15 Property: mp 202-10°C. Source: CHAI HU. Ref: 2, 403.

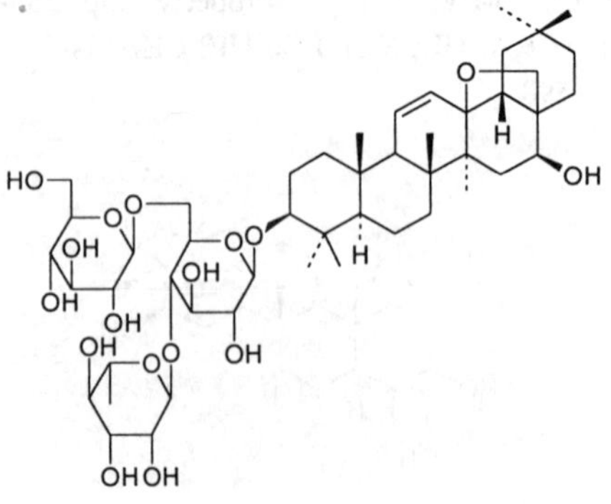

5665 Saikosaponin d

CAS: 20874-52-6 $C_{42}H_{68}O_{13}$ MW: 781.00 Property: mp 212-8°C. Source: CHAI HU, XIAO YE HEI CHAI HU. Ref: 5, 403, 598.

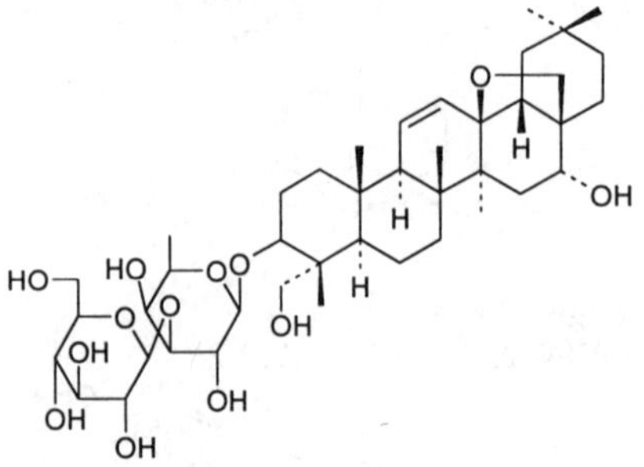

5666 Saikosaponin k

3β,16β,23,28-Tetrahydroxyoleana-11,13(18)-dien-3-O-β-D-xylopyranosyl-(1→2)-β-D-glucopyranosyl-(1→3)-β-D-fucopyranoside. $C_{47}H_{76}O_{17}$ MW: 913.12 Property: white powder, mp 241-245°C, $[\alpha]_D^{21}$ -20.9° (c=0.12, EtOH). Source: HEI CHAI HU. Ref: 264.

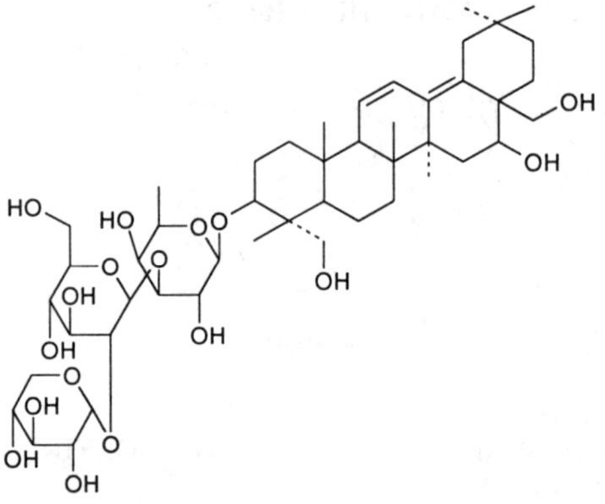

5667 Saikosaponin l

3β,16α,23,28,30-Pentahydroxyoleana-11,13(18)-dien-3-O-β-D-glucopyranosyl-(1→3)-β-D-fucopyranoside. $C_{42}H_{68}O_{14}$ MW: 797.00 Property: white powder, mp 208-212°C. Source: HEI CHAI HU. Ref: 264, 407.

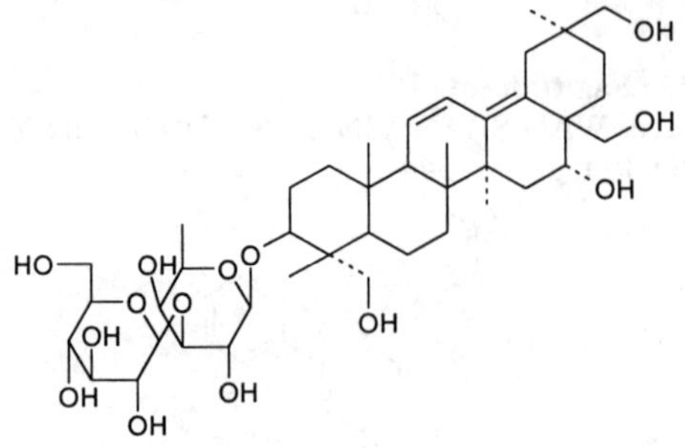

5668 Saikosaponin m
3β,23,28-trihydroxyoleana-11,13(18)-dien-3-O-β-D-glucopyranosyl-(1→3)-β-D-fucopyranoside. $C_{42}H_{68}O_{12}$ MW: 765.00 Property: white powder, mp 205-10°C, $[\alpha]_D^{21}$ -117.6° (c=0.03, ethanol). Source: HEI CHAI HU. Ref: 313.

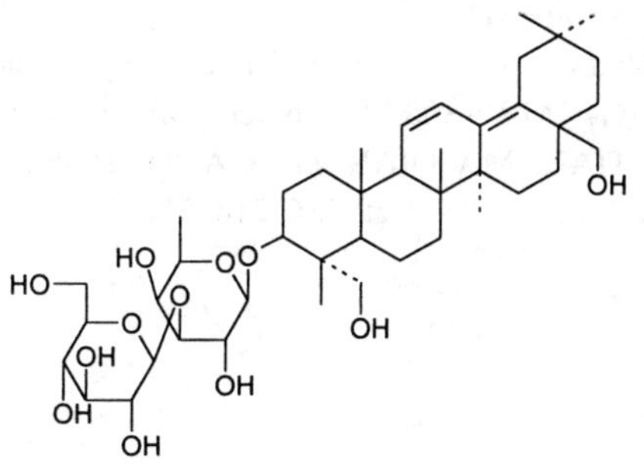

5669 Saikosaponin n
3β,16β,23,28-Tetrahydroxyoleana-11,13(18)-dien-3-O-β-D-glucopyranosyl-(1→6)-[α-L-rhamnopyranosyl(1→4)]-β-D-glucopyranoside. $C_{48}H_{78}O_{18}$ MW: 943.15 Property: white powder, mp 217-21°C, $[\alpha]_D^{21}$ +81.6° (c=0.10, ethanol). Source: HEI CHAI HU. Ref: 313.

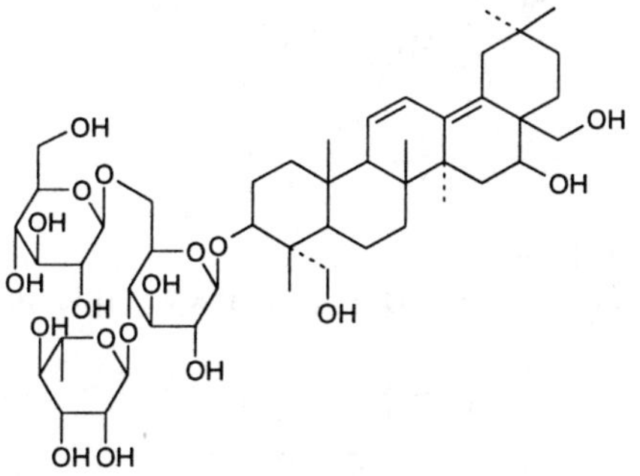

5670 Saikosaponin q
3β,16β,23,28,30-pentahydroxyoleana-11,13,(18)-diene-3β-D-glucopyranosyl-(1→6)-[α-L-rhamnopyranosyl(1→4)]-β-D-glucopyranoside. $C_{48}H_{78}O_{19}$ MW: 959.15 Property: white powder, mp 224-7°C. Source: XIAO YE HEI CHAI HU. Ref: 327.

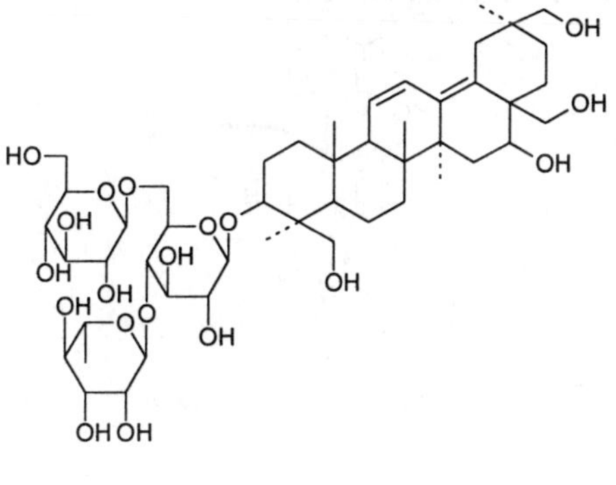

5671 Saikosaponin t
3β,16β,28-Trihydroxy-11-α-β-methoxy-olean-12-ene-3-O-β-D-glucosyl-(1→3)-β-D-fucoside. $C_{43}H_{72}O_{13}$ MW: 813.04 Property: white powder, mp 223-5°C. Source: BEI CHAI HU. Ref: 403.

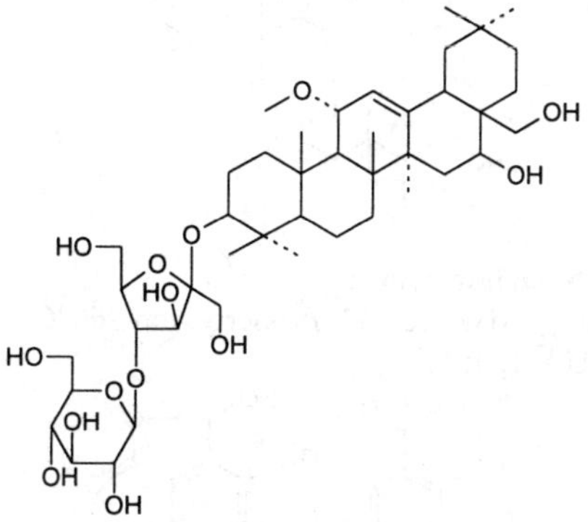

5672 Saikosaponin V
3-O-[β-D-glucopyranosyl(1→3)-β-D-fucopyranosyl] - 3β,16α,23,28-tetrahydroxy-olean-11,13(18)-dien-30-oic acid 30-O-[xylityl(1→1)]-β-D-glucopyranosyl -6-ester. $C_{53}H_{86}O_{24}$ MW: 1107.26 Property: white powder, mp 198-201°C. Source: BEI CHAI HU. Ref: 407.

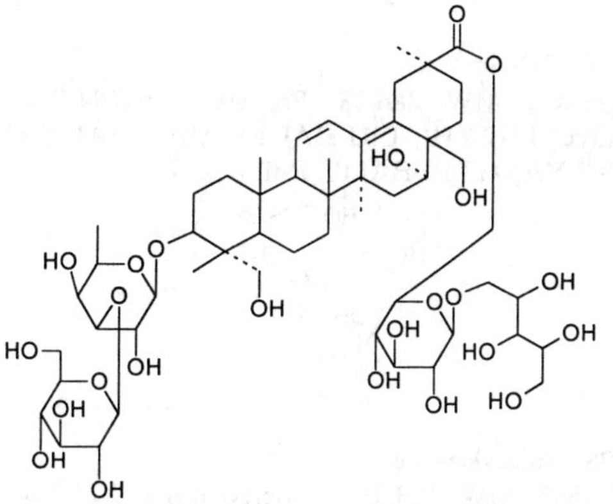

5673 Sakuranetin
$C_{16}H_{14}O_5$ MW: 286.29 Property: mp 152-154°C. Source: YING TAO. Ref: 6.

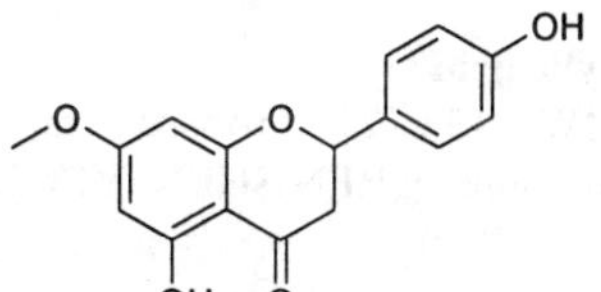

5674 Salaspermic acid
$C_{30}H_{48}O_4$ MW: 472.71 Source: LEI GONG TENG. Ref: 2.

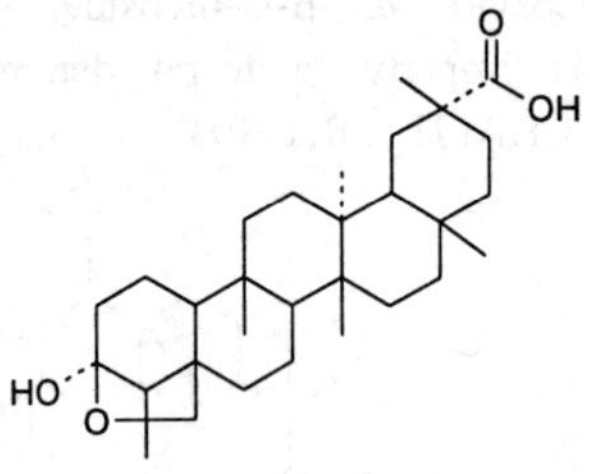

5675 Salazinic acid
$C_{19}H_{14}O_{10}$ MW: 402.32 Property: mp 260°C. Source: SHI HUA. Ref: 6.

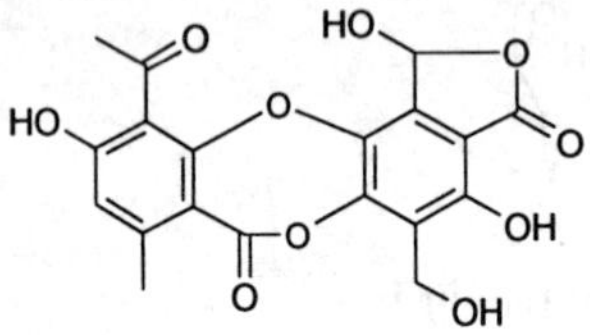

5676 Salicifoline
$C_{12}H_{20}NO_2$ MW: 210.30 Source: BAI LAN HUA, HOU PU, MU LAN PI, YE HE HUA. Ref: 6, 625.

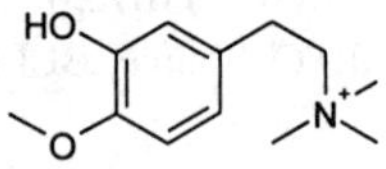

5677 Salicin
$C_{13}H_{18}O_7$ MW: 286.28 Property: mp 204.7-8.7°C. Source: LIU ZHI, LIU BAI PI, MAO BAI YANG, SHUI YANG MU BAI PI. Ref: 6, 269.

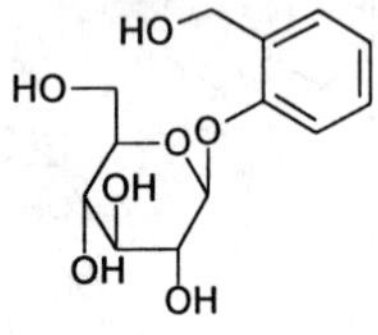

5678 Salicylamine
C_7H_9NO MW: 123.16 Property: mp 129°C. Source: QIAO MAI. Ref: 6.

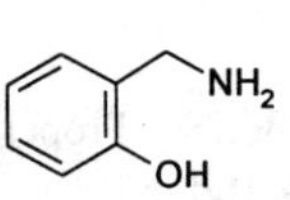

5679 Salicylic acid
$C_7H_6O_3$ MW: 138.12 Property: mp 159°C, bp 211°C/20mm. Source: REN SHEN, YIN CHEN HAO. Ref: 2.

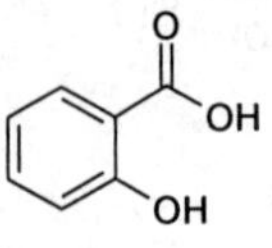

5680 N-Salicylidene-salicylamine
$C_{14}H_{13}NO_2$ MW: 227.27 Source: QIAO MAI. Ref: 6.

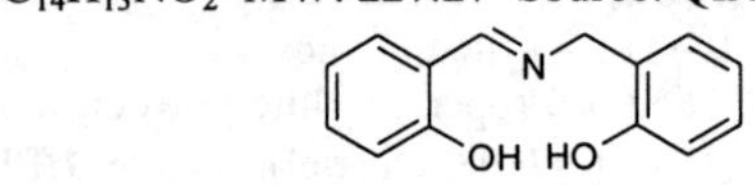

5681 Salidroside
2-[4-Hydroxyphenyl]ethanol-β-D-glucopyranoside.
$C_{14}H_{20}O_7$ MW: 300.31 Source: DA HUA, HONG JING TIAN, MA QIAN ZI, XIA YE HONG JING TIAN, YUE JU YE. Ref: 2, 6, 218, 516.

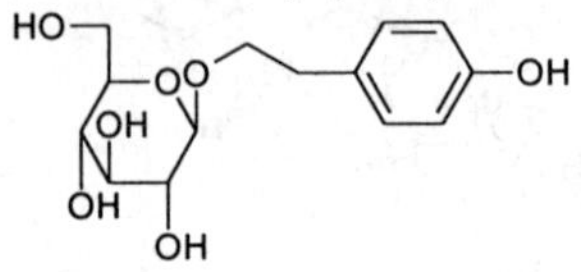

5682 Salipurposide
$C_{21}H_{22}O_{10}$ MW: 434.40 Property: mp 227°C. Source: SHUI YANG MU BAI PI, TAO ZHI. Ref: 6.

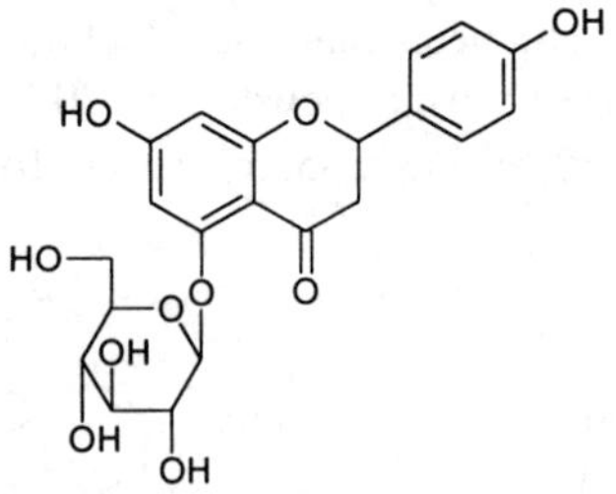

5683 Saloilenone
$C_{20}H_{20}O_2$ MW: 292.38 Source: DAN SHEN. Ref: 2.

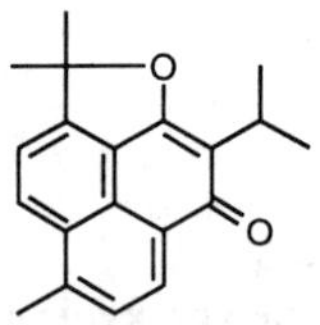

5684 Salutaridine
$C_{19}H_{21}NO_4$ MW: 327.38 Property: mp 197-8°C. Source: YA PIAN. Ref: 6.

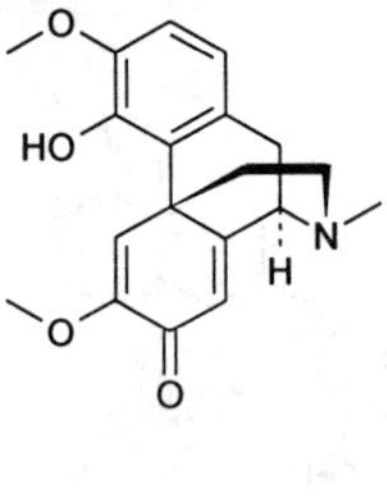

5685 Salviol
$C_{20}H_{30}O_2$ MW: 302.46 Property: mp 108°C. Source: DAN SHEN. Ref: 2.

5686 Sanchinoside B1
dammar-20(22)-en-3β,12β,25triol-6-O-β-D-glucopyranoside. $C_{36}H_{62}O_9$ MW: 638.89 Property: white powder, mp 144-6°C. Source: SAN QI. Ref: 28.

5687 Sandaracopimaric acid
Source: CI GU, JI MAO SONG. Ref: 520, 544.

5688 Sandaracopimarinol
$C_{20}H_{32}O$ MW: 288.48 Property: mp 63-5°C. Source: LIU SHAN. Ref: 6.

5689 Sanguinarine
ψ-Cheierythrine; Pseudochelerythrine. CAS: 2447-54-3. Property: mp 242-3°C (dec). Source: BAI QU CAI, BO LUO HUI, HE BAO MU DAN GEN, HE QING HUA, JU HUA HUANG LIAN, LI CHUN HUA, XI GUO JIAO HUI XIANG, YA PIAN, YING SU KE, ZI HUA YU DENG CAO (LIE BAO ZI JING). Ref: 4, 6.

5690 Sanleng acid
$C_{18}H_{34}O_5$ MW: 330.47 Property: white amorphous crystal, mp 116-8°C, soluble in ethanol, ethyl acetate. Source: SAN LENG. Ref: 480.

5691 Sanshool
$C_{16}H_{25}NO$ MW: 247.38 Property: mp 69°C. Source: YE HUA JIAO YE. Ref: 6.

5692 Santal aldehyde
$C_{15}H_{22}O$ MW: 218.34 Property: bp (+): 152-5°C/10 mm, (-): 105°C/0.3 mm. Source: TAN XIANG. Ref: 6.

5693 α-Santalene
$C_{15}H_{24}$ MW: 204.36 Property: bp 252°C/753 mm. Source: FENG DOU CAI, TAN XIANG, ZHANG MU. Ref: 6.

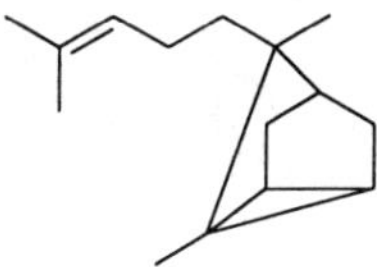

5694 β-Santalene
$C_{15}H_{24}$ MW: 204.36 Property: bp 125-7°C/9 mm, 263-4°C. Source: TAN XIANG, ZHANG MU. Ref: 6.

5695 Santalic acid
$C_{15}H_{22}O_2$ MW: 234.34 Property: mp β: 202°C γ: 189°C, bp α: 193°C/9 mm. Source: TAN XIANG. Ref: 6.

5696 α-Santalol
$C_{15}H_{24}O$ MW: 220.36 Property: bp 166-7°C/14mm. Source: HOU PO, REN SHEN, WU WEI ZI. Ref: 6.

5697 β-Santalol
$C_{15}H_{24}O$ MW: 220.36 Property: bp 177-8°C/17mm. Source: SHENG JIANG. Ref: 6.

5698 Santene
C_9H_{14} MW: 122.21 Property: bp 140-1°C. Source: TAN XIANG, YU XIANG CAO. Ref: 6.

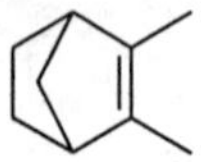

5699 Santenone
$C_9H_{14}O$ MW: 138.21 Property: mp (-): 58-61°C, (±): 55-7°C, bp (-): 193-5°C, (±): 197°C. Source: TAN XIANG. Ref: 6.

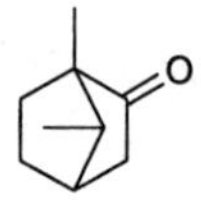

5700 Santenone alcohol
$C_9H_{16}O$ MW: 140.23 Property: mp 86°C (58-62°C). Source: TAN XIANG. Ref: 6.

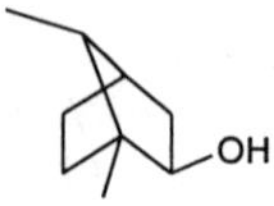

5701 α-Santonin
$C_{15}H_{18}O_3$ MW: 246.31 Property: mp (-): 174-6°C. Source: SHAN DAO NIAN HAO (HUI HAO). Ref: 6.

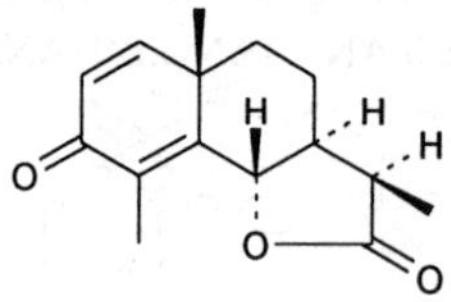

5702 β-Santonin
$C_{15}H_{18}O_3$ MW: 246.31 Property: mp (-): 216-8°C. Source: DONG BEI HUI HAO, HUANG HUA HAO. Ref: 6.

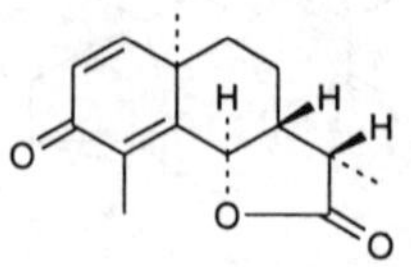

5703 Sapindoside A
$C_{41}H_{66}O_{12}$ MW: 750.98 Property: mp 214-6°C. Source: WU HUAN ZI YE, WU HUAN ZI PI. Ref: 6.

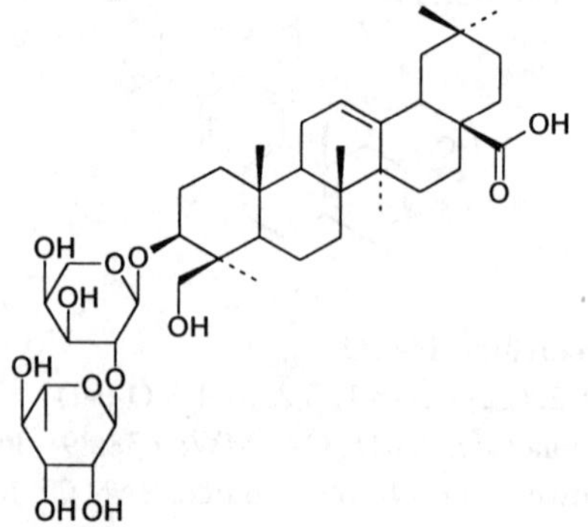

5704 Sapindoside B
$C_{46}H_{74}O_{16}$ MW: 883.09 Property: mp 276-8°C. Source: WU HUAN ZI YE, WU HUAN ZI PI. Ref: 6.

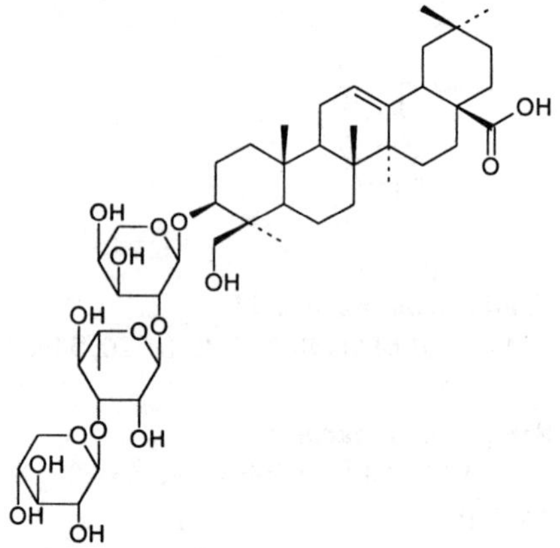

5705 Sapindoside C
$C_{52}H_{84}O_{21}$ MW: 1045.24 Property: mp 235°C. Source: WU HUAN ZI PI. Ref: 6.

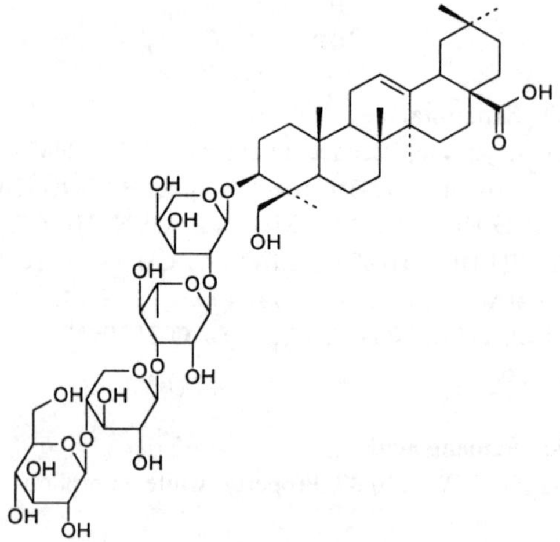

5706 Sapindoside D

$C_{64}H_{104}O_{30}$ MW: 1353.52 Source: WU HUAN ZI PI. Ref: 6.

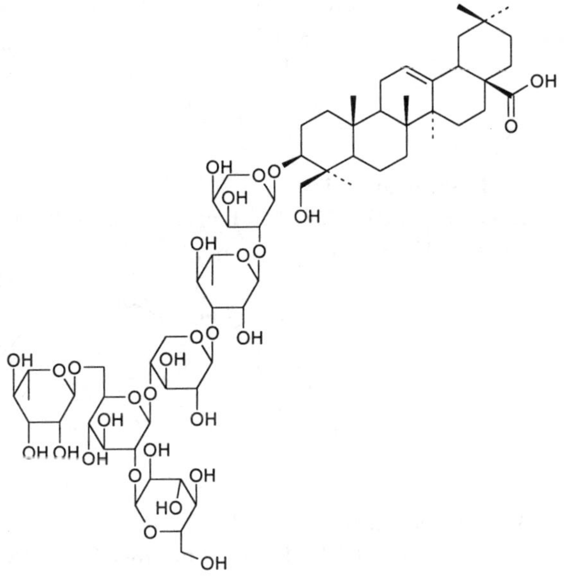

5707 Sapindoside E

$C_{80}H_{130}O_{42}$ MW: 1763.90 Source: WU HUAN ZI PI. Ref: 6.

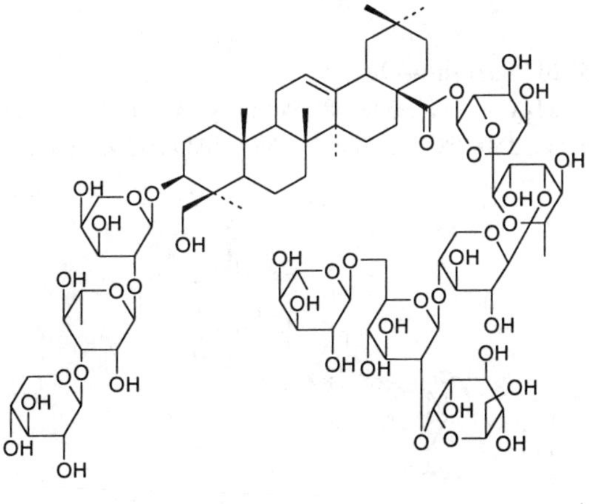

5708 Sapogenin ST-I

$C_{30}H_{50}O_3$ MW: 458.73 Property: mp 279-82°C. Source: CHA ZI XIN. Ref: 6.

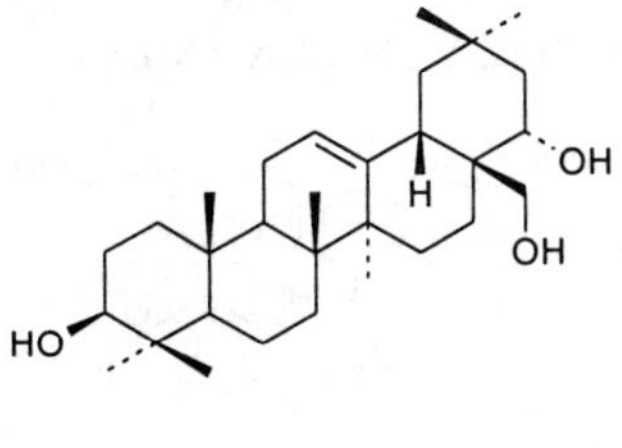

5709 Saponarin

$C_{27}H_{30}O_{15}$ MW: 594.53 Property: mp 231-2°C (dec). Source: MU JIN HUA, SHUI MU CAO. Ref: 6.

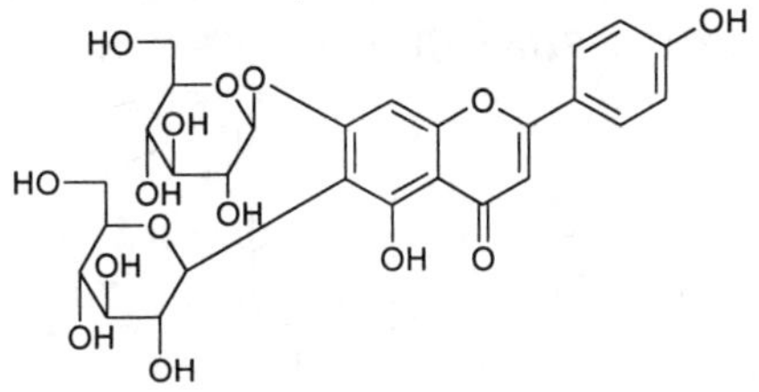

5710 Sappanin

2,4,3',4'-Tetrahydroxybiphenyl. $C_{12}H_{10}O_4$ MW: 218.21 Property: mp 210-1°C. Source: SU MU. Ref: 6.

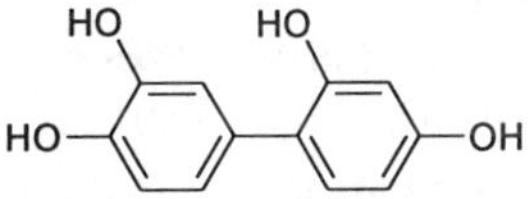

5711 Sarcosine

$C_3H_7NO_2$ MW: 89.09 Property: mp 212-3°C (dec). Source: LI YU, MO GU. Ref: 6.

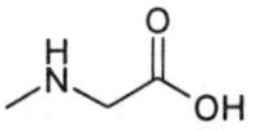

5712 Sarcostin

$C_{21}H_{34}O_6$ MW: 382.50 Source: BAI SHOU WU, LUO MO, XU CHANG QING. Ref: 6.

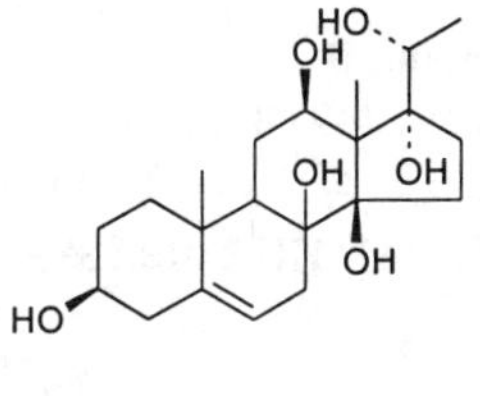

5713 Sarcovaging A

$C_{28}H_{48}N_2O_3$ MW: 460.71 Property: white acicular crystal, mp 277-8 °C, $[\alpha]_D^{25}$ +21.2° (c=0.11, chloroform). Source: HAI NAN YE SHAN HUA. Ref: 399.

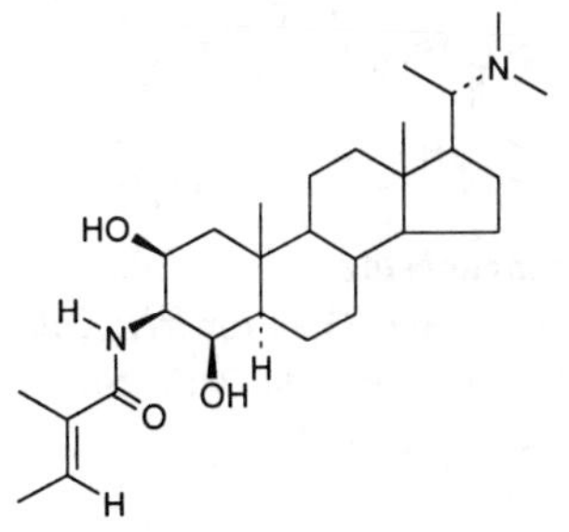

5714 Sarcovaging B

$C_{30}H_{50}N_2O_4$ MW: 502.74 Property: white crystal, mp 205-6 °C, $[\alpha]_D^{25}$ +19.6 ° (c=0.06, chloroform). Source: HAI NAN YE SHAN HUA. Ref: 399.

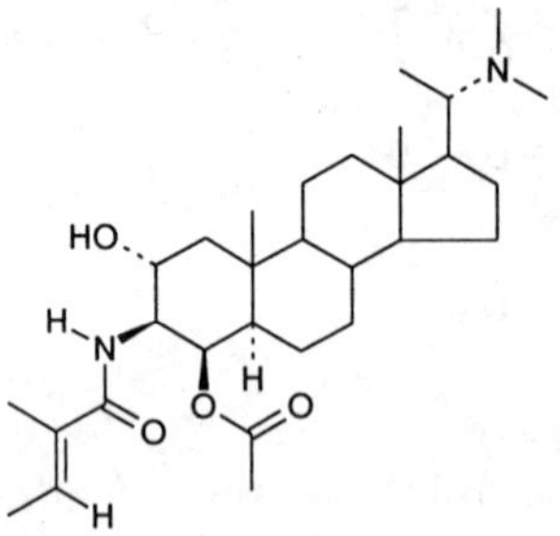

5715 Sarcovaging C

$C_{30}H_{50}N_2O_3$ MW: 486.74 Property: white acicular crystal, mp 192-4°C, $[\alpha]_D^{13}$ -9.01° (c=0.122, chloroform). Source: HAI NAN YE SHAN HUA. Ref: 399.

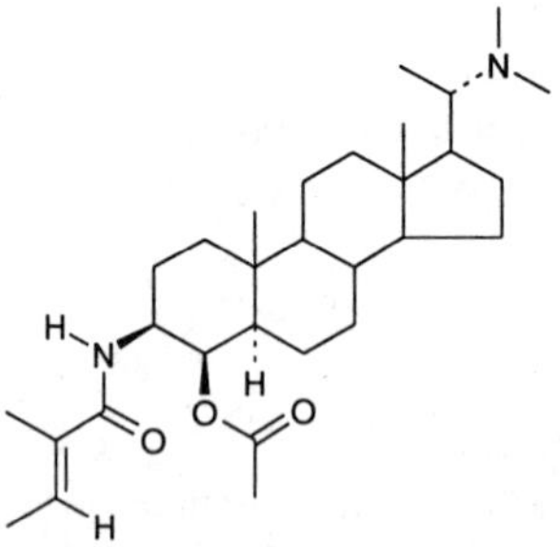

5716 Sarcovaging D

$C_{28}H_{44}N_2O_2$ MW: 440.68 Property: white crystal, mp 170-2°C, $[\alpha]_D^{25}$ +39.5° (c=0.07, chloroform). Source: HAI NAN YE SHAN HUA. Ref: 399.

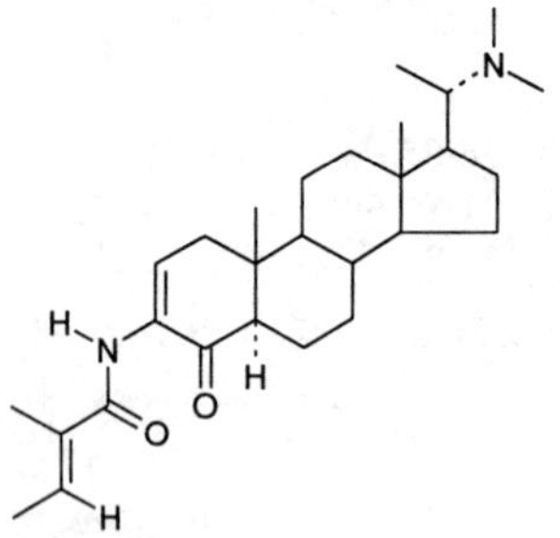

5717 Sargencuneside

$C_{14}H_{20}O_7$ MW: 300.31 Property: colorless acicular crystal (ethanol), mp 161-2°C. Source: DA XUE TENG. Ref: 481.

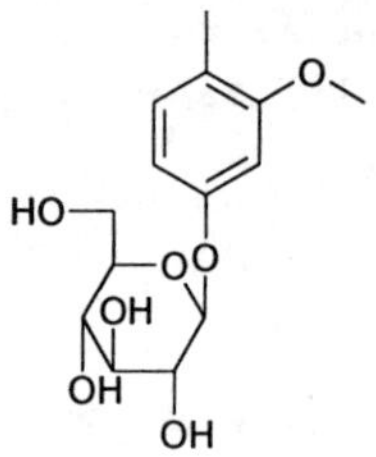

5718 Saringosterol

$C_{29}H_{48}O_2$ MW: 428.70 Property: mp 160-1°C. Source: KUN BU. Ref: 6.

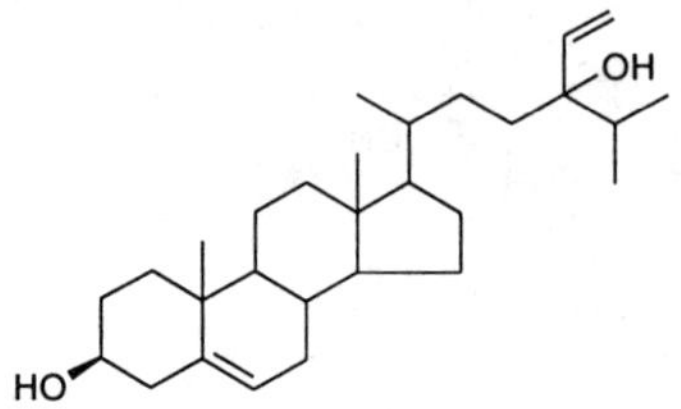

5719 Sarmentose

$C_7H_{14}O_4$ MW: 162.19 Property: mp 78-9°C. Source: FU SHOU CAO, LUO MO ZI. Ref: 6.

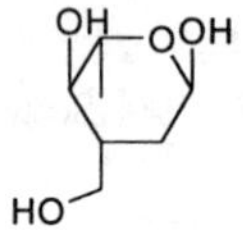

5720 Sarmutoside

$C_{30}H_{44}O_9$ MW: 548.68 Property: mp 150-2°C, 233-45°C, 250-2°C. Source: YANG JIAO AO ZI. Ref: 6.

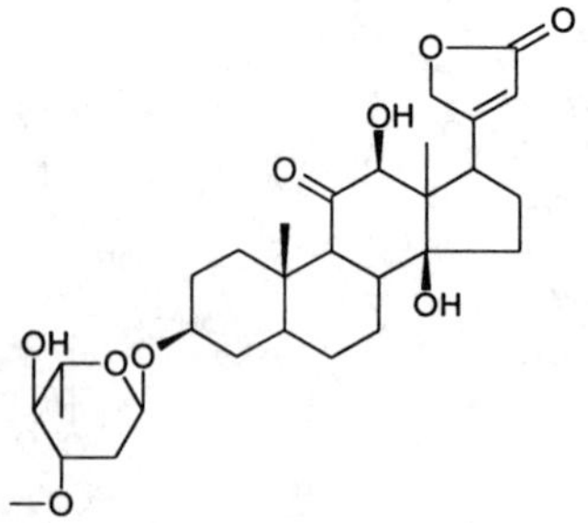

5721 Sarpagine

$C_{19}H_{22}N_2O_2$ MW: 310.40 Property: white prismatic crystal, mp 300-10°C, $[\alpha]_D^{24.4}$ +48.65° (c=1.483, pyridine). Source: YANG JIAO MIAN. Ref: 633.

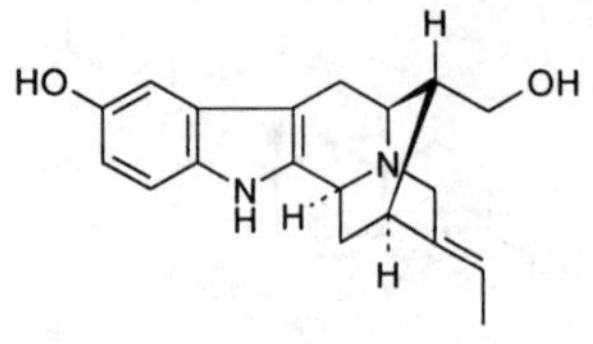

5722 Sarracenin

CAS: 59653-37-1 $C_{11}H_{14}O_5$ MW: 226.23 Property: mp 127-8°C (dec). Source: *Sarracenia flava* L. Ref: 5.

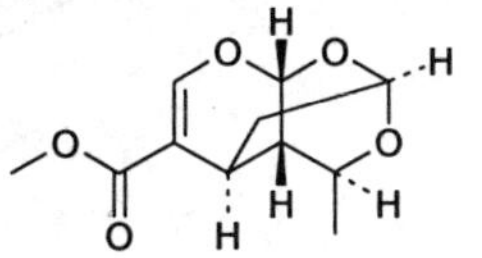

5723 Sarracine

CAS: 2492-09-3 $C_{18}H_{27}NO_5$ MW: 337.42 Property: mp 45-6°C, 51-2°C. Source: DA BAI DING CAO, HUANG WAN. Ref: 5, 6.

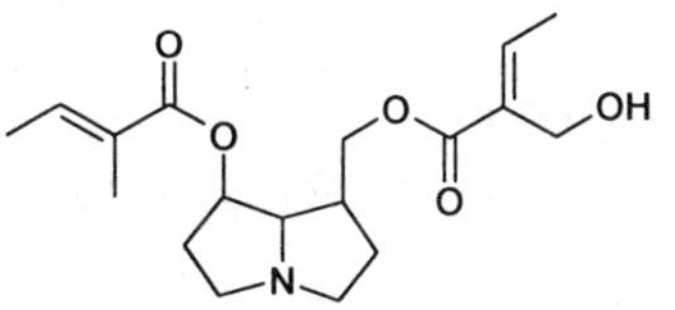

5724 Sarsasapogenin

$C_{27}H_{44}O_3$ MW: 416.65 Source: ZHI MU. Ref: 2.

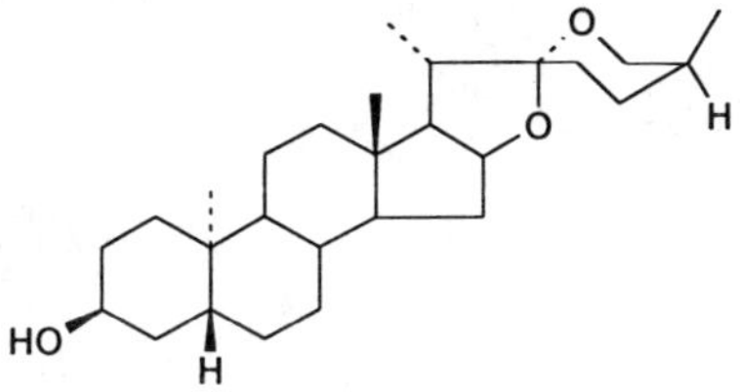

5725 Sarsasapogenone

$C_{27}H_{42}O_3$ MW: 414.63 Property: 176-8°C, $[\alpha]_D^{29}$ -56.0° (c=0.30, $CHCl_3$), existing in moldy source plant only. Source: CHA RUI SHU PIN, CHA RUI SHU YU. Ref: 10, 24.

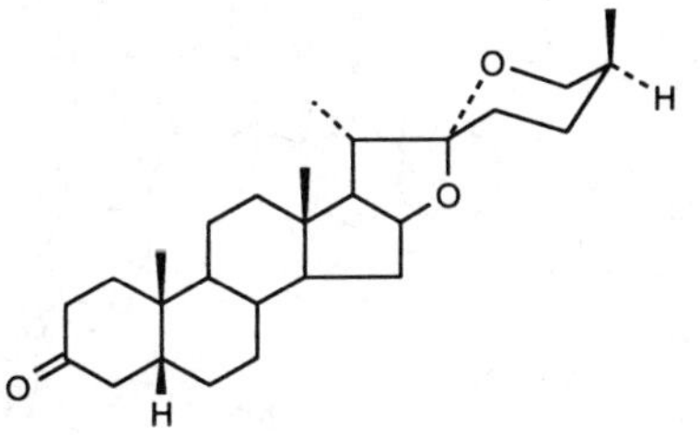

5726 Sativol

$C_{16}H_{10}O_6$ MW: 298.25 Property: mp 303°C. Source: MU XU. Ref: 6.

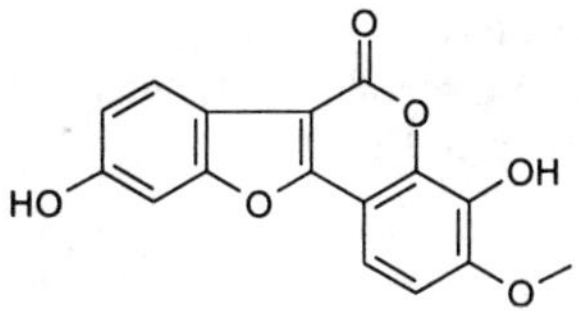

5727 Sativoside R1

Source: DA SUAN. Ref: 2.

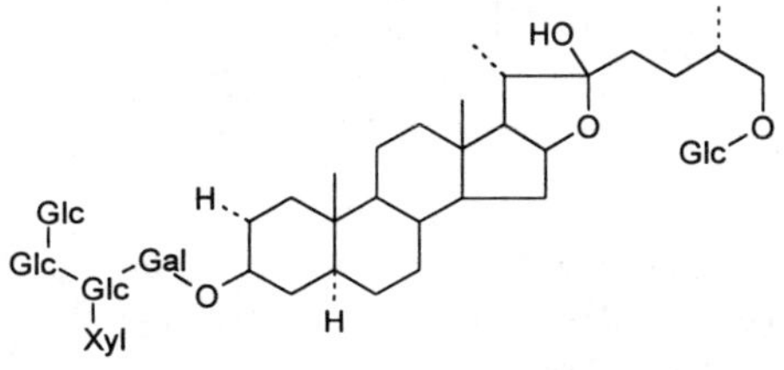

5728 Sativoside R2

Source: DA SUAN. Ref: 2.

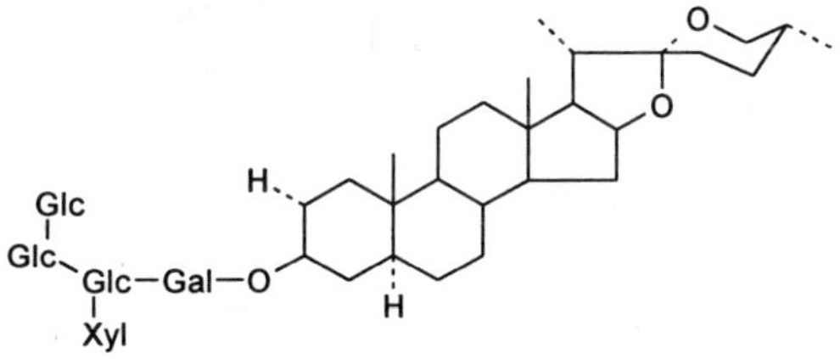

5729 Saussurea lactone

$C_{15}H_{22}O_2$ MW: 234.34 Property: mp 148-9°C. Source: MU XIANG. Ref: 2, 6.

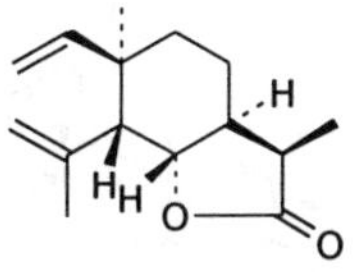

5730 Sauvissimoside R

Property: mp 256-8°C. Source: MAO MEI. Ref: 509.

5731 Savinin

Saussurine. $C_{20}H_{16}O_6$ MW: 352.35 Property: mp 146.4-8.4°C. Source: CHOU CAO, MU XIANG, WU JIA PI. Ref: 2, 6.

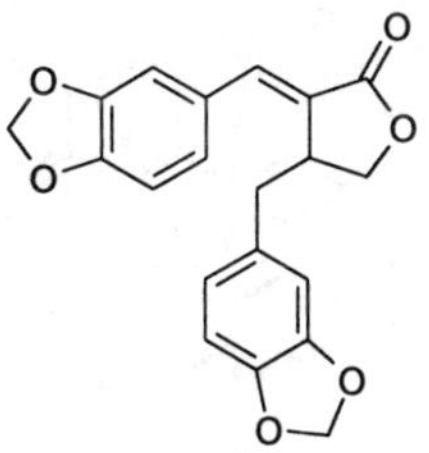

5732 Scabioside A
$C_{35}H_{56}O_8$ MW: 604.83 Property: mp 216-9°C. Source: BAI JIANG. Ref: 2, 6.

5733 Scabioside B
$C_{41}H_{66}O_{12}$ MW: 750.98 Property: mp 210-2°C. Source: BAI JIANG. Ref: 2.

5734 Scabioside C
$C_{41}H_{66}O_{13}$ MW: 766.98 Property: mp 216-9°C. Source: BAI JIANG. Ref: 2.

5735 Scabioside D
$C_{46}H_{74}O_{16}$ MW: 883.09 Property: mp 224-6°C. Source: BAI JIANG. Ref: 2.

5736 Scabioside E
$C_{52}H_{84}O_{20}$ MW: 1029.24 Property: mp 224-7°C. Source: BAI JIANG. Ref: 2.

5737 Scabioside F
$C_{57}H_{92}O_{24}$ MW: 1161.35 Source: BAI JIANG. Ref: 2.

5738 Scabioside G
$C_{63}H_{102}O_{29}$ MW: 1323.50 Property: mp 235-6°C. Source: BAI JIANG. Ref: 2.

5739 Scabroside
$C_{40}H_{44}O_{20}$ MW: 844.78 Source: LONG DAN. Ref: 2.

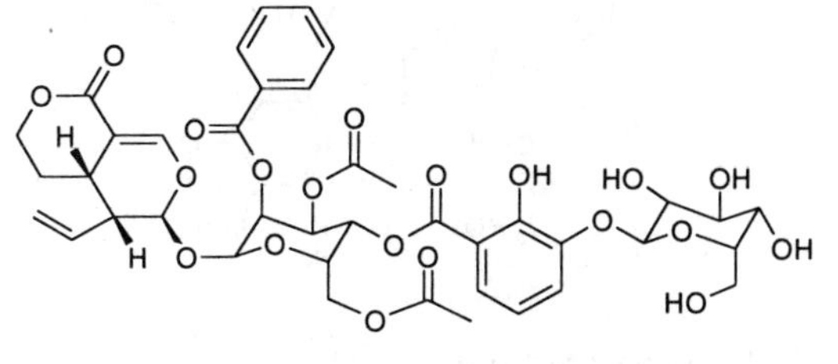

5740 Scandoside
$C_{16}H_{22}O_{11}$ MW: 390.35 Property: mp 139-43°C. Source: JI SHI TENG. Ref: 6.

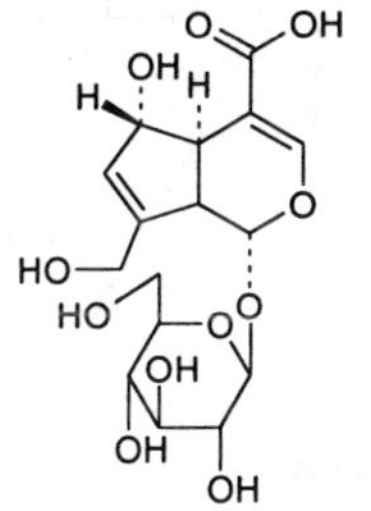

5741 Scandoside methyl ester
$C_{17}H_{24}O_{11}$ MW: 404.37 Source: ZHI ZI. Ref: 2, 626.

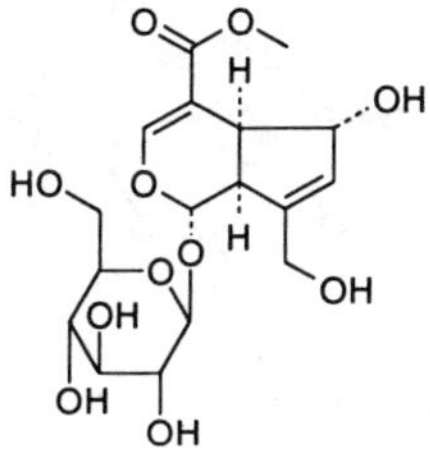

5742 Scatole
C_9H_9O MW: 131.18 Property: mp 95°C, bp 265-6°C/755 mm. Source: LING MAO XIANG. Ref: 6.

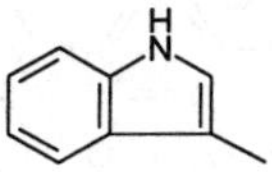

5743 Schicandrin
$C_{24}H_{32}O_7$ MW: 432.52 Source: WU WEI ZI. Ref: 2.

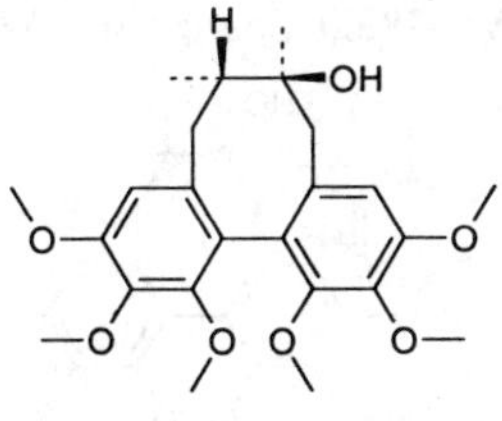

5744 Schikonin
d-Aikanin. CAS: 517-89-5 $C_{16}H_{16}O_5$ MW: 288.30 Property: mp 147-9°C. Source: ZI CAO. Ref: 5.

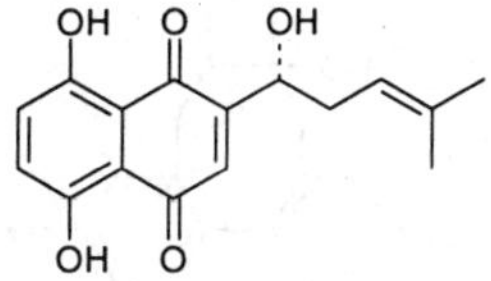

5745 Schinifoline
N-methyl-2-heptyl-4-quinolone. $C_{17}H_{23}NO$ MW: 257.38 Property: white acicular crystal, mp 81-2°C. Source: QING HUA JIAO. Ref: 207.

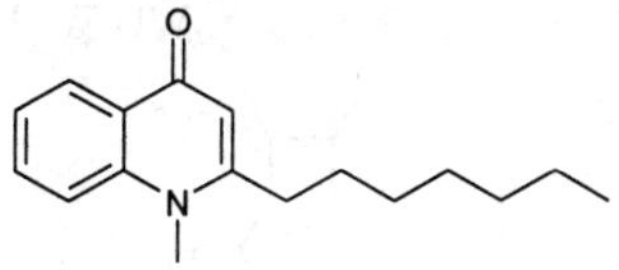

5746 Schisandrin
Schizandrin; γ-Schizandrin, Wuweizi alcohol A. $C_{24}H_{32}O_7$ MW: 432.52 Property: mp 118-9°C, 133 °C. Source: HU LU BA, WU WEI ZI. Ref: 4, 6, 588.

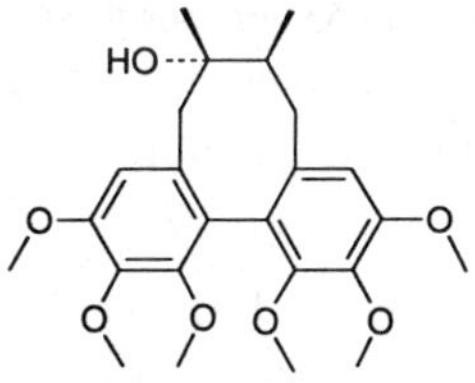

5747 γ-Schisandrin
(-)-Rubshisandrin; Schisandrin B; γ-Schizandrin; Wuweizisu. CAS: 61281-37-6 $C_{23}H_{28}O_6$ MW: 400.48 Property: rhombic crystal (methanol), mp 117-9°C, $[\alpha]_D^{17}$ -32° (ethanol). Source: HONG HUA WU WEI ZI, WU WEI ZI. Ref: 4, 39.

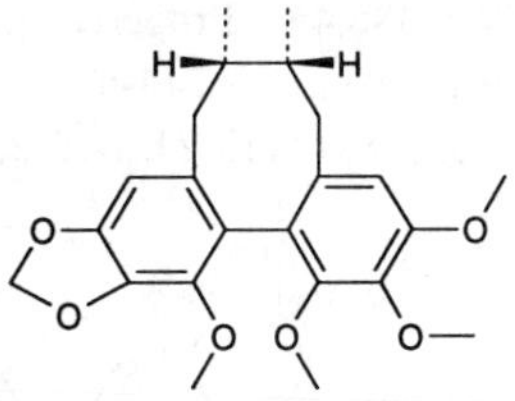

5748 Schisandrol
$C_{22}H_{28}O_7$ MW: 404.46 Source: WU WEI ZI. Ref: 2.

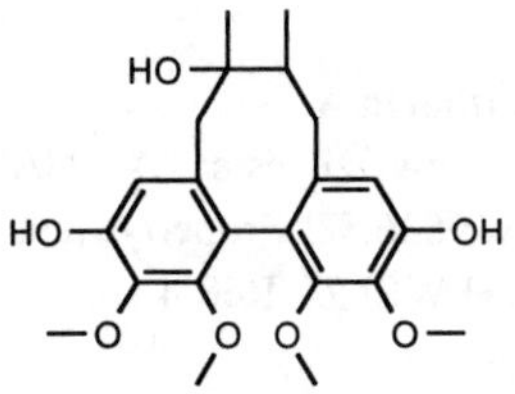

5749 Schisandrol A
$C_{24}H_{32}O_7$ MW: 432.52 Source: WU WEI ZI. Ref: 2.

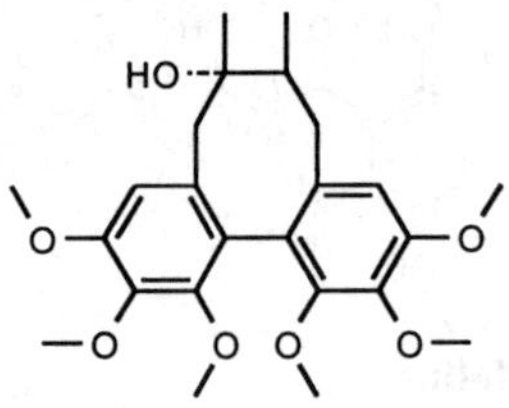

5750 Schisanhenol
$C_{23}H_{30}O_6$ MW: 402.49 Source: WU WEI ZI. Ref: 2.

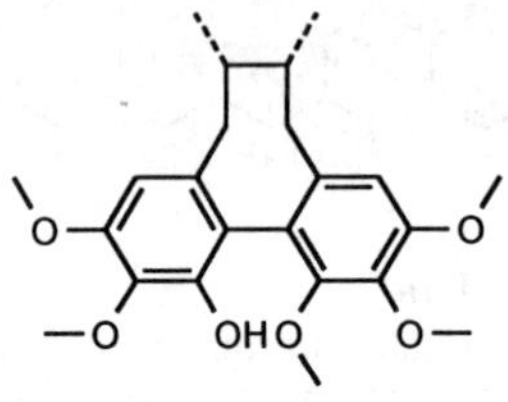

5751 Schisanhenol acetate
$C_{25}H_{32}O_7$ MW: 444.53 Property: acicular crystal, mp 157-9°C, $[\alpha]_D^{35}$ +31.6° (ethanol). Source: HONG HUA WU WEI ZI, WU WEI ZI. Ref: 2, 39.

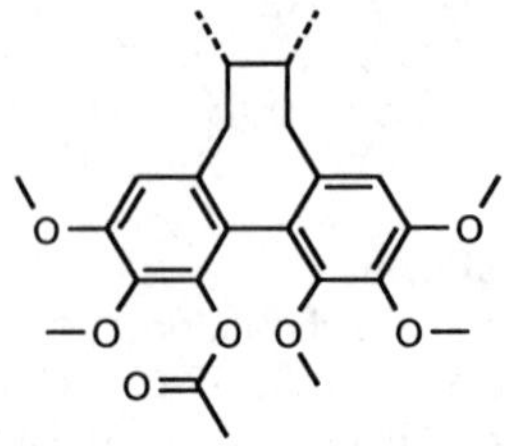

5752 Schisanhenol B
$C_{22}H_{26}O_6$ MW: 386.45 Property: granular crystal (petroleum spirit-ether), mp 144-6°C. Source: HONG HUA WU WEI ZI, WU WEI ZI. Ref: 2, 39.

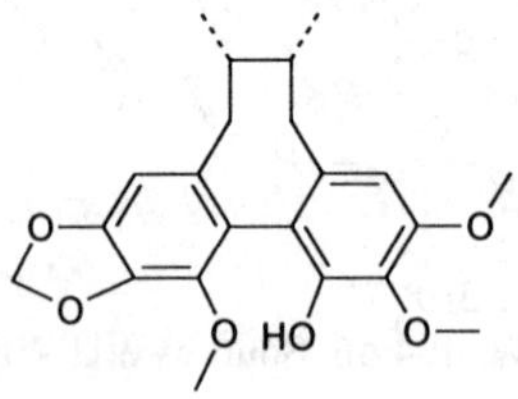

5753 Schisantherin A
Gomisin C; Wuweizi ester A. CAS: 58546-56-8 $C_{30}H_{32}O_9$ MW: 536.58 Property: mp 116-8°C, 122-4 °C. Source: WU WEI ZI. Ref: 4.

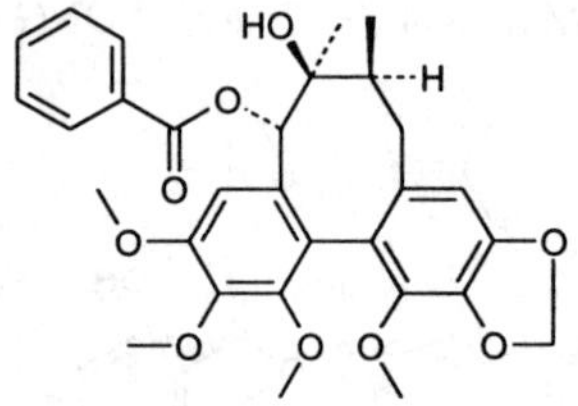

5754 Schisantherin B
Gomisin B; Wuweizi ester B. $C_{28}H_{34}O_9$ MW: 514.58 Property: mp 97-9°C Source: WU WEI ZI. Ref: 4.

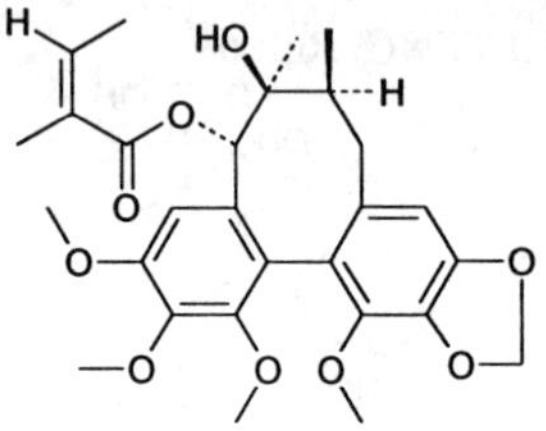

5755 Schisantherin C
$C_{28}H_{34}O_9$ MW: 514.58 Source: WU WEI ZI. Ref: 2.

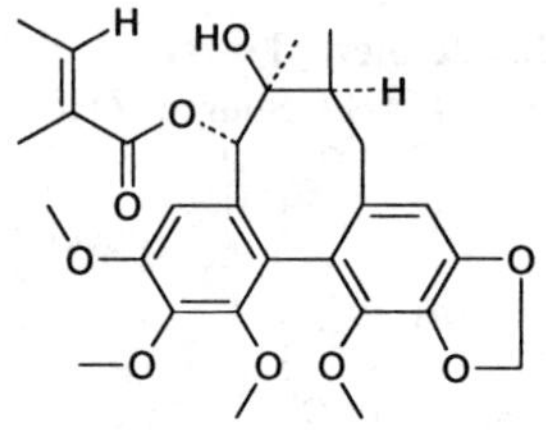

5756 Schisantherin D
$C_{29}H_{28}O_9$ MW: 520.54 Source: WU WEI ZI. Ref: 2.

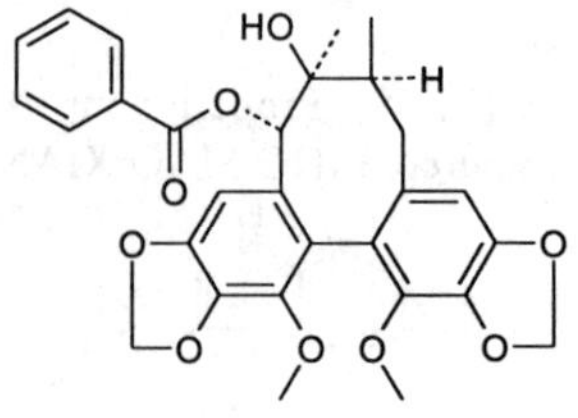

5757 Schisantherin E
$C_{30}H_{34}O_9$ MW: 538.60 Source: WU WEI ZI. Ref: 2.

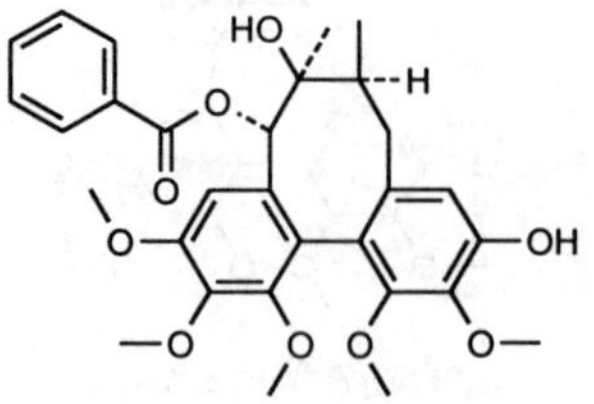

5759 Schizonepetoside A
$C_{16}H_{26}O_7$ MW: 330.38 Source: JIN JIE. Ref: 2.

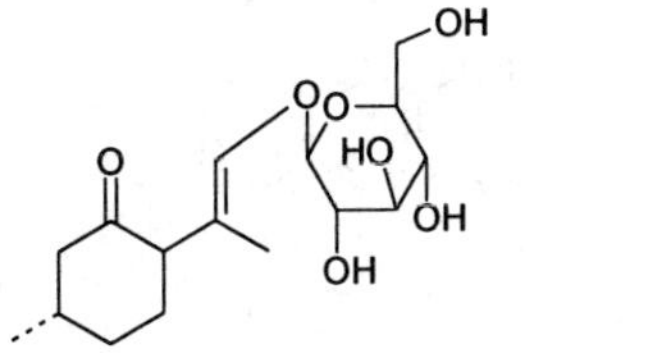

5760 Schizonepetoside B
Source: JIN JIE. Ref: 2.

5761 Schizonepetoside C
$C_{16}H_{26}O_7$ MW: 330.38 Source: JIN JIE. Ref: 2.

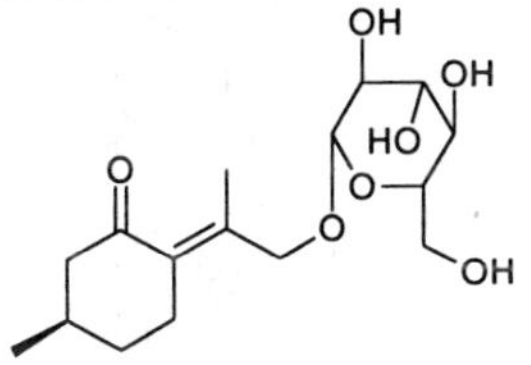

5762 Schizonodiol
$C_{10}H_{16}O_3$ MW: 184.24 Source: JIN JIE. Ref: 2.

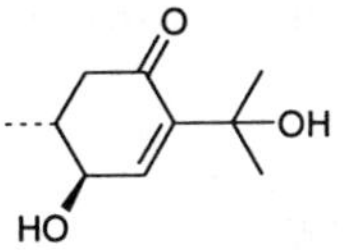

5763 Schizonol
$C_{10}H_{16}O_2$ MW: 168.24 Source: JIN JIE. Ref: 2.

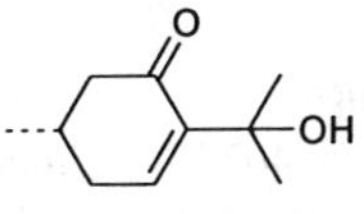

5764 Schkuhrin I
CAS: 38458-58-1 $C_{22}H_{28}O_8$ MW: 420.46 Source: *Schkuhria pinnata* (Lam.) Kuntze. Ref: 5.

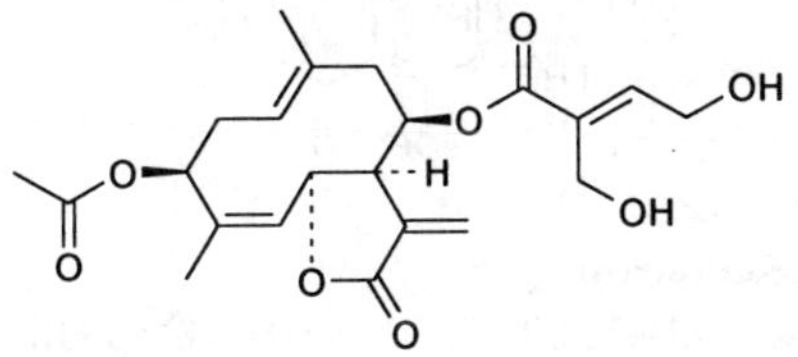

5765 Schkuhrin II
CAS: 70434-09-2 $C_{25}H_{34}O_9$ MW: 478.52 Source: *Schkuhria pinnata* (Lam.) Kuntze. Ref: 5.

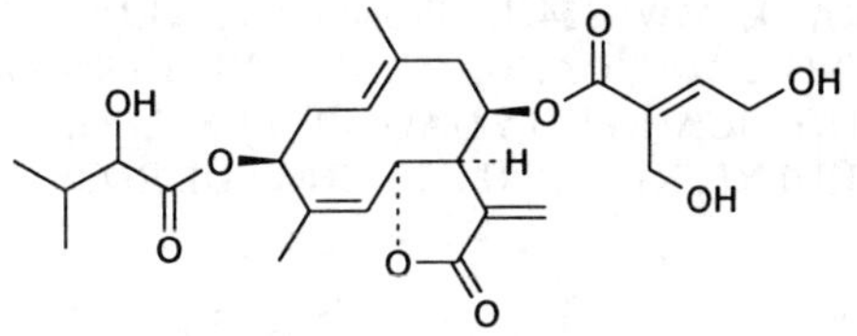

5766 Sciadopitysin
$C_{33}H_{24}O_9$ MW: 564.55 Property: mp 295-7°C. Source: BAI GUO, SAN JIAN SHAN. Ref: 2.

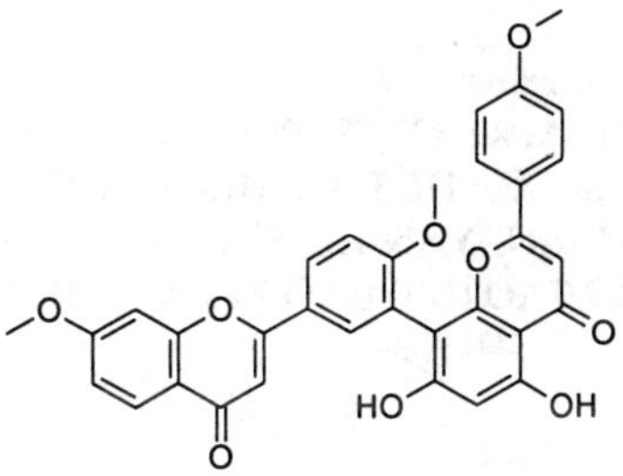

5767 Scoparone
Escoparone. CAS: 120-08-1 $C_{11}H_{10}O_4$ MW: 206.20 Property: mp 144-5°C. Source: LONG YAN DU HUO, YIN CHEN HAO. Ref: 4, 571.

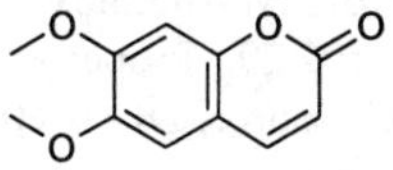

5768 Scopine
$C_8H_{13}NO_2$ MW: 155.20 Property: mp 76°C. Source: SAI LANG DANG. Ref: 6.

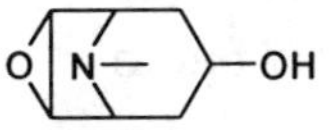

5769 Scoplatin
Property: light yellow acicular crystal, mp 202-4°C. Source: MAO LIAN HAO. Ref: 474.

5770 Scopoletin
Chrysatroic acid; Escoopoletin; Gelseminic acid; Scopoletol.$C_{10}H_8O_4$ MW: 192.17 Property: mp 204°C, 207-8°C. Source: BAI ZHI, DU HUO, DANG GUI, GOU QI ZI, HU LU BA, JIU LI XIANG, LONG YAN DU HUO, GUANG YE DING GONG TENG, QIN PI, QING HAO, YIN CHEN HAO. Ref: 2, 4, 11, 415, 571, 585, 588.

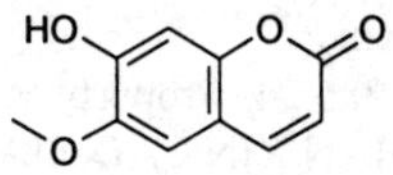

5771 Scopolin
$C_{16}H_{18}O_9$ MW: 354.32 Property: mp 219°C. Source: DONG LANG DANG, GUANG YE DING GONG TENG, HUANG HUA HAO, JIU LI XIANG, XIANG RI KUI YE, XIANG RI KUI JING SUI. Ref: 6, 11.

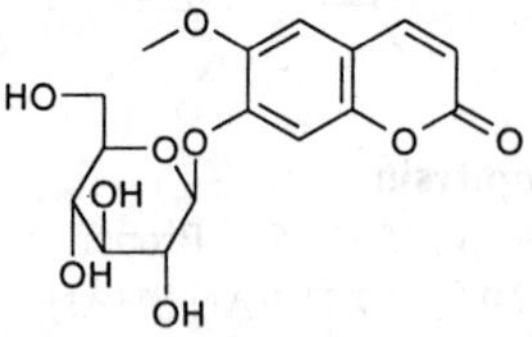

5772 Scoulerine
$C_{19}H_{21}NO_4$ MW: 327.38 Property: mp (+): 197°C, (-): 204°C. Source: HE BAO MU DAN GEN, JU HUA HUANG LIAN, YAN HU SUO, YA PIAN, ZI HUA YU DENG CAO (LIE BAO ZI JING). Ref: 6.

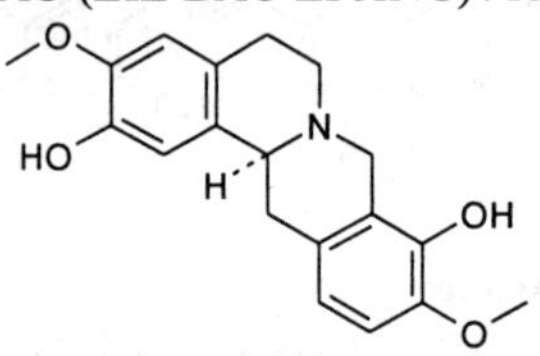

5773 Scuteamoenin
(2S)-2',5,6'-Trihydroxy-7-methoxyflavanone.
$C_{16}H_{14}O_6$ MW: 302.29 Property: colorless acicular crystal, mp 250°C. Source: DIAN HUANG QI N. Ref: 153.

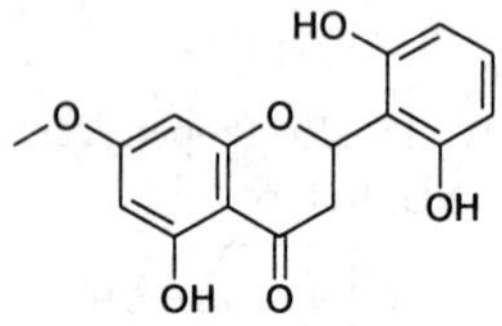

5774 Scuteamoenoside
(2S)-2',5,6'-trihydroxy-7-methoxyflavanone-2'-O-β-D-glucopyranoside. $C_{22}H_{24}O_{11}$ MW: 464.43 Property: colorless crystalline powder, mp 236-9°C. Source: DIAN HUANG QIN. Ref: 124.

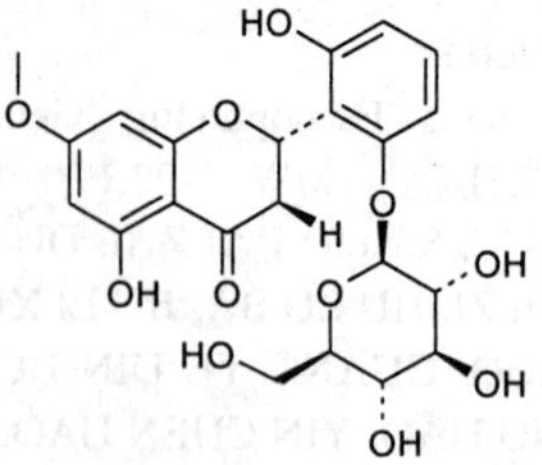

5775 Scutellarein
$C_{15}H_{10}O_6$ MW: 286.24 Property: mp 350°C. Source: CHOU MO LI, HAN XIN CAO, JIA LIAN QIAO YE, MU HU DIE, MU HU DIE SHU PI, ZI MEI SHU. Ref: 6.

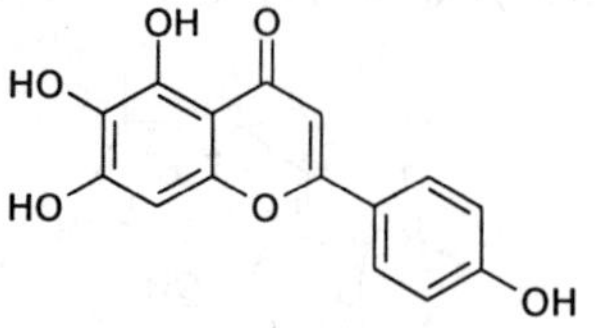

5776 Scutellarein-5-galactoside
$C_{21}H_{20}O_{11}$ MW: 448.39 Source: ZI MEI SHU. Ref: 6.

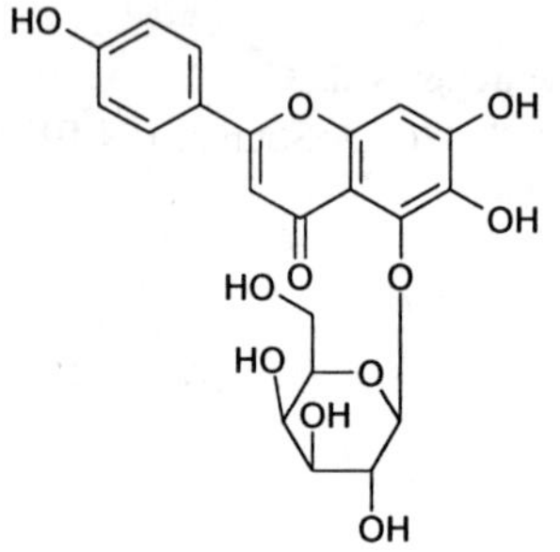

5777 Scutellarein-7-rutinoside
$C_{27}H_{30}O_{15}$ MW: 488.71 Source: MU HU DIE SHU PI. Ref: 6.

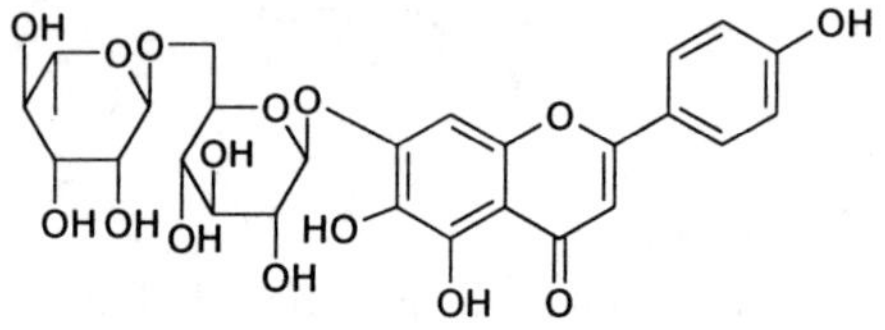

5778 Scutellarin
$C_{21}H_{18}O_{12}$ MW: 462.37 Property: mp >300°C. Source: CHOU MO LI, HUANG QIN, ZHEN ZHU MEI. Ref: 6.

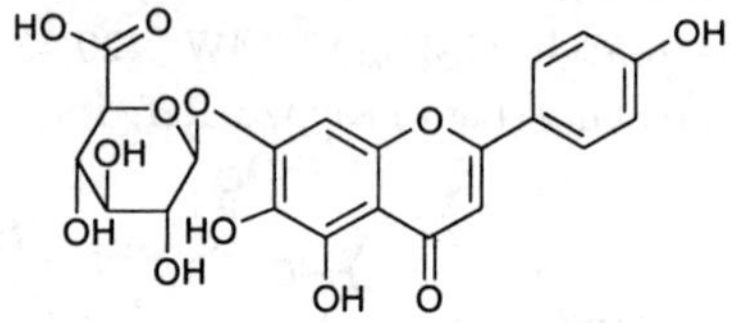

5779 Scutevulin
$C_{16}H_{12}O_6$ MW: 300.27 Source: HUANG QIN. Ref: 2.

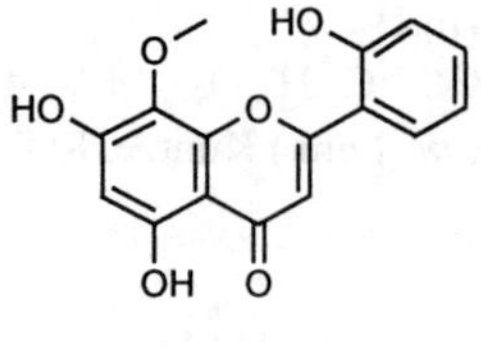

5780 Sebacic acid
$C_{10}H_{18}O_4$ MW: 202.25 Source: DANG GUI. Ref: 2.

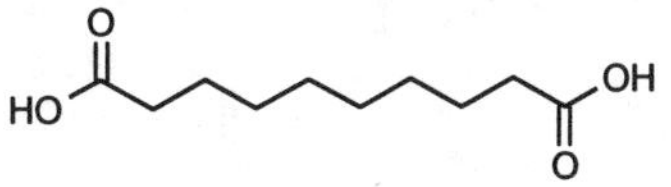

5781 Sebiferic acid
$C_{30}H_{48}O_2$ MW: 440.72 Property: mp 178-80°C. Source: WU JIU MU GEN PI. Ref: 6.

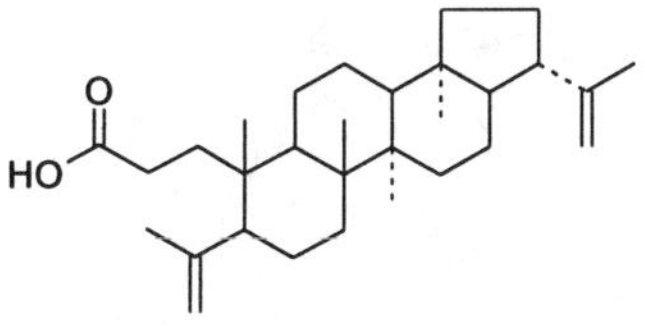

5782 Secalonic acid A
$C_{32}H_{30}O_{14}$ MW: 638.59 Property: mp 246-7°C (dec). Source: MAI JIAO. Ref: 6.

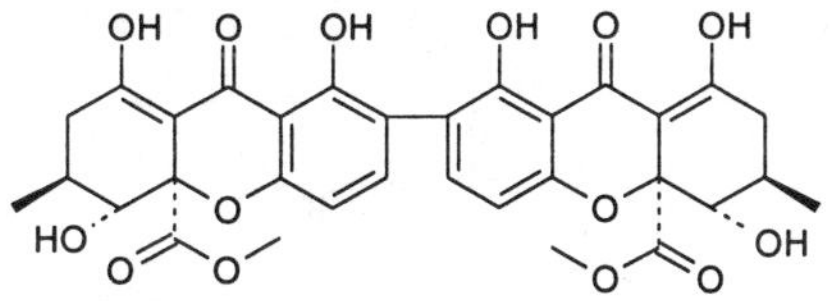

5783 Secalonic acid B
$C_{32}H_{30}O_{14}$ MW: 638.59 Property: mp 254-6°C (dec). Source: MAI JIAO. Ref: 6.

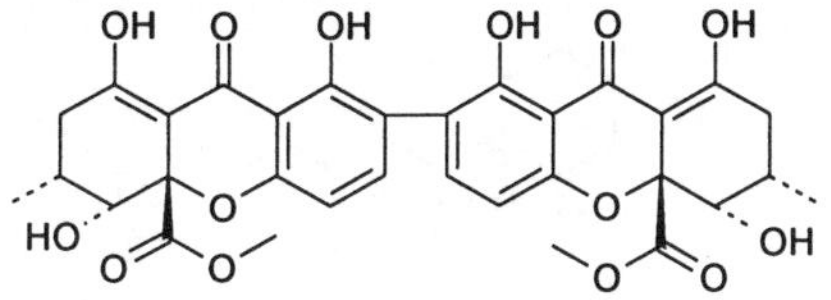

5784 Secalonic acid C
$C_{32}H_{30}O_{14}$ MW: 638.59 Property: mp 159-61°C. Source: MAI JIAO. Ref: 6.

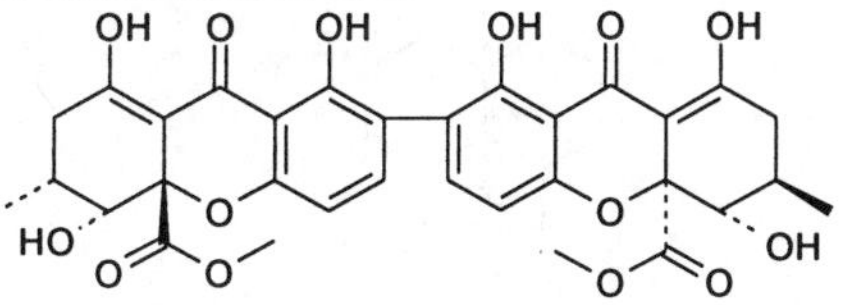

5785 Secalonic acid D
$C_{32}H_{30}O_{14}$ MW: 638.59 Property: mp 253-5°C. Source: MAI JIAO. Ref: 6.

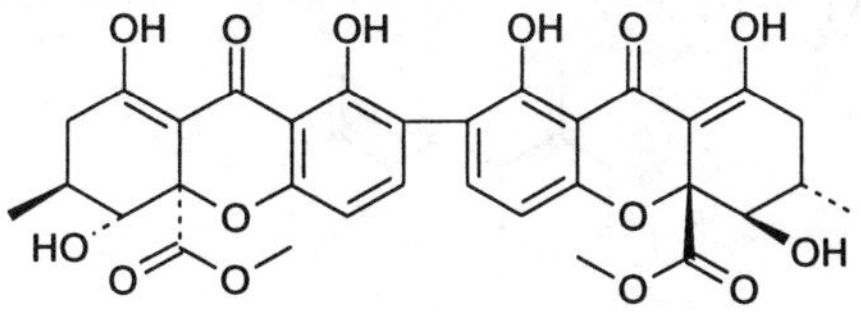

5786 Secologanic acid
$C_{16}H_{22}O_{10}$ MW: 374.35 Source: CHANG CHUN HUA. Ref: 2.

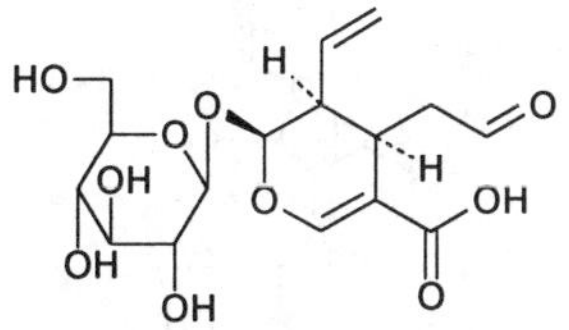

5787 Secologanin
$C_{17}H_{24}O_{10}$ MW: 388.37 Source: SHUI CAI. Ref: 6.

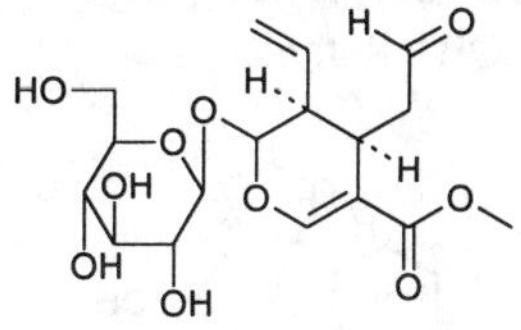

5788 Secologanoside
$C_{25}H_{32}O_{14}$ MW: 556.53 Property: mp 140.5°C. Source: CHANG CHUN HUA. Ref: 2.

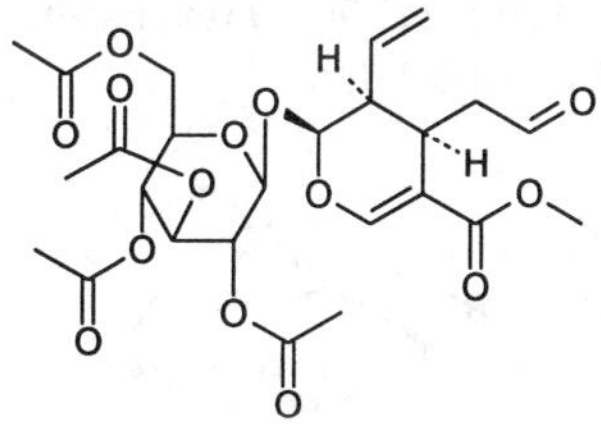

5789 Securinine
CAS: 5610-40-2 $C_{13}H_{15}NO_2$ MW: 217.27 Property: mp 142-3°C. Source: YI YE QIU. Ref: 6.

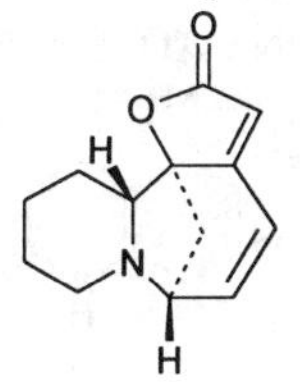

5790 Securinol A
$C_{13}H_{17}NO_3$ MW: 235.29 Property: mp (+): 135-6°C. Source: YI YE QIU. Ref: 6.

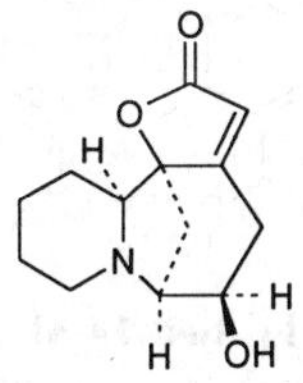

5791 Securinol B
$C_{13}H_{17}NO_3$ MW: 235.29 Property: mp (+): 158-60°C. Source: YI YE QIU. Ref: 6.

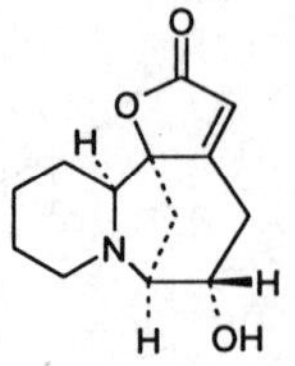

5792 Securinol C
$C_{13}H_{17}NO_3$ MW: 235.29 Property: mp (-): 114-5°C. Source: YI YE QIU. Ref: 6.

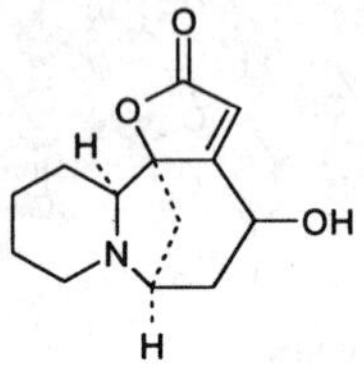

5793 Securitinine
$C_{14}H_{17}NO_3$ MW: 247.30 Property: mp 129-30°C. Source: YI YE QIU. Ref: 6.

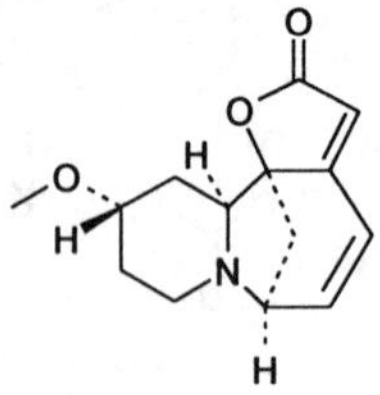

5794 Selagine
$C_{15}H_{20}N_2O$ MW: 244.34 Property: mp 224-6°C. Source: XIAO JIE JIN CAO. Ref: 6.

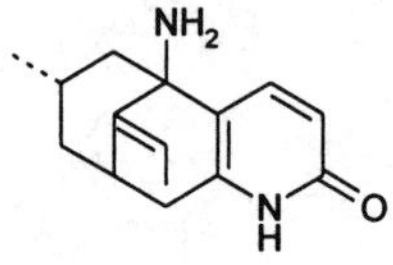

5795 (-)-Selina-3,11-dien-14-al
$C_{15}H_{22}O$ MW: 218.34 Source: CHEN XIANG. Ref: 13.

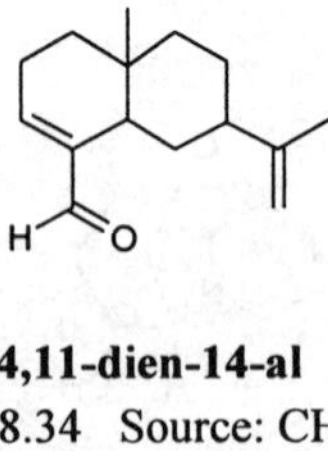

5796 (+)-Selina-4,11-dien-14-al
$C_{15}H_{22}O$ MW: 218.34 Source: CHEN XIANG. Ref: 13.

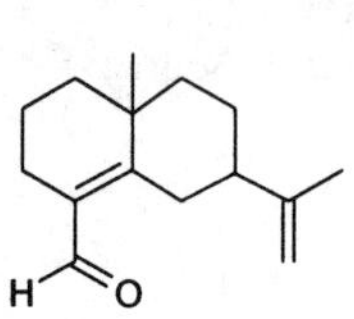

5797 (+)-Selina-3,11-dien-9-ol
$C_{15}H_{24}O$ MW: 220.36 Source: CHEN XIANG. Ref: 13.

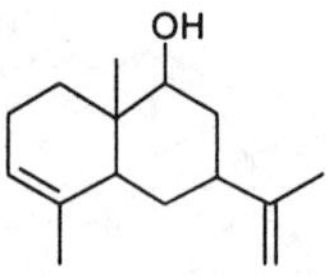

5798 (-)-Selina-3,11-dien-9-one
$C_{15}H_{22}O$ MW: 218.34 Source: CHEN XIANG. Ref: 13.

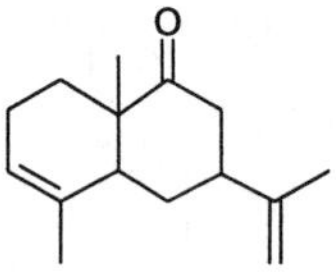

5799 Selinane
$C_{16}H_{30}$ MW: 222.42 Source: CHEN XIANG, MAN SHAN HONG. Ref: 6.

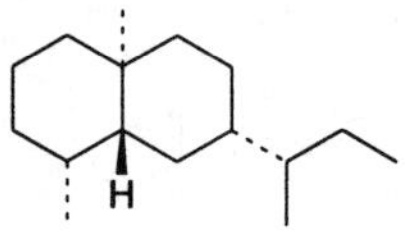

5800 α-Selinene
$C_{16}H_{26}$ MW: 218.39 Property: bp 268-72°C. Source: REN SHEN. Ref: 2.

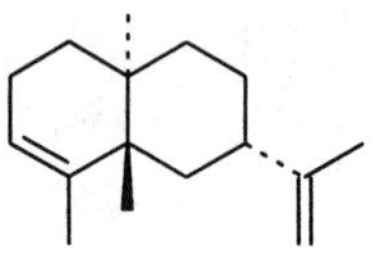

5801 β-Selinene
$C_{15}H_{24}$ MW: 204.36 Source: CANG ZHU, MU XIANG, MU XIANG, QIANG HUO, REN SHEN, WU WEI ZI. Ref: 2.

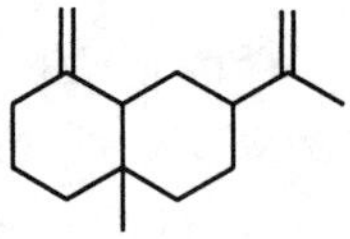

5802 γ-Selinene
$C_{15}H_{24}$ MW: 204.36 Source: REN SHEN. Ref: 2.

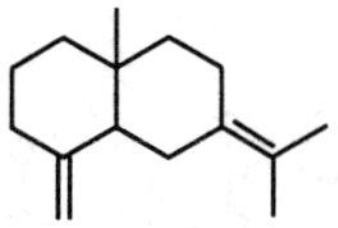

5803 Semi-α-carotenone
$C_{40}H_{56}O_2$ MW: 568.89 Property: mp 135°C. Source: JIU LI XIANG. Ref: 6.

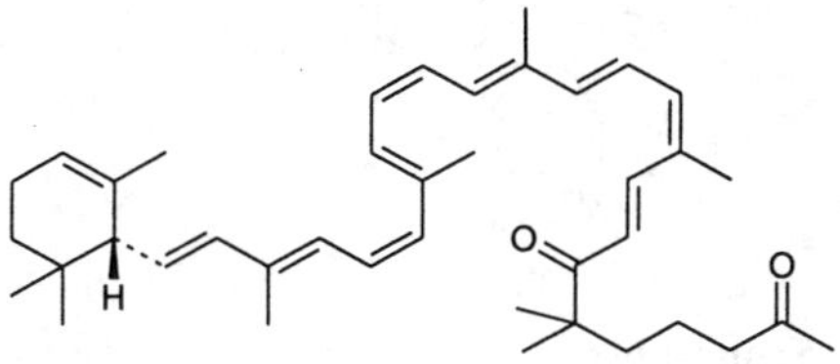

5804 Sempervine
Sempervirine. $C_{19}H_{16}N_2$ MW: 272.35 Property: mp 223°C (chloroform), 260-1°C. Source: GOU WEN, HU MAN TENG. Ref: 6, 14.

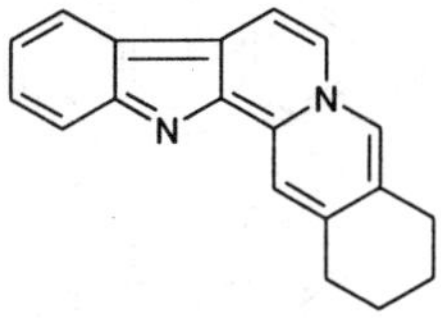

5805 Senbyak-angelicole
$C_{21}H_{22}O_7$ MW: 386.41 Source: BAI ZHI. Ref: 2.

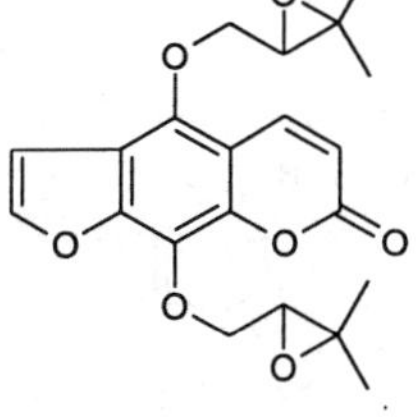

5806 Sendanone acetate
$C_{32}H_{48}O_5$ MW: 512.74 Property: mp 184-6°C. Source: KU LIAN PI. Ref: 6.

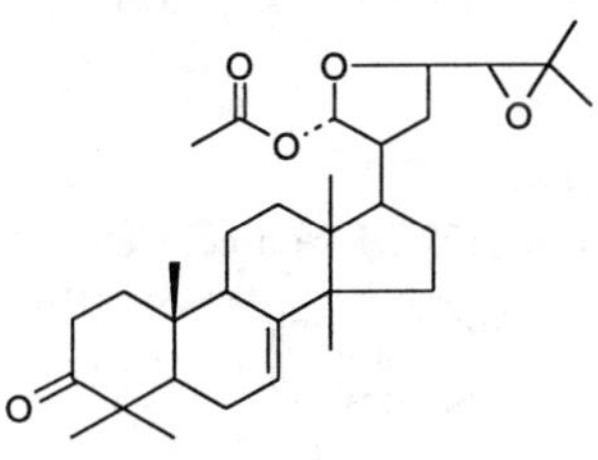

5807 Senecionine
$C_{18}H_{25}NO_5$ MW: 335.40 Property: mp 232-3°C. Source: DA BAI DING CAO. Ref: 6.

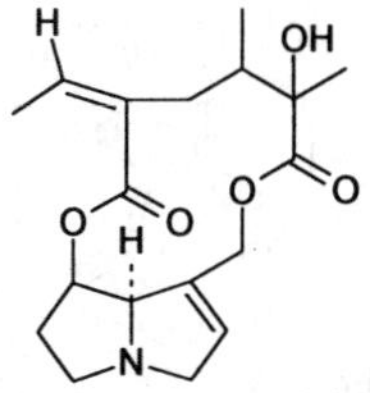

5808 (E)-Seneciphylline (IV)
$C_{18}H_{23}NO_5$ MW: 333.39 Property: white acicular crystal, mp 165°C. Source: JU YE SAN QI. Ref: 151.

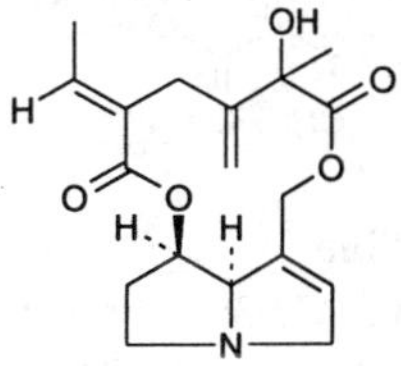

5809 Sengosterone
$C_{29}H_{44}O_9$ MW: 536.67 Property: mp 159-61°C. Source: CHUAN NIU XI. Ref: 6.

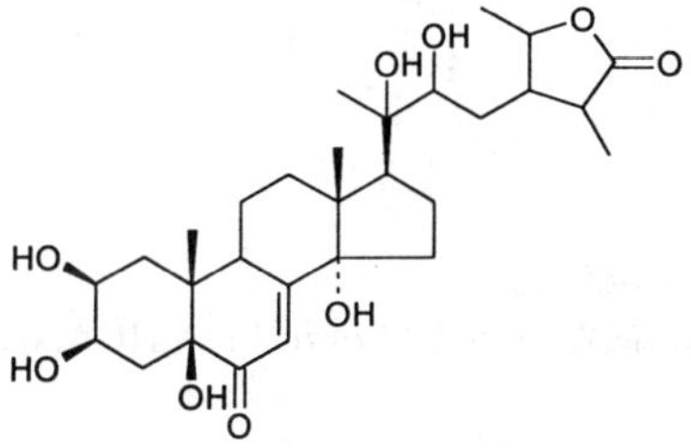

5810 Senkyunolide A
Source: CHA XIONG. Ref: 531.

5811 Senkyunolide G
Source: CHA XIONG. Ref: 531.

5812 Senkyunolide H
Source: CHA XIONG. Ref: 531.

5813 Senkyunolide I
Source: CHA XIONG. Ref: 531.

5814 Senkyunolide K
$C_{12}H_{16}O_3$ MW: 208.26 Source: CHUAN XIONG. Ref: 2.

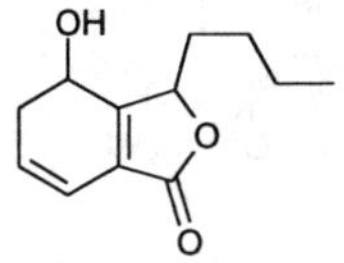

5815 Senkyunolide L
$C_{12}H_{15}ClO_3$ MW: 242.70 Source: CHUAN XIONG. Ref: 2.

5816 Senkyunolide M
$C_{16}H_{22}O_4$ MW: 278.35 Source: CHUAN XIONG. Ref: 2.

5817 Senlciphylline
$C_{18}H_{23}NO_5$ MW: 333.39 Property: mp 217-8°C. Source: DA BAI DING CAO, TU SAN QI. Ref: 6.

5818 Sennidin A
$C_{30}H_{18}O_{10}$ MW: 538.47 Source: DA HUANG. Ref: 2.

5819 Sennidin C
$C_{30}H_{20}O_9$ MW: 524.49 Source: DA HUANG. Ref: 2.

5820 Sennoside A
$C_{42}H_{38}O_{20}$ MW: 862.76 Source: DA HUANG. Ref: 2.

5821 Sennoside C
$C_{42}H_{40}O_{19}$ MW: 848.78 Source: DA HUANG. Ref: 2.

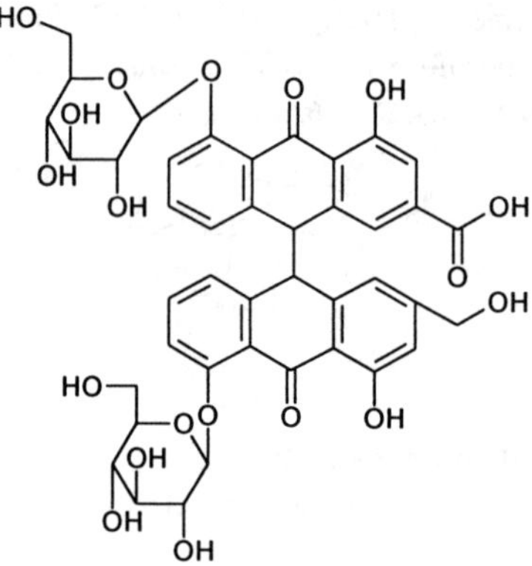

5822 Sennoside E
Source: DA HUANG. Ref: 2.

5823 Serotonine
$C_{10}H_{14}N_2O$ MW: 178.24 Source: CHAN SU. Ref: 2.

5824 Serpentine
$C_{21}H_{22}N_2O_3$ MW: 350.42 Source: CHANG CHUN HUA. Ref: 2.

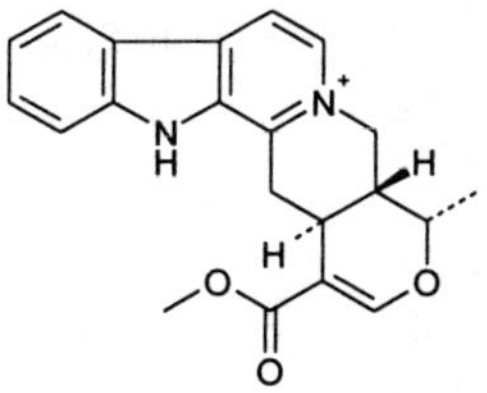

5825 Serpentineiue
$C_{42}H_{46}N_4O_6$ MW: 702.86 Property: mp 265-70°C. Source: LUO FU MU. Ref: 6.

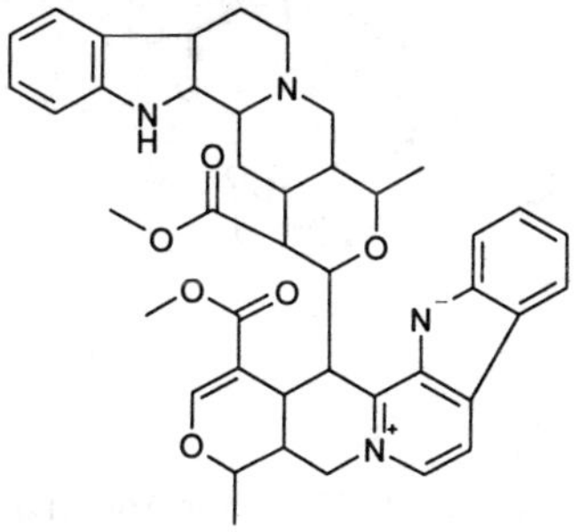

5826 Serratagenic acid
$C_{30}H_{46}O_5$ MW: 486.70 Property: mp >310°C. Source: SAN TAI HONG HUA. Ref: 6.

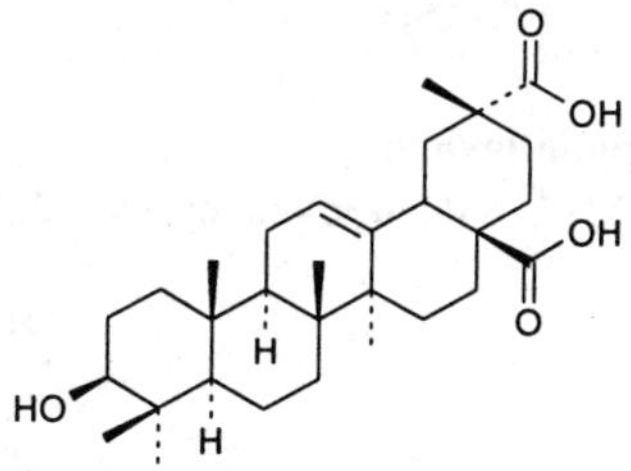

5827 Serratanidine
$C_{16}H_{25}NO_4$ MW: 295.38 Property: mp 210-1°C. Source: QIAN CENG TA. Ref: 6.

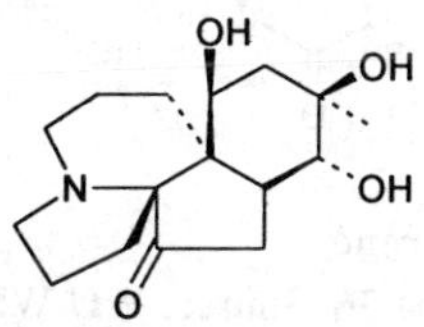

5828 Serratene
$C_{30}H_{50}$ MW: 410.73 Property: mp 239.5-40°C. Source: SHUI LONG GU. Ref: 6.

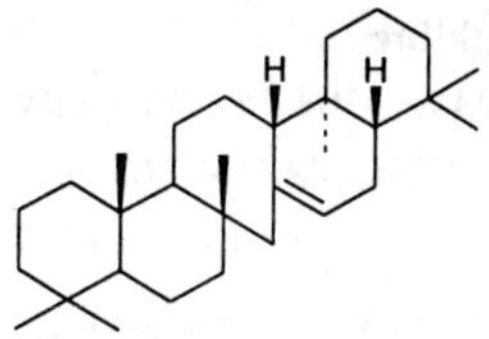

5829 Serratenediol
$C_{30}H_{50}O_2$ MW: 442.73 Property: mp 302.5-4.5°C. Source: GUO JIANG LONG, PU DI WU GONG, QIAN CENG TA. Ref: 6.

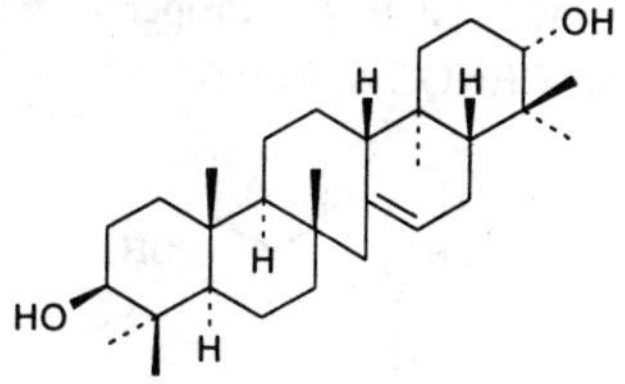

5830 Serratenediol-3-acetate
$C_{32}H_{52}O_3$ MW: 484.77 Property: mp 317-9°C. Source: QIAN CENG TA. Ref: 6.

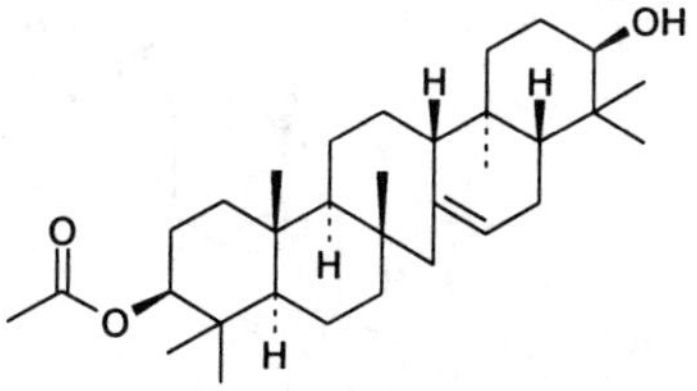

5831 Serratenediol-21-acetate
$C_{32}H_{52}O_3$ MW: 484.77 Property: white lamellar crystal, mp >300°C. Source: QIAN CENG TA. Ref: 109.

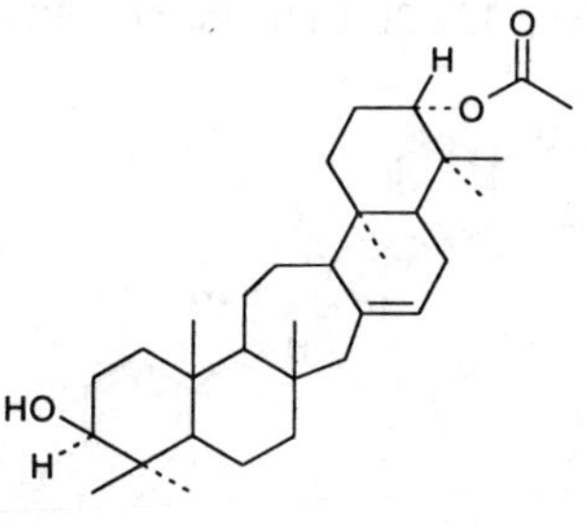

5832 Serratine
$C_{16}H_{25}NO_3$ MW: 279.38 Property: mp 253°C. Source: QIAN CENG TA. Ref: 6.

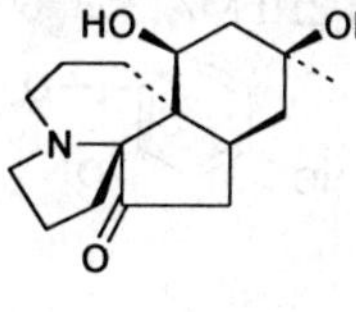

5833 Serratinidine

$C_{18}H_{28}N_2O_2$ MW: 304.44 Property: mp 232-4°C. Source: QIAN CENG TA. Ref: 6.

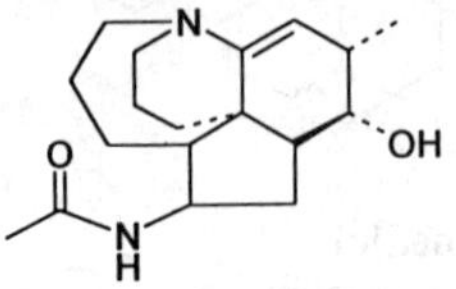

5834 Serratinine

$C_{16}H_{25}NO_3$ MW: 279.38 Property: mp 244-5°C. Source: QIAN CENG TA. Ref: 6.

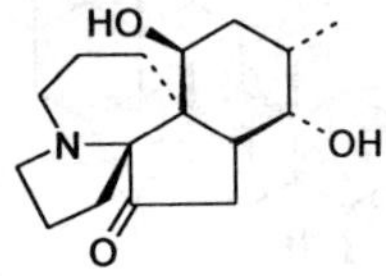

5835 Serratriol

$C_{30}H_{50}O_3$ MW: 458.73 Property: mp 335-6°C. Source: PU DI WU GONG, QIAN CENG TA. Ref: 6.

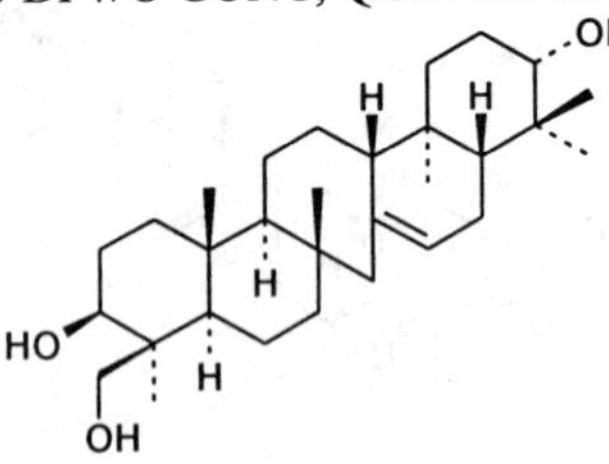

5836 Sesamin

$C_{20}H_{18}O_6$ MW: 354.36 Property: mp (+): 123-4°C, (-): 122-4°C, (±): 129-30°C. Source: CI WU JIA. Ref: 2.

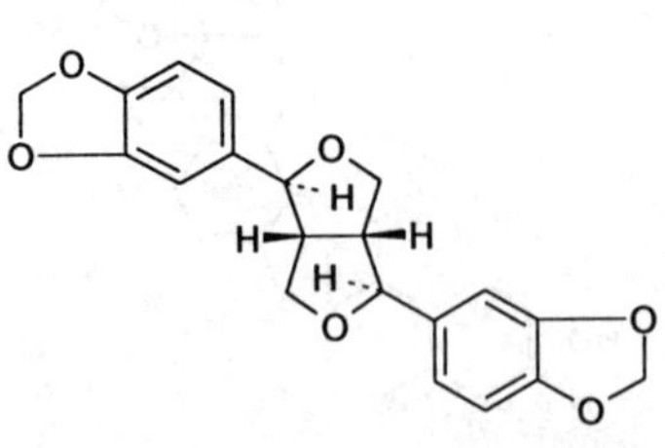

5837 Sesamol

$C_7H_6O_3$ MW: 138.12 Property: mp 65.8°C. Source: BAI ZHI MA, HEI ZHI MA. Ref: 6.

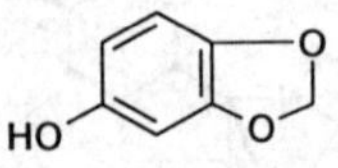

5838 Sesamolin

$C_{20}H_{18}O_7$ MW: 370.36 Property: mp 94°C. Source: HEI ZHI MA. Ref: 6.

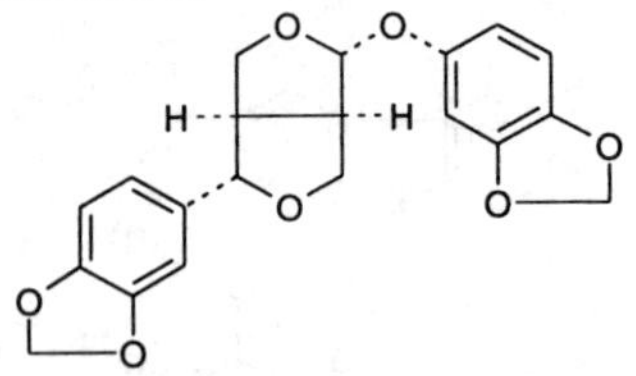

5839 Sesamoside

$C_{17}H_{24}O_{12}$ MW: 420.37 Source: MENG GU CAO SU, XIAN SHENG MA XIAN HAO. Ref: 560, 579.

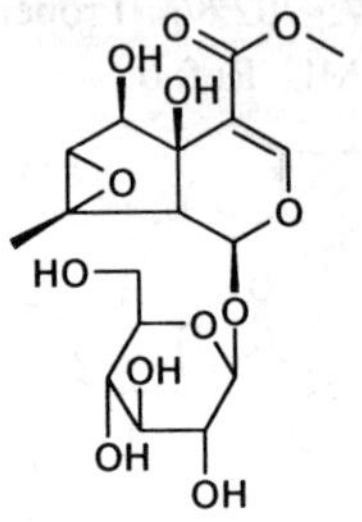

5840 Seselin

$C_{14}H_{12}O_3$ MW: 228.25 Property: mp 119-20°C. Source: ZHI GEN PI. Ref: 6.

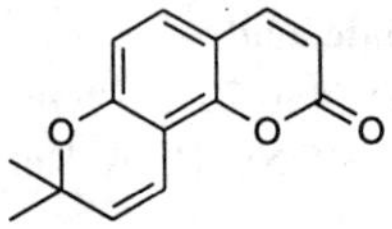

5841 Sesguoiaflavone

$C_{31}H_{20}O_9$ MW: 536.50 Source: SAN JIAN SHAN. Ref: 2.

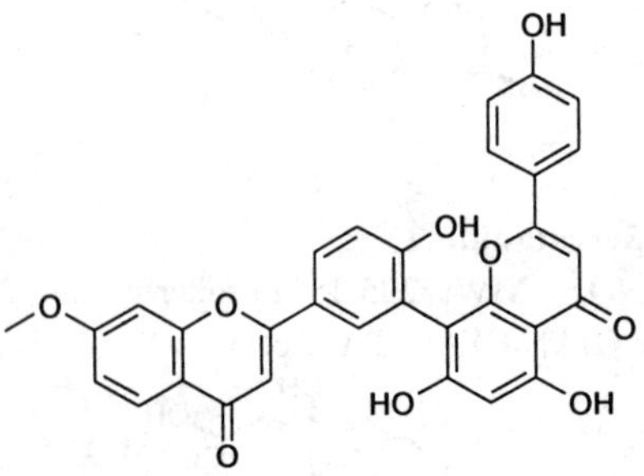

5842 Sesquicarene

$C_{15}H_{24}$ MW: 204.36 Source: WU WEI ZI. Ref: 2.

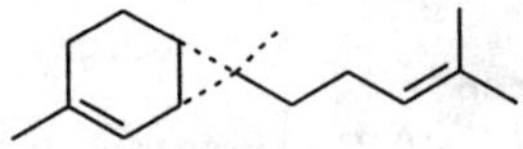

5843 β-Sesquiphellandrene
$C_{15}H_{24}$ MW: 204.36 Source: GAN JIANG. Ref: 2.

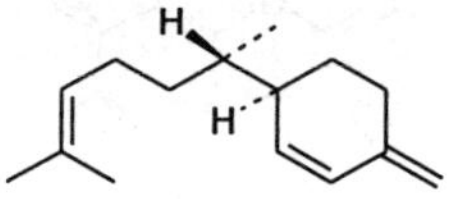

5844 Shakuchirin
$C_{25}H_{28}O_{11}$ MW: 504.50 Property: mp 100-10°C. Source: HUO TAN MU CAO,TIAN QIAO MAI GEN. Ref: 6.

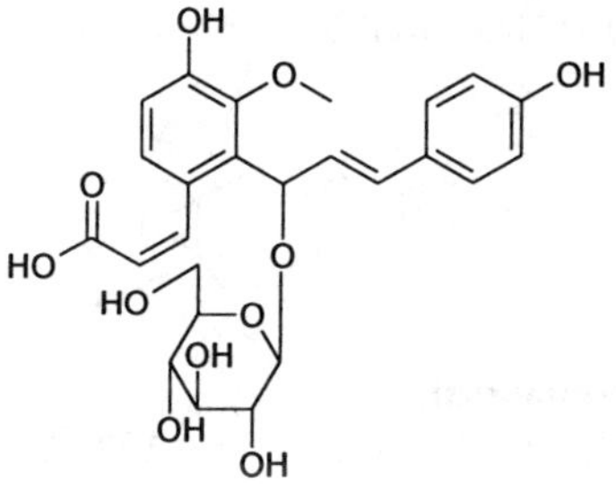

5845 Shanzhiside
$C_{16}H_{24}O_{11}$ MW: 392.36 Property: mp 82-90°C. Source: ZHI ZI. Ref: 2.

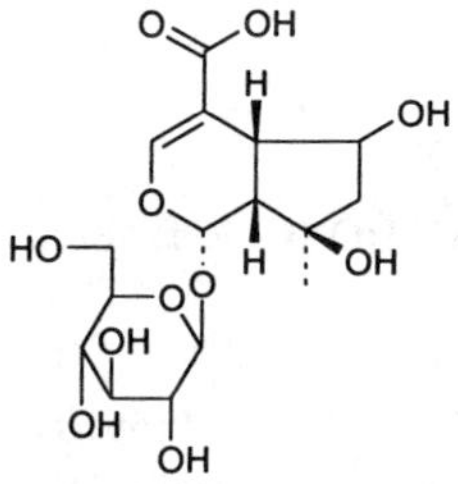

5846 Shihunidine
$C_{12}H_{14}N_2O$ MW: 202.26 Property: colorless columnar crystal (C_6H_6), mp 173-4°C, $[\alpha]_D^{20}$ 0°. Source: FEN HUA SHI HU. Ref: 189.

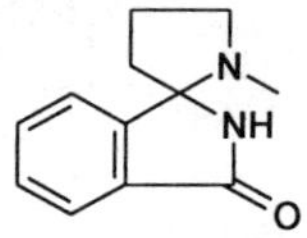

5847 Shihunine
$C_{12}H_{13}NO_2$ MW: 203.24 Property: mp 79°C. Source: FEN HUA SHI HU, SHI HU. Ref: 6, 189.

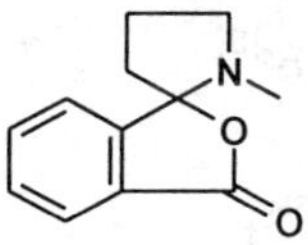

5848 Shikimic acid
$C_7H_{10}O_5$ MW: 174.15 Source: BAI GUO, MIN WAN BA JIAO GUO. Ref: 2, 315.

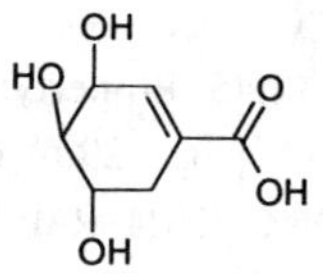

5849 Shikokianin
Source: MAO YE XIANG CHA CAI. Ref: 575.

5850 Shikonin
$C_{16}H_{16}O_5$ MW: 288.30 Source: ZI CAO. Ref: 2.

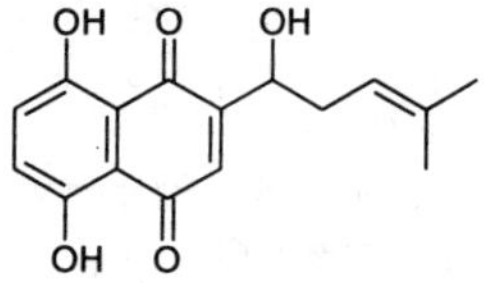

5851 Shionone
$C_{30}H_{50}O$ MW: 426.73 Property: mp 161-2°C. Source: ZI WAN. Ref: 6.

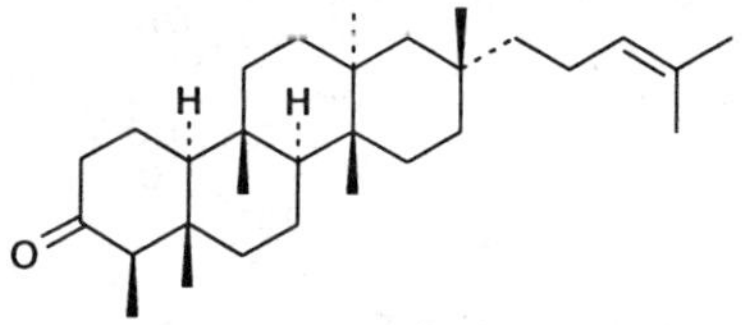

5852 6-Shogaol
$C_{17}H_{24}O_3$ MW: 276.38 Source: GAN JIANG, SHENG JIANG. Ref: 2.

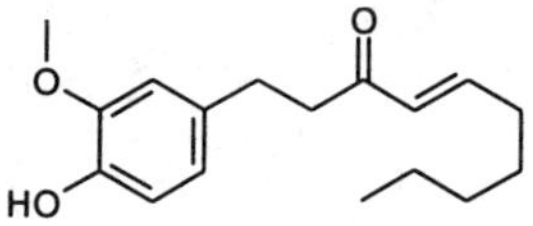

5853 Shyobunone
$C_{15}H_{24}O$ MW: 220.36 Source: BAI CHANG. Ref: 6.

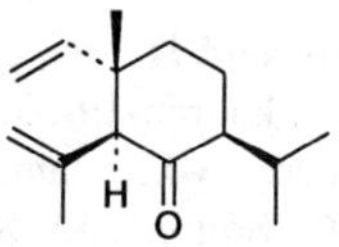

5854 Siaresinolic acid
$C_{30}H_{48}O_4$ MW: 472.71 Property: mp 274-5°C. Source: AN XI XIANG. Ref: 6.

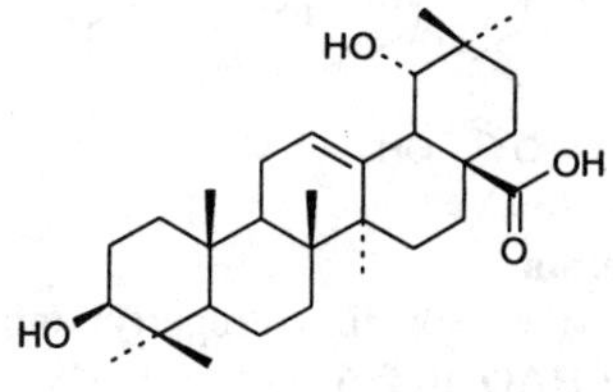

5855 Sibirioside A
$C_{21}H_{28}O_{12}$ MW: 472.45 Property: colorless prismatic crystal, mp 110-2°C, $[\alpha]_D$ -29.6° (c=0.20, methanol). Source: ZHAN LONG JIAN. Ref: 337.

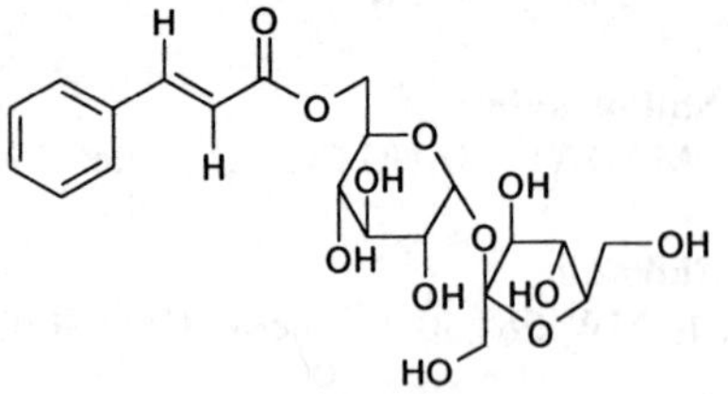

5856 Sibirioside B
$C_{22}H_{30}O_{13}$ MW: 502.48 Property: colorless prismatic crystal, mp 108-10°C, $[\alpha]_D$ -20.18° (c=0.34, methanol). Source: ZHAN LONG JIAN. Ref: 337.

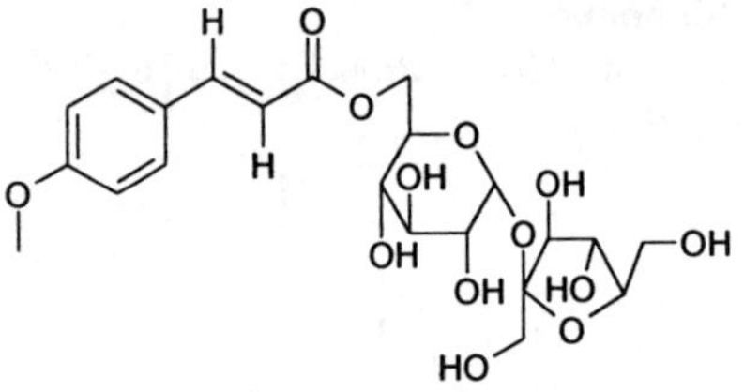

5857 Siegesesteric acid I
Ent-17-acetoxy-18-isobutyryloxy-16(α)-kauran-19-oic acid. $C_{26}H_{40}O_6$ MW: 448.61 Property: white acicular crystal (acetic ester), mp 152-3°C. Source: XI XIAN ZHI SUAN. Ref: 377.

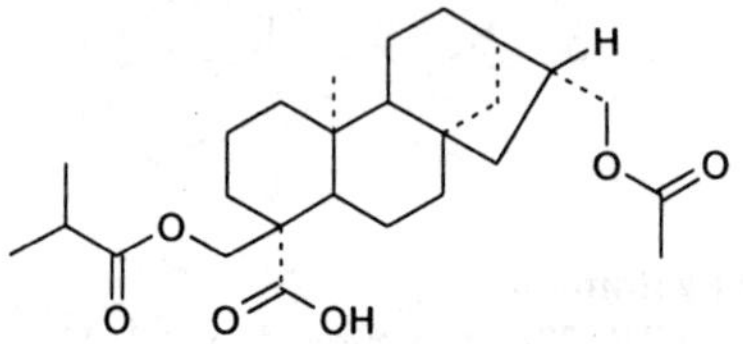

5858 Siegesetheric acid II
Ent-17-ethoxy-16(α)-kauran-19-oic acid. $C_{22}H_{36}O_3$ MW: 348.53 Property: white lamellar crystal (acetic ester), mp 202-4°C. Source: XI XIAN ZHI SUAN. Ref: 377.

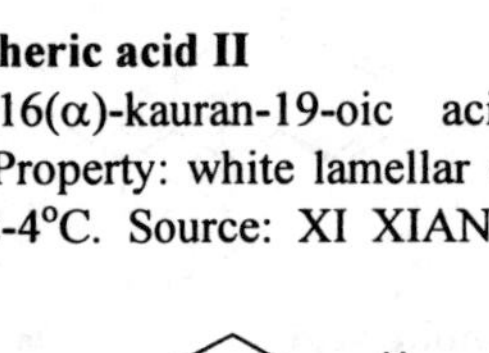

5859 Sieversin
$C_{17}H_{22}O_5$ MW: 306.36 Property: mp 128-31°C. Source: BAI HAO. Ref: 6.

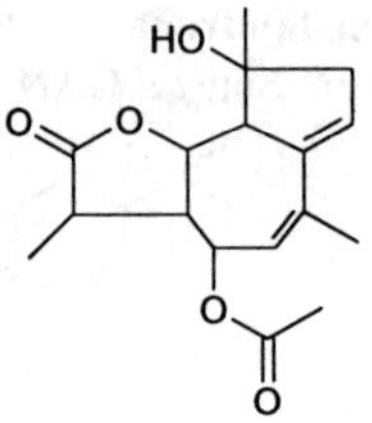

5860 Sieversinin
$C_{15}H_{20}O_3$ MW: 248.32 Property: mp 141-2°C. Source: BAI HAO. Ref: 6.

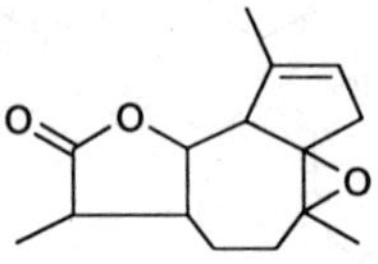

5861 Sikkimotoxin
CAS: 18651-67-7 Property: mp 120°C. Source: XI JIN GUI JIU. Ref: 5.

5862 Simalikalactone D
CAS: 35321-80-3 Property: mp 228-30°C. Source: KU SHU PI. Ref: 5.

5863 Simiral
Source: YI DIAN HONG. Ref: 522.

5864 Sinactine
$C_{20}H_{21}NO_4$ MW: 339.39 Property: mp (-): 175°C, (±): 168°C. Source: LI CHUN HUA, QING FENG TENG. Ref: 6.

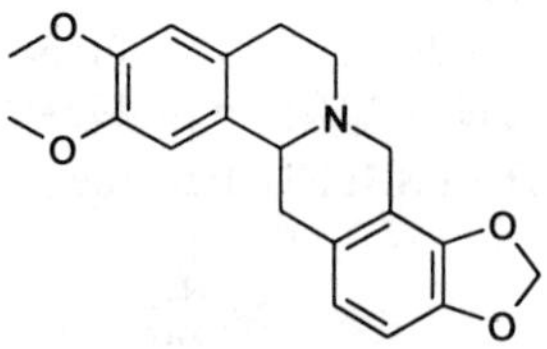

5865 Sinalbin
$C_{14}H_{18}NO_{10}S_2 \cdot C_{16}H_{24}NO_5$ MW: 424.43 • 310.37 Property: mp 139°C (anhydrate). Source: BAI JIE ZI, BAN LAN GEN, TING LI ZI. Ref: 6.

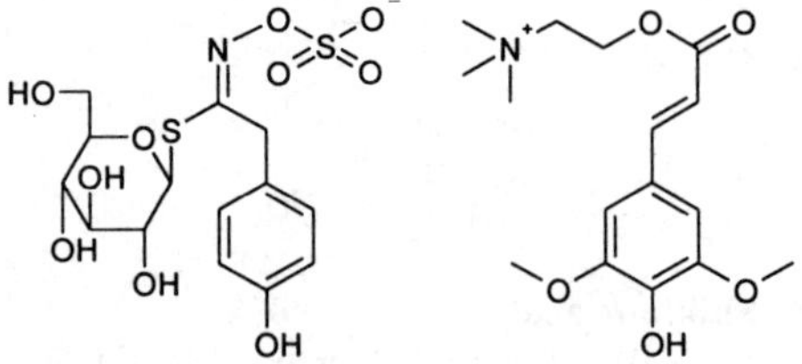

5866 Sinapic acid

$C_{11}H_{12}O_5$ MW: 224.22 Property: mp 192°C. Source: DI SHAO GUA, HUI XIANG JING YE, JIE ZI, LAO SHU GUA, NING MENG, NING MENG GEN, NING MENG YE, YANG CONG. Ref: 6.

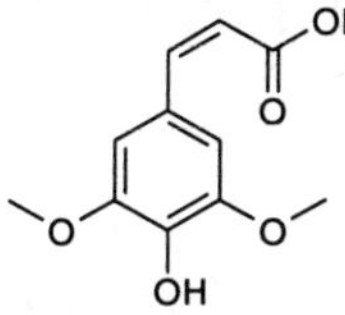

5867 Sinapic aldehyde

$C_{11}H_{12}O_4$ MW: 208.22 Source: HOU PU. Ref: 2.

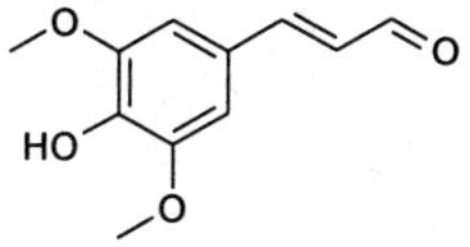

5868 Sinapine

$C_{16}H_{25}NO_6$ MW: 327.38 Property: mp 179°C. Source: BAI JIE ZI, JIE ZI. Ref: 6.

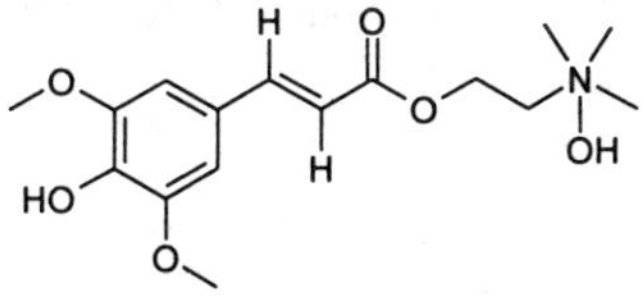

5869 6-Sinapoylspinosin

Source: DA ZAO, SUAN ZAO REN. Ref: 2.

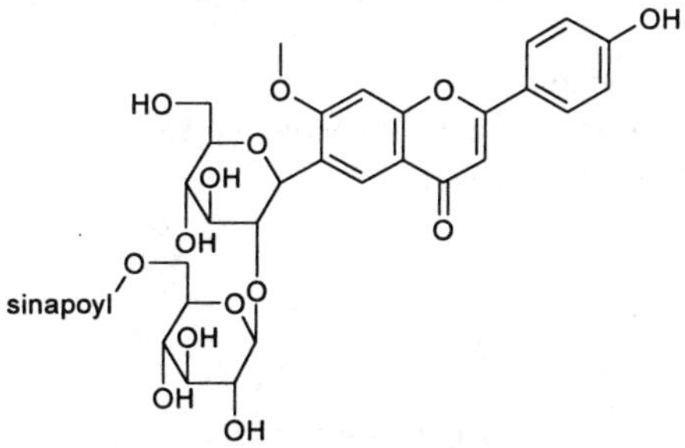

5870 Sineciphyllinine

$C_{20}H_{25}NO_6$ MW: 375.43 Property: white acicular crystal, mp 82-82.5°C. Source: JU YE SAN QI. Ref: 151.

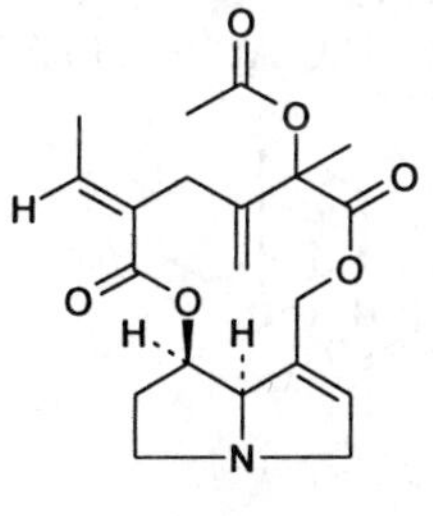

5871 Sinenofuranal

$C_{15}H_{24}O_2$ MW: 236.36 Source: BAI MU XIANG. Ref: 13.

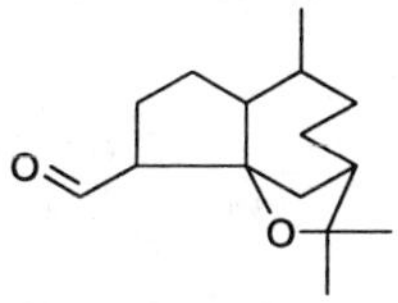

5872 Sinenofuranol

$C_{15}H_{26}O_2$ MW: 238.37 Source: BAI MU XIANG. Ref: 13.

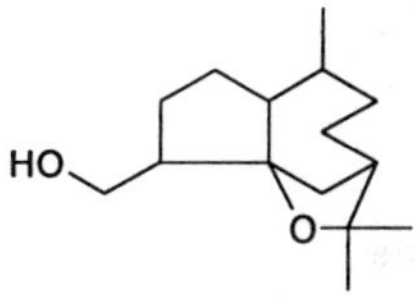

5873 Sinigrin

$C_{10}H_{16}NO_9S{\bullet}K^+$ MW: 358.37•39.10 Property: mp 127-9°C. Source: BAI JIANG, JIE ZI, JI CAI, XI MING, XIMINGZI. Ref: 4, 6.

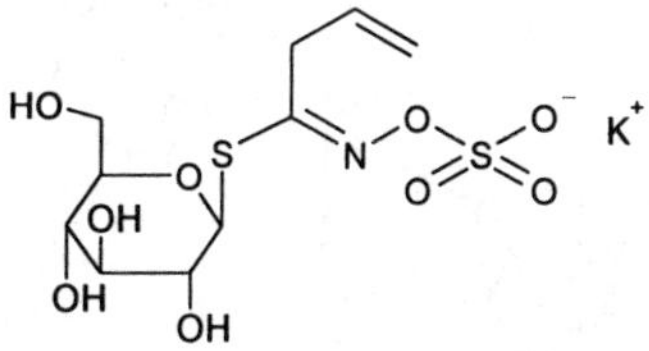

5874 Sinoacutine

$C_{19}H_{21}NO_4$ MW: 327.38 Property: mp 198°C. Source: JU HUA HUANG LIAN, QING FENG TENG, ZI HUA YU DENG CAO (LIE BAO ZI JING). Ref: 6.

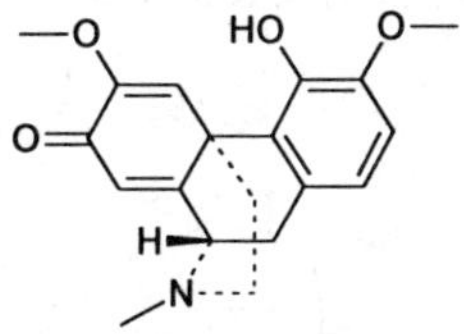

5875 Sinomenine

Coculine; Cucoline; Kukoline. CAS: 115-53-7 $C_{19}H_{23}NO_4$ MW: 329.40 Property: mp 162°C. Source: BIAN FU GE, BIAN FU GE GEN, QING FENG TENG. Ref: 4, 6.

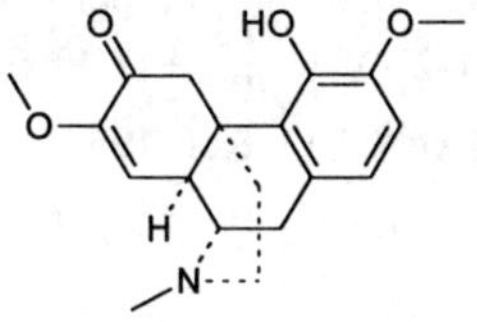

5876 Sinoside

$C_{30}H_{44}O_9$ MW: 548.68 Property: mp 197-202°C, 233-44°C. Source: YANG JIAO AO ZI. Ref: 6.

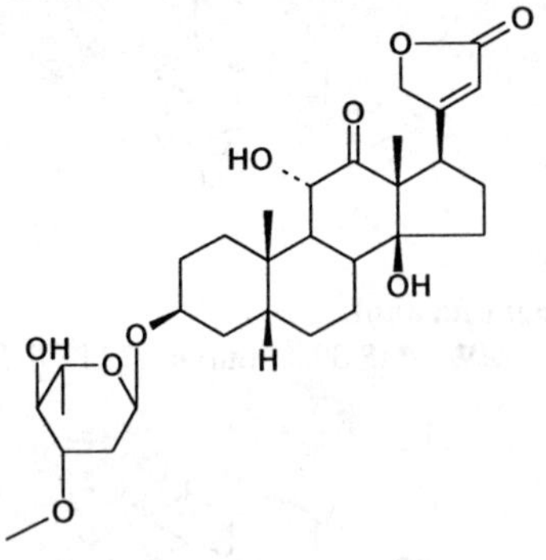

5877 Sinostroside

$C_{30}H_{44}O_9$ MW: 548.68 Property: mp 183-93°C. Source: YANG JIAO AO ZI. Ref: 6.

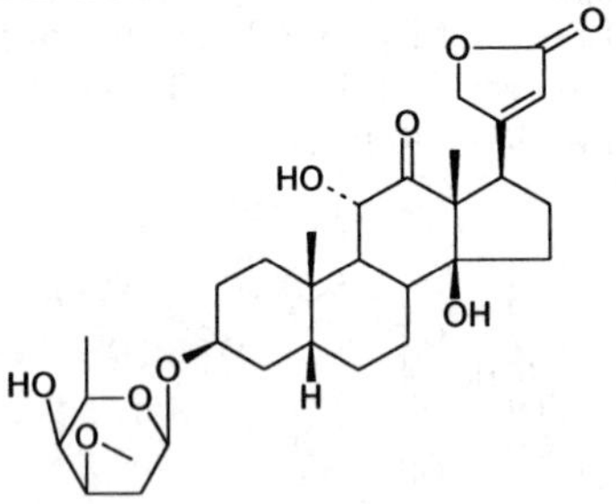

5878 Siraitic acid A

$C_{29}H_{44}O_5$ MW: 472.67 Property: white column crystal, mp 210-1°C, $[\alpha]_D^{22}$ +58.6° (c=0.50, EtOH). Source: LUO HAN GUO. Ref: 495.

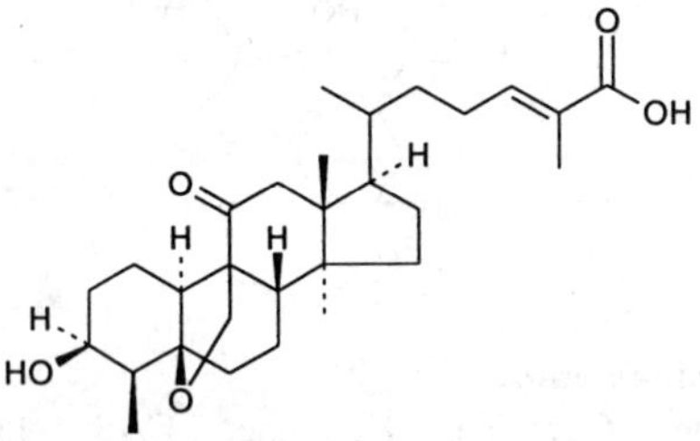

5879 Siraitic acid B

$C_{29}H_{42}O_5$ MW: 470.66 Property: white column crystal, mp 171-2°C, $[\alpha]_D^{22}$ +41.4° (c=0.50, EtOH). Source: LUO HAN GUO. Ref: 495.

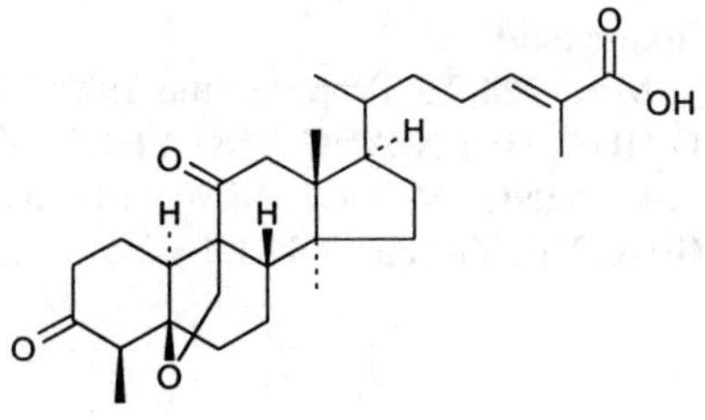

5880 Sisalagenin

$C_{27}H_{42}O_4$ MW: 430.63 Source: JIAN MA. Ref: 10.

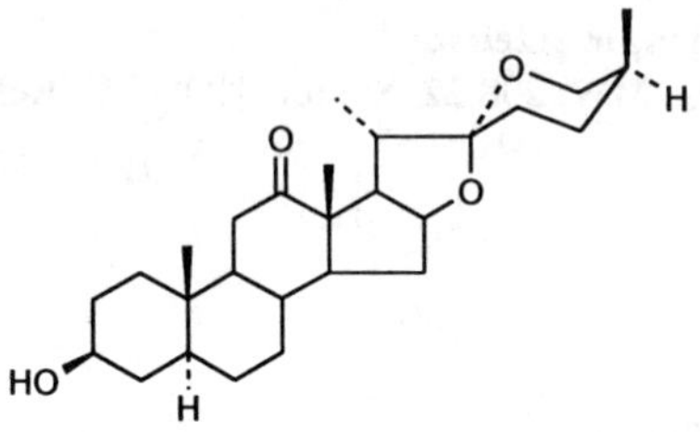

5881 Sisalagenone

$C_{27}H_{40}O_4$ MW: 428.62 Source: SHUI QIE. Ref: 6.

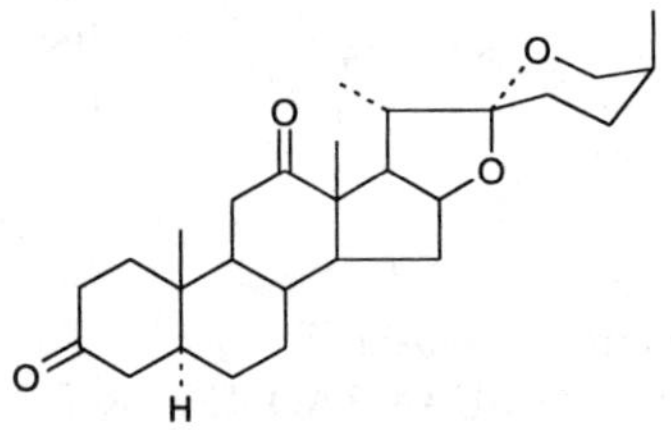

5882 α1-Sitosterol

$C_{29}H_{48}O$ MW: 412.71 Property: mp 164-6°C. Source: CHUAN XIN LIAN. Ref: 2.

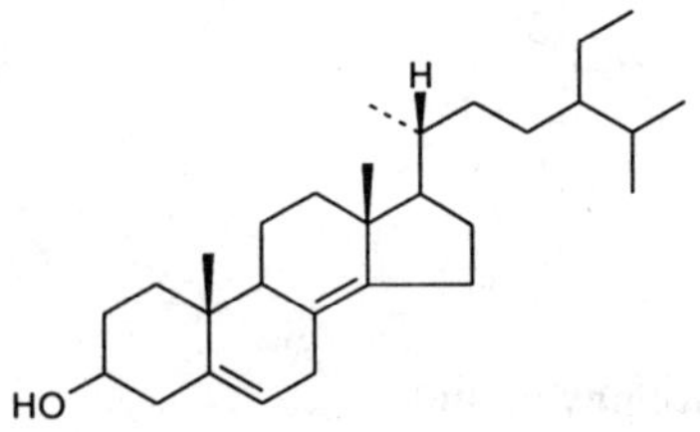

5883 γ-Sitosterol

$C_{29}H_{50}O$ MW: 414.72 Property: mp 147-8°C. Source: DA QING YE, YUN QIAN HU. Ref: 2, 177.

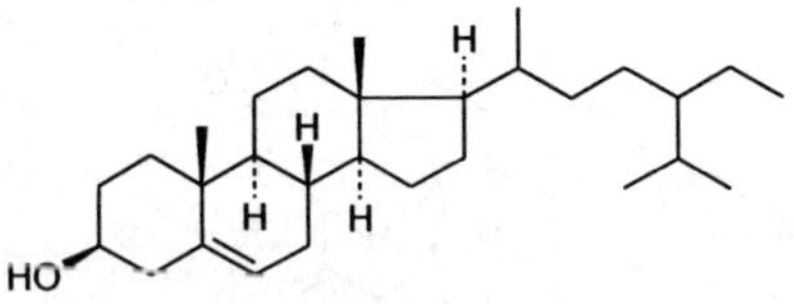

5884 β-Sitosterol

$C_{29}H_{50}O$ MW: 414.72 Property: mp 136-7°C. Source: BA DOU, BAI GUO, BAI SHAO YAO, BAN XIA, CHAN SU, CHUAN XIONG, CI WU JIA, CU LIU GUO(SHA JI), DA QING YE, DAN SHEN, DI GU PI, DONG CHONG XIA CAO, DU ZHONG, FANG FENG, GAN CAO, GAN DI HUANG, GE GEN, GOU QI ZI, GUI ZHI, HE SHOU WU, HONG HUA, HUANG BAI, HUANG QI, JU PI, LONG DAN, MU JIN PI, PU HUANG, QIANG HUO, QING HAO, REN SHEN, ROU CONG RONG, SAN QI, TIAN MA, TIAN NAN XING, XIAN HE CAO, YIN CHEN HAO, YU XING CAO, ZHI ZI, etc. Ref: 2, 4, 377, 519.

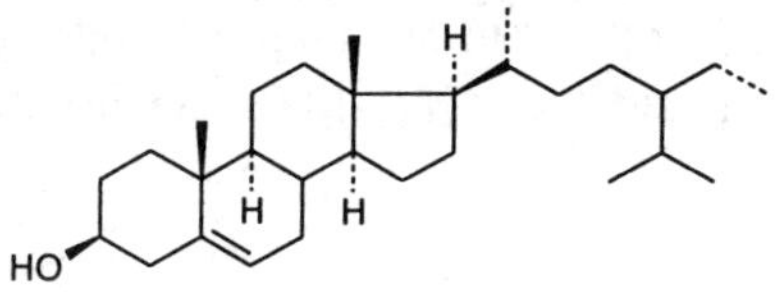

5885 β–Sitosterol-α-glucoside

$C_{35}H_{60}O_6$ MW: 576 Property: 300-2°C. Source: CHUAN CHI SHAO. Ref: 448.

5886 β-Sitosterol-β-D-glucoside

$C_{35}H_{60}O_6$ MW: 576.86 Property: mp 283-6°C (dec). Source: BAI JIANG, BAN XIA, CHUAN XIN LIAN, DONG FANG GOU JI, FANG JI YE BA QIA, GOU QI YE, HONG SAN QI, HUANG KUI, KU GUA, LI MU, MAN JING ZI, MU TONG, MU TONG GEN, SANG YE , SHUI QIE, XIANG JIA PI, YA PIAN, YU BAI FU, YUAN CAN SHA, ZHANG LIU TOU. Ref: 6, 377, 535, 562.

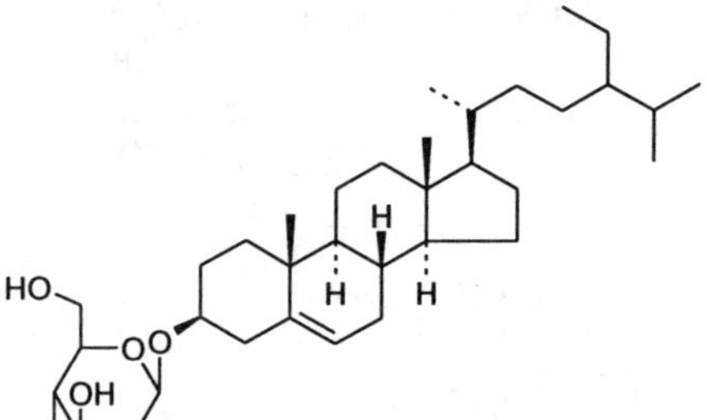

5887 β-Sitosterol-3-O-β-D-xylopyranoside

$C_{34}H_{58}O_5$ Property: colorless acicular crystal (methanol), mp 285-7°C, $[\alpha]_D$ -55.2° (c=0.39, pyridine). Source: NAN FANG TU SI ZI. Ref: 468.

5888 β-Sitosteryl acetate

$C_{31}H_{52}O_2$ MW: 456.76 Property: mp 134°C. Source: QIAO MU ZI ZHU. Ref: 6.

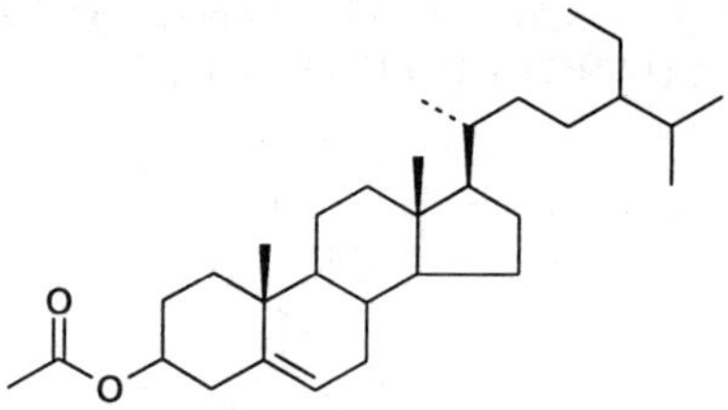

5889 β-Sitosteryl ferulate

$C_{39}H_{58}O_4$ MW: 590.89 Property: mp 131-1.5°C. Source: MI PI KANG. Ref: 6.

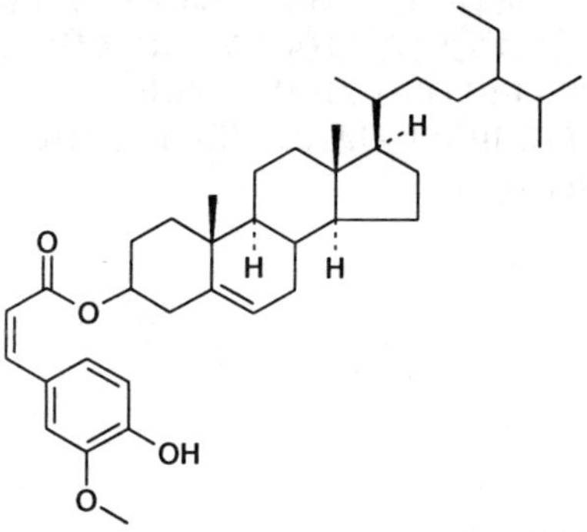

5890 β-Sitosteryl-D-glucoside-6'-palmitate

$C_{51}H_{90}O_7$ MW: 815.28 Source: DONG FANG GOU JI, YA PIAN. Ref: 6.

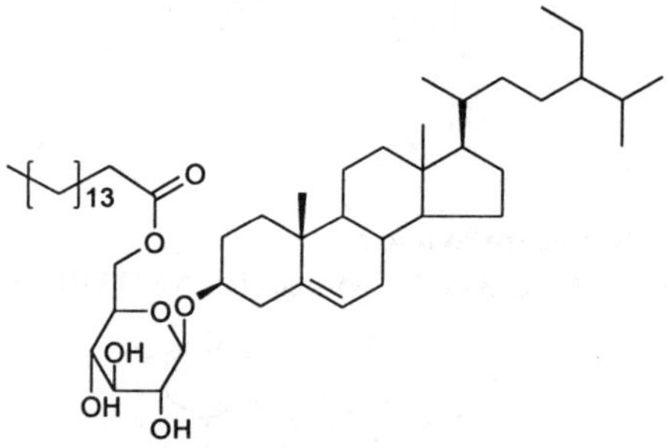

5891 Sitosteryl heptadecoate

Source: JI MAO SONG. Ref: 580.

5892 β-Sitosteryl palmitate

$C_{45}H_{80}O_2$ MW: 853.14 Property: mp 89°C. Source: PU HUANG. Ref: 2.

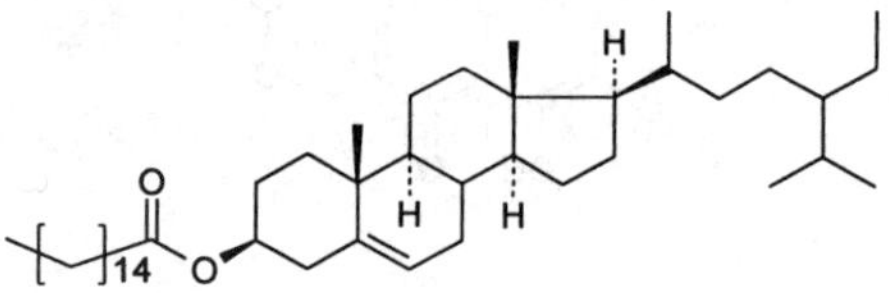

5893 Sitsirikine
$C_{21}H_{26}N_2O_3$ MW: 354.45 Property: mp 206-8°C. Source: CHANG CHUN HUA. Ref: 2.

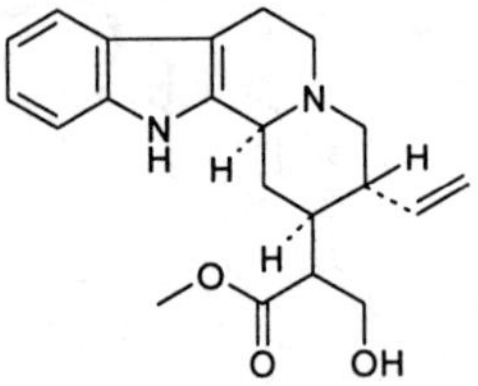

5894 Skimmianine
$C_{14}H_{13}NO_4$ MW: 259.26 Property: mp 176°C. Note: commonly in family *Rutaceae*. Source: BAI XIAN PI, CHOU CAO, CHOU SHAN YANG, CHU YE HUA JIAO PI, FEI LONG ZHANG XUE, GOU JU, HUA JIAO GEN, JIU LI XIANG, YIN YU, ZHU YE JIAO GEN. Ref: 6, 11.

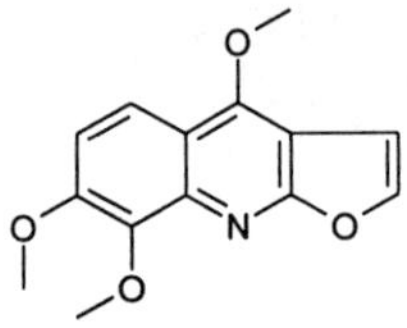

5895 Skimmin
$C_{15}H_{16}O_8$ MW: 324.29 Property: mp 219-21°C. Source: YIN YU. Ref: 6.

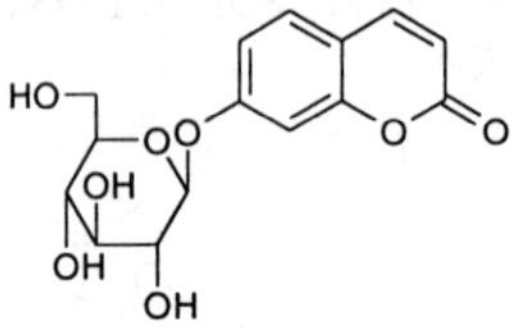

5896 Skullcapflavone I
$C_{17}H_{14}O_6$ MW: 314.30 Source: HUANG QIN. Ref: 2.

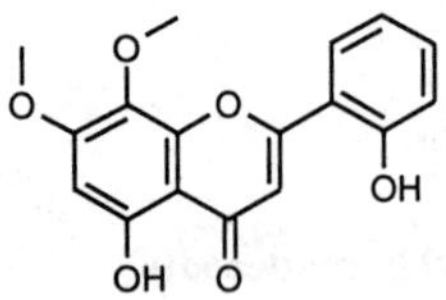

5897 Skullcapflavone II
$C_{19}H_{18}O_8$ MW: 374.35 Source: HUANG QIN. Ref: 2.

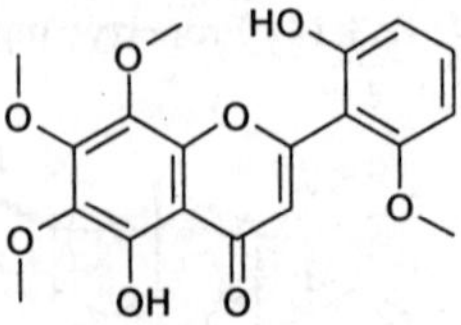

5898 Smilagenin
$C_{27}H_{44}O_3$ MW: 416.65 Property: mp 183-4°C. Source: ZHI MU. Ref: 2.

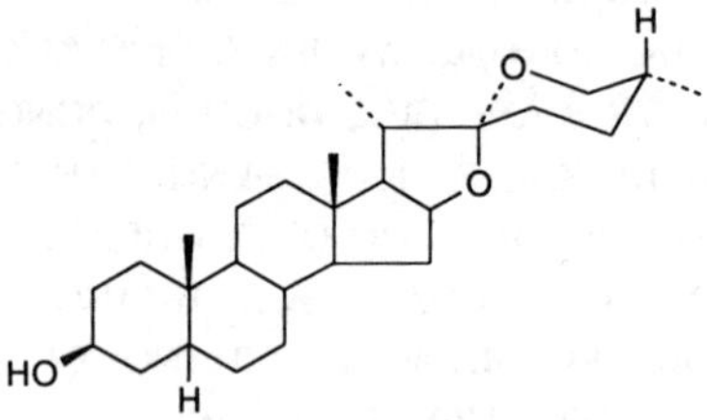

5899 Smilagenin-3-O-[β-D-glucopyranosyl (1→2)]-β-D-mannopyranoside
$C_{39}H_{64}O_{13}$ MW: 740.94 Property: white granular crystal, mp 265-7°C, $[\alpha]_D^{12}$ -189.3°. Source: ZHI MU. Ref: 199.

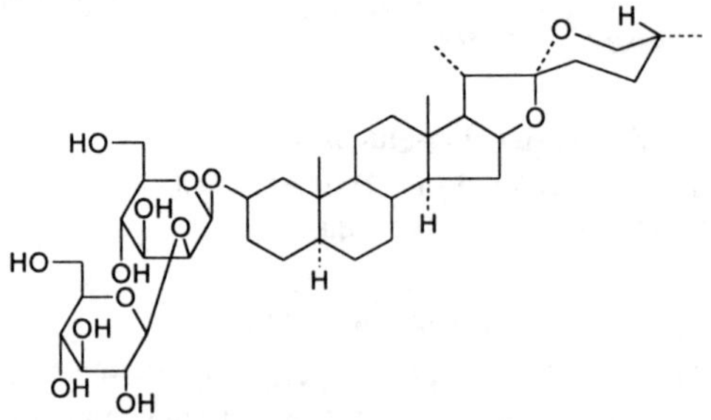

5900 Smilagenone
$C_{27}H_{42}O_3$ MW: 414.63 Property: It only exists in moldy source plants and leads to quality decreasing of the Diosgenin products. Source: CHUNG LONG SHU YU, CHA RUI SHU YU, DUN YE SHU YU, FUZHOU SHUYU, SHU KUI YE. Ref: 10.

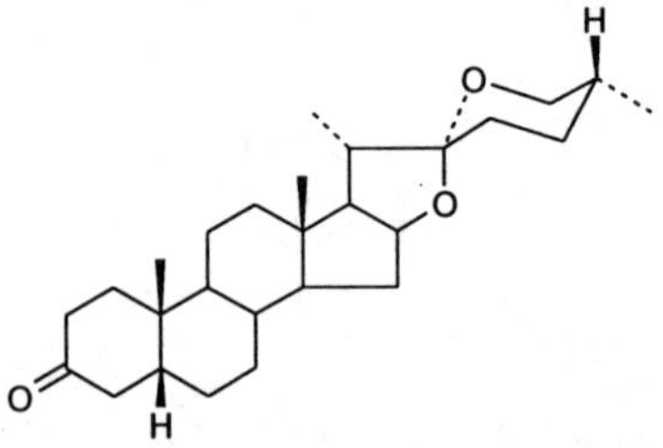

5901 Sodium tauropythocholate
$C_{26}H_{44}NNaO_7S$ MW: 537.70 Property: white powder, mp 192-4°C. Source: MANG SHE. Ref: 240.

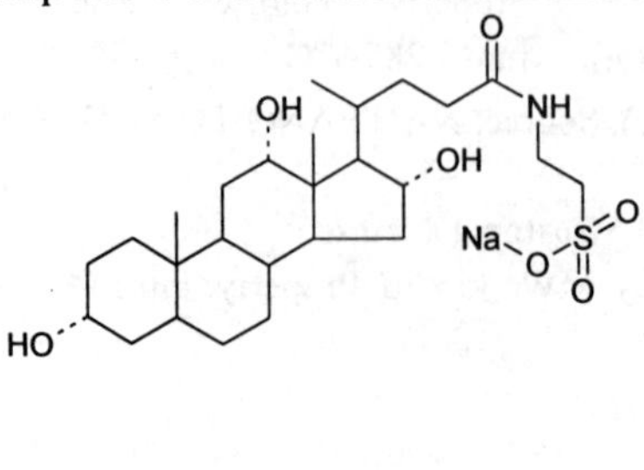

5902 Sodium tauro-α-trihydroxy-coprostanate
$C_{29}H_{50}NNaO_7S$ MW: 579.78 Property: mp 185°C. Source: QING WA DAN. Ref: 6.

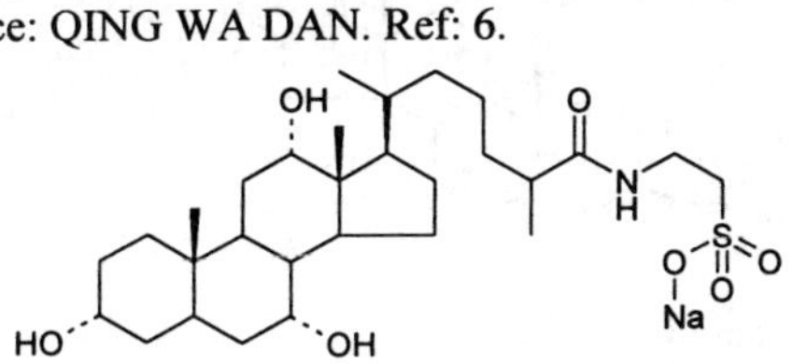

5903 Soladulcidine
$C_{27}H_{45}NO_2$ MW: 415.67 Property: mp 209-11°C. Source: BAI MAO TENG, KU QIE. Ref: 6.

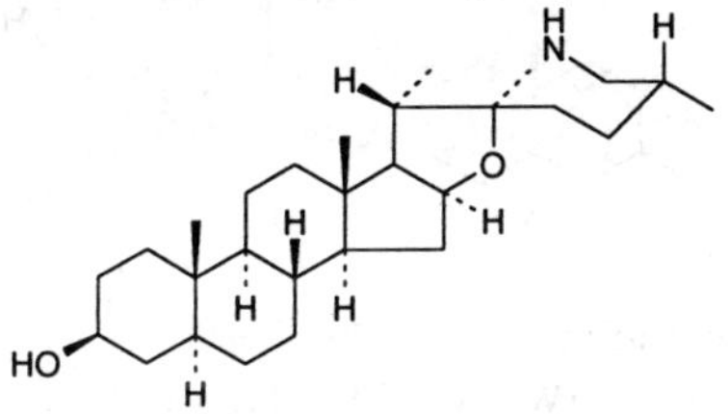

5904 Solamargine
$C_{45}H_{73}NO_{15}$ MW: 868.08 Property: mp 293-5°C. Source: BAI MAO TENG, CI TIAN QIE, KU QIE, LONG KUI, LA JIAO. Ref: 6.

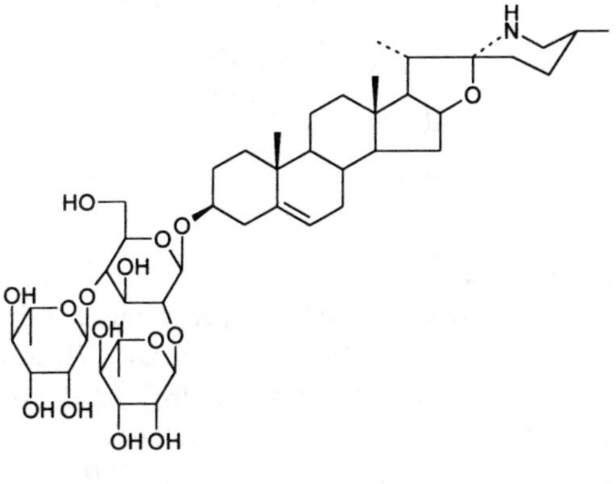

5905 β-Solamargine
$C_{39}H_{63}NO_{11}$ MW: 721.94 Source: YE DIAN QIE. Ref: 6.

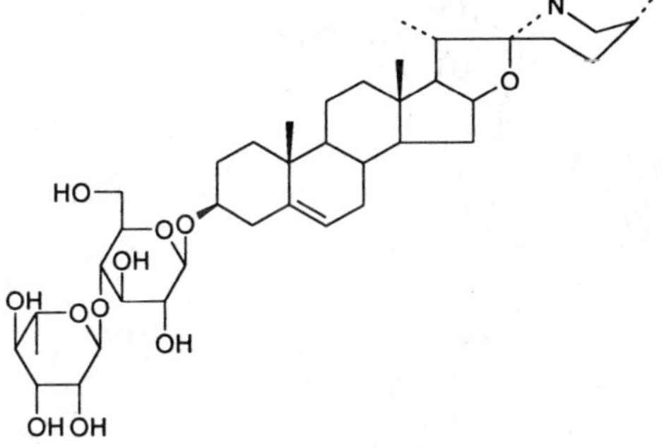

5906 α-Solamarine
$C_{45}H_{73}NO_{16}$ MW: 884.08 Property: mp 278-81°C (dec). Source: BAI MAO TENG, KU QIE. Ref: 6.

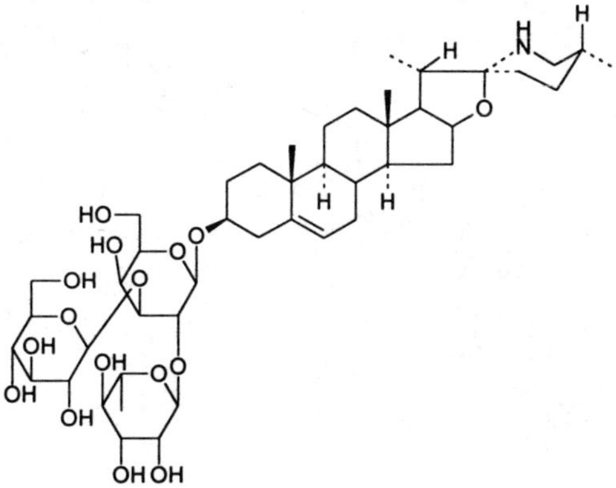

5907 γ1-Solamarine
$C_{39}H_{63}NO_{11}$ MW: 721.94 Property: mp 268-71°C (dec). Source: KU QIE. Ref: 6.

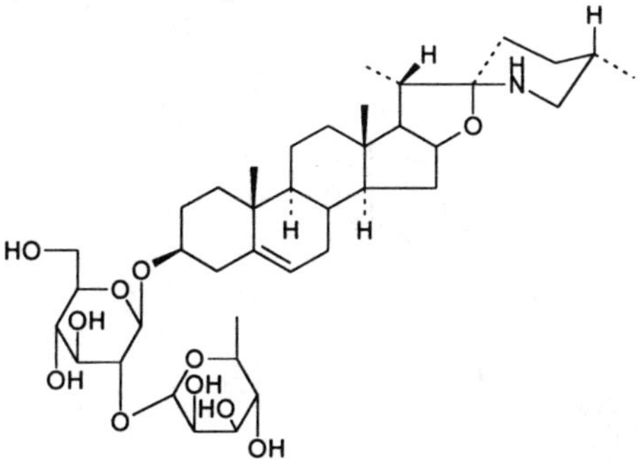

5908 β-Solamarine
CAS: 3671-38-3 $C_{45}H_{73}NO_{15}$ MW: 868.08 Property: mp 275-7°C (dec). Source: BAI MAO TENG, KU QIE. Ref: 5, 6.

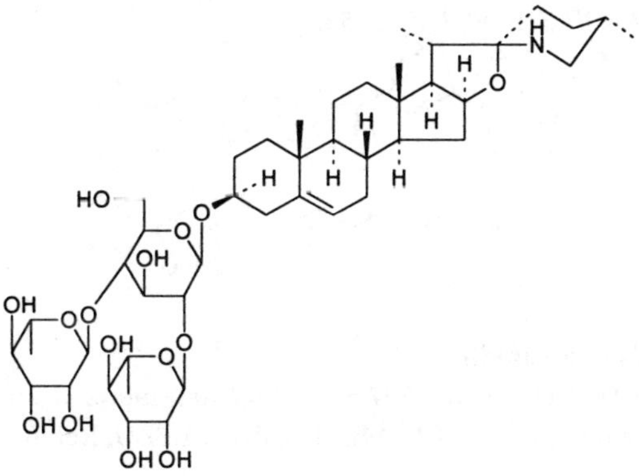

5909 γ2-Solamarine
$C_{39}H_{63}NO_{11}$ MW: 721.94 Property: mp 243-8°C (dec). Source: KU QIE. Ref: 6.

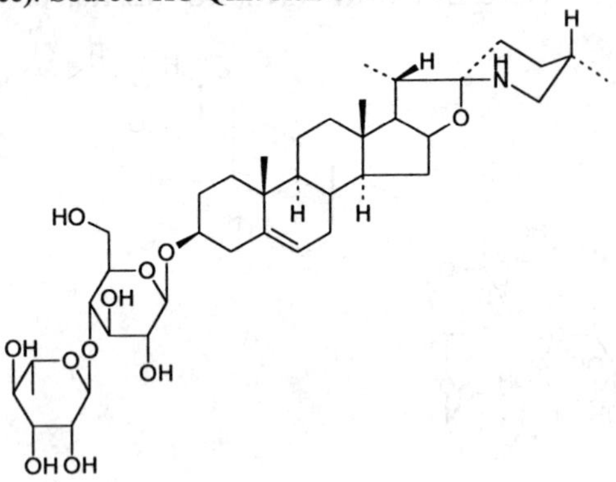

5910 δ-Solamarine
$C_{39}H_{63}NO_{12}$ MW: 737.94 Property: mp 265-9°C (dec). Source: KU QIE. Ref: 6.

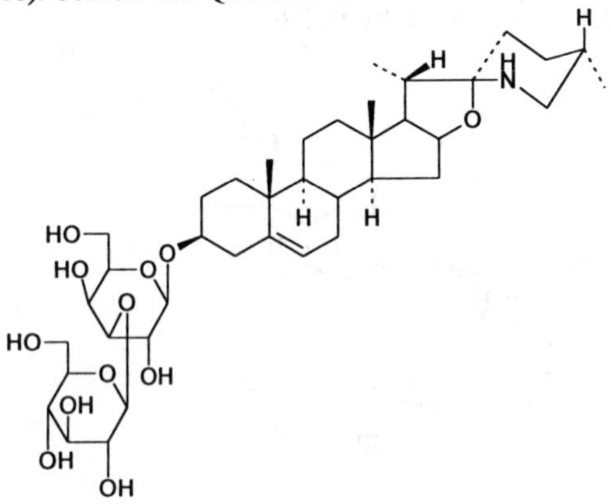

5911 Solamin
$C_{35}H_{64}O_5$ MW: 564.90 Property: white crystal, mp 74-5°C. Source: GUANG YE ZI YU PAN, NIU XIN PAN LI ZHI. Ref: 432, 355.

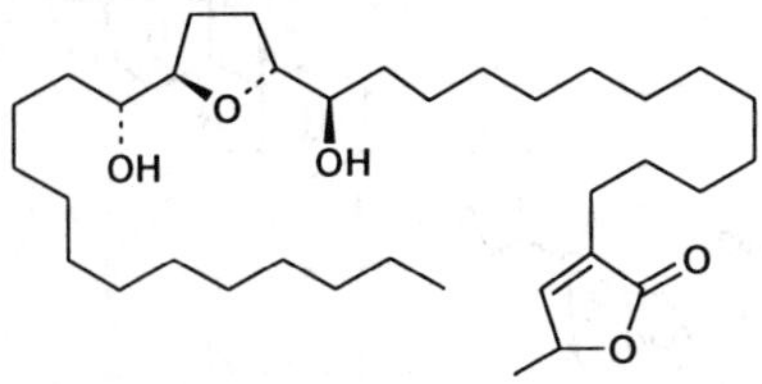

5912 Solanidine
$C_{27}H_{43}NO$ MW: 397.65 Property: mp 218-9°C. Source: CHUAN BEI MU, LA JIAO, LI LU. Ref: 6.

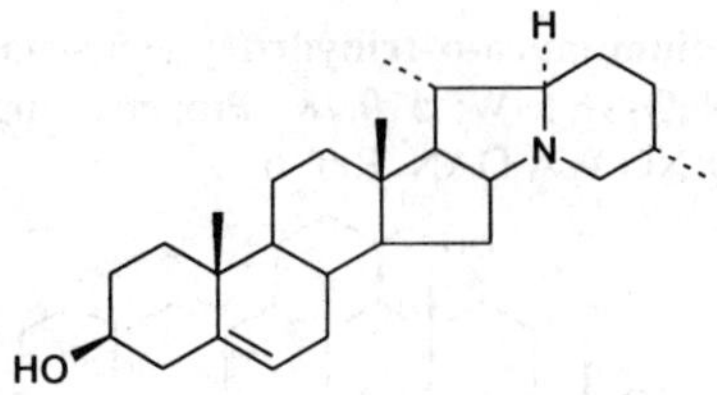

5913 Solanocapsine
$C_{27}H_{46}N_2O_2$ MW: 430.68 Property: mp 222°C. Source: YU SHAN HU GEN, YE HAI JIAO. Ref: 6.

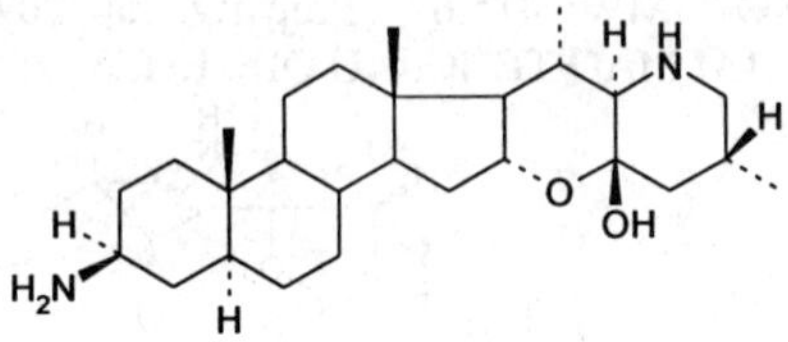

5914 Solasodine
$C_{27}H_{43}NO_2$ MW: 413.65 Property: mp 202°C. Source: BAI MAO TENG, CI TIAN QIE, KU QIE, LA JIAO, LONG KUI, QIE YE, TIAN QIE ZI. Ref: 6.

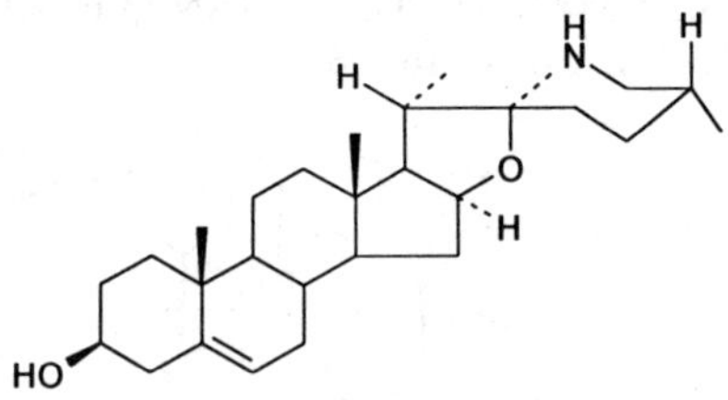

5915 Solasonine
$C_{45}H_{73}NO_{16}$ MW: 884.08 Property: mp 301-3°C. Source: BAI MAO TENG, CI TIAN QIE, HUANG GUO QIE, KU QIE, LA JIAO, LONG KUI, SHUI QIE, YE DIAN QIE, YE YAN YE. Ref: 6.

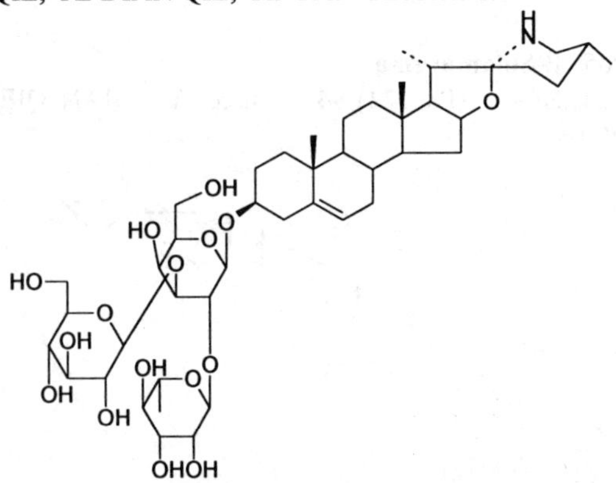

5916 Somalin
$C_{30}H_{46}O_8$ MW: 534.70 Property: mp 240-6°C. Source: FU SHOU CAO. Ref: 6.

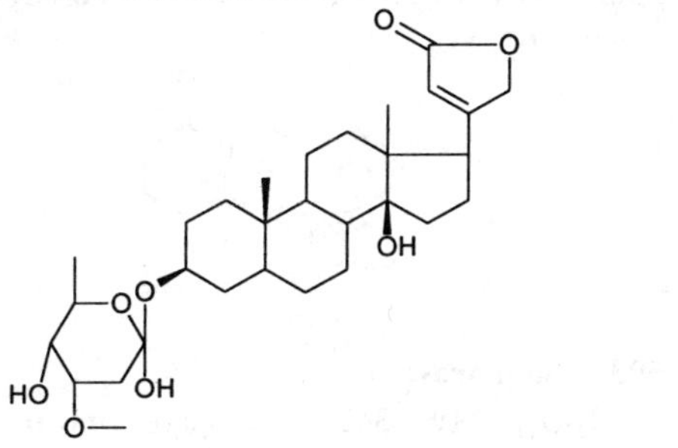

5917 Songbeisine
$C_{27}H_{41}NO_3$ MW: 427.63 Source: CHUAN BEI MU. Ref: 2.

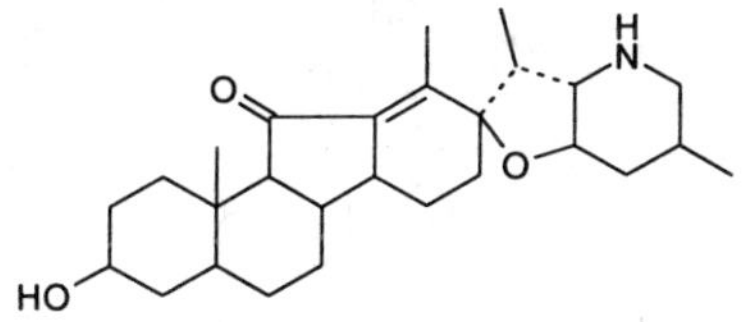

5918 Songoramine
$C_{22}H_{39}NO_3$ MW: 453.27 Property: mp 211-2°C colorless oleaginous substance, $[\alpha]_D^{26}$ -44.2° (c=0.266, $CHCl_3$). Source: E ZHANG YE FU ZI. Ref: 461.

5919 Sonpeimine
$C_{27}H_{43}NO_4$ Source: CHUAN BEI MU. Ref: 2.

5920 Sophocarpine
CAS: 6483-15-4 $C_{15}H_{22}N_2O$ MW: 246.36 Property: mp 52-3°C, 57-8°C. Source: BAI CI HUA, KU SHEN, KU DOU ZI. Ref: 4, 546, 564, 593.

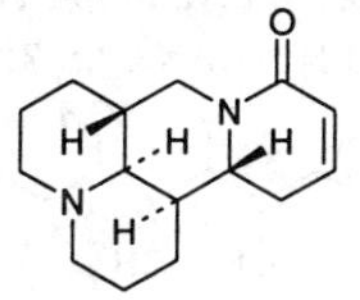

5921 Sophorabioside
$C_{27}H_{30}O_{14}$ MW: 578.53 Property: mp 247°C. Source: HUAI JIAO. Ref: 6.

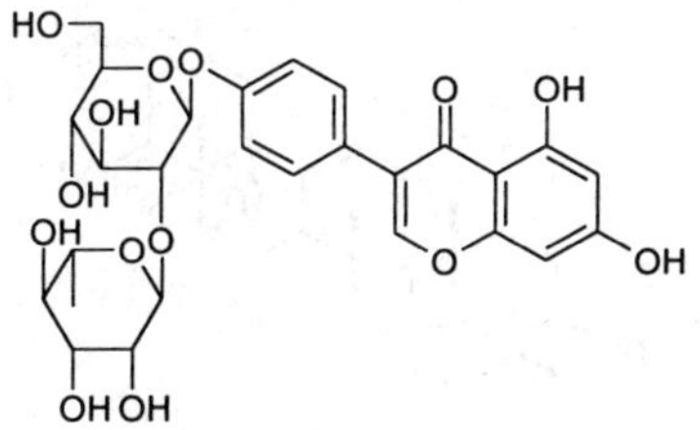

5922 Sophoradin
$C_{30}H_{36}O_4$ MW: 460.62 Property: mp 161°C. Source: SHAN DOU GEN. Ref: 6.

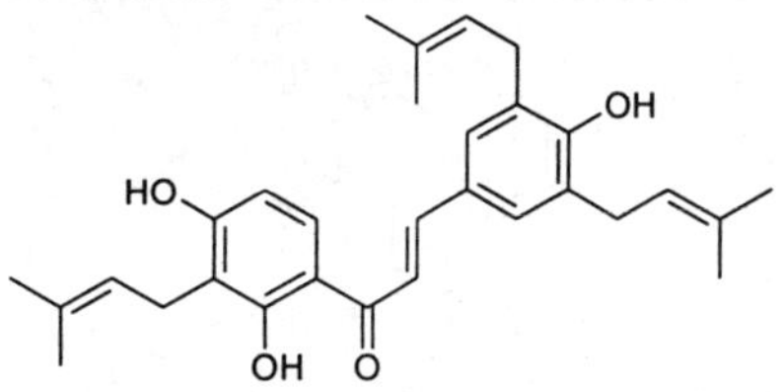

5923 Sophoradochromene
$C_{30}H_{34}O_4$ MW: 458.60 Property: mp 154°C. Source: SHAN DOU GEN. Ref: 6.

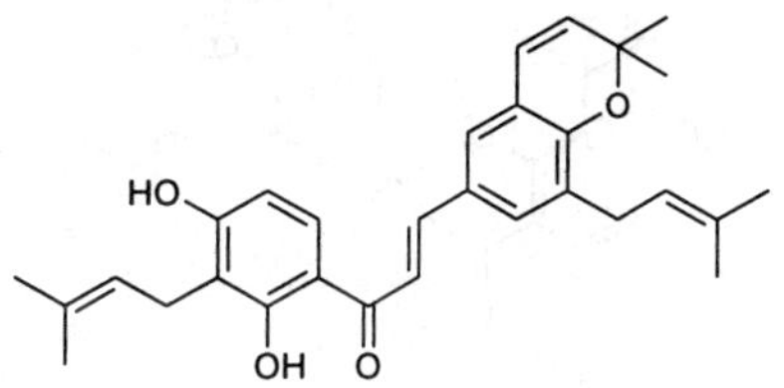

5924 Sophoraflavonoloside
$C_{27}H_{30}O_{16}$ MW: 610.53 Property: mp 207-8°C. Source: HUAI JIAO. Ref: 6.

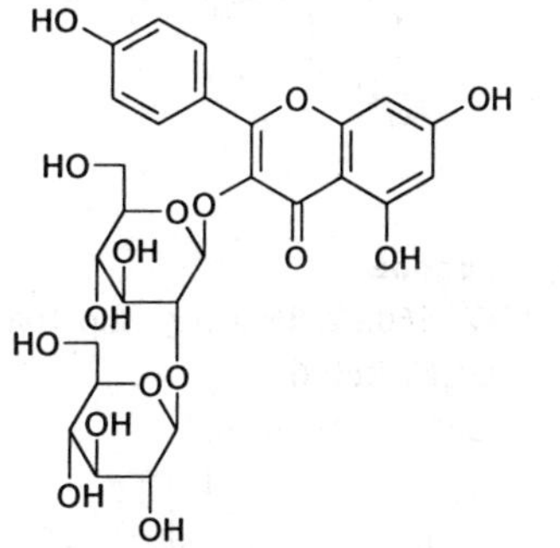

5925 Sophoraflavoside
$C_{58}H_{94}O_{27}$ MW: 1223.38 Source: KU SHEN. Ref: 2.

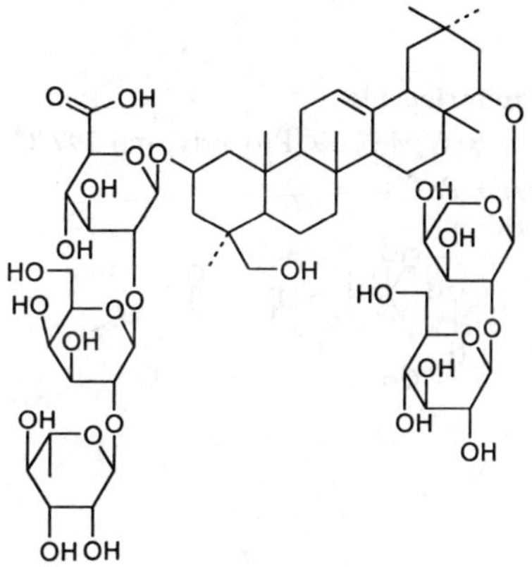

5926 Sophoramine
$C_{15}H_{20}N_2O$ MW: 244.34 Property: mp 163-5°C. Source: BAI CI HUA, KU SHEN. Ref: 2, 6, 546, 564.

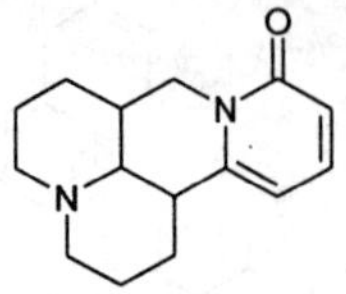

5927 Sophoranochromene
$C_{30}H_{34}O_4$ MW: 458.60 Property: mp 152°C. Source: SHAN DOU GEN. Ref: 6.

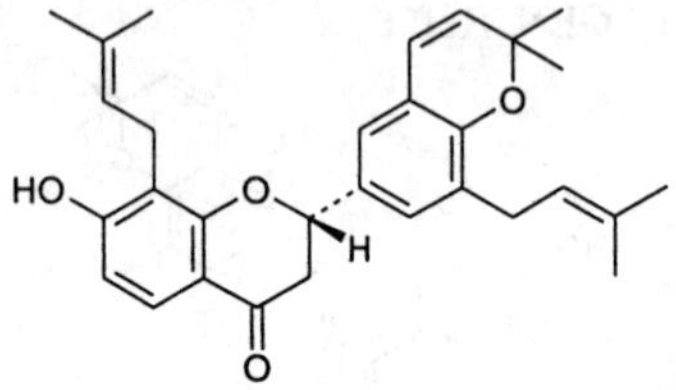

5928 Sophoranol N-oxide
$C_{15}H_{24}N_2O_3$ MW: 280.37 Source: KU SHEN. Ref: 2.

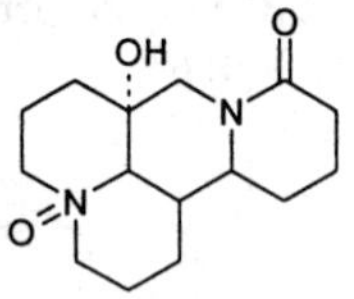

5929 Sophoranone
$C_{30}H_{36}O_4$ MW: 460.62 Property: mp 108°C. Source: SHAN DOU GEN. Ref: 6.

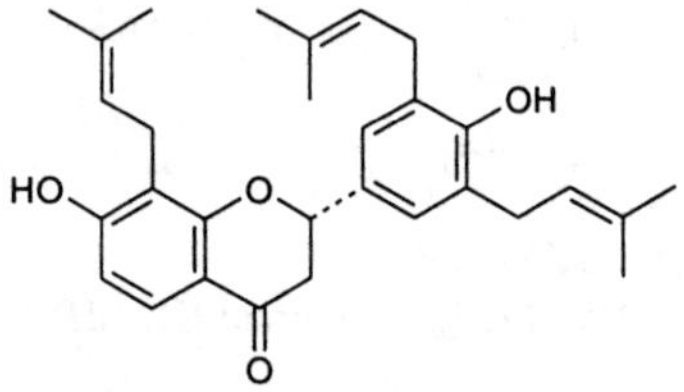

5930 Sophoricoside
$C_{21}H_{20}O_{10}$ MW: 432.39 Property: mp 297°C. Source: HUAI JIAO. Ref: 6.

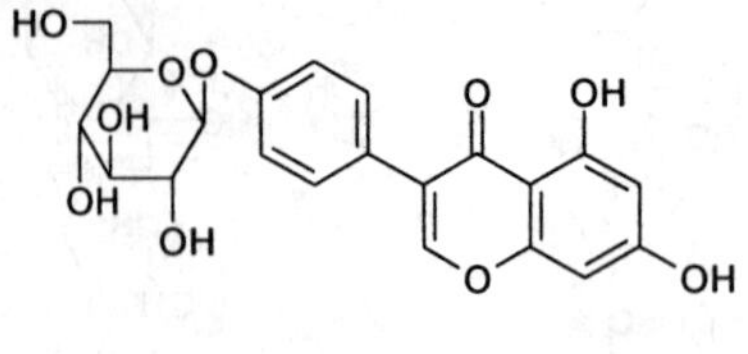

5931 Sophoridine
$C_{15}H_{24}N_2O$ MW: 248.37 Property: mp 108-10°C. Source: BAI CI HUA, KU DOU ZI, KU SHEN. Ref: 2, 546, 564, 593.

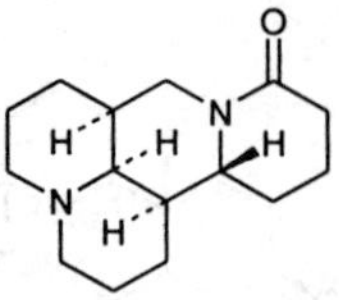

5932 Sophorose
$C_{12}H_{22}O_{11}$ MW: 342.30 Property: mp α: 196-8°C. Source: HUAI JIAO. Ref: 6.

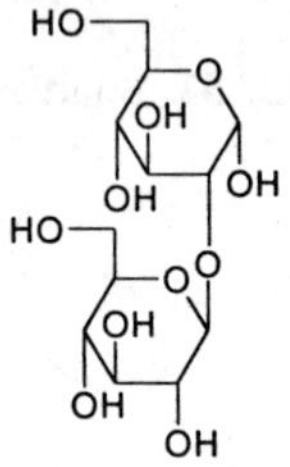

5933 Sorbarin
$C_{21}H_{20}O_{10}$ MW: 432.39 Property: mp >300°C. Source: ZHEN ZHU MEI. Ref: 6.

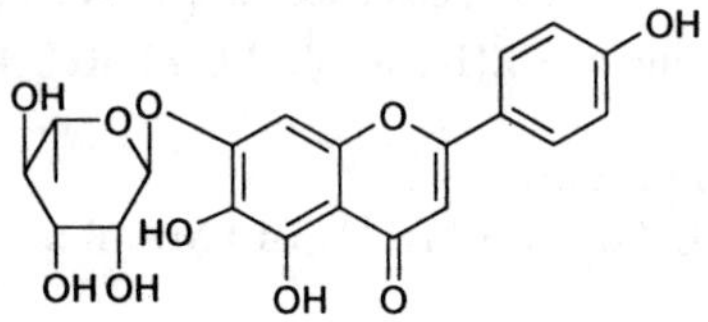

5934 Sorbitol
$C_6H_{14}O_6$ MW: 182.17 Property: mp 110-1°C (anhydrate). Source: JI CAI, PI PA YE, SHUI ZHI, SHUI ZHI YE, SHI LIU GEN, YUAN CAN ZI. Ref: 6.

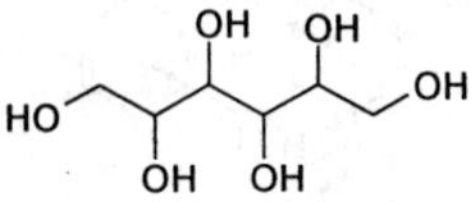

5935 Soyasapogenol A
$C_{30}H_{50}O_4$ MW: 474.73 Property: mp 308-12°C. Source: HEI DA DOU. Ref: 6.

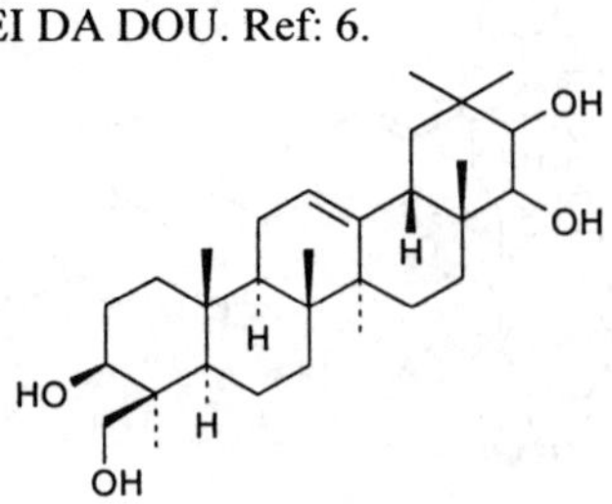

5936 Soyasapogenol B

$C_{30}H_{50}O_3$ MW: 458.73 Property: mp 258-9°C. Source: HEI DA DOU. Ref: 6.

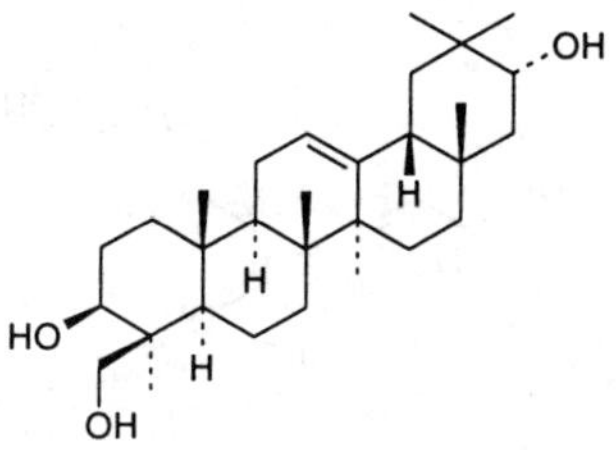

5937 Soyasapogenol C

$C_{30}H_{48}O_2$ MW: 440.72 Property: mp 238-9°C. Source: HEI DA DOU. Ref: 6.

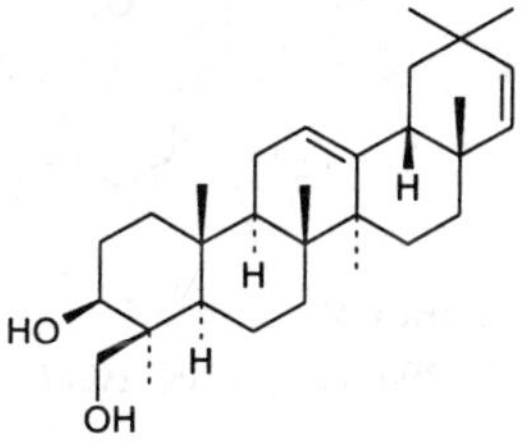

5938 Soyasapogenol D

$C_{30}H_{50}O_3$ MW: 458.73 Property: mp 298-9°C. Source: HEI DA DOU. Ref: 6.

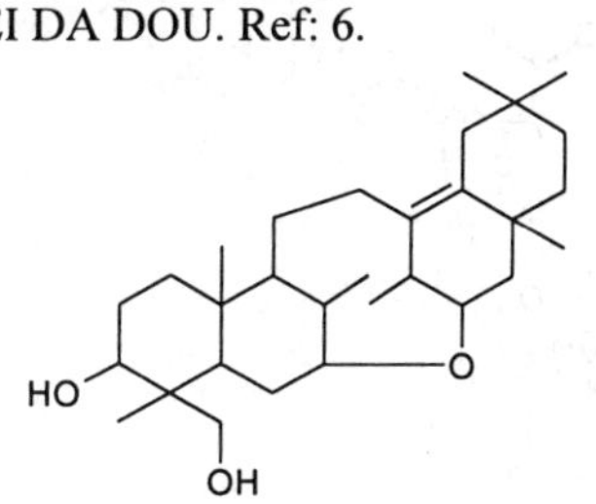

5939 Soyasapogenol E

$C_{30}H_{48}O_3$ MW: 456.72 Source: HEI DA DOU. Ref: 6.

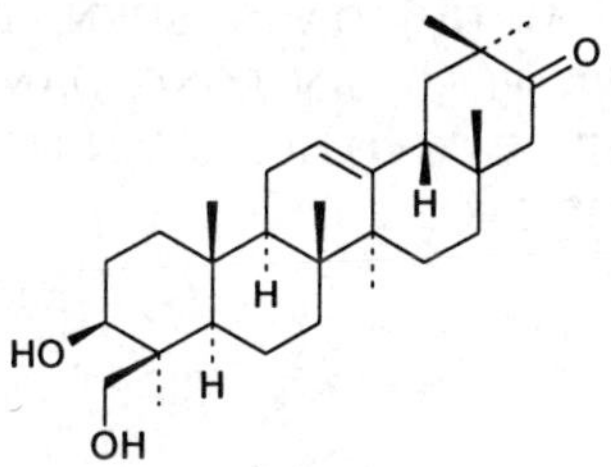

5940 Soyasaponin

$C_{48}H_{78}O_{17}$ MW: 927.15 Source: KU SHEN. Ref: 2.

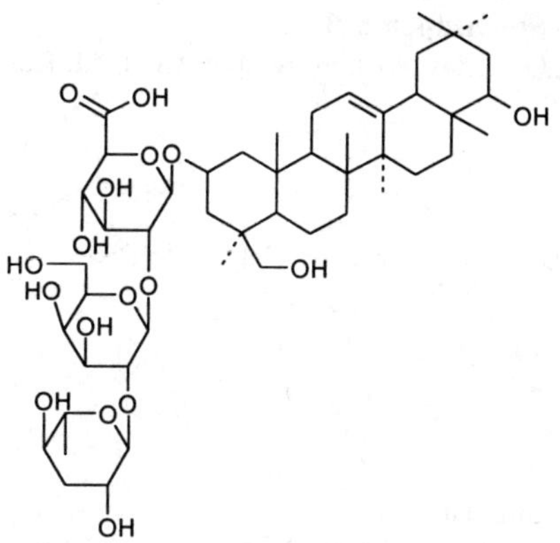

5941 Sparassol

$C_{10}H_{12}O_4$ MW: 196.20 Property: mp 67-8°C. Source: NAO YANG HUA. Ref: 6.

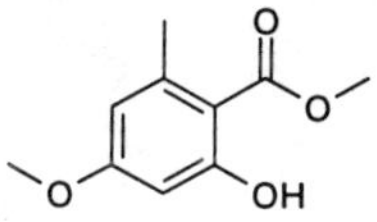

5942 Sparteine

$C_{15}H_{26}N_2$ MW: 234.39 Property: bp (-): 188°C/18 mm. Source: BAI QU CAI, MU MA DOU. Ref: 6.

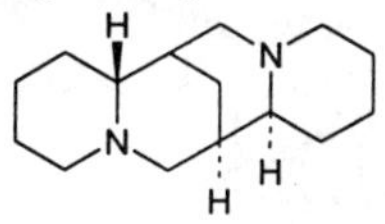

5943 Spathulenol

$C_{15}H_{24}O$ MW: 220.36 Source: CHUAN XIONG. Ref: 2.

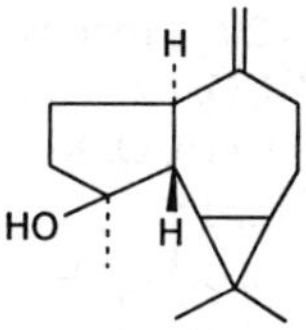

5944 Specneuzhenide

$C_{31}H_{42}O_{17}$ MW: 686.67 Property: colorless powder, mp 152-5°C. Source: NU ZHEN ZI. Ref: 386.

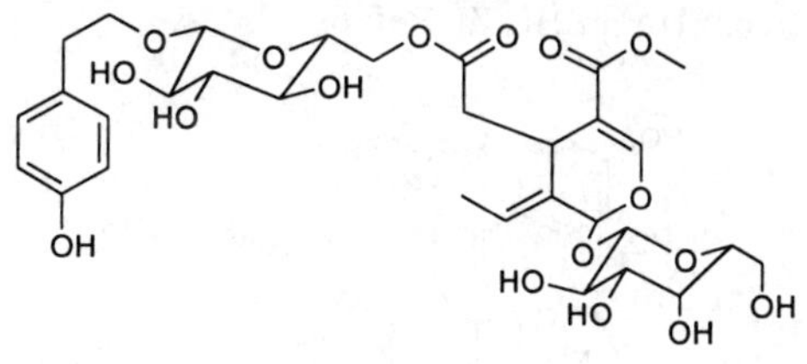

5945 Spinasaponin B

$C_{42}H_{66}O_{15}$ MW: 810.99 Source: BO CAI. Ref: 6.

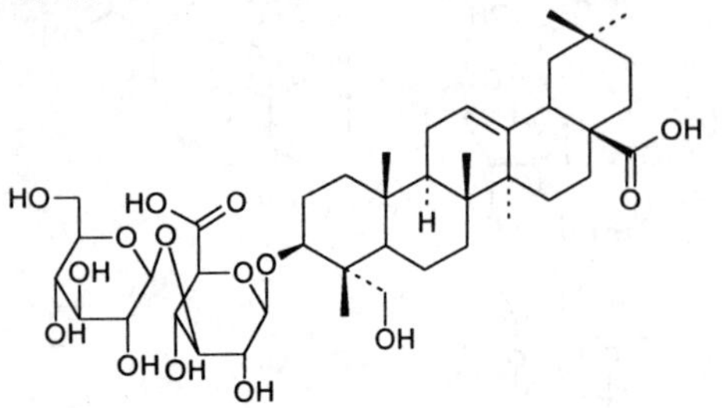

5946 Spherosinin

$C_{22}H_{24}O_5$ MW: 368.43 Property: mp 97-8°C. Source: NIAO PAO CAO. Ref: 6.

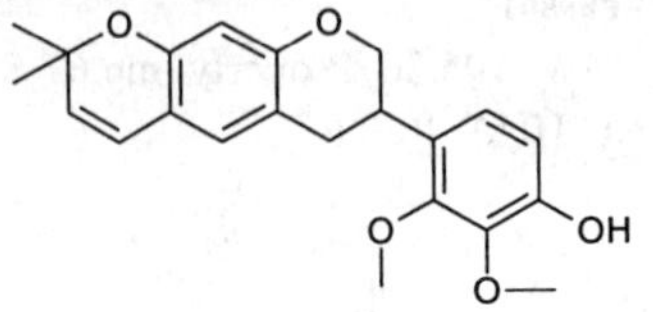

5947 Sphingomyelin

$C_{57}H_{117}N_2O_7P$ MW: 973.55 Property: mp 196-8°C. Source: MU ER, ZHANG YU. Ref: 6.

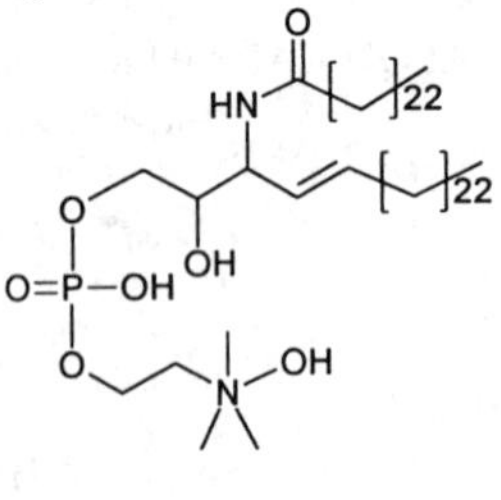

5948 Sphondin

$C_{12}H_8O_4$ MW: 216.20 Property: mp 183-6°C, 189-91°C. Source: DU HUO, LANG DU LI JIANG QIAN HU, YONG NING DU HUO. Ref: 6.

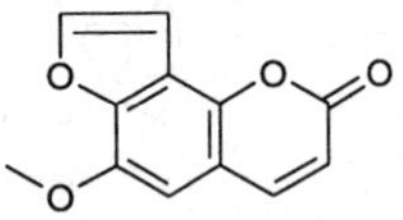

5949 Spicataside

$C_{36}H_{30}O_{15}$ MW: 702.63 Property: mp 232-3°C (dec). Source: SHAN ZHU ZI. Ref: 6.

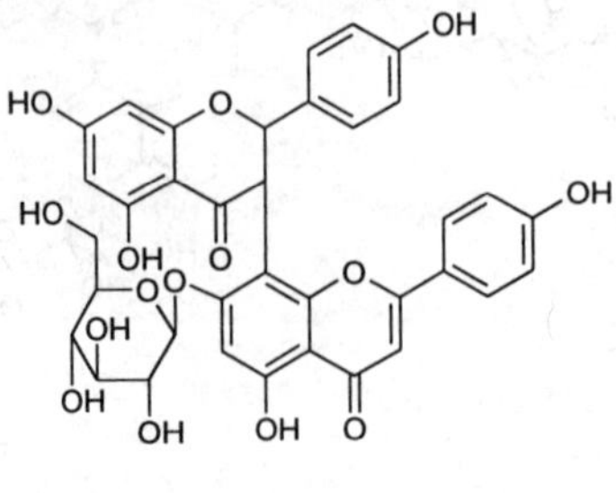

5950 Spinacetin

$C_{17}H_{14}O_8$ MW: 346.30 Property: mp 235-6°C. Source: BO CAI. Ref: 6.

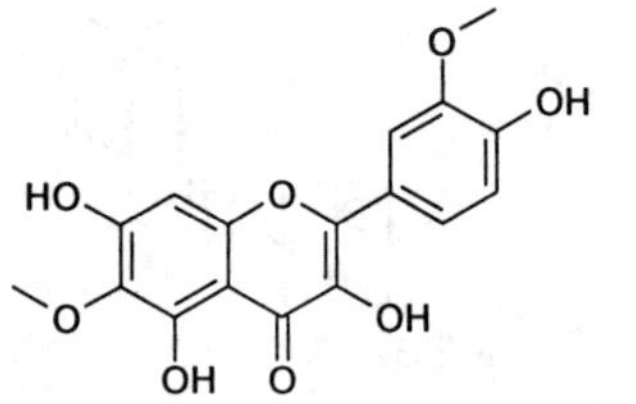

5951 Spherosin

$C_{17}H_{18}O_5$ MW: 302.33 Property: mp 151°C. Source: NIAO PAO CAO. Ref: 6.

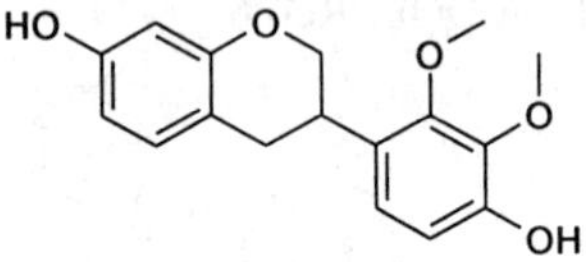

5952 Spinasaponin A

$C_{42}H_{66}O_{14}$ MW: 794.99 Source: BO CAI. Ref: 6.

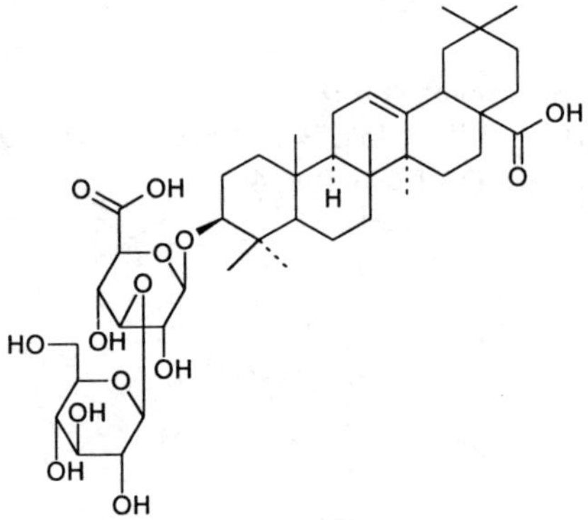

5953 α-Spinasterol

Chondrillasterol. $C_{29}H_{48}O$ MW: 412.71 Property: coloeless acicular crystal (ethanol), mp 159-60°C. Source: CHAI HU, DANG SHEN, GUA LOU, HUANG JIN FENG, JIN LONG DAN CAO, KU CAO (I), NIU XI, XIAO HUA SUAN TENG ZI. Ref: 2, 6, 437, 548, 582, 604.

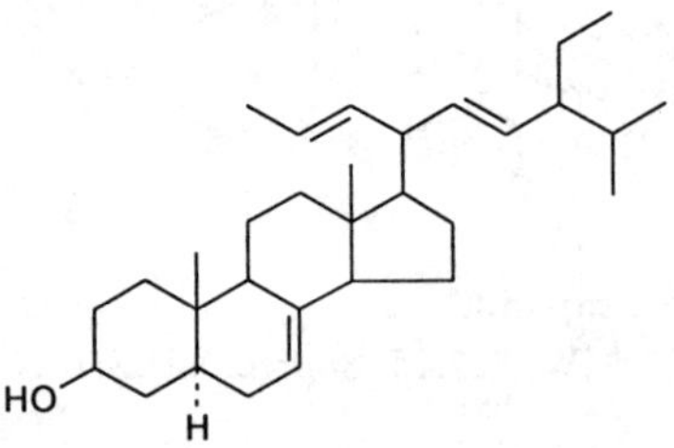

5954 α-Spinasterol-β-D-glucoside
$C_{35}H_{60}O_6$ MW: 576.86 Source: DANG SHEN, NIU XI, TIAN HUA FEN. Ref: 2, 582.

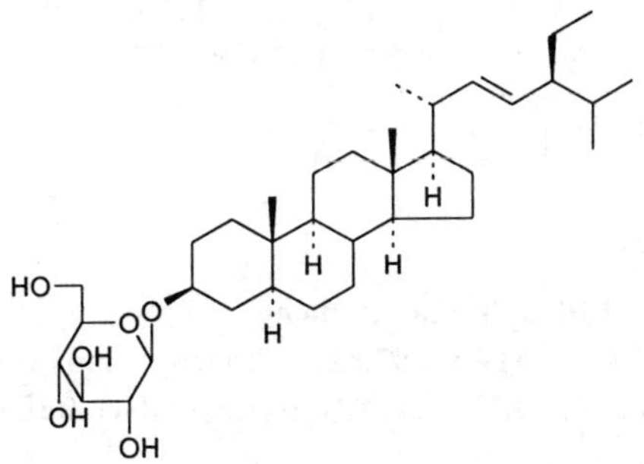

5955 Spinosin
$C_{28}H_{32}O_{15}$ MW: 608.56 Source: DA ZAO, SUAN ZAO REN. Ref: 2.

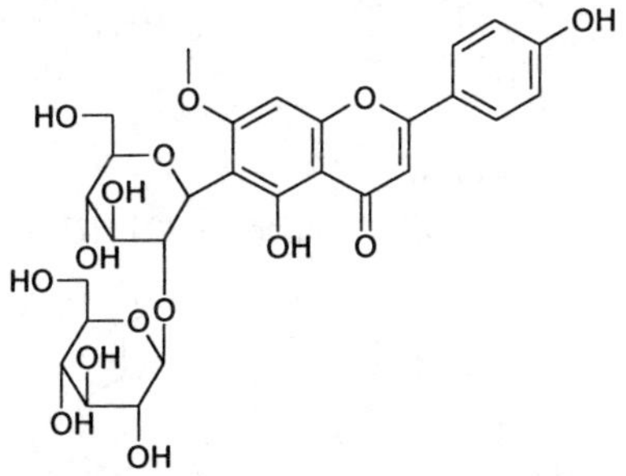

5956 Spiradine A
$C_{20}H_{25}NO_2$ MW: 311.43 Property: mp 281-2°C. Source: XIU XIAN JU YE. Ref: 6.

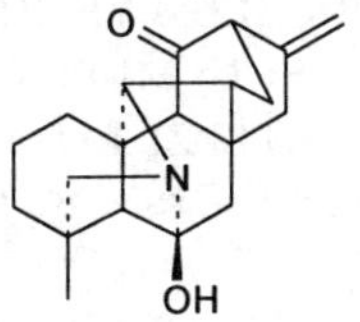

5957 Spiradine B
$C_{20}H_{27}NO_2$ MW: 313.44 Property: mp 259-60°C. Source: XIU XIAN JU YE. Ref: 6.

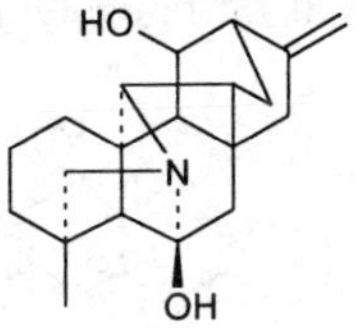

5958 Spiradine C
$C_{22}H_{29}NO_3$ MW: 355.48 Property: mp 248-9°C. Source: XIU XIAN JU YE. Ref: 6.

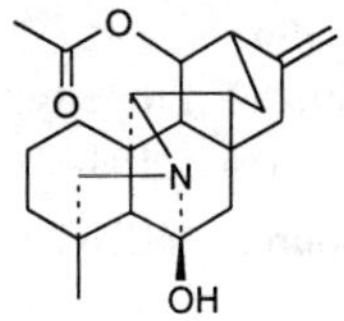

5959 Spiradine D
$C_{21}H_{27}NO_2$ MW: 325.45 Property: mp 134-5°C. Source: XIU XIAN JU YE. Ref: 6.

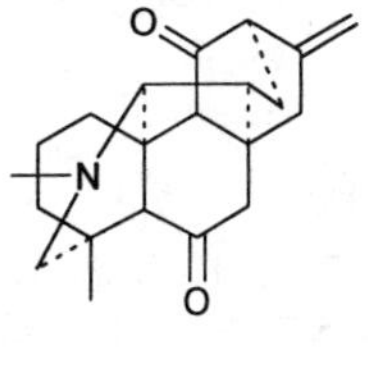

5960 Spiradine F
$C_{24}H_{33}NO_4$ MW: 399.53 Source: XIU XIAN JU YE. Ref: 6.

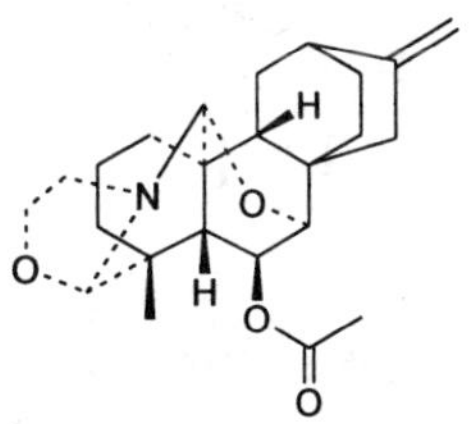

5961 Spiradine G
$C_{22}H_{31}NO_3$ MW: 357.50 Property: mp 168-70°C. Source: XIU XIAN JU YE. Ref: 6.

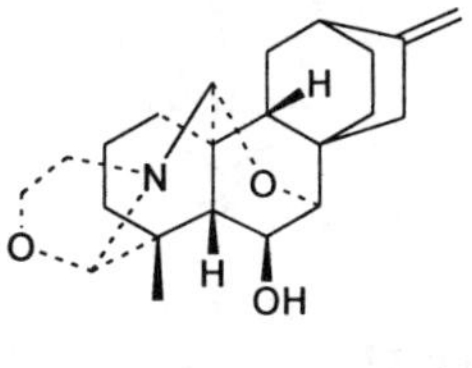

5962 Spiraeoside
$C_{21}H_{20}O_{12}$ MW: 464.39 Property: mp 209-11°C Source: HU CONG, MU FU RONG HUA. Ref: 6.

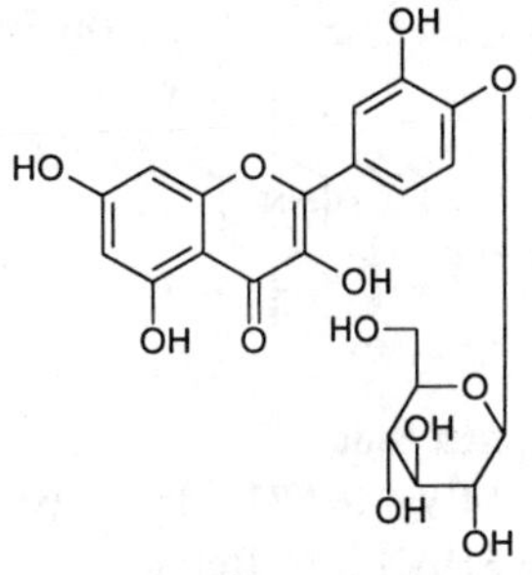

5963 Spiramongolin
$C_{20}H_{22}O_8$ MW: 390.39 Property: colorless rhomboid crystal (EtOH), mp 194-6°C, $[\alpha]_D^{20}$ +70.7° (c=0.3,MeOH). Source: MENG GU XIU XIAN JU. Ref: 421.

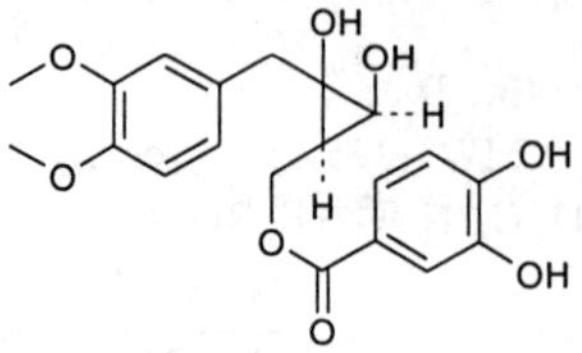

5964 Spirasine IV
$C_{20}H_{27}NO$ MW: 297.44 Property: amorphous white powder, $[\alpha]_D^{17}$ -95.7° (c=1.1, chloroform). Source: GUANG YE FEN HUA XIU XIAN JU. Ref: 43

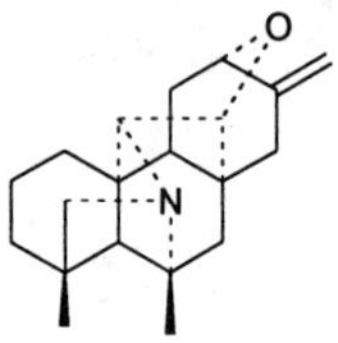

5965 Spirasine IX
$C_{20}H_{25}NO$ MW: 295.43 Property: colorless columnar crystal, mp. 157-8°C, $[\alpha]_D^{21}$ +135.5° (c=1.0, chloroform). Source: GUANG YE FEN HUA XIU XIAN. Ref: 43

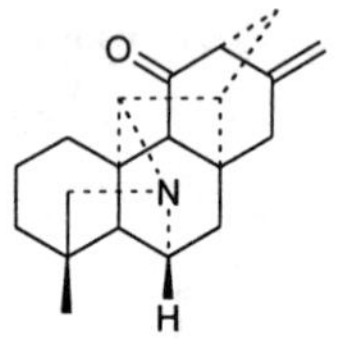

5966 Spirasine XI
$C_{21}H_{29}NO$ MW: 311.47 Property: white acicular crystal, mp 286-8°C, $[\alpha]_D^{11}$ -23.8° (c=0.84, chloroform) Source: GUANG YE FEN HUA XIU XIAN. Ref: 43.

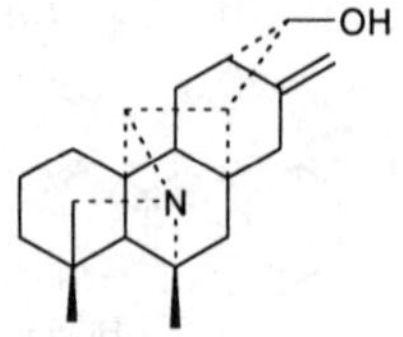

5967 Spiropachysine
$C_{31}H_{46}N_2O$ MW: 462.73 Property: mp 290-2°C. Source: XUE SHAN LIN. Ref: 6.

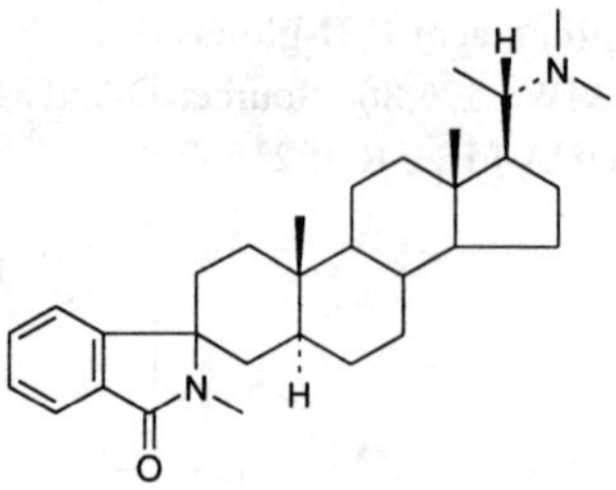

5968 25D-Spirosta-3,5-diene
$C_{27}H_{40}O_2$ MW: 392.62 Property: mp 164-5°C. Source: BEI XIE, CHUAN SHAN LONG. Ref: 6.

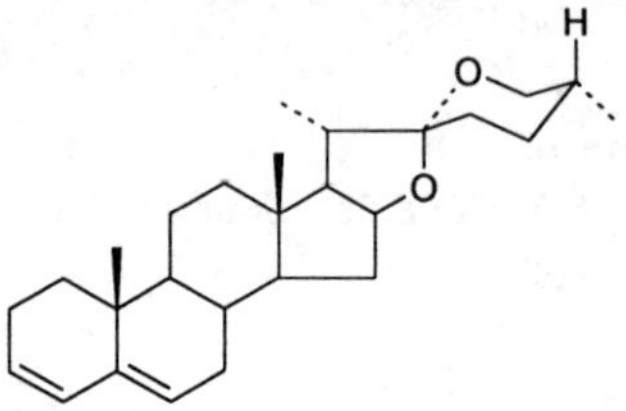

5969 Spongesterol
$C_{27}H_{46}O$ MW: 386.67 Source: QIAN HU. Ref: 6.

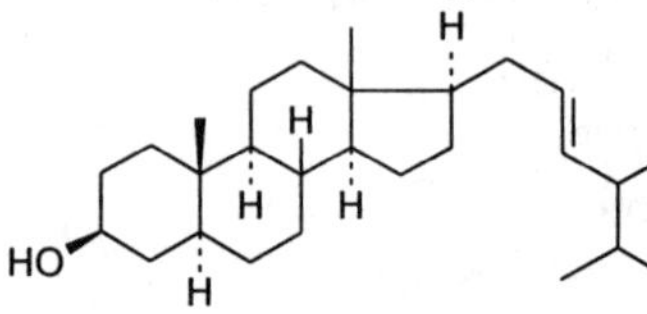

5970 Squalene
$C_{30}H_{50}$ MW: 410.73 Property: bp 284-5°C/25 mm. Source: A LI HONG (LUO YE SONG XUN), DONG FENG CAI, DOU YOU, MI PI KANG, SI GUA ZI, TONG YOU, XIANG SI ZI. Ref: 6.

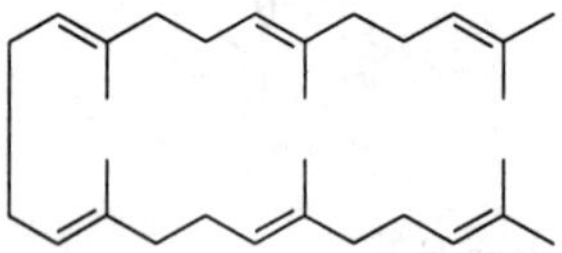

5971 Squamatic acid
$C_{19}H_{18}O_9$ MW: 390.35 Property: mp 219°C. Source: XUE CHA. Ref: 6.

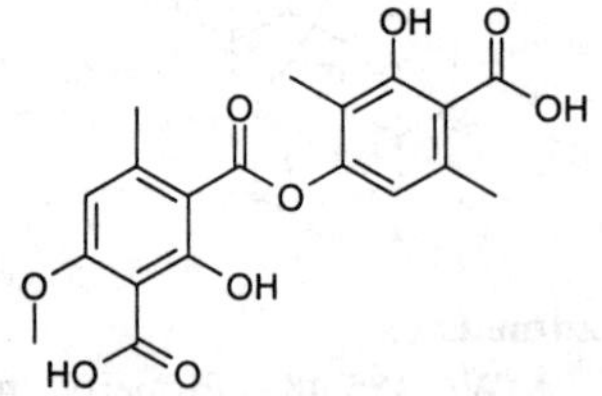

5972 Squamone (1)
$C_{35}H_{62}O_7$ MW: 594.88 Property: white crystal, mp 95-7°C, $[\alpha]_D^{25}$ +29° (c=0.1, methanol). Source: NIU XIN FAN LI ZHI. Ref: 401.

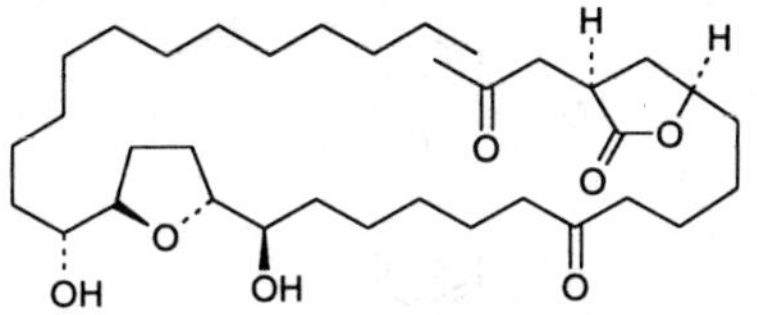

5973 Squamosamide
$C_{26}H_{27}NO_7$ MW: 465.51 Property: light yellow crystal, mp 200-2°C. Source: FAN LI ZHI. Ref: 221.

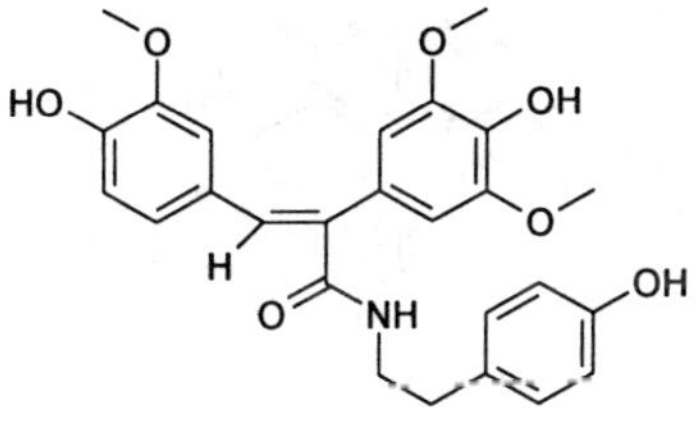

5974 Squamostatin B
$C_{37}H_{66}O_8$ MW: 638.93 Property: white crystal, mp 105-6°C, $[\alpha]_D^{20}$+13.5° (c=0.14, chloroform). Source: FAN LIZ HI. Ref: 303.

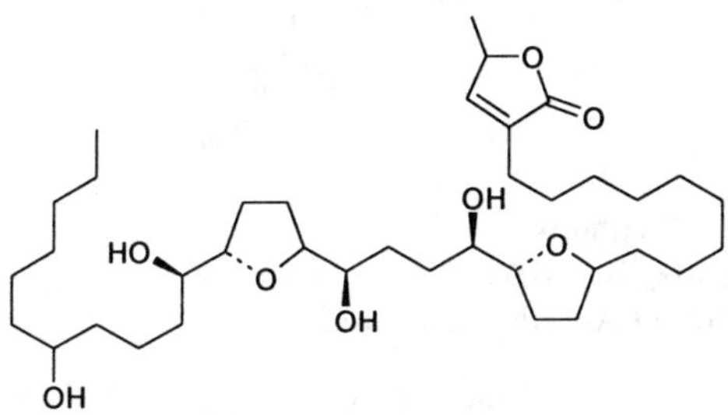

5975 Squasapogenol
Olean-11,13(18)-diene-3β,22β-diol. $C_{34}H_{52}O_4$ MW: 524.79 Property: colorless acicular crystal, mp >300°C. Source: YUAN GUO GAN CAO. Ref: 257.

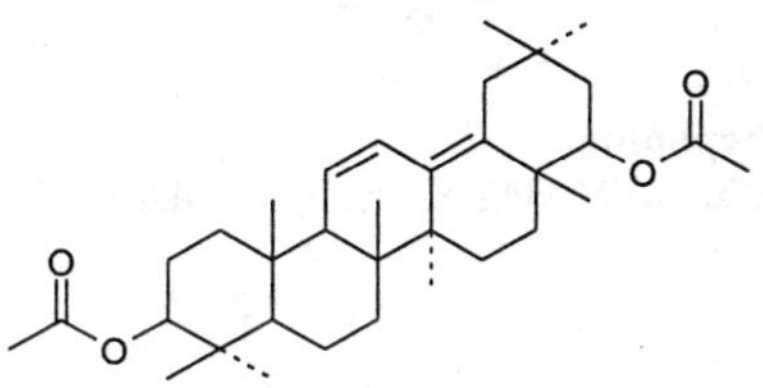

5976 Stachydrine
Cadabine. CAS: 471-87-4 $C_7H_{15}NO_2$ MW: 145.20 Property: mp 235-40°C (dec). Source: YI MU CAO, etc. Ref: 4.

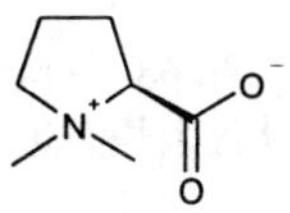

5977 Stachyose
$C_{24}H_{42}O_{21}$ MW: 666.59 Source: GAN DI HUANG, MAYING DAN. Ref: 2, 234.

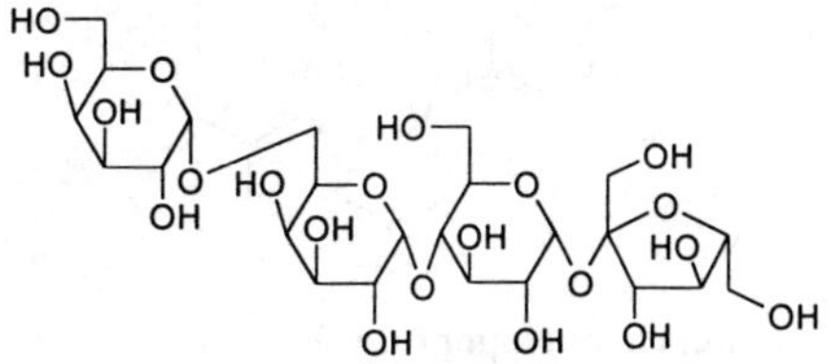

5978 Staphylin
$C_{16}H_{18}O_9$ MW: 354.32 Property: mp 248-51°C. Source: SHENG GU YOU. Ref: 6.

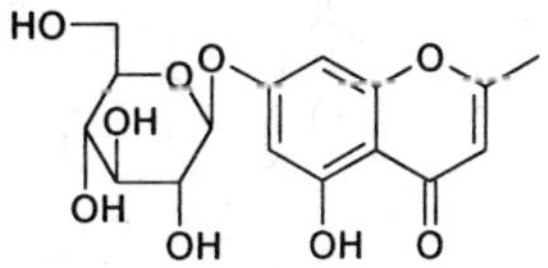

5979 Stearic acid
$C_{18}H_{36}O_2$ MW: 284.49 Property: mp 71.5-2.0°C. Source: BA DOU, BING LANG, BU GU ZHI, CHAI HU, CI WU JIA, CU LIU GUO (SHA JI), DA ZAO, DONG CHONG XIA CAO, GAN DI HUANG, GUA LOU, HONG HUA, GUANG JIN QIAN CAO, LI JIANG QIAN HU, LU HUI, PU HUANG, QIANG HUO, QUAN XIE, ROU CONG RONG, SHAN ZHA, XI YANG SHEN, XING REN, YA DAN ZI, YIN YANG HUO, YONG NING DU HUO, YU XING CAO, YUN QIAN HU, etc. Ref: 2, 177, 260, 530, 541, 557.

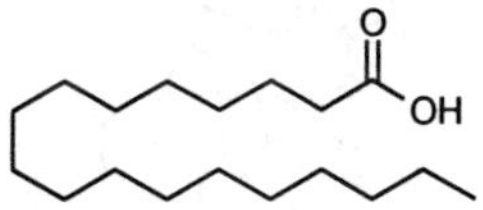

5980 Stearin
$C_{57}H_{110}O_6$ MW: 891.51 Property: mp α: 55°C, β: 73°C, β': 64°C. Source: BAI E GAO. Ref: 6.

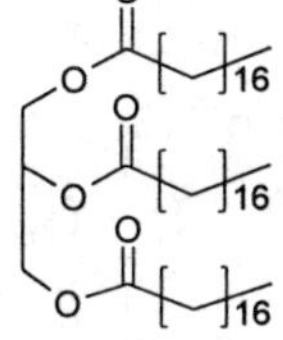

5981 Stebisimine
$C_{36}H_{34}N_2O_6$ MW: 590.68 Property: mp 233-5°C. Source: QIAN JIN TENG. Ref: 6.

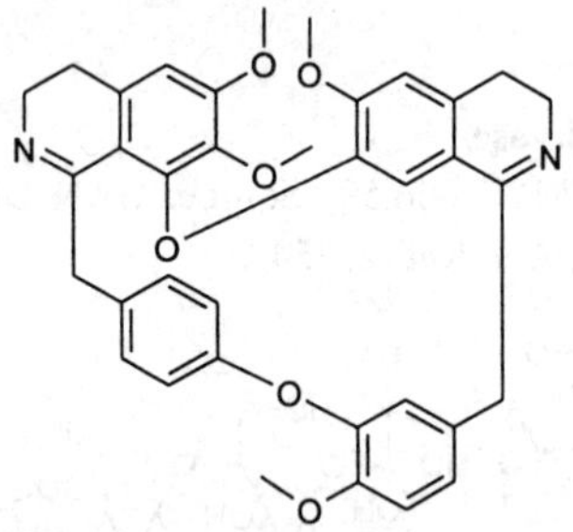

5982 Stellarria cyclopeptide
$C_{24}H_{34}N_6O_7$ MW: 518.57 Property: white lamellar crystal, mp >300°C, $[\alpha]_D^{20}$ +0.151° (c=1.0, C_5H_5N). Source: YIN CHAI HU. Ref: 238.

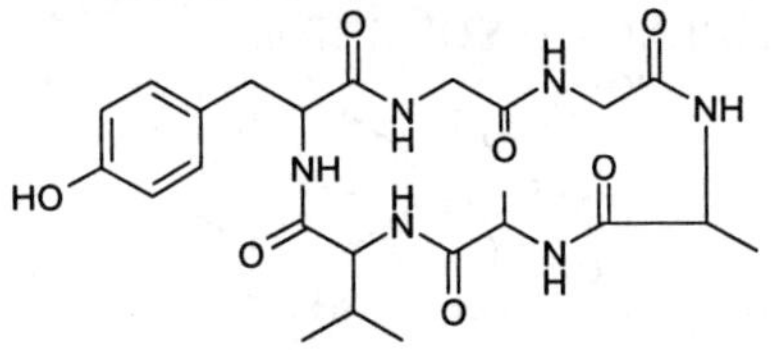

5983 Stemonine
$C_{17}H_{25}NO_4$ MW: 307.39 Property: mp 169°C. Source: BAI BU. Ref: 6.

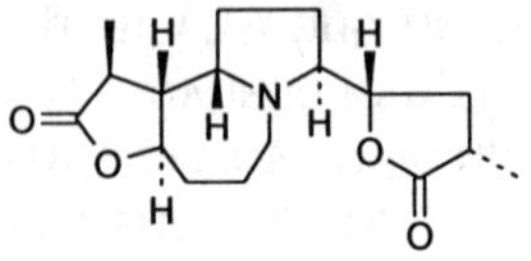

5984 Stenine
$C_{17}H_{27}NO_2$ MW: 277.41 Property: mp 65-7°C. Source: BAI BU. Ref: 6.

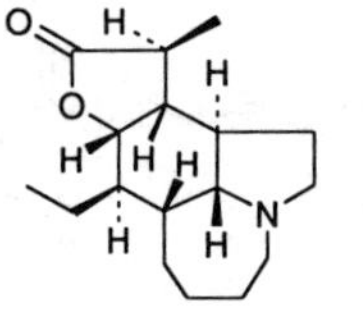

5985 Stephanine
CAS: 517-63-5 $C_{19}H_{19}NO_3$ MW: 309.37 Property: mp (-): 160-1°C, (±): 131-3°C. Source: DI BU RONG, QIAN JIN TENG, YE HE HUA. Ref: 4.

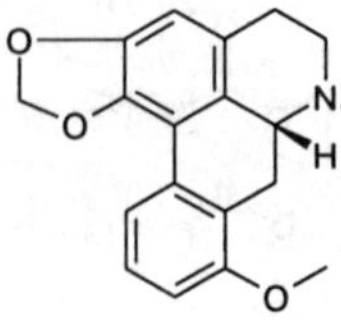

5986 Stephanthrine
$C_{19}H_{19}NO_2$ MW: 293.37 Property: white acicular crystal (methanol), mp 234-6°C (HBr). Source: FEN FANG JI, FANG JI. Ref: 2, 44.

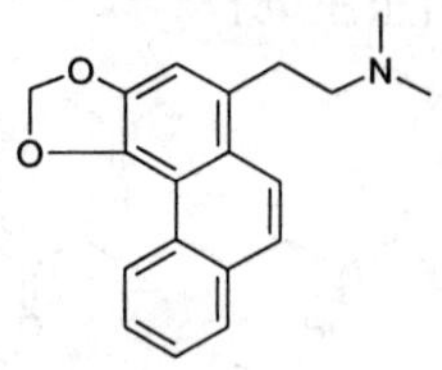

5987 Stepharine
$C_{18}H_{19}NO_3$ MW: 297.36 Property: mp 179-81°C. Source: Ref: 2.

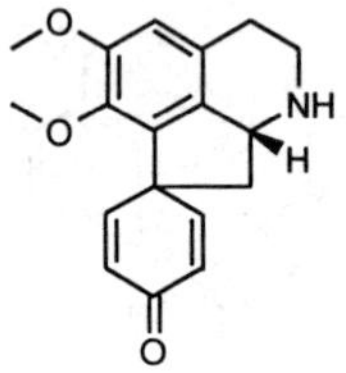

5988 Stepholidine
$C_{19}H_{21}NO_4$ MW: 327.38 Property: mp 126-8°C, 161-3°C. Source: BIAN FU GE GEN. Ref: 6.

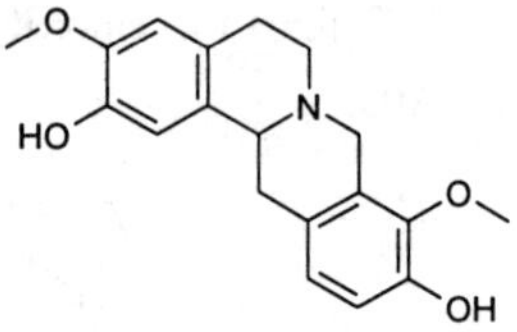

5989 Stepholine
$C_{36}H_{38}N_2O_4$ MW: 594.71 Property: mp 164-6°C. Source: QIAN JIN TENG. Ref: 6.

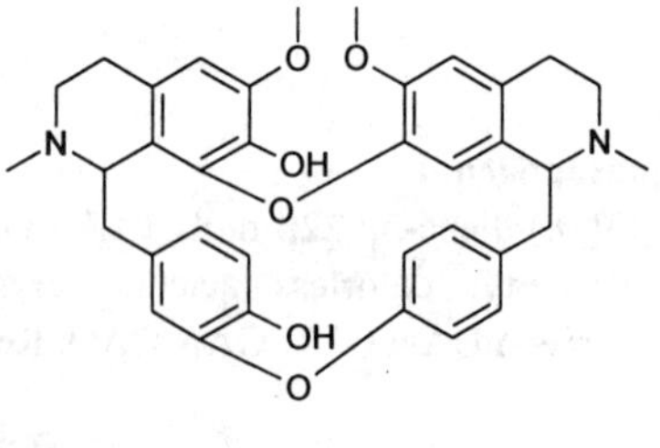

5990 Steponine
$C_{20}H_{24}NO_4$ MW: 342.42 Source: QIAN JIN TENG. Ref: 6.

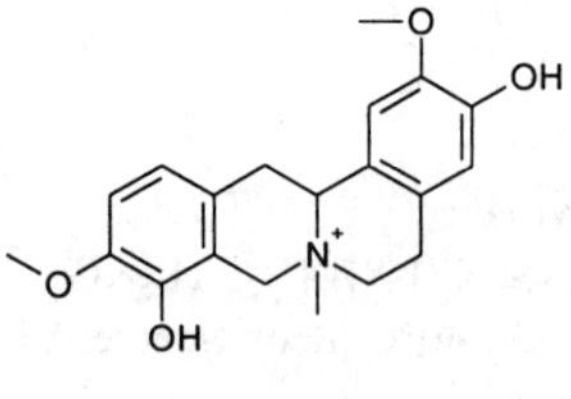

5991 Sterculic acid
$C_{19}H_{34}O_2$ MW: 294.48 Property: mp 18.2-8.3°C. Source: MU JIN ZI, WU TONG ZI. Ref: 6.

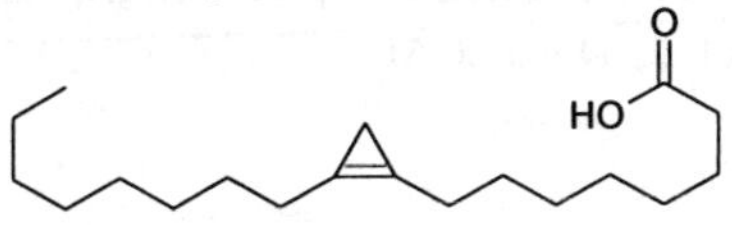

5992 5,25-Stigmastadienol
$C_{29}H_{48}O$ MW: 412.71 Source: GUA LOU. Ref: 2.

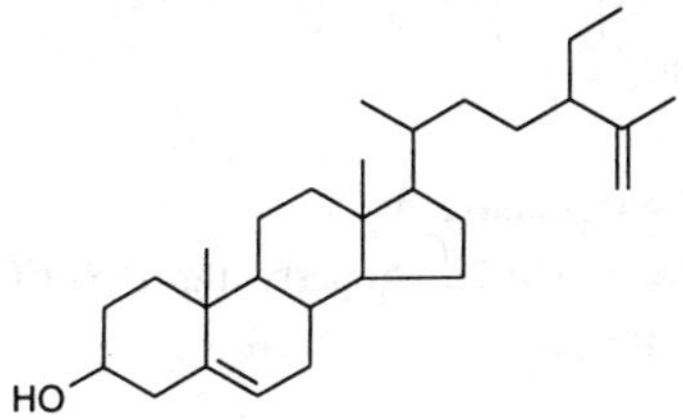

5993 7,24-Stigmastadienol
$C_{29}H_{48}O$ MW: 412.71 Source: GUA LOU. Ref: 2.

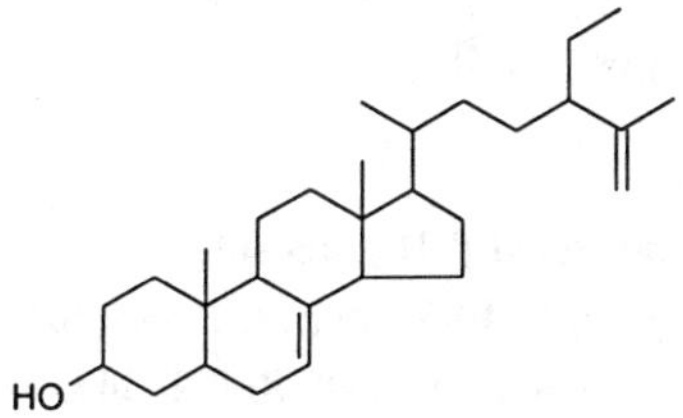

5994 7,25-Stigmastadienol
$C_{29}H_{48}O$ MW: 412.71 Source: GUA LOU. Ref: 2.

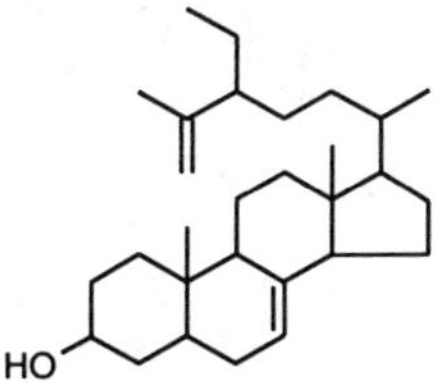

5995 5,25-Stigmastadien-3β-ol β-D-glucoside
$C_{35}H_{58}O_6$ MW: 574.85 Source: KU GUA. Ref: 6.

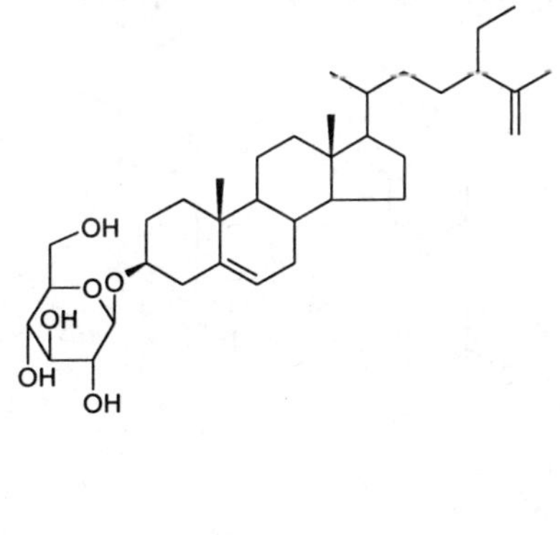

5996 Stigmasta-5, 22-dien-3-one
$C_{29}H_{46}O$ MW: 410.69 Source: Ref: 2.

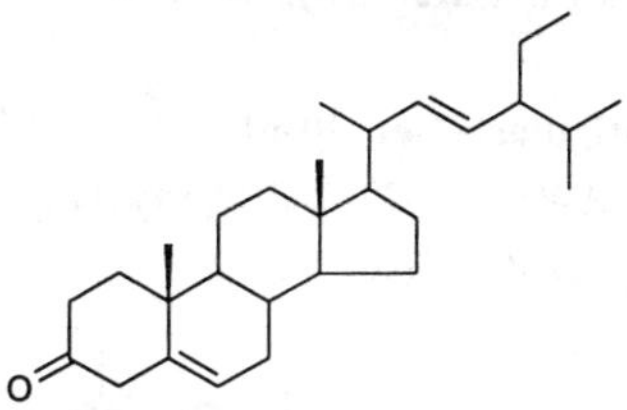

5997 α-Stigmasta-7,22-dien-3-one
$C_{29}H_{46}O$ MW: 410.69 Source: Ref: 2.

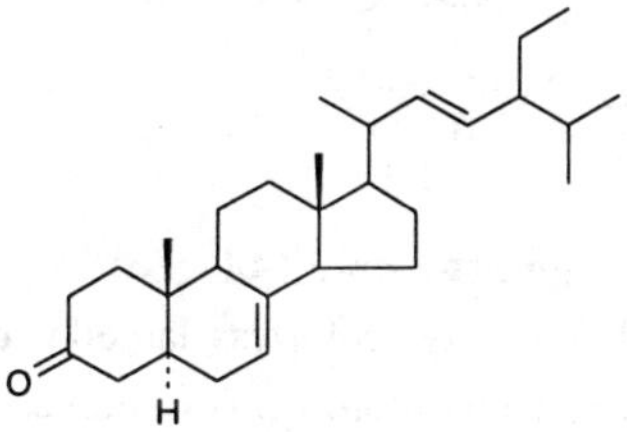

5998 5α-Stigmastan-3,6-dione
$C_{29}H_{48}O_2$ MW: 428.70 Source: BAO XING WEI MAO, PU HUANG. Ref: 2, 278.

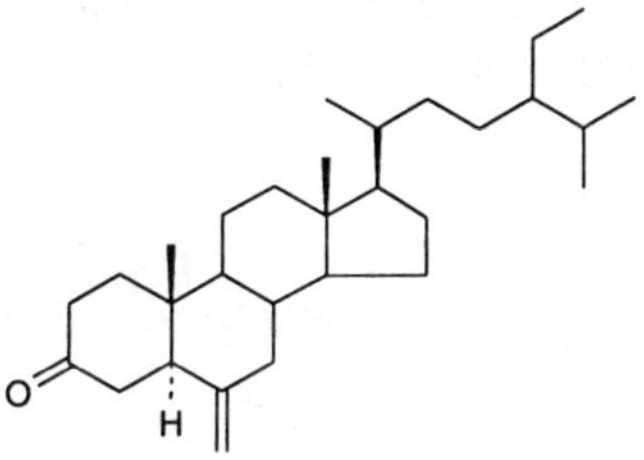

5999 Stigmastanol
$C_{29}H_{52}O$ MW: 416.74 Source: GUA LOU. Ref: 2.

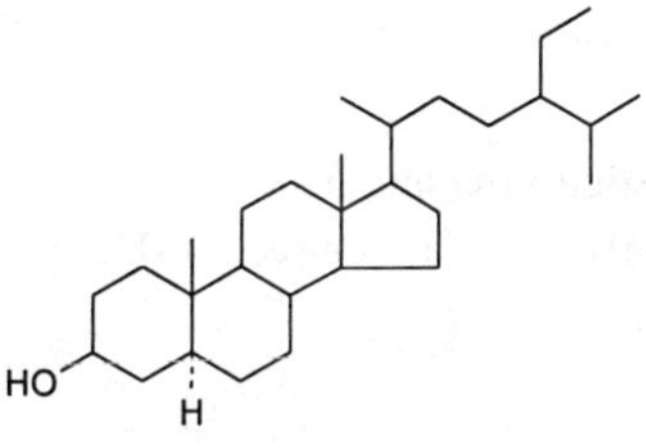

6000 7,22,25-Stigmastatrienol
$C_{29}H_{46}O$ MW: 410.69 Source: GUA LOU. Ref: 2.

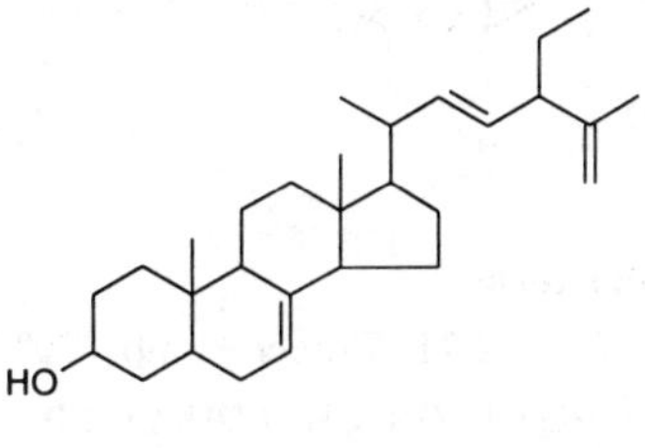

6001 Stigmast-4-ene-1,3-dione
Source: SHA REN. Ref: 518.

6002 5α-Stigmast-7-en-3β-ol
$C_{29}H_{50}O$ MW: 414.72 Property: mp 137-40°C. Source: PU GONG YING. Ref: 6.

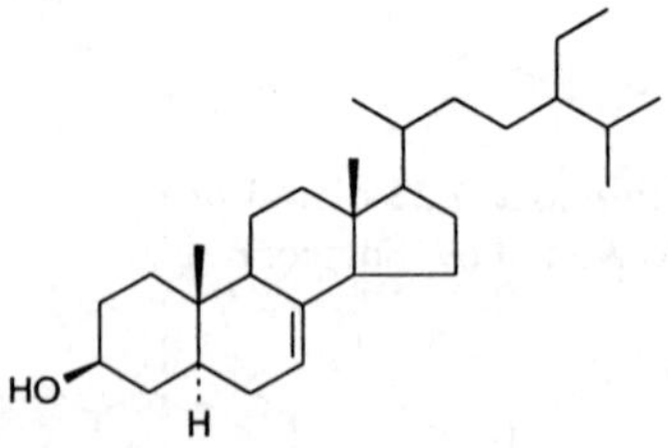

6003 24S-Stigmast-5-en-3β-ol
Clionasterol. Property: colorless lamellar crystal, mp 146-7°C (methanol-chloroform). Source: TOU JIE HAI MIAN. Ref: 459.

6004 Δ7-Stigmastenol-3-O-β-D-glucoside
$C_{35}H_{60}O_6$ MW: 576.9 Source: DANG SHEN, GUA LOU, TIAN HUA FEN. Ref: 2.

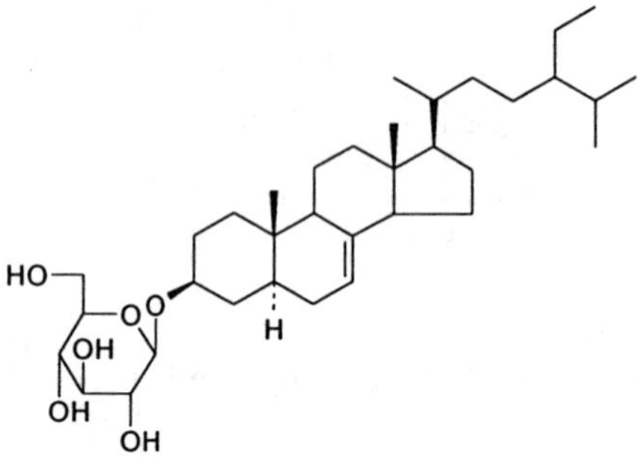

6005 Δ7-Stigmastenone-3
$C_{29}H_{48}O$ MW: 412.71 Source: DANG SHEN, GUA LOU. Ref: 2.

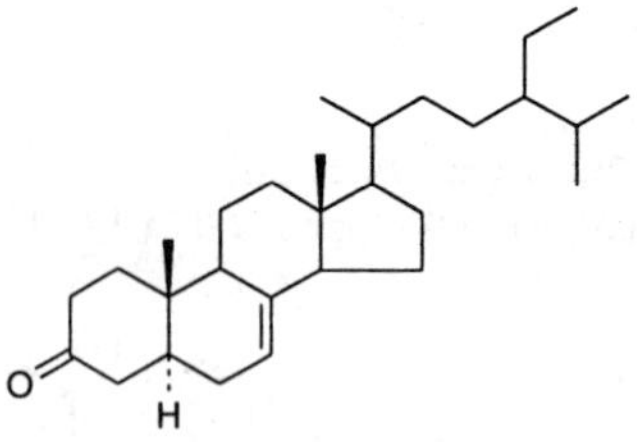

6006 Stigmasterol
$C_{29}H_{48}O$ MW: 412.71 Property: mp 170°C. Source: BAI HE HUA, BU GU ZHI, CHAI HU, CU LIU GUO (SHA JI), DA ZAO, DANG GUI, DANG SHEN, GAN DI HUANG, GUA LOU, HUANG HUA YUAN ZHI, HUANG QIN, MU XIANG, QING HAO, REN SHEN, SAN QI, XI XIAN. Ref: 2, 345, 372, 511.

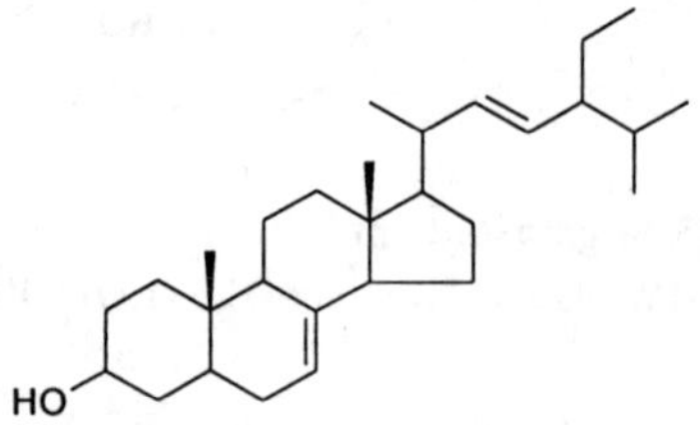

6007 Δ22-Stigmasterol
$C_{29}H_{50}O$ MW: 414.72 Property: mp 158-9°C. Source: CHAI HU. Ref: 6.

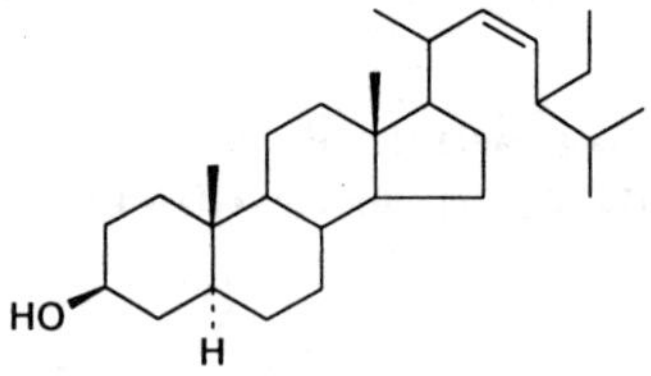

6008 Stigmasterol-β-D-glucoside
$C_{35}H_{58}O_6$ MW: 574.85 Source: DANG SHEN, DANG GUI, HUANG HUA YUAN ZHI. Ref: 2, 345.

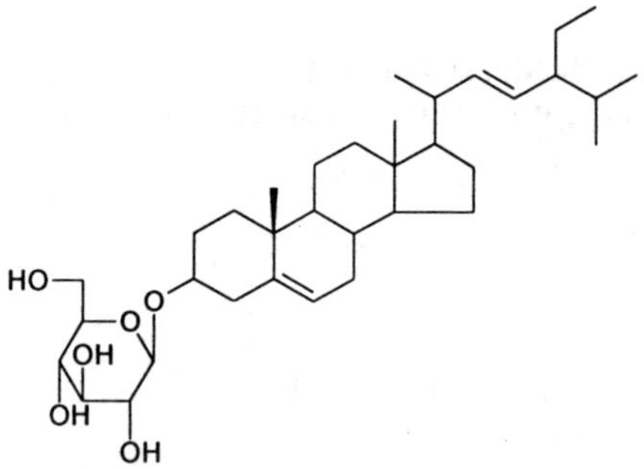

6009 Stigmasteryl ferulate
$C_{39}H_{56}O_4$ MW: 588.88 Source: MI PI KANG. Ref: 6.

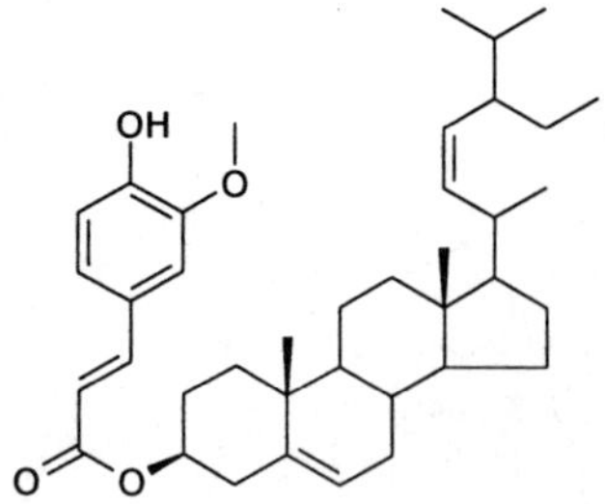

6010 Stigmasteryl palmitate
$C_{45}H_{78}O_2$ MW: 651.12 Source: CHE QIAN (CHE QIAN CAO), HUI XIANG GEN. Ref: 6.

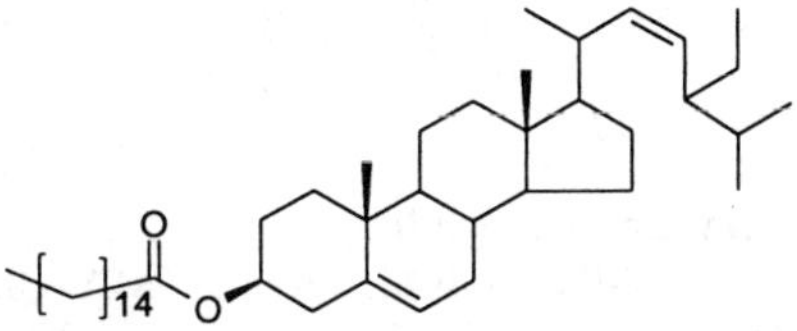

6011 Stigmast-3-O-β-D-glucopyranosyl-6-hexadecanoate
$C_{51}H_{88}O_7$ MW: 813.27 Property: white amorphous powder (methanol). Source: JI YE QIU HAI TANG. Ref: 431.

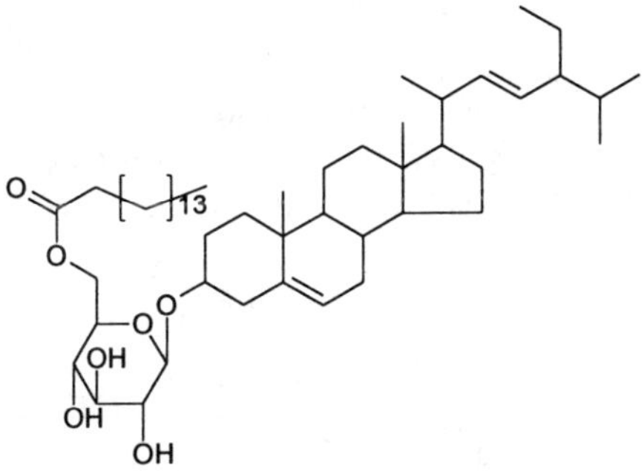

6012 Stilbene
Source: YIN XING. Ref: 579.

6014 Strictosamide
$C_{26}H_{30}N_2O_8$ MW: 498.54 Source: GOU TENG. Ref: 2.

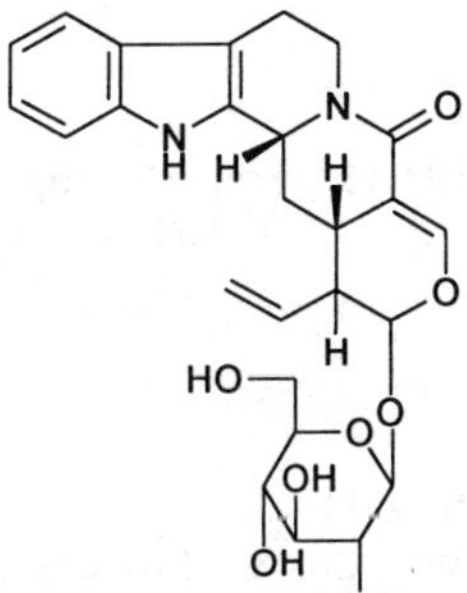

6015 Strobilanthin
5,7-Dimethoxy-4'-hydroxyflavone-4'-O-apioside. $C_{22}H_{22}O_9$ MW: 430.42 Property: light yellow crystalline powder, mp 214-6°C. Source: HONG ZE LAN. Ref: 654.

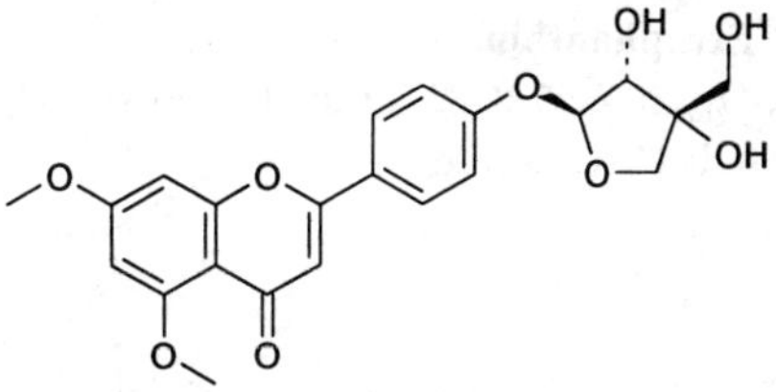

6016 Strophanthidin
Apocynamarin; Corchogenin; Corchorin; Corchortoxin; Cymarigenim. CAS: 66-28-4 $C_{23}H_{32}O_6$ MW: 404.51 Property: mp 235°C (anhydride). Source: LUO BU MA, GUI ZHU TANG JIE, FU SHOU CAO. Ref: 5.

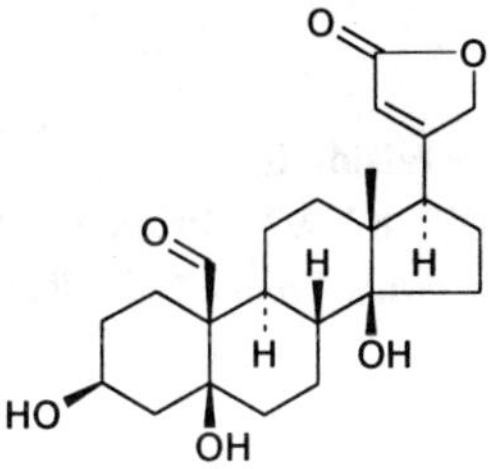

6017 Strophanthidin-β-D-digitaloside
$C_{30}H_{44}O_{10}$ MW: 564.68 Source: LUO BU MA. Ref: 2.

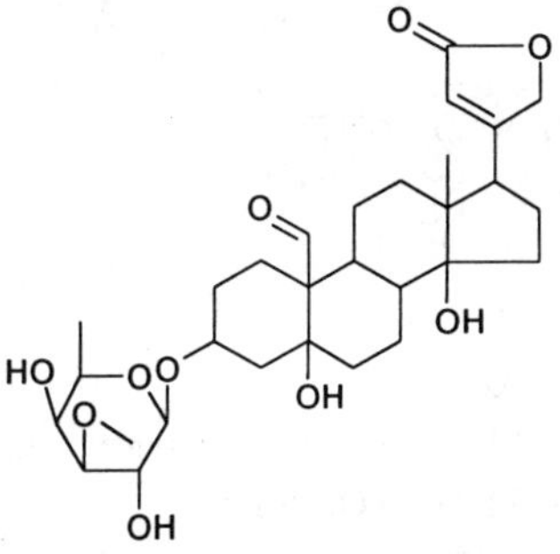

6018 Strophanthidin-β-D-glucosyl-(1→4)-β-D-digitaloside
$C_{36}H_{54}O_{15}$ MW: 726.82 Source: LUO BU MA. Ref: 2.

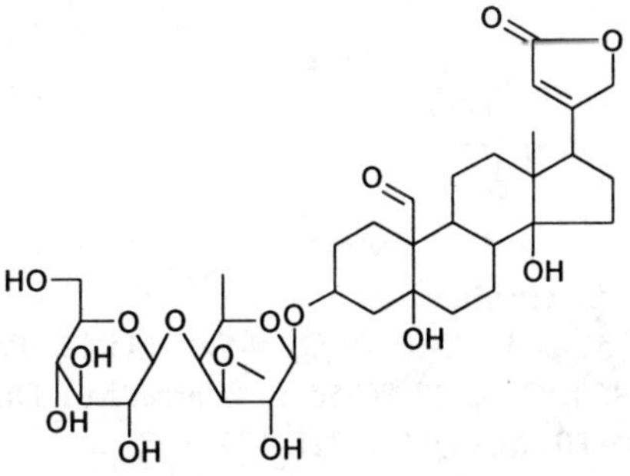

6019 Strophanthin
$C_{36}H_{54}O_{15}$ MW: 726.82 Property: mp 195°C. Source: FU SHOU CAO. Ref: 6.

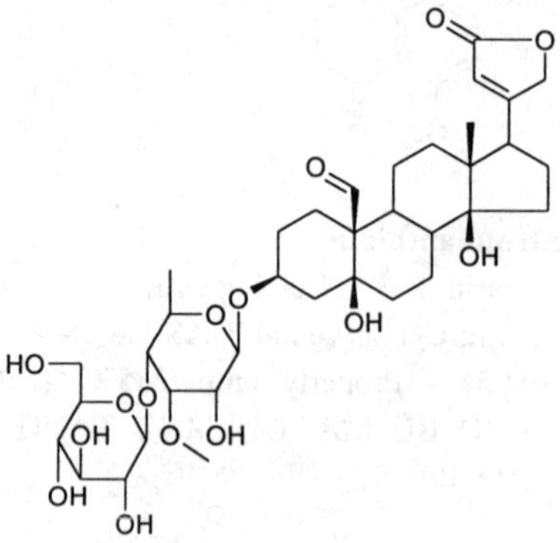

6020 Strophantylside K
$C_{42}H_{64}O_{19}$ MW: 872.97 Property: mp 199-200°C. Source: *Strophanthus Kombe* Oliv. Ref: 4.

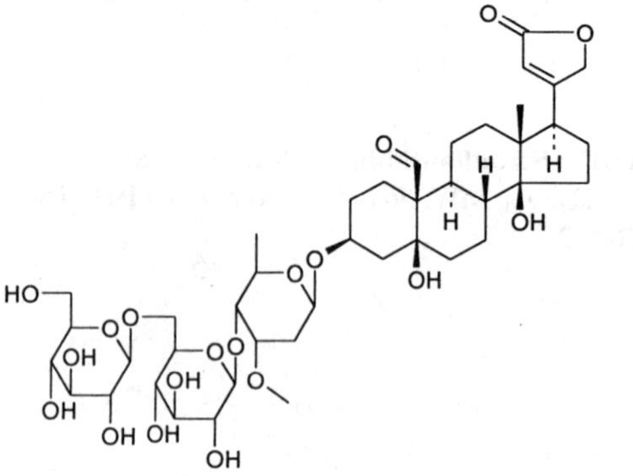

6021 Strospeside
$C_{30}H_{46}O_9$ MW: 550.70 Property: mp 246-50°C. Source: JIA ZHU TAO. Ref: 6.

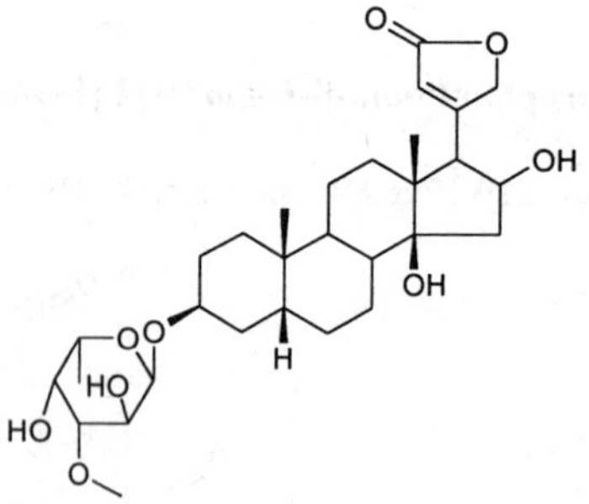

6022 Strychnine
CAS: 57-24-9 $C_{21}H_{22}N_2O_2$ MW: 334.42 Property: mp 286-8°C, bp 270°C/5mm. Source: MA QIAN ZI, MAO ZHU MA QIAN. Ref: 4, 542, 576.

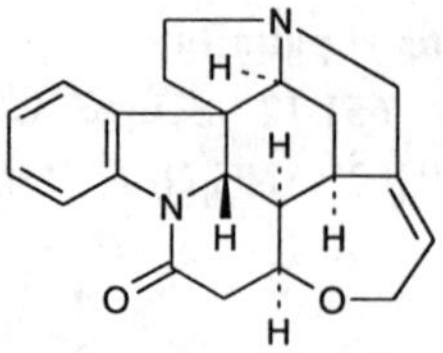

6023 Strychnine N-oxide
$C_{21}H_{22}N_2O_3$ MW: 350.42 Source: MA QIAN ZI. Ref: 542.

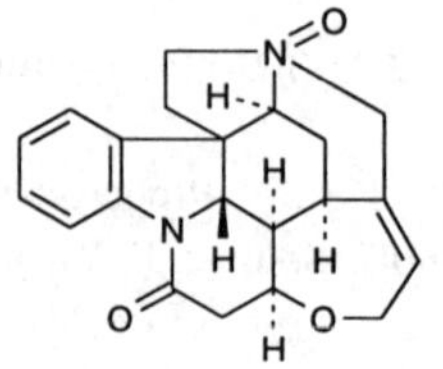

6024 Stylopine
$C_{19}H_{17}NO_4$ MW: 323.35 Property: mp (-): 204°C, (±): 222-3°C. Source: BAI QU CAI, HE QING HUA, JU HUA HUANG LIAN, YAN HU SUO. Ref: 6.

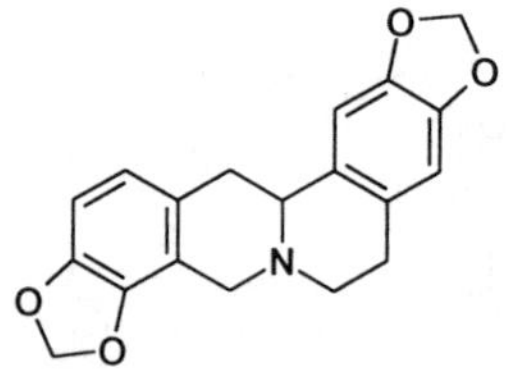

6025 Stylosin
Source: QIN PI. Ref: 2.

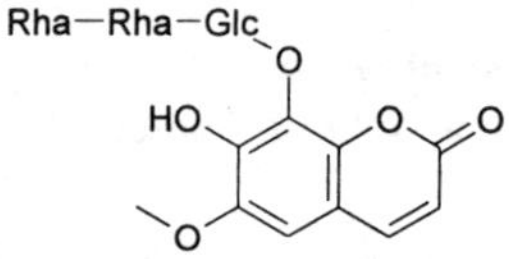

6026 Styrene
C_8H_8 MW: 104.15 Property: mp -55°C, bp 145-5.8°C. Source: AN XI XIANG. Ref: 6.

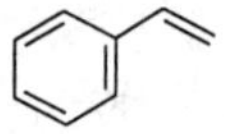

6027 Suaveolic acid
$C_{20}H_{32}O_3$ MW: 320.48 Property: mp 198-201°C (dec). Source: SHE BAI ZI. Ref: 6.

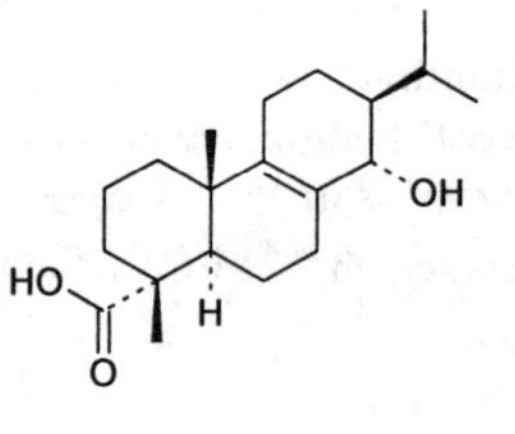

6028 Suaveolol

$C_{20}H_{34}O_2$ MW: 306.49 Property: mp 186-7°C. Source: SHE BAI ZI. Ref: 6.

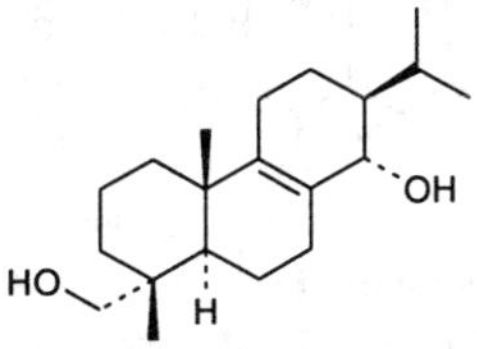

6029 Suavissimoside R1

Source: CU YE XUAN GOU ZI. Ref: 606.

6030 Suberenon

$C_{14}H_{12}O_4$ MW: 244.25 Source: CHOU CAO. Ref: 6.

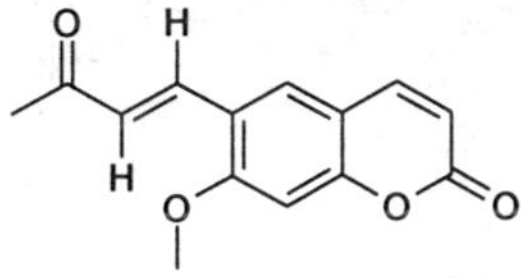

6031 Suberic acid

$C_8H_{14}O_4$ MW: 174.20 Property: mp 144°C. Source: CHAN SU, MU JIN PI. Ref: 2, 6, 519.

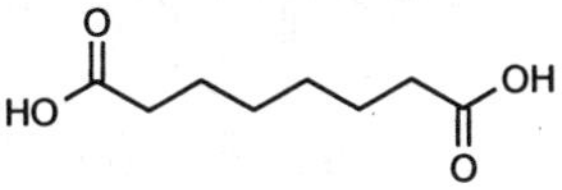

6032 Succinic acid

Butanedioic acid. CAS: 110-15-6 $C_4H_6O_4$ MW: 118.09 Property: mp 150°C, 185-9°C, bp 235°C. Source: CU LIU GUO (SHA JI), DANG GUI, LU HUI, GAN DI HUANG, JIN LONG DAN CAO, JIN QIAO MAI, MAO GENG XI XIAN, MU ZEI, PU HUANG, QUE MEI TENG, REN SHEN, ROU CONG RONG, SHAN ZHA, TIAN MA. Ref: 2, 4, 411, 476, 502, 515, 529, 594, 604.

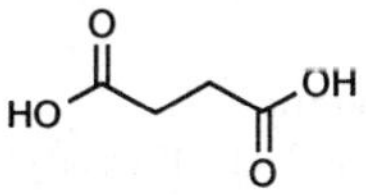

6033 Suchilactone

$C_{21}H_{20}O_6$ MW: 368.39 Source: DA JIN NIU CAO. Ref: 6.

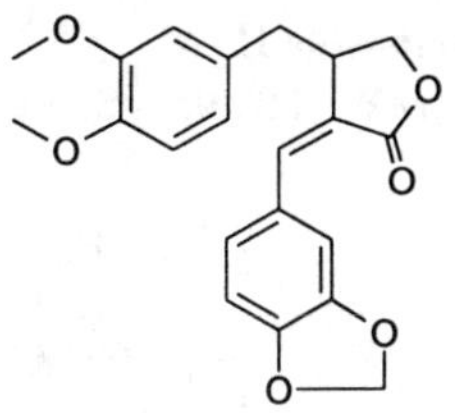

6034 Sucrose

$C_{12}H_{22}O_{11}$ MW: 342.30 Property: mp 184-5°C. Source: CI WU JIA, DA QING YE, FANG FENG, HUANG QI, HUANG QIN, LU HUI, QIANG HUO, REN SHEN, TIAN MA, XI YANG SHEN. Ref: 2.

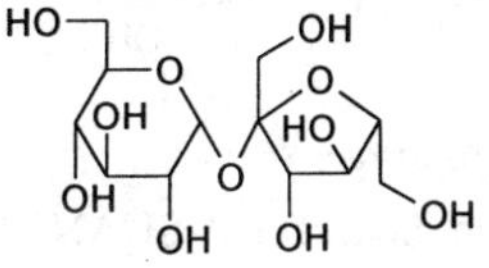

6035 Sugiol

$C_{20}H_{28}O_2$ MW: 300.44 Property: mp (+): 298-9°C (dec). Source: DU SONG SHI, SAN YE SHU WEI CAO. Ref: 6, 182.

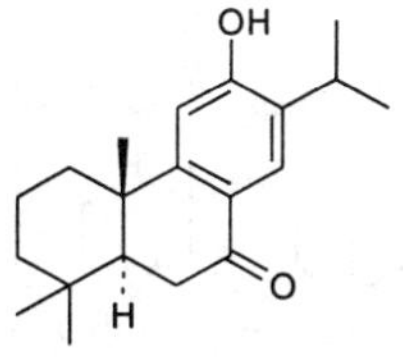

6036 Sulfanilic acid

$C_6H_7NO_3S$ MW: 173.19 Source: JI CAI. Ref: 6.

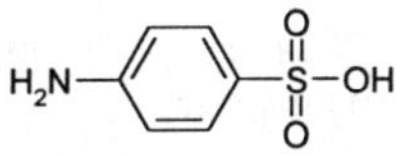

6037 Sulfopatrinoside I

$C_{42}H_{67}NaO_{17}S$ MW: 899.05 Source: BAI JIANG. Ref: 2.

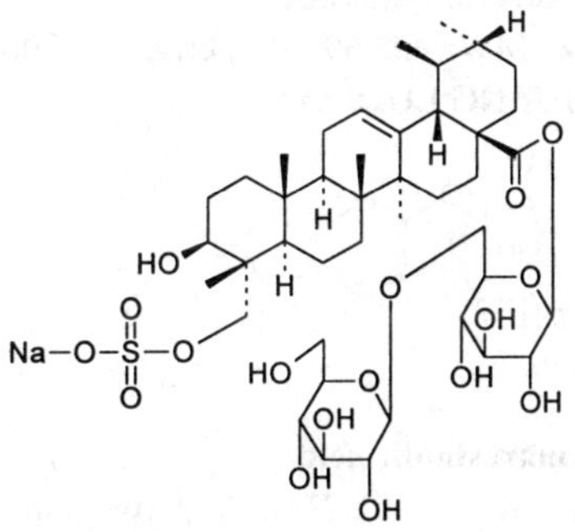

6038 Sulfopatrinoside II
$C_{42}H_{67}NaO_{17}S$ MW: 899.05 Source: BAI JIANG. Ref: 2.

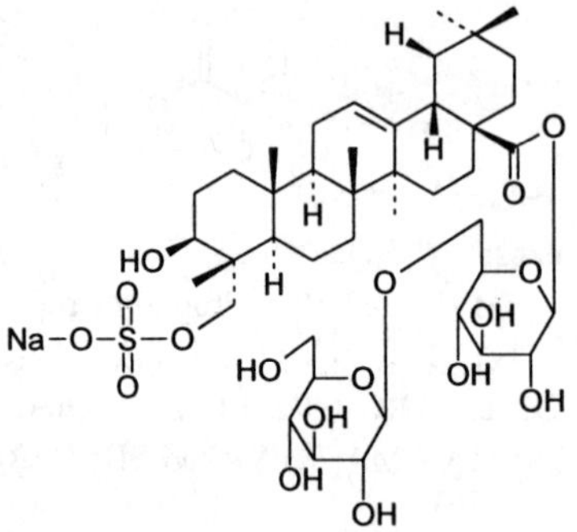

6039 Sulfur dioxide
O_2S MW: 64.06 Source: DA SUAN. Ref: 2.

O=S=O

6040 Sulfurenic acid
$C_{31}H_{50}O_4$ MW: 486.74 Property: mp 252-4°C. Source: A LI HONG (LUO YE SONG XUN) . Ref: 6.

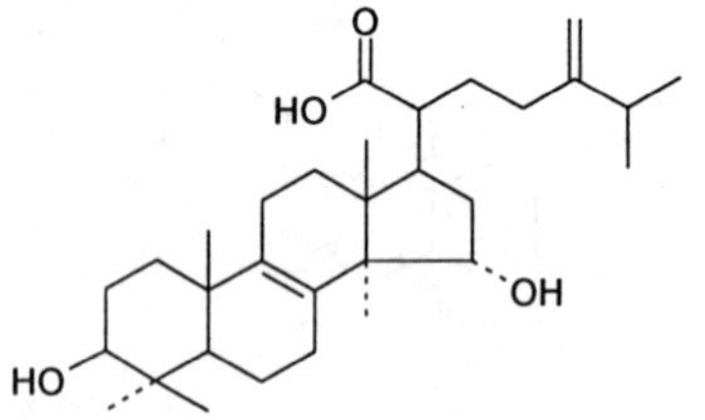

6041 Sulfuretin
$C_{15}H_{10}O_5$ MW: 270.24 Property: mp 280-5°C (dec). Source: HUANG LU. Ref: 6.

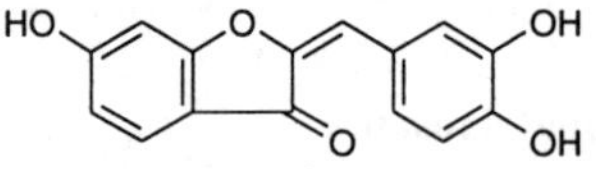

6042 Sulfuretin glucoside
$C_{21}H_{20}O_{10}$ MW: 432.39 Property: mp 200°C (dec). Source: HUANG LU. Ref: 6.

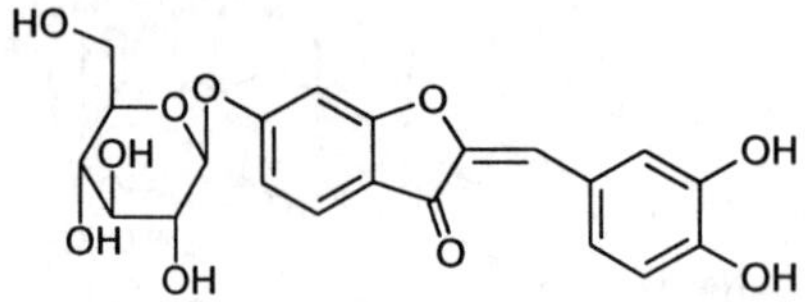

6043 Sumaresinolic acid
$C_{30}H_{48}O_4$ MW: 472.71 Property: mp 298-9°C. Source: AN XI XIANG. Ref: 6.

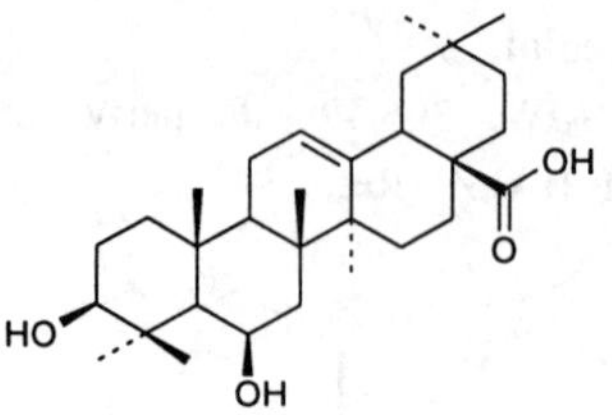

6044 Sutchuenensine IV
$C_{38}H_{42}N_2O_6$ MW: 622.77 Property: colorless powder, $[\alpha]_D^{27}$ -110° (c= 0.13, EtOH). Source: LUN HUAN TENG. Ref: 274.

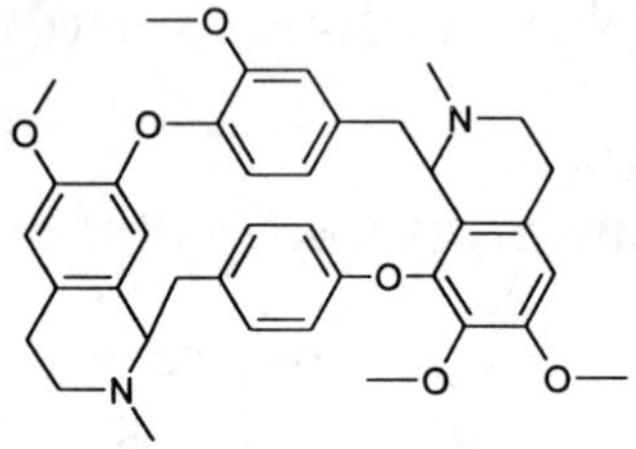

6045 Swerchirin
$C_{15}H_{12}O_6$ MW: 288.26 Property: yellow acicular crystal, mp 194-5°C. Source: BAO E ZHANG YA CAI. Ref: 634.

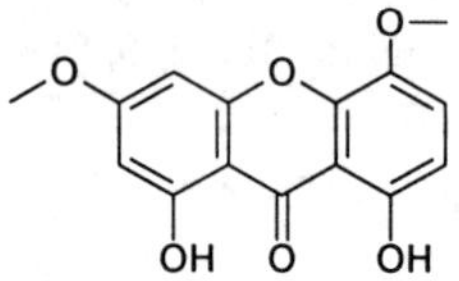

6046 Sweroside
$C_{16}H_{22}O_9$ MW: 358.35 Source: CHANG CHUN HUA, LONG DAN, SHAN ZHU YU, XIA YE ZHANG YA CAI, ZHANG YA CAI, ZI HONG ZHANG YE CAI. Ref: 2, 6, 220, 272.

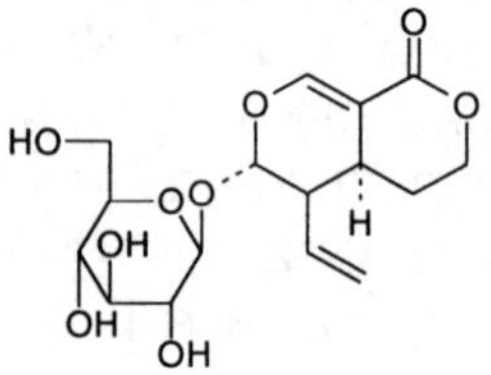

6047 Swertiajaponin
$C_{22}H_{22}O_{11}$ MW: 462.41 Property: mp 265°C (dec). Source: DOU CHI CAO. Ref: 6.

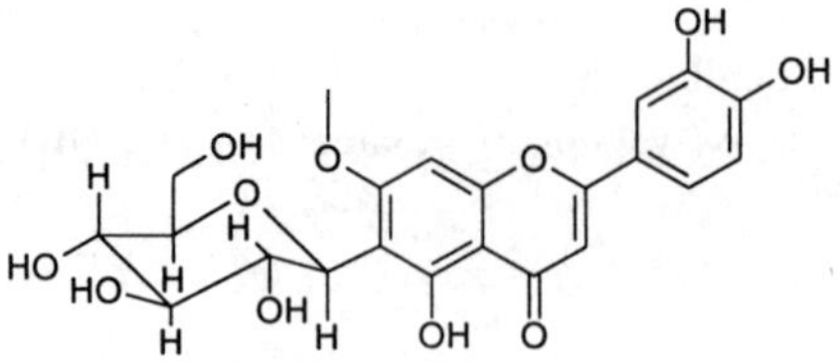

6048 Swertiamacroside
trans Caffeic acid-1-O-rutinose ester. $C_{21}H_{28}O_{13}$ MW: 488.45 Property: light yellow amorphous powder. Source: DA ZI ZHANG YA CAI. Ref: 149.

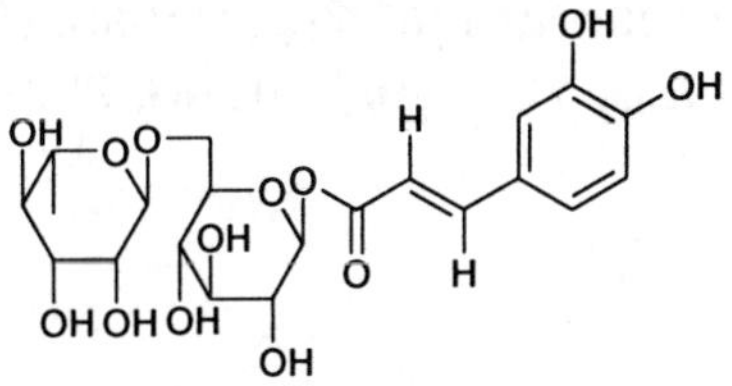

6049 Swertiamarin
$C_{16}H_{22}O_{10}$ MW: 374.35 Property: mp 103-4°C. Source: XIA YE ZHANG YA CAI, ZHANG YA CAI, ZI HONG ZHANG YE CAI. Ref: 6, 220, 272.

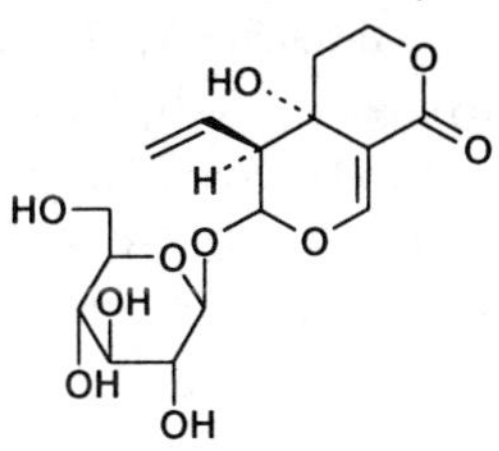

6050 Swertianolin
$C_{20}H_{20}O_{11}$ MW: 436.38 Property: light yellow powder, mp 227-9°C. Source: BAO E ZHANG YA CAI. Ref: 634.

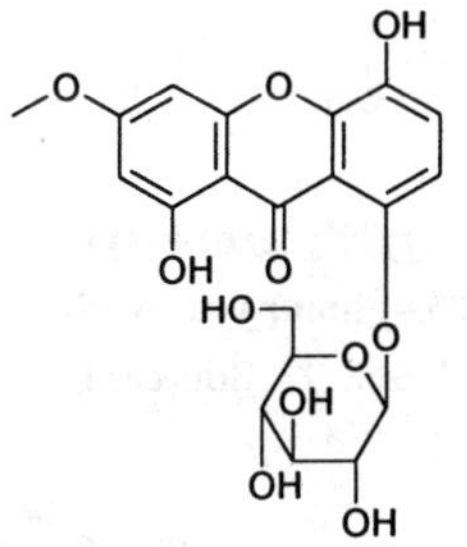

6051 Swertiapunimarin
6'-O-β-D-glucopyranosylsweroside. $C_{22}H_{32}O_{14}$ MW: 520.49 Property: white powder, mp 95-7 °C, $[\alpha]_D^{26}$ -169° (H_2O). Source: ZI HONG ZHANG YA CAI. Ref: 272.

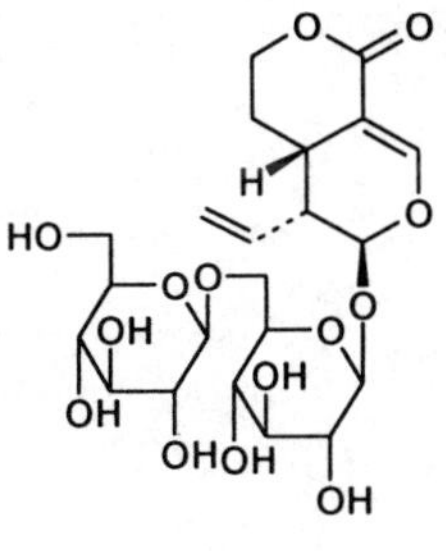

6052 Swertisin
$C_{22}H_{22}O_{10}$ MW: 446.41 Property: mp 248°C (dec). Source: DA ZAO, SUAN ZAO REN. Ref: 2.

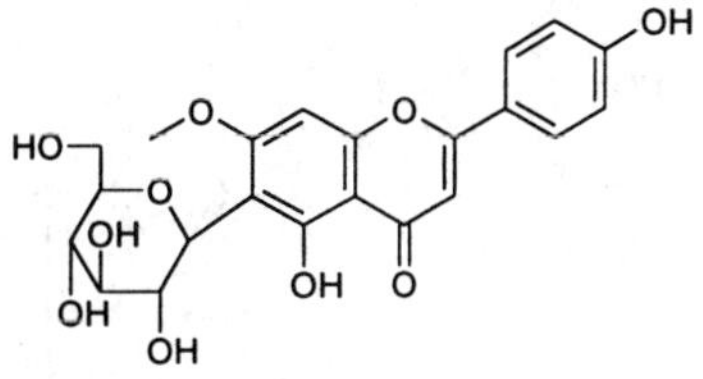

6053 Sylvestrene
$C_{10}H_{16}$ MW: 136.24 Source: DU HUO. Ref: 2.

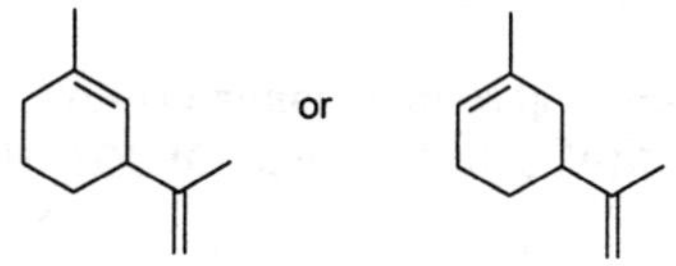

6054 Synephrine
Sympathol; Oxedrine. CAS: 94-07-5 $C_9H_{13}NO_2$ MW: 167.21 Property: mp 151-2°C, 184-5°C, 118-9°C (dec). Source: WU ZHU YU. Ref: 4.

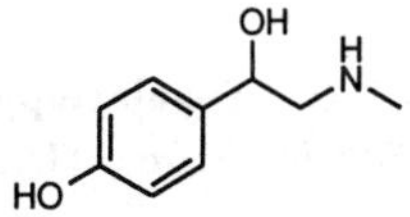

6055 Syringaldehyde
$C_9H_{10}O$ MW: 182.18 Source: DANG SHEN. Ref: 2.

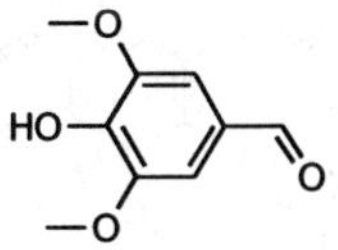

6056 dl-Syringaresinol
$C_{22}H_{26}O_8$ MW: 418.45 Source: HOU PO. Ref: 2.

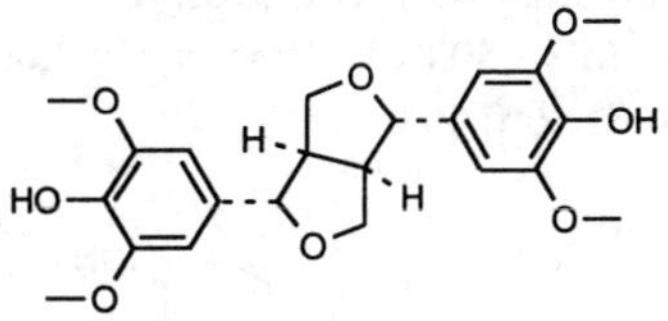

6057 (+)-Syringaresinol-di-O-β-D-glucoside
$C_{34}H_{46}O_{18}$ MW: 742.73 Source: CI WU JIA. Ref: 2.

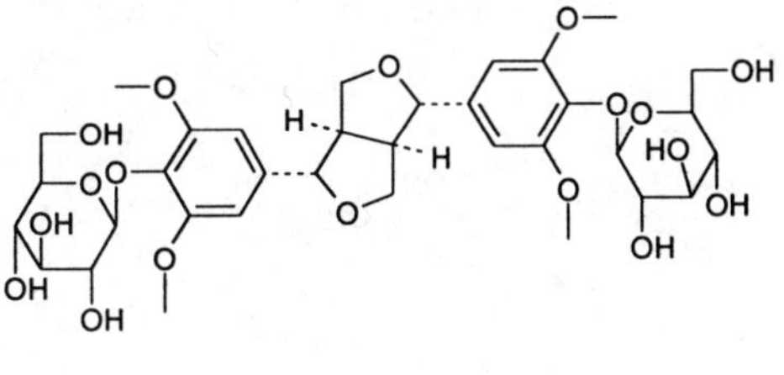

6058 Syringaresinol-4'-O-β-D-glucopyranoside
$C_{28}H_{36}O_{13}$ MW: 580.59 Source: HOU PO. Ref: 2.

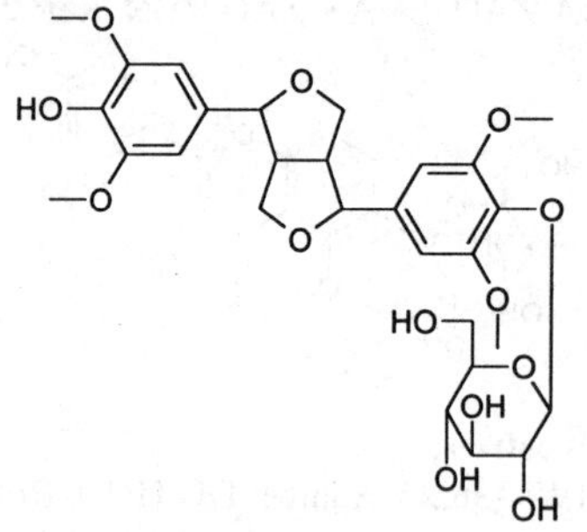

6059 (+)-Syringaresinol monoglucoside
$C_{28}H_{36}O_{13}$ MW: 580.59 Source: DU ZHONG. Ref: 2.

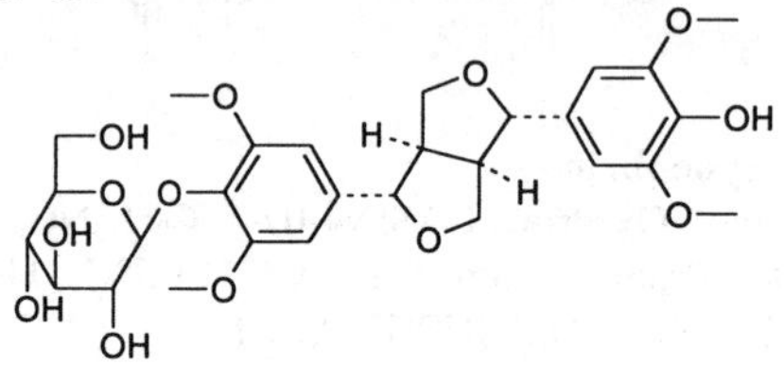

6060 Syringetin-3-O-β-D-galactopyranoside
$C_{23}H_{24}O_{13}$ MW: 508.44 Source: TIAN CONG. Ref: 6.

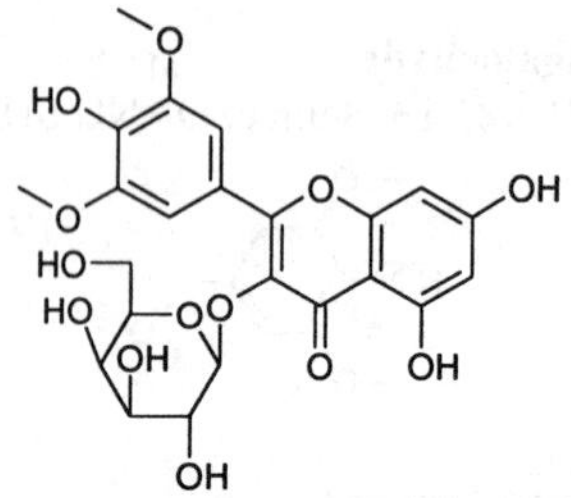

6061 Syringetin-3-O-β-D-glucoside
$C_{23}H_{24}O_{13}$ MW: 508.44 Property: yellow powder. Source: CI MI. Ref: 498.

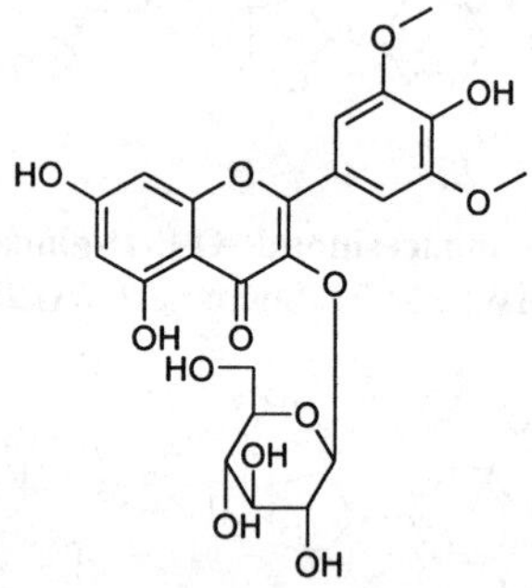

6062 Syringic acid
$C_9H_{10}O_5$ MW: 198.18 Property: mp 204-5°C. Source: BAI HUA YING SHAN HONG, DA YE JIN HUA CAO, HUI XIANG JING YE, MAN SHAN HONG, TU FU LING, YING SHAN HONG, ZHAO SHAN BAI. Ref: 6, 336.

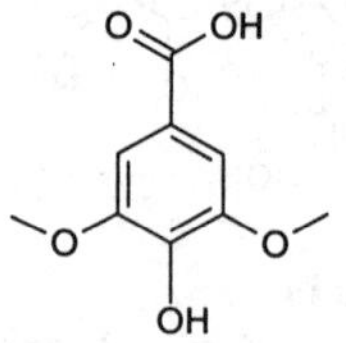

6063 Syringin
Eleutheroside B; Ilexanin A; Ligustrin; Lilacin; Magnolenin; Syringine. $C_{17}H_{24}O_9$ MW: 372.38 Property: white granular crystal, mp 192°C (MeOH). Source: CI WU JIA, DANG SHEN, DONG BEI CI REN SHEN, DU ZHONG, QIN PI, SI JI QING, WU JIA PI. Ref: 2, 6, 523, 527, 450.

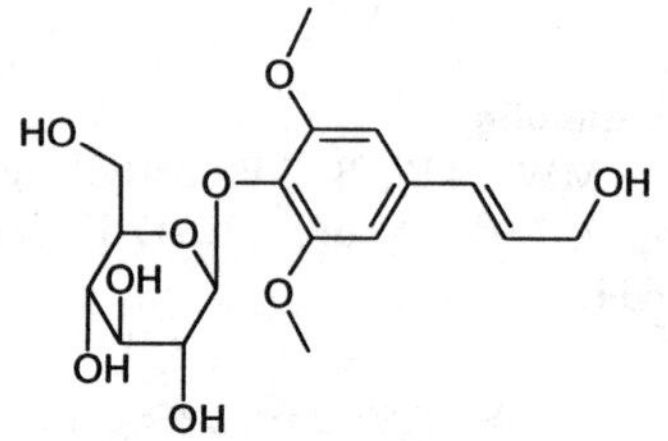

6064 Syringylglycerol-β-syringaresinol ether-4'',4'''-di-O-β-D-glucopyranoside
$C_{45}H_{60}O_{23}$ MW: 968.97 Source: DU ZHONG. Ref: 2.

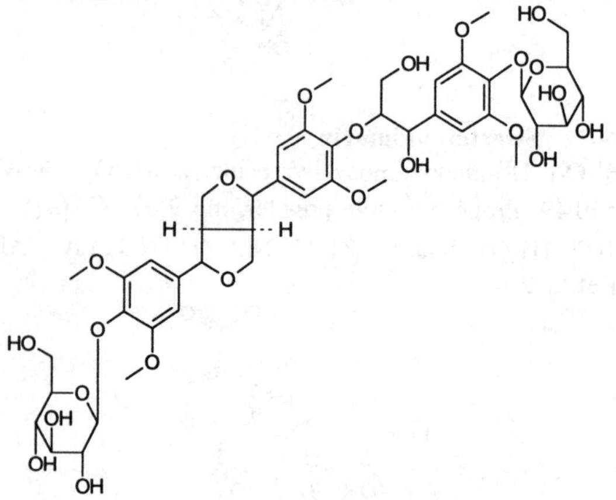

6065 19-(Z)-Taberpsychine
$C_{20}H_{26}N_2O$ MW: 310.44 Property: oil, $[\alpha]_D$ -180°. Source: HU MAN TENG. Ref: 14, 411, 416.

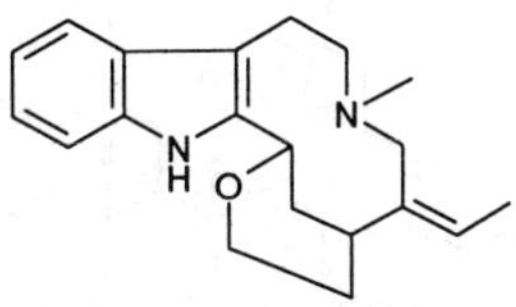

6066 Tabersonine
$C_{21}H_{24}N_2O_2$ MW: 336.44 Source: CHANG CHUN HUA. Ref: 2.

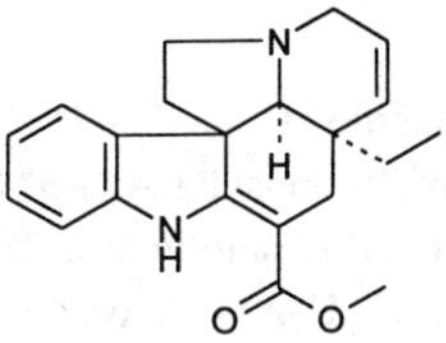

6067 Taccalonolide E
$C_{33}H_{42}O_{12}$ MW: 630.70 Source: LIE GUO SHU. Ref: 293.

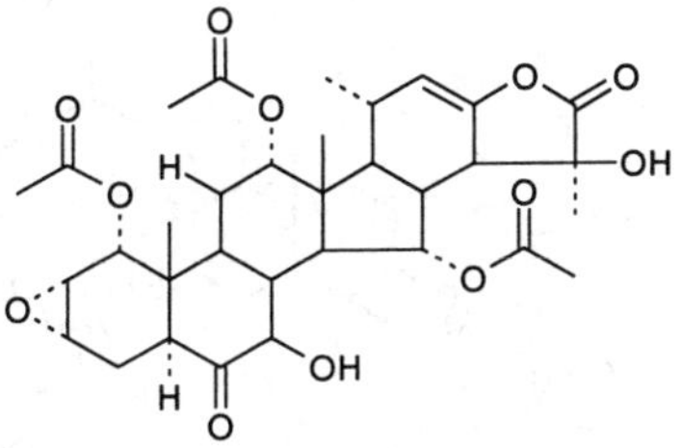

6068 Taccalonolide F
$C_{33}H_{42}O_{13}$ MW: 646.69 Source: LIE GUO SHU. Ref: 293.

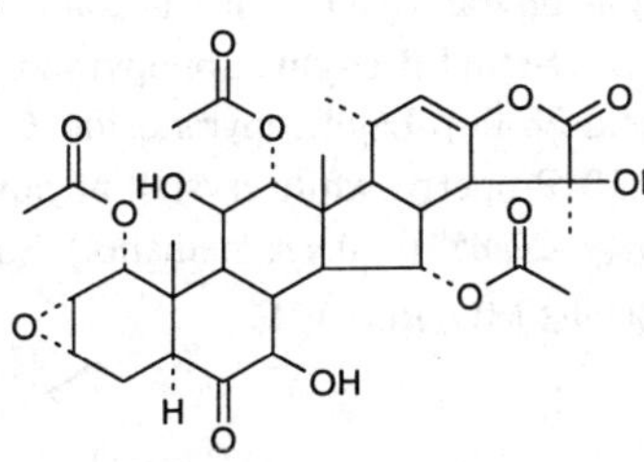

6069 Taccalonolide G
$C_{31}H_{42}O_{11}$ MW: 588.66 Source: LIE GUO SHU. Ref: 293.

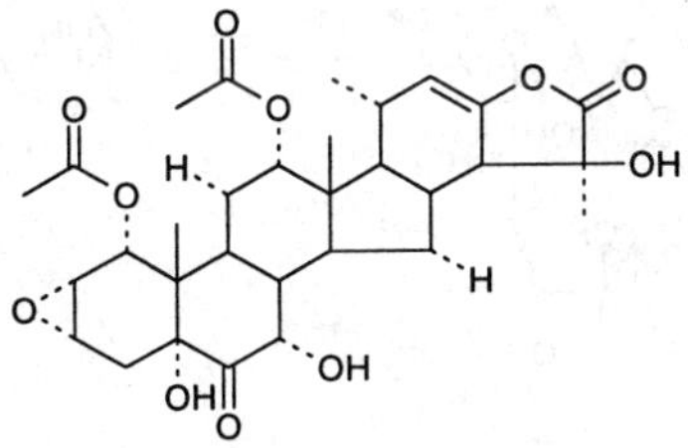

6070 Taccalonolide H
$C_{36}H_{44}O_{14}$ MW: 700.74 Source: LIE GUO SHU. Ref: 293.

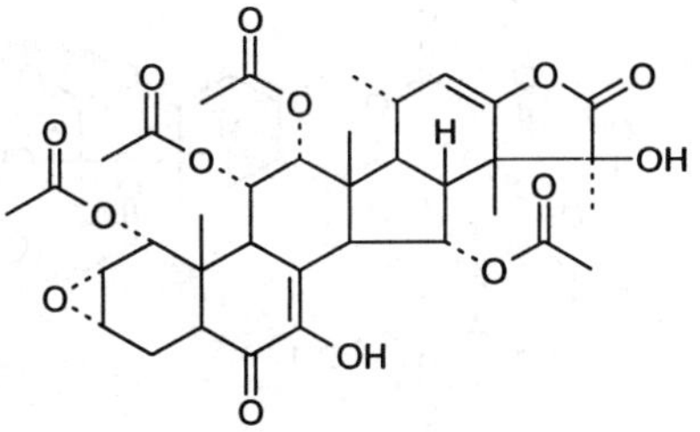

6071 Taccalonolide I
$C_{36}H_{46}O_{14}$ MW: 702.76 Source: LIE GUO SHU. Ref: 293.

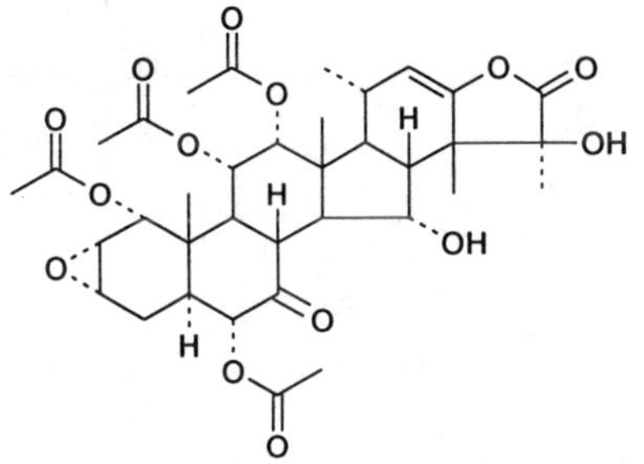

6072 Taccalonolide J
$C_{34}H_{44}O_{13}$ MW: 660.72 Source: LIE GUO SHU. Ref: 293.

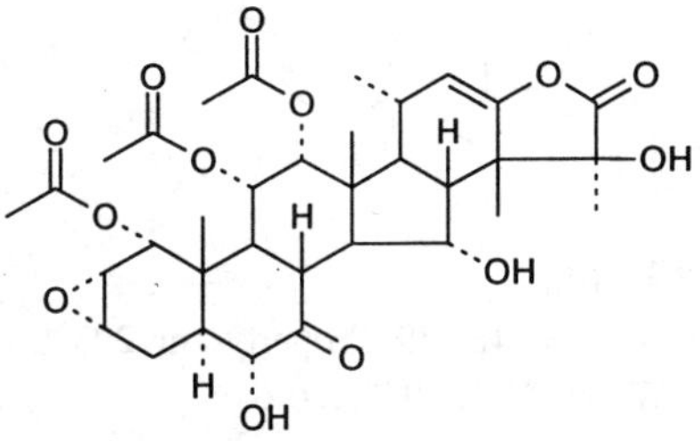

6073 Taccalonolide K
$C_{34}H_{44}O_{14}$ MW: 676.72 Source: LIE GUO SHU. Ref: 293.

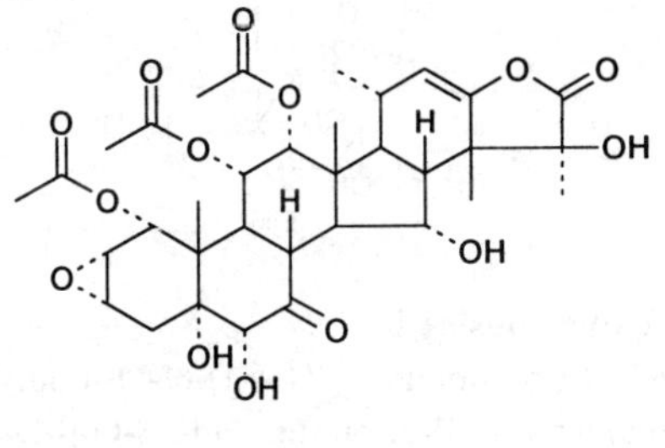

6074 Taccalonolide L
$C_{36}H_{46}O_{15}$ MW: 718.76 Source: LIE GUO SHU. Ref: 293.

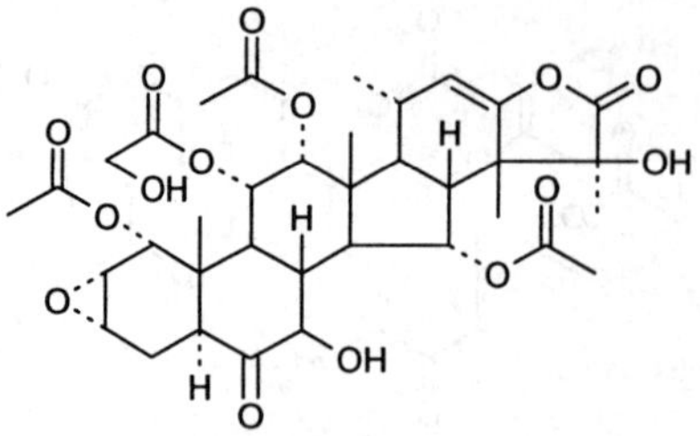

6075 Taccalonolide M
$C_{32}H_{42}O_{12}$ MW: 618.68 Source: LIE GUO SHU. Ref: 293.

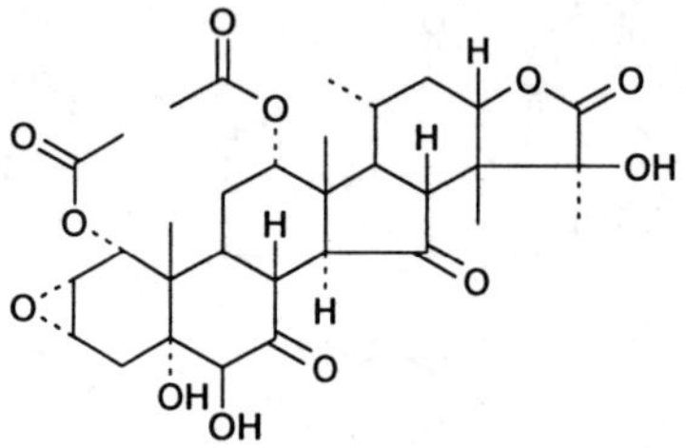

6076 Tadeonal
$C_{15}H_{22}O_2$ MW: 234.34 Property: mp 57°C, bp 138-40°C/0.8 mm. Source: SHUI LIAO. Ref: 6.

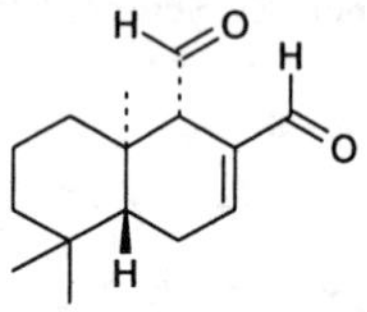

6077 Tagetiin
$C_{21}H_{20}O_{13}$ MW: 480.39 Property: mp 203°C (dec). Source: WAN SHOU JU. Ref: 6.

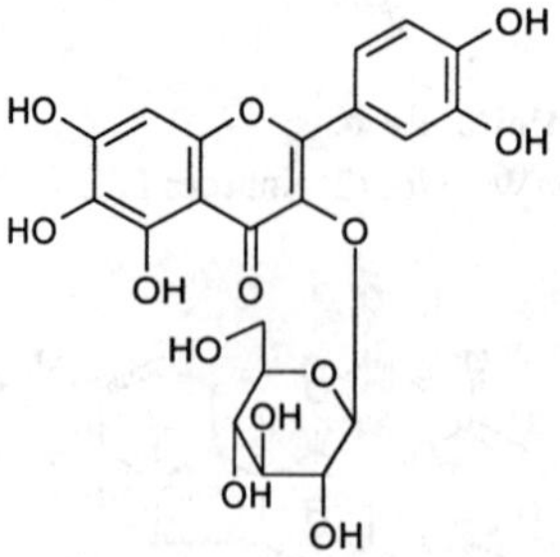

6078 Taibaienoside I
3-O-[α-L-Arabinofuranosyl(1→4)-6'-O-n-butyl-β-D-glucuronopyranosyl]-oleanolic acid-28-O-β-D-glucopyranoside. $C_{51}H_{82}O_{18}$ MW: 983.21 Property: white acicular crystal (chloroform-methanol), mp 177-80°C, $[\alpha]_D^{20}$ -20.23° (c=0.54, methanol). Source: TAI BAI SONG MU. Ref: 394.

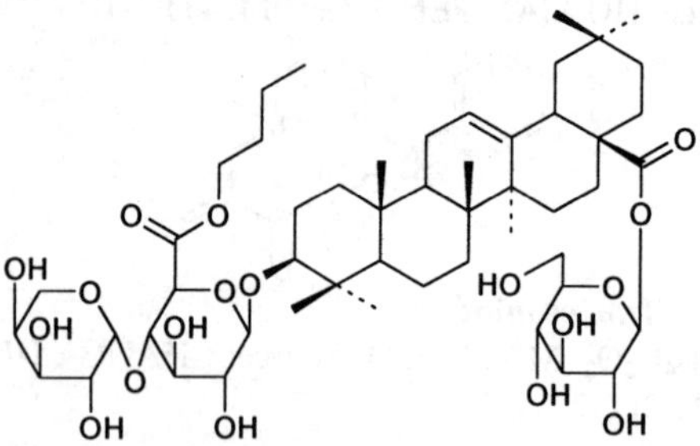

6079 Taibaienoside II
3-O-[α-L-Arabinofuranosyl(1→4)-6'-O-ethyl-β-D-glucuronopyranosyl]-oleanolic acid-28-O-β-D-glucopyranoside. $C_{49}H_{78}O_{18}$ MW: 955.16 Property: white crystalline powder, mp 194-5°C, $[\alpha]_D^{20}$ -22.85° (c=0.41, methanol). Source: TAI BAI SONG MU. Ref: 394.

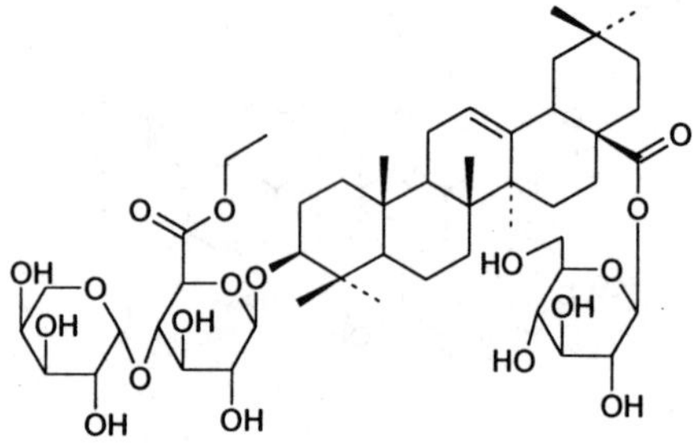

6080 Taibaienoside III
3-O-{β-D-glucopyranosyl(1→3)[α-L-arabinofuranosyl(1→4)]-6'-O-ethyl-β-D-glucuronopyranosyl}-oleanolic acid-28-O-β-D-glucopyranoside. $C_{55}H_{88}O_{23}$ MW: 1117.30 Property: white crystalline powder, mp 194-5°C, $[\alpha]_D^{20}$ -22.85° (c=0.41, methanol). Source: TAI BAI SONG MU. Ref: 394.

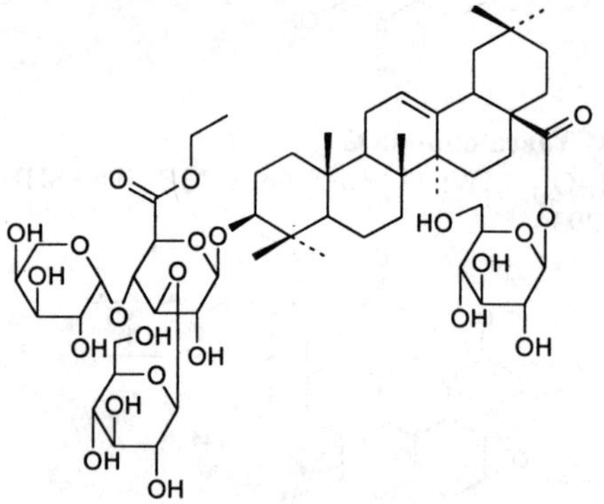

6081 Taibaienoside V

$C_{52}H_{86}O_{14}$ MW: 935.26 Property: white crystalline powder, mp 162-4°C. Source: TAI BAI SONG MU. Ref: 470.

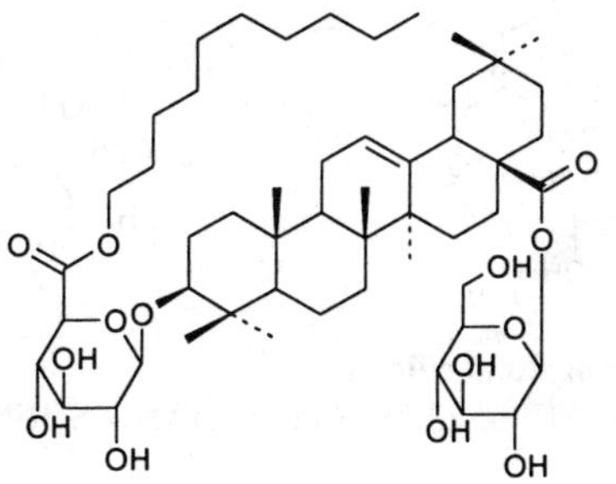

6082 Taibaienoside IV

$C_{46}H_{74}O_{14}$ MW: 851.09 Property: white crystalline powder, mp 181-4°C, $[\alpha]_D^{20}$ +8.12° (c=0.23, MeOH). Source: TAI BAI SONG MU. Ref: 470.

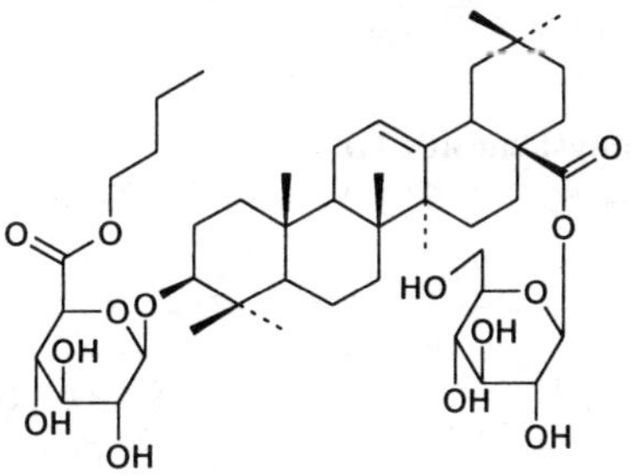

6083 Taibaienoside VII

3-O-{β-D-xylopyranosyl (1→2)[β-D-glucopyranosyl (1→3)]-6'-O-ethyl-β-D-glucuronopyranosyl} oleanolic acid-28-O-β-D-glucopyranoside. $C_{55}H_{88}O_{23}$ MW: 1117.30 Property: white crystalline powder, mp 207-9 °C. Source: TAI BAI SONG MU. Ref: 359.

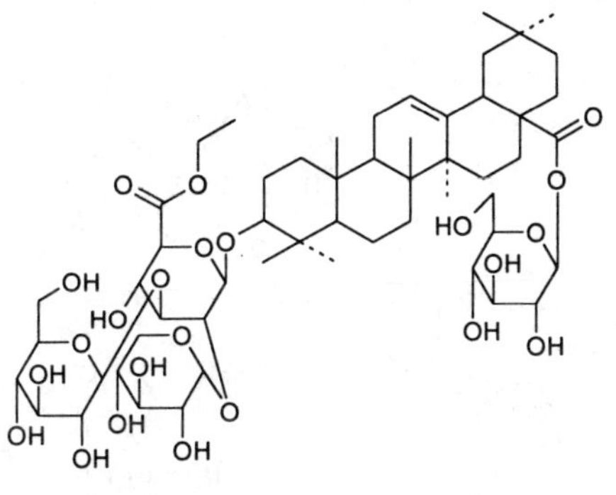

6084 Taibaienoside VIII

3-O-{β-D-xylopyranosyl(1→2)[β-D-glucopyranosyl (1→3)]-6'-O-butyl-β-D-glucuronopyranosyl}oleanolic acid-28-O-β-D-glucopyranoside. $C_{57}H_{92}O_{23}$ MW: 1145.55 Property: white crystalline powder, mp 212-3°C, $[\alpha]_D^{20}$ +4.90° (c=0.82, methanol). Source: TAI BAI SONG MU. Ref: 359.

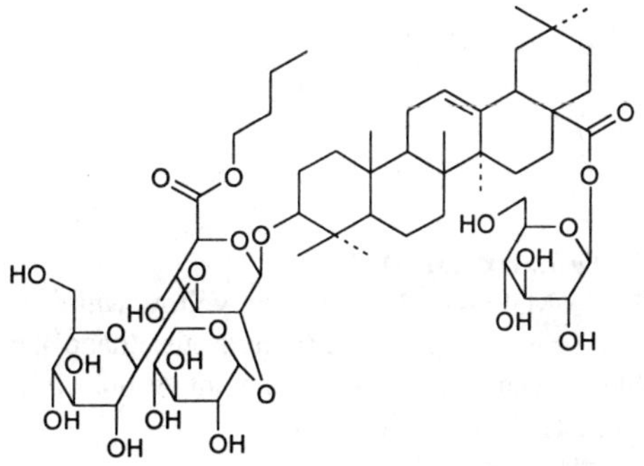

6085 Taipaienine I

$C_{27}H_{43}NO_3$ MW: 429.65 Property: acicular crystal, mp 120-2°C, $[\alpha]_D^{28}$ +12.9° (c=0.31, MeOH). Source: NING XIA BEI MU. Ref: 271.

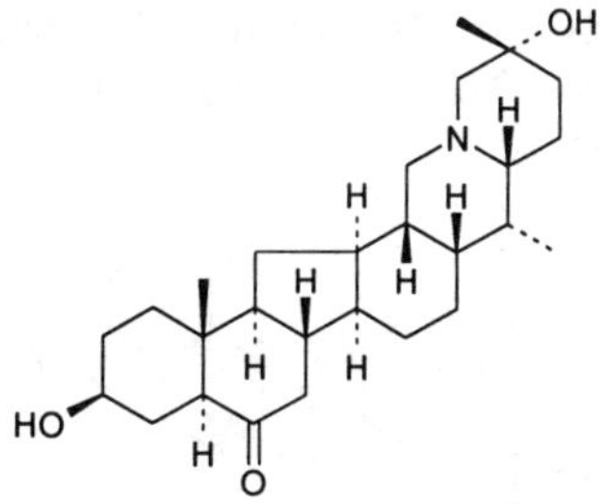

6086 Taiwanin E methyl ether

$C_{21}H_{14}O_7$ MW: 378.34 Property: mp 227-30°C. Source: JUE CHUANG. Ref: 6.

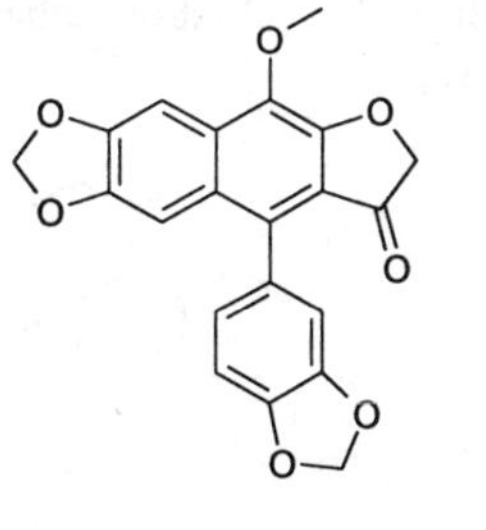

6087 Takatonine

$C_{21}H_{24}NO_4$ MW: 354.43 Source: YAN GUO CAO. Ref: 6.

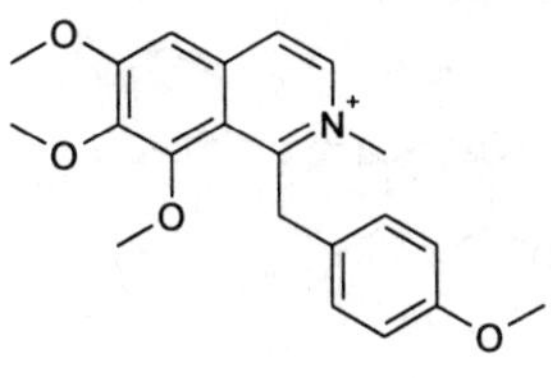

6088 Talatisamine
$C_{25}H_4NO_5$ MW: 435.61 Source: FU ZI. Ref: 2.

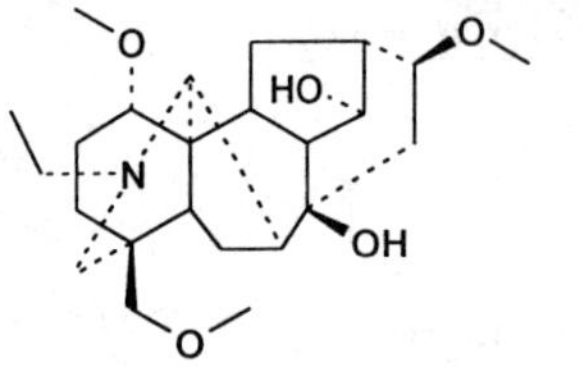

6089 Tamarixinol (I)
$C_{30}H_{52}O_2$ MW: 446.75 Property: yellow white granular crystal, mp 77-8°C (anhydrous ethanol), easy soluble in hexane, chloroform and anhydrous ethanol. Source: CHENG LIU. Ref: 115.

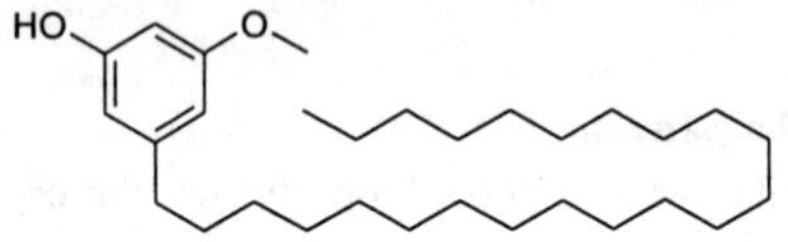

6090 Tamarixol (IV)
$C_{30}H_{50}O_2$ MW: 442.72 Property: white acicular crystal, mp 252-3°C (acetic ester). Source: CHENG LIU. Ref: 115.

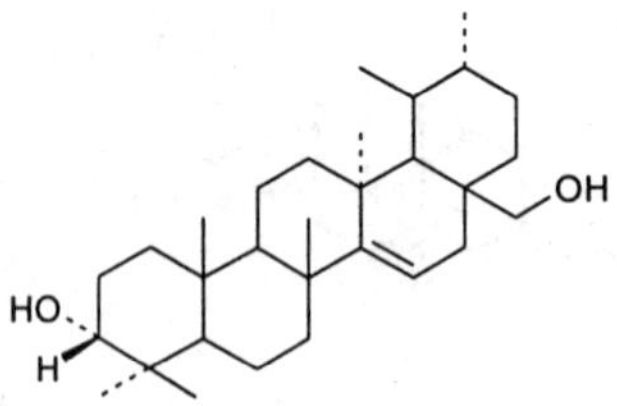

6091 Tamarixone (III)
$C_{30}H_{48}O_2$ MW: 440.72 Property: white crystalline powder, mp 238-40°C (anhydrous ethanol). Source: CHENG LIU. Ref: 115.

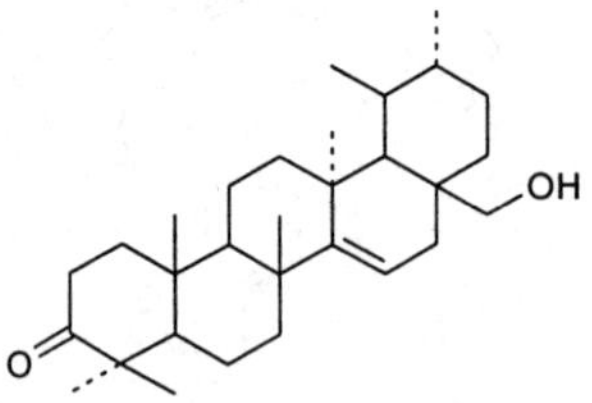

6092 Tangeretin
$C_{20}H_{20}O_7$ MW: 372.38 Property: mp 150-1°C. Source: JIN JU. Ref: 6.

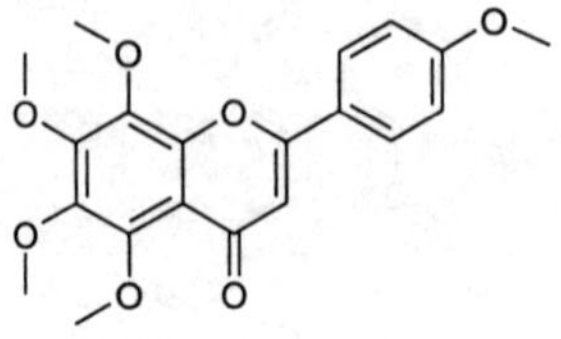

6093 Tangshenoside I
$C_{29}H_{42}O_{18}$ MW: 678.65 Source: DANG SHEN. Ref: 2.

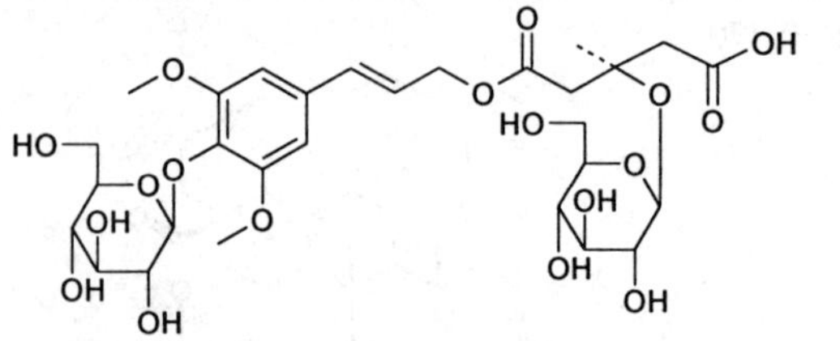

6094 Tangshenoside II
$C_{17}H_{24}O_9$ MW: 372.38 Source: DANG SHEN. Ref: 2.

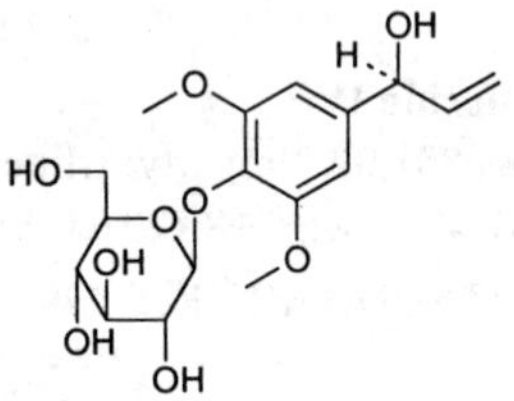

6095 Tangshenoside III
$C_{34}H_{46}O_{17}$ MW: 726.74 Source: DANG SHEN. Ref: 2.

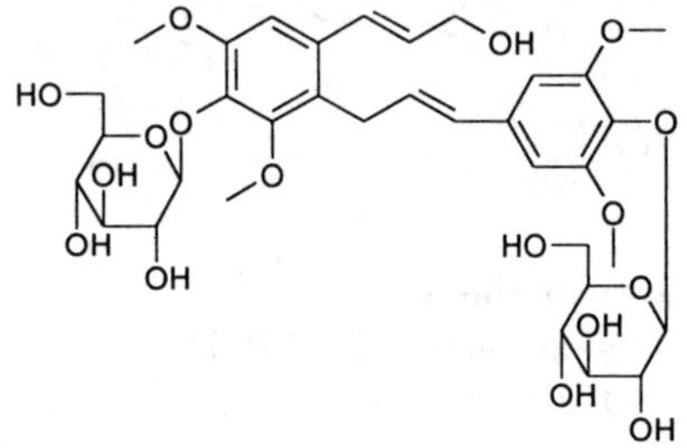

6096 Tangshenoside IV
$C_{46}H_{64}O_{26}$ MW: 103.01 Source: DANG SHEN. Ref: 2.

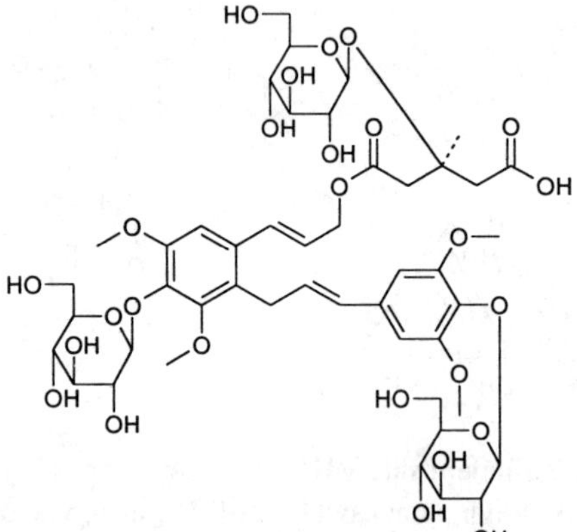

6097 Tanshidiol A
$C_{19}H_{24}O_3$ MW: 264.28 Source: DAN SHEN. Ref: 2.

6098 Tanshilactone
$C_{17}H_{12}O_3$ MW: 264.28 Source: DAN SHEN. Ref: 2.

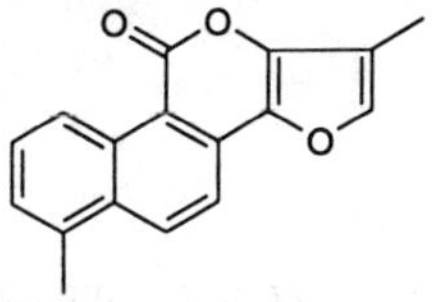

6099 Tanshinaldehyde II
$C_{19}H_{16}O_4$ MW: 308.34 Property: dark red acicular crystal, mp 223-5°C. Source: BAI HUA DAN SHEN. Ref: 185.

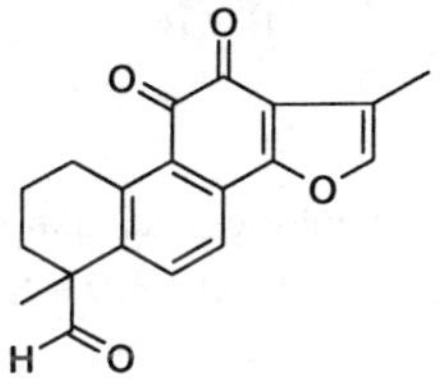

6100 Tanshinone I
$C_{18}H_{12}O_3$ MW: 276.29 Property: mp 233-4°C. Source: DAN SHEN. Ref: 4.

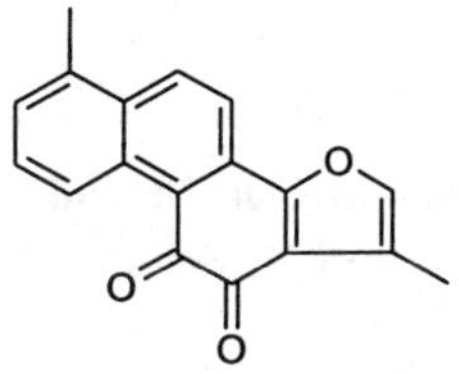

6101 Tanshinone II A
$C_{19}H_{18}O_3$ MW: 294.35 Property: mp 198-200°C. Source: DAN SHEN. Ref: 2, 4.

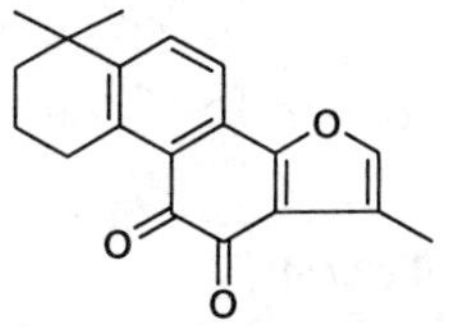

6102 Tanshinone II B
$C_{19}H_{18}O_4$ MW: 310.35 Property: mp 200-4°C. Source: DAN SHEN. Ref: 2, 4.

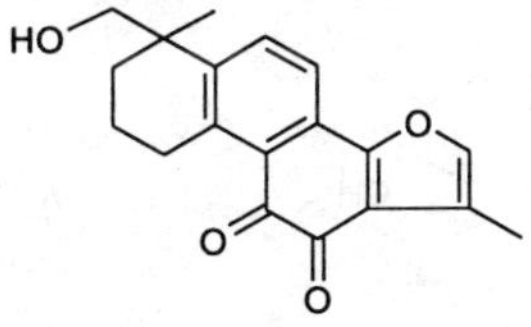

6103 Tanshiquinone A
$C_{18}H_{16}O_4$ MW: 296.33 Source: DAN SHEN. Ref: 2.

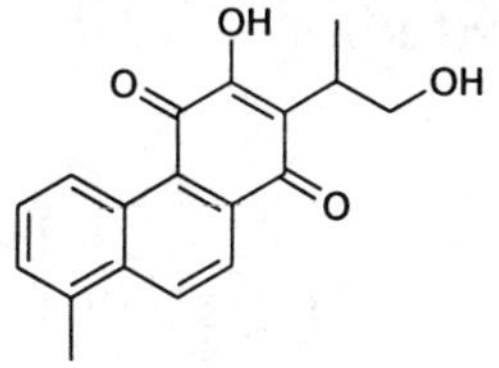

6104 Tanshiquinone B
$C_{18}H_{16}O_3$ MW: 280.33 Source: DAN SHEN. Ref: 2.

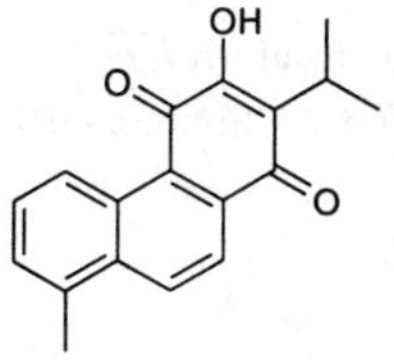

6105 Tanshiquinone C
$C_{16}H_{12}O_3$ MW: 252.27 Source: DAN SHEN. Ref: 2.

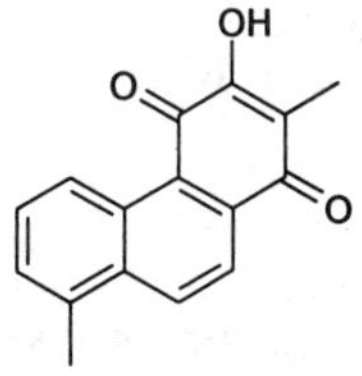

6106 Taraxanthin
$C_{40}H_{56}O_3$ MW: 584.89 Property: mp 184-5°C. Source: DAO CAO, KUAN DONG HUA, TU SI ZI. Ref: 6.

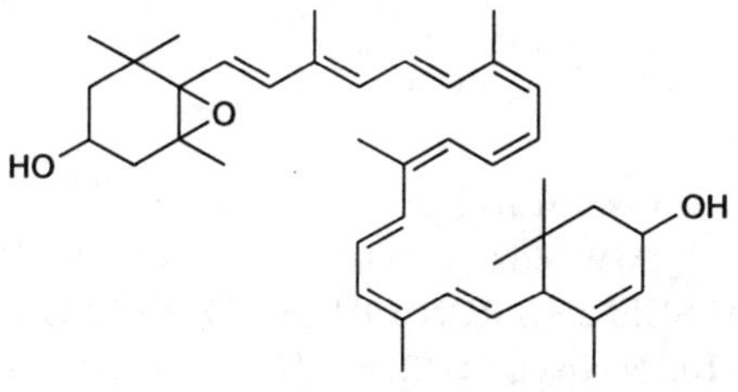

6107 Taraxasterol
$C_{30}H_{50}O$ MW: 426.73 Source: MU XIANG. Ref: 2.

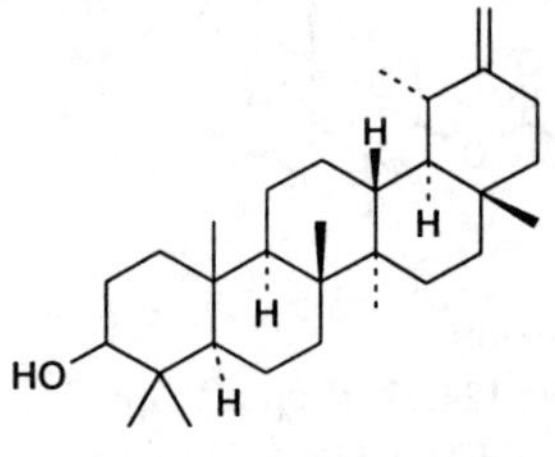

6108 φ-Taraxasterol
$C_{30}H_{50}O$ MW: 427.73 Property: mp 217-9°C. Source: PU GONG YING. Ref: 6.

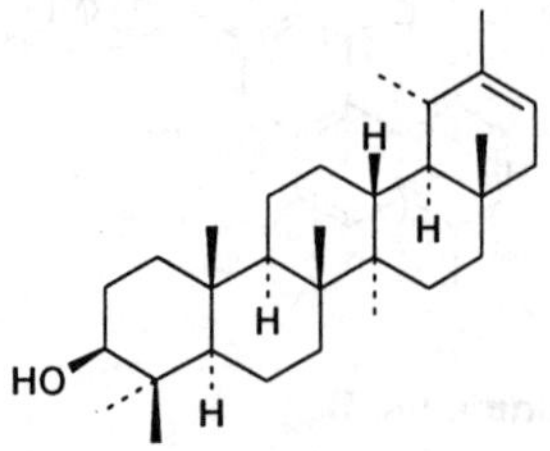

6109 Taraxasterol palmitate
$C_{32}H_{52}O_2$ MW: 468.77 Source: CHENG GAN CAO. Ref: 6.

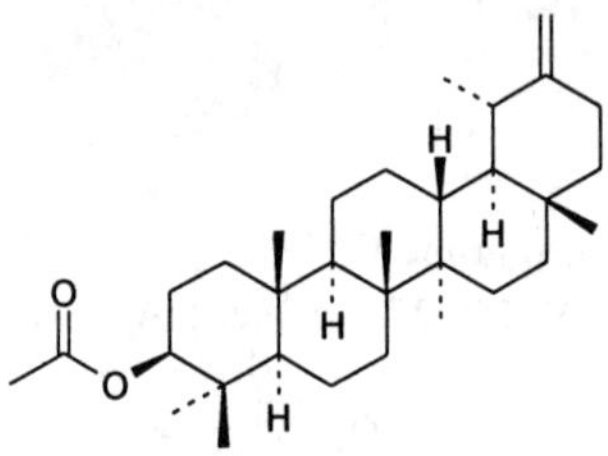

6110 Taraxerol
$C_{30}H_{50}O$ MW: 426.73 Property: mp 282-3°C. Source: BIAN TAO, DANG SHEN, QUE MEI TENG. Ref: 2, 515, 550.

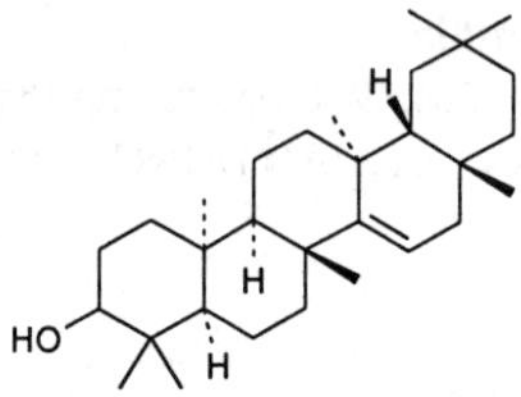

6111 Taraxerol acetate
$C_{32}H_{52}O_2$ MW: 468.77 Source: BI LI, CI SAN JIA, DANG SHEN, FU RONG JU GEN, FU SANG YE, MAO LIAN HAO. Ref: 2, 6, 474.

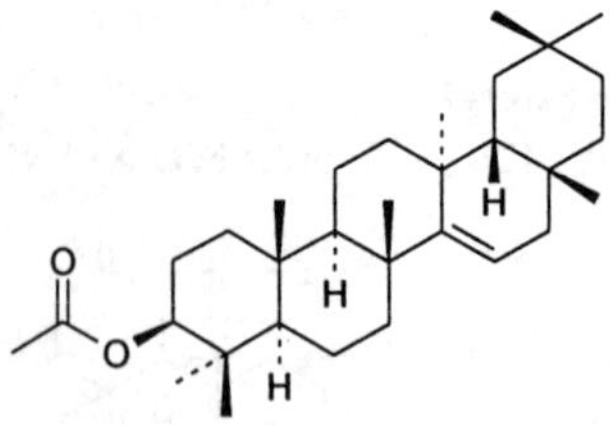

6112 Taraxerone
$C_{30}H_{48}O$ MW: 424.72 Property: mp 242-4°C. Source: FU RONG JU GEN, HUO YANG LE, JU JU. Ref: 6, 620.

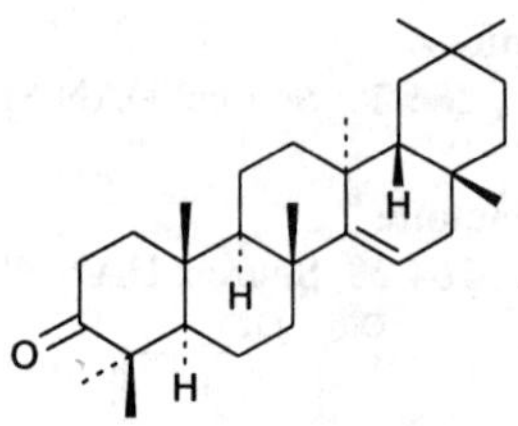

6113 Tartaric acid
$C_4H_6O_6$ MW: 150.09 Property: mp L: 170°C. Source: CU LIU GUO(SHA JI), DA ZAO, DU ZHONG, REN SHEN, SHAN ZHU YU. Ref: 2.

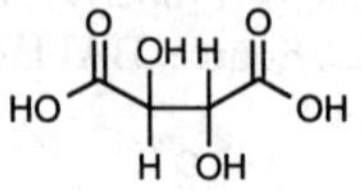

6114 Taurin
MW: 248 Property: colorless acicular crystal, mp 110-3°C. Source: MAO LIAN HAO. Ref: 474.

6115 Taurine
$C_2H_7NO_3S$ MW: 125.15 Property: mp 317°C (dec), 328°C. Source: QUAN XIE. Ref: 2.

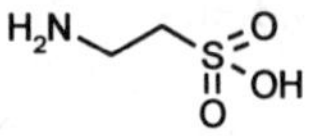

6116 Taurochenodeoxycholic acid
$C_{26}H_{45}NO_6S$ MW: 499.72 Source: XIONG DAN. Ref: 2.

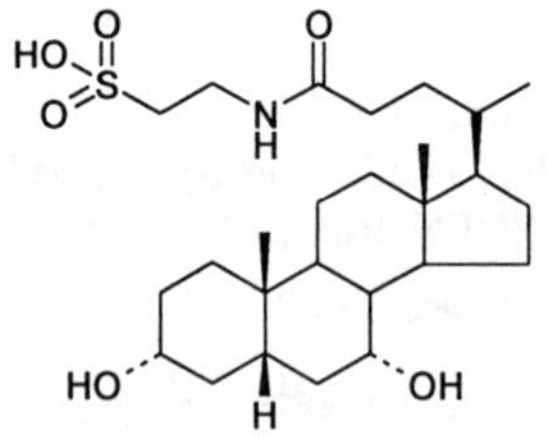

6117 Taurocholic acid
$C_{28}H_{49}NO_7S$ MW: 543.77 Property: mp 125°C(dec). Source: XIONG DAN. Ref: 2.

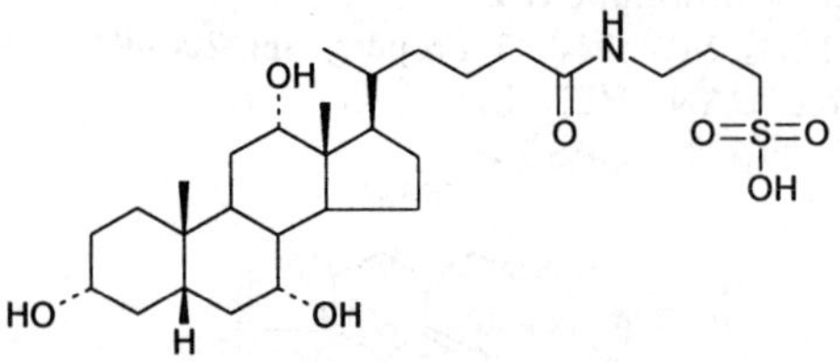

6118 Taurodeoxycholic acid

$C_{26}H_{45}NO_6S$ MW: 499.72 Source: XIONG DAN. Ref: 2.

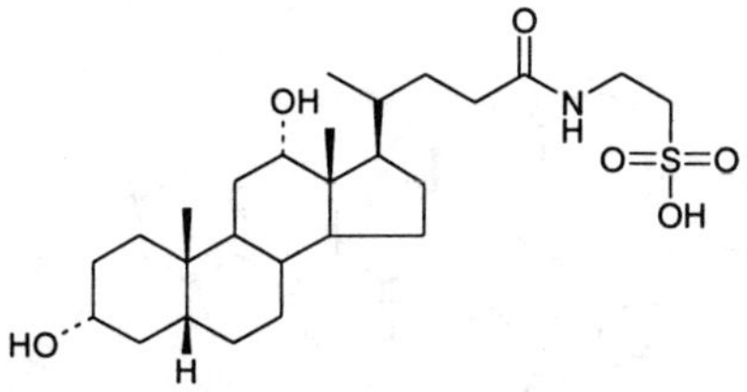

6119 Tauroursodeoxy cholic acid

$C_{26}H_{45}NO_5S$ MW: 483.72 Source: XIONG DAN. Ref: 2.

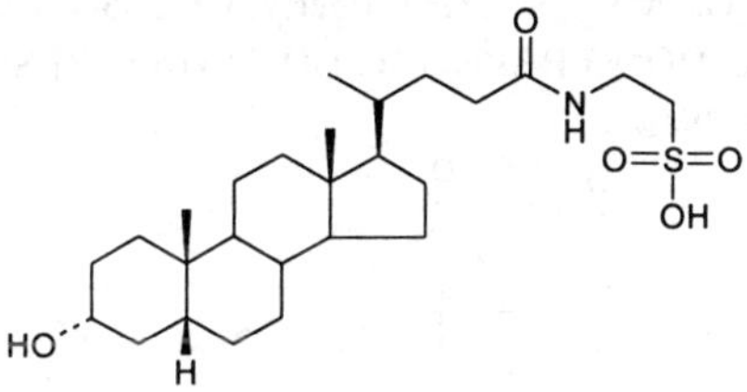

6120 Taxacustin XII

$C_{28}H_{40}O_{12}$ MW: 568.62 Property: colorless massive crystal, mp 225-7°C, $[\alpha]_D^{15}$ -38.4° (c=0.11, chloroform). Source: DONG BEI HONG DOU SHAN. Ref: 291.

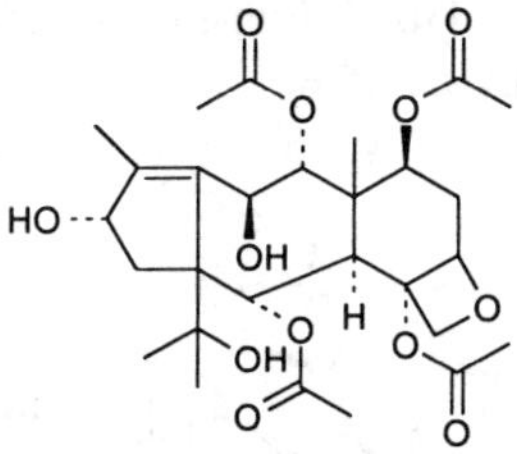

6121 Taxayuntin

$C_{35}H_{44}O_{13}$ MW: 672.73 Property: massive crystal colorless , mp 249-50°C (CH_3CO), $[\alpha]_D^{27}$ -53.3° (methanol). Source: YUN NAN HONG DOU SHAN. Ref: 300.

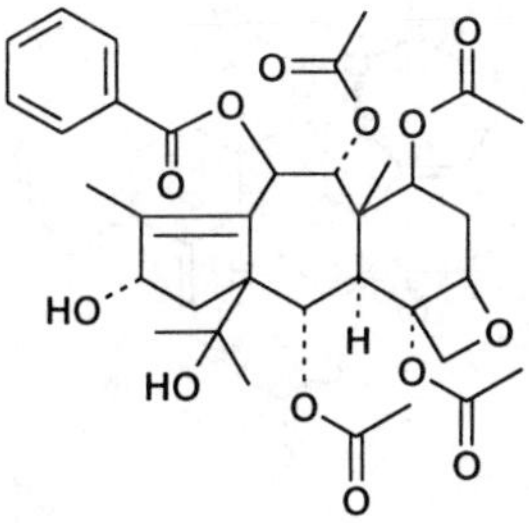

6122 Taxayuntin A

2α,7β,9α-trideacetyl-2α,7βdibenzoyl-10β-debenzoyl taxayuntin. $C_{36}H_{42}O_{11}$ MW: 650.73 Property: white powder, mp 160-3 °C, $[\alpha]_D^{22}$ ±0 °(c=0.05,chloroform). Source: YUN NAN HONG DOU SHAN. Ref: 383.

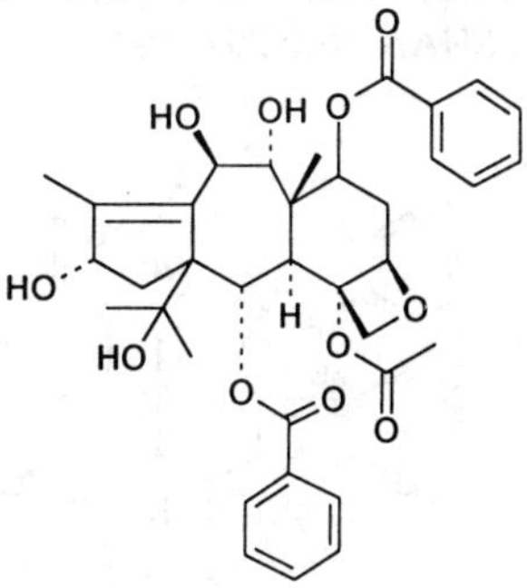

6123 Taxayuntin B

2α-Debenzoyl-2α-acetyl taxayuntin. $C_{31}H_{40}O_{11}$ MW: 588.66 Property: white acicular crystal, mp 225-8°C (methanol), $[\alpha]_D^{12}$ +25.1° (c=0.13, chloro-form). Source: YUN NAN HONG DOU SHAN. Ref: 383.

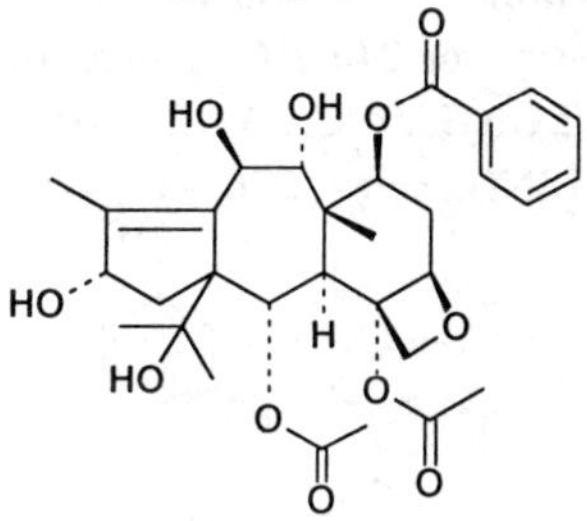

6124 Taxayuntin C

2α-deacetyl-2α-debenzoyl-13α-acetyl taxayuntin. $C_{42}H_{48}O_{14}$ MW: 776.84 Property: white granular crystal, mp 226-30°C (Abs ethanol), $[\alpha]_D^{17}$ -36.2° (c=0.17, methanol). Source: YUN NAN HONG DOU SHAN. Ref: 383.

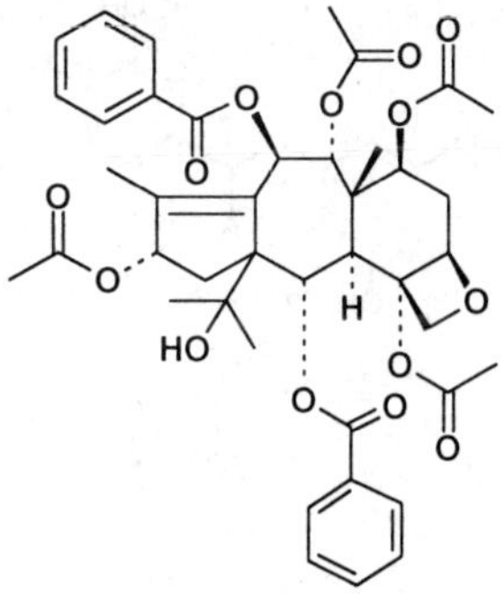

6125 Taxayuntin D

9α-deacetyl-9α-debenzoyl taxayuntin. $C_{47}H_{50}O_{14}$ MW: 838.91 Property: white granular crystal, mp 210-4°C (methanol), $[\alpha]_D^{17}$ -40.4° (c=0.16, methanol). Source: DONG BEI HONG DOU SHAN, YUN NAN HONG DOU SHAN. Ref: 291, 383.

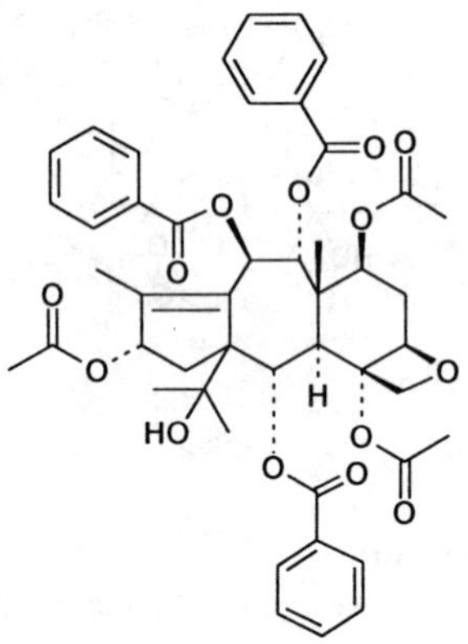

6126 Taxifolin

Distylin; Taxifoliol. CAS: 480-18-2 $C_{15}H_{12}O_7$ MW: 304.26 Property: mp 240-2°C. Source: BA DAN XING REN, LONG YA CAO GEN, HUANG LIAN YA, TU FU LING. Ref: 4, 336, 411, 416.

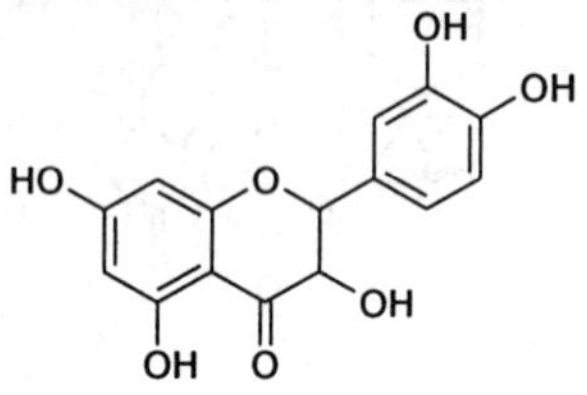

6127 (2S, 3S)-(-)-Taxifolin-3-O-β-D-glucopyranoside (X)

$C_{21}H_{22}O_{12}$ MW: 466.40 Property: white acicular crystal, mp 166-8°C, $[\alpha]_D^{14}$ -119.4° (c=0.5, methanol). Source: XIAN HE CAO. Ref: 152.

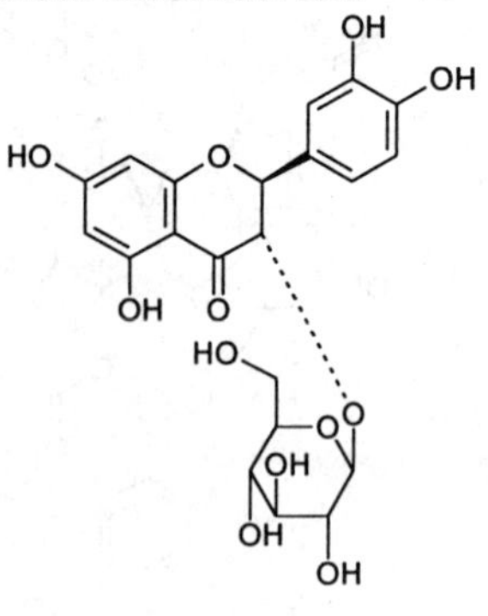

6128 Taxine A

$C_{37}H_{49}NO_{10}$ MW: 667.80 Property: mp 121-4°C. Source: ZI SHAN. Ref: 6.

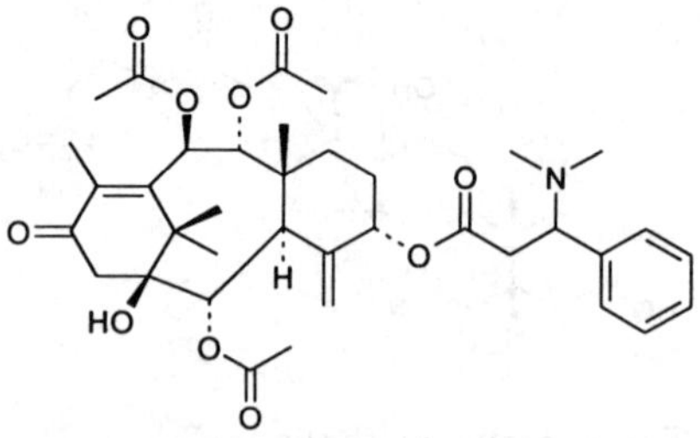

6129 Taxinine

$C_{35}H_{42}O_9$ MW: 606.72 Property: mp 265-7°C. Source: DONG BEI HONG DOU SHAN, ZI SHAN. Ref: 6, 291.

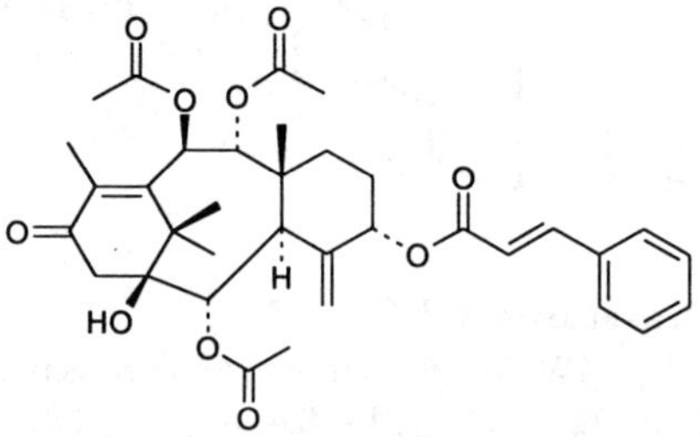

6130 Taxinine A

$C_{26}H_{36}O_8$ MW: 476.57 Property: mp 254-5°C. Source: ZI SHAN. Ref: 6.

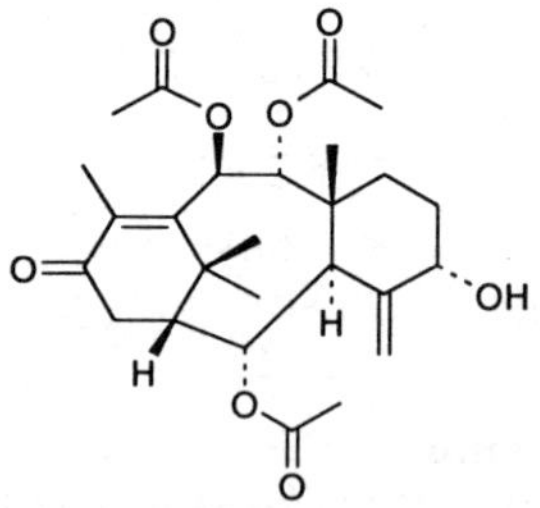

6131 Taxinine H

$C_{28}H_{38}O_9$ MW: 518.61 Property: mp 166-7°C. Source: ZI SHAN. Ref: 6.

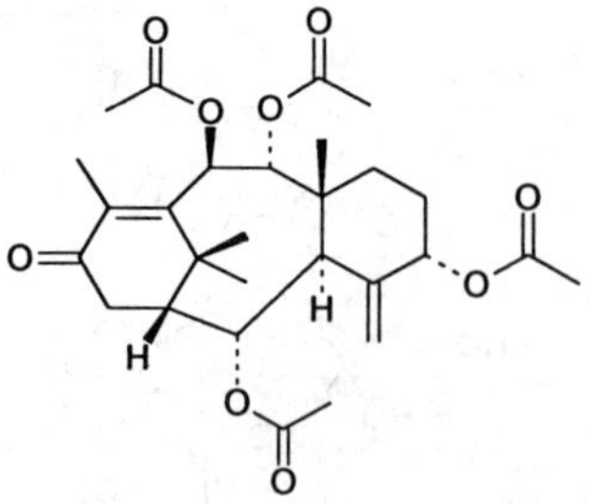

6132 Taxinine K
$C_{26}H_{36}O_8$ MW: 476.57 Property: mp 167-8°C. Source: ZI SHAN. Ref: 6.

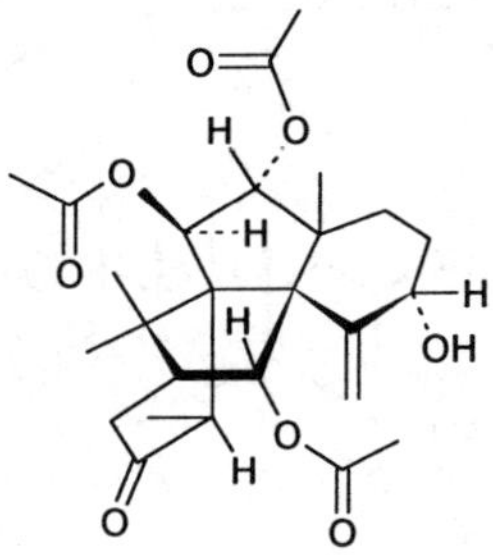

6133 Taxinine L
$C_{28}H_{38}O_9$ MW: 518.61 Property: mp 159-60°C. Source: ZI SHAN. Ref: 6.

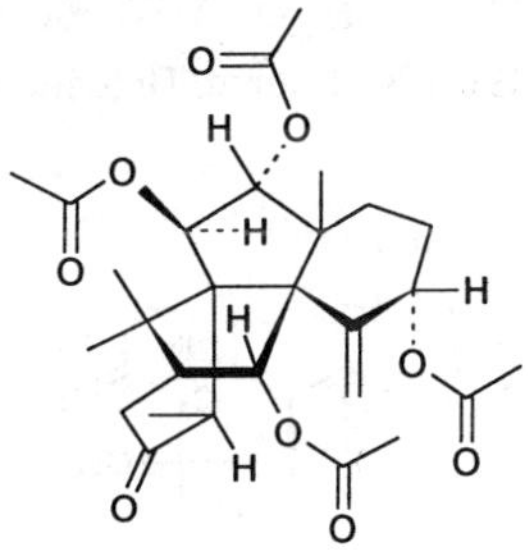

6134 Taxodine
$C_{19}H_{25}NO_3$ MW: 315.42 Source: SAN JIAN SHAN. Ref: 2.

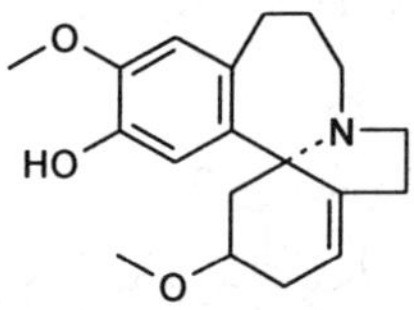

6135 Taxodione
CAS: 19026-31-4 $C_{20}H_{26}O_3$ MW: 314.43 Property: mp 115-6°C. Source: *Taxodium distichum* Rich. Ref: 5.

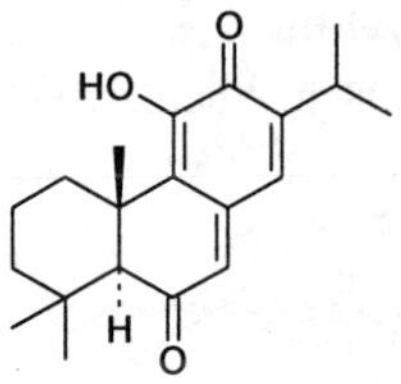

6136 Taxodone
CAS: 19039-02-2 $C_{20}H_{28}O_3$ MW: 316.44 Property: mp 164-6°C. Source: *Taxodium distichum* Rich. Ref: 5.

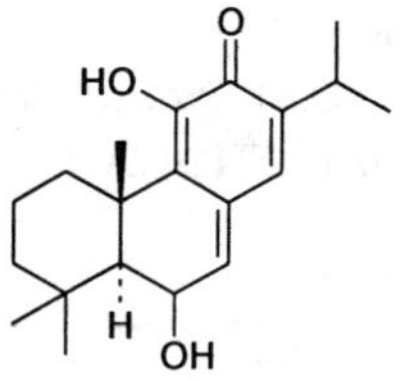

6137 Taxol
CAS: 33069-62-4 $C_{47}H_{51}NO_{14}$ MW: 853.93 Property: mp 213-6°C (dec). Source: YUN NAN HONG DOU SHAN, ZI SHAN. Ref: 5, 6, 202.

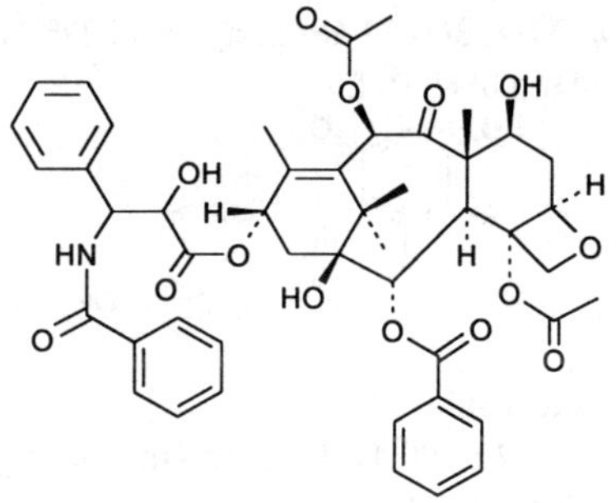

6138 Taxol B
Source: YUN NAN HONG DOU SHAN (bark). Ref: 563.

6139 Taxol C-7-xylose
Source: YUN NAN HONG DOU SHAN (bark). Ref: 563.

6140 Taxusin
$C_{28}H_{40}O_8$ MW: 504.63 Property: mp 126°C. Source: YUN NAN HONG DOU SHAN (bark), ZI SHAN. Ref: 6, 563.

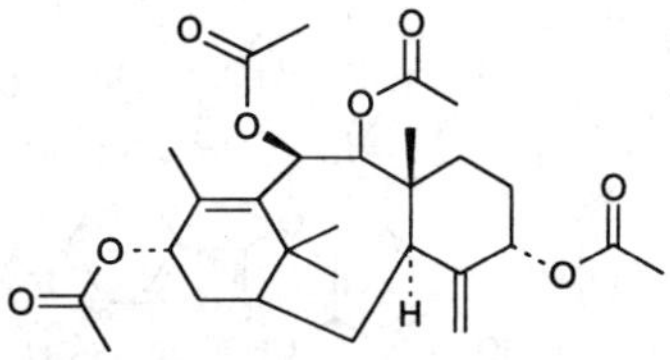

6141 Tazettine
$C_{18}H_{21}NO_5$ MW: 331.37 Property: mp 210-1°C. Source: DA YI ZHI JIAN, GAN FENG CAO, LUO QUN DAI GEN, SHUI XIAN GEN, SHUI GUI JIAO YE, SHI SUAN. Ref: 6.

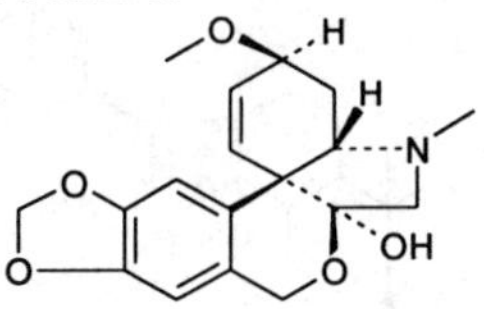

6142 Tectoridin

$C_{22}H_{22}O_{11}$ MW: 462.41 Property: mp 258°C. Source: BAI HUA SHE GAN, SHE GAN, YUAN WEI. Ref: 6.

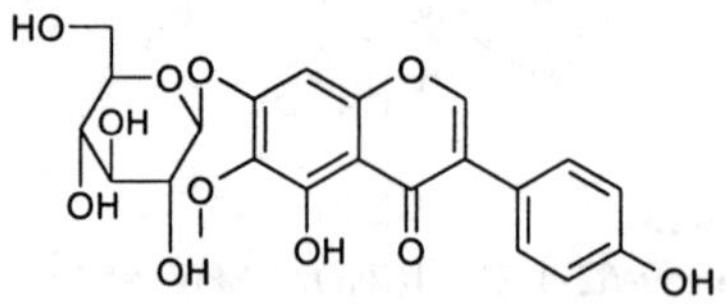

6143 Tectorigenin

$C_{16}H_{12}O_6$ MW: 300.27 Property: mp 227°C (dec). Source: SHE GAN. Ref: 6.

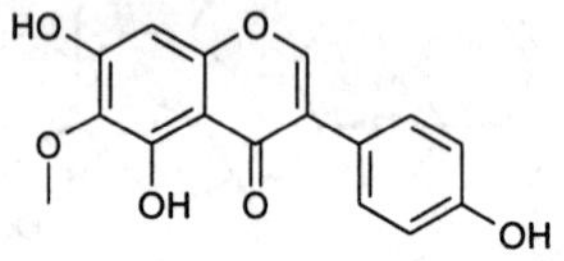

6144 Tectoruside

$C_{21}H_{30}O_{13}$ MW: 490.47 Property: mp 207-9°C. Source: YUAN WEI. Ref: 6.

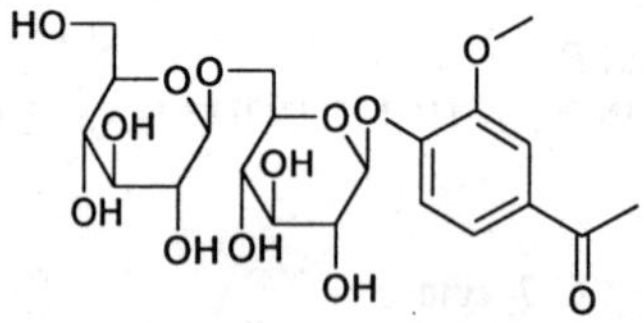

6145 Tellimagrandin II

$C_{41}H_{30}O_{26}$ MW: 938.68 Source: SHAN ZHU YU. Ref: 2.

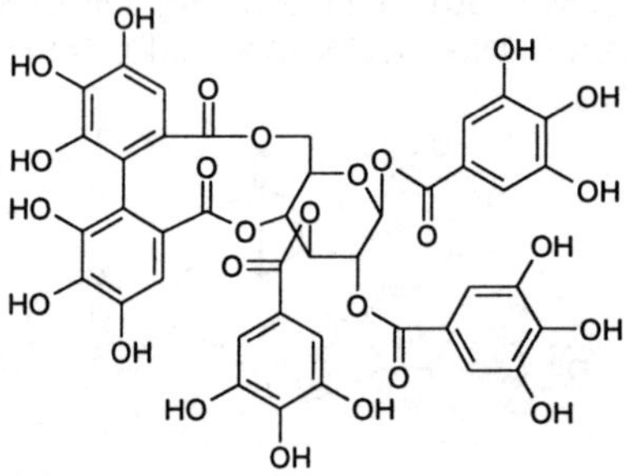

6146 Telocinobufagin

$C_{24}H_{34}O_5$ MW: 0402.54 Property: mp 160°C, 207-11°C. Source: CHAN SU. Ref: 2.

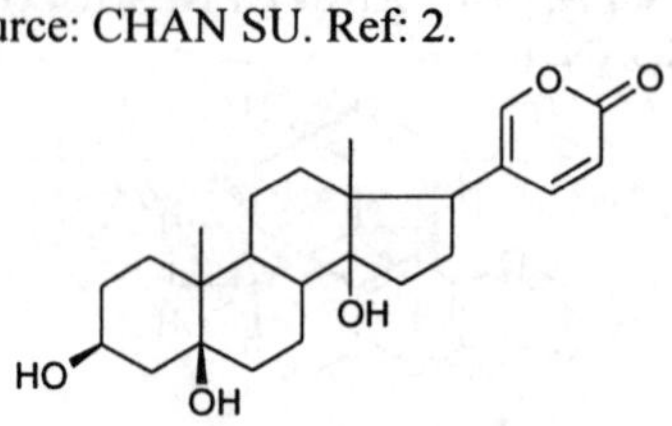

6147 Tenuifolin

$C_{36}H_{56}O_{12}$ MW: 680.84 Property: mp 298-300°C. Source: YUAN ZHI. Ref: 2.

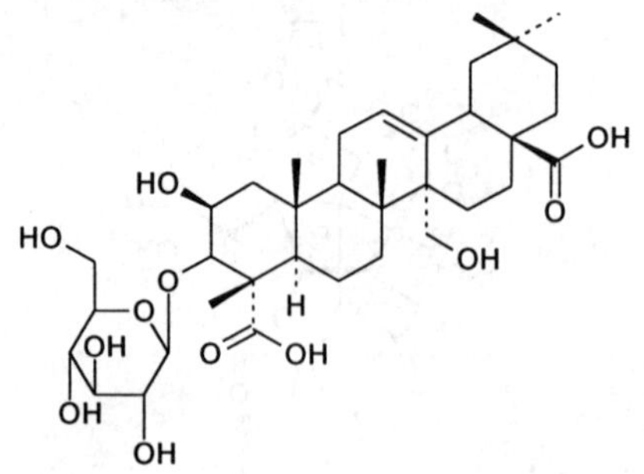

6148 Tenulin

CAS: 19202-92-7 $C_{17}H_{22}O_5$ MW: 306.36 Property: mp 188-9°C, 196-8°C. Source: Helenium tenuifolium Nutt. Ref: 5.

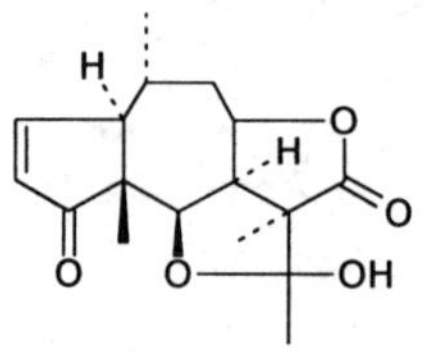

6149 Tephrosin

$C_{23}H_{22}O_7$ MW: 410.43 Property: mp 198°C. Source: HUI YE GEN, YU TENG. Ref: 6.

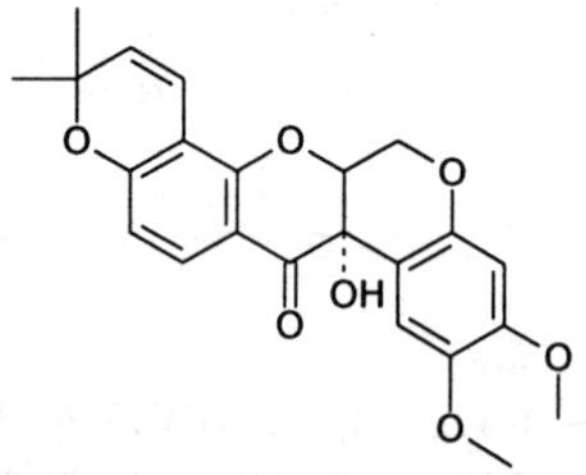

6150 3,4-Teracrylshikonin

$C_{23}H_{26}O_6$ MW: 398.46 Source: ZI CAO. Ref: 2.

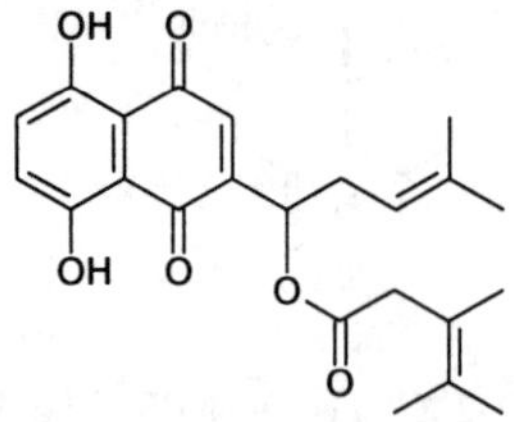

6151 Terchebin
$C_{41}H_{30}O_{26}$ MW: 938.68 Source: AN MO LE, HE ZI. Ref: 6.

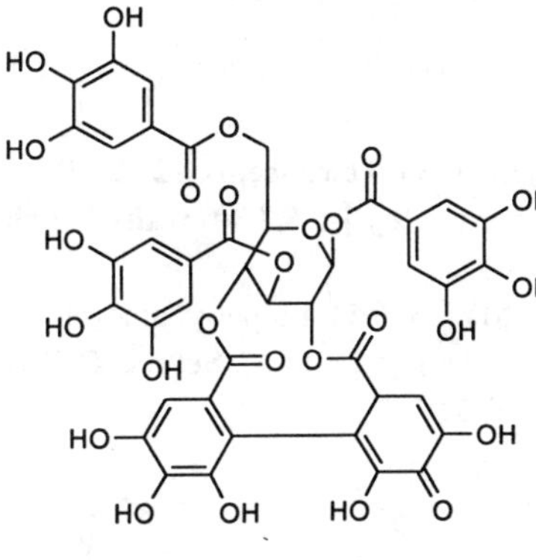

6152 Terephthalate dimethyl ester
Property: mp 137-8.5°C. Source: CHA XIONG. Ref: 531.

6153 Teresautalic acid
$C_{10}H_{14}O_2$ MW: 166.22 Property: mp 158°C. Source: TAN XIANG. Ref: 6.

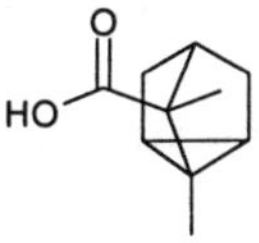

6154 Terminaline
$C_{23}H_{41}NO_2$ MW: 363.59 Property: mp 243-4°C. Source: XUE SHAN LIN. Ref: 6.

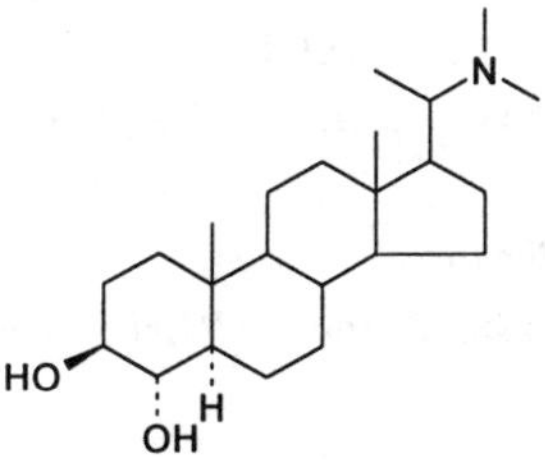

6155 α-Terpinene
$C_{10}H_{16}$ MW: 136.24 Property: bp 173.5-4.8°C/755mm. Source: DU HUO, JU PI, WU WEI ZI. Ref: 2.

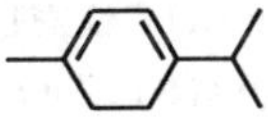

6156 β-Terpinene
$C_{10}H_{16}$ MW: 136.24 Property: bp 173-4°C. Source: CHAI HU. Ref: 2.

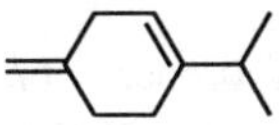

6157 γ-Terpinene
$C_{10}H_{16}$ MW: 136.24 Property: bp 183°C. Source: JU PI, LIAN QIAO, QIANG HUO, QING HAO, SHENG JIANG, WU WEI ZI, XI XIN. Ref: 2.

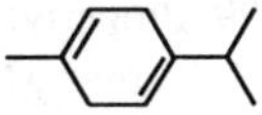

6158 Terpinen-4-ol
$C_{10}H_{18}O$ MW: 154.25 Source: LIAN QIAO, HOU PO, QIANG HUO, SHENG JIANG, XI XIN, WU WEI ZI. Ref: 2.

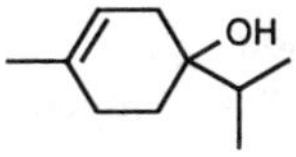

6159 α-Terpineol
$C_{10}H_{18}O$ MW: 154.25 Property: mp (+): 36.9°C, (-): 37°C, (±): 40-1°C, bp (+): 104°C/15mm, (±): 218.8-9.4°C/752mm. Source: CHAI HU, HOU PO, JIN YIN HUA, JU PI, LIAN QIAO, MA HUANG, QIANG HUO, QING HAO, SHENG JIANG, WU WEI ZI, XI XIN, XING REN, YIN CHEN HAO. Ref: 2.

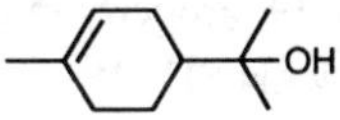

6160 cis-β-Terpineol
$C_{10}H_{18}O$ MW: 154.25 Property: mp 32-3°C. Source: CHAI HU, MI DIE XIANG, MA HUANG. Ref: 2, 6.

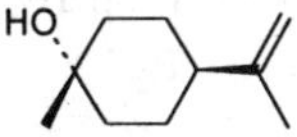

6161 trans-β-Terpineol
$C_{10}H_{18}O$ MW: 154.25 Property: mp 32-3°C. Source: CHAI HU, MI DIE XIANG, MA HUANG. Ref: 2, 6.

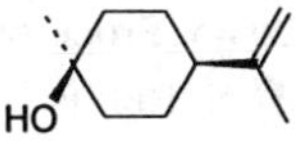

6162 δ-Terpineol
$C_{10}H_{18}O$ MW: 154.25 Source: BAI DOU KOU. Ref: 6.

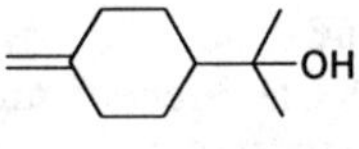

6163 Terpinolene
$C_{10}H_{16}$ MW: 136.24 Property: bp 186°C. Source: JU PI, QIANG HUO, SHENG JIANG, XI XIN. Ref: 2.

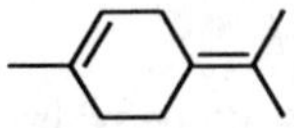

6164 Terpinyl acetate
$C_{12}H_{20}O_2$ MW: 196.29 Property: bp (+): 140/40 mm, (±): 104-6°C/11mm°C. Source: MAN JING ZI YE. Ref: 6.

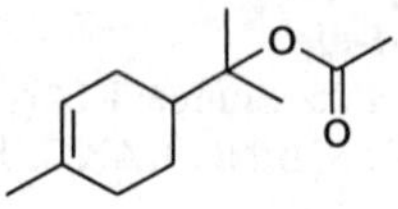

6165 Terrestriamide
$C_{18}H_{17}NO_5$ MW: 327.34 Property: light yellow crystal, mp 218-220°C. Source: CI LIJ I. Ref: 295.

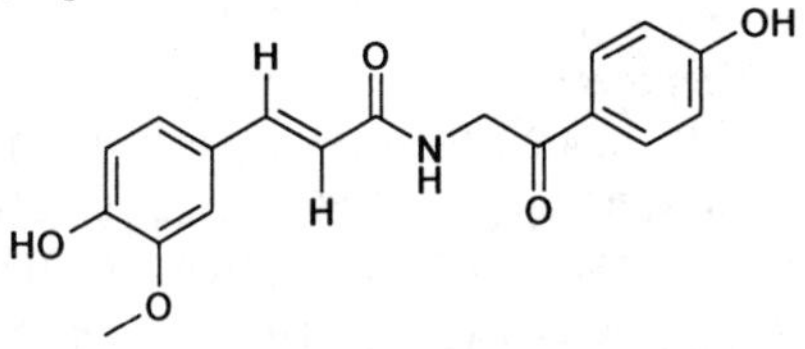

6166 α-Terthienyl
$C_{12}H_8S_3$ MW: 248.39 Property: mp 92-3°C. Source: MO HAN LIAN, WAN SHOU JU. Ref: 6, 619.

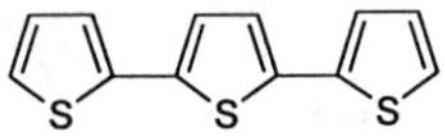

6167 α-Terthienyl methanol
$C_{13}H_{10}OS_3$ MW: 278.42 Property: mp 150-1°C. Source: MO HAN LIAN. Ref: 6.

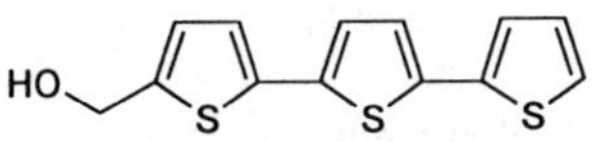

6168 α-Terthienyl methyl acetate
$C_{15}H_{12}O_2S_3$ MW: 320.45 Property: mp 114-6°C. Source: MO HAN LIAN. Ref: 6.

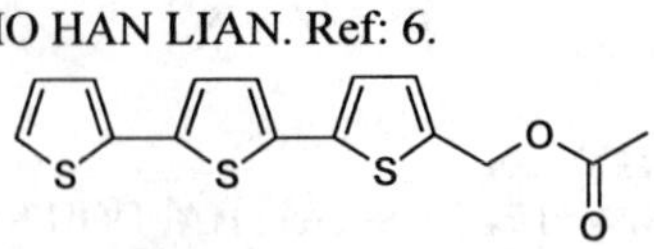

6169 Testosterone
$C_{19}H_{28}O_2$ MW: 288.43 Property: mp 154-4.5°C. Source: SHE XIANG. Ref: 2.

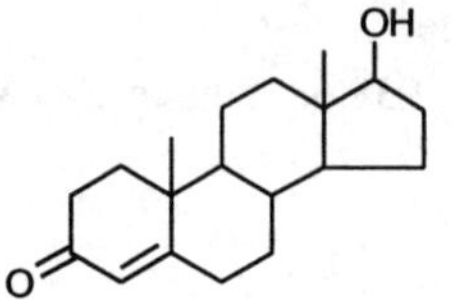

6170 5α,6β,7β,8α-Tetraacetoxy-2-[2-(4'-methoxyphenyl)ethyl]-5,6,7,8-tetrahydro-chromone (AH1a)
$C_{26}H_{28}O_{11}$ MW: 516.51 Property: amorphous crystal, mp 58-60°C (dec), $[\alpha]_D$ -14.3°. Source: CHEN XIANG. Ref: 13.

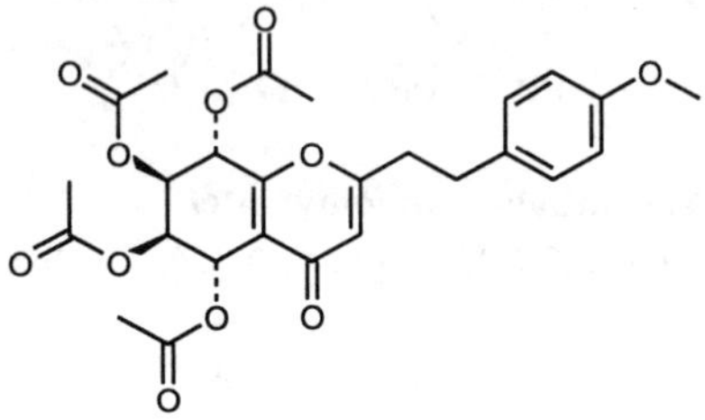

6171 Tetraacetylbrazilin
Property: mp 155-7°C. Source: SU MU. Ref: 508.

6172 n-Tetracosanoic acid
$C_{24}H_{48}O_2$ MW: 368.65 Source: DANG GUI, QIANG HUO. Ref: 2.

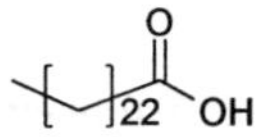

6173 Tetracosanyl ferulate
Source: GUANG XI XUE JIE. Ref: 616.

6174 Tetradecane
$C_{14}H_{30}$ MW: 198.40 Source: REN SHEN, SAN QI. Ref: 2.

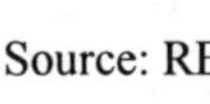

6175 Tetradecanoic acid
$C_{14}H_{28}O_2$ MW: 228.38 Property: mp 58°C, bp 250.5°C/mm. Source: BU GU ZHI, BING LANG, GAN DI HUANG, QIANG HUO, XING REN. Ref: 2.

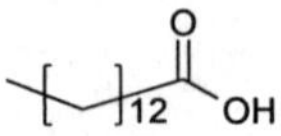

6176 1-Tetradecanol
$C_{14}H_{30}O$ MW: 214.39 Source: BAI ZHI, DANG GUI. Ref: 2.

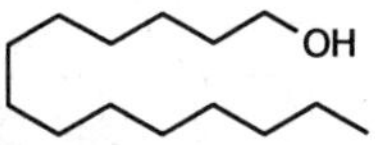

6177 1-Tetradecene
$C_{14}H_{28}$ MW: 196.38 Source: BAI ZHI, DU HUO. Ref: 2.

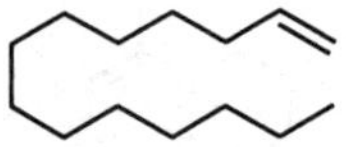

6178 cis-4-Tetradecenoic acid
$C_{14}H_{26}O_2$ MW: 226.36 Property: mp 18-8.5°C, bp 185-8°C/13 mm. Source: ZHEN CAI. Ref: 6.

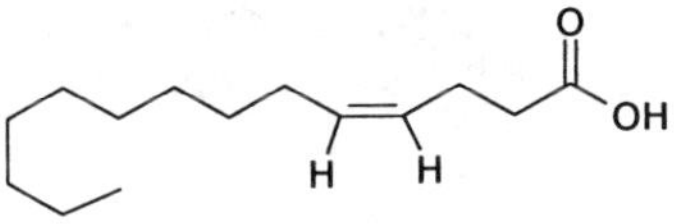

6179 Tetradecenoic acid A
Tsuzuic aicd. $C_{14}H_{26}O_2$ MW: 226.36 Source: BING LANG. Ref: 2.

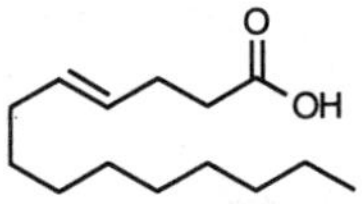

6180 Tetradecenoic acid B
Physeteric acid. $C_{14}H_{26}O_2$ MW: 226.36 Source: BING LANG. Ref: 2.

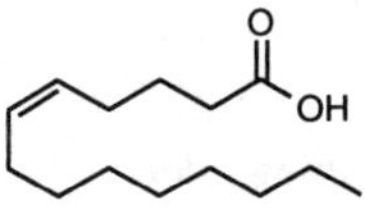

6181 Tetradecenoic acid C
Myristoleic acid. $C_{14}H_{26}O_2$ MW: 226.36 Source: BING LANG. Ref: 2.

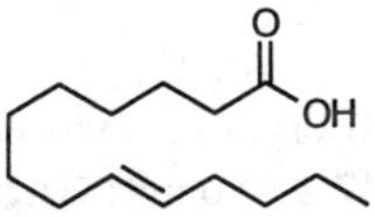

6182 Tetradec-8,10,12-triyne-6-ene-3-one
$C_{14}H_{14}O$ MW: 198.27 Source: AI YE. Ref: 6.

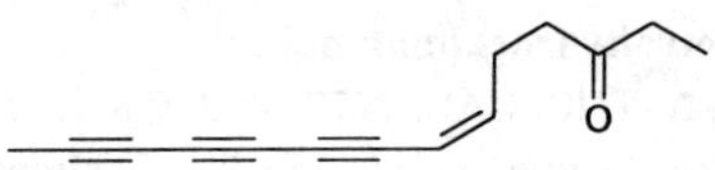

6183 1,2,9,10-Tetradehydroaristolane
$C_{15}H_{22}$ MW: 202.32 Source: GAN SONG. Ref: 6.

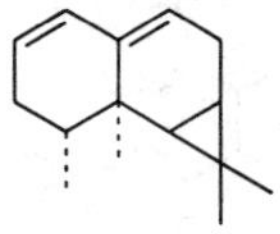

6184 1,2,3,6-Tetra-O-galloyl-β-D-glucose
$C_{34}H_{28}O_{22}$ MW: 788.59 Source: SHAN ZHU YU. Ref: 2.

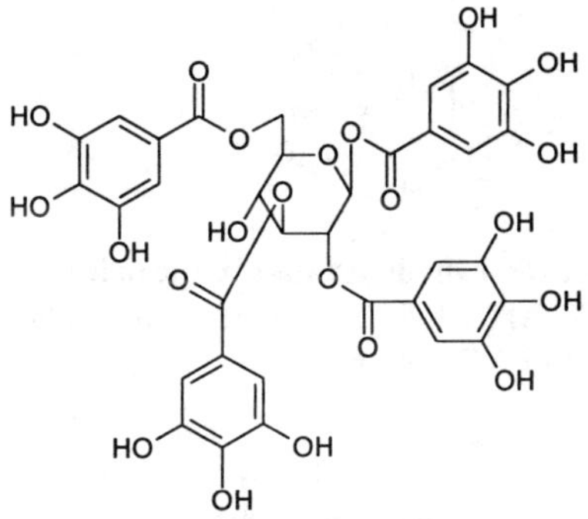

6185 Tetrahydroalstonine
(3α)-3,4,5,6-Tetrahydroalstonine. CAS: 6974-90-4
$C_{21}H_{24}N_2O_3$ MW: 352.44 Property: white crystal, mp 300-10°C, $[\alpha]_D^{23.2}$ -106.77° (c=0.48, $CHCl_3$). Source: CHANG CHUN HUA, YANG JIAO MIAN.
Ref: 4, 633.

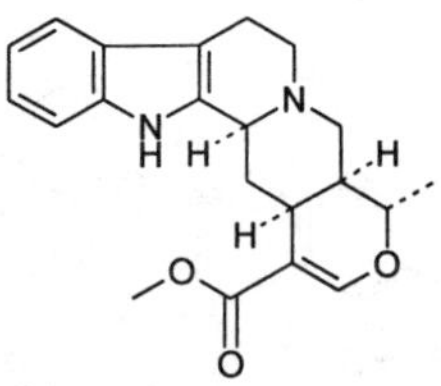

6186 (-)-Tetrahydroberberine
$C_{20}H_{21}NO_4$ MW: 339.39 Source: YAN HU SUO. Ref: 2.

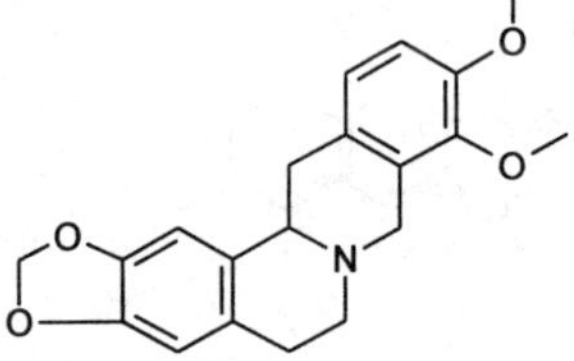

6187 Tetrahydrocannabinol Δ9
Δ^9-THC; Δ^1-THC. CAS: 1972-08-3 $C_{21}H_{30}O_2$ MW: 314.47 Property: bp D -(-): 155-7°C/0.05mm, 200°C/0.05 mm. Source: MA HUA. Ref: 4.

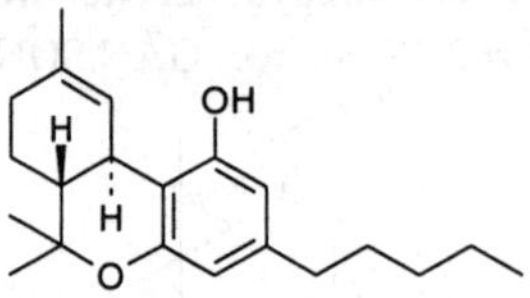

6188 Tetrahydrocannabinol Δ8
Δ^8-THC. $C_{21}H_{30}O_2$ MW: 314.47 Source: MA HUA. Ref: 6.

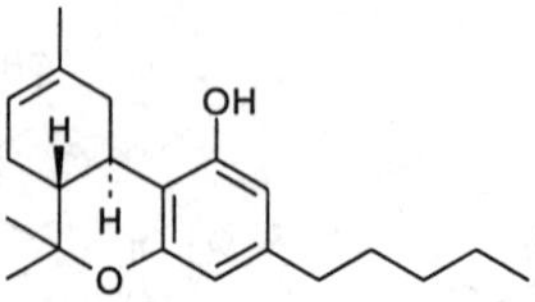

6189 Δ2-Tetrahydrocannabinolic acid
$C_{22}H_{30}O_4$ MW: 358.48 Property: mp 158-60°C (dec). Source: MA YE. Ref: 6.

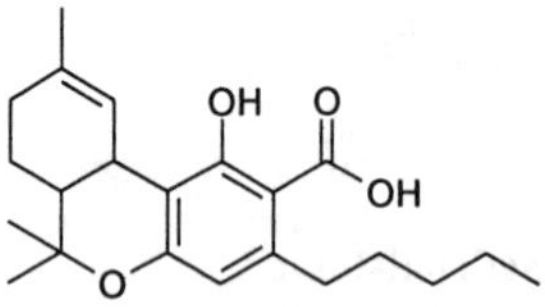

6190 (-)-Tetrahydrocoptisine
$C_{19}H_{17}NO_4$ MW: 323.35 Property: mp (-):204°C, (±): 222-3°C, bp (±): 260°C/0.01mm. Source: YAN HU SUO. Ref: 2, 6.

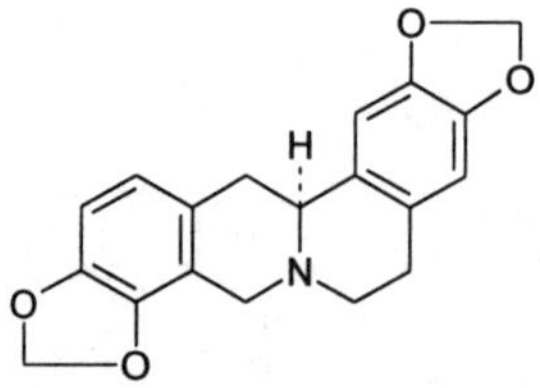

6191 Tetrahydrocorysamine
$C_{20}H_{19}NO_4$ MW: 337.38 Property: mp (-): 136-7°C, (±): 202-3°C. Source: JU HUA HUANG LIAN, YAN HU SUO, ZI HUA YU DENG CAO (LIE BAO ZI JING) . Ref: 6.

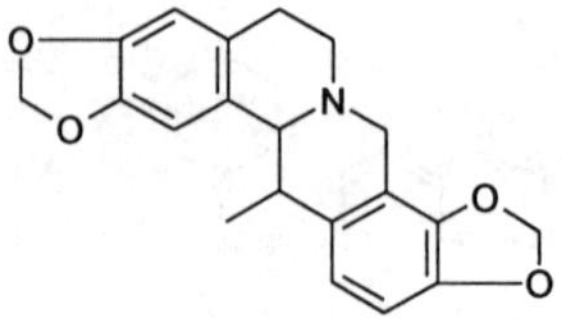

6192 Tetrahydrocyperaguinone
$C_{14}H_{14}O_4$ MW: 246.27 Property: mp 138-40°C. Source: PIAO FU CAO. Ref: 6.

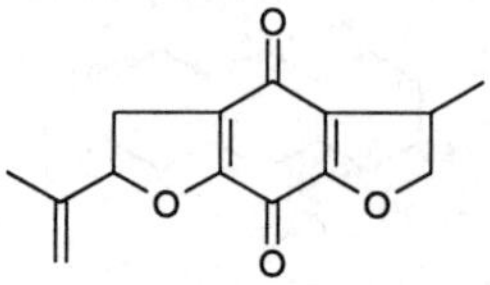

6193 5,6,7,8-Tetrahydro-2,4-dimethylquinoline
$C_{11}H_{15}N$ MW: 161.25 Source: GAN CAO. Ref: 2.

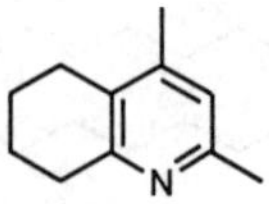

6194 Tetrahydroharman
$C_{12}H_{14}N_2$ MW: 186.26 Property: mp 178-80°C. Source: SHA ZAO SHU PI. Ref: 6.

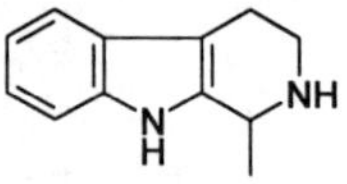

6195 Tetrahydroharmine
$C_{13}H_{16}N_2O$ MW: 219.29 Property: mp (+): 198.4-9.8°C. Source: LUO TUO PENG ZI. Ref: 6.

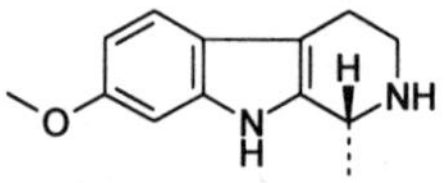

6196 Tetrahydroharmol
$C_{12}H_{14}N_2O$ MW: 202.26 Property: mp 254-5°C. Source: SHA ZAO SHU PI. Ref: 6.

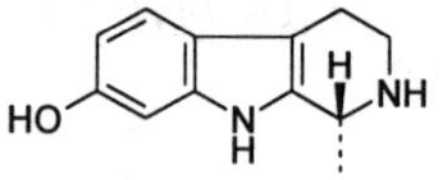

6197 Tetrahydromagnolol
$C_{18}H_{22}O_2$ MW: 270.37 Source: HOU PO. Ref: 2.

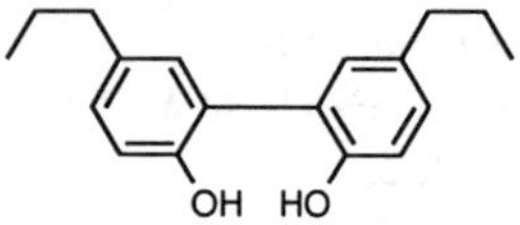

6198 5,6,7,8-Tetrahydro-4-methylquinoline
$C_{10}H_{13}N$ MW: 147.22 Source: GAN CAO. Ref: 2.

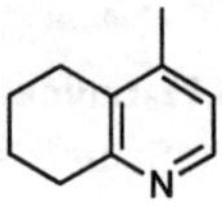

6199 1,2,3,4-Tetrahydro-1-oxo-β-carboline
$C_{11}H_{10}N_2O$ MW: 186.22 Property: white acicular crystal, mp 168-70°C. Source: WU ZHU YU. Ref: 347.

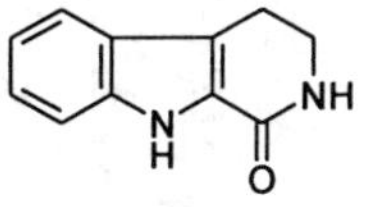

6200 Tetrahydropalmatine
Caseanine; Corydalis; Hyndarine; Rotundine; $C_{21}H_{25}NO_4$ MW: 355.44 Property: mp (+): 143°C, (-): 141-2°C, (±): 148°C. Source: HUANG BAI, HUANG JIN, JU HUA HUANG LIAN, JIN BU HUAN,YAN HU SUO, XIA TIAN WU. Ref: 4, 6.

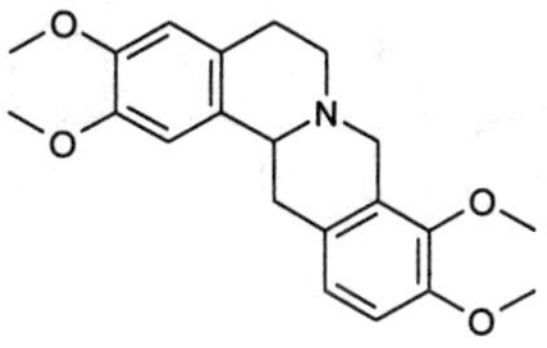

6201 Tetrahydropiperic acid
$C_{12}H_{14}O_4$ MW: 222.24 Source: BI BA. Ref: 6.

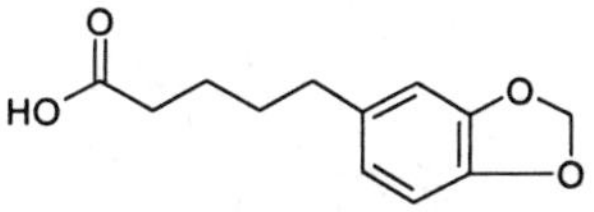

6202 1,2,15,16-Tetrahydrotanshiquinone
$C_{18}H_{16}O_3$ MW: 280.33 Property: violet red columnar crystal (methanol), mp 140-2°C. Source: BAI HUA DAN SHEN. Ref: 185.

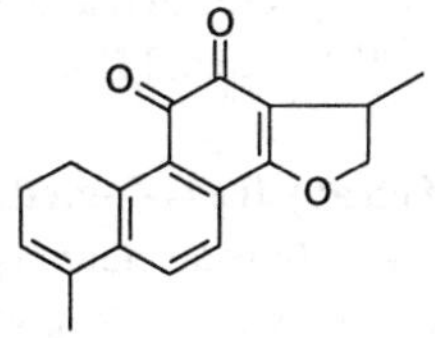

6204 3β,5β,11α,14β-Tetrahydroxy-5β-card-20(22) enolide-3α-L-rhamnoside
$C_{29}H_{44}O_{10}$ MW: 552.67 Source: LING LAN. Ref: 6.

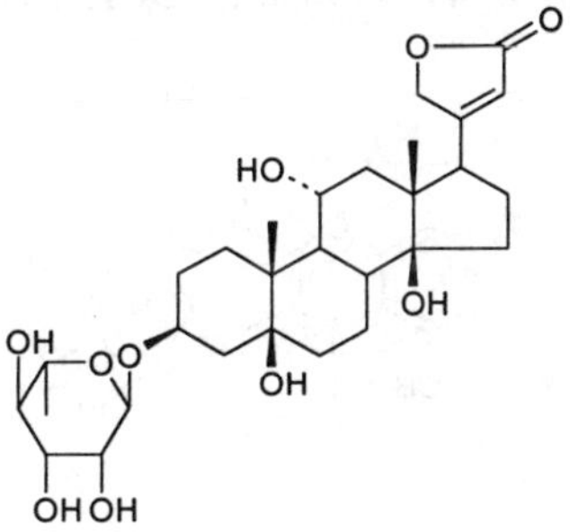

6205 3,2',4',6'-Tetrahydroxy-4,3'-dimethoxy chalcone
$C_{17}H_{16}O_7$ MW: 332.31 Source: DA JIN QIAN CAO. Ref: 2.

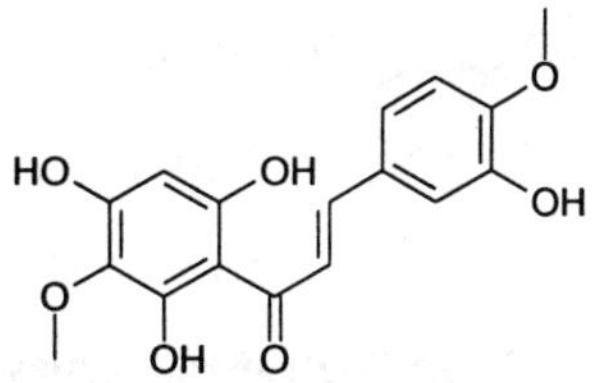

6206 5,7,2',5'-Tetrahydroxy-8,6'-dimethoxy flavone
$C_{17}H_{14}O_8$ MW: 346.30 Source: HUANG QIN. Ref: 2.

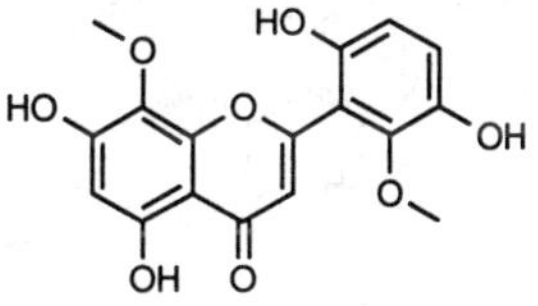

6207 5,7,3',4'-Tetrahydroxy-6,8-dimethoxy flavone
MW: 346 Property: yellow acicular crystal, mp 254-6°C. Source: MAO LIAN HAO. Ref: 474.

6208 5,7,8,3'-Tetrahydroxy-3,4'-dimethoxy flavone
$C_{17}H_{14}O_8$ MW: 346.30 Source: QING HAO. Ref: 2.

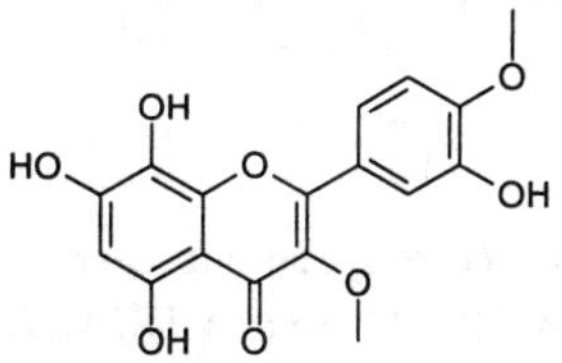

6209 7β,11β,14β,20-Tetrahydroxy-ent-kaur-16-en-6,15-dione
$C_{20}H_{26}O_6$ MW: 362.43 Property: colorless acicular crystal, mp 262-4°C. Source: ZI MAO XIANG CHA CAI. Ref: 653.

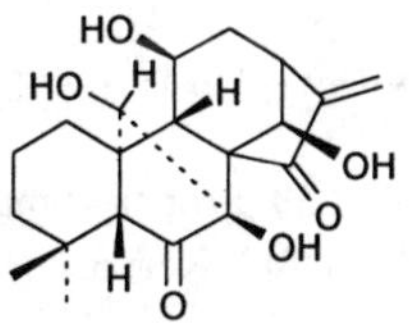

6210 3',4',5,7-Tetrahydroxyflavanol
$C_{15}H_{14}O_6$ MW: 290.28 Source: LING LAN. Ref: 6.

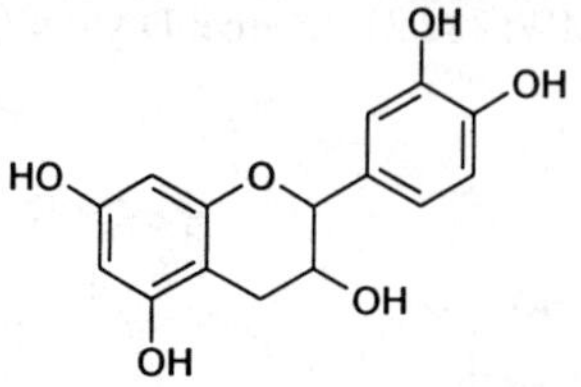

6211 (2R,3R)-2',3,5,7-tetrahydroxyflavanone
$C_{15}H_{12}O_6$ MW: 288.26 Property: light yellow rhomboid crystal, mp 119-20°C. Source: DIAN HUANG QIN. Ref: 124.

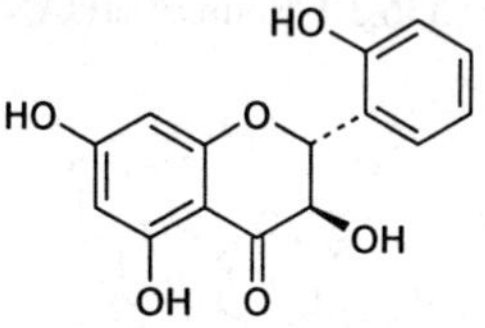

6212 5,7,3',5'-Tetrahydroxy-flavanonol-3-O-β-D-glu
Source: SAN LING. Ref: 573.

6213 5,7,2',3'-Tetrahydroxyflavone
$C_{15}H_{10}O_6$ MW: 286.24 Source: HUANG QIN. Ref: 2.

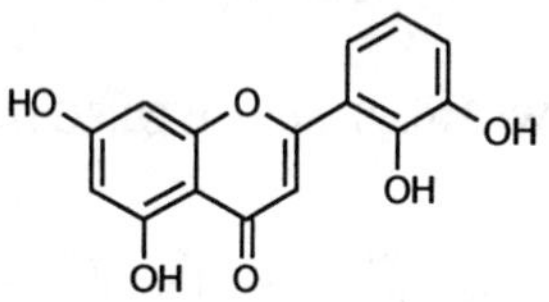

6214 5,7,2',6'-Tetrahydroxyflavone
$C_{15}H_{10}O_6$ MW: 286.24 Source: HUANG QIN. Ref: 2.

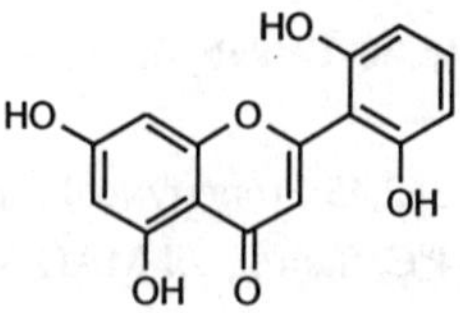

6215 3,4',5,7-Tetrahydroxyflavone-3-L-rhamnoside
$C_{21}H_{20}O_{10}$ MW: 432.39 Property: mp 172-4°C. Source: MAO YAN CAO. Ref: 6.

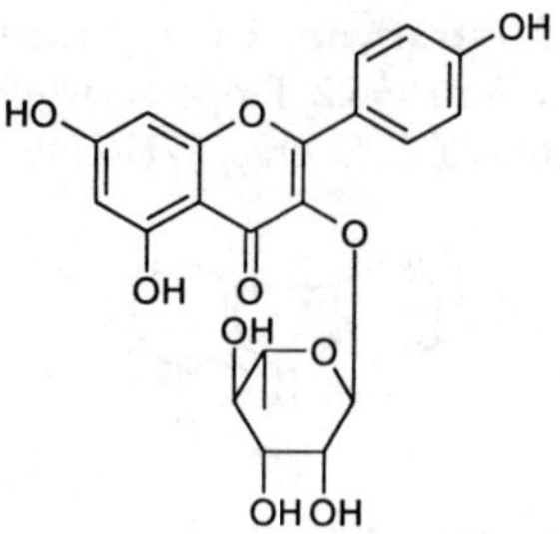

6216 5α,6β,7β,8α-Tetrahydroxy-2-[2-(2'-hydroxy phenyl)ethyl]-5,6,7,8-tetrahydrochromone (AH23)
$C_{17}H_{18}O_7$ MW: 334.33 Property: colorless acicular crystal, mp 143-5°C. Source: CHEN XIANG. Ref: 13.

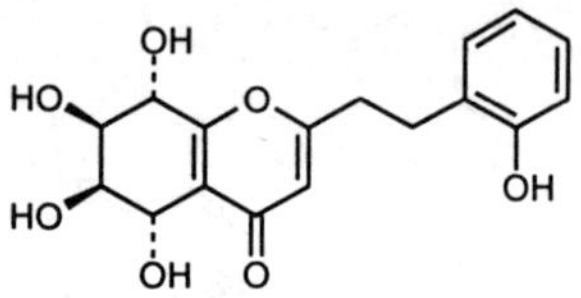

6217 2,6,2',4'-Tetrahydroxy-6'-methoxychal-cone
$C_{16}H_{14}O_6$ MW: 302.29 Source: HUANG QIN. Ref: 2.

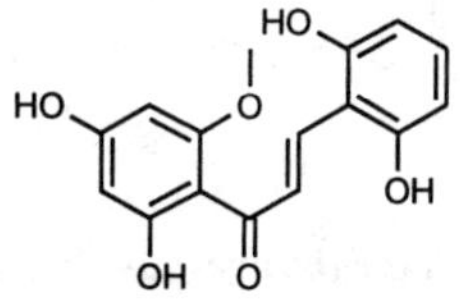

6218 5,7,3',4'-Tetrahydroxy-6-methoxy flavone MW: 316 Property: yellow acicular crystal, mp 257-9oC. Source: MAO LIAN HAO. Ref: 474.

6219 5,6,3',4'-Tetrahydroxy-7-methoxy flavone
MW: 316 Property: yellow acicular crystal, mp 300-1°C. Source: MAO LIAN HAO. Ref: 474.

6220 5,7, 3',4'-Tetrahydroxy-8-methoxy-flavonol-3-O-β-D-galactoside
$C_{22}H_{22}O_{13}$ MW: 494.41 Source: DI YANG QUE. Ref: 6.

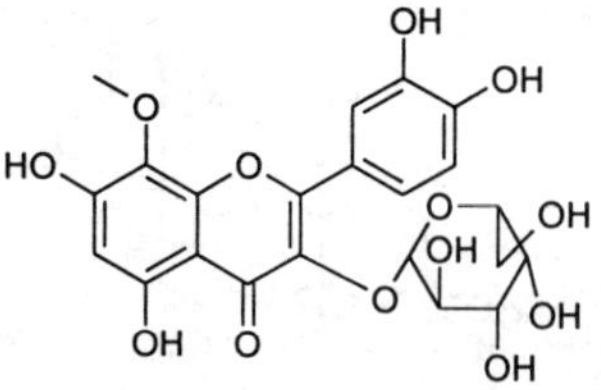

6221 5α,6β,7β,8α-Tetrahydroxy-2-[2-(4'-methoxyphenyl)ethyl]-5,6,7,8-tetrahydro chromone (AH2a)

$C_{18}H_{20}O_7$ MW: 348.36 Property: colorless acicular crystal, mp 198-9°C (dec), $[\alpha]_D$ -67.7°. Source: CHEN XIANG. Ref: 13.

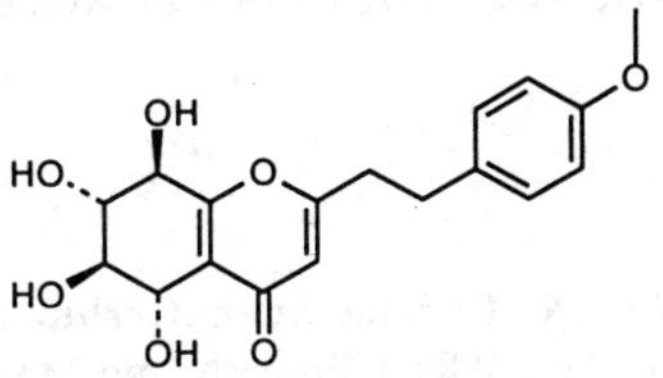

6222 5α,6β,7β,8α-Tetrahydroxy-2-[2-(2'-methoxyphenyl) ethyl]-5,6,7,8-tetrahydro-chromone (AH2b)

$C_{17}H_{18}O_7$ MW: 334.33 Property: colorless acicular crystal, mp 135-7°C (dec), $[\alpha]_D$ -40.0°. Source: CHEN XIANG. Ref: 13.

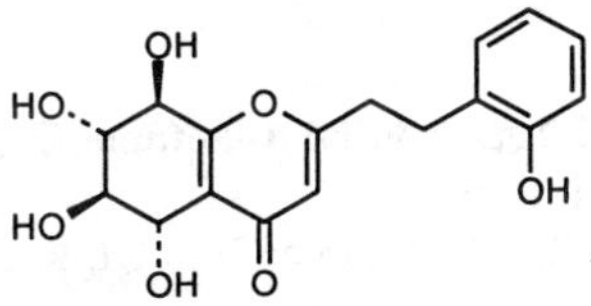

6223 Tetrahydroxynorbufostane

$C_{26}H_{46}O_4$ MW: 422.65 Property: mp 148°C. Source: CHAN CHU DAN. Ref: 6.

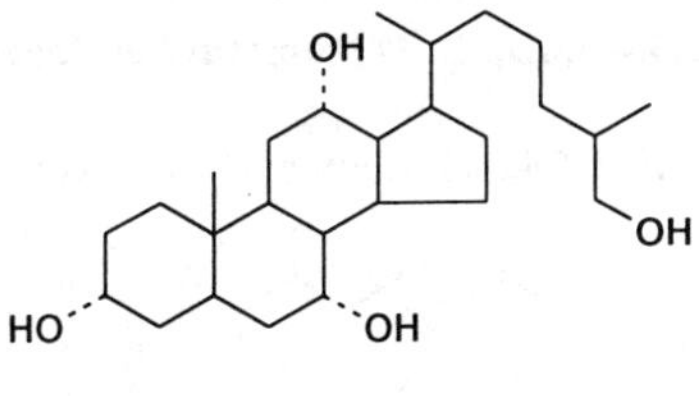

6224 Tetrahydroxystilbene (1)

$C_{14}H_{12}O_4$ MW: 244.25 Property: mp 229°C (dec). Source: FANG JI YE BA QIA, SANG ZHI. Ref: 6, 535.

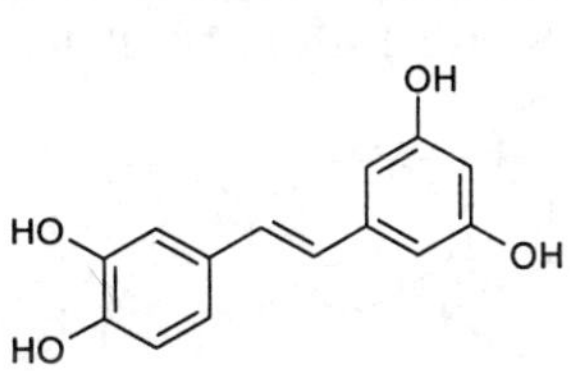

6225 Tetrahydroxystilbene (2)

$C_{14}H_{12}O_4$ MW: 244.25 Property: mp 202°C. Source: SANG ZHI. Ref: 6.

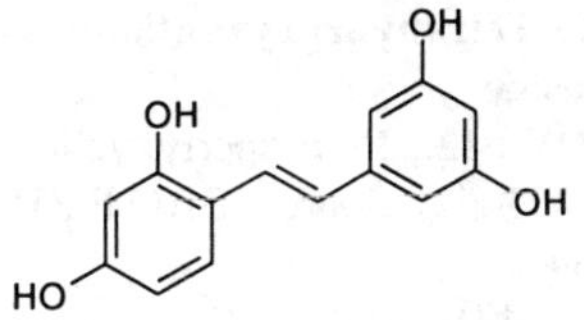

6226 2,3,5,4'-Tetrahydroxystilbene-2-O-β-D-glucoside

$C_{20}H_{22}O_9$ MW: 406.39 Source: HE SHOU WU. Ref: 2.

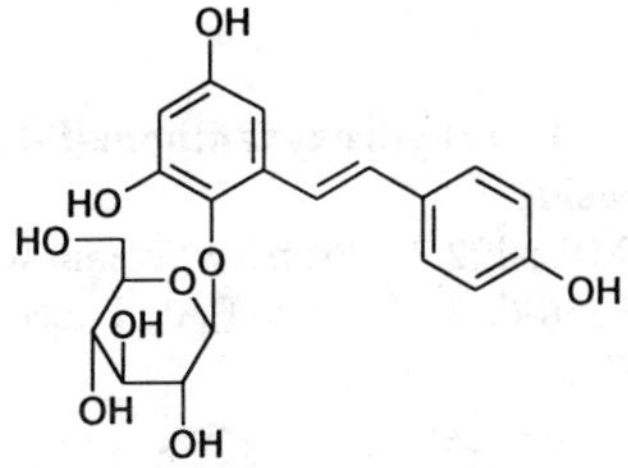

6227 3,4,3',5'-Tetrahydroxystilbene-3-glucoside

$C_{20}H_{22}O_9$ MW: 406.39 Source: DA HUANG. Ref: 2.

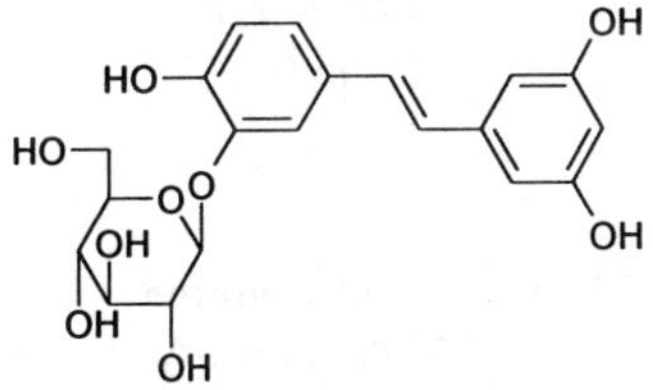

6228 2,3,5,4'-tetrahydroxystilbene-2,3-O-β-D-glucoside

$C_{26}H_{32}O_{14}$ MW: 568.54 Property: colorless acicular crystal, mp 265-7°C. Source: HE SHOU WU. Ref: 292.

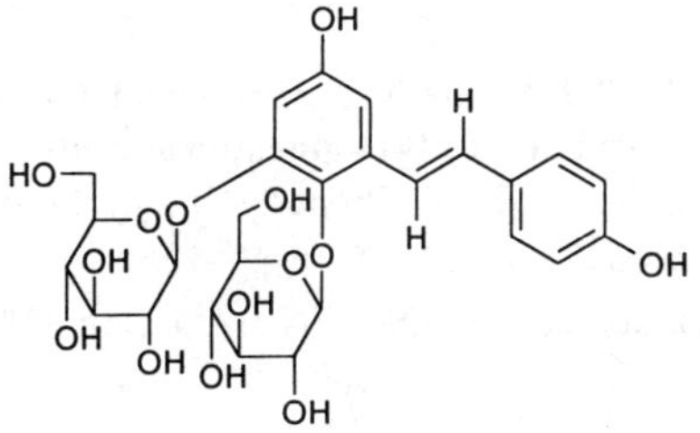

6229 1,3,6,7-Tetrahydroxyxanthone

$C_{13}H_8O_6$ MW: 260.61 Source: SHAN ZHU ZI. Ref: 6.

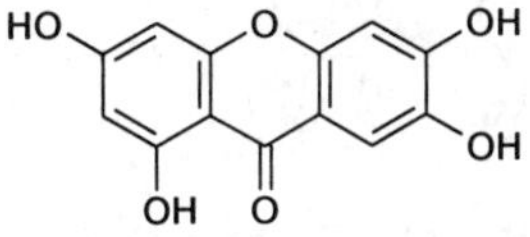

6230 1,3,7,8-Tetrahydroxyxanthone-1-O-β-D-glucopyranoside
$C_{19}H_{18}O_{11}$ MW: 422.35 Property: yellow crystalline powder, mp 255-8°C. Source: BAO E ZHANG YA CAI. Ref: 634.

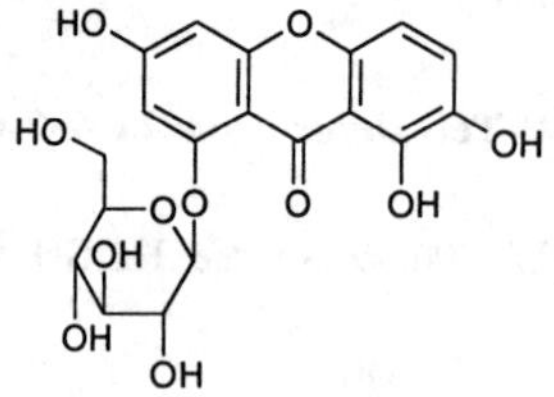

6231 1,3,7,8-Tetrahydroxyxanthone-8-O-β-D-glucopyranoside
$C_{19}H_{18}O_{11}$ MW: 422.35 Property: cream white powder, mp 256-60°C. Source: BAO E ZHANG YA CAI. Ref: 634.

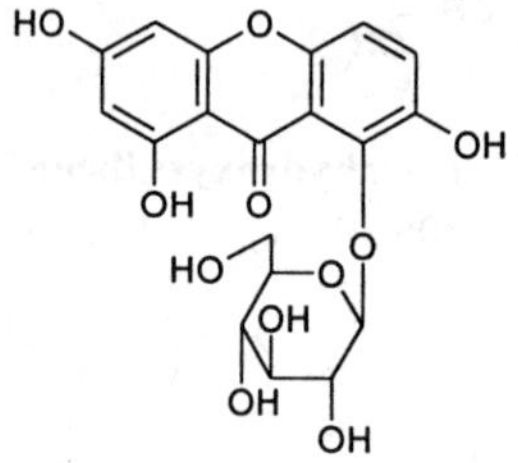

6232 3,5,3',5'-Tetraiodothyronine
$C_{15}H_{11}I_4NO_4$ MW: 776.88 Property: mp (-): 235°C, (±): 220°C(changing black), 231-3°C (dec). Source: NIU YE. Ref: 6.

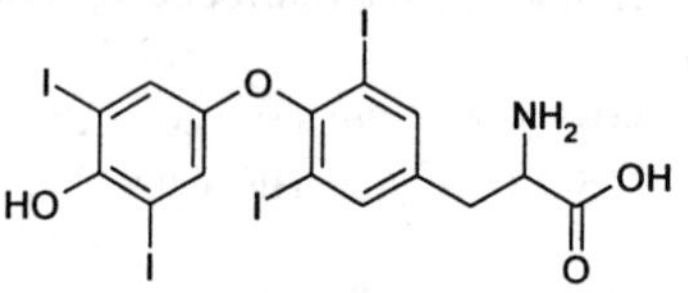

6233 2,3,4,7-Tetramethoxyxanthone-1-O-β-D-xylopyranosyl-(1→6)-β-D-glucopyranoside
$C_{28}H_{34}O_{16}$ MW: 626.57 Property: light yellow acicular crystal, mp 134-5°C, $[\alpha]_D^{25}$ -125 (c=0.4%, pyridine). Source: HUANG JIN JIAO. Ref: 328.

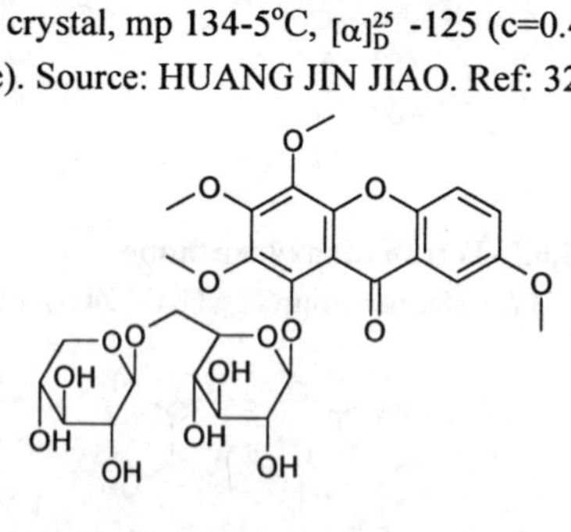

6234 (-)2D,4D,6D,8D-Tetramethyl decanoic acid
$C_{14}H_{28}O_2$ MW: 228.38 Source: E CUI. Ref: 6.

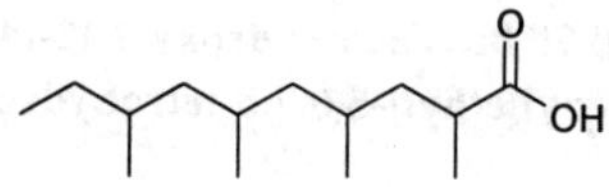

6235 Tetramethyl diaminobutane
$C_8H_{20}N_2$ MW: 144.26 Property: bp 169°C. Source: LANG DANG GEN, TIAN XIAN ZI. Ref: 6.

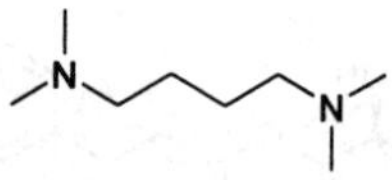

6236 N,N,N',N'-Tetramethyl-holarrhimine
$C_{25}H_{44}N_2O$ MW: 388.64 Property: mp 233-5°C. Source: ZHI XIE MU PI. Ref: 6.

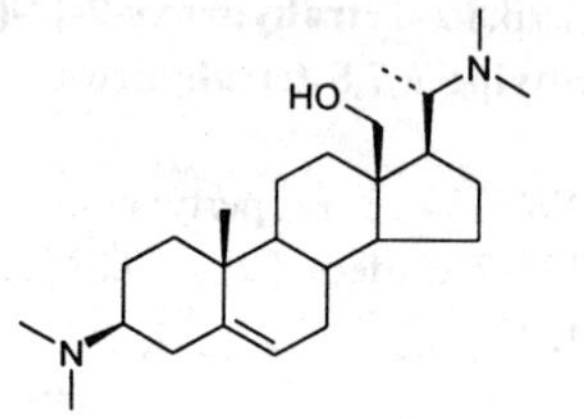

6237 1,1,5,5-Tetramethyl-4-methano-2,3,4,6,7, 10-hexahydronaphthalene
$C_{15}H_{24}$ MW: 204.36 Source: SAN QI. Ref: 2.

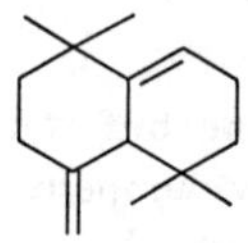

6238 (-)2D,4D,6D,8D-Tetramethyl undecanoic acid
$C_{15}H_{30}O_2$ MW: 242.41 Source: E CUI. Ref: 6.

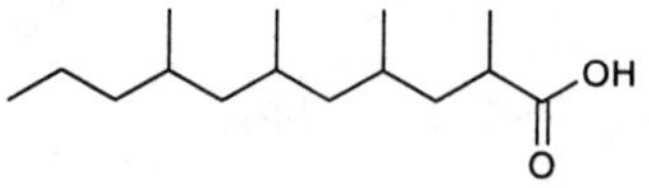

6239 Tetrandrine
Fanchinin; Hanfangchin A. CAS: 518-34-3
$C_{38}H_{42}N_2O_6$ MW: 622.77 Property: mp (+): 217-8°C, (±): 257-8°C. Source: HAN FANG JI. Ref: 5.

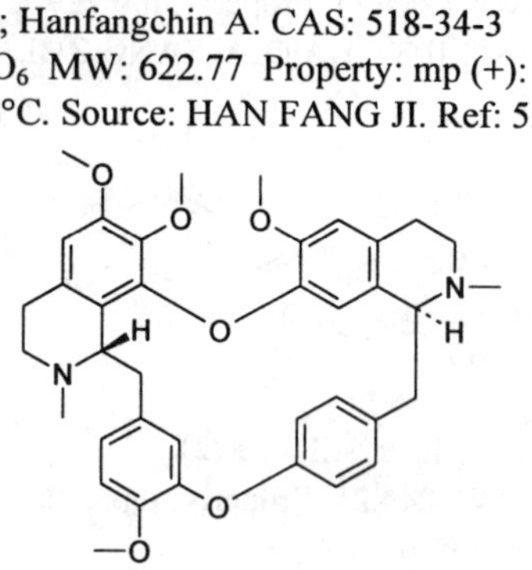

6240 Tetrodonic acid
$C_{12}H_{17}N_3O_8$ MW: 331.28 Source: HE TUN. Ref: 6.

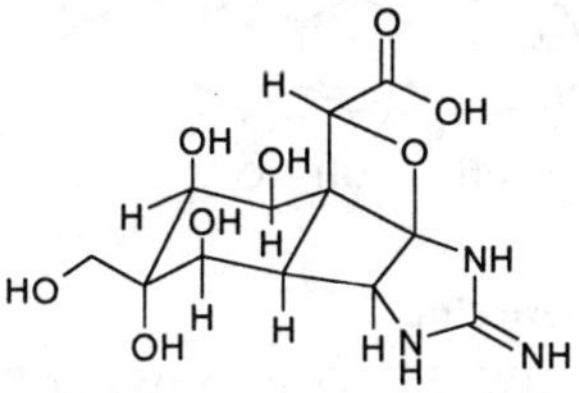

6241 Tetrodotoxin
$C_{11}H_{17}N_3O_8$ MW: 319.27 Source: HE TUN. Ref: 6.

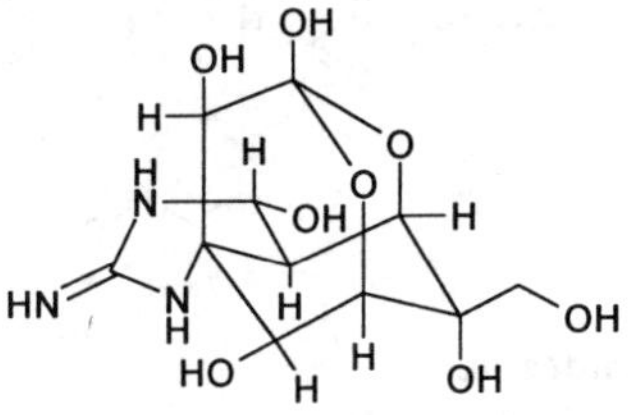

6242 Tetuin
$C_{21}H_{20}O_{10}$ MW: 432.39 Property: mp 114°C. Source: MU HU DIE. Ref: 6.

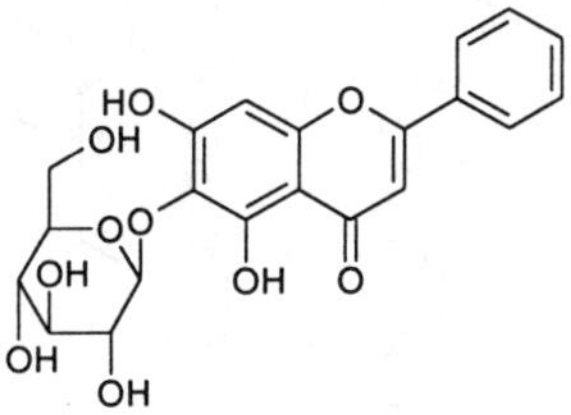

6243 Teucvin
Source: ER CHI XIANG KE KE. Ref: 577.

6244 Teuperinin A
Source: ER CHI XIANG KE KE. Ref: 577.

6245 Teuquadrin B
$C_{22}H_{26}O_7$ MW: 402.45 Property: colorless acicular crystal, mp 236-9°C, $[\alpha]_D^{26}$ +46.27°(c=0.13,$CHCl_3$). Source: TIE ZHOU CAO. Ref: 277.

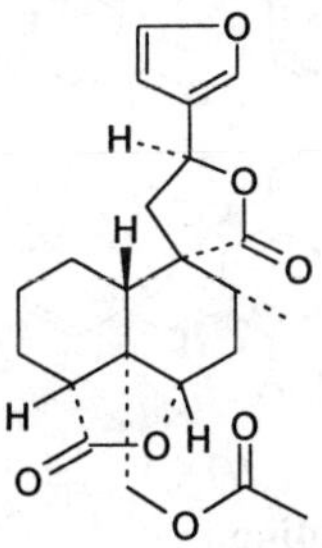

6246 Thalcimine
Thalsimine. $C_{38}H_{40}N_2O_7$ MW: 636.75 Property: mp 140-2°C. Source: MA WEI LIAN, YING SHUI HUANG LIAN. Ref: 5, 6.

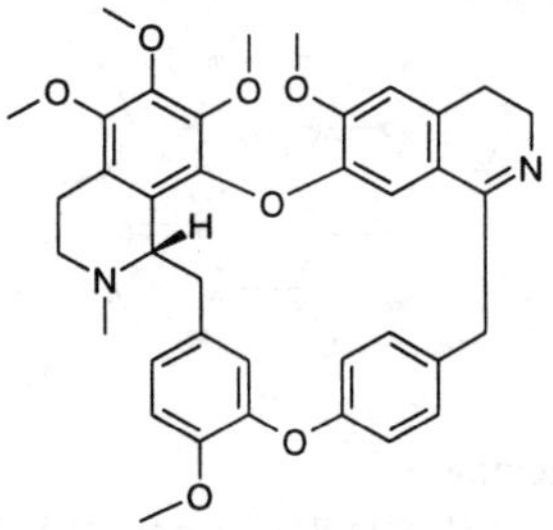

6247 Thalfoetidine
$C_{38}H_{42}N_2O_7$ MW: 638.77 Property: mp 168-70°C. Source: MA WEI LIAN. Ref: 6.

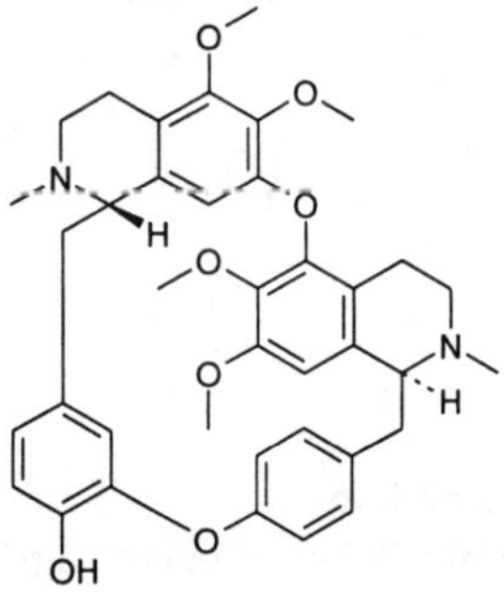

6248 Thalicberine
$C_{37}H_{40}N_2O_6$ MW: 608.74 Property: mp 161°C. Source: YAN GUO CAO. Ref: 6.

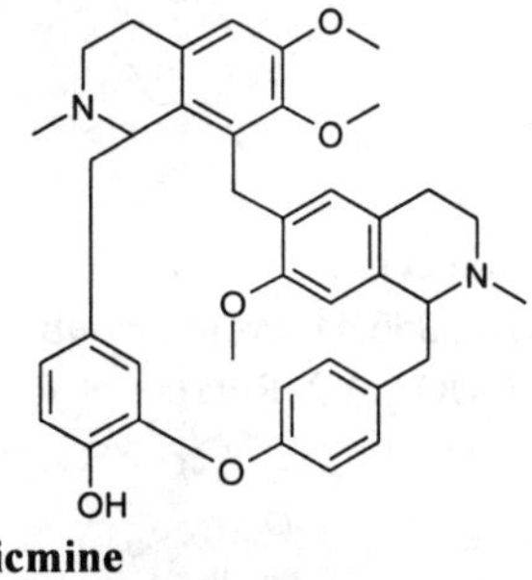

6249 Thalicmine
Ocoteine. CAS: 3246-21-7 $C_{21}H_{23}NO_5$ MW: 369.42 Property: mp 137-38°C. Source: YING SHUI HUANG LIAN. Ref: 5, 6.

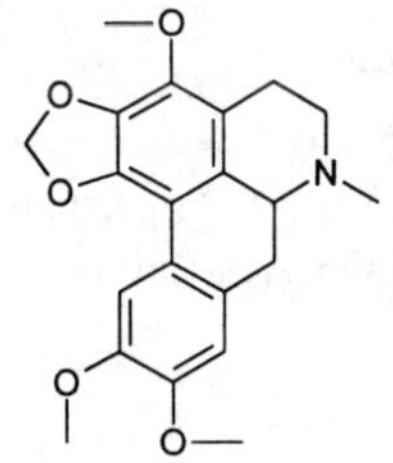

6250 Thalicminine
$C_{20}H_{15}NO_6$ MW: 365.35 Property: mp 263-5°C (chloroform), 274-5°C (chloroform-ethanol). Source: YING SHUI HUANG LIAN. Ref: 6.

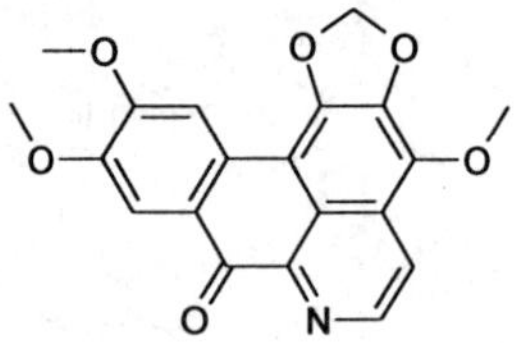

6251 Thalicrine
$C_{36}H_{38}N_2O_6$ MW: 594.71 Source: YAN GUO CAO. Ref: 6.

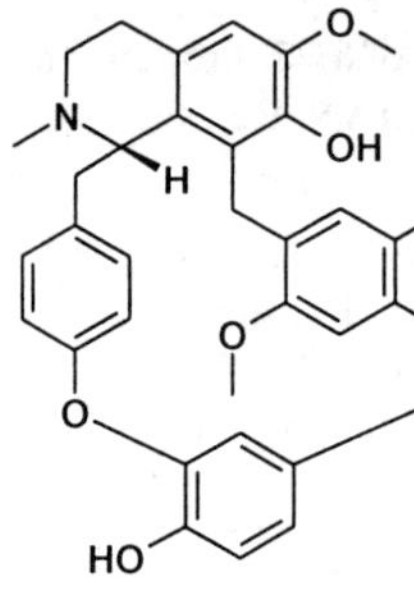

6252 Thalicsimidine
$C_{22}H_{27}NO_5$ MW: 385.46 Property: mp 131-2°C. Source: YING SHUI HUANG LIAN.Ref: 6.

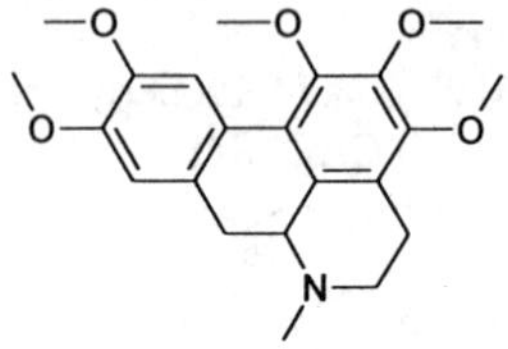

6253 Thalicthuberine
$C_{21}H_{25}NO_4$ MW: 355.44 Property: mp 126-7°C. Source: YAN GUO CAO. Ref: 6.

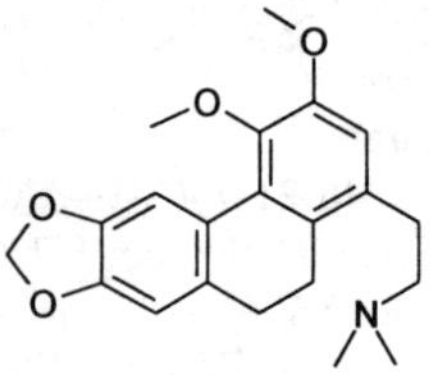

6254 Thalictiin
$C_{21}H_{20}O_{10}$ MW: 432.39 Property: mp 238-9.5°C. Source: YAN GUO CAO. Ref: 6.

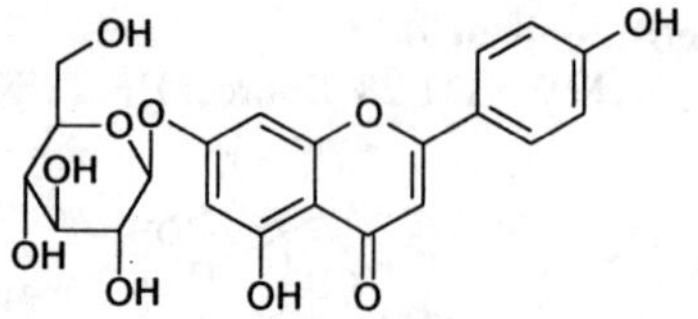

6255 Thalictircine
$C_{20}H_{21}NO_5$ MW: 355.39 Property: mp 261-3°C. Source: YING SHUI HUANG LIAN. Ref: 6.

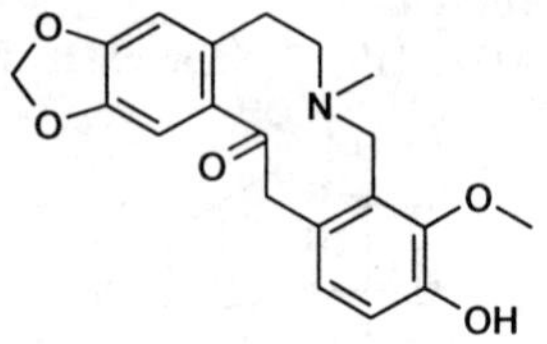

6256 Thalidezine
$C_{38}H_{42}N_2O_7$ MW: 638.77 Property: mp 158-9°C. Source: YING SHUI HUANG LIAN. Ref: 6.

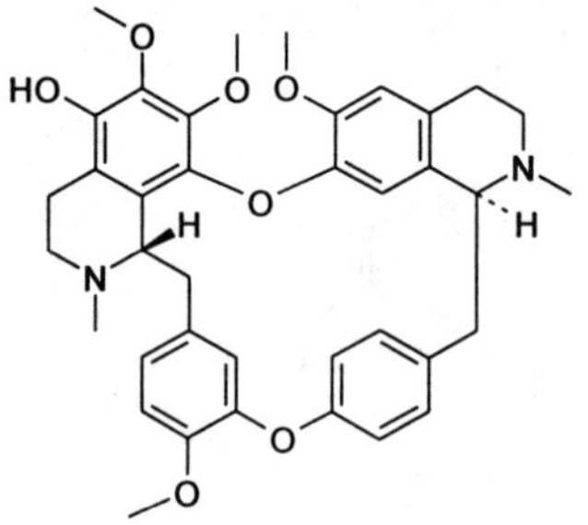

6257 Thalifendine
Source: HE NAN TANG SONG CAO. Ref: 537.

6258 Thalisamine
$C_{39}H_{44}N_2O_7$ MW: 652.79 Property: mp 191-4°C. Source: YING SHUI HUANG LIAN. Ref: 6.

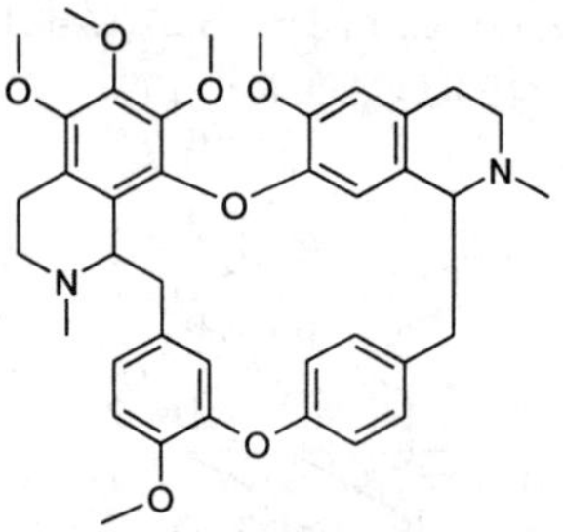

6259 Thalmelatidine
Source: HE NAN TANG SONG CAO. Ref: 537.

6260 Thalphinine
$C_{39}H_{42}N_2O_8$ MW: 666.78 Source: MA WEI LIAN. Ref: 6.

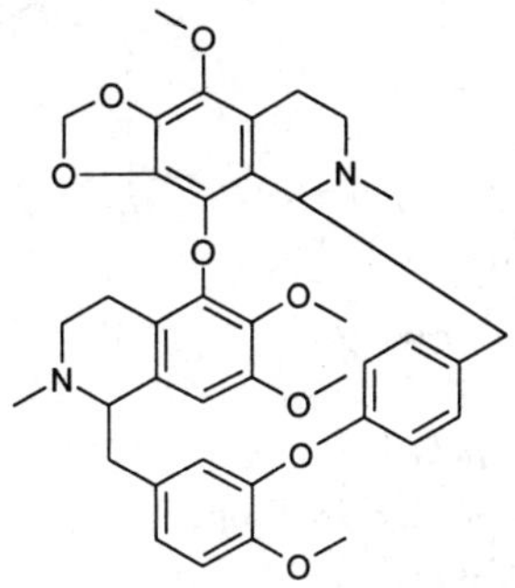

6261 Thalpine
$C_{38}H_{36}N_2O_8$ MW: 648.72 Source: MA WEI LIAN. Ref: 6.

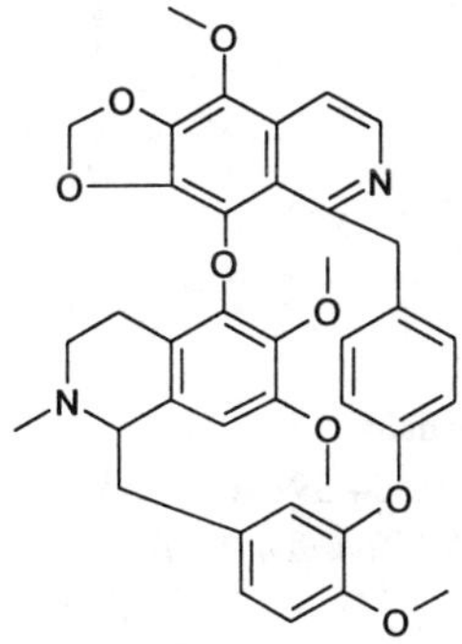

6263 Thamnolic acid
$C_{19}H_{16}O_{11}$ MW: 420.33 Property: mp 223°C. Source: XUE CHA. Ref: 6.

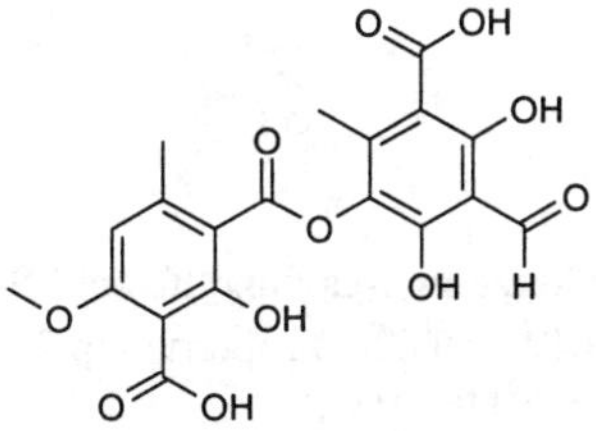

6264 Thaspine
Taspine. Source: HONG MAO QI. Ref: 6.

6265 Theanine
$C_7H_{14}N_2O_3$ MW: 174.20 Property: mp 217-8°C(dec). Source: CHA ZI XIN, CHA ZI, YOU CHA GEN PI. Ref: 6.

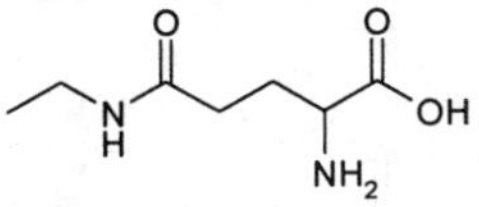

6266 Theaspirone
$C_{13}H_{20}O_2$ MW: 208.30 Source: CHA YE. Ref: 6.

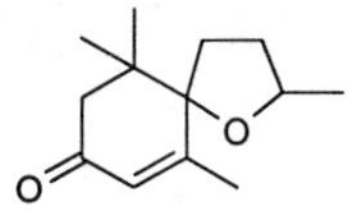

6267 Thebaine
$C_{19}H_{21}NO_3$ MW: 311.38 Property: mp 193°C. Source: LI CHUN HUA, LI CHUN HUA, YA PIAN, YING SU, YING SU KE. Ref: 6.

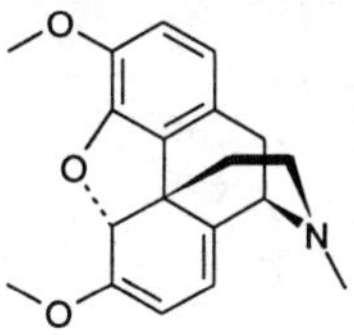

6268 Theobromine
$C_7H_8N_4O_2$ MW: 180.17 Property: mp 351°C, 290°C (sub). Source: CHA YE. Ref: 6.

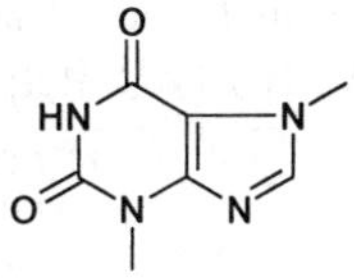

6269 Theophylline
$C_7H_8N_4O_2$ MW: 180.17 Property: mp 264°C. Source: CHA YE. Ref: 6.

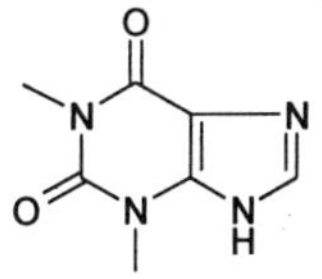

6270 Thermopsamine
$C_{15}H_{26}N_2O$ MW: 250.39 Property: mp 154-5°C. Source: MU MA DOU. Ref: 6.

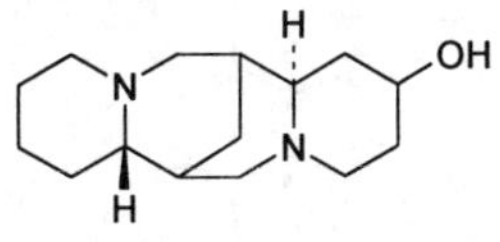

6271 Thermopsine
$C_{15}H_{20}N_2O$ MW: 244.34 Property: mp (+): 207°C, (-): 206.5°C, (±): 171-2°C. Source: GAO SHAN HUANG HUA, MU MA DOU, YE JUE MING. Ref: 6.

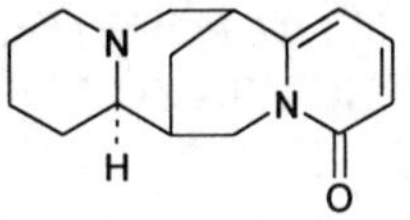

6272 Thevebioside
$C_{36}H_{56}O_{13}$ MW: 696.84 Source: HUANG HUA JIA ZHU TAO. Ref: 6.

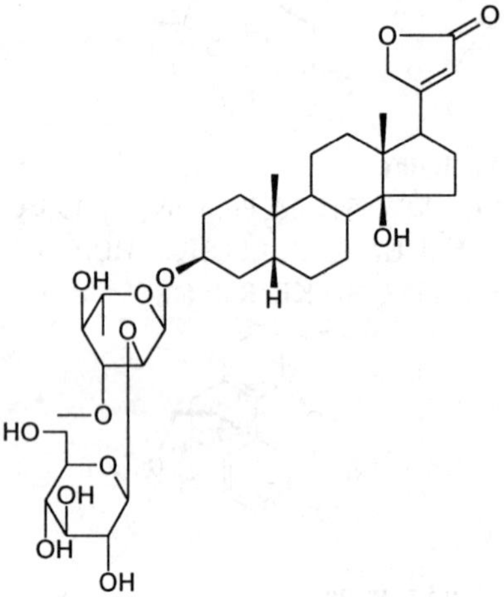

6273 Thevefolin
$C_{30}H_{46}O_8$ MW: 534.70 Property: mp 260°C. Source: HUANG HUA JIA ZHU TAO. Ref: 6.

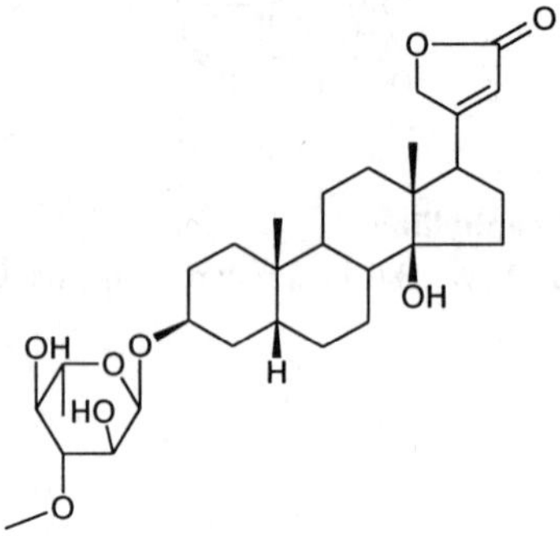

6274 Thevesid
$C_{16}H_{22}O_{11}$ MW: 390.35 Source: HUANG HUA JIA ZHU TAO. Ref: 6.

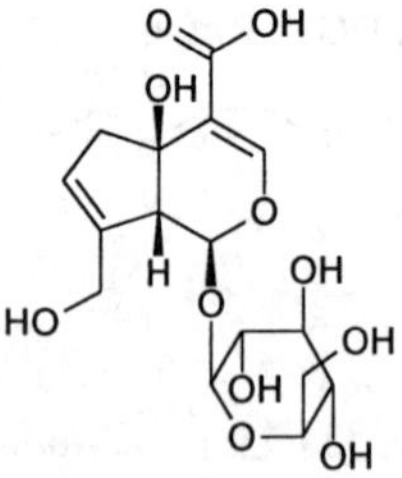

6275 Thevetin A
$C_{42}H_{64}O_{19}$ MW: 872.97 Property: mp 208-10°C. Source: HUANG HUA JIA ZHU TAO. Ref: 6.

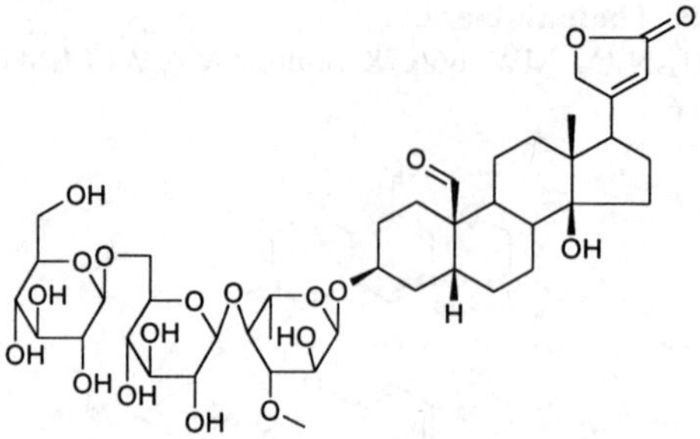

6276 Thevetin B
$C_{42}H_{66}O_{18}$ MW: 858.98 Property: mp 197-201°C. Source: HUANG HUA JIA ZHU TAO. Ref: 6.

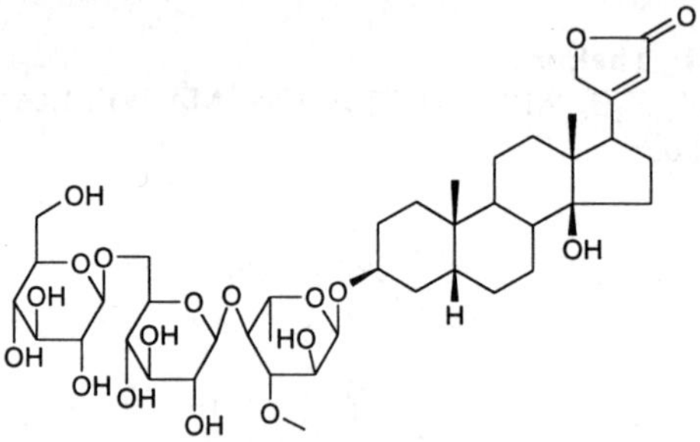

6277 Theviridoside
$C_{17}H_{24}O_{11}$ MW: 404.39 Source: HUANG HUA JIA ZHU TAO, MA YING DAN. Ref: 6, 234.

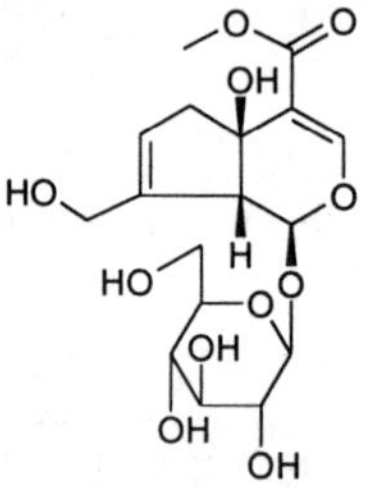

6278 1,4-Thiazane-3-carboxylic acid S-oxide
$C_5H_{9N}O_3S$ MW: 163.20 Property: mp 248-50°C (dec). Source: KUN BU. Ref: 6.

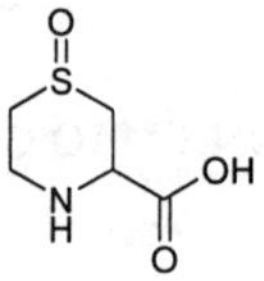

6279 3-(2-Thienyl) propargyl aldehyde
C_7H_4OS MW: 136.17 Source: YANG SHI CAO. Ref: 6.

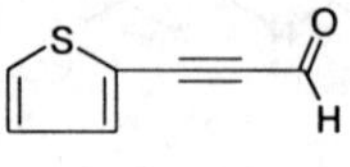

6280 1-Thiocyano-2-hydroxy-3-butene
C_5H_7NOS MW: 129.18 Source: DA QING YE. Ref: 2.

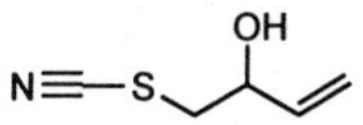

6281 Thladioside H1
Property: white powder, mp 220°C (dec). Source: DA BAO CHI BO. Ref: 425.

6282 Threitol
$C_4H_{10}O_4$ MW: 122.12 Property: mp D (+): 88.5-9°C, L (-): 88°C, DL: 72°C. Source: ZHEN MO. Ref: 6.

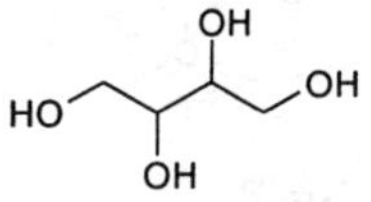

6283 Threo-dihydroxydehydrodiconiferyl alcohol
$C_{20}H_{24}O_8$ MW: 392.41 Source: DU ZHONG. Ref: 2.

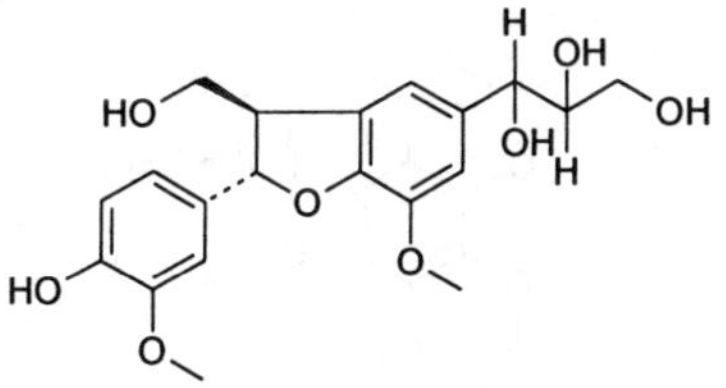

6284 (±)-Threo-guaiacylglycerol
$C_{10}H_{14}O_5$ MW: 214.22 Source: DU ZHONG. Ref: 2.

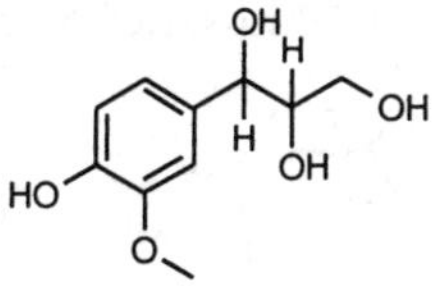

6285 Thujanol-4
$C_{10}H_{18}O$ MW: 154.25 Property: *cis*-: (+): mp 36.5-7.2°C, trans-: (+): mp 60-1°C, bp 193-8°C. Source: SHE XIANG CAO. Ref: 6.

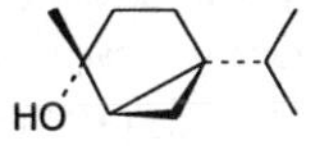

6286 α-Thujaplicin
$C_{10}H_{12}O_2$ MW: 162.21 Property: mp 82°C. Source: SHAN CI BAI. Ref: 6.

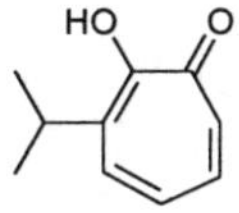

6287 β-Thujaplicin
$C_{10}H_{12}O_2$ MW: 162.21 Property: mp 52-2.5°C. Source: SHAN CI BAI. Ref: 6.

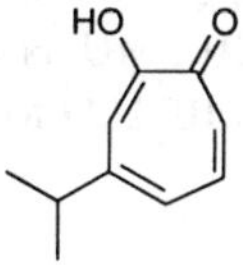

6288 Thujene
$C_{10}H_{16}$ MW: 136.24 Property: bp (+): 152-2.5°C, (-): 151°C. Source: JU PI, QIANG HUO, SHENG JIANG. Ref: 2.

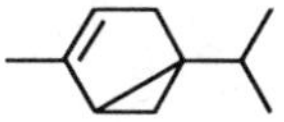

6289 1-Thujone
$C_{10}H_{16}O$ MW: 152.24 Source: YIN CHEN HAO. Ref: 2.

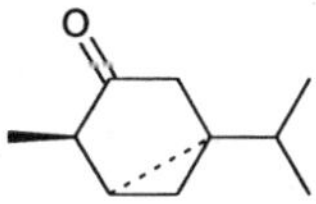

6290 Thujopsadiene
$C_{15}H_{22}$ MW: 202.34 Property: bp 115°C/10 mm. Source: BAI ZHI JIE. Ref: 6.

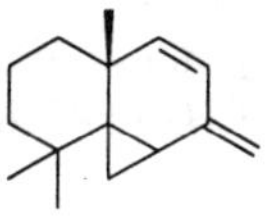

6291 Thujopsene
$C_{15}H_{24}$ MW: 204.36 Property: bp 121-2°C/12mm. Source: WU WEI ZI. Ref: 2.

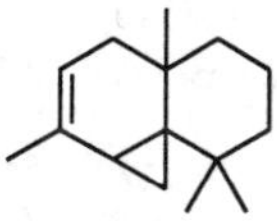

6292 Thujyalcohol
$C_{10}H_{16}O$ MW: 152.24 Property: mp (-): 66-7°C. Source: YIN CHEN HAO. Ref: 2.

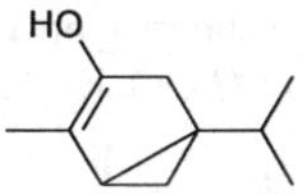

6293 Thymidine
$C_{10}H_{14}N_2O_5$ MW: 242.09 Property: colorless acicular crystal, mp 184-6.5°C (methanol). Source: AN HUI BEU MU, GAN SU BEI MU, NAN FANG TU SI ZI, PING BEI MU, TOU JIE HAI MIAN, ZHE BEI MU. Ref: 459, 569, 689

6294 Thymine
$C_5H_6N_2O_2$ MW: 126.12 Property: mp 326°C. Source: MU ZEI. Ref: 2.

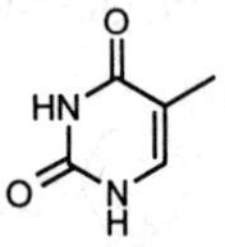

6295 Thymohydroquinone
$C_{10}H_{14}O_2$ MW: 154.25 Property: mp 143°C, bp 290°C. Source: PEI LAN. Ref: 6.

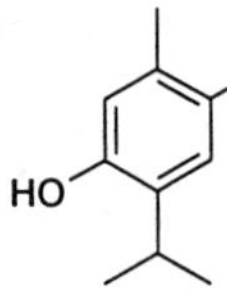

6296 Thymol
Thyme camphor; M-Thymol. CAS: 89-83-8 $C_{10}H_{14}O$ MW: 150.22 Property: mp 51.5°C, bp 211-2°C/745mm. Source: CHAI HU, DU HUO, JU PI. Ref: 2, 4.

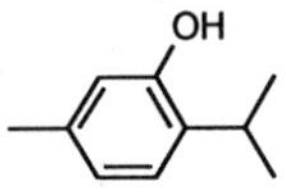

6297 Thymol methyl ether
$C_{11}H_{16}O$ MW: 164.25 Source: WU WEI ZI. Ref: 2.

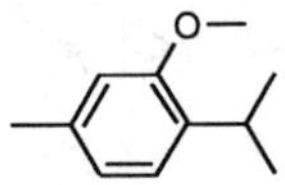

6298 Tiglaldehyde
C_5H_8O MW: 84.12 Property: bp 116.5-7.5°C/738 mm. Source: XI XIANG CONG. Ref: 6.

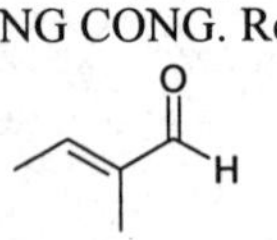

6299 Tiglic acid
$C_5H_8O_2$ MW: 100.12 Source: BA DOU, DU HUO. Ref: 2.

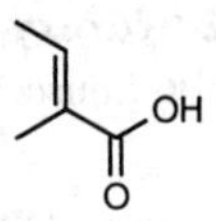

6300 Tigloylgomisin H
Source: WU WEI ZI. Ref: 2.

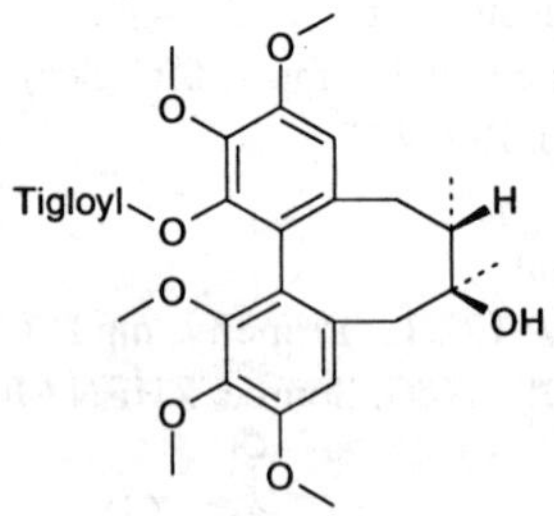

6301 Tigloylgomisin P
Source: WU WEI ZI. Ref: 2.

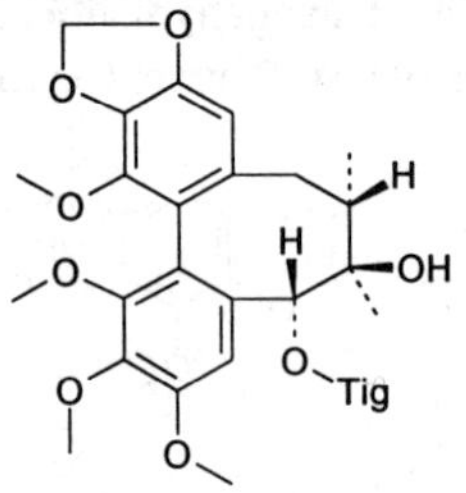

6302 3α-Tigloyloxytropane
$C_{13}H_{21}NO_2$ MW: 223.32 Property: mp 181.5-3°C. Source: SUAN JIANG GEN. Ref: 6.

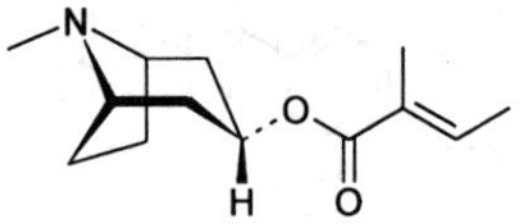

6303 Tigogenin
$C_{27}H_{44}O_3$ MW: 416.65 Property: mp 205-6°C, raw material for synthesis of steroid cortical hormones drugs. Source: BAI MAO TENG, DONG YI HAO JIAN MA, DUAN YE LONG SHE LAN, FAN MA, HU LU BA, JIAN MA, KU QIE, NIAN YU XU, WU CI FAN MA, XIA YE LONG SHE LAN, ZHANG LIU TOU. Ref: 6, 10.

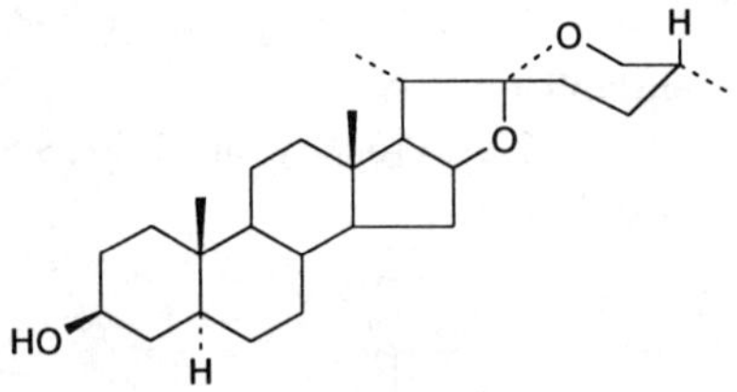

6304 Tigogenone
$C_{27}H_{42}O_3$ MW: 414.63 Class: B1, 5α-sapogenin.
Source: WU CI FAN MA. Ref: 10.

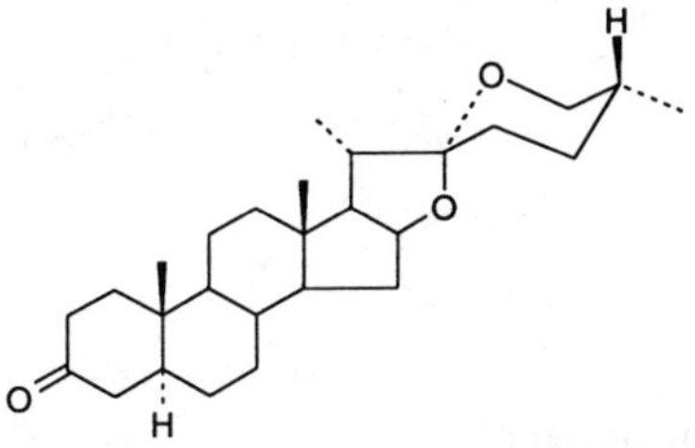

6305 Tilianine
$C_{22}H_{22}O_{10}$ MW: 446.41 Source: HUO XIANG.
Ref: 2.

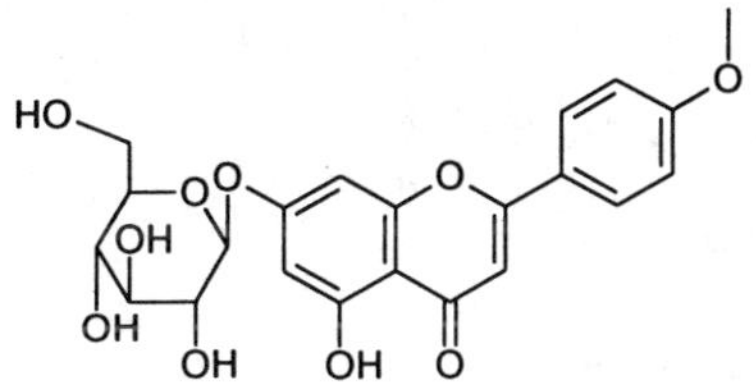

6306 Timobiose
$C_{12}H_{22}O_{11}$ MW: 342.30 Property: mp 164-70°C.
Source: ZHI MU. Ref: 2.

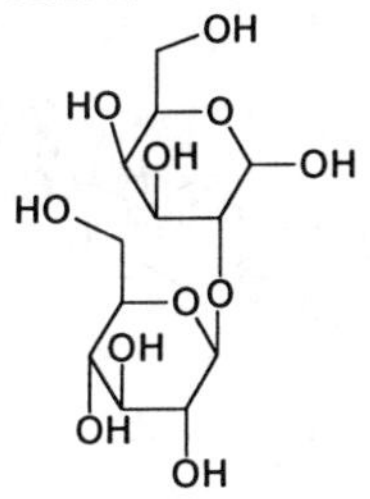

6307 Timosaponin A-1
$C_{33}H_{54}O_8$ MW: 578.79 Source: ZHI MU. Ref: 2.

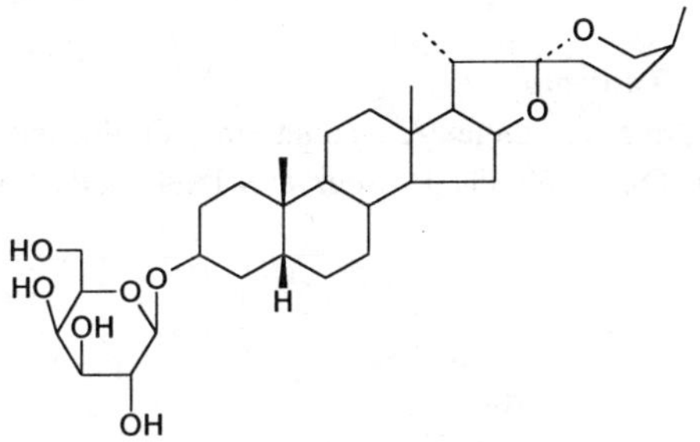

6308 Timosaponin A-III
$C_{39}H_{64}O_{13}$ MW: 740.94 Property: mp 317-22°C (dec). Source: ZHI MU. Ref: 6.

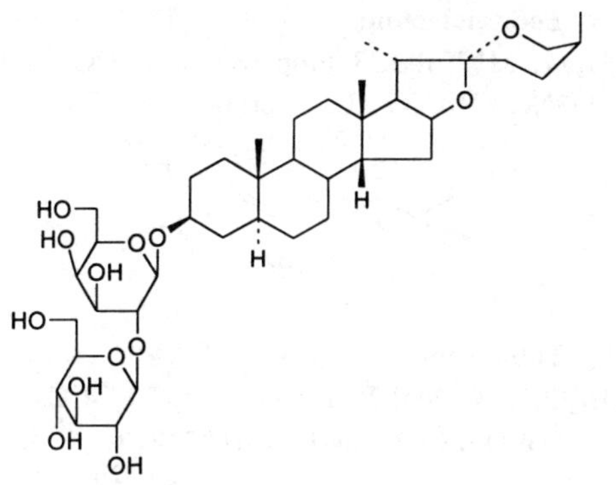

6309 (24Z)-7,24-Tirucalladien-3β,27-diol
$C_{30}H_{50}O_2$ MW: 442.73 Source: KU SHU PI. Ref: 12.

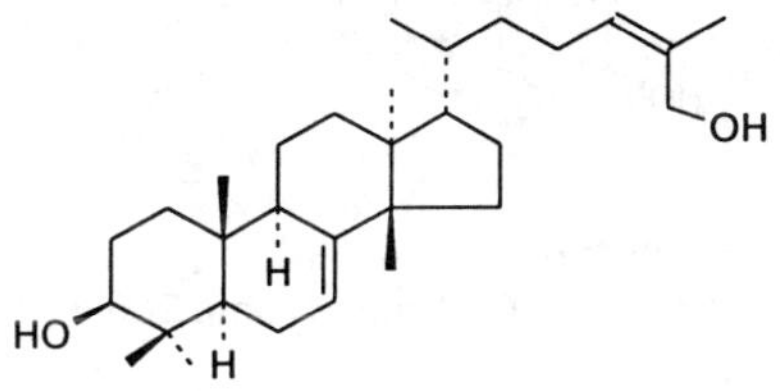

6310 TN-1
$C_{35}H_{60}O_8$ MW: 608.86 Source: QI YE DAN. Ref: 2.

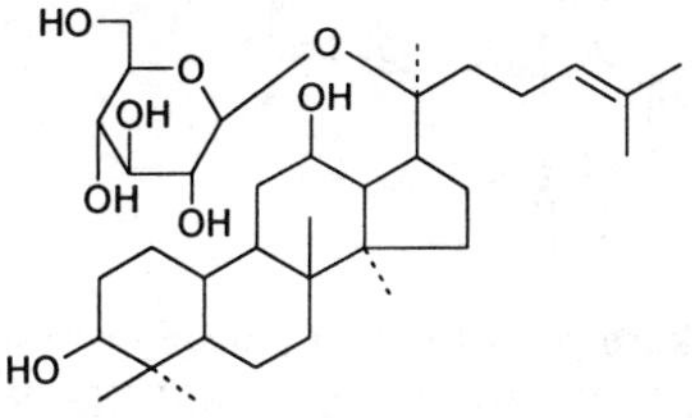

6311 TN-2
Source: QI YE DAN. Ref: 2.

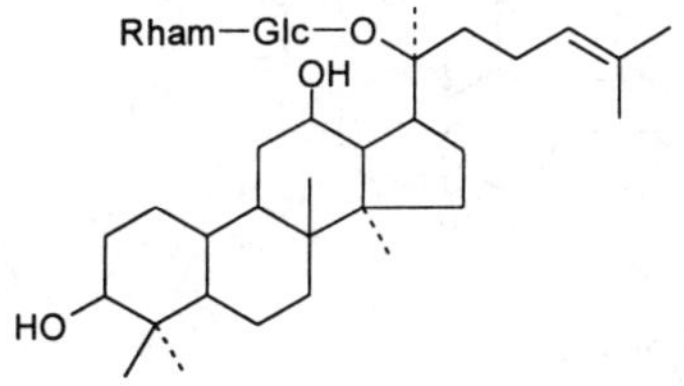

6312 Toddaculine
$C_{16}H_{18}O_4$ MW: 274.32 Property: mp 95°C. Source: FEI LONG ZHANG XUE. Ref: 6.

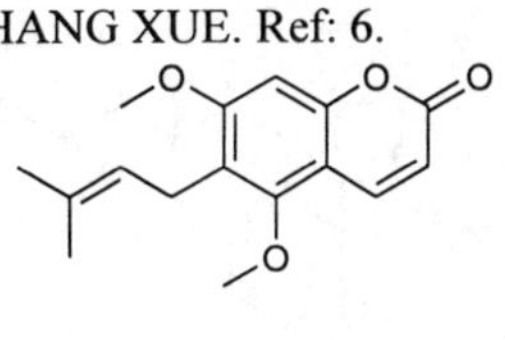

6313 Toddalolactone
$C_{16}H_{20}O_6$ MW: 308.33 Property: mp 132°C. Source: FEI LONG ZHANG XUE. Ref: 6.

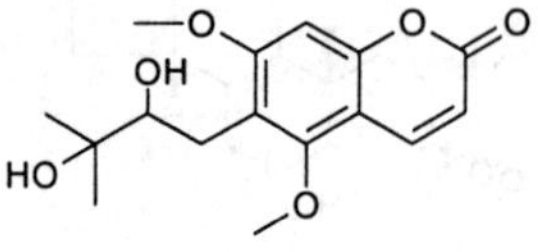

6314 Tohogenol
$C_{30}H_{52}O_3$ MW: 460.75 Property: mp 242-4°C. Source: GUO JIANG LONG, QIAN CENG TA. Ref: 6.

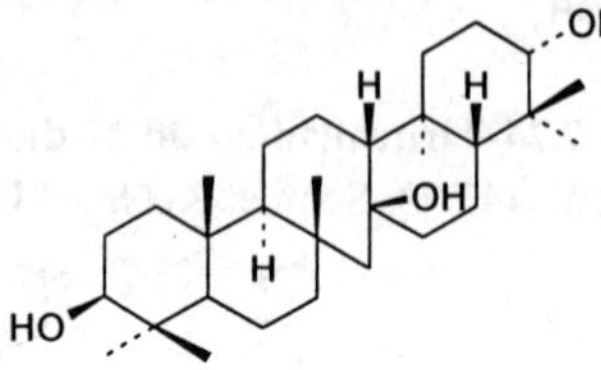

6315 Tokorogenin
$C_{27}H_{44}O_5$ MW: 448.65 Property: mp 266-8°C. Source: BEI XIE. Ref: 6.

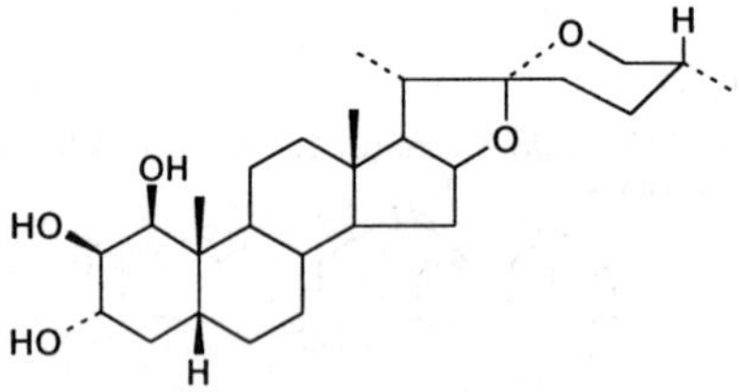

6316 Tokorogenin-l-O-β-D-glucopyranoside
$C_{33}H_{54}O_{10}$ MW: 610.79 Source: BEI XIE. Ref: 6.

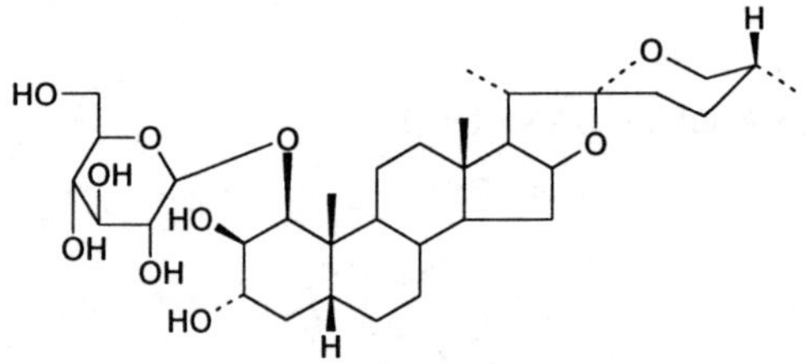

6317 Tokoronin
$C_{33}H_{54}O_9$ MW: 594.79 Property: mp 270-4°C (dec). Source: BEI XIE. Ref: 6.

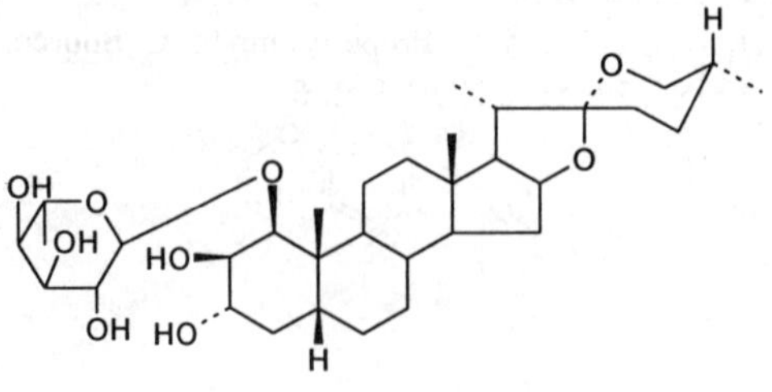

6318 p-Tolyl-methyl carbinol diferuloyl methane
$C_{30}H_{30}O_7$ MW: 502.57 Source: YU JIN. Ref: 6.

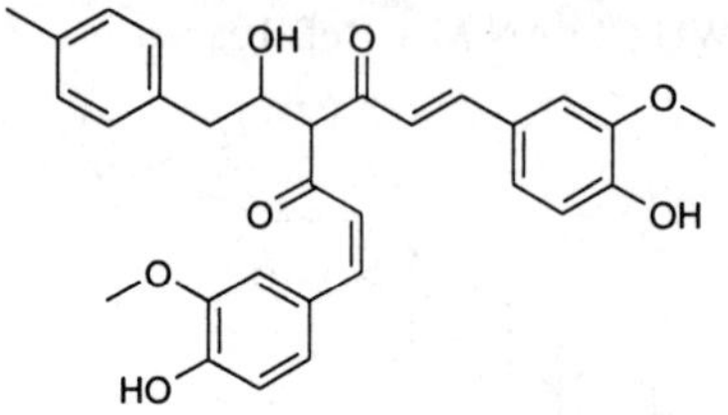

6319 Tomatidenol
$C_{27}H_{43}NO_2$ MW: 413.65 Property: mp 235-8°C, 206°C. Source: BAI MAO TENG, KU QIE. Ref: 6.

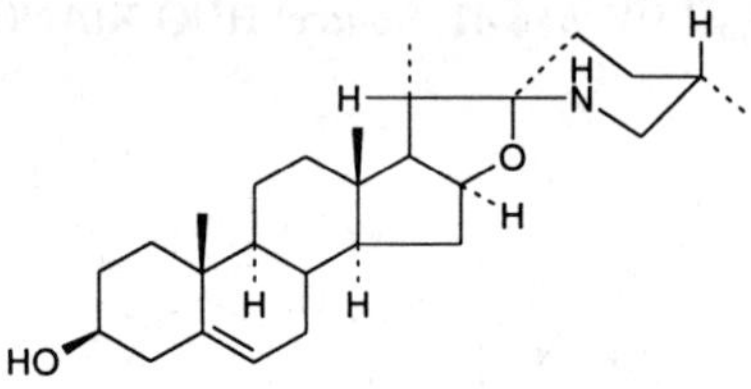

6320 Tomatine
Lycopersidin; Tomatin; α-Tomatin. CAS: 17406-45-0
$C_{50}H_{83}NO_{21}$ MW: 1034.21 Property: mp 263-8°C. Source: FAN QIE. Ref: 4.

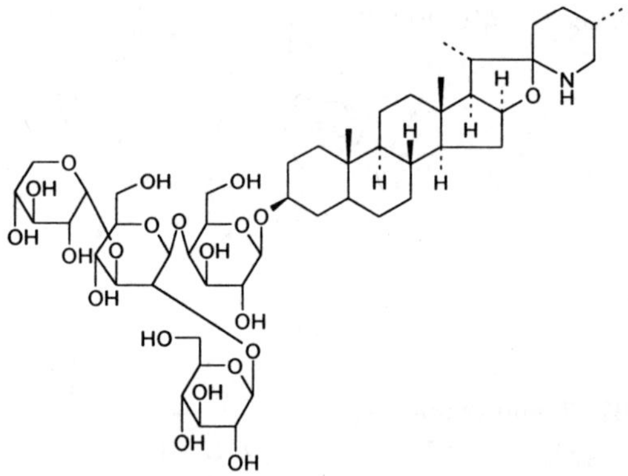

6321 Tomenin
5-Hydroxy-6,7-dimethoxy-coumarin-5-O-glucoside.
$C_{17}H_{20}O_{10}$ MW: 384.34 Source: SHAN YING TAO. Ref: 6.

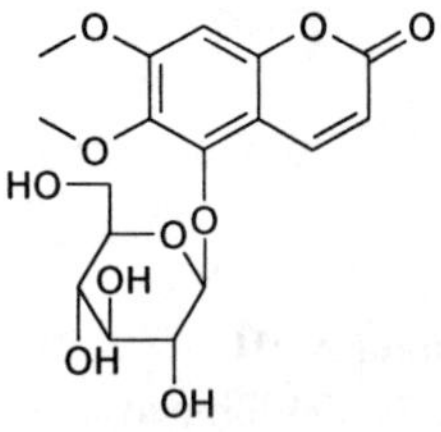

6323 Tomentogenin

$C_{21}H_{36}O_5$ MW: 368.52 Property: mp 256.5-9.5°C. Source: XU CHANG QING. Ref: 6.

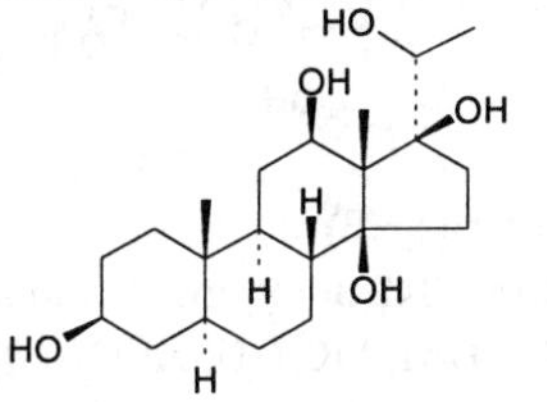

6324 Tomentosin

$C_{34}H_{24}O_{22}$ MW: 784.56 Property: brown amorphous powder easy soluble in MeOH and Me_2CO. Source: TAO JIN NIANG. Ref: 429.

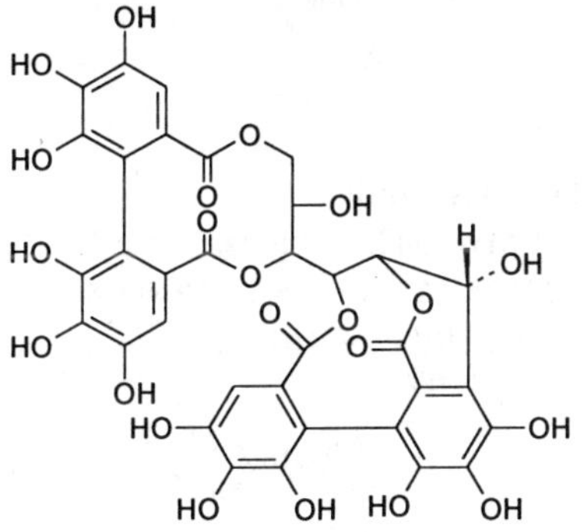

6325 Toosendanin

Azedarachin; Chuanliansu. $C_{30}H_{38}O_{11}$ MW: 574.63 Property: mp 178-80°C. Source: CHUAN LIAN ZI, CHUN BAI PI, KU LIAN PI. Ref: 4.

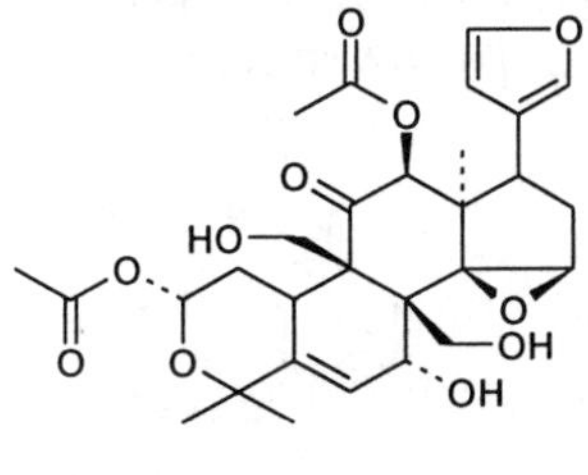

6326 Torachrysone

$C_{14}H_{14}O_4$ MW: 246.27 Source: JUE MING ZI. Ref: 2.

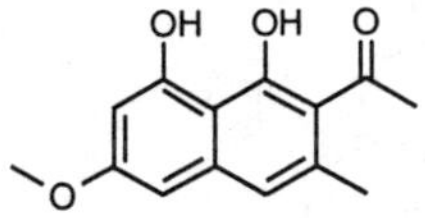

6327 Torachrysone-8-O-β-D-glucoside

$C_{20}H_{24}O_9$ MW: 408.41 Source: DA HUANG, HU ZHANG. Ref: 2.

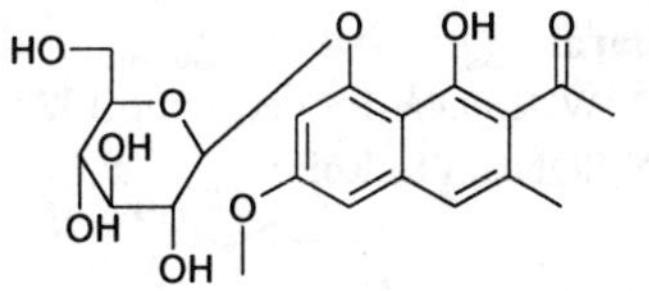

6328 Torachrysone-8-O-β-D-(6'-oxayl)-gluco-side

$C_{22}H_{24}O_{12}$ MW: 480.43 Source: DA HUANG. Ref: 2.

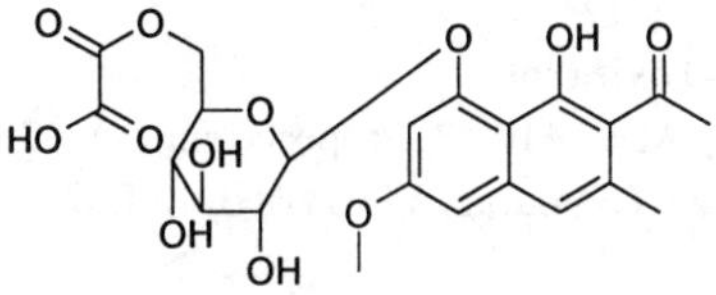

6329 Toralactone

$C_{15}H_{12}O_5$ MW: 272.26 Property: mp 253-4°C. Source: JUE MING ZI. Ref: 2, 6.

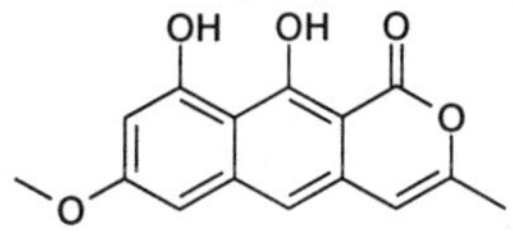

6330 Torilin

$C_{22}H_{34}O_5$ MW: 378.51 Property: mp 77-8°C. Source: HE SHI. Ref: 6.

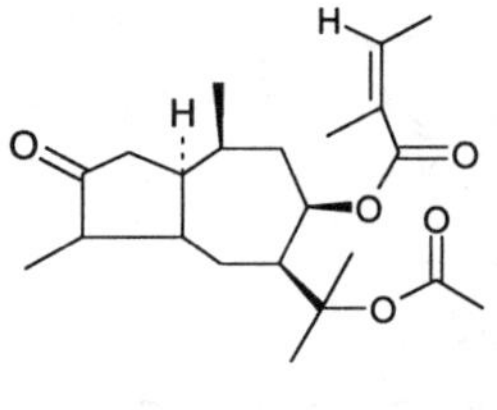

6331 Torilolone

$C_{15}H_{24}O_3$ MW: 252.36 Property: mp 136-7°C. Source: HE SHI. Ref: 6.

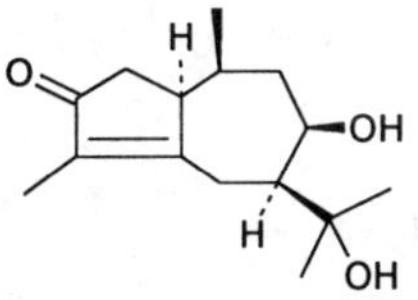

6333 Torvogenin

$C_{27}H_{42}O_4$ MW: 430.63 Source: SHUI QIE. Ref: 6.

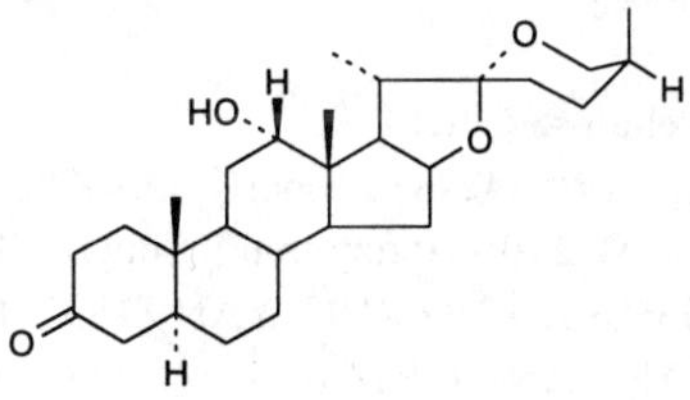

6334 Totarol
$C_{20}H_{30}O$ MW: 286.46 Property: mp 132°C. Source: LUO HAN SONG YE. Ref: 6.

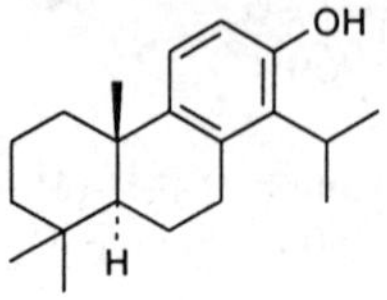

6335 α-Toxicarol
$C_{23}H_{22}O_7$ MW: 410.43 Property: mp (-): 125-7°C, (±): 219-23°C. Source: YU TENG. Ref: 6.

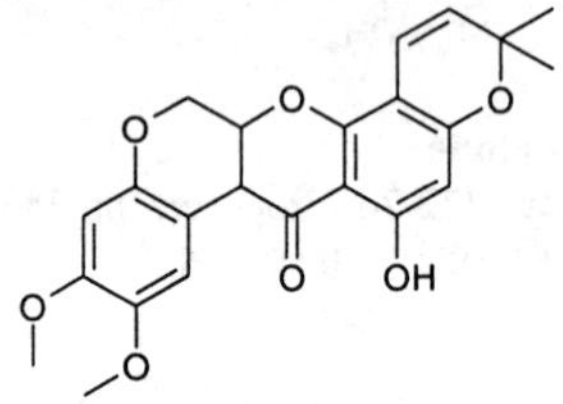

6336 β-Toxicarol
$C_{23}H_{22}O_7$ MW: 410.43 Property: mp (±): 169-70°C. Source: YU TENG. Ref: 6.

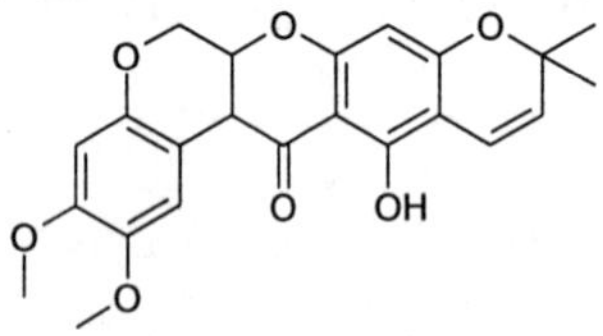

6337 Tracheloside
$C_{27}H_{34}O_{12}$ MW: 550.56 Property: mp 168-70°C. Source: LUO SHI TENG. Ref: 6.

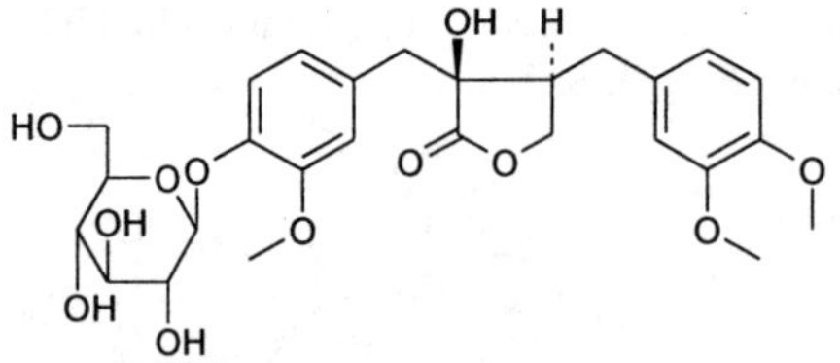

6338 Trachelosperoside E-1
Property: mp 252-4°C. Source: CU YE XUAN GOU ZI. Ref: 606.

6339 Trehalose (α:α)
$C_{12}H_{22}O_{11}$ MW: 342.30 Property: mp 97°C (containing water), 210°C (anhydrate). Source: JUAN BAI, MO GU, XIANG XUN, YAN ZHOU JUAN BAI, YUAN CAN ZI. Ref: 6.

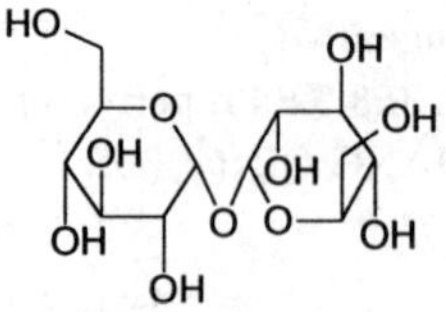

6340 Trehalose (α:β)
$C_{12}H_{22}O_{11}$ MW: 342.30 Property: mp 210-20°C. Source: JUAN BAI, MO GU, XIANG XUN, YUAN CAN ZI, ZHOU JUAN BAI. Ref: 6.

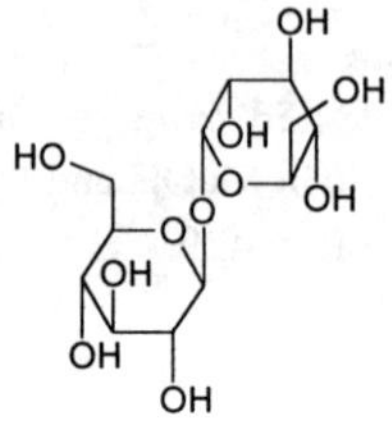

6341 Trehalose (β:β)
$C_{12}H_{22}O_{11}$ MW: 342.30 Property: mp 135-40°C. Source: JUAN BAI, MO GU, XIANG XUN, YUAN CAN ZI, ZHOU JUAN BAI. Ref: 6.

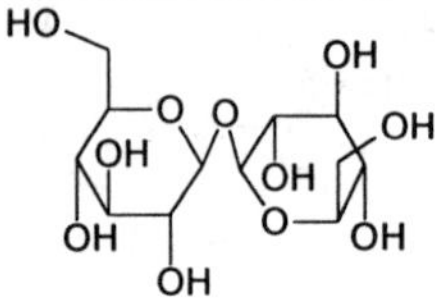

6342 Triacanthine
Triacanthin. CAS: 10091-84-6 $C_{10}H_{13}O_5$ MW: 203.25 Property: mp 228-9°C. Source: ZAO JIA, ZAO JIA YE, ZAO JIA GEN PI. Ref: 4.

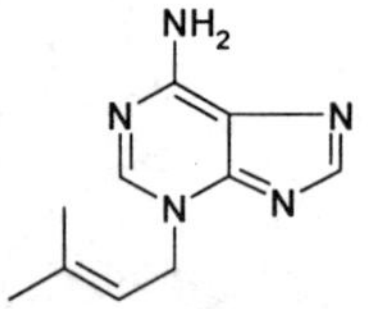

6343 Triacetylhispidulin
$C_{22}H_{18}O_9$ MW: 426.38 Property: mp 168.7°C. Source: CHANG GUAN JIA MO LI. Ref: 6.

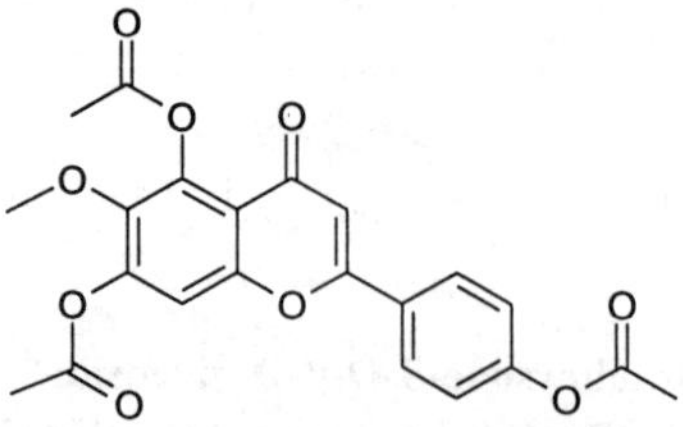

6344 Triacontane

$C_{30}H_{62}$ MW: 422.83 Source: BU GU ZHI. Ref: 2.

6345 Triacontanedioic acid

$C_{30}H_{58}O_4$ MW: 482.79 Property: mp 108°C, 123-5°C. Source: WEN JING. Ref: 6.

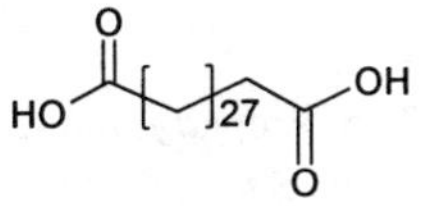

6346 Triacontanedioic acid dimethyl ester

$C_{32}H_{62}O_4$ MW: 510.85 Source: WEN JING. Ref: 6.

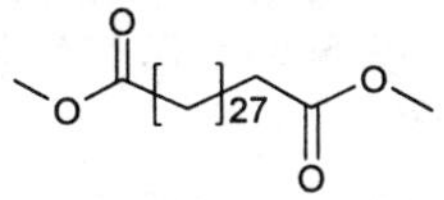

6347 n-Triacontanoic acid

Property: coloeless crystalline powder (ethanol), mp 82-3°C. Source: XIAO HUA SUAN TENG ZI. Ref: 437.

6348 n-Triacontanol

$C_{30}H_{62}O$ MW: 438.83 Property: mp 76-8°C, 83-4°C. Source: DU ZHONG, JIN LONG DAN CAO, MA HUANG, ROU CONG RONG. Ref: 2, 529, 614.

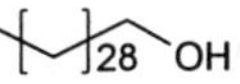

6349 16-Triacontanol

$C_{30}H_{62}O$ MW: 438.83 Source: LONG YAN YE. Ref: 6.

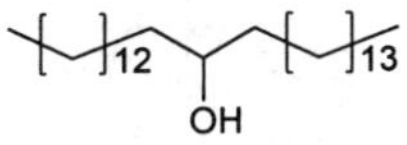

6350 Tribuloside

$C_{30}H_{26}O_{13}$ MW: 594.53 Source: CI JI LI. Ref: 6.

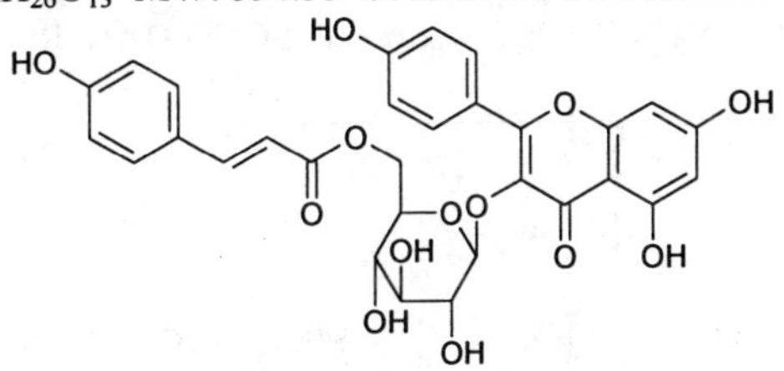

6351 Trichodesmine

$C_{18}H_{27}NO_6$ MW: 353.42 Property: mp 160-1°C. Source: HUA JIN DAN. Ref: 6.

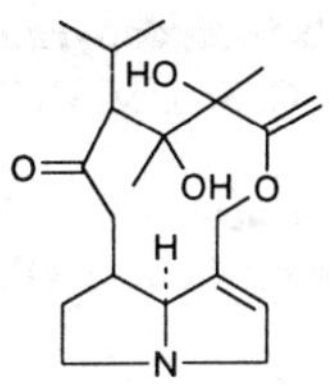

6352 Trichorabdal B

$C_{22}H_{28}O_7$ MW: 404.46 Property: colorless acicular crystal, mp 160-2°C. Source: ZI MAO XIANG CHA CAI. Ref: 653.

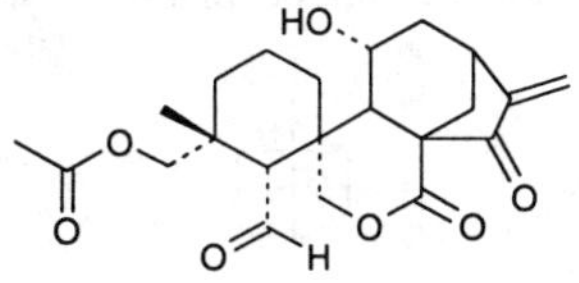

6353 Trichorabdal H

Source: MAO YE XIANG CHA CAI. Ref: 575.

6354 Trichosanatine

3-[(1-phenyl) ethylidene] amino-2-hydroxy-propyl α-(benzoylamino)-benzenepropanoate. $C_{27}H_{28}N_2O_4$ MW: 444.54 Property: colorless acicular crystal, mp 175.5-6.0 °C. Source: SHUANG BIAN GUA LOU. Ref: 331.

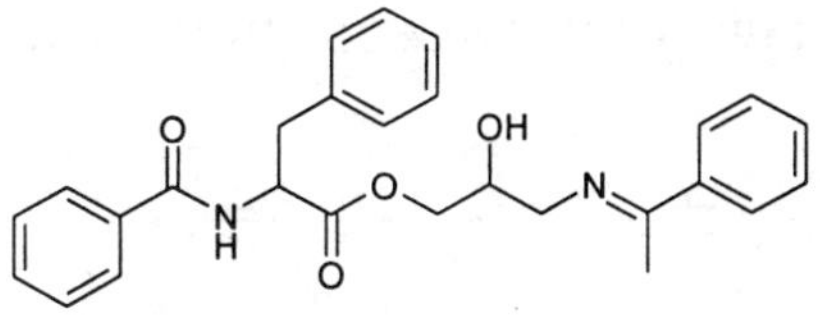

6355 Trichosanic acid

$C_{18}H_{30}O_2$ MW: 278.44 Property: mp 44°C. Source: GUA LOU. Ref: 2.

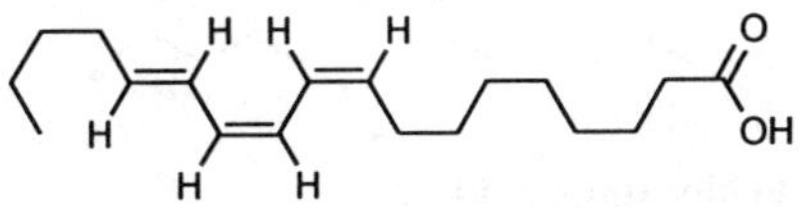

6356 Tricin

CAS: 520-32-1 $C_{17}H_{14}O_7$ MW: 330.30 Property: yellow powder. Source: CHAO XIAN YIN YANG HUO, CU MAO YIN YANG HUO, HU LU BA, GUA LOU. Ref: 4, 458, 539, 615.

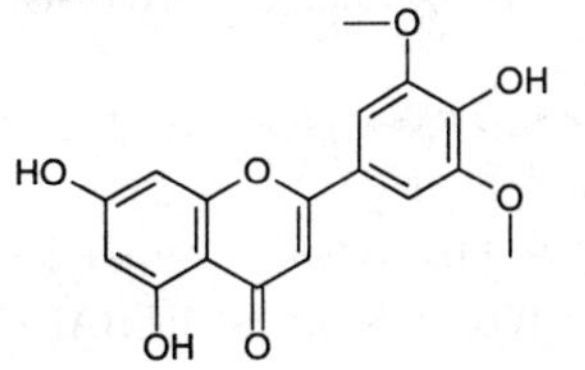

6357 Tricin-7-O-β-D-glucopyranoside
Property: mp 246-8°C. Source: HU LU BA. Ref: 615.

6358 n-Tricosanoic acid
$C_{23}H_{46}O_2$ MW: 354.62 Source: QIANG HUO. Ref: 2.

6359 Tricyclene
$C_{10}H_{16}$ MW: 136.24 Source: SHENG JIANG. Ref: 2.

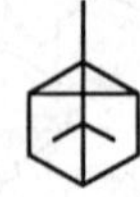

6360 Tricyclovetivene
$C_{15}H_{24}$ MW: 204.36 Property: bp 120-2°C/10 mm. Source: HUA JIN DAN. Ref: 6.

6361 1,11-Tridecadiene-3,5,7,9-tetrayne
$C_{13}H_8$ MW: 164.21 Source: NIU BANG GEN. Ref: 6.

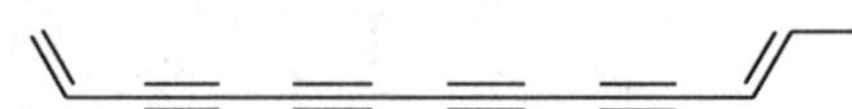

6362 n-Tridecane
$C_{13}H_{28}$ MW: 184.37 Source: CHAI HU, REN SHEN. Ref: 2.

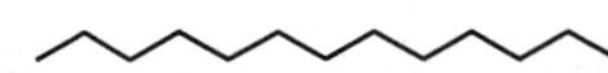

6363 Tridecanoic acid
$C_{13}H_{26}O_2$ MW: 214.35 Source: BAI ZHI. Ref: 2.

6364 1,4,7-Tridecatriene
$C_{13}H_{22}$ MW: 178.32 Source: FENG DOU CAI. Ref: 6.

6365 1,3,11-Tridecatriene-5,7,9-triyne
$C_{13}H_{10}$ MW: 166.22 Source: NIU BANG GEN. Ref: 6.

6366 Trideca-1,3,5-triene-7,9,11-triyne
$C_{13}H_{10}$ MW: 166.22 Property: mp 88-93°C. Source: YANG SHI CAO. Ref: 6.

6367 Tridecene
$C_{13}H_{26}$ MW: 182.35 Property: mp -22.2°C, bp 102°C/10mm. Source: SAN QI. Ref: 2.

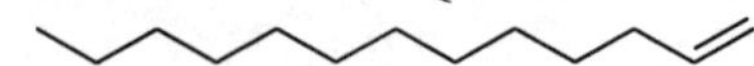

6368 1-Tridecene-3,5,7,9,11-pentyne
$C_{13}H_6$ MW: 162.19 Source: BI MA GEN, HONG TOU CAO. Ref: 6.

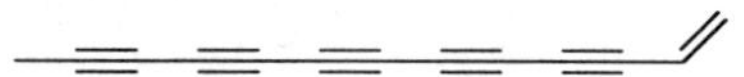

6369 1,3,4-Tridehydrofangchinolium hydroxide
$C_{37}H_{39}N_2O_6$ MW: 607.73 Source: FANG JI. Ref: 2.

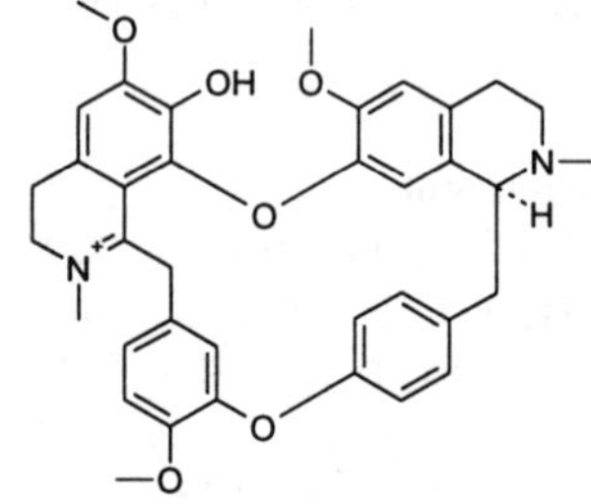

6370 2,2,2-Tri-ethoxyl-ethanol
$C_8H_{18}O_4$ MW: 178.23 Source: SAN QI. Ref: 2.

6371 Trifloroside
$C_{35}H_{42}O_{20}$ MW: 782.71 Source: LONG DAN. Ref: 2.

6372 Trifolin

$C_{21}H_{20}O_{11}$ MW: 448.39 Property: mp 260°C. Source: CI BO, GOU TENG, HONG CHE ZHOU CAO, HU ZHI ZI, REN SHEN, SAN XIAO CAO, TAO HUA, XIAO XUE REN SHEN, ZHEN ZHU MEI. Ref: 2, 6.

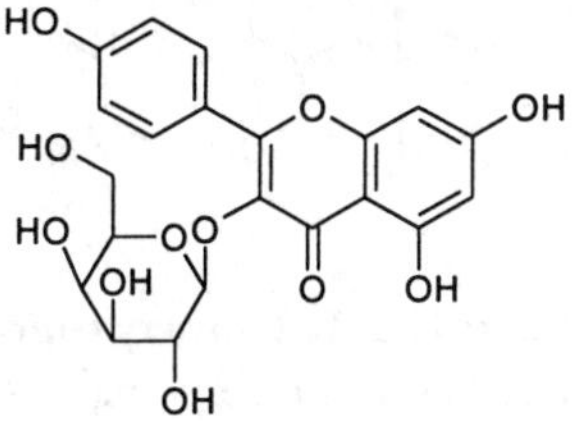

6373 Trifolirhizin

CAS: 6807-83-6 $C_{22}H_{22}O_{10}$ MW: 446.41 Property: mp 142-4°C (dec). Source: HONG CHE ZHOU CAO, SHAN DOU GEN. Ref: 5.

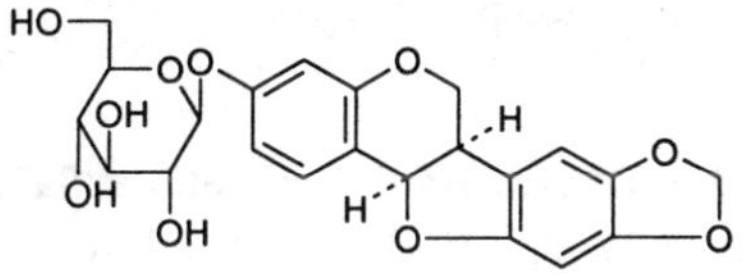

6374 1,2,3-Tri-O-galloyl-β-D-glucose

$C_{27}H_{24}O_{18}$ MW: 636.48 Source: SHAN ZHU YU. Ref: 2.

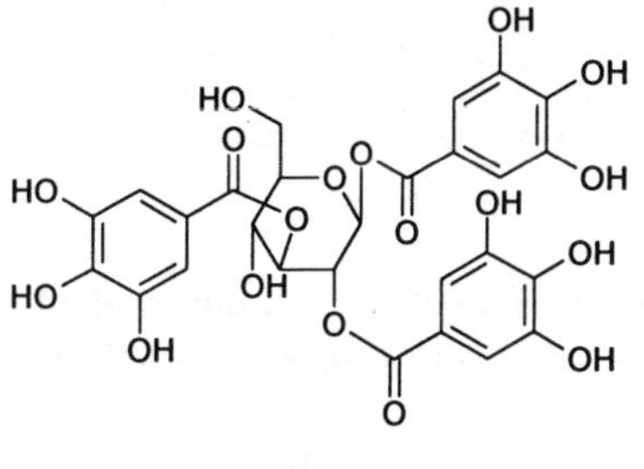

6375 1,2,6-Tri-O-galloyl-glucose

$C_{27}H_{24}O_{18}$ MW: 636.48 Source: DA HUANG, SHAN ZHU YU. Ref: 2.

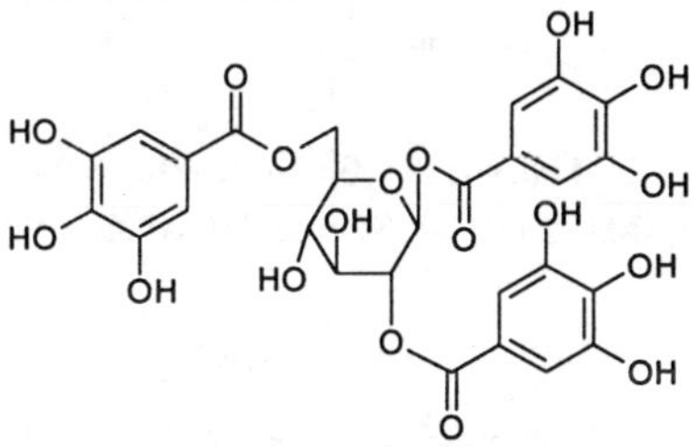

6376 1,3,6-Trigalloyl-β-glucose

$C_{27}H_{24}O_{18}$ MW: 636.48 Source: HE ZI. Ref: 6.

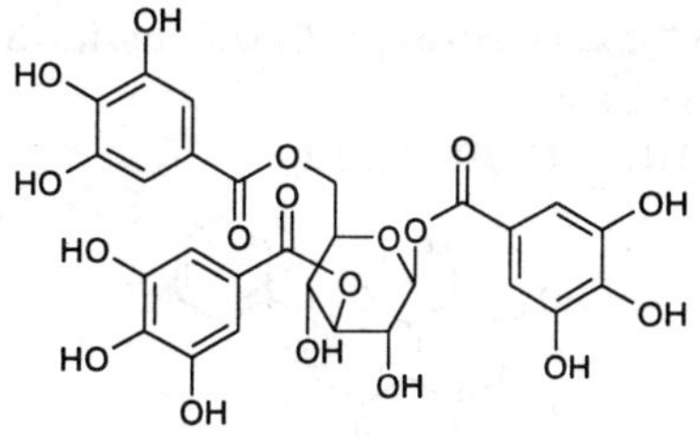

6377 Triglochinin

$C_{14}H_{17}NO_{10}$ MW: 359.29 Source: HAI JIU CAI. Ref: 6.

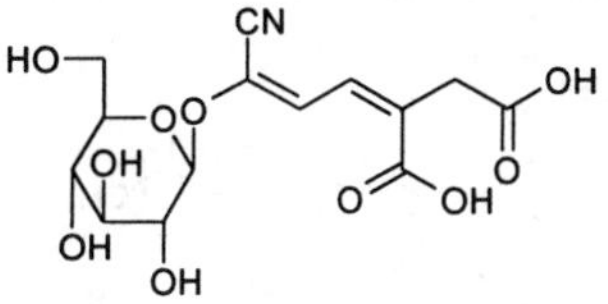

6378 Triglyceride

Source: REN SHEN. Ref: 2.

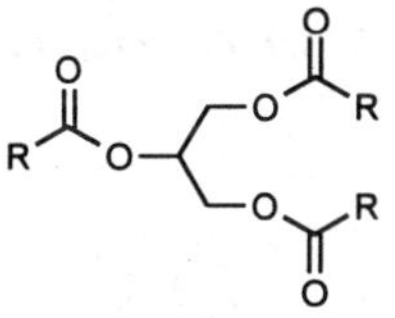

R=hydrocarbon

6379 Trigonelline

$C_7H_7NO_2$ MW: 137.14 Property: mp 218°C (dec). Source: BAI XIAN PI, DONG GUA ZI, FAN QIE, HONG HUA CAI, HU LU BA, MA HUA, NAN GUA, QIE YE, QIE ZI, SANG YE, SHI JUN ZI, SHI JUN ZI YE, XIANG SI ZI, ZI MO LI YE. Ref: 6.

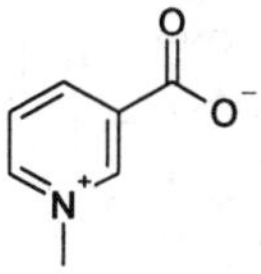

6380 7α,21S,25-Trihydroxy-3β-acetoxy-21S, 23 R-epoxy-9(11)-en-dammarane

$C_{32}H_{52}O_6$ MW: 532.77 Property: colorless acicular crystal($CHCl_3$), mp 201°C, $[\alpha]_D^{21.5}$ -32°(c=1.0,$CHCl_3$). Source: XIANG GANG JIAN MU. Ref: 422.

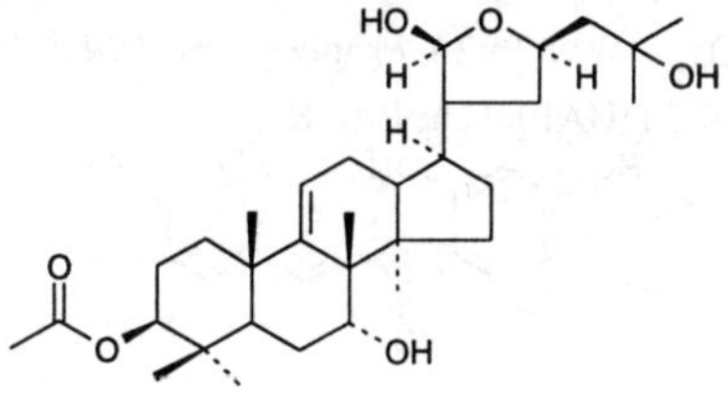

6381 5,7,4'-Trihydroxy-6-C-arabinoside-8-C-glucoside flavone
Source: HUANG QIN. Ref: 2.

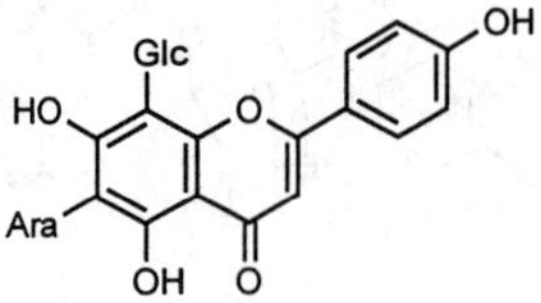

6382 2,3,4-Trihydroxy-benzenepropanoic acid
$C_9H_{10}O_5$ MW: 198.18 Source: HUANG LIAN. Ref: 2.

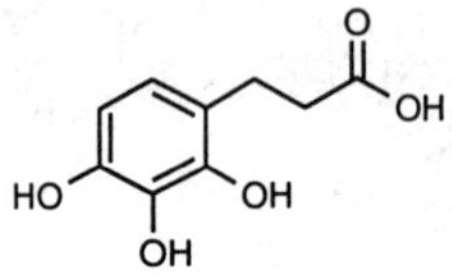

6383 Trihydroxybufosterocholanic acid
$C_{28}H_{48}O_5$ MW: 464.69 Property: mp 200°C. Source: CHAN CHU DAN. Ref: 6.

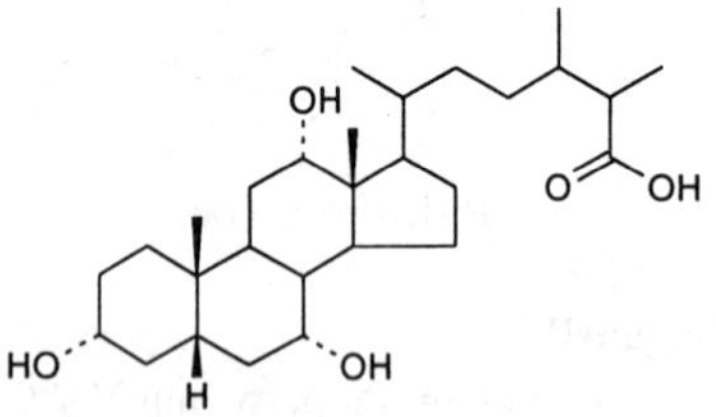

6384 Trihydroxybufosterocholenic acid
$C_{28}H_{46}O_5$ MW: 462.68 Property: mp 160°C. Source: CHAN CHU DAN. Ref: 6.

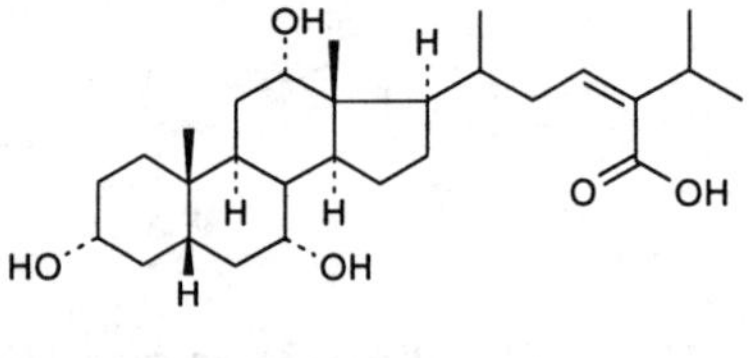

6385 2,4,4'-Trihydroxychalcone
Isoliquiritigenin. Source: GAN CAO. Ref: 6.

6386 4,2',4'-Trihydroxychalcone
$C_{15}H_{12}O_4$ MW: 526.26 Property: mp 199.5-200.5°C. Source: CI HUAI HUA. Ref: 6.

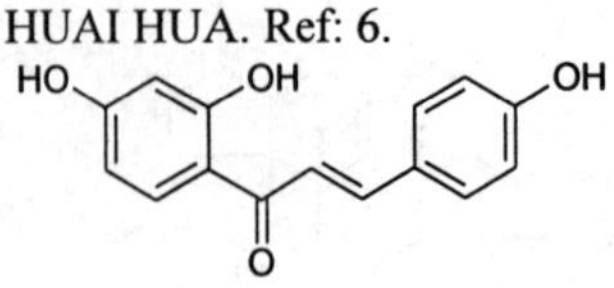

6387 α-Trihydroxy coprostanic acid
$C_{26}H_{44}O_5$ MW: 436.64 Property: mp 174-6°C. Source: QING WA DAN. Ref: 6.

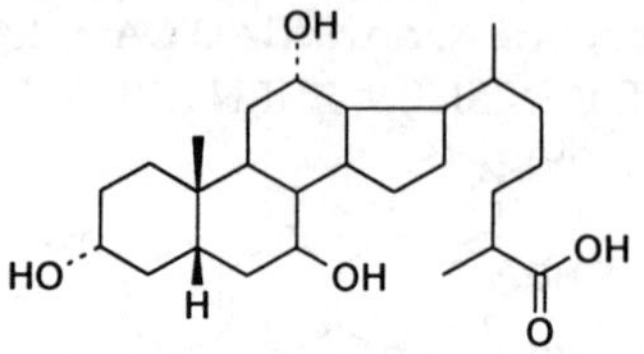

6388 Δ23-3α,7α,12α-Trihydroxy coprostenic acid
$C_{27}H_{44}O_5$ MW: 448.65 Property: mp 176-9°C. Source: CHAN CHU DAN. Ref: 6.

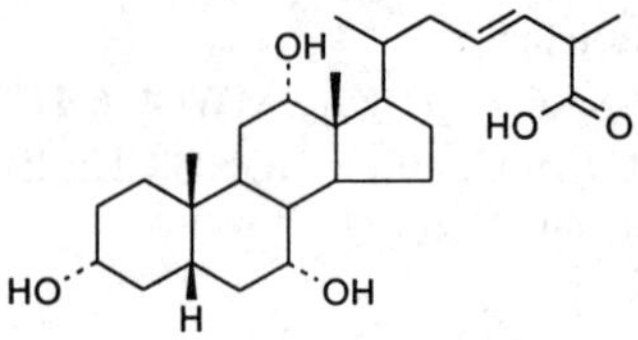

6389 3,5,6-Trihydroxy-4',7-dimethoxyflavone
$C_{17}H_{14}O_7$ MW: 330.30 Property: yellow crystal, mp 234-5°C, soluble in acetone and methanol, hardly soluble in chloroform and water. Source: FO SHOU GAN. Ref: 31.

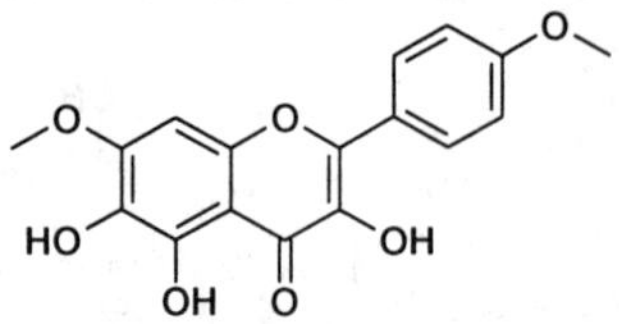

6390 5,2',6'-Trihydroxy-7,8-dimethoxyflavone
$C_{17}H_{14}O_7$ MW: 330.30 Source: HUANG QIN. Ref: 2.

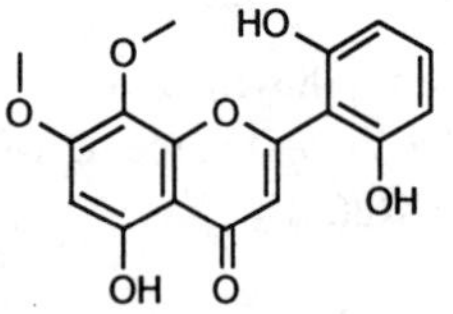

6391 5,7,2'-Trihydroxy-8,6'-dimethoxyflavone
$C_{17}H_{14}O_7$ MW: 330.30 Source: HUANG QIN. Ref: 2.

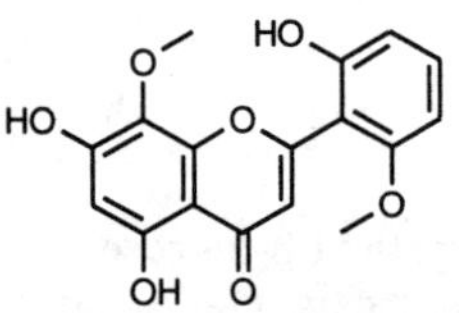

6392 5,8,2'-Trihydroxy-6,7-dimethoxyflavone
$C_{17}H_{14}O_7$ MW: 330.30 Source: HUANG QIN. Ref: 2.

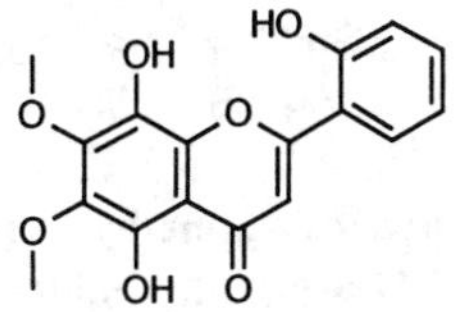

6393 1,6,7-Trihydroxy-2,3-dimethoxyxanthone
$C_{15}H_{12}O_7$ MW: 304.26 Property: light yellow acicular crystal (chloroform-methanol), mp 232-4°C. Source: HUANG HUA YUAN ZHI. Ref: 345.

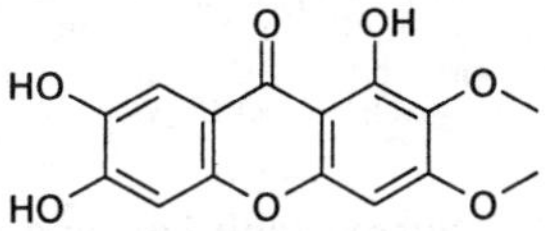

6394 5,7,2'-Trihydroxyflavone
$C_{15}H_{10}O_5$ MW: 270.24 Source: HUANG QIN. Ref: 2.

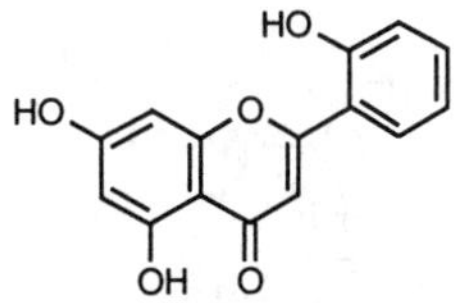

6395 7,3',4'-Trihydroxyflavone
$C_{15}H_{10}O_5$ MW: 270.24 Source: BAI CI HUA (seed). Ref: 561.

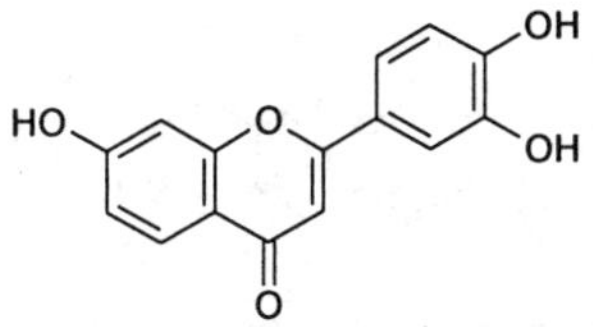

6396 5,7,4'-Trihydroxy-6-C-glucoside-8-C-arabinoside flavone
Source: HUANG QIN. Ref: 2.

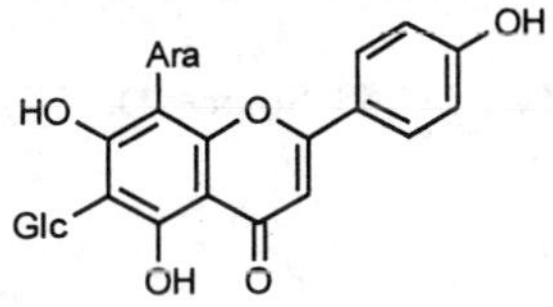

6397 3β,15ξ,16-Trihydroxy isopimaric acid
$C_{20}H_{32}O_5$ MW: 352.48 Property: white acicular crystal, mp 256-8°C, $[\alpha]_D^{21}$ +27.9° (c=0.05, methanol). Source: WULINGZHI. Ref: 88.

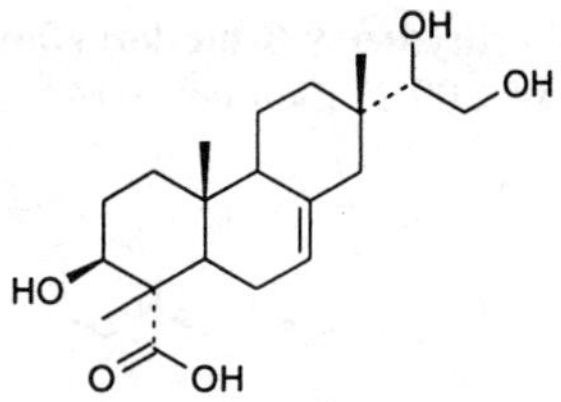

6398 Trihydroxy isosterocholenic acid
$C_{27}H_{44}O_5$ MW: 448.65 Property: mp 227°C. Source: CHAN CHU DAN. Ref: 6.

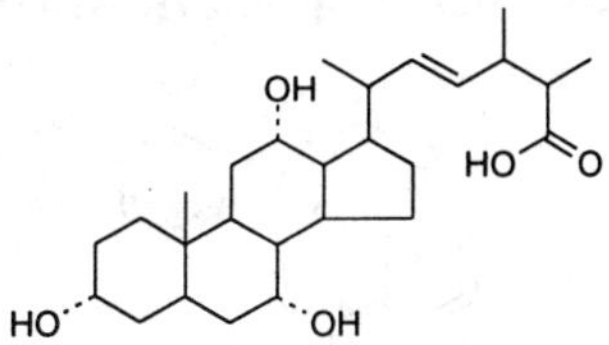

6399 7,2',6'-Trihydroxy-5-methoxychalcone
$C_{16}H_{14}O_6$ MW: 302.29 Source: Ref: 2.

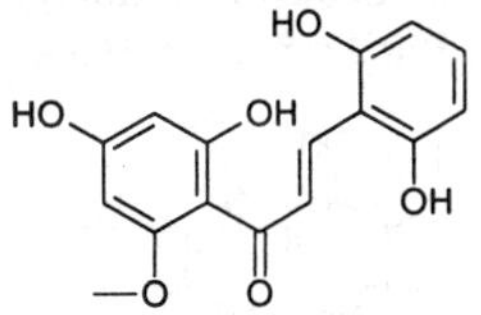

6400 5,7,4'-Trihydroxy-6-methoxyflavanone
$C_{16}H_{14}O_6$ MW: 302.29 Source: HUANG QIN. Ref: 2.

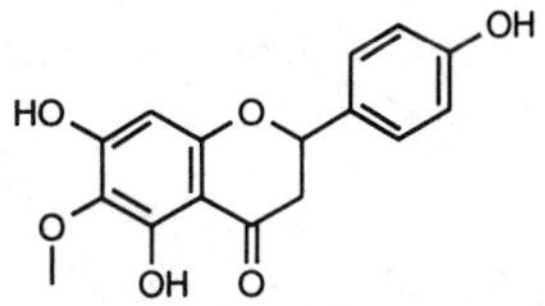

6401 7,2'6'-Trihydroxy-5-methoxyflavanone
$C_{16}H_{14}O_6$ MW: 302.27 Source: HUANG QIN. Ref: 2.

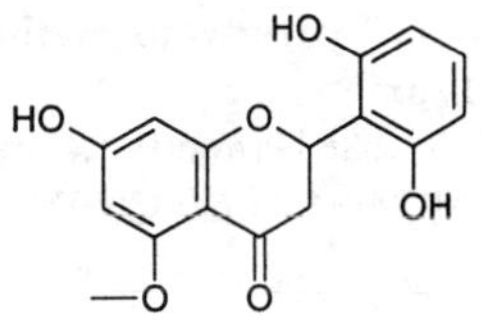

6402 5,7,2'-Trihydroxy-6-methoxyflavone
$C_{16}H_{12}O_6$ MW: 300.27 Source: HUANG QIN. Ref: 2.

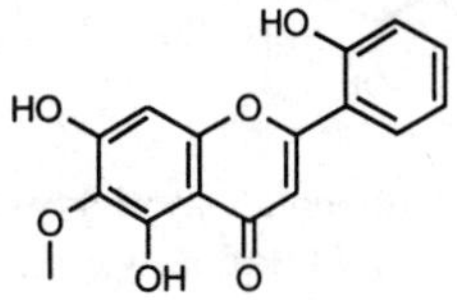

6403 5,7,2'-Trihydroxy-8-methoxyflavone
$C_{16}H_{12}O_6$ MW: 300.27 Source: HUANG QIN. Ref: 2.

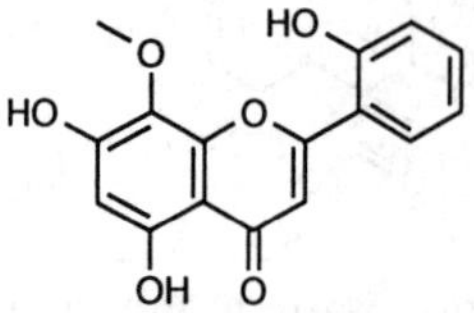

6404 5,7,4'-Trihydroxy-8-methoxyflavone
$C_{16}H_{12}O_6$ MW: 300.27 Source: HUANG QIN. Ref: 2.

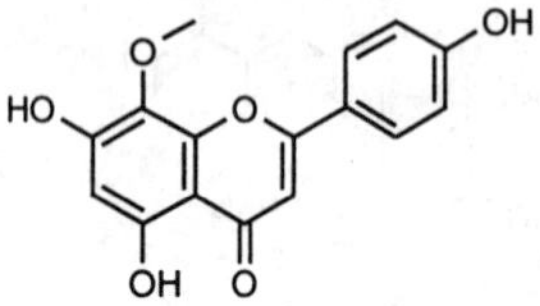

6405 5,8,2'-Trihydroxy-7-methoxyflavone
$C_{16}H_{12}O_6$ MW: 300.27 Source: HUANG QIN. Ref: 2.

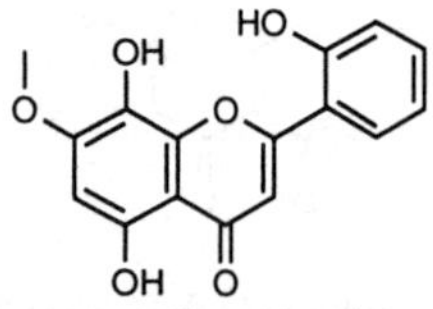

6406 3,4',5-Trihydroxy-7-methoxy-8-isopentenylflavone
$C_{21}H_{20}O_6$ MW: 368.39 Source: KU SHEN. Ref: 6.

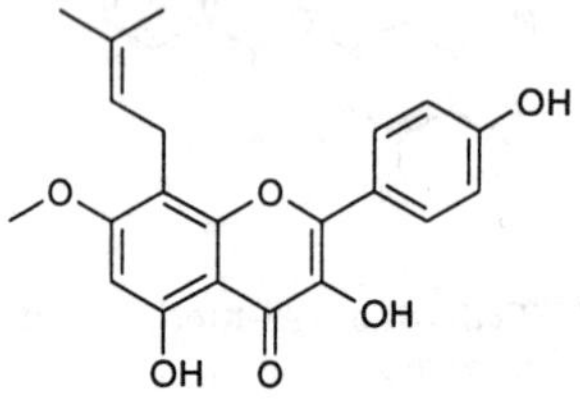

6407 5α,6β,7β-Trihydroxy-8α-methoxy-2-(2-phenylethyl) chromone
$C_{18}H_{20}O_6$ MW: 332.36 Property: white powder, mp 130-5°C, $[\alpha]_D$ +1.94°. Source: CHEN XIANG. Ref: 13.

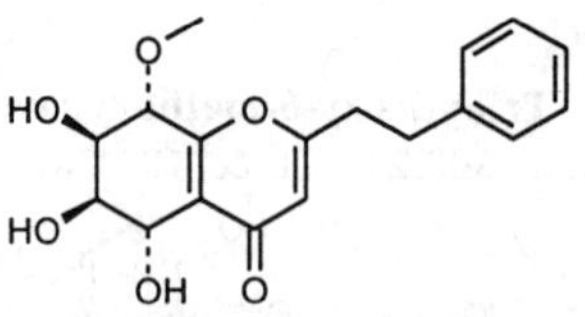

6408 1,3,7-Trihydroxyl-8-methoxyxanthone
$C_{14}H_{10}O_6$ MW: 274.43 Property: yellow long acicular crystal, mp 224-5°C. Source: BAO E ZHANG YA CAI. Ref: 634.

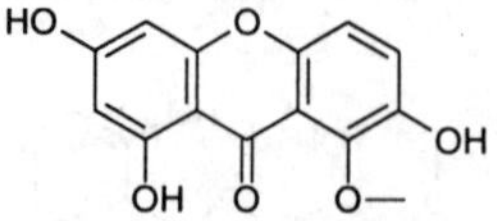

6409 1,3,6-Trihydroxy-2-methyl-9,10-anthraquinone-3-O-(6'-O-acetyl)-β-D-glucoside
$C_{23}H_{22}O_{11}$ MW: 474.43 Property: yellow crystalline powder (methanol), mp 263-4°C. Source: QIAN CAO GEN. Ref: 174.

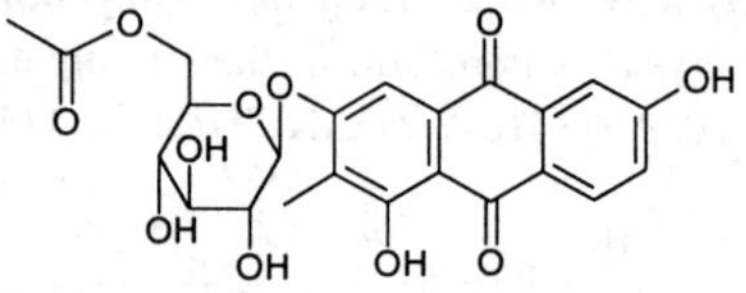

6410 1,2,4-Trihydroxynaphthalene-4-glucoside
$C_{16}H_{18}O_8$ MW: 338.32 Source: TOU GU CAO. Ref: 6.

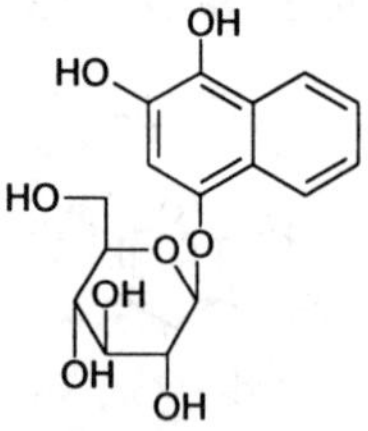

6411 Trihydroxypropylpterisin
$C_9H_{11}N_5O_4$ MW: 253.22 Property: mp 250°C (dec). Source: CHAN PI. Ref: 6.

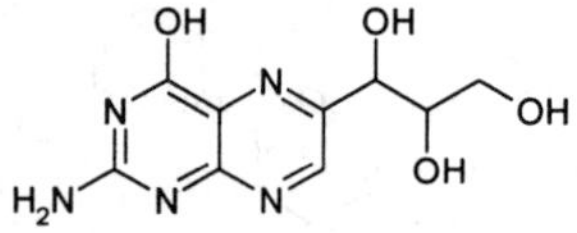

6412 3,5,4'-Trihydroxystilbene
Property: mp 244-6°C. Source: FANG JI YE BA QIA, TIAN SHAN DA HUANG. Ref: 535, 609.

6413 3,5,4'-Trihydroxystilbene-4'-(6''-galloyl)-glucoside
$C_{27}H_{26}O_{12}$ MW: 542.50 Source: DA HUANG. Ref: 2.

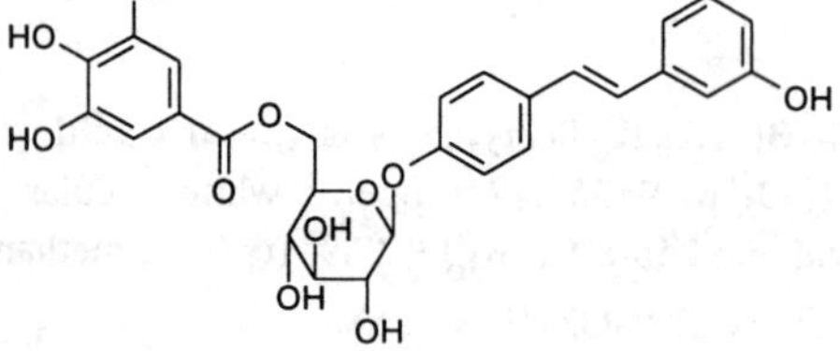

6414 3,5,4'-Trihydroxystilene-4'-glucoside
$C_{20}H_{22}O_8$ MW: 390.39 Source: DA HUANG. Ref: 2.

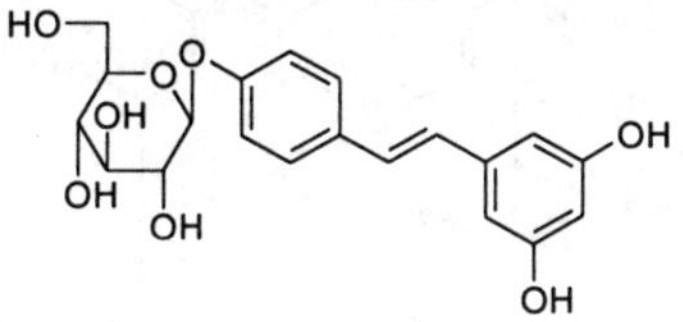

6415 3,6,7-Trihydroxy-4,5,6,7-tetrahydro-3-butylphthalide
$C_{12}H_{18}O_5$ MW: 242.27 Source: CHUAN XIONG. Ref: 2.

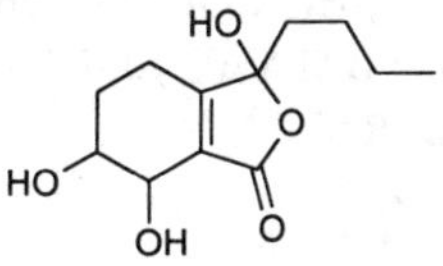

6416 3,5,3'-Trihydroxy-6,7,4'-trimethoxy flavone
$C_{18}H_{16}O_8$ MW: 360.32 Source: Ref: 2.

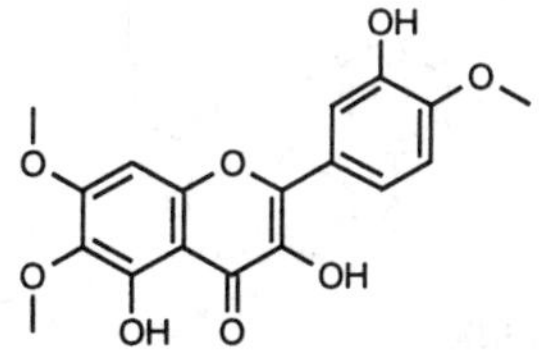

6417 3,5,6-Trihydroxy-3',4',7-trimethoxy flavone
$C_{18}H_{16}O_8$ MW: 360.32 Property: orange crystal, mp 272°C (decomposition), soluble in acetone and methanol, hardly soluble in chloroform and water. Source: FE SHOU GAN. Ref: 31.

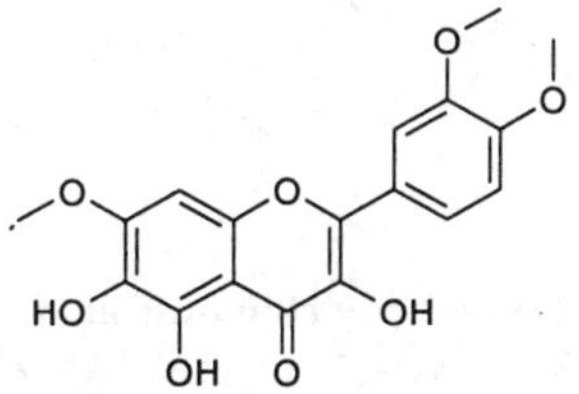

6418 5,2',4'-Trihydroxy-6,7,5'-trimethoxy flavone
$C_{18}H_{16}O_8$ MW: 360.32 Source: QING HAO. Ref: 2.

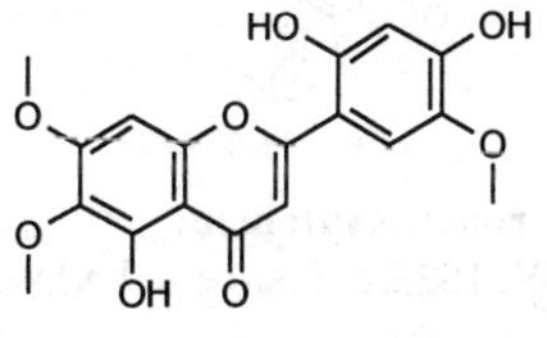

6419 5,2',5'-Trihydroxy-6,7,8-trimethoxy flavone
$C_{18}H_{16}O_9$ MW: 376.32 Source: HUANG QIN. Ref: 2.

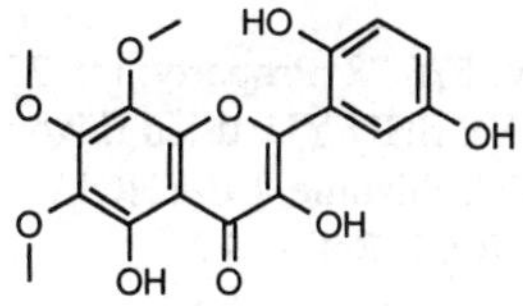

6421 3,3',5'-Triiodothyronine
$C_{15}H_{12}I_3O_4$ MW: 650.98 Source: NIU YE. Ref: 6.

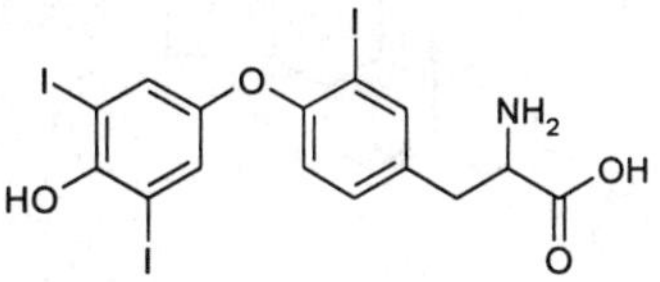

6422 3,5,3'-Triiodothyronine
$C_{15}H_{12}I_3O_4$ MW: 650.98 Property: mp 236-7°C (dec). Source: NIU YE. Ref: 6.

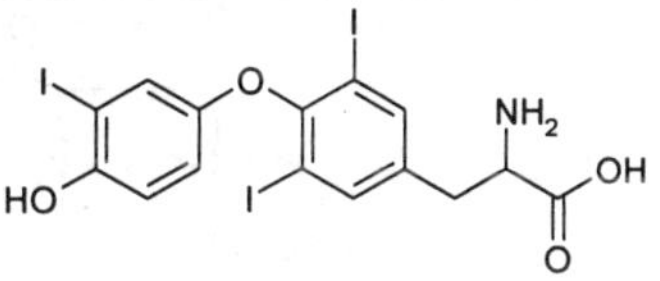

6423 1,3,5-Triisopropylphene
$C_{15}H_{24}$ MW: 204.36 Source: XI YANG SHEN. Ref: 2.

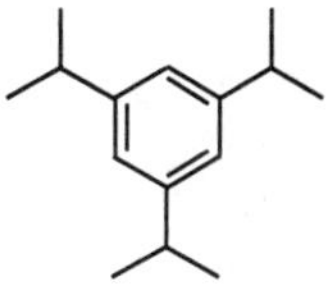

6424 Trillarin
$C_{39}H_{62}O_{13}$ MW: 738.92 Property: mp 197-200°C. Source: YU ER QI. Ref: 6.

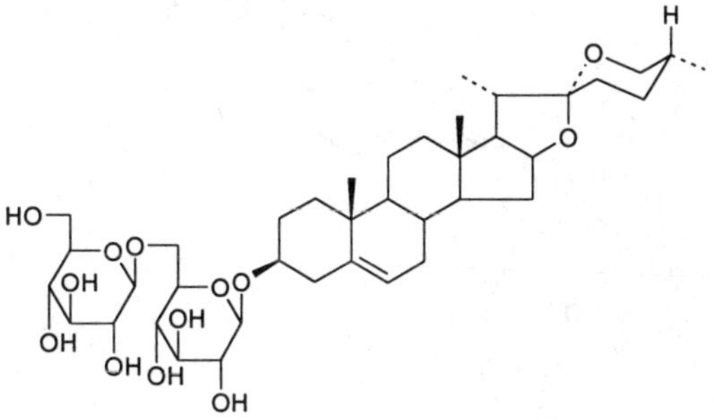

6425 Trillin
$C_{33}H_{52}O_8$ MW: 576.78 Property: mp 275-80°C. Source: DUN YE SHU YU, dried rhizome, CHUNG LONG SHU YU, rhizome, FU ZHOU SHU YU, dried rhizome, YU ER QI. Ref: 6, 10.

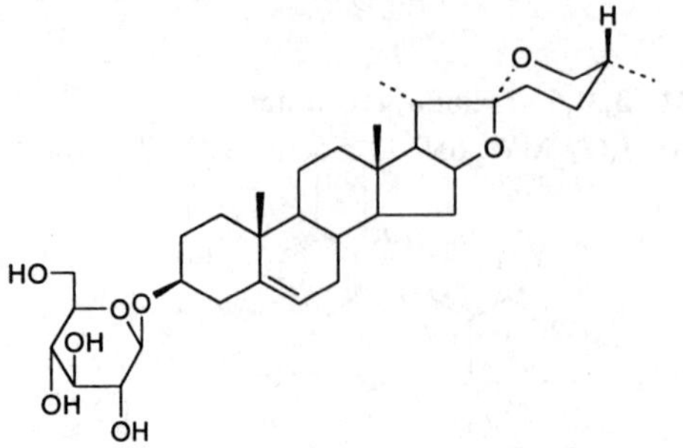

6426 Trilloside A
$C_{45}H_{72}O_{17}$ MW: 885.07 Source: YU ER QI. Ref: 6.

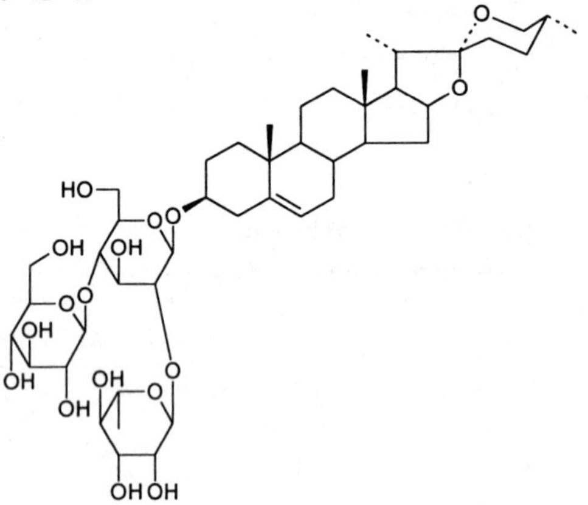

6427 Trilloside B
$C_{45}H_{72}O_{18}$ MW: 901.06 Source: YU ER QI. Ref: 6.

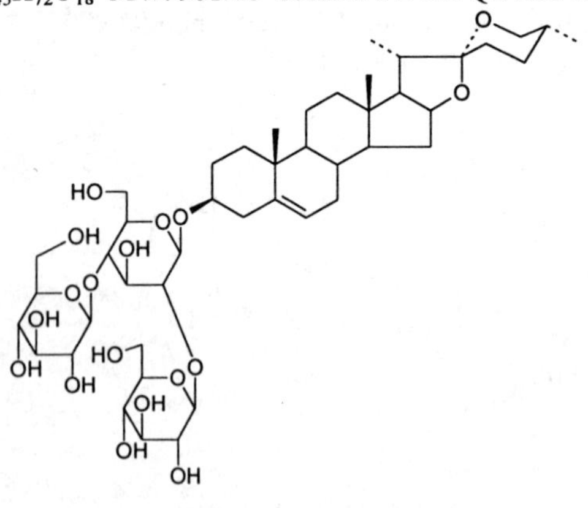

6428 Trilobamine
$C_{35}H_{36}N_2O_6$ MW: 580.69 Property: mp 194-6°C. Source: FANG JI. Ref: 6.

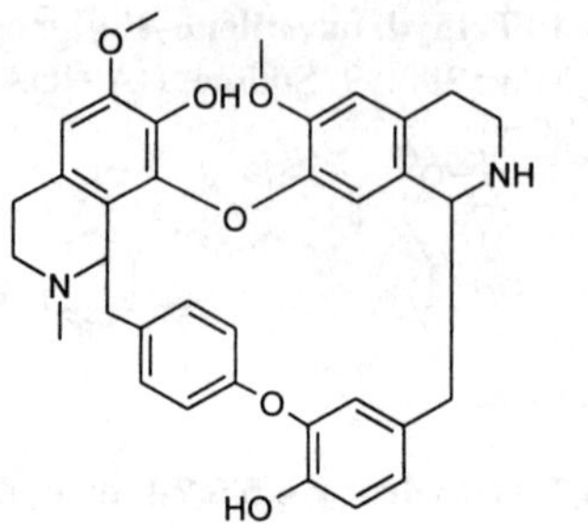

6429 Trilobine
CAS: 6138-73-4 $C_{35}H_{34}N_2O_5$ MW: 562.67 Property: mp 237°C. Source: BAI YAO ZI, FANG JI, HENG ZHOU WU YAO. Ref: 4.

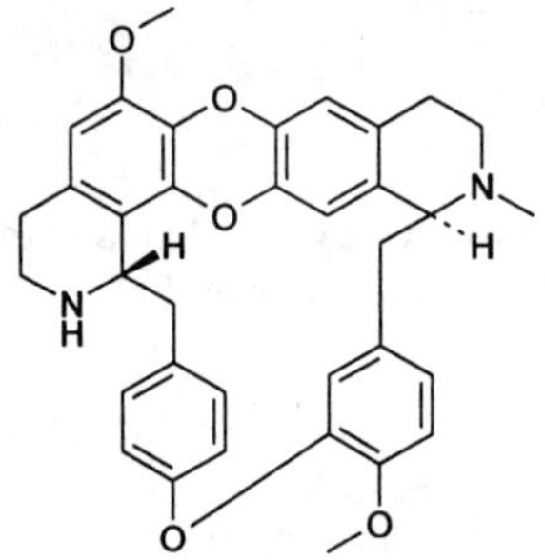

6430 Trilobolide
$C_{27}H_{38}O_{10}$ MW: 522.60 Property: mp 191-2°C. Source: *Laser trilobum* L. Ref: 5.

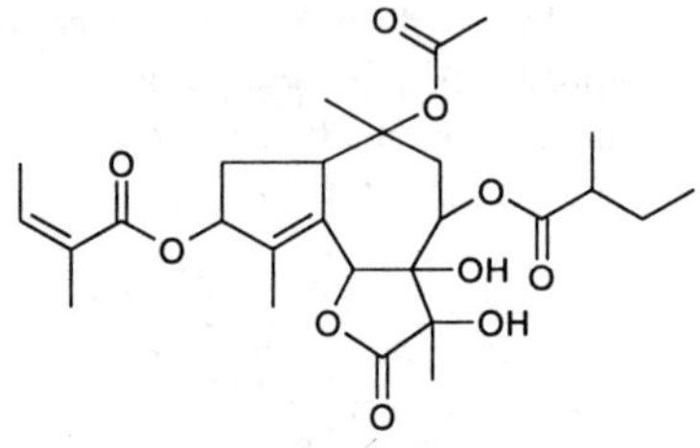

6431 3,4,5-Trimethoxy cinnamic acid
$C_{12}H_{14}O_5$ MW: 238.24 Source: YUAN ZHI. Ref: 2.

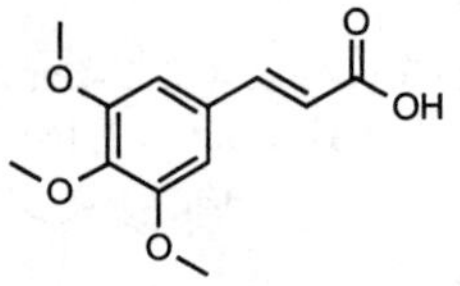

6432 2,3,5-Trimethoxytoluene
$C_{10}H_{14}O_3$ MW: 182.22 Source: XI XIN. Ref: 2.

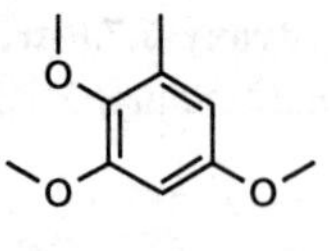

6433 3,4,5-Trimethoxytoluene
$C_{10}H_{14}O_3$ MW: 182.22 Source: XI XIN. Ref: 2.

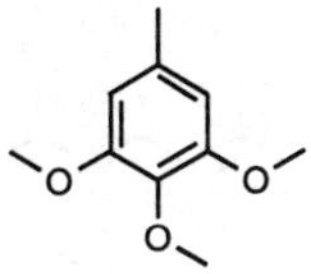

6434 Trimethylamine
C_3H_9N MW: 59.11 Source: CHUAN XIONG, QUAN XIE. Ref: 2.

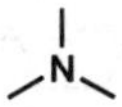

6435 Trimethylamine oxide
C_3H_9NO MW: 75.11 Property: mp 255-7°C. Source: HAI XIA. Ref: 6.

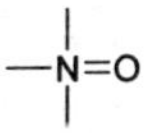

6436 1,2,3-Trimethyl-benzene
C_9H_{12} MW: 120.20 Source: SHAN ZHA. Ref: 2.

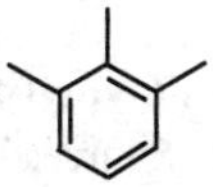

6437 3,6,6-Trimethyl-bicyclo[3,1, 1]hept-2-ene
$C_{10}H_{16}$ MW: 136.24 Source: BAI ZHI. Ref: 2.

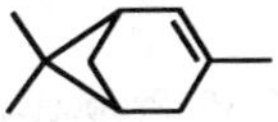

6438 1,2,3-Trimethyl-cyclohexane
C_9H_{18} MW: 126.24 Source: SHAN ZHA. Ref: 2.

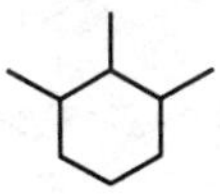

6439 1,3,5-Trimethyl-cyclohexane
C_9H_{18} MW: 126.24 Source: SHAN ZHA. Ref: 2.

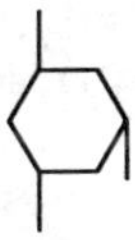

6440 1, 3,4-Trimethyl-3-cyclohexene-1-carboxaldehyde
$C_{10}H_{16}O$ MW: 152.24 Source: MA HUANG. Ref: 2.

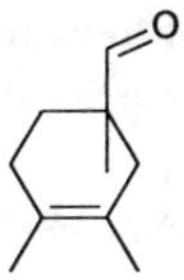

6441 1,1,3-Trimethyl-cyclopentane
C_8H_{16} MW: 112.22 Source: Ref: 2.

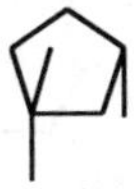

6442 3,7,11-Trimethyldodeca-1,7,10-trien-3-ol-9-one
$C_{15}H_{24}O_2$ MW: 236.36 Source: ZHANG SHU YE. Ref: 6.

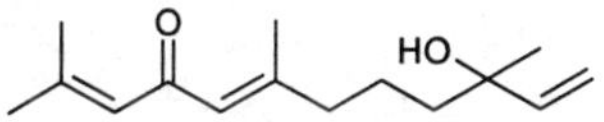

6443 3,3',4-Tri-O-methyl ellagic acid
$C_{17}H_{12}O_8$ MW: 344.28 Property: mp 297°C (dec). Source: XI SHU, ZI WEI GEN. Ref: 6.

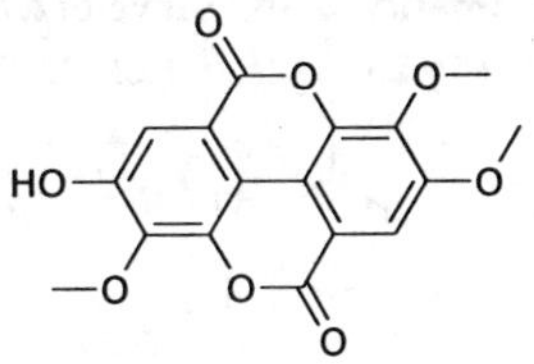

6444 Trimethyl ester dehydrochebulic acid
$C_{17}H_{16}O_{11}$ MW: 396.31 Property: white acicular crystal, mp 204-6°C, $[\alpha]_D$ +28.5° (MeOH). Source:YE XIA ZHU. Ref: 283.

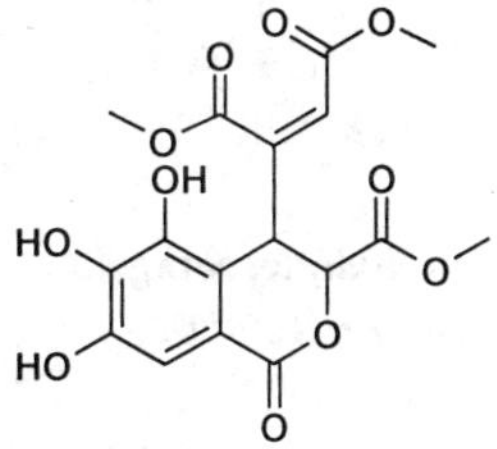

6445 Trimethylgalloylglucose
$C_{16}H_{22}O_{10}$ MW: 374.35 Source: HUANG LU ZHI YE. Ref: 6.

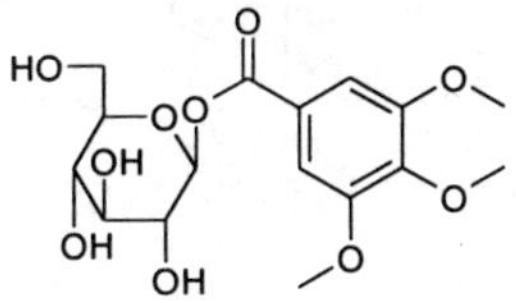

6446 2,3,4-Trimethyl-hexane
C_9H_{20} MW: 128.26 Source: SHAN ZHA. Ref: 2.

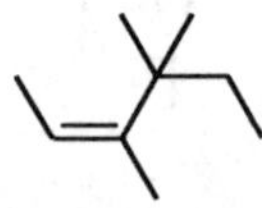

6447 3,4,4-Trimethyl-2-hexene
C_9H_{18} MW: 126.24 Source: SHAN ZHA. Ref: 2.

6448 4,11,11-Trimethyl-methylene bicyclo[7.2.0] undec-4-ene
$C_{15}H_{24}$ MW: 204.36 Source: BAI ZHI. Ref: 2.

6449 1,3,3-Trimethyl-2-oxybicyclo[2.2.2]octane
$C_{10}H_{18}O$ MW: 154.25 Source: Ref: 2.

6450 2,3,4-Trimethyl-5-phenyloxazolidine
$C_{12}H_{17}NO$ MW: 191.28 Source: MA HUANG. Ref: 2.

6451 3,6,7-Trimethylquercetagenin
Source: MAN JING ZI. Ref: 562.

6452 1,3,3-Trimethyltricyclo[2.2.1.02,6]heptane
$C_{10}H_{16}$ MW: 136.24 Source: SHENG JIANG. Ref: 2.

6453 4,8,12-Trimethyl tridecanoic acid
$C_{16}H_{32}O_2$ MW: 256.43 Source: QIANG HUO. Ref: 2.

6454 [Z,E]-4,8,12-Trimethyl-3,7,11-tridecatrienoate
$C_{14}H_{22}O_2$ MW: 222.33 Source: DU HUO. Ref: 2.

6455 4,4,8-Trimethyl-3β,7α,23-trihydroxy chola-14,24-dien-21-oic acid-21,23-lactone
$C_{30}H_{46}O_4$ MW: 470.70 Source: KU LIAN PI. Ref: 6.

6456 2,2,6-Trimethyl-6-vinyl-tetrahydropyran
$C_{10}H_{18}O$ MW: 154.25 Source: XIANG YE. Ref: 6.

6457 Triolein
$C_{57}H_{104}O_6$ MW: 885.46 Property: mp -4°C, bp 235-40°C/18 mm. Source: BAI E GAO, TONG YOU. Ref: 6.

6458 Tripdiolide
$C_{20}H_{24}O_7$ MW: 376.41 Property: mp 210-1°C, 226-8°C. Source: LEI GONG TENG. Ref: 4, 256.

6459 Tripdiotolnide

$C_{20}H_{24}O_6$ MW: 360.41 Property: colorless hyaloid rabdiod crystal, mp 222-4°C. Source: LEI GONG TENG. Ref: 256.

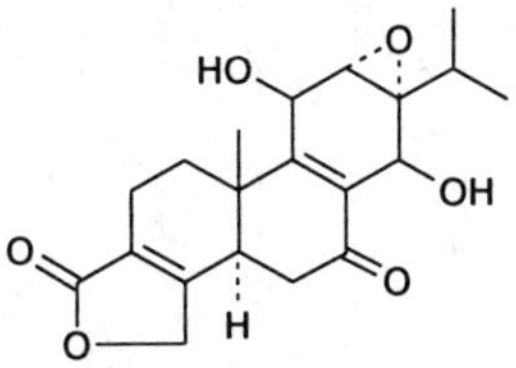

6460 Triptodihydroxy acid methyl ester

$C_{31}H_{50}O_4$ MW: 486.74 Source: LEI GONG TENG. Ref: 2.

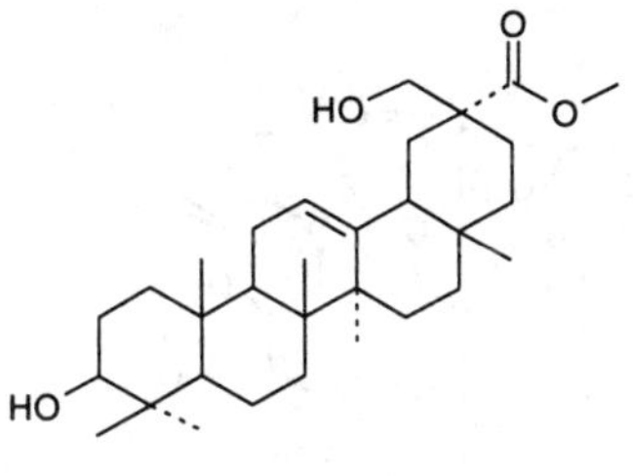

6461 Triptoditerpenic acid B

$C_{21}H_{28}O_3$ MW: 328.46 Property: white acicular crystal, mp 209-11°C. Source: KUN MING SHAN HAI TANG. Ref: 252.

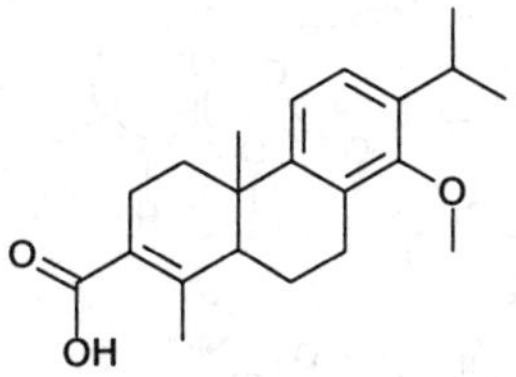

6462 Triptofordin A

$C_{31}H_{36}O_6$ MW: 504.63 Source: LEI GONG TENG. Ref: 2.

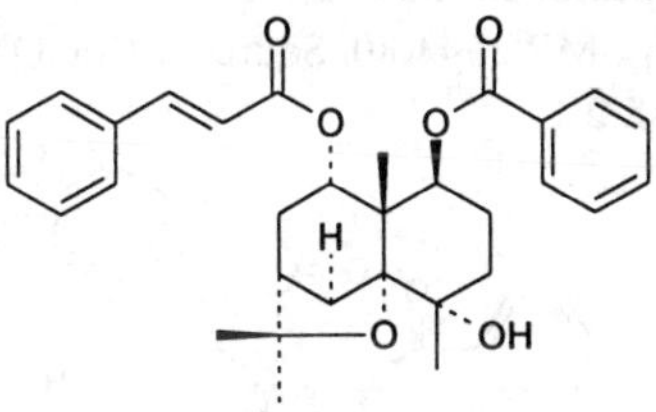

6463 Triptofordin B1

$C_{29}H_{34}O_6$ MW: 478.59 Source: LEI GONG TENG. Ref: 2.

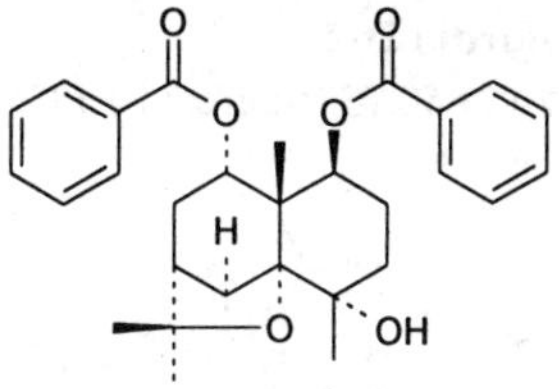

6464 Triptofordin B2

$C_{33}H_{36}O_{11}$ MW: 608.65 Source: LEI GONG TENG. Ref: 2.

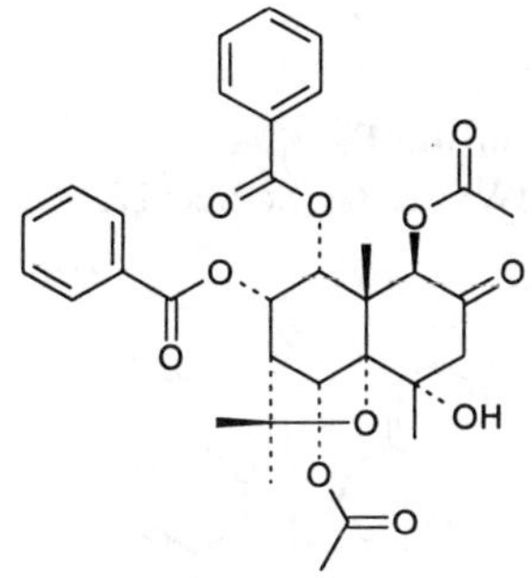

6465 Triptofordin C-2

$C_{33}H_{38}O_{11}$ MW: 610.66 Source: LEI GONG TENG. Ref: 2.

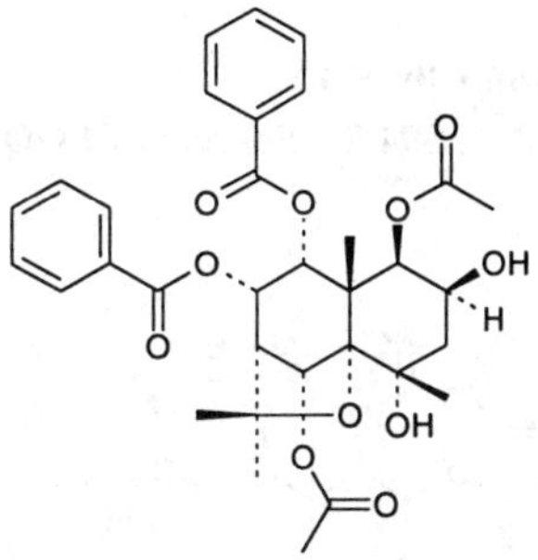

6466 Triptofordin D-1

$C_{34}H_{38}O_{10}$ MW: 606.68 Source: LEI GONG TENG. Ref: 2.

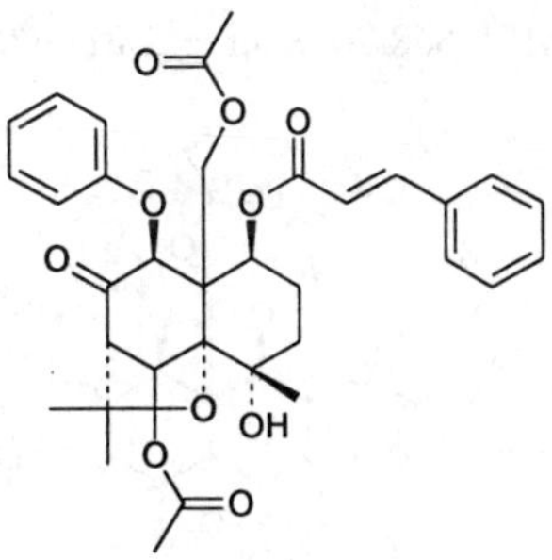

6467 Triptofordin D-2
$C_{36}H_{42}O_{11}$ MW: 650.73 Source: LEI GONG TENG. Ref: 2.

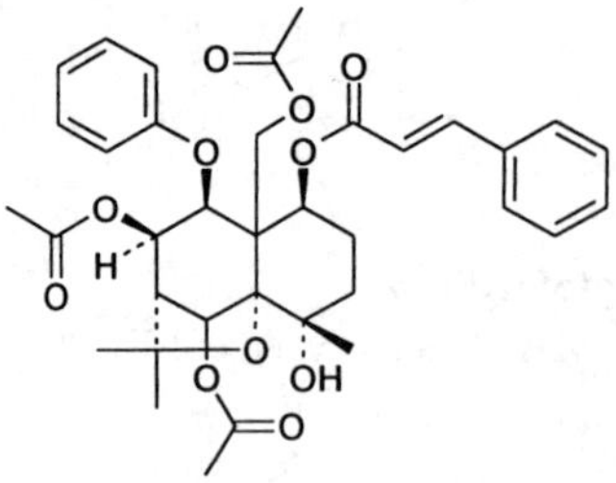

6468 Triptofordin E
$C_{33}H_{38}O_{11}$ MW: 610.66 Source: LEI GONG TENG. Ref: 2.

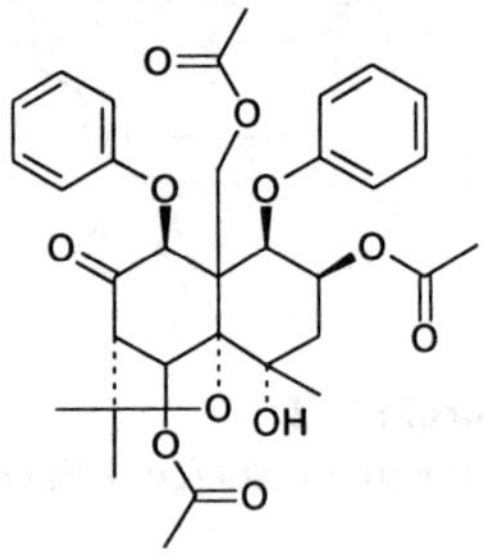

6469 Triptofordin F-1
$C_{37}H_{42}O_{13}$ MW: 694.74 Source: LEI GONG TENG. Ref: 2.

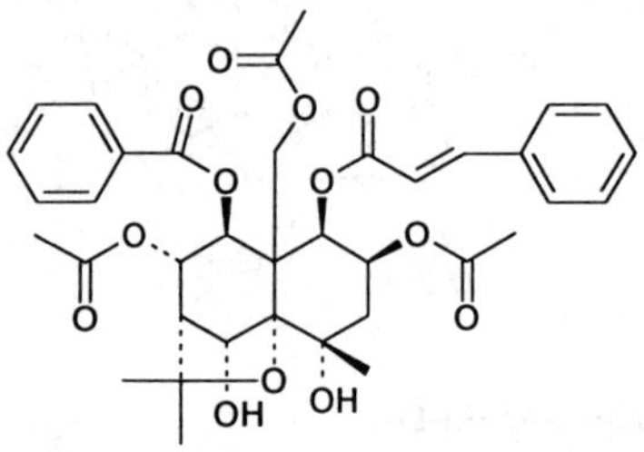

6470 Triptofordin F-2
$C_{35}H_{40}O_{13}$ MW: 668.70 Source: LEI GONG TENG. Ref: 2.

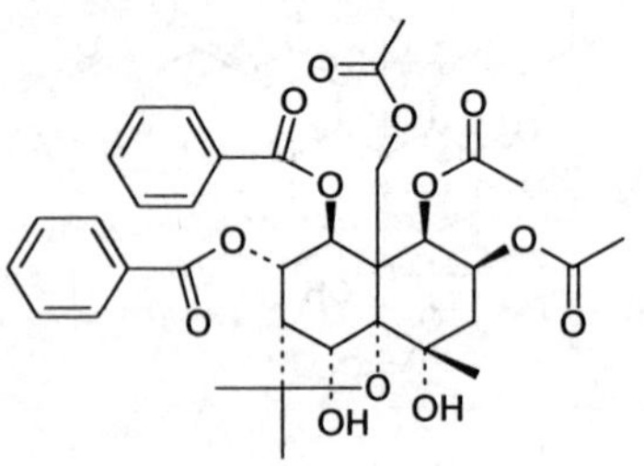

6471 Triptofordin F-3
$C_{37}H_{42}O_{14}$ MW: 710.74 Source: LEI GONG TENG. Ref: 2.

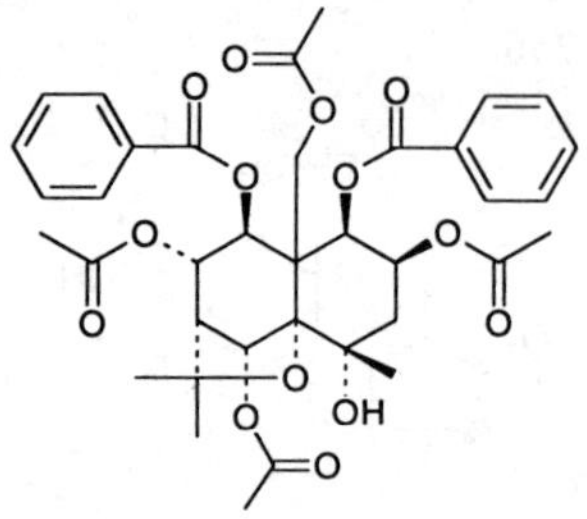

6472 Triptofordin F-4
$C_{35}H_{40}O_{12}$ MW: 652.70 Source: LEI GONG TENG. Ref: 2.

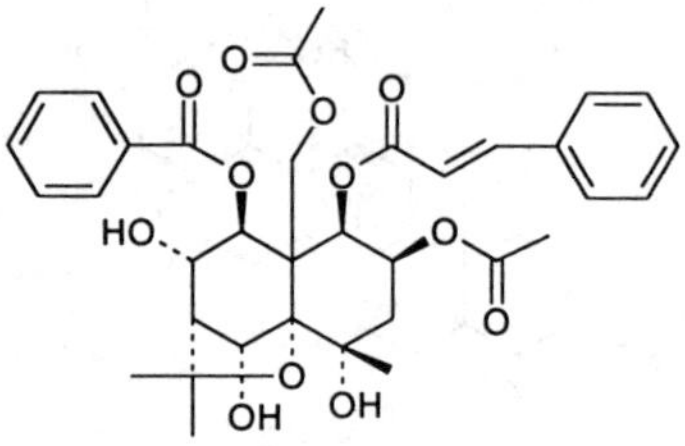

6473 Triptofordinine A-1
$C_{41}H_{43}NO_{12}$ MW: 741.80 Source: LEI GONG TENG. Ref: 2.

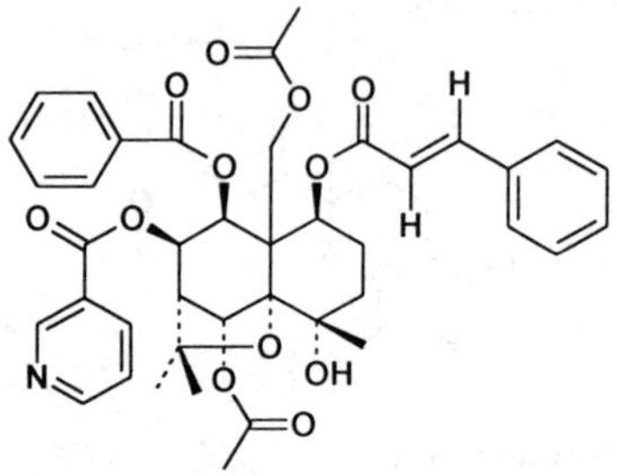

6474 Triptofordinine A-2
$C_{41}H_{43}NO_{12}$ MW: 741.80 Source: LEI GONG TENG. Ref: 2.

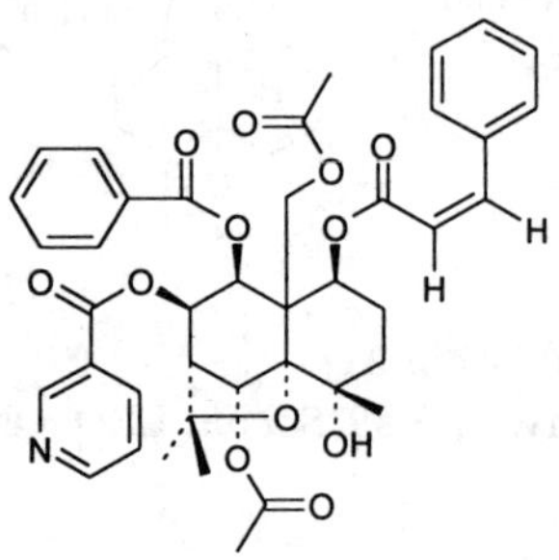

6475 Triptolide
$C_{20}H_{24}O_6$ MW: 360.41 Property: 227-8°C. Source: KUN MING SHAN HAI TANG, LEI GONG TENG. Ref: 4.

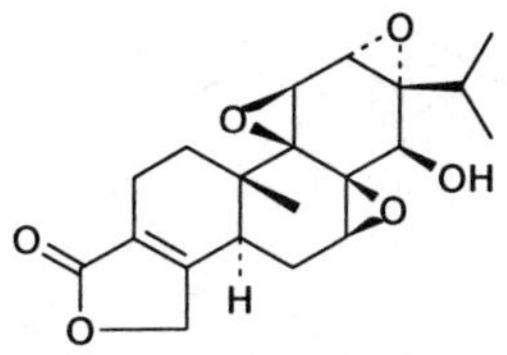

6476 Triptolidenol
$C_{20}H_{24}O_7$ MW: 376.41 Source: LEI GONG TENG. Ref: 256.

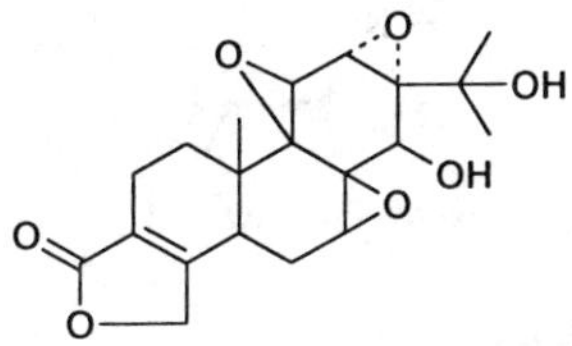

6477 Triptonide
CAS: 38647-11-9 $C_{20}H_{22}O_6$ MW: 358.39 Property: mp 226-8°C. Source: LEI GONG TENG. Ref: 5.

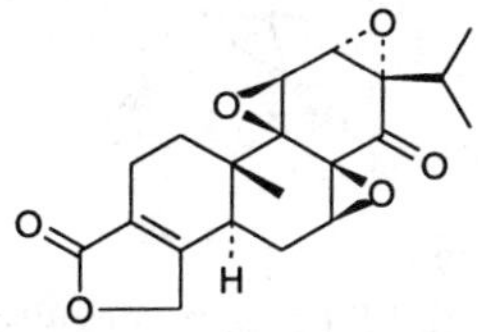

6478 Triptonoditerpenic acid
$C_{21}H_{28}O_4$ MW: 344.45 Property: white acicular crystal, mp 189-91°C. Source: KUN MING SHAN HAI TANG. Ref: 197.

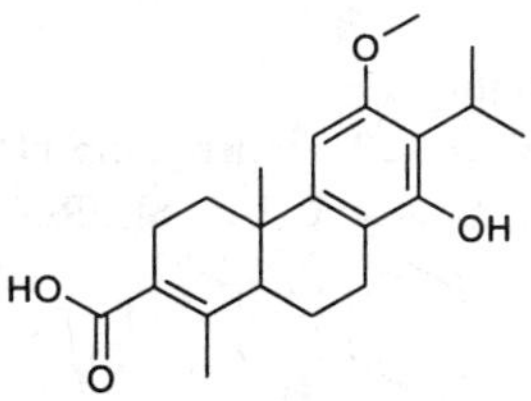

6479 Triptonolide
$C_{20}H_{22}O_4$ MW: 326.40 Source: Ref: 2.

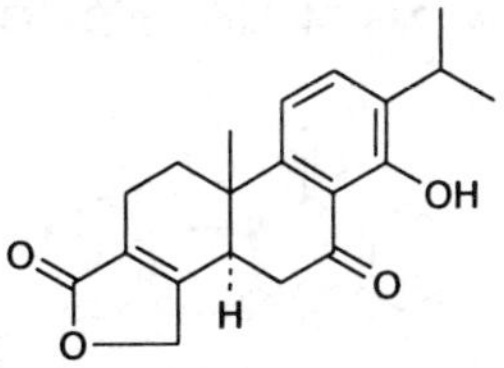

6480 Triptonoterpene
$C_{20}H_{28}O_2$ MW: 300.45 Source: LEI GONG TENG. Ref: 2.

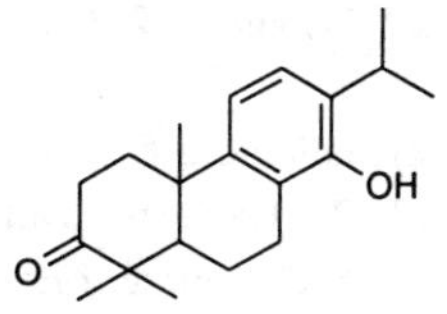

6481 Triptonoterpene methyl ether
$C_{21}H_{30}O_3$ MW: 330.47 Source: LEI GONG TENG. Ref: 2.

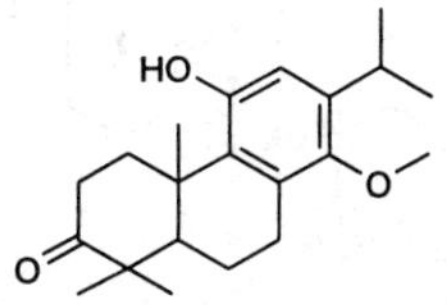

6482 Triptonoterpenol
$C_{21}H_{30}O_4$ MW: 346.47 Property: colorless columnar crystal, mp 197-9°C. Source: LEI GONG TENG. Ref: 78.

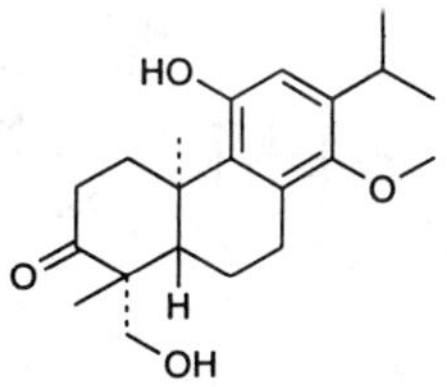

6483 Triptophenolide
Source: LEI GONG TENG. Ref: 655.

6484 Triptophenolide methyl ether
$C_{21}H_{26}O_3$ MW: 326.44 Source: LEI GONG TENG. Ref: 2.

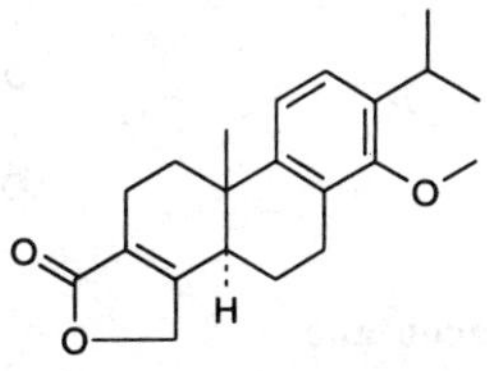

6485 Triptotriterpenic acid A
$C_{30}H_{48}O_4$ MW: 472.71 Source: LEI GONG TENG. Ref: 2.

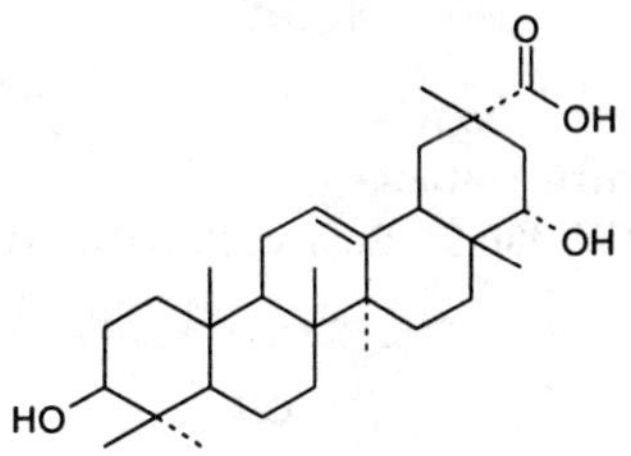

6486 Triptotriterpenic acid B
Source: LEI GONG TENG. Ref: 2.

6487 Triptotriterpenic acid C
$C_{30}H_{48}O_4$ MW: 472.71 Property: white amorphous powder, mp 247.5-9.5°C. Source: LEI GONG TENG. Bioactivity: having antiinflammatory. Ref: 125.

6488 Triptotriterpenoidel lactone A
$C_{31}H_{48}O_2$ MW: 452.73 Source: LEI GONG TENG. Ref: 2.

6489 Triricinolein
$C_{57}H_{104}O_9$ MW: 933.46 Source: BI MA YOU. Ref: 6.

6490 n-Tritriacontane
$C_{33}H_{68}$ MW: 464.91 Property: mp 72°C, bp 208°C/0 mm. Source: GUANG JIN QIAN CAO, JI CHANG LANG DU. Ref: 6.

6491 6-Tritriacontanol
$C_{33}H_{68}O$ MW: 480.91 Source: PU HUANG. Ref: 2.

6492 Tropic acid
$C_9H_{10}O_3$ MW: 166.18 Property: mp (±): 118°C. Source: MAN TUO LUO GEN. Ref: 6.

6493 Tropine
$C_8H_{15}NO$ MW: 141.21 Property: mp 63°C, bp 229°C. Source: LANG DANG GEN, MAN TUO LUO ZI, MAN TUO LUO GEN, SAI LANG DANG, ZANG QIE. Ref: 6.

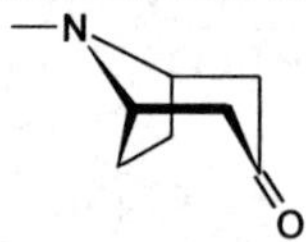

6494 Tropinone
$C_8H_{13}NO$ MW: 1139.20 Property: mp 42°C, bp 224-5°C. Source: JIA SUAN JIANG. Ref: 6.

6495 Tropolone
$C_7H_6O_2$ MW: 122.12 Property: mp 49-50°C. Source: SHAN CI BAI. Ref: 6.

6496 Tryptamine
$C_{10}H_{12}N_2$ MW: 160.22 Property: mp 116-7°C, bp 137°C/0.15mm. Source: CHAN SU. Ref: 2.

6497 Tryptanthrin
$C_{15}H_8N_2O_2$ MW: 248.24 Source: DA QING YE. Ref: 2.

6498 Tryptophane
$C_{11}H_{12}N_2O_2$ MW: 204.23 Property: mp (+): 275-82°C, (-): 289°C (dec), (±): 283-5°C. Source: DA QING YE, CAN JIAN, GUI GAI. Ref: 6.

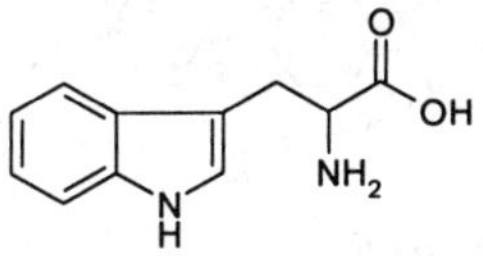

6499 Tuberostemonine
$C_{22}H_{33}NO_4$ MW: 375.51 Property: mp 86-8°C. Source: BAI BU. Ref: 6.

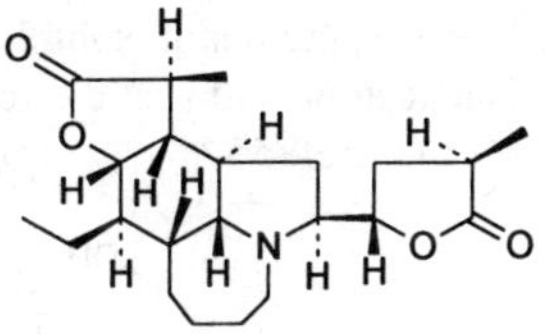

6500 Tuduranine
$C_{18}H_{19}NO_3$ MW: 297.36 Source: QING FENG TENG. Ref: 6.

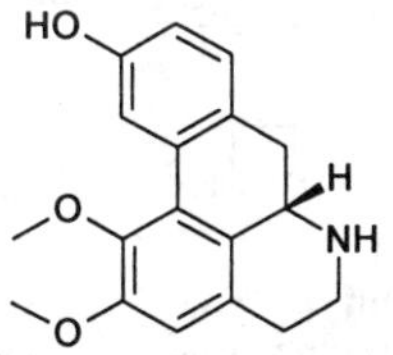

6501 Tufulingoside
5,7-Dihydroxyl-chromone-3-α-L-rhamnopyranoside. $C_{15}H_{16}O_9$ MW: 340.29 Property: lignt yellow cluster crystal (MeOH/CHCl3), mp 227-9°C. Source: TU FU LING. Ref: 499.

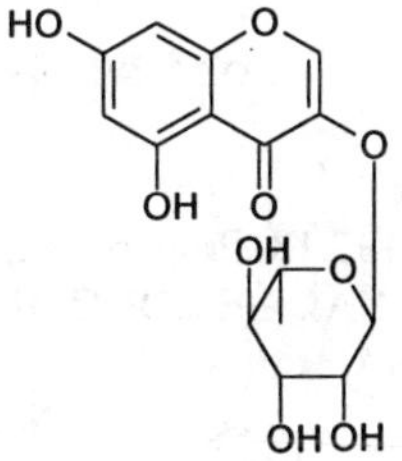

6502 Tulipalin
Tulipalin A. CAS: 547-65-9 $C_5H_6O_2$ MW: 98.10 Property: mp 85-6°C. Source: YU JIN XIANG. Ref: 5.

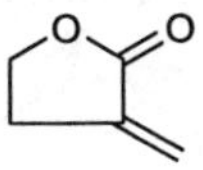

6503 Tulipinolide
CAS: 24164-12-3 $C_{17}H_{22}O_4$ MW: 290.36 Property: mp 181°C (dec). Source: *Liriodendron tulipifera* L. Ref: 5.

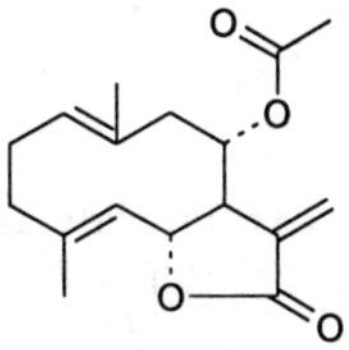

6504 Tuliposide A
$C_{11}H_{18}O_8$ MW: 278.26 Source: YU JIN XIANG. Ref: 6.

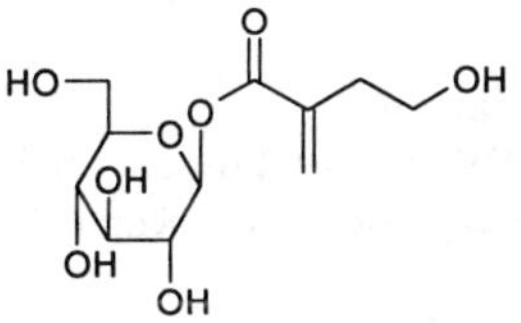

6505 Tuliposide B
$C_{11}H_{18}O_9$ MW: 294.26 Source: YU JIN XIANG. Ref: 6.

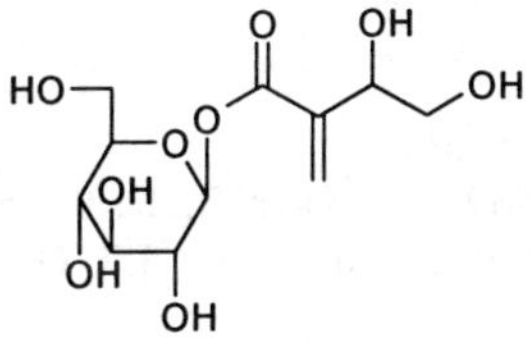

6506 Tumulosic acid
$C_{31}H_{50}O_4$ MW: 486.74 Property: mp 306°C (dec). Source: FU LING. Ref: 2, 6.

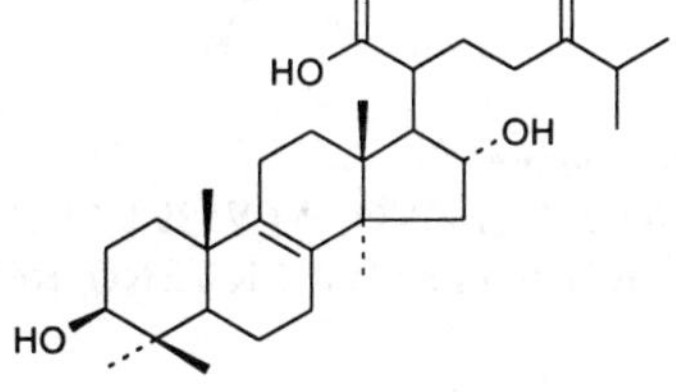

6507 Turanose
$C_{12}H_{22}O_{11}$ MW: 342.30 Property: mp 157°C (dec). Source: PU HUANG. Ref: 6.

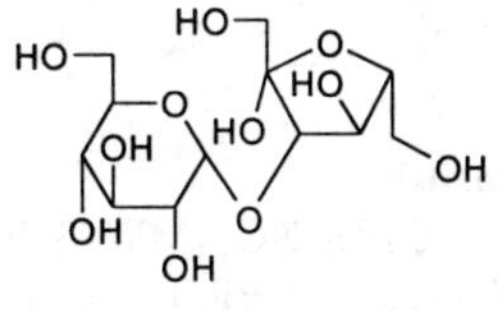

6508 Turmerone
$C_{15}H_{20}O$ MW: 216.33 Property: bp 159-60°C/10 mm. Source: YU JIN. Ref: 6.

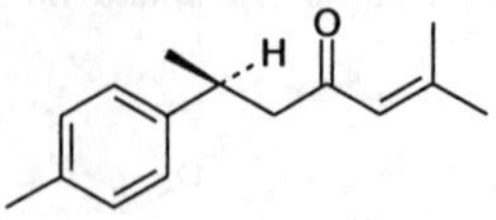

6509 Tutin
$C_{15}H_{18}O_6$ MW: 294.31 Property: mp 211-3°C. Source: MA SANG YE. Ref: 4, 6.

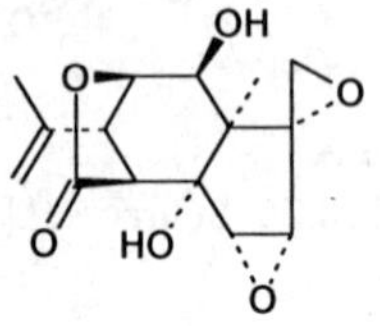

6510 Tylocrebrine
$C_{24}H_{27}NO_4$ MW: 393.49 Property: mp (-): 218-20°C (dec). Source: WA ER TENG. Ref: 6.

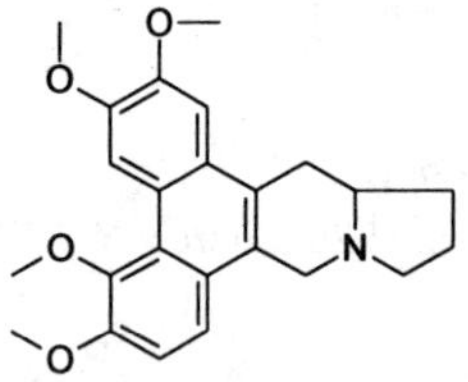

6511 Tylophoridine
CAS: 325223-69-6 $C_{22}H_{23}NO_4$ MW: 365.43 Property: mp 213-4°C. Source: WA ER TENG. Ref: 5.

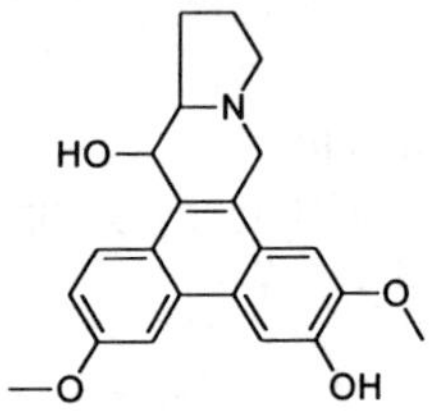

6512 Tylophorine
CAS: 482-02-2 $C_{24}H_{27}NO_4$ MW: 393.49 Property: mp 292°C (dec). Source: WA ER TENG. Ref: 4.

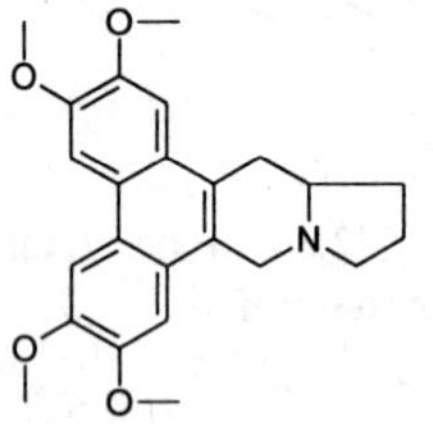

6513 Tylophorinine
CAS: 6794-27-5 $C_{23}H_{25}NO_4$ MW: 379.46 Property: mp 248-9°C. Source: WA ER TENG. Ref: 5.

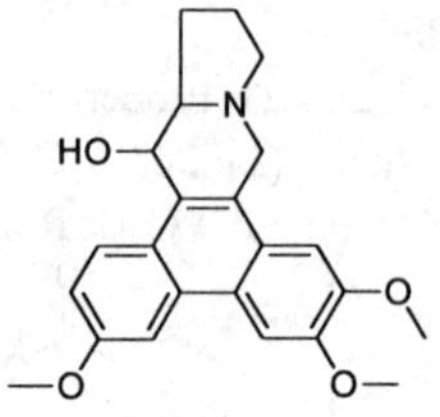

6514 Typhaneoside
Isorhamnetin-3-O-(2^G-α-L-rhamnopyranosyl)-α-L-rhamnopyranosyl-(1→6)-β-D-glncopyranoside. $C_{34}H_{42}O_{20}$ MW: 770.70 Property:yellow amorphous powder, mp 148-50°C, $[\alpha]_D^{20}$ -58° (c=1.3, methanol), easily soluble in water, methanol; soluble in ethanol; slightly soluble in acetone and acetic ester. Source: XIA YE XIANG PU. Ref: 55.

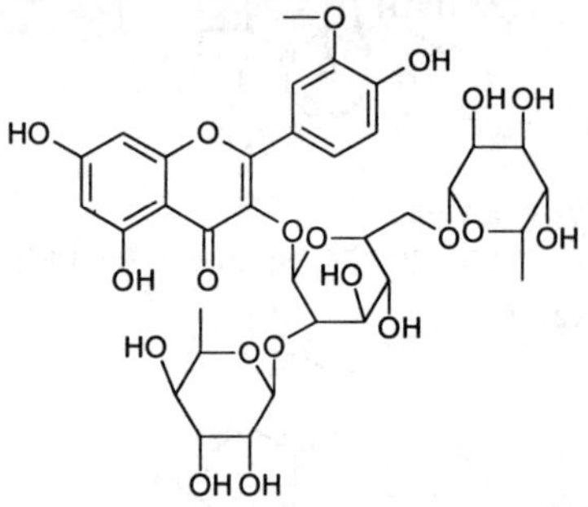

6515 Typhic acid
$C_{19}H_{20}O_7$ MW: 360.37 Property: white massive crystal, mp 248-50°C. Source: PU HUANG, XIA XIANG PU. Ref: 2, 80.

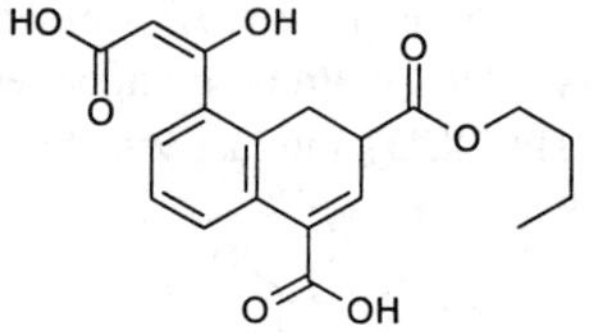

6516 Tyramine
$C_8H_{11}NO$ MW: 137.18 Property: mp 164-4.5°C. Source: BAI QU CAI, GE CONG, JIANG, MAI JIAO, YE ZHI MA. Ref: 6.

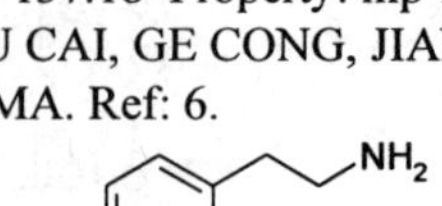

6517 Tyrosol
$C_8H_{10}O_2$ MW: 138.17 Property: mp 93°C. Source: DA HUA HONG JING TIAN, XIA YE HONG JING TIAN. Ref: 218, 516.

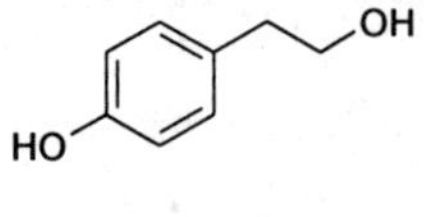

6518 Ugonin A
$C_{25}H_{26}O_6$ MW: 422.48 Property: mp 225-6°C. Source: RU DI WU GONG. Ref: 6.

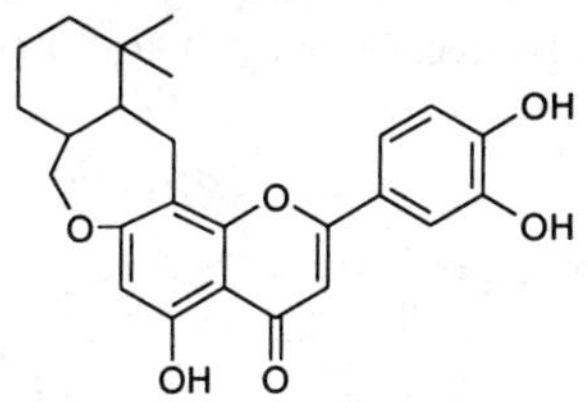

6519 Ugonin B
$C_{26}H_{28}O_6$ MW: 436.51 Property: mp 252-4°C. Source: RU DI WU GONG. Ref: 6.

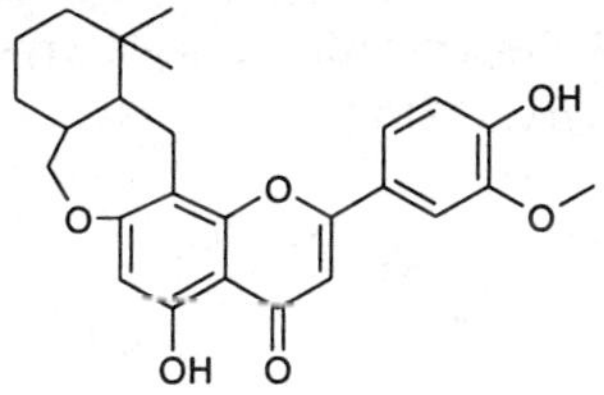

6520 Ugonin C
$C_{21}H_{20}O_6$ MW: 368.39 Property: mp (-): 236-7°C. Source: RU DI WU GONG. Ref: 6.

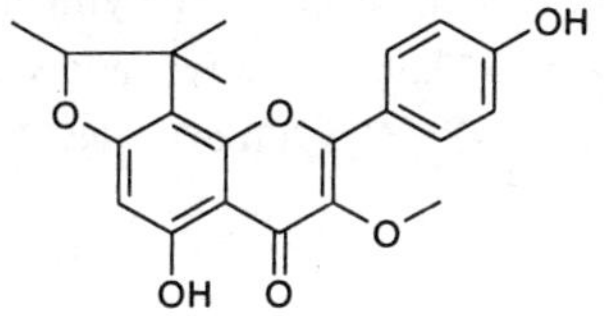

6521 Ugonin D
$C_{20}H_{20}O_5$ MW: 340.38 Property: mp 183°C. Source: RU DI WU GONG. Ref: 6.

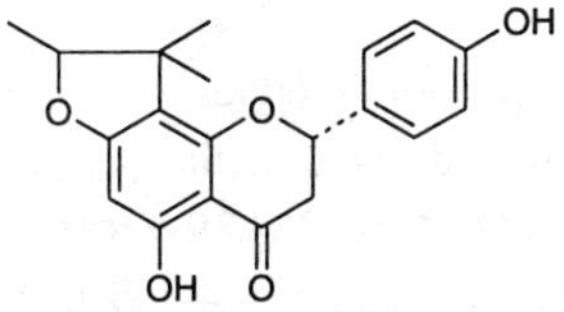

6522 Ulmoprenol
Source: DU ZHONG. Ref: 2.

6523 Ulmoside
Source: DU ZHONG. Ref: 2.

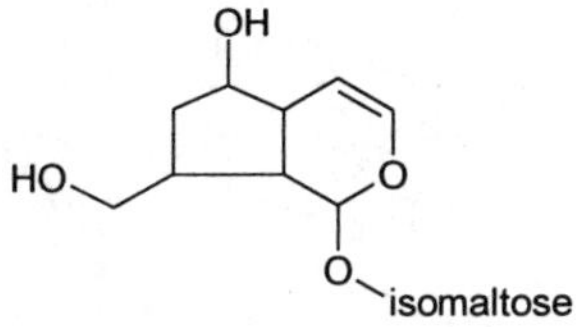

6524 Umbelliferone
7-Hydroxycoumarin. CAS: 93-35-6 $C_9H_6O_3$ MW: 162.15 Property: mp 225-8°C. Source: BAI ZHI, DU HUO, HUI XIANG, LANG DU, LONG YAN DU HUO, QIAN HUA JIAO, PI HAN CAO, ZANG YAN XUN DAO NIU. Ref: 4, 207, 324, 556, 571.

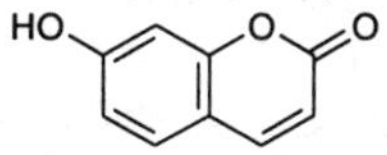

6525 Umbelliprenin
7-Hydroxycoumarin farnesyl ether. $C_{24}H_{30}O_3$ MW: Property: mp 61-3°C. Source: SHI LUO ZI. Ref: 6.

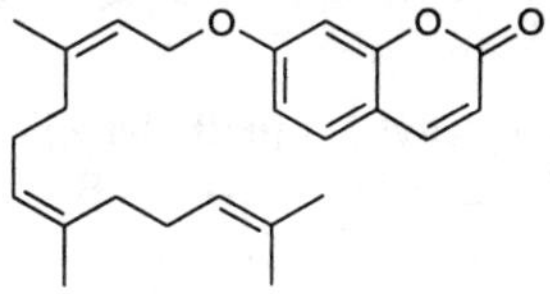

6526 Undecanoic acid
$C_{11}H_{22}O_2$ MW: 186.30 Source: FU LING. Ref: 2.

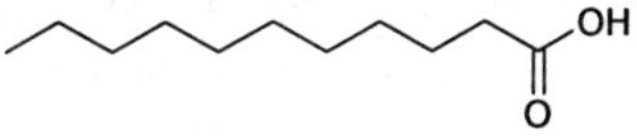

6527 Undecan-2-ol
$C_{11}H_{24}O$ MW: 172.31 Property: mp (+): 12°C, bp (-): 231-3°C, (±): 228-9°C. Source: CHOU CAO. Ref: 6.

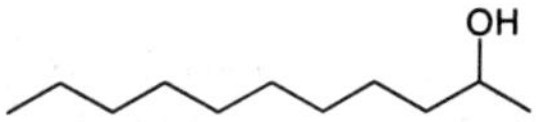

6528 2-Undecanone
$C_{11}H_{22}O$ MW: 170.30 Source: YU XING CAO. Ref: 2.

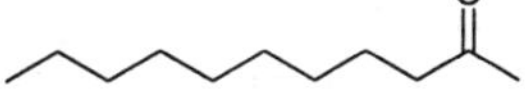

6529 Undecene
$C_{11}H_{22}$ MW: 154.30 Property: bp 192-5°C. Source: BAI ZHI. Ref: 2.

6530 10-Undecenoic acid
$C_{11}H_{20}O_2$ MW: 184.28 Source: BAI ZHI. Ref: 2.

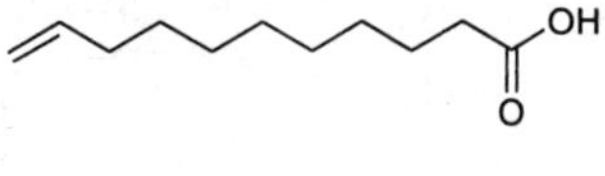

6531 n-Undecyl acetate
$C_{13}H_{26}O_2$ MW: 214.35 Source: HEI MA YI. Ref: 6.

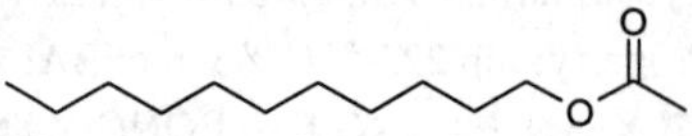

6532 2-Undecyl acetate
$C_{13}H_{26}O_2$ MW: 214.35 Source: CHOU CAO. Ref: 6.

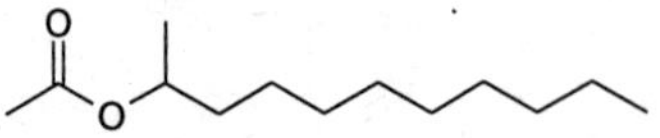

6533 Undecyl alcohol
$C_{11}H_{24}O$ MW: 172.31 Property: mp 19-11°C, bp 147°C/25mm. Source: HEI MA YI. Ref: 6.

6534 1-Undecylenyl-3,4-methylenedioxy benzene
$C_{18}H_{28}O_2$ MW: 276.42 Source: BI BA. Ref: 6.

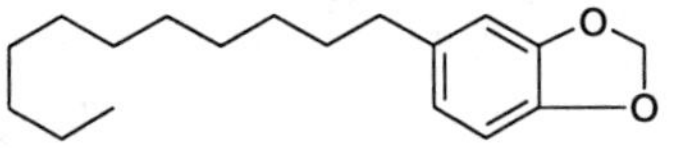

6535 Ungeremine
Lecobetaine. $C_{16}H_{12}NO_3$ MW: 266.28 Property: mp 270-2°C. Source: *Ungernia* minor. Ref: 4.

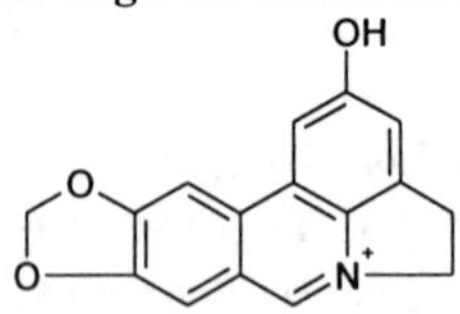

6536 Uracil
$C_4H_4N_2O_2$ MW: 112.09 Property: 335°C. Source: DANG GUI, DONG CHONG XIA CAO, SI CHUAN JIANG YOU FU ZI. Ref: 2, 239.

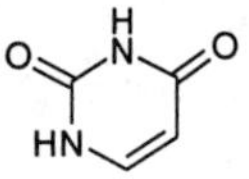

6537 Uralene
5,6,3',4'-tetrahydroxy-3-methoxy-6'-isoprenyl flavone. $C_{21}H_{20}O_7$ MW: 384.39 Property: light yellow lamellar crystal, mp 216-218°C. Source: WU LA ER GAN CAO. Ref: 251.

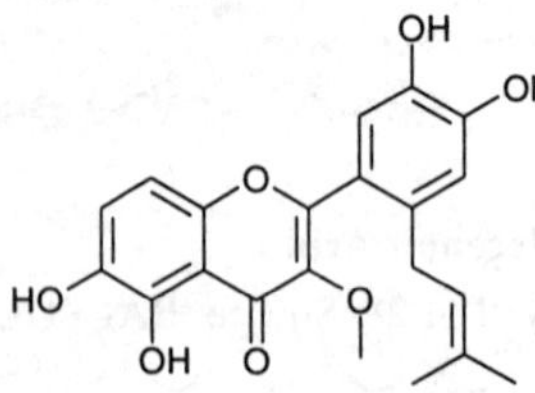

6539 Uralenin
5,7,3',4'-Tetrahydroxy-5'-isoprenylflavone. $C_{20}H_{18}O_7$ MW: 370.36 Property: white crystalline powder, mp 212.5-4.0°C. Source: GAN CAO. Ref: 171.

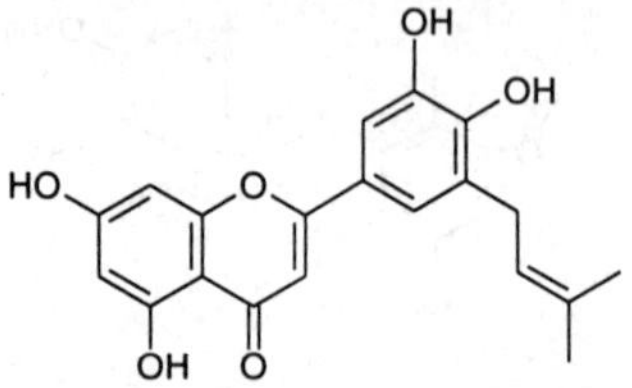

6540 Uralenneoside
1-O-Protocatechuyl-β-D-xylopyranose. $C_{12}H_{14}O_8$ MW: 286.24 Property: white granular crystal, mp 185-7°C. Source: GANCAO. Ref: 231.

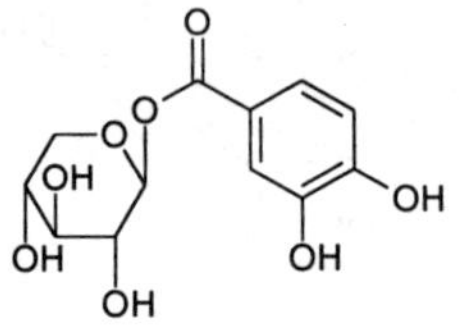

6541 Uralenol
3,5,7,3',4'-Pentahydroxy-5'-isoprenylflavone. $C_{20}H_{18}O_7$ MW: 370.36 Property: yellow acicular crystal, mp 170.5-2.5°C. Source: GANCAO. Ref: 171.

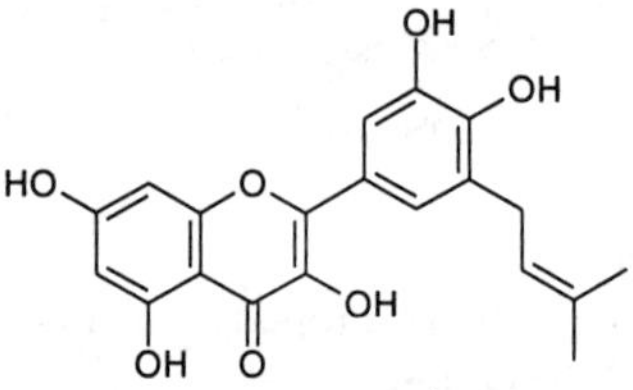

6542 Uralenol-3-methylether
5,7,3',4'-4-tetrahydroxy-3-methoxy-5'-isoprenyl flavone. $C_{21}H_{20}O_7$ MW: 384.39 Property: dark yellow lamellar crystal, mp 104-109°C. Source: WU LA ER GAN CAO. Ref: 251.

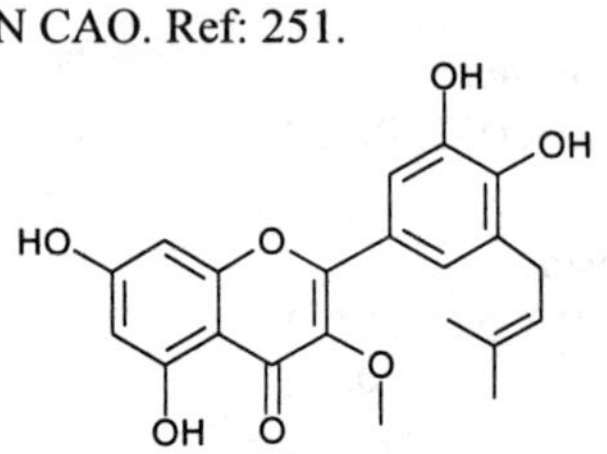

6543 Uralsaponin A
3β-Hydroxy-11-oxo-olean-12-en-30-oic acid-3-O -β-D-glucuronopyranosyl-(1-2)-β-D-glucurono-pyranoside(I). $C_{42}H_{66}O_{14}$ MW: 794.99 Property: white granular crystal, mp 235°C, $[\alpha]_D^{18}$ +42.7° (c=0.45, 90% methanol). Source: WU LA ER GAN CAO. Ref: 57.

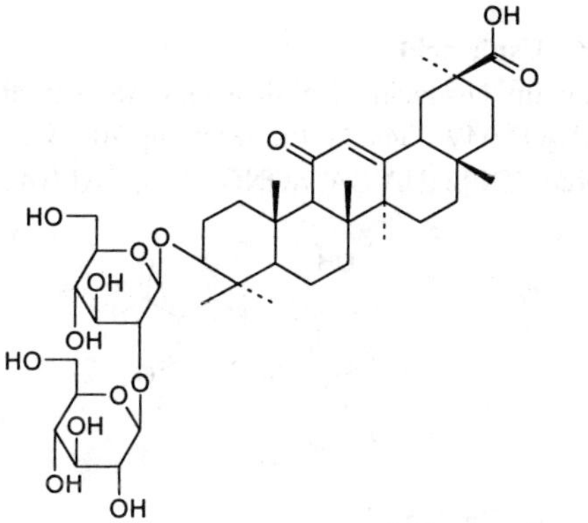

6544 Uralsaponin B
3β-Hydroxy-11-oxo-olean-12-en-30-oic acid-3-O -β-D-glucuronopyranosyl-(1-3)-β-D-glucurono-pyranoside(II). $C_{42}H_{66}O_{14}$ MW: 794.99 Property: white granular crystal, mp 244°C, $[\alpha]_D^{18}$ +31.0° (c=0.29, 90% methanol). Source: HUANG GAN CAO, WU LA ER GAN CAO. Ref: 57, 195.

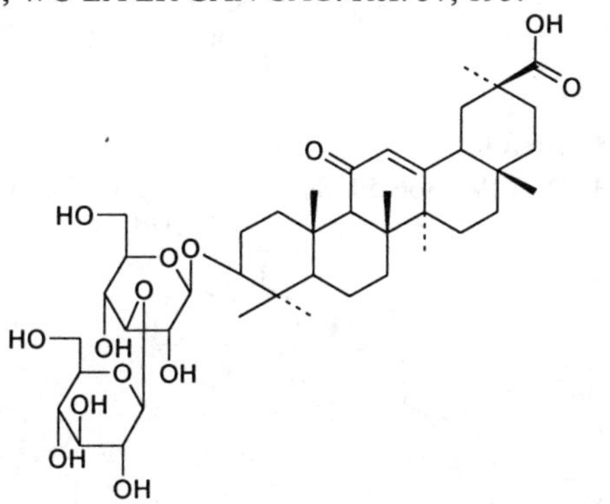

6545 Urea
C_3H_6O MW: 58.08 Property: mp 132°C. Source: DONG GUA ZI, LI SHU PI, MA BO, NIU DAN, NIU XUE, REN NIAO, REN ZHONG BAI, WU LING ZHI, XIA TIAN GAO, YE MING SHA. Ref: 6.

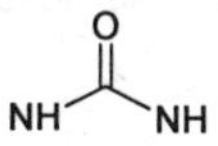

6546 Uric acid
$C_5H_4N_4O_3$ MW: 168.11 Property: not mp °C, >400°C (dec). Source: MA BO, NIU XUE, REN NIAO, REN ZHONG BAI, XIA TIAN GAO, YE MING SHA, YUAN CAN ZI. Ref: 6.

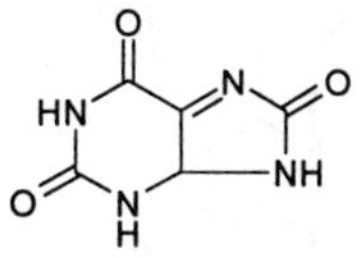

6547 Uridine monophosphate
$C_9H_{13}N_2O_9P$ MW: 324.19 Property: mp 198.5°C. Source: MO GU. Ref: 6.

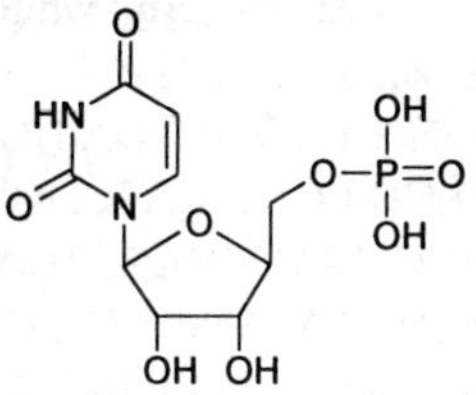

6548 Uridylic acid
$C_9H_{13}N_2O_9P$ MW: 324.19 Property: mp 195°C (dec). Source: GOU QI YE. Ref: 6.

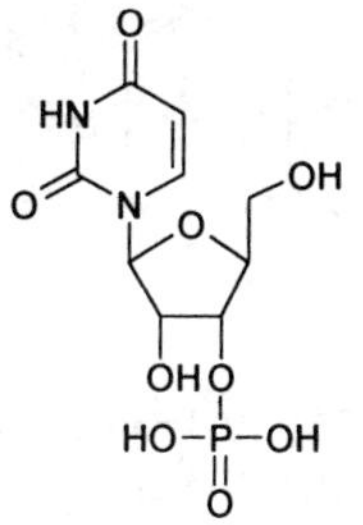

6549 Urobilin
$C_{33}H_{42}N_4O_6$ MW: 590.73 Property: mp 177°C. Source: REN NIAO. Ref: 6.

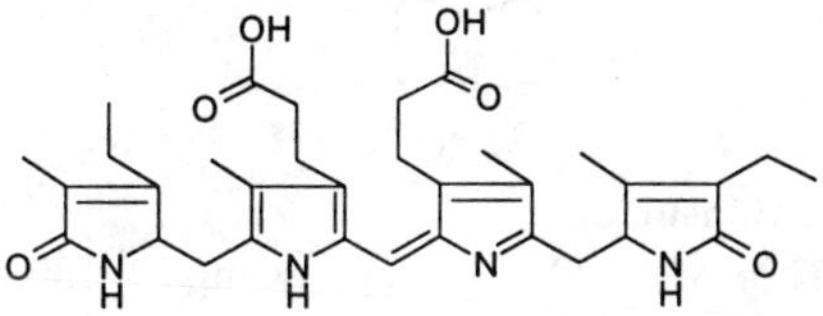

6550 Urocanic acid
$C_6H_6N_2O_2$ MW: 138.13 Property: mp α:(trans) 218-24°C, β: (cis) 175-6°C. Source: GUI GAI. Ref: 6.

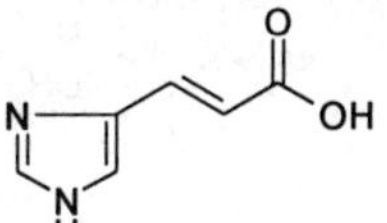

6551 Ursodeoxycholic acid
$C_{24}H_{40}O_4$ MW: 392.58 Source: XIONG DAN. Ref: 2.

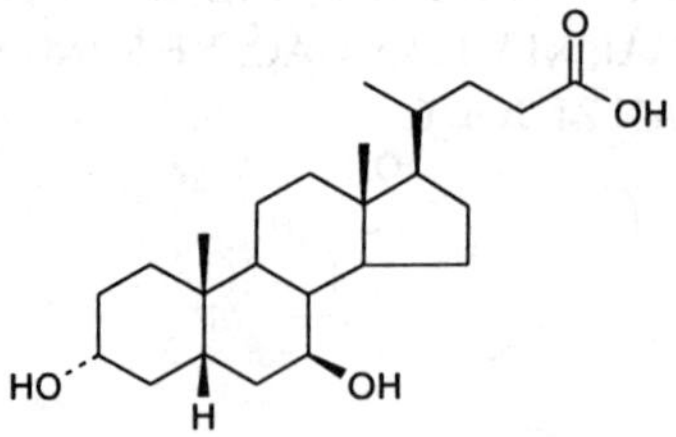

6552 Ursolic acid
Malol; Prunol; β-Ursolic acid, Urson, CAS: 77-52-1 $C_{30}H_{48}O_3$ MW: 456.72 Property: white solid powder (chloroform-methanol), mp 298-4°C, 265-7°C. Source: CHI NAN, CHONG YA YAO, DA HONG PAO, DAN SHEN, DENG LONG CAO, DONG LING CAO, DU ZHONG, LIAN QIAO, RUAN ZAO MI HOU TAO, SHAN DI XIANG CHA CAI, SHAN ZHA, SHAN ZHU YU, ZHI ZI. Ref: 4, 454, 367, 428, 501, 592, 595, 600.

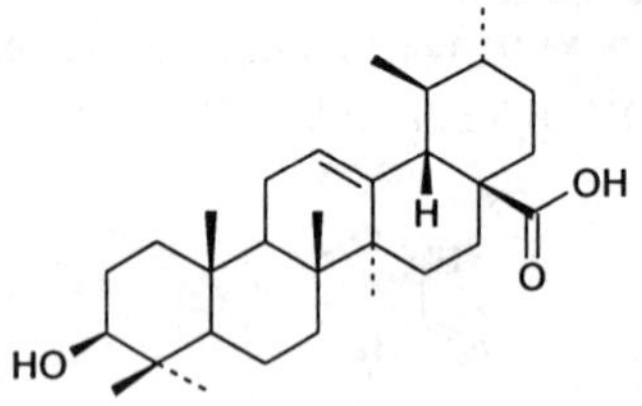

6553 Usaramine
$C_{18}H_{25}NO_6$ MW: 351.40 Property: mp (trans): 182.5-3.5°C. Source: XIANG LING CAO. Ref: 6.

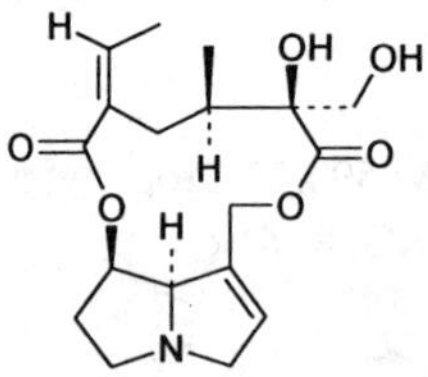

6554 Ushinsunine
$C_{18}H_{17}NO_3$ MW: 295.34 Property: mp (-): 180-1°C. Source: BAI LAN HUA, HUANG MIAN GUI. Ref: 6.

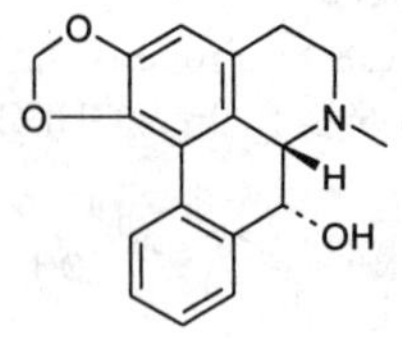

6555 Usnetic acid
$C_{13}H_{14}O_6$ MW: 266.25 Source: SHI HUA. Ref: 6.

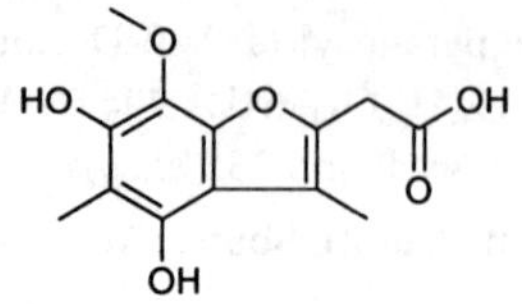

6556 Usnic acid
Usmneim; Usniacin; Usninic acid. CAS: 125-46-2 $C_{18}H_{16}O_7$ MW: 344.32 Property: mp 202-4°C. Source: JIN SHUA BA, SONG LUO, TAI BAI HUA. Ref: 4.

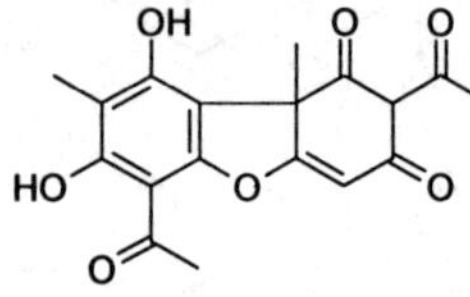

6557 Ustilaginoidin A
$C_{28}H_{18}O_{10}$ MW: 514.45 Property: mp >300°C. Source: JING GU NU. Ref: 6.

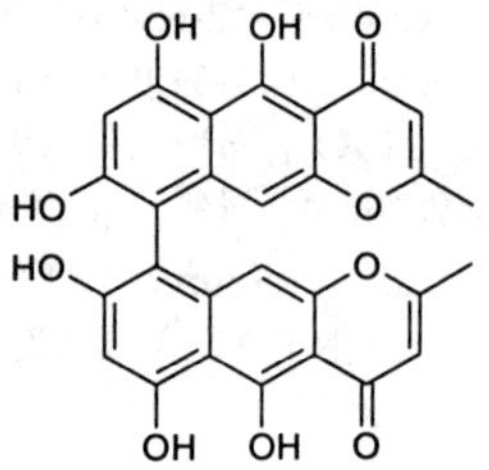

6558 Utendin
$C_{21}H_{34}O_5$ MW: 366.50 Source: LUO MO. Ref: 6.

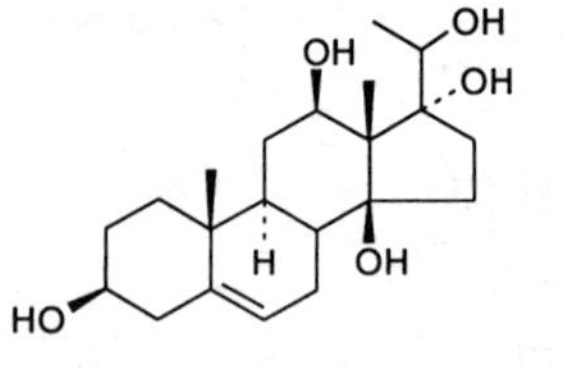

6559 Uvaol
$C_{30}H_{50}O_2$ MW: 442.73 Property: mp 233°C. Source: KU DING CHA. Ref: 6.

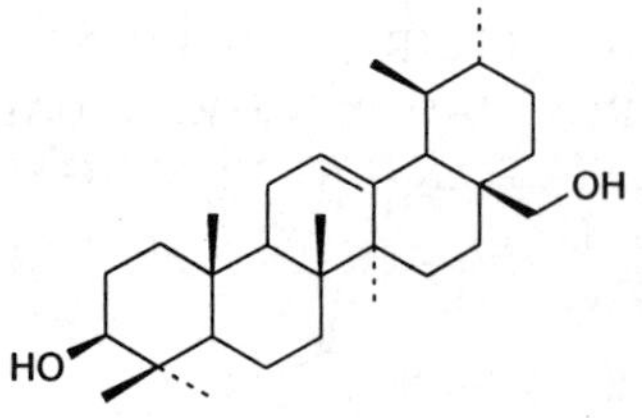

6560 Uvaribonianin III
$C_{37}H_{66}O_7$ MW: 622.93 Property: colorless gelatinoid, $[\alpha]_D^{15}$ +13° (c=0.01, chloroform). Source: GUANG YE ZI YU PAN. Ref: 355.

6561 Uvaribonin II
$C_{39}H_{70}O_8$ MW: 666.99 Property: white wax solid, mp 50-2°C, $[\alpha]_D^{15}$ +13° (c=0.02, chloroform). Source: GUANG YE ZI YU PAN. Ref: 355.

6562 Uvaribonol D
$C_{21}H_{20}O_7$ MW: 384.39 Property: white solid, mp 65-7°C, $[\alpha]_D^{20}$ +40.1° (c=0.02, Methanol). Source: GUANG YE ZI YU PAN. Ref: 406.

6563 Uvaribonol E
$C_{21}H_{20}O_7$ MW: 347.39 Property: white solid, mp 125-7°C, $[\alpha]_D^{24}$ -33.4° (c=0.04, Methanol). Source: GUANG YE ZI YU PAN. Ref: 406.

6564 Uvaribonol F
$C_{18}H_{20}O_8$ MW: 364.36 Property: white acicular crystal, mp 148-9°C, $[\alpha]_D^{24}$ +40.0° (c=0.02, Methanol). Source: GUANG YE ZI YU PAN. Ref: 406.

6565 Uvaribonol G
$C_{18}H_{20}O_8$ MW: 364.32 Property: white prismatic crystal, mp 98-100°C, $[\alpha]_D^{24}$ -120.6° (c=0.07, Methanol). Source: GUANG YE ZI YU PAN. Ref: 406.

6566 Uvaribonone I
$C_{39}H_{68}O_8$ MW: 664.97 Property: white wax solid, mp 42-4°C, $[\alpha]_D^{15}$ +15°(c=0.06, chloroform) Source: GUANG YE ZI YU PAN. Ref: 355.

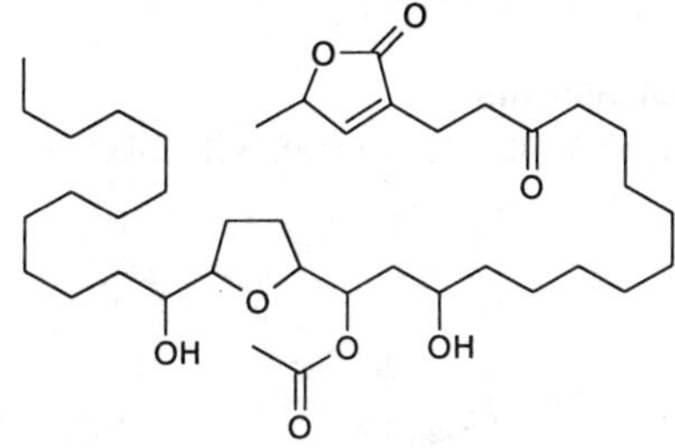

6567 Uvarigrandin A
$C_{37}H_{66}O_7$ MW: 622.93 Property: white wax solid. Source: DA HUA ZI YU PAN. Ref: 378.

6568 Uvarigrin
$C_{37}H_{68}O_6$ MW: 608.95 Property: colorless lame-llar crystal (acetone), mp 85-6°C, $[\alpha]_D^{21}$ +30.5° (c= 0.02, methanol). Source: DA HUA ZI YU PAN. Ref: 378.

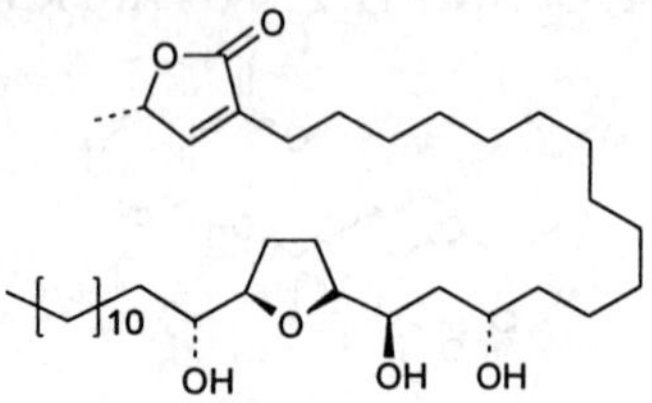

6569 Uzarigenin
CAS: 466-09-1 $C_{23}H_{34}O_4$ MW: 374.53 Property: mp 246°C. Source: LIAN SHENG GUI ZI HUA. Ref: 5, 6.

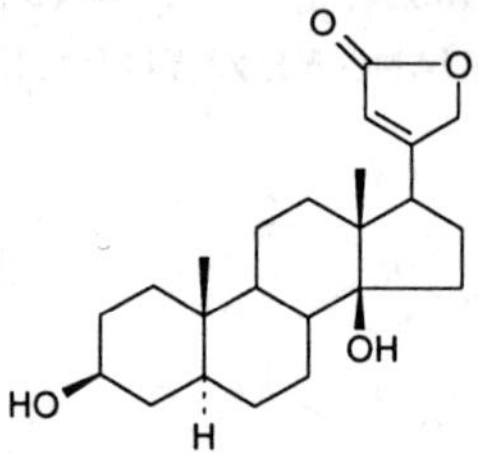

6570 Valencene
$C_{16}H_{26}$ MW: 218.39 Property: bp 123°C/11mm. Source: HUO XIANG. Ref: 2.

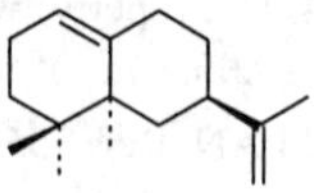

6571 Valepotriate
$C_{22}H_{30}O_8$ MW: 422.48 Source: XIE CAO. Ref: 6.

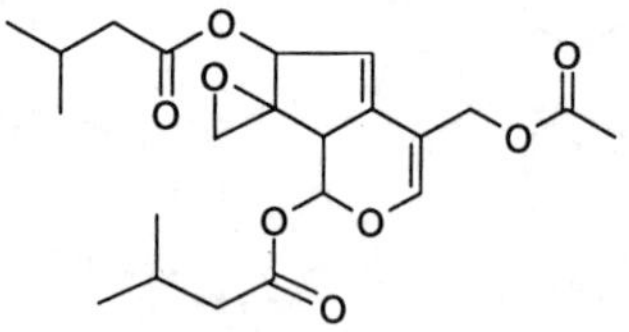

6572 Valeranone
Jatamansone. $C_{15}H_{26}O$ MW: 222.37 Property: bp (-): 155-6°C/11mm. Source: GAN SONG, XIE CAO. Ref: 6.

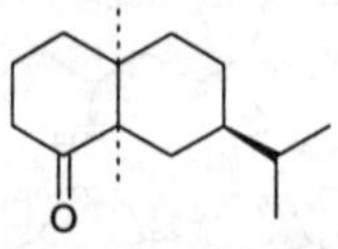

6573 Valerenic acid
$C_{15}H_{22}O_2$ MW: 234.34 Property: mp 140-2°C. Source: XIE CAO. Ref: 6.

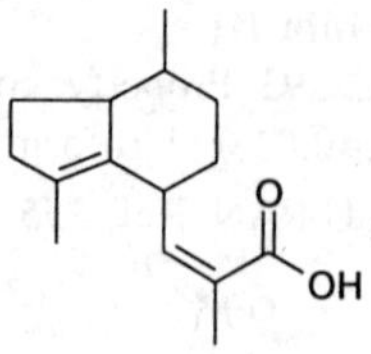

6574 Valerenolic acid
$C_{16}H_{24}O_2$ MW: 248.37 Property: mp 171-3°C. Source: XIE CAO. Ref: 6.

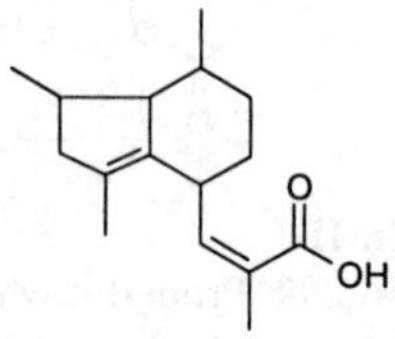

6575 Valerenone
$C_5H_{22}O$ MW: 218.34 Property: bp 87-9°C/0.05mm. Source: XIE CAO. Ref: 6.

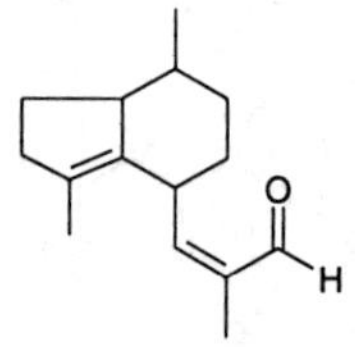

6576 Valerianae alkaloid A
$C_{18}H_{22}NO \bullet Cl$ MW: 268.38•35.45 Property: mp 201-3°C (dec). Source: XIE CAO. Ref: 6.

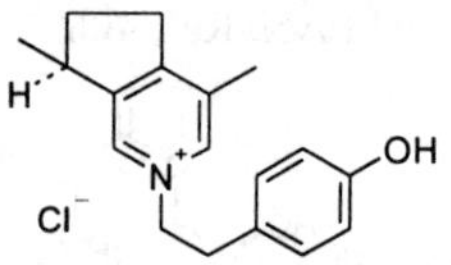

6577 Valerianae alkaloid B
$C_{18}H_{22}NO_2 \bullet Cl$ MW: 284.38•35.5 Property: mp 220-7°C (dec). Source: XIE CAO. Ref: 6.

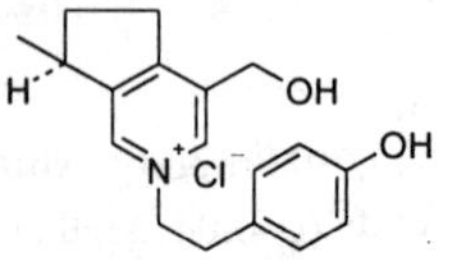

6578 Valerianine
$C_{11}H_{15}NO$ MW: 177.25 Property: mp 134°C. Source: XIE CAO. Ref: 6.

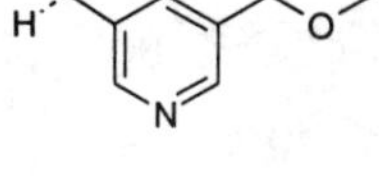

6579 Valerianol
$C_{15}H_{26}O$ MW: 222.37 Property: bp 120°C/0.01mm. Source: XIE CAO. Ref: 6.

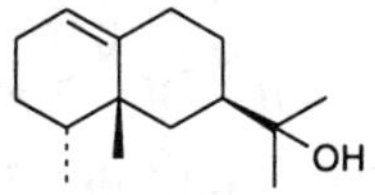

6580 Valeric aldehyde
$C_5H_{10}O$ MW: 86.13 Property: bp 103°C. Source: DA SUAN. Ref: 6.

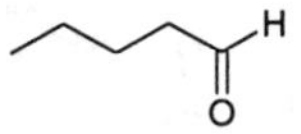

6581 Valerine
$C_8H_{15}NO_2$ MW: 157.21 Property: mp 209-10°C. Source: XIE CAO. Ref: 6.

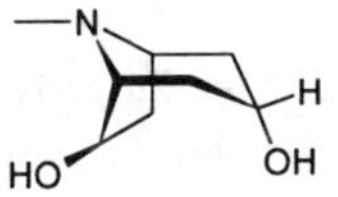

6582 n-Valerophenone-O-carboxylic acid
$C_{12}H_{14}O_3$ MW: 206.24 Source: DANG GUI. Ref: 2.

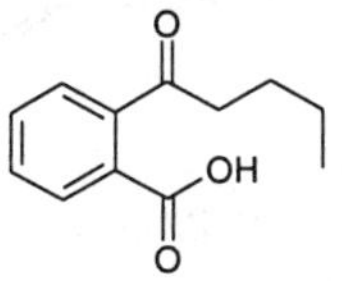

6583 Valerosidatum
$C_{21}H_{34}O_{11}$ MW: 426.50 Property: mp 78-80°C. Source: XIE CAO, ZHI ZHU XIANG. Ref: 6.

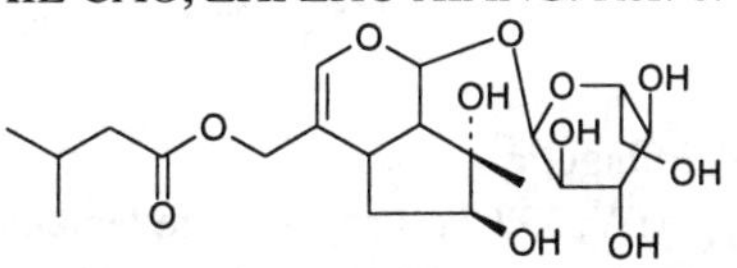

6584 L-Valine-L-valine anhydride
$C_{10}H_{20}N_2O_3$ MW: 216.28 Source: CHUAN XIONG. Ref: 2.

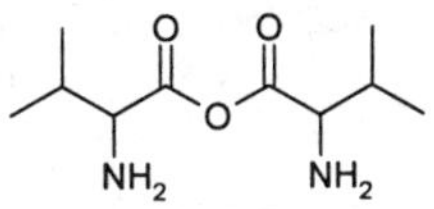

6585 Vallesiachotamine
$C_{21}H_{22}N_2O_3$ MW: 350.42 Source: Ref: 2.

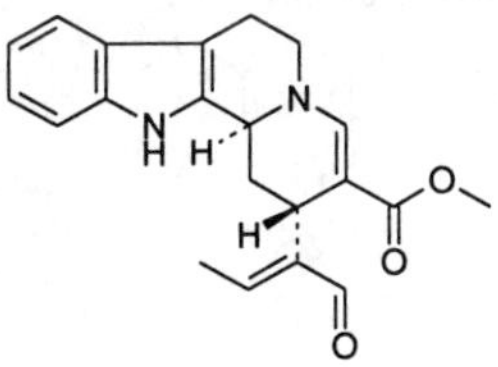

6586 Vanillic acid
$C_8H_8O_4$ MW: 168.15 Property: mp 210°C (sub). Source: BAI HUA QIAN HU, CHUAN XIONG, DANG GUI, DANG SHEN, DU ZHONG, GUA LOU, KU LIAN, MA HUANG, MU ZEI, PU HUANG, REN SHEN, SHE PU TAO. Ref: 2, 297, 415, 552, 648.

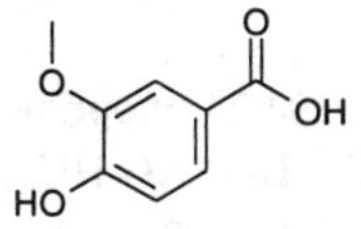

6587 Vanillin
CAS: 121-33-5 $C_8H_8O_3$ MW: 152.15 Property: mp 80-1°C. Source: CHUAN XIONG, DANG GUI, KU LIAN, MU ZEI, TIAN MA, XIN JIANG GAO BEN, YIN CHEN HAO. Ref: 2, 4, 333, 648.

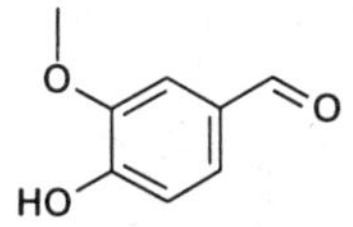

6588 Vanillin acetate
$C_{10}H_{10}O_4$ MW: 194.19 Source: CHAI HU. Ref: 2.

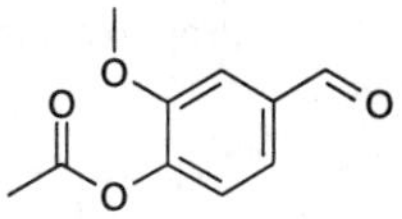

6589 6-O-Vanilloylajugol
Source: GAN DI HUANG. Ref: 2.

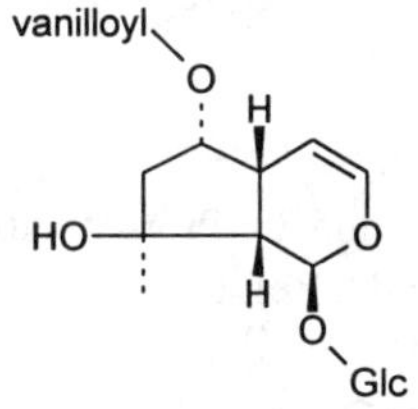

6590 Vanilloyl calleryanin
$C_{21}H_{24}O_{11}$ MW: 452.42 Source: YE LI ZHI YE. Ref: 6.

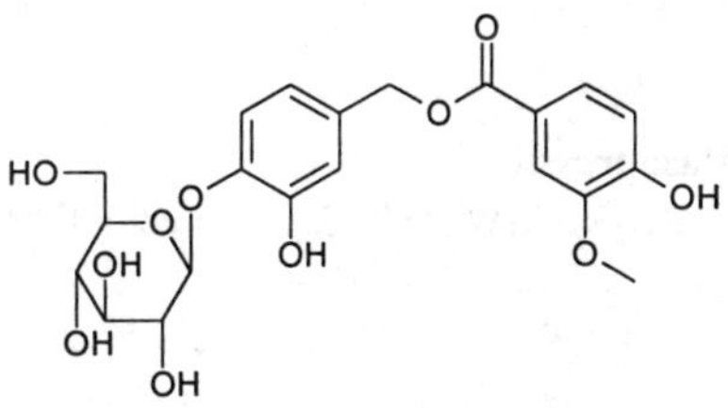

6591 Vanillyl alcohol
CAS: 498-00-0 $C_8H_{10}O_3$ MW: 154.17 Property: mp 115°C. Source: TIAN MA. Ref: 4.

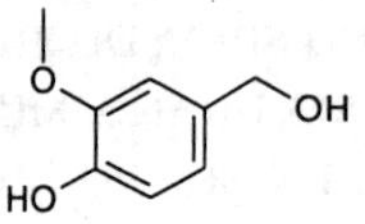

6592 Vasicinol
$C_{11}H_{12}N_2O_2$ MW: 204.23 Property: mp 260°C. Source: DA BO GU, HUANG HUA ZI. Ref: 6.

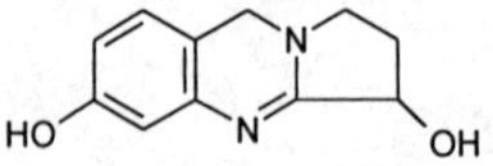

6593 Vasicinone
$C_{11}H_{10}N_2O_2$ MW: 202.21 Property: mp (-): 200-1°C, (±): 211-2°C. Source: DA BO GU, HUANG HUA ZI, LUO TUO PENG, LUO TUO PENG ZI. Ref: 6.

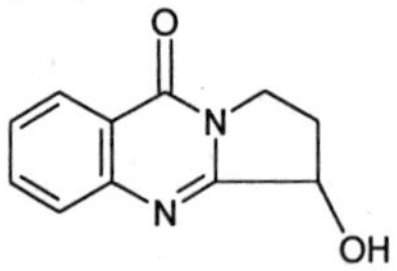

6594 Vasicoline
$C_{19}H_{21}N_3$ MW: 291.40 Property: mp 135°C. Source: DA BO GU. Ref: 6.

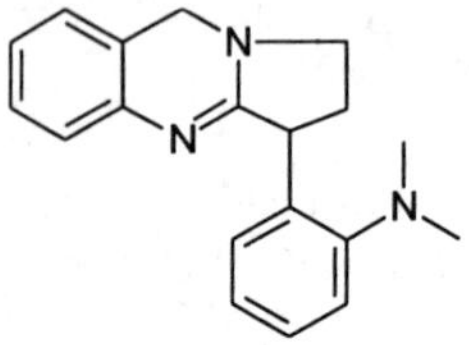

6595 Vasicolinone
$C_{19}H_{19}N_3O$ MW: 305.38 Property: mp 152°C. Source: DA BO GU. Ref: 6.

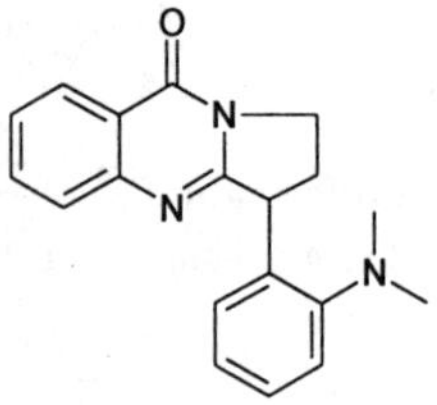

6596 Vasopressin
$C_{46}H_{65}N_{15}O_{12}S_2$ MW: 1084.25 Source: NIU NAO. Ref: 6.

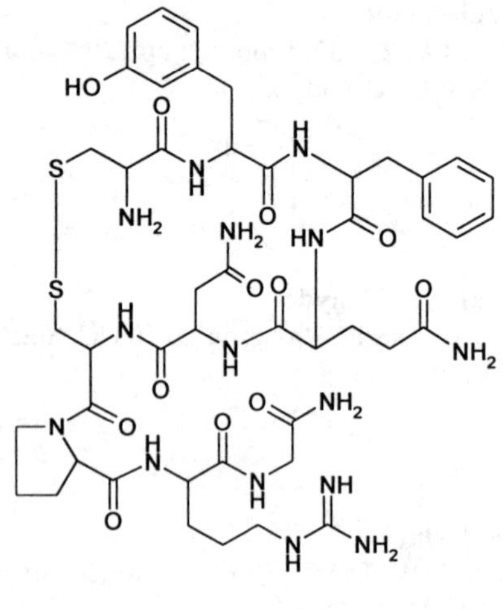

6597 Vellosimine
$C_{19}H_{20}N_2O$ MW: 292.38 Property: mp 305-6°C. Source: LUO FU MU. Ref: 6.

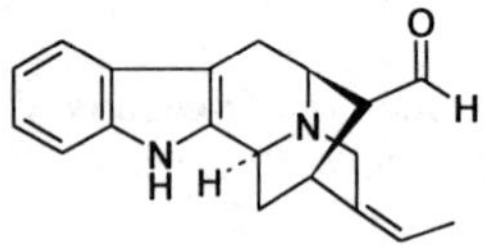

6598 Venoterpine
$C_9H_{11}NO$ MW: 149.19 Property: mp 129-30°C. Source: XI SHU. Ref: 6.

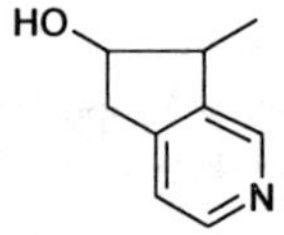

6599 Ventilagolin
$C_{17}H_{16}O_7$ MW: 332.31 Property: red lamellar crystal, mp 165-7°C. Source: YI HE GUO. Ref: 258.

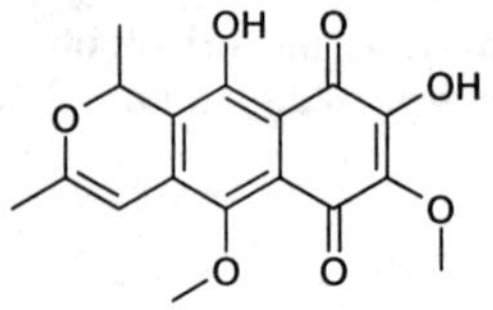

6600 Veratrole
$C_8H_{10}O_2$ MW: 138.17 Property: mp 22.5°C. Source: FENG DOU CAI. Ref: 6.

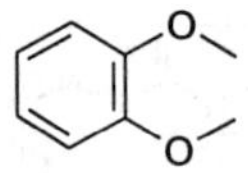

6601 Veratroyl zygadenine
$C_{36}H_{51}NO_{10}$ MW: 657.81 Property: mp 270-1°C. Source: LI LU. Ref: 6.

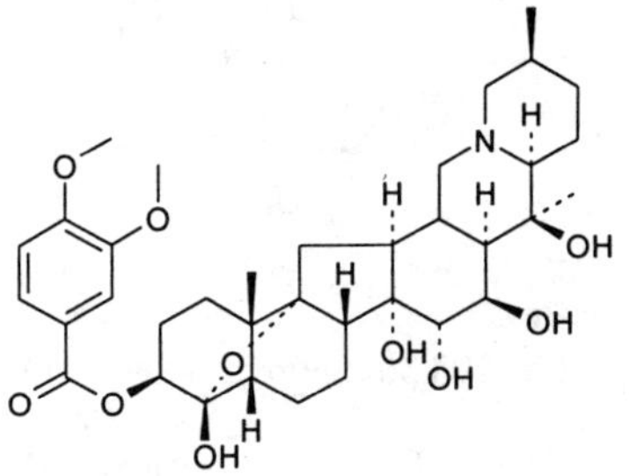

6602 Verbascose
$C_{30}H_{52}O_{26}$ MW: 828.73 Property: mp 219-220°C. Source: GAN DI HUANG, MA YING DAN. Ref: 2, 234.

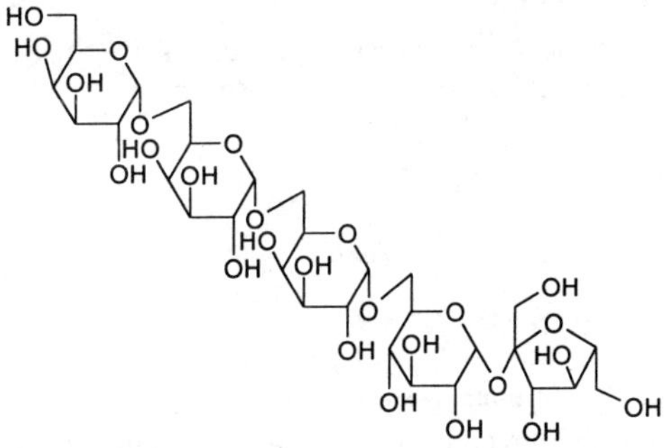

6604 Verbenol
$C_{10}H_{16}O$ MW: 152.24 Property: (+) cis: mp 15.5°C, bp 90°C/10mm, (+) trans: mp 24°C, bp 92°C/10mm. Source: MI DIE XIANG. Ref: 6.

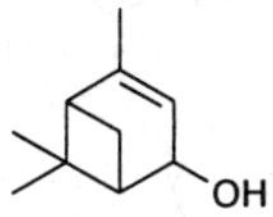

6605 Vernodalin
CAS: 21871-10-3 Source: *Vernonia amygdalina* Del. Ref: 5.

6606 Vernolepin
CAS: 18542-37-5 Property: mp 181-2°C. Source: *Vernonia hymenolepis* A. Rich. Ref: 5.

6607 Vernolide
CAS: 27428-86-0 $C_{19}H_{22}O_7$ MW: 362.38 Property: mp 180-3°C. Source: *Vernonia amygdalina* Del. Ref: 5.

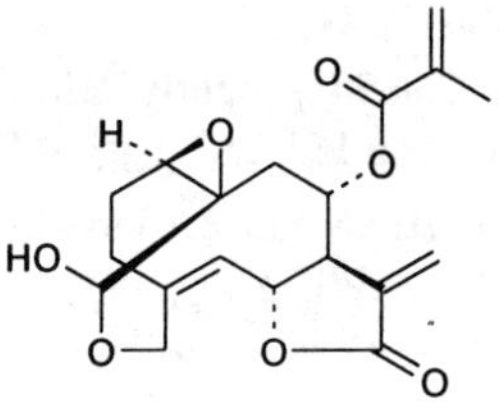

6608 Vernomenin
CAS: 20107-26-0 $C_{15}H_{16}O_5$ MW: 276.29 Source: *Vernonia hymenolepis* A. Rich. Ref: 5.

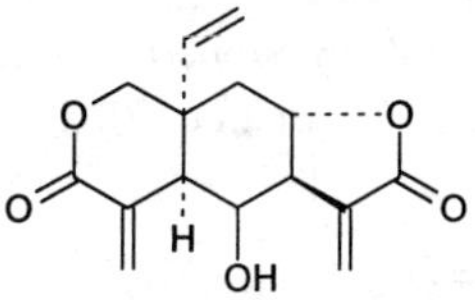

6609 Vernomygdin
CAS: 21871-14-7 $C_{19}H_{24}O_7$ MW: 364.40 Property: mp 208-10°C. Source: *Vernonia amygdalina* Del. Ref: 5.

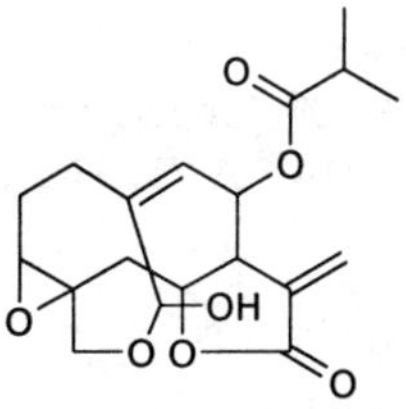

6610 Versicolactone A
$C_{15}H_{20}O_2$ MW: 232.33 Property: colorless rhombic crystal, mp 130-2°C, $[\alpha]_D^6$ +486° (c=0.1276, chloroform). Source: BIAN SE MA DOU LING. Ref: 209.

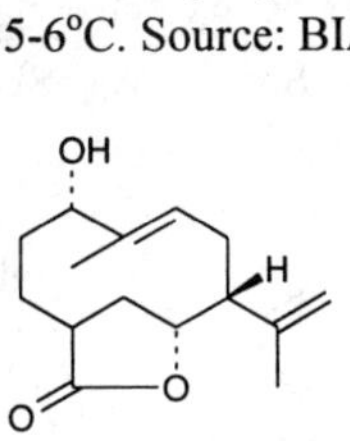

6611 Versicolactonc B
$C_{15}H_{20}O_3$ MW: 250.34 Property: white iceflower - like crystal, mp 135-6°C. Source: BIAN SE MA DAI LING. Ref: 51.

6612 Versicolactone C
$C_{15}H_{22}O_4$ MW: 266.34 Property: white short claviform crystal, mp 181-2°C $[\alpha]_D^{36}$ -11.4° (c=2.6, ethanol). Source: BIAN SE MA DAI LING. Ref: 51.

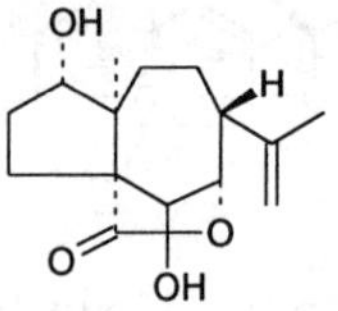

6613 Versicolactone D
$C_{30}H_{40}O_3$ MW: 448.65 Property: Colorless hyaloid crystal, mp 172-2.5°C. Source: BIAN SE MA DOU LING. Ref: 146.

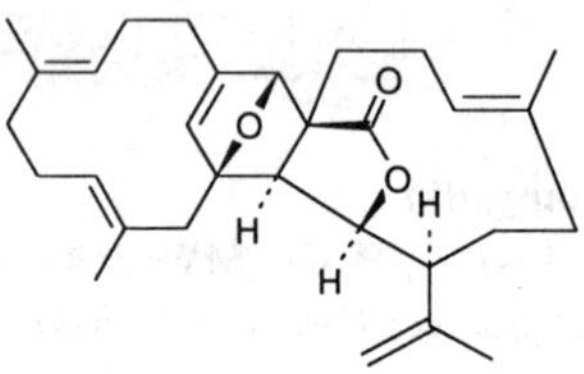

6614 Vertia flavone
$C_{16}H_{12}O_5$ MW: 284.27 Property: mp 325-7°C. Source: HUANG HUA JIA ZHU TAO. Ref: 6.

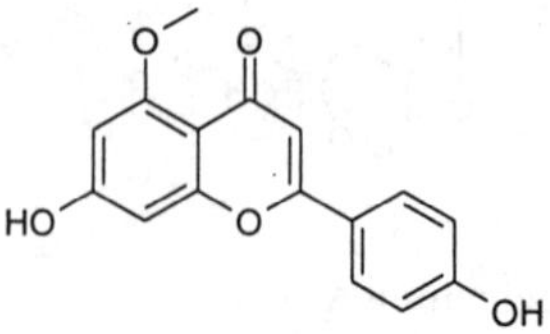

6615 Verticillatine
$C_{20}H_{25}N_2O_3^+ \bullet Cl^-$ MW: 341.43•35.45 Property: colorless acicular crystal, mp 324-6°C (decomposition). Source: HONG GUO LUO FU MU. Ref: 26.

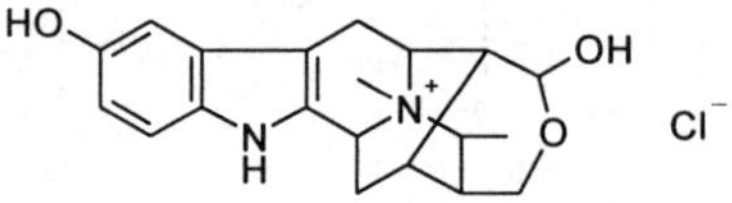

6616 Verussustilbene
trans-3-Methoxy-2,3',4,5'-tetrahydroxystilbene. $C_{15}H_{14}O_5$ MW: 274.28 Property: light yellow amorphous powder. Source: WU SU LI LI LU. Ref: 438.

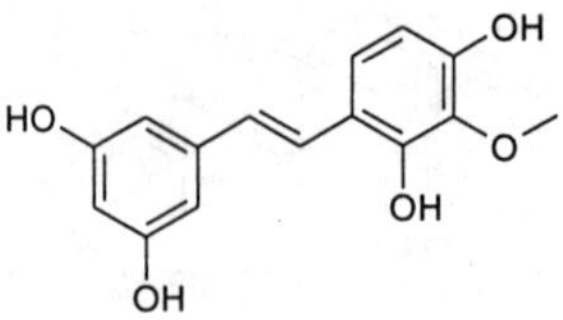

6617 Viburnitol
$C_6H_{12}O_5$ MW: 164.16 Property: mp 180-1°C. Source: YANG SHI CAO. Ref: 6.

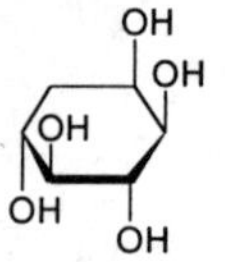

6618 Vicenin-2
$C_{17}H_{14}O_5$ MW: 298.30 Source: GAN CAO. Ref: 2.

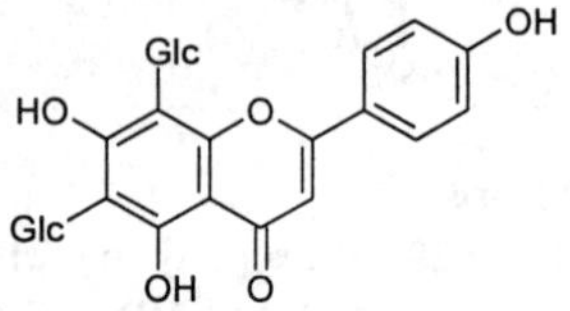

6619 Vicianin
$C_{19}H_{25}NO_{10}$ MW: 427.41 Property: mp 147-8°C. Source: WANG BU LIU XING. Ref: 6.

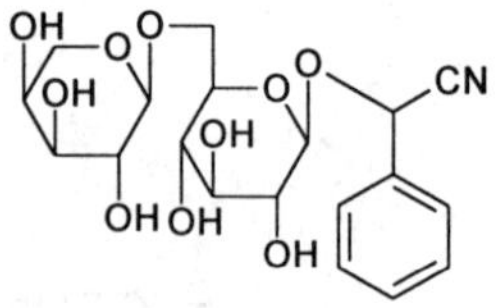

6620 β-Vicianosyl-3-quercetin
α-L-Arabinopyranosido-(1→6)-β-D-glucopyranosyl-3-quercetin. $C_{26}H_{28}O_{16}$ MW: 596.50 Property: mp 200-2°C. Source: XING CAI. Ref: 6.

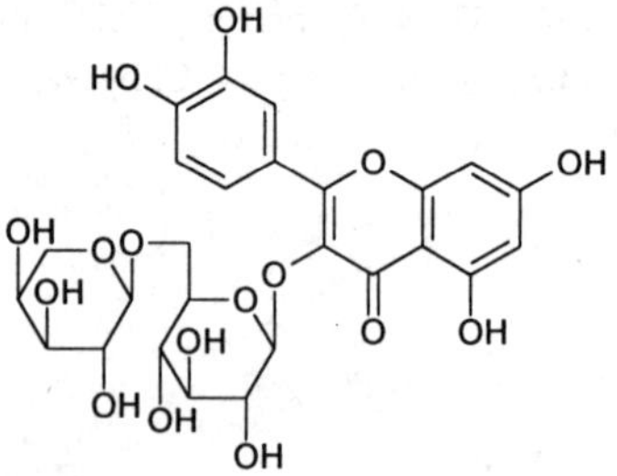

6621 Vicine
2,6-Diamino-4,5-dihydroxy pyrimidine-5-β-glucoside. $C_{10}H_{18}N_4O_7$ MW: 306.28 Property: mp 243-4°C (dec). Source: CAN DOU, KU GUA. Ref: 6, 176.

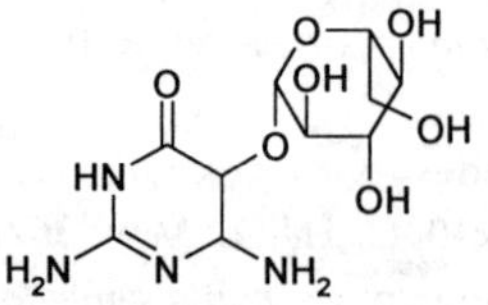

6622 Vilangin
$C_{35}H_{52}O_8$ MW: 600.80 Property: mp 264-5°C (dec). Source: XIAN SUAN QIANG. Ref: 6.

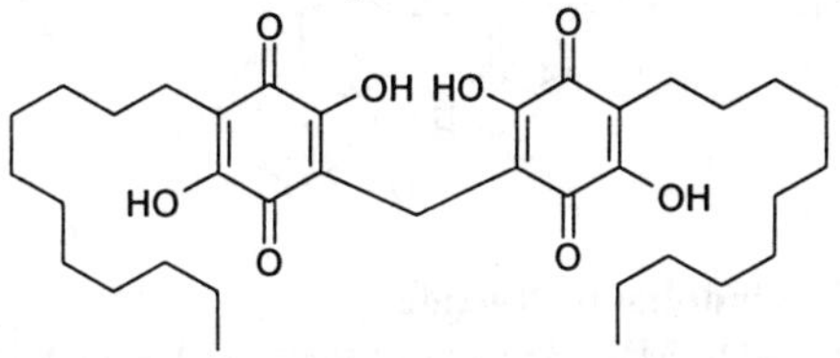

6623 Villoside
$C_{16}H_{28}O_8$ MW: 346.38 Source: BAI JIANG. Ref: 2.

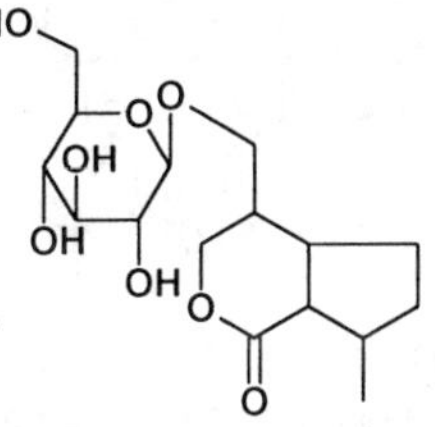

6624 Villosol
$C_{10}H_{16}O_4$ MW: 200.24 Property: white crystal, mp 143-5°C, $[\alpha]_D^{18}$ +170.73° (c=0.5, MOH). Source: BAI HUA BAI JIANG. Ref: 34.

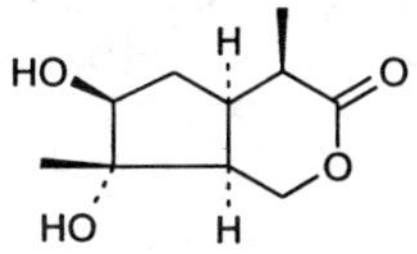

6625 Villosolside
$C_{16}H_{26}O_9$ MW: 262.38 Property: white crystal, mp 228-30°C, $[\alpha]_D^{35}$ +93.37° (c=0.5, H_2O). Source: BAI HUA BAI JIANG. Ref: 36.

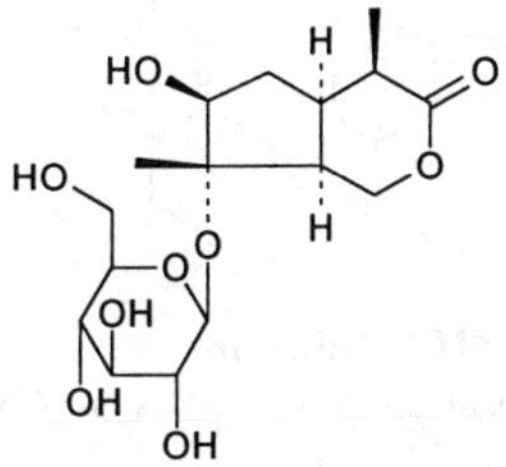

6626 Vilmorrianine C
Source: DIAN XI WU TOU. Ref: 618.

6627 Vinamidine
$C_{45}H_{58}N_4O_9$ MW: 798.99 Source: CHANG CHUN HUA. Ref: 2.

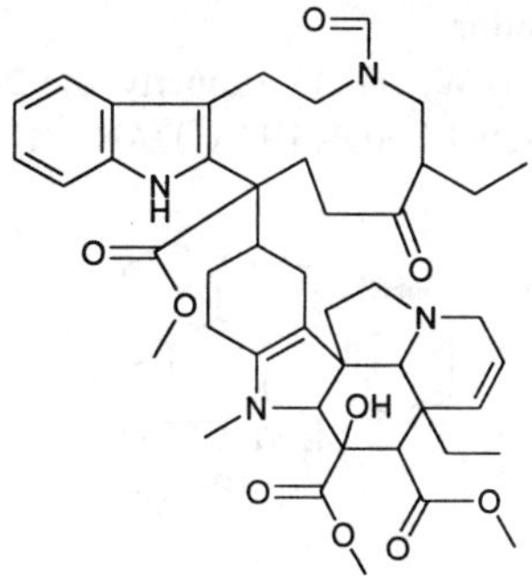

6628 Vinblastine
Vincaleukoblastine. CAS: 865-21-4 $C_{46}H_{58}N_4O_9$ MW: 811.00 Property: mp 211-6°C. Source: CHANG CHUN HUA. Ref: 5.

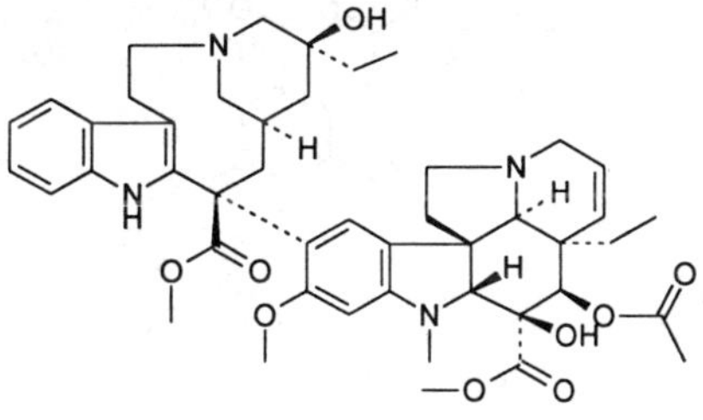

6629 Vincadioline
3α-Hydroxy-Vincaleukoblastine. CAS: 56897-74-6 $C_{46}H_{58}N_4O_{10}$ MW: 827.00 Property: mp 218-21°C. Source: CHANG CHUN HUA. Ref: 5.

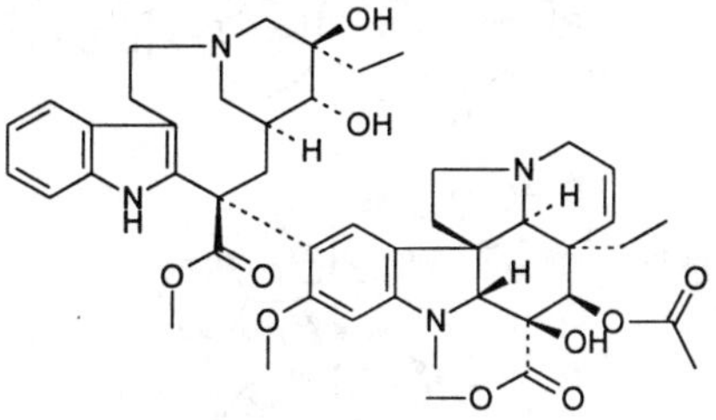

6630 Vincamine
Minorine. CAS: 1617-90-9 Property: mp 232-3°C. Source: CHANG CHUN HUA. Ref: 4.

6631 Vincarin
$C_{21}H_{24}N_2O_3$ MW: 352.44 Property: mp 263-4°C. Source: CHANG CHUN HUA. Ref: 4.

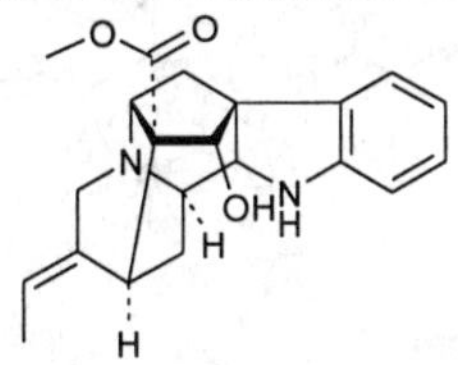

6632 Vincoline
$C_{21}H_{24}N_2O_4$ MW: 368.44 Property: mp 230-3°C. Source: CHANG CHUN HUA, DAN MU. Ref: 2, 118.

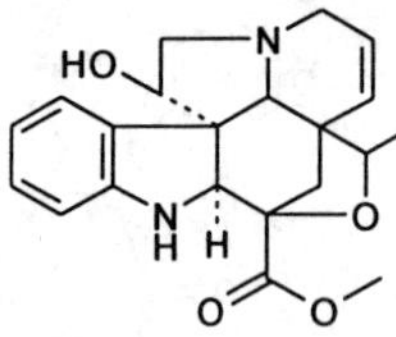

6633 Vincoside lactam
$C_{26}H_{30}N_2O_8$ MW: 498.54 Property: mp 210°C. Source: GOU TENG. Ref: 2.

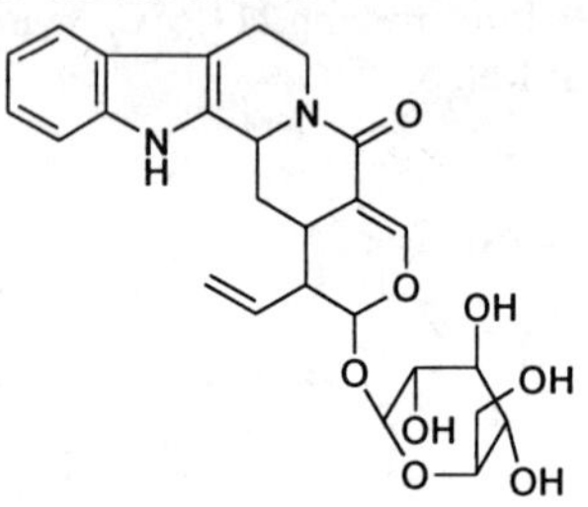

6634 Vincristine
Leuroristine. CAS: 57-22-7 $C_{46}H_{56}N_4O_{10}$ MW: 824.98 Property: mp 218-20°C (dec). Source: CHANG CHUN HUA. Ref: 4.

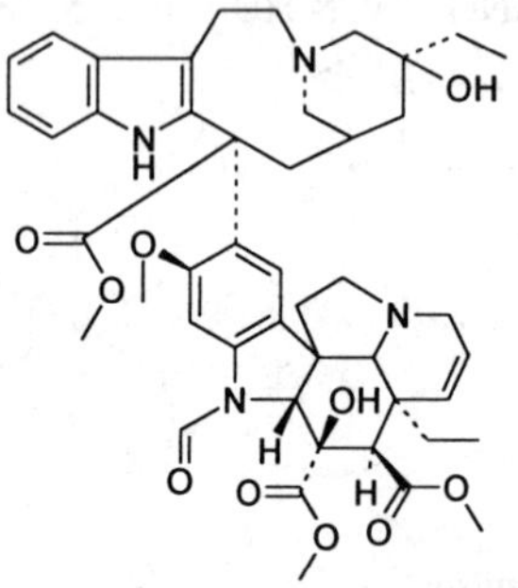

6635 Vindoline
$C_{25}H_{32}N_2O_6$ MW: 456.54 Property: mp 154-5°C. Source: CHANG CHUN HUA. Ref: 2.

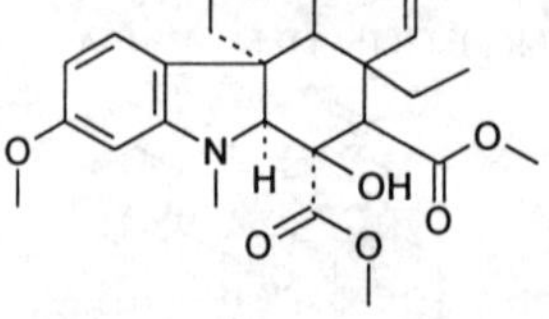

6636 Vindolinine
$C_{21}H_{24}N_2O_2$ MW: 336.44 Property: mp 214-8°C. Source: CHANG CHUN HUA. Ref: 2.

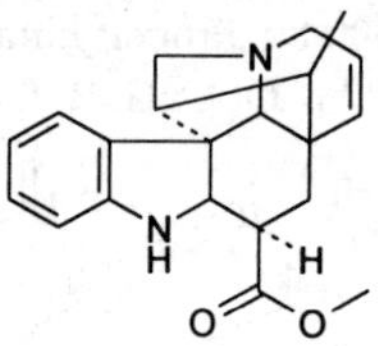

6637 Vindolinine-N-oxide
$C_{21}H_{26}N_2O_3$ MW: 354.45 Source: CHANG CHUN HUA. Ref: 2.

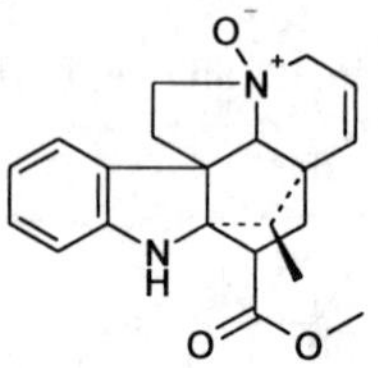

6638 Vindorosine
Vindolidine. $C_{24}H_{30}N_2O_5$ MW: 426.52 Property: 244-50°C (dec). Source: CHANG CHUN HUA. Ref: 2.

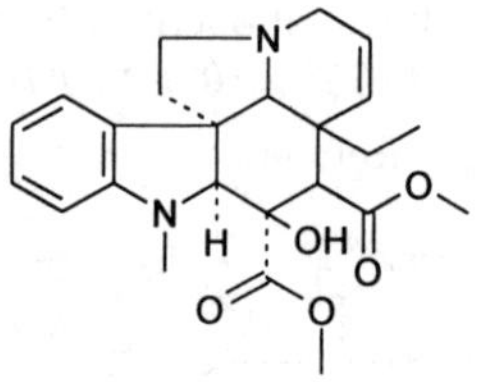

6639 1-Vinyl-4,8-dimethoxy-β-carboline
$C_{15}H_{14}N_2O_2$ MW: 254.29 Property: yellowish prismatic crystal, mp 158-9°C. Source: KU SHU PI. Ref: 12.

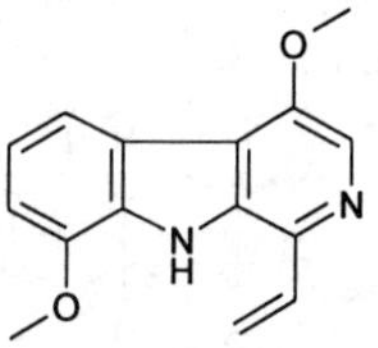

6640 2-Vinyl-4H-1,2-dithiin
$C_6H_8S_2$ MW: 144.26 Source: DA SUAN. Ref: 2.

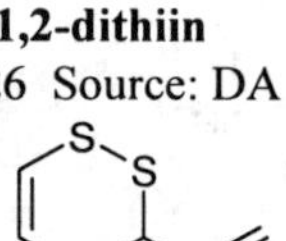

6641 2-Vinyl-4H-1,3-dithiin
$C_6H_8S_2$ MW: 144.26 Source: DA SUAN. Ref: 2.

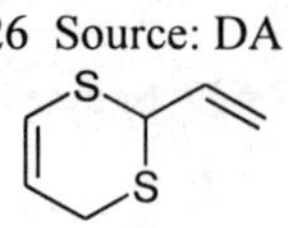

6642 3-Vinyl-1,2-dithio-4-cyclohexene
$C_6H_8S_2$ MW: 144.26 Source: DA SUAN. Ref: 2.

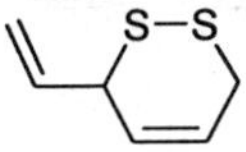

6643 3-Vinyl-1, 2-dithio-5-cyclohexene
$C_6H_8S_2$ MW: 144.26 Source: DA SUAN. Ref: 2.

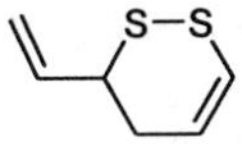

6644 1-Vinyl-4-methoxy-β-carboline
$C_{14}H_{12}N_2O$ MW: 224.26 Source: KU SHU PI. Ref: 12.

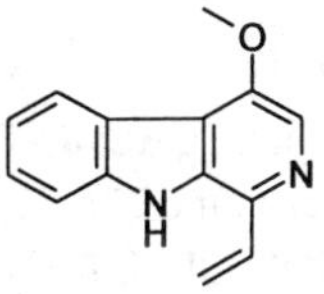

6645 l-5-Vinyl-2-thiooxazolidone
C_5H_7NOS MW: 129.18 Source: GAN LAN. Ref: 6.

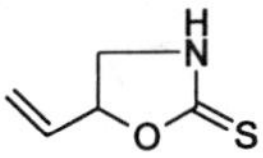

6646 4-Vinyl-1, 2,3-trithio-5-cyclohexene
$C_5H_6S_3$ MW: 162.30 Source: DA SUAN. Ref: 2.

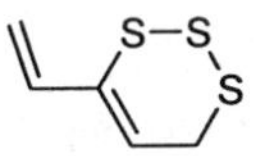

6647 Violaxanthin
$C_{40}H_{56}O_4$ MW: 600.89 Property: mp 208°C. Source: DAO CAO, FAN MU GUA, IN ZHAN JU, KONG QUE CAO, MANG GUO, JNING MENG YE, PU GONG YING, SUAN MO YE, SUAN SHUI CAO. Ref: 6.

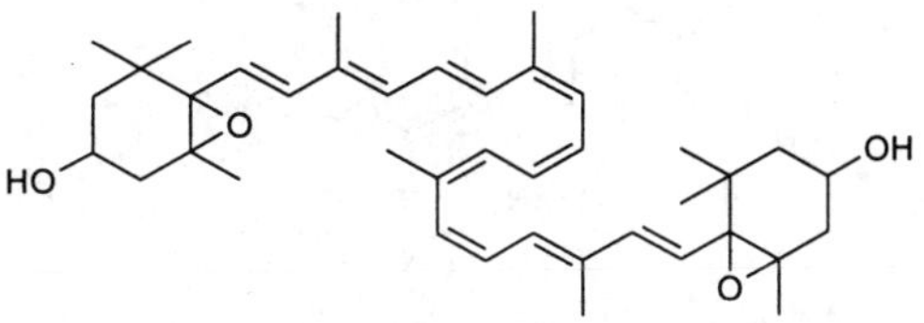

6648 Violutoside
$C_{19}H_{26}O_{12}$ MW: 446.41 Property: mp 173°C (dec). Source: SAN SE JIN. Ref: 6.

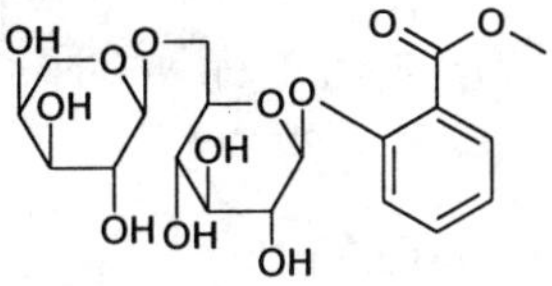

6649 Virensic acid
$C_{18}H_{14}O_8$ MW: 358.31 Property: mp 245-7°C. Source: JIN SI DAI. Ref: 6.

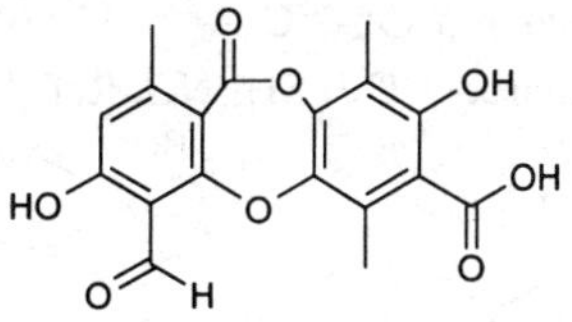

6650 Viridiflorine
$C_{17}H_{31}NO_4$ MW: 313.44 Property: mp 102.5-3.5°C. Source: YAO YONG DAO TI HU. Ref: 6.

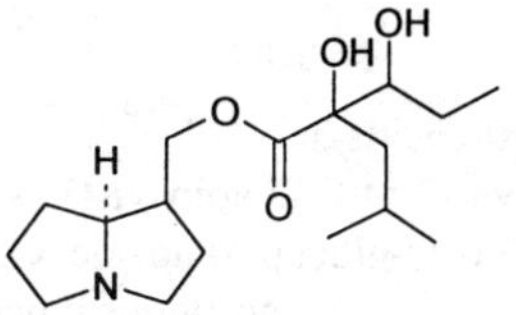

6651 Viscumneoside
Rhamnazin-3-O-β-D-apisoyl-(1→2)-[6"-O-(3-hydroxy-3-methylglutarate)]-glucoside. $C_{34}H_{40}O_{20}$ MW: 768.69 Property: yellow ropy liquid, $[\alpha]_D^{23}$ -31.0° (c=0.32, methanol). Source: HU JI SHENG. Ref: 163.

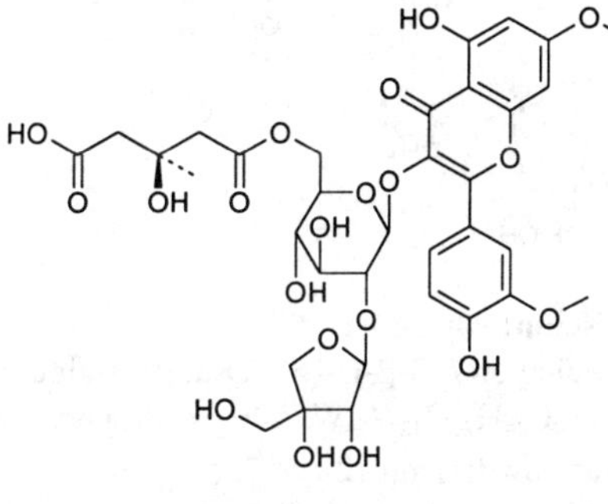

6652 Viscumneoside III
Homoeriodictyol-7-O-β-D-apiosyl-(1→2)-β-D-glucopyranoside. $C_{27}H_{32}O_{15}$ MW: 596.55 Property: white amorphous powder, mp 208-10°C, $[\alpha]_D^{18}$ -67.3° (c=0.42, methanol). Source: HU JI SHENG. Ref: 111.

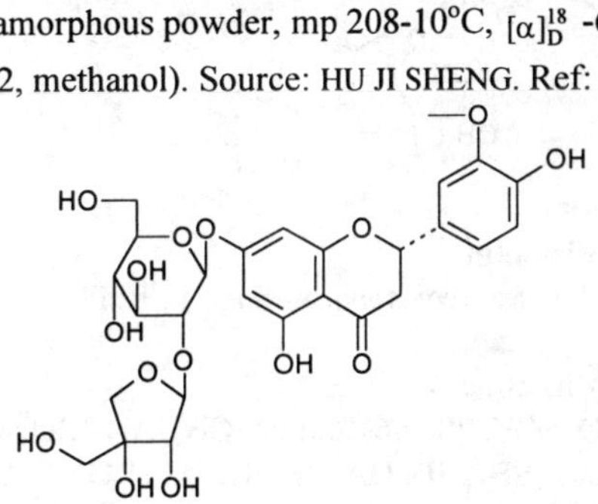

6653 Viscumneoside IV
Rhamnazin-O-β-D-(6"-β-hydroxy-β-methylglu-taryl) glucoside. $C_{29}H_{32}O_{16}$ MW: 637.57 Property: yellow acicular crystal, mp 195-7°C, $[\alpha]_D^{20}$ +14.64° (c=0.25, methanol). Source: HU JI SHENG. Ref: 113.

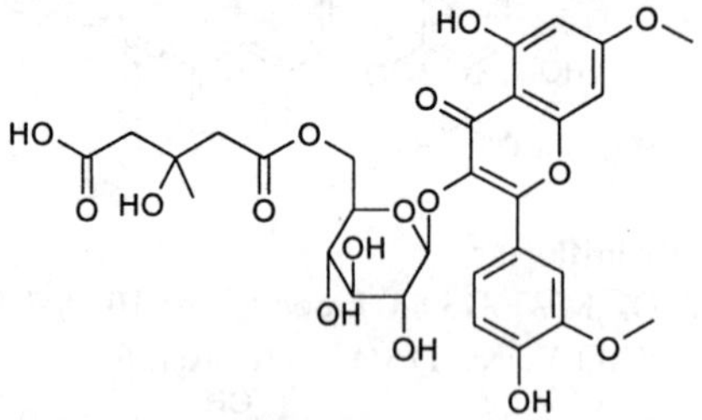

6654 Viscumneoside V
Homoeriodictyol-7-O-β-D-apiosyl-(1→5)-β-D-apiosyl-(1→2)-β-D-glucopyranoside. $C_{32}H_{40}O_{19}$ MW: 728.66 Property: white amorphous powder, mp 136-9°C, $[\alpha]_D^{20}$ -127.0° (c=0.42, methanol). Source: HU JI SHENG. Ref: 111.

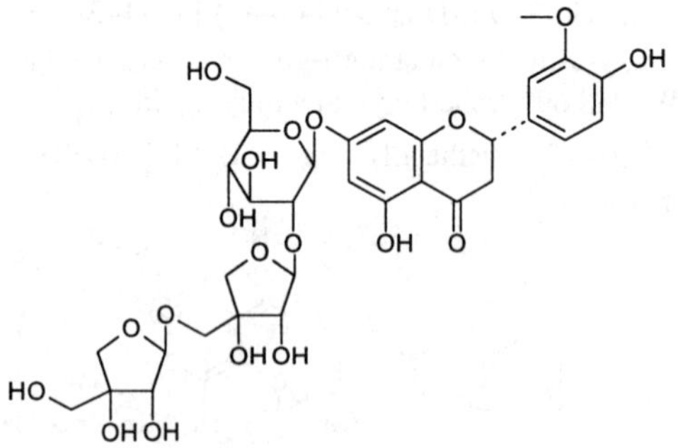

6655 Viscumneoside VI
Homoeriodictyol-7-O-β-D-(6''-O-acetyl)-gluco-pyranoside. $C_{24}H_{26}O_{12}$ MW: 506.47 Property: white amorphous powder, mp 124-6°C, $[\alpha]_D$ -78.2° (c= 0.29, methanol). Source: HU JI SHENG. Ref: 111.

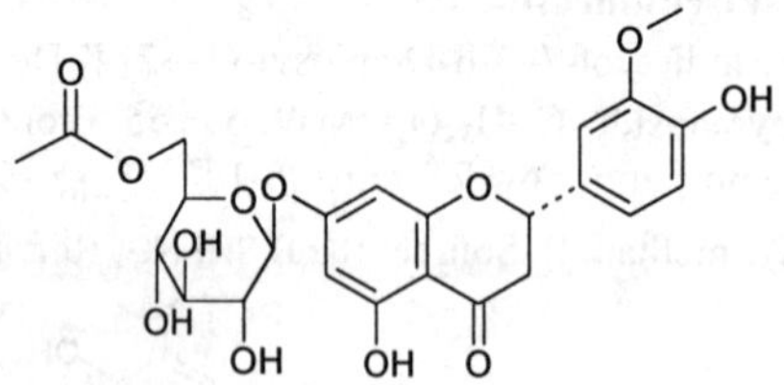

6656 Visnadin
Visnamine. Source: *Ammi visnage* L. Ref: 4.

6657 Vitamine A
$C_{20}H_{30}O$ MW: 286.46 Source: CHUAN XIONG, CU LIU GUO (SHA JI), DANG GUI, LU RONG, SHAN ZHU YU. Ref: 2.

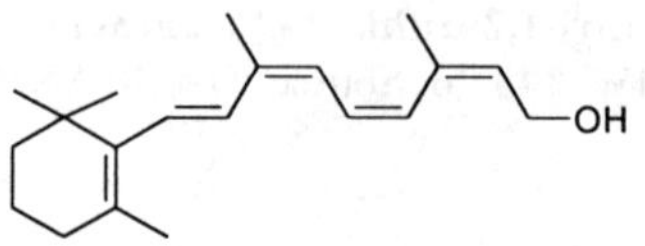

6658 Vitamin B1
Thiamine. Source: CU LIU GUO (SHA JI), DA ZAO, DONG CHONG XIA CAO, GOU QI ZI, REN SHEN, ZI SU. Ref: 2.

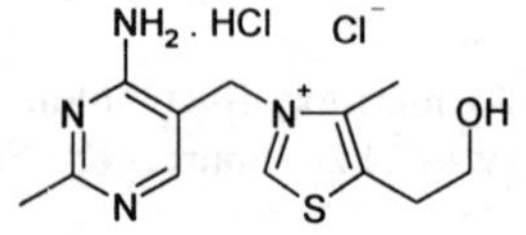

6659 Vitamin B2
Riboflavine; Vitamin G. CAS: 83-88-5 $C_{17}H_{20}N_4O_6$ MW: 376.37 Property: mp 278-82°C. Source: BAI GUO, DA ZAO, GOU QI ZI, REN SHEN. Ref: 2, 5.

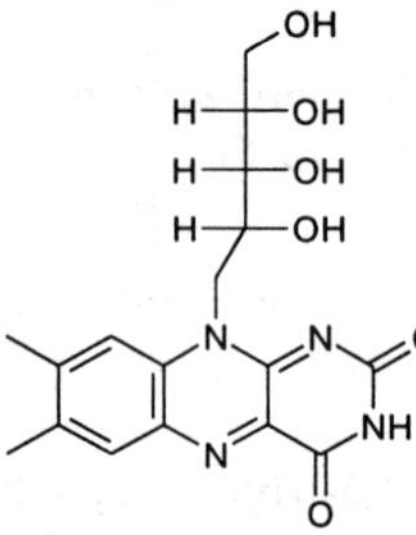

6660 Vitamin B5
Pantothenic acid. Property: mp 271°C (dec). Source: YE ZI RANG. Ref: 6.

6661 Vitamine B12
Source: CU LIU GUO (SHA JI), DANG GUI, DONG CHONG XIA CAO, REN SHEN. Ref: 2.

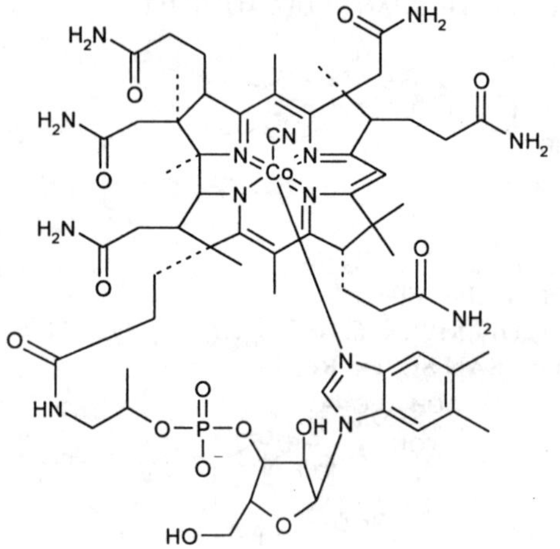

6662 Vitamin B15
$C_{20}H_{40}N_2O_8$ MW: 436.55 Source: MI PI KANG. Ref: 6.

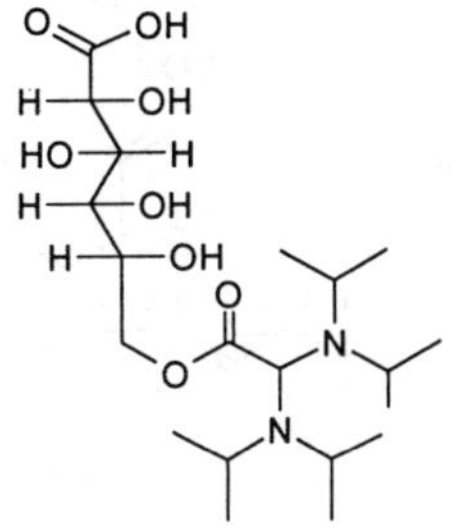

6663 Vitamine C
$C_6H_8O_6$ MW: 176.13 Source: CU LIU GUO (SHA JI), DONG CHONG XIA CAO, QI YE DAN, REN SHEN, SHAN YAO, SUAN ZAO REN, WU WEI ZI, ZHI SHI. Ref: 2.

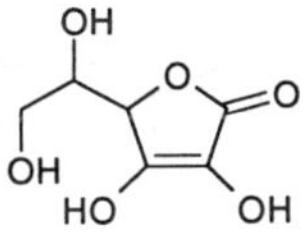

6664 Vitamin D2
$C_{28}H_{44}O$ MW: 396.66 Property: mp 115-6°C. Source: MAI JIAO, SONG XUN. Ref: 6.

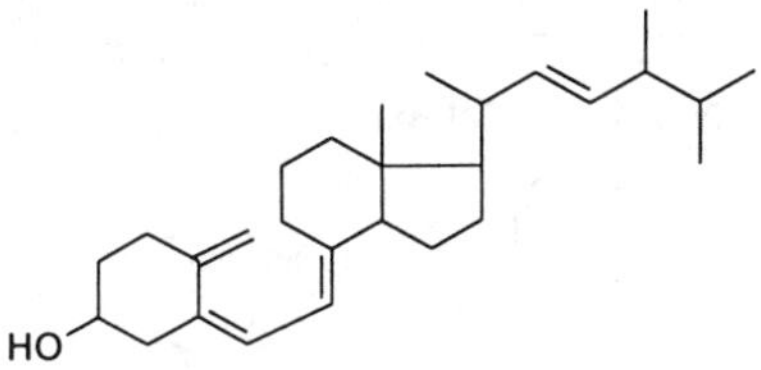

6665 Vitamine E(α)
α-Tocopherol. $C_{29}H_{50}O_2$ MW: 430.72 Property: bp (+): 140°C/10^{-6}mm. Source: BO CAI, CU LIU GUO (SHA JI), LUO HUA SHENG, MU JIN ZI, WU WEI ZI, YE ZI RANG. Ref: 2, 6.

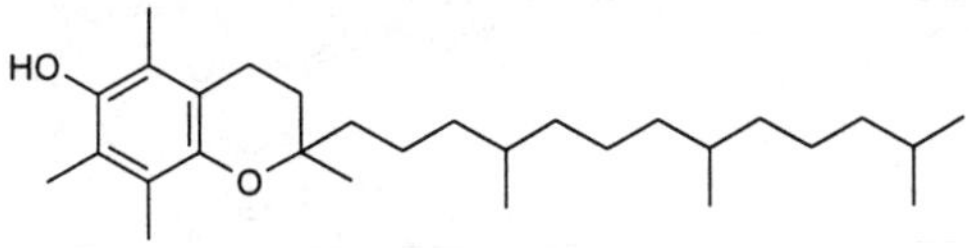

6666 Vitamine E(β)
β-Tocopherol. $C_{28}H_{48}O_2$ MW: 416.69 Source: CU LIU GUO (SHA JI), MU JIN ZI, WU WEI ZI. Ref: 2, 6.

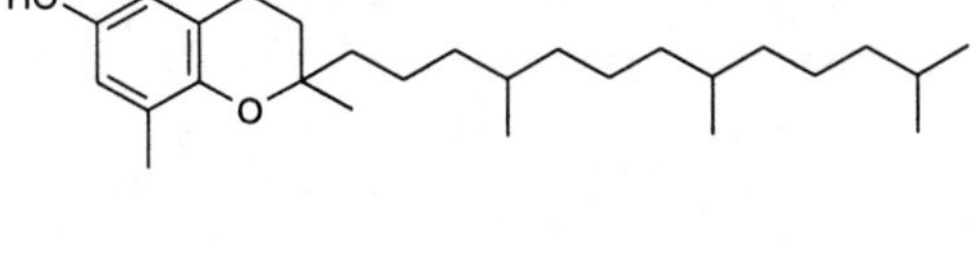

6667 Vitamine E(γ)
γ-Tocopherol. $C_{28}H_{48}O_2$ MW: 416.69 Property: mp -3 to -2°C. Source: CU LIU GUO (SHA JI), LUO HUA SHENG, WU WEI ZI, YE ZI RANG. Ref: 2, 6.

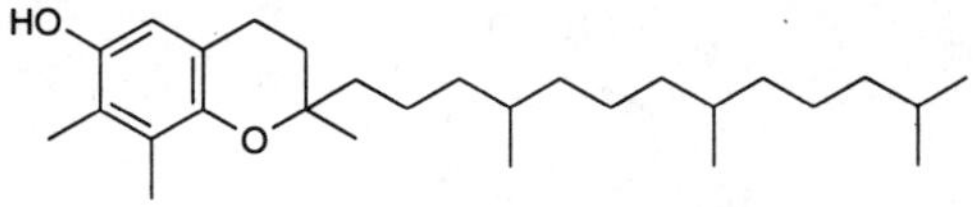

6668 Vitamine E(δ)
δ-Tocopherol $C_{27}H_{46}O_2$ MW: 402.67 Phylloqui-none Property: bp (+): 150°C/10^{-3}mm. Source: CU LIU GUO (SHA JI), MU JIN ZI, WU WEI ZI. Ref: 2, 6.

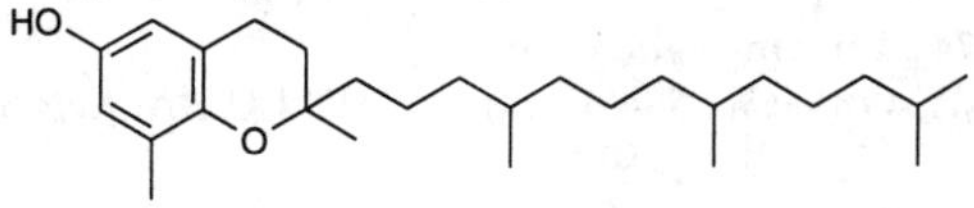

6669 Vitamine K1
Phylloquinone. $C_{31}H_{48}O_2$ MW: 452.73 Property: mp -20°C. Source: CU LIU GUO (SHA JI). Ref: 2.

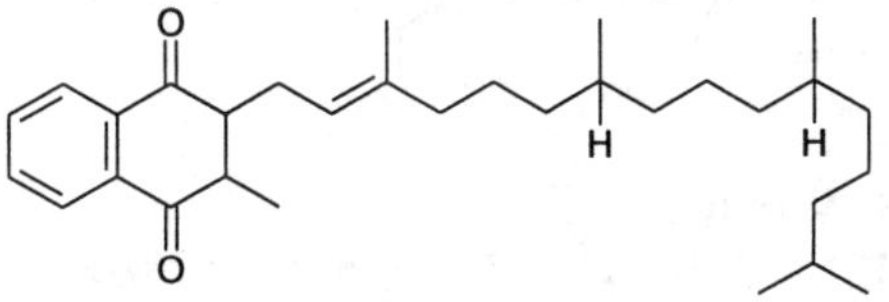

6670 Vitamine K2
Farnoquinone. $C_{41}H_{58}O_2$ MW: 582.92 Source: CU LIU GUO (SHA JI). Ref: 2.

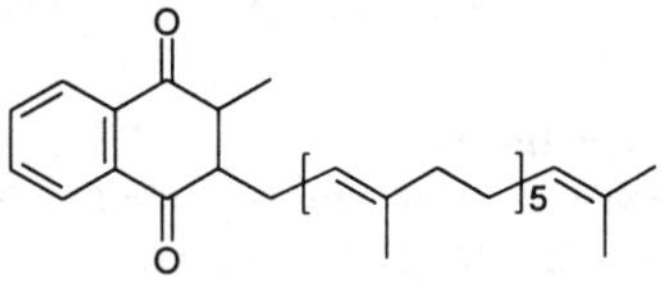

6671 Vitamin U
$C_6H_{14}NO_2S•Cl$ MW: 164.25•35.45 Source: GAN LAN. Ref: 6.

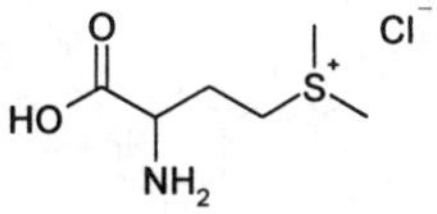

6672 Vitexicarpin
$C_{19}H_{18}O_8$ MW: 374.35 Source: MAN JING ZI. Ref: 6.

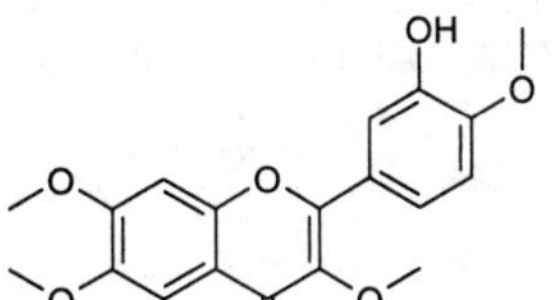

6673 Vitexin
$C_{21}H_{20}O_{10}$ MW: 432.39 Property: mp 258-9°C, 263°C. Source: CHANG BAN JIN LIAN HUA, HU LU BA, SHAN ZHA. Ref: 2, 245, 615.

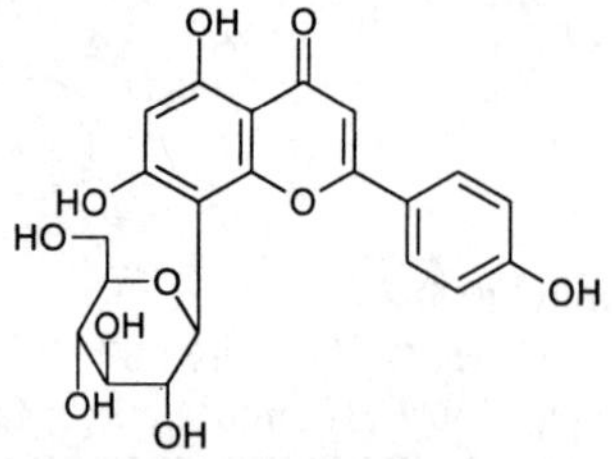

6674 Vitexin-7-glucoside
$C_{27}H_{30}O_{15}$ MW: 594.53 Source: HU LU BA. Ref: 6.

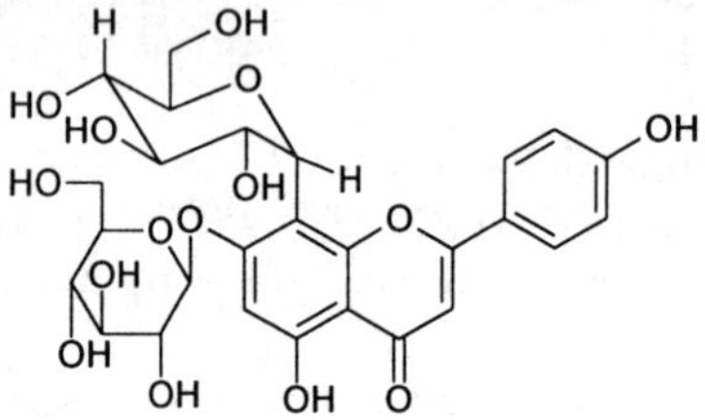

6675 Vittatine
$C_{16}H_{17}NO_3$ MW: 271.32 Property: mp 207-8°C (sub). Source: SHI SUAN. Ref: 6.

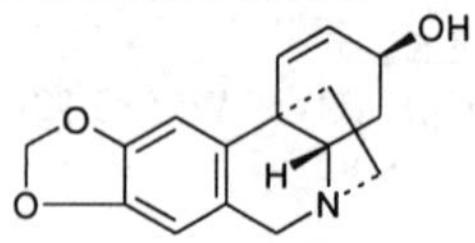

6676 Volkensiflavone
$C_{30}H_{20}O_{10}$ MW: 540.49 Property: mp (+): 300°C (dec). Source: SHAN ZHU ZI. Ref: 6.

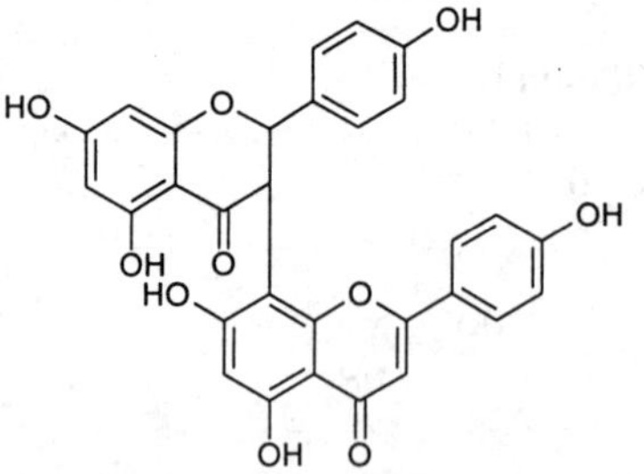

6677 Vomicine
$C_{22}H_{24}N_2O_4$ MW: 380.45 Property: mp 278-80°C. Source: MA QIAN ZI. Ref: 2, 542.

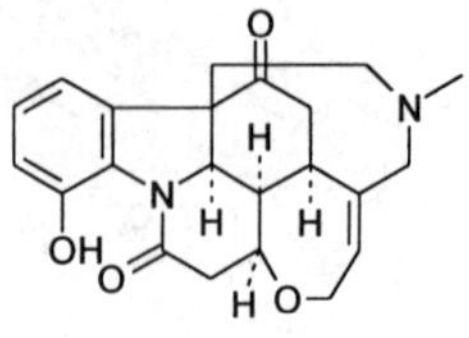

6678 Vulgarobufalin 3-suberoye-L-arginine ester
Source: CHAN SU. Ref: 2.

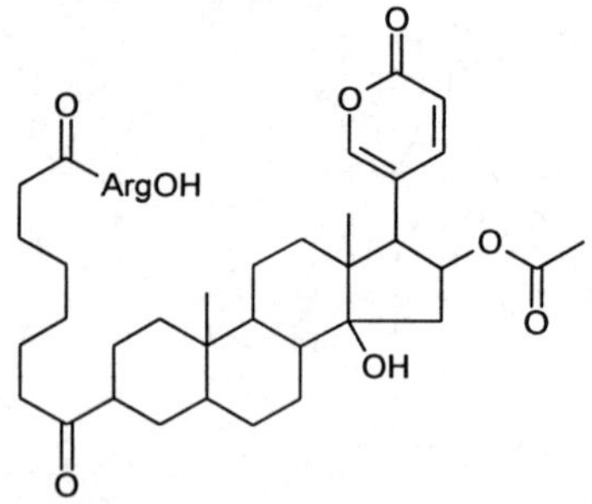

6679 Vulgaxanthin I
$C_{14}H_{17}N_3O_7$ MW: 339.31 Source: ZI MO LI GEN. Ref: 6.

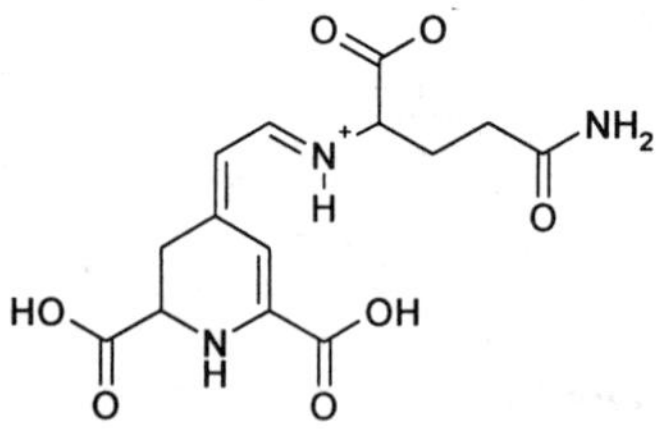

6680 Vulpinic acid
$C_{19}H_{14}O_5$ MW: 322.32 Property: mp 148-9°C. Source: JIN SI DAI. Ref: 6.

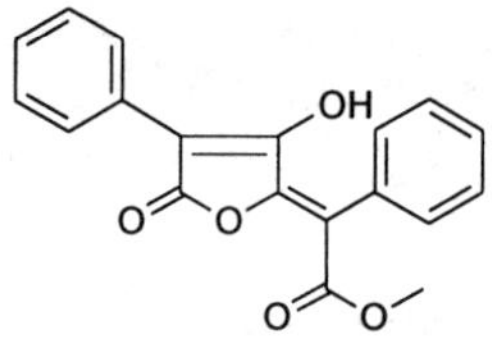

6681 Wallichoside
$C_{30}H_{46}O_7$ MW: 518.70 Property: mp 193-6°C. Source: PAO DAN GUO. Ref: 6.

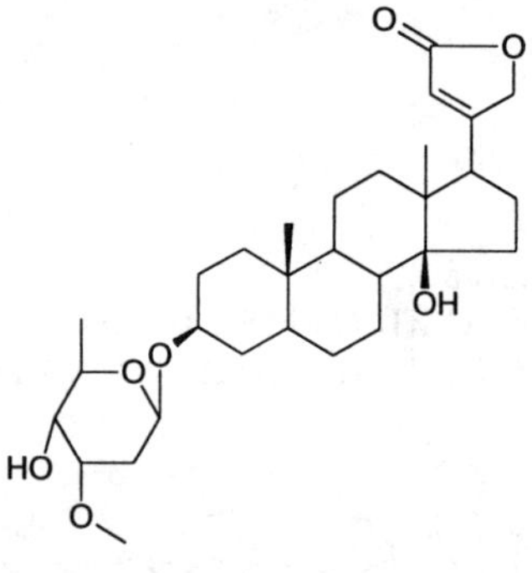

6682 Wanepimedoside A
Source: YIN YANG HUO. Ref: 635.

6683 Wanpeinine A
5α,14α,22β-Cevanine-3β,6α,20β-triol. $C_{27}H_{45}NO_3$ MW: 431.66 Property: white clustered crystal, mp 281-3°C (d), $[\alpha]_D$ -8.71°. Source: AN HUI BEI MU. Ref: 65.

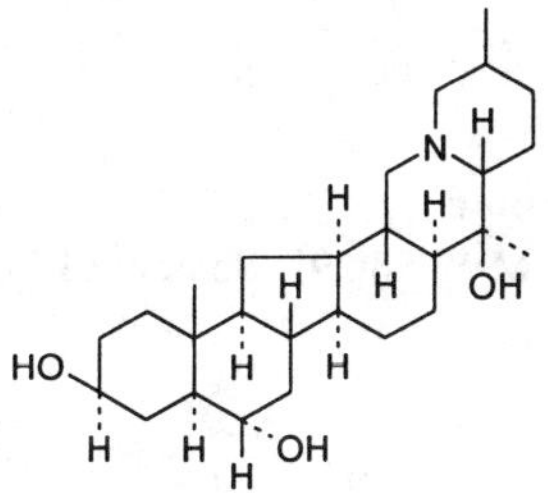

6685 Wedelolactone
$C_{16}H_{12}O_7$ MW: 316.27 Property: mp 327-30°C (dec). Source: BAI ZHI JIE. Ref: 6.

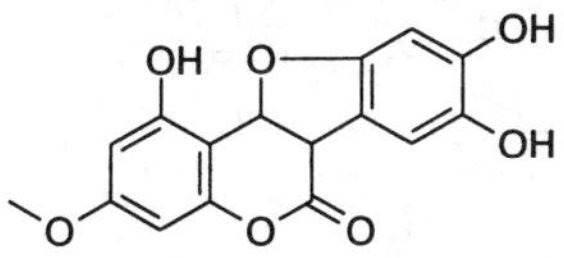

6686 Widdrol
$C_{15}H_{26}O$ MW: 222.37 Property: mp (+): 98°C, (±): 86-7°C. Source: BAI ZHI JIE, REN SHEN. Ref: 2, 6.

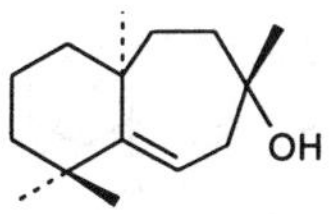

6687 cis-Widdrol α-epoxide
$C_{15}H_{26}O_2$ MW: 238.37 Property: mp cis-: 154°C. Source: BAI ZHI JIE. Ref: 6.

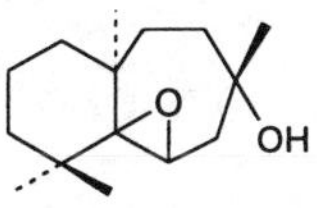

6688 trans-Widdrol α-epoxide
$C_{15}H_{26}O_2$ MW: 238.37 Property: mp trans-: 119°C. Source: BAI ZHI JIE. Ref: 6.

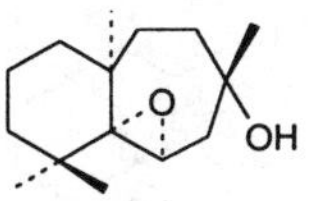

6689 Wikstroemin
$C_{28}H_{32}O_{15}$ MW: 608.56 Property: mp 200-2°C/270-2°C. Source: LIAO GE WANG GEN. Ref: 6.

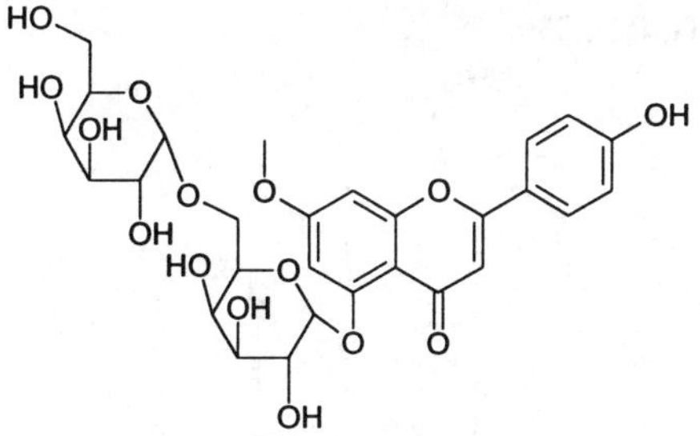

6690 Wikstromol
(+)(-)-Nortrac helogenin. CAS: 61521-74-2 $C_{20}H_{22}O_7$ MW: 374.39 Source: *Daphne odora* Thunb., etc. Ref: 5.

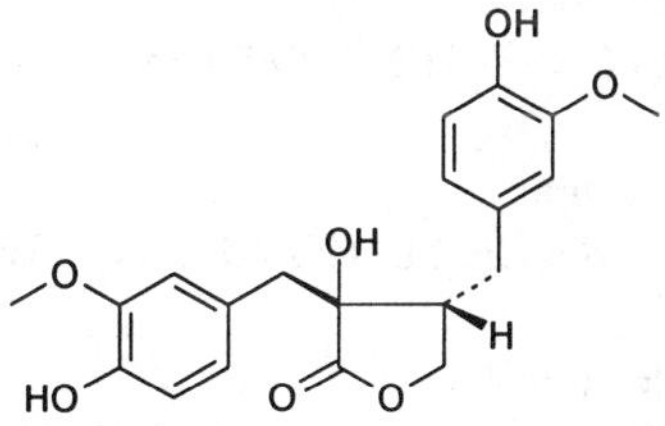

6691 Wilfordic acid
$C_{11}H_{13}NO_4$ MW: 223.23 Source: LEI GONG TENG. Ref: 2.

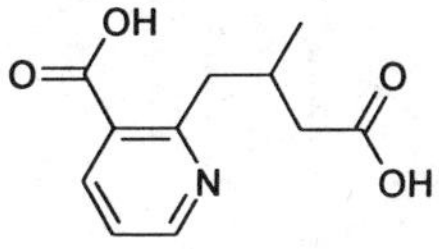

6692 Wilfordine
$C_{43}H_{49}NO_{19}$ MW: 883.87 Property: mp 175-6°C. Source: LEI GONG TENG. Ref: 2, 655.

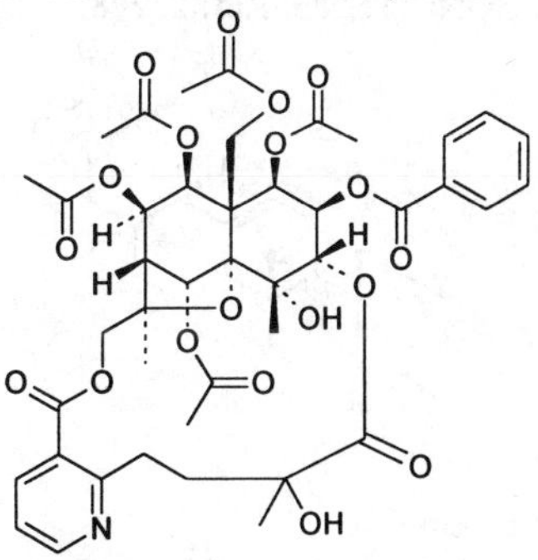

6693 Wilfordside
$C_{43}H_{49}NO_{19}$ MW: 883.87 Property: colorless columnar crystal, mp 176-8°C. Source: LEI GONG TENG. Ref: 330.

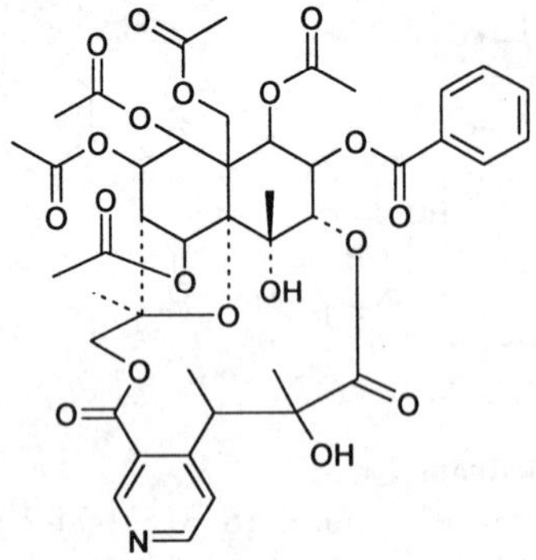

6694 Wilforgine
Source: LEI GONG TENG. Ref: 655.

6695 Wilforine
$C_{43}H_{49}O_{18}N$ Source: LEI GONG TENG. Ref: 2, 655.

6696 Wilforlide A
$C_{30}H_{46}O_3$ MW: 454.70 Source: BAO XING WEI MAO, LEI GONG TENG. Ref: 2, 278.

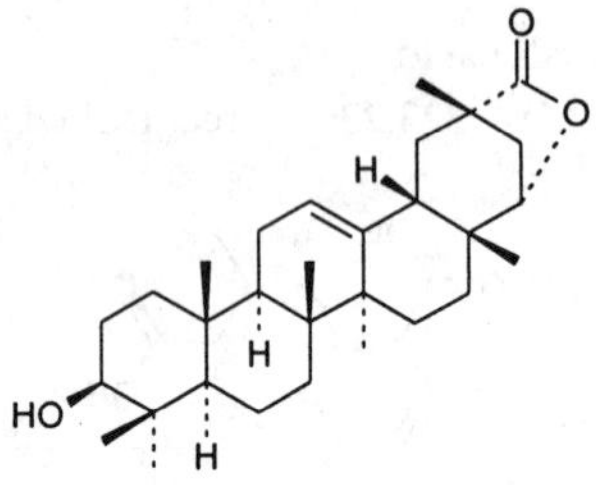

6697 Wilforlide B
$C_{30}H_{44}O_3$ MW: 452.68 Source: BAO XING WEI MAO, LEI GONG TENG. Ref: 2, 278.

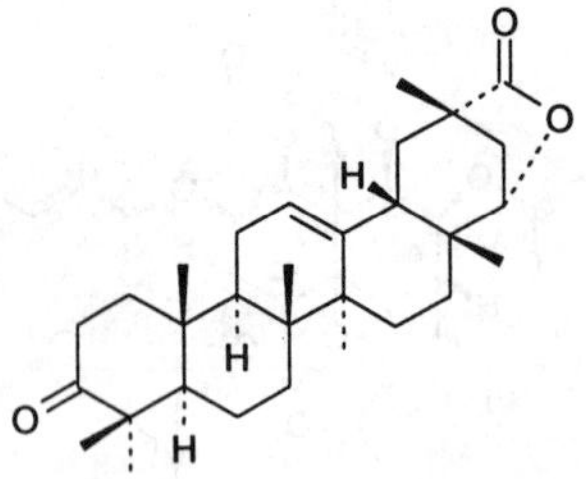

6698 Wilformine
$C_{39}H_{49}NO_{18}$ MW: 819.82 Source: LEI GONG TENG. Ref: 2.

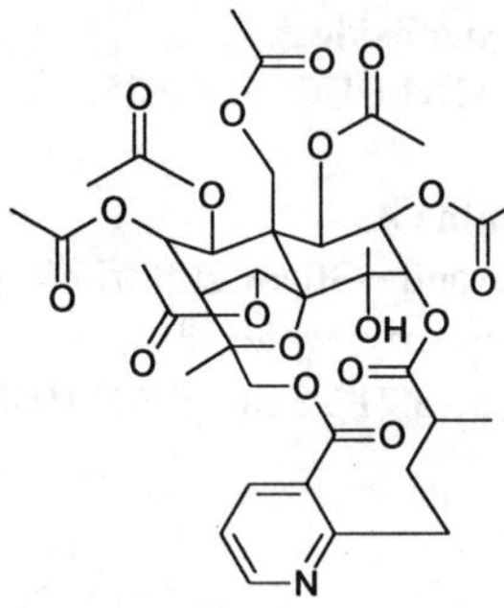

6699 Wilfornine
$C_{44}H_{52}N_2O_{17}$ MW: 880.91 Source: LEI GONG TENG. Ref: 2.

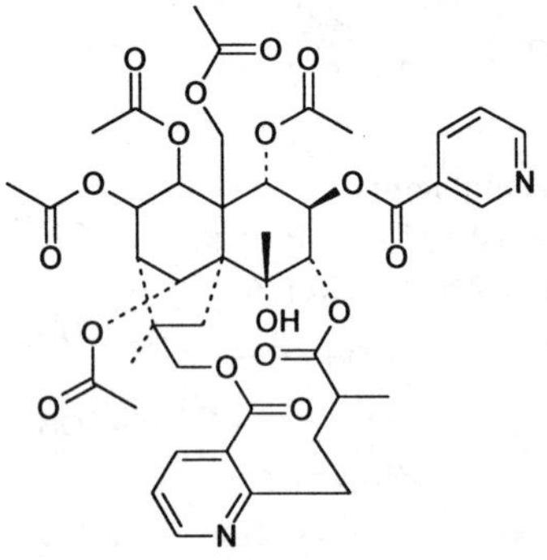

6700 Wilforonide
$C_{13}H_{16}O_3$ MW: 220.27 Source: LEI GONG TENG. Ref: 2.

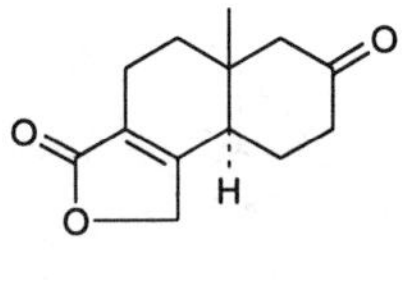

6701 Wilforzine
$C_{41}H_{47}O_{17}N$ Source: LEI GONG TENG. Ref: 2, 655.

6702 Wilfotrine
$C_{41}H_{47}O_{20}N$ Source: LEI GONG TENG. Ref: 2, 655.

6703 Wilsonine
$C_{20}H_{25}NO_4$ MW: 343.43 Source: SAN JIAN SHAN. Ref: 2.

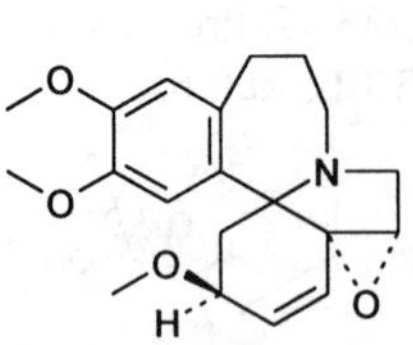

6704 Withaferin A
CAS: 5119-48-2 $C_{28}H_{38}O_6$ MW: 470.61 Property: mp 252-3°C. Source: *Withania somnifera* Dun. Ref: 5.

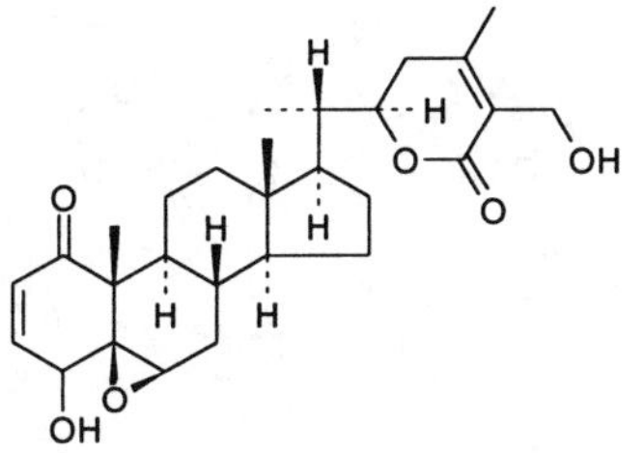

6705 Withametelin
$C_{26}H_{32}O_4$ MW: 408.54 Source: YANG JIN HUA. Ref: 2.

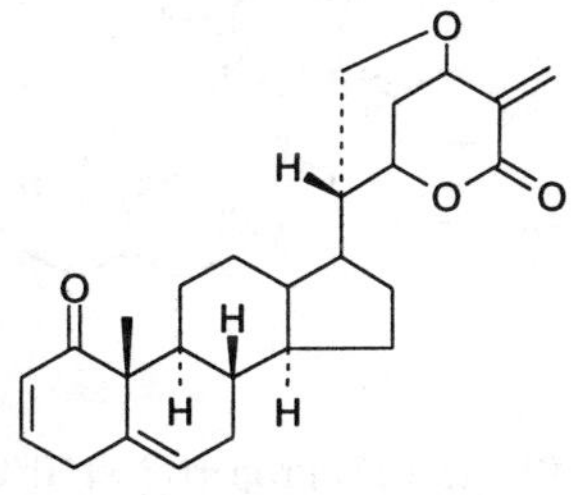

6706 Withanicandrin
$C_{28}H_{36}O_6$ MW: 468.60 Property: mp 267-9°C. Source: JIA SUAN JIANG. Ref: 6.

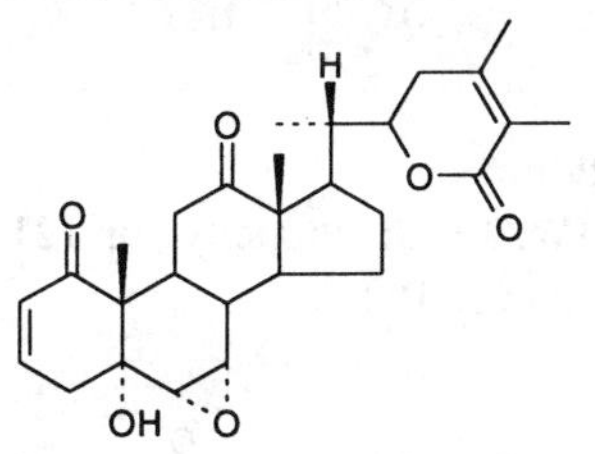

6707 Withanolide D
CAS: 30655-48-2 $C_{28}H_{38}O_5$ MW: 454.61 Property: mp 253-5°C. Source: *Withania somnifera* Dun. Ref: 5.

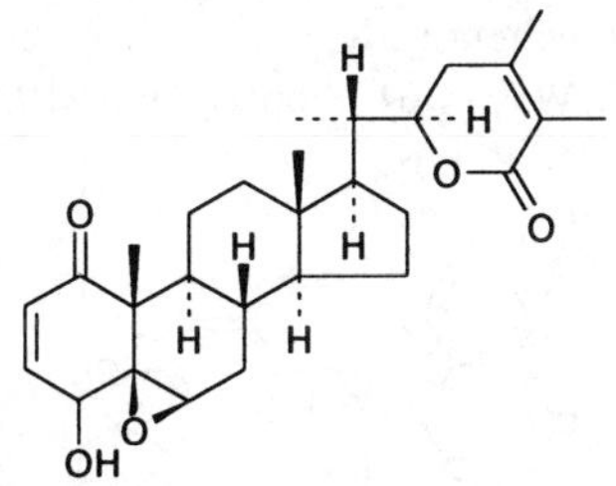

6708 Withaphysalin A
$C_{28}H_{34}O_6$ MW: 466.58 Source: TIAN PAO ZI. Ref: 6.

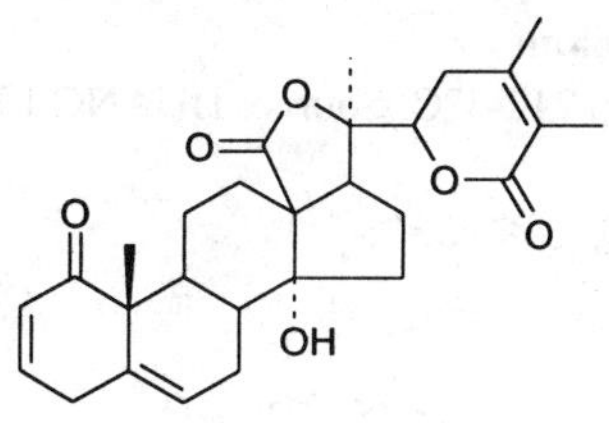

6709 Withaphysalin B
$C_{28}H_{34}O_6$ MW: 466.58 Source: TIAN PAO ZI. Ref: 6.

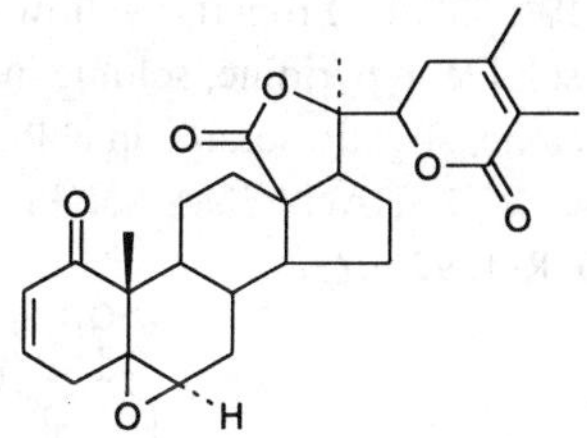

6710 Wogonin
$C_{16}H_{12}O_5$ MW: 284.27 Property: mp 203°C. Source: HUANG QIN. Ref: 2.

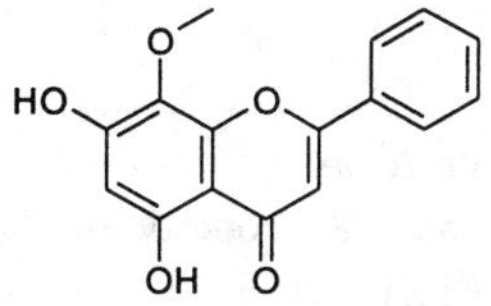

6711 Wogonoside
$C_{22}H_{20}O_{11}$ MW: 460.40 Source: HUANG QIN. Ref: 2.

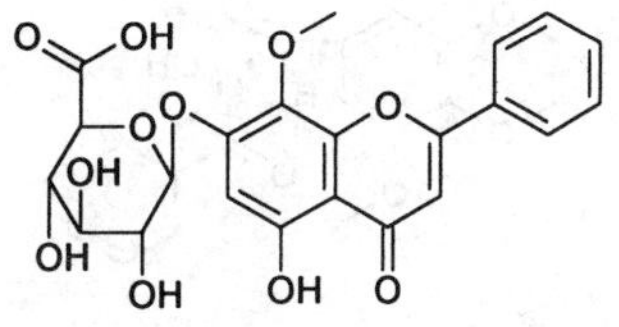

6712 Woodwardic acid
$C_{30}H_{48}O_3$ MW: 456.72 Property: mp 273-4°C (dec). Source: DONG FANG GOU JI. Ref: 6.

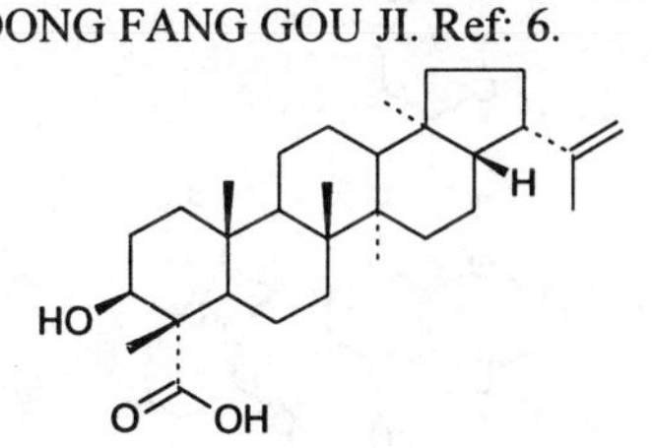

6713 Worenine
Property: mp 212-3°C. Source: HUANG LIAN. Ref: 2.

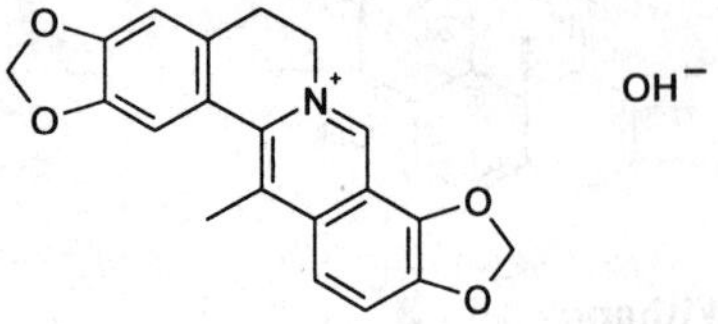

OH⁻

6714 Wushanicariin
$C_{27}H_{30}O_{11}$ MW: 530.53 Property: yellow acicular crystal, easy soluble in pyridine, soluble in ethanol , methanol, acetone, slightly soluble in chloro-form, mp 252°C. Source: WU SHAN YIN YANG HUO, YIN YANG HUO. Ref: 92, 623.

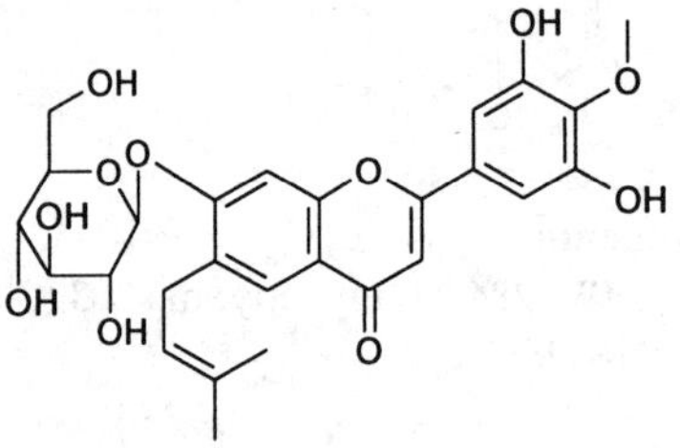

6715 Wuweizi ester A
$C_{30}H_{32}O_{9}$ MW: 536.58 Property: mp 122-4°C. Source: WU WEI ZI. Ref: 6.

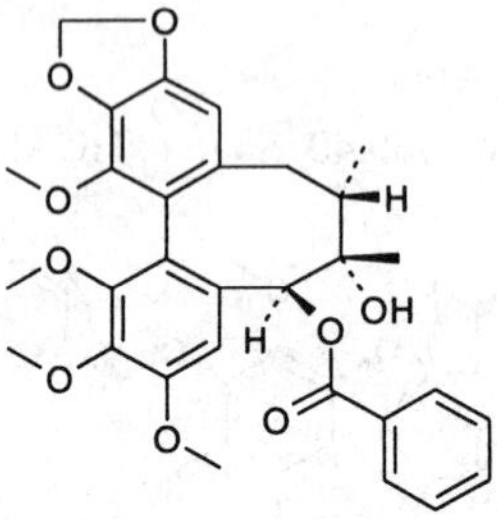

6716 Wuweizi ester B
$C_{27}H_{32}O_{10}$ MW: 516.55 Property: mp 97-9°C. Source: WU WEI ZI. Ref: 6.

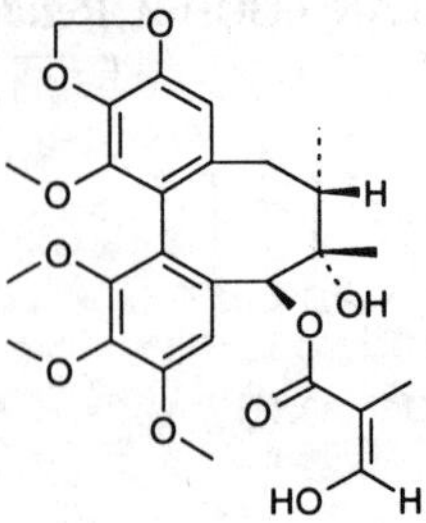

6717 Wuweizisu C
$C_{22}H_{24}O_{6}$ MW: 384.43 Source: WU WEI ZI. Ref: 2, 39.

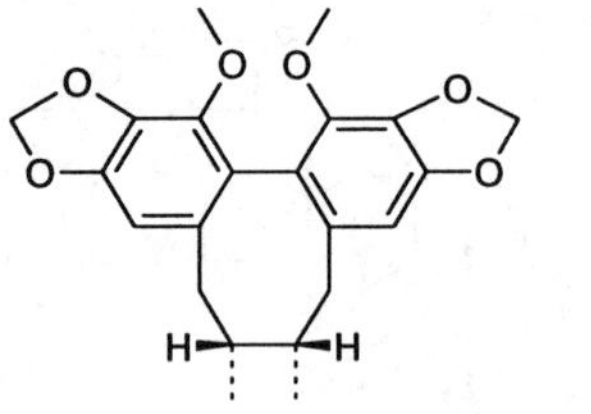

6718 Xanthaline
$C_{20}H_{19}NO_{5}$ MW: 535.38 Property: mp 210°C. Source: YA PIAN. Ref: 6.

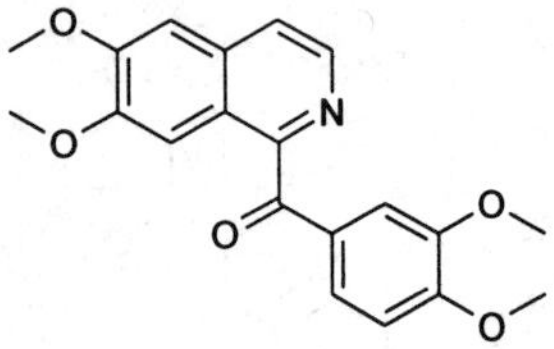

6719 Xanthine
$C_{5}H_{6}N_{4}O_{2}$ MW: 154.13 Property: >150°C, dec. Source: CHA YE, QIU YIN, XIA TIAN GAO. Ref: 6.

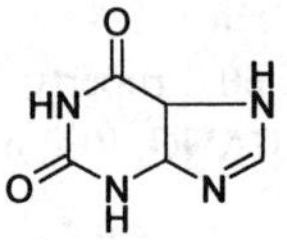

6720 Xanthinin
$C_{17}H_{22}O_{5}$ MW: 306.36 Property: mp 121-2°C. Source: CANG ER. Ref: 6.

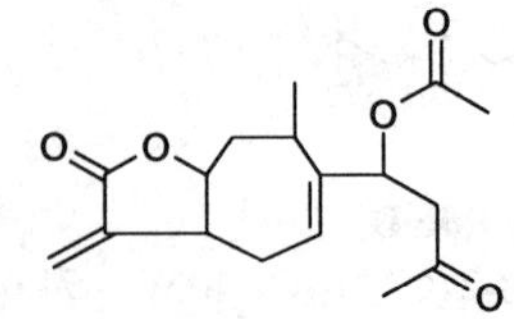

6721 Xanthochymuside
$C_{37}H_{30}O_{15}$ MW: 714.64 Property: mp 219°C. Source: SHAN ZHU ZI. Ref: 6.

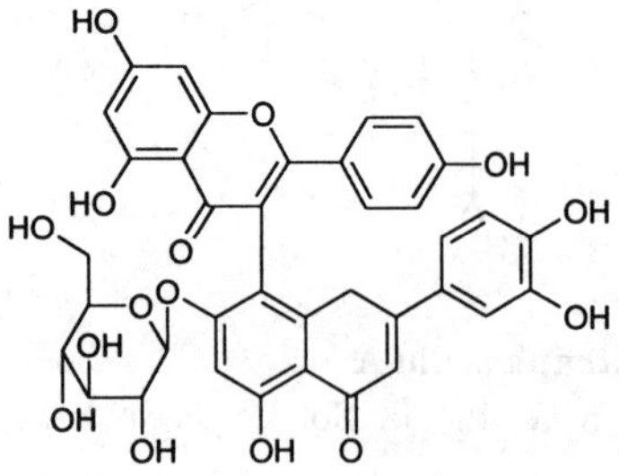

6722 Xanthohumol
$C_{21}H_{22}O_5$ MW: 354.41 Property: mp 172°C. Source: KU SHEN. Ref: 6.

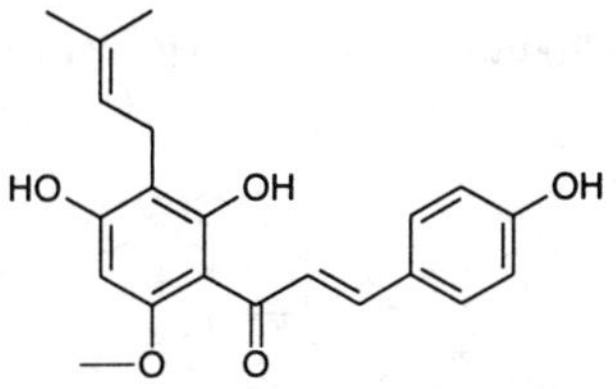

6723 Xanthomicrol
$C_{18}H_{16}O_7$ MW: 344.32 Property: mp 227-30°C. Source: MEI SHANG LU. Ref: 6.

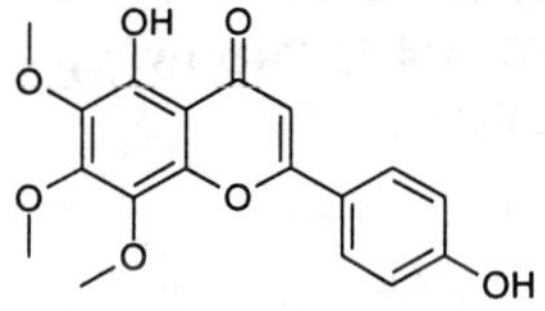

6724 Xanthommatin
$C_{20}H_{13}N_3O_8$ MW: 423.32 Source: YUAN CAN ZI. Ref: 6.

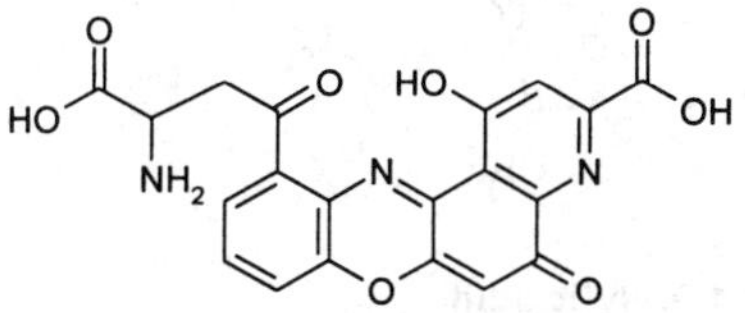

6725 Xanthoperol
$C_{20}H_{26}O_3$ MW: 314.43 Property: mp (+): 255-70°C (dec). Source: DU SONG SHI. Ref: 6.

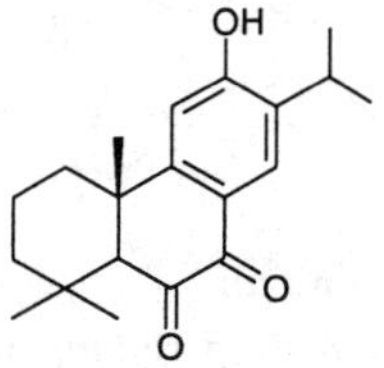

6726 Xanthoplanine
$C_{21}H_{26}NO_4$ MW: 356.45 Source: ZHU YE JIAO, ZHU YE JIAO GEN. Ref: 6.

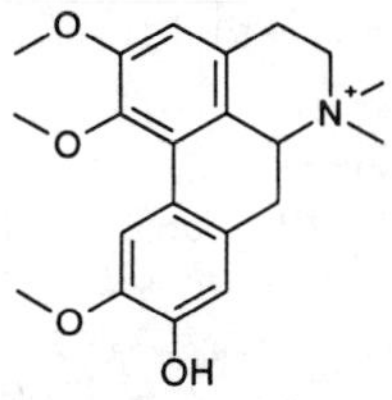

6727 Xanthopterin
$C_6H_5N_5O_2$ MW: 179.14 Property: mp >410°C, (>360°C, carbonization). Source: JIN YU. Ref: 6.

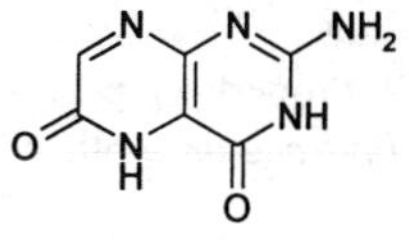

6728 Xanthotoxin
CAS: 298-81-7 $C_{12}H_8O_4$ MW: 216.20 Property: mp 148°C. Source: BAI ZHI, BU GU ZHI, DU HUO, YUN NAN QIANG HUO. Ref: 5, 558.

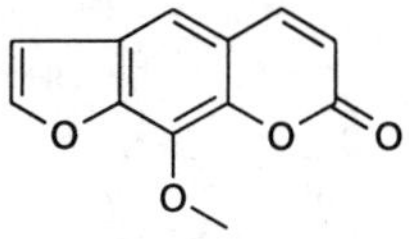

6729 Xanthotoxol
$C_{11}H_6O_4$ MW: 202.17 Property: mp 251-2°C. Source: BAI ZHI, QIANG HUO, YUN NAN QIANG HUO, YUN QIAN HU. Ref: 2, 177, 325, 507, 558.

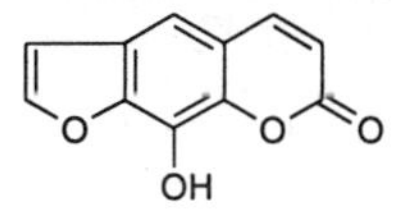

6730 Xanthoxylin
$C_{10}H_{12}O_4$ MW: 196.20 Property: bp 86°C Source: WU JIU MU GEN PI. Ref: 6.

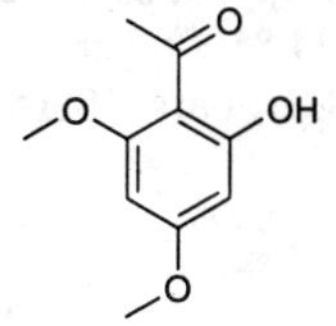

6731 Xanthumin
$C_{17}H_{22}O_5$ MW: 306.36 Property: mp 101°C (ether-chloroform), 97-8.5°C (ether). Source: CANG ER. Ref: 6.

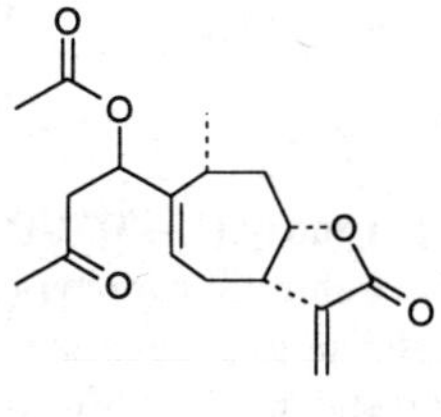

6732 Xanthyletin
CAS: 553-19-5 $C_{14}H_{12}O_3$ MW: 228.25 Property: mp 131.5°C, bp 140-5°C/0.1mm. Source: CHOU CAO, CHU YE HUA JIAO PI, GAN, NING MENG GEN. Ref: 5, 6.

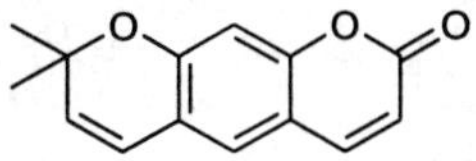

6733 Xerantholide
CAS: 65017-97-2 Property: mp 175-7°C. Source: *Xeranthemum cylindraceum* Sibth. et Smith. Ref: 5.

6734 Xuelianlactone
$C_{15}H_{20}O_3$ MW: 248.32 Property: colorless acicular crystal, mp 129-31°C, $[\alpha]_D$ +32.34°. Source: XUE LIAN. Ref: 62.

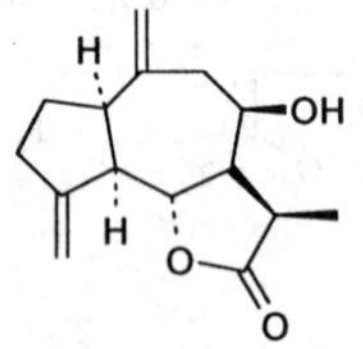

6735 Xylitol
$C_7H_{16}O_5$ MW: 180.20 Property: mp 93-4°C, bp 215-7°C/1mm. Source: MO GU. Ref: 6.

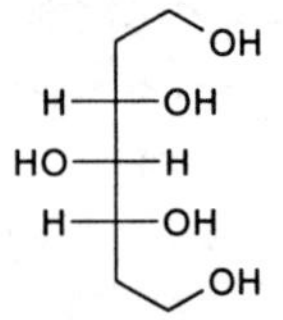

6736 3-O-β-D-Xylopyranosyl-esculentic acid
$C_{35}H_{54}O_{10}$ MW: 634.85 Property: white acicular crystal, mp 219-21°C. Source: SHANG LU. Ref: 169.

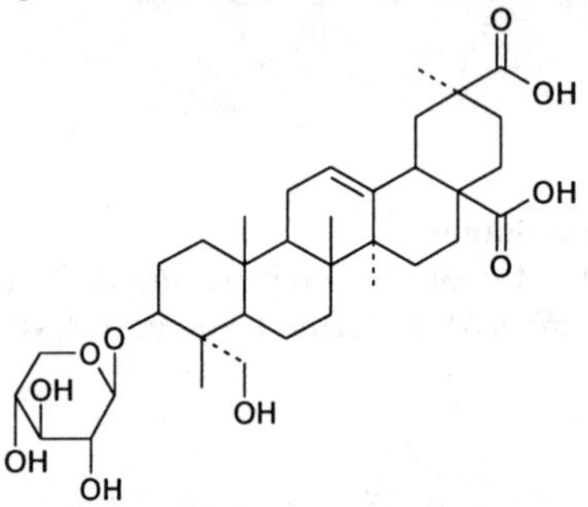

6737 β-D-Xylopyranosyl(1→3)-β-D-xyloyranosyl(1→4)-α-L-rhamnopyranosyl-(1→2)-β-D-xylopyranosyl ester of gypsogenin
Property: white crystal, mp 210-5°C. Source: DA BAO CHI BO. Ref: 425.

6738 Xylose
$C_5H_{10}O_5$ MW: 150.13 Source: LU HUI, REN SHEN. Ref: 2.

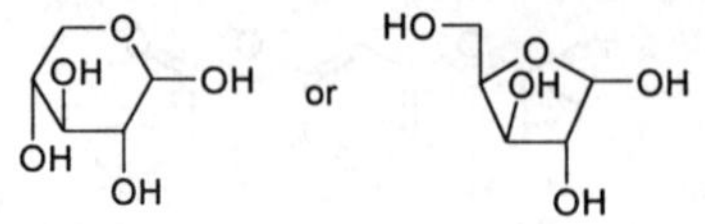

6739 7-Xylosyl-10-deacetyl baccatin III
$C_{34}H_{44}O_{14}$ MW: 676.72 Property: white crystalline powder, mp 244-6°C (methanol), $[\alpha]_D^{30}$ -26.9° (methanol). Source: YUN NAN HONG DOU SHAN. Ref: 296.

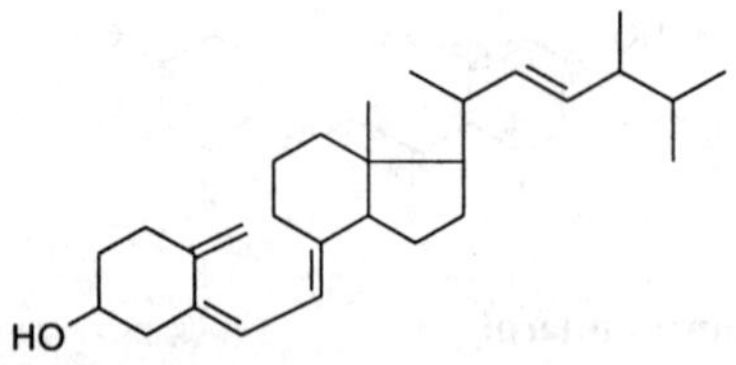

6740 O-D-Xylosylvitexin
$C_{26}H_{28}O_{14}$ MW: 564.50 Property: mp 210°C. Source: TIAN CHEN. Ref: 6.

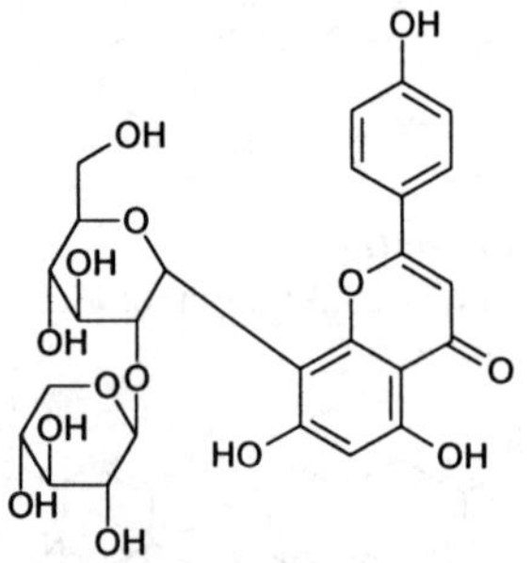

6741 3,4-Xylylic acid
$C_9H_{10}O_2$ MW: 150.18 Property: mp 166°C. Source: MU TIAN LIAO. Ref: 6.

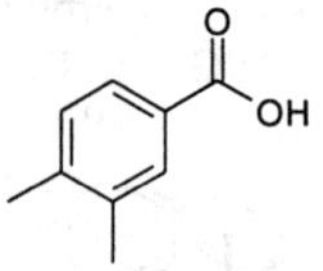

6742 Xylylic acid nitrile
C_9H_9N MW: 131.18 Property: mp 66°C. Source: MU TIAN LIAO. Ref: 6.

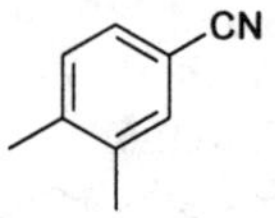

6743 Yadanziolide D
$C_{19}H_{24}O_9$ MW: 396.40 Source: YA DAN ZI. Ref: 2.

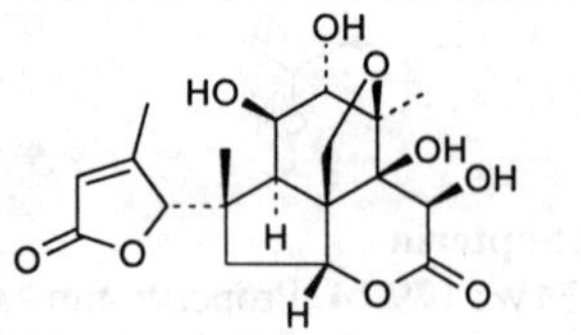

6744 Yadanzioside A
$C_{23}H_{30}O_{10}$ MW: 466.49 Source: YA DAN ZI. Ref: 2.

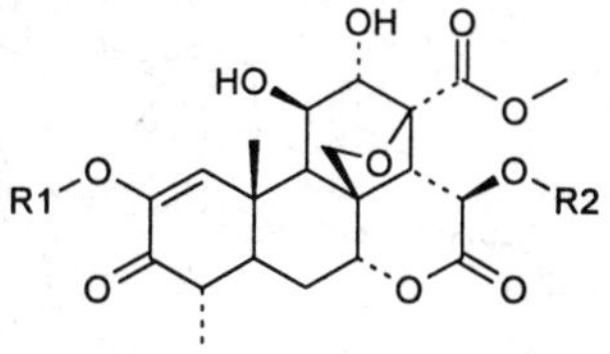

R1=Glucosyl
R2=3,4-dimethyl-4-hydroxy-2-pentenoyl

6745 Yadanzioside C
Source: YA DAN ZI. Ref: 2.

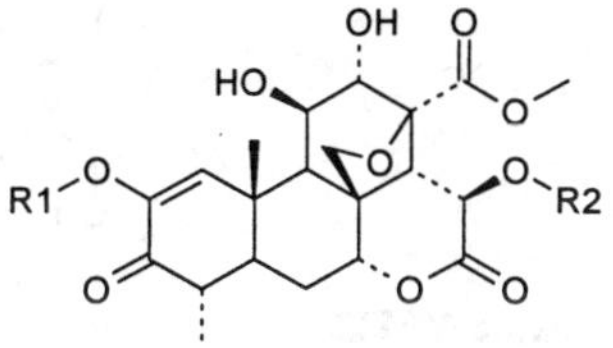

R1=Glucosyl
R2=3,4-dimethyl (4-acetoxy-2-pentenoyl)

6746 Yadanzioside F
Source: YA DAN ZI. Ref: 2.

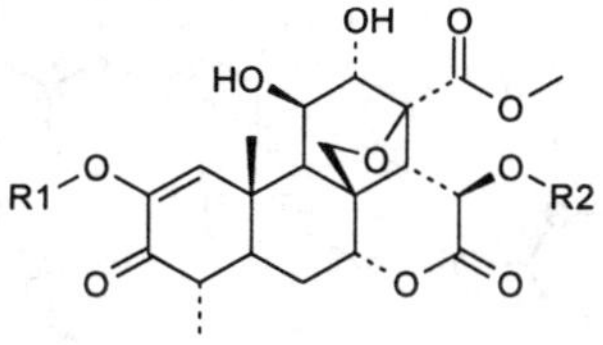

R1=Glucosyl R2=2-methylbutanoyl

6747 Yadanzioside G
Source: YA DAN ZI. Ref: 2.

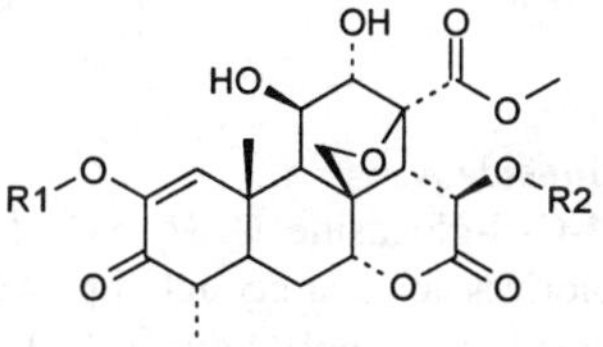

R1=Glucosyl R2=AcO

6748 Yadanzioside I
Source: YA DAN ZI. Ref: 2.

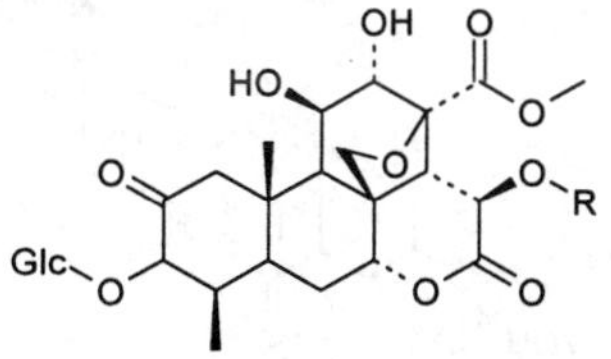

R=3,4-dimethyl-4-hydroxy-2-pentenic acid residue

6749 Yadanzioside K
Source: YA DAN ZI. Ref: 2.

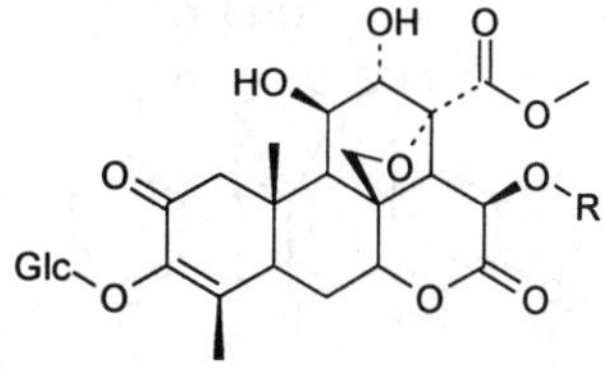

R=acetic acid residue

6750 Yadanzioside L
Source: YA DAN ZI. Ref: 2.

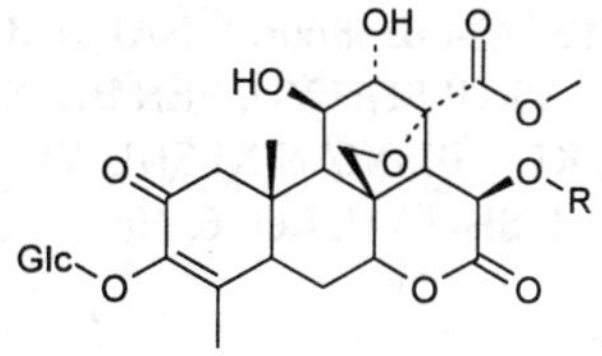

R=3,4-dimethyl-4acyloxy-2-pentenic acid residue

6751 Yadanzioside M
$C_{33}H_{40}O_{15}$ MW: 676.68 Source: YA DAN ZI. Ref: 2.

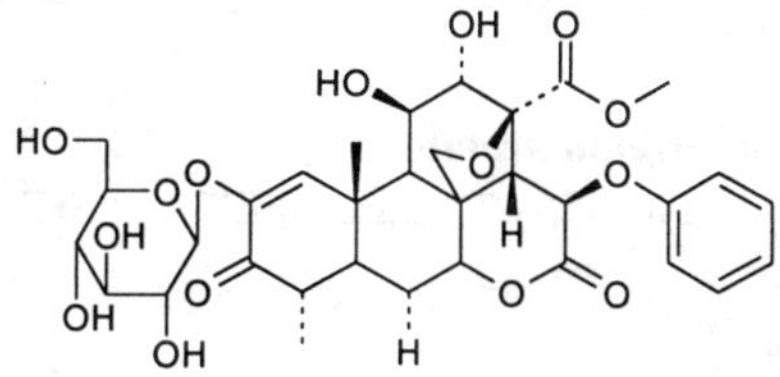

6752 Yadanzioside N
$C_{34}H_{46}O_{16}$ MW: 710.74 Source: YA DAN ZI. Ref: 2.

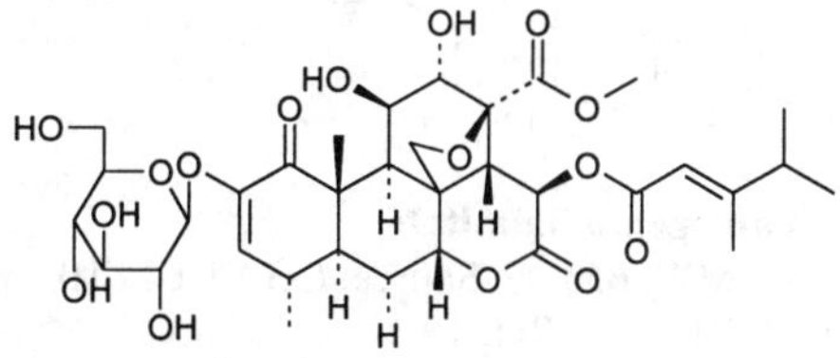

6753 Yadanzioside O
$C_{36}H_{48}O_{18}$ MW: 768.77 Source: YA DAN ZI. Ref: 2.

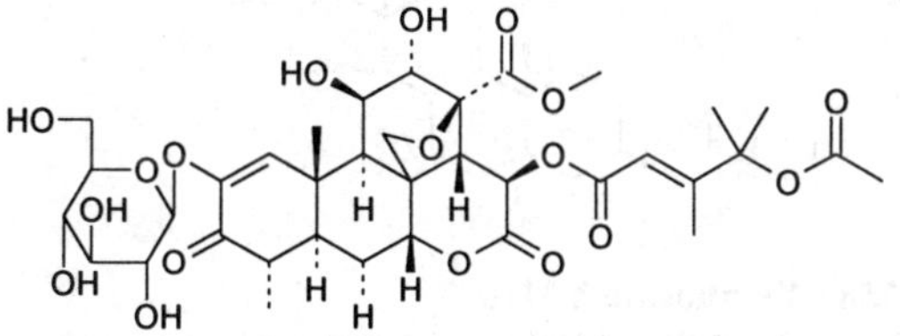

6754 Yadanzioside P
$C_{34}H_{46}O_{16}$ MW: 710.74 Source: YA DAN ZI. Ref: 2.

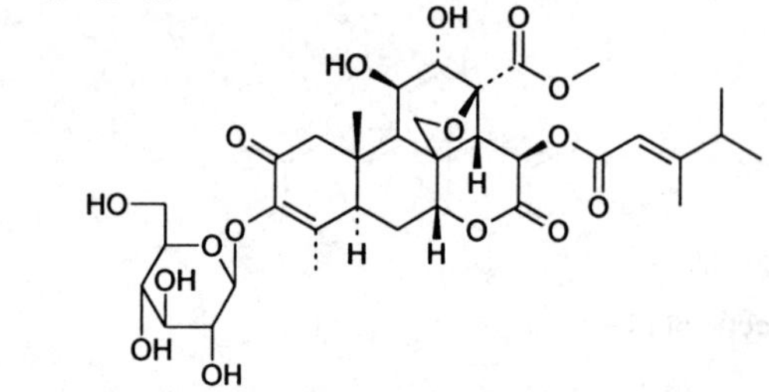

6755 Yamogenin
$C_{27}H_{42}O_3$ MW: 414.63 Source: BAI MAO TENG, BEI XIE, CHA RUI SHU YU, FEN BEI SHU YU, HU LU BA, KU QIE, XIAN XI SHU YU, XIAO HUA DUN YE SHU YU. Ref: 6, 10.

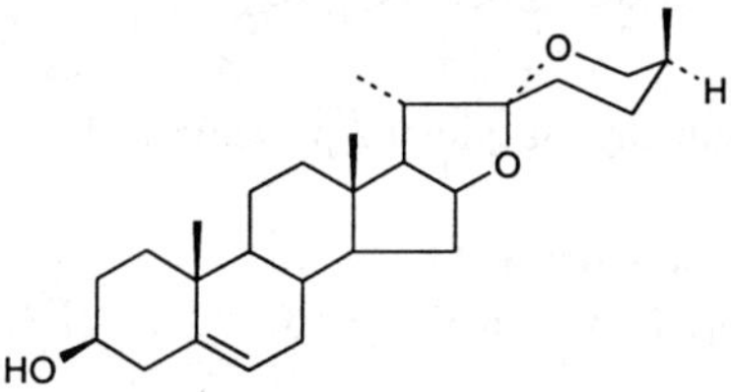

6756 Yamogenin acetate
$C_{29}H_{44}O_4$ MW: 456.67 Source: FEN BEI SHU YU. Ref: 10.

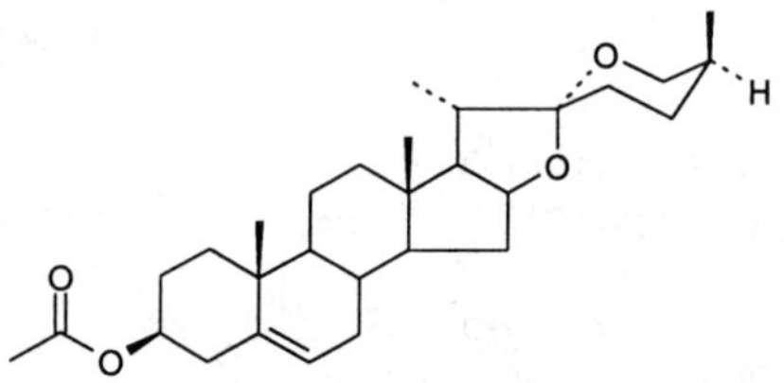

6757 Yamogenin palmitate
$C_{43}H_{72}O_4$ MW: 653.05 Source: CHA RUI SHU YU, FEN BEI SHU YU. Ref: 10.

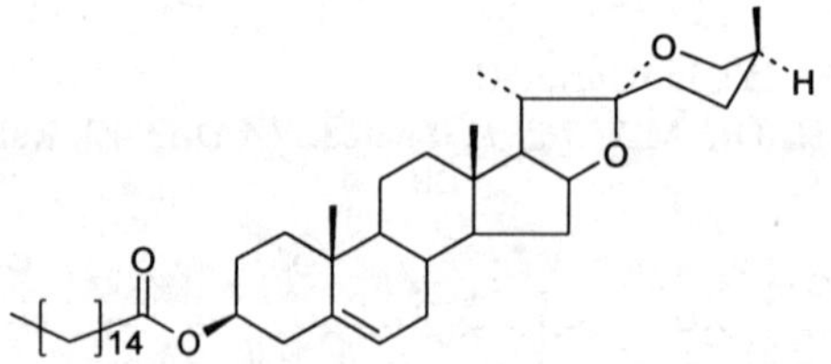

6758 Yemuoside YM10
$C_{58}H_{92}O_{25}$ MW: 1189.36 Property: white powder, mp 215-9°C(dec), $[\alpha]_D^{20}$ -4.41°(c=0.272, MEOH). Source: YE MU GUA. Ref: 131.

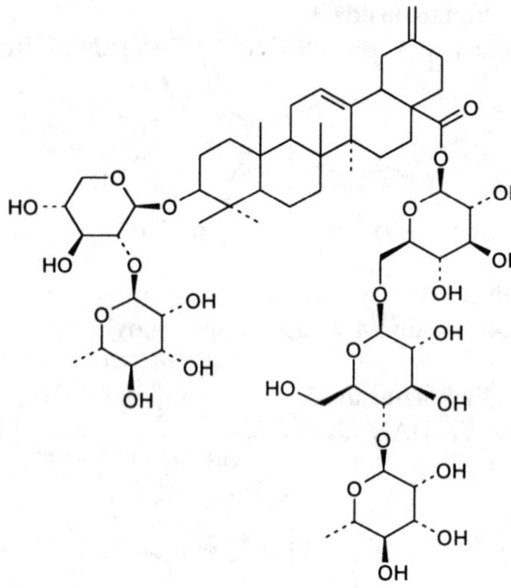

6759 Yemuoside YM12
$C_{52}H_{82}O_{21}$ MW: 1043.22 Property: white powder, mp 200-4°C, $[\alpha]_D^{20}$ +10.12° (c=0.346, MeOH). Source: YE MU GUA. Ref: 131.

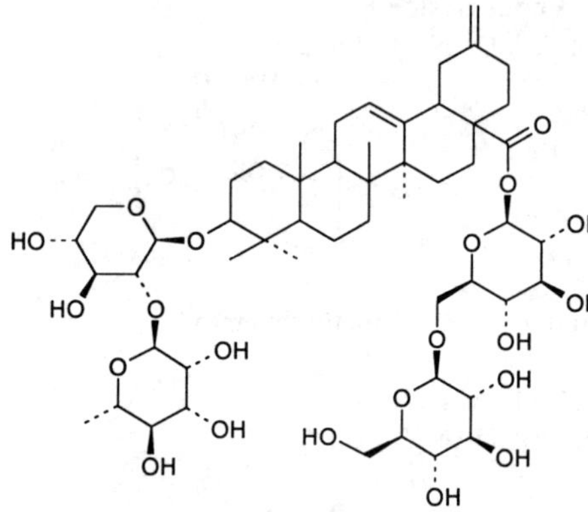

6760 Yibeinoside A
Sinpeinine-3-O-β-glucoside. $C_{33}H_{53}NO_7$ MW: 575.79 Property: colorless acicular crystal, mp 248-50°C, $[\alpha]_D^{15}$ -59° (c=0.1, methanol). Source: YI BEI MU. Ref: 172.

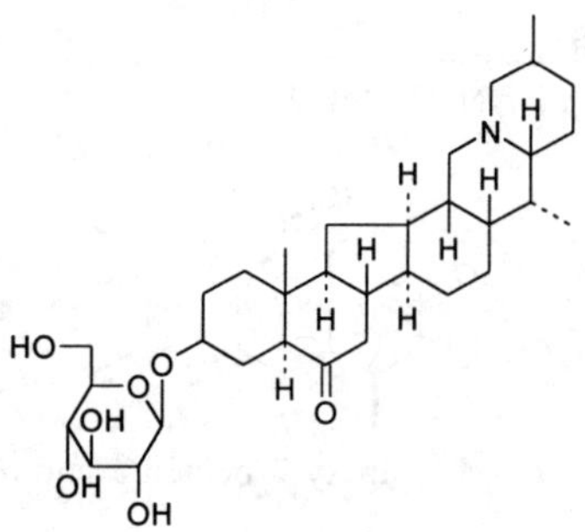

6761 Yibeinoside B

$C_{33}H_{53}NO_7$ MW: 575.79 Property: colorless acicular crystal (MeOH), mp 202-204°C. Source: YI BEI MU. Ref: 259.

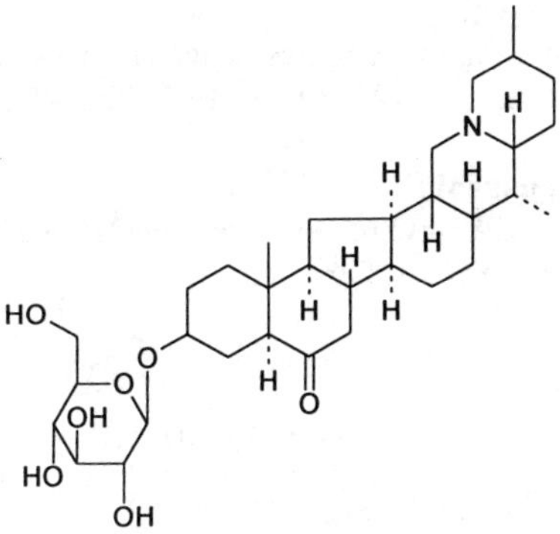

6762 Yibeinoside C

22,26-epiminocholest-6-one-3-O-β-D-glucopyrano-syl (1→4)-β-D-galactopyranoside. $C_{39}H_{65}NO_{12}$ MW: 739.95 Property: colorless acicular crystal, mp 209-11°C. Source: YI BEI MU. Ref: 656.

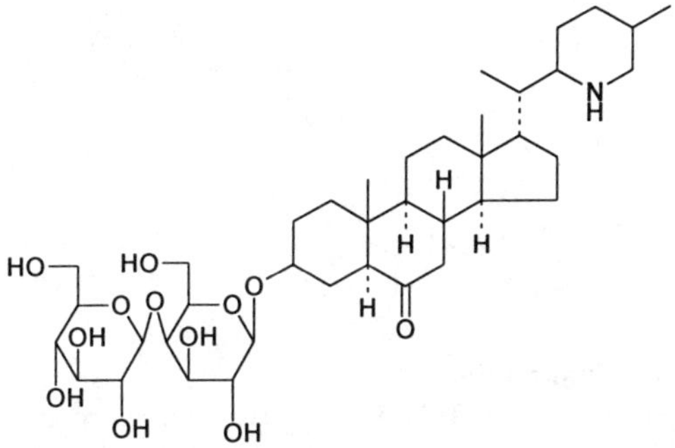

6763 Yibeissine

22,26-Imino-17,23-oxidojerv-12-en-6-oxo-3β, 11α-diol. $C_{27}H_{41}NO_4$ MW: 443.63 Property: colorless acicular crystal, mp 164.5-6°C, $[\alpha]_D^{25}$ -47.6° (c=0.13, ethanol). Source: YI BEI MU. Ref: 219.

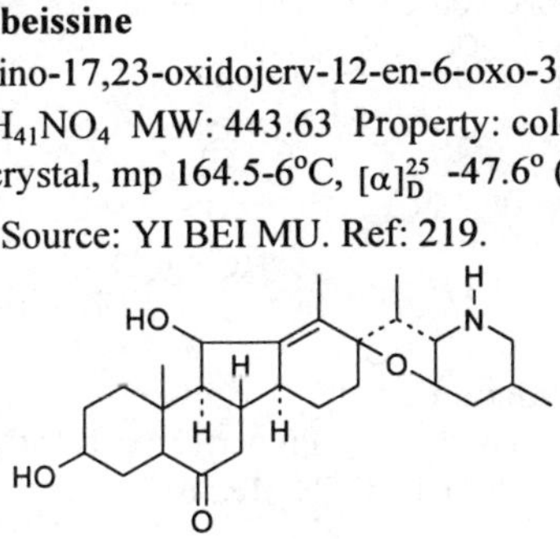

6764 Yingyanghuo A

$C_{25}H_{24}O_6$ MW: 420.47 Source: YIN YANG HUO. Ref: 635.

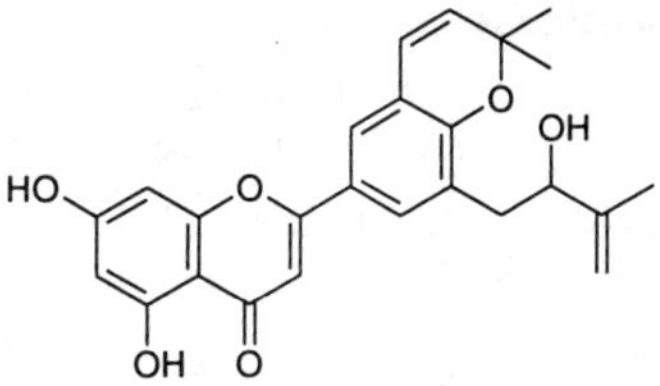

6765 Yingyanghuo B

$C_{25}H_{26}O_6$ MW: 422.48 Source: YIN YANG HUO. Ref: 635.

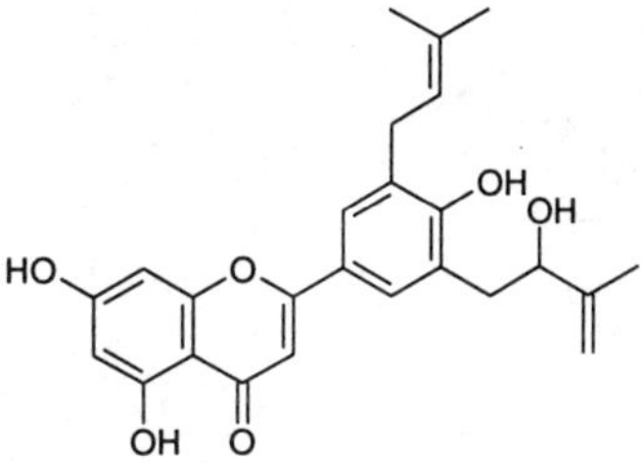

6766 Yingyanghuo C

$C_{20}H_{16}O_5$ MW: 336.35 Source: YIN YANG HUO. Ref: 635.

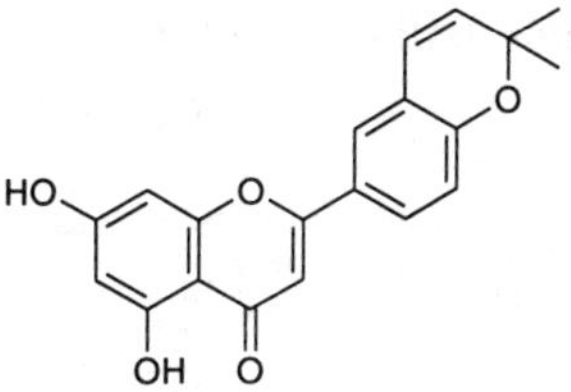

6767 Yingyanghuo D

$C_{20}H_{18}O_5$ MW: 338.36 Source: YIN YANG HUO. Ref: 635.

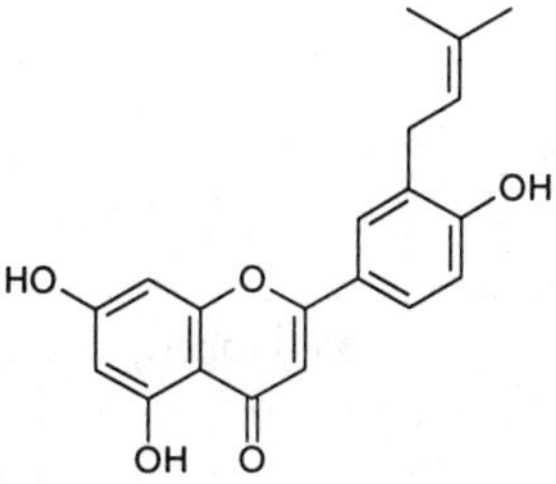

6768 Yingyanghuo E

$C_{20}H_{16}O_6$ MW: 352.35 Source: YIN YANG HUO. Ref: 635.

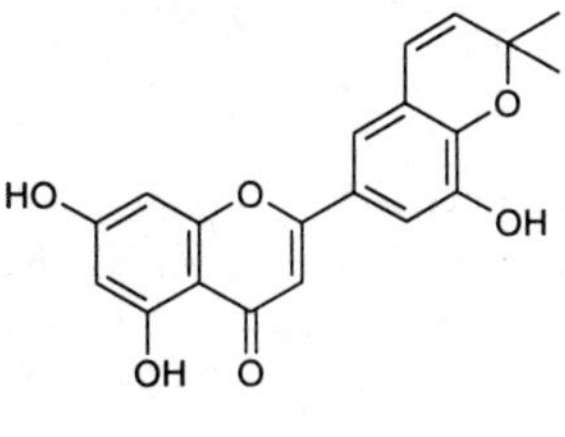

6769 Yixinoside A
$C_{54}H_{92}O_{23}$ MW: 1109.32 Property: white powder, mp 201-202°C, $[\alpha]_D^{14}$ +11.28° (c=0.98, methanol). Source: HUI GUO JIAO GU LAN. Ref: 329.

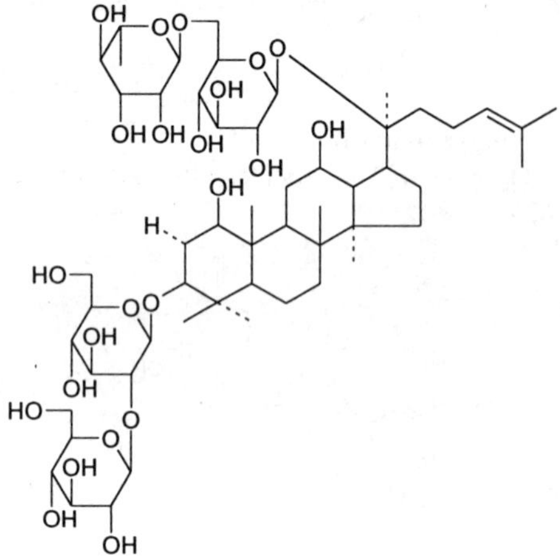

6770 Yixinoside B
$C_{42}H_{72}O_{14}$ MW: 801.03 Property: white powder, mp 181-4°C. Source: HUI GUO JIAO GU LAN. Ref: 329.

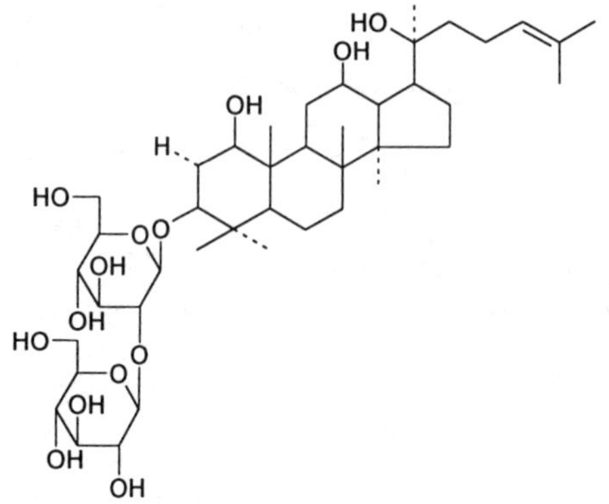

6771 Yohimbine
$C_{21}H_{26}N_2O_3$ MW: 354.45 Property: mp 241°C. Source: LUO FU MU. Ref: 6.

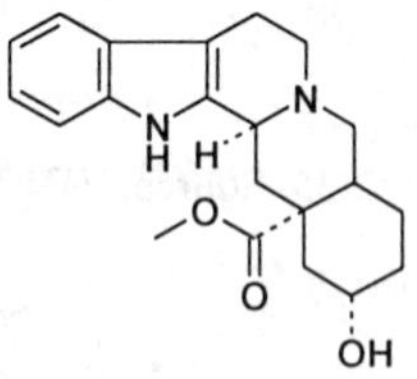

6772 Yomogi alcohol A
$C_{10}H_{18}O$ MW: 154.25 Source: AI YE. Ref: 6.

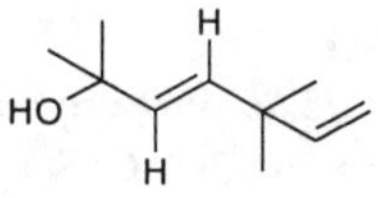

6773 Yomogin
MW: 244 Property: colorless acicular crystal, mp 202-4°C. Source: MAO LIAN HAO. Ref: 474.

6774 Yonogenin
$C_{27}H_{44}O_4$ MW: 432.65 Property: mp 210-3°C. Source: BEI XIE. Ref: 6.

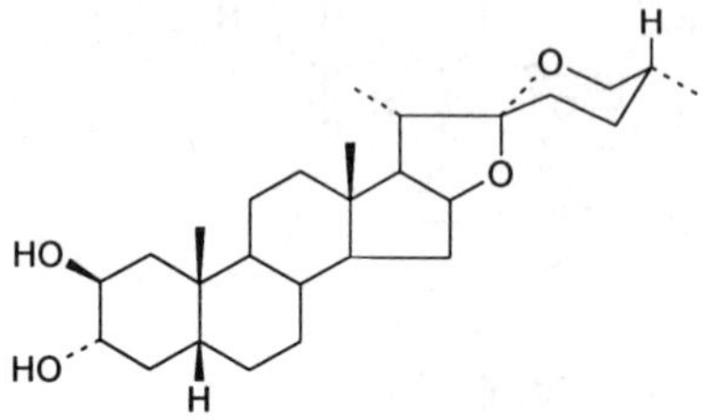

6775 Yononin
$C_{32}H_{52}O_8$ MW: 564.77 Property: mp 238-40°C (dec). Source: BEI XIE. Ref: 6.

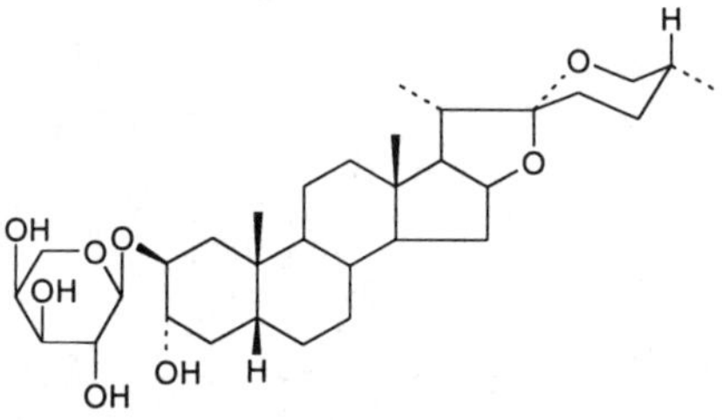

6776 Yuanhunine
$C_{21}H_{25}NO_4$ MW: 355.44 Property: colorless rhomboid crystal, mp 166-8°C, $[\alpha]_D^{23}$ +229.7° (c= 0.16, 95% ethanol). Source: YAN HU SUO. Ref: 56.

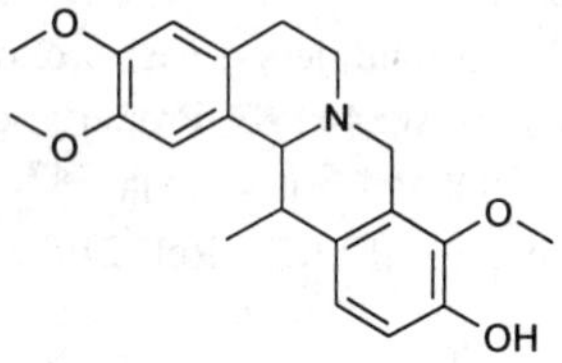

6777 Yuenkanin
$C_{27}H_{30}O_{14}$ MW: 578.53 Property: mp 180°C/270°C. Source: YUAN HUA GEN. Ref: 6.

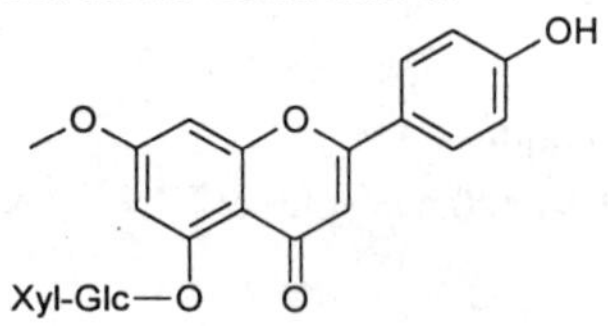

Xyl-Glc—O

6778 Yunaconitine
Source: DIAN XI WU TOU. Ref: 618.

6779 Yunnanxamine
9-Deoxo-9α-hydroxytaxol. $C_{47}H_{51}NO_{14}$ MW: 853.93 Property: white powder, mp 174-6°C, $[\alpha]_D^{22}$ -13.1° (c=0.08, chloroform). Source: YUN NAN HONG DOU SHAN. Ref: 316.

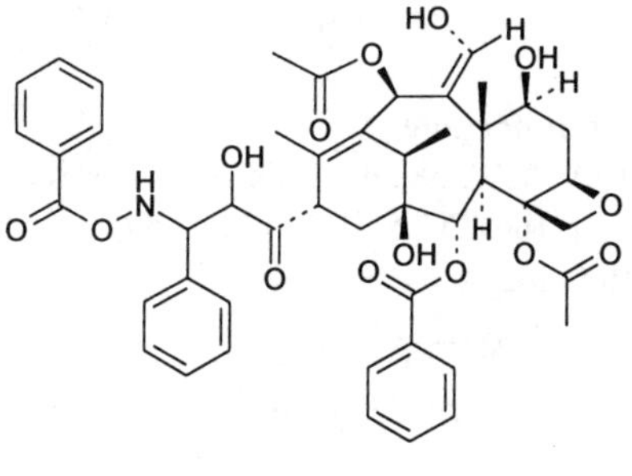

6780 Yunnanxane
Taxa-4(20),11-diene-2α,5α10β,14β-tetraol-2α,5α, 10β-triacetate-14β-α-methyl-β-hydroxyl butyrate. $C_{31}H_{46}O_9$ MW: 562.71 Property: colorless transparent massive crystal, mp 165-7°C, $[\alpha]_D^{17}$ +41.6° (methanol). Source: YUN NAN HONG DOU SHAN. Ref: 202.

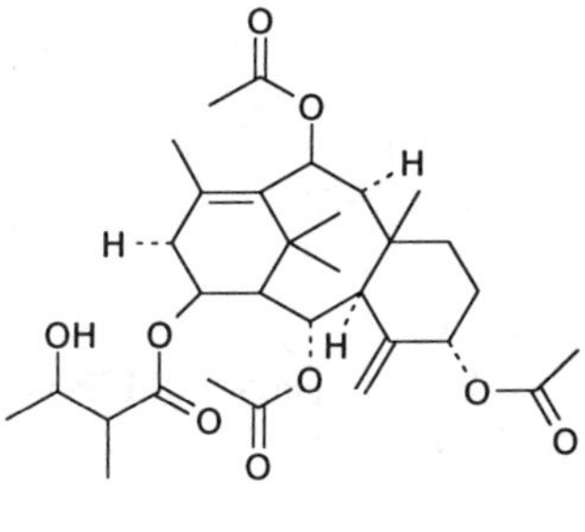

6781 Yunnanxol
13(2',3'-Dihydroxy-3'-phenyl)-propionyl bacca-tin. $C_{39}H_{44}O_{13}$ MW: 720.78 Property: white powder, mp 154-7°C, $[\alpha]_D^{12}$ -75.2° (c=0.055, chloroform). Source: YUN NAN HONG DOU SHAN. Ref: 316.

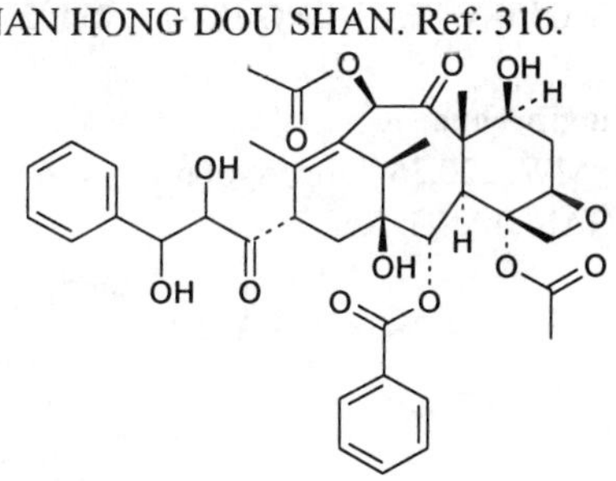

6782 Yuzhizioside
3-O-β-D-xylopyranosyl-(1→2)-α-L-arabinopyranosyl oleanolic acid 28-O-β-D-glucopyranosyl-(1→6)-β-D-glucopyranoside. $C_{52}H_{84}O_{21}$ MW: 1045.24 Property: white acicular crystal, mp 213-6°C. Source: BAI MU TONG. Ref: 299.

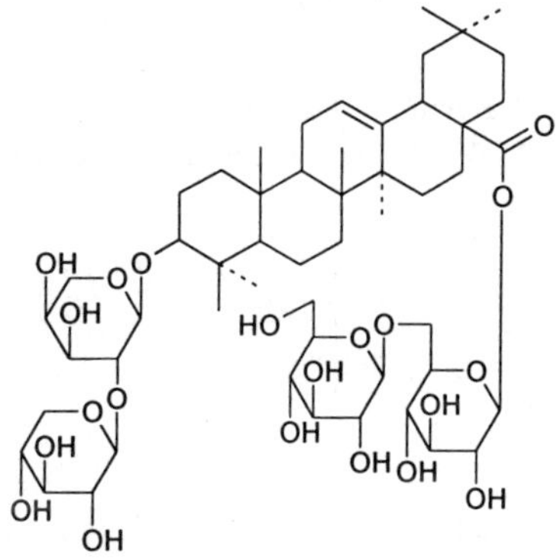

6783 Zaluzanin C
CAS: 16868-87-2 $C_{15}H_{18}O_3$ MW: 246.31 Property: mp 94-5°C. Source: *Zaluzanin robinsonii* Sharp, *Pertya robusta* Beauv, etc. Ref: 5.

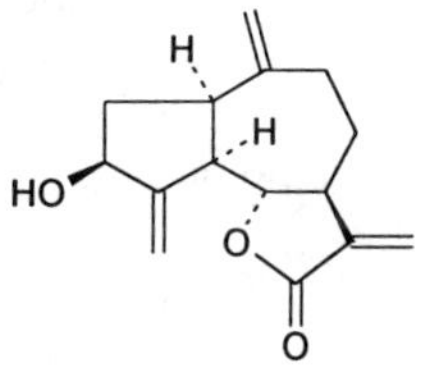

6784 Zeatin
$C_{10}H_{13}N_5O$ MW: 219.25 Property: mp 207-8°C. Source: TAO NAN GUA, YU SHU SHU. Ref: 6.

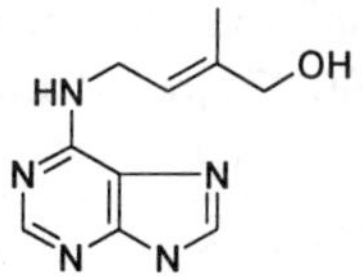

6785 Zeaxanthine
$C_{40}H_5O$ MW: 568.89 Property: mp 215.5°C. Source: GOU QI ZI. Ref: 2.

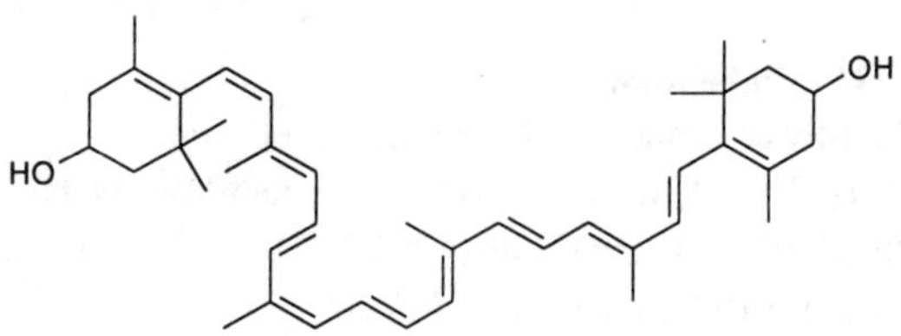

6787 Zederone
$C_{15}H_{18}O_3$ MW: 246.31 Property: mp 153.5-4°C. Source: PENG E SHU. Ref: 6.

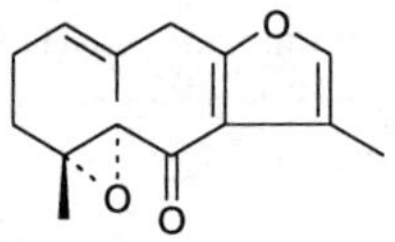

6788 Zedoarone
$C_{15}H_{18}O_2$ MW: 230.31 Source: PENG E SHU. Ref: 6.

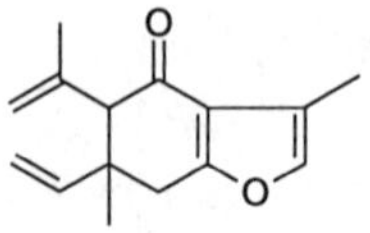

6789 Zhebeinine
5α,14α-Cevanine-3β,6α,20β-triol. $C_{27}H_{45}NO_3$ MW: 431.66 Property: white acicular crystal, mp 222-4°C, $[\alpha]_D^{25}$ -21.3° (c=0.5, ethanol). Source: ZHE BEI MU. Ref: 186, 528.

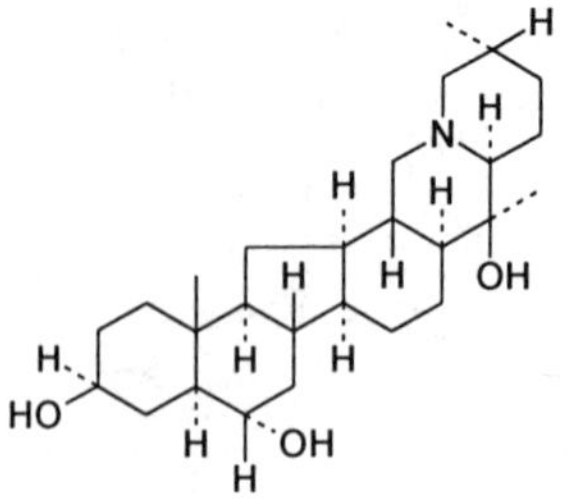

6790 Zhebeiresinol
2-(3',5'-Dimethoxy-4'-hydroxyphenyl)-3,7-dioxabicyclo[3,3,0]octan-6-one. $C_{14}H_{16}O_6$ MW: 280.28 Property: light yellow prismatic crystal, mp 193-194°C. Source: ZHE BEI MU. Ref: 262.

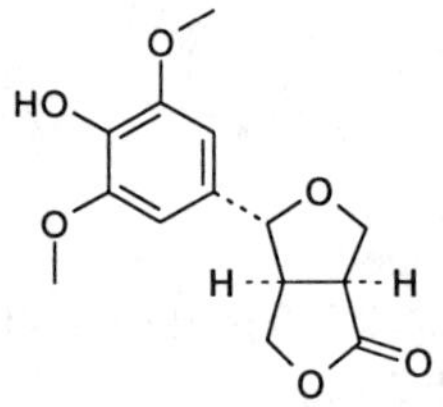

6791 Ziebeimine
5α,14α-cevanine-13,17-dehydro-3α,6β-diol. $C_{27}H_{43}NO_2$ MW: 413.65 Property: colorless crystal, mp 186-8°C, $[\alpha]_D^{23}$ +10.6°(c=0.09 $CHCl_3$). Source: ZI HUA E BEI BEI MU. Ref: 136.

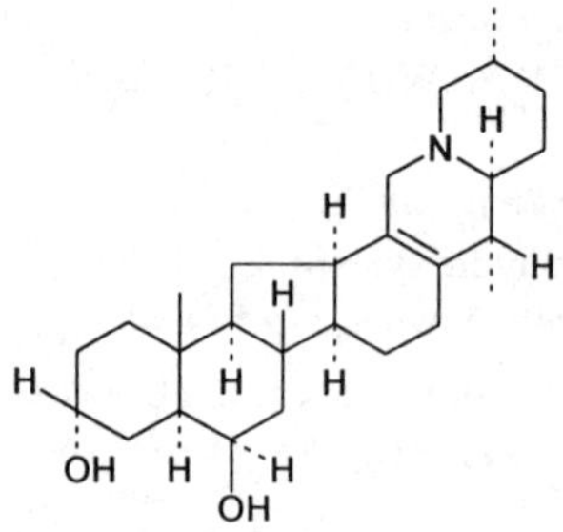

6791b Zijinlongine
$C_{21}H_{21}NO_6$ MW: 383.40 Property: colorless lamellar crystal, mp 166-7°C. Source: DA TENG LING ER CAO. Ref: 162.

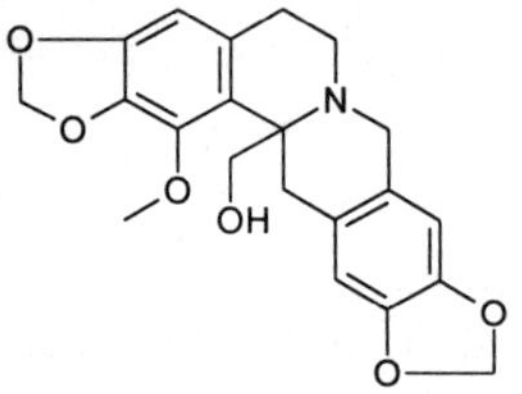

6792 Zingerone
$C_{11}H_{14}O_3$ MW: 194.23 Property: mp 40-1°C, bp 190°C/16mm. Source: GAN JIANG, SHENG JIANG. Ref: 2.

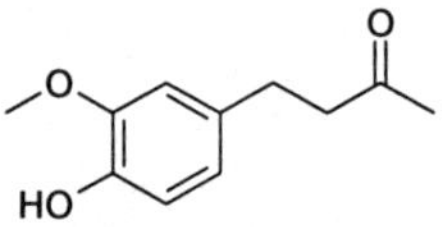

6793 Zingiberene
$C_{15}H_{24}$ MW: 204.36 Property: (-): 134°C/14mm. Source: GAN JIANG. Ref: 2.

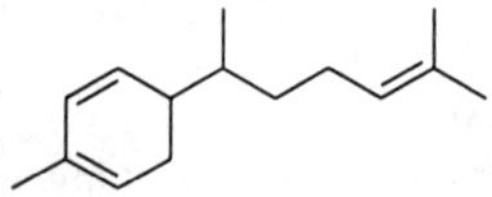

6794 Zingiberol
Source: GAN JIANG, SHENG JIANG. Ref: 2.

6795 Zingiberone
$C_{15}H_{24}O$ MW: 220.36 Property: bp 156°C/6mm. Source: GAN JIANG. Ref: 2.

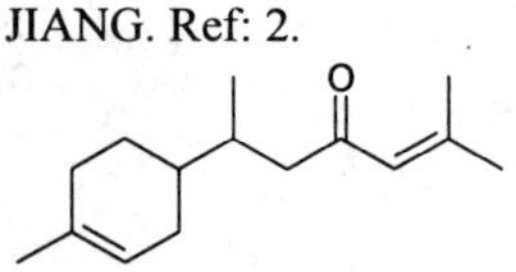

6796 Zivulgarin

4"-β-O-Glucopyranosyl swertisin. $C_{28}H_{32}O_{15}$ MW: 608.56 Property: light yellow acicular crystal, mp 275-7°C (methanol). Source: SUAN ZAO REN. Ref: 73.

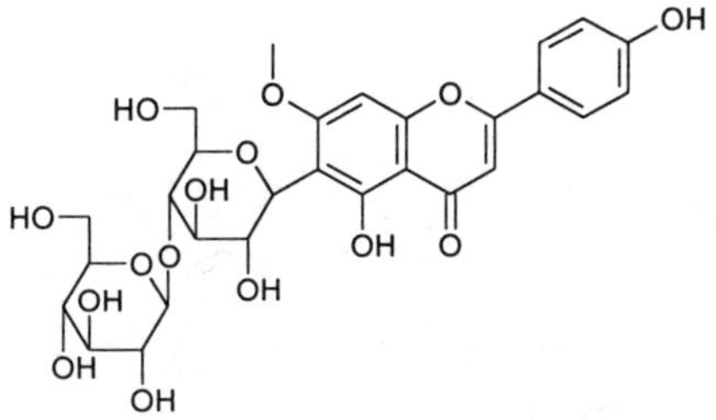

6797 Ziyu glycoside I

$C_{41}H_{66}O_{13}$ MW: 766.98 Property: mp 256-60°C. Source: DI YU. Ref: 6.

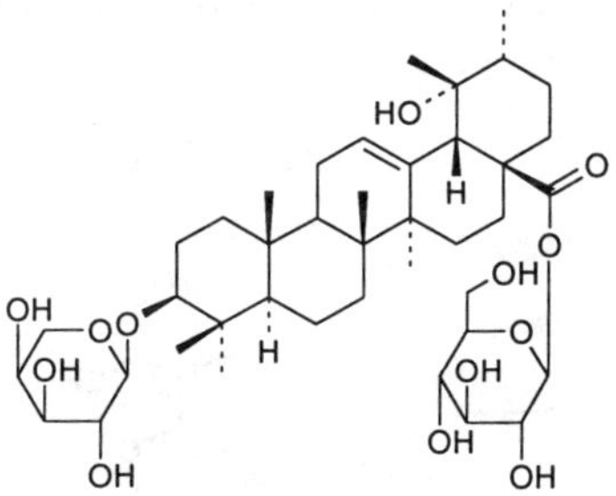

6798 Ziyu glycoside II

$C_{35}H_{56}O_{8}$ MW: 604.83 Source: DI YU. Ref: 6.

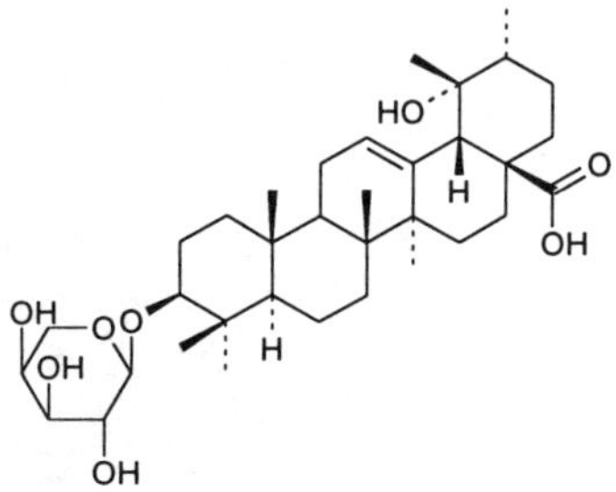

6799 Zizybeoside I

$C_{19}H_{28}O_{11}$ MW: 432.43 Source: DA ZAO. Ref: 2.

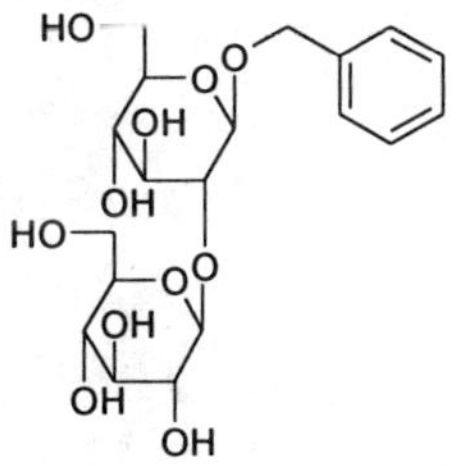

6800 Zizybeoside II

Source: DA ZAO. Ref: 2.

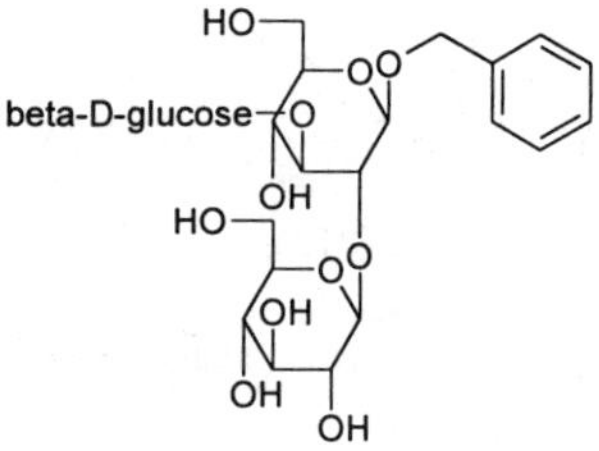

6801 Zizyphus saponin I

$C_{47}H_{76}O_{17}$ MW: 913.12 Source: DA ZAO. Ref: 2.

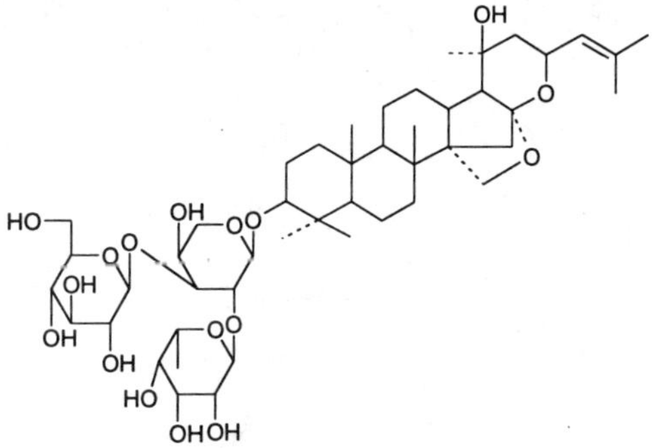

6802 Zizyphus saponin II

$C_{47}H_{76}O_{17}$ MW: 913.12 Source: DA ZAO. Ref: 2.

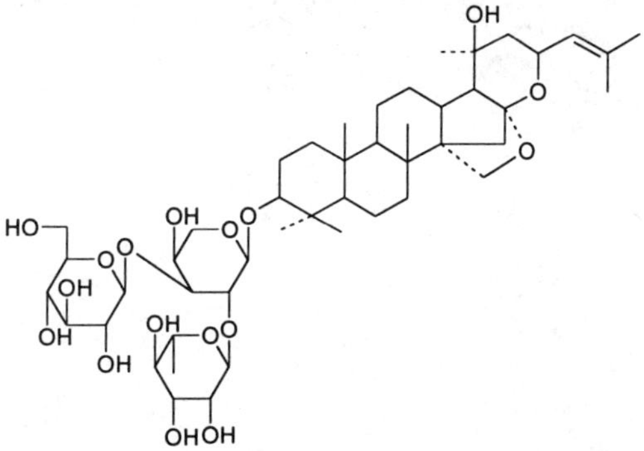

6803 Zizyphus saponin III

$C_{53}H_{86}O_{20}$ MW: 1043.26 Source: DA ZAO. Ref: 2.

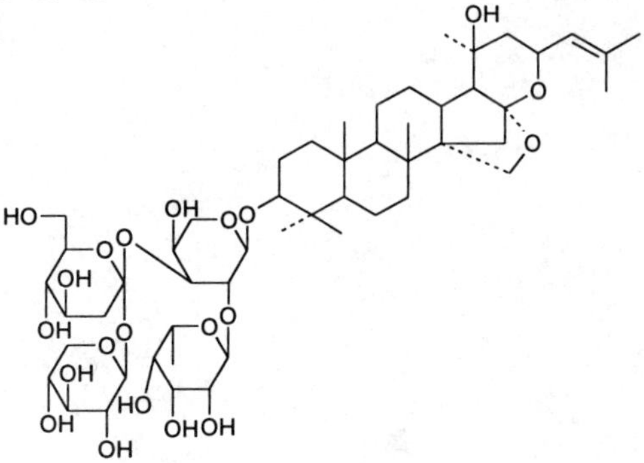

6804 Zizyvoside I
Source: DA ZAO. Ref: 2.

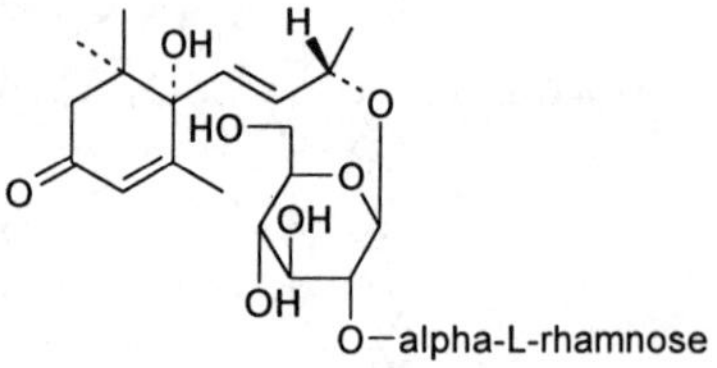

6805 Zizyvoside II
$C_{31}H_{50}O_{18}$ MW: 710.73 Source: DA ZAO. Ref: 2.

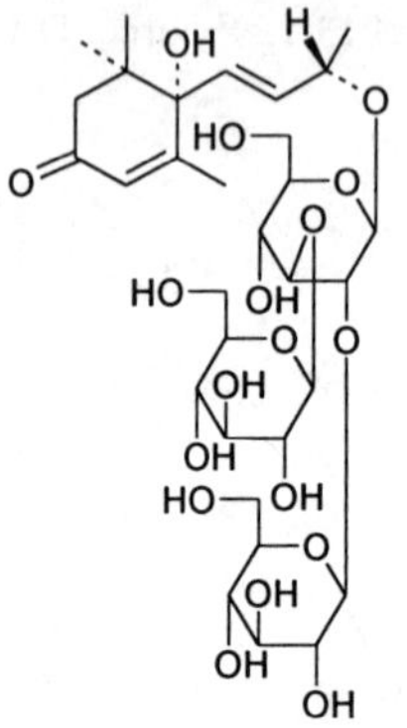

6806 Zonarene
$C_{15}H_{24}$ MW: 204.36 Source: SHENG JIANG. Ref: 2.

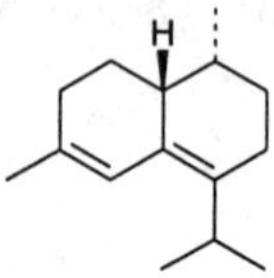

6807 Zygacine
$C_{29}H_{45}NO_8$ MW: 535.68
Source: LI LU. Ref: 6.

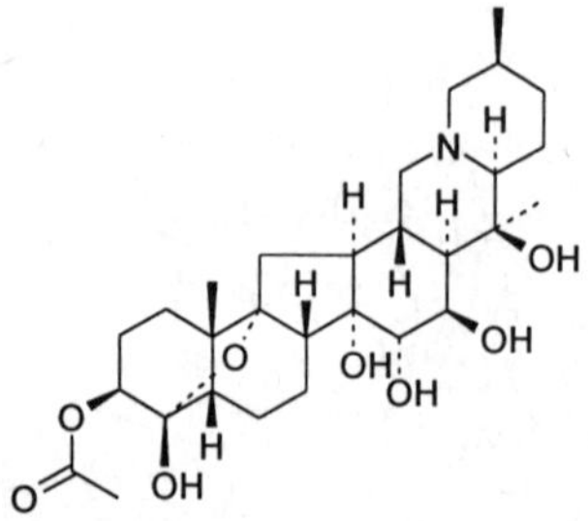

6808 Zygadenilic acid δ-lactone-16-angelate
$C_{32}H_{47}NO_8$ MW: 573.73 Property: mp 235°C.
Source: LI LU. Ref: 6.

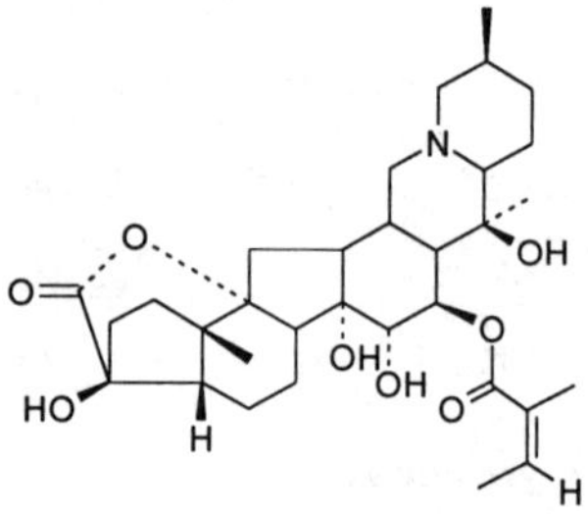

Part II

NATURAL SOURCES, EFFECTS AND INDICATIONS OF TRADITIONAL CHINESE MEDICINES

Natural Sources, Effects and Indications of Traditional Chinese Medicines

Abelmusk; SHE XIANG Origin: *Moschus moschiferus* L.; *Moschus berezovskii* Flerov.; *Moschus sifanicus* Przewalski (all *Cervidae*). Part: dried secretion obtained from the musk gland of the musk deer. Effects: To open the orifices, repel foulness, free the network vessels, and dissipate stasis. Indications: Unconsciousness and convulsion syncope, phlegm-induced syncope, apoplexy and epilepsy; sores, carbuncles and other suppurative cutaneous infections; sudden gastric and abdominal pain, pain caused by ecchymoma in traumatic injuries, and pain of impediment-syndrome (arthralgia-syndrome); bind in the abdomen, menstrual block, retention of dead fetus or retained placenta.

Acutangular Scopolia; SAN FEN SAN Origin: *Scopolia acutangula* C. Y. Wu *et* C. Chen [= *Anisodus acutangulus* C. Y. Wu *et* C. Chen] (*Solanaceae*). Part: root, leaf or seed. Effects: To anesthetize and settle pain. Indications: Stomach pain, fracture, wind-damp pain (rheumatalgia), knocks and falls.

Acute Common Perilla Leaf; ZI SU YE Origin: *Perilla frutescens* (L.) Britt. var. *acuta* (Thunb.) Kudo (*Labiatae*). See Crisped Common Perilla Leaf.

Acute Common Perilla Seed; ZI SU ZI Origin: *Perilla frutescens* (L.) Britt. var. *acuta* (Thunb.) Kudo (*Labiatae*). See Crisped Common Perilla Seed.

Acute Common Perilla Stem; ZI SU GENG Origin: *Perilla frutescens* (L.) Britt. var. *acuta* (Thunb.) Kudo (*Labiatae*). See Crisped Common Perilla Stem.

Acutifoliate Podocarpium Herb; SHAN MA HUANG Origin: *Desmodium racemosum* (Thunb.) DC. [= *Podocarpium podocarpum* var. *oxyphyllum* (DC.) Yang *et* Huang] (*Leguminosae*). Part: herb. Effects: To dispel wind-damp, dissipate stasis, and disperse swelling. Indications: Asthma, wind-damp pain (rheumatalgia), flooding and vaginal discharge, mammary welling abscess, knocks and falls.

Adder's Tongue; PING ER XIAO CAO Origin: *Ophioglossum vulgatum* L. (*Ophioglossaceae*). Part: herb. Effects: To clear heat and cool blood, settle pain and resolve toxin. Indications: Lung heat cough, taxation damage and blood ejection, pulmonary welling abscess, jaundice, stomachache, abdomen pain from sand, strangury-turbidity, swelling and toxin of welling abscess and sores, snake or insect bites, knocks and falls.

Adhesive Rehmannia Dried Root; GAN DI HUANG Origin: *Rehmannia glutinosa* (Gaertn.) Libosch *ex* Mey. (*Scrophulariaceae*). Part: dried root. Effects: To remove heat from the blood, nourish *yin* and promote secretion. Indications: Epidemic febrile diseases marked by fever, dryness in the mouth, red or deep red tongue; blood ejection, spontaneous external bleeding, bloody urine, flooding and spotting; febrile diseases in the later stage with lingering lowgrade fever; chronic diseases with fever due to deficiency of *yin*; diabetes from *yin* deficiency.

African Myrsine; DA HONG PAO Origin: *Myrsine africana* L. (*Leguminosae*). Part: root or herb. Effects: To quicken the blood, dispel wind, and rectify damp. Indications: Wind-damp impediment (arthralgia-syndrome), diarrhea, dysentery, blood strangury, taxation damage coughing blood.

Ailanthus-like Pricklyash Bark; CHU YE HUA JIAO PI Origin: *Zanthoxylum ailanthoides* Sieb. *et* Zucc. (*Rutaceae*). Part: bark. Indications: Postpartum wind pain in joints.

Ailanthus-like Pricklyash; SHI ZHU YU (CHU YE HUA JIAO) Origin: *Zanthoxylum ailanthoides* Sieb. *et* Zucc. (*Rutaceae*). Part: fruit. Effects: To worm the center, dry damp, kill worms, and relieve pain. Indications: Cold pain in heart region and abdomen, cold rheum, diarrhea, cold dysentery, damp impediment, red and white vaginal discharge, toothache.

Air-plant Herb; LUO DI SHENG GEN Origin: *Bryophyllum pinnatum* (L. f.) Oken (*Crassula-ceae*). Part: root or herb. Effects: To cool blood and stanch bleeding, disperse swelling and resolve toxin. Indications: Blood ejection, bleeding from wounds, stomachache, arthralgia, sore swollen throat, mam-mary welling abscess, clove sore, ulcerating sore, scalds.

Airpotato Yam; HUANG YAO ZI Origin: *Dioscorea bulbifera* L (*Dioscoreaceae*). Part: tuber. Effects: To dissipate bind and disperse goiter, clear heat and resolve toxin, cool the blood and stanch bleeding. Indications: Goiter; swelling and toxin of sores, sore swollen throat, snake bite; blood ejection, nosebleed, counging of blood.

Aizoon Stonecrop Root; JING TIAN SAN QI GEN Origin: *Sedum aizoon* L. (*Crassulaceae*). Part: root. Effects: To stanch bleeding, disperse swelling and settle pain. Indications: Blood ejection, sponta-neous external bleeding, bleeding of external injury, painful injury of sinews and bones.

Alfalfa Root; MU XU GEN Origin: *Medicago sativa* L. (*Leguminosae*). Part: root. Effects: To clear damp-heat and disinhibit urine. Indications: Jaundice, urethral stone, night blindness.

Alfalfa; MU XU Origin: *Medicago sativa* L. (*Leguminosae*). Part: herb. Effects: To clear spleen and stomach, disinhibit large intestine and small intestine. Indications: Vesical calculus.

Alligator Alternanthera; KONG XIN XIAN Origin: *Alternanthera philoxeroides* (Mart.) Griseb. (*Amaranthaceae*). Part: fresh aerial parts. Effects: To clear heat and cool the blood, disinhibit urine and resolve toxin. Indications: Measles papules, encepha-litis B, pulmonary tuberculosis with hemoptysis, strangury-turbidity, herpes zoster, clove and boil, snakebite.

Alpine Yallow; YI ZHI HAO Origin: *Achillea alpina* L. (*Compositae*). Part: herb. Effects: To quicken the blood, dispel wind, relieve pain and resolve toxin. Indications: Knocks and falls, wind-damp pain (rheumatalgia), glomus, swollen welling abscess.

Alplne Thermopsis; GAO SHAN HUANG HUA Origin: *Thermopsis alpina* Ledeb. (*Legumi-nosae*). Part: flower and fruit. Indications: Rabid dog bite.

Altai Heteropappus; A ER TAI ZI WAN Origin: *Heteropappus altaicus* (Willd.) Novopokr. (*Compositae*). Part: herb. Effects: To clear heat and downbear fire, expel pus. Indications: Infective febrile disease, effulgent liver-gallbladder fire, papules, sore and boil.

American Ginseng; XI YANG SHEN Origin: *Panax quinquefolium* L. (*Araliaceae*). Part: root. Effects: To boost the lung and spleen, to clear vacuity fire, and to engender liquid and allay thirst. Indications: Lung vacuity and enduring cough, blood loss, dry throat and thirst, vacuity heat and vexation and fatigue.

American Maidenhair Fern; TIE SI QI Origin: *Adiantum pedatum* L. (*Adiantaceae*). Part: whole plant. Effects: To disinhibit water and free strangury, eliminate damp, regulate menstruation and relieve pain. Indications: Inhibited urination, strangury, bloody urine, dysentery, wind-damp swelling and pain, menstrual disorder, flooding and spotting, white vaginal discharge, toothache.

American Pokeweed; MEI SHANG LU Origin: *Phytolacca americana* L. (*Phytolaccaceae*). Part: root. Effects: To drain precipitation and disinhibit water, disperse swelling and dissipate bind. Indications: Edema with feeling of fullness and distention, constipation and inhibited urination; swollen welling abscess.

Ammbergris; LONG XIAN XIANG Origin: *Physeter catodon* L. (*Physeteridae*). Part: dried secretion in the intestines of spern whales. Effects: To move *qi* and quicken the blood, dissipate bind and relieve pain, disinhibit water and free strangury, and used as a fixative in perfumes. Indications: Cough and panting with *qi* counterflow, *qi* binding with concretion and accumulation, pain in the heart region and abdomen, strangury.

Amphibious Knotweed; LIANG QI LIAO Origin: *Polygonum amphibium* L. (*Polygonaceae*). Part: herb. Effects: To clear heat and disinhibit dampness. Indications: Dysentery, puffy swelling in the foot, clove sore.

Amur Adonis; FU SHOU CAO Origin: *Adonis amurensis* Reg. *et* Radde (*Ranunculaceae*). Part: herb. Effects: To strengthen the heart and disinhibit urine. Indications: Heart palpitation, edema, epilepsy.

Natural Sources, Effects and Indications of Traditional Chinese Medicines

Amur Barerry; XIAO BO Origin: *Berberis amurensis* Rupr. (*Berberidaceae*). Part: root and branchlet. Effects: To clear heat and dry dampness, drain fire and resolve toxin. Indications: Acute enteritis, dysentery, jaundice, heat impediment, scrofula, pneumonia, conjunctivitis, swollen welling abscess sore and boil, flooding.

Amur Corktree; HUANG BAI Origin: *Phellodendron amurene* Rupr. (*Rutaceae*). Part: bark. Effects: To drain fire and dispel damp and toxin. Indications: Various damp-heat syndromes shown as dysentery (fever, abdominal pain, diarrhea, purulent and bloody stool, and temesmus), jaundice, yellow thick foul leukorrhagia,, swelling pain in the knees and feet, urinary tract infections with difficulty and pain in micturition; infections on the body surface such as boils, sores, swelling, ulcers, eczema, canker sores, hemorrhoids, burns, and scalds; exuberance of fire with tidal fever, hectic fever and night sweat, emission.

Amur Jackinthepulpit; TIAN NAN XING Origin: *Arisaema amurense* Maxim. (*Araceae*). See Reddish Jackinthepulpit.

Amygdalate Apricot Seed; BA DAN XING REN Origin: *Prunum amygdalus* Batsch (*Rosaceae*). Part: fried seed. Effects: To moisten the lung and suppress cough, transform phlegm and precipitate *qi*. Indications: Vacuity-taxation cough, oppression and counterflow in the heart region and abdomen.

Ancients Euphorbia; HUO YANG LE Origin: *Euphorbia antiquorum* L. (*Euphorbiaceae*). Part: stem. Effects: To disperse swelling, free the stool, and kill worms. Indications: Drum distention, toxin swelling, scab and *lai*, acute gastroenteritis.

Angled Bittersweet; DIAO GAN MA Origin: *Celastrus angulata* Maxim. (*Celastraceae*). Part: root or root bark. Effects: To clear heat and outthrust papules, soothe sinew and quicken the network vessels,resolve toxin and kill worms, regulate menstruation. Indications: Bald sores, yellow-water sore, swelling and pain from fracture, vagina itch.

Annual Fleabane; YI NIAN PENG Origin: *Erigeron annuus* (L.) Pers. (*Compositae*). Part: root and herb. Effects: To clear heat and resolve toxin, to promote digestion. Indications: Indigestion, enteritis and diarrhea, infective hepatitis, lymphnoditis, bloody urine.

Ansu Apricot Seed; XING REN Origin: *Prunus armeniaca* L. var. *ansu* Maxim. (*Rosaceae*). See Apricot Seed.

Ansu Apricot; XING ZI Origin: *Prunus armeniaca* L. var. *ansu* Maxim. (*Rosaceae*). See Apricot.

Antifebrile Dichroa; CHANG SHAN Origin: *Dichroa febrifuga* Lour. (*Saxifragaceae*). Part: root. Effects: To eliminate phlegm and interrupt malaria. Indications: Malaria, scrofula.

Apisin; FENG DU Origin: *Apis cerana* Fabricius (*Apidae*). Part: apisin. Effects: To dispel wind-damp. Indications: Rheumatic arthritis, bron-chial asthma, goiter, rheumatism, purulent swelling.

Apple Mint Herb; YU XIANG CAO Origin: *Mentha rotundifolia* (L.) Huds. (*Labiatae*). Part: herb. Effects: To dissipate wind-heat, eliminate swollen toxin. Indications: Wind damage cold, stomach *qi* pain, nosebleed, red eyes, clove sore and heat boil.

Apricot Seed; XING REN Origin: *Prunus armeniaca* L. (*Rosaceae*). Part: bitter seed. Effects: To dispel phlegm, suppress cough, calm panting, and moisten the intestines. Indications: Cough due to external contraction, panting and fullness, throat impediment, intestinal dryness with constipation.

Apricot; XING ZI Origin: *Prunus armeniaca* L. (*Rosaceae*). Part: fruit. Effects: To moisten the lung and stabilize panting, engender liquid and allay thirst.

Arabian Jasmine; MO LI HUA Origin: *Jasminum sambac* (L.) Ait. (*Oleaceae*). Part: flower. Effects: To rectify *qi* and open depression, repel foulness and harmonize the center. Indications: Dysentery and abdominal pain, conjunctivitis, toxin of sores.

Argy Wormwood Leaf; AI YE Origin: *Artemisia argyl* Levl. *et* Vant (*Compositae*). Part: leaf. Effects: To warm the channels and stanch bleeding, disperse cold and relieve pain. Indications: flooding and spotting, menstrual pain, hemoptysis, pruritus, eczema, and also used for moxibustion.

Armillariella Tabescens; LIANG JUN Origin: *Armillariella tabescens* (Scop. *ex* Fr.) Sing. (*Tricholomataceae*). Part: mycelium. Effects: To expel inflammation. Indications: Inflamation of the gallbladder, hepatitis, appendicitis, otitis media.

Aromatic turmeric; YU JIN Origin: *Curcuma aromatica* Salisb. (*Zingiberaceae*). See Common turmaric.

Arrowshaped Tinospora; JIN GUO LAN Origin: *Tinospora sagittata* Gagn. (*Menispermaceae*). See Hairystalk Tinospora.

Asafetida Giantfennel Resin; A WEI Origin: *Ferula asafoetida* L. (*Umbelliferae*). Part: gum resin. Effects: To promote digestion and as an anthelmintic. Indications: Concretions and conglomerations, glomus and mass, worm accumulation, meat-type food accumulation, cold pain in heart region and abdomen, malaria, dysentery.

Asia White Birch Bark; BAI HUA PI (one of the **HUA MU PI**) Origin: *Betula platyphylla* Suk. (*Betulaceae*). See Japanese White Birch Bark.

Asian Tetracera; XI YE TENG Origin: *Tetracera asiatica* (Lour.) Hoogl. (*Dilleniaceae*). Part: root or leaf. Indications: Enteritis, dysentery, prolapse of the rectum, seminal emission, knocks and falls.

Asiatic Cornelian Cherry (Common Macro-carpium); SHAN ZHU YU Origin: *Cornus Officinalis* Sieb. *et* Zucc. [=*Macrocarpium officinalis* (Sieb. *et* Zucc.) Nakai] (*Cornaceae*). Part: scrcocarp. Effects: To supplement the liver and the kidney, and arrest spontaneous emission and sweating. Indications: Dizziness, lassitude of the loins and knees, impotence, seminal emission, frequent urination, enuresis; incessant hidrorrhea; metrorrhagia, metrostaxis, and menorrhagia.

Asiatic Moonseed Root; BIAN FU GE GEN Origin: *Menispermum dauricum* DC. (*Menisperma-ceae*). Part: rhizome. Effects: To dispel wind and clear heat, rectify *qi* and transform damp. Indications: Pain from wind-damp impediment (arthralgia-syndrome), numbness, edema, leg *qi* (beriberi), tonsillitis, pharyngolaryngitis, dysentery, enteritis, stomachache with abdominal distention.

Asiatic Moonseed; BIAN FU GE Origin: *Menispermum dauricum* DC. (*Menispermaceae*). Part: stem. Indications: Lumbar pain, scrofula.

Asiatic Pennywort Herb; JI XUE CAO Origin: *Centella asiatica* (L.) Urban (*Umbelliferae*). Part: herb (with root). Effects: To clear heat and disinhibit damp, disperse swelling and resolve toxin. Indications: Sand *qi* abdominal pain, summerheat diarrhea, dysentery, damp-heat jaundice, sand strangury, blood strangury, blood ejection, spontaneous external bleeding, coughing of blood, red eyes, swollen throat, wind papules, scab and lichen, swelling and toxin of clove welling abscess, knocks and falls.

Asiatic Plantain; CHE QIAN Origin: *Plantago asiatica* L. (*Plantaginaceae*). Part: herb. Effects: To disinhibit water and free strangury, to clear heat and improve acuity of sight. Indications: Urinary stoppage, strangury-turbidity, bloody urine, heat dysentery; vaginal discharge; jaundice, edema, diarrhea; nosebleed, sore red swollen eyes, throat impediment and nipple moth, ulcerating sore of the skin; cough.

AsiaticToddalia; FEI LONG ZHANG XUE Origin: *Toddalia asiatica* (L.) Lam. (*Rutaceae*). Part: root or root bark. Effects: To dispel wind and relieve pain, dissipate stasis and stanch bleeding. Indications: Wind-damp pain (rheumatalgia), stomach pain, knocks and falls, blood ejection, spontaneous external bleeding, knife wound, menstrual block, menstrual pain.

Aspongopus; JIU XIANG CHONG Origin: *Aspongopus chinensis* Dallas (*Pentatomidae*). Part: dried body. Effects: To rectify *qi* and relieve pain, to warm the kidney and reinforce *yang*. Indications: *Qi* stagnation in the chest, pain and oppression in the stomach dust, spleen-kidney depletion detriment, aching lumbus and knees, impotence.

Assam Crotalaria; ZI XIAO RONG Origin: *Crotalaria assamica* Benth. (*Leguminosae*). Part: stem and leaf. Indications: Cough with blood ejection, toothache, swelling and distention, child head sore.

Austral Akebia Root; MU TONG GEN Origin: *Akebia trifoliata* (Thunb.) Koidz. var. *australis* (Diels) Rehd. (*Lardizabalaceae*). Part: root. Effects: To dispel wind and disinhibit urination, to move *qi* and quicken the blood. Indications: Wind-damp (rheumatism) with painful joints, inhibited urination, gastrointestinal *qi* distention, mounting *qi,* menstrual block, knocks and falls.

Austral Akebia; BAI MU TONG (one of the **MU TONG)** Origin: *Akebia trifoliata* (Thunb.) Koidz. var. *australis* (Diels) Rehd. (*Lardizabalaceae*). Part: stem. Effects: To remove intense heat from the heart to purge off intense heat from the body, and to promote diuresis and milk secretion. Indications: Dump-heat in the urinary bladder, scanty dark urine, dribbling and painful micturition; canker sores, vexation and dark urine; hypogalactia after delivery.

Autumn Zephyrlily Herb; GAN FENG CAO Origin: *Zephyranthes candida* Herb. (*Amaryllidaceae*). Part: herb. Effects: To calm the liver and extinguish wind. Indications: Epilepsy, acute fright wind in children.

Avicenna's Pricklyash; YING BU BO Origin: *Zanthoxylum avicennae* (Lam.) DC. (*Rutaceae*). Part: root. Effects: To dispel wind and transform damp, disperse swelling and free the network vessels. Indications: Sore swollen throat, yellow swelling, malaria, wind-damp bone pain, contusion from knocks and falls.

Aweto (Chinese Caterpillar Fungus); DONG CHONG XIA CAO Origin: *Cordyceps sinensis* (Berk.) Sacc. (*Clavicipitaceae*). Part: a drug consisting of the dried fungus growing on the larva of a caterpillar. Effects: To supplement vacuity detriment, boost essential *qi*, suppress cough and transform phlegm. Indications: Phlegm-rheum panting and cough, vacuity panting, consumption cough, hacking of blood, spontaneous sweating, night sweating, impotence, seminal emission, aching lumbus and knees, enduring vacuity after illness.

Aztec Marigold Leaf; WAN SHOU JU YE Origin: *Rohdea japonica* Roth. (*Compositae*). Part: leaf. Indications: Welling abscess, sore, *gan*, clove sore, and innominate toxin swelling.

Aztec Marigold; WAN SHOU JU Origin: *Tagetes erecta* L. (*Compositae*). Part: Inflorescence. Effects: To calm the liver and clear heat, dispel wind and transform phlegm. Indications: Dizzy head and vision, wind-fire eye pain, fright wind in children, common cold and cough, pertussis, mammary, mumps.

Babylon Weeping Willow Branch; LIU ZHI Origin: *Salix babylonica* L. (*Salicaceae*). Part: branchlet. Effects: To dispel wind, disinhibit urine, relieve pain, and disperse swelling. Indications: Pain from wind-damp impediment (arthralgia-syndrome), strangury, white turbidity, urinary stoppage, infectious hepatitis, wind swelling, clove sore, cinnabar toxin, tooth decay, gum swelling.

Babylon Weeping Willow Root-bast; LIU BAI PI Origin: *Salix babylonica* L. (*Salicaceae*). Part: root bast. Effects: To dispel wind and disinhibit dampness, disperse swelling and relieve pain. Indications: Wind-damp bone pain, wind swelling and pruritus, jaundice, strangury-turbidity, mammary welling abscess, toothache, burns and scalds.

Baikal Meadowrue; MA WEI LIAN Origin: *Thalictrum baicalense* Turcz. (*Ranunculaceae*). See Manyleaf Meadowrue.

Baikal Skullcap; HUANG QIN Origin: *Scutellaria baicalensis* Georgi (*Labiatae*). Part: root. Effects: To remove heat dampness and toxin, drain intense heat, stanch bleeding, and prevent miscarriage. Indications: Fever, feeling of fullness in the chest, and greasy tongue coating; jaundice, damp-heat in the lower-*jiao* with difficult and painful micturition; suppurative infections on the body surface; acute febrile diseases with high fever, restlessness, yellow tongue coating, rapid purse; cough with yellow sputum of lung-heat; blood ejection, spontaneous external bleeding, bloody urine, bloody stool, flooding and spotting.

Bailan Flower; BAI LAN HUA Origin: *Michelia alba* DC. (*Magnoliaceae*). Part: flower. Effects: To suppress cough and transform turbidity. Indications: Chronic bronchitis, prostatitis, white vaginal discharge.

Balloonflower; JIE GENG Origin: *Platycodon grandiflorum* (Jacq.) A. DC. (*Campanulaceae*). Part: root. Effects: To dispel heat-phlegm and keep the lung well ventilated, to relieve sore-throat and to promote pus discharge. Indications: Affection by wind-heat exopathogens shown as cough, sore throat, hoarseness, unsmooth expectoration; pulmonary abscess and chest pain, purulent and bloody expectoration.

Balloonvine Heartseed; JIA KU GUA Origin: *Cardiospermum halicacabum* L. (*Sapinda-ceae*). Part: herb. Effects: To clear heat and disinhibit water, cool the blood and resolve toxin. Indications: Jaundice, strangury, clove sore, vesicle sore, scab and *lai*, snakebite.

Balsamiferous Blumea; AI NA XIANG Origin: *Blumea balsamifera* DC. (*Compositae*). Part: leaf and branchlet. Effects: Warm the center and quicken the blood, dispel wind and eliminate damp, kill worms. Indications: Cold-damp diarrhea and dysentery, abdominal pain with rumbling intestines, swelling and distention, sinew and bone pain, knocks and falls, lichen.

Balsampear Seed; KU GUA ZI Origin: *Momordica charantia* L. (*Cucurbitaceae*). Part: seed. Effects: To boost *qi* and invigorate *yang*.

Balsampear; KU GUA Origin: *Momordica charantia* L. (*Cucurbitaceae*). Part: fruit. Effects: To clear summerheat heat, brighten the eyes, and resolve toxin. Indications: Febrile disease with vexation and thirst, summerheat stroke, dysentery, painful red eyes, swollen welling abscess, cinnabar toxin, malign sore.

Bambooleaf Pricklyash Root; ZHU YE JIAO GEN Origin: *Zanthoxylum planispinum* Sieb. *et* Zucc. (*Rutaceae*). Part: root. Effects: To dispel wind and quicken the blood, dissipate cold and relieve pain. Indications: Headache and common cold, cough, vomiting and diarrhea, wind-damp (rheumatism) with painful joints, knocks and falls, toothache.

Bambooleaf Pricklyash; ZHU YE JIAO Origin: *Zanthoxylum planispinum* Sieb. *et* Zucc. (*Rutaceae*). Part: fruit. Effects: To dissipate cold, resolve pain, and dispel roundworm. Indications: Stomach cold, stomachache due to roundworm, toothache, damp sore.

Barbary Wolfberry Fruit; ZI Origin: *Lycium barbarum* L. (*Solanaceae*). See Chinese Wolfberry Fruit.

Barbary Wolfberry Leaf; GOU QI YE Origin: *Lycium barbarum* L. (*Solanaceae*). See Chinese Wolfberry Leaf.

Barbary Wolfberry Root-bark; DI GU PI (GOU QI GEN PI) Origin: *Lycium barbarum* L. (*Solanaceae*). See Chinese Wolfberry Root-bark.

Barbate Cyclea; YIN BU HUAN Origin: *Cyclea barbata* (Wall.) Miers (*Menispermaceae*). Part: root and stem. Effects: To clear heat and resolve toxin, disinhibit damp and free strangury, disperse stasis and relieve pain. Indications: Wind heat common cold, sore throat, dysentery, sand strangury, knocks and falls.

Barbate Deadnettle; YE ZHI MA Origin: *Lamium barbatum* Sieb. *et* Zucc. (*Labiatae*). Part: flower or herb. Indications: Lung heat coughing of blood, blood strangury, white vaginal discharge, menstrual irregularities, vacuity fever in children, knocks and falls, toxin swelling.

Barkless Puff-ball; MA BO Origin: *Saliosphaera fenzlii* Reich. (*Lycoperdaceae*). Part: sporophore. Effects: To clear the lung, disinhibit throat, resolve toxin, and to stanch bleeding. Indications: Lung heat cough, loss of voice, sore swollen throat; blood ejection, nosebleed due to blood-heat.

Barley Germinating Fruit; MAI YA Origin: *Hordeum vulgare* L. (*Gramineae*). Part: germinated fruit. Effects: To promote digestion, strengthen the spleen and to stop milk secretion. Indications: Anorexia, feeling of fullness in the stomach and abdominal distention caused by food retention and indigestion; for stopping milk secretion.

Basil Fruit; LUO LE ZI Origin: *Ocimum basilicum* L. (*Labiatae*). Part: fruit. Indications: Red eyes and profuse eye discharge, ingrown eyelash, eye screen, galloping *gan* of the teeth and gum.

Basil Herb; LUO LE Origin: *Ocimum basilicum* L. (*Labiatae*). Part: herb. Effects: To course wind and move *qi*, transform damp and disperse food, quicken the blood and resolve toxin. Indications: External contraction and headache, food distention and *qi* stagnation, stomach duct pain, diarrhea, menstrual irregularities, knocks and falls, snake or insect bites, damp sore of skin, dormant papules with pruritus.

Bastard Speedwell; YI ZHI XIANG Origin: *Veronica spuria* L. (*Scrophulariaceae*). Part: herb. Effects: To settle cough, transform phlegm, and calm panting. Indications: Chronic trachitis.

Bastardtoadflaxlike Swallowwort; DI SHAO GUA Origin: *Cynanchum thesioides* (Freyn) K. Schum. (*Asclepiadaceae*). Part: herb and fruit. Effects: To supplement lung-*qi*, clear heat and downbear fire, engender liquid and allay thirst, expel inflammation and relieve pain. Indications: Vacuity and depletion of *qi*-blood, brain neurosism, sore throat.

Bat Dung; YE MING SHA Origin: *Vespertilio superans* Thomas (*Vespertilionidae*). Part: dried feces. Effects: To clear heat and brighten the eyes, dissipate blood and eliminate accumulation. Indications: Clear-eye blindness, night blindness, internal or external obstruction and screen, scrofula, *gan* accumulation, malaria.

Bean Blister Beetle; GE SHANG TING CHANG Origin: *Epicauta gorhami* Mars. (*Meloidae*). Part: body. Effects: To expel stasis and break accumulation. Indications: Menstrual block, concretions and conglomerations, accumulation and gathering, swollen fistula.

Bear Gall; XIONG DAN Origin: *Selenarctos thibetanus* G. Cuvier; *Ursus arctos* L. (*Ursidae*). Part: dried gall. Effects: To remove heat, subdue hyperfunction of the liver and brighten the eyes. Indications: Fright wind, epilepsy, and convulsion due to liver heat and liver wind; sore red swollen eyes due to liver heat, aversion to light, eye screen; swelling and pain of welling abscess and sores, swelling and pain of hemorrhoid.

Bear's Paw; XIONG ZHANG Origin: *Selenarctos thibetanus* G. Cuvier; *Ursus arctos* L. (*Ursidae*). Part: paw. Effects: To tonify *qi* and blood, dispel wind and eliminate impediment, fortify the spleen and stomach. Indications: Vacuity weakness of the spleen and stomach, vacuitr detriment.

Beautiful Galangal; DA CAO KOU Origin: *Alpinia speciosa* K. Schum. (*Zingiberaceae*). Part: seed. Effects: To dry dampness and dissipate cold, eliminate phlegm and interrupt malaria, fortify the spleen and worm the stomach. Indications: Cold pain in heart regain and abdomen, distention and fullness of the chest and abdomen, phlegm-damp accumulation and obstruction, indigestion, vomiting and diarrhea.

Beautiful Phyllodium Root; PAI QIAN CAO GEN Origin: *Desmodium pulchellum* (L.) Benth. (*Leguminosae*). Part: root. Effects: To move blood and break stasis, eliminate damp and disperse swelling. Indications: Swelling of the liver and spleen, arthritis, menstrual disorder, menstrual block, prolapse of uterus, welling abscess and flat abscess, clove sore, knocks and falls.

Beautiful Phyllodium; PAI QIAN CAO Origin: *Desmodium pulchellum* (L.) Benth. (*Legumi-nosae*). Part: aerial parts. Effects: To dispel wind and disinhibit water, dissipate stasis and disperse swelling. Indications: Common cold, pain from wind-damp impediment (arthralgia-syndrome), edema with drum distention, throat wind, toothache, painful swelling from knocks and falls.

Beautiful Sweetgum Leaf; FENG XIANG SHU YE (b) Origin: *Liquidambar taiwaniana* Hance (*Hamamelidaceae*). Part: leaf. Indications: Acute gastroenteritis, dysentery, postpartum wind, evil, child umbilical wind, swollen welling abscess effusion of the back.

Bee Wax; MI LA Origin: *Apis cerana* Fabricius (*Apidae*). Part: bee wax. Effects: To resolve toxin, engender flesh, settle pain. Indications: Acute heart pain, dysentery with pus and blood, enduring diarrhea, stirring fetus with bleeding, internal attack from sore and welling abscess, enduring ulceration, burns and scalds.

Belgaum Walnut Seed; SHI LI ZI Origin: *Aleurites moluccana* (L.) Willd. (*Labiatae*). Part: seed. Effects: To free the channels and clear stasis heat. Indications: Menstrual block.

Benzoin; AN XI XIANG Origin: *Styrax benzoin* Dryand. (*Styracaceae*). Part: balsam. Effects: To promote the circulation of *qi* and blood, to relieve pain;, and as an aromatic stimulant for resurrection. Indications: Sudden stroke and fulminant reversal, pain in heart region and abdomen, postpartum blood dizziness, child fright epilepsy, wind impediment and pain in the lumbus.

Berry-bearing Campion; BAI NIU XI Origin: *Cucubalus baccifer* L. (*Caryophyllaceae*). Part: root. Effects: To cool the blood and quicken the blood, disinhibit damp and disperse swelling. Indications: Menstrual block, inverted menstruation, knocks and falls, wind-damp with painful joints, strangury, edema, scrofula, swelling and toxin of welling abscess and flat abscess.

Betel Pepper Leaf; JU JIANG YE Origin: *Piper betle* L. (*Piperaceae*). Part: leaf. Effects: To dispel wind and dry dampness, kill worms and relieve itching. Indications: Wind cold cough, stomachache, wind toxin leg *qi* (beriberi), scab and lai, eczema, foot lichen, scalds.

Betenutpalm; BING LANG Origin: *Areca catechu* L. (*Palmae*). Part: seed. Effects: To expel parasites, promote digestion and the circulation of *qi* and water. Indications: Many kinds of parasitosis in the intestinal tract (cestodiasis, fasciolopsiasis, ascariasis, ancylostomiasis, enterobiasis); abdominal distention, constipation or diarrhea with tenesmus; edema and pain of beriberi, repletion edema.

Bigflower Cape Jasmine Leaf; SHUI ZHI YE Origin: *Gardenia jasminoides* Ellis var. *grandiflora* Nakai (*Rubiaceae*). Part: leaf. Effects: To disperse swelling. Indications: Knocks and falls.

Bigflower Cape Jasmine; SHUI ZHI Origin: *Gardenia jasminoides* Ellis var. *grandiflora* Nakai (*Rubiaceae*). Part: fruit. Effects: To dissipate heat-toxin. Indications: Sprain.

Bigleaf Beautyberry; DA YE ZI ZHU Origin: *Callicarpa macrophylla* Vahl. (*Verbenaceae*). Part: root or leaf. Effects: To stanch bleeding and relieve pain, dissipate stasis and eliminate swelling. Indications: Hacking of blood, spontaneous external bleeding, bleeding from wounds, bleeding from dental extraction, painful swelling from knocks and falls, wind-damp bone pain.

Bignay Chinalaurel; WU YUE CHA Origin: *Antidesma bunius* (L.) Spr. (*Euphorbiaceae*). Part: root, leaf and fruit. Effects: To engender liquid and allay thirst, to quicken blood and resolve toxin. Indications: Cough with thirst, knocks and falls, toxin of sores.

Birchleaf Pear; TANG LI Origin: *Pyrus betulaefolia* Bge. (*Rosaceae*). Part: fruit. Effects: To constrain the lung and astringe the intestines. Indications: Cough, diarrhea, dysentery.

Bird Rape; YUN TAI ZI Origin: *Brassica campestris* L. [= *Brassica campestris* L. var. *oleifera* DC.] (*Cruciferae*). Part: seed. Effects: To promote circulation of blood and *qi*, to reduce swelling and resolve mass. Indications: Postpartum blood stagnation and abdominal pain, blood dysentery, toxin swelling, hemorrhoids and fistulas.

Birdsfoot Trefoil; DI YANG QUE Origin: *Lotus corniculatus* L. (*Leguminosae*). Part: herb and flower. Effects: To clear heat and suppress cough, calm panting, disperse glomus and fullness, promote lactation. Indications: Wind-heat cough without phlegm, pain in stomach with glomus and fullness, hemorrhoid, nebulous eye screen.

Bistort; QUAN SHEN Origin: *Polygonum bistorta* L. (*Polygonaceae*). Part: rhizome. Effects: To clear heat and resolve toxin, dispel dampness and dissipate swollen welling abscess. Indications: Diarrhea due to damp-heat, dysentery with pus and blood, tenesmus; welling abscess and open sore due to heat-toxin, mouth and tongue sores; disperse edema.

Bitter Citrus; DAI DAI HUA Origin: *Citrus aurantium* L. var. *amara* Engl. (*Rutaceae*). Part: dried flower-bud. Effects: To regulate *qi* , soothe the liver, and harmonize the stomach. Indications: Oppression in the chest due to glomus, distention and pain in stomach duct and abdomen, vomiting, reduced eating.

Bitter Nightshade; BAI MAO TENG Origin: *Solanum dulcamara* L. (*Solanaceae*). See Bittersweet.

Bitter Nightshade; KU QIE Origin: *Solanum dulcamara* L. (*Solanaceae*). Part: fruit. Effects: To disinhibit urine and disperse swelling. Indications: Neuralgia.

Bitter Willow Bast; SHUI YANG MU BAI PI Origin: *Salix purpurea* L. (*Salicaceae*). Part: bast. Indications: Incised wound.

Bitter Willow Branch and Leaf; SHUI YANG ZHI YE Origin: *Salix purpurea* L. (*Salicaceae*). Part: branchlet and leaf. Effects: To clear heat and resolve toxin. Indications: Enduring dysentery, swelling and toxin of welling abscess and sores.

Bittersweet; BAI MAO TENG Origin: *Solanum lyratum* Thunb. (*Solanaceae*). Part: herb. Effects: To clear heat and disinhibit damp, dispel wind and resolve toxin. Indications: Malaria, jaundice, edema, strangury, wind-damp with painful joints, cinnabar toxin, clove sore.

Black Falsehellebore; LI LU Origin: *Veratrum nigrum* L. (*Liliaceae*). Part: root and rhizome. Indications: Wind phlegm, insect toxin, wind stroke and phlegm congestion, wind epilepsy and madness, jaundice, enduring malaria, diarrhea, headache, throat impediment, nasal polyp, scab and lichen, malign sore.

Black Henbane Root; LANG DANG GEN Origin: *Hyoscyamus niger* L. (*Solanaceae*). Part: root. Effects: To kill worms. Indications: Evil malaria, lichen and scab.

Black Henbane Seed; TIAN XIAN ZI (LANG DANG ZI) Origin: *Hyoscyamus niger* L. (*Solana-ceae*). Part: seed. Effects: Used as a spasmolytic, anodyne, anticonvulsive, antipantingtic and antidiarrheic. Indications: Mania and withdrawal, wind epilepsy, wind impediment and reversal pain, panting and cough, stomach pain, dysentery, enduring diarrhea, prolapse of the rectum, toothache, swollen welling abscess, malign sore.

Black Locust Flower; CI HUAI HUA Origin: *Robinia pseudoacacia* L. (*Leguminosae*). Part: flower. Indications: Precipitate blood of large intestine, hacking of blood, red flooding.

Black Nightshade; LONG KUI Origin: *Solanum nigrum* L. (*Solanaceae*). Part: aerial parts. Effects: To clear heat and resolve toxin, quicken the blood and eliminate swelling. Indications: Clove sore, swollen welling abscess, cinnabar toxin, sprain from knocks and falls, chronic trachitis, acute nephritis.

Black Pepper; HU JIAO Origin: *Piper nigrum* L. (*Piperaceae*). Part: fruit. Effects: To warm the center and relieve pain. Indications: Gastrointeestinal cold, pain in the stomach duct and abdomen, vomiting and diarrhea.

Black Soyabean Leaf; HEI DA DOU YE Origin: *Glycine max* (L.) Merr. (*Leguminosae*). Part: leaf. Indications: Blood strangury, snakebite.

Black Soyabean Spermoderm; HEI DA DOU PI Origin: *Glycine max* (L.) Merr. (*Leguminosae*). Part: spermoderm. Effects: To nourish the blood and soothe wind. Indications: *Yin* vacuity and heat vexation, night sweating, dizziness, headache.

Black Soyabean; HEI DA DOU Origin: *Glycine max* (L.) Merr. (*Leguminosae*). Part: lackcolored seed. Effects: To quicken the blood and disinhibit water, dispel wind and resolve toxin. Indications: Edema with distention and fullness, wind toxic wind and leg *qi* (beriberi), jaundice and general edema, wind impediment and contracture of sinews, postpartum wind tetany, clenched jaw, swelling and toxin of welling abscess and sores, drug's toxin.

Blackberrylily; SHE GAN Origin: *Belam-canda chinensis* (L.) DC. (*Iridaceae*). Part: rhizome. Effects: To clear heat and resolve toxin, dispel phlegm and disinhibit throat. Indications: Sore swollen throat with heat phlegm congesting the lung; cough and panting with phlegm congestion.

Blackflower Fritillary; WU HUA BEI MU (one of the **CHUAN BEI MU**) Origin: *Fritillaria cirrhosa* D. Don var. *ecirrhosa* Franch. (*Liliaceae*). See Tendrilleaf Fritillary.

Blister Beetle; BAN MAO Origin: *Mylabris phalerata* Pall. ; *Mylabris cichorii* Linnaeus (all *Meloidae*). Part: dried body. Effects: To attack toxin and dispel blood stasis. Indications: External use: malign sore, stubborn lichen, deviated eyes and mouth, throat moth; oral: scrofula, rabid dog bite.

Bloodflower Milkweed; LIAN SHENG GUI ZI HUA Origin: *Asclepias curassavica* L. (*Asclepiadaceae*). Part: herb. Effects: To expel inflammation and clear heat, quicken the blood and stanch bleeding. Indications: Tonsillitis, pneumonia, bronchitis, urinary tract infection, flooding and spotting with vaginal discharge, bleeding from wounds.

Bloodred Iris; DOU CHI CAO Origin: *Iris sanguinea* Hornem. [= *Iris sanguinea* Donn] (*Iridaceae*). Part: rhizome and root. Effects: To disperse accumulation and move water. Indications: Stromach-ache, abdominal pain.

Blushred Rabdosia; DONG LING CAO Origin: *Rabdosia rubescens* (Hemsl.) Hara (*Labiatae*). Part: aerial parts. Effects: To clear heat and resolve toxin, expel inflammation and relieve pain, fortify the stomach, quicken the blood, and inhibit tumor. Indications: (modern clinical) Acute pyogenic tonsillitis, liver cencer, carcinoma of esophagus, epithelial proliferayion of esophagus.

Bogbean Gen; SHUI CAI GEN Origin: *Menyanthes trifoliata* L. (*Gentianaceae*). Part: rhizome. Effects: To moisten the lung and suppress cough, suppress cough, lower blood pressure.

Bogbean; SHUI CAI Origin: *Menyanthes trifoliata* L. (*Gentianaceae*). Part: leaf or herb. Effects: To fortify the spleen and disperse food, nourish the heart and quiet the spirit. Indications: Gastritis, stomachache, indigestion, heart palpitation and insomnia, disquieted heart spirit.

Boor's Mustardd Seed; XI MING ZI Origin: *Thlaspi arvense* L. (*Cruciferae*). Part: seed. Indica-tions: Sore red swollen eyes and tearing.

Boor's Mustardd; XI MING Origin: *Thlaspi arvense* L. (*Cruciferae*). Part: herb. Effects: To harmonize the center and boost *qi,* disinhibit liver and brighten the eyes. Indications: Nephritis, inflamma-tion of endometrium.

Boreal Wild Chrysanthemum Flower; YE JU HUA Origin: *Chrysanthemum boreale* Mak. (*Com-positae*). See Indian Wild Chrysanthemum Flower.

Boreal Wild Chrysanthemum; BEI YE JU (one of the **YE JU**) Origin: *Chrysanthemum boreale* Mak. (*Compositae*). See Indian Wild Chrysanthe-mum.

Borneol; BING PIAN Origin: *Dryobalanops aromatica* Gaertn. f. (*Dipterocarpaceae*). Part: resin. Effects: As an aromatic stimulant for resuscitation, and as an antipyretic and analgesic agent. Indications: Phlegm syncope, apoplexy, coma, convulsion; swollen and sore throat, canker sores, blood-shot, swollen and painful eyes, sores, ulcers; angina pectoris of coronary heart disease.

Bottle Gourd; HU LU Origin: Lagenaria siceraria (Molina) Standl. var. *depressa* Ser. (*Cucurbitaceae*). Part: fruit. Effects: To disinhibit water and free strangury, disperse swelling. Indications: Edema, abdominal distention, ascites, jaundice, strangury,.

Bottle-brush; WEN JING Origin: *Equisetum arvense* L. (*Equisetaceae*). Part: aerial parts. Effects: To clear heat and cool the blood, suppress cough and disinhibit urine. Indications: Blood ejection, spon-taneous external bleeding, bloody stool, inverted menstruation, cough and panting, strangury.

Bouquet Larkspur; CUI QUE HUA Origin: *Delphinium grandiflorum* L. (*Ranunculaceae*). Part: herb or root. Effects: To drain fire, relieve pain, kill worms.

Bower Actinidia; MI HOU LI Origin: *Actinidia arguta* (Sieb. *et* Zucc.) Planch. (*Actinidia-ceae*). Part: root or leaf. Effects: To fortify the stomach, clear heat, disinhibit damp. Indications: Indigestion, vomiting, diarrhea, jaundice, wind-damp with painful joints.

Brainea; GUAN ZHONG Origin: *Brainea insignis* (Hook.) J. Sm. (*Blechnaceae*). See Male Fern Rhizome.

Bretschneider Pear Leaf; LI YE Origin: *Pyrus bretschneideri* Rehd. (*Rosaceae*). Part: leaf. Effects: To resolve toxin of mushrooms. Indications: Child mounting *qi*.

Bridalwreath Spiraea; XIAO YE HUA Origin: *Spiraea prunifolia* Sieb. *et* Zucc. (*Rosaceae*). Part: root. Indications: Sore swollen throat.

British Inula Herb; JIN FO CAO Origin: *Inula britannica* L. (*Compositae*). See Japanese Inula Herb.

British Inula Flower; XUAN FU HUA Origin: *Inula britannica* L. (*Compositae*). See Chinese Inula Flower.

Broadbean Leaf; CAN DOU YE Origin: *Vicia faba* L. (*Leguminosae*). Part: leaf. Indications: Pulmonary tuberculosis with hemoptysis, bleeding of digestive tract, bleeding of external injury, shank sore.

Broadbean Pericarp; CAN DOU JIA KE Origin: *Vicia faba* L. (*Leguminosae*). Part: pericarp. Indications: Hacking of blood, nosebleed, bloody urine, bleeding of digestive tract, heaven-borne sore, scalds.

Broadbean Spermoderm; CAN DOU KE Origin: *Vicia faba* L. (*Leguminosae*). Part: spermoderm. Effects: To disinhibit urine percolate damp. Indications: Edema, leg *qi* (beriberi), inhibited urination, heaven-borne sore, yellow-water sore.

Broadbean Stem; CAN DOU JING Origin: *Vicia faba* L. (*Leguminosae*). Part: stem. Effects: To stanch bleeding, check diarrhea. Indications: Internal bleeding, water diarrhea, scalds.

Broadbean; CAN DOU Origin: *Vicia faba* L. (*Leguminosae*). Part: seed. Effects: To fortify the spleen and disinhibit damp. Indications: Diaphragm food, edema.

Broadleaf Cattail Pollen; PU HUANG Origin: *Typha latifolia* L. (*Typhaceae*). See Longbract Cattail Pollen.

Broadleaf Common Valeriana; ZHI ZHU XIANG Origin: *Valeriana officnalis* L. var. *latifolia* Miq. (*Valerianaceae*). See Jatamans Valeriana.

Broadleaf Giantfennel Resin; A WEI Origin: *Ferula conocaula* Eug. (*Umbelliferae*). See Catchweed Bedstraw.

Broadleaf Globethistle; HUA ZHOU LOU LU (one of the **LOU LU**) Origin: *Echinops latifolus* Tausch (*Compositae*). See Uniflower Swisscentaury.

Broadleaf Holly; KU DING CHA Origin: *Ilex latafolia* Thunb. (*Aquifoliaceae*). Part: leaf. Effects: To dissipate wind heat, clear head and eyes, eliminate vexation and thirst. Indications: Headache, toothache, red eyes, purulent ear, Febrile disease with vexation and thirst, dysentery.

Broomcorn Millet; SHU MI Origin: *Panicum miliaceum* L (*Gramineae*). Part: seed. Effects: To supplement the spleen and boost *qi.* Indications: Diarrhea and dysentery, vexation thirst, vomiting with counterflow, cough, stomachache, goose mouth sore in children, scalds.

Buddha's Lamp; SHAN GAN CAO Origin: *Mussaenda pubescens* Ait. f. (*Rubiaceae*). Part: stem and leaf. Effects: To resolve the exterior, clear summerheat, disinhibit dampness, resolve toxin, and quicken blood. Indications: Common cold, summer-heat stroke, fever, cough, sore swollen throat, summerheat-damp diarrhea, dysentery, swelling and pus of sores, knocks and falls, snake bite.

Buffalo Horn; SHUI NIU JIAO Origin: *Bubalus bubalis* L. (*Bovidae*). Part: horn. Effects: To clear heat, resolve toxin, and cool the blood. Indications: Headache due to febrile disease, vigorous fever and clouded spitit, macular eruption, blood ejection and spontaneous external bleeding, child fright wind, throat impediment and swollen throat.

Bulbiferous Stonecrop; XIAO JIAN CAO Origin: *Sedum bulbiferum* Mak. (*Crassulaceae*). Part: herb. Effects: To dissipate cold and rectify *qi*. Indications: Cold-heat malaria, food accumulation and abdominal pain, wind-damp paralysis, scourge epidemic and papules.

Bumalda Bladdernut; SHENG GU YOU Origin: *Staphylea bumalda* DC. (*Staphyleaceae*). Part: fruit or root. Indications: Dry cough, postpartum blood stasis.

Bunga Ash Bark; QIN PI Origin: *Fraxinus bungeana* DC. (*Oleaceae*). See Largeleaf Chinese Ash Bark.

Bunge Giantfennel; SHA QIAN HU Origin: *Ferula borealis* Kuan (*Umbelliferae*). Part: root. Effects: To resolve the exterior and clear heat, dispel phlegm and settle cough. Indications: Common cold, fever, headache, pneumonia, trachitis, cough and panting with oppression in the chest, tonsillitis, tuberculosis of the lymphnode.

Bunge Hackberry; BANG BANG MU Origin: *Celtis bungeana* Bl. (*Ulmaceae*). Part: bark and branchlet. Effects: To suppress cough and dispel phlegm. Indications: Chronic bronchitis.

Bunge Pricklyash Root; HUA JIAO GEN Origin: *Zanthoxylum bungeanum* Maxim. (*Rutaceae*). Part: root. Effects: To kill worm. Indications: Vacuity and cold of the kidney and bladder, blood strangury, leg *qi* (beriberi), damp sore.

Bunge Pricklyash; HUA JIAO Origin: *Zanthoxylum bungeanum* Maxim. (*Rutaceae*). Part: pericarp. Effects: To warm the middle-*jiao* and relieve pain, to remove dampness and kill parasites. Indications: Spleen-stomach vacuity cold, cold pain in the stomach duct and abdomen, vomiting, diarrhea; abdomen pain and vomiting due to roundworm, vomiting of roundworm.

Bunge Swallowwort; BAI SHOU WU Origin: *Cynanchum bungei* Decne. (*Asclepiadaceae*). Part: tuber root. Effects: To enrich and nourish, strengthen, and supplement blood. Indications: Vacuity and weakness due to enduring illness, anaemia, premature graying, chronic wind impediment, limp aching lumbus and knees, hemorrhoid, intestinal bleeding, enduring malaria due to *yin* vacuity, enduring ulcerating sore, constipation in senile patients.

Burmacoast Padauk; ZI TAN Origin: *Pterocarpus indicus* Willd. (*Leguminosae*). Part: wood. Effects: To disperse swelling, stanch bleeding, and settle pain. Indications: Toxin swelling, bleeding from incised wound.

Bush Redpepper; LA JIAO Origin: *Capsicum frutescens* L. (*Solanaceae*). Part: ripe fruit. Effects: To warm the center amd dispel cold, invigorate the stomach and promote digestion. Indications: Cold stagnation and abdominal pain, vomiting, diarrhea, frostbite, scab and lichen.

Cabbage; GAN LAN Origin: *Brassica oleracea* L. var. *capiata* L. (*Cruciferae*). Part: leaf. Effects: To boost the kidney, supplement bone marrow, benefit five viscera and six bowels, benefit joints,free the channels and network vessels, brighten the eyes and nourish the ears, fortify human and reduced sleep, boostthe heart, invigorate sinew and bones.

Cablin Potchouli; GUANG HUO XIANG (one of the **HUO XIANG)** Origin: *Pogostemon cablin* (Blanco) Benth. (*Labiatae*). Part: aerial parts. Effects: To quicken *qi*, harmonize the center, repel foulness, and dispel dampness. Indications: Disturbance of the middle-*jiao* with epigastric dullness, abdominal distention, anorexia, nausea and vomiting; Affection by exopathogenic wind-cold in summer or impairment of the viscera by eating uncooked food with fever, headache, chest oppression, abdominal disstemsion, nausea, vomiting, diarrhea; various kinds of vomiting.

Cairo Morningglory; WU ZHAO LONG Origin: Ipomoea cairica (L.) Swe*et* (*Convolvulaceae*). Part: root, or stem and leaf. Effects: To clear heat and disinhibit water, to resolve toxin. Indications: Lung-heat cough, inhibited urination, strangury, bloody urine, swelling and toxin of welling abscess and flat abscess.

California Burclover Root; MU XU GEN Origin: *Medicago hispida* Gaertn. (*Leguminosae*). See Alfalfa Root.

California Burclover; MU XU Origin: *Medicago hispida* Gaertn. (*Leguminosae*). See Alfalfa.

Callery Pear Branch and Leaf; YE LI ZHI YE Origin: *Pyrus calleryana* Decne. (*Rosaceae*). Part: branchlet and leaf. Indications: Enduring vomiting and diarrhea, abdomen pain and cramp, stomach reflux vomiting.

Calyx-shaped Daphniphyllum Fruit; NIU ER FENG ZI Origin: *Daphniphyllum calycinum* Benth. (*Daphniphyllaceae*). Part: fruit. Indications: Chronic dysentery.

Calyx-shaped Daphniphyllum Leaf; NIU ER FENG ZHI YE Origin: *Daphniphyllum calycinum* Benth. (*Daphniphyllaceae*). Part: leaf. Effects: To expel wind, relieve pain and disperse swelling. Indications: Wind-damp bone pain, edema.

Camphortree Leaf; ZHANG SHU YE Origin: *Cinnamomum camphora* (L.) Presl (*Lauraceae*). Part: leaf. Effects: To dispel wind and eliminate dampness, relieve pain and kill worms. Indications: Wind-damp bone pain, scab and lichen, knocks and falls.

Camphortree; ZHANG MU (ZHANG SHU) Origin: *Cinnamomum camphora* (L.) Presl. (*Laura-ceae*). Part: wood. Effects: To dispel wind-damp, move *qi* blood, disinhibit joints. Indications: Disten-tion and pain in heart region and abdomen, leg *qi* (beriberi), pain wind, scab and lichen, knocks and falls.

Canereed Spiralflagg; ZHANG LIU TOU Origin: *Costus speciosus* (Koen.) Smith. (*Zingibera-ceae*). Part: rhizome. Effects: To move water and disperse swelling. Indications: Edema and drum distention, white turbidity, swollen welling abscess, malign sore.

Canton Abrus Herb; JI GU CAO Origin: *Abrus fruticulosus* Wall. *ex* Wight *et* Arn. [= *Abrus cantoniensis* Hance] (*Leguminosae*). Part: herb. Effects: To remove heat and damp, to relieve the depressed liver *qi* and relieve pain. Indications: Interohepatitis, stomachache, mammary welling abscess, scrofula, painful stasis blood due to knocks and falls.

Canton Buttercup Herb; ZI KOU CAO Origin: *Ranunculus cantoniensis* DC. (*Ranunculaceae*). Part: herb. Indications: Nebulous eye screen, jaundice.

Cape Jasmine Fruit; ZHI ZI Origin: *Gardenia jasminoides* Ellis (*Rubiaceae*). Part: ripe fruit. Effects: To drain fire and relieve dysphoria, clear heat and disinhibit urine, remove heat from the blood and stanch bleeding. Indications: Febrile diseases shown as vexation, melancholia, and restlessness; stagnation of damp-heat in the liver and gall shown as fever, jaundice, scanty dark urine; blood ejection, spontaneous external bleeding, dysentery with bloody stool and bloody urine.

Cape of Good Hope Aloe Dried Juice; HAO WANG JIAO LU HUI (one of the **LU HUI**) Origin: *Aloe ferox* Mill. (*Liliaceae*). See Kulaso Aloe Dried Juice.

Caper Euphorbia Latex; XU SUI ZI JING ZHONG BAI ZHI Origin: *Euphorbia lathyris* L. (*Euphorbiaceae*). Part: white juice in stem. Indica-tions: White patch.

Caper Euphorbia Seed; QIAN JIN ZI Origin: *Euphorbia lathyris* L. (*Euphorbiaceae*). Part: ripe seed without seed coat. Effects: For internal use, the seed kernel should be defatted; used to remove edema, eliminate blood stasis and resolve bind. Indications: Edema and abdominal fullness, inhibited urine and stool; stasis, concretions and conglomerations; menstrual block; stubborn lichen, wart, poisonous snake bite.

Capillary Wormwood; YIN CHEN HAO Origin: *Artemisia capillaris* Thunb. (*Compositae*). Part: young shoot. Effects: To remove heat, damp and treat jaundice. Indications: Juandice with obvious yellow eyes and skin, fever, scanty dark urine due to damp-heat.

Capitate Cyathula; CHUAN NIU XI Origin: *Cyathula capitata* (Wall.) Moq. (*Amaranthaceae*). See Mediinal Cyathula.

Capitateflower Velvetbean; LI DOU Origin: *Stizolobium capitatum* (Sweet) O. Ktze. (*Legumino-sae*). Part: seed. Effects: To worm the center and boost *qi.*

Carp Gall; LI YU DAN Origin: *Cyprinus carpio* L. (*Cyprinidae*). Part: gall. Effects: To clear heat and brighten the eyes, dissipate screen and disperse swelling. Indications: Sore red swollen eyes, clear-eye blindness, eye screen, sore throat, throat impediment.

Carp Skin; LI YU PI Origin: *Cyprinus carpio* L. (*Cyprinidae*). Part: skin. Indications: Dormant papules, bones stuck in the throat.

Carp; LI YU Origin: *Cyprinus carpio* L. (*Cyprinidae*). Part: meat. Effects: To disinhibit water and disperse swelling, precipitate *qi and* free milk. Indications: Edema with distention and fullness, leg *qi* (beriberi), jaundice, cough and panting, breast milk stoppage.

Carrot Seed; HU LUO BO ZI Origin: *Daucus carota* L. var. *sativa* DC. (*Umbelliferae*). Part: seed. Indications: Enduring dysentery, phlegm panting.

Carrot; HU LUO BO Origin: *Daucus carota* L. var. *sativa* DC. (*Umbelliferae*). Part: root. Effects: To reinforce the spleen and remove food stagnancy. Indications: Indigestion, enduring dysentery, cough.

Cassiabarktree Twig; GUI ZHI Origin: *Cinnamomum cassia* Presl (*Lauraceae*). Part: twig. Effects: To induce diaohoresis, warm the channels for ensuring flow of *yang-qi.* Indications: Externally contracted wind-cold with symptoms as aversion to cold, fever, headache; impediment, aching joints; irregular menstruation, menstrual block and abdominal pain, bind in the abdomen; vague pain in the epigastric region; cold in the back, hypochondriac distention, cough, dyspnea and vertigo; obstruction of *qi* in the chest and chest pain, palpitation and slow pulse with irregular intervals.

Cassiabarktree; ROU GUI Origin: *Cinna-momum cassia* Presl (*Lauraceae*). Part: bark. Effects: To supplement the kidney-yang, warm the spleen and stomach, remove internal cold and obstruction in the channels. Indications: *Yang* deficiency syndromes: aversion to cold, cold limbs, impotence and frequent micturition; gastric and abdominal cold pain, poor appetite and loose stool; various pains due to stagnation of *qi*, lumbago, menstrual block, and menorrhalgia.

Castorbean Leaf; BI MA YE Origin: *Ricinus communis* L. (*Euphorbiaceae*). Part: leaf. Effects: To draw out pus and relieve itching, and relieve cough and calm asthma. Indications: Leg *qi* (beriberi), swelling and pain of scrotum, coughing of phlegm panting, goose-foot wind, sores and boils.

Castorbean Oil; BI MA YOU Origin: *Ricinus communis* L. (*Euphorbiaceae*). Part: oil expressed from the seeds. Indications: Dry bound stool, sore and scab, burns.

Castorbean Root; BI MA GEN Origin: *Ricinus communis* L. (*Euphorbiaceae*). Part: root. Effects: To dispel wind and dissipate stasis, resolve tetany, and as a sedative. Indications: Lockjaw, epilepsy, rheumatalgia, stasis and pain from knocks and falls, scrofula.

Castorbean Seed; BI MA ZI Origin: *Ricinus communis* L. (*Euphorbiaceae*). Part: ripe seed. Effects: To disperse swelling and draw out toxin, drain precipitation and free stagnation. Indications: Swelling and toxin of welling abscess and flat abscess, scrofula, throat impediment, scab, *lai*, lichen, sore, edema with full abdomen, dry bound stool.

Catchweed Bedstraw; BA XIAN CAO Origin: *Galium aparine* L. (*Rubiaceae*). Part: herb. Effects: To clear damp-heat, dissipate stasis, disperse swelling, and resolve toxin. Indications: Strangury-turbidity, bloody urine, knocks and falls, intestinal welling abscess, swollen boil, otitis media.

Catnip; JIA JING JIE Origin: *Nepeta cataria* L. (*Labiatae*). Part: herb. Effects: To dispel wind and effuse sweat, resolve heat, outthrust papules, stanch bleeding. Indications: Wind damage and common cold, headache, fever and aversion to cold, sore swollen throat, conjunctivitis.

Caudate Milkwort; SHUI HUANG YANG MU Origin: *Polygala caudata* Rehd. *et* Wils. (*Polygalaceae*). Part: root. Effects: To clear heat, disinhibit dampness, and free strangury. Indications: Icterohepatitis, bloody urine, wheezing and panting.

Caudate Sweetleaf Leaf; SHAN FAN YE Origin: *Symplocos caudata* Wall. (*Symplocaceae*). Part: leaf. Effects: To clear heat and promote contraction. Indications: Blood ejection due to pulmonary tuberculosis, bloody stool, enduring dysentery, acute tonsillitis, acute otitis media, wind eye with ulceration of the eyelid rim.

Celery Wormwood; QING HAO Origin: *Artemisia apiacea* Hance (*Compositae*). Part: aerial parts. Effects: Used as a febrifuge to treat heatstroke and malaria. Indications: Febrile diseases at the later stage with nocturnal fever or lingering low-grade fever, or steaming bone with tidal fever, night fever, feverish sensation in the palms and soles; malaria with alternate fevers and chills; externally contracted summerheat-heat with fever with or without sweating, dizziness and headache; infantile fever in summer.

Centipede; WU GONG Origin: *Scolopendra subspinipes mutians* L. Koch (*Scolopendridae*). Part: dried body. Effects: To extinguish wind and check tetany, resolve toxin and dissipate bind, free the network vessels and relieve pain. Indications: Acute and chronic fright wind, lockjaw, spasm and convulsion; swelling and toxin of sores and open sores, scrofula with ulceration; intractable headache with pulling sensation, pain from wind-damp impediment (arthralgia-syndrome).

Cera Chinensis Wax; CHONG BAI LA Origin: *Ericerus pela* (Chavannes) (*Coccidae*). Part: insect wax. Effects: To arrest bleeding, promote tissue regeneration and settle pain. Indications: Bleeding from incised wound, bloody urine, precipitate blood, enduring ulcerating sore, lower body *gan*.

Cernuous Clubmoss Herb; PU DI WU GONG Origin: *Lycopodium cernnum* L. (*Lycopo-diaceae*). Part: herb. Effects: To dispel wind-damp, soothe sinews and network vessels, quicken the blood and stanch bleeding. Indications: Rheumatism with painful hypertonicity and numb, hepatitis, dysentery, wind papules, red eyes, blood ejection, spontaneous external bleeding, bloody stool, knocks and falls, burns and scalds.

Ceylon Helminthostachys; RU DI WU GONG Origin: *Helminthostachys zeylanica* (L.) Hook. (*Helminyhostachyaceae*). Part: rhizome. Effects: To remove heat, eliminate damp, and relieve pain. Indications: Taxation fever with cough, dysentery, internal injury, stasis blood and pain.

Ceylon Persimmon Sawdust; WU MU XIE Origin: *Diospyros ebenum* Koen. (*Ebenaceae*). Part: sawdust. Effects: To resolve toxin. Indications: Cholera with vomiting.

Chachi Citrus Pericarp; GAN PI Origin: *Citrus chachiensis* Hort. (*Rutaceae*). Part: pericarp. Effects: To precipitate *qi* and regulate the center, transform phlegm, and dispel the effects of liquor. Indications: Dietary imbalance after illness, *qi* ascent with vexation and fullness, liquor damage and thirst.

Chachi Citrus; GAN Origin: *Citrus chachiensis* Hort. (*Rutaceae*). Part: fruit. Effects: To engender liquid and allay thirst, dispel the effects of liquor, disinhibit urine.

Champac Michelia; HUANG MIAN GUI Origin: *Michelia champaca* L (*Magnoliaceae*). Part: root. Effects: To dispel wind-damp, benefit the throat. Indications: Wind-damp bone pain, bones stuck in the throat.

Champignon; XIANG XUN Origin: *Lentinus edodes* (Berk.) Sing. (*Tricholomataceae*). Part: sporophore. Effects: To boost stomach *qi*. Indications: Pox, papules.

Champion Wood Fern; MAO GUAN ZHONG Origin: *Dryopteris championii* (Benth.) C. Chr. *ex* Ching (*Dryopteridaceae*). Part: dried rhizome. Effects: To clear heat and resolve toxin, suppress cough and calm panting. Indications: Hookworm, common cold, panting, bloody stool.

Chaulmoogratree Seed; DA FENG ZI Origin: *Hydrocarpus anthelmintica* Pierr. *ex* Less. (*Flacourticeae*). Part: seed. Effects: To dispel wind and dry dampness, attack toxic substances and kill parasites. Indications: Numbing wind (leprosy), scab and lichen, red bayberry sore.

Chicken Brain; JI NAO Origin: *Gallus gallus domesticus* Brisson (*Phasianidae*). Part: brain. Indications: Difficult delivery, child epilepsy.

Chicken; JI ROU Origin: *Gallus gallus domesticus* Brisson (*Phasianidae*). Part: meat. Effects: To warm the center and boost *qi,* supplement essence and replenish the marrow. Indications: Vacuity taxation with emaciation and weakness, torpid stomach and poor appetite, diarrhea, dysentery, diabetes, edema, frequent urination, flooding and spotting, vaginal discharge, postpartum scant breast milk, vacuity and weakness after illness.

Chicken's Gizzard Endothelium; JI NEI JIN Origin: *Gallus gallus domesticus* Brisson (*Phasianidae*). Part: dried lining membrane of the gizzard. Effects: As a stomachic, digestant and as a drug to induce decomposition of calculi. Indications: Abdominal distention and anorexia, infantile dyspepsia and malnutrition; enuresis and seminal emission; lithiasis.

Chinaberry-tree Bark; KU LIAN PI Origin: *Melia azedarach* L. (*Meliaceae*). Part: dried stem or root bark. Effects: To kill worms and to treat lichen and scab. Indications: Roundworm, hookworm; lichen in the head, scab sore.

Chinaberry-tree Flower; LIAN HUA Origin: *Melia azedarach* L. (*Meliaceae*). See Szechwan China-berry Flower.

Chinese Aloe Dried Juice; BAN WEN LU HUI (one of the **LU HUI**) Origin: *Aloe vera* L. var. *chinensis* (Haw.) Berger (*Liliaceae*). See Kulaso Aloe Dried Juice.

Chinese Angelica; DANG GUI Origin: *Angelica sinensis* (Oliv.) Diels (*Umbelliferae*). Part: root. Effects: To nourish blood and regulate menstrua-tion, to quicken the blood, relieve pain, and to moisten the intestines and relieve constipation. Indications: Blood deficiency syndrome; irregular menstruation, menstrual block and menorrhalgia; various kinds of pains due to blood stasis and rheumatic impediment; sores, carbuncles; and constipation.

Chinese Arborvitae Branch; BAI ZHI JIE (CE BAI ZHI JIE) Origin: *Thuja orientalis* (L.) Endl. [= *Platycladus orientalis* (L.) Franco] (*Cupressaceae*). Part: branchlet. Indications: Wind impediment, joint-running wind, cholera cramps, painful swelling of tooth decay.

Chinese Arborvitae Leaf; CE BAI YE Origin: *Thuja orientalis* (L.) Endl. [= *Platycladus orientalis* (L.) Franco] (*Cupressaceae*). Part: leaf. Effects: To cold blood and stanch bleeding, to dispel wind, eliminate damp, and dissipate toxin swelling. Indications: Blood ejection, spontaneous external bleeding, bloody urine, blood dysentery, intestinal wind, flooding and spotting, pain from wind-damp impediment (arthralgia-syndrome), hypertension, bacillary dysentery, cough, cinnabar toxin, mumps, and scald.

Chinese Ash Bark; QIN PI Origin: *Fraxinus chinensis* Roxb. (*Oleaceae*). See Largeleaf Chinese Ash Bark.

Chinese Astilbe Root; LUO XIN FU GEN Origin: *Astilbe chinensis* (Maxim.) Franch. *et* Sav. (*Saxifragaceae*). Part: root. Effects: To quicken blood and dispel stasis, relieve pain and resolve toxin. Indications: Knocks and falls, pain in joints, pain in sinew and bone, stomachache, pain after the operation.

Chinese Astilbe; LUO XIN FU Origin: *Astilbe chinensis* (Maxim.) Franch. *et* Sav. (*Saxifra-gaceae*). Part: herb. Effects: To dispel wind, clear heat, and suppress cough. Indications: Wind heat common cold, pain in head and body, cough.

Chinese Atractylodes; CANG ZHU Origin: *Atractylodes chinensis* Koidz. (*Compositae*). See Swordlike Atractylodes.

Chinese Aucuba; TIAN JIAO BAN Origin: *Aucuba chinensis* Benth. (*Cornaceae*). Part: leaf. Indications: Rub damage, burns and scalds, hemorrhoid.

Chinese Azalea Flower; NAO YANG HUA Origin: *Rhododendron molle* (Bl.) G. Don (*Ericaceae*). Part: flower. Effects: To expel wind-evil and settle pain, eliminate dampness. Indications: Intractable wind-damp impediment (arthralgia-syndrome), pain from fracture, intrac-table skin lichen.

Chinese Box Juvenile Leaf; HUANG YANG MU YE Origin: *Buxus microphylla* Sieb. *et* Zucc. var. *sinica* Rehd. *et* Wils. (*Buxaceae*). Part: juvenile leaf. Indications: Difficult delivery, summerheat boil.

Chinese Buckeye Seed; SUO LUO ZI Origin: *Aesculus chinensis* Bge. (*Hippocastanaceae*). Part: ripe fruit without shell. Effects: To rectify *qi*, relieve stuffiness and pain in the epigastrium. Indications: Oppression in the chest, rib-side pain, stomach pain abdominal distention due to liver stomach *qi* stagnation; premenstrual distention and pain of the breasts.

Chinese Cedar; LIU SHAN Origin: *Crypto-meria fortunei* Hooibrenk (*Taxodiaceae*). Part: root bark. Indications: Lichen.

Chinese Clematis; WEI LING XIAN Origin: *Clematis chinensis* Osbeck (*Ranunculaceae*). Part: root. Effects: To dispel wind and eliminate damp, free the channels and the network vessels, and relieve pain due to impediment. Indications: Pain from wind-damp impediment (arthralgia-syndrome), bones stuck in the throat, dysphagia-occlusion, glomus.

Chinese Coriaria Leaf; MA SANG YE Origin: *Coriaria sinica* Maxim. (*Coriariaceae*). Part: leaf. Indications: Welling abscess and flat abscess, toxin swelling, scab and *lai,* yellow-water sore, scalds.

Chinese Corktree; HUANG BAI Origin: *Phellodendron chinense* Schneid. (*Rutaceae*). See Amur Corktree.

Chinese Cricket; XI SHUAI Origin: *Gryllulus chinensis* Weber (*Gryllidae*). Part: dried body. Effects: To disinhibit urine. Indications: Urinary block, edema, drum distention.

Chinese Crinum Root; LUO QUN DAI GEN Origin: *Crinum asiaticum* L. var. *sinicum* Bak. (*Amaryllidaceae*). Part: root and bulb. Indications: Cough, pain in the throat, knocks and falls, toothache.

Chinese Crossostephium Root; FU RONG JU GEN Origin: *Crossostephium chinense* (L.) Mak. *ex* Cham. *et* Schltr. (*Compositae*). Part: root. Effects: To dispel wind and damp. Indications: Rheumatic arthritis, stomach duct cold pain.

Chinese Diploclisia; QING FENG TENG Origin: *Diploclisia chinensis* Merr. (*Menispermaceae*). See Orientvine.

Chinese Dodder Seed; TU SI ZI Origin: *Cuscuta chinensis* Lam. (*Convolvulaceae*). Part: ripe seed. Effects: To supplement the liver and kidney, boost essence-marrew, brighten eyes (to improve acuity of sight). Indications: Aching lumbus and knees, seminal emission, diabetes (wasting-thirst disease), dribble after voiding, dim vision.

Chinese Dwarf Cherry Seed; YU LI REN Origin: *Prunus humilis* Bge. (*Rosaceae*). See Dwarf Flowering Cherry Seed.

Chinese Eaglewood; BAI MU XIANG (one of the **CHEN XIANG**) Origin: *Aquilaria sinensis* (Lour.) Gilg (*Thymelaeaceae*). See Eaglewood.

Chinese Elm Bark; LANG YU PI Origin: Ulmus paruifolia Jacq. (*Ulmaceae*). Part: bark. Effects: To disinhibit water and free strangury, eliminate welling abscess.

Chinese Ephedra; MA HUANG Origin: *Ephedra sinica* Stapf (*Ephedraceae*). Part: herbaceous twigs. Effects: To induce diaphoresis, relieve panting and facilitate the lung-*qi* and disinhibit urine. Indications: Syndrome of exterior repletion shown as aversion to cold, fever, headache, nosal congestion, anhidrosis, floating and tense pulse; cough; edema.

Chinese Fevervine Fruit; JI SHI TENG GUO Origin: *Paederia scandens* (Lour.) Merr. (*Rubiaceae*). Part: fruit. Indications: Insect sting, frostbite.

Chinese Fevervine; JI SHI TENG Origin: *Paederia scandens* (Lour.) Merr. (*Rubiaceae*). Part: aerial parts. Effects: To dispel wind and activate blood flow, to remove damp, food stagnancy and toxin and to relieve pain. Indications: Wind-damp pain (rheumatalgia), abdominal diarrhea and dysentery, pain in stomach duct and abdomen, *qi* vacuity and puffy swelling, heavy head and low food intake, swollen liver and spleen, scrofula, intestinal welling abscess, innominate toxin swelling, knocks and falls.

Chinese Forgetmenot; GOU SHI HUA Origin: *Cynoglossum amabile* Stapf *et* Drumm. (*Boraginaceae*). Part: herb. Effects: To clear the lung and transform phlegm, stanch bleeding. Indications: Cough, blood ejection, scrofula, knife wound.

Chinese Galangal; LIAN JIANG Origin: *Alpinia chinensis* Rosc. (*Zingiberaceae*). Part: rhizome. Effects: To warm the stomach and disperse cold, disperse food and relieve pain. Indications: Stomachache with distention and oppression, dysphagia-occlusion and vomiting counterflow, abdominal pain and diaarrhea, rheumatism and cold pain of joints.

Chinese Gambirplant; HUA GOU TENG (one of the **GOU TENG**) Origin: *Uncaria sinensis* (Oliv.) Havil. (*Rubiaceae*). See Sharpleaf Gambir-plant.

Chinese Goldthread; HUANG LIAN Origin: *Coptis chinensis* Franch. (*Ranunculaceae*). Part: rhizome. Effects: To clear heat and dry damp, drain fire, and clear away toxin. Indications: Damp-heat syndrome of the large intestine shown as diarrhea, dysentery, tenesmus; acute febrile diseases manifested as high fever, dysphoric, unconsciousness and delirium; blood ejection, spontaneous external bleeding; sores, carbuncles, furuncles and boils, septicemia, swellings and pain in the ears and eyes; canker sores in the mouth, exudative skin infections and pruritus.

Chinese Hawthorn Leaf ; SHAN ZHA YE Origin: *Crataegus pinnatifida* Bge. (*Rosaceae*). Part: leaf. Indications: Hypertension.

Chinese Hawthorn; SHAN ZHA Origin: *Crataegus pinnatifida* Bge. (*Rosaceae*). Part: fruit. Effects: To remove food stagnancy and blood stasis. Indications: Indigestion and retention of food, abdominal distention, anorexia, abdominal pain and diarrhea; postpartum abdominal pain and lochiorrhea due to blood retention; hypertension; hyperlipemia; angina pectoris of coronary heart disease.

Chinese Hibiscus Flower; FU SANG HUA Origin: *Hibiscus rosasinensis* L. (*Malvaceae*). Part: flower. Effects: To clear the lung and transform phlegm, cool the blood and resolve toxin. Indications: Phlegm-fire cough, nosebleed, dysentery, red and white turbidity, swollen welling abscess, toxin sore.

Chinese Hibiscus Leaf; FU SANG YE Origin: *Hibiscus rosasinensis* L. (*Malvaceae*). Part: leaf. Effects: To cool the blood and resolve toxin. Indications: Swollen welling abscess, toxin sore, spontaneous external bleeding.

Chinese Holly Bark; GOU GU SHU PI Origin: *Ilex cornuta* Lindl. (*Aquifoliaceae*). Part: bark. Effects: To supplement yin, boost the liver and kidney, and strengthen lumbus and legs.

Chinese Holly Leaf; GOU GU YE Origin: *Ilex cornuta* Lindl. (*Aquifoliaceae*). Part: leaf. Effects: To supplement the liver and kidney, nourish *qi*-blood, and dispel wind-damp. Indications: Lung taxation and cough, taxation and loss of blood, weakness in the lumbus and knees, pain from wind-damp impediment (arthralgia-syndrome), knocks and falls.

Chinese Holly; KU DING CHA Origin: *Ilex cornuta* Lindl. (*Aquifoliaceae*). See Broadleaf Holly.

Chinese Honeylocust Leaf; ZAO JIA YE Origin: *Gleditsia sinensis* Lam. (*Leguminosae*). Part: leaf. Indications: Wind sore.

Chinese Honeylocust Root-bark; ZAO JIA GEN PI Origin: *Gleditsia sinensis* Lam. (*Leguminosae*). Part: root bark. Effects: Root: to free the orifices, eliminate wind and resolve toxin; root-bark: kill worms. Indications: Root: painful bone due to wind-damp, itch, toxin of sores, innominate toxin swelling; root-bark: wind-heat phlegm *qi.*

Chinese Honeylocust; ZAO JIA Origin: *Gleditsia sinensis* Lam. (*Leguminosae*). Part: fruit. Effects: To dispel wind-phlegm, to eliminate damp-toxin, and to kill worms. Indications: Wind stroke with deviated eyes and mouth, head wind and headache, coughing of phlegm and panting , intestinal wind bleeding, food-denying dysentery, swollen welling abscess and toxin in the stool; sore, lichen, scab and *lai.*

Chinese Inula Flower; XUAN FU HUA Origin: *Inula britannica* L. var. *chinensis* (Rupr.) Reg. (*Compositae*). Part: capitulum. Effects: To disperse phlegm and precipitate *qi,* soften hardness, move water. Indications: Cough with dyspnea and profuse spuutum; epigastric fullness, vomiting and eructation.

Chinese Ivy; CHANG CHUN TENG Origin: *Hedera ncpalensis* K. Koch var. *sinensis* (Tobl.) Rehd. (*Araliaceae*). Part: stem and leaf. Effects: To dispel wind and disinhibit dampness, calm the liver and resolve toxin. Indications: Rheumatic arthritis, hepatitis, dizzy head, deviated eyes and mouth, spontaneous external bleeding, spontaneous external bleeding, swelling and toxin of welling abscess and flat abscess.

Chinese Juniper Leaf; GUI YE Origin: *Sobina chinensis* (L.) Antoine (*Cupressaceae*). Part: leaf. Effects: To expel wind and dissipate cold, quicken the blood and resolve toxin. Indications: Wind-cold common cold, wind-damp (rheumatism) with painful joints, urticaria, early stage of toxin swelling.

Chinese Knotweed Herb; HUO TAN MU CAO Origin: *Polygonum chinense* L. (*Polygonaceae*). Part: herb. Effects: To clear heat and disinhibit damp, cool the blood and resolve toxin. Indications: Diarrhea, dysentery, jaundice, wind-heat throat pain, summer infixation in children, fright convulsion, white vaginal discharge, swelling of welling abscess and damp sore, knocks and falls.

Chinese Ligusticum; GAO BEN Origin: *Ligusticum sinense* Oliv. (*Umbelliferae*). Part: rhizome and root. Effects: To dissipate cold and resolve the exterior, dispel wind and eliminate dampness, relieve pain. Indications: Headache due to external contraction of wind and cold, vertex headache, pain in tooth and cheek, hemilateral headache; wind-cold-damp impediment and pain in the limbs.

Chinese Lizardtail; SAN BAI CAO Origin: *Saururus chinensis* (Lour.) Baill. (*Saururaceae*). Part: rhizome or whole plant. Effects: To clear heat and disinhibit damp, disperse swelling and resolve toxin, used as an antipyretic, detoxicant, diuretic, and detumescence. Indications: Edema, beriberi (leg *qi*), jaundice, strangury-turbidity, vaginal discharge, swollen welling abscess, clove sore.

Chinese Lobelia; BAN BIAN LIAN Origin: *Lobelia chinensis* Lour. [= *Lobelia radicans* Thunb.] (*Campanulaceae*). Part: herb. Effects: To disinhibit water, disperse swelling, and resolve toxin. Indications: Poisonous snake bite, bee or scorpion sting, clove sore with swelling and pain in the early stage; edema with greater abdomen, swelling of the face and feet.

Chinese Loropetalum; JI HUA YE Origin: *Loropetalum chinense* (R. Br.) Oliv. (*Hamameli-daceae*). Part: leaf or stem. Effects: To clear heat and check diarrhea, quicken the blood and stanch bleeding. Indications: Summer-heat diarrhea and dysentery, Sinew sprain and wrenching, bleeding from wounds, eye pain, sore throat.

Chinese Magnolia Flower; YE HE HUA Origin: *Magnolia coco* (Lour.) DC. (*Magnoliaceae*). Part: flower. Indications: Liver depression and *qi* pain, knocks and falls, concretions and conglomerations, white vaginal discharge.

Chinese Magnoliavine; WU WEI ZI Origin: *Schisandra chinensis* (Turcz.) Baill. (*Schisandra-ceae*). Part: ripe fruit. Effects: To relieve dry cough, supplement the kidney, promote secretion and arrest diarrhea. Indications: Chronic cough and panting; impairment of the body fluid manifested as thirst, spontaneous or night sweating; emission and spermatorrhea; diarrhea; fidget, palpitation, insomnia and dreaminess; high level of GPT.

Chinese Mahonia Fruit; SHI DA GONG LAO ZI Origin: *Mahonia fortunei* (Lindl.) Fedde (*Berberidaceae*). See Leatherleaf Mahonia Fruit.

Chinese Mahonia Leaf; SHI DA GONG LAO YE Origin: *Mahonia fortunei* (Lindl.) Fedde (*Berberidaceae*). See Leatherleaf Mahonia Leaf.

Chinese Mahonia; SHI DA GONG LAO MU Origin: *Mahonia fortunei* (Lindl.) Fedde (*Berberida-ceae*). See Leatherleaf Mahonia.

Chinese Milkvetch Seed; ZI YUN YING ZI Origin: *Astragalus sinicus* L. (*Leguminosae*). Part: seed. Effects: To quicken the nlood and brighten the eyes. Indications: Eye disease.

Chinese Milkvetch; HONG HUA CAI (ZI YUN YING) Origin: *Astragalus sinicus* L. (*Legu-minosae*). Part: herb. Effects: To clear heat and resolve toxin. Indications: Wind phlegm cough, throat pain, fire eye, clove sore, herpes zoster, bleeding due to external injury.

Chinese Milkwort Herb; DA JIN NIU CAO Origin: *Polygala chinensis* L. (*Polygalaceae*). Part: herb with root or root. Effects: To suppress cough, disperse accumulation, quicken the blood and dissipate stasis. Indications: Consumption cough with phlegm, dysentery, *gan* accumulation, , snake bite, knocks and falls.

Chinese Narcissus Bulb; SHUI XIAN GEN Origin: *Narcissus tazeyya* L. var. *chinensis* Roem. (*Amaryllidaceae*). Part: bulb. Indications: Swelling and toxin of welling abscess and sores, insect bites, fish bones stuck in the throat.

Chinese Narcissus Flower; SHUI XIAN HUA Origin: *Narcissus tazeyya* L. var. *chinensis* Roem. (*Amaryllidaceae*). Part: flower. Effects: To dispel wind and eliminate heat, quicken the blood and regulate menstruation. Indications: Wind *qi*, menstrual irregularities.

Chinese nardostachys; GAN SONG Origin: *Nardostachys chinensis* Batal. (*Valeria-naceae*). Part: root and rhizome. Effects: To rectify *qi* and relieve pain, to arouse spleen and fortify the stomach. Indications: Stomachache, distention and fullness in the chest and abdomen, headache, hysteria, beriberi.

Chinese Orthodon; SHI XIANG ROU Origin: *Orthodon chinensis* (Maxim.) Kudo (*Labiatae*). Part: herb. Effects: To dispel summerheat, quicken the blood, rectify *qi*, and transform dampness. Indications: Common cold in the summer, summer-heat stroke with vomiting and nausea, abdominal pain and diarrhea, stasis and pain from knocks and falls, eczema, swollen boil.

Chinese Photinia Leaf; SHI NAN YE Origin: *Photinia serrulata* Lindl. (*Rosaceae*). Part: leaf. Effects: To dispel wind, free the network vessels, and boost the kidney. Indications: Wind impediment, aching pain of the lumbus and back, kidney vacuity and leg weakness, hemilateral headache, wind papules.

Chinese Pink; QU MAI Origin: *Dianthus chinensis* L. (*Caryophyllaceae*). See Lilac Pink.

Chinese Plumyew Brench and Leaf; SAN JIAN SHAN Origin: *Cephalotaxus sinesis* (Rehd. *et* Wils.) Li (*Cephalotaxaceae*). See Fortune Plumyew Brench and Leaf.

Chinese Plumyew Seed; TU XIANG FEI (SAN JIAN SHAN ZI) Origin: *Cephalotaxus sinesis* (Rehd. *et* Wils.) Li (*Cephalotaxaceae*). See Fortune Plumyew.

Chinese Podocarpus Leaf; LUO HAN SONG YE Origin: *Podocarpus macrophyllus* (Thunb.) D. Don var. *maki* (Sieb.) Endl. (*Podocar-paceae*). Part: branchlet and leaf. Indications: Blood ejection, coughing of blood.

Chinese Podocarpus Seed; LUO HAN SONG SHI Origin: *Podocarpus macrophyllus* (Thunb.) D. Don var. *maki* (Sieb.) Endl. (*Podocar-paceae*). Part: seed and receptacle. Effects: To supplement the kidney and boost the lung, greatly supplement original *qi*. Indications: Blood vacuity, withered-yellow facial complexion, pain in the region of the heart and stomach.

Chinese pulsatilla; BAI TOU WENG Origin: *Pulsatilla chinensis* (Bge.) Reg. (*Ranuncu-laceae*). Part: root. Effects: To remove heat and toxin, eliminate pathogenic heat in the blood and arrest dysentery and diarrhea. Indications: Diarrhea and dysentery with bloody stool; abdominal pain and tenesmus; trichomoniasis vaginalis.

Chinese Pyrola Herb; LU XIAN CAO Origin: *Pyrola rotundifolia* L. subsp. *chinensis* H. Andres (*Pyrolaceae*). Part: herb. Effects: To supplement vacuity and boost the kidney, dispel wind and eliminate dampness, quicken the blood and regulate menstruation. Indications: Vacuity and weakness with cough, taxation damage and blood ejection, rheumatism with painful joints, flooding and spotting, white vaginal discharge, bleeding of external injury.

Chinese Seriphidium; SHAN DAO NIAN HAO (HUI HAO) Origin: *Artemisia cina* (Berg. *ex* Poljak) Poljak [= *Seriphidium cinum* (Berg. *ex* Poljak) Poljak] (*Compositae*). Part: inflorescence and leaf. Effects: To expel worms. Indications: Roundworm disease, pinworm disease.

Chinese Silkvine Root-bark; XIANG JIA PI Origin: *Periploca sepium* Bge. (*Asclepiadaceae*). Part: root bark. Effects: To dispel wind and damp, strengthen sinews and bones. Indications: Rheumatic arthritis, weakness of sinews and bones in children, slowness to walk due to infantile wilting pattern, edema and inhibited urination.

Chinese Silvergrass; MANG JING Origin: *Miscanthus sinensis* Anderss. (*Gramineae*). Part: stem. Effects: To dissipate bliid, disinhibit urine, resolve heat ahd toxin. Indications: Wind evil.

Chinese Soapberry Fruit; WU HUAN ZI PI Origin: *Sapindus mukorossi* Gaertn. (*Sapindaceae*). Part: fruit. Effects: To clear heat and transform phlegm, to relieve pain and disperse accumulation. Indications: Swelling and pain from throat impediment, stomachache, mounting pain, (rheumatalgia), worm accumulation, retention of food, innominate toxin swelling.

Chinese Soapberry Leaf; WU HUAN ZI YE Origin: *Sapindus mukorossi* Gaertn. (*Sapindaceae*). Part: branchlet and leaf. Indications: Snake bite, whooping cough.

Chinese St. John'swort Fruit; JIN SI TAO GUO SHI Origin: *Hypericum chinense* L. (*Guttiferae*). Part: fruit. Indications: Lung disease, whooping cough.

Chinese Starjasmine; LUO SHI TENG Origin: *Trachelospermum jasminoides* (Lindl.) Lem. (*Apocynaceae*). Part: leafy stem. Effects: To relieve rigidity of muscles, ensure normal flow of *qi* and blood in the collaterals, dispel blood stasis and stanch bleeding. Indications: Wind-damp impediment (arthralgia-syndrome), hypertonicity of the sinews; throat impediment, swollen welling abscess.

Chinese Stauntonvine; YE MU GUA Origin: *Stauntonia hexaphylla* Decne. (*Lardizabalaceae*). Part: stem and leaf. Effects: To expel wind, relieve pain, and promote circulation of *qi* and blood.

Chinese Stellera; RUI XIANG LANG DU (one of the **LANG DU**) Origin: *Stellera chamaejasme* L. (*Thymelaeaceae*). Part: root. Effects: To expel water and dispel phlegm, break break accumulation and kill worms. Indications: Edema and abdominal distention, accumulation from phlegm, food and worms, pain in heart region and abdomen, chronic trachitis, cough, panting, scab and lichen, hemorrhoids and fistulas, tuberculosis of the lymphnode, skin, bone and epididymis.

Chinese Stephania; JIN BU HUAN Origin: *Stephania sinica* Diels (*Menispermaceae*). Part: root. Effects: To clear heat and resolve toxin, fortify the stomach and relieve pain, dissipate stasis and disperse swelling. Indications: External contraction and cough, sore throat, mough and tongue sores, vomiting and diarrhea, dysentery, stomachache, swelling and toxin of welling abscess and flat abscess, knocks and falls.

Chinese Sumac Leaf; YAN FU YE Origin: *Rhus chinensis* Mill. (*Anacardiaceae*). Part: fresh leaf. Effects: To transform phlegm and relieve cough, promote contraction and resolve toxin. Indications: Phlegm cough, bloody stool, blood dysentery, night sweating, sore.

Chinese Tallowtree Bark; WU JIU MU GEN PI Origin: *Sapium sebiferum* (L.) Roxb. (*Euphorbiaceae*). Part: root bark. Effects: To disinhibit water and disperse accumulation, kill worms and resolve toxin. Indications: Concretion, conglomeration, accumulation and gathering; edema, drum distention, urinary and fecal stoppage, damp sore, toxin of clove sore, scab and lichen.

Chinese Thorowax; BEI CHAI HU (one of the **CHAI HU**) Origin: *Bupleurum chinense* DC. (*Umbelliferae*). Part: root. Effects: To harmonize the exterior and interior, soothe the liver and upbear *yang*. Indications: Fever of common cold, feeling of fullness and discomfort in the chest and hypochondrium, bitter taste and dryness in the throat; stagnation of the liver-*qi* shown as feeling of fullness and oppression in the chest and disphraum, distending pain in the hypochondrium; proctoptosis, hysteroptosis, gastroptosis, short breath, fatigue and lassitude; malaria.

Chinese Toona Root-bast; CHUN BAI PI Origin: *Toona sinensis* (A. Juss.) Roem. (*Meliaceae*). Part: root bast. Effects: To eliminate heat and dry dampness, astringe the intestines and stanch bleeding, and kill worms. Indications: Enduring dysentery, enduring drainage, intestinal wind bleeding, flooding and spotting, vaginal discharge, seminal emission, white turbidity, *gan* accumulation, roundworm disease, sore and lichen.

Chinese Umbrellaleaf; WO ER QI Origin: *Diphylleia sinensis* Li (*Berberidaceae*). Part: rhizome. Effects: To dispel wind-damp, clear heat and cool the blood, quicken the blood and relieve pain, drain precipitation. Indications: Rheumatic arthritis, lumbar and leg pain, steaming bone and taxation fever, knocks and falls, menstrual irregularities, painful bind in the lesser-abdomen, swollen welling abscess.

Chinese Waxgourd Seed; DONG GUA ZI Origin: *Benincasa hispida* (Thunb.) Cogn. (*Cucurbita-ceae*). Part: seed. Effects: To clear heat and resolve phlegm, to disperse welling abscess and disinhibit water. Indications: Phlegm-heat cough, welling abscess of the lung, intestinal welling abscess, strangury, edema, leg *qi* (beriberi), hemorrhoid.

Chinese Waxmyrtle Bark; YANG MEI SHU PI Origin: *Murica rubra* (Lour.) Sieb. *et* Zucc. (*Myricaceae*). Part: bark. Indications: Dysentery, knocks and falls, nebulous eye screen, toothache, burns and scalds, malign scab and *lai* sore.

Chinese Waxmyrtle; YANG MEI Origin: *Murica rubra* (Lour.) Sieb. *et* Zucc. (*Myricaceae*). Part: fruit. Effects: To engender liquid and allay thirst, harmonize stomach and disperse food. Indications: Vexation and thirst, vomiting and diarrhea, dysentery, abdominal pain.

Chinese Weeping Cypress Leaf; BAI SHU YE Origin: *Cupressus funebris* Endl. (*Cupressaceae*). Part: leaf. Effects: To harmonize the blood, stanch bleeding, and engender flesh. Indications: Blood ejection, blood dysentery, hemorrhoid, scalds.

Chinese Wisteria Seed; ZI TENG ZI Origin: *Wisteria sinensis* Sweet (*Leguminosae*). Part: seed. Effects: To killworm, relieve pain, and resolve toxin. Indications: Sinew and bone pain.

Chinese Wisteria; ZI TENG Origin: *Wisteria sinensis* Sweet (*Leguminosae*). Part: stem and leaf.

Chinese Wolfberry Fruit; ZI Origin: *Lycium chinense* Mill. (*Solanaceae*). Part: fruit. Effects: To replenish the vital essence and the blood and improve acuity of sight. Indications: Lassitude of the loins and legs, seminal emission; dizziness and blurred vision; phthisical cough; diabetes.

Chinese Wolfberry Leaf; GOU QI YE Origin: *Lycium chinense* Mill. (*Solanaceae*). Part: leaf. Effects: To supplement vacuity and boost essence, clear heat and allay thirst, dispel wind and brighten the eyes. Indications: Fever of vacuity taxation, vexation and thirst, sore red eyes and clouded vision, eye screen, night blindness, flooding and vaginal discharge, heat toxin swollen sore.

Chinese Wolfberry Root-bark; DI GU PI (GOU QI GEN PI) Origin: *Lycium chinense* Mill (*Solanaceae*). Part: root bark. Effects: To remove heat from the blood and lower the asthenic heat. Indications: Hectic or tidal fever with night sweat; infantile malnutrition (*gan* accumulation) with fever; cough with dyspnea or hemoptysis; profuse urination in wasting-thirst disease (diabetes); blood ejection and spontaneous external bleeding.

Chive; XI XIANG CONG Origin: Allium schoenoprasum L. (*Liliaceae*). Part: herb or root head. Effects: To free *qi* and effuse sweat, resolve the exterior. Indications: Wind-heat common cold with headache, cold-damp red swelling, pain wind, sore.

Christina Loosestrife Herb; DA JIN QIAN CAO Origin: *Lysimachia christinae* Hance (*Primulaceae*). Part: herb. Effects: To induce diuresis and remove calculi, reduce heat and swelling, and remove damp and treat jaundice. Indications: Stranguria, lithiasis in the liver, gallbladder, kidney, urinary bladder, and ureter; jaundice due to damp-heat; boils, furuncles and other infections on the body surface.

Chrusanthemum-like Groundsel Herb; TU SAN QI Origin: *Senecio chrysanthemoides* DC. (*Compositae*). Part: herb or root. Effects: To quicken blood and disperse swelling. Indications: Knocks and falls, stasis swelling and pain, swollen and opening of welling abscess, mammary welling abscess.

Chu-lan Tree; MI ZI LAN Origin: *Aglaia odorata* Lour. (*Meliaceae*). Part: flower or leaf. Effects: Flower: resolve depression and loosen the center, hasten delivery, dispel the effects of liquor, clear the lung, arouse the brain and eyes, allay vexation and thirst. Indications: Flower: distention and fullness in the chest and diaphragm, early stage of dysphagia-occlusion, cough and heavy head; leaf: knocks and falls, flat abscess.

Chuanxiong (Wallich Ligusticum) ; CHUAN XIONG Origin: *Ligusticum wallichii* Franch. (*Umbelliferae*). Part: rhizome. Effects: To quicken thc blood, dispel blood stasis, move *qi* and relieve pain. Indications: Irregular menstruation, menstrual pain, menstrual block, dystocia, postpartum lochiostasis, abdominal pain; pain in the hypochondrium, numbness, extremities, traumatic injuries, sores; headache, rheumatic impediment; angina pectoris of coronary heart disease; ischemic cerebrovascular diseases.

Civet; LING MAO XIANG Origin: *Viverra zibetha* L. (*Viverridae*). Part: secretion with a musky odor secreted from the anal scent glands. Effects: To promote the flow of *qi,* repel foulness, and relieve pain. Indications: Sudden pain in heart region and abdomen, mounting pain.

Cladonia fallax Lichen; JIN SHUA BA Origin: *Cladonia fallax* Abbayes (*Cladoniaceae*). Part: lichen. Effects: Sedation, anti-inflammation, and relieveing pain. Indications: Epilepsy, schizophrenia, neurasthenia, dizzy head and vision.

Clammy Hopseedbush Leaf; CHE SANG ZI YE Origin: *Dodonaea viscosa* (L.) Jacq. (*Sapindaceae*). Part: leaf. Effects: To clear heat and percolate damp, to eliminate swelling and resolve toxin. Indications: Dribbling urination, dribbing urinary block, shoulder swelling, clove sore and boil, swelling and pain in the perineum, burns and scalds.

Clethra Loosestrife; ZHEN ZHU CAI (ZHEN ZHU YE) Origin: *Lyaimachia Clethroides* Duby (*Primulaceae*). Part: root or herb. Effects: To quicken blood and regulate menstruation, disinhibit water and disperse swelling. Indications: Menstrual disorder, white vaginal discharge, child *gan* accumulation, edema, dysentery, knocks and falls, sore throat, mammary welling abscess.

Climbing Entada Seed; KE TENG ZI Origin: *Entada phaseoloides* (L.) Merr. (*Leguminosae*). Part: seed. Indications: Bloody stool, blood dysentery, jaundice, prolapse of the rectum, hemorrhoid, throat impediment.

Climbing Fig; BI LI Origin: *Ficus pumila* L. (*Moraceae*). Part: leafy stem. Effects: To dispel wind and disinhibit dampness, quicken the blood and resolve toxin. Indications: Pain from wind-damp impediment (arthralgia-syndrome), diarrhea, strangury, knocks and falls, swollen welling abscess, sore and boil.

Climbing Groundsel; QIAN LI GUANG Origin: *Senecio scandens* Buch.-Ham. (*Compositae*). Part: aerial parts. Effects: Used as an antipyretic and detoxicant to clear the liver and improve acuity of sight. Indications: Wind-fire red eye, eye screen, typhoid fever, bacillary dysentery, lobar pneumonia, tonsillitis, enteritis, jaundice, influenza, toxemia, hematosepsis, swelling and toxin of welling abscess and boil, dry or damp lichen, cinnabar toxin, eczema, scalds, trichomonal vaginitis.

Clove; DING XIANG Origin: *Syzygium aromaticum* (L.) Merr. *et* Perry (*Myrtaceae*). Part: flower bud. Effects: To warm the middle-*jiao,* send down the upward adverse flow of *qi* and to warm the kidney and reinforce its vital function. Indications: Vomiting and hiccough due to stomach-cold, reduced eating and diarrhea; impotence and limp legs due to insufficiency of kidney *yang*.

Cochinchinese Asparagus; TIAN MEN DONG Origin: *Asparagus cochinchinensis* (Lour.) Merr. (*Liliaceae*). Part: root tuber. Effects: To replenish vital essence and moisten dryness, and to remove heat from the lung and relieve coughing. Indications: *Yin* vacuity fever, cough and blood ejection, lung wilting, pulmonary welling abscess, sore swollen throat, diabetes, constipation.

Cochinhina Momordica Root; MU BIE GEN Origin: *Momordica cochinchinensis* (Lour.) Spr. (*Cucurbitaceae*). Part: tuber root. Effects: To resolve toxin and expel inflammation, to eliminate swelling and relieve pain. Indications: Welling abscess and sore, toxin clove sore, innominate toxin swelling, lymphnoditis.

Cochinhina Momordica Seed; MU BIE ZI Origin: *Momordica cochinchinensis* (Lour.) Spr. (*Cucurbitaceae*). Part: ripe seed. Effects: To disperse swelling and dissipate bind, to dispel toxin. Indications: Swollen welling abscess, clove sore, scrofula, hemorrhoid, innominate toxin swelling, lichen, wind damp impediment, hypertonicity of sinews and vessels.

Cockroach; ZHANG LANG Origin: *Blatta orientalis* L. (*Blattidae*). Part: body. Effects: To break stasis and transform accumulation, disperse swelling and resolve toxin. Indications: Child *gan* accumulation, concretion, conglomeration, accumulation, gathering, clove sore, throat moth, swollen welling abscess, snake or insect bites.

Coconut Albumen; YE ZI RANG Origin: *Cocos nucifera* L. (*Palmae*). Part: albumen. Effects: To boost *qi* and dispel wind. Indications: Fascio-lopsiasis, *gan* accumulation.

Coconut Oil; YE ZI YOU Origin: *Cocos nucifera* L. (*Palmae*). Part: oil. Indications: Scab and lichen, frostbite.

Coconut Root-bark; YE ZI PI Origin: *Cocos nucifera* L. (*Palmae*). Part: root bark. Effects: To stanch bleeding, relieve pain. Indications: Nosebleed, stomachache, vomiting and diarrhea.

Coffee Senna; WANG JIANG NAN Origin: *Cassia occidentalis* L. (*Leguminosae*). Part: stem and leaf. Effects: To depurate the lung, clear the liver, harmonize stomach, disperse swelling and resolve toxin. Indications: Cough, asthma, glomus pain in stomach duct and abdomen, blood strangury, constipation, headache, red eyes, swelling and toxin of clove and sores, insect and snake bite.

Collett Yam; CHA RUI SHU YU (one of the **BEI XIE**) Origin: *Dioscorea collettii* Hook. f. (*Dioscoriaceae*). See Hypoglaucous Collett Yam.

Colophony; SONG XIANG Origin: *Pinus massoniana* Lamb. (*Pinaceae*). Part: residue left after the distillation of the turpentine oil from the crude oleo-resin of various spp of *Pinus.* Effects: Used as an antirheumatic, diuretic, anodyne, and as a drug to expel pus, remove toxin and promote granulation. Indications: Welling abscess and flat abscess, clove toxin, hemorrhoids and fistulas, malign sore, scab and lichen, bald white scalp sore, incised wound, sprain, pain from wind-damp impediment (arthralgia-syndrome), leprosy and itching.

Colored Mistletoe; HU JI SHENG (one of the **SANG JI SHENG**) Origin: *Viscum coloratum* (Kom.) Nakai (*Lorantha-ceae*). Part: foliferous stem. Effects: To dispel wind-damp and supplement the liver and kidney, strengthen sinew and bone, and quiet the fetus. Indications: Wind-damp impediment (arthralgia-syndrome), pain in the loins and legs; threatencd abortion, vaginal bleeding during pregnancy; hypertension.

Combined Spicebush; WU YAO Origin: *Lindera strychnifolia* (Sieb. *et* Zucc.) Villar [= *Lindera aggregata* (Sims) Kosterm.] (*Lauraceae*). Part: root tuber. Effects: To rectify *qi* and ease pain, to dispel cold and warm the kidney. Indications: Distention and pain in the chest and abdomen with *qi* counterflow, stagnation of abiding food, stomach reflux and vomiting, cold mounting, beriberi, frequent urination.

Common Alstonia; XIANG PI MU Origin: *Alstonia scholaris* (L.) R. Br. (*Apocynaceae*). Part: bark or leaf. Effects: To clear heat and resolve toxin, stanch bleeding and disperse swelling. Indications: Common cold, pneumonia, whooping cough, sand *qi* with stomachache and diarrhea, vomiting inpregnancy, knocks and falls, ulcerative bleeding.

Common Andrographis; CHUAN XIN LIAN Origin: *Andrographis paniculata* (Burm.f.) Nees (*Acanthaceae*). Part: dried aerial parts. Effects: To clear heat, resolve toxin, and dry dampness. Indications: Warm disease in the initial stage, fever, headache; lung heat cough, pulmonary welling abscess, sore swollen throat; swollen boil, poisonous snake bite; diarrhea due to damp-heat, heat strangury, damp papule.

Common Anemarrhena; ZHI MU Origin: *Anemarrhena asphodeloides* Bge. (*Liliaceae*). Part: rhizome. Effects: To clear away heat, to drain fire, to replenish *yin* essence and moisten the viscera, to promote the production of body fluid to resolve thirst. Indications: Epidemic febrile diseases with high fever, dire thirst, full and forceful pulse; cough due to lung heat, dry cough with thick sputum; hyperactivity of fire with hectic fever, vexation and night sweat; diabetes shown as thirst, polydipsia, polyuria.

Common Anisodus; SAI LANG DANG Origin: *Anisodus luridus* Link *et* Otto (*Solanaceae*). Part: root. Effects: To resolve tetany and relieve pain. Indications: Stomachache, gallbladder gripping pain, acute and chronic gastroenteritis.

Common Aspidistra; ZHI ZHU BAO DAN Origin: *Aspidistra elatior* Bl. (*Liliaceae*). Part: rhizome. Effects: To quicken the blood and free the network vessels, drain heat and disinhibit urine. Indications: Knocks and falls, lumbar pain, menstrual block and abdominal pain, headache, toothache, heat cough and summerheat damage, diarrhea, sand strangury.

Common Atlantic Octopus; ZHANG YU Origin: *Octopus vulgaris* Lamarck (*Octopodidae*). Part: meat. Effects: To nourish the blood and boost *qi,* promote contraction and engender flesh. Indications: Vacuity of *qi* and blood, swelling and toxin of welling abscess and flat abscess, ulceration of enduring sore.

Common Aucklandia (Costustoot); MU XIANG Origin: *Saussurea lappa* Clarke [= *Aucklandia lappa* Decne] (*Compositae*). Part: root. Effects: To rectify *qi* and relieve pain, warm the center and restore normal functioning of the stomach. Indications: Abdominal distention and pain, anorexia, borborygmus, diarrhea and dysentery.

Common Banana; XIANG JIAO Origin: *Musa paradisiaca* L. var. *sapientum* O. Ktze. [= *Musa sapientum* L.] (*Musaceae*). Part: fruit. Effects: To clear heat, moisten the intestines, and resolve toxin. Indications: Febrile disease with vexation and thirst, constipation, blood hemorrhoid.

Common Baphicacanthus Leaf; DA QING YE Origin: *Baphicacanthus cusia* (Nees) Bremek (*Acanthaceae*). See Indigo-coloured Woad Leaf.

Common Baphicacanthus Root; BAN LAN GEN Origin: *Baphicacanthus cusia* (Nees) Brem. (*Cruciferae*). See Dyers Woad Root.

Common Bombax Flower; MU MIAN HUA Origin: *Gossampinus malabarica* (DC.) Merr. (*Bombacaceae*). Part: flower. Effects: To clear heat and disinhibit damp, to resolve toxin and stanch bleeding. Indications: Diarrhea, dysentery, flooding, sore-toxin, bleeding from incised wound.

Common Broadlily; LEI GONG QI Origin: *Clintonia alpina* (Royle) Kunth (*Liliaceae*). Part: herb. Effects: To dispel wind, vanguish toxin, dissipate stasis, and relieve pain. Indications: Knocks and falls, taxation damage.

Common Buckwheat Stem; QIAO MAI JIE Origin: *Fagopyrum esculentum* Moench (*Polygonaceae*). Part: stem and leaf. Effects: To lubricate the intestines and precipitate *qi*, stanch bleeding, consume malign flesh. Indications: Dysphagia, swollen welling abscess.

Common Buckwheat; QIAO MAI Origin: *Fagopyrum esculentum* Moench (*Polygonaceae*). Part: seed. Effects: To open the stomach and loosen the intestines, precipitate *qi* and disperse accumulation. Indications: Intestine-gripping sand, gastrointestinal accumulation, chronic diarrhea, food-denying dysentery, red wandering cinnabar toxin, welling abscess and flat abscess effusion of the back, scrofula, burns and scalds.

Common Butterbush; FENG XIANG SHU YE (a) Origin: *Cephalanthus occidentalis* L. (*Rubiaceae*). Part: leaf or bud. Effects: To clear heat and resolve toxin, contract damp and relieve itching. Indications: Itching sore of skin, heaven-borne sore, foot rot, knocks and falls, toothache, dysentery, enteritis.

Common Camptotheac; XI SHU Origin: *Camptotheca acuminata* Decne. (*Nyssaceae*). Part: fruit or root. Indications: (Trying to used for) cancer, acute and chronic leukemia, psoriasis, swollen liver and spleen due to schistosomiasis,

Common Caper; LAO SHU GUA Origin: *Capparis spinosa* L. (*Capparidaceae*). Part: root bark, leaf and fruit. Effects: To dispel wind, dissipate cold, and eliminate dampness. Indications: Acute and chronic rheumatic arthritis.

Common Carpesium Fruit; HE SHI (TIAN MING JING GUO) Origin: *Carpesium abrota-noides* L. (*Compositae*). Part: fruit. Effects: To kill worms. Indications: Ascariasis, enterobiasis and teniasis.

Common Carpesium; TIAN MING JING Origin: *Carpesium abrotanoides* L. (*Compositae*). Part: root, stem and leaf. Effects: To dispel cough, clear heat, break blood, stanch bleeding, resolve toxin, kill worms. Indications: Nipple moth, throat impediment, malaria, acute hepatitis, acute or chronic fright wind, worm accumulation, blood conglomera-tion, spontaneous external bleeding, blood strangury, swelling and toxin of clove and sores, skin itchy papules.

Common Cashew Fruit; DU XIAN ZI Origin: *Anacardium occidentale* L. (*Anacardiaceae*). Part: fruit. Indications: Cough and counterflow, vexation and thirst.

Common Cerberustree; NIU XIN QIE ZI Origin: *Cerbera manghas* L. (*Apocynaceae*). Part: kernel. Indications: Narcotic (for external use only).

Common Chicory; JU QU Origin: *Cichorium intybus* L. (*Compositae*). Part: herb. Effects: To clear liver and disinhibit gallbladder. Indications: Icterohepatitis.

Common Cissampelos; XI SHENG TENG Origin: *Cissampelos pareira* L. (*Menispermaceae*). Part: herb. Effects: To relieve pain, stanch bleeding, and engender flesh. Indications: Knocks and falls.

Common Cnidium; SHE CHUANG ZI Origin: *Cnidium monnieri* (L.) Cusson (*Umbelliferae*). Part: fruit. Effects: To warm the kidney and rainforce *yang,* dispel wind, dry damp, kill worms. Indications: Impotence, scrotal damp itch, vaginal discharge, pudendal itch, infertility due to uterus cold, pain from wind-damp impediment (arthralgia-syndrome), scab and lichen, damp sore.

Common Coltsfoot; KUAN DONG HUA Origin: *Tussilago farfara* L. (*Compositae*). Part: flower bud. Effects: To moisten the lung and precipitate *qi*, suppress cough and transform phlegm. Indications: Cough, cough with panting, cold cough, cough with phlegm and blood, fulminant cough.

Common Crapemyrtle Flower; ZI WEI HUA Origin: *Lagerstroemia indica* L. (*Lythraceae*). Part: flower. Indications: Postpartum flooding, concretions and conglomerations, flooding, vaginal discharge, scab and lichen, *lai* and sore.

Common Crapemyrtle Leaf; ZI WEI YE Origin: *Lagerstroemia indica* L. (*Lythraceae*). Part: leaf. Indications: Dysentery, eczema, bleeding from wounds.

Common Crapemyrtle Root; ZI WEI GEN Origin: *Lagerstroemia indica* L. (*Lythraceae*). Part: root. Effects: To move the blood. Indications: Swelling and toxin of welling abscess and sores, toothache, dysentery.

Common Cyanotis; LU SHUI CAO (II) Origin: *Cyanotis vaga* (Lour.) Roem. *et* Schult. (*Commelinaceae*). Part: root. Effects: To supplement vacuity, eliminate damp, soothe sinew and quicken the network vessels. Indications: Incessint vacuity fever, nephritis with edema, rheumatism with painful joints, eczema.

Common Dayflower Herb; YA ZHI CAO Origin: *Commelina communis* L. (*Commelinaceae*). Part: aerial parts. Effects: To clear heat and resolve toxin, disinhibit urine. Indications: Fever; heat strangury and short voidingss of reddish urine, edema with fever; sore swollen throat, swelling and toxin of welling abscess and sores, poisonous snake bite.

Common Devilpepper Stem and LeafLUO FU MU JING YE Origin: *Rauwolfia verticillata* (Lour.) Baill. (*Apocynaceae*). Part: stem and leaf. Effects: To dispel wind, lower blood pressure, move stasis, and resolve toxin. Indications: Common cold, hypertension, sand with vomiting and diarrhea, sore throat, swollen welling abscess, sore and scab, knocks and falls.

Common Devilpepper; LUO FU MU Origin: *Rauwolfia verticillata* (Lour.) Baill. (*Apocynaceae*). Part: root. Effects: To clear wind-heat, reduce the liver fire, and eliminate swelling and toxin. Indications: Common cold with fever, sore swollen throat, hypertension with headache and dizziness, sand with abdomen pain and vomiting-diarrhea, wind itch of sore and scab.

Common Ducksmeat; FU PING Origin: *Spirodela polyrrhiza* Schleid. (*Lemnaceae*). Part: herb. Effects: To effuse sweat, dispel wind, move water, clear heat and resolve toxin. Indications: External contraction of wind-heat, fever and without sweating; inhibited eruption of measles papules; dormant papules of wind-heat, itchy skin; edema with exterior pattern.

Common Duckwood; FU PING Origin: *Lemna minor* L. (*Lemnaceae*). See Common Ducksmeat.

Common Dysosma; GUI JIU Origin: *Dysosma versipellis* (Hance) M. Cheng (*Berberida-ceae*). Part: rhizome. Effects: To dispel phlegm and dissipate bind, resolve toxin and remove stasis. Indications: Consumption damage, cough, blood ejection, stomachache, goiter, scrofula, swollen welling abscess, clove sore, knocks and falls, snakebite.

Common Elsholtzia; BAN BIAN SU Origin: *Elsholtzia ciliata* (Yhunb.) Hyland (*Labiatae*). Part: herb. Effects: To expel wind and effuse sweat. Indications: Paralysis, blood ejection due to consumption damage, common cold, menstruant's morbidity, toxin of sores.

Common Evolvulus; TU DING GUI Origin: *Evolvulus alsinoides* L. (*Convolvulaceae*). Part: herb. Effects: To clear heat and disinhibit dampness. Indications: Jaundice, strangury-turbidity, vaginal discharge, clove sore, scab sore.

Common Fenugreek; HU LU BA Origin: *Trigonella foenumgraecum* L. (*Leguminosae*). Part: seed. Effects: To supplement kidney *yang*, to dispel cold dampness. Indications: Cold mounting, distention and fullness in abdomen and rib-side, cold-damp leg *qi* (beriberi) (beriberi), kidney vacuity aching lumbus, impotence.

Common Flax Seed; YA MA ZI Origin: *Linum usitatissimum* L. (*Linaceae*). Part: ripe seed. Effects: To expel wind and remove dryness. Indications: Leprosy (numbing wind), itchy papules, hair loss, dry stool.

Common Flax; YA MA Origin: *Linum usitatissimum* L. (*Linaceae*). Part: herb. Effects: Root: Calm the liver, supplement vacuity and quicken the blood. Indications: Root: chronic hepatitis, testitis, sprain from knocks and falls; Stem and leaf: headache due to liver-wind, bleeding from wounds.

Common Floweringquince; MU GUA Origin: *Chaenomeles lagenaria* (Loisel.) Koidz. (*Rosaceae*). Part: fruit. Effects: To restore normal functioning of the stomach and remove damp, to relieve rigidity of muscles and promote circulation of *qi* and blood in the collaterals. Indications: Wind-damp impediment (arthralgia-syndrome), hypertonicity of the sinew and vessels, leg *qi* (beriberi) puffy swelling and pain; both vomiting and diarrhea withcramp; indigestion.

Common Floweringquince; QIU MU GUA Origin: *Chaenomeles speciosa* (Sweet) Nakai (*Rosaceae*). Part: fruit. Effects: To soothe the liver and harmonize the stomach, eliminate damp and relieve pain. Indications: Vomiting and diarrhea with oppression in the chest, wind-damp pain in sinews and bones, leg *qi* (beriberi).

Common Four-o'clock Leaf; ZI MO LI YE Origin: *Mirabilis jalapa* L. (*Nyctaginaceae*). Part: leaf. Indications: Welling abscess, boil, scab, lichen, wounds.

Common Four-o'clock Root; ZI MO LI GEN Origin: *Mirabilis jalapa* L. (*Nyctaginaceae*). Part: root. Effects: To disinhibit urine, drain heat, quicken the blood, and dissipate stasis. Indications: Strangury-turbidity, vaginal discharge, lung taxation and blood ejection, swollen welling abscess effusion of the back, acute arthritis.

Common Ginger Dried Rhizome; GAN JIANG Origin: *Zingiber officinale* Rosc. (*Zingibera-ceae*). Part: dried rhizome. Effects: To warm the middle-*jiao* and restore *yang*, and to warm the channels ad remove water retention Indications: Gastric and abdominal cold pain, nausea, vomiting, diarrhea, anorexia; cough, dyspnea, chilly sensation in the back, profuse thin clear sputum.

Common Goldenrod; YI ZHI HUANG HUA Origin: *Solidago virgaurea* L. var. *leiocarpa* (Benth.) A. Gray [= *Solidago decurrens* Lour.] (*Compositae*). Part: herb. Effects: To expel wind and as an antipy-retic, antibacterial and antiphlogistic. Indications: Common cold and headache, sore swollen throat, jaundice, whooping cough, child fright wind, knocks and falls, swollen welling abscess in the back, goose-foot wind.

Common Heron's Bill Herb; LAO GUAN CAO Origin: *Erodium stephanianum* Willd. (*Geraniaceae*). Part: aerial parts. Effects: To dispel wind and quicken the blood, clear heat and resolve toxin. Indications: Wind-damp pain (rheumatalgia), hypertonicity and numbness, welling abscess and flat abscess, knocks and falls, enteritis, dysentery.

Common Hogfennel; QIAN HU Origin: *Peucedanum decursivum* (Miq.) Maxim. (*Umbellife-rae*). See Whiteflower Hogfennel.

Common Houndstongue; YAO YONG DAO TI HU Origin: *Cynoglossum officinale* L. (*Boragina-ceae*). Part: root. Effects: To nourish *yin* and moisten the lung, clear heat and relieve cough. Indications: pulmonary tuberculosis and cough, loss of voice, nosebleed, blood ejection.

Common Indianmulberry; YANG JIAO TENG Origin: *Morinda umbellata* L. (*Rubiaceae*). Part: root or bark. Effects: To dispel wind and dampness. Indications: Swelling and pain in joints, kidney vacuity and lumbar pain.

Common Japanese Clubmoss; SHEN JIN CAO Origin: *Lycopodium clavatum* L. (*Lycopodiaceae*). Part: whole plant. Effects: To dispel wind and remove damp, and to relieve rigidity of muscles and joints. Indications: Wind-cold-damp impediment, aching pain in joints, numbness of the skin, weakness of the limbs, edema, knocks and falls.

Common Jasminorange; JIU LI XIANG Origin: *Murraya paniculata* (L.) Jacks. (*Rutaceae*). Part: leaf and branchlet. Effects: To move *qi* and relieve pain, quicken the blood to remove the stasis, expel wind and remove damp, anesthesia and relieving convulsion; oxytocic and abortion. Indications: Chronic gastritis, duodenal ulcer, stomachache, rheumatic arthritis, traumatic injury and pain caused by ecchymoma, eczema, toothache, snakebite. Pharmacological actions: local anesthesia, antifertility activity in white rat due to estrin-like action, but no effects in golden hamster.

Common Jujube (Chinese Date); DA ZAO Origin: *Ziziphus jujuba* Mill. (*Rhamnaceae*). Part: ripe fruit. Effects: To supplement the spleen and harmonize the stomach, boost *qi* and engender liquid, harmonize construction and defense. Indications: Stomach vacuity and reduced food intake, spleen weak and sloppy stool, insufficiency of *qi*-blood-fluids, construction-defense disharmony, heart palpitation and fearful throbbing, visceral agitation.

Common Jujube Seed; SUAN ZAO REN Origin: *Ziziphus jujuba* Mill. var. *spinosa* (Bunge) Hu *ex* H. F. Chow (*Rhamnaceae*). Part: seed. Effects: To nourish the liver, quiet the heart, quiet the spirit, constrain sweat. Indications: Vacuity vexation and insomnia, dreaminess, fright palpitation and fearful throbbing, vexation and thirst, vacuity sweating, night sweating.

Common Knotgrass; BIAN XU Origin: *Polygonum aviculare* L. (*Polygonaceae*). Part: dried aerial parts. Effects: To clear heat, disinhibit urine and kill parasites. Indications: Short voidings of reddish urine, strangury with inhibited painful urination, blood strangury; damp ecsema, pudendal itch.

Common Lantana; WU SE MEI Origin: *Lantana camara* L. (*Verbenaceae*). Part: leaf or branchlet. Effects: To disperse swelling and resolve toxin, dispel wind and relieve itching. Indications: Swollen welling abscess, damp-toxin, scab and *lai*, toxin of sores.

Common Lophatherum Root; SUI GU ZI (DAN ZHU YE GEN) Origin: *Lophatherum gracile* Brongn. (*Gramineae*). Part: rhizome and root. Effects: To clear heat and disinhibit urine, hasten delivery.

Common Lophatherum; DAN ZHU YE Origin: *Lophatherum gracile* Brongn. (*Gramineae*). Part: aerial parts. Effects: To clear heart fire, eliminate heat vexation, disinihibit urine. Indications: Mouth and tongue sores, inhibited urination with stinging pain; vexation and thirst.

Common Marsharigold; MA TI YE Origin: *Caltha palustris* L. (*Ranunculaceae*). Part: herb. Effects: To eliminate wind and dissipate cold. Indications: Dizzy head and vision, pain in whole body.

Common Monkshood; CHUAN WU TOU (one of the **CAO WU TOU**) Origin: *Aconitum carmichaeli* Debx. (*Ranunculaceae*). Part: yuberous root. Effects: To track wind and overcome damp, disperse cold and relieve pain, open phlegm, disperse swelling. Indications: Wind-cold-damp impediment, wind stroke apralysis, lockjaw, head wind, cold pain in stomach duct and abdomen, phlegm impediment, *qi* lump, cold dysentery, throat impediment, welling abscess and flat abscess, clove sore, scrofula.

Common Nandina Fruit; NAN TIAN ZHU ZI Origin: *Nandina domestica* Thunb. (*Berberidaceae*). Part: ripe fruit. Effects: To constrain the lung and suppress cough, clear the liver and brighten the eyes. Indications: Enduring cough, panting, whooping cough, malaria, body *gan* ulceration.

Common Nandina Root; NAN TIAN ZHU GEN Origin: *Nandina domestica* Thunb. (*Berberidaceae*). Part: root. Effects: To dispel wind and eliminate dampness, clear heat and transform phlegm. Indications: Wind-heat headache, lung heat cough, damp heat jaundice, pain from wind-damp impediment (arthralgia-syndrome), fire eyes, sore, scrofula.

Common Nandina Stem; NAN TIAN ZHU GENG Origin: *Nandina domestica* Thunb. (*Berberidaceae*). Part: branchlet. Effects: To settle cough and check panting,

Common Nasturtium; HAN LIAN HUA Origin: *Tropaeolum majus* L. (*Tropaeolaceae*). Part: herb. Effects: To clear heat and resolve toxin. Indications: Toxin of sores, sore red swollen eyes, malign sore.

Common onion; YANG CONG Origin: *Allium cepa* L. (*Liliaceae*). Part: bulb. Indications: Wound, ulcerating sore, trichomonal vaginitis.

Common Origanum; TU XIANG RU Origin: *Origanum vulgare* L. (*Labiatae*). Part: herb. Effects: To resolve the exterior, rectify *qi*, and transform dampness. Indications: Wind damage and cold, fever, vomiting, distention and fullness in the chest and diaphragm, diarrhea, jaundice, child *gan* accumulation.

Common Pearleverlasting; DA YE BAI TOU WENG Origin: *Anaphalis margaritacea* (L.) Benth. *et* Hook. f. (*Compositae*). Part: herb (with root). Effects: To clear heat, drain fire, and dry dampness. Indications: Blood ejection, dysentery, toothache, mammary welling abscess, scrofula.

Common Peganum Herb; LUO TUO PENG Origin: *Peganum harmala* L. (*Zygophyllaceae*). Part: herb. Effects: To diffuse lung *qi*, dispel wind-damp, and disperse toxin swelling. Indications: Cough and shortness of breath, pain from wind-damp impediment (arthralgia-syndrome), itchy skin, innominate toxin swelling.

Common Peganum Seed; LUO TUO PENG ZI Origin: *Peganum harmala* L. (*Zygophyllaceae*). Part: seed. Effects: To diffuse lung, relieving cough and asthma, dispel wind-damp. Indications: Cough and panting, inhibited urination, numbness of the limbs, aching pain in joints.

Common Peony (wild); SHAO YAO (one of the **CHI SHAO YAO**) Origin: *Paeonia lactiflora* Pall. (*Ranunculaceae*). Part: root. Effects: To remove pathogenic heat and eliminate pathogenic heat from the blood, to activate blood circulation and dispel blood stasis. Indications: Epidemic febrile diseases manifested as fever, maculas or eruptions, or bleeding such as blood ejection, spontaneous external bleeding; menstrual block and menorrhalgia; blood-shot eyes with swelling pain from liver-heat, suppurative infections on the body surface; painful swelling of traumatic injuries.

Common peony; BAI SHAO YAO Origin: *Paeonia lactiflora* Pall. (*Ranunculaceae*). Part: root. Effects: To check hyperactivity of the liver, to soften the liver and relieve pain, and to astringe *yin* and nourish blood. Indications: Irregular menstruation, menstrual pain, flooding and spotting; spontaneous or night sweating; pain in the hypochondrium, stomach and abdomen, and pain in the extremities; headache and vertigo.

Common Perilla Fruit; BAI SU ZI Origin: *Perilla frutescens* (L.) Britt. (*Labiatae*). Part: fruit. Effects: To lower body *qi* and disperse phlegm, relieve cough and panting, moisten intestines and loosen the bowels. Indications: Stagnation of phlegm, cough, panting, constipation.

Common Pheasant; ZHI Origin: *Phasianus colchicus* Gmelin (*Phasianidae*). Part: meat. Effects: To supplement the spleen and boost *qi.* Indications: Dysentery, diabetes, frequent urination.

Common Physochlaina; PAO NANG CAO Origin: *Physochlaina physaloides* (L.) G. Don (*Solanaceae*). Part: root or herb. Effects: Root: to supplement vacuity and worm the center, quiet the spirit and stabilize panting; herb: to clear heat and resolve toxin, dispel damp and kill worms. Indications: Root: vacuity cold diarrhea, taxation damage, coughing of phlegm panting, disquieted heart spirit; herb: otitis media, paranasal sinusitis, sore swollen throat, swelling and toxin of sore and welling abscess, headache.

Common Pistache; HUANG LIAN YA Origin: *Pistacia chinensis* Bge. (*Anacardiaceae*). Part: leaf, bud. Effects: To clear heat, resolve toxin, and allay thirst. Indications: Summerheat thirst, sand, dysentery, sore swollen throat, ulceration of the mouth and tongle, wind-damp sore, lacquer sore.

Common Quince; WEN PO Origin: *Cydonia oblonga* Mill. (*Rosaceae*). Part: fruit. Effects: To precipitate *qi* disperse food. Indications: Vomiting of sour water, food accumulation and chest oppression.

Common Reed Rhizome; LU GEN Origin: *Phragmites communis* Trin. (*Gramineae*). Part: rhizome. Effects: To remove heat, promote secretion, arrest vomiting, relieve fidgets and induce diuresis. Indications: Heat damaging liquid, heat vexation and thirst; stomach heat and retching; lung heat cough, cough due to external contraction of wind and heat; dribbling urination with reddish urine and stinging pain.

Common Rue Herb; CHOU CAO Origin: *Ruta graveolens* L. (*Rutaceae*). Part: herb. Effects: To dispel wind, abate heat, disinhibit urine, quicken the blood, resolve toxin, and disperse swelling. Indications: Common cold with fever, wind-damp bone pain, fright wind in children, inhibited urination, diarrhea, mounting *qi,* menstrual block, knocks and falls, heat toxin sore, eczema.

Common Sage Herb; LI ZHI CAO Origin: *Salvia plebeia* R. Br. (*Labiatae*). Part: aerial parts. Effects: To cool the blood, disinhibit water, resolve toxin, and kill worms. Indications: Coughing of blood, blood ejection, bloody urine, flooding and spotting, ascites, white turbidity, swelling and pain in the throat, swollen welling abscess, hemorrhoid.

Common Scouring Rush; MU ZEI Origin: *Equisetum hiemale* L. (*Equisetaceae*). Part: aerial parts. Effects: To course wind and dissipate heat, to brighten eyes and eliminate nebulous eye screens, to stanch bleeding. Indications: Red eyes and tearing, nebulous eye screens; bloody stool, hemorrhoidal bleeding.

Common Selfheal; XIA KU CAO Origin: *Prunella vulgaris* L. (*Labiatae*). Part: spike. Effects: To clear liver fire, dissipate stasis and bind, and lower blood pressure. Indications: Liver fire flaming upward, sore red swollen eyes, headache, dizziness; phlegm-fire depression, scrofula, goiter; hypertension.

Common Sinopodophyllm; TAO ER QI Origin: *Podophyllum emodi* Wall. var. *chinense* Sprague (*Berberidaceae*). Part: root and rhizome. Effects: To relieve rheumatism, promote circulation of *qi* and blood, relieve pain and stanch bleeding, and externally as an anticancer drug. Indications: Wind-damp pain (rheumatalgia), cough and panting, stomachache, knocks and falls.

Common Smoketree Branch and Leaf; HUANG LU ZHI YE Origin: *Cotinus coggygria* Scop. (*Anacardiaceae*). Part: branchlet and leaf. Effects: To eliminate dampness and heat. Indications: Jaundice, burns and scalds, lacquer sore.

Common Smoketree; HUANG LU Origin: *Cotinus coggygria* Scop. (*Anacardiaceae*). Part: wood. Effects: To eliminate heat vexation, resolve liquor jaundice. Indications: Yellow eyes, red eyes, lacquer sore, burns and scald.

Common Spiderflower Seed; BAI HUA CAI ZI Origin: *Cleome gynandra* L. (*Capparidaceae*). Part: seed. Effects: To dissipate wind and eliminate dampness, quicken the blood and relieve pain. Indications: Wind-damp impediment (arthralgia-syndrome), hemorrhoid, malaria.

Common Squill; MIAN ZAO ER Origin: *Scilla sinensis* (Lour.) Merr. (*Liliaceae*). Part: bulb or herb. Effects: To quicken the blood and resolve toxin, disperse swelling and relieve pain. Indications: Mammary welling abscess, intestinal welling abscess, knocks and falls, lumbar and leg pain.

Common St. John'swort; GUAN YE LIAN QIAO Origin: *Hypericum perforatum* L. (*Guttife-rae*). Part: herb (with root). Effects: To clear heat and resolve toxin, stanch bleeding by promoting contraction, and disinhibit damp. Indications: Hacking of blood, blood ejection, intestinal wind bleeding, bleeding of external injury, wind-damp bone pain, mouth and nose sores, toxin of sores, burns and scalds.

Common St. Paulswort; XI XIAN Origin: *Siegesbeckia orientalis* L. (*Compositae*). Part: aerial parts. Effects: To dispel wind-damp, to relieve rigidity of muscles and joints and as a sedative to relieve mantle strain. Indications: Wind-damp impediment (arthralgia-syndrome), pain in the joints, numbness or paralysis of the limbs due to wind stroke; swelling and toxin of welling abscess and sores, eczema with itching; hypertension.

Common Stelmatocrypton; SHENG TENG Origin: *Stelmatocrypton khasianum* (Benth.) H. Baill. (*Asclepiadaceae*). Part: lianoid stem or herb. Effects: To resolve the exterior and warm the center, dispel wind and free the network vessels. Indications: Common cold, trachitis, stomachache, glomus and distention, pain due to wind-damp.

Common Threewingnut; LEI GONG TENG Origin: *Tripterygium wilfordii* Hook. f. (*Celastraceae*). Part: root, leaf and flower. Effects: To kill worms, expel inflammation, resolve toxin; with high toxicity.

Common Tobacco; YAN CAO Origin: *Nicotiana tabacum* L. (*Solanaceae*). Part: leaf. Effects: To move *qi* and relieve pain, resolve toxin and kill worms. Indications: Food stagnation bloating, *qi* bind pain, welling abscess and flat abscess, clove sore, scab and lichen, snake bite, dog bite.

Common Tulip Root; YU JIN XIANG GEN Origin: *Tulipa gesneriana* L. (*Liliaceae*). Part: root. Effects: Sedation. Indications: Visceral agitation.

Common Tulip; YU JIN XIANG Origin: *Tulipa gesneriana* L. (*Liliaceae*). Part: flower. Indications: Malign *qi*.

Common turmeric; JIANG HUANG (one of the **YU JIN**) Origin: *Curcuma longa* L. (*Zingibera-ceae*). Part: tuber root. Effects: To promote blood circulation for relieving pain, to invigorate the flow of *qi* for soothing depressed liver, to clear away heat in the blood and heart, to normalize the gall and remove jaundice. Indications: Pain in the chest, hypochond-rium, stomach, abdomen; distending pain in the breasts and menstrual pain, bind in the abdomen; damp-warm syndrome, including restlessness, melancholia, epilepsy and madness, unconsciousness with feeling of stuffiness and fullness in the chest and upper abdomen; blood ejection, epiataxis, hematuria, spontaneous external bleeding during menstruation; jaundice.

Common Turmeric; JIANG HUANG Origin: *Curcuma longa* L. (*Zingiberaceae*). Part: rhizome. Effects: To break blood and move *qi*, to free menstruation and relieve pain. Indications: Pain in the chest and rib-side, menstrual block with abdominal pain due to *qi* stagnation and blood stasis, pain from wind-damp impediment (arthralgia-syndrome), early stage of swelling abscess, open sores, sores and boil.

Common Valeriana; XIE CAO Origin: *Valeriana officinalis* L. (*Valerianaceae*). Part: root and rhizome. Indications: Disquieted heart spirit, weak of stomach, lumbar pain, menstrual irregularities, knocks and falls.

Common Vetch; DA CHAO CAI Origin: *Vicia sativa* L. (*Leguminosae*). Part: herb. Effects: To clear heat and disinhibit dampness, to harmonize blood and eliminate stasis. Indications: Jaundice, edema, malaria, nosebleed, heart palpitation, dream emission, menstrual irregularities.

Common Vladimiria; MU XIANG Origin: *Vladimiria souliei* (Franch.) Ling (*Compositae*). See Common Aucklandia (Costustoot).

Common Waterhyacinth; SHUI HU LU Origin: *Eichhornia crassipes* Solms (*Pontederiaceae*). Part: herb or root. Effects: To resolve toxin and eliminate dampness, dispel wind-heat. Indications: heat sore.

Common Watershield; CHUN Origin: *Brasenia schreberi* J. F. Gmel. (*Nymphaeaceae*). Part: stem and leaf. Effects: To clear heat and disinhibit water, disperse swelling and resolve toxin. Indications: Heat dysentery, jaundice, swollen welling abscess, clove sore.

Common Wedgelet Fern; DA YE JIN HUA CAO Origin: *Stenoloma chusanum* (L.) Ching (*Lindsaeaceae*). Part: herb or rhizome. Effects: To clear heat, resolve toxin, disinhibit dampness, and stanch bleeding. Indications: Wind-heat common cold, summerheat stroke and sand, diarrhea, dysentery, white turbidity, white vaginal discharge, cough, blood ejection, bloody stool, bloody urine, *gan* of the teeth and gums, swollen welling abscess.

Common Yam; SHAN YAO Origin: *Dioscorea opposita* Thunb. (*Dioscoreaceae*). Part: rhizome. Effects: To strengthen the spleen and alleviate diarrhea, and supplement the lung and replenish vital essence. Indications: Poor appetite, lassitude or loose stool and diarrhea; cough and dyspnea due to lung deficiency; spermatorrhea, leucorrhagia, frequent urination; diabetes.

Common Yarrow Herb; YANG SHI CAO Origin: *Achillea millefolium* L. (*Compositae*). Part: herb. Effects: To clear heat and resolve toxin, harmonize the blood and regulate menstruation. Indications: Swelling and toxin of welling abscess and boil, knocks and falls, bleeding from hemorrhoids, irregular menses.

Complanate Clubmoss; GUO JIANG LONG Origin: *Lycopodium complanatum* L. (*Lycopodiaceae*). Part: herb. Effects: To course wind and overcome damp, soothe sinew and quicken the network vessels, disinhibit urine, dissipate stasis. Indications: Numbness due to damp-impediment, sinew and bone pain, strangury, knocks and falls.

Concentrated Beef Extract; XIA TIAN GAO Origin: *Bos taurus domesticus* Gmelin (*Bovidae*). Part: beef extract. Effects: To supplement *qi* and boost blood, fortify the spleen and quiet the center. Indications: Vacuity taxation with marked emaciation , wind stroke, hemiplegia, spleen vacuity and glomus accumulation, diabetes.

Conic Gymnadenia; SHOU ZHANG SHEN Origin: *Gymnadenia conopsea* R. Br. (*Orchidaceae*). Part: tuber. Effects: To supplement and boost *qi*-blood, engender liquid and allay thirst. Indications: Lung vacuity cough-panting, vacuity taxation with marked emaciation, neurosism, enduring diarrhea, loss of blood, vaginal discharge, scant breast milk, chronic hepatitis.

Contorted Tanglehead; DI JIN Origin: *Heteropogon contortus* (L.) Beauv. (*Gramineae*). Part: rhizome or herb. Effects: To clear heat and allay thirst, dispel wind and eliminate dampness. Indications: Febrile disease, diabetes, cough, vomiting and diarrhea, joint pain.

Coprinus Sporophore; GUI GAI Origin: *Coprinus atramentarius* (Bull.) Fr. (*Agaricaceae*). Part: sporophore. Indications: Child epilepsy, swollen clove, malign sore.

Coralhead Plant Seed; XIANG SI ZI Origin: *Abrus precatorium* L. (*Leguminosae*). Part: seed. Effects: Used as an antiemetic, expectorant, and parasiticide. Indications: Heart and abdomen *qi,* heat oppression headache, wind phlegm, scab, stubborn lichen.

Coralhead Plant; XIANG SI TENG Origin: *Abrus precatorium* L. (*Leguminosae*). Part: stem with leaf. Effects: To engender liquid and moisten the lung, clear heat and disinhibit urine. Indications: Sore throat, hepatitis, bronchitis.

Cordateleaf Sida; HUANG HUA ZI Origin: *Sida cordifolia* L. (*Malvaceae*). See Slimyhair Sida.

Coriander Seed; HU SUI ZI Origin: *Coriandrum sativum* L. (*Umbelliferae*). Part: dried ripe fruit. Effects: To outthrust papules, fortify the stomach. Indications: Inability to taste food, dysentery, hemorrhoid.

Corn Poppy Fruit; LI CHUN HUA GUO SHI Origin: *Papaver rhoeas* L. (*Papaveraceae*). Part: fruit. Effects: To check diarrhea, settle pain, and suppress cough.

Corn Poppy; LI CHUN HUA Origin: *Papaver rhoeas* L. (*Papaveraceae*). Part: flower or herb. Indications: Dysentery.

Corniculate Spurgentian; HUA MAO Origin: *Halenia corniculata* (L.) Cornaz. (*Gentianaceae*). Part: herb. Effects: To clear heat and resolve toxin, cool the blood and stanch bleeding. Indications: Hepatitis, angiitis, infective fever due to external injury, bleeding due to external injury.

Coromandel Lannea; HOU PI SHU Origin: *Lannea grandis* (Dennst.) Engl. (*Anacardiaceae*). Part: bark. Effects: To set a fracture, and resolve toxin. Indications: Fracture, toxin of puffer fish.

Coronarious Gingerlily; TU QIANG HUO Origin: *Hedychium Coronarium* Koen. (*Zingibera-ceae*). Part: rhizome. Effects: To eliminate wind and dissipate cold, resolve the exterior and effuse sweat. Indications: Headache, body pains, sinew and bone pain from wind-dampness, knocks and falls.

Cottonrose Hibiscus Flower; MU FU RONG HUA Origin: *Hibiscus mutabilis* L. (*Malvaceae*). Part: flower. Effects: To clear heat and cool blood, to disperse swelling and resolve toxin. Indications: Swollen welling abscess, clove sore, scalds, lung-heat cough, blood ejection, flooding and spotting, white vaginal discharge.

Cow Milk; NIU RU Origin: *Bos taurus domesticus* Gmelin or *Bubalus bubalis* Linnaeus (*Bovidae*). Part: milk. Effects: To supplement vacuity and detriment, boost the lung and stomach, engender liquid and moisten the intestine. Indications: vacuity, weak, taxation and detriment; stomach reflux and dysphagia-occlusion, diabetes, constipation.

Cow-bezoar (Ox-gallstone); NIU HUANG Origin: *Bos taurus domesticus* Gmelin or *Bubalus bubalis* Linnaeus (*Bovidae*). Part: gallstone. Effects: To remove heat from the heart, induce resuscitation, eliminate phlegm, relieve convulsion, and remove heat and toxic substance. Indications: High fever and unconsciousness, spasm and convulsion, or acute infantile convulsion; unconsciousness and delirium, apoplexy, infantile convulsion and epilepsy due to retention of phlegm-heat in the interior; sore throat, ulcers in the throat, canker sores in the mouth and on the tongue, carbuncles, boils and other pyogenic skin infections due to accumulation of toxic heat.

Cowberry Fruit Leaf; YUE JU YE Origin: *Vaccinium vitis-idaea* L. (*Ericaceae*). Part: leaf. Effects: To disinhibit urine and resolve toxin. Indications: Gonorrheal urethritis, cystitis, acute rheumatism.

Cowherb; WANG BU LIU XING Origin: *Vaccaria segetalis* (Neck.) Garcke (*Caryophyllaceae*). Part: seed. Effects: To quicken the blood and promote milk secretion, to disperse swelling and close sores. Indications: Menstrual block, breast milk stoppage, difficult delivery, blood strangury, swollen welling abscess, incised wound pain.

Crassnerve Gymnadenia; SHOU ZHANG SHEN Origin: *Gymnadenia crassinervis* Finet (*Orchidaceae*). See Conic Gymnadenia.

Creeping Rockfoil; HU ER CAO Origin: *Saxifraga stolonifera* (L.) Meerb. (*Saxifragaceae*). Part: herb. Effects: To dispel wind and clear heat, cool the blood and resolve toxin. Indications: Wind papules, eczema, otitis media, cinnabar toxin, cough with blood ejection, pulmonary welling abscess, flooding and spotting, hemorrhoid.

Creeping Rostellularia; JUE CHUANG Origin: *Rostellularia procumbens* (L.) Nees (*Acanthaceae*). Part: dried whole plant. Effects: To clear heat and resolve toxin, disinhibit dampness and disperse stagnation, quicken the blood and relieve pain. Indications: Common cold with fever, cough, sore throat, malaria, dysentery, jaundice, nephritis and general edema, sinew and bone pain, child *gan* accumulation and malnutrition, welling abscess and flat abscess, clove sore, knocks and falls.

Creeping Skyflower Leaf; JIA LIAN QIAO YE Origin: *Duranta repena* L. (*Verbenaceae*). Part: leaf. Effects: To quicken stasis and disperse swelling.

Crescent-shaped Euphorbia Herb; MAO YAN CAO Origin: *Euphorbia lunulata* Bge. (*Euphorbiaceae*). Part: whole herb. Effects: To expel phlegm, settle cough, calm asthma, draw out toxin, relieve itching. Indications: Scrofula.

Crispateleaf Ardisia Leaf; BAI LIANG JIN YE Origin: *Ardisia crispa* (Thunb.) A. DC. (*Myrsinaceae*). Part: leaf. Effects: To free strangury. Indications: Sores, injury.

Crispateleaf Ardisia; BAI LIANG JIN Origin: *Ardisia crispa* (Thunb.) A. DC. (*Myrsinaceae*). Part: root and rhizome. Effects: To clear heat, dispel phlegm, and disinhibit damp. Indications: Sore swollen throat, lung disease with cough, inhibited coughing of phlegm, damp-heat jaundice, nephritis with edema, dysentery, white turbidity, wind-damp bone pain, toothache, swelling and pain in testis.

Crisped Common Perilla Leaf; ZI SU YE Origin: *Perilla frutescens* (L.) Britt. var. *crispa* (Thunb.) Hand. -Mazz. (*Labiatae*). Part: leaf. Effects: To dissipate cold and resolve the exterior, move *qi* and loosen center, resolve toxin. Indications: Wind-cold common cold, fever, aversion to cold, headache, nosal congestion, cough and oppression in the chest; spleen-stomach *qi* stagnation, oppression in the chest and vomiting; vomiting in pregnancy and fullness and oppression in the chest and abdomen; abdominal pain, vomiting and diarrhea due to eating fish or crab, verruca vulgaris.

Crisped Common Perilla Seed; ZI SU ZI Origin: *Perilla frutescens* (L.) Britt. var. *crispa* (Thunb.) Hand. -Mazz. (*Labiatae*). Part: seed. Effects: Downbear *qi* and transform phlegm, calm asthma, moisten the intestines. Indications: Phlegm congestion and *qi* counterflow, cough and panting, intestinal dryness with constipation,chronic trachitis,

Crisped Common Perilla Stem; ZI SU GENG Origin: *Perilla frutescens* (L.) Britt. var. *crispa* (Thunb.) Hand. -Mazz. (*Labiatae*). Part: stem. Effects: Loosen the center and rectify *qi,* relieve pain, quiet the fetus. Indications: Glomus and oppression in the chest and diaphragm, stomach duct pain, belching and vomiting, stirring fetus.

Crisped Dock; NIU ER DA HUANG Origin: *Rumex crispus* L. (*Polygonaceae*). Part: root. Effects: To clear heat and cool blood, transform phlegm and suppress cough, free stool and kill worms. Indications: Acute hepatitis, chronic trachitis, blood ejection, flooding, purple patches due to thrombopenia, dry bound stool, dysentery, scab and lichen, bald sores, clove sore, boil.

Crownofhorns Euphorbia; TIE HAI TANG Origin: *Euphorbia milii* Ch. des Moulins (*Euphorbia-ceae*). Part: stem, leaf and root. Effects: To expel the pus, resolve toxin, and expel water. Indications: Welling abscess, bubo sore, hepatitis, greater abdonem edema,

Crucian Carp; JIN YU Origin: *Carassium auratus* (L.) (*Cyprinidae*). Part: meat or body. Effects: To clear heat, disinhibit water, and resolve toxin. Indications: Water drum distention, jaundice, cough.

Cubeba Piper; BI CHENG QIE Origin: *Piper cubeba* L. (*Lauraceae*). Part: fruit. Effects: To warm up the spleen and kidney, and to promote the circulation of *qi* and relieve pain. Indications: Pain due to stomach-cold, vomiting, hiccough; inhibited urination due to cold pattern; turbid urine in children.

Cucumber; HUANG GUA Origin: *Cuccumis sativus* L. (*Cucurbitaceae*). Part: fruit. Effects: To remove heat, disinhibit water, and resolve toxin. Indications: Vexation and thirst, sore swollen throat, fire eyes, burns and scald.

Cudweed; SHU QU CAO Origin: *Gnaphalium affine* D. Don (*Compositae*). Part: herb. Effects: To suppress cough and transform phlegm, dispel wind cold. Indications: Cough with profuse phlegm, asthma, wind-cold common cold, sinew and bone pain, white vaginal discharge, welling abscess and open sore.

Cuneate Lespedeza; YE GUAN MEN Origin: *Lespedeza cuneata* (Dum.Cours.) G. Don (*Leguminosae*). Part: herb with root. Effects: To tonify the liver and kidney, boost lung yin, dissipate stasis and eliminate swelling. Indications: Emission, enuresis, white turbidity, white vaginal discharge, asthma, stomachache, taxation damage, child *gan* accumulation, diarrhea, knocks and falls, loss of visual acuity, red eyes, mammary welling abscess.

Curly Bristlethistle; FEI LIAN Origin: *Carduun crispus* L. (*Compositae*). Part: root or herb. Effects: To dispel wind, clear heat, disinhibit damp, cool the blood and dissipate stasis. Indications: Wind-heat common cold, head wind dizziness, wind-heat impediment, itchy skin, urethral infection, chyluria, bloody urine, vaginal discharge, stasis and swelling from knocks and falls, swelling and toxin of clove sore, burns and scalds.

Cushaw Seed; NAN GUA ZI Origin: *Cucurbita moschata* (Duch.) Poiret (*Cucurbitaceae*). Part: seed. Effects: To expel worms. Indications: Cestodiasis, ascariasis; schistosomiasis.

Cushaw; NAN GUA Origin: *Cucurbita moschata* (Duch.) Poiret (*Cucurbitaceae*). Part: fruit. Effects: To supplement the spleen and boost *qi,* expel inflammation and relieve pain, resolve toxin and kill worms.

Cuspidate Mnium Herb; SHUI MU CAO Origin: *Mnium cuspidatum* Hedw. (*Mniaceae*). Part: herb. Effects: To stanch bleeding. Indications: Nosebleed, flooding and spotting.

Cutechu; HAI ER CHA Origin: *Acacia catechu* (L.) Willd (*Leguminosae*). Part: stem and leaf. Effects: To clear heat and transform phlegm, stanch bleeding, disperse food, engender flesh, and settle pain. Indications: Phlegm heat cough, diabetes, blood ejection, spontaneous external bleeding, bloody urine, blood dysentery, flooding, child indigestion, *gan* of the teeth and gum, mouth sore, throat impediment, wet sore.

Daghestan Sweetclover Herb; PI HAN CAO Origin: *Melilotus suaveolens* Ledeb. (*Leguminosae*). Part: herb. Effects: To clear heat and resolve toxin, transform dampness, kill worms. Indications: Summerheat-heat and oppression in the chest, malaria, dysentery, strangury, sore of the skin.

Dahuria Gentian; QIN JIAO Origin: *Gentiana dahurica* Fisch. (*Gentianaceae*). See Largeleaf Gentian.

Dahurian Angelica; BAI ZHI Origin: *Angelica dahurica* (Fisch. *ex* Hoffm.) Benth. *et* Hook. f. *ex* Franch. *et* Sav. (*Umbelliferae*). Part: root. Effects: To expel pathogenic wind from the body surface, to remove dampness, arrest pain, and to reduce swelling and promote pus discharge. Indications: Wind-cold common cold with headache and nosal congestion; headache, toothache, especially in the forehead and superciliary region; infections on the body surface, acute mastitis, sores, swellings; leukorrhagia; stomachache.

Dahurian Angelica; XING AN BAI ZHI (one of the **DU HUO**) Origin: *Angelica dahurica* (Fisch. *ex* Hoffm.) Benth. *et* Hook. f. *ex* Franch. *et* Sav. (*Umbelliferae*). See Doubleteeth Pubescent Angelica.

Dahurian Patrinia; HUANG HUA BAI JIANG (one of the **BAI JIANG**) Origin: *Patrinia scabiosaefolia* Fisch. (*Valerianaceae*). See Whiteflo-wer Patrinia.

Dahurian Rhododendron; MAN SHAN HONG Origin: *Rhododendron dauricum* L. (*Ericaceae*). Part: leaf. Effects: To suppress cough and dispel phlegm. Indications: Cough, chronic bronchitis, bronchial asthma.

Danshen; DAN SHEN Origin: *Salvia miltiorrhiza* Bge. (*Labiatae*). Part: root. Effects: To quicken the blood and dispel blood stasis, to remove heat and cool the blood and to tranquilize the mind. Indications: Gynecological diseases (menstruation disorders, obstetrical problems), ectopic pregnancy, epigastric and abdominal pain, bind in the abdomen, hepatosplenomegaly, traumatic injuries, arthritis of heat type; sores, carbuncles; vexation and insomnia; coronary heart disease; thromboangitiites obliterans (Buerger's disease).

Dateplum Persimmon; JUN QIAN ZI Origin: *Diaspyros lotus* L. (*Ebenaceae*). Part: fruit. Effects: To allay heat-vexation and thirst, settle the heart, moisturize the complexion. Indications: Heat-vexation, diabetes.

David Peach Bast; TAO JING BAI PI Origin: *Prunus davidiana* (Carr.) Franch. (*Rosaceae*). See Peach Bast.

David Peach Flower; TAO HUA Origin: *Prunus davidiana* (Carr.) Franch. (*Rosaceae*). See Peach Flower.

David Peach Juvenile Branch; TAO ZHI Origin: *Prunus davidiana* (Carr.) Franch. (*Rosaceae*). See Peach Juvenile Branch.

David Peach Leaf; TAO YE Origin: *Prunus davidiana* (Carr.) Franch. (*Rosaceae*). See Peach Leaf.

David Peach Root; TAO GEN Origin: *Prunus davidiana* (Carr.) Franch. (*Rosaceae*). See Peach Root.

David's Maidenhair Fern; ZHU ZONG CAO Origin: *Adiantum davidii* Franch. (*Adiantaceae*). See Maidenhair Fern.

Decumbent Bugle Herb; BAI MAO XIA KU CAO Origin: *Ajuga decumbens* Thunb. (*Labiatae*). Part: herb. Effects: To suppress cough and transform phlegm, clear heat and cool the blood, eliminate swelling and resolve toxin. Indications: Sore swollen throat, swelling of welling abscess, sores, and boil, pulmonary welling abscess, intestinal welling abscess; lung-heat cough with yellow and concentrated phlegm; coughing of blood due to blood-heat, spontaneous external bleeding, or bleeding due to external injury.

Decumbent Corydalis; XIA TIAN WU Origin: *Corydalis decumbens* (Thunb.) Pers. (*Papaveraceae*). Part: rhizome. Effects: To lower the blood pressure and settle tetany, move *qi* and relieve pain, quicken the blood and dispel stasis. Indications: Hypertension, hemiplegia, rheumatic arthritis, sciatica, sequel of infantile paralysis (Heine-Medin disease).

Delavay Fritillary; LENG SHA BEI MU (one of the **CHUAN BEI MU**) Origin: *Fritillaria delavayi* Franch. (*Liliaceae*). See Tendrilleaf Fritillary.

Delavay Larkspur; XIAO CAO WU Origin: *Delphinium delavayi* Franch. (*Ranunculaceae*). See Yunnan Larkspur.

Delavay Stephania; DI BU RONG Origin: *Stephania delavayi* Diels (*Menispermaceae*). Part: tuber. Effects: To clear heat and resolve toxin, eliminate phlegm, interrupt malaria, and relieve pain. Indications: Swelling and toxin of welling abscess and flat abscess, throat block, malaria, stomachache.

Deltoid Goldthread; HUANG LIAN Origin: *Coptis deltoidea* C. Y. Cheng *et* Hsiao (*Ranuncula-ceae*). See Chinese Goldthread.

Densefruit Pittany Root-bark; BAI XIAN PI Origin: *Dictamnus dasycarpus* Turcz. (*Rutaceae*). Part: root bark. Effects: To dispel and remove dampness, heat and toxins. Indications: Damp-heat sore and papules, profuse pus or yellow-water sore, damp ulceration on the skin, itchy skin; damp-heat jaundice, damp-heat impediment.

Denticulate Vladimiria; MU XIANG Origin: *Vladimiria denticulata* Ling (*Compositae*). See Common Aucklandia (Costustoot).

Depressed Plantain; CHE QIAN Origin: *Plantago depressa* Willd. (*Plantaginaceae*). See Asiatic Plantain.

Desertliving Cistanche; ROU CONG RONG Origin: *Cistanche deserticola* Y. C. Ma (*Orobancha-ceae*). See Saline Cistanche.

Dichotomous Fimbristylis; PIAO FU CAO Origin: *Fimbristylis dichotoma* (L.) Vahl (*Cyperaceae*). Part: herb. Effects: To disinhibit urine.

Diels Millettia; JI XUE TENG Origin: *Millettia dielsiana* Harms *ex* Diels (*Leguminosae*). See Suberect Spatholobus.

Diels Trema; SHAN YOU MA Origin: *Trema dielsiana* Hard.-Mazz. (*Ulmaceae*). Part: leaf. Effects: To relieve pain, stanch bleeding. Indications: Boil toxin.

Diffract Usnea Filament; SONG LUO Origin: *Usnea diffracta* Vain. (*Usneaceae*). See Long Usnea Filament.

Diffuse Erysimum; TANG JIE Origin: *Erysimum diffusum* Ehrh. (*Cruciferae*). Part: seed. Effects: To clear the heat in blood, suppress cough, strengthen the heart, and resolve toxin of meat. Indications: Vacuity consumption with fever, pulmonary tuberculosis with cough, insufficiency of heart force.

Dill Fruit; SHI LUO ZI Origin: *Anethum graveolens* L. (*Umbelliferae*). Part: fruit. Effects: To worm the spleen and the kidney, open the stomach, move *qi*, disperse cold, and resolve toxin of fish andmeat. Indications: Sand foulness retching, cold pain in the abdomen, cold mounting, glomus and fullness with reduced eating.

Diluteyellow Crotalaria; HUANG HUA DI DING Origin: *Crotalaria albida* Heyne (*Legumino-sae*). Part: herb. Effects: To clear heat, resolve toxin, and disinhibit urine. Indications: Enduring cough with phlegm and diarrhea, urethritis, cystitis, welling abscess and flat abscess, clove sore.

Divaricate Saposhnikovia; FANG FENG Origin: *Saposhnikovia divaricata* (Turcz.) Schischk. (*Umbelliferae*). Part: root. Effects: To induce diaphoresis, dispel wind, remove damp and relieve pain. Indications: Exterior syndromes due to affection by exopathogens shown as headache and pantalgia; impediment, joint pain and muscular spasm; tetanus with opisthotonus, trismus, spasm and convulsion.

Divaricate Strophanthus; YANG JIAO AO ZI Origin: *Strophanthus divaricatus* (Lour.) Hook. *et* Arn. (*Apocynaceae*). Part: seed. Effects: To quicken the blood and disperse swelling, relieve itching and kill worms. Indications: Wind-damp, scab and lichen, knocks and falls, swollen sores.

Diversileaf Artocarpus; BO LUO MI Origin: *Artocarpus heterophyllus* Lam. (*Moraceae*). Part: fruit. Effects: To allay vexation and thirst, dispel the effects of liquor, boost *qi,* increase the appetite.

Diversileaf Jackinthepulpit; TIAN NAN XING Origin: *Arisaema heterophyllum* Bl. (*Araceae*). See Reddish Jackinthepulpit.

Dog Heart; GOU XIN Origin: *Canis familiaris* L. (*Canidae*). Part: heart. Effects: To eliminate *qi* evil. Indications: Wind impediment, rabid dog bite, nosebleed, sore in lower body.

Dog Meat; GOU ROU Origin: *Canis familiaris* L. (*Canidae*). Part: meat. Effects: To supplement the spleen and boost *qi,* warm the kidney and reinforce *yang.* Indications: Spleen-kidney *qi* vacuity, distention and fullness in the chest and abdomen, drum distention, puffy swelling, weakness in the lumbus and knees, cold malaria, enduring vanquished sore.

Dogbane Herb; LUO BU MA Origin: *Apoynum venetum* L. (*Apocynaceae*). Part: herb. Effects: To clear heat, lower blood pressure, strengthen the heart, and disinhibit urine. Indications: Heart diseases, hypertension, neurosism, hepatitis with abdominal distention, nephritic edema.

Dolphin; HAI TUN YU Origin: *Delphinus delphis* L. (*Delphinidae*). Part: meat or fat. Indications: Meat: miasmic malaria; fat in the skin: miasmic malaria, scab and lichen, hemorrhoids and fistulas.

Doubleteeth Pubescent Angelica; ZHONG CHI MAO DANG GUI (one of the **DU HUO**) Origin: *Angelica pubescens* Maxim. f. *biserrata* Shan *et* Yuan (*Umbelliferae*). Part: root. Effects: To dispel wind and eliminate dampness, disperse cold and relieve pain. Indications: Impediment due to wind-damp, especially in the lower part of the body, unable to walk due to pains in the waist and legs, placidity and impediment of the feet; external contraction of wind-cold and damp evil in the interior shown as headache, aching joints all over the body, slight aversion to cold.

Downy Cherry; SHAN YING TAO Origin: *Prunus tomentosa* Thunb. (*Rosaceae*). Part: fruit. Effects: To boost *qi* and secure essence. Indications: Diarrhea, seminal emission.

Downy Groundcherry; KU ZHI Origin: *Physalis pubescens* L. (*Solanaceae*). Part: herb. Effects: To clear heat and resolve toxin, disinhibit urine. Indications: Common cold, lung heat and cough, painful swelling of throat, gum swelling, damp-heat jaundice, dysentery, edema, heat strangury, heaven-borne sore, clove sore.

Downy Rosemyrtle Leaf; SHAN REN YE Origin: *Rhodomyrtus tomentosa* (Ait.) Hassk. (*Myrtaceae*). Part: leaf. Indications: Headache, diarrhea, *gan* accumulation, bleeding due to external injury, scab sore.

Dried Chinese (or Amur) Woodfrog; HA SHI MA Origin: *Rana temporaria chensinensis* David; *Rana amurensis* Boulenger (*Ranidae*). Part: dried body. Effects: To nourish the lung and the kidney. Indications: Cough from vacuity and taxation, cough due to consumptive disease.

Droughtdysentery Holarrhena Bark; ZHI XIE MU PI Origin: *Holarrhena antidysenterica* Wall. (*Apocynaceae*). Part: bark. Effects: To check diarrhea and kill worms. Indications: Diarrhea, dysentery, hypertension.

Drug Sweetflag; BAI CHANG Origin: *Acorus calamus* L. (*Araceae*). Part: rhizome. Effects: To resolve phlegm, cause resuscitation, promote digestion and remove dampness. Indications: Epilepsy, fright palpitation and forgetfulness, unclear spirit-mind, damp- stagnation glomus and distention, diarrhea, dysentery, pain due to wind-damp, swollen welling abscess, boil and sores.

Duhat Fruit; YE DONG QING QUO Origin: *Syzygium brachyantherum* Merr. *et* Perry (*Myrtaceae*). Part: fruit. Effects: To suppress cough and calm asthma. Indications: Cold asthma, anaphylactic asthma.

Dunn Wampee; YE HUANG PI Origin: *Clausena dentata* (Willd.) Roem. (*Rutaceae*). Part: leaf and root. Effects: To soothe wind and rectify *qi,* eliminate damp and harmonize stasis. Indications: Common cold, measles papules, asthma, stomachache, rheumatism, edema, sprain and contusion, fracture, dislocation.

Dwarf Flowering Cherry Seed; YU LI REN Origin: *Prunus japonica* Thunb. (*Rosaceae*). Part: ripe seed. Effects: To moisten the bowels and to relieve constipation, and to induce diuresis for eliminating edema. Indications: Constipation; edema with ascites, edema due to beriberi, difficulty in micturition.

Dwarf Lilyturf; MAI MEN DONG Origin: *Ophiopogon japonicus* (Thunb.) Ker-Gawl. (*Lilia-ceae*). Part: tuberous root. Effects: To nourish vital essence, to remove heat from the heart, and to remove dryness from the lung. Indications: Dry cough with sticky sputum or phthisical cough with hemoptysis; dry tongue and thirst; vexation and insomnia; constipation due to dryness of the bowels.

Dyers Woad Leaf; DA QING YE Origin: *Isatis tinctoria* L. (*Cruciferae*). See Indigo-coloured Woad Leaf.

Dyers Woad Root; BAN LAN GEN Origin: *Isatis tinctoria* L. (*Cruciferae*). Part: root. Effects: To clear heat and resolve toxin, to cool the blood and disinhibit throat. Indications: Fever due to warm-heat disease, headache, sore throat, maculopapular eruption, mumps, swelling and toxin of welling abscess and sores.

Eaglewood; CHEN XIANG Origin: *Aquilaria agallocha* Roxb. (*Thymelaeaceae*). Part: resinous wood. Effects: To rectify *qi* and relieve pain, to warm the center and send down flatulence. Indications: *Qi* counterflow and panting, vomiting and hiccough, pain and distention in stomach duct and abdomen, vacuity cold lumbus and knees, large intestinal vacuity constipation, *qi* strangury of urination, seminal cold. Pharmacological action: Baimuxinic acid and agarospirol in volatile oil show high bioactivity for some pharmacological models of nervous system.

Earthworm; QIU YIN Origin: *Pheretima aspergillum* (E. Perrier) (*Megascolecidae*); *Allolo-bophora caliginosa trapezoides* (Ant. Duges) (*Lumbricidae*). Part: body. Effects: To clear heat, calm the liver, check panting, free the network vessels. Indications: High fever and manic agitation, fright wind and convulsion, wind heat headache, red eyes, wind stroke and half-body paralysis (hemiplegia), panting, throat impediment, arthralgia, bleeding gums, urinary stoppage, scrofula, mumps, sore.

East-Asia Low Meadowrue; YAN GUO CAO Origin: *Thalictrum thunbergii* DC. (*Ranunculaceae*). Part: root. Effects: To clear heat and resolve toxin. Indications: Toothache, acute dermitis, eczema.

Easter Heraldtrumpet; PAO DAN GUO Origin: *Beaumontia grandiflora* Wall. (*Apocynaceae*). Part: root and leaf. Effects: To dispel wind-damp, dissipate stasis and quicken the blood, join bone. Indications: Fracture, knocks and falls, rheumatic pain in the lumbus and legs, muscular strain of the lumbar region, rheumatic arthritis.

Eastern Bracken Fern; JUE Origin: *Pteridium aquilinum* (L.) Kuhn var. *latiusculum* (Desv.) Underw (*Pteridaceae*). Part: epicormic leaf. Effects: To clear heat, transform phlegm, lubricate the intestines, downbear *qi*. Indications: Food occlusion, *qi* occlusion, intestinal wind heat toxin.

Ebracteolate Euphorbia; YUE XIAN DA JI (one of the **LANG DU**) Origin: *Euphorbia ebracteolata* Hayata (*Euphorbiaceae*). See Chinese Stellera.

Edible Tulip; GUANG CI GU Origin: *Tulipa edulis* (Miq.) Bak. (*Liliaceae*). Part: bulb. Effects: To remove heat and counteract toxins, to reduce swelling and resolve mass. Indications: Sore swollen throat, scrofula, welling abscess and flat abscess, swollen sore, postpartum stasis.

Eelgrass Herb; KU CAO (I) Origin: *Vallisneria spiralis* L. (*Hydrocharitaceae*). Part: herb. Effects: To rectify the blood of *qi*. Indications: White vaginal discharge, lochia.

Ehrenberg Myrrh; MO YAO Origin: *Balsamodendron ehrenbergianum* Berg. (*Bursera-ceae*). See Myrrh.

Elecampane Inula; TU MU XIANG Origin: *Inula helenium* L. (*Compositae*). Part: root. Effects: To fortify the spleen and harmonize the stomach, to promote circulation of *qi* and relieve pain. Indications: Distention, fullness and pain in the chest and abdomen, vomiting and diarrhea, dysentery, malaria.

Elephant Bone; XIANG GU Origin: *Elephas maximus* L. (*Elephantidae*). Part: bone. Effects: To resolve toxin.

Elephant Gall; XIANG DAN Origin: *Elephas maximus* L. (*Elephantidae*). Part: gall. Effects: To clear the liver, brighten the eyes, disperse swelling. Indications: Eye screen, *gan* accumulation, swelling of sores.

Elephant Meat; XIANG ROU Origin: *Elephas maximus* L. (*Elephantidae*). Part: meat. Indications: Bald sore.

Ellgrass; HAI DAI (DA YE ZAO) Origin: *Zostera marina* L. (*Potamogetonaceae*). Part: herb. Effects: To softenhard bind and transform phlegm, disinhibit water and drain heat. Indications: Goiter, mounting-conglomeration, edema, leg *qi* (beriberi).

Emblic Leafflower Bark; YOU GAN MU PI Origin: *Phyllanthus emlica* L. (*Euphorbiaceae*). Part: bark. Indications: Mouth sore, clove sore, hemorrhoid, eczema of scrotum, bleeding of external injury.

Emblic Leafflower Leaf; YOU GAN YE Origin: *Phyllanthus emlica* L. (*Euphorbiaceae*). Part: leaf. Indications: Skin eczema, clove sore, hemorrhoids and fistulas.

Emblic Leafflower Root; YOU GAN GEN Origin: *Phyllanthus emlica* L. (*Euphorbiaceae*). Part: root. Effects: To clear heat and resolve toxin. Indications: Diarrhea, hypertension, syphills, body *gan,* centipede bite.

Emblic Leafflower; AN MO LE Origin: *Phyllanthus emblica* L. (*Euphorbiaceae*). Part: fruit. Effects: To transform phlegm and relieve cough, engender liquid and allay thirst, resolve toxin. Indications: Common cold with fever, cough with sore throat, diphtheria, heat vexation and thirst.

English Walnut Exocarp; HU TAO QING PI Origin: *Juglans regia* L. (*Juglandaceae*). Part: exocarp. Effects: To resolve toxin and disperse swelling. Indications: Stomachache, abdominal pain, water dysentery, swelling and toxin of welling abscess and sores, oxhide lichen, fish scale lichen, lotus leaf lichen, bald sores.

English Walnut Leaf; HU TAO YE Origin: *Juglans regia* L. (*Juglandaceae*). Part: leaf. Effects: To resolve toxin and kill worms. Indications: White vaginal discharge, scab, elephant hide legs.

English Walnut Seed; HU TAO REN Origin: *Juglans regia* L. (*Juglandaceae*). Part: seed. Effects: To supplement the kidney and secure essence, warm the lung and stabilize panting, and moisten the intestines. Indications: Kidney vacuity panting and cough, lumbar pain and weak leg, impotence, seminal emission, frequent urination, stone strangury, dry bound stool.

Erect St. John's wort; XIAO LIAN QIAO Origin: *Hypericum erectum* Thunb. (*Guttiferae*). Part: herb. Effects: To quicken the blood and stanch bleeding, to regulate menstruation and free milk, to disperse swelling and relieve pain. Indications: Blood ejection, spontaneous external bleeding, endome-trorrhagia, menstrual irregularities, breast milk stoppage, swollen boil, knocks and falls, bleeding wound.

Ergot; MAI JIAO Origin: *Claviceps purpurea* (Fr.) Turasne (*Clavicipitaceae*). Part: sclerotium. Effects: To stanch bleeding. Indications: Uterine bleeding, incessant postpartum bleeding, hemilateral headache.

Eucalyptus Leaf; AN YE Origin: *Eucalyptus gloulus* Labill. (*Myrtaceae*). Part: leaf. Effects: To resolve heat. Indications: Common cold, influenza, dysentery, enteritis, arthralgia, cystitis, scalds, scab and lichen, cinnabar toxin, neurodermatitis, eczema, swelling and toxin of welling abscess and sore.

Eucommia; DU ZHONG Origin: *Eucommia ulmoides* Oliv. (*Eucommiaceae*). Part: bark. Effects: To supplement the liver and the kidney, reinforce muscles and bones, and to prevent abortion and lower blood pressure. Indications: Aches in the loins and knees, lassitude of the muscles, impotence, frequent urination; flooding and spotting, orthreatened abortion and vaginal bleeding; hypertension with deficiency of the kidney.

Eumenol Angelica; BAI ZHI Origin: *Angelica anomala* Lallem. (*Umbelliferae*). See Dahurian Angelica.

European Grape Stem and Leaf; PU TAO TENG YE Origin: *Vitis vinifera* L. (*Vitaceae*). Part: stem and leaf. Indications: Edema, inhibited urination, red eyes, swollen welling abscess.

European Grape; PU TAO Origin: *Vitis vinifera* L. (*Vitaceae*). Part: fruit. Effects: To supplement *qi* and blood, strengthen sinew and bone, disinhibit urine. Indications: Vacuity of *qi* and blood, lung vacuity and cough, heart palpitation and night sweating, pain from wind-damp impediment (arthralgia-syndrome), strangury, general edema.

European Hop Female-flower; PI JIU HUA Origin: *Humulus lupulus* L. (*Moraceae*). Part: female-flower. Effects: To fortify the stomach and disperse food, disinhibit urine and quiet the spirit. Indications: Indigestion, abdominal distention, general edema, cystitis, pulmonary tuberculosis, insomnia.

European Pyrola Herb; LU XIAN CAO Origin: *Pyrola rotundifolia* L. (*Pyrolaceae*). See Chinese Pyrola Herb.

European Verbena Herb; MA BIAN CAO Origin: *Verbena officinalis* L. (*Verbenaceae*). Part: herb (with root). Effects: To remove heat, induce diuresis, eliminate blood stasis and reduce swelling. Indications: Externally contracted fever, damp-heat jaundice, edema, dysentery, malaria, diphtheria, throat impediment, strangury, menstrual block, concretions and conglomerations, swelling and toxin of welling abscess and sores, *gan* of the teeth and gums.

European Waterhemlock Root; DU QIN GEN Origin: *Cicuta virosa* L. (*Umbelliferae*). Part: root. Indications: Medullitis (external use only, with high toxicity)

Evergreen Dogwood; JI SU ZI Origin: *Cornus capitata* Wall. [= *Dendrobenthamia capitata* (Wall.) Hutch] (*Cornaceae*). Part: leaf and fruit. Effects: To clear heat and resolve toxin, disinhibit water and kill worms. Indications: Hepatitis, ascites, roundworm, burns and scalds.

Evergreen Euonymus; DIAO JING CAO Origin: *Euonymus japonicus* Thunb. (*Celastraceae*). Part: root. Effects: To regulate menstruation and transform stasis. Indications: Menstrual irregularities, menstrual pain

Eyeshaped Dendrobium; LIU SU SHI HU (one of the **SHI HU**) Origin: *Dendrobium fimbriatum* Hook. var. *oculatum* Hook. (*Orchidaceae*). See Noble Dendrobium.

False Chinese Swertia; ZHANG YA CAI Origin: *Swertia pseudochinensis* Hara (*Gentianaceae*). Part: herb. Effects: To clear heat, fortify the stomach, disinhibit dampness. Indications: Indigestion, gastritis, Jaundice, fire eyes, toothache, mouth sore.

Falsesour Cherry; YING TAO Origin: *Prunus pseudocerasus* Lindl. (*Rosaceae*). Part: fruit. Effects: To boost *qi,* dispel wind-damp. Indications: Paralysis, numbness of the limbs, rheumatic pain in the lumbus and legs, frostbite.

Fangchi; GUANG FANG JI (one of the **FANG JI**) Origin: *Aristolochia fangchi* Wu (*Aristolochiaceae*). See Fourstamen Stephania.

Felthair pyrrosia frond; SHI WEI Origin: *Pyrrosia drakeana* (Franch.) Ching (*Polypodiaceae*). See Japanese Felt Fern Frond.

Fennel Fruit; HUI XIANG Origin: *Foeniculum vulgare* Mill. (*Umbelliferae*). Part: fruit. Effects: To warm the kidney and disperse cold, harmonize the stomach and rectify *qi.* Indications: Cold mounting, cold pain in the lesser-abdomen, kidney vacuity and lumbar pain, stomachache, vomiting, dry or wet leg *qi* (beriberi).

Fennel Root; HUI XIANG GEN Origin: *Foeniculum vulgare* Mill. (*Umbelliferae*). Part: root. Effects: To warm the kidney and harmonize the center, move *qi* and relieve pain. Indications: Cold mounting, stomach cold retching, abdominal pain, wind-damp (rheumatism) with painful joints.

Fennel Stem and Leaf; HUI XIANG JING YE Origin: *Foeniculum vulgare* Mill. (*Umbelliferae*). Part: stem and leaf. Effects: To expel wind, normalize *qi,* and relieve pain. Indications: Sand *qi,* mounting *qi,* swollen welling abscess.

Field Bindweed; TIAN XUAN HUA Origin: *Convolvulus arvensis* L. (*Convolvulaceae*). Part: herb and flower. Effects: To dispel wind and relieve pain, relieve itching. Indications: Neurodermatitis, tooth-ache, rheumatic arthritis.

Field Grounsel Herb; DA BAI DING CAO Origin: *Senecio orgzetorum* Diels (*Compositae*). Part: herb. Effects: To clear heat and resolve toxin. Indications: White mouth sore in children, clove sore.

Field Lacquertree; LIN BEI ZI Origin: *Toxicodendron succedaneum* (L.) O. Kuntze [= *Rhus succedanea* L.] (*Anacardiaceae*). Part: root or root bark. Effects: To clear heat and resolve toxin, stanch bleeding. Indications: Bloody urine, flooding, vaginal discharge, sore and lichen.

Field Sowthistle Herb; NIU SHE TOU Origin: *Sonchus arvensis* L. (*Compositae*). Part: herb. Effects: To clear heat and resolve toxin. Indications: Appendicitis, dysentery, hemorrhoid, emission, white turbidity, mastitis, swelling and toxin of sore and boil, burns and scalds.

Fig Leaf; WU HUA GUO YE Origin: *Ficus carica* L. (*Moraceae*). Part: leaf. Effects: To eliminate damp-heat and resolve sore and toxin. Indications: Pain in heart region, swelling and toxin, hemorrhoid.

Fig; WU HUA GUO Origin: *Ficus carica* L. (*Moraceae*). Part: succuylent receptacle. Effects: Used as a gastrotonic, laxative, antiphlogistic and detoxicant. Indications: Enteritis, dysentery, constipation, hemorrhoid, throat pain, welling abscess and sores, scab and lichen.

Figwortflower Picrorhiza; HU HUANG LIAN Origin: *Picrorrhiza scrophulariaeflora* Pennell (*Scrophulariaceae*). See Picrorhiza..

Filiform Cassytha; WU YE TENG Origin: *Cassytha filiformis* L. (*Lauraceae*). Part: herb. Effects: To clear heat and disinhibit damp, to cool blood and resolve toxin. Indications: Liver-heat emaciation, lung-heat cough, jaundice, dysentery, nosebleed, blood strangury, swollen welling abscess, scab sore, scalds.

Fineleaf Schizonepeta; JING JIE Origin: *Schizonepeta tenuifolia* (Benth.) Briq. (*Labiatae*). Part: aerial parts. Effects: To cause diaphoresis and expel wind, and promote eruption. Indications: Externally contracted wind-cold shown as aversion to cold, fever, headache, no sweating; exterior syndrome due to wind-heat shown as fever, headache, bloodshot eyes, sore throat; German measles, pruritus, measles without adequate eruption; blood ejection, spontaneous external bleeding, bloody stool, flooding and spotting.

Fingerleaf Rodgersflower; MU HE Origin: *Rodgersia aesculifolia* Batal. (*Saxifragaceae*). Part: rhizome. Effects: To clear heat and transform damp, stanch bleeding and engender flesh. Indications: Damp-heat dysentery, enduring diarrhea, white turbidity, vaginal discharge, flooding and spotting, blood ejection, spontaneous external bleeding, bloody stool, toxin of sores, incised wound.

Fischer Euphorbia; LANG DU DA JI (one of the **LANG DU**) Origin: *Euphorbia fischeriana* Steud. (*Euphorbiaceae*). See Chinese Stellera..

Fistular Onion; CONG BAI Origin: *Allium fistulosum* L. (*Liliaceae*). Part: fresh bulb. Effects: To effuse the exterior, free *yang*, resolve toxin. Indications: Wind-cold common cold; abdominal drarrhea, reversal cold and faint pulse due to *yin* cold; sore, welling abscess, and clove.

Fiveleaf Akebia Root; MU TONG GEN Origin: *Akebia quinata* (Thunb.) Decne. (*Lardizabala-ceae*). See Austral Akebia Root.

Fiveleaf Akebia; MU TONG Origin: *Akebia quinata* (Thunb.) Decne. (*Lardizabalaceae*). See Austral Akebia.

Fiveleaf Gynostemma; QI YE DAN (JIAO GU LAN) Origin: *Gynostemma pentaphylla* (Thunb.) Makino (*Cucurbitaceae*). Part: herb. Effects: To expel inflammation and resolve toxin, suppress cough and transform phlegm. Indications: Chronic trachitis.

Flannel Mullein; MAO RUI HUA Origin: *Verbascum thapsus* L. (*Scrophulariaceae*). Part: herb. Effects: To clear heat and resolve toxin, stanch bleeding and dissipate stasis. Indications: Pneumonia, chronic appendicitis, toxin of sores, sprain from knocks and falls, bleeding from wounds.

Flatshoot Mistletoe; FENG XIANG JI SHENG Origin: *Viscum articulatum* Burm. f. (*Loranthaceae*). Part: branchlet and leaf. Effects: To dispel wind and quicken the blood, eliminate dampness, suppress cough and dispel phlegm. Indications: Aching pain of the lumbus and limbs, wind-damp bone pain, taxation damage and cough, red and white dysentery, flooding and spotting, vaginal discharge, postpartum blood-*qi* pain, sore and scab.

Flatspine Pricklyash Leaf; YE HUA JIAO YE Origin: *Zanthoxylum simulans* Hance (*Rutaceae*). Part: leaf. Effects: To dispel wind and dissipate cold, fortify the stomach and expel worms, eliminate damp and check diarrhea, quicken the blood and free the. Indications: Knocks and falls, rheumatalgia, pain of blood stasis, menstrual block, hacking of blood, blood ejection, pain wind in joints.

Fleshfingered Citron; FO SHOU (FO SHOU GAN) Origin: *Citrus medica* L. var. *sarcodactylis* (Noot.) Swingle (*Rutaceae*). Part: fruit. Effects: To rectify *qi* and relieve pain, to fortify the stomach and resolve phlegm. Indications: Stomach pain, rib-side distention, vomiting, dysphagia-occlusion, phlegm-rheum cough and panting.

Flixweed Tansymustard Seed; TING LI ZI Origin: *Lepidium sophia* (L.) Schur (*Cruciferae*). See Pepperweed Seed.

Florida Waltheria; HE TA CAO Origin: *Waltheria americana* L. (*Sterculiaceae*). Part: root and stem. Effects: To expel wind-evil and dispel damp, expel inflammation and resolve toxin. Indications: White vaginal discharge, welling abscess and boil, mastitis.

Florists Chrysanthemum Flower; JU HUA Origin: *Chrysanthemum morifolium* Ramat. (*Compositae*). Part: capitulum. Effects: To dispel wind and heat, remove the heat from the liver and brighten the eyes, and as an antipyretic and detoxicant. Indications: Externally contracted wind-heat or epidemic febrile diseases, fever, dizziness, headache; conjunctival congestion with swelling pain; hyperactivity of the liver-yang shown as headache, dizziness, feeling of fullness in the head.

Fomes Officinalis Sporophore; A LI HONG (LUO YE SONG XUN) Origin: *Fomes officinalis* (Vill. *et* Fr.) Ames (*Polyporaceae*). Part: sporophore. Effects: To warm the lung and resolve phlegm, activate blood and disperse swelling, downbear *qi* and calm panting, dispel wind and eliminate dampness. Indications: Cough, asthma, stomachache, urethral stone, nephritis, chronic rheumatic arthritis, laryngopharyngitis, peridentitis, poisonous snake bites.

Forbes Notopterygium; KUAN YE QIANG HUO (one of the **QIANG HUO**) Origin: *Notoptery-gium forbesii* Boiss. (*Umbelliferae*). See Incised Notopterygium.

Forest Gray Gum Leaf; XI YE AN YE Origin: *Eucalyptus tereticornis* Smith (*Myrtaceae*). Part: leaf. Indications: Common cold, cough, *qi* distention abdominal pain, diarrhea and dysentery, knocks and falls; toxin sore, ulcerating sore.

Fortune Eupatorium; PEI LAN Origin: *Eupatorium fortunei* Turcz. (*Compositae*). Part: aerial parts. Effects: To remove dump and relieve heat-stroke. Indications: Damp obstructing the middle-*jiao*; external contraction summer-heat.

Fortune Paulownia Fruit; PAO TONG GUO Origin: *Paulownia fortunei* (Seem.) Hemsl. (*Scrophulariaceae*). Part: fruit. Effects: To eliminate the phlegm, suppress cough, and relieve asthma. Indications: Chronic trachitis.

Fortune Paulownia; TONG MU (PAO TONG) Origin: *Paulownia fortunei* (Seem.) Hemsl. (*Scrophulariaceae*). Part: wood. Indications: Swelling starting from the feet.

Fortune Plumyew Brench and Leaf; SAN JIAN SHAN Origin: *Cephalotaxus fortunei* Hook. f. (*Cephalotaxaceae*). Part: branchlet and leaf. Effects: Antitumour activity. Indications: Malignant tumour.

Fortune Plumyew Seed; TU XIANG FEI (SAN JIAN SHAN ZI) Origin: *Cephalotaxus fortunei* Hook. f. (*Cephalotaxaceae*). Part: seed. Indications: Food accumulation, roundworm disease; malignant tumour.

Fortune's Holly Fern; HUN JI TOU Origin: *Cyrtomium fortunei* J. Sm. (*Dryopteridaceae*). Part: rhizome. Effects: To clear heat and resolve toxin, cool the blood and extinguish wind, dissipate stasis and stanch bleeding, expel worms. Indications: Common cold, febrile disease, maculopapular eruption, sand foulness, malaria, hepatitis, liver *yang* dizziness and headache, blood ejection, flooding, vaginal discharge, mammary welling abscess, scrofula, knocks and falls.

Forture Euonymus; FU FANG TENG Origin: *Euonymus fortunei* (Turcz.) Hand.-Mazz. (*Celastraceae*). Part: stem and leaf. Effects: To soothe sinew and quicken the network vessels, stanch bleeding and disperse stasis. Indications: Taxation detriment of lumbar flesh, pain from wind-damp impediment (arthralgia-syndrome), hacking of blood, flooding, menstrual irregularities, traumatic injury with fracture, bleeding from wounds.

Fourstamen Stephania; FEN FANG JI (one of the **FANG JI**) Origin: *Stephania tetrandra* S. Moore (*Menispermaceae*). Part: root. Effects: To dispel wind-damp, relieve, and disinhibit water. Indications: Arthralgia due to wind-damp, joint pain due to cold-damp, placidity and swelling pain of the lower limbs; beriberi; edema, ascites and difficulty in micturition.

Foxtail Millet; SU MI Origin: *Setaria italica* (L.) Beauv. (*Gramineae*). Part: seed. Effects: To harmonize the center and benefit the kidney, eliminate heat and resolve toxin. Indications: Vacuity heat of the spleen and stomach, stomach reflux vomiting, diabetes, diarrhea.

Foxtail-like Sophora; KU DOU ZI Origin: *Sophora alopecuroides* L. (*Leguminosae*). Part: herb and seed. Effects: To clear heat and dry dampness, relieve pain and kill worms.

Fragile Codium Frond; SHUI SONG Origin: *Codium fragile* (Sur.) Har. (*Codiaceae*). Part: frond. Indications: Edema, stream toxin, hasten delivery.

Fragrant Citrus Seed; CHEN ZI HE Origin: *Citrus junos* Tanaka (*Rutaceae*). Part: seed. Indications: Mounting *qi*, stranguries, lumbar pain.

Fragrant Eupatorium Herb; FEI JI CAO Origin: *Eupatorium adoratum* L. (*Compositae*). Part: herb. Effects: To kill worms and stanch bleeding, Indications: Dry leech bite.

Fragrant Glorybower; CHOU MO LI Origin: *Clerodendron fragrans* Vent. (*Verbenaceae*). Part: root and leaf. Effects: To dispel wind and eliminate dampness, quicken the blood and disperse swelling. Indications: Wind-damp bone pain, leg *qi* (beriberi), edema, hemorrhoid, prolapse of the rectum, itchy papules, scab sore, chronic medullitis.

Fragrant Solomonseal; YU ZHU Origin: *Polygonatum odoratum* (Mill.) Druce (*Liliaceae*). Part: rhizome. Effects: To nourish yin, moisten dryness, eliminate vexation, and allay thirst. Indications: Febrile disease wearing *yin*, cough with vexation and thirst, vacuity-taxation with fever, swift digestion with rapid hungering, frequent urination.

Franchet Groundcherry Root; SUAN JIANG GEN Origin: *Physalis alkekengi* L. var. *franchetii* (Mast.) Mak. (*Solanaceae*). Part: root. Effects: To clear heat and disinhibit water. Indications: Malaria, jaundice, mounting *qi*.

Franchet Groundcherry; SUAN JIANG Origin: *Physalis alkekengi* L. var. *franchetii* (Mast.) Mak. (*Solanaceae*). Part: herb. Effects: To clear heat and resolve toxin, disinhibit urine. Indications: Heat cough, sore throat, jaundice, dysentery, edema, clove sore, cinnabar toxin.

French Marigold Herb; KONG QUE CAO Origin: *Tagetes patula* L. (*Compositae*). Part: herb. Effects: To clear heat and disinhibit damp, suppress cough. Indications: Cough, dysentery.

Fresh Common Ginger; SHENG JIANG Origin: *Zingiber officinale* Rosc. (*Zingiberaceae*). Part: fresh rhizome. Effects: To cause diaphoresis, to warm the middle-*jiao* and arrest vomiting, and to warm the lung and arrest cough. Indications: External contraction of wind and cold, aversion to cold with fever, headache, nosal congestion; stomach cold, vomiting; cough due to wind-cold invading the lung.

Fringed Iris; HU DIE HUA Origin: *Iris japonica* Thunb. (*Iridaceae*). Part: herb. Effects: To clear heat and resolve toxin, fortify the spleen and disperse accumulation. Indications: Child *gan* accu-mulation, lymphnoditis.

Fungus-infected Rice Spike; JING GU NU Origin: *Oryza sativa* L.[pathogen is *Ustilaginoidea virens* (Cke.) Tak.] (*Gramineae*). Part: spike. Indications: Galloping throat impediment.

Furcate Gloiopeltis Frond; LU JIAO CAI Origin: *Gloiopeltis furcata* (Post. *et* Rupr.) J. Ag. (*Endocladiaceae*). Part: alga. Effects: To clear heat, disperse food, and transform phlegm. Indications: Taxation fever, phlegm bind, glomus accumulation, hemorrhoid.

Galanga Galangal; DA LIANG JIANG Origin: *Alpinia galanga* (L.) Swartz. (*Zingiberaceae*). Part: rhizome. Effects: To worm stomach, dissipate cold, and relieve pain. Indications: *Qi* pain in the regain of the heart and stomach, stomach cold, food damage vomiting and drainage.

Galanga Resurrectionlily; SHAN NAI Origin: *Kaempferia galanga* L. (*Zingiberaceae*). Part: rhizome. Effects: To promote *qi* circulation, warm the middle-*jiao* and relieve pain. Indications: Cold pain in heart region and abdomen, stagnation of food, knocks and falls, toothache.

Gambier Gambirplant; HAI ER CHA Origin: *Uncaria gambier* Roxb. (*Rubiaceae*). See Cutechu.

Gamboge Tree Resin; TENG HUANG Origin: *Garcinia morella* Desv. (*Guttiferae*). Part: gum resin. Effects: To disperse swelling and transform toxin, stanch bleeding and kill worms. Indications: Swelling and toxin of welling abscess and flat abscess, stubborn lichen, malign sore, bleeding from damage, *gan* of the teeth and gum, burns and scalds.

Garden Balsam Seed; JI XING ZI Origin: *Impatiens balsamina* L. (*Balsaminaceae*). Part: ripe seed. Effects: To softenhard bind and remove food stagnancy, break the blood. Indications: Menstrual block, accumulation lamp, dysphagia-occlusion, swollen and harden open sore, bones stuck in the throat.

Garden Balsam; TOU GU CAO Origin: *Impatiens balsamina* L. (*Balsaminaceae*). See Tuberculate Speranskia.

Garden Balsum Flower; FENG XIAN HUA Origin: *Impatiens balsamina* L. (*Balsaminaceae*). Part: flower. Effects: To dispel wind and quicken the blood, disperse swelling and relieve pain. Indications: Wind-damp hemiplegia, lumber and rib-side pain, menstrual block and abdominal pain, posttpartum bloodstasis, knocks and falls, welling abscess and flat abscess, clove sore, goose-foot wind, ashen nail.

Garden Balsum Root; FENG XIAN GEN Origin: *Impatiens balsamina* L. (*Balsaminaceae*). Part: root. Effects: To quicken the blood and free the channels, soften hardness and disperse swelling. Indications: Sinew and bone pain due to wind-damp, painful swelling from knocks and falls, bones stuck in the throat.

Garden Burnet; DI YU Origin: *Sanguisorba officinalis* L. (*Rosaceae*). Part: root. Effects: To remove the heat from the blood and stanch bleeding, to treat carbuncle and promote tissue regeneration. Indications: Various kinds of bleeding, especially for hemorrhoidal bleeding, hemafetic, flooding and spotting, dysentery with bloody stool; eczema, skin ulceration and scalds.

Garden Eggplant Leaf; QIE YE Origin: *Solanum melongena* L. (*Solanaceae*). Part: leaf. Indications: Blood strangury, blood dysentery, intestinal wind bleeding, swollen welling abscess, frostbite.

Garden Eggplant; QIE ZI Origin: *Solanum melongena* L. (*Solanaceae*). Part: fruit. Effects: To clear heat and quicken the blood, relieve pain and disperse swelling. Indications: Intestinal wind bleeding, heat toxin welling abscess and sore, uncerating sore of skin.

Garden Euphorbia Herb; DA FEI YANG CAO Origin: *Euphorbia hirta* L. (*Euphorbiaceae*). Part: herb (with root). Effects: To clear heat and resolve toxin, **percolate** dampness and relieve itching, free milk. Indications: Acute enteronitis, bacillary dysentery, strangury, bloody urine, welling abscess of the lung, mammary welling abscess, clove sore, toxin swelling, eczema, foot lichen, itchy skin.

Garden Lettuce; WO JU Origin: *Lactuca sativa* L. (*Compositae*). Part: seed. Effects: To promote lactation and as a diuretic. Indications: Inhibited urination, bloody urine, breast milk stoppage.

Garden Millingtonia; ZI MEI SHU Origin: *Millingtonia hortensis* L. f. (*Bignoniaceae*). Part: bark or leaf. Effects: To eliminate wind and relieve itching, expel worm and resolve toxin, suppress cough and transform phlegm. Indications: Urticaria, eczema, leptochroa, roundworm, cough with phlegm and panting.

Garden Pansy; SAN SE JIN Origin: *Viola tricolor* L. (*Violaceae*). Part: herb. Effects: To suppress cough. Indications: Cough, scrofula in children, inflammation in respiratory.

Garden Pea; WAN DOU Origin: *Pisum sativum* L. (*Leguminosae*). Part: seed. Effects: To harmonize the center and precipitate *qi,* disinhibit urine, resolve sore toxin. Indications: Cholera cramps, leg *qi* (beriberi), swollen welling abscess.

Garden Radish Seed; LAI FU ZI Origin: *Raphanus sativus* L. (*Cruciferae*). Part: seed. Effects: To precipitate *qi* and stabilize panting, disperse food and transform phlegm. Indications: Abdominal distention, eructation with fetid odour and acid regurgitation; abdominal pain, diarrhea with tenesums; retention of excessive phlegm, cough, dyspnea.

Garden Radish; LAI FU Origin: *Raphanus sativus* L. (*Cruciferae*). Part: fresh root. Effects: To disperse accumulation and stagnation, transform phlegm heat, precipitate *qi,* loosen the center, and resolve toxin. Indications: Food accumulation with distention and fullness, phlegm cough with loss of voice, blood ejection, spontaneous external bleeding, diabetes, dysentery, hemilateral headache, headache.

Garden Sorrel Leaf; SUAN MO YE Origin: *Rumex acetosa* L. (*Polygonaceae*). Part: leaf. Indica-tions: Sore swollen throat, bleeding of the gum, spleen vacuity with diarrhea, painful stasis from knocks and falls, hemorrhoid.

Garden Sorrel; SUAN MO Origin: *Rumex acetosa* L. (*Polygonaceae*). Part: root. Effects: To clear heat, disinhibit urine, cool the blood, and kill worms. Indications: Heat dysentery, strangury, urinary stoppage, blood ejection, malign sore, scab and lichen.

Garlic; DA SUAN Origin: *Allium sativum* L. (*Liliaceae*). Part: bulb. Effects: To resolve toxin, fortify the stomach, move *qi*, disperse concretions and accumulations, and kill worms. Indications: Accumulated food, cold pain in the stomach duct and abdomen, water swelling with distention and fullness, diarrhea, dysentery, malaria, whooping cough, swelling, toxin of welling abscess and flat abscess, bald white scalp sore, snake or insect bites.

Ghostplant Wormwood; YA JIAO AI Origin: *Artemisia lactiflora* Wall. *ex* DC. (*Compositae*). Part: herb. Effects: To dispel wind and relieve cough, quicken blood and harmonize stasis. Indications: Headache, cough, diarrhea, bloody stool, bloody urine, menstrual block, white vaginal discharge, postpartum abdomen pain, swelling and pain of welling abscess and flat abscess, knocks and falls, burns and scalds.

Giant Typhonium; YU BAI FU Origin: *Typhoniun giganteum* Engl. (*Araceae*). Part: tuber root. Effects: To dry dampness and transform phlegm, dispel wind and check tetany, resolve toxin and dissipate bind. Indications: Wind-phlegm congestion, deviated eyes and mouth, lockjaw, hemilateral headache; snake bite, scrofula and phlegm node.

Giantreed Rhizome; LU ZHU GEN Origin: *Arundo donax* L. (*Gramineae*). Part: rhizome. Effects: To clear heat and disinhibit water. Indications: Febrile disease and mania, vacuity taxation with steaming bone, strangury, inhibited urination, wind-fire toothache.

Gigantic Angelica; TU DANG GUI (II) Origin: *Angelica gigas* Nakai (*Umbelliferae*). Part: root. Effects: To extinguish wind and harmonize the blood. Indications: Pain in joints, wrenching and spraining.

Ginkgo Bark; BAI GUO SHU PI Origin: *Ginkgo biloba* L. (*Ginkgoaceae*). Part: bark. Indications: Oxhide lichen, copper coin lichen.

Ginkgo Leaf; BAI GUO YE Origin: *Ginkgo biloba* L. (*Ginkgoaceae*). Part: leaf. Effects: To boost the heart and constrain the lung, transform damp and check diarrhea. Indications: Oppression in the chest and pain in the heart region, heart palpitation and fearful throbbing, phlegm panting with cough, diarrhea, white vaginal discharge.

Ginkgo Nut; BAI GUO Origin: *Ginkgo biloba* L. (*Ginkgoaceae*). Part: nut. Effects: To constrain the lung and stabilize panting, stop vaginal discharge and turbidity, reduce urination. Indications: Cough with phlegm, wheezing and panting, white vaginal discharge, white turbidity, seminal emission, strangury, frequent urination.

Ginkgo Root; BAI GUO GEN Origin: *Ginkgo biloba* L. (*Ginkgoaceae*). Part: root. Effects: To boost *qi* and supplement vacuity. Indications: White vaginal discharge, seminal emission.

Ginseng; REN SHEN Origin: *Panax ginseng* C. A. Mey. (*Araliaceae*). Part: root. Effects: To reinforce *qi* and restore pulse from collapse, to supplement the lung and the spleen, to promote secretion of body fluid and relieve mental stress. Indications: Prodromal manifestations of prostration syndrome due to deficiency of *qi*; deficiency syndrome of the spleen; syndrome of deficiency of the lung-*qi*; thirst and diabetes due to impairment of body fluid; irritability, insomnia, dreaminess, palpitation induced by fright, forgetfulness, listlessness, lassitude and others due to deficiency of both the heart and spleen; syndromes of deficiency of the blood or both the *qi* and blood.

Glabrous Sarcandra; JIU JIE CHA Origin: *Sarcandra glabra* (Thunb.) Nakai (*Chloranthaceae*). Part: leaf and branchlet. Effects: To clear away heat, eliminate wind and blood stasis, and to set a fracture. Indications: Pneumonia, acute appendicitis, acute gastroenteritis, bacillary dysentery, wind-damp pain (rheumatalgia), knocks and falls, bone fracture.

Glabrousleaf Chinese Corktree; HUANG BAI Origin: *Phellodendron chinense* Schneid. var. *glabriusculum* Schneid. (*Rutaceae*). See Amur Corktree..

Glandularstalk St. Paulswort; XIAN GENG XI XIAN (one of the **XI XIAN**) Origin: *Siegesbeckia orientalis* L. var. *pubescens* Mak. (*Compositae*). See Common St. Paulswort.

Glaucousback Honeysuckle; JIN YIN HUA Origin: *Lonicera hypoglauca* Miq. (*Captifoliaceae*). See Japanese Honeysuckle.

Globeamaranth; QIAN RI HONG Origin: *Gomphrena globosa* L. (*Amaranthaceae*). Part: inflorescence or herb. Effects: To clear liver, dissipate bind, suppress cough and calm panting. Indications: Head wind, eye pain, panting (asthma) and cough, dysentery, whooping cough, fright in children, scrofula, sore.

Globefish; HE TUN Origin: *Fugu ocellatus* (Osbeck) (*Tetraodontidae*). Part: meat. Effects: To supplement vacuity and remove damp, an extremely toxic substance.

Glossy Privet Fruit; NU ZHEN ZI Origin: *Ligustrum lucidum* Ait. (*Oleaceae*). Part: fruit. Effects: To supplement the liver and kidney, strengthen lumbus and knees, brighten the eyes. Indications: *Yin* vacuity internal heat, dizzy head, flowery vision, ringing in the ears, limp aching lumbus and knees, premature graying.

Gmelin Sealavender Herb; BU XUE CAO Origin: *Limonium gmelinii* (Willd.) O. Ktze. (*Plumbaginaceae*). Part: herb. Effects: To stanch bleeding and dissipate stasis. Indications: Dysfunctional uterine bleeding, cervical carcinoma.

Goat Hide; YANG PI Origin: *Capra hircus* L.; *Ovis aries* L. (*Bovidae*). Part: hide. Effects: To supplement vacuity and and taxation. Indications: Wind, vacuity wind in the lung.

Goat Milk; YANG RU Origin: *Capra hircus* L.; *Ovis aries* L. (*Bovidae*). Part: milk. Effects: To warm and supplement vacuity. Indications: Vacuity taxation with emaciation and weakness, diabetes, stomach reflux, vomiting, mouth sore, lacquer sore.

Goat Pancreas; YANG YI Origin: *Capra hircus* L.; *Ovis aries* L. (*Bovidae*). Part: pancreas. Effects: To moisten the lung and dispel phlegm. Indications: Enduring cough, vaginal discharge, sores.

Goering Lemongrass; YE XIANG MAO Origin: *Cymbopogon goeringii* (Steud.) A. Camus (*Gramineae*). Part: herb. Effects: To relieve cough and calm asthma, expel inflammation and relieve pain, check diarrhea, stanch bleeding, dispel wind-damp, disperse swelling, free the channels and network vessels, and increase the appetite. Indications: Acute and chronic bronchitis, bronchial asthma, rheumatic arthritis, headache, knocks and falls, diarrhea, *qi* pain in the region of the heart and stomach, abdominal pain.

Golden Buckwheat Root; TIAN QIAO MAI GEN Origin: *Fagopyrum cymosum* Meisr. (*Polygo-naceae*). Part: root and rhizome. Effects: To resolve toxin, to dispel wind and. Indications: Sore swollen throat, and sores, scrofula, hepatitis, pulmonary welling abscess, aching sinews and bones, head wind, stomachache, bacillary dysentery, white vaginal discharge.

Golden Lycoris; DA YI ZHI JIAN Origin: *Lycoris aurea* Herb. (*Amaryllidaceae*). Part: burb. Effects: To resolve sore toxin, eliminate swollen welling abscess, and kill worms. Indications: Swollen welling abscess, clove sore with subcutaneous nodes, burns and scalds.

Goldenflower Dendrobium; SHU HUA SHI HU (one of the **SHI HU**) Origin: *Dendrobium chrysanthum* Wall. (*Orchidaceae*). See Noble Dendrobium.

Goldenshower Senna Fruit; PO LUO MEN ZAO JIA Origin: *Cassia fistula* L. (*Leguminosae*). Part: fruit. Indications: Heat wind in region of the heart and diaphragm, steaming bone fever and chills, three worms.

Goldsaxifrage Herb; JIN QIAN KU YE CAO Origin: *Chrysosplenium grayanum* Maxim. (*Saxifra-gaceae*). Part: herb. Indications: Clove sore.

Goose Fat; BAI E GAO Origin: *Anser domestica* Geese (*Anatidae*). Part: fat of goose. Effects: To moisten the skin and disperse swollen welling abscess. Indications: Erosion of the skin.

Goose Tail-meat; E CUI Origin: *Anser domestica* Geese (*Anatidae*). Part: tail meat. Indications: Purulent ear, deafness.

Graceful Jessamine; GOU WEN Origin: *Gelsemium elegans* Benth (*Loga-niaceae*). Part: herb. Effects: To dispel wind and attack toxin, eliminate swelling and relieve pain; with high toxicity. Indications: Scab and *lai*, eczema, scrofula, clove sore, knocks and falls, pain from wind-damp impediment (arthralgia-syndrome), neurodynia. In clinic: for hepatoma, carcinoma, cancer of the esooophagus with moderate effects.

Gram Chickpea; HUI HUI DOU Origin: *Cicer arietinum* L. (*Leguminosae*). Part: seed. Indications: Diabetes.

Grassleaf Sweetflag Leaf; SHI CHANG PU YE Origin: Acorus gramineus Soland. (*Araceae*). Part: leaf. Indications: Scab, great wind sore.

Grassleaf Sweetflag; SHI CHANG PU Origin: *Acorus gramineus* Soland. (*Araceae*). Part: rhizome. Effects: To induce resuscitation, expel phlegm, remove dump and normalize the functioning of the stomach. Indications: Loss of consciousness and confusion of the mind; palpitation, insomnia, amnesia and tinnitus; oppressed feeling in the chest, abdominal distention, anorexia and poor appetite.

Great Burdock Fruit; NIU BANG ZI Origin: *Arctium lappa* L. (*Compositae*). Part: fruit. Effects: To course wind and dissipate heat, to resolve toxin and outthrust papules, and to relieve sore-throat. Indications: External contraction of wind-heat, cough and difficulty in coughing of phlegm, sore swollen throat; inhibited eruption of measles papules, wind-heat papules; heat-toxin sore and swelling, mumps.

Great Burdock Root; NIU BANG GEN Origin: *Arctium lappa* L. (*Compositae*). Part: root. Effects: To dispel wind-heat, to eliminate swelling and toxin. Indications: swollen face due to wind-toxin, dizzy head, heat-swollen throat, toothache, cough, diabetes, welling abscess and flat abscess, sore and scab.

Great Willowherb (Firewood); HONG KUAI ZI Origin: *Chamaenerion angustifolium* (L.) Scop. [= *Epilobium angustifolium* L.] (*Onagraceae*). Part: herb. Effects: To moisten the intestines and promote lactation. Indications: *Qi* vacuity and puffy swelling, intestinal efflux diarrhea, food accumulation with distention and fullness, swollen kidney sac.

Greater Celandine; BAI QU CAI Origin: *Chelidonium majus* L. (*Papaveraceae*). Part: herb. Effects: To settle pain and suppress cough, disinhibit urine and resolve toxin. Indications: Gastroin-testinal pain, jaundice, edema, scab and lichen, swelling of sores, snake bite, insect bite.

Grecian Laurel; YUE GUI ZI Origin: *Laurus nobilis* L. (*Lauraceae*). Part: fruit. Effects: To resolve toxin. Indications: Child intertrigo behind ear, scab and lichen.

Green Alectoria Filament; JIN SI DAI Origin: *Alectoria vivens* Tayl. (*Usneaceae*). Part: filament. Effects: To eliminate wind-damp, stanch bleeding and relieve pain, regulate menstruation and quicken the blood, quiet the spirit with sedation, fortify the spleen and stomach. Indications: Taxation damage with lumbar and leg pain, bleeding due to external injury, menstrual irregularities, prolapse of uterus, white vaginal discharge, mental disease, epilepsy, hemiplegia, impotence, dizzy head and vision.

Greenish Lily; BAI HE Origin: *Lilium brownii* F. E. Brown var. *colchesteri* Wils. (*Liliaceae*). Part: bulb. Effects: To moisten the lung and arrest cough, to ease mental anxiety and to promote digestion. Indications: Cough due to dryness of the lung, phthisical cough with hemoptysis, and for the later stage of febrile diseases.

Guava Bark; FAN SHI LIU PI Origin: *Psidium guajava* L. (*Myrtaceae*). Part: bark. Indications: Damp toxin of scab sore, toothache, sore and boil in children.

Guava Immature Fruit; FAN SHI LIU GAN Origin: *Psidium guajava* L. (*Myrtaceae*). Part: unripe fruit. Effects: To stop drain. Indications: Dysentery

Guava Leaf; FAN SHI LIU YE Origin: *Psidium guajava* L. (*Myrtaceae*). Part: leaf. Effects: To promote contraction and stop drain. Indications: Diarrhea, enduring dysentery, eczema, bleeding from wounds, itchy skin, prickly heat.

Gypsophila; HUANG JIE GU DAN Origin: *Gypsophila acutifolia* Fisch. (*Caryophyllaceae*). Part: root. Effects: To quicken blood and dissipate stasis, disperse swelling and relieve pain, transform putridity and engender flesh. Indications: Knocks and falls, fracture, traumatic injury.

Gypsum Fibrosum; SHI GAO Origin: Calcium sulphate, $CaSO_4$symbol 215 \f "Symbol" \s 9·}H_2O. Effects: To remove intense heat and dysphoria and to quench thirst, and, when calcined, used externally as an astringent to promote tissue regeneration. Indications: Acute febrile diseases shown as high fever, dysphoria, thirst, sweating, full pulse; panting, shortness of breath, vexation, thirst; headache, swollen and painful gum; slow-healing uncerated sores, eczema, burns, scalds.

Haichow Elsholtzia; XIANG RU Origin: *Elsholtzia splendens* Nakai *ex* F. Maekawa (*Labiatae*). Part: aerial parts. Effects: To induce diaphoresis, eliminate summer-heat and remove damp, disinhibit water and disperse swelling. Indications: Fever, aversion to cold, headache, no sweating, abdominal pain, vomiting and diarrhea due to external contraction of wind-cold or summer-dampness; edema and inhibited urination.

Hairstalk St. Paulswort; MAO GENG XI XIAN (one of the **XI XIAN**) Origin: *Siegesbeckia orientalis* L. var. *glabrescens* Mak. [=*Siegesbeckia glabrescens* Mak.] (*Compositae*). See Common St. Paulswort.

Hairy Antler; LU RONG Origin: *Cervus nippon* Temminck; *Cervus elaphus* L. (all *Cervidae*). Part: hairy young horn of mail deer or stag. Effects: To invigorate the kidney-*yang*, replenish vital essence and blood and strengthen muscles and bones. Indications: Aversion to cold, coldness in the extremities, impotence, spermatorrhea, sterility due to uterine coldness, frequent urination, soreness of the loins and knees, dizziness, tinnitus, listlessness; placidity of extremities, infantile maldevelopment, delayed walking and dentition, infantile metopism; metrorrhagia, metrostaxis and profuse leucorrhea; deep-rooted carbuncle.

Hairy Chestnut Bast; LI SHU PI Origin: *Castanea mollissima* Bl. (*Fagaceae*). Part: bast. Indications: Cinnabar toxin, *lai*, mouth sore, lacquer sore, knocks.

Hairy Datura Flower; YANG JIN HUA Origin: *Datura innoxia* Mill. (*Solanaceae*). See Hindu Datura Flower.

Hairy Datura Leaf; MAN TUO LUO YE Origin: *Datura inoxia* Mill. (*Solanaceae*). See Hindu Datura Leaf.

Hairy Datura Root; MAN TUO LUO GEN Origin: *Datura inoxia* Mill. (*Solanaceae*). See Hindu Datura Root.

Hairy Datura Seed; MAN TUO LUO ZI Origin: *Datura inoxia* Mill. (*Solanaceae*). See Hindu Datura Seed.

Hairy Willowweed; SHUI JIE GU DAN Origin: *Epilobium hirsutum* L. (*Onagraceae*). Part: flower, root, or herb with root. Effects: To quicken the blood and stanch bleeding, expel inflammation and relieve pain, eliminate putridity and engender flesh. Indications: Profuse menstruation, bone fracture, knocks and falls, sores and boils, wollen welling abscess, scalds.

Hairystalk Tinospora; JIN GUO LAN Origin: *Tinospora capillipes* Gagn. (*Menispermaceae*). Part: root. Effects: To remove heat and toxic substance, to relieve sore-throat and reduce swelling. Indications: Acute or chronic tonsillitis, acute pharyngolaryngitis, stomatitis, mumps, mastitis, appendicitis, acute or chronic enteritis, welling abscess and flat abscess, clove sore, bacillary dysentery, stomachache, heat cough and loss of voice.

Hairyvein Agrimonia Root; LONG YA CAO GEN (XIAN HE CAO GEN) Origin: *Agrimonia pilosa* Ledeb. var. *japonica* (Miq.) Nakai (*Rosaceae*). Part: root. Indications: Red and white dysentery, menstrual block, toxin swelling, tapeworm.

Hairyvein Argimonia Rhizome; XIAN HE CAO GEN YA Origin: *Argimonia pilosa* Ledeb. var. *japonica* (Miq.) Nakai (*Rosaceae*). Part: rhizome. Effects: To expel tapeworm. Indications: Tapeworm.

Hairyvein Argimonia; XIAN HE CAO Origin: *Argimonia pilosa* Ledeb. var. *japonica* (Miq.) Nakai (*Rosaceae*). Part: aerial parts. Effects: To stanch bleeding and fortify the stomach. Indications: Hacking and ejecting of blood, bloody urine, bloody stool, red and white dysentery, flooding, spotting and vaginal discharge; taxation damage, swollen welling abscess, bleeding from knocks and falls.

Hard Bluegrass; LONG XU CAO (II) Origin: *Poa sphondylodes* Trin. (*Labiatae*). Part: aerial parts. Effects: To clear heat and resolve toxin, disinhibit urine, relieve pain. Indications: Dribbling and difficult urination, yellow-water sore.

Hard Clam Shell; WEN GE Origin: *Meretrix meretrix* L. (*Veneridae*). Part: shell. Effects: To clear heat and disinhibit damp, transform phlegm and soften hardness. Indications: Thirst and heat vexation, cough and counterflow, chest impediment, scrofula, phlegm node, flooding and spotting, hemorrhoids and fistulas.

Harlequin Glorybower Leaf; CHOU WU TONG Origin: *Clerodendron trichotomum* Thunb. (*Verbenaceae*). Part: leaf. Effects: To dispel wind and dampness, lower bleed pressure. Indications: Wind-damp impediment (arthralgia-syndrome), numbness of the limbs, hemiplegia, hypertension, hemicrania, malaria, dysentery, hemorrhoid, welling abscess and flat abscess, scab sore.

Harlequin Glorybower Root; CHOU WU TONG GEN Origin: *Clerodendron trchotomum* Thunb. (*Verbenaceae*). Part: root. Indications: Malaria, pain from wind-damp impediment (arthralgia-syndrome), hypertension, food accumulation bloating, child *gan* accumulation, knocks and falls.

Heartleaf Houttuynia Herb; YU XING CAO Origin: *Houttuynia cordata* Thunb. (*Saururaceae*). Part: aerial parts. Effects: To clear heat and resolve toxin, to expel pus and disinhibit urine. Indications: Pulmonary welling abscess with coughing of pus and blood, lung-heat cough with concentrated phlegm; sore due to heat and toxin; heat strangury, inhibited and painful urination.

Hedgehog Brain; WEI NAO Origin: *Erinaceus europaeus* L.; *Hemiechinus dauuricus* Sundevall (*Erinaceidae*). Part: brain. Indications: Wolf-fistula.

Hedgehog Heart and Liver; WEI XIN GAN Origin: *Erinaceus europaeus* L.; *Hemiechinus dauuricus* Sundevall (*Erinaceidae*). Part: heart and liver. Indications: Ant-fistula, bee-fistula, scrofula, malign sore.

Hedgehog Hide; CI WEI PI (WEI PI) Origin: *Erinaceus europaeus* L.; *Hemiechinus dauuricus* Sundevall (*Erinaceidae*). Part: dried sprind skin. Effects: To downbear *qi* and settle pain, to cool the blood and stanch bleeding. Indications: Stomach reflux vomiting, abdominal pain and mounting *qi*, intestinal wind hemorrhoids and fistulas, seminal emission.

Hemp Fimble Leaf; MA YE Origin: *Cannabis sativa* L. (*Moraceae*). Part: leaf. Indications: Malaria, asthma, roundworm.

Hemp Fimble Seed; HUO MA REN Origin: *Cannabis sativa* L. (*Moraceae*). Part: ripe seed. Effects: To moisten the bowels and to relieve constipation. Indications: Intestinal dry constipation.

Hemp Fimble; MA HUA Origin: *Cannabis sativa* L. (*Moraceae*). Part: male-flower. Effects: To dispel wind and quicken the blood. Indications: Numbness of the limbs, itching in whole body, menstrual block.

Hemsley Cowparsnip; HIU WEI DU HUO (one of the **DU HUO**) Origin: *Heracleum hemsleya-num* Diels (*Umbelliferae*). See Doubleteeth Pubescent Angelica.

Hen's Egg Yolk; JI ZI HUANG Origin: *Gallus gallus domesticus* Brisson (*Phasianidae*). Part: egg yolk. Effects: To enrish *yin* and moisten dryness, nourish the blood and extinguish wind. Indications: Sleepless due to vexation, febrile disease tetanic reversal, vacuity-taxation blood ejection, retching counterflow, dysentery, fetal bleeding, scalds, hepatitis, child indigestion.

Hen's Egg-albumen; JI ZI BAI Origin: *Gallus gallus domesticus* Brisson (*Phasianidae*). Part: egg white. Effects: To moisten the lung and disinhibit throat, clear heat and resolve toxin. Indications: Sore throat, red eyes, cough and counterflow, dysentery, malaria, burns, heat toxin painful swelling.

Henbit Deadnettle Herb; BAO GAI CAO Origin: *Lamium amplexicaule* L. (*Labiatae*). Part: whole plant. Effects: To dispel wind and free the network vessels, disperse swelling and relieve pain. Indications: Sinew and bone pain, numbness of the limbs, knocks and falls, scrofula.

Henna Leaf; ZHI JIA HUA YE Origin: *Lawsonia inermis* L. (*Lythraceae*). Part: leaf. Effects: To promote contraction and clear heat. Indications: external use: wounds.

Henry Acanthopanax Leaf; CAO YE WU JIA YE (one of the **WU JIA YE**) Origin: *Acanthopanax henryi* (Oliv.) Harms (*Araliaceae*). See Slenderstyle Acanthopanax Leaf.

Henry Acanthopanax Root-bark ; CAO YE WU JIA PI (one of the **WU JIA PI**) Origin: *Acan-thopanax henryi* (Oliv.) Harms (*Araliaceae*). See Slenderstyle Acanthopanax Root-bark.

Hernandialeaf Stephania; RU LAN Origin: *Stephania hernandifolia* (Willd.) Walp. (*Menisperma-ceae*). Part: root. Effects: To dispel wind and eliminate dampness, clear heat and resolve toxin. Indications: Wind-damp (rheumatism) with painful joints, summerheat stroke, dysentery, sore and toxin of welling abscess and boil.

Heterophylla Falsestarwort; TAI ZI SHEN Origin: *Pseudostellaria heterophylla* (Miq.) Pax *ex* Pax *et* Hoffm. (*Caryophyllaceae*). Part: root. Effects: To supplement the lung and replenish *qi,* strengthen the spleen, and producing the body fluid. Indications: lung vacuity cough, spleen vacuity and reduced food intake, heart palpitation with spontaneous sweating, lassitude of essence-spirit.

Himalayan Coralbean; QIAO MU CI TONG Origin: *Erythrina arborescens* Roxb. (*Leguminosae*). Part: root, leaf and fruit. Effects: To clear heat and dispel wind, fortify the spleen and disinhibit dampness. Indications: Distention and pain in the head, dysentery.

Hindu Datura Flower; YANG JIN HUA Origin: *Datura metel* L. (*Solanaceae*). Part: flower. Effects: To suppress cough and calm panting, to relieve pain and settle tetany. Indications: Cough and panting without phlegm; cold pain in heart region and abdomen, pain from wind-damp impediment (arthralgia-syndrome), knocks and falls; epilepsy, spasm and convulsion due to chronic fright wind.

Hindu Datura Leaf; MAN TUO LUO YE Origin: *Datura metel* L. (*Solanaceae*). Part: leaf. Indications: Cough and panting, impediment pain, leg *qi* (beriberi), prolapse of the rectum.

Hindu Datura Root; MAN TUO LUO GEN Origin: *Datura metel* L. (*Solanaceae*). Part: root. Indications: Malign sore, rabid dog bite.

Hindu Datura Seed; MAN TUO LUO ZI Origin: *Datura metel* L. (*Solanaceae*). Part: seed or fruit. Effects: To calm asthma, dispel wind, and relieve pain. Indications: Cough and panting, fright epilepsy, wind-cold-damp impediment, dysentery, prolapse of the rectum, knocks and falls.

Hindu Lotus Large Rhizome; OU Origin: *Nelumbo nucifera* Gaertn. (*Nymphaeaceae*). Part: rhizome. Effects: To promote traction and stanch bleeding. Indications: Various kinds of bleeding.

Hindu Lotus Leaf-base; HE YE DI Origin: *Nelumbo nucifera* Gaertn. (*Nymphaeaceae*). Part: leaf-base. Effects: To clear summerheat and remove damp, harmonize the blood and quiet the fetus. Indications: Blood dysentery, diarrhea, stirring fetus.

Hindu Lotus Leaf; HE YE Origin: *Nelumbo nucifera* Gaertn. (*Nymphaeaceae*). Part: leaf. Effects: To clear summerheat and disinhibit damp, upbear the clear and *yang*, and stanch blood. Indications: Summerheat-damp diarrhea, dizziness, water-*qi* general edema, thunder head wind, blood ejection, spontaneous external bleeding, spontaneous external bleeding, bloody stool, postpartum blood dizziness.

Hindu Lotus Petiole; HE GENG Origin: *Nelumbo nucifera* Gaertn. (*Nymphaeaceae*). Part: dried petiole and pedicel. Effects: To remove summer-heat, to promote circulation of *qi* and water. Indications: Summerheat-damp and oppression in the chest, diarrhea, dysentery, strangury, vaginal discharge.

Hindu Lotus Plumule; LIAN ZI XIN Origin: *Nelumbo nucifera* Gaertn. (*Nymphaeaceae*). Part: dried plumule and radicle in the seed. Effects: To remove heat from the heart, stanch bleeding and astringe essence, and as a tranquilizer and antihypertensive. Indications: Vexation and thirst, blood ejection, seminal emission, sore red swollen eyes, hypertension.

Hindu Lotus Seed; LIAN ZI Origin: *Nelumbo nucifera* Gaertn. (*Nymphaeaceae*). Part: seed. Effects: To relieve mental strain and strengthen the kidney, and as a stomachic and antidiarrheic. Indications: Chronic diarrhea, poor appetite; seminal emission, and spermatorrhea; restlessness, fright-induced palpitation, and insomnia; metrorrhagia, metrostaxis, and leukorrhagia.

Hirsute Respberry; CI BO Origin: *Rubus hirsutus* Thunb. (*Rosaceae*). Part: root or leaf. Effects: To clear heat and resolve toxin. Indications: Summer-heat damage with vomiting and diarrhea, wind-fire headache, common cold, jaundice.

Hispid Arthraxon Herb; JIN CAO Origin: *Arthraxon hispidus* (Thunb.) Mak. (*Gramineae*). Part: herb. Effects: To relievie cough and asthma, kill worms.

Hispid Yam; BAI SHU LANG Origin: *Dioscorea hispida* Dennst. (*Dioscoreaceae*). Part: tuber. Effects: To dissipate heat, disperse swelling, and resolve toxin. Indications: Swelling and toxin of welling abscess and flat abscess, syphilis, body *gan*, knocks and falls.

Hollowed Wampee; SHAN HUANG PI Origin: *Clausena excavata* Burm. f. (*Rutaceae*). Part: branchlet and leaf. Effects: To course wind and resolve the exterior, move *qi* and relieve pain, interrupt malaria, and kill worms. Indications: Upper respiratory track infection, influenza, malaria, abdominal pain, knocks and falls, fracture.

Hollyhock Flower; SHU KUI HUA Origin: *Althaea rosea* (L.) Cav. (*Malvaceae*). Part: flower. Effects: To harmonize the blood and moisten dryness. Indications: Dysentery, blood ejection, blood flooding, vaginal discharge, urinary and fecal stoppage, malaria, child wind papules.

Honey; FENG MI Origin: *Apis cerana* Fabricius (*Apidae*). Part: honey. Effects: To supplement the stomach and spleen, moisten the lung and lubricate the intestines, and resolve toxin. Indications: Spleen-stomach vacuity, fatigue and reduced food intake, pain in the stomach duct and abdomen; lung vacuity and enduring cough, lung dryness cough, dry throat; intestinal dryness with constipation; sores and open sores, scalds.

Hookedhairypod Tickclover; HONG MU JI CAO Origin: *Desmodium gangeticum* (L.) DC. (*Leguminosae*). Part: stem and leaf. Effects: To stanch bleeding and relieve pain, disperse stasis and dissipate swelling. Indications: Knocks and falls.

Hookedspine Bittersweet; CI NAN SHE TENG Origin: *Celastrus flagellaris* Rupt. (*Cela-straceae*). Part: root, fruit or stem. Effects: To dispel wind-damp, strengthen sinew and bone. Indications: Wind-damp pain (rheumatalgia), arthritis, painful swelling due to knocks and falls, innominate toxin swelling.

Horseweed Fleabane; QI ZHOU YI ZHI HAO Origin: *Erigeron canadensis* L. (*Compositae*). Part: herb. Effects: To clear heat and resolve toxin, dispel wind and relieve itching. Indications: Stomatitis, otitis media, conjunctivitis, wind-fire toothache, wind-damp bone pain.

Hosie Ormosia Seed; HONG DOU Origin: *Ormosia hosiei* Hemsl. *et* Wils. (*Leguminosae*). Part: seed. Effects: To rectify *qi* and free the channels. Indications: Mounting *qi*, abdominal pain, blood stagnation and menstrual block.

Human Hair; XUE YU Origin: *Homo sapiens* L. Part: human hair. Effects: To eliminate stasis and stanch bleeding. Indications: Blood ejection, nosebleed, bleeding in gums, blood dysentery, blood strangury, flooding and spotting.

Human Placenta; ZI HE CHE Origin: *Homo sapiens* L. Part: human placenta. Effects: To supplement *qi*, nourish the blood, and boost essence. Indications: Vacuity detriment, marked emaciation, taxation fever steaming bone, cough and panting, hacking of blood, night sweating, seminal emission, impotence; insufficiency of *qi* and blood, infertility, scant breast milk.

Human Urine Sediment; REN ZHONG BAI Origin: *Homo sapiens* L. Part: sediment of human urine. Effects: To clear heat, downbear fire, and disperse stasis. Indications: Taxation fever, lung wilting, spontaneous external bleeding, blood ejection, throat impediment, *gan* of the teeth and gums, mouth and tongue sores.

Human Urine; REN NIAO Origin: *Homo sapiens* L. Part: human urine. Effects: To enrich *yin* and downbear fire, to stanch bleeding and disperse stasis. Indications: *Yin*-vacuity fever, taxation damage coughing of blood, blood ejection, spontaneous external bleeding, postpartum blood stasis, blood dizziness, knocks and falls, blood stasis pain.

Humifuse Euphorbia; DI JIN CAO Origin: *Euphorbia humifusa* Willd. (*Euphorbiaceae*). Part: herb. Effects: To clear heat and resolve toxin, quicken the blood and stanch bleeding, disinhibit damp and free milk. Indications: Diarrhea due to heat toxin, swollen welling abscess, poisonous snake bite; bloody stool, bloody urine, flooding and spotting, bleeding due to external injury; damp-heat jaundice, inhibited urination.

Hyacinth Dolichos Seed; BIAN DOU Origin: *Dolichos lablab* L. (*Leguminosae*). Part: seed. Effects: Fortify the spleen and transform dampness. Indications: Spleen vacuity with damp, fatigue and lack of strength, reduced food intake and sloppy stool, or diarrhea; spleen vacuity and downpour of damp-turbidity, heavy profuse of white vaginal discharge; summerheat-damp vomiting and diarrhea.

Hypoglaucous Collett Yam; FEN BEI SHU YU (one of the **BEI XIE**) Origin: *Dioscorea hypoglauca* Palib. (*Dioscoriaceae*). Part: rhizome. Effects: To dispel wind and disinhibit dampness. Indications: Unctuous strangury; white vaginal discharge due to prevalence of damp; pain from wind-damp impediment (arthralgia-syndrome), lumbar pain.

Ignat Poisonnut Seed; LU SONG GUO Origin: *Strychnos ignatii* Berg. (*Loganiaceae*). Part: ripe seed. Indications: Stomachache, diarrhea, dysentery, malaria, worm accumulation, bleeding from wounds, centipede bite.

Bitter Orange; ZHI SHI Origin: *Citrus aurantium* L. (*Rutaceae*). Part: immature fruit. Effects: To relieve stagnation of *qi* to remove food stagnation, to resolve phlegm to relieve feeling of fullness. Indications: Abdominal distention and pain; feeling of stiffness and fullness in the chest and upper abdomen; gastroptosis; gastric dilatation; prolapse of rectum and hysteroptosis.

Immature Persimmon Fruit Juice; SHI QI Origin: *Diospyros kaki* L. f. (*Ebenaceae*). Part: fruit juice. Indications: Hypertension.

Incised Corydalis; ZI HUA YU DENG CAO Origin: *Corydalis incusa* (Thunb.) Pers. (*Papavera-ceae*). Part: herb or root. Effects: To resolve toxin and kill worms. Indications: Scab and *lai*, lichen sore.

Incised Notopterygium; QIANG HUO Origin: *Notopterygium incisum* Ting *ex* H. T. Chang (*Umbelliferae*). Part: rhizome or root. Effects: To induce diaphoresis and dispel cold, relieve rheumatism and pain. Indications: Fever, aversion to cold, headache, and pains from affection of exopathogenic wind-cold; impediment, pains in limbs and joints, especially in upper part of the body.

India Madder Root; QIAN CAO GEN Origin: *Rubia cordifolia* L. (*Rubiaceae*). Part: root. Effects: To remove heat from blood and stanch bleeding, activate blood flow and dispel blood stasis. Indications: Many kinds of bleeding due to blood heat, blood stagnation menstrual block, knocks and falls, pain from stasis, joint pain from impediment.

India Mustart Seed; JIE ZI Origin: *Brassica juncea* (L.) Czern. *et* Coss. (*Cruciferae*). Part: seed. Effects: To warm and resolve cold phlegm, to promote circulation of *qi* and relieve pain. Indications: Stomach cold and vomiting of food, pain in heart region and abdomen, lung cold and cough, painful impediment, throat impediment, flowing phlegm, knocks and falls.

Indian Abutilon Herb; MO PAN CAO Origin: *Abutilon indicum* (L.) Sweet (*Malvaceae*). Part: herb. Effects: To clear heat and disinhibit damp, open the orifices and quicken the blood. Indications: Diarrhea, strangury, tinnitus, deafness, mounting *qi,* swollen welling abscess, urticaria.

Indian Aeginetia; YE GU Origin: *Aeginetia indica* L. (*Orobanchaceae*). Part: whole plant. Indications: Sore swollen throat, urethral infection, medullitis, clove sore.

Indian Azalea Leaf; DU JUAN HUA YE Origin: *Rhododendron simsii* Planch. (*Ericaceae*). Part: leaf. Effects: To clear heat and resolve toxin, stanch bleeding. Indications: Swollen welling abscess and clove sores, bleeding due to external injury, urticaria.

Indian Azalea; DU JUAN HUA Origin: *Rhododendron simsii* Planch. (*Ericaceae*). Part: flower or fruit. Effects: To harmonize the blood and regulate menstruation, dispel wind and damp. Indications: Menstrual irregularities, menstrual block, flooding and spotting, knocks and falls, wind-damp pain (rheumatalgia), blood ejection, spontaneous external bleeding.

Indian Bread; FU LING Origin: *Poria cocos* (Schw.) Wolf (*Polyporaceae*). Part: dried sclerotium of the fungus. Effects: To promote water metabolism and remove damp, reinforce the function of the spleen and relieve mental stress. Indications: Dysuria, edema, and phlegm retention; lassitude, anorexia, and loose stool; fright palpitation and insomnia.

Indian Damnacanthus; HU CI Origin: *Dammacanthus indicus* Gaertn. f. (*Rubiaceae*). Part: herb. Effects: To dispel wind and disinhibit dampness, quicken the blood and disperse swelling. Indications: Pain wind, pain from wind-damp impediment (arthralgia-syndrome), phlegm -rheum cough, pulmonary welling abscess, edema, lump glomus, jaundice, menstrual block, child *gan* accumulation, urticaria, knocks and falls.

Indian Glorybower; CHANG GUAN JIA MO LI Origin: *Clerodendron indicum* (L.) O. Ktze. (*Verbenaceae*). Part: herb. Effects: To expel inflammation and disinhibit urine, quicken the blood and disperse swelling, dispel wind-damp. Indications: Urethral infection, cystitis, sprain from knocks and falls, wind-damp bone pain.

Indian Heliotrope; DA WEI YAO Origin: *Heliotropium indicum* L. (*Boraginaceae*). Part: herb or root. Effects: To clear heat, disinhibit urine, eliminate swelling and resolve toxin. Indications: Pneumonia, pyothorax, sore throat, vesical calculus, child acute fright wind, putrescence, swollen welling abscess.

Indian Iphigenia; CAO BEI MU Origin: *Iphigenia indica* Kunth *et* Benth (*Liliaceae*). Part: bulb. Effects: To relieve cough and asthma, settle pain, and as an anticancer. Indications: Bronchitis, asthma, carcinoma of breast, nasopharyngeal carcinoma.

Indian Jujube; MIAN ZAO Origin: *Ziziphus mauritiana* Lam. (*Rhamnaceae*). Part: bark. Effects: To expel inflammation and engender flesh. Indications: Burns and scalds.

Indian Leadword; ZI XUE HUA Origin: *Plumbago indica* L. (*Plumbaginaceae*). Part: stem, leaf or flower. Effects: To break the blood, relieve pain, and regulate menstruation. Indications: Menstrual block, abdominal pain during menstruation, damp lichen, ulcerating sore.

Indian Lettuce; SHAN WO JU Origin: *Lactuca indica* L. (*Compositae*). Part: herb. Effects: To resolve heat. Indications: Wart.

Indian Nightshade; TIAN QIE ZI Origin: *Solanum indicum* L. (*Solanaceae*). Part: fruit, seed and leaf. Effects: To dispel wind and eliminate evil. Indications: Toothache, headache, deep-source nasal congestion.

Indian Quassiawood; KU SHU PI Origin: *Picrasma quassioides* (D.Don) Benn. (*Simaroubaceae*). Part: bark, root bark, and stem. Effects: To clear heat and damp, resolve toxin and expel inflammation, kill worms. Indication: Bacterial dysentery, alimentary inflammation, infection of biliary tract, acute pyogenic infection, scabies and tinea, eczema, and snake-bite. Pharmacological action: Bacteriostasis of KU SHU PI total alkaloid against 9β-hemolytic *Streptococcus* 816, *Staphylococcus aureus* 209P, *Shigella sonnei* 51334, *Bacillus subtitis* 6633, and sarcina. antifungal (see canthin-6-one), lowering blood pressure, anti-venin.

Indian Skullcap; HAN XIN CAO Origin: *Scutellaria indica* L. (*Labiatae*). Part: herb with root. Effects: To dispel wind and quicken the blood, resolve toxin and relieve pain. Indications: Knocks and falls, blood ejection, coughing of blood, swollen welling abscess, clove toxin, throat wind, toothache.

Indian Stringbush Root; LIAO GE WANG GEN Origin: *Wikstroemia indica* (L.) C. A. Mey. (*Thymelaeaceae*). Part: root. Effects: To clear heat, disinhibit urine, resolve toxin, kill worms and break accumulation. Indications: Pneumonia, mumps, water swelling and distention, scrofula, swelling and toxin of sores (and open sores), knocks and falls.

Indian Trumpetflower Bark; MU HU DIE SHU PI Origin: *Oroxylum indicum* (L.) Vent. (*Bignoniaceae*). Part: bark. Effects: To clear heat and disinhibit damp, to disperse swelling and resolve toxin. Indications: Infective hepatitis, cystitis, sore swollen throat, eczema, ulcerating welling abscess and sores.

Indian Trumpetflower; MU HU DIE Origin: *Oroxylum indicum* (L.) Vent. (*Bignoniaceae*). Part: seed. Effects: To remove heat from the lung, relieve sore-throat, facilitate the flow of the liver-*qi* and regulate the functioning of the stomach. Indications: Cough, throat impediment, loss of voice, *qi* pain in the liver and stomach, enduring opening of a sore.

Indian Wild Chrysanthemum Flower; YE JU HUA Origin: *Chrysanthemum indicum* L. (*Compositae*). Part: flower-head. Effects: To soothe wind and clear heat, disperse swelling and resolve toxin. Indications: Wind heat common cold, pneumo-nia, diphtheria, gastroenteritis, hypertension, clove sore, welling abscess, mouth sore, cinnabar toxin, eczema, heaven-borne sore.

Indian Wild Chrysanthemum; YE JU Origin: *Chrysanthemum indicum* L. (*Compositae*). Part: herb and root. Effects: To clear heat and resolve toxin. Indications: Swollen welling abscess, clove sore, red eyes, scrofula, heaven-borne sore, eczema.

Indianpipe; SHUI JINGLAN Origin: *Monotropa uniflora* L. (*Pyrolaceae*). Part: root. Effects: To supplement vacuity and weakness. Indications: Vacuity cough.

Indigo-coloured Woad Leaf; DA QING YE Origin: *Isatis indigotica* Fort. (*Cruciferae*). Part: leaf. Effects: To clear away heat and detoxication, to cool the blood and remove ecchymosis. Indications: Epidemic febrile diseases with high fever, restlessness, maculas and eruptions, unconsciousness and delirium; erysipelas, canker sores, swollen, and sore throat.

Indigoplant Leaf; DA QING YE Origin: *Polygonum tinctorium* Ait (*Polygonaceae*). See Indigo-coloured Woad Leaf.

Indigowoad Root; BAN LAN GEN Origin: *Isatis indigotica* Fort. (*Cruciferae*). See Dyers Woad Root

Inflated Licorice; ZHANG GU GAN CAO (one of the **GAN CAO**) Origin: *Glycyrrhiza inflata* Batal. (*Leguminosae*). See Ural Licorice.

Inflatedfruit Senna; JIANG MANG Origin: *Cassia sophera* L. (*Leguminosae*). Part: seed. Effects: To remove phlegm and allay thirst, regulate the center.

Intermediate Ephedra; MA HUANG Origin: *Ephedra intermeddia* Schrenk *et* Mey. (*Ephedraceae*). See Chinese Ephedra.

Involute Spikemoss; YAN ZHOU JUAN BAI Origin: *Selaginella involvens* (Sw.) Spring (*Selagi-nellaceae*). Part: herb. Effects: To cool the blood and stanch bleeding, transform phlegm and stabilize panting, disinhibit water and eliminate swelling. Indications: Blood ejection, spontaneous external bleeding, bleeding and prolapse of the rectum, cough with phlegm, asthma, jaundice, edema, strangury, vaginal discharge, scalds.

Ivy Glorybind; MIAN GEN TENG Origin: *Calystegia hederacea* Wall. (*Convolvulaceae*). Part: herb or root. Indications: Strangury, white vaginal discharge, menstrual irregularities, child *gan* accumulation.

Japanese Alder; CHI YANG Origin: *Alnus japonica* Sieb. *et* Zucc. (*Betulaceae*). Part: bark, tender twig and leaf. Effects: To clear heat and downbear the fire. Indications: Incessant nosebleed, bleeding due to external injury, provention of water diarrhea.

Japanese Ampelopsis; BAI LIAN Origin: *Ampelopsis japonica* (Thunb.) Mak. (*Vitaceae*). Part: tuberous root. Effects: As an antipyretic, antiphlogistic and detoxicant. Indications: Swelling and toxin of welling abscess and sores, burn and scald.

Japanese Apricot; WU MEI Origin: *Prunus mume* (Sieb.) Sieb. *et* Zucc. (*Rosaceae*). Part: unripe fruit. Effects: Used for astringing the lung to relieve cough, astringing the bowels to stop diarrhea, promoting the production of body fluid to quench thirst, and regulation the stomach to alleviate colic caused by ascariasis. Indications: To relieve cough; to arrest chronic diarrhea and dysentery; to relieve abdominal colic and vomiting caused by ascariasis; used for diabetes; in treating bloody stool, hematuria, flooding and spotting; used externally to subdue swellings and to cure ophthalmic pterygium.

Japanese Aralia; CI LAO YA Origin: *Aralia elata* (Miq.) Seem. (*Araliaceae*). Part: bark. Effects: To supplement *qi* and quiet the spirit, nourish the essence and enrich the kidney, dispel wind and quicken the blood. Indications: Neurosism, rheumatic arthritis, diabetes, *yang* vacuity and *qi* weakness, insufficiency of kidney *yang*.

Japanese Ardisia Root; ZI JIN NIU GEN Origin: *Ardisia japonica* (Hornst.) Bl. (*Myrsinaceae*). Part: root. Effects: To eliminate wind phlegm. Indications: Seasonal diaphragm *qi.*

Japanese Ardisia; ZI JIN NIU Origin: *Ardisia japonica* (Hornst.) Bl. (*Myrsinaceae*). Part: stem and leaf. Effects: To settle cough, dispel phlegm, quicken the blood, disinhibit urine, qnd resolve toxin. Indications: Chronic trachitis, pulmonary tuberculosis with cough and hemoptysis, blood ejection, taxation damage and strength desertion, aching sinews and bones, hepatitis, dysentery, acute and chronic nephritis, hypertension, mounting *qi,* toxin swelling.

Japanese Avens Root; SHUI YANG MEI (I) GEN Origin: *Geum japonicum* Thunb. (*Rosaceae*). Part: root. Indications: Kidney vacuity and dizziness, common cold due to wind-cold, diarrhea and dysentery with abdominal pain.

Japanese Avens; SHUI YANG MEI (I) Origin: *Geum japonicum* Thunb. (*Rosaceae*). Part: herb. Effects: To supplement vacuity and boost kidney, quicken the blood and resolve toxin. Indications: Dizzy head and vision, forceless of the limbs, seminal emision and impotence, exterior vacuity and common cold, cough and blood ejection, vacuity cold and abdominal pain, menstrual disorder, swelling of sores, bone fracture.

Japanese balanophora; GE XUN Origin: *Balanophora japonica* Mak. (*Balanophoraceae*). Part: herb. Effects: To clear heat and resolve toxin, dispel the effects of liquor. Indications: Wind heat macular eruption, lung heat cough, blood ejection, flooding, hemorrhoid.

Japanese Barerry; XIAO BO Origin: *Berberis thunbergii* DC. (*Berberidaceae*). See Amur Barerry.

Japanese Buckeye Seed; SUO LUO ZI Origin: *Aesculus Turbinata* BL. (*Hippocastanaceae*). See Chinese Buckeye Seed.

Japanese Butterbur; FENG DOU CAI Origin: *Petasites japoniaus* (Sieb. *et* Zucc.) F. Schmidt (*Compositae*). Part: rhizome. Effects: To resolve toxin and dispel stasis, disperse swelling and relieve pain. Indications: Tonsillitis, swelling and toxin of welling abscess and clove sore, knocks and falls, snakebite.

Japanese Buttercup; MAO GEN Origin: *Ranunculus japonicus* Thunb. (*Ranunculaceae*). Part: herb and root. Indications: Malaria, jaundice, hemilateral headache, stomachache, wind-damp (rheumatism) with painful joints, crane's knee wind, swollen welling abscess, malign sore, scab and lichen, toothache, fire-eye.

Japanese Cayratia; WU LIAN MEI Origin: *Cayratia japonica* (Thunb.) Gagn. (*Vitaceae*). Part: herb or root. Effects: To clear heat and disinhibit damp, resolve toxin and disperse swelling. Indications: Swollen welling abscess, clove sore, mumps, cinnabar toxin, wind-damp pain (rheumatalgia), jaundice, dysentery, bloody urine, white turbidity.

Japanese Chain Fern; GUAN ZHONG Origin: *Woodwardia japonica* (L. f.) Sm (*Blechnaceae*). See Male Fern Rhizome.

Japanese Creeper; DI JIN Origin: *Parthenocissus tricuspidata* (Sieb. *et* Zucc.) Planch. (*Vitaceae*). Part: root and stem. Effects: To quicken the blood, dispel wind, and relieve pain. Indications: Postpartum blood stasis, abdominal lump, red and white vaginal discharge, wind-damp sinew and bone pain, hemilateral headache.

Japanese Cryptotaenia; YA ER QIN Origin: *Cryptoaenia japonica* Hassk. (*Umbelliferae*). Part: stem and leaf. Effects: To resolve toxin and expel inflammation, quicken the blood and disperse swelling. Indications: Pneumonia, pulmonary abscess, strangury, mounting *qi,* wind-fire toothache, swollen abscess and clove sore, herpes zoster, itchy skin.

Japanese Dock; YANG TI Origin: *Rumex japonicus* Houtt. (*Polygonaceae*). Part: root. Effects: To clear heat, free the stool, disinhibited water, stanch bleeding, and kill worms. Indications: Dry bound stool, strangury-turbidity, jaundice, blood ejection, intestinal wind, functional uterine bleeding, bald sores, scab and lichen, swollen welling abscess, knocks and falls.

Japanese Dodder Seed; DA TU SI ZI (one of the **TU SI ZI**) Origin: *Cuscuta japonica* Choisy (*Convolvulaceae*). See Chinese Dodder Seed.

Japanese Eel; MAN LI YU Origin: *Anguilla japonica* Temminck *et* Schlegel (*Anguillidae*). Part: meat or whole fish. Effects: To supplement vacuity emaciation, dispel wind-damp, kill worms. Indications: Vacuity taxation with steaming bone, pain from wind-damp impediment (arthralgia-syndrome), leg *qi* (beriberi), wind papules, child *gan,* flooding and spotting, intestinal wind, hemorrhoids and fistulas, sore.

Japanese Eupatorium; CHENG GAN CAO Origin: *Eupatorium japonicum* Thunb. (*Compositae*). Part: herb or root. Effects: To effuse the exterior and disperse cold, outthrust papules. Indications: Non-eruption of measles papules, cold damp laubar pain, wind-cold cough.

Japanese Eurya; LING MU Origin: *Eurya Japonica* Thunb. (*Theaceae*). Part: leaf or fruit. Effects: To dispel wind and eliminate dampness, disperse swelling and relieve pain.

Japanese Farfugium Herb; LIAN PENG CAO Origin: *Farfugium japonicum* (L.) Kitam. (*Compositae*). Part: whole plant. Effects: To clear heat, resolve toxin, and quicken the blood. Indications: Wind-heat common cold, sore swollen throat, sore swollen throat, clove sore, scrofula, knocks and falls.

Japanese Felt Fern Frond; SHI WEI Origin: *Pyrrosia lingua* (Thunb.) Farw. (*Polypodiaceae*). Part: leaf. Effects: To disinhibit water and free strangury, and to relieve cough. Indications: Strangury-turbidity and bloody urine, stone strangury, edema; cough and panting due to lung-heat; flooding and spotting, blood ejection, nosebleed.

Japanese Fleeceflower (Giant Knotweed); HU ZHANG Origin: *Polygonum cuspidatum* Sieb. *et* Zucc. (*Poligonaceae*). Part: rhizome. Effects: To remove heat, damp and toxic substances from the body and to promote blood circulation. Indications: Wind-damp with sinew and bone pain, damp-heat jaundice, strangury-turbidity and vaginal discharge, menstrual block, postpartum retention of the lochia, concretions and gatherings, numbness, paralysis, and precipitate blood, knocks and falls, scald, malign sore and lichen.

Japanese Galangal; TU SHA REN Origin: *Alpinia japonica* Miq. (*Zingiberaceae*). Part: fruit or seed. Effects: To move *qi* , regulate the center, and fortify the stomach. Indications: Glomus, distention and abdominal pain; vomiting, diarrhea.

Japanese Ginseng; ZHU JIE SAN QI Origin: *Panax pseudoginseng* Wall. var. *japonicus* (Mey.) Hoo *et* Tseng (*Araliaceae*). Part: rhizome. Effects: To suppress cough and transform phlegm, dissipate stasis and quicken the blood. Indications: Cough with profuse phlegm, blood ejection due to taxation damage, knocks and falls, swollen welling abscess, bleeding due to external injury.

Japanese Honeysuckle; JIN YIN HUA Origin: *Lonicera japonica* Thunb. (*Captifoliaceae*). Part: flower bud. Effects: To remove heat and toxic substance and to dispel wind-heat. Indications: Externally contracted wind-heat or epidemic febrile diseases of early stage shown as fever, slight aversion to wind and cold; high fever, dire thirst, and full pulse; sores and carbuncles, furuncles and swellings; diarrhea and dysentery with purulent and bloody stool.

Japanese Hop Herb; LU CAO Origin: *Humulus scandens* (Lour.) Merr. (*Moraceae*). Part: herb. Effects: To clear heat and resolve toxin, disperse stasis, disinhibit urine. Indications: Strangury, inhibited urination, malaria, abdominal diarrhea, dysentery, pulmonary tuberculosis, pulmonary purulent sore, pneumonia, *lai* sore, hemorrhoid, toxin of welling abscess, scrofula.

Japanese Hylomecon; HE QING HUA Origin: *Hylomecon japonica* (Thunb.) Prantl *et* Kündig (*Papaveraceae*). Part: root. Effects: To dispel wind-damp, soothe sinew and quicken the network vessels, dissipate stasis and disperse swelling, relieve pain and stanch blood. Indications: Rheumatic arthritis, taxation damage, knocks and falls.

Japanese Inula Herb; JIN FO CAO Origin: *Inula japonica* Thunb. (*Compositae*). Part: aerial parts. Effects: To dissipate wind-heat, transform phlegm-rheum, and eliminate swelling and toxin. Indications: Wind-cold cough, deep-lying rheum and phlegm panting, distending pain in the rib-side, clove sore, toxin swelling.

Japanese Kerria Flower; DI TANG HUA Origin: *Kerria japonica* (L.) DC. (*Rosaceae*). Part: flower or branchlet and leaf. Effects: To dispel wind and moisten the lung, suppress cough and transform phlegm. Indications: Enduring cough, indigestion, edema, rheumatalgia, heat toxin sore.

Japanese Maesa; DU JING SHAN Origin: *Maesa japonica* (Thunb.) Moritzi (*Myrsinaceae*). Part: root and leaf. Effects: To dispel wind, resolve toxin, and disperse swelling. Indications: Common cold, headache, dizziness, cold-heat agitation and thirst, edema, pain in the lumbus.

Japanese Mahonia Fruit; SHI DA GONG LAO ZI Origin: *Mahonia japonica* (Thunb.) DC. (*Berberidaceae*). See Leatherleaf Mahonia Fruit.

Japanese Mahonia Leaf; SHI DA GONG LAO YE Origin: *Mahonia japonica* (Thunb.) DC. (*Berberidaceae*). See Leatherleaf Mahonia Leaf.

Japanese Mahonia; SHI DA GONG LAO MU Origin: *Mahonia japonica* (Thunb.) DC. (*Berberidaceae*). See Leatherleaf Mahonia.

Japanese Mallotus; YE WU TONG Origin: *Mallotus japonicus* Muell.-Arg. (*Euphorbiaceae*). Part: bark. Effects: To regulate functions of the digestive system. Indications: Gastric ulcer, duodenal ulcer.

Japanese Metaplexis Seed; LUO MO ZI Origin: *Metaplexis japonica* (Thunb.) Mak. (*Asclepiadaceae*). Part: seed. Effects: To supplement essence and benefit *qi,* engender flesh and stanch bleeding, resolve toxin. Indications: Vacuity taxation, impotence, bleeding from incised wound.

Japanese Metaplexis; LUO MO Origin: *Metaplexis japonica* (Thunb.) Mak. (*Asclepiadaceae*). Part: herb or root. Effects: To supplement essence and benefit *qi,* free milk and resolve toxin. Indications: Vacuity-detriment taxation damage, impotence, vaginal discharge, breast milk stoppage, cinnabar toxin, swelling of sores.

Japanese Orixa; CHOU SHAN YANG Origin: *Orixa japonica* Thunb. (*Rutaceae*). Part: root. Effects: To clear heat and resolve the exterior, move *qi* and relieve pain, dispel wind and disinhibit dampness. Indications: Wind-heat common cold, cough, sore throat, toothache, stomachache, wind-damp with painful joints, dysentery, innominate toxin swelling.

Japanese Osmunda Fern; GUAN ZHONG Origin: *Osmunda japonica* Thunb. (*Osmundaceae*). See Male Fern Rhizome.

Japanese Pachysandra; XUE SHAN LIN Origin: *Pachysandra terminalis* Sieb. *et* Zucc. (*Buxaceae*). Part: herb with root. Effects: To clear heat and resolve toxin, eliminate wind damp, regulate menstruation, and quicken the blood. Indications: Wind-damp pain in sinews and bones, white vaginal discharge, profuse menstruation, vexation.

Japanese Pagodatree Fruit; HUAI JIAO Origin: *Sophora japonica* L. (*Leguminosae*). Part: fruit. Effects: To clear heat and moisten the liver, cool the blood and stanch bleeding. Indications: Intestinal wind bleeding, bleeding from hemorrhoids, flooding and spotting, blood strangury, blood dysentery, vexation and oppression in the heart and chest, wind dizziness and desiring fall, genital sore with damp itch.

Japanese Pagodatree Root; HUAI GEN Origin: *Sophora japonica* L. (*Leguminosae*). Part: root. Indications: Hemorrhoid, throat impediment, roundworm.

Japanese Polypody; SHUI LONG GU Origin: *Polypodium* niponicum Mett. (*Polypodiaceae*). Part: rhizome. Effects: To transform damp and clear heat, To dispel wind and free the network vessels. Indications: Sand foulness and diarrhea, dysentery, strangury, white turbidity, wind impediment, lumbar pain, fire eye, swelling of sores.

Japanese Pyrola Herb; LU SHOU CAO Origin: *Pyrola japonica* Klenze *ex* Alef. (*Pyrolaceae*). Part: herb. Effects: To regulate menstruation. Indications: *Yin* vacuity, white vaginal discharge.

Japanese Raisin Tree Root; ZHI JU GEN Origin: *Hovenia dulcis* Thunb. (*Rhamnaceae*). Part: root. Indications: Vacuity taxation with blood ejection, pain in sinews and bones due to wind-damp.

Japanese Rose Root; QIANG WEI GEN Origin: *Rosa multiflora* Thunb. (*Rosaceae*). Part: root. Effects: To clear heat and disinhibit damp, dispel wind and quicken the blood, and resolve toxin. Indications: Pulmonary welling abscess, diabetes, dysentery, arthritis, paralysis, blood ejection, spontaneous external bleeding, bloody stool, frequent urination, enuresis, menstrual irregularities, knocks and falls, sores and boils, scab and lichen.

Japanese Sabia; QING FENG TENG Origin: *Sabia japonica* Maxim. (*Sabiaceae*). See Orientvine.

Japanese Scopolia; DONG LANG DANG Origin: *Scopolia japonica* Maxim. (*Solanaceae*). Part: rhizome. Effects: To resolve tetany and settle pain, constrain sweat and astringe the intestines. Indications: Various pain, manic agitation of essence-spirit, swelling and toxin of welling abscess and sore, anthrax, bleeding due to external injury, body lichen.

Japanese Snailseed; MU FANG JI (one of the **FANG JI**) Origin: *Cocculus trilobus* (Thunb.) DC. (*Menispermaceae*). See Fourstamen Stephania.

Japanese Snailseed Stem; QING TAN XIANG Origin: *Cocculus trilobus* (Thunb.) DC. (*Menispermaceae*). Part: stem and leaf. Effects: To climinate wind and damp, eliminate swelling. Indications: Paralysis due to wind, phlegm-damp streaming sore, itching in legs and knees, stomachache, sand and *qi* pain.

Japanese Snakegourd Seed; WANG GUA ZI Origin: *Trichosanthes cucumeroides* (Ser.) Maxim. (*Cucurbitaceae*). Part: seed. Effects: To clear heat and cool the blood. Indications: Lung wilting and blood ejection, jaundice, dysentery, intestinal wind bleeding.

Japanese Snakegourd; WANG GUA Origin: *Trichosanthes cucumeroides* (Ser.) Maxim. (*Cucurbitaceae*). Part: fruit. Effects: To remove heat, promote fluid secretion, to dispel blood stasis and promote lactation. Indications: Diabetes, jaundice, dysphagia-occlusion and stomach reflux, menstrual block, scant breast milk, swollen welling abscess, chronic laryngopharyngitis.

Japanese Spicebush; SAN ZUAN FENG Origin: *Lindera obtusiloba* Bl. (*Lauraceae*). Part: bark. Effects: To soothe sinew and quicken blood, dissipate stasis and disperse swelling. Indications: Knocks and falls, stasis swelling and pain.

Japanese Spiraea Leaf; XIU XIAN JU YE Origin: *Spiraea japonica* L. f. (*Rosaceae*). Part: leaf. Effects: To disperse swelling and resolve toxin, eliminate putridity and engender flesh. Indications: Chronic medullitis.

Japanese Staphania; QIAN JIN TENG Origin: *Stephania japonica* (Thunb.) Miers (*Menispermaceae*). Part: root or stem and leaf. Effects: Clear heat and resolve toxin, dispel wind and disinhibit damp. Indications: Dysentery, malaria, pain from wind-damp impediment (arthralgia-syndrome), edema, strangury-turbidity, sore swollen throat, swollen welling abscess, sores and boils.

Japanese Stemona; BAI BU Origin: *Stemona japonica* (Bl.) Miq. (*Stemonaceae*). See Sessile Stemona.

Japanese Thistle; DA JI (b) Origin: *Cirsium japonicum* DC. (*Compositae*). Part: aerial parts or root. Effects: To remove heat from the blood and stanch bleeding, to disinhibit urine and lower blood pressure and to treat carbuncle. Indications: Blood ejection and spontaneous external bleeding, bloody urine, blood strangury, flooding, vaginal discharge, intestinal wind and intestinal welling abscess, ulcerating welling abscess and sores, clove sore.

Japanese White Birch Bark; HONG HUA PI (one of the **HUA MU PI**) Origin: *Betula platyphylla* Suk. var. *japonica* (Sieb.) Hara (*Betulaceae*). Part: bark. Effects: To clear heat and disinhibit damp, dispel phlegm and relieve cough, disperse swelling and resolve toxin. Indications: Pneumonia, dysentery, diarrhea, jaundice, nephritis, urinary tract infection, chronic trachitis, acute tonsillitis, periodontitis, acute mastitis, swollen boil, itchy papules, scalds.

Japanese Wormwood; MU HAO Origin: *Artemisia japonica* Thumb. (*Compositae*). Part: herb. Effects: To resolve the exterior, clear heat, and kill worms. Indications: Common cold and generalized fever, taxation damage and cough, tidal fever, child *gan* fever, malaria, mouth sore, scab and lichen, eczema.

Japanese Yew; ZI SHAN Origin: *Taxus cuspidata* Sieb. *et* Zucc. (*Taxaceae*). Part: branchlet and leaf. Effects: To disinhibit urine and free the channels. Indications: Kidney disease, diabetes.

Japonese Ganoderma; ZI ZHI (one of the **LING ZHI CAO**) Origin: *Ganoderma japonicum* (Fr.) Lloyd (*Polyporaceae*). Part: dried sporophore. Effects: Used as a tonic, roborant, sedative, and stomachic. Indications: Vacuity and taxation, cough, panting, insomnia, indigestion.

Jatamans Valeriana; ZHI ZHU XIANG Origin: *Valeriana jatamansii* Jones (*Valerianaceae*). Part: rhizome. Effects: To move *qi* and disperse cold, quicken the blood and regulate menstruation. Indications: Sand and painful distention in stomach duct and abdomen, vomiting and diarrhea, lung *qi* edema, wind-cold common cold, menstrual irregularities, consumption damage and cough.

javan Bishopwood; QIU FENG MU Origin: *Bischofia javanica* Bl. (*Euphorbiaceae*). Part: Root bark, Branchlet and Leaf. Effects: Root-bark, branchlet and leaf: to expel wind, quicken the blood, and eliminate swelling; leaf: move *qi* and quicken the blood, eliminate swelling and vanquish toxin. Indications: Root-bark, branchlet and leaf: wind-damp bone pain; leaf: depression of *qi* and blood, abscess and sore; root: red and white dysentery.

Java Brucea; YA DAN ZI Origin: *Brucea javanica* (L.) Merr. (*Simaroubaceae*). Part: fruit. Effects: To clear heat and dry damp, kill worms and resolve toxin. Indications: Malaria; blood dysentery due to heat and toxin, dysentery with pus and blood, tenesmus; corn and common wart.

Javan Waterdropwort Flower; QIN HUA Origin: *Oenanthe javanica* (Bl.) DC. (*Umbelliferae*). Part: flower.

Javan Waterdropwort; SHUI QIN Origin: *Oenanthe javanica* (Bl.) DC. (*Umbelliferae*). Part: herb. Effects: To clear heat and disinhibit water. Indications: Fulminant fever with vexation and thirst, jaundice, edema, strangury, vaginal discharge, scrofula, mumps.

Jehol Ligusticum; LIAO GAO BEN (one of the **GAO BEN**) Origin: *Ligusticum jeholense* Nakai *et* Kitag. (*Umbelliferae*). See Chinese Ligusticum.

Jerusalemcherry Root; YU SHAN HU GEN Origin: *Solanum pseudocapsicum* L. (*Solanaceae*). Part: root. Effects: To relieve pain. Indications: Consumption damage and lumbar pain.

Jobstears Root; YI YI GEN Origin: *Coix lachrymajobi* L. (*Gramineae*). Part: root. Effects: To clear heat and disinhibit damp, fortify the spleen and kill worms. Indications: Jaundice, edema, strangury, mounting *qi,* menstrual block, vaginal discharge, abdomen pain from insect accumulation.

Jobstears; YI YI REN Origin: *Coix lachrymajobi* L. (*Gramineae*). Part: seed. Effects: To remove heat and damp, disinhibit urination and expel the pus, strengthen the spleen and check diarrhea. Indications: Inhibited urination, edema, leg *qi* (beriberi), spleen vacuity and diarrhea,; pain from wind-damp impediment (arthralgia-syndrome), hy-pertonicity of the sinews; welling abscess in the lung, intestinal welling abscess.

Jointwood Senna; SHEN HUANG DOU Origin: *Cassia nodosa* L. (*Leguminosae*). Part: fruit. Effects: To resolve toxin. Indications: Papules, pox.

Kadsura Pepper Stem; HAI FENG TENG Origin: *Piper kadsura* (Choisy) Ohwi [=*Piper futo-kadsura* Sieb.] (*Piperaceae*). Part: stem. Effects: To dispel wind-damp, free the channels and network vessels, rectify *qi.* Indications: Wind-damp impedi-ment, inhibited joints, inhibited sinew movement, pain in the lumbus and knees, pain from knocks and falls.

Kaempfer Dutchmanspipe; ZHU SHA LIAN Origin: *Aristolochia kaempferi* Willd. (*Aristolochia-ceae*). Part: tuber. Effects: To clear fire and disperse swelling, dissipate blood and relieve pain, resolve snake-toxin. Indications: Red and white dysentery, pain in chest, abdomen or throat, poisonous snake bite.

Kamalatree Pericarpial Glandular Hairs; LU SONG QIU MAO Origin: *Mallotus philippinensis* (Lam.) Muell.-Arg. (*Euphorbiaceae*). Part: pericarpial glandular hairs. Effects: To kill worm. Indications: Tapeworm disease, injury, putrefying sore, swelling in foot, rheumatism.

Kamchatka Bugbane; YE SHENG MA Origin: *Cimicifuga simplex* Wormsk. (*Ranunculaceae*). Part: rhizome. Effects: To dissipate wind, resolve toxin, upbear *yang, and* outthrust papules. Indications: *Yang* brightness headache, sore throat, maculopapular eruption, wind heat sore, enduring diarrhea and prolapse of the rectum, flooding and vaginal discharge, child measles papules.

Kansui Euphoria; GAN SUI Origin: *Euphorbia kansui* Liou (*Euphorbiaceae*). Part: tuberous root. Effects: As hydragogue and purgative for hydrothorax and ascites. Indications: Edema in the face and body, ascites, and hydrothorax; suppurative infections on the body surface; epilepsy of wind-phlegm.

Katsumada Galangal; CAO DOU KOU Origin: *Alpinia katsumadai* Hayata (*Zingiberaceae*). Part: seed. Effects: To remove dampness and strengthen the spleen, and to warm the stomach and arrest vomiting. Indications: Cold-damp encumbering the spleen and stomach; distention, fullness and pain in the stomach duct and abdomen, vomiting, diarrhea.

Kelp Thallus; KUN BU Origin: *Laminaria japonica* Aresch. (*Laminariaceae*). Part: dried thallus. Effects: To soften and resolve bind, to eliminate phlegm and move water. Indications: Scrofula, goiter, dysphagia-occlusion, water swelling (edema), painful swollen testicles, vaginal discharge.

Khasi Nightshade Fruit; CI TIAN QIE Origin: *Solanum khasianum* C. B. Clarke (*Solanaceae*). Part: fruit. Effects: To resolve toxin and expel inflammation, relieve pain with sedation. Indications: Pain from wind-damp or traumatic injury, nervous headache, stomachache, toothache, mastitis, mumps.

Kidney Bean Seed; BAI FAN DOU Origin: *Phaseolus vulgaris* L. (*Leguminosae*). Part: seed. Effects: To enrich and nourish, resolve heat, disinhibit urine, and disperse swelling. Indications: Edema, leg *qi* (beriberi).

kidneyleaf Goldenray; HU LU QI Origin: *Ligularia fischeri* (Ledeb.) Turcz. (*Compositae*). See Toothleaf Goldenray.

King Solomonseal; HUANG JING Origin: *Polygonatum kingianum* Coll. *et* Hemsl. (*Liliaceae*). See Siberian Solomonseal.

Kirilow Groundsel Herb; GOU SHE CAO Origin: *Tephroseris kirilowii* (Turcz. *ex* DC.) Holub [= *Senecio integrifolius* (L.) Clairvill var. *fauriei* (Levl. *et* Vant.) Kitam.] (*Compositae*). Part: herb. Effects: To clear heat and disinhibit water, kill worms. Indications: Open pus sore of the lung, nephritis with edema, swollen boil, scab sore.

Knotteflower Phyla Herb; PENG LAI CAO Origin: *Lippia nodiflora* (L.) L. C. Rich. (*Verbena-ceae*). Part: herb. Effects: To dispel wind and clear heat, disperse swelling and resolve toxin. Indications: Sore throat moth, swelling and toxin of welling abscess and flat abscess, heat dysentery, strangury, *gan* of the teeth and gum, herpes zoster.

Korean Pine Seed; HAI SONG ZI Origin: *Pinus koraiensis* Sieb. *et* Zucc. (*Pinaceae*). Part: seed. Effects: To nourish fluids, extinguish wind, moisten the lung and lubricate the intestines. Indications: Wind impediment, dizzy head, dry cough, blood ejection, constipation.

Korean Rhododendron; YING SHAN HONG Origin: *Rhododendron mucronulatum* Turcz. (*Erica-ceae*). Part: leaf. Effects: To resolve the exterior, clear the lung, and suppress cough. Indications: Common cold, headache, cough, bronchitis.

Kulaso Aloe Dried Juice; KU LA SUO LU HUI (one of the **LU HUI**) Origin: *Aloe vera* L. (*Liliaceae*). Part: solid residue obtained by evaporating the liquid which drains from the leaves. Effects: To clear the liver and relieve constipation. Indications: Constipation due to heat bind, habitual constipation; child *gan* accumulation, roundworm; lichen.

Kusamaki Broadleaved PodocarpusLeaf; LUO HAN SONG YE Origin: *Podocarpus macrophyllus* (Thunb.) D. Don (*Podocarpaceae*). See Chinese Podocarpus Leaf.

Kusamaki Broadleaved Podocarpus Seed; LUO HAN SONG SHI Origin: *Podocarpus macrophyllus* (Thunb.) D. Don (*Podocarpaceae*). See Chinese Podocarpus Seed.

Kusnezoff Monkshood; BEI WU TOU (one of the **CAO WU TOU**) Origin: *Aconitum kusnezoffii* Rchb. (*Ranunculaceae*). See Common Monkshood

Lac; ZI CAO RONG Origin: *Laccifer lacca* Kerr. (*Lacciferidae*). Part: gum of the lac insect. Effects: To clear heat, cool the blood, and resolve toxin. Indications: Measles papules, non-eruption of measles papules, postpartum blood dizziness, vaginal discharge, swelling and toxin of sore and scab.

Lalang Grass Leaf; MAO CAO YE Origin: *Imperata cylindrica* (L.) P. Beauv. var. *major* (Nees) C. E. Hubb. (*Gramineae*). Part: leaf. Effects: To free the channels and network vessels. Indications: Postpartum wind-damp pain.

Lalang Grass Rhizome; BAI MAO GEN Origin: *Imperata cylindrica* (L.) P. Beauv. var. *major* (Nees) C. E. Hubb. (*Gramineae*). Part: rhizome. Effects: To remove heat, especially heat from the blood and to promote secretion and urination. Indications: Febrile disease with vexation and thirst, blood ejection and spontaneous external bleeding, lung heat rapid panting, stomach heat hiccough, strangury, inhibited urination, edema, jaundice.

Lambsquarters Juvenile; LI Origin: *Chenopodium album* L. (*Chenopodiaceae*). Part: juvenile herb. Effects: To clear heat, disinhibit damp, and kill worms. Indications: Dysentery, abdominal diarrhea, damp sore, itchy papules, insect bite.

Lance Coreopsis; XIAN YE JIN JI JU Origin: *Coreopsis lanceolata* L. (*Compositae*). Part: leaf. Effects: To transform stasis and disperse swelling, clear heat and resolve toxin. Indications: Innominate toxin swelling, knife wound.

Lanceleaf Lily; BAI HE Origin: *Lilium longiflorum* Thunb. (*Liliaceae*). See Greenish Lily.

Lanceleaf Thermopsis; MU MA DOU Origin: *Thermopsis lanceolata* R. Br. (*Leguminosae*). Part: herb. Effects: To eliminate the phlegm and suppress cough. Indications: Coughing of phlegm panting.

Lanceolate Starwort; YIN CHAI HU Origin: *Stellaria dichotoma* L. var. *lanceolata* Bge. (*Caryophyllaceae*). Part: root. Effects: To remove fever due to vacuity of *qi*, essence of blood, and that due to infantile malnutrition. Indications: *Yin* vacuity with fever, taxation fever steaming bone, night sweating; clear *gan* (malnutrition) heat, child worm accumulation with fever, enlarged abdomen, emaciation, thirst, and red eyes due to *gan* of the liver.

Large Puff-ball; MA BO Origin: *Calvatia gigantea* (Batsch *ex* Pers.) Lloye (*Lycoperdaceae*). See Bark-less Puff-ball.

Largeflower Epimedium Root; YIN YANG HUO GEN Origin: *Epimedium grandiflorum* Morr. (*Berberidaceae*). Part: root. Indications: Men: vacuity strangury, white turbidity, dizzy head; women: white vaginal discharge, menstrual disorder; asthma.

Largeflower Epimedium; YIN YANG HUO Origin: *Epimedium grandiflorum* Morr. (*Berberida-ceae*). Part: aerial parts. Effects: To supplement the kidney, invigorate *yang*, atrengthen muscles and bones, and as an antirheumatic. Indications: Impotence, lassitude of the loins and knees, frequent urination, female sterility; impediment, muscular spasm, numb hands and feet due to wind-cold-damp; climacteric hypertension; cough due to deficiency of *yang*.

Largeflower Euonymus; YE DU ZHONG Origin: *Euonymus grandiflorus* Wall. (*Celastraceae*). Part: root or bark. Indications: Lumbar pain, blood stasis and menstrual block, menstrual pain.

Largeflower Paniculate Hydrangea; FEN TUAN HUA Origin: *Hydrangea paniculata* Sieb. var. *grandiflora* Sieb. (*Saxifragaceae*). See Paniculate Hydrangea.

Largeflower Purslane; BAN ZHI LIAN Origin: *Portulaca grandiflora* Hook. (*Labiatae*). Part: herb. Effects: To remove pathogenic heat and toxin, to eliminate blood stasis and stanch bleeding, and to disinhibit urine and treat cancer. Indications: Sore swollen throat, scalds, knocks and falls, damp sore.

Largehead Atractylodes; BAI ZHU Origin: *Atractylodes macrocephala* Koidz. [= *Atractylis macrocephala* (Koidz.) Hand.-Mazz.] (*Compositae*). Part: root. Effects: To reinforce the spleen and replenish *qi*, to promote diuresis and arrest profuce or spontaneous sweating. Indications: Poor appetite, loose stool, epigastric and abdominal distention, lassitude and asthenia; phlegm retention and edema; spontaneous sweating; threatened abortion.

Largeleaf Chinese Ash Bark; QIN PI Origin: *Fraxinus rhynchophylla* Hance (*Oleaceae*). Part: bark. Effects: To clear heat and resolve toxin, clear the liver and improve acuity of sight. Indications: Diarrhea due to heat toxin, blood dysentery, tenesmus; depression and heat of liver channel, sore red swollen eyes, eye screen.

Largeleaf Gamirplant; DA YE GOU TENG Origin: *Uncaria macrophylla* Wall. (*Rubiaceae*). Part: stem with hooks. Effects: To clear heat and calm liver, extinguish wind and settle fright. Indications: Convulsion, hypertension, nervous headache, osteomyelitis.

Largeleaf Gentian; QIN JIAO Origin: *Gentiana macrophylla* Pall. (*Gentianaceae*). Part: dried root. Effects: To dispel wind and eliminate dampness, harmonize the blood and soothe sinew, clear heat and disinhibit urine. Indications: Wind-damp impediment (arthralgia-syndrome), hypertonicity in whole body or joints, steaming bone tidal fever; dump-heat jaundice.

Largeleaf Hydrangea; BA XIAN HUA Origin: *Hydrangea macrophylla* (Thunb.) Ser. (*Saxifragaceae*). Part: root, leaf and flower. Effects: To interrupt malaria. Indications: Malaria, heart heat fright palpitation, vexation and agitation.

Largeleaf Spicebush Root-bark; DIAO ZHANG GEN PI Origin: *Lindera umbellate* Thunb. (*Lauraceae*). Part: root bark. Indications: Running piglet, leg *qi* (beriberi), edema, scab and lichen, bleeding from wounds.

Largeseed Hemsleya; LUO GUO DI Origin: *Hemsleya macrosperma* C. Y. Wu (*Cucurbitaceae*). Part: tuber root. Effects: To clear heat and resolve toxin, disperse swelling and relieve pain. Indications: Swelling and pain in the throat, toothache, the eye to be red and gall, bacillary dysentery, enteritis, stomachache, hepatitis, urinary tract infection, swelling of clove sore.

Largeserrate Mosla; JI NING Origin: *Mosla grosseserrata* Maxim. (*Labiatae*). Part: stem and leaf. Effects: To kill worms. Indications: Diarrhea and dysentery due to cold *qi,* acid vomiting.

Lateripening Bartsia Herb; CHI YE CAO Origin: *Odontites serotina* Reich. (*Scrophulariaceae*). Part: herb. Effects: To clear heat and dry dampness, cold the blood and relieve pain. Indications: Febrile infectious disease, depressed liver-gallbladder heat, pain of static blood.

Laurelleaf Snailseed; HENG ZHOU WU YAO Origin: *Cocculus laurifolius* DC. (*Menisper-maceae*). Part: root or whole herb. Indications: Hypertension, headache, mounting *qi,* abdominal pain, rheumatic pain in the legs.

Lavandulaleaf Chrysanthemum Flower; YE JU HUA Origin: *Chrysanthemum lavandulaefolium* (Fisch.) Mak. (*Compositae*). See Indian Wild Chrysanthemum Flower.

Lavandulaleaf Chrysanthemum; YAN XIANG JU (one of the **YE JU**) Origin: *Chrysanthe-mum lavandulaefolium* (Fisch.) Mak. (*Compositae*). See Indian Wild Chrysanthemum.

Laver; ZI CAI Origin: *Porphyra tenera* Kjellm. (*Bangiaceae*). Part: thallospore. Effects: To transform phlegm and soften hardness, clear heat and disinhibit urine. Indications: Goiter, leg *qi* (beriberi), edema, strangury.

Laxleaf Sweetroot; XIANG GEN QIN Origin: *Osmorhiza aristata* (Thunb.) Mak. *et* Yabe var. *laxa* (Royle) Constance *et* Shan (*Umbelliferae*). Part: root. Effects: To disperse cold and effuse the exterior, relieve pain. Indications: Wind-cold common cold, headache in the nape,pain in whole body.

Leafy Euphorbia; JI CHANG LANG DU Origin: *Euphorbia esula* L. (*Euphorbiaceae*). Part: root. Effects: To disinhibit water, disperse edema, kill worms, and attack gastrointestinal accumulation.

Leatherleaf Mahonia Fruit; SHI DA GONG LAO ZI Origin: *Mahonia bealei* (Fort.) Carr. (*Berberidaceae*). Part: fruit. Effects: To clear heat and rectify dampness. Indications: Steaming bone tidal fever, diarrhea, flooding and vaginal discharge, strangury-turbidity.

Leatherleaf Mahonia Leaf; SHI DA GONG LAO YE Origin: *Mahonia bealei* (Fort.) Carr. (*Berberidaceae*). Part: leaf. Effects: To clear heat and supplement vacuity, to suppress cough and transform phlegm. Indications: Pulmonary consumption with coughing of blood, steaming bone tidal fever, dizzy head and ringing in the ears, limp aching lumbus and legs, vexation, red eyes.

Leatherleaf Mahonia; SHI DA GONG LAO MU Origin: *Mahonia bealei* (Fort.) Carr. (*Berberidaceae*). Part: stem. Effects: To clear the lung and supplement *yin*, cool the blood, allay thirst, kill worms, and free the stool. Indications: Consumption cough.

Leatherleaf Millettia Root; KUN MING JI XUE TENG GEN Origin: *Millettia reticulata* Benth. (*Leguminosae*). Part: root. Effects: Sedation.

Ledger Cinchona; JIN JI LE Origin: *Cinchona ledgeriana* Moens. (*Rubiaceae*). See Redbark Cinchona.

Lemon eucalyptus Leaf; NING MENG AN YE Origin: *Eucalyptus citriodora* Hook f. (*Myrtaceae*). Part: leaf. Effects: To disperse swelling and dissipate toxin. Indications: Abdominal pain and diarrhea, sore and boil, skin diseases, wind-damp bone pain.

Lemon Leaf; NING MENG YE Origin: *Citrus limon* Burm. (*Rutaceae*). Part: leaf. Effects: To relieve cough and reduce sputum, rectify *qi* and increase the appetite. Indications: Cough and panting, abdominal distention, diarrhea.

Lemon Root; NING MENG GEN Origin: *Citrus limon* Burm. (*Rutaceae*). Part: root. Effects: To relieve pain and dispel stasis. Indications: Knocks and falls, rabid dog bite.

Lemon; NING MENG Origin: *Citrus limon* Burm. (*Rutaceae*). Part: fruit. Effects: To engender liquid and allay thirst, dispel summerheat, quiet the fetus.

Lemonlike Citrus Leaf; NING MENG YE Origin: *Citrus limonia* Osbeck (*Rutaceae*). See Lemon Leaf.

Lemonlike Citrus Root; NING MENG GEN Origin: Citrus limonia Osbeck (*Rutaceae*). See Lemon Root.

Lemonlike Citrus; NING MENG Origin: *Citrus limonia* Osbeck (*Rutaceae*). See Lemon.

Leprieur Caloglossa Frond; ZHE GU CAI Origin: *Caloglossa leprieurii* (Mont.) J. Ag. (*Delesseriaceae*). Part: frond. Effects: To kill worms. Indications: Child insect accumulation.

Lesser Galangal; GAO LIANG JIANG Origin: *Alpinia officinarum* Hance (*Zingiberaceae*). Part: rhizome. Effects: To warm the stomach, dispel wind, dissipate cold, move *qi*, and relieve pain. Indications: Cold pain in the stomach duct and abdomen, vomiting, and diarrhea.

Lettuce Ulva Frond; SHI CHUN Origin: *Ulva lactuca* L. (*Ulvaceae*). Part: frond. Effects: To disinhibit urine. Indications: Inhibited urination, *qi* bind below the umbilicus.

Levant Cotton Oil; MIAN ZI YOU Origin: *Gossypium herbaceum* L. (*Malvaceae*). Part: seed oil. Indications: Malign sore, scab and lichen.

Levant Cotton Root; MIAN HUA GEN Origin: *Gossypium herbaceum* L. (*Malvaceae*). Part: root bark. Effects: To supplement vacuity, calm asthma, and regulate menstruation. Indications: Vacuity and cough-asthma, mounting *qi,* flooding and vaginal discharge, prolapse of uterus.

Levant Cotton; MIAN HUA Origin: *Gossypium herbaceum* L. (*Malvaceae*). Part: tomentum of the seed. Effects: To stanch bleeding. Indications: Blood ejection, precipitate blood, flooding, bleeding from incised wound.

Licorice; GUANG GUO GAN CAO (one of the **GAN CAO**) Origin: *Glycyrrhiza glabra* L. (*Leguminosae*). See Ural Licorice.

Lightyellow Sophora Seed; KU SHEN SHI Origin: *Sophora flavescens* Ait. (*Leguminosae*). Part: seed. Effects: To brighten the eyes, fortify the stomach, and expel roundworms. Indications: Acute bacillary dysentery, constipation.

Lightyellow Sophora; KU SHEN Origin: *Sophora flavescens* Ait. (*Leguminosae*). Part: dried root. Effects: To clear heat and dry dampness, and as anthelmintic and antipruritic. Indications: Jaundice, diarrhea, vaginal discharge and pudendal itch caused by damp-heat; itchy skin, purulent nest sore, scab and lichen, leprosy; damp-heat brewing, inhibited urination with hot pain.

Lilac Daphne Root; YUAN HUA GEN Origin: *Daphne genkwa* Sieb. *et* Zucc. (*Thymelaea-ceae*). Part: root. Indications: Edema, scrofula, breast abscess, homorrhoids and scab.

Lilac Daphne; YUAN HUA Origin: *Daphne genkwa* Sieb. *et* Zucc. (*Thymelaeaceae*). Part: flower bud. Effects: To remove retained water and fluid, and externally as parasiticide and treating cutaneous infections. Indications: Edema in the face and body, ascites, and hydrothorax; profuse sputum and cough, chronic bronchitis; scalp infection, tinea capitis, and neuro-dermatitis.

Lilac Pink; QU MAI Origin: *Dianthus superbus* L. (*Caryophyllaceae*). Part: aerial parts. Effects: To disinhibit water and relieve strangury. Indications: Short voidings of reddish urine, strangury with inhibited painful urination, menstrual block.

Lily Magnolia Bark; MU LAN PI Origin: *Magnolia liliflora* Desr. (*Magnoliaceae*). Part: bark. Indications: Liquor jaundice, damp-itch in the genital region, *Lai* disease, double tongue, welling abscess and flat abscess, edema.

Lily Magnolia Flower; MU LAN HUA Origin: *Magnolia liliflora* Desr. (*Magnoliaceae*). Part: flower. Indications: Bones of fish or other food stuck in the throat.

Lily Magnolia; XIN YI Origin: *Magnolia liliflora* Desr. (*Magnoliaceae*). Part: flower buds. Effects: To dissipate wind-cold and relieve stuffed nose. Indications: External contraction of wind-cold, headache and nosal congestion, especially for deep-source nosal congestion and headache, loss of smell, profuse turbid snivel.

Lily of the valley; LING LAN Origin: *Convallaria keiskei* Miq. [= *Convallaria majalis* L.] (*Liliaceae*). Part: herb with root. Effects: To warm yang and dishibit water, quicken the blood and dispel wind. Indications: Cardiac failure, general edema, taxation damage, flooding and spotting, white vaginal discharge, knocks and falls.

Lindley Eupatorium; CHENG GAN SHENG MA Origin: *Eupatorium lindleyanum* DC. (*Compo-sitae*). Part: root. Effects: To exterior cold and abate fever. Indications: Common cold, malaria, intestinal parasitic disease.

Linearleaf Gentian; LONG DAN Origin: *Gentiana manshurica* Kitagawa (*Gentianaceae*). See Rough Gentian.

Linearleaf Inula Flower; XUAN FU HUA Origin: *Inula linariaefolia* Turcz. (*Compositae*). See Chinese Inula Flower.

Linearleaf Inula Herb; JIN FO CAO Origin: *Inula linariifolia* Turcz. (*Compositae*). See Japanese Inula Herb.

Linearleaf Thistle; KU AO Origin: *Cirsium chinense* Gardn. *et* Champ. (*Compositae*). Part: herb. Effects: To clear heat and resolve toxin, cool the blood and quicken the blood. Indications: Vexation and oppression due to summerheat heat, flooding and spotting, blood ejection from knocks and falls, hemorrhoid, clove sore.

Little Groundcherry; TIAN PAO ZI Origin: *Physalis minima* L. (*Solanaceae*). Part: herb or fruit. Effects: To percolate dampness and kill worms. Indications: Jaundice, inhibited urination, chronic cough and panting, *gan* disease, scrofula, heaven-borne sore, damp sore.

Littleflower Plumbagella Herb; JI WA CAO Origin: *Plumbagella micrantha* (Ledeb.) Spach (*Plumbaginaceae*). Part: herb. Indications: Neurodermatitis, oxhide lichen, tinea capitis, tinea manuum, tinea pedis, wart.

Littleleaf Lemmaphyyllum Herb; LUO YAN CAO Origin: *Lemmaphyllum microphyllum* Presl (*Polypodiaceae*). Part: herb (with root). Effects: To clear the lung and suppress cough, cool the blood and resolve toxin. Indications: Pulmonary welling abscess, coughing of blood, blood ejection, spontaneous external bleeding, bloody urine, swollen welling abscess, scab and *lai*, knocks and falls, wind-fire toothache.

Lobed Kudzuvine Leaf; GE YE Origin: *Pueraria lobata* (Willd.) Ohwi (*Leguminosae*). Part: leaf. Indications: Bleeding from incised wound.

Lobed Kudzuvine Root; GE GEN Origin: *Pueraria lobata* (Willd.) Ohwi (*Leguminosae*). Part: root. Effects: To dispel pathogenic factors from the superficial muscles and reduce heat, reinforce *yang* and promote eruption, and promote salivation and relieve thirst. Indications: Exterior syndromes: fever, headache, no sweating, stiffness and pain in the neck and back; dire thirst in febrile diseases, polydipsia of diabetes; early stage of measles, diarrhea.

Lobedleaf Pharbitis Seed; QIAN NIU ZI Origin: *Pharbitis nil* (L.) Choisy (*Convolvulaceae*). Part: seed. Effects: To drain water, precipitate *qi,* and kill worms. Indications: Collection of water-rheum, swelling and distention of water abdomen; damp-heat accumulation and stagnation in the stomach and intestines, constipation; worm accumulation and abdomen pain.

lobster; HAI XIA Origin: *Panulirus ornatus* (Fabricius) (*Palinuridae*). See Prawn.

Loddiges Dendrobium; MEI HUA SHI HU (one of the **SHI HU**) Origin: *Dendrobium loddigesii* Rolfe. (*Orchidaceae*). See Noble Dendrobium.

Long Pepper; BI BA Origin: *Piper longum* L. (*Piperaceae*). Part: fruit-spike. Effects: To warm the center and relieve pain. Indications: Vomiting due to stomach-cold, hiccough, pain in the abdomen, and diarrhea.

Long Usnea Filament; SONG LUO Origin: *Usnea longissima* Ach. (*Usneaceae*). Part: filament. Effects: To clear the livet and transform phlegm, stanch bleeding and resolve toxin. Indications: Headache, red eyes, cough with profuse phlegm, malaria, scrofula, white vaginal discharge, flooding and spotting, bleeding due to external injury, swollen welling abscess, poisonous snake bites.

Longan Leaf; LONG YAN YE Origin: *Euphoria longan* (Lour.) Steud. (*Sapindaceae*). Part: leaf. Indications: Common cold, malaria, swollen clove sore, hemorrhoid.

Longbract Cattail Pollen; PU HUANG Origin: *Typha angustata* Bory *et* Chaub. (*Typhaceae*). Part: pollen. Effects: To cool the blood and stanch bleeding, quicken the blood and disperse stasis. Indications: Various kinds of bleeding, including hemoptysis, spontaneous external bleeding, blood ejection, bloody stool, bloody urine, flooding and spotting, and traumatic bleeding; cardiac or abdominal pains, menstrual pain and afterpains; blood strangury with inhibited pain..

Longpedicel Chinese Buscherry Seed; YU LI REN Origin: *Prunus japonica* Thunb. var. *nakaii* (Lévl.) Rehd. (*Rosaceae*). See Dwarf Flowering Cherry Seed.

Longroot Onion; GE CONG Origin: *Allium victorialis* L. (*Liliaceae*). Part: bulb. Effects: To eliminate miasmic toxin.

LongtubeGround Ivy; JIN QIAN CAO Origin: *Glechoma longituba* (Nakai) Kurp. (*Labiatae*). Part: aerial parts. Effects: To clear heat, disinhibit urine, suppress cough, disperse swelling, and resolve toxin. Indications: Jaundice, edema, vesical calculus, malaria, welling abscess of the lung, cough, blood ejection, strangury-turbidity, vaginal discharge, pain from wind-damp impediment (arthralgia-syndrome), child *gan* accumulation, fright epilepsy, swollen welling abscess, sore and lichen, eczema.

Lopseed Herb; LAO PO ZI ZHEN XIAN Origin: *Phryma leptostachya* L. (*Phrymataceae*). Part: herb or root. Effects: To resolve toxin and kill worms. Indications: Scab sore, yellow-water sore, infection and fever of sore toxin.

Loquat Leaf; PI PA YE Origin: *Eriobotrya japonica* (Thunb.) Lindl. (*Rosaceae*). Part: leaf. Effects: To clear the lung and harmonize the stomach, to downbear *qi* and transform phlegm. Indications: Cough with phlegm due to lung-heat, coughing of blood, nosebleed, vomiting due to stomach heat.

Loquat Seed; PI PA HE Origin: *Eriobotrya japonica* (Thunb.) Lindl. (*Rosaceae*). Part: seed. Effects: To transform phlegm and suppress cough, soothe the liver and rectify *qi.* Indications: Cough, mounting *qi,* edema, scrofula.

Lovely Hemsleya; LUO GUO DI Origin: *Hemsleya amabilis* Diels (*Cucurbitaceae*). See Largeseed Hemsleya.

Low Lily; BAI HE Origin: *Lilium pumilum* DC. (*Liliaceae*). See Greenish Lily.

Lucid Ganoderma; CHI ZHI (one of the **LING ZHI CAO**) Origin: *Ganoderma lucidum* (Leyss. *ex* Fr.) Karst. (*Polyporaceae*). See Japonese Ganoderma.

Lunate Peltate Sundew; MAO GAO CAI Origin: *Drosera peltata* Smith var. *lunata* (Buch.-Ham.) C. B. Clarke (*Droseraceae*). Part: herb. Indications: Stomachache, red and white dysentery, child *gan* accumulation, knocks and falls.

Lunathyrium Fern; GUAN ZHONG Origin: *Lunathyrium acrostichoides* (Sw.) Ching (*Athyria-ceae*). See Male Fern Rhizome.

Lychee Seed; LI ZHI HE Origin: *Litchi chinensis* Sonn. (*Sapindaceae*). Part: seed. Effects: To rectify *qi,* dispel cold, relieve pain, and resolve bind. Indications: Painful mounting *qi* or painful swollen testicles due to reverting *yin* liver channel and congealing cold *qi* stagnation; premenstrual abdominal pain, postpartum abdominal pain.

Macropodous Solomonseal; HUANG JING Origin: *Polygonatum macropodium* Turcz. (*Liliaceae*). See Siberian Solomonseal.

Madagascar Periwinkle; CHANG CHUN HUA Origin: *Catharanthus roseus* (L.) G. Don. (*Apocyna-ceae*). Part: herb. Effects: To settle fright and quite the spirit, to calm the liver and lower the blood pressure. Indications: Hypertension, Hodgkin's disease, malignant tumor, leukemia, lung cancer, chronic epithelioma, lymphoma.

Maidenhair Fern; ZHU ZONG CAO Origin: *Adiantum capillusveneris* L. (*Adiantaceae*). Part: herb. Effects: To clear heat, dispel wind, disinhibit urine, disperse swelling. Indications: Cough with bleed ejection, pain from wind-damp impediment (arthralgia-syndrome), strangury-turbidity, vaginal discharge, dysentery, swelling of breast, wind itchy papules, wind eczema.

Maize Style; YU MI XU Origin: *Zea mays* L. (*Gramineae*). Part: style and stigma. Effects: To disinhibit urine, drain heat, calm the liver and disinhibit the gallbladder. Indications: Nephritis with edema, leg *qi* (beriberi), icterohepatitis, hypertension, inflamation of the gallbladder, gallstones, diabetes, blood ejection, spontaneous external bleeding, deep-source nasal congestion, mammary welling abscess.

Maize; YU SHU SHU Origin: *Zea mays* L. (*Gramineae*). Part: seed. Effects: To regulate center and increase the appetite, boost the lung and quiet the heart, disinhibit urine.

Malabanut; DA BO GU Origin: *Adhatoda vasica* Nees (*Acanthaceae*). Part: branchlet and leaf. Effects: To quicken the blood and dissipate stasis. Indications: Wind-damp impediment (arthralgia-syndrome), knocks and falls, blood stasis swelling and pain, menstrual irregularities.

Malay Blumea Herb; HONG TOU CAO Origin: *Blumea lacera* (Burm. f.) DC. (*Compositae*). Part: aerial parts. Effects: To clear heat and resolve toxin, expel inflammation. Indications: Child pneumonia, tonsillitis, mumps, stomatitis, innominate toxin swelling, itchy skin.

Malaytea Scurfpea; BU GU ZHI Origin: *Psoralea corylifolia* L. (Leguminosae). Part: fruit. Effects: To invigorate the kidney-*yang* and to warm the spleen and treat diarrhea. Indications: Impotence, seminal emission, cold pain in the loins and knees, frequent urination and enuresis; diarrhea before dawn; externally for vitiligo and alopecia areata.

Male Fern Rhizome; GUAN ZHONG Origin: *Dryopteris crassirhizoma* Nakai (*Dryopteri-daceae*). Part: rhizome. Effects: To clear heat and resolve toxin, stanch blood and kill worms. Indications: Hookworm , tapeworm, pinworm; wind-heat common cold, maculopapular eruption due to warm heat, mumps.

Manaplant Alhagi Sweet Secretion; CI MI (LUO TUO CI) Origin: *Alhagi pseudalhagi* Desv. (*Leguminosae*). Part: sweet secretion. Indications: Steaming bone with vexation and thirst, blood dysentery, abdominal diarrhea, pain in abdomen, headache.

Manchurian Dutchmanspipe; GUAN MU TONG Origin: *Aristolochia manshuriensis* Kom. (*Aristolochiaceae*). Part: stem. Effects: To clear heat and drain fire,to promote diuresis and milk secration. Indications: Dump-heat in the urinary bladder, scanty dark urine, dribbling and painful micturition; canker sores, vexation and dark urine; hypogalactia after delivery.

Manchurian Rhododendron; ZHAO SHAN BAI Origin: *Rhododendron micranthum* Turcz. (*Ericaceae*). Part: branchlet, leaf or flower. Effects: To dispel wind, free the network vessels, stanch bleeding. Indications: Bronchitis, dysentery, postpartum generalized pain, fracture.

Manchurian Wildginger; XI XIN Origin: *Asarum heterotropoides* F. Schm. var. *mandshuricum* (Maxim.) Kitag. (*Aristolochiaceae*). Part: whole plant. Effects: To induce diaphoresis and dispel cold and wind, relieve pain, warm the lung and reduce phlegm. Indications: Headache, toothache, and impediment; exterior pattern due to external contraction of wind and cold; cold rheum lying latent in the lung, cough and panting; deep-source nasal congestion.

Mango Bark; MANG GUO SHU PI Origin: *Mongifera indica* L. (*Anacardiaceae*). Part: bark. Indications: Summerheat damage, generalized fever and aversion to cold.

Mango Leaf; MANG GUO YE Origin: *Mongifera indic*a L. (*Anacardiaceae*). Part: leaf. Effects: To move *qi* and course stagnation. Indications: Abdominal pain due to heat stagnation, *qi* distention, sand accumulation, putrefying sore, child *gan* accumulation, diabetes.

Mango Seed; MANG GUO HE Origin: *Mongifera indica* L. (*Anacardiaceae*). Part: seed. Indications: Mounting *qi,* food stagnation.

Mango; MANG GUO Origin: *Mongifera indica* L. (*Anacardiaceae*). Part: fruit. Effects: To boost the stomach and check vomiting, allay thirst and disinhibit urine. Indications: Menstrual block in woman, men's inhibited blood vessel.

Manyflower Garcinia; SHAN ZHU ZI Origin: *Garcinia multiflora* Champ. (*Guttiferae*). Part: bark or fruit. Effects: To disperse inflammation and relieve pain, to promote contraction and engender flesh. Indications: Burns and scalds, eczema, stomatitis, periodontitis, ulcerating welling abscess and sores.

Manyflower Glorybower Leaf; DA QING YE Origin: *Clerodendron cyrtophyllum* Turcz. (*Verbena-ceae*). See Indigo-coloured Woad Leaf.

Manyflower Solomonseal; HUANG JING Origin: *Polygonatum cyrtonema* Hua (*Liliaceae*). See Siberian Solomonseal.

Manyflower Tylophora; WA ER TENG Origin: *Tylophora floribunda* Miq. (*Asclepiadaceae*). Part: root. Effects: To dispel wind and transform phlegm, resolve toxin and dissipate stasis. Indications: Fright wind in children, summerheat stroke and abdomen pain, asthma with phlegm and cough, swelling and pain in the throat, stomachache, toothache, wind-damp pain (rheumatalgia), knocks and falls.

Manyleaf Meadowrue; MA WEI LIAN Origin: *Thalictrum foliolosum* DC. (*Ranunculaceae*). Part: rhizome and root. Effects: To clear heat and dry dampness, to resolve toxin. Indications: Dysentery, enteritis, infective hepatitis, common cold, measles, swollen welling abscess sore and boil, conjunctivitis.

Manyleaf Paris; ZAO XIU Origin: *Paris polyphlla* Smith (*Liliaceae*). Part: rhizome. Effects: To clear heat and resolve toxin, disperse swelling and relieve pain, extinguish wind and settle fright. Indications: Swelling and toxin of welling abscess and sores, poisonous snake bite; lever heat induced wind, fright epilepsy, clouded spirit due to febrile disease, convulsion; bleeding due to external injury, stasis swelling and pain.

Manynerve Embelia; MA GUI HUA Origin: *Embelia oblongifolia* Hemsl. (*Myrsinaceae*). Part: fruit. Effects: To expel worms, dispel wind-dampness. Indications: Tapeworm disease.

Manyprickle Acanthopanax Leaf; CI WU JIA YE (one of the **WU JIA YE**) Origin: *Acantho-panax senticosus* (Rupr. *et* Maxim.) Harms (*Aralia-ceae*). See Slenderstyle Acanthopanax Leaf.

Manyprickle Acanthopanax Root-bark; CI WU JIA PI (one of the **WU JIA PI**) Origin: *Acanthopanax senticosus* (Rupr. *et* Maxim.) Harms (*Araliaceae*). See Slenderstyle Acanthopanax Root-bark.

Manyprickle Acanthopanax Root; CI WU JIA (WU JIA GEN) Origin: *Acanthopanax senticosus* (Rupr. *et* Maxim.) Harms (*Araliaceae*). Part: root and rhizome. Effects: To boost *qi* and fortify the spleen, supplement the kidney and quiet the spirit. Indications: Spleen-kidney *yang* vacuity, body vacuity and lack of strength, poor appetite, aching pain in the lumbus and knees, insomnia and profuse dreaming; Modern clinical: melancholia, leucopenia, cerebral embolism, hyperlipemia, hypopiesia, coronary heart disease, angina pectoris, diabetes, acute altitude sickness.

Manyspike Knotweed; DUO SUI LIAO Origin: *Polygonum polystachyum* Wall. *ex* Meisn (*Polygonaceae*). Part: herb. Effects: To dispel wind and disinhibit damp, kill worm and check dysentery, clear heat and resolve toxin. Indications: Bacillary dysentery, enteronitis, child indigestion, knocks and falls, wind-damp swelling and pain, eczema.

Manyspike Tanoak Leaf; DUO SUI SHI KE YE Origin: *Lithocarpus polystachyus* Rehd. (*Fagaceae*). Part: leaf. Indications: Hypertension.

Marchantia Polymorpha Lichen ; DI SUO LUO Origin: *Marchantia polymorpha* L. (*Marchantiaceae*). Part: lichen. Effects: To ingender flesh, draw out toxin, and clear heat. Indications: Scalds, lichen, knife wound, fracture, foot rot for many years.

Marginate American Agave; JIN BIAN LONG SHE LAN Origin: *Agave americana* L. var. *marginata* Hort. (*Agavaceae*). Part: leaf. Effects: To moisten the lung, transform phlegm, and suppress cough. Indications: Vacuity taxation with cough, blood ejection, asthma.

Marsh Horsetail Herb; GU JIE CAO Origin: *Equisetum palustre* L. (*Equisetaceae*). Part: herb. Effects: To soothe wind and brighten the eyes, soothe sinew and quicken the blood. Indications: Tearing on exposure to wind, eye screen, knocks and falls, intestinal wind, blood hemorrhoid.

Marshy Betony; GUANG YE SHUI SU Origin: *Stachys palustris* L. (*Labiatae*). Part: root or herb. Effects: To clear heat and transform phlegm, and as an antibacterial and anti-inflammatory. Indications: Wind-heat cough, swelling and pain in the throat, whooping cough, dysentery, zoster.

Matteuccia Fern; GUAN ZHONG Origin: *Matteuccia struthiopteris* (L.) Todaro (*Onocleaceae*). See Male Fern Rhizome.

Maywood; MU JU Origin: *Matricaria chamomilla* L. [= *Matricaria recutita* L.] (*Compo-sitae*). Part: flower or herb. Effects: To dispel wind and resolve the exterior. Indications: Common cold, wind-damp pain (rheumatalgia).

Meadow Cranesbill Herb; CAO YUAN LAO GUAN CAO Origin: *Geranium pratense* L. (*Geraniaceae*). Part: herb. Indications: Acute bacillary dysentery.

Medicinal Citron Leaf; XIANG YUAN YE Origin: *Citrus medica* L. (*Rutaceae*). Part: leaf. Indications: Cold damage cough.

Medicinal Citron; XIANG YUAN Origin: *Citrus medica* L. (*Rutaceae*). Part: fruit. Effects: To rectify *qi* and relieve depression, strengthen the spleen, and reduce phlegm. Indications: Oppression in the chest, rib-side pain, pain and distention in stomach duct and abdomem, belching and low food intake, vomiting due to liver stomach *qi* stagnation; phlegm-damp congestion, cough and profuse phlegm.

Medicinal Evodia; WU ZHU YU Origin: *Evodia rutaecarpa* (Juss.) Benth. (*Rutaceae*). Part: fruit. Effects: To dispel cold, to dry damp, to soothe the liver, to lower the adverse flow of *qi*, and to relieve pain. Indications: Pathogenic cold in the interior: gastric and abdominal cold pain, periumbilical colic, headache and salivation, chronic diarrhea and diarrhea before dawn; placidity and pain of the lower limbs; vomiting and acid regurgitation; canker sores; hypertension.

Medicinal Indianmulberry; BA JI TIAN Origin: *Morinda officinalis* How (*Rubiaceae*). Part: root. Effects: To invigorate the kidney-yang, strengthen muscles and bones, and as an antirheumatic. Indications: Impotence, lesser-abdominal cold pain, urinary incontinence, vacuity and cold of the uterus, wind-cold-damp impediment, aching lumbus and knees.

Medicinal Rhubarb; DA HUANG Origin: *Rheum officinale* Baill. (*Polygonaceae*). Part: root and rhizome. Effects: To induce precipitation, to remove heat and toxin and to quicken the blood and dispel blood stasis. Indications: Constipation; dysentery, loose but unsmooth discharge of stool; blood ejection and spontaneous external bleeding; blood-shot eyes, gum swelling and pain, and sore throat; sores, carbuncles and burns; postpartum abdominal pain caused by blood stasis, bind in the abdomen, injuries; jaundice and stranguria.

Medicine Terminalia Fruit; HE ZI Origin: *Terminalia chebula* Retz. (*Combretaceae*). Part: fruit. Effects: To constrain the lung and astringe the intestines, precipitate *qi*. Indications: Enduring cough and loss of voice, enduring diarrhea, enduring dysentery, prolapse of the rectum, bloody stool, flooding and spotting, vaginal discharge, seminal emission, frequent urination.

Medicine Terminalia Leaf; HE ZI YE Origin: *Terminalia chebula* Retz. (*Combretaceae*). Part: leaf. Effects: To precipitate *qi,* disperse phlegm, allay thirst, and check dysentery. Indications: Same as Medicine Terminalia Fruit (HE ZI, *1006*).

Mediinal Cyathula; CHUAN NIU XI Origin: *Cyathula officinalis* Kuan (*Amaranthaceae*). Part: root. Effects: To promote blood circulation and dispel blood stasis, to ease joint movement and ensure proper down-ward flow of the blood. Indications: Wind-damp pain in the lumbus and knees, flaccid paralysis of limbs and hypertonicity of the sinews, blood strangury, bloody urine, menstrual block, concretions and conglomerations.

Meiwa Kumquat Leaf; JIN JU YE Origin: *Fortunella crassifolia* Swingle (*Rutaceae*). See Oval Kumquat Leaf.

Meiwa Kumquat; JIN JU Origin: *Fortunella crassifolia* Swingle (*Rutaceae*). See Oval Kumquat.

Mellea Armillaria Sporophore; ZHEN MO Origin: *Armillaria mellea* (Vahl *ex* Fr.) Quél. (*Tricholomataceae*). Part: sporophore. Effects: To dispel wind and quicken the network vessels, strengthen bones and muscles. Indications: Epilepsy, lumbar and leg pain.

Membranous Milkvetch; HUANG QI Origin: *Astragalus membranaceus* (Fisch.) Bge. (*Leguminosae*). Part: root. Effects: To replenish *qi* and keep *yang-qi* ascending, consolidate superficial resistance, disinhibit urine, promote pus discharge, and tissue regeneration. Indications: Deficiency of the spleen-*qi* and lung-*qi* or syndrome of sinking of *qi* of the middle-*jiao*; spontaneous and night sweating; non-rupture of carbuncles or slow healing long after ulceration of carbuncles; facial edema, scanty urine, palpitation and shortness of breath; numb extremities or hemiplegia after apoplexy with full consciousness and weak pulse; diabetes.

Mexican Tea; TU JING JIE Origin: *Chenopodium ambrosioides* L. (*Chenopodiaceae*). Part: fruiting aerial parts. Effects: To expel wind, kill parasites, stimulate menstrual discharge and relieve pain. Indications: Wind-damp impediment (arthralgia-syndrome) of the skin, menstrual block, painful menstruation, hookworm, roundworm, skin eczema, snake or insect bites.

Mitten Crab Chelae; XIE KE Origin: *Eriocheir sinensis* H. Milne-Edwards (*Grapsidae*). Part: shell. Effects: To break stasis and disperse accumulation. Indications: Accumulation and stagnation of stasis blood, pain in the rib-side, pain in abdomen, mammary welling abscess, frostbite.

Moderate Asiabell; DANG SHEN Origin: *Codonopsis pilosula* Nannf. var. *modesta* (Nannf.) L.T. Shen [= *Codonopsis Modesta* Nannf.] (*Campanulaceae*). *See* Pilose Asiabell.

Mongolian Dandelion; PU GONG YING Origin: *Taraxacum mongolicum* Hand.-Mazz. (*Compositae*). Part: aerial parts. Effects: To clear heat and resolve toxin, disinhibit urine and expel node. Indications: Swollen welling abscess, open sore, and clove sores due to heat-toxin, mammary welling abscess, pulmonary welling abscess with concentrated phlegm and chest pain, intestinal welling abscess with exuberant heat toxin, sore swollen throat; sore red swollen eyes; jaundice due to damp-heat, dribbing urination and stinging pain.

Mongolian Ephedra; MA HUANG Origin: *Ephedra equisetina* Bge. (*Ephedraceae*). See Chinese Ephedra

Mongolian Milkvetch; MENG GU HUANG QI (one of the **HUANG QI**) Origin: *Astragalus mongholicus* Bge. (*Leguminosae*). See Membranous Milkvetch.

Mongolian Snakegourd Root; TIAN HUA FEN (GUA LOU GEN) Origin: *Trichosanthes kirilowii* Maxim. (*Cucurbitaceae*). Part: tuber root. Effects: To clear heat and engender liquid, to disperse swelling and expel pus. Indications: Heat damaging liquid, dry mouth and thirst, thirst with liking for fluids due to wasting-thirst disease; lung heat cough, dryness cough with phlegm, coughing of blood; swelling of welling abscess and open sore, exuberant heat toxin, red swelling and scorching pain; malignant grape mole, chronic epithelioma.

Mongolian Snakegourd; GUA LOU Origin: *Trichosanthes kirilowii* Maxim. (*Cucurbitaceae*). Part: fruit. Effects: To remove heat and reduce heat-phlegm, relieve stuffiness of the chest and as a laxative to relieve constipation. Indications: Cough of lung -heat with yellow and thick sputum, unsmooth expectoration, fullness in the chest, and dry stool; chest pain; carbuncles of breast and pulmonary abscess; dry of the intestines with constipation.

Mountain Spicy Tree; BI CHENG QIE Origin: *Litsea cubeba* (Lour.) Pers. (*Lauraceae*). See Cubeba Piper.

Mountain Yam; SHAN BEI XIE (one of the **BEI XIE**) Origin: *Dioscorea tokoro* Mak. (*Dioscoria-ceae*). See Hypoglaucous Collett Yam.

Moupin Dutchmanspipe; HUAI TONG Origin: *Aristolochia moupinensis* Franch. (*Aristolochiaceae*). Part: stem or root. Effects: To clear heat and eliminate damp, expel pus and relieve pain, move water and promote lactation. Indications: Inhibited urination, bloody urine, trichomonal vaginitis, eczema, urticaria, rheumatism with painful joints, swollen welling abscess, malign sore, five stranguries.

Mullein Nightbrier Leaf; YE YAN YE Origin: *Solanum verbascifolium* L. (*Solanaceae*). Part: leaf. Indications: Yellow swelling, pain wind, flooding, painful swelling from knocks and falls, toothache, scrofula, welling abscess, eczema, dermatitis.

Mung Bean Blister Beetle; QING NIANG ZI Origin: Lytta caraganae Pallas (*Meloidae*). Part: dried body. Effects: To attack toxin and expel stasis. Indications: Scrofula, rabid dog bite.

Muriculate Eucheuma Frond; QI LIN CAI Origin: *Eucheuma muricatum* (Gmel.) Web. V. Bos. (*Solieriaceae*). Part: frond. Effects: To eliminate phlegm.

Mushroom; MO GU Origin: *Agaricus campestris* L. *ex* Fr. (*Agaricaceae*). Part: sporophore. Effects: To raise the spirit, promote the appetite, check diarrhea, check vomiting, transform phlegm, rectify*qi,*andbenefit the intestines and stomach.

Muskmallow; HUANG KUI Origin: *Abelmoschus moschatus* (L.) Medic. (*Malvaceae*). Part: root or leaf. Effects: To resolve toxin and disperse swelling, expel pus and relieve pain. Indications: Swelling and pain of welling abscess and sore, innominate toxin swelling, snake's-head sore.

Muskmelon Fruit Pedicel; GUA DI Origin: *Cucumis melo* L. (*Cucurbitaceae*). Part: fruit pedicel. Effects: Vomiting wind-phlegm abiding food, drain water-damp collecting rheum. Indications: Abiding food with phlegm-drool, congest upper stomach duct, hard glomus in the chest, wind-phlegm epilepsy, damp-heat jaundice, puffy swelling in four limbs, nasal congestion, throat impediment.

Myrrh; MO YAO Origin: *Commiphora myrrha* Engl. (*Burseraceae*). Part: gum resin. Effects: To quicken the blood, relieve pain, and promote tissue regeneration. Indications: Pain from knocks and falls, incised wound., pain in sinew and bone, heart region and abdomen, concretions and conglomerations, menstrual block, swelling and pain of welling abscess and flat abscess, hemorrhoidal and fistulas, eye screen.

Nanmu Lignum; NAN MU Origin: *Phoebe nanmu* (Oliv.) Gamble (*Lauraceae*). Part: wood, branchlet and leaf. Indications: Vomiting and diarrhea with cramp, edema.

Narrowleaf Cattail Pollen; PU HUANG Origin: *Typha angustifolia* L. (*Typhaceae*). See Longbract Cattail Pollen.

Narrowleaf Euphorbia; XI YE DA JI Origin: *Euphorbia esula* L. var. *cyparissoides* Boiss. (*Euphorbiaceae*). Part: whole plant. Indications: Swollen sore.

Narrowleaf Scabious; MENG GU SHAN LUO BO Origin: *Scabiosa comosa* Fisch. (*Dipsacaceae*). Part: flower. Effects: To clear heat and drain fire. Indications: Liver fire headache, fever, lung heat cough, jaundice.

Narrowleaf Senna Leaf; FAN XIE YE Origin: *Cassia angustifolia* Vahl (*Leguminosae*). Part: leaf. Effects: To drain heat and abduct stagnation. Indications: Constipation due to heat bind.

Negundo Chastetree Leaf; HUANG JING YE Origin: *Vitex negundo* L. (*Verbenaceae*). Part: leaf. Effects: To clear heat and resolve the exterior, disinhibit dampness and resolve toxin. Indications: Common cold, summerheat stroke, vomiting and diarrhea, dysentery, malaria, jaundice, rheumatism, painful swelling from knocks and falls, sore and welling abscess, scab and lichen.

Nepal Dock; YANG TI Origin: *Rumex nepalensis* Spr. (*Polygonaceae*). See Japanese Dock.

Nervate Twayblade; JIAN XUE QING Origin: *Liparis nervosa* (Thunb.) Lindl. (*Orchida-ceae*). Part: herb. Effects: To cool blood and stanch bleeding, to clear hear and resolve toxin. Indications: Blood ejection, hacking of blood, intestinal wind bleeding, flooding, bleeding during the operation, fright wind in children, heat-toxin sores and open sores, snake bite.

Nippon Hawthorn Leaf; SHAN ZHA YE Origin: *Crataegus cuneata* Sieb. *et* Zucc. (*Rosaceae*). See Chinese Hawthorn Leaf.

Nippon Hawthorn; SHAN ZHA Origin: *Crataegus cuneata* Sieb. *et* Zucc. (*Rosaceae*). See Chinese Hawthorn.

Nippon Yam; CHUAN SHAN LONG (CHUAN LONG SHU YU) Origin: *Dioscorea nipponica* Mak. (*Dioscoreaceae*). Part: rhizome. Effects: To dispel wind and remove dump, quicken the blood and relieve pain, expel phlegm and arrest coughing. Indications: Wind-cold-damp impediment, chronic trachitis, indigestion, taxation detriment and sprain, malaria, swollen welling abscess.

Noble Dendrobium; SHI HU Origin: *Dendrobium nobile* Lindl. (*Orchidaceae*). Part: stem. Effects: To replenish *yin* essence and nourish the stomach, and to remove heat and promote the production of fluid. Indications: Dry mouth; fever of deficiency; improving acuity of vision, and strengthening the loins and knees.

Northeast Seriphidium; DONG BEI HUI HAO Origin: *Seriphidium finitum* (Kitag.) Ling *et* Y. R. Ling [= *Artemisia finita* Kitag.] (*Compositae*). Part: flower. Effects: To quiet worm. Indications: Roundworm.

Northern Dutchmanspipe; BEI MA DOU LING (one of the **MA DOU LING**) Origin: *Aristolochia contorta* Bge. (*Aristolochiaceae*). Part: fruit. Effects: To clear the lung and downbear *qi*, to transform phlegm and suppress cough. Indications: Lung heat cough and panting, cough of blood, loss of voice, hemorrhoids and fistulas with swelling and pain.

Northern Dutchmanspipe Root; QING MU XIAN (MA DOU LING GEN) Origin: *Aristolochia contorta* Bge. (*Aristolochiaceae*). Part: root. Effects: To promote the flow of *qi,* resolve toxin, and disperse swelling. Indications: Distention and pain in the chest and abdomen, sand, enteritis and dysentery, hypertension, mounting *qi,* snakebite, swollen welling abscess, clove sore, itchy or damp-erosion of the skin.

Nude Fern; SHI SHUA BA Origin: *Psilotum nudum* (L.) Griseb. (*Psilotaceae*). Part: herb. Effects: To quicken the blood and free the channels, dispel wind-damp. Indications: Wind-damp impendment, menstrual block, blood ejection, knocks and falls.

Nudicaulous Grounsel Herb; ZI BEI TIAN KUI CAO Origin: *Senecio nudicaulis* Buch.-Ham. (*Compositae*). Part: herb. Effects: To quicken blood and dispel stasis, regulate menstruation. Indications: Menstrual irregularities, profuse white vaginal discharge, rheumatism, internal and external injury from knocks and falls.

Nut-vomitive Poisonnut; MA QIAN ZI Origin: *Strychnos nux-vomica* L. (*Loganiaceae*). Part: seed. Effects: To remove obstruction of the channels and relieve pain, to disperse swelling and dissipate bind. Indications: Throat impediment, sore throat, swelling and toxin of welling abscess and flat abscess, wind impediment with pain, bone fracture.

Nutgrass Galingale; XIANG FU Origin: *Cyperus rotundus* L. (*Cyperaceae*). Part: rhizome. Effects: To soothe the liver and rectify *qi,* to regulate menstruation and relieve pain. Indications: Distention and pain in the chest, hypochondrium and abdomen; irregular menstruation and menstrual pain.

Obovate Peony; CAO SHAO YAO (one of the **CHI SHAO YAO**) Origin: *Paeonia obovata* Maxim. (*Ranunculaceae*). See Common Peony (wild).

Odorate Rosewood; JIANG ZHEN XIANG Origin: *Dalbergia odorifera* T. Chen (*Leguminosae*). Part: heart wood. Effects: To quicken the blood, relieve pain and stanch bleeding. Indications: Blood ejection, hemoptysis, bleeding from incised wound, knocks and falls, swelling of abscess and sore, wind-damp pain in the lumbus and leg *qi* pain in the region of the heart and stomach.

Officinal Asparagus; XIAO BAI BU Origin: *Asparagus officinalis* L. (*Liliaceae*). Part: tuber root. Effects: To moisten the lung and settle cough, dispel phlegm and kill worms. Indications: Lung heat, scab and lichen, all kinds of parasites.

Officinal Mangolia; HOU PO Origin: *Magnolia officinalis* Rehd. *et* Wils. (*Magnoliaceae*). Part: bark. Effects: To rectify *qi* and remove dampness, and relieve panting. Indications: Gastric and abdominal distention; cough and panting due to phlegm in the lung.

Oiltea Camellia Root-bark; YOU CHA GEN PI Origin: *Camellia oleifera* Abel (*Theaceae*). Part: root bark. Effects: To dissipate stasis and disperse swelling, quicken the blood and join bones. Indications: Fracture, sprain and contusion, abdominal pain, itchy skin, burns and scalds.

Oiltea Camellia; CHA ZI XIN Origin: *Camellia oleifera* Abel (*Theaceae*). Part: seed. Effects: To move *qi* and soothe stagnation. Indications: *Qi* stagnation with abdominal pain and diarrhea, itchy skin, burns and scalds.

Oldham Bamboo Shoot; LU SUN PIAN Origin: *Sinocalamus oldhami* (Munro) Mcclure (*Gramineae*). Part: shoot. Indications: Cough and panting.

Oldworld Arrowhead Corm; CI GU Origin: *Sagittaria sagittifolia* L. (*Alismataceae*). Part: corm. Effects: To move the blood and free strangury. Indications: Postpartum blood stasis, retention of the placenta, strangury, cough with phlegm and blood.

Olibanum; RU XIANG Origin: *Boswellia carterii* Birdw. (*Anacardiaceae*). Part: gum resin. Effects: To quicken the blood, relieve pain and promote tissue regeneration. Indications: *Qi*-blood congealing and stagnation, pain in the heart and abdomen, swelling and toxin of welling abscess and sores, knocks and falls, menstrual pain, postpartum blood stasis with stabbing pain.

Olive; GAN LAN Origin: *Canarium album* (Lour.) Raeusch. (*Burseraceae*). Part: fruit. Effects: To clear the lung, disinhibit throat, engender liquid, and resolve toxin. Indications: Sore swollen throat, vexation and thirst, cough and blood ejection, bacillary dysentery, epilepsy.

Omei Mountain Goldthread; HUANG LIAN Origin: *Coptis omeiensis* (Chen) C. Y. Cheng (*Ranunculaceae*). See Chinese Goldthread.

Omoto Nipponlily Root; WAN NIAN QING GEN Origin: *Rohdeajaponica* Roth. (*Liliaceae*). Part: root, rhizome and leaf. Effects: Used as a cardiatonic, diuretic, antipyretic, detoxicant, and hemostatic. Indications: Cardiac failure, sore swollen throat, diphtheria, edema, drum distention, hacking of blood, blood ejection, clove sore, cinnabar toxin, snake bite, scald.

Opium Poppy Pericarp; YING SU KE Origin: *Papaver somniferum* L. (*Papaveraceae*). Part: capsule. Effects: To astringe intestines and check diarrhea, astringe the lung and suppress cough, and relieve pain. Indications: Enduring cough, enduring dysentery, enduring drainage; prolapse of the rectum, bloody stool; pain in heart, abdomen, sinew and bone; seminal efflux, profuse urination, white vaginal discharge.

Opium Poppy; YING SU Origin: *Papaver somniferum* L. (*Papaveraceae*). Part: seed. Indica-tions: Stomach reflux, abdominal pain, diarrhea, prolapse of rectum.

Opium; YA PIAN Origin: *Papaver sommiferum* L. (*Papaveraceae*). Part: latex from the unripe capsules. Effects: To constrain the lung and astringe the intestines, suppress cough, relieve pain. Indications: Enduring cough, enduring diarrhea, enduring dysentery, prolapse of the rectum, pain in heart region and abdomen, pain of sinews and bones.

Orange Daylily; XUAN CAO GEN Origin: *Hemerocallis fulva* L. (*Liliaceae*). Part: root. Effects: To disinhibit water and cool the blood. Indications: Edema, inhibited urination, strangury-turbidity, vaginal discharge, jaundice, spontaneous external bleeding, bloody stool, flooding and spotting, mammary welling abscess.

Orange Stonecrop; FEI CAI Origin: *Sedum kamtschaticum* Fisch. (*Crassulaceae*). Part: herb or root. Effects: To quicken the blood and stanch bleeding, restful heart, disinhibit dampness, disperse swelling and resolve toxin. Indications: Knocks and falls, coughing of blood, blood ejection, bloody stool, heart palpitation, swollen welling abscess.

Oriental Bittersweet Leaf; NAN SHE TENG YE Origin: *Celastrus orbiculatus* Thunb. (*Celastraceae*). Part: leaf. Indications: Poisonous snake bites.

Oriental Bittersweet Root; NAN SHE TENG GEN Origin: *Celastrus orbiculatus* Thunb. (*Celastraceae*). Part: root. Effects: To dispel wind and overcome dampness, move *qi* and dissipate the blood, relieve swelling and resolve toxin. Indications: Pain in sinews and bones due to wind-damp, knocks and falls, sand *qi* with vomiting and abdominal pain, swelling and toxin of welling abscess and flat abscess.

Oriental Blechnum Frond; GUAN ZHONG Origin: *Blechnum orientale* L. (*Blechnaceae*). See Male Fern Rhizome.

Oriental Blueberry Leaf; NAN ZHU YE Origin: *Vaccinium bracteatum* Thunb. (*Ericaceae*). Part: leaf. Effects: To boost essence *qi,* strengthen sinew and bone, brighten the eyes, check diarrhea.

Oriental Buckthorn Root; LI LA GEN Origin: *Rhamnus crenata* Sieb. *et* Zucc. (*Rhamnaceae*). Part: root or root bark. Effects: To clear heat and disinhibit damp, kill worms and resolve toxin. Indications: Scab, lichen, lai, clove sore, scalds, roundworm.

Oriental Chain Fern; DONG FANG GOU JI Origin: *Woodwardia orientalis* Sm. (*Blechnaceae*). Part: rhizome. Effects: To dispel wind-damp, invigorate the lumbus and knees. Indications: Lumbar and leg pain, dysentery, snake bite.

Oriental Sesame Leaf; HU MA YE Origin: *Sesamum indicum* DC. (*Pedaliaceae*). Part: leaf. Indications: Wind-cold-damp impediment, flooding, blood ejection, wet-itching in the genital region.

Oriental Sesame; BAI ZHI MA (HU MA ZI) Origin: *Sesamum indicum* DC. (*Pedaliaceae*). Part: white seed. Effects: To moisten dryness and lubricate the intestines. Indications: Straitened spleen and difficult defecation, child head sore.

Oriental sesame; HEI ZHI MA Origin: *Sesamum indicun* DC (*Pedaliaceae*). Part: seed. Effects: To supplement the liver and kidney, moisten the five viscera (heart, lung, spleen, liver, and kidney) Indications: Insufficiency of the liver and kidney, vacuity wind dizziness, wind impediment, paralysis, dry bound stool, vacuity and marked emaciation afterillness, premature graying, scant breast milk.

Oriental Stephania; BAI YAO ZI Origin: *Stephania cepharantha* Hayata (*Menispermaceae*). Part: tuberous root. Effects: To clear heat and disperse phlegm, cool the blood and resolve toxin, relieve pain. Indications: Sore throat and throat impediment, cough, blood ejection, spontaneous external bleeding, bleeding from incised wound, heat toxin swollen welling abscess, scrofula.

Oriental Sweetgum Resin; SU HE XIANG Origin: *Liquidambar orientalis* Mill. (*Hamamelidaceae*). Part: balsam from the trunk. Effects: To induce resuscitation and expectorate phlegm. Indications: Sudden faint and syncope due to phlegm blockage, apoplexy or epilepsy due to pathogenic cold or phlegm blockage in the interior; cold pain and sensation of fullness and tightness in the chest and abdomen; angina pectoris of coronary heart disease.

Oriental variegated Coralbean Bark; HAI TONG PI Origin: *Erythrina variegata* L. var. *orentalis* (L.) Merr. (*Leguminosae*). Part: bark. Effects: To dispel wind-damp, to promote circulation of *qi* and to induce diuresis and relieve edema. Indications: Wind-damp impediment (arthralgia-syndrome), pain in the lumbus and knees; scab, lichen, and eczema.

Oriental Waterplantain; ZE XIE Origin: *Alisma orientale* (Sam.) Juzepcz. [= *Alisma plantagoaquatica* L. var. *orientale* Samuels] (*Alisma-taceae*). Part: leaf. Effects: To induce diuresis to excrete damp, and to expel heat. Indications: Dysuria, edema, phlegm retention, diarrhea, stranguria with turbid urine, and leukorrhagia.

Orientvine; QING FENG TENG Origin: *Sinomenium acutum* (Thunb.) Rehd. *et* Wils. (*Menispermaceae*). Part: stem. Effects: Used as an antirheumatic and analgesic agent for rheumatic arthritis, articular swelling and pain. Indications: Rheumatic arthritis, articular swelling and pain.

Oval Kumquat Leaf; JIN JU YE Origin: *Fortunella margarita* (Lour.) Swingle (*Rutaceae*). Part: leaf. Effects: To soothe depressed liver *qi,* open stomach *qi,* dissipate lung *qi*. Indications: Dysphagia-occlusion, scrofula.

Oval Kumquat; JIN JU Origin: *Fortunella margarita* (Lour.) Swingle (*Rutaceae*). Part: fruit. Effects: To rectify *qi* and resolve depression, transform phlegm and rectify *qi* and resolve depression. Indications: Oppression and depression in the chest, liquor damage with thirst, food stragnation in torpid stomach.

Ovate Catalpa Fruit; ZI SHI Origin: *Catalpa ovata* G. Don (*Bignoniaceae*). Part: fruit. Effects: To disinhibit urine, kill worms. Indications: General edema.

Ovate Catalpa Leaf; ZI YE Origin: *Catalpa ovata* G. Don (*Bignoniaceae*). Part: leaf. Indications: Vigorous fever in children, scab and sore, itchy skin.

Ovate Catalpa; ZI MU Origin: *Catalpa ovata* G. Don (*Bignoniaceae*). Part: wood. Indications: Pain wind in the extremities, cholera without spitting and purging.

Ovateleaf Holly; JIU BI YING Origin: *Ilex rotunda* Thunb. (*Aquifoliaceae*). Part: bark. Effects: To clear heat and resolve toxin, disinhibit damp and relieve pain. Indications: Common cold with fever, tonsillitis, sore swollen throat, acute and chronic hepatitis, acute gastroenteritis, gastric and duodenal ulcer, wind-damp with painful joints, knocks and falls, burns and scald.

Ovateleaf Knotweed; HONG SAN QI Origin: *Polygonum suffultum* Maxim. (*Leguminosae*). Part: rhizome. Effects: To dissipate blood and stanch bleeding, move *qi* and regulate menstruation. Indications: Knocks and falls, taxation damage and blood ejection, bloody stool, flooding and spotting, menstrual irregularities.

Ox Blood; NIU XUE Origin: *Bos taurus domesticus* Gmelin; *Bubalus bubalis* Linnaeus (*Bovidae*). Part: blood. Effects: To rectify blood and center. Indications: bloody stool, blood dysentery, menstrual block, blood.

Ox Brain; NIU NAO Origin: *Bos taurus domesticus* Gmelin; *Bubalus bubalis* Linnaeus (*Bovidae*). Part: brain. Indications: Head wind dizziness, diabetes, glomus *qi*.

Ox Gall; NIU DAN Origin: *Bos taurus domesticus* Gmelin; *Bubalus bubalis* Linnaeus (*Bovidae*). Part: gall. Effects: To clear liver and brighten the eyes, disinhibit gallbladder and free intestine, resolve toxin and eliminate swelling. Indications: Wind-heat eye disease, jaundice, constipation, fright wind in children, swollen welling abscess, hemorrhoid.

Ox Kidney; NIU SHEN Origin: *Bos taurus domesticus* Gmelin; *Bubalus bubalis* Linnaeus (*Bovidae*). Part: kindey. Effects: To supplement kidney and boost essence. Indications: Damp impediment.

Ox Liver; NIU GAN Origin: *Bos taurus domesticus* Gmelin; *Bubalus bubalis* Linnaeus (*Bovidae*). Part: liver. Effects: To nourish blood, supplement liver, and brighten the eyes. Indications: Blood vacuity and withered-yellow, vacuity taxation and marked emaciation, clear-eye blindness, night blindness.

Ox Lung; NIU FEI Origin: *Bos taurus domesticus* Gmelin; *Bubalus bubalis* Linnaeus (*Bovidae*). Part: lung. Effects: To supplement lung. Indications: Cough and counterflow.

Ox Teeth; NIU CHI Origin: *Bos taurus domesticus* Gmelin; *Bubalus bubalis* Linnaeus (*Bovidae*). Part: teeth. Indications: Ox epilepsy in children.

Ox Thyroid; NIU YE Origin: *Bos taurus domesticus* Gmelin; *Bubalus bubalis* Linnaeus (*Bovidae*). Part: thyroid. Indications: Throat impediment, *qi* goiter.

Oxhide Gelatin; HUANG MING JIAO Origin: *Bos taurus domesticus* Gmelin (*Bovidae*). Part: gelatin made from the hide of ox. Effects: To enrich *yin* and moisten dryness, stanch bleeding and disperse swelling. Indications: Vacuity taxation lung wilting, cough and hacking of blood, blood ejection, spontaneous external bleeding, flooding and spotting, knocks and falls, swollen welling abscess, scalds.

Oyster Meat; MU LI ROU Origin: *Ostrea rivularis* Gould; *Ostrea talienwhanensis* Crosse; *Ostrea gigas* Thunberg (all *Osteridae*). Part: meat. Effects: To enrish *yin* and nourish the blood. Indications: Heat vexation and insomnia, disquieted heart spirit, cinnabar toxin.

Pale Bittersweet; MIAN TENG Origin: *Celastrus hypoleucus* (Oliv.) Warb. (*Celastraceae*). Part: root. Effects: To transform stasis and disperse swelling. Indications: Red swelling from knocks and falls.

Palmatipartiteleaf Neocheiropteris; SHAN JUE Origin: *Neocheiropteris palmatopedata* (Bak.) Christ (*Polypodiaceae*). Part: rhizome or herb. Effects: To disperse bloating, dispel wind damp. Indications: Wind damp leg *qi* (beriberi).

Paniculate Goldraintree; LUAN HUA Origin: *Koelreuteria paniculata* Laxm. (*Sapindaceae*). Part: flower. Indications: Eye pain, eye swelling, red eye sand tearing.

Paniculate Hydrangea; FEN TUAN HUA Origin: *Hydrangea paniculata* Sieb. (*Saxifragaceae*). Part: flower. Effects: To disperse damp, break the blood. Indications: Kidney sac wind.

Paniculate Onosma; ZI CAO Origin: *Onosma paniculatum* Bur. *et* Franch. (*Boraginaceae*). See Redroot Gromwell.

Paniculate Spotflower; TIAN WEN CAO Origin: *Spilanthes acmella* (L.) Dalz. *et* Gibs. (*Compositae*). Part: herb. Effects: To suppress cough and stabilize panting, disperse swelling and relieve pain, resolve toxin and dissipate bind. Indications: Common cold and cough, chronic bronchitis, asthma, whooping cough, pulmonary tuberculosis, snake bite, toxin swelling of cores, toothache, malaria, abdominal diarrhea, pain in abdomen, knocks and falls, rheumatic arthritis.

Paniculate Swallowwort; XU CHANG QING Origin: *Cynanchum paniculatum* (bge.) Kitag. (*Asclepiadaceae*). Part: root. Effects: To dispel wind and settle pain, suppress cough, disinhibit water and disperse swelling, quicken the blood and resolve toxin, and relieve itching. Indications: Wind-damp impediment (arthralgia-syndrome), lumbar pain, pain from knocks and falls, pain in the abdomen and stomach duct, toothache; damp ecsema, urticaria, stubborn lichen; poisonous snake bite.

Papaya Fruit; FAN MU GUA Origin: *Carica papaya* L. (*Caricaceae*). Part: fruit. Indications: Stomachache, dysentery, inhibited urine and stool, wind impediment, foot rot.

Papaya Leaf; FAN MU GUA YE Origin: *Carica papaya* L. (*Caricaceae*). Part: leaf. Effects: To disperse swelling. Indications: Ulcerating sore.

Parasite Scurrula; SANG JI SHENG Origin: *Loranthus parasiticus* (L.) Merr. (*Lorantha-ceae*). See Colored Mistletoe.

Parmelia Lichen; SHI HUA Origin: *Parmelia saxatilis* Ach. (*Parmeliaceae*). Part: lichen. Effects: To nourish the blood and brighten the eyes, supplement the kidney and disinhibit urine, clear heat and resolve toxin. Indications: Blurred vision, blood ejection, flooding, pain in the lumbus and knees, painful voidings of hot urine, white turbidity, white vaginal discharge, burns and scalds.

Pashi Pear Fruit; CHUAN LI GUO Origin: *Pyrus pashia* Buch.-Ham. *ex* D. Don (*Rosaceae*). Part: fruit. Effects: To disperse food accumulation, transform stasis and stagnation. Indica-tions: Meat-type food accumulation, indigestion, diarrhea, menstrual pain, postpartum blood stasis with pain, hypertension.

Passionflower; XI FAN LIAN Origin: *Passiflora caerulea* L. (*Passifloraceae*). Part: herb. Effects: To eliminate wind and clear heat, suppress cough and transform the phlegm, and as narcosis and sedative. Indications: Heavy head due to wind-heat, nasal congestion and runny nose, neurodynia, sleepless, menstrual pain, dysentery.

Patience Dock; NIU XI XI Origin: *Rumex patientia* L. (*Polygonaceae*). Part: root. Effects: To clear heat and resolve toxin, quicken the blood and stanch bleeding, free stool and kill worms. Indications: Dysentery, hepatitis, chronic enteritis, knocks and falls, bleeding from internal damage, thrombopenia, constipation, welling abscess and sores, scab and lichen, pus blister sore,

Pax Ash Bark; QIN PI Origin: *Fraxinus paxiana* Lingelsh (*Oleaceae*). See Largeleaf Chinese Ash Bark.

Peach Bast; TAO JING BAI PI Origin: *Prunus persica* (L.) Batsch (*Rosaceae*). Part: bast. Indications: Edema, sand *qi* and abdomen pain, lung heat panting and oppression, welling abscess and flat abscess, scrofula, wet sore.

Peach Flower; TAO HUA Origin: *Prunus persica* (L.) Batsch. (*Rosaceae*). Part: flower. Effects: To disinhibit water, quicken the blood, and free the stool. Indications: Edema, leg *qi* (beriberi), phlegm-rheum, phlegm-rheum, inhibited urine and stool, menstrual block.

Peach Juvenile Branch; TAO ZHI Origin: Prunus persica (L.) Batsch (*Rosaceae*). Part: branchlet. Indications: Pain in heart region and abdomen, invisible worm sores.

Peach Leaf; TAO YE Origin: *Prunus persica* (L.) Batsch. (*Rosaceae*). Part: leaf. Effects: To dispel wind-damp, clear heat, and kill worms. Indications: Head wind, headache, wind impediment, malaria, eczema, sore, lichen and scab.

Peach Root; TAO GEN Origin: *Prunus persica* (L.) Batsch. (*Rosaceae*). Part: root. Effects: To break blood and move blood. Indications: Jaundice, ejection, spontaneous external bleeding, menstrual block, swollen welling abscess, hemorrhoid.

Peachliking Pumpkin; TAO NAN GUA Origin: *Cucurbita pepo* L. var. *akoda* Mak. (*Cucurbi-taceae*). Part: fruit. Indications: Bronchial asthma.

Peanut Branch and Leaf; LUO HUA SHENG ZHI YE Origin: *Arachis hypogaea* L. (*Leguminosae*). Part: branchlet and leaf. Indications: Knocks and falls, toxin of sores.

Peanut Oil; LUO HUA SHENG YOU Origin: *Arachis hypogaea* L. (*Leguminosae*). Part: oil. Effects: To lubricate the intestines and precipitate accumulation.

Peanut; LUO HUA SHENG Origin: *Arachis lypogaea* L. (*Leguminosae*). Part: seed. Effects: To moisten the lung and harmonize stomach. Indications: Dry cough, stomach reflux, leg *qi* (beriberi), scant breast milk.

Pedunculate Acronychia; SHA TANG MU Origin: *Acronychia pedunculata* (L.) Miq. (*Rutaceae*). Part: wood or root. Effects: To move *qi* and quicken the blood, fortify the spleen and suppress cough. Indications: Wind-damp pain in the lumbus and legs, stasis pain from knocks and falls, *qi* pain in the region of the heart and stomach, bronchitis, common cold, cough.

Peking Euphorbia; DA JI (a) Origin: *Euphorbia pekinensis* Rupr. (*Euphorbiaceae*). Part: tuberous root. Effects: As a hydragogue, and externally to reduce swelling and resolve bind. Indications: Edema in the face and body, ascites, and hydrothorax; suppurative infections on the body surface.

Peking pyrrosia frond; SHI WEI Origin: *Pyrrosia davidii* (Gies.) Ching (*Polypodiaceae*). See Japanese Felt Fern Frond.

Peppertree Pricklyash Root; HUA JIAO GEN Origin: *Zanthoxylum schinifolium* Sieb. *et* Zucc. (*Rutaceae*). See Bunge Pricklyash Root.

Peppertree Pricklyash; QING HUA JIAO (one of the **HUA JIAO**) Origin: *Zanthoxylum schinifolium* Sieb. *et* Zucc. (*Rutaceae*). See Bungc Pricklyash.

Pepperweed Seed; TING LI ZI Origin: *Lepidium apetalum* Willd. (*Cruciferae*). Part: seed. Effects: To remove heat from the lung, relieve panting, disinhibit urine and remove edema. Indications: Phlegm accumulation; pleural effusion, ascites, scanty urination.

Perfoliate Knotweed Root; GANG BAN GUI GEN Origin: *Polygonum perfoliatum* L. (*Polygona-ceae*). Part: root. Indications: Mough-level nape flat abscess, hemorrhoid and fistula.

Pericarp; CHEN ZI PI Origin: *Citrus junos* Tanaka (*Rutaceae*). Part: peel. Effects: To transform phlegm, disinhibit diaphragm, disperse food, check vomiting. Indications: Toxin of fish and crab.

Persimmon Leaf; SHI YE Origin: *Diospyros kaki* L. f. (*Ebenaceae*). Part: leaf. Indications: Cough and panting, lung-*qi* distention, internal bleeding.

Persimmon Root; SHI GEN Origin: *Diospyros kaki* L. f. (*Ebenaceae*). Part: root. Effects: To cool blood and stanch bleeding. Indications: Flooding, blood dysentery, hemorrhoid.

Persimmon; SHI ZI Origin: *Diospyros kaki* L. f. (*Ebenaceae*). Part: fruit. Effects: To clear heat, allay thirst, and moisten the lung. Indications: Heat thirst, cough, blood ejection, mouth sore.

Pertusate Ulva Frond; SHI CHUN Origin: *Ulva pertusa* Kjellm. (*Ulvaceae*). See Lettuce Ulva Frond.

Peru Balmtree Resin; BI LU XIANG JIAO Origin: *Myroxylon pereirae* (Royle) Klotzsch (*Leguminosae*). Part: resin. Effects: dispelling phlegm and sterilization Indications: Scab sore, coin lichen.

Peru Herb; JIA SUAN JIANG Origin: *Nicandra physaloides* (L.) Gaerth. (*Solanaceae*). Part: herb. Effects: To clear heat and resolve toxin, dispel phlegm, and as a sedative. Indications: Rabid dog bite, mental disease, epilepsy, rheumatalgia, sore and boil, common cold.

Peruvian Groundcherry Herb; DENG LONG CAO Origin: *Physalis peruviana* L. (*Solanaceae*). Part: whole plant. Effects: To clear heat and move *qi,* relieve pain and disperse swelling. Indications: Common cold, mumps, throat pain, cough, abdominal distention, mounting *qi* , heaven-borne sore.

Petioled pyrrosia frond; SHI WEI Origin: *Pyrrosia petiolosa* (Christ) Ching (*Polypodiaceae*). See Japanese Felt Fern Frond.

Phellinus Igniarius; SANG HUANG Origin: *Phellinus igniarius* (L. *ex* Fr.) Quél. (*Polyporaceae*). Part: sporophore. Indications: Flooding, blood strangury, prolapse of the rectum with bleeding, vaginal discharge, menstrual block.

Phoenix Date; WU LOU ZI Origin: *Phoenix dactylifera* L. (*Palmae*). Part: fruit. Effects: To worm center and boost *qi,* to supplement vacuity and detriment. Indications: Cough with phlegm, vacuity and detriment.

Phoenix Tree Bast; WU TONG BAI PI Origin: *Firmiana simplex* (L.) W. F. Wight (*Stercu-liaceae*). Part: bast. Effects: To dispel wind and eliminate dampness, quicken the blood and relieve pain. Indications: Pain from wind-damp impediment (arthralgia-syndrome), knocks and falls, menstrual irregularities, hemorrhoid, cinnabar toxin.

Phoenix Tree Leaf; WU TONG YE Origin: *Firmiana simplex* (L.) W. F. Wight (*Sterculiaceae*). Part: leaf. Effects: To dispel wind and eliminate dampness, clear heat and resolve toxin. Indications: Rheumatalgia, numbness, swelling and toxin of welling abscess and sore, hemorrhoid, shank sore, bleeding from wounds, hypertension.

Phoenix Tree Seed; WU TONG ZI Origin: *Firmiana simplex* (L.) W. F. Wight (*Sterculiaceae*). Part: seed. Effects: To normalize *qi,* harmonize stomach and disperse food. Indications: Food damage, stomachache, mounting *qi,* mouth sore in children.

Picrorhiza; HU HUANG LIAN Origin: *Picrorrhiza kurrooa* Royle *ex* Benth. (*Scrophularia-ceae*). Part: rhizome. Effects: To relieve fever due to vacuity of *qi,* essence and blood, treat infantile malnutrition with fever and remove damp-heat. Indications: Steaming bone tidal fever due to *yin* vacuity, night sweating; child *gan* accumulation, indigestion, abdominal distention and emaciation, dysentery, fever; gastroin-testinal damp-heat and diarrhea, hemorrhoid with swelling and pain.

Pig Gall; ZHU DAN Origin: *Sus scrofa domestica* Brisson (*Suidae*). Part: gall. Effects: To clear heat and resolve toxin, moisten dryness. Indications: Febrile disease vexation and thirst, constipation, jaundice, whooping cough, asthma, diarrhea, dysentery, red eyes, throat impediment, purulent ear, swollen welling abscess and clove sores.

Pigeon Vetch; XIAO CHAO CAI Origin: *Vicia hirsuta* (L.) S. F. Gray (*Leguminosae*). Part: herb. Effects: To resolve the exterior and disinhibit damp, to quicken the blood and stanch bleeding. Indications: Jaundice, malaria, nosebleed, white vaginal discharge.

Pilose Asiabell; DANG SHEN Origin: *Codonopsis pilosula* (Franch.) Nannf. (*Campanula-ceae*). Part: root. Effects: To supplement the middle-*jiao* and reinforce *qi,* engender liquid and nourish the blood. Indications: The syndrome of deficiency of the spleen; short breath, cough, dyspnea, weak and low voice due to deficiency of the lung-*qi; for consumption of both qi* and body fluid in febrile diseases with symptoms such as short breath and thirst; dizziness or sallow complexion and edema due to blood deficiency.

Pilose Gerbera; MAO DA DING CAO Origin: *Gerbera piloselloides* Cass. (*Compositae*). Part: herb. Effects: To diffuse lung and suppress cough, effuse sweat and disinhibit water, move *qi* and quicken blood. Indications: Wind damage and cough, asthma, distention and fullness, urinary stoppage, child food accumulation, menstrual block, knocks and falls, welling abscess and flat abscess, clove sore, streaming sore.

Pilular Adina; SHUI TUAN HUA Origin: *Adina pilulifera* (Lam.) Franch. *ex* Drake (*Rubiaceae*). Part: herb, or flower and fruit. Effects: To clear heat and disinhibit damp, disperse stasis and settle pain, stanch bleeding and engender flesh. Indications: Dysentery, enteronitis, puffy swelling due to damp-heat, swelling and toxin of welling abscess and sores, eczema, foot rot, ulcerating sore, bleeding from wounds.

Pine Mushroom; SONG XUN Origin: *Armillaria matsutake* Ito *et* Imai (*Tricholomataceae*). Part: sporophore. Indications: Incessint urinary turbidity.

Pink Plumepoppy; BO LUO HUI Origin: *Macleaya cordata* (Willd.) R. Br. (*Papaveraceae*). Part: herb with root. Effects: To disperse swelling and resolve toxin, kill worms. Indications: Clove sore of the finger, purulent swelling, acute tonsillitis, otitis media, trichomonal vaginitis, lower limb ulcerating sore, scalds, stubborn lichen.

Pink Reineckea Herb; JI XIANG CAO Origin: *Reineckea carnea* (Andr.) Kunth (*Liliaceae*). Part: herb with root. Effects: To clear the lung and suppress cough, rectify blood and resolve toxin. Indications: Cough due to lung heat, blood ejection, spontaneous external bleeding, bloody stool, toxin sore, knocks and falls, fire eye, *gan* accumulation.

Plum Flower; BAI MEI HUA Origin: *Prunus mume* (Sieb.) Sieb. *et* Zucc. (*Rosaceae*). Part: bud. Effects: To soothe the depressed liver, normalize the function of the stomach and resolve phlegm. Indications: Plum-pit *qi*, liver-stomach *qi* pain, poor appetite, dizzy head, scrofula.

Poiret Barerry; XIAO BO Origin: *Berberis poiretii* Schneid. (*Berberidaceae*). See Amur Barerry.

Poisonous Buttercup; SHI LONG RUI Origin: *Ranunculus sceleratus* L. (*Ranunculaceae*). Part: herb. Indications: Swelling and toxin of welling abscess and boil, scrofula, malaria, ulcerating sore of the leg.

Pomegranate Root; SHI LIU GEN Origin: *Punica granatum* L. (*Punicaceae*). Part: root. Effects: To kill worms, astringe the intestines, and check discharge. Indications: Roundworm, tapeworm, enduring diarrhea, enduring dysentery, red and white vaginal discharge.

Pomegranate; SUAN SHI LIU Origin: *Punica granatum* L. (*Punicaceae*). Part: fruit. Indications: Efflux diarrhea, enduring dysentery, flooding and spotting with vaginal discharge.

Pond Frog Gall; QING WA DAN Origin: *Rana nigromaculata* Hallowell; *Rana plancyi* Lataste (all *Ranidae*). Part: gall. Indications: measles papules with complicated pneumonia.

Pond Frog; QING WA Origin: *Rana nigromaculata* Hallowell; *Rana plancyi* Lataste (all *Ranidae*). Part: body. Effects: To clear heat and resolve toxin, supplement vacuity, disinhibit water and disperse swelling. Indications: Taxation heat, puffy swelling, *gan*, water drum distention, dysphagia-occlusion, dysentery, toad head scourge, child heat sore.

Poongaoil Pongamia; SHUI LIU DOU Origin: *Pongamia pinnata* (L.) Merr. (*Leguminosae*). Part: seed. Indications: Scab and *lai*, lichen, pus sore.

Popyporus Agaric; ZHU LING Origin: *Polyporus umbellatus* (Pers.) Fries (*Polyporaceae*). Part: dried sclerotium. Effects: To disinhibit urine percolate damp. Indications: Dysuria, edema, diarrhea, stranguria with turbid urine, and leukorrhagia.

Potmarigold Calendula; JIN ZHAN JU Origin: *Calendula officinalis* L. (*Compositae*). Part: flower and root. Effects: Root: to move *qi* and quicken the blood; flower: to cool the blood and stanch bleeding. Indications: Root: cold pain of stomach, mounting *qi,* concretions and conglomera-tions; flower: intestinal wind bleeding.

Prawn; HAI XIA Origin: *Penaeus orientalis* Kishinouye (*Penaeidae*). Part: meat or body. Effects: To supplement the kidney and strengthen *yang,* open the stomach and transform phlegm.

Prepared Common Monkshood Daughter Root; FU ZI Origin: *Aconitum carmichaeli* Debx. (*Ranunculaceae*). Part: daughter root. Effects: As an cardiotonic to restore *yang* for the treatment of collapse and shock, to warm the kidney and reinforce*yang*, and to warm the middle-*jiao* and relieve pain. Indications: *Yang* depletion syndrome marked by spontaneous cold sweating, cold limbs, and pulse as faint as none; *yang* deficiency syndromes -- aversion to cold, cold limbs, impotence and frequent micturition; gastric and abdominal cold pain, poor appetite and loose stool; palpitation, shortness of breath, obstruction of *qi* and pain in the chest; difficulty in micturition and edema of the limbs; impediment syndrome marked by joint pains all over the body; spontaneous sweating.

Prince's-feather Herb; HONG CAO Origin: *Polygonum orientale* L. (*Polygonaceae*). Part: herb (with root). Indications: Rheumatic arthritis, malaria, mounting *qi,* leg *qi* (beriberi), swollen sore.

Prinos-like salacia; SUO LA MU Origin: *Salacia prinoides* DC. (*Hippocrateaceae*). Part: root. Effects: To free the channels and network vessels, dispel wind damp. Indications: Rheumatic arthritis, taxation detriment of lumbar flesh, weak constitution and leck of strength.

Pubescent Angelica; MAO DANG GUI (one of the **DU HUO**) Origin: *Angelica pubescens* Maxim. (*Umbelliferae*). See Doubleteeth Pubescent Angelica.

Pummelo Seed; YOU HE Origin: *Citrus grandis* (L.) Osbeck (*Rutaceae*). Part: seed. Indications: Small intestinal mounting *qi.*

Pummelo; YOU Origin: *Citrus grandis* (L.) Osbeck (*Rutaceae*). Part: fruit. Indications: Low food intake and inability to taste food in pregnant woman, malign *qi* in the stomach.

Puncturevine Caltrap Root; JI LI GEN Origin: *Tribulus terrestris* L. (*Zygophyllaceae*). Part: root. Indications: Toothache due to beaten.

Puncturevine Caltrap; CI JI LI Origin: *Tribulus terrestris* L. (*Zygophyllaceae*). Part: fruit. Effects: To dissipate wind and brighten the eyes, precipitate *qi* and move blood. Indications: Headache, itchy body, red swollen eyes and eye screen, fullness in the chest, cough and counterflow, concretions and conglomerations, difficult lactation, welling abscess and flat abscess, scrofula.

Pungent Litse; ZHEN CAI Origin: *Litsea pungens* Hemsl. [= *Lindera umbellata* Thunb.] (*Lauraceae*). Part: wood. Indications: Coughing of phlegm-rheum, accumulation-gathering and distention-fullness, leg *qi* (beriberi), child sore and scab in children.

Purging Croton; BA DOU Origin: *Croton tiglium* L. (*Euphorbiaceae*). Part: dried seed. Effects: To eliminate the accumulation of cold and stagnated food, to dispel retained water and clear phlegm, and as a drastic precipitating medicinal. caution: for internal administration, the defatted powder of croton seed should be used. Indications: Abdominal fullness and distending pain, fecal stoppage, and even rapid breathing and fulminant reversal; child feeding accumulation, profuse phlegm and frignt palpitation; enlarged abdomen with edema; throat impediment, phlegm-drool congestion, hasty breathing; swollen welling abscess and ripe pus without open, scab, lichen and malign sore.

Purple Bergenia; YAN BAI CAI Origin: *Bergenin purpurascens* (Hook. f. *et* Thoms.) Engl. (*Saxifragaceae*). Part: rhizome or whole plant. Indications: Vacuity and weakness with dizzy head, taxation damage and cough, blood ejection, hacking of blood, strangury-turbidity, white vaginal discharge, toxin swelling.

Purple Puff-ball; MA BO Origin: *Calvatia linacina* (Mont. *et* Berk.) Lloye (*Lycoperdaceae*). See Bark-less Puff-ball.

Purple Tephrosia Root; HUI YE GEN Origin: *Tephrosia purpurea* (L.) Pers. (*Leguminosae*). Part: root. Effects: To clear heat and disperse stagnation. Indications: Distention of stomach, *qi* distention, indigestion, gastritis with stomachache.

Purpleflower Crotalaria; YE BAI HE Origin: *Crotalaria sessiliflora* L. (*Leguminosae*). Part: herb. Effects: To clear heat, resolve toxin, and disinhibit dampness. Indications: Dysentery, sore and boil, child *gan* accumulation.

Purplestem Angelica; ZI JING DU HUO (one of the **DU HUO**) Origin: *Angelica porphyrocaulis* Nakai *et* Kitag. (*Umbelliferae*). See Doubleteeth Pubescent Angelica.

Purslane; MA CHI XIAN Origin: *Portulaca oleracea* L. (*Portulacaceae*). Part: aerial parts. Effects: To remove heat, dampness and toxic substance, and to remove heat from the blood and stanch bleeding. Indications: Damp-heat diarrhea, diarrhea with pus and blood, tenesmus; red and white vaginal discharge, fire toxin welling abscess and boil; heat strangury, blood strangury.

Racemose Corydalis; HUANG JIN Origin: *Corydalis racemosa* (Thunb.) Pers. (*Papaveraceae*). Part: herb or root. Effects: To clearheat, disinhibit urine, resolve toxin, and kill worms. Indications: Scab and lichen, swelling pain of toxin sore, red eyes, fire flow, summerheat heat diarrhea and dysentery, lung disease with coughing of blood, fright wind in children.

Rangooncreeper Leaf; SHI JUN ZI YE Origin: *Quisqualis indica* L. (*Combretaceae*). Part: leaf. Effects: To kill worms and disperse *gan*, increase the appetite. Indications: Child *gan* accumulation.

Rangooncreeper; SHI JUN ZI Origin: *Quisqualis indica* L. (*Combretaceae*). Part: ripe fruit. Effects: To poison and expel parasites and to remove stagnation of food. Indications: Ascariasis, enterobiasis; infantile indigestion with food retention.

Red Clover; HONG CHE ZHOU CAO Origin: Trifolium pratense L. (*Leguminosae*). Part: flower and inflorescence. Effects: To settle tetany, suppress cough, and check panting. Indications: Local ulcerating sore.

Red Fruit Leaf; SHAN ZHA YE Origin: *Crataegus pinnatifida* Bge. var. *major* N. E. Br. (*Rosaceae*). See Chinese Hawthorn Leaf.

Red Fruit; SHAN ZHA Origin: *Crataegus pinnatifida* Bge. var. *major* N. E. Br. (*Rosaceae*). See Chinese Hawthorn.

Red Knoxia; HONG YA DA JI (one of the **DA JI (a)**) Origin: *Knoxia valerianoides* Thorel *ex* Pitard (*Rubiaceae*). See Peking Euphorbia.

Red Lady-bug; HONG NIANG ZI Origin: *Huechys sanguinea* De Geer. (*Cicadidae*). Part: dried body Effects: To attack toxin, free stasis, and break accumulation. Indications: Scrofula, lichen, blood stasis and menstrual block, rabid dog bite.

Red Nanmu Bark; HONG NAN PI Origin: *Machilus thunbergii* Sieb. *et* Zucc. (*Lauraceae*). Part: bark. Indications: Sinew sprain and contusion, incessant vomiting and diarrhea, cramp and swelling of the feet.

Red Thorowax; HONG CHAI HU (one of the **CHAI HU**) Origin: *Bupleurum scorzonerifolium* Willd. (*Umbelliferae*). See Chinese Thorowax.

Red-knees; SHUI LIAO Origin: *Polygonum hydropiper* L. (*Polygonaceae*). Part: herb. Effects: To transform damp and move *qi*, dispel wind and disperse swelling. Indications: Sand foulness and abdominal pain, vomiting and diarrhea with cramp, diarrhea, dysentery, wind-damp (rheumatism), leg *qi* (beriberi), swollen welling abscess, scrofula, knocks and falls.

Redbark Cinchona; JIN JI LE Origin: *Cinchona succirubra* Pav. (*Rubiaceae*). Part: bark. Effects: To resolve heat and used as an antimalarial drug. Indications: Malaria.

Redcalyx Glotybower; GUI DENG LONG Origin: *Clerodendron fortunatum* L. (*Verbenaceae*). Part: herb. Effects: To clear heat and resolve toxin, suppress cough and dispel wind. Indications: Common cold, sore throat, cough, lung disease, stomachache, abdominal pain, swollen boil, knocks and falls, rheumatism.

Reddish Jackinthepulpit; TIAN NAN XING Origin: *Arisaema consanguineum* Schott (*Araceae*). Part: root tuber. Effects: To dry dampness and transform phlegm, to dispel wind and relieve convulsion, and externally to reduce swelling and resolve bind. Indications: Wind stroke with phlegm congestion, deviated eyes and mouth, hemiplegia, epilepsy, fright wind, lockjaw, wind-phlegm dizziness, throat impediment, scrofula, swollen welling abscess, knocks and falls, snake bite, insect bite.

Redroot Gromwell; ZI CAO Origin: *Lithospermum erythrhizon* Sieb. *et* Zucc. (*Boragina-ceae*). Part: root. Effects: To clear heat from the blood, resolve toxin, quicken the blood and cool the blood. Indications: Febrile diseases marked by maculas and eruptions; suppurative infections on body surface, eczema, vulvitis, scalding.

Reeves Skimmia; YIN YU Origin: *Skimmia reevesiana* Fortune (*Rutaceae*). Part: stem and leaf. Indications: Pain from wind-damp impediment (arthralgia-syndrome), hypertonicity of the limbs, weakness of legs.

Reindeer Moss; SHI RUI Origin: *Cladonia rangiferina* Web. (*Cladoniaceae*). Part: herb. Effects: To clear heat and transform phlegm, cool the liver and scrofula. Indications: Heat vexation, mouth sore and coughing of blood, blood ejection, headache or hemilateral headache, eye screen and flowery or clouded vision, heat strangury, jaundice, bleeding from wounds.

Remote Lemongrass; YUN XIANG CAO Origin: *Cymbopogon distans* (Nees) A. Camus (*Gramineae*). Part: aerial parts. Effects: To dispel cold and remove damp, treat panting and arrest cough, and promote circulation of *qi*, and relieve depression. Indications: Summerheat damage and common cold, strangury, aching sinews and bones due to wind-damp, chronic trachitis.

Rhinoceros Horn; XI JIAO Origin: *Rhinoceros unicornis* L.; *Rhinoceros sondaicus* Desmarest; *Rhinoceros sumatrensis* (Fischer) (all *Rhinocerotidae*). Part: horn. Effects: To clear heat and cool the blood, resolve toxin, stabilize fright. Indications: Blood ejection, spontaneous external bleeding due to blood heat; acute febrile diseases shown as persistent high fever, unconsciousness and delirium; blood ejection; epidemic febrile diseases marked by fever, dark purple maculas or eruptions.

Rice Frog Gall; XIA MA DAN Origin: *Rana limnocharis* Boie (*Ranidae*). Part: gall juice. Indications: Loss of voice in children.

Rice Spermoderm; MI PI KANG Origin: *Oryza sativa* L. (*Gramineae*). Part: spermoderm. Indications: Dysphagia-occlusion, leg *qi* (beriberi).

Rice Straw; DAO CAO Origin: *Oryza sativa* L. (*Gramineae*). Part: stem and leaf. Effects: To loosen the center and precipitate *qi,* disperse food accumulation. Indications: Dysphagia-occlusion, stomach reflux, food stagnation, diarrhea, abdominal pain, diabetes, jaundice, white turbidity, hemorrhoid, scalds.

Rice; JING MI Origin: *Oryza sativa* L. (*Gramineae*). Part: seed. Effects: To supplement the spleen and boost *qi.* Indications: Vexation and thirst, diarrhea.

Rigescent Gentian; LONG DAN Origin: *Gentiana rigescens* Franch. (*Gentianaceae*). See Rough Gentian.

Robust Leontice; HONG MAO QI Origin: *Leontice robustum* (Maxim.) Diels (*Berberidaceae*). Part: root and rhizome. Effects: To dispel blood stasis and stanch bleeding, to dispel wind and relieve pain. Indications: Sinew and bone pain due to wind-damp, knocks and falls, menstrual irregularities.

Roce Pelargonium; XIANG YE Origin: *Pelargonium graveolens* Lsymbol 162 \f "Symbol" \s 9′}Herit (*Geraniaceae*). Part: herb. Indications: Rheumatism, mounting *qi,* scrotal eczema, scab and lichen.

Rocket Consolida; FEI YAN CAO Origin: *Consolida ajacis* (L.) Schur (*Ranunculaceae*). Part: root and seed. Effects: similar with WU TOU. Indications: Panting, edema, abdominal pain.

Roof Iris; YUAN WEI Origin: *Iris tectorum* Maxim. (*Iridaceae*). Part: rhizome. Effects: To disperse accumulation and break stasis, move water and resolve toxin. Indications: Distention and fullness due to food stagnation, concretion and gathering, drum distention, toxin swelling, hemorrhoids and fistulas, knocks and falls.

Rorippa; HAN CAI Origin: *Rorippa montana* (Wall.) Small (*Cruciferae*). Part: herb. Effects: To dispel phlegm and suppress cough, clear heat and resolve toxin, disinhibit damp and abate jaundice. Indications: Coughing of phlegm and panting; red swollen throat with pain, swelling and toxin of welling abscess; damp-heat jaundice.

Rosemary; MI DIE XIANG Origin: *Rosmarinus officinalis* L. (*Labiatae*). Part: herb. Effects: To fortify the stomach and effuse sweat. Indications: Headache.

Rosthorn Snakegourd Root; TIAN HUA FEN (GUA LOU GEN) Origin: *Trichosanthes rosthornii* Harms (*Cucurbitaceae*). See Mongolian Snakegourd Root.

Rosthorn Snakegourd; GUA LOU Origin: *Trichosanthes rosthornii* Harms (*Cucurbitaceae*). See Mongolian Snakegourd.

Rough Gentian; LONG DAN Origin: *Gentiana scabra* Bunge (*Gentianaceae*). Part: root and rhizome. Effects: To remove damp-heat from the liver and the gallbladder and as a stomachic. Indications: Jaundice from damp-heat; repletion fire in the liver and gall shown as headache, fullness in the head, blood shot, swollen and painful eyes, pain in the hypochondriac region, bitter taste, and deafness; persistent high fever, spasm and convulsion.

Roughleaf Bedstraw; BA XIAN CAO Origin: *Galium asperifolium* Wall. (*Rubiaceae*). See Catchweed Bedstraw.

Round Cardamom; BAI DOU KOU Origin: *Amomun kravanh* Pierre *ex* Gagnep. [= *Amomum cardamomum* L.] (*Zingiberaceae*). Part: seed. Effects: To dispel damp-cold from the stomach and eliminate flatulence and arrest vomiting. Indications: Spleen-stomach *qi* stagnation due to damp obstructing the middle-jiao; vomiting with stomach-cold, vomiting of milk in infants with stomach-cold.

Roundleaf Pharbitis Seed; QIAN NIU ZI Origin: *Pharbitis purpurea* (L.) Voigt (*Convolvula-ceae*). See Lobedleaf Pharbitis Seed.

Roundpod Jute Leaf; HUANG MA YE Origin: *Corchorus capsularis* L. (*Tiliaceae*). Part: leaf. Effects: To rectify *qi* and stanch bleeding, expel pus and engender flesh. Indications: Abdominal pain, dysentery, flooding, sore and welling abscess.

Roundpod Jute Seed; HUANG MA ZI Origin: *Corchorus capsularis* L. (*Tiliaceae*). Part: seed. Effects: To strengthen the heart, anesthetize. Indications: Flooding, cough damage lung.

Royal Jelly; FENG RU Origin: *Apis cerana* Fabricius (*Apidae*). Part: royal jelly. Effects: To nourish and strengthen, boost the liver and fortify the spleen. Indications: Weakness after illness, dystrophy in children, senile weak constitution, infective hepatitis, hypertension, rheumatic arthritis, duodenal ulcer.

Royal Paulownia Fruit; PAO TONG GUO Origin: *Paulownia tomentosa* (Thunb.) Steud. (*Scrophulariaceae*). See Fortune Paulownia Fruit.

Royal Paulownia; TONG MU (PAO TONG) Origin: *Paulownia tomentosa* (Thunb.) Steud. (*Scrophulariaceae*). See Fortune Paulownia.

Royle Euphorbia Latex; BA WANG BIAN Origin: *Euphorbia royleana* Boiss. (*Euphorbiaceae*). Part: stem and leaf or white juice in stem. Indications: Toxin of sores, skin lichen, edema.

Rufous Turtle Dove; BAN JIU Origin: *Streptopelia orientalis* (Latham) (*Columbidae*). Part: meat. Effects: To boost *qi*, brighten the eyes, strengthen sinew and bone. Indications: Vacuity-detriment, hiccough.

Rugose Rose; MEI GUI HUA Origin: *Rosa rugosa* Thunb. (*Rosaceae*). Part: flower. Effects: To normalize the flow of *qi* and nourish the blood in the liver. Indications: Liver-stomach *qi* pain, wind impediment, ejection and hacking of blood, menstrual disorder, red and white vaginal discharge, dysentery, mammary welling abscess, toxin swelling.

Russian Boschniakia; CAO CONG RONG Origin: *Boschniakia rossica* Fedtsch. *et* Flerov (*Orobanchaceae*). Part: whole herb. Effects: To supplement the kidney and strengthen *yang,* moisten the intestines and stanch bleeding. Indications: Kidney vacuity and impotence, cold pain in the lumbus and knees, cold pain in the lumbus and knees, senile habitual constipation, cystitis.

Russian olive Bark; SHA ZAO SHU PI Origin: *Elaeagnus angustifolia* L. (*Elaeagnaceae*). Part: bark. Effects: To promote contraction and relieve pain, clear heat, cool the blood, and stanch bleeding. Indications: White vaginal discharge, burns.

Russianolive; SHA ZAO Origin: *Elaeagnus angustifolia* L. (*Elaeagnaceae*). Part: fruit. Effects: To strengthen and tranquilize, secure essence, fortify the stomach, check diarrhea, regulate menstruation, anddisinhibit urine. Indications: Stomachache, abdominal diarrhea, vacuity and weakness, lung heat cough.

Rust-coloured Crotalaria; XIANG LING CAO Origin: *Crotalaria ferruginea* Grah. (*Legumi-nosae*). Part: herb (with root). Effects: To constrain lung *qi,* supplement the spleen and kidney, disinhibit urine, and disperse swelling and toxin. Indications: Enduring cough with bloody phlegm, tinnitus, deafness, dream emission, chronic nephritis, cystitis, calculus of kindey, calculus of kindey, lymphnoditis, clove toxin, malign sore.

Safflower; HONG HUA Origin: *Carthamus tinctrius* L. (*Compositae*). Part: flower. Effects: To quicken the blood, dispel blood stasis and restore normal menstruation. Indications: Menstrual block, menstrual pain, afterpains, pains due to blood stasis (chest, hypochondrium, traumatic injuries, sores, carbuncles)

Saffron Crocus Stigma; ZANG HONG HUA Origin: *Crocus sativus* L. (*Iridaceae*). Part: stigma. Effects: To quicken blood and transform stasis, dissipate depression and open bind. Indications: Anxiety and depression, glomus and oppression in the chest and diaphragm, blood ejection, cold damage mania, fright temerity, menstrual block, postpartum blood stasis and abdominal pain, painful swelling from knocks and falls.

Sagittate Epimedium Root; YIN YANG HUO GEN Origin: *Epimedium sagittatum* (Sieb. *et* Zucc.) Maxim. (*Berberidaceae*). See Largeflower Epimedium Root.

Sagittate Epimedium; JIAN YE YIN YANG HUO (one of the **YIN YANG HUO**) Origin: *Epimedium sagittatum* (Sieb. *et* Zucc.) Maxim. (*Berberidaceae*). See Largeflower Epimedium.

Sago Frond; FENG WEI JIAO YE (SU TIE YE) Origin: *Cycas revoluta* Thunb. (*Cycadaceae*). Part: leaf. Effects: To rectify *qi* and quicken the blood. Indications: Liver-stomach *qi* pain, menstrual block, difficult delivery, cough, blood ejection, knocks and falls, knife wound.

Sago Seed; TIE SHU GUO (SU TIE SHU GUO) Origin: *Cycas revoluta* Thunb. (*Cycada-ceae*). Part: seed. Effects: To promote contraction, settle cough and dispel phlegm, increase the appetite, stanch bleeding, expel inflammation. Indications: Dysentery, hiccough, cough with profuse phlegm, knocks and falls, knife wound.

Saline Cistanche; ROU CONG RONG Origin: *Cistanche salsa* (C. A. Mey.) G. Beck (*Orobanchaceae*). Part: fleshy stem. Effects: To supplement the kidney and invigorate *yang* and also as a laxative. Indications: Impotence, cold pain in the loins and knees, female sterility; constipation.

Saline Swainsonia; NIAO PAO CAO Origin: *Swainsonia salsula* Taub. (*Leguminosae*). Part: fruit. Effects: To disinhibit urine. Indications: Ascites due to cirrhosis, angioneurotic edema, chronic hepatitis with edema.

Sanchi; SAN QI Origin: *Panax pseudo-ginseng* Wall. var. *notoginseng* (Burk.) Hoo *et* Tseng [=*Panax notoginseng* (Burk.) F. H. Chen] (*Aralia-ceae*). Part: root. Effects: To stanch bleeding, dispel blood stasis, and relieve pain. Indications: Many kinds of bleeding; traumatic injuries; angina pectoris of coronary heart disease.

Sand Pear Leaf; LI YE Origin: *Pyrus pyrifolia* (Burm. F.) Nakai (*Rosaceae*). See Bretschneider Pear Leaf.

Sandal Beadtree Seed; HAI HONG DOU Origin: *Adenanthera pavonina* L. (*Leguminosae*). Part: seed. Indications: Wandering wind of the head and face.

Sandalwood; TAN XIANG Origin: *Santalum album* L. (*Santalaceae*). Part: heart wood. Effects: To rectify *qi* and harmonize the stomach. Indications: Pain in the chest and abdomen, cold-pain in the stomach, vomiting of water due to congealing cold *qi* stagnation; coronary heart disease with pattern of *qi* stagnation and blood stasis.

Sappan Caesalpinia; SU MU Origin: *Caesalpinia sappan* L. (*Leguminosae*). Part: heart wood. Effects: To quicken the blood, break stasis, reduce swelling and relieve pain. Indications: Menstrual block, postpartum abdominal pain due to blood stasis and *qi* stagnation, swollen welling abscess, lockjaw, dysentery.

Savin; CHOU BAI Origin: *Sabina vulgaris* Antoine (*Cupressaceae*). Part: branchlet or cone. Effects: To dispel wind-damp, quicken blood and relieve pain, and as a sedative. Indications: Rheumatic arthritis.

Savoury Rhododendron; XIAO YE PI PA Origin: *Rhododendron anthopogonoides* Maxim. (*Ericaceae*). Part: leaf. Effects: To suppress cough, calm panting, dispel phlegm. Indications: Senile chronic trachitis, cough, panting.

Scabrous Cowparsnip; BAI ZHI Origin: *Heracleum scabridum* Franch. (*Umbelliferae*). See Dahurian Angelica.

Scabrous Doellingeria; DONG FENG CAI Origin: *Doellingeria scaber* (Thunb.) Nees (*Compositae*). Part: herb. Indications: Knocks and falls, snake bite.

Scabrous Elephantfoot; KU DI DAN Origin: *Elephantopus scaber* L. (*Compositae*). Part: herb. Effects: To cool the blood, clear heat, disinhibit water, and resolve toxin. Indications: Nosebleed, jaundice, strangury, leg *qi* (beriberi), edema, swollen welling abscess, clove sore, snake or insect bites.

Scabrous Mosla; SHI JI NING Origin: *Mosla scabra* (Thunb.) C. Y. Wu *et* H. W. Li (*Labiatae*). Part: herb. Effects: To clear summerheat-heat, dispel wind-damp, disperse swelling, and resolve toxin. Indications: Summerheat sand, spontaneous external bleeding, blood dysentery, common cold and cough, chronic trachitis, swelling of welling abscess, flat abscess and sore, wind papules, prickly heat.

Scapose Marsharigold; MA TI YE Origin: *Caltha scaposa* Hook. f. *et* Thoms (*Ranunculaceae*). See Common Marsharigold.

Scorpion; QUAN XIE Origin: *Buthus martensi* Karsch (*Buthidae*). Part: body. Effects: As an anticonvulsive and to counteract toxin, resolve mass, remove obstruction of the channels and ease pain. Indications: Spasm and convulsion due to many causes; sores, carbuncles, poisoning swellings, scrofula and subcutaneous nodes; stubborn headache and migraine or rheumatic impediment.

Seabuckthorn Fruit; CU LIU GUO (SHA JI) Origin: *Hippophae rhamnoides* L. (*Elaeagnaceae*). Part: fruit. Effects: To quicken blood and dissipate stasis, transform phlegm and loosen the chest, invigorate the spleen and fortify the stomach. Indications: Knocks and falls, stasis swelling, cough with profuse phlegm, difficult breath, indigestion.

Selago-like Climbing Fern; XIAO JIE JIN CAO Origin: *Huperzia selago* (L.) Bernh. *ex* Schrank *et* Mart. [= *Lycopodium selago* L.] (*huper-ziaceae*). Part: herb. Effects: To dissipate wind and harmonize blood, to stanch bleeding and restore muscles and tendons, and to dispel swelling and relieve pain. Indications: Knocks and falls, bleeding due to external injury, wind-damp pain (rheumatalgia).

Sensitiveplant Herb; HAN XIU CAO Origin: *Mimosa pudica* L. (*Leguminosae*). Part: herb. Effects: To clear heat and quite the spirit, disperse accumulation and resolve toxin. Indications: Enteritis, gastritis, insomnia, child *gan* accumulation, sore heat swollen eyes, pus swelling in deep part, herpes zoster.

Septemlobate Kalopanax Bark; CI QIU SHU PI Origin: *Kalopanax septemlobus* (Thunb.) Koidz. (*Araliaceae*). Part: bark. Effects: To dispel wind and eliminate dampness, quicken the blood, and kill worms. Indications: Pain from wind-damp impediment (arthralgia-syndrome), pain in the lumbus and knees, welling abscess and flat abscess, sore and lichen.

Sericeous Cinquefoil; JIN JIN BANG Origin: *Potentilla reptons* L.var. *sericophylla* Franch. (*Rosaceae*). Part: root. Effects: To engender liquid and allay thirst, supplement *yin* and eliminate vacuity heat. Indications: Vacuity taxation with leukorrhea, vacuity panting.

Serpent-head; LI YU Origin: *Ophiocephalus argus* Cantor *(Ophiocephalidae).* Part: meat or whole fish. Effects: To supplement spleen, disinhibit water. Indications: Edema, damp impediment, leg *qi* (beriberi), hemorrhoid, scab and lichen.

Serrate Clubmoss; QIAN CENG TA Origin: *Huperzia serrata* (Thunb.) Trev. [=*Lycopodium serrayum* Thunb.] (*Huperziaceae*). Part: herb. Effects: To abate fever, eliminate damp, disperse stasis, stanch bleeding. Indications: Pneumonia, pulmonary welling abscess, taxation damage and blood ejection, bleeding from hemorrhoids, white vaginal discharge, knocks and falls, toxin swelling.

Serrate Glorybower; SAN TAI HONG HUA Origin: *Clerodendron serratum* (L.) Spr. (*Verbena-ceae*). Part: herb. Effects: To join bone, relieve pain, and interrupt malaria. Indications: Fracture, knocks and falls, wind-damp pain (rheumatalgia), malaria.

Sessile Stemona; BAI BU Origin: *Stemona sessilifolia* (Miq.) Franch. *et* Sav. (*Stemonaceae*). Part: root. Effects: To moisten the lung, arrest cough and as a parasiticite. Indications: Wind-cold cough, whooping cough, pulmonary tuberculosis, cough and panting in senile patients; roundworm disease, pinworm disease; scab and lichen of the skin, eczema.

Sessileflower Acanthopanax Leaf; WU GENG WU JIA YE (one of the **WU JIA YE**) Origin: *Acanthopanax sessiliflorus* (Rupr. *et* Maxim.) Seem (*Araliaceae*). See Slenderstyle Acanthopanax Leaf.

Sessileflower Acanthopanax Root-bark; WU GENG WU JIA PI (one of the **WU JIA PI**) Origin: *Acanthopanax sessiliflorus* (Rupr. *et* Maxim.) Seem (*Araliaceae*). See Slenderstyle Acanthopanax Root-bark.

Setose Asparagus; WEN ZHU Origin: *Asparagus setaceus* (Kunth) Jessop [= *Asparagus plumosus* Bak.] (*Liliaceae*). Part: herb. Effects: To cool the blood and resolve toxin, disinhibit urine and free strangury.

Shady Groundsel; HUANG WAN Origin: *Senecio nemorensis* L (*Compositae*). Part: herb. Effects: To clear heat and resolve toxin. Indications: Heat dysentery, swollen eyes, toxin of welling abscess, boil and clove sore.

Shagspine Peashrub; GUI JIAN JIN JI ER Origin: *Caragana jubata* (Pall.) Poir. (*Leguminosae*). Part: bark, stem and leaf. Effects: To join sinew and bone, dispel wind and eliminate dampness, quicken the blood and free the network vessels, disperse swelling and relieve pain. Indications: Knocks and falls, wind-damp pain in sinews and bones, irregular menses, mastitis.

Shallot; HU CONG Origin: *Allium ascalonicum* L. (*Liliaceae*). Part: bulb. Effects: To worm the center and precipitate *qi*. Indications: Edema, distention and fullness, toxin swelling.

Sharpleaf Gambirplant; GOU TENG Origin: *Uncaria rhynchophylla* (Miq.) Jacks. (*Rubiaceae*). Part: hooked stem. Effects: To remove heat, check hyperfunction of the liver and subdue endogenous wind, i.e., to relieve dizziness. Indications: Epilepsy induced by terror and convulsion; feeling of fullness in the head, headache and blood-shot, swollen and painful eyes due to the flaring-up of liver-fire; dizziness due to hyperactivity of the liver-*yang*.

Sharpleaf Senna Leaf; FAN XIE YE Origin: *Cassia acutifolia* Del. (*Leguminosae*). See Narrowleaf Senna Leaf.

Shearer's Pyrrosia Frond; SHI WEI Origin: *Pyrrosia sheareri* (Bak.) Ching (*Polypodiaceae*). See Japanese Felt Fern Frond.

Shepherdspurse Seed; JI CAI ZI Origin: *Capsella bursapastoris* (L.) Medic. (*Cruciferae*). Part: seed. Effects: To remove wind and brighten the eyes. Indications: Eye pain, eye screen, clear-eye blindness.

Shepherdspurse; JI CAI Origin: *Capsella bursapastoris* (L.) Medic. (*Cruciferae*). Part: herb with root. Effects: To harmonize the spleen, disinhibit water, stanch bleeding, and brighten the eyes. Indications: Dysentery, edema, strangury, chyluria, blood ejection, bloody stool, flooding, profuse menstruation, pain with red eyes.

Shield Floatingheart; XING CAI Origin: *Nymphoides peltatum* (Gmel.) O. Ktze. (*Gentiana-ceae*). Part: herb. Effects: To clear heat and disinhibit urine, disperse swelling and resolve toxin. Indications: Fever and chills, heat strangyru, swollen welling abscess, fire cinnabar.

Shiningleaf Birch Bark; LIANG YE HUA PI Origin: *Betula luminifera* H. Winkl. (*Betulaceae*). Part: bark. Effects: To eliminate damp, disperse food, and resolve toxin. Indications: Food accumulation and stagnation, mammary welling abscess with red swelling, seasonal heat toxin sore, wind papules, short voidings of reddish urine, bloating in the chest and abdomen, jaundice.

Shiningleaf Millettia; JI XUE TENG Origin: *Millettia nitida* Benth. (*Leguminosae*). See Suberect Spatholobus.

Shiny Bugleweed Root; DI SUN (ZE LAN GEN) Origin: *Lycopus lucidus* Turcz. (*Labiatae*). Part: rhizome. Effects: To quicken the blood, boost *qi*, and disperse water. Indications: Blood ejection, spontaneous external bleeding, postpartum abdominal pain, vaginal discharge.

Shiny Bugleweed Stem and Leaf; ZE LAN Origin: *Lycopus lucidus* Turcz. (*Labiatae*). Part: stem with leaf. Effects: To quicken the blood and move water. Indications: Menstrual block, concretions and conglomerations, postpartum stasis and stagnation with abdominal pain, puffy swelling in the body and face, knocks and falls, incised wound, swollen.

Shinyleaf Pricklyash; RU DI JIN NIU Origin: *Zanthoxylum nitidum* (Roxb.) DC. (*Rutaceae*). Part: root or branchlet with leaf. Effects: To dispel wind and free the network vessels, disperse swelling and relieve pain. Indications: Wind-damp bone pain, throat impediment, scrofula, stomach pain, toothache, burns and scalds.

Shore Podgrass; HAI JIU CAI Origin: *Triglochin maritimum* L. (*Juncaginaceae*). Part: herb and fruit. Effects: Herb: to clear heat and nourish *yin,* engender liquid and allay thirst; fruit: enrichng and supplement, checking diarrhea, and sedation. Indications: Fruit: eye pain.

Shortanther Syzygium Fruit; YE DONG QING QUO Origin: *Syzygium cumini* (L.) Skeels (*Myrtaceae*). See Duhat Fruit.

Shortclustered Plantainlily; DA YU BIAO HUA Origin: *Hosta sieboldiana* Engl. (*Liliaceae*). Part: root or flower. Indications: Toxin sore, headache.

Shorthorned Epimedium Root; YIN YANG HUO GEN Origin: *Epimedium brevicornum* Maxim. (*Berberidaceae*). See Largeflower Epimedium Root.

Shorthorned Epimedium; XIN YE YIN YANG HUO (one of the **YIN YANG HUO**) Origin: *Epimedium brevicornum* Maxim. (*Berberidaceae*). See Largeflower Epimedium.

Shortscape Fleabane; DENG ZHAN XI XIN Origin: *Erigeron breviscapus* (Vant.) Hand.-Mazz. (*Compositae*). Part: herb. Effects: To eliminate cold and superficial evil, to dispel wind and damp, to activate collaterals and relieve pain. Indications: Common cold with headache and nasal congestion, pain from wind-damp impediment (arthralgia-syndrome), paralysis, acute gastritis, child *gan* accumulation, knocks and falls.

Shortstalk Monkshood; XUE SHANG YI ZHI HAO Origin: *Aconitum brachypodum* Diels (*Ranunculaceae*). Part: root. Effects: To expel inflammation and relieve pain, dispel wind and eliminate dampness. Indications: Knocks and falls, fracture, wind-damp bone pain, toothache, swelling and toxin of sores, poisonous snake bites.

Shortstalk Slimtop Meadowrue; YING SHUI HUANG LIAN Origin: *Thalictrum simplex* L. var. brevipes Hara (*Ranunculaceae*). Part: root. Effects: To clear damp-heat and resolve toxin. Indications: Jaundice, dysentery, asthma, measles papules with complicated pneumonia, *gan* of the nose, red eyes, heat sore.

Shorttube Lycoris; SHI SUAN Origin: *Lycoris radiata* (L'Her.) Herb. (*Amaryllidaceae*). Part: bulb. Effects: To dispel phlegm, disinhibit urine, resolve toxin, and promote ejection. Indications: Throat wind, edema, swelling and toxin of welling abscess and flat abscess, clove sore, scrofula.

Showy Bleedingheart; HE BAO MU DAN GEN Origin: *Dicentra spectabilis* (L.) Lem. (*Papaveraceae*). Part: rhizome. Effects: To dissipate the blood, eliminate toxin of sores, remove wind, and harmonize the blood. Indications: Incised wound.

Shrub Lespedeza; HU ZHI ZI Origin: *Lespedeza bicolor* Turcz. (*Leguminosae*). Part: stem and leaf. Effects: To moisten the lung and clear heat, disinhibit water and free strangury. Indications: Lung heat cough, whooping cough, nosebleed, strangury.

Shrubalthea Flower; MU JIN HUA Origin: Hibiscus syriacus L. (*Malvaceae*). Part: flower. Effects: To remove damp-heat and to cool the blood. Indications: Intestinal wind bleeding, dysentery, white vaginal discharge.

Shrubalthea Fruit; MU JIN ZI Origin: *Hibiscus syriacus* L. (*Malvaceae*). Part: fruit. Effects: To clear lung and transform phlegm. Indications: Lung-wind phlegm and panting, cough and loss of voice, hemilateral head wind, head wind, yellow-water pus sore.

Shrubby Baeckea; GANG SONG Origin: *Baeckea frutescens* L. (*Myrtaceae*). Part: leaf, flower and fruit. Effects: To eliminate damp-heat, eliminate stasis and releive pain, disinhibit urine, and kill worms. Indications: Knocks and falls, wind-damp pain (rheumatalgia), strangury, scab, foot lichen.

Siberian Cocklebur; CANG ER Origin: *Xanthium sibiricus* Patr. *ex* Widd. (*Compositae*). Part: stem and leaf. Effects: To dispel wind and dissipate heat, resolve toxin and kill worms. Indications: Head wind, dizzy head, damp impediment and hypertonicity, red eyes, eye screen, wind *lai*, swollen clove sore, heat toxin sore, itchy skin.

Siberian Nitraria; KA MI Origin: *Nitraria Sibirica* Pall. (*Zygophyllaceae*). Part: fruit. Effects: To fortify the spleen and the stomach, enrich and supplement for health promotion, regulate menstruation and quicken the blood. Indications: Emaciation and weakness, dual depletion of *qi* and blood, spleen-stomach disharmony, indigestion, menstrual irregularities, pain in the lumbus and abdomen.

Siberian Solomonseal; HUANG JING Origin: *Polygonatum sibiricum* Redoute (*Liliaceae*). Part: rhizome. Effects: To supplement the spleen and moisten the lung, replenish vital essence and promote body fluid production. Indications: Vacuity detriment cold and heat, pulmonary consumption with coughing of blood, weak constitution and reduced food intake, weak sinews and bones, wind-damp pain (rheuma-talgia), wind lichen and wind *lai.*

Sickle Senna Seed; JUE MING ZI Origin: *Cassia tora* L. (*Leguminosae*). Part: seed. Effects: To clear the liver and brighten the eyes, disinhibit water and free the stool. Indications: Red eyes due to wind-heat, clear-eye blindness, night blindness, hypertension, hepatitis, ascites due to cirrhosis, habitual constipation.

Siebold Greenbrier; NIAN YU XU Origin: *Smilax sieboldi* Miq. (*Liliaceae*). Part: rhizome and root. Effects: To dispel wind and quicken the blood, disperse swelling and relieve pain. Indications: Wind-damp pain in sinews and bones, clove sore, toxin swelling.

Siebold Wildginger; XI XIN Origin: *Asarum sieboldii* Miq. (*Aristolochiaceae*). See Manchurian Wildginger.

Sievers Wormwood; BAI HAO Origin: *Artemisia sieversiana* Ehrh. *ex* Willd. (*Compositae*). Part: herb. Indications: Wind-cold-damp impediment, jaundice, heat dysentery, scab and *lai*.

Silk Cocoon; CAN JIAN Origin: *Bombyx mori* L. (*Bombycidae*). Part: silk covering spun by larva. Indications: Bloody stool, bloody urine, flooding, diabetes, stomach reflux, *gan* sore, swollen welling abscess.

Silktree Albizia Bark; HE HUAN PI Origin: *Albizzia julibrissin* Durazz. (*Leguminosae*). Part: bark. Effects: To resolve depression, harmonize the blood, quite the heart, and to disperse swollen welling abscess. Indications: Disquieted heart spirit, anxiety and insomnia, pulmonary welling abscess, swollen welling abscess, scrofula, damage to sinew and bone.

Silkworm Egg; YUAN CAN ZI Origin: *Bombyx mori* L. (*Bombycidae*). Part: silkworm egg. Indications: Heat blood strangury, footling presentation.

Silkworm Feculae; YUAN CAN SHA Origin: *Bombyx mori* L. (*Bombycidae*). Part: silkworm feculae. Effects: To dispel wind and eliminate damp, harmonize the stomach and transform turbidity. Indications: Wind-damp impediment (arthralgia-syndrome), paralysis of the body or limbs, eczema with itching; vomiting, diarrhea, and cramp due to internal damp and turbidity, hypertonicity of the limbs.

Silkworm King; YUAN CAN E Origin: *Bombyx mori* L. (*Bombycidae*). Part: silkworm king. Effects: To tonify liver and kidney, invigorate yang and astringe essence. Indications: Impotence, seminal emission, white turbidity, bloody urine, white turbidity, ulcerating sore, scalds.

Silkworm Larva; BAI JIANG CAN Origin: *Bombyx mori* L. (*Bombycidae*). Part: dried larva. Effects: To dispel wind and resolve tetany, to transform phlegm and dissipate binds. Indications: Wind stroke and loss of voice, fright epilepsy, head wind, throat wind, throat impediment, scrofula and subcutaneous nodes, wind sore and dormant papules, cinnabar toxin, mastitis.

Silky Ant; HEI MA YI Origin: *Formica fusca* L. (*Formicidae*). Part: body. Indications: Snakebite, painful swelling of clove toxin.

Silvervine Actinidia; MU TIAN LIAO Origin: *Actinidia polygama* (Sieb. *et* Zucc.) Maxim. (*Actinidiaceae*). Part: branchlet and leaf. Indications: Concretion, bind, accumulation and gathering; wind taxation and vacuity-cold.

Silvery Aleuritopteris; TONG JING CAO Origin: *Aleuritopteris argentea* (Gmel.) Fée (*Sinopte-ridaceae*). Part: herb. Effects: To regulate menstrua-tion, suppress cough, and dispel damp. Indications: Cough, menstrual disorder, red and white vaginal discharge.

Simple Digenea Frond; HAI REN CAO Origin: *Digenea simplex* (Wulf.) C. Ag. (*Rhodomela-ceae*). Part: algal frond. Indications: Roundworms.

Simpleleaf Shrub Chastetree Leaf; MAN JING ZI YE Origin: *Vitex rotundifolia* L. (*Verbena-ceae*). Part: leaf. Effects: To disperse swelling and relieve pain. Indications: Head wind, knocks and falls.

Simpleleaf Shrub Chastetree; MAN JING ZI Origin: *Vitex rotundifolia* L. (*Verbenaceae*). Part: seed. Effects: To dispel wind and heat, to clear and disinhibit head and eyes. Indications: External contraction of wind-heat, clouded heavy head, headache, hemilateral headache; clouded vision, sore red swollen eyes, profuse tearing; pain from wind-damp impediment (arthralgia-syndrome) with pain, hypertonicity of limbs.

Singharanut; LING Origin: *Trapa bispinosa* Roxb (*Trapaceae*). Part: pulp. Effects: Eaten raw: clear summerheat and resolve heat, eliminate vexation and allay thirst; cooked eat: boost *qi* and fortify the spleen.

Singkwa Towelgourd Seed; SI GUA ZI Origin: *Luffa acutangula* Roxb (*Cucurbitaceae*). See Suakwa Vegetalesponge Seed.

Singkwa Towelgourd; SI GUA Origin: *Luffa acutangula* Roxb (*Cucurbitaceae*). See Suakwa Vegetalesponge.

Sinkiang Giantfennel Resin; A WEI Origin: *Ferula caspica* Marsh.-Bieb. (*Umbelliferae*). See Asafetida Giantfennel Resin.

Sinkiang-Tibet Arnebia; ZI CAO Origin: *Arnebia euchroma* (Royle) Johnst. (*Boraginaceae*). See Redroot Gromwell.

Sisal Hemp-plant (Sisal Agave); JIAN MA Origin: *Agave sisalana* Perr. *ex* Engelm. (*Agavaceae*). Part: leaf. Effects: To dissipate toxin with clearing coolness and expel pus. Indications: Swollen welling abscess and sore.

Sixangular Dysosma; BA JIAO LIAN Origin: *Dysosma pleiantha* (Hance) Woods. (*Berberidaceae*). Part: rhizome and root. Effects: To clear heat and resolve toxin, transform phlegm and dissipate binds, dispel stasis and reduce swelling. Indications: Swollen welling abscess, clove sore, scrofula, throat moth, knocks and falls, snake bite.

Skin-carp; CHONG CHUN YU Origin: *Hemibarbus labeo* (Pallas) (*Cyprinidae*). Part: meat. Indications: Pain of the lumbar spine (lested ten years), aching and numbness in the lumbus and knees, inability to walk.

Skyblue Broomrape; LIE DANG Origin: *Orobanche coerulescens* Steph. (*Orobanchaceae*). Part: whole plant. Effects: To supplement the kidney and invigorate *yang*. Indications: Kidney vacuity, cold pain in the lumbus and knees, impotence, seminal emission.

Slender Dutchmanspipe; MA DOU LING Origin: *Aristolochia debilis* Sieb. *et* Zucc. (*Aristolo-chiaceae*). See Northern Dutchmanspipe.

Slender Dutchmanspipe Root; QING MU XIAN (MA DOU LING GEN) Origin: *Aristolochia debilis* Sieb. *et* Zucc. (*Aristolochiaceae*). See Northern Dutchmanspipe Root.

Slenderleaf Ligusticum; HUO GAO BEN (one of the **GAO BEN**) Origin: *Ligusticum tenuissimum* (Nakai) Kitag. (*Umbelliferae*). See Chinese Ligusticum.

Slenderstyle Acanthopanax Leaf; WU JIA YE Origin: *Acanthopanax gracilistylus* W. W. Smith (*Araliaceae*). Part: leaf. Effects: To disperse swelling and pain. Indications: Skin wind, knocks and falls.

Slenderstyle Acanthopanax Root-bark; WU JIA PI Origin: *Acanthopanax gracilistylus* W. W. Smith (*Araliaceae*). Part: root bark. Effects: To dispel wind-damp and strengthen bone, tendon and muscle, quicken blood and dispel stasis. Indications: Hypertonicity of the limbs, limp lumbus and knees, slowness in learning to walk; edema.

Slimyhair Sida; HUANG HUA ZI Origin: *Sida mysorensis* Wight *et* Arn. (*Malvaceae*). Part: leaf or root. Effects: To quicken the blood and move *qi,* clear heat and resolve toxin. Indications: Hepatitis, dysentery, taxation detriment of lumbar flesh, lack of strength, purulent open sore.

Small Bugbane; SAN MIAN DAO Origin: *Cimicifuga acerina* (Sieb. *et* Zucc.) Tanaka (*Ranun-culaceae*). Part: rhizome. Effects: To clear heat, quicken the blood, and relieve toxin. Indications: Sore dry throat, taxation detriment, lumbar and leg pain due to wind-damp, swollen boil.

Small Centipeda Herb; E BU SHI CAO Origin: *Centipeda minima* (L.) A. Br. *et* Aschers (*Compositae*). Part: herb with flower. Effects: To dispel wind and dissipate cold, overcome damp, remove eye screen, free nasal congestion. Indications: Common cold, cold asthma, throat impediment, whooping cough, sand *qi* and abdominal pain, amebic dysentery, malaria, *gan* diarrhea, deep-source nasal congestion, nasal polyp, eye screen with dry itching, shank sore, scab and lichen, knocks and falls.

Small Yellow Daylily; XUAN CAO GEN Origin: *Hemerocallis minor* Mill. (*Liliaceae*). See Orange Daylily.

Snake Sansevieria; HU WEI LAN Origin: *Sansevieria trifasciata* Prain (*Agavaceae*). Part: leaf. Effects: To clear heat and resolve toxin. Indications: Common cold, bronchitis, traumatic injury, sore.

Snake Slough; SHE TUI Origin: *Elaphe taeniurus* Cope; *Elaphe carinata*; *Zaocys dhumnades*; *Dinodon rufozonatum* (all *Colubredae*). Part: dried membrane of the snakes. Effects: To dispel wind, stabilize fright, eliminate eye screens, disperse swelling, and kill worms. Indications: Child fright epilepsy, throat wind and mouth sore, wooden tongue, double tongue, eye screen, clove sore, swollen welling abscess, scrofula, mumps, hemorrhoids and fistulas, scab and lichen.

Snow Azalea; BAI HUA YING SHAN HONG Origin: *Rhododendron mucronatum* G. Don (*Ericaceae*). Part: flower, root and leaf. Effects: To armonize blood and dissipate stasis. Indications: Blood ejection, intestinal wind bleeding, dysentery, flooding, knocks and falls.

Soda-apple Nightshade; YE DIAN QIE Origin: *Solanum surattense* Burm. f. (*Solanaceae*). Part: whole plant. Effects: To suppress cough and calm asthma, dissipate stasis and relieve pain. Indications: Asthma, chronic bronchitis, stomachache, rheumatalgia, scrofula, cold purulent sore, knocks and falls.

Soft-hair Cowparsnip; RUAN MAO DU HUO (one of the **DU HUO**) Origin: *Heracleum lanatum* Michx. (*Umbelliferae*). See Doubleteeth Pubescent Angelica.

Sorghum; GAO LIANG Origin: *Sorghum vulgare* Pers (*Gramineae*). Part: seed. Effects: To worm the center and disinhibit *qi*, check diarrhea and astringe the intestines, and dispel wind. Indications: Cholera, dysentery, damp heat inhibited urination, visiting wind and intractable impediment.

Sorrel Rhubarb; DA HUANG Origin: *Rheum palmatum* L. (*Polygonaceae*). See Medicinal Rhubarb.

Southwest pyrrosia frond; SHI WEI Origin: *Pyrrosia gralla* (Gies.) Ching (*Polypodiaceae*). See Japanese Felt Fern Frond.

Soy Sauce; JIANG Origin: Legume crop. (*Leguminosae*). Part: seed of beans Effects: To remove heat, resolve toxin. Indications: Bee sting and insect bites.

Soybean Oil; DOU YOU Origin: *Glycine max* (L.) Merr. (*Leguminosae*). Part: seed oil. Effects: To expel worms and moisten the intestines. Indications: Dry bound stool.

Spicate Clerodendranthus; MAO XU CAO Origin: *Clerodendranthus spicatus* (Thunb.) C. Y. Wu (*Labiatae*). Part: herb. Effects: To clear heat and dispel damp, expel the stone and disinhibit water. Indications: Acute and chronic nephritis, cystitis, urethral stone, rheumatic arthritis.

Spiced Juice of Mature Winter-vegetable; CHEN DONG CAI LU ZHI Origin: *Brassica chinensis* L. (*Cruciferae*). Part: juice from whole herb. Effects: To clear lung-fire, phlegm and cough; resolve swelling and pain in throat. Indications: Phlegm and cough due to lung-fire, swelling and pain in throat.

Spiked Gingerlily; TU LIANG JIANG Origin: *Hedychium spicatum* Ham (*Zingiberaceae*). Part: rhizome. Effects: To worm the stomach, dissipate cold, dry dampness. Indications: *Qi* pain, stomach pain, abdomen pain, stomach cold pain, indigestion, malaria.

Spiked Loosestrife; QIAN QU CAI Origin: *Lythrum salicaria* L. (*Lythraceae*). Part: herb. Effects: To clear heat and cool blood. Indications: Dysentery, flooding, ulcerating sore.

Spineless Common Jujube; DA ZAO Origin: *Ziziphus jujuba* Mill. var. *inermis* (Bge.) Rehd. (*Rhamnaceae*). See Common Jujube (Chinese Date).

Spinach; BO CAI Origin: *Spinacia oleracea* L. (*Chenopodiaceae*). Part: herb with root. Effects: To nourish blood, stanch bleeding, constrain yin, and moisten dryness. Indications: Spontaneous external bleeding, bloody stool, scurvy, diabetes conduct rheum, dry and stagnational stool.

Star Anise; BA JIAO HUI XIANG Origin: *Illicium verum* Hook. f. (*Magnoliaceae*). Part: fruit. Effects: To warm the middle-*jiao* and expel cold, ensure normal flow of *qi* and relieve pain. Indications: Cold mounting with pain, sagging of one testicle; stomach cold vomiting and reduced eating, pain and distention in stomach duct and abdomen; abdomen pain with cold pattern.

Stellate Cladonia Fruticose Thallus; TAI BAI HUA Origin: *Cladonia stellaris* (Opiz.) Pouzar *et* Vezda [= *Cladonia alpestris* (L.) Rabht.] (*Clado-niaceae*). Part: branch-like body. Effects: To supplement vacuity, fortify spleen and stomach, expel inflammation and relieve pain. Indications: Vacuous body, stomach vacuity and steaming bone tidal fever, pain in joints, no thought of food and drink.

Stiffleaf Juniper Fruit; DU SONG SHI Origin: *Juniperus rigida* Sieb. *et* Zucc. (*Cupressaceae*). Part: fruit. Effects: To dispel wind and eliminate dampness, disinhibit urine, effuse sweat, fortify the stomach , and settle pain. Indications: Edema, pain wind.

Straw-coloured Gentian; QIN JIAO Origin: *Gentiana straminea* Maxim. (*Gentianaceae*). See Largeleaf Gentian.

Strictleaf Dracaena Leaf; JIAN YE TIE SHU YE Origin: *Cordyline strcta* Endl. (*Agavaceae*). Part: leaf. Indications: Knocks and falls, cough with blood ejection, nosebleed, bloody stool and urine, bleeding wound, child *gan* accumulation, asthma, dysentery.

Stringy Stonecrop; SHI ZHI JIA Origin: *Sedum sarmentosum* Bge. (*Crassulaceae*). Part: herb. Effects: To clear heat, disperse swelling, and resolve toxin. Indications: Sore swollen throat, hepatitis, heat strangury, swollen welling abscess, burns and scalds, snake bite, insect bite.

Suakwa Vegetalesponge Seed; SI GUA ZI Origin: *Luffa cylindrica* (L.) Roem. (*Cucurbitaceae*). Part: seed. Effects: To remove heat and dryness, expel intestinal parasites. Indications: Puffy swelling of limbs or face, stone strangury, intestinal wind hemorrhoids and fistulas.

Suakwa Vegetablesponge; SI GUA Origin: *Luffa cylindrica* (L.) Roem. (*Cucurbitaceae*). Part: dried vascular bundles of the mature fruit. Effects: To quicken the blood, remove obstruction of the channels, induce diuresis and relieve edema. Indications: Generalized fever with vexation and thirst, phlegm panting with cough, intestinal wind hemorrhoids and fistulas, flooding and vaginal discharge, blood strangury, clove sore, breast milk stoppage, swollen welling abscess.

Suberect Spatholobus; JI XUE TENG Origin: *Spatholobus suberectus* Dunn (*Leguminosae*). Part: stem. Effects: To supplement the blood and activate blood flow, and to relieve rigidity of muscles and joints. Indications: Aching lumbus and knees, numbness and paralysis, menstrual disorder.

Subshrubby Peony Bark; MU DAN PI Origin: *Paeonia suffruticosa* Andr. (*Ranunculaceae*). Part: root bark. Effects: To remove heat, especially from blood, to activate blood flow, and to dispel blood stasis. Indications: Epidemic febrile diseases marked by maculas and eruptions; blood ejection, spontaneous external bleeding; febrile diseases in the later stage; fever prior to menstruation, menstrual block, menorrhalgia, abdominal mass; acute appendicitis with abdominal pain and constipation; suppurative infections on the body surface.

Suffrutescent Securinega; YI YE QIU Origin: *Securinega suffruticosa* (Pall.) Rehd. (*Euphor-biaceae*). Part: root and tender twigs. Effects: To quicken the blood and soothe the sinews, to fortify the spleen and boost kidney. Indications: Wind-damp lumbar pain, numbness of the limbs, hemiplegia, impotence, facial paralysis, sequel of infantile paralysis.

Sugary Citrus Pericarp; GAN PI Origin: Citrus suavissima Hort. *ex* Tanaka (*Rutaceae*). See Chachi Citrus Pericarp.

Sugary Citrus; GAN Origin: *Citrus suavissima* Hort. *ex* Tanaka (*Rutaceae*). See Chachi Citrus.

Sun Euphorbia; ZE QI Origin: *Euphorbia helioscopia* L. (*Euphorbiaceae*). Part: whole plant. Effects: To disinhibit water and disperse swelling, transform phlegm, suppress cough, and dissipate bind. Indications: Greater abdomen and edema, puffy swelling of the face and limbs; cough due to lung-heat, phlegm-rheum cough; scrofula.

Sunflower Leaf; XIANG RI KUI YE Origin: *Helianthus annuus* L. (*Compositae*). Part: leaf. Effects: To fortify the stomach. Indications: Hypertension.

Sunflower Seed; XIANG RI KUI ZI Origin: *Helianthus annuus L.* (*Compositae*). Part: seed. Indications: Blood dysentery, welling abscess with pus.

Sunflower Stem Pith; XIANG RI KUI JING SUI Origin: *Helianthus annuus L.* (*Compositae*). Part: stem pith. Indications: Blood strangury, urethral stone, chyluria, inhibited urination.

Sunflower; XIANG RI KUI HUA Origin: *Helianthus annuus* L. (*Compositae*). Part: flower. Effects: To dispel wind and brighten the eyes, hasten delivery. Indications: Heavy head, swollen face.

Sweet Broomwort; YE GAN CAO Origin: *Scoparia dulcis* L. (*Scrophulariaceae*). Part: herb. Effects: To clear heat and resolve toxin, disinhibit urine and disperse swelling. Indications: Lung heat cough, summerheat-heat diarrhea, leg *qi* (beriberi) with general edema, child measles papules, eczema, prickly heat, laryngitis, cinnabar toxin.

Sweet Orange; TIAN CHEN Origin: *Citrus sinensis* (L.) Osbeck (*Rutaceae*). Part: ripe fruit. Effects: To move *qi,* precipitate *qi, relieve pain,* disperse distention, and free milk. Indications: Breast milk stoppage.

Sweet Osmanthus Flower; GUI HUA Origin: *Osmanthus fragrans* Lour. (*Oleaceae*). Part: flower. Effects: To transform phlegm and dissipate stasis. Indications: Phlegm-rheum cough panting, intestinal wind blood dysentery, mounting and conglomeration, toothache, bad breath.

Sweet Wormwood; QING HAO Origin: *Artemisia annua* L. (*Compositae*). Same as *1363*; See Celery Wormwood.

Sweet Wormwood; HUANG HUA HAO Origin: *Artemisia annua* L. (*Compositae*). Part: herb. Effects: To clear heat and resolve malaria, expel wind and resolve itch. Indications: Summerheat damage, malaria, tidal fever, fright wind in children, heat diarrhea, malign sore, lichen and scab.

Sweetcane Culm; GAN ZHE Origin: *Saccharum sinensis* Roxb. (*Gramineae*). Part: stem. Effects: To clear heat and engender liquid, precipitate *qi* and moisten dampness. Indications: Damage to fluids due to febrile disease, vexation and thirst, stomach reflux vomiting, lung damp cough, dry bound stool.

Sweetscented Oleander; JIA ZHU TAO Origin: *Nerium indicum* Mill. (*Apocynaceae*). Part: leaf or bark. Effects: To strengthen the heart and disinhibit urine, dispel phlegm and stabilize panting, eliminate stasis and settle pain. Indications: Heart failure, panting and cough, epilepsy, swelling and pain from knocks and falls, menstrual block.

Sword Jackbean; DAO DOU Origin: *Canavalia gladiata* (Jacq.) DC. (*Leguminosae*). Part: seed. Effects: To warm the middle-*jiao,* keep the adverse energy downward and to supplement the kidney. Indications: Vacuity cold and hiccough, vomiting, abdominal distention, kidney vacuity lumbar pain, phlegm panting.

Swordlike Atractylodes; CANG ZHU Origin: *Atractylodes lancea* (Thunb.) DC. (*Compositae*). Part: rhizome. Effects: To remove dampness and strengthen the spleen and to dispel wind. Indications: Disturbance of the middle-*jiao* with epigastric dullness, abdominal distention, anorexia, nausea and vomiting, lassitude; wind-cold-dump impediment, pain in the joints and extremities; eye problems such as external or internal oculopathy, optic atrophy, night blindness.

Szechuan Lovage; CHUAN XIONG Origin: *Ligusticum chuanxiong* Hort. (*Umbelliferae*). See Chuan-xiong (Wallich Ligusticum).

Szechwan Chinaberry Bark; KU LIAN PI Origin: *Melia toosendan* Sieb. *et* Zucc. (*Meliaceae*). See Chinaberry-tree Bark.

Szechwan Chinaberry Flower; LIAN HUA Origin: *Melia toosendan* Sieb. *et* Zucc. (*Meliaceae*). Part: flower. Indications: Prickly heat.

Szechwan Chinaberry Fruit; CHUAN LIAN ZI (KU LIAN) Origin: *Melia toosendan* Sieb. *et* Zucc. (*Meliaceae*). Part: fruit. Effects: To rectify *qi* , to relieve pain, to clear liver-heat, and to expel intestinal parasites. Indications: Heat reversal heart pain, pain in the rib-side, pain from mounting *qi*, abdominal pain due to worm accumulation.

Szechwan Notopterygium; CHUAN QIANG HUO (one of the **QIANG HUO**) Origin: *Notoptery-gium franchetii* Boiss. (*Umbelliferae*). See Incised Notopterygium.

Szechwon Tangshen; DANG SHEN Origin: *Codonopsis tangshen* Oliv. (*Campanulaceae*). See Pilose Asiabell.

Taiwan Angelika; BAI ZHI Origin: *Angelica taiwaniana* Boiss. (*Umbelliferae*). See Dahurian Angelica.

Taiwan Juniper; SHAN CI BAI Origin: *Juniperus taiwaniana* Hayata (*Cupressaceae*). Part: root or fruit. Indications: Lichen of skin, enduring low fever.

Tall Gastrodia; TIAN MA Origin: *Gastrodia elata* Blume (*Orchidaceae*). Part: stem tuber. Effects: To subdue the exuberant *yang* of the liver, calm the internal wind, and relieve convulsion and fainting. Indications: Epilepsy induced by fright and convulsion ; headache and light-headedness; rheumatic impediment, numbness of the limbs or tetraplegia.

Tall Hymenodictyon; TU LIAN QIAO Origin: *Hymenodictyon excelsum* (Roxb.) Wall. (*Rubiaceae*). Part: bark. Effects: To clear heat and resolve toxin, suppress cough and interrupt malaria. Indications: Malaria, malign malaria, common cold, high fever, cough with profuse phlegm.

Tamarind Fruit; SUAN JIAO Origin: *Tamarindus indica* L. (*Leguminosae*). Part: fruit. Effects: To clear summerheat-heat, transform accumulation and stagnation. Indications: Poor appetite due to summerheat-heat, vomiting in pregnancy, child *gan* accumulation.

Tamariskoid Spikemoss; JUAN BAI Origin: *Selaginella tamariscina* (Beauv.) Spring (*Selaginella-ceae*). Part: dried whole plant. Effects: To break blood, and to arrest bleeding when charred. Indications: Raw: menstrual block, concretions and conglomerations, knocks and falls, abdominal pain, asthma; scorch-fry: blood ejection, bloody urine, bloody stool, prolapse of the rectum.

Tangerine Pericarp; JU PI (CHEN PI) Origin: *Citrus reticulata* Blanco (*Rutaceae*). Part: pericarp. Effects: To rectify *qi* and harmonize the center (digestion), dispel damp and transform phlegm. Indications: Abdominal distention, belching, nausea and vomiting; oppressed feeling in the chest, abdominal distention, poor appetite, lassitude, loose stool, and thick greasy fur on the tongue; accumulation of phlegm-dampness in the lung marked by cough, profuse sputum, full and oppressed feeling of the chest.

Tangerine Seed; JU HE Origin: *Citrus reticulata* Blanco (*Rutaceae*). Part: seed. Effects: To rectify *qi* and relieve pian, resolve bind. Indications: Mounting *qi,* painful swollen testicles, mammary welling abscess, lumbar pain, bladder *qi* pain.

Tangle Thallus; KUN BU Origin: *Ecklonia kurome* Okam. (*Alariaceae*). See Kelp Thallus.

Tangut Anisodus; ZANG QIE Origin: *Anisodus tanguticus* (Maxim.) Pascher (*Solanaceae*). Part: root and seed. Effects: To settle pain and anesthetize, resolve tetany and disperse swelling.

Tangut Rhubarb; DA HUANG Origin: *Rheum tanguticum* Maxim. *ex* Balf. (*Polygonaceae*). See Medicinal Rhubarb.

Taro; YE YU Origin: *Colocasia antiquorum* Schott *et* Endl. (*Araceae*). Part: rhizome. Indications: Mammary welling abscess, toxin swelling, leprosy, scab and lichen, knocks and falls, bee sting.

Tatarion Aster; ZI WAN Origin: *Aster tataricus* L. f. (*Compositae*). Part: root and rhizome. Effects: To transform phlegm and suppress cough, worm the lung and precipitate *qi.* Indications: Cough and counterflow *qi* ascent, cough with inhibited feeling, enduring cough due to lung vacuity, phlegm containing blood.

Tea Root; CHA SHU GEN Origin: *Camellia sinensis* O. Ktze. (*Theaceae*). Part: root. Indications: Heart disease, mouth sore, oxhide lichen.

Tea Seed; CHA ZI Origin: *Camellia sinensis* O. Ktze. (*Theaceae*). Part: seed. Indications: Rapid panting and cough.

Tea; CHA YE Origin: *Camellia sinensis* O. Ktze. (*Theaceae*). Part: tender leaf. Effects: To refresh oneself, relieve thirst and fatigue, and as a digestant, diuretic and detoxicant. Indications: Headache, clouded vision, profuse sleeping, vexation and thirst, food accumulation and phlegm stagnation, malaria, dysentery.

Tendrilleaf Fritillary; JUAN YE BEI MU (one of the **CHUAN BEI MU**) Origin: *Fritillaria cirrhosa* D. Don (*Liliaceae*). Part: bulb. Effects: To moisten the lung, arrest cough and resolve heat-phlegm. Indications: Cough, scanty sputum and dry throat; scrofula, sores, and abscesses.

Tendrilleaf Solomonseal; HUANG JING Origin: *Polygonatum cirrhifolium* (Wall.) Royle (*Liliaceae*). See Siberian Solomonseal.

Ternate Pinellia; BAN XIA Origin: *Pinellia ternata* (Thunb.) Breit. (*Araceae*). Part: tuber. Effects: To remove dampness and resolve cold-phlegm, to smooth the upward adverse flow of *qi* and arrest vomiting. Indications: Profuse sputum, cough, adverse upward flow of *qi* and vertigo; nausea and vomiting; feeling of stuffiness and distention in the chest and upper abdomen, globus hystericus, goiter, subcutaneous nodules, carbuncles, deep-rooted carbuncles, lumbodorsal cellulitis, and breast furuncles.

Tetragonal Crotalaria; HUA JIN DAN Origin: *Crotalaria tetragona* Roxb.[= *Crotalaria tetragona* Andr.] (*Verbenaceae*). Part: herb or root. Effects: To transform stagnation and relieve pain. Indications: Abdominal pain, iron or wood intake .

Tetraphyllous Paris; WANG SUN Origin: *Paris tetraphylla* A. Gray (*Liliaceae*). Part: rhizome. Indications: Impediment, aching pain in the limbs, red and white dysentery.

Thatch Screwpine Flower; LU DOU LE HUA Origin: *Pandanus tectorius* Soland. (*Pandanaceae*). Part: flower. Effects: To clear heat and disinhibit water, eliminite damp-heat, check diarrhea. Indica-tions: Mounting *qi,* urinary stoppage, strangury-turbidity, mouth-level nape sore.

Thickfruit Millettia; KU TAN ZI Origin: *Millettia pachycarpa* Benth. (*Leguminosae*). Part: seed or fruit. Effects: To kill worms, attack toxin, and relieve pain. Indications: Scab sore, lichen, lai, sand *qi* with abdominal pain, child *gan* accumulation.

Thickleaf Bergenia; YAN BAI CAI Origin: *Bergenin crassifolia* (L.) Fritsch (*Saxifragaceae*). See Purple Bergenia.

Thickleaf Boea; YAN BAI CAI Origin: *Boea crassifolia* Hemsl. (*Gesneriaceae*). See Purple Bergenia.

Thickstemen Gentian; QIN JIAO Origin: *Gentiana crassicaulis* Duthie *ex* Burkill (*Gentiana-ceae*). See Largeleaf Gentian.

Thinfruit Hypecoum; XI GUO JIAO HUI XIANG Origin: *Hypecoum leptocarpum* Hook. f. *et* Thoms. (*Papaveraceae*). Part: whole plant. Effects: To resolve heat and settle pain, resolve toxin and expel inflammation. Indications: Wind damage and common cold, headache, pain in the joints of the limbs, inflamation of the gallbladder, food poisoning.

Thinleaf Buckthorn Root; JIANG LI MU GEN Origin: *Rhamnus leptophylla* Schneid. (*Rham-naceae*). Part: root. Effects: To disperse food, move water, and eliminate stasis. Indications: Food accumulation bloating, edema and drum distention, menstrual block.

Thinleaf Milkwort; YUAN ZHI Origin: Polygala tenuifolia Willd. (*Polygalaceae*). Part: root. Effects: As a sedative, expectorant and resuscitating agent. Indications: Irritability, palpitation, insomnia, forgetfulness; mental confusion, vague mind, epilepsy induced by terror; cough with profuse sputum, thick and difficult to spit; carbuncles, poisoning swelling, painful swelling in breasts.

Thinnest Yam; QIAN XI SHU YU (one of the **BEI XIE**) Origin: *Dioscorea gracillima* Miq. (*Dioscoriaceae*). See Hypoglaucous Collett Yam.

Thomson Kudzuvine Root; GE GEN Origin: *Pueraria thomsonii* Benth. (*Leguminosae*). See Lobed Kudzuvine Root.

Thorowort Pondweed; SUAN SHUI CAO Origin: *Potamogeton perfoliatus* L. (*Potamogetona-ceae*). Part: herb. Effects: To percolate damp and resolve the exterior. Indications: Eczema, itchy skin.

Three-coloured Amaranth; YAN LAI HONG Origin: *Amaranthus tricolor* L. (*Amaranthaceae*). Part: herb. Indications: Dysentery, blood ejection, flooding, eye screen.

Threeflower Clematis; BAI HUA TENG Origin: *Clematis terniflora* DC. [= *Clematis maximo-wicziana* Franch. *et* Sav.] (*Ranunculaceae*). Part: root. Effects: To disperse swelling and relieve pain. Indications: Pallas pit viper bite.

Threeflower Gentian; LONG DAN Origin: *Gentiana triflora* Pall. (*Gentianaceae*). See Rough Gentian.

Threeleaf Akebia Root; MU TONG GEN Origin: *Akebia trifoliata* (Thunb.) Koidz. (*Lardizaba-laceae*). See Austral Akebia Root.

Threeleaf Akebia; SAN YE MU TONG (one of the **MU TONG**) Origin: *Akebia trifoliata* (Thunb.) Koidz. (*Lardizabalaceae*). See Austral Akebia.

Threeleaf Chastetree Leaf; MAN JING ZI YE Origin: *Vitex trifolia* L. (*Verbenaceae*). See Simpleleaf Shrub Chastetree Leaf.

Threeleaf Chastetree; MAN JING ZI Origin: *Vitex trifolia* L. (*Verbenaceae*). See Simpleleaf Shrub Chastetree.

Thunberg Fritillary; ZHE BEI MU Origin: *Fritillaria verticillata* Willd. var. *thunbergii* Bak. [=*Fritillaria thunbergii* Miq.] (*Liliaceae*). Part: bulb. Effects: To moisten the lung, arrest cough and resolve heat-phlegm. Indications: Scrofula, sores, and abscesses; cough, scanty sputum and dry throat.

Thunberg Knotweed; SHUI MA TIAO Origin: *Polygonum thunbergii* Sieb. *et* Zucc. (*Polygonaceae*). Part: herb. Indications: Sand.

Thunberg's Lepisorus; WA WEI Origin: *Lepisorus thunbergianus* (Kaulf.) Ching (*Polypodia-ceae*). Part: herb. Effects: To disinhibit urination and stanch bleeding. Indications: Strangury, dysentery, cough with blood ejection, *gan* of the teeth and gums.

Thyme; SHE XIANG CAO Origin: *Thymus vulgaris* L. (*Labiatae*). Part: herb. Effects: To suppress cough and expel wind. Indications: Whooping cough, acute bronchitis, pharyngolaryn-gitis.

Thymifolious Euporbia; XIAO FEI YANG CAO Origin: *Euphorbia thymifolia* L. (*Euphorbia-ceae*). Part: herb. Effects: To clear heat and disinhibit damp, to disperse swelling and resolve toxin. Indications: Malaria, dysentery, diarrhea, eczema, mammary welling abscess, hemorrhoid.

Tianshan Mountain Mountainash; TIAN SHAN HUA QIU Origin: *Sorbus tianschanica* Rupr. (*Rosaceae*). Part: branchlet and fruit. Effects: To clear lung and suppress cough, to supplement spleen and engender liquids. Indications: Pulmonary tuberculosis, cough and asthma, gastritis, vitaminosis A and C.

Tibet Gentian; QIN JIAO Origin: *Gentiana tibetica* King (*Gentianaceae*). See Largeleaf Gentian.

Tibet Lyonia; LI MU Origin: *Lyonia ovalifolia* (Wall.) Drude (*Ericaceae*). Part: branchlet, leaf and fruit. Effects: To dispel wind, resolve toxin, supplement the lumbus and legs, boost *yang*. Indications: Wind blood marked emaciation.

Tibetan Hellebore; TIE KUAI ZI (II) Origin: *Helleborus thibetanus* Franch. (*Ranunculaceae*). Part: root. Effects: To clear heat and resolve toxin, quicken blood and dissipate stasis, disperse swelling and relieve pain. Indications: Cystitis, urethritis, swelling and toxin of sores and boils, swelling and toxin of sores and boils, taxation damage.

Tiger Fat; HU GAO Origin: *Panthera tigris* L. (*Felidae*). Part: fat. Indications: Stomach reflux, head sore and bald white scalp sore, hemorrhoid with precipitation of blood.

Tithymalus-like Pedilanthus; YU DAI GEN Origin: *Pedilanthus tithymaloides* (L.) Poit. (*Euphor-biaceae*). Part: herb. Effects: To clear heat and resolve toxin, stanch bleeding and settle pain. Indications: Swelling and toxin of sores, painful swelling from knocks and falls, bleeding due to external injury, fire eye.

Toad Gall; CHAN CHU DAN Origin: *Bufo bufo gargarizans* Cantor; *Bufo melanostictus* Schneider (*Bufonidae*). Part: gall. Indications: Tracheitis.

Toad Skin Secretion Cake; CHAN SU Origin: *Bufo bufo gargarizans* Cantor; *Bufo melanostictus* Schneider (*Bufonidae*). Part: dried secretion of the skin glands. Effects: To resolve toxin, disperse swelling, strengthen the heart, and relieve pain. Indications: Clove sore, welling abscess and flat abscess, effusion of the back, scrofula, chronic medullitis, sore swollen throat, child *gan* accumulation, cardiac failure, toothache of wind and insect.

Toad Skin; CHAN PI Origin: *Bufo bufo gargarizans* Cantor; *Bufo melanostictus* Schneider (*Bufonidae*). Part: skin. Effects: To clear heat and resolve toxin, disinhibit water and disperse distention. Indications: Swelling and toxin of welling abscess and flat abscess, scrofula, neoplasm, *gan* accumulation and abdominal distention, chronic trachitis.

Tomato; FAN QIE Origin: *Lycopersicon esculentum* Mill. (*Solanaceae*). Part: fresh fruit. Effects: To engender liquid and allay thirst, fortify the stomach and disperse food. Indications: Thirst, poor appetite.

Tomentose Caudate Croton; MAO YE BA DOU Origin: *Croton caudatus* Geisel. var. *tomentosus* Hook. (*Euphorbiaceae*). Part: herb. Effects: To settle fright and dispel wind, abate heat and relieve pain, soothe sinew and quicken the network vessels. Indications: Malaria, high fever, fright epilepsy and convulsion, rheumatic arthritis, numbness.

Tonkin Snowbell; AN XI XIANG Origin: *Styrax tonkinensis* (Pier.) Craib *ex* Hart. (*Styracaceae*). See Benzoin.

Tonkin Sophora Root; SHAN DOU GEN Origin: *Sophora subprostrata* Chun *et* T. Chen (*Leguminosae*). Part: root and rhizome. Effects: Used as an antipyretic, detoxicant, antiphlogistic, anodyne, and to relieve sore-throat. Indications: Heat-toxin brewing, sore swollen throat; Jaundice due to damp-heat, swelling and toxin of welling abscess and sores.

Toothleaf Goldenray; HU LU QI Origin: *Ligularia dentata* (A. Gray.) Hara (*Compositae*). Part: root and rhizome. Effects: To rectify *qi* and quicken the blood, relieve pain, suppress cough and dispel phlegm. Indications: Knocks and falls, taxation damage, lumbar and leg pain, cough and panting, cough and panting, pulmonary welling abscess with hacking of blood.

Tortedfruit Screwtree; HUO SUO MA Origin: *Helicteres isora* L. (*Sterculiaceae*). Part: root. Effects: To move *qi* and relieve pain. Indications: Chronic gastritis, gastric ulcer.

Tree Beautyberry; QIAO MU ZI ZHU Origin: *Callicarpa arborea* Roxb. (*Verbenaceae*). Part: root and leaf. Effects: To cool the blood and stanch bleeding. Indications: Bleeding due to external injury, bleeding of digestive tract, spontaneous external bleeding, flooding and spotting.

Tree Falsespiraea; ZHEN ZHU MEI Origin: *Sorbaria arborea* Schneid. (*Rosaceae*). Part: bark. Effects: To quicken blood and dispel stasis, disperse swelling and relieve pain. Indications: Fracture, knocks and falls.

Tree of Heaven Ailanthus Bast; CHU BAI PI Origin: *Ailanthus altissima* (Mill.) Swingle (*Simarou-baceae*). Part: bast. Effects: To eliminate heat and dry dampness, astringe the intestines and stanch bleeding, and kill worms. Indications: Enduring dysentery, enduring drainage, intestinal wind bleeding, flooding and spotting, vaginal discharge, seminal emission, white turbidity, roundworm disease.

Trifoliate Acanthopanax; CI SAN JIA Origin: *Acanthopanax trifoliatus* (L.) Merr. (*Aralia-ceae*). Part: root or root bark. Effects: To clear heat and resolve toxin, dispel wind and disinhibit dampness, soothe sinew and quicken the blood. Indications: Common cold with high fever, coughing of phlegm and blood, wind-damp (rheumatism) with painful joints, jaundice, white vaginal discharge, urethral stone, knocks and falls, swollen boil and sore.

Trifoliate Jewelvine; YU TENG Origin: Derris trifoliata Lour. (*Leguminosae*). Part: root or herb. Indications: Painful swelling from knocks and falls, lichen.

Trifoliate Orange; ZHI SHI Origin: *Poncirus trifoliata* (L.) Raf. (*Rutaceae*). See Bitter Orange.

Trifoliate-orange Leaf; GOU JU YE Origin: *Poncirus trifoliata* (L.) Raf. (*Rutaceae*). Part: leaf. Effects: To rectify *qi* and dispel wind, disperse swelling and dissipate bind.

Trifoliate-orange Root-bark; ZHI GEN PI Origin: *Poncirus trifoliata* (L.) Raf. (*Rutaceae*). Part: root bark. Indications: Toothache, hemorrhoids, bloody stool.

Trifoliate-orange Seed; GOU JU HE Origin: *Poncirus trifoliata* (L.) Raf. (*Rutaceae*). Part: seed. Indications: Incessant intestinal wind bleeding.

Trifoliate-orange; GOU JU Origin: *Poncirus trifoliata* (L.) Raf. (*Rutaceae*). Part: unripe fruit. Effects: To break *qi* and dissipate bind, to course the liver and resolve depression. Indications: Binding depression of liver *qi,* mammary consumption, mounting *qi* with pain; non-transformation of food, *qi* stagnation, distention and fullness in the stomach duct and abdomen.

Trogopterus Dung; WU LING ZHI Origin: *Trogopterus xanthipes* Milne-Edwords; *Pteromys volans* L. (*Petauristidae*). Part: dried feces. Effects: To quicken the blood, dispel blood stasis and to relieve pain. Indications: Menstrual block, post-partum blood stasis with pain, flooding, excessive menstrual flow, incessant red vaginal discharge; snake bite, scorpion bite, centipede bite.

Tropical American Hymenocallis Leaf; SHUI GUI JIAO YE Origin: *Hymenocallis ameri-cana* Roem. (*Amaryllidaceae*). Part: leaf. Effects: To sooth sinew and quicken the blood. Indications: Painful swelling from knocks and falls.

True Indigo; MU LAN Origin: *Indigofera tinctoria* L. (*Leguminosae*). Part: stem and leaf. Effects: To clear heat and resolve toxin, to eliminate stasis and stanch bleeding. Indications: Encephalitis B, mumps, red eye, swollen sores, blood ejection.

True Lacquertree Seed; QI ZI Origin: *Rhus verniciflua* Stokes (*Anacardiaceae*). Part: seed. Effects: To precipitate blood.

Tschonosk Trillium; YU ER QI Origin: *Trillum tschonoskii* Maxim. (*Liliaceae*). Part: rhizome. Effects: To dispel wind and soothe the liver, quicken the blood and stanch bleeding. Indications: Hyper-tension, dizziness and headache, knocks and falls, fracture, lumbar and leg pain, bleeding due to external injury.

Tube Fleeceflower Stem; YE JIAO TENG Origin: *Polygonum multiflorum* Thunb. (*Polygona-ceae*). Part: stem. Effects: To relieve mental stress, dispel wind and remove obstruction of the channels. Indications: Insomnia, taxation damage, profuse sweating, blood vacuity and body pain, welling abscess and flat abscess, scrofula, wind sore and scab lichen.

Tuber Fleeceflower; HE SHOU WU Origin: *Polygonum multiflorum* Thunb. (*Polygonaceae*). Part: tuberous root. Effects: The raw drug is used as a laxative for constipation and detoxicant for boils; the prepared drug is used to replenish the vital essence of the liver and kidney and to nourish the blood for the treatment of anemia, early greying of hair, aching back and knees, neurasthenia and hypercholesteremia. Indications: Dizziness, blurred vision, premature grey hair, lassitude of the loins and legs, seminal emission and spermatorrhea; chronic malaria; sores, swellings and scrofula; constipation.

Tuber Onion; JIU CAI Origin: *Allium tuberosum* Rottler (*Liliaceae*). Part: leaf. Effects: To warm the center, *move qi,* eliminate blood stasis, and remove toxin. Indications: Chest impediment, dysphagia-occlusion, stomach reflux, blood ejection, spontaneous external bleeding, bloody urine, dysentery, diabetes, hemorrhoids and fistulas, prolapse of the rectum, knocks and falls, insect and scorpion stings.

Tuber Stemona; BAI BU Origin: *Stemona tuberosa* Lour. (*Stemonaceae*). See Sessile Stemona.

Tuberculate Speranskia; TOU GU CAO Origin: *Speranskia tuberculata* (Bge.) Baill. (*Euphorbiaceae*). Part: herb. Effects: To dispel wind and eliminate dampness, soothe sinew and quicken the blood, relieve pain. Indications: Pain from wind-damp impediment (arthralgia-syndrome), contracture of muscles and joints, cold damp leg *qi* (beriberi), swelling and toxin of sore and lichen.

Tuberousroot Jerusalemsage; KUAI JING CAO SU Origin: *Phlomis tuberosa* L. (*Labiatae*). Part: herb or root. Effects: To resolve toxin and expel syphills. Indications: Menstrual disorder, syphills, purulent wounds.

Tungoiltree Seed Oil; TONG YOU Origin: *Aleurites fordii* Hemsl. (*Euphorbiaceae*). Part: seed oil. Indications: Scab and lichen, shank sore, burns and scalds, cracking from frostbite.

Twoanther Mosla; DA YE XIANG RU Origin: *Mosla dianthera* (Ham.) Maxim. (*Labiatae*). Part: herb. Effects: To dispel wind and normalize *qi*, warm the center and relieve pain, kill worms and relieve itching. Indications: Summerheat damage and abdominal distention, sand *qi* pain, hemorrhoids and fistulas with bleeding, common cold with fever, eczema, itchy skin, miliaria alba, trichomonal vaginitis.

Twoflower Jerusalemcherry; YE HAI JIAO Origin: *Solanum capsicastrum* Link (*Solanaceae*). Part: herb. Effects: To disperse accumulation, disinhibit diaphragm, precipitate heat toxin. Indications: Rheumatism and paralysis, damp heat itchy sore, clove sore, menstruant's morbidity.

Twolobed Officinal Mangolia; HOU PO Origin: *Magnolia biloba* (Rehd. *et* Wils.) Cheng (*Magnoliaceae*). See Officinal Mangolia.

Twotooth Achyranthes; TU NIU XI Origin: *Achyranthes bidentata* Bl. (*Amaranthaceae*). Part: root and rhizome. Effects: To quicken blood and dissipate stasis, dispel damp and disinhibit urine, clear heat and resolve toxin. Indications: Strangury, bloody urine, menstrual block, concretions and conglomerations, wind-damp (rheumatism) with painful joints, beriberi (leg *qi*), edema, dysentery, malaria, diphtheria, swollen welling abscess, knocks and falls.

Twotooth Achyranthes; NIU XI Origin: *Achyranthes bidentata* Bl. (*Amaranthaceae*). Part: root. Effects: To quicken the blood and dispel blood stasis. Indications: Irregular menstruation, menstrual block, menstrual pain, dystocia, retention of placenta, afterpains, traumatic injuries; lassitude of the legs, aching pain in the loins and knees; difficulty in urination, hematuria, urethra pain during micturition; hematuresis, spontaneous external bleeding, canker sores, toothache, headache, vergito.

Udo; TU DANG GUI (I) Origin: *Aralia cordata* Thunb. (*Araliaceae*). Part: rhizome and root. Effects: To extinguish wind and harmonize the blood, effuse sweat and settle pain, disinhibit urine and disperse swelling, course wind and supplement vacuity. Indications: Wrenching and spraining of the limbs, hemilateral head wind.

Unarmed Glorybower; SHUI HU MAN Origin: *Clerodendron inerme* (L.) Gaertn. (*Verbenaceae*). Part: branchlet and leaf. Effects: To eliminate stasis, disperse swelling, eliminate dampness, and kill worms. Indications: Stasis and swelling from knocks and falls, eczema, sore and scab.

Undaria; KUN BU Origin: *Undaria pinnatifida* (Harv.) Sur. (*Alariaceae*). See Kelp Thallus.

Unibract Fritillary; LENG SHA BEI MU (one of the **CHUAN BEI MU**) Origin: *Fritillaria unibracteata* Hsiao *et* K. C. Hsiao (*Liliaceae*). See Tendrilleaf Fritillary.

Uniflower Swisscentaury; QI ZHOU LOU LU (one of the **LOU LU**) Origin: *Rhaponticum uniflorum* (L.) DC. (*Compositae*). Part: root. Effects: To clear heat and resolve toxin, disperse swelling and expel the pus, promote lactation, free the sinews and vessels. Indications: Swelling and pain of welling abscess and sores, mammary welling abscess; heat evil congesting, distention of the breasts, breast milk stoppage.

Ural Falsespiraea; ZHEN ZHU MEI Origin: *Sorbaria sorbifolia* (L.) A. Br. (*Rosaceae*). See Tree Falsespiraea.

Ural Licorice; GAN CAO Origin: *Glycyrrhiza uralensis* Fisch. (*Leguminosae*). Part: root and rhizome. Effects: To supplement the center and replenish *qi,* clear the heat and resolve the toxin, moisturize the lung and arrest cough, relieve spasm and pain. Indications: Short breath, asthenia, poor appetite and loose stool; cough and dyspnea; sores, ulcers and other pyogenic skin infections, swollen and sore throat, and food or drug poisoning; epigastric and abdominal pains and muscular spasm and pain.

Ussurian Pear Leaf; LI YE Origin: *Pyrus ussuriensis* Maxim. (*Rosaceae*). See Bretschneider Pear Leaf.

Vanillagrass; MAO XIANG HUA Origin: *Hierochloe odorata* (L.) Beauv. (*Gramineae*). Part: inflorescence. Effects: To warm the stomach, check vomiting. Indications: Cold pain in heart region and abdomen.

Veitch Peony; CHUAN CHI SHAO (one of the **CHI SHAO YAO**) Origin: *Paeonia veitchii* Lynch (*Ranunculaceae*). See Common Peony (wild).

Vermiculate Thamnolia Thallus; XUE CHA Origin: *Thamnolia vermicularis* (Ach.) Asahina (*Thamnoliaceae*). Part: lichen body. Effects: To clear heat and allay thirst, arouse the brain and quiet spirit. Indications: Vacuity taxation with steaming bone, pneumonia with cough, epilepsy with manic agitation, neurasthenia, hypertension.

Verticillate Acanthopanax Leaf; LUN SAN WU JIA YE (one of the **WU JIA YE**) Origin: *Acanthopanax verticillatus* Hoo (*Araliaceae*). See Slenderstyle Acanthopanax Leaf.

Verticillate Acanthopanax Root-bark; WU JIA PI Origin: *Acanthopanax verticillatus* Hoo (*Araliaceae*). See Slenderstyle Acanthopanax Root-bark.

Verticillate Cladonia; XIAO LA BA Origin: *Cladonia verticillata* Hoffm. (*Cladoniaceae*). Part: herb. Effects: To stanch bleeding and clear heat. Indications: coughing of blood, knife wound, burns and scalds.

Vesper Iris; BAI HUA SHE GAN Origin: *Iris dichotoma* Pall. (*Iridaceae*). Part: root or herb. Effects: To clear heat and resolve toxin, quicken the blood and disperse swelling. Indications: Sore swollen throat, hepatitis, stomachache, hepatitis, painful swollen gums.

Vetchleaf Sophora Leaf; BAI CI HUA YE Origin: *Sophora viciifolia* Hance (*Leguminosae*). Part: leaf. Effects: To clear heat and resolve toxin. Indications: Toxin swelling.

Vinegar; CU Effects: To dissipate stasis and stanch bleeding, resolve toxin and kill worms. Indications: Postpartum blood dizziness, concretion and conglomeration, jaundice, yellow sweating, blood ejection, spontaneous external bleeding, bloody stool, itching in the genital region, swelling of abscess and sore.

Virgate Wormwood; YIN CHEN HAO Origin: *Artemisia scoparia* Wldst. *et* Kitaibel (*Compositae*). See Capillary Wormwood.

Virginia Pepperweed Seed; TING LI ZI Origin: *Lepidium virginicum* L. (*Cruciferae*). See Pepperweed Seed .

Walking Maidenhair; BIAN YE TIE XIAN JUE Origin: *Adiantum caudatum* L. (*Adiantaceae*). Part: herb. Effects: To clear heat and resolve toxin, disinhibit water and disperse swelling. Indications: Edema, yellow-water sore, mammary welling abscess.

Water Nightshade; SHUI QIE Origin: *Solanum torvum* Sw. (*Solanaceae*). Part: root. Effects: To quicken blood, dissipate stasis and relieve pain. Indications: Pain with stasis from knocks and falls, taxation detriment in lumbar muscle, coughing of blood, sand, stomachache, clove sore, swollen welling abscess.

Watermelon Seed; XI GUA ZI REN Origin: *Citrullus vulgaris* Schrad. (*Cucurbitaceae*). Part: seed. Effects: To clear the lung and moisten the intestine, harmonize the center and allay thirst. Indications: Blood ejection, enduring cough.

Watermelon; XI GUA Origin: *Citrullus vulgaris* Schrad. (*Cucurbitaceae*). Part: fruit. Effects: To clear heat and resolve summerheat, eliminate vexation and allay thirst, disinhibit urine. Indications: Summerheat-heat, vexation and thirst, damage to liquid by the exuberant heat, inhibited urination, throat impediment, mouth sore.

Wayaka Yambean Seed; DI GUA ZI Origin: *Pachyrhizus erosus* (L.) Urban (*Leguminosae*). Part: seed. Indications: Scab and lichen, swollen welling abscess.

Weeping Forsythia; LIAN QIAO Origin: *Forsythia suspensa* (Thunb.) Vahl (*Oleaceae*). Part: dried fruit. Effects: To dispel wind-heat, remove heat and toxic substances, treat carbuncles and resolve bind. Indications: Externally contracted wind-heat or epidemic febrile diseases of early stage manifested as fever, headache, thirst; suppurative infections on the body surface, or scrofula and tuberculous adenitis.

White Chinaure Herb; YAN JIAO CAO Origin: *Boenninghausenia albiflora* (Hook.) Meissn. (*Rutaceae*). Part: herb. Effects: To clear heat and cool the blood, soothe sinew and quicken the blood, expel inflammation. Indications: Common cold, laryngo-pharyngitis, hepatitis, hacking of blood, spontaneous external bleeding, pain in the lumbus, knocks and falls, subcutaneous static blood.

White Clover Herb; SAN XIAO CAO Origin: Trifolium repens L. (*Leguminosae*). Part: herb. Effects: To clear heat and cool the blood. Indications: Madness (disorder of head).

White Dendrobium; TIE PI SHI HU (one of the **SHI HU**) Origin: *Dendrobium candidum* Wall. *ex* Lindl. (*Orchidaceae*). See Noble Dendrobium.

White Mulberry Bast; SANG BAI PI Origin: *Morus alba* L. (*Moraceae*). Part: root bast. Effects: To drain the lung and calm panting, disinhibit urine and disperse swelling. Indications: Cough and panting with profuse phlegm due to lung-heat; puffy swelling, edema due to inhibited urination; hypertension.

White Mulberry Branch; SANG ZHI Origin: *Morus alba* L. (*Moraceae*). Part: young twig. Effects: To dispel wind and free the network vessels. Indications: Wind-damp impediment (arthralgia-syndrome), hypertonicity in whole body or joints, edema.

White Mulberry; SANG YE Origin: *Morus alba* L. (*Moraceae*). Part: leaf. Effects: To dispel wind, remove heat from the liver and brighten the eyes. Indications: Externally contracted wind-heat or epidemic febrile diseases, fever, dizziness, headache, cough, swollen and sore throat; cough with thick sputum, dryness in the nose and throat; conjunctival congestion with dryness, pain and delacrimation.

White Mustard Seed; BAI JIE ZI Origin: *Sinapis alba* L. [= *Brassica alba* (L.) Boiss.] (*Cruciferae*). Part: seed. Effects: To warm the lung and dispel cold-phlegm, remove obstruction and relieve pain. Indications: Accumulation of cold-phlegm in the lung shown as cough, panting, watery and thin sputum; deep-rooted carbuncle of *yin* nature.

White Sweetclover Root; CHOU MU XU GEN Origin: *Melilotus suaveolens* Ledeb. (*Legumi-nosae*). Part: root. Effects: To clear heat and resolve toxin. Indications: Tuberculosis of the lymphnode (scrofula).

Whiteflower Embelia; XIAN SUAN QIANG Origin: *Embelia ribes* Burm. f. (*Myrsinaceae*). Part: root. Effects: To relieve swelling, expel toxin, and relieve pain. Indications: Menstrual block, child head sore, knocks and falls.

Whiteflower Hogfennel; BAI HUA QIAN HU (one of the **QIAN HU**) Origin: *Peucedanum prae-ruptorum* Dunn (*Umbelliferae*). Part: root. Effects: To downbear *qi* and transform phlegm, diffuse wind-heat. Indications: Non-diffusion of lung *qi*, panting and cough with thick phlegm; external contraction of wind-heat.

Whiteflower Leadword; BAI HUA DAN Origin: *Plumbago zeylanica* L. (*Plumbaginaceae*). Part: herb and root. Effects: To dispel wind and dissipate stasis, resolve toxin and kill worms. Indications: Wind-damp with painful joints, blood stasis and menstrual block, knocks and falls, toxin swelling and malign sore, scab and lichen.

Whiteflower Mucuna; JI XUE TENG Origin: *Mucuna birdwoodiana* Tutcher (*Leguminosae*). See Suberect Spatholobus.

Whiteflower Patrinia; BAI HUA BAI JIANG (one of the **BAI JIANG**) Origin: *Patrinia villosa* Juss. (*Valerianaceae*). Part: herb. Effects: To clear heat and resolve toxin, expel pus and break stasis. Indications: Intestinal welling abscess, dysentery, red and white vaginal discharge, postpartum stasis and abdominal pain, red eyes with painful swelling, swollen welling abscess, scab and lichen.

Whiteflower Trillium; YU ER QI Origin: *Trillum camtschaticum* Pall. (*Liliaceae*). See Tscho-nosk Trillium.

Whorlleaf Litse; DIE DA LAO Origin: *Litsea verticillata* Hance (*Lauraceae*). Part: stem, leaf or root. Effects: To dissipate stasis blood and disperse swelling. Indications: Knocks and falls, toxin swelling.

Wild Boar Gall; YE ZHU DAN Origin: *Sus scrofa* L. (*Suidae*). Part: gall. Effects: To clear heat and resolve toxin. Indications: Clove sore, toxin swelling, scalds.

Wild Carrot; HE SHI FENG Origin: *Daucus carota* L. (*Umbelliferae*). Part: herb. Effects: To kill worms, disperse swelling, disperse *qi*, and transform phlegm.

Wild Honeysuckle; JIN YIN HUA Origin: *Lonicera confusa* DC. (*Captifoliaceae*). See Japanese Honeysuckle.

Wild Mint; BO HE Origin: *Mentha haplocalyx* Briq. (*Labiatae*). Part: dried aerial parts. Effects: To dispel wind and heat and promote eruption. Indications: Externally contracted wind-heat or epidemic febrile diseases shown as fever, slight aversion to cold, headache, anhidrosis; common cold, headache, conjunctival congestion, swollen and sore throat; measles at the early stage, incomplete eruption of measles, German measles, pruritus; stagnation of the liver-*qi*.

Wild Spikenard; SHE BAI ZI Origin: *Hyptis suaveolens* Poit (*Labiatae*). Part: stem and leaf. Effects: To soothe wind and dissipate stasis, resolve toxin and settle pain. Indications: Common cold, rheumatism, eczema, knocks and falls.

Wild Thermopsis; YE JUE MING Origin: *Thermopsis lupinoides* (L.) Link. (*Leguminosae*). Part: herb and seed. Effects: To resolve toxin, disperse swelling, dispel phlegm, and promote vomiting. Indications: Malign sore, scab and lichen.

Wildcelery; HAN QIN Origin: *Apium graveolens* L. var. *dulce* DC. (*Umbelliferae*). Part: herb. Effects: To quite the liver and clear heat, dispel wind and disinhibit dampness. Indications: Hyperten-sion, headache and dizzy, red face and eyes, blood strangury, swollen welling abscess.

Wilford Cranesbill Herb; LAO GUAN CAO Origin: *Geranium wilfordii* Maxim. (*Geraniaceae*). See Common Heron's Bill Herb.

Willmott Ceratostigma; ZI JIN LIAN Origin: *Ceratostigma willmottianum* Stapf (*Plumba-ginaceae*). Part: root. Effects: To quicken the blood and relieve pain, transform stasis and engender flesh. Indications: Knocks and falls, fracture.

Willowleaf Achyranthes; TU NIU XI Origin: *Achyranthes longgifolia* Mak. (*Amaranthaceae*). See Twotooth Achyranthes.

Wilson Buckeye Seed; SUO LUO ZI Origin: *Aesculus wilsonee* Rehd. (*Hippocastanaceae*). See Chinese Buckeye Seed.

Wilson Citron Fruit; ZHI SHI Origin: *Citrus wilsonii* Tanaka (*Rutaceae*). See Bitter Orange.

Wilson Citron; XIANG YUAN Origin: *Citrus wilsonii* Tanaka (*Rutaceae*). See Medicinal Citron.

Wine; JIU Effects: To quicken the blood and free vessels, dissipate cold, free the medicinal strength. Indications: Pain from wind cold impediment, hypertonicity of sinews and vessels, chest impediment, cold pain in heart region and abdomen.

Winged Euonymus; GUI JIAN YU Origin: *Euonymus alatus* (Thunb.) Sieb. (*Celastraceae*). Part: winged branchlet. Effects: To break the blood, treat menstrual disturbances and dispel wind, and kill worms. Indications: Menstrual block, concretions and conglomerations, postpartum stasis and stagnation with abdominal pain, abdomen pain from insect accumulation.

Winged Yam; SHAN YAO Origin: *Diosco-rea alata* L. (*Dioscoreaceae*). Same as *1516*. See Common Yam.

Winged Yam; MAO SHU Origin: *Dioscorea alata L.* (*Dioscoreaceae*). Part: rhizome. Effects: To impediment spleen and kidney, rough essence and *qi*, disperse swelling and relieve pain. Indications: Burns and scalds, putrefying sore on the face, crab-eye.

Winter Daphne Flower; RUI XIANG HUA Origin: *Daphne odora* Thunb. (*Thymelaeaceae*). Part: flower. Indications: Sore swollen throat, toothache, rheumatalgia.

Winter Daphne Root; RUI XIANG GEN Origin: *Daphne odora* Thunb. (*Thymelaeaceae*). Part: root. Indications: Acute throat wind.

Winterberry Euonymus; SI MIAN MU Origin: *Euonymus bungeanus* Maxim. (*Celastraceae*). Part: root, bark, fruit, or branchlet and leaf. Effects: To dispel wind-damp, quicken the blood, and stanch bleeding. Indications: Rheumatic arthritis, lumbar pain, thromboangiitis obliterans (Buerger's disease), spontaneous external bleeding, lacquer sore, hemorrhoids.

Wintergreen Barberry; TU HUANG LIAN Origin: *Berberis Julianae* Schneid. (*Berberidaceae*). Part: root or herb. Effects: To clear heat and resolve toxin, to disinhibit urine. Indications: Diarrhea, red dysentery, fire eye pain, painful swollen gums sore, pharyngolaryngitis, heat strangury, mumps, cinnabar toxin, eczema.

Wintersweet Immayure Flower; LA MEI HUA Origin: *Chimonanthus praecox* (L.) Link (*Calycanthaceae*). Part: flower bud. Effects: To resolve summerheat and engender liquid. Indications: Febrile disease with vexation and thirst, oppression in the chest, cough, burns and scalds.

Woodland Beakchervil; E SHEN Origin: Anthriscus sylvestris (L.) Hoffm. (*Umbelliferae*). Part: root. Effects: To supplement the spleen and boost *qi,* disperse edema. Indications: Spleen vacuity and food distention, stomachache, lack of strength in the limbs, lung vacuity and cough panting, senile nocturia, blood ejection from knocks and falls.

Woods Lacquertree Leaf; YE QI SHU YE Origin: *Rhus sylvestris* Sieb. *et* Zucc. (*Anacardiaceae*). Part: leaf. Effects: To break blood and free the channels, disperse accumulation and kill worms. Indications: Roundworm, bleeding from wounds, callus.

Woolly Lespedeza; XIAO XUE REN SHEN Origin: *Lespedeza tomentosa* (Thunb.) Sieb. (*Legumi-nosae*). Part: root. Effects: To quicken the blood and dissipate stasis, to eliminate inflammation and resolve toxin, to engender flesh and promote bone growth, and to dispel wind and eliminate damp. Indications: Knocks and falls, bone fracture, swelling and pain of sores and boils, rheumatic arthritis.

Woolly Philydrum; TIAN CONG Origin: *Philydrum lanuginosum* Banks (*Phylydraceae*). Part: herb. Indications: Foot rot, lichen.

Wormseed Mustard; GUI ZHU TANG JIE Origin: *Erysimum cheranthoides* L. (*Cruciferae*). Part: herb. Effects: To strengthen the heart and disinhibit urine, fortify the spleen and harmonize the stomach. Indications: Heart palpitation, puffy swelling, indigestion.

Wormwood-like Motherwort Herb; YI MU CAO Origin: *Leonurus heterophyllus* Sweet (*Labia-tae*). Part: aerial parts. Effects: To quicken the blood and dispel blood stasis, disinhibit urine, normalize menstruation, clear away heat and toxins. Indications: Irregular menstruation, distending pain in the lower abdomen, menstrual block, afterpains, lochiorrhea; traumatic injuries; difficult urination, edema; sores and carbuncles, pruritus and skin urticaria; acute or chronic nephritic edema; angina pectoris of coronary heart disease.

Wrinkled Gianthyssop; HUO XIANG Origin: *Agastache rugosa* (Fisch. *et* Mey.) O. Ktze. (*Labiatae*). See Cablin Potchouli.

Yadirik Scurrula; MAO YE SANG JI SHENG (one of the **SANG JI SHENG**) Origin: *Loranthus yadoriki* Sieb. (*Loranthaceae*). See Colored Mistletoe.

Yangtao Actinidia; MI HOU TAO Origin: *Actinidia chinensis* Planch. (*Actinidiaceae*). Part: fruit. Effects: To resolve heat, allay thirst, free strangury. Indications: Heat vexation, diabetes, jaundice, stone strangury, hemorrhoid.

Yanhusuo; YAN HU SUO Origin: *Corydalis yanhusuo* W. T. Wang [=*Corydalis turtschaninovii* Bess. f. *yanhusuo* Y. H. Chou *et* C. C. Hsu] (*Papaveraceae*). Part: rhizome. Effects: To quicken the blood, promote circulation of *qi,* and relieve pain. Indications: Pains in the chest, hypochondrium, stomach, abdomen, extremities; menstrual pain, traumatic injuries.

Yellow Bedstraw; PENG ZI CAI Origin: *Galium verum* L. (*Rubiaceae*). Part: herb. Effects: To clear heat and resolve toxin, move the blood and relieve itching. Indications: Heaptitis, painful swelling throat moth, swelling of clove sore and boil, paddy field dermatitis, urticaria, knocks and falls, blood *qi* pain.

Yellow Daylily; XUAN CAO GEN Origin: *Hemerocallis flava* L. (*Liliaceae*). See Orange Daylily.

Yellow Licorice; HUANG GAN CAO (one of the **GAN CAO**) Origin: *Glycyrrhiza kansuensis* Chang *et* Peng (*Leguminosae*). See Ural Licorice.

Yellow Oleander; HUANG HUA JIA ZHU TAO Origin: *Thevetia peruviana* (Pers.) K. Schum. (*Apocynaceae*). Part: seed. Effects: To strengthen the heart. Indications: Cardiac failure, paroxysmal supra-ventricular tachycardia, paroxysmal auricular fibrillation.

Yellow Toadflax; LIU CHUAN YU Origin: *Linaria vulgaris* Mill. (*Scrophulariaceae*). Part: herb. Effects: To clear heat and resolve toxin, dissipate stasis and disperse swelling. Indications: Headache, head dizziness, jaundice, hemorrhoid, constipation, skin disease, burns and scalds.

Yellowflower Broomrape; LIE DANG Origin: *Orobanche pycnostachya* Hance (*Orobancha-ceae*). See Skyblue Broomrape.

Yellowflower Corydalis; JU HUA HUANG LIAN Origin: *Corydalis pallida* (Thunb.) Pers. (*Papaveraceae*). Part: root. Effects: To clear heat, draw out toxin, and disperse swelling. Indications: Welling abscess, heat boil, innominate toxin swelling, wind-fire eye pain.

Yellowfruit Nightshade; HUANG GUO QIE Origin: *Solanum xanthocarpum* Schrad. *et* Wendl. (*Solanaceae*). Part: root, fruit and seed. Effects: To clear heat and disinhibit damp, disperse stasis and relieve pain.

Yellowmouth Dutchmanspipe; HAN FANG JI (one of the **ANG JI**) Origin: *Aristolochia hetero-phylla* Hemsl. (*Aristolochiaceae*). See Fourstamen Stephania.

Yerbadetajo; MO HAN LIAN Origin: *Eclipta prostrata* L. [=*Eclipta alba* (L.) Hassk](*Compositae*). Part: aerial parts. Effects: To cool blood and stanch bleeding, supplement the kidney and boost *yin*. Indications: Blood ejection, coughing of blood, nosebleed, bloody urine, bloody stool, blood dysentery, and bleeding knife wound; premature graying, diphtheria, strangury-turbidity, vaginal discharge, pudendal itch.

Yulan Magnolia; YU LAN (one of the **XIN YI**) Origin: *Magnolia denudata* Desr. (*Magnoliaceae*). See Lily Magnolia.

Yunnan Alstonia; DIAN JI GU CHANG SHAN Origin: *Alstomia yunnanensis* Diels (*Apocy-naceae*). Part: branchlet and leaf. Effects: To expel inflammation, stanch bleeding, join bones, and relieve pain. Indications: Malaria, hepatitis.

Yunnan Goldthread; HUANG LIAN Origin: *Coptis teetoides* C. Y. Cheng [= *Coptis teeta* Wall.] (*Ranunculaceae*). See Chinese Goldthread.

Yunnan Larkspur; XIAO CAO WU Origin: *Delphinium yunnanense* Franch. (*Ranunculaceae*). Part: tuber root. Effects: To dispel wind and eliminate damp, dissipate cold and relieve pain, free the network vessels and dissipate stasis. Indications: Wind-damp (rheumatism) with painful joints, stomach cold pain, knocks and falls.

Yunnan Wintergreen; TOU GU XIANG Origin: *Gaulthcria yunnanensis* (Franch.) Rehd. (*Ericaceae*). Part: stem and leaf. Effects: To dispel wind and eliminate dampness, quicken the blood and free the network vessels. Indications: Wind-damp (rheumatism) with painful joints, water drum distention, knocks and falls, toothache, eczema.

Zedoary turmeric; PENG E SHU (one of the **YU JIN**) Origin: *Curcuma zedoaria* (Berg.) Rosc. (*Zingiberaceae*). See Common turmaric.

Zedoary Turmeric; PENG E SHU Origin: *Curcuma zedoaria* (Berg.) Rosc. (*Zingiberaceae*). Part: rhizome. Effects: To break blood and dispel stasis, move *qi* and relieve pain. Indications: Menstrual block with abdominal pain, concretions, conglomerations, accumulations and gatherings due to *qi* stagnation and blood stasis; accumulated food, fullness and pain in the stomach duct and abdomen.

Part III

INDEXES

Index of
Traditional Chinese Medicines
by Chinese Name

Index of Traditional Chinese Medicines by Chinese Name

TCM Name	Name in English	Origin Latin Name	Family
A ER TAI ZI WAN	Altai Heteropappus	Heteropappus altaicus (Willd.) Novopokr.	Compositae
A LI A LI HONG	Fomes Officinalis Sporophore	Fomes officinalis (Vill. et Fr.) Ames	Polyporaceae
A WEI	Asafetida Giantfennel Resin	Ferula asafoetida L.	Umbelliferae
	Broadleaf Giantfennel Resin	Ferula conocaula Eug.	Umbelliferae
	Sinkiang Giantfennel Resin	Ferula caspica Marsh.-Bieb.	Umbelliferae
AI NA XIANG	Balsamiferous Blumea	Blumea balsamifera DC.	Compositae
AI YE	Argy Wormwood Leaf	Artemisia argyl Lévl. et Vant	Compositae
AI ZI YU PAN	Low Uvaria	Uvaria Chamae P. Beauv.	Annonaceae
AN HUI BEI MU	Anhwei Fritillary	Fritillaria anhuiensis S. Chen et S. Yin	Liliaceae
AN HUI SONG MU	Subcapitate Aralia	Aralia subcapitata Hoo	Araliaceae
AN MO LE	Emblic Leafflower	Phyllanthus emblica L.	Euphorbiaceae
AN XI XIANG	Benzoin	Styrax benzoin Dryand.	Styracaceae
	Tonkin Snowbell	Styrax tonkinensis (Pier.) Craib ex Hart.	Styracaceae
AN YE	Eucalyptus Leaf	Eucalyptus gloulus Labill.	Myrtaceae
AN ZI BEI MU (of CHUAN BEI MU)	Unibract Fritillary	Fritillaria unibracteata Hsiao et K. C. Hsiao	Liliaceae
BA DAN XING REN	Amygdalate Apricot Seed	Prunum amygdalus Batsch	Rosaceae
BA DOU	Purging Croton	Croton tiglium L.	Euphorbiaceae
BA JI TIAN	Medicinal Indianmulberry	Morinda officinalis How	Rubiaceae
BA JIAO HUI XIANG	Star Anise	Illicium verum Hook. f.	Magnoliaceae
BA JIAO LIAN	Sixangular Dysosma	Dysosma pleiantha (Hance) Woods.	Berberidaceae
BA QIA	Chinaroot Greenbrier	Smilax china L.	Liliaceae
BA WANG BIAN	Royle Euphorbia Latex	Euphorbia royleana Boiss.	Euphorbiaceae
BA XIAN CAO	Catchweed Bedstraw	Galium aparine L.	Rubiaceae
	Roughleaf Bedstraw	Galium asperifolium Wall.	Rubiaceae
BA XIAN HUA	Largeleaf Hydrangea	Hydrangea macrophylla (Thunb.) Ser.	Saxifragaceae
BAI BU	Japanese Stemona	Stemona japonica (Bl.) Miq.	Stemonaceae
	Sessile Stemona	Stemona sessilifolia (Miq.) Franch. et Sav.	Stemonaceae
	Tuber Stemona	Stemona tuberosa Lour.	Stemonaceae
BAI CHANG	Drug Sweetflag	Acorus calamus L.	Araceae
BAI CI HUA	Vetchleaf Sophora	Sophora viciifolia Hance	Leguminosae
BAI CI HUA YE	Vetchleaf Sophora Leaf	Sophora viciifolia Hance	Leguminosae
BAI CI HUA ZI	Vetchleaf Sophora Seed	Sophora viciifolia Hance	Leguminosae
BAI DOU KOU	Round Cardamom	Amomun kravanh Pierre ex Gagnep. [= Amomum cardamomum L.]	Zingiberaceae
BAI E GAO	Goose Fat	Anser domestica Geese	Anatidae
BAI FAN DOU	Kidney Bean Seed	Phaseolus vulgaris L.	Leguminosae
BAI GUO	Ginkgo Nut	Ginkgo biloba L.	Ginkgoaceae
BAI GUO GEN	Ginkgo Root	Ginkgo biloba L.	Ginkgoaceae
BAI GUO SHU PI	Ginkgo Bark	Ginkgo biloba L.	Ginkgoaceae
BAI GUO YE	Ginkgo Leaf	Ginkgo biloba L.	Ginkgoaceae
BAI HAO	Sievers Wormwood	Artemisia sieversiana Ehrh. ex Willd.	Compositae
BAI HE	Greenish Lily	Lilium brownii F.E. Brown var. colchesteri Wils.	Liliaceae
	Lanceleaf Lily	Lilium longiflorum Thunb.	Liliaceae

Index of Traditional Chinese Medicines by Chinese Name

TCM Name	Name in English	Origin Latin Name	Family
	Lily	Lilium brownii F.E. Brown var. viridulum Baker	Liliaceae
	Low Lily	Lilium pumilum DC.	Liliaceae
BAI HOU WU TOU	Whitethroat Monkshood	Aconitum leucostomum Worosch.	Ranunculaceae
BAI HUA	see BAI HUA PI		
BAI HUA BAI JIANG (of BAI JIANG)	Whiteflower Patrinia	Patrinia villosa Juss.	Valerianaceae
BAI HUA CAI ZI	Common Spiderflower Seed	Cleome gynandra L.	Capparidaceae
BAI HUA DAN	Whiteflower Leadword	Plumbago zeylanica L.	Plumbaginaceae
BAI HUA DAN SHEN	Whiteflower Danshen	Salvia miltiorrhiza f. alba C. Y. Wu	Labiatae
BAI HUA HAO	see YA JIAO AI		
BAI HUA LONG DAN	Alpine Gentian	Gentiana algida Pall.	Gentianaceae
BAI HUA PI (of HUA MU PI)	Asia White Birch Bark	Betula platyphylla Suk.	Betulaceae
BAI HUA QIAN HU (of QIAN HU)	Whiteflower Hogfennel	Peucedanum praeruptorum Dunn	Umbelliferae
BAI HUA SHE GAN	Vesper Iris	Iris dichotoma Pall.	Iridaceae
BAI HUA SHE SHE CAO	Spreading Hedyitis	Oldenlandia diffusa (Willd.) Roxb. [= Hedyotis diffusa Willd.]	Rubiaceae
BAI HUA TENG	Threeflower Clematis	Clematis terniflora DC. [= Clematis maximowicziana Franch. et Sav.]	Ranunculaceae
BAI HUA YING SHAN HONG	Snow Azalea	Rhododendron mucronatum G. Don	Ericaceae
BAI JIAN MU	Campus-belu Aspidosperma	Aspidosperma campus-belus A. P. Duarte.	
BAI JIANG	See BAI HUA BAI JIANG,	Patrinia villosa Juss.;	Valerianaceae
	HUANG HUA BAI JIANG:	Patrinia scabiosaefolia Fisch.	Valerianaceae
BAI JIANG CAN	Silkworm Larva	Bombyx mori L.	Ombycidae
BAI JIE ZI	White Mustard Seed	Sinapis alba L. [= Brassica alba (L.) Boiss.]	Cruciferae
BAI LAI SHI JU	Bailai's Chrysanthemum	Baileya multiratiata Harv. et Gray.	
BAI LAN HUA	Bailan Flower	Michelia alba DC.	Magnoliaceae
BAI LIAN	Japanese Ampelopsis	Ampelopsis japonica (Thunb.) Mak.	Vitaceae
BAI LIANG JIN	Crispateleaf Ardisia	Ardisia crispa (Thunb.) A. DC.	Myrsinaceae
BAI LIANG JIN YE	Crispateleaf Ardisia Leaf	Ardisia crispa (Thunb.) A. DC.	Myrsinaceae
BAI MAO GEN	Lalang Grass Rhizome	Imperata cylindrica (L.) P. Beauv. var. major (Nees) C. E. Hubb.	Gramineae
BAI MAO TENG	Bitter Nightshade	Solanum dulcamara L.	Solanaceae
	Bittersweet	Solanum lyratum Thunb.	Solanaceae
BAI MAO XIA KU CAO	Decumbent Bugle Herb	Ajuga decumbens Thunb.	Labiatae
BAI MEI HUA	Plum Flower	Prunus mume (Sieb.) Sieb. et Zucc.	Rosaceae
BAI MU TONG (of MU TONG)	Austral Akebia	Akebia trifoliata (Thunb.) Koidz. var. australis (Diels) Rehd.	Lardizabalaceae
BAI MU XIANG (of CHEN XIANG)	Chinese Eaglewood	Aquilaria sinensis (Lour.) Gilg	Thymelaeaceae
BAI NIU XI	Berry-bearing Campion	Cucubalus baccifer L.	Caryophyllaceae
BAI QU CAI	Greater Celandine	Chelidonium majus L.	Paraveraceae
BAI SHAO YAO	Common peony	Paeonia lactiflora Pall.	Ranunculaceae
BAI SHOU WU	Bunge Swllowwort	Cynanchum bungei Decne.	Asclepiadaceae
BAI SHU LANG	Hispid Yam	Dioscorea hispida Dennst.	Dioscoreaceae

Index of Traditional Chinese Medicines by Chinese Name

TCM Name	Name in English	Origin Latin Name	Family
BAI SHU YE	Chinese Weeping Cypress Leaf	Cupressus funebris Endl.	Cupressaceae
BAI SU ZI	Common Perilla Fruit	Perilla frutescens (L.) Britt.	Labiatae
BAI TOU WENG	Chinese pulsatilla	Pulsatilla chinensis (Bge.) Reg.	Ranunculaceae
BAI XIAN PI	Densefruit Pittany Root-bark	Dictamnus dasycarpus Turcz.	Rutaceae
BAI YA MA	White Flax	Linum album Kotschy ex Boiss	Linaceae
BAI YAO ZI	Oriental Stephania	Stephania cepharantha Hayata	Menispermaceae
BAI ZHI	Dahurian Angelica	Angelica dahurica (Fisch. ex Hoffm.) Benth. et Hook. f. ex Franch. et Sav.	Umbelliferae
	Eumenol Angelica	Angelica anomala Lallem.	Umbelliferae
	Scabrous Cowparsnip	Heracleum scabridum Franch.	Umbelliferae
	Taiwan Angelika	Angelica taiwaniana Boiss.	Umbelliferae
BAI ZHI JIE (CE BAI ZHI JIE)	Chinese Arborvitae Branch	Thuja orientalis (L.) Endl. [= Platycladus orientalis (L.) Franco]	Cupressaceae
BAI ZHI MA (HU MA ZI)	Oriental Sesame	Sesamum indicum DC.	Pedaliaceae
BAI ZHU	Largehead Atractylodes	Atractylodes macrocephala Koidz. [= Atractylis macrocephala (Koidz.) Hand.-Mazz.]	Compositae
BAN BIAN LIAN	Chinese Lobelia	Lobelia chinensis Lour. [= Lobelia radicans Thunb.]	Campanulaceae
BAN BIAN SU	Common Elsholtzia	Elsholtzia ciliata (Yhunb.) Hyland	Labiatae
BAN JIU	Rufous Turtle Dove	Streptopelia orientalis (Latham)	Columbidae
BAN LAN GEN	Common Baphicacanthus Root	Baphicacanthus cusia (Nees) Brem.	Cruciferae
	Dyers Woad Root	Isatis tinctoria L.	Cruciferae
	Indigowoad Root	Isatis indigotica Fort.	Cruciferae
BAN MAO	Blister Beetle	Mylabris phalerata Pall. ; Mylabris cichorii Linnaeus	Meloidae Meloidae
BAN WEN LU HUI (of LU HUI)	Chinese Aloe Dried Juice	Aloe vera L. var. chinensis (Haw.) Berger	Liliaceae
BAN XIA	Ternate Pinellia	Pinellia ternata (Thunb.) Breit.	Araceae
BAN ZHI LIAN	Largeflower Purslane	Portulaca grandiflora Hook.	Labiatae
BANG BANG MU	Bunge Hackberry	Celtis bungeana Bl.	Ulmaceae
BAO E ZHANG YA CAI	Calycin Swertia	Swertia calycina Franch.	Gentianaceae
BAO GAI CAO	Henbit Deadnettle Herb	Lamium amplexicaule L.	Labiatae
BAO GAI LING ZHI	Cape Ganoderma	Ganoderma capense (Lloyd) Teng	Polyproraceae
BAO MA ZI	Amur Lilac	Syringa amurensis Rupr.	Oleaceae
BAO PI JUN	Amanita	Amanita panthorina	Amanitaceae
BAO XING WEI MAO	Paohsing Euonymus	Euonymus mupinensis Loes. et Rehd.	Celastraceae
BEI CHAI HU (of CHAI HU)	Chinese Thorowax	Bupleurum chinense DC.	Umbelliferae
BEI MA DOU LING (of MA DOU LING)	Northern Dutchmanspipe	Aristolochia contorta Bge.	Aristolochiaceae
BEI WU TOU (of CAO WU TOU)	Kusnezoff Monkshood	Aconitum kusnezoffii Rchb.	Ranunculaceae
BEI XIE	See FEN BEI SHU YU,	Dioscorea hypoglauca Palib.;	Dioscoriaceae
	CHA RUI SHU YU,	Dioscorea collettii Hook. f.;	Dioscoriaceae
	SHAN BEI XIE,	Dioscorea tokoro Mak.;	Dioscoriaceae
	XIAN XI SHU YU,	Dioscorea gracillima Miq.;	Dioscoriaceae
	FU ZHOU SHU YU:	Dioscorea futschauensis R. Kunth	Dioscoriaceae

Index of Traditional Chinese Medicines by Chinese Name

TCM Name	Name in English	Origin Latin Name	Family
BEI YE JU (of YE JU)	Boreal Wild Chrysanthemum	Chrysanthemum boreale Mak.	Compositae
BI BA	Long Pepper	Piper longum L.	Piperaceae
BI BA GEN	Long Pepper Root	Piper longum L.	Piperaceae
BI CHENG QIE	Cubeba Piper	Piper cubeba L.	Lauraceae
	Mountain Spicy Tree	Litsea cubeba (Lour.) Pers.	Lauraceae
BI LI	Climbing Fig	Ficus pumila L.	Moraceae
BI LU XIANG JIAO	Peru Balmtree Resin	Myroxylon pereirae (Royle) Klotzsch	Leguminosae
BI MA GEN	Castorbean Root	Ricinus communis L.	Euphorbiaceae
BI MA YE	Castorbean Leaf	Ricinus communis L.	Euphorbiaceae
BI MA YOU	Castorbean Oil	Ricinus communis L.	Euphorbiaceae
BI MA ZI	Castorbean Seed	Ricinus communis L.	Euphorbiaceae
BIAN DOU	Hyacinth Dolichos Seed	Dolichos lablab L.	Leguminosae
BIAN FU GE	Asiatic Moonseed	Menispermum dauricum DC.	Menispermaceae
BIAN FU GE GEN	Asiatic Moonseed Root	Menispermum dauricum DC.	Menispermaceae
BIAN GUO JIAO GU LAN	Flatfruit Gynostemma	Gynostemma compressum X. X. Chen et D. R. Liang	Cucurbitaceae
BIAN JING HUANG QI	Flatstem Milkvetch	Astragalus complanatus R. Br.	Leguminosae
BIAN SE MA DOU LING	Versicolorous Dutchmanspipe	Aristolochia versicolar S. M. Hwang	Aristolochiaceae
BIAN TAO	Peachform Mango	Mangifera persiciformis C.Y. Wu et T. L. Ming	Anacardiaceae
BIAN XU	Common Knotgrass	Polygonum aviculare L.	Polygonaceae
BIAN YE TIE XIAN JUE	Walking Maidenhair	Adiantum caudatum L.	Adiantaceae
BING GUO HUA JIAO	Stalkedfruit Pricklyash	Zanthoxylum podocarpum Hemsl.	Rutaceae
BING LANG	Betenutpalm	Areca catechu L.	Palmae
BING PIAN	Borneol	Dryobalanops aromatica Gaertn. f.	Dipterocarpaceae
BO CAI	Spinish	Spinacia oleracea L.	Chenopodiaceae
BO HE	Wild Mint	Mentha haplocalyx Briq.	Labiatae
BO LUO HUI	Pink Plumepoppy	Macleaya cordata (Willd.) R. Br.	Papaveraceae
BO LUO MI	Diversileaf Artocarpus	Artocarpus heterophyllus Lam.	Moraceae
BU GU ZHI	Malaytea Scurfpea	Psoralea corylifolia L.	Papilionaceae
BU XUE CAO	Gmelin Sealavender Herb	Limonium gmelinii (Willd.) O. Ktze.	Plumbaginaceae
CAN DOU	Broadbean	Vicia faba L.	Leguminosae
CAN DOU JIA KE	Broadbean Pericarp	Vicia faba L.	Leguminosae
CAN DOU JING	Broadbean Stem	Vicia faba L.	Leguminosae
CAN DOU KE	Broadbean Spermoderm	Vicia faba L.	Leguminosae
CAN DOU YE	Broadbean Leaf	Vicia faba L.	Leguminosae
CAN JIAN	Silk Cocoon	Bombyx mori L.	Bombycidae
CANG ER	Siberian Cocklebur	Xanthium sibiricus Patr. ex Widd.	Compositae
CANG ZHU	Chinese Atractylodes	Atractylodes chinensis Koidz.	Compositae
	Swordlike Atractylodes	Atractylodes lancea (Thunb.) DC.	Compositae
CAO BEI MU	Indian Iphigenia	Iphigenia indica Kunth et Benth	Liliaceae
CAO CONG RONG	Russian Boschniakia	Boschniakia rossica Fedtsch. et Flerov	Orobanchaceae
CAO DOU KOU	Katsumada Galangal	Alpinia katsumadai Hayata	Zingiberaceae
CAO SHAN HU (JIU JIE CHA)	Glabrous Sarcandra	Sarcandra glabra (Thunb.) Nakai	Chloranthaceae
CAO SHAO YAO (of CHI SHAO YAO)	Obovate Peony	Paeonia obovata Maxim.	Ranunculaceae
CAO WU TOU	See CHUAN WU TOU, BEI WU TOU:	Aconitum carmichaeli Debx.; Aconitum kusnezoffii Rchb.	Ranunculaceae Ranunculaceae

Index of Traditional Chinese Medicines by Chinese Name

TCM Name	Name in English	Origin Latin Name	Family
CAO YE WU JIA PI (of WU JIA PI)	Henry Acanthopanax Root-bark	Acanthopanax henryi (Oliv.) Harms	Araliaceae
CAO YE WU JIA YE (of WU JIA YE)	Henry Acanthopanax Leaf	Acanthopanax henryi (Oliv.) Harms	Araliaceae
CAO YUAN LAO GUAN CAO	Meadow Cranesbill Herb	Geranium pratense L.	Geraniaceae
CE BAI YE	Chinese Arborvitae Leaf	Thuja orientalis (L.) Endl. [= Platycladus orientalis (L.) Franco]	Cupressaceae
CE BAI ZHI JIE (BAI ZHI JIE)	Chinese Arborvitae Branch	Thuja orientalis (L.) Endl. [= Platycladus orientalis (L.) Franco]	Cupressaceae
CHA RUI SHU YU (of BEI XIE)	Collett Yam	Dioscorea collettii Hook. f.	Dioscoriaceae
CHA SHU	Common Sassafras	Sassafras tzumu Hemsl.	Lauraceae
CHA SHU GEN	Tea Root	Camellia sinensis O. Ktze.	Theaceae
CHA XIONG	Chaxiong Ligusticum	Ligusticum sinense Oliv. cv. chaxiong	Umbelliferae
CHA XUONG	Chaxiong Ligusticum	Ligusticum sinense Oliv. cv. chaxiong	Umbelliferae
CHA YE	Tea	Camellia sinensis O. Ktze.	Theaceae
CHA ZI	Tea Seed	Camellia sinensis O. Ktze.	Theaceae
CHA ZI XIN	Oiltea Camellia	Camellia oleifera Abel	Theaceae
CHAI HU	See BEI CHAI HU, HONG CHAI HU, DA YE CHAI HU:	Bupleurum chinense DC.; Bupleurum scorzonerifolium Willd.; Bupleurum longiradiatum Turcz.	Umbelliferae Umbelliferae Umbelliferae
CHAI HUANG JIANG	Rosthorn Yam Rhizome	Dioscorea nipponica Makino subsp rosthornii (Prain et Burk) Ting	Dioscoreaceae
CHAN CHU (GAN CHAN CHU)	Toad	Bufo bufo gargarizans Cantor; Bufo melanostictus Schneider	Bufonidae Bufonidae
CHAN CHU DAN	Toad Gall	Bufo bufo gargarizans Cantor; Bufo melanostictus Schneider	Bufonidae Bufonidae
CHAN PI	Toad Skin	Bufo bufo gargarizans Cantor; Bufo melanostictus Schneider	Bufonidae Bufonidae
CHAN SU	Toad Skin Secretion Cake	Bufo bufo gargarizans Cantor; Bufo melanostictus Schneider	Bufonidae Bufonidae
CHANG BAN JIN LIAN HUA	Langpetal Globeflower	Trollius macropetalus (Franch.) Schmidt	Ranunculaceae
CHANG BAO XIANG PU (of XIANG PU)	Longbract Cattail	Typha angustata Bory et Chaub.	Typhaceae
CHANG CHUN HUA	Madagascar Periwinkle	Catharanthus roseus (L.) G. Don.	Apocynaceae
CHANG CHUN TENG	Chinese Ivy	Hedera ncpalensis K. Koch var. sinensis (Tobl.) Rehd.	Araliaceae
CHANG GENG JIAO GU LAN	longstalk Gynostemma	Gynostemma longipes C. Y. Wu	Cucurbhitaceae
CHANG GENG NAN WU WEI ZI	Longpeduncle Kadsura	Kadsura longepedunculata Finet et Gagnep.	Schisandraceae
CHANG GUAN JIA MO LI	Indian Glorybower	Clerodendron indicum (L.) O. Ktze.	Verbenaceae
CHANG GUAN XIANG CHA CAI	Longtube Rabdosia	Rabdosia longituba (Miquel) Hara.	Labiatae
CHANG SHAN	Antifebrile Dichroa	Dichroa febrifuga Lour.	Saxifragaceae
CHANG YE XIANG CHA CAI	Longleaf Rabdosia	Rabdosia stracheyi (Benth. ex Hook. f.) Hara	Labiatae
CHAO TIAN JIAO	Conical Redpepper	Capsicum annuum L. var. conoides (Mill.) Irish	Solanaceae

Index of Traditional Chinese Medicines by Chinese Name

TCM Name	Name in English	Origin Latin Name	Family
CHAO XIAN YIN YANG HUO	Korean Epimedium	Epimedium koreanum Nakai	Berberidaceae
CHE QIAN	Asiatic Plantain	Plantago asiatica L.	Plantaginaceae
	Depressed Plantain	Plantago depressa Willd.	Plantaginaceae
CHE SANG ZI YE	Clammy Hopseedbush Leaf	Dodonaea viscosa (L.) Jacq.	Sapindaceae
CHEN DONG CAI LU ZHI	Spiced Juice of Mature Winter-vegetable	Brassica chinensis L.	Cruciferae
CHEN PI (PI JU)	Tangerine Pericarp	Citrus reticulata Blanco	Rutaceae
CHEN XIANG	Eaglewood	Aquilaria agallocha Roxb.	Thymelaeaceae
CHEN ZI	Fragrant Citrus	Citrus junos Tanaka	Rutaceae
CHEN ZI HE	Fragrant Citrus Seed	Citrus junos Tanaka	Rutaceae
CHEN ZI PI	Pericarp	Citrus junos Tanaka	Rutaceae
CHENG GAN CAO	Japanese Eupatorium	Eupatorium japonicum Thunb.	Compositae
CHENG GAN SHENG MA	Lindley Eupatorium	Eupatorium lindleyanum DC.	Compositae
CHENG LIU	Chinese Tamarisk	Tamarix chinensis Lour.	Tamaricaceae
CHI NAN	Boxleaf Syzygium	Syzygium buxifolium Hook. et Arn.	Myrtaceae
CHI SHAO YAO	See SHAO YAO,	Paeonia lactiflora Pall.;	Ranunculaceae
	CAO SHAO YAO,	Paeonia obovata Maxim.;	Ranunculaceae
	CHUAN CHI SHAO:	Paeonia veitchii Lynch.	Ranunculaceae
CHI YANG	Japanese Alder	Alnus japonica Sieb. et Zucc.	Betulaceae
CHI YE CAO	Lateripening Bartsia Herb	Odontites serotina Reich.	Scrophulariaceae
CHI ZHI (of LING ZHI CAO)	Lucid Ganoderma	Ganoderma lucidum (Leyss. ex Fr.) Karst.	Polyporaceae
CHI ZI SHU	see ZHAI YE BAN FENG HE		
CHONG BAI LA	Cera Chinensis Wax	Ericerus pela (Chavannes)	Coccidae
CHONG CHUN YU	Skin-carp	Hemibarbus labeo (Pallas)	Cyprinidae
CHONG LOU PAI CAO	Parisshape Loosestrife	Lysimachia paridiformis Franch.	Primalaceme
CHONG YA YAO	Ternateleaf Rabdosia	Isodon ternifolius (D. Don) Kudo	Labiatae
CHOU BAI	Savin	Sabina vulgaris Antoine	Cupressaceae
CHOU CAO	Common Rue Herb	Ruta graveolens L.	Rutaceae
CHOU MO LI	Fragrant Glorybower	Clerodendron fragrans Vent.	Verbenaceae
CHOU MU XU GEN	White Sweetclover Root	Melilotus suaveolens Ledeb.	Leguminosae
CHOU SHAN YANG	Japanese Orixa	Orixa japonica Thunb.	Rutaceae
CHOU WU TONG	Harrlequin Glorybower Leaf	Clerodendron trichotomum Thunb.	Verbenaceae
CHOU WU TONG GEN	Harrlequin Glorybower Root	Clerodendron trichotomum Thunb.	Verbenaceae
CHU BAI PI	Tree of Heaven Ailanthus Bast	Ailanthus altissima (Mill.) Swingle	Simaroubaceae
CHU YE HUA JIAO (SHI ZHU YU)	Ailanthus-like Pricklyash	Zanthoxylum ailanthoides Sieb. et Zucc.	Rutaceae
CHU YE HUA JIAO PI	Ailanthus-like Pricklyash Bark	Zanthoxylum ailanthoides Sieb. et Zucc.	Rutaceae
CHUAN BAI HE	Uniclor Divid Lily	Lilium davidii Duch. var. uniclor Cotton	Liliaceae

Index of Traditional Chinese Medicines by Chinese Name

TCM Name	Name in English	Origin Latin Name	Family
CHUAN BEI MU	See JUAN YE BEI MU, WU HUA BEI MU, LENG SHA BEI MU, AN ZI BEI MU, YI BEI MU, PING BEI MU, GAN SU BEI MU:	Fritillaria cirrhosa D. Don; F. cirrhosa D. Don var. ecirrhosa Franch.; Fritillaria delavayi Franch.; Fritillaria unibracteata Hsiao et K. C. Hsiao; Fritillaria pallidiflora Schrenk; Fritillaria ussuriensis Maxim.; Fritillaria przewalskii Maxim. ex Batal.	Liliaceae Liliaceae Liliaceae Liliaceae Liliaceae Liliaceae Liliaceae
CHUAN CHAN JIU JIE LONG	Tiny Ardisia	Ardisia pusilla A. DC.	Myrsinaceae
CHUAN CHI SHAO (of CHI SHAO YAO)	Veitch Peony	Paeonia veitchii Lynch	Ranunculaceae
CHUAN DIAN YIN YANG HUO	David Epimedium	Epimedium davidii Franch.	Berberidaceae
CHUAN E YIN YANG HUO	Fargesi Epimedium	Epimedium fargesii Franch.	Berberidaceae
CHUAN JIN PI (MU JIN PI)	Shrubalthea Bark	Hibiscus syriacus L.	Malvaceae
CHUAN LI GUO	Pashi Pear Fruit	Pyrus pashia Buch.-Ham. ex D. Don	Rosaceae
CHUAN LIAN ZI (KU LIAN)	Szechwan Chinaberry Fruit	Melia toosendan Sieb. et Zucc.	Meliaceae
CHUAN LONG SHU YU (CHUAN SHAN LONG)	Nippon Yam	Dioscorea nipponica Mak.	Dioscoreaceae
CHUAN NIU XI	Capitate Cyathula	Cyathula capitata (Wall.) Moq.	Amaranthaceae
	Mediinal Cyathula	Cyathula officinalis Kuan	Amaranthaceae
CHUAN QIANG HUO (of QIANG HUO)	Szechwan Notopterygium	Notopterygium franchetii Boiss.	Umbelliferae
CHUAN SHAN CHENG	Hemsley Melodinus	Melodinus hemsleyanus Diels	Apocynaceae
CHUAN SHAN JIA	Pangolin	Manis pentadactyla Linnaeus	Manidae
CHUAN SHAN LONG (CHUAN LONG SHU YU)	Nippon Yam	Dioscorea nipponica Mak.	Dioscoreaceae
CHUAN WU TOU (of CAO WU TOU)	Common Monkshood	Aconitum carmichaeli Debx.	Ranunculaceae
CHUAN XIN LIAN	Common Andrographis	Andrographis paniculata (Burm.f.) Nees	Acanthaceae
CHUAN XIONG	Chuanxiong (Wallich Ligusticum)	Ligusticum wallichii Franch.	Umbelliferae
	Szechuan Lovage	Ligusticum chuanxiong Hort.	Umbelliferae
CHUAN XU DUAN (of XU DUAN)	Himalayan Teasel	Dipsacus asperoides C. Y. Cheng et T. M. Ai	Dipsacaceae
CHUAN ZANG XIANG CHA CAI	Szechwan-Tibet Rabdosia	Isodon pharicus (Prain) Murata	Labiatae
CHUN	Common Watershield	Brasenia schreberi J. F. Gmel.	Nymphaeaceae
CHUN BAI PI	Chinese Toona Root-bast	Toona sinensis (A. Juss.) Roem.	Meliaceae
CI BO	Hirsute Respberry	Rubus hirsutus Thunb.	Rosaceae
CI GU	Oldworld Arrowhead Corm	Sagittaria sagittifolia L.	Alismataceae
CI GUO FAN LI ZHI	Guanabana	Annona muricata L.	Annonaceae
CI GUO GAN CAO	Pricklyfruit Licorice	Glycyrrhiza pallidiflora Maxim.	Leguminosae
CI HUAI HUA	Black Locust Flower	Robinia pseudoacacia L.	Leguminosae

Index of Traditional Chinese Medicines by Chinese Name

TCM Name	Name in English	Origin Latin Name	Family
DA JI (a)	Peking Euphorbia	Euphorbia pekinensis Rupr.	Euphorbiaceae
DA JI (b)	Japanese Thistle	Cirsium japonicum DC.	Conpositae
DA JIN NIU CAO	Chinese Milkwort Herb	Polygala chinensis L.	Polygalaceae
DA JIN QIAN CAO	Christina Loosestrife Herb	Lysimachia christinae Hance	Primulaceae
DA LANG DU	Large Euphorbia Root	Euphorbia nematocypha Hand.-Mazz.	Euphorbiaceae
DA LIANG JIANG	Galanga Galangal	Alpinia galanga (L.) Swartz.	Zingiberaceae
DA PO WAN WAN HUA	Hupeh Anemone	Anemone hupehensis Lem.	Ranunculaceae
DA QING YE	Common Baphicacanthus Leaf	Baphicacanthus cusia (Nees) Bremek	Acanthaceae
	Dyers Woad Leaf	Isatis tinctoria L.	Cruciferae
	Indigo-coloured Woad Leaf	Isatis indigotica Fort.	Cruciferae
	Indigoplant Leaf	Polygonum tinctorium Ait	Polygonaceae
	Manyflower Glorybower Leaf	Clerodendron cyrtophyllum Turcz.	Verbenaceae
DA SUAN	Garlic	Allium sativum L.	Liliaceae
DA TENG LING ER CAO	Torulosous Dactylicapnos	Dactylicapnos torulosa (Hook. f. et Thoms.) Hutch.	Fumariaceae
DA TU SI ZI (of TU SI ZI)	Japanese Dodder Seed	Cuscuta japonica Choisy	Convolvulaceae
DA WEI YAO	Indian Heliotrope	Heliotropium indicum L.	Boraginaceae
DA XUE TENG	Sargentgloryvine	Sargentodoxa cuneata (Oeiv.) Rehd. et Wils.	Sargentodoxacea e
DA YE BAI TOU WENG	Common Pearleverlasting	Anaphalis margaritacea (L.) Benth. et Hook. f.	Compositae
DA YE CAI	Doederlein's Spikemoss Herb	Selaginella doederleinii Hieron.	Selaginellaceae
DA YE CHAI HU (of CHAI HU)	Bigleaf Thorowax	Bupleurum longiradiatum Turcz.	Umbelliferae
DA YE GOU TENG	Largeleaf Gamirplant	Uncaria macrophylla Wall.	Rubiaceae
DA YE HOU PU (DA YE MU LAN)	Bigleaf Magnolia	Magnolia rostrata W. W. Smith	Magnoliaceae
DA YE JIN HUA CAO	Common Wedgelet Fern	Stenoloma chusanum (L.) Ching	Lindsaeaceae
DA YE MU LAN (DA YE HOU PU)	Bigleaf Magnolia	Magnolia rostrata W. W. Smith	Magnoliaceae
DA YE NIU NAI CAI	Ko Condorvine	Marsdenia koi Tsiang	Asclepiadaceae
DA YE XIANG CHA CAI	Largeleaf Rabdosia	Rabdosia macrophylla (Migo) C. Wu et H. Li	Labiatae
DA YE XIANG RU	Twoanther Mosla	Mosla dianthera (Ham.) Maxim.	Labiatae
DA YE ZAO (HAI DAI)	Ellgrass	Zostera marina L.	Potamogetonacea e
DA YE ZI ZHU	Bigleaf Beautyberry	Callicarpa macrophylla Vahl.	Verbenaceae
DA YI ZHI JIAN	Golden Lycoris	Lycoris aurea Herb.	Amaryllidaceae
DA YU BIAO HUA	Shortclustered Plantainlily	Hosta sieboldiana Engl.	Liliaceae
DA ZAO	Common Jujube (Chinese Date)	Ziziphus jujuba Mill.	Rhamnaceae
	Spineless Common Jujube	Ziziphus jujuba Mill. var. inermis (Bge.) Rehd.	Rhamnaceae
DA ZI ZHANG YA CAI	Bigseed Swertia	Swertia macrosperma C. B. Clarke	Gentianaceae
DAI DAI HUA	Bitter Citrus	Citrus aurantium L. var. amara Engl.	Rutaceae
DAI YA XIAO DENG TAI	see PEN JIA SHU		
DAN MU	Medicinal Fatheadtree	Nauclea officinalis Pierre ex Pitard	Rubiaceae

Index of Traditional Chinese Medicines by Chinese Name

TCM Name	Name in English	Origin Latin Name	Family
DAN SHEN	Danshen	Salvia miltiorrhiza Bge.	Labiatae
DAN ZHU YE	Common Lophatherum	Lophatherum gracile Brongn.	Gramineae
DAN ZHU YE GEN (SUI GU ZI)	Common Lophatherum Root	Lophatherum gracile Brongn.	Gramineae
DANG GUI	Chinese Angelica	Angelica sinensis (Oliv.) Diels	Umbelliferae
DANG SHEN	Moderate Asiabell	Codonopsis pilosula Nannf. var. modesta (Nannf.) L. T. Shen [= Codonopsis Modesta Nannf.]	Campanulaceae
	Pilose Asiabell	Codonopsis pilosula (Franch.) Nannf.	Campanulaceae
	Szechwon Tangshen	Codonopsis tangshen Oliv.	Campanulaceae
DAO CAO	Rice Straw	Oryza sativa L.	Gramineae
DAO DOU	Sword Jackbean	Canavalia gladiata (Jacq.) DC.	Leguminosae
DAS YE AN YE	Swamp Mahogany	Eucalyptus robusta Smith	Myrtaceae
DAYE QIAN CAO	Smoothstalk Madder	Rubia schumannina Pritz	Rubiaceae
DENG LONG CAO	Manyhead Clinopodium	Clinopodium polycephalum (Vant.) C. Y. Wu et Hsuan	Labiatae
DENG LONG CAO	Peruvian Groundcherry Herb	Physalis peruviana L.	Solanaceae
DENG ZHAN XI XIN	Shortscape Fleabane	Erigeron breviscapus (Vant.) Hand.-Mazz.	Compositae
DI BU RONG	Delavay Stephania	Stephania delavayi Diels	Menispermaceae
DI FENG PI	Difengpi Anisetree	Illicium difengpi K. I. B. et K. I. M.	Illiciaceae
DI GU PI (GOU QI GEN PI)	Barbary Wolfberry Root-bark	Lycium barbarum L.	Solanaceae
	Chinese Wolfberry Root-bark	Lycium chinense Mill.	Solanaceae
DI GUA ZI	Wayaka Yambean Seed	Pachyrhizus erosus (L.) Urban	Leguminosae
DI JIN	Contorted Tanglehead	Heteropogon contortus (L.) Beauv.	Gramineae
	Japanese Creeper	Parthenocissus tricuspidata (Sieb. et Zucc.) Planch.	Vitaceae
DI JIN CAO	Humifuse Euphorbia	Euphorbia humifusa Willd.	Euphorbiaceae
DI SHAO GUA	Bastardtoadflaxlike Swallowwort	Cynanchum thesioides (Freyn) K. Schum.	Asclepiadaceae
DI SUN (ZE LAN GEN)	Shiny Bugleweed Root	Lycopus lucidus Turcz.	Labiatae
DI SUO LUO	Marchantia Polymorpha Lichen	Marchantia polymorpha L.	Marchantiaceae
DI TANG HUA	Japanese Kerria Flower	Kerria japonica (L.) DC.	Rosaceae
DI YANG QUE	Birdsfoot Trefoil	Lotus corniculatus L.	Leguminosae
DI YU	Garden Burnet	Sanguisorba officinalis L.	Rosaceae
DIAN HUANG QIN	Yunnan Skullcap	Scutellaria amoena C. H. Wright	Labiatae
DIAN JI GU CHANG SHAN	Yunnan Alstonia	Alstomia yunnanensis Diels	Apocynaceae
DIAN XI WU TOU	Yunnanwest Monkshood	Aconitum bulleyanum Diels	Ranunculaceae
DIAO GAN MA	Angled Bittersweet	Celastrus angulata Maxim.	Celastraceae
DIAO JING CAO	Evergreen Euonymus	Euonymus japonicus Thunb.	Celastraceae
DIAO ZHANG GEN PI	Largeleaf Spicebush Root-bark	Lindera umbellate Thunb.	Lauraceae
DIE DA LAO	Whorlleaf Litse	Litsea verticillata Hance	Lauraceae
DING XIANG	Clove	Syzygium aromaticum (L.) Merr. et Perry	Myrtaceae
DONG BEI CI REN SHEN	see CI REN SHEN		

Index of Traditional Chinese Medicines by Chinese Name

TCM Name	Name in English	Origin Latin Name	Family
DONG BEI CI REN SHEN (CI REN SHEN)	Tall Oplopanax	Oplopanax elatus Nakai	Arliaceae
DONG BEI HE SHI	European Stickseed	Lappula echinata Gilib.	Boraginaceae
DONG BEI HONG DOU SHAN	see ZI SHAN		
DONG BEI HUI HAO	Northeast Seriphidium	Seriphidium finitum (Kitag.) Ling et Y. R. Ling [= Artemisia finita Kitag.]	Compositae
DONG BEI PING BEI MU	see PING BEI MU		
DONG CHONG XIA CAO	Aweto (Chinese Caterpillar Fungus)	Cordyceps sinensis (Berk.) Sacc.	Clavicipitaceae
DONG FANG GOU JI	Oriental Chain Fern	Woodwardia orientalis Sm.	Blechnaceae
DONG FENG CAI	Scabrous Doellingeria	Doellingeria scaber (Thunb.) Nees	Compositae
DONG FENG JU	Boxleaf Atalantia	Atalantia buxifolia (Poir.) Oliv.	Rutaceae
DONG FENG JU GEN	Boxleaf Atalantia Root	Atalantia buxifolia (Poir.) Oliv.	Rutaceae
DONG FENG JU YE	Boxleaf Atalantia Leaf	Atalantia buxifolia (Poir.) Oliv.	Rutaceae
DONG GUA ZI	Chinese Waxgourd Seed	Benincasa hispida (Thunb.) Cogn.	Cucurbitaceae
DONG LANG DANG	Japanese Scopolia	Scopolia japonica Maxim.	Solanaceae
DONG LING CAO	Blushred Rabdosia	Rabdosia rubescens (Hemsl.) Hara	Labiatae
DONG QING (SI JI QING)	Purpleflower Holly	Ilex chinensis Sims [= Ilex purpurea]	Aquifoliaceae
DONG YI HAO JIAN MA	Cultivate Sisalan Agave East-1	Agave east-one	Agavaceae
DOU CHI CAO	Bloodred Iris	Iris sanguinea Hornem. [= Iris sanguinea Donn]	Iridaceae
DOU YE JIU LI XIANG	Euchretaleaf Common Jasminorange	Murraya euchrestifolia Hayata	Rutaceae
DOU YOU	Soybean Oil	Glycine max (L.) Merr.	Leguminosae
DU HENG	Forbes Wildginger	Asarum forbesii Maxim.	Aristolochiaceae
DU HUO	See ZHONG CHI MAO DANG GUI,	Angelica pubescens Maxim. f. biserrata Shan et Yuan;	Umbelliferae
	MAO DANG GUI,	Angelica pubescens Maxim.;	Umbelliferae
	XING AN BAI ZHI,	Angelica dahurica (Fisch. ex Hoffm.) Benth. et Hook. f. ex Franch. et Sav.;	Umbelliferae
	ZI JING DU HUO,	Angelica porphyrocaulis Nakai et	Umbelliferae
	HIU WEI DU HUO,	Kitag.; Heracleum hemsleyanum	Umbelliferae
	RUAN MAO DU HUO,	Diels;	Umbelliferae
	YONG NING DU HUO:	Heracleum lanatum Michx.; Heracleum yungningense Hand.-Mass	Umbelliferae
DU JING SHAN	Japanese Maesa	Maesa japonica (Thunb.) Moritzi	Myrsinaceae
DU JUAN HUA	Indian Azalea	Rhododendron simsii Planch.	Ericaceae
DU JUAN HUA YE	Indian Azalea Leaf	Rhododendron simsii Planch.	Ericaceae
DU QIN GEN	European Waterhemlock Root	Cicuta virosa L.	Umbelliferae
DU SONG SHI	Stiffleaf Juniper Fruit	Juniperus rigida Sieb. et Zucc.	Cupressaceae
DU XIAN ZI	Common Cashew Fruit	Anacardium occidentale L.	Anacardiaceae
DU YI WEI	Common Lamiophlomis	Lamiophlomis rotata (Benth.) Kudo [= Phlomis rotata Benth.]	Labiatae
DU ZHONG	Eucommia	Eucommia ulmoides Oliv.	Eucommiaceae
DUAN CI HU CI	Shortspine Damnacanthus	Damnacanthus subspinosus Hand.-Mazz.	Rubiaceae
DUAN JU	Globular Pepper	Piper mullesua D. Don.	Piperaceae

Index of Traditional Chinese Medicines by Chinese Name

TCM Name	Name in English	Origin Latin Name	Family
DUAN YE LONG SHE LAN	Narrowleaf Agave	Agave angustifolia Haw	Agavaceae
DUN YE GUI JIU	Common Mayapple	Podophyllum peltatum L.	Berberidaceae
DUN YE SHU YU	Peltate Yam Rhizome	Dioscorea zingiberensis C. H. Wright	Dioscoreaceae
DUO SHE FEI PENG	Multiradiate Fleabane	Erigeron multiradiatus (Wall.) Benth.	Compositae
DUO SUI LIAO	Manyspike Knotweed	Polygonum polystachyum Wall. ex Meisn	Polygonaceae
DUO SUI LUO HAN SONG SHI	Manyspike Podocarpus	Podocarpus polystachyus R. Br.	Podocarpaceae
DUO SUI SHI KE YE	Manyspike Tanoak Leaf	Lithocarpus polystachyus Rehd.	Fagaceae
E BU SHI CAO	Small Centipeda Herb	Centipeda minima (L.) A. Br. et Aschers	Compositae
E CUI	Goose Tail-meat	Anser domestica Geese	Anatidae
E GAO XUN	Amanita Fungus	Amanita strobilifomis (Paul.) Quél.	Amanitaceae
E RONG TENG	Chinese Swallowwort	Cynanchum chinense R. Br.	Asclepiadaceae
E SHEN	Woodland Beakchervil	Anthriscus sylvestris (L.) Hoffm.	Umbelliferae
E ZHANG YE FU ZI	see FU ZI		
EN SHI BA JI	Medicinal Damnacanthus	Damnacanthus officinarum Huang	Rubiaceae
ER CHI XIANG KE	Twodenntate Germander	Teucrium bidentatum Hemsl.	Labiatae
ER YE NIU PI XIAO	Auriculate Swallowwort	Cynanchum auriculatum Royle ex Wight	Asclepiadaceae
FAN LI ZHI	Custardapple	Annona squamosa L.	Annonaceae
FAN MA	American Agave	Agave americana L.	Agavaceae
FAN MU GUA	Papaya Fruit	Carica papaya L.	Caricaceae
FAN MU GUA YE	Papaya Leaf	Carica papaya L.	Caricaceae
FAN QIE	Tomato	Lycopersicon esculentum Mill.	Solanaceae
FAN SHI LIU GAN	Guava Immature Fruit	Psidium guajava L.	Myrtaceae
FAN SHI LIU PI	Guava Bark	Psidium guajava L.	Myrtaceae
FAN SHI LIU YE	Guava Leaf	Psidium guajava L.	Myrtaceae
FAN XIE YE	Narrowleaf Senna Leaf Sharpleaf Senna Leaf	Cassia angustifolia Vahl Cassia acutifolia Del.	Leguminosae Leguminosae
FANG FENG	Divaricate Saposhnikovia	Saposhnikovia divaricata (Turcz.) Schischk.	Umbelliferae
FANG JI	See FEN FANG JI, MU FANG JI, GUANG FANG JI, HAN FANG JI:	Stephania tetrandra S. Moore; Cocculus trilobus (Thunb.) DC.; Aristolochia fangchi Wu; Aristolochia heterophylla Hemsl.	Menispermaceae Menispermaceae Aristolochiaceae Aristolochiaceae
FEI CAI	Orange Stonecrop	Sedum kamtschaticum Fisch.	Crassulaceae
FEI JI CAO	Fragrant Eupatorium Herb	Eupatorium adoratum L.	Compositae
FEI LIAN	Curly Bristlethistle	Carduun crispus L.	Compositae
FEI LONG ZHANG XUE	AsiaticToddalia	Toddalia asiatica (L.) Lam.	Rutaceae
FEI YAN CAO	Rocket Consolida	Consolida ajacis (L.) Schur	Ranunculaceae
FEN BEI SHU YU (of BEI XIE)	Hypoglaucous Collett Yam	Dioscorea hypoglauca Palib.	Dioscoriaceae
FEN FANG JI (of FANG JI)	Fourstamen Stephania	Stephania tetrandra S. Moore	Menispermaceae
FEN TUAN HUA	Largeflower Paniculate Hydrangea Paniculate Hydrangea	Hydrangea paniculata Sieb. var. grandiflora Sieb. Hydrangea paniculata Sieb.	Saxifragaceae Saxifragaceae
FENG DOU CAI	Japanese Butterbur	Petasites japoniaus (Sieb. et Zucc.) F. Schmidt	Compositae
FENG DU	Apisin	Apis cerana Fabricius	Apidae

Index of Traditional Chinese Medicines by Chinese Name

TCM Name	Name in English	Origin Latin Name	Family
FENG JIAO	Propolis	Apis mellifera ligustica Spin.	Apidae
FENG LUN CAI	Chinese Clinopodium	Clinopodium chinense (Benth.) O. Ktze.	Labiatae
FENG MI	Honey	Apis cerana Fabricius	Apidae
FENG RU	Royal Jelly	Apis cerana Fabricius	Apidae
FENG WEI JIAO YE (SU TIE YE)	Sago Frond	Cycas revoluta Thunb.	Cycadaceae
FENG WEI PA SHAN HU	Mary Arthromeris	Arthromeris mairei (Brause) Ching [= Polypodium mairei Brause]	Polypodiaceae
FENG XIAN GEN	Garden Balsum Root	Impatiens balsamina L.	Balsaminaceae
FENG XIAN HUA	Garden Balsum Flower	Impatiens balsamina L.	Balsaminaceae
FENG XIANG JI SHENG	Flatshoot Mistletoe	Viscum articulatum Burm. f.	Loranthaceae
FENG XIANG SHU	Beautiful Sweetgum	Liquidambar formosana Hance	Hamamelidaceae
FENG XIANG SHU YE (a)	Common Butterbush	Cephalanthus occidentalis L.	Rubiaceae
FENG XIANG SHU YE (b)	Beautiful Sweetgum Leaf	Liquidambar taiwaniana Hance	Hamamelidaceae
FO SHOU (FO SHOU GAN)	Fleshfingered Citron	Citrus medica L. var. sarcodactylis (Noot.) Swingle	Rutaceae
FO SHOU GAN (FO SHOU)	Fleshfingered Citron	Citrus medica L. var. sarcodactylis (Noot.) Swingle	Rutaceae
FU FANG TENG	Forture Euonymus	Euonymus fortunei (Turcz.) Hand.-Mazz.	Celastraceae
FU LING	Indian Bread	Poria cocos (Schw.) Wolf	Polyporaceae
FU PING	Common Ducksmeat	Spirodela polyrrhiza Schleid.	Lemnaceae
	Common Duckwood	Lemna minor L.	Lemnaceae
FU RONG JU GEN	Chinese Crossostephium Root	Crossostephium chinense (L.) Mak. ex Cham. et Schltr.	Compositae
FU SANG HUA	Chinese Hibiscus Flower	Hibiscus rosasinensis L.	Malvaceae
FU SANG YE	Chinese Hibiscus Leaf	Hibiscus rosasinensis L.	Malvaceae
FU SHOU CAO	Amur Adonis	Adonis amurensis Reg. et Radde	Ranunculaceae
FU ZHOU SHU YU (of BEI XIE)	Foochow Yam Rhizome	Dioscorea futschauensis R. Kunth	Dioscoreaceae
FU ZI	Prepared Common Monkshood Daughter Root	Aconitum carmichaeli Debx.	Ranunculaceae
GAN	Chachi Citrus	Citrus chachiensis Hort.	Rutaceae
GAN	Sugary Citrus	Citrus suavissima Hort. ex Tanaka	Rutaceae
GAN CAO	Ural Licorice	Glycyrrhiza uralensis Fisch.	Leguminosae
GAN CHAN CHU (CHAN CHU)	Toad	Bufo bufo gargarizans Cantor; Bufo melanostictus Schneider	Bufonidae Bufonidae
GAN DI HUANG	Adhesive Rehmannia Dried Root	Rehmannia glutinosa (Gaertn.) Libosch ex Mey.	Scrophulariaceae
GAN FENG CAO	Autumn Zephyrlily Herb	Zephyranthes candida Herb.	Amaryllidaceae
GAN JIANG	Common Ginger Dried Rhizome	Zingiber officinalc Rosc.	Zingiberaceae
GAN JU	Lavandulaleaf Dendranthema	Dendranthema lavandulifolium (Fisch.) Ling et Shih	Compositae
GAN LAN	Cabbage	Brassica oleracea L. var. capiata L.	Cruciferae
	Olive	Canarium album (Lour.) Raeusch.	Burseraceae
GAN PI	Chachi Citrus Pericarp	Citrus chachiensis Hort.	Rutaceae
	Sugary Citrus Pericarp	Citrus suavissima Hort. ex Tanaka	Rutaceae
GAN SONG	Chinese nardostachys	Nardostachys chinensis Batal.	Valerianaceae

Index of Traditional Chinese Medicines by Chinese Name

TCM Name	Name in English	Origin Latin Name	Family
GAN SU BEI MU (of CHUAN BEI MU)	Przewalsk Fritillary	Fritillaria przewalskii Maxim. ex Batal.	Liliaceae
GAN SUI	Kansui Euphoria	Euphorbia kansui Liou	Euphorbiaceae
GAN ZHE	Sweetcane Culm	Saccharum sinensis Roxb.	Gramineae
GANG BAN GUI GEN	Perfoliate Knotweed Root	Polygonum perfoliatum L.	Polygonaceae
GANG SONG	Shrubby Baeckea	Baeckea frutescens L.	Myrtaceae
GAO BEN	Chinese Ligusticum	Ligusticum sinense Oliv.	Umbelliferae
GAO LIANG	Sorghum	Sorghum vulgare Pers	Gramineae
GAO LIANG JIANG	Lesser Galangal	Alpinia officinarum Hance	Zingiberaceae
GAO SHAN HUANG HUA	Alpine Thermopsis	Thermopsis alpina Ledeb.	Leguminosae
GE CONG	Longroot Onion	Allium victorialis L.	Liliaceae
GE GEN	Lobed Kudzuvine Root	Pueraria lobata (Willd.) Ohwi	Leguminosae
	Thomson Kudzuvine Root	Pueraria thomsonii Benth.	Leguminosae
GE SHANG TING CHANG	Bean Blister Beetle	Epicauta gorhami Mars.	Meloidae
GE XUN	Japanese balanophora	Balanophora japonica Mak.	Balanophoraceae
GE YE	Lobed Kudzuvine Leaf	Pueraria lobata (Willd.) Ohwi	Leguminosae
GOU GU SHU PI	Chinese Holly Bark	Ilex cornuta Lindl.	Aquifoliaceae
GOU GU YE	Chinese Holly Leaf	Ilex cornuta Lindl.	Aquifoliaceae
GOU JU	Trifoliate-orange	Poncirus trifoliata (L.) Raf.	Rutaceae
GOU JU HE	Trifoliate-orange Seed	Poncirus trifoliata (L.) Raf.	Rutaceae
GOU JU YE	Trifoliate-orange Leaf	Poncirus trifoliata (L.) Raf.	Rutaceae
GOU QI GEN PI (DI GU PI)	Barbary Wolfberry Root-bark	Lycium barbarum L.	Solanaceae
	Chinese Wolfberry Root-bark	Lycium chinense Mill	Solanaceae
GOU QI YE	Barbary Wolfberry Leaf	Lycium barbarum L.	Solanaceae
	Chinese Wolfberry Leaf	Lycium chinense Mill.	Solanaceae
GOU QI ZI	Barbary Wolfberry Fruit	Lycium barbarum L.	Solanaceae
	Chinese Wolfberry Fruit	Lycium chinense Mill.	Solanaceae
GOU ROU	Dog Meat	Canis familiaris L.	Canidae
GOU SHE CAO	Kirilow Groundsel Herb	Tephroseris kirilowii (Turcz. ex DC.) Holub [= Senecio integrifolius (L.) Clairvill var. fauriei (Lévl. et Vant.) Kitam.]	Compositae
GOU SHI HUA	Chinese Forgetmenot	Cynoglossum amabile Stapf et Drumm.	Boraginaceae
GOU TENG	Sharpleaf Gambirplant	Uncaria rhynchophylla (Miq.) Jacks.	Rubiaceae
GOU WEN	Graceful Jessamine	Gelsemium elegans Benth	Loganiaceae
GOU XIN	Dog Heart	Canis familiaris L.	Canidae
GU CHUI SHI HU	Yellowbow Dendrobium	Dendrobium chrysotoxum Lindl.	Orchidaceae
GU JIE CAO	Marsh Horsetail Herb	Equisetum palustre L.	Equisetaceae
GU SUI BU	Baron's Drynaria Rhizome	Drynaria baronii (Christ) Diels	Polypodiaceae
	Fortune's Drynaria Rhizome	Drynaria fortunei (Kunze) J. Sm.	Polypodiaceae
GUA DI	Muskmelon Fruit Pedicel	Cucumis melo L.	Cucurbitaceae
GUA LOU	Mongolian Snakegourd	Trichosanthes kirilowii Maxim.	Cucurbitaceae
	Rosthorn Snakegourd	Trichosanthes rosthornii Harms	Cucurbitaceae
GUA LOU GEN (TIAN HUA FEN)	Mongolian Snakegourd Root	Trichosanthes kirilowii Maxim.	Cucurbitaceae
	Rosthorn Snakegourd Root	Trichosanthes rosthornii Harms	Cucurbitaceae
GUAI QIN	Polymorphic Angelica	Angelica polymorpha Maxim.	Umbelliferae

Index of Traditional Chinese Medicines by Chinese Name

TCM Name	Name in English	Origin Latin Name	Family
GUAN HUA MA DOU LING	Tubeflower Dutchmanspipe	Aristolochia tubiflora Dunn	Aristolochiaceae
GUAN JIN TENG	Corrugate Chinese Dregea	Dregea sinensis Hemsl. var. corrugata (Schneid) Tsiang et P. T. Li	Asclepiadaceae
GUAN MU TONG	Manchurian Dutchmanspipe	Aristolochia manshuriensis Kom.	Aristolochiaceae
GUAN YE LIAN QIAO	Common St. John'swort	Hypericum perforatum L.	Guttiferae
GUAN ZHONG	Brainea	Brainea insignis (Hook.) J. Sm.	Blechnaceae
	Japanese Chain Fern	Woodwardia japonica (L. f.) Sm.	Blechnaceae
	Japanese Osmunda Fern	Osmunda japonica Thunb.	Osmundaceae
	Lunathyrium Fern	Lunathyrium acrostichoides (Sw.) Ching	Athyriaceae
	Male Fern Rhizome	Dryopteris crassirhizoma Nakai	Dryopteridaceae
	Matteuccia Fern	Matteuccia struthiopteris (L.) Todaro	Onocleaceae
	Oriental Blechnum Frond	Blechnum orientale L.	Blechnaceae
GUANG CI GU	Edible Tulip	Tulipa edulis (Miq.) Bak.	Liliaceae
GUANG FANG JI (of FANG JI)	Fangchi	Aristolochia fangchi Wu	Aristolochiaceae
GUANG GUO GAN CAO (of GAN CAO)	Licorice	Glycyrrhiza glabra L.	Leguminosae
GUANG HUO XIANG (of HUO XIANG)	Cablin Potchouli	Pogostemon cablin (Blanco) Benth.	Labiatae
GUANG JIN QIAN CAO	Snowbellleaf Tickclover	Desmodium styracifolium (Osbeck) Merr.	Leguminosae
GUANG XI XUE JIE (JIAN YE LONG XUE SHU)	Swordleaf Dracaena	Dracaena cochinchinensis (Lour.) S. C. Chen	Liliaceae
GUANG YE DING GONG TENG	Glabrousleaf Erycibe	Erycibe schmidtii Craib	Convolvulaceae
GUANG YE FEN HUA XIU XIAN JU	Fortune Japanese Spiraea	Spiraea japonica L. f. var. fortunei (Phanch.) Rehd.	Rosaceae
GUANG YE SHUI SU	Marshy Betony	Stachys palustris L.	Labiatae
GUANG YE ZI YU PAN	Glabrousleaf Uvaria	Uvaria boniana Finet et Gagnep.	Annonaceae
GUI DENG LONG	Redcalyx Glotybower	Clerodendron fortunatum L.	Verbenaceae
GUI GAI	Coprinus Sporophore	Coprinus atramentarius (Bull.) Fr.	Agaricaceae
GUI HUA	Sweet Osmanthus Flower	Osmanthus fragrans Lour.	Oleaceae
GUI JIAN JIN JI ER	Shagspine Peashrub	Caragana jubata (Pall.) Poir.	Leguminosae
GUI JIAN YU	Winged Euonymus	Euonymus alatus (Thunb.) Sieb.	Celastraceae
GUI JIU	Common Dysosma	Dysosma versipellis (Hance) M. Cheng	Berberidaceae
GUI PI	Japanese Cinnamon	Cinnamomum japonicum Sieb.	Lauraceae
GUI YE	Chinese Juniper Leaf	Sobina chinensis (L.) Antoine	Cupressaceae
GUI ZHI	Cassiabarktree Twig	Cinnamomum cassia Presl	Lauraceae
GUI ZHU TANG JIE	Wormseed Mustard	Erysimum cheranthoides L.	Cruciferae
GUO CHAN CHEN XIANG	see BAI MU XIANG		
GUO JIANG LONG	Complanate Clubmoss	Lycopodium complanatum L.	Lycopodiaceae
GUO YE GE	Mirifica Kudzuvine	Pueraria mirifica	Leguminosae
HA SHI MA	Dried Chinese Woodfrog	Rana temporaria chensinensis David;	Ranidae
	Dried Amur Woodfrog	Rana amurensis Boulenger	Ranidae
HAI DAI (DA YE ZAO)	Ellgrass	Zostera marina L.	Potamogetonaceae

Index of Traditional Chinese Medicines by Chinese Name

TCM Name	Name in English	Origin Latin Name	Family
HAI ER CHA	Cutechu	Acacia catechu (L.) Willd	Leguminosae
	Gambier Gambirplant	Uncaria gambier Roxb.	Rubiaceae
HAI FENG TENG	Kadsura Pepper Stem	Piper kadsura (Choisy) Ohwi [= Piper futo-kadsura Sieb.]	Piperaceae
HAI HONG DOU	Sandal Beadtree Seed	Adenanthera pavonina L.	Leguminosae
HAI JIU CAI	Shore Podgrass	Triglochin maritimum L.	Juncaginaceae
HAI NAN GE NA XIANG	Hainan Goniothalamus	Goniothalamus howii Merr.	Annonaceae
HAI NAN LUO FU MU	Hainan Devilpepper	Rauvolfia verticillata (Lour) Baill. var. hainanensis Tsiang	Apocynaceae
HAI NAN QING NIU DAN	Hainan Tinospora	Tinospora hainanesis H. S. Lo et Z. X. Li	Menispermaceae
HAI NAN YE SHAN HUA	Hainan Sarcococca	Sarcococca vagans Stapf	Buxaceae
HAI REN CAO	Simple Digenea Frond	Digenea simplex (Wulf.) C. Ag.	Rhodomelaceae
HAI SHEN CHANG	Sea-cucunber Intestines	Stichopus japonicus Selenka	Stichopodidae
HAI SONG ZI	Korean Pine Seed	Pinus koraiensis Sieb. et Zucc.	Pinaceae
HAI TONG PI	Oriental variegated Coralbean Bark	Erythrina variegata L. var. orentalis (L.) Merr.	Leguminosae
HAI TUN YU	Dolphin	Delphinus delphis L.	Delphinidae
HAI XIA	Lobster	Panulirus ornatus (Fabricius)	Palinuridae
	Prawn	Penaeus orientalis Kishinouye	Penaeidae
HAI ZAO	Fusiform Sargasum	Sargassum fusiforme (Harv.) Setch.	Sargassaceae
	Palli Sargasum	Sargassum pallidum (Turn.) C. Ag.	Sargassaceae
HAN CAI	Rorippa	Rorippa montana (Wall.) Small	Cruciferae
HAN FANG JI (of FANG JI)	Yellowmouth Dutchmanspipe	Aristolochia heterophylla Hemsl.	Aristolochiaceae
HAN LIAN CAO (MO HAN LIAN)	Yerbadetajo	Eclipta prostrata L. [= Eclipta alba (L.) Hassk]	Compositae
HAN LIAN HUA	Common Nasturtium	Tropaeolum majus L.	Tropaeolaceae
HAN QIN	Wildcelery	Apium graveolens L. var. dulce DC.	Umbelliferae
HAN XIN CAO	Indian Skullcap	Scutellaria indica L.	Labiatae
HAN XIU CAO	Sensitiveplant Herb	Mimosa pudica L.	Leguminosae
HAO WANG JIAO LU HUI (of LU HUI)	Cape of Good Hope Aloe Dried Juice	Aloe ferox Mill.	Liliaceae
HE BAO MU DAN GEN	Showy Bleedingheart	Dicentra spectabilis (L.) Lem.	Papaveraceae
HE GENG	Hindu Lotus Petiole	Nelumbo nucifera Gaertn.	Nymphaeaceae
HE HUAN PI	Silktree Albizia Bark	Albizzia julibrissin Durazz.	Leguminosae
HE NAN TANG SONG CAO	Honan Meadowrue	Thalictrum honanenae W.T. Wang et S. H. Wang	Ranunculaceae
HE QING HUA	Japanese Hylomecon	Hylomecon japonica (Thunb.) Prantl et Kündig	Papaveraceae
HE SHI (TIAN MING JING)	Common Carpesium Fruit	Carpesium abrotanoides L.	Compositae
HE SHI FENG	Wild Carrot	Daucus carota L.	Umbelliferae
HE SHOU WU	Tuber Fleeceflower	Polygonum multiflorum Thunb.	Polygonaceae
HE TA CAO	Florida Waltheria	Waltheria americana L.	Sterculiaceae
HE TUN	Globefish	Fugu ocellatus (Osbeck)	Tetraodontidae
HE YE	Hindu Lotus Leaf	Nelumbo nucifera Gaertn.	Nymphaeaceae
HE YE DI	Hindu Lotus Leaf-base	Nelumbo nucifera Gaertn.	Nymphaeaceae
HE ZI	Medicine Terminalia Fruit	Terminalia chebula Retz.	Combretaceae
HE ZI YE	Medicine Terminalia Leaf	Terminalia chebula Retz.	Combretaceae

Index of Traditional Chinese Medicines by Chinese Name

TCM Name	Name in English	Origin Latin Name	Family
HEI CHAI HU	Black Thorowax	Bupleurum smithii Wolff	Umbelliferae
HEI DA DOU	Black Soyabean	Glycine max (L.) Merr.	Leguminosae
HEI DA DOU PI	Black Soyabean Spermoderm	Glycine max (L.) Merr.	Leguminosae
HEI DA DOU YE	Black Soyabean Leaf	Glycine max (L.) Merr.	Leguminosae
HEI MA YI	Silky Ant	Formica fusca L.	Formicidae
HEI MAN	Regel Threewingnut	Tripterygium regelii Sprague et Takeda.	Celastraceae
HEI SHUI CUI QUE	Potanin Larkspur	Delphinium potaninii W. T. Wang	Ranunculaceae
HEI ZHI MA	Oriental sesame	Sesamum indicum DC.	Pedaliaceae
HENG ZHOU WU YAO	Laurelleaf Snailseed	Cocculus laurifolius DC.	Menispermaceae
HIU WEI DU HUO (of DU HUO)	Hemsley Cowparsnip	Heracleum hemsleyanum Diels	Umbelliferae
HONG CAO	Prince's-feather Herb	Polygonum orientale L.	Polygonaceae
HONG CHAI HU (of CHAI HU)	Red Thorowax	Bupleurum scorzonerifolium Willd.	Umbelliferae
HONG CHE ZHOU CAO	Red Clover	Trifolium pratense L.	Leguminosae
HONG DOU	Hosie Ormosia Seed	Ormosia hosiei Hemsl. et Wils.	Leguminosae
HONG GEN CAO	Hispid Sage	Salvia prionitis Hance	Labiatae
HONG GUO LUO FU MU	Redfruit Devilpepper	Rauvolfia verticillata (Lour.) Baill. f. rubrocarpa H. T. Chang.	Apocynaceae
HONG HUA	Safflower	Carthamus tinctrius L.	Compositae
HONG HUA CAI (ZI YUN YING)	Chinese Milkvetch	Astragalus sinicus L.	Leguminosae
HONG HUA PI (of HUA MU PI)	Japanese White Birch Bark	Betula platyphylla Suk. var. japonica (Sieb.) Hara	Betulaceae
HONG HUA WU WEI ZI	Redflower Magnoliavine	Schisandra rubriflora Rhed et Wils	Schisandraceae
HONG HUI XIANG	Henry Anisetree	Illicium henryi Diels	Illiciaceae
HONG KUAI ZI	Great Willowherb (Firewood)	Chamaenerion angustifolium (L.) Scop. [= Epilobium angustifolium L.]	Onagraceae
HONG MAO QI	Robust Leontice	Leontice robustum (Maxim.) Diels	Berberidaceae
HONG MU JI CAO	Hookedhairypod Tickclover	Desmodium gangeticum (L.) DC.	Leguminosae
HONG NAN PI	Red Nanmu Bark	Machilus thunbergii Sieb. et Zucc.	Lauraceae
HONG NIANG ZI	Red Lady-bug	Huechys sanguinea De Geer.	Cicadidae
HONG SAN QI	Ovateleaf Knotweed	Polygonum suffultum Maxim.	Leguminosae
HONG SHEN	see REN SHEN		
HONG TOU CAO	Malay Blumea Herb	Blumea lacera (Burm. f.) DC.	Compositae
HONG YA DA JI (of DA JI (a))	Red Knoxia	Knoxia valerianoides Thorel ex Pitard	Rubiaceae
HONG YAO ZI	Ciliatenerve Knotweed Root	Polygonum ciliinerve (Nakai) Ohwi	Polygonaceae
HONG ZE LAN	Japanese Conehead	Strobilanthes japonicus (Thunb.) Miq.	Acanthaceae
HOU GU JUN	see HOU TOU JUN		
HOU PI SHU	Coromandel Lannea	Lannea grandis (Dennst.) Engl.	Anacardiaceae
HOU PO	Officinal Mangolia	Magnolia officinalis Rehd. et Wils.	Magnoliaceae
	Twolobed Officinal Mangolia	Magnolia biloba (Rehd. et Wils.) Cheng	Magnoliaceae

Index of Traditional Chinese Medicines by Chinese Name

TCM Name	Name in English	Origin Latin Name	Family
HOU TOU JUN	Bearded Tooth Carpophore	Hericium erinaceus (Bull. ex Fr.) Pers. [= Hydnum erinaceus Bull. ex Fr.]	Hydnaceae
HOU ZHANG	Bodinier Cinnamon	Cinnamomum bodinieri Lévl.	Lauraceae
HU BEI BEI MU	Hupeh Fritillary	Fritillaria hupehensis Hsiao et K. C. Hsiao	Liliaceae
HU BEI GUA LOU	Hupeh Snakegourd	Trichosanthes hupehensis C.Y.Cheng et Yueh.	Cucurbitaceae
HU BEI SHAN MAI DONG	Hubei Liriope	Liriope spicata (Thunb.) Lour. var. prolifera Y. T. Ma	Liliaceae
HU BEI YANG TI JIA	Hupeh Bauhinia	Bauhinia hupehara Craib	Leguminosae
HU CI	Indian Damnacanthus	Dammacanthus indicus Gaertn. f.	Rubiaceae
HU CONG	Shallot	Allium ascalonicum L.	Liliaceae
HU DIE HUA	Fringed Iris	Iris japonica Thunb.	Iridaceae
HU ER CAO	Creeping Rockfoil	Saxifraga stolonifera (L.) Meerb.	Saxifragaceae
HU GAO	Tiger Fat	Panthera tigris L.	Felidae
HU HUANG LIAN	Figwortflower Picrorhiza	Picrorrhiza scrophulariaeflora Pennell	Scrophulariaceae
	Picrorhiza	Picrorrhiza kurrooa Royle ex Benth.	Scrophulariaceae
HU JI SHENG (of SANG JI SHENG)	Colored Mistletoe	Viscum coloratum (Kom.) Nakai	Loranthaceae
HU JIAO	Black Pepper	Piper nigrum L.	Piperaceae
HU LU	Bottle Gourd	Lagenaria siceraria (Molina) Standl. var. depressa Ser.	Cucurbitaceae
HU LU BA	Common Fenugreek	Trigonella foenum-graecum L.	Leguminosae
HU LU QI	kindeyleaf Goldenray	Ligularia fischeri (Ledeb.) Turcz.	Compositae
	Toothleaf Goldenray	Ligularia dentata (A. Gray.) Hara	Compositae
HU LUO BO	Carrot	Daucus carota L. var. sativa DC.	Umbelliferae
HU LUO BO ZI	Carrot Seed	Daucus carota L. var. sativa DC.	Umbelliferae
HU MA YE	Oriental Sesame Leaf	Sesamum indicum DC.	Pedaliaceae
HU MA ZI (BAI ZHI MA)	Oriental Sesame	Sesamum indicum DC.	Pedaliaceae
HU SUI ZI	Coriander Seed	Coriandrum sativum L.	Umbelliferae
HU TAO QING PI	English Walnut Exocarp	Juglans regia L.	Juglandaceae
HU TAO REN	English Walnut Seed	Juglans regia L.	Juglandaceae
HU TAO YE	English Walnut Leaf	Juglans regia L.	Juglandaceae
HU WEI LAN	Snake Sansevieria	Sansevieria trifasciata Prain	Agavaceae
HU ZHANG	Japanese Fleeceflower (Giant Knotweed)	Polygonum cuspidatum Sieb. et Zucc.	Poligonaceae
HU ZHI ZI	Shrub Lespedeza	Lespedeza bicolor Turcz.	Leguminosae
HUA BEI BAI QIAN	Hancock Swallowwort	Cynanchum hancockianum (Maxim) Al. Iljinski	Asclepiadaceae
HUA GOU TENG (of GOU TENG)	Chinese Gambirplant	Uncaria sinensis (Oliv.) Havil.	Rubiaceae
HUA JIAO	Bunge Pricklyash	Zanthoxylum bungeanum Maxim.	Rutaceae
HUA JIAO GEN	Bunge Pricklyash Root	Zanthoxylum bungeanum Maxim.	Rutaceae
	Peppertree Pricklyash Root	Zanthoxylum schinifolium Sieb. et Zucc.	Rutaceae
HUA JIN DAN	Tetragonal Crotalaria	Crotalaria tetragona Roxb. [= Crotalaria tetragona Andr.]	Verbenaceae
HUA LIAN XI XIN	Largeflower Wildginger	Asarum maximum Hemsl.	Aristolochiaceae
HUA MAO	Corniculate Spurgentian	Halenia corniculata (L.) Cornaz.	Gentianaceae
HUA MU PI	See HONG HUA PI, BAI HUA PI:	Betula platyphylla Suk. var. japonica (Sieb.) Hara; Betula platyphylla Suk.	Betulaceae Betulaceae

Index of Traditional Chinese Medicines by Chinese Name

TCM Name	Name in English	Origin Latin Name	Family
HUA NAN MA WEI SHAN	Fordi Phlegmariurus	Phlegmariurus fordii (Baker) Ching	Huperziaceae
HUA XI BEI MU	Huaxi Fritillary	Fritillaria siechuanica	Liliaceae
HUA XIANG SHU YE	Dyetree Leaf	Platycarya strobilacea Sieb. et Zucc.	Juglandaceae
HUA ZHOU LOU LU (of LOU LU)	Broadleaf Globethistle	Echinops latifolus Tausch	Compositae
HUAI GEN	Japanese Pagodatree Root	Sophora japonica L.	Leguminosae
HUAI JIAO	Japanese Pagodatree Fruit	Sophora japonica L.	Leguminosae
HUAI QING DI HUANG (of GAN DI HUANG)	Hueiching Rehmannia	Rehmannia glutinosa Libosch. f. hueichingensis (Chao et Schih) Hsiao	Scrophulariaceae
HUAI TONG	Moupin Dutchmanspipe	Aristolochia moupinensis Franch.	Aristolochiaceae
HUANG BAI	Amur Corktree	Phellodendron amurene Rupr.	Rutaceae
	Chinese Corktree	Phellodendron chinense Schneid.	Rutaceae
	Glabrousleaf Chinese Corktree	Phellodendron chinense Schneid. var. glabriusculum Schneid.	Rutaceae
HUANG GAN CAO	Eurycapa Licorice	Glycyrrhiza eurycapa P. C. Li.	Leguminosae
HUANG GAN CAO (of GAN CAO)	Yellow Licorice	Glycyrrhiza kansuensis Chang et Peng	Leguminosae
HUANG GUA	Cucumber	Cuccumis sativus L.	Cucurbitaceae
HUANG GUO QIE	Yellowfruit Nightshade	Solanum xanthocarpum Schrad. et Wendl.	Solanaceae
HUANG HE MAO REN DONG	Yellowhair Honeysuckle	Lonicera fulvotomentosa Hsu et S. C. Cheng	Caprifoliaceae
HUANG HUA BAI JIANG (of BAI JIANG)	Dahurian Patrinia	Patrinia scabiosaefolia Fisch.	Valerianaceae
HUANG HUA DI DING	Diluteyellow Crotalaria	Crotalaria albida Heyne	Leguminosae
HUANG HUA HAO	Sweet Wormwood	Artemisia annua L.	Compositae
HUANG HUA JIA ZHU TAO	Yellow Oleander	Thevetia peruviana (Pers.) K. Schum.	Apocynaceae
HUANG HUA REN	Acute Sida	Sida acuta Burm. f.	Malvaceae
HUANG HUA YUAN ZHI	Yellowflower Milkwort	Polygala arillata Buch.-Ham.	Polygalaceae
HUANG HUA ZI	Cordateleaf Sida	Sida cordifolia L.	Malvaceae
	Slimyhair Sida	Sida mysorensis Wight et Arn.	Malvaceae
HUANG JIE GU DAN	Gypsophila	Gypsophila acutifolia Fisch.	Caryophyllaceae
HUANG JIN	Racemose Corydalis	Corydalis racemosa (Thunb.) Pers.	Papaveraceae
HUANG JIN FENG	Incurvedspur Snapweed	Impatiens siculifer Hook. F.	Balsaminaceae
HUANG JING	King Solomonseal	Polygonatum kingianum Coll. et Hemsl.	Liliaceae
	Macropodous Solomonseal	Polygonatum macropodium Turcz.	Liliaceae
	Manyflower Solomonseal	Polygonatum cyrtonema Hua	Liliaceae
	Siberian Solomonseal	Polygonatum sibiricum Redoute	Liliaceae
	Tendrilleaf Solomonseal	Polygonatum cirrhifolium (Wall.) Royle	Liliaceae
HUANG JING YE	Negundo Chastetree Leaf	Vitex negundo L.	Verbenaceae
HUANG KUI	Muskmallow	Abelmoschus moschatus (L.) Medic.	Malvaceae
HUANG LIAN	Chinese Goldthread	Coptis chinensis Franch.	Ranunculaceae
	Deltoid Goldthread	Coptis deltoidea C. Y. Cheng et Hsiao	Ranunculaceae
	Omei Mountain Goldthread	Coptis omeiensis (Chen) C. Y. Cheng	Ranunculaceae
	Yunnan Goldthread	Coptis teetoides C. Y. Cheng [= Coptis teeta Wall.]	Ranunculaceae
HUANG LIAN YA	Common Pistache	Pistacia chinensis Bge.	Anacardiaceae

Index of Traditional Chinese Medicines by Chinese Name

TCM Name	Name in English	Origin Latin Name	Family
HUANG LU	Common Smoketree	Cotinus coggygria Scop.	Anacardiaceae
HUANG LU ZHI YE	Common Smoketree Branch and Leaf	Cotinus coggygria Scop.	Anacardiaceae
HUANG MA YE	Roundpod Jute Leaf	Corchorus capsularis L.	Tiliaceae
HUANG MA ZI	Roundpod Jute Seed	Corchorus capsularis L.	Tiliaceae
HUANG MAO WU TOU	Yellowhail Monkshood	Aconitum chrysotrichum W. T. Wang	Ranunculaceae
HUANG MIAN GUI	Champac Michelia	Michelia champaca L	Magnoliaceae
HUANG MING JIAO	Oxhide Gelatin	Bos taurus domesticus Gmelin	Bovidae
HUANG PI	see HUANG PI YE		
HUANG PI YE	Chinese Wampee Leaf	Clausena lansium (Lour) Skeels	Rutaceae
HUANG QI	Membranous Milkvetch	Astragalus membranaceus (Fisch.) Bge.	Leguminosae
HUANG QIN	Baikal Skullcap	Scutellaria baicalensis Georgi	Labiatae
HUANG QIN JIAO	Baillon Veratrilla	Veratrilla baillonii Franch	Gantianaceae
HUANG SHAN YAO	Yellow Yam Rhizome	Dioscorea panthaica Prain et Burkill	Dioscoreaceae
HUANG WAN	Shady Groundsel	Senecio nemorensis L	Compositae
HUANG XIAO BO	Yellow Barberry	Berberis tschonoskiana Regel	Berberidaceae
HUANG YANG MU YE	Chinese Box Juvenile Leaf	Buxus microphylla Sieb. et Zucc. var. sinica Rehd. et Wils.	Buxaceae
HUANG YAO ZI	Airpotato Yam	Dioscorea bulbifera L	Dioscoreaceae
HUI BAO HAO	Roxburgh Wormwood	Artemisia roxbugiana Bess.	Compositae
HUI GUO JIAO GU LAN	Rostratefruit Gynostemma	Gynostemma yixingense C. Y. Wu et SSK Chen	Cucurbhitaceae
HUI HAO (SHAN DAO NIAN HAO)	Chinese Seriphidium	Artemisia cina (Berg. ex Poljak) Poljak [= Seriphidium cinum (Berg. ex Poljak) Poljak]	Compositae
HUI HUI DOU	Gram Chickpea	Cicer arietinum L.	Leguminosae
HUI XIANG	Fennel Fruit	Foeniculum vulgare Mill.	Umbelliferae
HUI XIANG GEN	Fennel Root	Foeniculum vulgare Mill.	Umbelliferae
HUI XIANG JING YE	Fennel Stem and Leaf	Foeniculum vulgare Mill.	Umbelliferae
HUI YE GEN	Purple Tephrosia Root	Tephrosia purpurea (L.) Pers.	Leguminosae
HUI ZHAN MAO REN DONG	see DA HUA REN DONG		
HUI ZHU NIU NAI CAI	Beakstyle Condorvine	Marsdenia oreophila Smith	Asclepiadaceae
HUN JI TOU	Fortune's Holly Fern	Cyrtomium fortunei J. Sm.	Dryopteridaceae
HUO GAO BEN (of GAO BEN)	Slenderleaf Ligusticum	Ligusticum tenuissimum (Nakai) Kitag.	Umbelliferae
HUO MA REN	Hemp Fimble Seed	Cannabis sativa L.	Moraceae
HUO SUO MA	Tortedfruit Screwtree	Helicteres isora L.	Sterculiaceae
HUO TAN MU CAO	Chinese Knotweed Herb	Polygonum chinense L.	Polygonaceae
HUO XIANG	Wrinkled Gianthyssop	Agastache rugosa (Fisch. et Mey.) O. Ktze.	Labiatae
HUO YANG LE	Ancients Euphorbia	Euphorbia antiquorum L.	Euphorbiaceae
JI CAI	Shepherdspurse	Capsella bursapastoris (L.) Medic.	Cruciferae
JI CAI ZI	Shepherdspurse Seed	Capsella bursapastoris (L.) Medic.	Cruciferae
JI CHANG LANG DU	Leafy Euphorbia	Euphorbia esula L.	Euphorbiaceae
JI GU CAO	Canton Abrus Herb	Abrus fruticulosus Wall. ex Wight et Arn. [= Abrus cantoniensis Hance]	Leguminosae
JI GU CHANG SHAN	see DIAN JI GU CHANG SHAN		

TCM Name	Name in English	Origin Latin Name	Family
JI HUA YE	Chinese Loropetalum	Loropetalum chinense (R. Br.) Oliv.	Hamamelidaceae
JI LI GEN	Puncturevine Caltrap Root	Tribulus terrestris L.	Zygophyllaceae
JI MAO SONG	Imbricate Podocarpus	Podocarpus imbricatus Bl.	Podocarpaceae
JI NAO	Chicken Brain	Gallus gallus domesticus Brisson	Phasianidae
JI NEI JIN	Chicken's Gizzard Endothelium	Gallus gallus domesticus Brisson	Phasianidae
JI NI	Apricotleaf Ladybell	Adenophora trachelioides Maxim.	Campanulaceae
JI NING	Largeserrate Mosla	Mosla grosseserrata Maxim.	Labiatae
JI ROU	Chicken	Gallus gallus domesticus Brisson	Phasianidae
JI SHI TENG	Chinese Fevervine	Paederia scandens (Lour.) Merr.	Rubiaceae
JI SHI TENG GUO	Chinese Fevervine Fruit	Paederia scandens (Lour.) Merr.	Rubiaceae
JI SU ZI	Evergreen Dogwood	Cornus capitata Wall. [= Dendrobenthamia capitata (Wall.) Hutch]	Cornaceae
JI WA CAO	Littleflower Plumbagella Herb	Plumbagella micrantha (Ledeb.) Spach	Plumbaginaceae
JI XIANG CAO	Pink Reineckea Herb	Reineckea carnea (Andr.) Kunth	Liliaceae
JI XING ZI	Garden Balsam Seed	Impatiens balsamina L.	Balsaminaceae
JI XUE CAO	Asiatic Pennywort Herb	Centella asiatica (L.) Urban	Umbelliferae
JI XUE TENG	Diels Millettia	Millettia dielsiana Harms ex Diels	Leguminosae
JI XUE TENG	Shiningleaf Millettia	Millettia nitida Benth.	Leguminosae
JI XUE TENG	Suberect Spatholobus	Spatholobus suberectus Dunn	Leguminosae
JI XUE TENG	Whiteflower Mucuna	Mucuna birdwoodiana Tutcher	Leguminosae
JI YE QIU HAI TANG	Limpricht Begonia	Begonia limprichtii Irmsch.	Begoniaceae
JI ZI BAI	Hen's Egg-albumen	Gallus gallus domesticus Brisson	Phasianidae
JI ZI HUANG	Hen's Egg Yolk	Gallus gallus domesticus Brisson	Phasianidae
JI ZONG	Collybia Albuminosa Sporophore	Collybia albuminosa (Berk.) Petch	Tricholomataceae
JIA BAI HE	Hyacinth Falselily	Notholirion hyacinthinum (Wils.) Stapf	Liliaceae
JIA JING JIE	Catnip	Nepeta cataria L.	Labiatae
JIA KU GUA	Balloonvine Heartseed	Cardiospermum halicacabum L.	Sapindaceae
JIA LIAN QIAO YE	Creeping Skyflower Leaf	Duranta repena L.	Verbenaceae
JIA SUAN JIANG	Peru Herb	Nicandra physaloides (L.) Gaerth.	Solanaceae
JIA XI ZHUI XIANG CHA CAI	Falselittleconical Rabdosia	Rabdosia coetsoides C. Y. Wu	Labiatae
JIA YING ZHUA	Chinese Desmos	Desmos cochinchinensis Lour. [= Desmos chinensis Lour.]	Annonaceae
JIA ZHU TAO	Sweetscented Oleander	Nerium indicum Mill.	Apocynaceae
JIAN DI PU GONG YING (of PU GONG YING)	Chinese Dandelion	Taraxacum sinicum Kitag.	Compositae
JIAN LIE HAI YING SU	Acutelobed Hornpoppy	Glaucium oxylobum Boiss. et Bushse	Papaveraceae
JIAN MA	Sisal Hemp-plant (Sisal Agave)	Agave sisalana Perr. ex Engelm.	Agavaceae
JIAN XUE QING	Nervate Twayblade	Liparis nervosa (Thunb.) Lindl.	Orchidaceae
JIAN YE LONG XUE SHU (GUANG XI XUE JIE)	Swordleaf Dracaena	Dracaena cochinchinensis (Lour.) S. C. Chen	Liliaceae
JIAN YE QING FENG TENG	Sharpleaf Sabia	Sabia swinhoei Hemsl. ex Forb. et Hemsl.	Sabiaceae
JIAN YE TIE SHU YE	Strictleaf Dracaena Leaf	Cordyline strcta Endl.	Agavaceae

Index of Traditional Chinese Medicines by Chinese Name

TCM Name	Name in English	Origin Latin Name	Family
JIAN YE YIN YANG HUO (of YIN YANG HUO)	Sagittate Epimedium	Epimedium sagittatum (Sieb. et Zucc.) Maxim.	Berberidaceae
JIANG	Soy Sauce	Legume crop.	Leguminosae
JIANG HUANG	Common Turmeric	Curcuma longa L.	Zingiberaceae
JIANG HUANG (of YU JIN)	Aromatic Turmeric	Curcuma aromatica Salisb.	Zingiberaceae
JIANG LI MU GEN	Thinleaf Buckthorn Root	Rhamnus leptophylla Schneid.	Rhamnaceae
JIANG MANG	Inflatedfruit Senna	Cassia sophera L.	Leguminosae
JIANG YOU FU ZI	see FU ZI		
JIANG ZHEN XIANG	Odorate Rosewood	Dalbergia odorifera T. Chen	Leguminosae
JIAO GU LAN (QI YE DAN)	Fiveleaf Gynostemma	Gynostemma pentaphylla (Thunb.) Makino	Cucurbitaceae
JIE GENG	Balloonflower	Platycodon grandiflorum (Jacq.) A. DC.	Campanulaceae
JIE ZI	India Mustart Seed	Brassica juncea (L.) Czern. et Coss.	Cruciferae
JIN BIAN LONG SHE LAN	Marginate American Agave	Agave americana L. var. marginata Hort.	Agavaceae
JIN BU HUAN	Chinese Stephania	Stephania sinica Diels	Menispermaceae
JIN CAO	Hispid Arthraxon Herb	Arthraxon hispidus (Thunb.) Mak.	Gramineae
JIN FO CAO	Brithsh Inula Herb	Inula britannica L.	Compositae
	Japanese Inula Herb	Inula japonica Thunb.	Compositae
	Linearleaf Inula Herb	Inula linariaefolia Turcz.	Compositae
JIN GANG DA	Japanese Croomia	Croomia japonica Miq.	Stemonaceae
JIN GUO LAN	Arrowshaped Tinospora	Tinospora sagittata Gagn.	Menispermaceae
	Hairystalk Tinospora	Tinospora capillipes Gagn.	Menispermaceae
JIN JI LE	Ledger Cinchona	Cinchona ledgeriana Moens.	Rubiaceae
	Redbark Cinchona	Cinchona succirubra Pav.	Rubiaceae
JIN JI' ER (JIN QUE GEN)	Chinese Peashrub Root	Caragana sinica (Buc'hoz) Rehd.	Leguminosae
JIN JIN BANG	Sericeous Cinquefoil	Potentilla reptons L.var. sericophylla Franch.	Rosaceae
JIN JU	Meiwa Kumquat	Fortunella crassifolia Swingle	Rutaceae
	Oval Kumquat	Fortunella margarita (Lour.) Swingle	Rutaceae
JIN JU YE	Meiwa Kumquat Leaf	Fortunella crassifolia Swingle	Rutaceae
	Oval Kumquat Leaf	Fortunella margarita (Lour.) Swingle	Rutaceae
JIN LONG DAN CAO	Blin Conyza	Conyza blinii Lévl.	Conpositae
JIN MAO ER CAO	Goldhair Hedyotis	Hedyotis chrysotricha (Polib.) Merr. [= Oldenlandia chrysotricha (Polib.) Chun]	Rubiaceae
JIN PING GE NA XIANG	Leiocarpus Goniothalamus	Goniothalamus leiocarpus	Annonaceae
JIN QIAN CAO	Longtube Ground Ivy	Glechoma longituba (Nakai) Kurp.	Labiatae
JIN QIAN KU YE CAO	Goldsaxifrage Herb	Chrysosplenium grayanum Maxim.	Saxifragaceae
JIN QUE GEN (JIN JI' ER)	Chinese Peashrub Root	Caragana sinica (Buc'hoz) Rehd.	Leguminosae
JIN SHUA BA	Cladonia fallax Lichen	Cladonia fallax Abbayes	Cladoniaceae
JIN SI DAI	Green Alectoria Filament	Alectoria vivens Tayl.	Usneaceae
JIN SI TAO GUO SHI	Chinese St. John'swort Fruit	Hypericum chinense L.	Guttiferae
JIN YIN HUA	Glaucousback Honeysuckle	Lonicera hypoglauca Miq.	Captifoliaceae
	Japanese Honeysuckle	Lonicera japonica Thunb.	Captifoliaceae
	Wild Honeysuckle	Lonicera confusa DC.	Captifoliaceae

Index of Traditional Chinese Medicines by Chinese Name

TCM Name	Name in English	Origin Latin Name	Family
JIN YING ZI	Cherokee Rose	Rosa laevigata Michx.	Rosaceae
JIN YU	Crucian Carp	Carassium auratus (L.)	Cyprinidae
JIN ZHAN JU	Potmarigold Calendula	Calendula officinalis L.	Compositae
JING GU NU	Fungus-infected Rice Spike	Oryza sativa L. (The pathogen is Ustilaginoidea virens (Cke.) Tak.)	Gramineae
JING HONG GE NA XIANG	Cheliensis Goniothalamus	Goniothalamus cheliensis	Annonaceae
JING JIE	Fineleaf Schizonepeta	Schizonepeta tenuifolia (Benth.) Briq.	Labiatae
JING MI	Rice	Oryza sativa L.	Gramineae
JING TIAN SAN QI GEN	Aizoon Stonecrop Root	Sedum aizoon L.	Crassulaceae
JIU	Wine	-	-
JIU BI YING	Ovateleaf Holly	Ilex rotunda Thunb.	Aquifoliaceae
JIU CAI	Tuber Onion	Allium tuberosum Rottler	Liliaceae
JIU JIE CHA (CAO SHAN HU)	Glabrous Sarcandra	Sarcandra glabra (Thunb.) Nakai	Chloranthaceae
JIU LI XIANG	Common Jasminorange	Murraya paniculata (L.) Jacks.	Rutaceae
JIU XIANG CHONG	Aspongopus	Aspongopus chinensis Dallas	Pentatomidae
JU HE	Tangerine Seed	Citrus reticulata Blanco	Rutaceae
JU HUA	Florists Chrysanthemum Flower	Chrysanthemum morifolium Ramat.	Compositae
JU HUA HUANG LIAN	Yellowflower Corydalis	Corydalis pallida (Thunb.) Pers.	Papaveraceae
JU JIANG YE	Betel Pepper Leaf	Piper betle L.	Piperaceae
JU NA HUA	Southern Crapemyrtle	Lagerstroemia subcostata Koehne	Lythraceae
JU PI (CHEN PI)	Tangerine Pericarp	Citrus reticulata Blanco	Rutaceae
JU QU	Common Chicory	Cichorium intybus L.	Compositae
JU YE SAN QI	see SAN QI CAO		
JUAN BAI	Tamariskoid Spikemoss	Selaginella tamariscina (Beauv.) Spring	Selaginellaceae
JUAN YE BEI MU (of CHUAN BEI MU)	Tendrilleaf	Fritillaria cirrhosa D. Don	Liliaceae
JUE	Eastern Bracken Fern	Pteridium aquilinum (L.) Kuhn var. latiusculum (Desv.) Underw	Pteridaceae
JUE CHUANG	Creeping Rostellularia	Rostellularia procumbens (L.) Nees	Acanthaceae
JUE MING ZI	Sickle Senna Seed	Cassia tora L.	Leguminosae
JUN QIAN ZI	Dateplum Persimmon	Diaspyros lotus L.	Ebenaceae
KA MI	Siberian Nitraria	Nitraria Sibirica Pall.	Zygophyllaceae
KE TENG ZI	Climbing Entada Seed	Entada phaseoloides (L.) Merr.	Leguminosae
KONG QUE CAO	French Marigold Herb	Tagetes patula L.	Compositae
KONG XIN XIAN	Alligator Alternanthera	Alternanthera philoxeroides (Mart.) Griseb.	Amaranthaceae
KOU TOU CHONG	Burrowed Click Beetle	Pleonomus canaliculatus Faldermann	Elateridae
KU AO	Linearleaf Thistle	Cirsium chinense Gardn. et Champ.	Compositae
KU CAO (I)	Eelgrass Herb	Vallisneria spiralis L.	Hydrocharitaceae
KU DI DAN	Scabrous Elephantfoot	Elephantopus scaber L.	Compositae
KU DING CHA	Broadleaf Holly	Ilex latafolia Thunb.	Aquifoliaceae
	Chinese Holly	Ilex cornuta Lindl.	Aquifoliaceae
KU DOU ZI	Foxtail-like Sophora	Sophora alopecuroides L.	Leguminosae
KU GUA	Balsampear	Momordica charantia L.	Cucurbitaceae
KU GUA ZI	Balsampear Seed	Momordica charantia L.	Cucurbitaceae
KU HONG GU	Bitter Russula	Russula rosacea (Bull) Grray	Russulaceae
KU LA SUO LU HUI (of LU HUI)	Kulaso Aloe Dried Juice	Aloe vera L.	Liliaceae

TCM Name	Name in English	Origin Latin Name	Family
KU LIAN (CHUAN LIAN ZI)	Szechwan Chinaberry Fruit	Melia toosendan Sieb. et Zucc.	Meliaceae
KU LIAN PI	Chinaberry-tree Bark	Melia azedarach L.	Meliaceae
	Szechwan Chinaberry Bark	Melia toosendan Sieb. et Zucc.	Meliaceae
KU QIE	Bitter Nightshade	Solanum dulcamara L.	Solanaceae
KU SHEN	Lightyellow Sophora	Sophora flavescens Ait.	Leguminosae
KU SHEN SHI	Lightyellow Sophora Seed	Sophora flavescens Ait.	Leguminosae
KU SHENG	Chinese Dregea	Dregea sinensis Hemsl.	Asclepiadaceae
KU SHU PI	Indian Quassiawood	Picrasma quassioides (D.Don) Benn.	Simaroubaceae
KU TAN ZI	Thickfruit Millettia	Millettia pachycarpa Benth.	Leguminosae
KU ZHI	Downy Groundcherry	Physalis pubescens L.	Solanaceae
KUAI JING CAO SU	Tuberousroot Jerusalemsage	Phlomis tuberosa L.	Labiatae
KUAN DONG	see KUAN DONG HUA		
KUAN DONG HUA	Common Coltsfoot	Tussilago farfara L.	Compositae
KUAN YE QIANG HUO (of QIANG HUO)	Forbes Notopterygium	Notopterygium forbesii Boiss.	Umbelliferae
KUN BU	Kelp Thallus	Laminaria japonica Aresch.	Laminariaceae
	Tangle Thallus	Ecklonia kurome Okam.	Alariaceae
	Undaria	Undaria pinnatifida (Harv.) Sur.	Alariaceae
KUN MING JI XUE TENG GEN	Leatherleaf Millettia Root	Millettia reticulata Benth.	Leguminosae
KUN MING SHAN HAI TANG	Glaucousback Threewingnut	Tripterygium hypoglaucum (Lévl.) Hutch	Celastraceae
LA JIAO	Bush Redpepper	Capsicum frutescens L.	Solanaceae
LA MEI HUA	Wintersweet Immayure Flower	Chimonanthus praecox (L.) Link	Calycanthaceae
LAI FU	Garden Radish	Raphanus sativus L.	Cruciferae
LAI FU ZI	Garden Radish Seed	Raphanus sativus L.	Cruciferae
LANG DANG GEN	Black Henbane Root	Hyoscyamus niger L.	Solanaceae
LANG DANG ZI (TIAN XIAN ZI)	Black Henbane Seed	Hyoscyamus niger L.	Solanaceae
LANG DU	See RUI XIANG LANG DU, LANG DU DA JI, YUE XIAN DA JI:	Stellera chamaejasme L.; Euphorbia fischeriana Steud.; Euphorbia ebracteolata Hayata	(Thymelaeaceae) (Euphorbiaceae) (Euphorbiaceae)
LANG DU DA JI (of LANG DU)	Fischer Euphorbia	Euphorbia fischeriana Steud.	Euphorbiaceae
LANG YU PI	Chinese Elm Bark	Ulmus paruifolia Jacq.	Ulmaceae
LAO GUAN CAO	Common Heron's Bill Herb	Erodium stephanianum Willd.	Geraniaceae
	Wilford Cranesbill Herb	Geranium wilfordii Maxim.	Geraniaceae
LAO PO ZI ZHEN XIAN	Lopseed Herb	Phryma leptostachya L.	Phrymataceae
LAO SHU GUA	Common Caper	Capparis spinosa L.	Capparidaceae
LEI GONG QI	Common Broadlily	Clintonia alpina (Royle) Kunth	Liliaceae
LEI GONG TENG	Common Threewingnut	Tripterygium wilfordii Hook. f.	Celastraceae
LENG SHA BEI MU (of CHUAN BEI MU)	Delavay Fritillary	Fritillaria delavayi Franch.	Liliaceae
LI	Lambsquarters Juvenile	Chenopodium album L.	Chenopodiaceae
LI CHUN HUA	Corn Poppy	Papaver rhoeas L.	Papaveraceae
LI CHUN HUA GUO SHI	Corn Poppy Fruit	Papaver rhoeas L.	Papaveraceae
LI DOU	Capitateflower Velvetbean	Stizolobium capitatum (Sweet) O. Ktze.	Leguminosae

Index of Traditional Chinese Medicines by Chinese Name

TCM Name	Name in English	Origin Latin Name	Family
LI HE REN	Japanese Plum Kernel	Prunus salicina Lindl.	Rosaceae
LI JIANG QIAN HU	Likiang Hogfennel	Peucedanum govanianum (Wall) Benth ex C. B. Clarke var. bicolo Wolff	Umbellifera
LI LA GEN	Oriental Buckthorn Root	Rhamnus crenata Sieb. et Zucc.	Rhamnaceae
LI LU	Black Falsehellebore	Veratrum nigrum L.	Liliaceae
LI MU	Tibet Lyonia	Lyonia ovalifolia (Wall.) Drude	Ericaceae
LI SHU PI	Hairy Chestnut Bast	Castanea mollissima Bl.	Fagaceae
LI YE	Bretschneider Pear Leaf	Pyrus bretschneideri Rehd.	Rosaceae
	Sand Pear Leaf	Pyrus pyrifolia (Burm. F.) Nakai	Rosaceae
	Ussurian Pear Leaf	Pyrus ussuriensis Maxim.	Rosaceae
LI YU	Carp	Cyprinus carpio L.	Cyprinidae
LI YU DAN	Carp Gall	Cyprinus carpio L.	Cyprinidae
LI YU PI	Carp Skin	Cyprinus carpio L.	Cyprinidae
LI ZHI	Lychee	Litchi chinensis Sonn.	Sapindaceae
LI ZHI CAO	Common Sage Herb	Salvia plebeia R. Br.	Labiatae
LI ZHI HAO	Forrest Bugle	Ajuga forrestii Diels	Labiatae
LI ZHI HE	Lychee Seed	Litchi chinensis Sonn.	Sapindaceae
LI ZI	Japanese Plum	Prunus salicina Lindl.	Rosaceae
LIAN HUA	Chinaberry-tree Flower	Melia azedarach L.	Meliaceae
	Szechwan Chinaberry Flower	Melia toosendan Sieb. et Zucc.	Meliaceae
LIAN JIANG	Chinese Galangal	Alpinia chinensis Rosc.	Zingiberaceae
LIAN PENG CAO	Japanese Farfugium Herb	Farfugium japonicum (L.) Kitam.	Compositae
LIAN QIAO	Weeping Forsythia	Forsythia suspensa (Thunb.) Vahl	Oleaceae
LIAN SHENG GUI ZI HUA	Bloodflower Milkweed	Asclepias curassavica L.	Asclepiadaceae
LIAN YI	Hindu Lotus Spermoderm	Nelumbo nucifera Gaertn.	Nymphaeaceae
LIAN ZI	Hindu Lotus Seed	Nelumbo nucifera Gaertn.	Nymphaeaceae
LIAN ZI XIN	Hindu Lotus Plumule	Nelumbo nucifera Gaertn.	Nymphaeaceae
LIANG JUN	Armillariella Tabescens	Armillariella tabescens (Scop. ex Fr.) Sing.	Tricholomataceae
LIANG QI LIAO	Amphibious Knotweed	Polygonum amphibium L.	Polygonaceae
LIANG YE HUA PI	Shiningleaf Birch Bark	Betula luminifera H. Winkl.	Betulaceae
LIAO GAO BEN (of GAO BEN)	Jehol Ligusticum	Ligusticum jeholense Nakai et Kitag.	Umbelliferae
LIAO GE WANG GEN	Indian Stringbush Root	Wikstroemia indica (L.) C. A. Mey.	Thymelaeaceae
LIAO LAN (QING DAI)	Indigoplant	Polygonum tinctorium Ait.	Polygonaceae
LIE BAO ZI JING (ZI HUA YU DENG CAO)	Incised Corydalis	Corydalis incusa (Thunb.) Pers.	Papaveraceae
LIE DANG	Skyblue Broomrape	Orobanche coerulescens Steph.	Orobanchaceae
	Yellowflower Broomrape	Orobanche pycnostachya Hance	Orobanchaceae
LIE GUO SHU	Lobedfruit Tacca	Tacca plantaginea (Hance) Drenth.	Taccaceae
LIN BEI ZI	Field Lacquertree	Toxicodendron succedaneum (L.) O. Kuntze [= Rhus succedanea L.]	Anacardiaceae
LIN QIN	Chinese Pearleaf Crabapple	Malus asiatica Nakai	Rosaceae
LING	Singharanut	Trapa bispinosa Roxb	Trapaceae
LING LAN	Lilyofthevalley	Convallaria keiskei Miq. [= Convallaria majalis L.]	Liliaceae
LING MAO XIANG	Civet	Viverra zibetha L.	Viverridae
LING MU	Japanese Eurya	Eurya Japonica Thunb.	Theaceae

TCM Name	Name in English	Origin Latin Name	Family
LING ZHI CAO	See ZI ZHI,	Ganoderma japonicum (Fr.) Lloyd;	Polyporaceae
	CHI ZHI:	Ganoderma lucidum (Leyss. ex Fr.) Karst.	Polyporaceae
LIU BAI PI	Babylon Weeping Willow Root-bast	Salix babylonica L.	Salicaceae
LIU CHUAN YU	Yellow Toadflax	Linaria vulgaris Mill.	Scrophulariaceae
LIU SHAN	Chinese Cedar	Cryptomeria fortunei Hooibrenk	Taxodiaceae
LIU SU SHI HU (of SHI HU)	Eyeshaped Dendrobium	Dendrobium fimbriatum Hook. var. oculatum Hook.	Orchidaceae
LIU YE BAI QIAN	Willowleaf Swallowwort	Cynanchum stauntoni (Decne.) Schltr. ex Lévl.	Asclepiadaceae
LIU ZHI	Babylon Weeping Willow Branch	Salix babylonica L.	Salicaceae
LONG DAN	Linearleaf Gentian	Gentiana manshurica Kitagawa	Gentianaceae
	Rigescent Gentian	Gentiana rigescens Franch.	Gentianaceae
	Rough Gentian	Gentiana scabra Bunge	Gentianaceae
	Threeflower Gentian	Gentiana triflora Pall.	Gentianaceae
LONG KUI	Black Nightshade	Solanum nigrum L.	Solanaceae
LONG XIAN XIANG	Ammbergris	Physeter catodon L.	Physeteridae
LONG XU CAO (II)	Hard Bluegrass	Poa sphondylodes Trin.	Labiatae
LONG YA CAO GEN (XIAN HE CAO GEN)	Hairyvein Agrimonia Root	Agrimonia pilosa Ledeb. var. japonica (Miq.) Nakai	Rosaceae
LONG YAN DU HUO	Farges Aralia	Aralia fargesii Franch.	Araliaceae
LONG YAN YE	Longan Leaf	Euphoria longan (Lour.) Steud.	Sapindaceae
LOU LU	See QI ZHOU,	Rhaponticum uniflorum (L.) DC.;	(Compositae)
	HUA ZHOU LOU LU:	Echinops latifolus Tausch	(Compositae)
LU CAO	Japanese Hop Herb	Humulus scandens (Lour.) Merr.	Moraceae
LU DOU LE HUA	Thatch Screwpine Flower	Pandanus tectorius Soland.	Pandanaceae
LU GEN	Common Reed Rhizome	Phragmites communis Trin.	Gramineae
LU HUI	See KU LA SUO LU HUI,	Aloe vera L.;	(Liliaceae)
	HAO WANG JIAO LU HUI,	Aloe ferox Mill.;	(Liliaceae)
	BAN WEN LU HUI:	Aloe vera L. var. chinensis (Haw.) Berger	(Liliaceae)
LU JIAO CAI	Furcate Gloiopeltis Frond	Gloiopeltis furcata (Post. et Rupr.) J. Ag.	Endocladiaceae
LU RONG	Hairy Antler	Cervus nippon Temminck;	Cervidae
		Cervus elaphus L.	Cervidae
LU RUI WU TOU	Nakedstamen Monkshood	Aconitum gymnandrum Maxim	Ranunculaceae
LU SHOU CAO	Japanese Pyrola Herb	Pyrola japonica Klenze ex Alef.	Pyrolaceae
LU SHUI CAO (II)	Common Cyanotis	Cyanotis vaga (Lour.) Roem. et Schult.	Commelinaceae
LU SONG GUO	Ignat Poisonnut Seed	Strychnos ignatii Berg.	Loganiaceae
LU SONG QIU MAO	Kamalatree Pericarpial Glandular Hairs	Mallotus philippinensis (Lam.) Muell.-Arg.	Euphorbiaceae
LU SUN PIAN	Oldham Bamboo Shoot	Sinocalamus oldhami (Munro) Mcclure	Gramineae
LU XIAN CAO	Chinese Pyrola Herb	Pyrola rotundifolia L. subsp. chinensis H. Andres	Pyrolaceae
LU XIAN CAO	European Pyrola Herb	Pyrola rotundifolia L.	Pyrolaceae
LU ZHU GEN	Giantreed Rhizome	Arundo donax L.	Gramineae
LUAN HUA	Paniculate Goldraintree	Koelreuteria paniculata Laxm.	Sapindaceae
LUN HUAN TENG	Racemose Cyclea	Cyclea racemosa Oliv.	Menispermaceae

Index of Traditional Chinese Medicines by Chinese Name

TCM Name	Name in English	Origin Latin Name	Family
LUN SAN WU JIA PI (of WU JIA PI)	Verticillate Acanthopanax Root-bark	Acanthopanax verticillatus Hoo	Araliaceae
LUN SAN WU JIA YE (of WU JIA YE)	Verticillate Acanthopanax Leaf	Acanthopanax verticillatus Hoo	Araliaceae
LUN YE PO PO NA (ZHAN LONG JIAN)	Siberian Veronicastrum	Veronicastrum sibirica (L.) Pennell	Scroophulariacea e
LUO BU MA	Dogbane Herb	Apoynum venetum L.	Apocynaceae
LUO DI SHENG GEN	Air-plant Herb	Bryophyllum pinnatum (L. f.) Oken	Crassulaceae
LUO FU MU	Common Devilpepper	Rauwolfia verticillata (Lour.) Baill.	Apocynaceae
LUO FU MU JING YE	Common Devilpepper Stem and Leaf	Rauwolfia verticillata (Lour.) Baill.	Apocynaceae
LUO GUO DI	Largeseed Hemsleya	Hemsleya macrosperma C. Y. Wu	Cucurbitaceae
	Lovely Hemsleya	Hemsleya amabilis Diels	Cucurbitaceae
LUO HAN GUO	Grosvenor Siraitia	Siraitia grosvenorii (Swingle) C. Jeffrey ex Lu et Z. Y. Zhang [= Momordica grosvenorii Swingle]	Cucurbitaceae
LUO HAN SONG SHI	Chinese Podocarpus Seed	Podocarpus macrophyllus (Thunb.) D. Don var. maki (Sieb.) Endl.	Podocarpaceae
	Kusamaki Broadleaved Podocarpus Seed	Podocarpus macrophyllus (Thunb.) D. Don	Podocarpaceae
LUO HAN SONG YE	Chinese Podocarpus Leaf	Podocarpus macrophyllus (Thunb.) D. Don var. maki (Sieb.) Endl.	Podocarpaceae
	Kusamaki Broadleaved Podocarpus Leaf	Podocarpus macrophyllus (Thunb.) D. Don	Podocarpaceae
LUO HUA SHENG	Peanut	Arachis hypogaea L.	Leguminosae
LUO HUA SHENG YOU	Peanut Oil	Arachis hypogaea L.	Leguminosae
LUO HUA SHENG ZHI YE	Peanut Branch and Leaf	Arachis hypogaea L.	Leguminosae
LUO KUI HUA	Red Vinespinach	Basella rubra L.	Basellaceae
LUO LE	Basil Herb	Ocimum basilicum L.	Labiatae
LUO LE ZI	Basil Fruit	Ocimum basilicum L.	Labiatae
LUO MO	Japanese Metaplexis	Metaplexis japonica (Thunb.) Mak.	Asclepiadaceae
LUO MO ZI	Japanese Metaplexis Seed	Metaplexis japonica (Thunb.) Mak.	Asclepiadaceae
LUO QUN DAI GEN	Chinese Crinum Root	Crinum asiaticum L. var. sinicum Bak.	Amaryllidaceae
LUO SHI TENG	Chinese Starjasmine	Trachelospermum jasminoides (Lindl.) Lem.	Apocynaceae
LUO TUO CI (CI MI)	Manaplant Alhagi Sweet Secretion	Alhagi pseudalhagi Desv.	Leguminosae
LUO TUO PENG	Common Peganum Herb	Peganum harmala L.	Zygophyllaceae
LUO TUO PENG ZI	Common Peganum Seed	Peganum harmala L.	Zygophyllaceae
LUO XIN FU	Chinese Astilbe	Astilbe chinensis (Maxim.) Franch. et Sav.	Saxifragaceae
LUO XIN FU GEN	Chinesc Astilbe Root	Astilbe chinensis (Maxim.) Franch. et Sav.	Saxifragaceae
LUO YAN CAO	Littleleaf Lemmaphyyllum Herb	Lemmaphyllum microphyllum Presl	Polypodiaceae
MA BIAN CAO	European Verbena Herb	Verbena officinalis L.	Verbenaceae
MA BO	Bark-less Puff-ball	Saliosphaera fenzlii Reich.	Lycoperdaceae
	Large Puff-ball	Calvatia gigantea (Batsch ex Pers.) Lloye	Lycoperdaceae

Index of Traditional Chinese Medicines by Chinese Name

TCM Name	Name in English	Origin Latin Name	Family
	Purple Puff-ball	Calvatia linacina (Mont. et Berk.) Lloye	Lycoperdaceae
MA CHI XIAN	Purslane	Portulaca oleracea L.	Portulacaceae
MA DOU LING	Slender Dutchmanspipe	Aristolochia debilis Sieb. et Zucc.	Aristolochiaceae
MA DOU LING GEN (QING MU XIAN)	Northern Dutchmanspipe Root	Aristolochia contorta Bge.	Aristolochiaceae
	Slender Dutchmanspipe Root	Aristolochia debilis Sieb. et Zucc.	Aristolochiaceae
MA GUI HUA	Manynerve Embelia	Embelia oblongifolia Hemsl.	Myrsinaceae
MA HUA	Hemp Fimble	Cannabis sativa L.	Moraceae
MA HUANG	Chinese Ephedra	Ephedra sinica Stapf	Ephedraceae
	Intermediate Ephedra	Ephedra intermeddia Schrenk et Mey.	Ephedraceae
	Mongolian Ephedra	Ephedra equisetina Bge.	Ephedraceae
MA LIU YE	Chinese Wingnut	Pterocarya stenoptera DC.	Juglandaceae
MA QIAN ZI	Nut-vomitive Poisonnut	Strychnos nux-vomica L.	Loganiaceae
MA SANG	Chinese Coriaria	Coriaria sinica Maxim. [= Coriaria nepalensis Wall.]	Coriariaceae
MA SANG YE	Chinese Coriaria Leaf	Coriaria sinica Maxim.	Coriariaceae
MA TI YE	Common Marsharigold	Caltha palustris L.	Ranunculaceae
	Scapose Marsharigold	Caltha scaposa Hook. f. et Thoms	Ranunculaceae
MA TONG HUA	Sharptooth Incarvillea	Incarvillea arguta Royle	Bignoniaceae
MA WEI LIAN	Baikal Meadowrue	Thalictrum baicalense Turcz.	Ranunculaceae
	Manyleaf Meadowrue	Thalictrum foliolosum DC.	Ranunculaceae
MA YE	Hemp Fimble Leaf	Cannabis sativa L.	Moraceae
MA YI DAN	see WU SE MEI		
MAI DONG (MAI MEN DONG)	Dwarf Lilyturf	Ophiopogon japonicus (Thunb.) Ker-Gawl.	Liliaceae
MAI JIAO	Ergot	Claviceps purpurea (Fr.) Turasne	Clavicipitaceae
MAI MEN DONG (MAI DONG)	Dwarf Lilyturf	Ophiopogon japonicus (Thunb.) Ker-Gawl.	Liliaceae
MAI YA	Barley Germinating Fruit	Hordeum vulgare L.	Gramineae
MAN JING ZI	Simpleleaf Shrub Chastetree	Vitex rotundifolia L.	Verbenaceae
	Threeleaf Chastetree	Vitex trifolia L.	Verbenaceae
MAN JING ZI YE	Simpleleaf Shrub Chastetree Leaf	Vitex rotundifolia L.	Verbenaceae
	Threeleaf Chastetree Leaf	Vitex trifolia L.	Verbenaceae
MAN LI YU	Japanese Eel	Anguilla japonica Temminck et Schlegel	Anguillidae
MAN SHAN HONG	Dahurian Rhododendron	Rhododendron dauricum L.	Ericaceae
MAN TUO LUO GEN	Hairy Datura Root	Datura inoxia Mill.	Solanaceae
	Hindu Datura Root	Datura metel L.	Solanaceae
MAN TUO LUO YE	Hairy Datura Leaf	Datura inoxia Mill.	Solanaceae
	Hindu Datura Leaf	Datura metel L.	Solanaceae
MAN TUO LUO ZI	Hairy Datura Seed	Datura inoxia Mill.	Solanaceae
	Hindu Datura Seed	Datura metel L.	Solanaceae
MAN XING QIAN JIN BA	Philippine Flemingia	Flemingia philippinensis (Merr. et Rolfe) Li	Leguminosae
MANG GUO	Mango	Mongifera indica L.	Anacardiaceae
MANG GUO HE	Mango Seed	Mongifera indica L.	Anacardiaceae
MANG GUO SHU PI	Mango Bark	Mongifera indica L.	Anacardiaceae
MANG GUO YE	Mango Leaf	Mongifera indica L.	Anacardiaceae
MANG JING	Chinese Silvergrass	Miscanthus sinensis Anderss.	Gramineae

Index of Traditional Chinese Medicines by Chinese Name

TCM Name	Name in English	Origin Latin Name	Family
MANG SHE	Indian Python	Python molurus bivittatus Schlegel	Boidae
MAO BAI YANG	Chinese White Poplar	Populus tomentosa Carr.	Salicaceae
MAO CAO YE	Lalang Grass Leaf	Imperata cylindrica (L.) P. Beauv. var. major (Nees) C. E. Hubb.	Gramineae
MAO DA DING CAO	Pilose Gerbera	Gerbera piloselloides Cass.	Compositae
MAO DANG GUI (of DU HUO)	Pubescent Angelica	Angelica pubescens Maxim.	Umbelliferae
MAO GAO CAI	Lunate Peltate Sundew	Drosera peltata Smith var. lunata (Buch.-Ham.) C. B. Clarke	Droseraceae
MAO GEN	Japanese Buttercup	Ranunculus japonicus Thunb.	Ranunculaceae
MAO GENG HONG MAO WU JIA	Hispidus Girald Acanthopanax	Acanthopanax giraldii Harms var. hispidus Hoo	Araliaceae
MAO GENG XI XIAN (of XI XIAN)	Hairstalk St. Paulswort	Siegesbeckia orientalis L. var. glabrescens Mak. [= Siegesbeckia glabrescens Mak.]	Compositae
MAO GUAN ZHONG	Champion Wood Fern	Dryopteris championii (Benth.) C. Chr. ex Ching	Dryopteridaceae
MAO LIAN HAO	Hairy Wormwood	Artemisia vestita Wall.	Compositae
MAO MEI	Japanese Raspberry	Rubus parviforlius L.	Rosaceae
MAO RUI HUA	Flannel Mullein	Verbascum thapsus L.	Scrophulariaceae
MAO SHU	Winged Yam	Dioscorea alata L.	Dioscoreaceae
MAO XIAN ZHU JU TAI	Hairy Rhynchotechum	Rhynchotechum vestitum Hook. f. et Thoms.	Gesneriaceae
MAO XIANG HUA	Vanillagrass	Hierochloe odorata (L.) Beauv.	Gramineae
MAO XU CAO	Spicate Clerodendranthus	Clerodendranthus spicatus (Thunb.) C. Y. Wu	Labiatae
MAO YAN CAO	Crescent-shaped Euphorbia Herb	Euphorbia lunulata Bge.	Euphorbiaceae
MAO YE BA DOU	Tomentose Caudate Croton	Croton caudatus Geisel. var. tomentosus Hook.	Euphorbiaceae
MAO YE SANG JI SHENG (of SANG JI SHENG)	Yadirik Scurrula	Loranthus yadoriki Sieb.	Loranthaceae
MAO YE XIANG CHA CAI	Japanese Rabdosia	Rabdosia japonica (Burm. f.) Hara.	Labiatae
MAO ZHU MA QIAN	Hairstyle Poisonnut	Strychnos nitida G. Don	Loganiaceae
MEI GUI HUA	Rugose Rose	Rosa rugosa Thunb.	Rosaceae
MEI HE REN	Mumeplant (Japanese Apricot)	Prunus mume (Sieb.) Sieb. et Zucc.	Rosaceae
MEI HUA SHI HU (of SHI HU)	Loddiges Dendrobium	Dendrobium loddigesii Rolfe.	Orchidaceae
MEI LI HONG DOU SHAN	Maire Yew	Taxus mairei (Lemée et Lévl.) S. Y. Hu	Taxaceae
MEI LI ZHU SHI DOU	Beautiful Crotalaria	Crotalaria spectabilis Roth.	Leguminosae
MEI SHANG LU	American Pokeweed	Phytolacca americana L.	Phytolaccaceae
MENG GU CAO SU	Mongolian Jjerusalemsage	Phlomis mongolica Turcz.	Labiatae
MENG GU HUANG QI (of HUANG QI)	Mongolian Milkvetch	Astragalus mongholicus Bge.	Leguminosae
MENG GU LI	Mongolian Oak	Quercus mongolica Fisch.	Fagaceae
MENG GU SHAN LUO BO	Narrowleaf Scabious	Scabiosa comosa Fisch.	Dipsacaceae
MENG GU XIU XIAN JU	Mongolian Spiraea	Spiraea mongolica Maxim.	Rosaceae

Index of Traditional Chinese Medicines by Chinese Name

TCM Name	Name in English	Origin Latin Name	Family
MU LAN	True Indigo	Indigofera tinctoria L.	Leguminosae
MU LAN HUA	Lily Magnolia Flower	Magnolia liliflora Desr.	Magnoliaceae
MU LAN PI	Lily Magnolia Bark	Magnolia liliflora Desr.	Magnoliaceae
MU LI ROU	Oyster Meat	Ostrea rivularis Gould;	Osteridae
		Ostrea talienwhanensis Crosse;	Osteridae
		Ostrea gigas Thunberg	Osteridae
MU MA DOU	Lanceleaf Thermopsis	Thermopsis lanceolata R. Br.	Leguminosae
MU MIAN HUA	Common Bombax Flower	Gossampinus malabarica (DC.) Merr.	Bombacaceae
MU TIAN LIAO	Silvervine Actinidia	Actinidia polygama (Sieb. et Zucc.) Maxim.	Actinidiaceae
MU TONG	Fiveleaf Akebia	Akebia quinata (Thunb.) Decne.	Lardizabalaceae
MU TONG GEN	Austral Akebia Root	Akebia trifoliata (Thunb.) Koidz. var. australis (Diels) Rehd.	Lardizabalaceae
	Fiveleaf Akebia Root	Akebia quinata (Thunb.) Decne.	Lardizabalaceae
	Threeleaf Akebia Root	Akebia trifoliata (Thunb.) Koidz.	Lardizabalaceae
MU TONG MA DOU LING	see GUAN MU TONG		
MU XIANG	Common Aucklandia (Costustoot)	Saussurea lappa Clarke [= Aucklandia lappa Decne]	Compositae
	Common Vladimiria	Vladimiria souliei (Franch.) Ling	Compositae
	Denticulate Vladimiria	Vladimiria denticulata Ling	Compositae
MU XU	Alfalfa	Medicago sativa L.	Leguminosae
	California Burclover	Medicago hispida Gaertn.	Leguminosae
MU XU GEN	Alfalfa Root	Medicago sativa L.	Leguminosae
	California Burclover Root	Medicago hispida Gaertn.	Leguminosae
MU ZEI	Common Scouring Rush	Equisetum hiemale L.	Equisetaceae
NAN FANG TU SI ZI (of TU SI ZI)	South Dodder	Cuscuta australis R. Br.	Convolvulaceae
NAN GUA	Cushaw	Cucurbita moschata (Duch.) Poiret	Cucurbitaceae
NAN GUA ZI	Cushaw Seed	Cucurbita moschata (Duch.) Poiret	Cucurbitaceae
NAN LING QIAN HU	Nanling Hogfennel	Peucedanum longshengense Shan et Sheh	Umbelliferae
NAN MU	Nanmu Lignum	Phoebe nanmu (Oliv.) Gamble	Lauraceae
NAN SHE TENG GEN	Oriental Bittersweet Root	Celastrus orbiculatus Thunb.	Celastraceae
NAN SHE TENG YE	Oriental Bittersweet Leaf	Celastrus orbiculatus Thunb.	Celastraceae
NAN TIAN ZHU GEN	Common Nandina Root	Nandina domestica Thunb.	Berberidaceae
NAN TIAN ZHU GENG	Common Nandina Stem	Nandina domestica Thunb.	Berberidaceae
NAN TIAN ZHU ZI	Common Nandina Fruit	Nandina domestica Thunb.	Berberidaceae
NAN ZHU YE	Oriental Blueberry Leaf	Vaccinium bracteatum Thunb.	Ericaceae
NAO YANG HUA	Chinese Azalea Flower	Rhododendron molle (Bl.) G. Don	Ericaceae
NEI ZHE XIANG CHA CAI	Inflexed Rabdosia	Rabdosia inflexa (Thunb.) Hara	Labiatae
NEN YE JIU LI XIANG (2807-JIU LI XIANG)	Juvenileleaf Common Jasminorange	Murraya microphylla	Rutaceae
NI YU LONG WU TOU	Pseudostapfia Monkshood	Aconitum pseudosta pfianum W. T. Wang	Ranunculaceae
NIAN YE YOU	Glutinose Bluebeard	Caryopteris glutinosa Rehd.	Verbenaceae
NIAN YU XU	Siebold Greenbrier	Smilax sieboldi Miq.	Liliaceae
NIAO PAO CAO	Saline Swainsonia	Swainsonia salsula Taub.	Leguminosae
NING GUO BEI MU	Ningguo Fritillary	Fritillaria ningguoensis S. C. Chen et S. F. Yin	Liliaceae
NING MENG	Lemon	Citrus limon Burm.	Rutaceae
	Lemonlike Citrus	Citrus limonia Osbeck	Rutaceae

TCM Name	Name in English	Origin Latin Name	Family
NING MENG AN YE	Lemon eucalyptus Leaf	Eucalyptus citriodora Hook f.	Myrtaceae
NING MENG GEN	Lemon Root	Citrus limon Burm.	Rutaceae
	Lemonlike Citrus Root	Citrus limonia Osbeck	Rutaceae
NING MENG YE	Lemon Leaf	Citrus limon Burm.	Rutaceae
	Lemonlike Citrus Leaf	Citrus limonia Osbeck	Rutaceae
NING XIA BEI MU	Ningxia Fritillary	Fritillaria taipaiensis P. Y. Li var. ningxiaensis Y.K. Yang et.J.K.Wu	Liliaceae
NIU BANG GEN	Great Burdock Root	Arctium lappa L.	Compositae
NIU BANG ZI	Great Burdock Fruit	Arctium lappa L.	Compositae
NIU CHI	Ox Teeth	Bos taurus domesticus Gmelin; Bubalus bubalis Linnaeus	Bovidae Bovidae
NIU DAN	Ox Gall	Bos taurus domesticus Gmelin; Bubalus bubalis Linnaeus	Bovidae Bovidae
NIU ER DA HUANG	Crisped Dock	Rumex crispus L.	Polygonaceae
NIU ER FENG ZHI YE	Calyx-shaped Daphniphyllum Leaf	Daphniphyllum calycinum Benth.	Daphniphyllaceae
NIU ER FENG ZI	Calyx-shaped Daphniphyllum Fruit	Daphniphyllum calycinum Benth.	Daphniphyllaceae
NIU FEI	Ox Lung	Bos taurus domesticus Gmelin; Bubalus bubalis Linnaeus	Bovidae Bovidae
NIU GAN	Ox Liver	Bos taurus domesticus Gmelin; Bubalus bubalis Linnaeus	Bovidae Bovidae
NIU HUANG	Cow-bezoar (Ox-gallstone)	Bos taurus domesticus Gmelin; Bubalus bubalis Linnaeus	Bovidae Bovidae
NIU NAO	Ox Brain	Bos taurus domesticus Gmelin; Bubalus bubalis Linnaeus	Bovidae Bovidae
NIU RU	Cow Milk	Bos taurus domesticus Gmelin; Bubalus bubalis Linnaeus	Bovidae Bovidae
NIU SHE CAO	Toothedfruit Dock	Rumex dentatus L.	Polygonaceae
NIU SHE TOU	Field Sowthistle Herb	Sonchus arvensis L.	Compositae
NIU SHEN	Ox Kindey	Bos taurus domesticus Gmelin; Bubalus bubalis Linnaeus	Bovidae Bovidae
NIU XI	Twotooth Achyranthes	Achyranthes bidentata Bl.	Amaranthaceae
NIU XI XI	Patience Dock	Rumex patientia L.	Polygonaceae
NIU XIN FAN LI ZHI	Bullocksheart Custardapple	Annona reticulata L.	Annonaceae
NIU XIN QIE ZI	Common Cerberustree	Cerbera manghas L.	Apocynaceae
NIU XUE	Ox Blood	Bos taurus domesticus Gmelin; Bubalus bubalis Linnaeus	Bovidae Bovidae
NIU YE	Ox Thyroid	Bos taurus domesticus Gmelin; Bubalus bubalis Linnaeus	Bovidae Bovidae
NU ZHEN ZI	Glossy Privet Fruit	Ligustrum lucidum Ait.	Oleaceae
OU	Hindu Lotus Large Rhizome	Nelumbo nucifera Gaertn.	Nymphaeaceae
PAI QIAN CAO	Beautiful Phyllodium	Desmodium pulchellum (L.) Benth.	Leguminosae
PAI QIAN CAO GEN	Beautiful Phyllodium Root	Desmodium pulchellum (L.) Benth.	Leguminosae
PAO DAN GUO	Easter Heraldtrumpet	Beaumontia grandiflora Wall.	Apocynaceae
PAO NANG CAO	Common Physochlaina	Physochlaina physaloides (L.) G. Don	Solanaceae
PAO PAO CAO	Mountain Crazyweed	Oxytropis oxyphylla DC.	Leguminosae
PAO TONG (TONG MU)	Fortune Paulownia	Paulownia fortunei (Seem.) Hemsl.	Scrophulariaceae
	Royal Paulownia	Paulownia tomentosa (Thunb.) Steud.	Scrophulariaceae
PAO TONG GUO	Fortune Paulownia Fruit	Paulownia fortunei (Seem.) Hemsl.	Scrophulariaceae
	Royal Paulownia Fruit	Paulownia tomentosa (Thunb.) Steud.	Scrophulariaceae

Index of Traditional Chinese Medicines by Chinese Name

TCM Name	Name in English	Origin Latin Name	Family
PEI LAN	Fortune Eupatorium	Eupatorium fortunei Turcz.	Compositae
PEN JIA SHU	Prettyleaf Winchia	Winchia calophylla A. DC.	Apocynaceae
PENG E SHU (of YU JIN)	Zedoary Turmeric	Curcuma zedoaria (Berg.) Rosc.	Zingiberaceae
PENG LAI CAO	Knotteflower Phyla Herb	Lippia nodiflora (L.) L. C. Rich.	Verbenaceae
PENG XIAN XUE DAN	Pengxian Hemsleya	Hemsleya pengxianensis W. J. Chang	Cucurbitaceae
PENG ZI CAI	Yellow Bedstraw	Galium verum L.	Rubiaceae
PI HAN CAO	Daghestan Sweetclover Herb	Melilotus suaveolens Ledeb.	Leguminosae
PI JIU HUA	European Hop Female-flower	Humulus lupulus L.	Moraceae
PI PA HE	Loquat Seed	Eriobotrya japonica (Thunb.) Lindl.	Rosaceae
PI PA YE	Loquat Leaf	Eriobotrya japonica (Thunb.) Lindl.	Rosaceae
PIAO FU CAO	Dichotomous Fimbristylis	Fimbristylis dichotoma (L.) Vahl	Cyperaceae
PING BEI MU (of CHUAN BEI MU)	Ussuri Fritillary	Fritillaria ussuriensis Maxim.	Liliaceae
PING ER XIAO CAO	Adder's Tongue	Ophioglossum vulgatum L.	Ophioglossaceae
PO LUO MEN ZAO JIA	Goldenshower Senna Fruit	Cassia fistula L.	Leguminosae
PU DI WU GONG	Cernuous Clubmoss Herb	Lycopodium cernnum L.	Lycopodiaceae
PU ER CHA	Assam Tea	Camellia sinensis var. assamica (Masters) Kitamura	Theaceae
PU GE WU TOU	Pukee Monkshood	Aconitum pukeese W. T. Wang	Ranunculaceae
PU GONG YING	Mongolian Dandelion	Taraxacum mongolicum Hand.-Mazz.	Compositae
PU HUANG	Broadleaf Cattail Pollen	Typha latifolia L.	Typhaceae
	Longbract Cattail Pollen	Typha angustata Bory et Chaub.	Typhaceae
	Narrowleaf Cattail Pollen	Typha angustifolia L.	Typhaceae
PU TAO	European Grape	Vitis vinifera L.	Vitaceae
PU TAO TENG YE	European Grape Stem and Leaf	Vitis vinifera L.	Vitaceae
PU TI SHU HUA	Miquel Linden	Tilia miqueliana Maxim.	Tiliaceae
QI DUN GUO (YOU GAN LAN)	Common Olive	Olea europaea L.	Oleaceae
QI LIN CAI	Muriculate Eucheuma Frond	Eucheuma muricatum (Gmel.) Web. V. Bos.	Solieriaceae
QI YE DAN (JIAO GU LAN)	Fiveleaf Gynostemma	Gynostemma pentaphylla (Thunb.) Makino	Cucurbitaceae
QI ZHOU LOU LU (of LOU LU)	Uniflower Swisscentaury	Rhaponticum uniflorum (L.) DC.	Compositae
QI ZHOU YI ZHI HAO	Horseweed Fleabane	Erigeron canadensis L.	Compositae
QI ZI	True Lacquertree Seed	Rhus verniciflua Stokes	Anacardiaceae
QIAN CAO GEN	India Madder Root	Rubia cordifolia L.	Rubiaceae
QIAN CENG TA	Serrate Clubmoss	Huperzia serrata (Thunb.) Trev. [= Lycopodium serrayum Thunb.]	Huperziaceae
QIAN HU	Common Hogfennel	Peucedanum decursivum (Miq.) Maxim.	Umbelliferae
QIAN JIN TENG	Japanese Staphania	Stephania japonica (Thunb.) Miers	Menispermaceae
QIAN JIN ZI	Caper Euphorbia Seed	Euphorbia lathyris L.	Euphorbiaceae
QIAN LI GUANG	Climbing Groundsel	Senecio scandens Buch.-Ham.	Compositae
QIAN MA	Hempleaf Nettle	Urtica cannabina L.	Urticaceae
	Narrowleaf Nettle	Urtica angustifolia Fisch. ex Hornem.	Urticaceae
QIAN NIU ZI	Lobedleaf Pharbitis Seed	Pharbitis nil (L.) Choisy	Convolvulaceae
	Roundleaf Pharbitis Seed	Pharbitis purpurea (L.) Voigt	Convolvulaceae
QIAN QU CAI	Spiked Loosestrife	Lythrum salicaria L.	Lythraceae

Index of Traditional Chinese Medicines by Chinese Name

TCM Name	Name in English	Origin Latin Name	Family
QIAN RI HONG	Globeamaranth	Gomphrena globosa L.	Amaranthaceae
QIANG HUO	Incised Notopterygium	Notopterygium incisum Ting ex H. T. Chang	Umbelliferae
QIANG WEI GEN	Japanese Rose Root	Rosa multiflora Thunb.	Rosaceae
QIAO MAI	Common Buckwheat	Fagopyrum esculentum Moench	Polygonaceae
QIAO MAI JIE	Common Buckwheat Stem	Fagopyrum esculentum Moench	Polygonaceae
QIAO MU CI TONG	Himalayan Coralbean	Erythrina arborescens Roxb.	Leguminosae
QIAO MU ZI ZHU	Tree Beautyberry	Callicarpa arborea Roxb.	Verbenaceae
QIE YE	Garden Eggplant Leaf	Solanum melongena L.	Solanaceae
QIE ZI	Garden Eggplant	Solanum melongena L.	Solanaceae
QIN HUA	Javan Waterdropwort Flower	Oenanthe javanica (Bl.) DC.	Umbelliferae
QIN JIAO	Dahuria Gentian	Gentiana dahurica Fisch.	Gentianaceae
	Largeleaf Gentian	Gentiana macrophylla Pall.	Gentianaceae
	Straw-coloured Gentian	Gentiana straminea Maxim.	Gentianaceae
	Thickstemen Gentian	Gentiana crassicaulis Duthie ex Burkill	Gentianaceae
	Tibet Gentian	Gentiana tibetica King	Gentianaceae
QIN LING ZHU ZI SHEN	Largeleaf JapaneseGinseng	Panax japonicus var. major (Burk.) Wu et Feng	Arliaceae
QIN PI	Bunga Ash Bark	Fraxinus bungeana DC.	Oleaceae
	Chinese Ash Bark	Fraxinus chinensis Roxb.	Oleaceae
	Largeleaf Chinese Ash Bark	Fraxinus rhynchophylla Hance	Oleaceae
	Pax Ash Bark	Fraxinus paxiana Lingelsh	Oleaceae
QING DAI (LIAO LAN)	Indigoplant	Polygonum tinctorium Ait.	Polygonaceae
QING FENG TENG	Chinese Diploclisia	Diploclisia chinensis Merr.	Menispermaceae
	Japanese Sabia	Sabia japonica Maxim.	Sabiaceae
	Orientvine	Sinomenium acutum (Thunb.) Rehd. et Wils.	Menispermaceae
QING HAO	Celery Wormwood	Artemisia apiacea Hance	Compositae
	Sweet Wormwood	Artemisia annua L.	Compositae
QING HUA JIAO (of HUA JIAO)	Peppertree Pricklyash	Zanthoxylum schinifolium Sieb. et Zucc.	Rutaceae
QING MU XIAN (MA DOU LING GEN)	Northern Dutchmanspipe Root	Aristolochia contorta Bge.	Aristolochiaceae
	Slender Dutchmanspipe Root	Aristolochia debilis Sieb. et Zucc.	Aristolochiaceae
QING NIANG ZI	Mung Bean Blister Beetle	Lytta caraganae Pallas	Meloidae
QING QIAN LIU (TIAN CHA SHU)	Roundwingfruit Cyclocarya	Cyclocarya paliurus (Batal.) Iljinskaja	Juglandaceae
QING TAN XIANG	Japanese Snailseed Stem	Cocculus trilobus (Thunb.) DC.	Menispermaceae
QING WA	Pond Frog	Rana nigromaculata Hallowell;	Ranidae
		Rana plancyi Lataste	Ranidae
QING WA DAN	Pond Frog Gall	Rana nigromaculata Hallowell;	Ranidae
		Rana plancyi Lataste	Ranidae
QIU FENG MU	javan Bishopwood	Bischofia javanica Bl.	Euphorbiaceae
QIU HUA NIU NAI CAI	Globose Condorvine	Marsdenia globifera Tsiang	Asclepiadaceae
QIU MU GUA	Common Floweringquince	Chaenomeles speciosa (Sweet) Nakai	Rosaceae
QIU YIN	Earthworm	Pheretima aspergillum (E. Perrier);	Megascolecidae
		Allolobophora caliginosa trapezoides (Ant. Duges)	Lumbricidae
QU MAI	Chinese Pink	Dianthus chinensis L.	Caryophyllaceae

Index of Traditional Chinese Medicines by Chinese Name

Index of Traditional Chinese Medicines by Chinese Name

TCM Name	Name in English	Origin Latin Name	Family
SHAN YAO	Common Yam	Dioscorea opposita Thunb.	Dioscoreaceae
	Winged Yam	Dioscorea alata L.	Dioscoreaceae
SHAN YE WAN DOU	Broadleaf Vetch	Vicia amoena Fisch.	Leguminosae
SHAN YING TAO	Downy Cherry	Prunus tomentosa Thunb.	Rosaceae
SHAN YOU MA	Diels Trema	Trema dielsiana Hard.-Mazz.	Ulmaceae
SHAN ZHA	Chinese Hawthorn	Crataegus pinnatifida Bge.	Rosaceae
	Nippon Hawthorn	Crataegus cuneata Sieb. et Zucc.	Rosaceae
	Red Fruit	Crataegus pinnatifida Bge. var. major N. E. Br.	Rosaceae
SHAN ZHA YE	Chinese Hawthorn Leaf	Crataegus pinnatifida Bge.	Rosaceae
	Nippon Hawthorn Leaf	Crataegus cuneata Sieb. et Zucc.	Rosaceae
	Red Fruit Leaf	Crataegus pinnatifida Bge. var. major N. E. Br.	Rosaceae
SHAN ZHI MA	Narrowleaf Screwtree	Helicteres angustifolia L.	Sterculiaceae
SHAN ZHI ZI	see ZHI ZI		
SHAN ZHU YU	Asiatic Cornelian Cherry (Common Macrocarpium)	Cornus Officinalis Sieb. et Zucc. [= Macrocarpium officinalis (Sieb. et Zucc.) Nakai]	Cornaceae
SHAN ZHU ZI	Manyflower Garcinia	Garcinia multiflora Champ.	Guttiferae
SHANG LU	Indian Pokeweed	Phytolacca esculenta Van Houtte [= Phytolacca acinosa Roxb.]	Phytolaccaceae
SHAO YAO (of CHI SHAO YAO)	Common Peony (wild)	Paeonia lactiflora Pall.	Ranunculaceae
SHE BAI ZI	Wild Spikenard	Hyptis suaveolens Poit	Labiatae
SHE CHUANG ZI	Common Cnidium	Cnidium monnieri (L.) Cusson	Umbelliferae
SHE GAN	Blackberrylily	Belamcanda chinensis (L.) DC.	Iridaceae
SHE GEN CAO	Japanese Ophiorrhiza	Ophiorrhiza japonica Bl.	Rubiaceae
SHE MEI	Indian Mockstrawberry	Duchesnea indica (Andr.) Focke	Rosaceae
SHE PU TAO	Ampelopsis	Ampelopsis brevipedunculata (Maxim.) Trautv.	Vitaceae
SHE TUI	Snake Slough	Elaphe taeniurus Cope;	Colubredae
		Elaphe carinata;	Colubredae
		Zaocys dhumnades;	Colubredae
		Dinodon rufozonatum	Colubredae
SHE XIANG	Abelmusk	Moschus moschiferus L.;	Cervidae
		Moschus berezovskii Flerov.;	Cervidae
		Moschus sifanicus Przewalski	Cervidae
SHE XIANG CAO	Thyme	Thymus vulgaris L.	Labiatae
SHEN HUANG DOU	Jointwood Senna	Cassia nodosa L.	Leguminosae
SHEN JIN CAO	Common Japanese Clubmoss	Lycopodium clavatum L.	Lycopodiaceae
SHENG GU YOU	Bumalda Bladdernut	Staphylea bumalda DC.	Staphyleaceae
SHENG HONG JI	Tropic Ageratum	Ageratum conyzoides L.	Compositae
SHENG JIANG	Fresh Common Ginger	Zingiber officinale Rosc.	Zingiberaceae
SHENG MA	Skunk Bugbane	Cimicifuga foetida L.	Ranunculaceae
SHENG QI	Lacquer	Rhus verniciflua Stokes	Anacardiaceae
SHENG TENG	Common Stelmatocrypton	Stelmatocrypton khasianum (Benth.) H. Baill.	Asclepiadaceae
SHI CHANG PU	Grassleaf Sweetflag	Acorus gramineus Soland.	Araceae
SHI CHANG PU YE	Grassleaf Sweetflag Leaf	Acorus gramineus Soland.	Araceae
SHI CHUN	Lettuce Ulva Frond	Ulva lactuca L.	Ulvaceae
	Pertusate Ulva Frond	Ulva pertusa Kjellm.	Ulvaceae

Index of Traditional Chinese Medicines by Chinese Name

TCM Name	Name in English	Origin Latin Name	Family
SHI DA GONG LAO MU	Chinese Mahonia	Mahonia fortunei (Lindl.) Fedde	Berberidaceae
	Japanese Mahonia	Mahonia japonica (Thunb.) DC.	Berberidaceae
	Leatherleaf Mahonia	Mahonia bealei (Fort.) Carr.	Berberidaceae
SHI DA GONG LAO YE	Chinese Mahonia Leaf	Mahonia fortunei (Lindl.) Fedde	Berberidaceae
	Japanese Mahonia Leaf	Mahonia japonica (Thunb.) DC.	Berberidaceae
	Leatherleaf Mahonia Leaf	Mahonia bealei (Fort.) Carr.	Berberidaceae
SHI DA GONG LAO ZI	Chinese Mahonia Fruit	Mahonia fortunei (Lindl.) Fedde	Berberidaceae
	Japanese Mahonia Fruit	Mahonia japonica (Thunb.) DC.	Berberidaceae
	Leatherleaf Mahonia Fruit	Mahonia bealei (Fort.) Carr.	Berberidaceae
SHI DI	Persimmon Persistent Calyx	Diospyros kaki L. f.	Ebenaceae
SHI DIAO LAN	Fewflower Lysionotus	Lysionotus paucylora Maxim.	Gesneriaceae
SHI GAO	Gypsum Fibrosum	Calcium sulphate, $CaSO_4$symbol 215 \f "Symbol" \s 8·}H_2O.	
SHI GEN	Persimmon Root	Diospyros kaki L. f.	Ebenaceae
SHI HU	Noble Dendrobium	Dendrobium nobile Lindl.	Orchidaceae
SHI HUA	Parmelia Lichen	Parmelia saxatilis Ach.	Parmeliaceae
SHI JI NING	Scabrous Mosla	Mosla scabra (Thunb.) C. Y. Wu et H. W. Li	Labiatae
SHI JUN ZI	Rangooncreeper	Quisqualis indica L.	Combretaceae
SHI JUN ZI YE	Rangooncreeper Leaf	Quisqualis indica L.	Combretaceae
SHI LA HONG	Fish Pelargonium	Pelargonium hortorum Bailey	Geraniaceae
SHI LI ZI	Belgaum Walnut Seed	Aleurites moluccana (L.) Willd.	Labiatae
SHI LIU GEN	Pomegranate Root	Punica granatum L.	Punicaceae
SHI LIU PI	Pomegranate Peel	Punica granatum L.	Punicaceae
SHI LONG RUI	Poisonous Buttercup	Ranunculus sceleratus L.	Ranunculaceae
SHI LUO ZI	Dill Fruit	Anethum graveolens L.	Umbelliferae
SHI NAN YE	Chinese Photinia Leaf	Photinia serrulata Lindl.	Rosaceae
SHI QI	Immature Persimmon Fruit Juice	Diospyros kaki L. f.	Ebenaceae
SHI RUI	Reindeer Moss	Cladonia rangiferina Web.	Cladoniaceae
SHI SHUA BA	Nude Fern	Psilotum nudum (L.) Griseb.	Psilotaceae
SHI SUAN	Shorttube Lycoris	Lycoris radiata (L'Her.) Herb.	Amaryllidaceae
SHI WEI	Felthair pyrrosia frond	Pyrrosia drakeana (Franch.) Ching	Polypodiaceae
	Japanese Felt Fern Frond	Pyrrosia lingua (Thunb.) Farw.	Polypodiaceae
	Peking pyrrosia frond	Pyrrosia davidii (Gies.) Ching	Polypodiaceae
	Petioled pyrrosia frond	Pyrrosia petiolosa (Christ) Ching	Polypodiaceae
	Shearer's Pyrrosia Frond	Pyrrosia sheareri (Bak.) Ching	Polypodiaceae
	Southwest pyrrosia frond	Pyrrosia gralla (Gies.) Ching	Polypodiaceae
SHI XIANG ROU	Chinese Orthodon	Orthodon chinensis (Maxim.) Kudo	Labiatae
SHI YE	Persimmon Leaf	Diospyros kaki L. f.	Ebenaceae
SHI ZHI JIA	Stringy Stonecrop	Sedum sarmentosum Bge.	Crassulaceae
SHI ZHU YU (CHU YE HUA JIAO)	Ailanthus-like Pricklyash	Zanthoxylum ailanthoides Sieb. et Zucc.	Rutaceae
SHI ZI	Persimmon	Diospyros kaki L. f.	Ebenaceae
SHOU ZHANG SHEN	Conic Gymnadenia	Gymnadenia conopsea R. Br.	Orchidaceae
	Crassnerve Gymnadenia	Gymnadenia crassinervis Finet	Orchidaceae
SHU HUA SHI HU (of SHI HU)	Goldenflower Dendrobium	Dendrobium chrysanthum Wall.	Orchidaceae
SHU KUI HUA	Hollyhock Flower	Althaea rosea (L.) Cav.	Malvaceae

Index of Traditional Chinese Medicines by Chinese Name

TCM Name	Name in English	Origin Latin Name	Family
SHU KUI YE	Hollyhock-like Yam Rhizome	Dioscorea althaeoira Kunth sp. Nov.	Dioscoreaceae
SHU LI	Davurian Buckthorn	Rhamnus davurica Pall.	Rhamnaceae
SHU MI	Broomcorn Millet	Panicum miliaceum L	Gramineae
SHU QU CAO	Cudweed	Gnaphalium affine D. Don	Compositae
SHU ZHANG LAO GUAN CAO	Siberian Cranesbill	Geranium sibiricum L.	Geraniaceae
SHUANG BIAN GUA LOU	Oneflower Snakegourd	Trichosanthes rosthornii Harms [= Trichosanthes Uniflora Hao]	Cucurbhitaceae
SHUI CAI	Bogbean	Menyanthcs trifoliata L.	Gentianaceae
SHUI CAI GEN	Bogbean Gen	Menyanthes trifoliata L.	Gentianaceae
SHUI CHAO YANG	Aquatic-sunflower Inula	Inula helianthus-aguatica C. Y. Wu ex Ling	Compositae
SHUI GUI JIAO YE	Tropical American Hymenocallis Leaf	Hymenocallis americana Roem.	Amaryllidaceae
SHUI HU LU	Common Waterhyacinth	Eichhornia crassipes Solms	Pontederiaceae
SHUI HU MAN	Unarmed Glorybower	Clerodendron inerme (L.) Gaertn.	Verbenaceae
SHUI HUANG YANG MU	Caudate Milkwort	Polygala caudata Rehd. et Wils.	Polygalaceae
SHUI HUI XIANG	Winked Marshweed	Limnophila rugosa (Roth) Merr.	Scrophulariaceae
SHUI JIE GU DAN	Hairy Willowweed	Epilobium hirsutum L.	Onagraceae
SHUI JINGLAN	Indianpipe	Monotropa uniflora L.	Pyrolaceae
SHUI LIAO	Red-knees	Polygonum hydropiper L.	Polygonaceae
SHUI LIU DOU	Poongaoil Pongamia	Pongamia pinnata (L.) Merr.	Leguminosae
SHUI LONG GU	Japanese Polypody	Polypodium niponicum Mett.	Polypodiaceae
SHUI MA TIAO	Thunberg Knotweed	Polygonum thunbergii Sieb. et Zucc.	Polygonaceae
SHUI MAN QING	Dilatata Speedwell	Veronica linariifolia Pall. ex Link. subsp. dilatata (Nakai et Kitagawa) Hong	Scroophulariacea e
SHUI MU CAO	Cuspidate Mnium Herb	Mnium cuspidatum Hedw.	Mniaceae
SHUI NIU JIAO	Buffalo Horn	Bubalus bubalis L.	Bovidae
SHUI QIE	Water Nightshade	Solanum torvum Sw.	Solanaceae
SHUI QIN	Javan Waterdropwort	Oenanthe javanica (Bl.) DC.	Umbelliferae
SHUI SONG	Fragile Codium Frond	Codium fragile (Sur.) Har.	Codiaceae
SHUI TUAN HUA	Pilular Adina	Adina pilulifera (Lam.) Franch. ex Drake	Rubiaceae
SHUI XIAN CAO	Corymbose Hedyotis	Oldenlandia corymbosa L. [= Hedyotis corymbosa (L.) Lam.]	Rubiaceae
SHUI XIAN GEN	Chinese Narcissus Bulb	Narcissus tazeyya L. var. chinensis Roem.	Amaryllidaceae
SHUI XIAN HUA	Chinese Narcissus Flower	Narcissus tazeyya L. var. chinensis Roem.	Amaryllidaceae
SHUI YANG MEI (I)	Japanese Avens	Geum japonicum Thunb.	Rosaceae
SHUI YANG MEI (I) GEN	Japanese Avens Root	Geum japonicum Thunb.	Rosaceae
SHUI YANG MEI (II)	Thinleaf Adina	Adina rubella (Sieb. et Zucc.) Hance	Rubiaceae
SHUI YANG MU BAI PI	Bitter Willow Bast	Salix purpurea L.	Salicaceae
SHUI YANG ZHI YE	Bitter Willow Branch and Leaf	Salix purpurea L.	Salicaceae
SHUI ZHI	Bigflower Cape Jasmine	Gardenia jasminoides Ellis var. grandiflora Nakai	Rubiaceae

Index of Traditional Chinese Medicines by Chinese Name

TCM Name	Name in English	Origin Latin Name	Family
SHUI ZHI YE	Bigflower Cape Jasmine Leaf	Gardenia jasminoides Ellis var. grandiflora Nakai	Rubiaceae
SI CHUAN LUN HUAN TENG	Szechwan Cyclea	Cyclea sutchuenensis Gagnep.	Menispermaceae
SI GUA	Singkwa Towelgourd	Luffa acutangula Roxb	Cucurbitaceae
	Suakwa Vegetablesponge	Luffa cylindrica (L.) Roem.	Cucurbitaceae
SI GUA TENG	Singkwa Towelgourd Stem	Luffa acutangula Roxb	Cucurbitaceae
	Suakwa Vegetalesponge Stem	Luffa cylindrica (L.) Roem.	Cucurbitaceae
SI GUA ZI	Singkwa Towelgourd Seed	Luffa acutangula Roxb	Cucurbitaceae
	Suakwa Vegetalesponge Seed	Luffa cylindrica (L.) Roem.	Cucurbitaceae
SI JI QING (DONG QING)	Purpleflower Holly	Ilex chinensis Sims [= Ilex purpurea]	Aquifoliaceae
SI MAO TENG	Longeared Epigynum	Epigynum auritum (Schneid.) Tsiang et P. T. Li	Apocynaceae
SI MIAN MU	Winterberry Euonymus	Euonymus bungeanus Maxim.	Celastraceae
SONG LUO	Diffract Usnea Filament	Usnea diffracta Vain.	Usneaceae
	Long Usnea Filament	Usnea longissima Ach.	Usneaceae
SONG MU BAI PI	Japanese Aralia	Aralia chinensis L.	Arliaceae
SONG PAN WU TOU	Sungpan Monkshood	Aconitum sungpanense Handsymbol 45 \f "Symbol" \s 8-Mazz	Ranunculaceae
SONG XIANG	Colophony	Pinus massoniana Lamb.	Pinaceae
SONG XUN	Pine Mushroom	Armillaria matsutake Ito et Imai	Tricholomataceae
SONG YE FANG FENG (of FANG FENG)	Yunnan Seseli	Seseli yunnanense Franch.	Umbelliferae
SONG YE QIAN LI GUANG	Pineleaf Groundsel	Senecio abrotanifolius L.	Compositae
SU HE XIANG	Oriental Sweetgum Resin	Liquidambar orientalis Mill.	Hamamelidaceae
SU MI	Foxtail Millet	Setaria italica (L.) Beauv.	Gramineae
SU MU	Sappan Caesalpinia	Caesalpinia sappan L.	Leguminosae
SU TIE SHU GUO (TIE SHU GUO)	Sago Seed	Cycas revoluta Thunb.	Cycadaceae
SU TIE YE (FENG WEI JIAO YE)	Sago Frond	Cycas revoluta Thunb.	Cycadaceae
SUAN JIANG	Franchet Groundcherry	Physalis alkekengi L. var. franchetii (Mast.) Mak.	Solanaceae
SUAN JIANG GEN	Franchet Groundcherry Root	Physalis alkekengi L. var. franchetii (Mast.) Mak.	Solanaceae
SUAN JIAO	Tamarind Fruit	Tamarindus indica L.	Leguminosae
SUAN MO	Garden Sorrel	Rumex acetosa L.	Polygonaceae
SUAN MO YE	Garden Sorrel Leaf	Rumex acetosa L.	Polygonaceae
SUAN SHI LIU	Pomegranate	Punica granatum L.	Punicaceae
SUAN SHUI CAO	Thorowort Pondweed	Potamogeton perfoliatus L.	Potamogetonaceae
SUAN ZAO	Spine Data	Ziziphus spinosus Hu	Rhamnaceae
SUAN ZAO REN	Common Jujube Seed	Ziziphus jujuba Mill. var. spinosa (Bunge) Hu ex H. F. Chow [= Zyziphs jujuba Miller]	Rhamnaceae
SUI GU ZI (DAN ZHU YE GEN)	Common Lophatherum Root	Lophatherum gracile Brongn.	Gramineae
SUO LA MU	Prinos-like salacia	Salacia prinoides DC.	Hippocrateaceae

Index of Traditional Chinese Medicines by Chinese Name

TCM Name	Name in English	Origin Latin Name	Family
SUO LUO ZI	Chinese Buckeye Seed	Aesculus chinensis Bge.	Hippocastanaceae
	Japanese Buckeye Seed	Aesculus Turbinata BL.	Hippocastanaceae
	Wilson Buckeye Seed	Aesculus wilsonee Rehd.	Hippocastanaceae
TAI BAI HUA	Stellate Cladonia Fruticose Thallus	Cladonia stellaris (Opiz.) Pouzar et Vezda [= Cladonia alpestris (L.) Rabht.]	Cladoniaceae
TAI BAI SONG MU	Taibaien Aralia	Aralia taibaiensis Z. Z. Wang et H. C. Zheng	Arliaceae
TAI SHAN YAN FU MU	Taishan Sumac	Rhus taishanensis S. B. Liang sp. nov	Anacardiaceae
TAI WAN JIU LI XIANG	Taiwan Common Jasminorange	Murraya crenulata	Rutaceae
TAI ZI SHEN	Heterophylla Falsestarwort	Pseudostellaria heterophylla (Miq.) Pax ex Pax et Hoffm.	Caryophyllaceae
TAN XIANG	Sandalwood	Santalum album L.	Santalaceae
TANG JIE	Diffuse Erysimum	Erysimum diffusum Ehrh.	Cruciferae
TANG LI	Birchleaf Pear	Pyrus betulaefolia Bge.	Rosaceae
TAO ER QI	Common Sinopodophyllm	Podophyllum emodi Wall. var. chinense Sprague	Berberidaceae
TAO GEN	David Peach Root	Prunus davidiana (Carr.) Franch.	Rosaceae
	Peach Root	Prunus persica (L.) Batsch.	Rosaceae
TAO HUA	David Peach Flower	Prunus davidiana (Carr.) Franch.	Rosaceae
	Peach Flower	Prunus persica (L.) Batsch.	Rosaceae
TAO JIAO	David Peach Resin	Prunus davidiana (Carr.) Franch.	Rosaceae
	Peach Resin	Prunus persica (L.) Batsch.	Rosaceae
TAO JIN NIANG	Rosemyrtle	Rhodomyrtus tomentosa (Ait.) Hassk.	Myrtaceae
TAO JING BAI PI	David Peach Bast	Prunus davidiana (Carr.) Franch.	Rosaceae
	Peach Bast	Prunus persica (L.) Batsch.	Rosaceae
TAO NAN GUA	Peachliking Pumpkin	Cucurbita pepo L. var. akoda Mak.	Cucurbitaceae
TAO REN	Peach	Prunus persica (L.) Batsch.	Rosaceae
TAO YE	David Peach Leaf	Prunus davidiana (Carr.) Franch.	Rosaceae
	Peach Leaf	Prunus persica (L.) Batsch.	Rosaceae
TAO ZHI	David Peach Juvenile Branch	Prunus davidiana (Carr.) Franch.	Rosaceae
	Peach Juvenile Branch	Prunus persica (L.) Batsch.	Rosaceae
TENG HUANG	Gamboge Tree Resin	Garcinia morella Desv.	Guttiferae
TIAN CHA SHU (QING QIAN LIU)	Roundwingfruit Cyclocarya	Cyclocarya paliurus (Batal.) Iljinskaja	Juglandaceae
TIAN CHEN	Sweet Orange	Citrus sinensis (L.) Osbeck	Rutaceae
TIAN CONG	Woolly Philydrum	Philydrum lanuginosum Banks	Phylydraceae
TIAN HUA FEN (GUA LOU GEN)	Mongolian Snakegourd Root	Trichosanthes kirilowii Maxim.	Cucurbitaceae
	Rosthorn Snakegourd Root	Trichosanthes rosthornii Harms	Cucurbitaceae
TIAN JIAO BAN	Chinese Aucuba	Aucuba chinensis Benth.	Cornaceae
TIAN MA	Tall Gastrodia	Gastrodia clata Blume	Orchidaceae
TIAN MEN DONG	Cochinchinese Asparagus	Asparagus cochinchinensis (Lour.) Merr.	Liliaceae
TIAN MING JING	Common Carpesium	Carpesium abrotanoides L.	Compositae
TIAN MING JING (HE SHI)	Common Carpesium Fruit	Carpesium abrotanoides L.	Compositae

Index of Traditional Chinese Medicines by Chinese Name

TCM Name	Name in English	Origin Latin Name	Family
TU SAN QI	Chrusanthemum-like Groundsel Herb	Senecio chrysanthemoides DC.	Compositae
TU SHA REN	Japanese Galangal	Alpinia japonica Miq.	Zingiberaceae
TU SI ZI	Chinese Dodder Seed	Cuscuta chinensis Lam.	Convolvulaceae
TU XIANG FEI (SAN JIAN SHAN ZI)	Chinese Plumyew Seed	Cephalotaxus sinesis (Rehd. et Wils.) Li	Cephalotaxaceae
	Fortune Plumyew Seed	Cephalotaxus fortunei Hook. f.	Cephalotaxaceae
TU XIANG RU	Common Origanum	Origanum vulgare L.	Labiatae
TUN CAO	Common Ragweed	Ambrosia artemisiifolia L.	Compositae
TUN XING GUO	Topeng Pygeum	Pygeum topengii Merr.	Rosaceae
WA ER TENG	Manyflower Tylophora	Tylophora floribunda Miq.	Asclepiadaceae
WA MAI DING GONG TENG	Wamai Erycibe	Erycibe elliptilimba Merr. et Chun	Convolvulaceae
WA WEI	Thunberg's Lepisorus	Lepisorus thunbergianus (Kaulf.) Ching	Polypodiaceae
WAN DOU	Garden Pea	Pisum sativum L.	Leguminosae
WAN NIAN QING GEN	Omoto Nipponlily Root	Rohdea japonica Roth.	Liliaceae
WAN SHAN YIN YANG HUO	Wanshan Epimedium	Epimedium wanshanense S. Z. He et Guo.	Berberidaceae
WAN SHOU JU	Aztec Marigold	Tagetes erecta L.	Compositae
WAN SHOU JU YE	Aztec Marigold Leaf	Rohdea japonica Roth.	Compositae
WAN ZHUO WU TOU	Curvebeak Monkshood	Aconitum campylorrhynchum Handsymbol 45 \f "Symbol" \s 8-Mazz	Ranunculaceae
WANG BU LIU XING	Cowherb	Vaccaria segetalis (Neck.) Garcke	Caryophyllaceae
WANG CHUN MU LAN (of XIN YI)	Biond Magnolia	Magnolia biondii Pamp. [= Magnolia fargesii Cheng]	Magnoliaceae
WANG GUA	Japanese Snakegourd	Trichosanthes cucumeroides (Ser.) Maxim.	Cucurbitaceae
WANG GUA ZI	Japanese Snakegourd Seed	Trichosanthes cucumeroides (Ser.) Maxim.	Cucurbitaceae
WANG JIANG NAN	Coffee Senna	Cassia occidentalis L.	Leguminosae
WANG JIANG NAN ZI	Coffee Senna Seed	Cassia occidentalis L.	Leguminosae
WANG SUN	Tetraphyllous Paris	Paris tetraphylla A. Gray	Liliaceae
WEI LING XIAN	Chinese Clematis	Clematis chinensis Osbeck	Ranunculaceae
WEI NAO	Hedgehog Brain	Erinaceus europaeus L.; Hemiechinus dauuricus Sundevall	Erinaceidae Erinaceidae
WEI PI (CI WEI PI)	Hedgehog Hide	Erinaceus europaeus L.; Hemiechinus dauuricus Sundevall	Erinaceidae Erinaceidae
WEI XIN GAN	Hedgehog Heart and Liver	Erinaceus europaeus L.; Hemiechinus dauuricus Sundevall	Erinaceidae Erinaceidae
WEN GE	Hard Clam Shell	Meretrix meretrix L.	Veneridae
WEN JING	Bottle-brush	Equisetum arvense L.	Equisetaceae
WEN PO	Common Quince	Cydonia oblonga Mill.	Rosaceae
WEN ZHU	Setose Asparagus	Asparagus setaceus (Kunth) Jessop [= Asparagus plumosus Bak.]	Liliaceae
WO ER QI (SHAN HE YE)	Chinese Umbrellaleaf	Diphylleia sinensis Li	Berberidaceae
WO JU	Garden Lettuce	Lactuca sativa L.	Compositae
WU CI FAN MA	Spineless Agave	Agave americana L. var. variegata Nichols	Agavaceae
WU GENG WU JIA PI (of WU JIA PI)	Sessileflower Acanthopanax Root-bark	Acanthopanax sessiliflorus (Rupr. et Maxim.) Seem	Araliaceae

Index of Traditional Chinese Medicines by Chinese Name

TCM Name	Name in English	Origin Latin Name	Family
WU GENG WU JIA YE (of WU JIA YE)	Sessileflower Acanthopanax Leaf	Acanthopanax sessiliflorus (Rupr. et Maxim.) Seem	Araliaceae
WU GONG	Centipede	Scolopendra subspinipes mutians L. Koch	Scolopendridae
WU HUA BEI MU (of CHUAN BEI MU)	Blackflower Fritillary	Fritillaria cirrhosa D. Don var. ecirrhosa Franch.	Liliaceae
WU HUA GUO	Fig	Ficus carica L.	Moraceae
WU HUA GUO GEN	Fig Root	Ficus carica L.	Moraceae
WU HUA GUO YE	Fig Leaf	Ficus carica L.	Moraceae
WU HUAN ZI PI	Chinese Soapberry Fruit	Sapindus mukorossi Gaertn.	Sapindaceae
WU HUAN ZI YE	Chinese Soapberry Leaf	Sapindus mukorossi Gaertn.	Sapindaceae
WU JIA GEN (CI WU JIA)	Manyprickle Acanthopanax Root	Acanthopanax senticosus (Rupr. et Maxim.) Harms	Araliaceae
WU JIA PI	Slenderstyle Acanthopanax Root-bark	Acanthopanax gracilistylus W. W. Smith	Araliaceae
WU JIA YE	Slenderstyle Acanthopanax Leaf	Acanthopanax gracilistylus W. W. Smith	Araliaceae
WU JIU MU GEN PI	Chinese Tallowtree Bark	Sapium sebiferum (L.) Roxb.	Euphorbiaceae
WU JIU YE	Chinese Tallowtree Leaf	Sapium sebiferum (L.) Roxb.	Euphorbiaceae
WU LA ER GAN CAO	Ural Licorice	Glycyrrhiza uralensis Fisch.	Leguminosae
WU LI	Serpent-head (Black Fish)	Ophiocephalus argus Cantor	Ophiocephalidae
WU LIAN MEI	Japanese Cayratia	Cayratia japonica (Thunb.) Gagn.	Vitaceae
WU LING ZHI	Trogopterus Dung	Trogopterus xanthipes Milne-Edwords; Pteromys volans L.	Petauristidae Petauristidae
WU LOU ZI	Phoenix Date	Phoenix dactylifera L.	Palmae
WU MEI	Japanese Apricot	Prunus mume (Sieb.) Sieb. et Zucc.	Rosaceae
WU MU XIE	Ceylon Persimmon Sawdust	Diospyros ebenum Koen.	Ebenaceae
WU SE MEI	Common Lantana	Lantana camara L.	Verbenaceae
WU SHAN YIN YANG HUO	Wushan Epimedium	Epimedium wushanense T. S. Ying	Berberidaceae
WU SU LI LI LU	Ussuri Falsehellebore	Veratrum nigrum L. var. ussuriense Nakai	Liliaceae
WU TONG BAI PI	Phoenix Tree Bast	Firmiana simplex (L.) W. F. Wight	Sterculiaceae
WU TONG YE	Phoenix Tree Leaf	Firmiana simplex (L.) W. F. Wight	Sterculiaceae
WU TONG ZI	Phoenix Tree Seed	Firmiana simplex (L.) W. F. Wight	Sterculiaceae
WU WEI ZI	Chinese Magnoliavine	Schisandra chinensis (Turcz.) Baill.	Schisandraceae
WU YAO	Combined Spicebush	Lindera strychnifolia (Sieb. et Zucc.) Villar [= Lindera aggregata (Sims) Kosterm.]	Lauraceae
WU YE TENG	Filiform Cassytha	Cassytha filiformis L.	Lauraceae
WU YUE CHA	Bignay Chinalaurel	Antidesma bunius (L.) Spr.	Euphorbiaceae
WU ZHAO LONG	Cairo Morningglory	Ipomoea cairica (L.) Sweet	Convolvulaceae
WU ZHU YU	Medicinal Evodia	Evodia rutaecarpa (Juss.) Benth.	Rutaceae
XI FAN LIAN	Passionflower	Passiflora caerulea L.	Passifloraceae
XI GUA	Watermelon	Citrullus vulgaris Schrad.	Cucurbitaceae
XI GUA ZI REN	Watermelon Seed	Citrullus vulgaris Schrad.	Cucurbitaceae
XI GUO JIAO HUI XIANG	Thinfruit Hypecoum	Hypecoum leptocarpum Hook. f. et Thoms.	Papaveraceae
XI HUA XUE DAN	Smallflower Hemsleya	Hemsleya graciliflora (Harms) cogn. [= Alsomitra graciliflora Harms]	Cucurbhitaceae
XI HUANG CAO	Serrate Rabdosia	Rabdosia serra (Maxim.) Hara	Labiatae

Index of Traditional Chinese Medicines by Chinese Name

TCM Name	Name in English	Origin Latin Name	Family
XI JIAO	Rhinoceros Horn	Rhinoceros unicornis L.;	Rhinocerotidae
		Rhinoceros sondaicus Desmarest;	Rhinocerotidae
		Rhinoceros sumatrensis (Fischer)	Rhinocerotidae
XI LUO HAN SONG	Musengerra Podocarpus	Podocarpus gracilior Pilg.	Podocarpaceae
XI MING	Boor's Mustardd	Thlaspi arvense L.	Cruciferae
XI MING ZI	Boor's Mustardd Seed	Thlaspi arvense L.	Cruciferae
XI NAN REN DONG	South-western Honeysuckle	Lonicera bournei Hemsl.	Caprifoliaceae
XI SHENG TENG	Common Cissampelos	Cissampelos pareira L.	Menispermaceae
XI SHU	Common Camptotheac	Camptotheca acuminata Decne.	Nyssaceae
XI SHUAI	Chinese Cricket	Gryllulus chinensis Weber	Gryllidae
XI XIAN	Common St. Paulswort	Siegesbeckia orientalis L.	Compositae
XI XIANG CONG	Chive	Allium schoenoprasum L.	Liliaceae
XI XIN	Manchurian Wildginger	Asarum heterotropoides F. Schm. var. mandshuricum (Maxim.) Kitag.	Aristolochiaceae
	Siebold Wildginger	Asarum sieboldii Miq.	Aristolochiaceae
XI YANG SHEN	American Ginseng	Panax quinquefolium L.	Araliaceae
XI YE AN YE	Forest Gray Gum Leaf	Eucalyptus tereticornis Smith	Myrtaceae
XI YE DA JI	Narrowleaf Euphorbia	Euphorbia esula L. var. cyparissoides Boiss.	Euphorbiaceae
XI YE TENG	Asian Tetracera	Tetracera asiatica (Lour.) Hoogl.	Dilleniaceae
XI YUAN TENG	Greyblue Pericampylus	Pericampylus glaucus (Lam.) Merr.	Menispermaceae
XIA KU CAO	Common Selfheal	Prunella vulgaris L.	Labiatae
XIA MA DAN	Rice Frog Gall	Rana limnocharis Boie	Ranidae
XIA TIAN GAO	Concentrated Beef Extract	Bos taurus domesticus Gmelin	Bovidae
XIA TIAN WU	Decumbent Corydalis	Corydalis decumbens (Thunb.) Pers.	Papaveraceae
XIA XIANG PU	see CHANG BAO XIANG PU		
XIA YE HONG JING TIAN	Kirilow Rhodiola	Rhodiola kirilowii (Reg.) Reg.	Crassulaceae
XIA YE LONG SHE LAN	Shortleaf Agave	Agave cantala Roxb.	Agavaceae
XIA YE TANG SONG CAO	Narrowleaf Meadowrue	Thalictrum Incidum L.	Ranunculaceae
XIA YE XIANG PU (of XIANG PU)	Narrowleaf Cattail	Typha angustifolia L.	Typhaceae
XIA YE ZHANG YA CAI	Narrowleaf Swertia	Swertia angustifolia Buch.-Ham. ex D. Don	Gentianaceae
XIAN CHI SHE PU TAO	Bigdentate Ampelopsis	Ampelopsis grossedentata (Hand. Mazz.) W.T. Wang [= Ampelopsis cantoniesis (H. et A.) Pl. var. grossedentata Hand.-Mazz.]	Vitaceae
XIAN GENG XI XIAN (of XI XIAN)	Glandularstalk St. Paulswort	Siegesbeckia orientalis L. var. pubescens Mak.	Compositae
XIAN HE CAO	Hairyvein Argimonia	Argimonia pilosa Ledeb. var. japonica (Miq.) Nakai	Rosaceae
XIAN HE CAO GEN (LONG YA CAO GEN)	Hairyvein Agrimonia Root	Agrimonia pilosa Ledeb. var. japonica (Miq.) Nakai	Rosaceae
XIAN HE CAO GEN YA	Hairyvein Argimonia Rhizome	Argimonia pilosa Ledeb. var. japonica (Miq.) Nakai	Rosaceae
XIAN HUA XIANG CHA CAI	Grandularflower Rabdosia	Isodon adenanthus (Diels.) Kudo	Labiatae
XIAN MAI XIANG CHA CAI	Veined Rabdosia	Rabdosia nervosa (Hemsl.) C. Y. Wu. et H. W. Li	Labiatae

TCM Name	Name in English	Origin Latin Name	Family
XIAN MAO	Common Cruculigo	Curculigo orchioides Gaertn.	Hypoxidaceae
XIAN SHENG MA	Muscicolous Woodbetony	Pedicularis muscicola Maxim.	Scrophulariaceae
XIAN HAO			
XIAN SUAN QIANG	Whiteflower Embelia	Embelia ribes Burm. f.	Myrsinaceae
XIAN XI SHU YU (of BEI XIE)	Thinnest Yam	Dioscorea gracillima Miq.	Dioscoriaceae
XIAN YE JIN JI JU	Lance Coreopsis	Coreopsis lanceolata L.	Compositae
XIANG DAN	Elephant Gall	Elephas maximus L.	Elephantidae
XIANG FU	Nutgrass Galingale	Cyperus rotundus L.	Cyperaceae
XIANG GANG JIAN MU	Hongkong Pencilwood	Dysoxylum hongkongense (Tufch.) Merr.	Meliaceae
XIANG GEN QIN	Laxleaf Sweetroot	Osmorhiza aristata (Thunb.) Mak. et Yabe var. laxa (Royle) Constance et Shan	Umbelliferae
XIANG GU	Elephant Bone	Elephas maximus L.	Elephantidae
XIANG JIA PI	Chinese Silkvine Root-bark	Periploca sepium Bge.	Asclepiadaceae
XIANG JIAO	Common Banana	Musa paradisiaca L. var. sapientum O. Ktze. [= Musa sapientum L.]	Musaceae
XIANG LING CAO	Rust-coloured Crotalaria	Crotalaria ferruginea Grah.	Leguminosae
XIANG MAO	Lemongrass	Cymbopogon citratus (DC.) Stapf	Gramineae
XIANG PI MU	Common Alstonia	Alstonia scholaris (L.) R. Br.	Apocynaceae
XIANG PU	See CHANG BAO XIANG PU, XIA YE XIANG PU:	Typha angustata Bory et Chaub.; Typha angustifolia L.	(Typhaceae) (Typhaceae)
XIANG RI KUI HUA	Sunflower	Helianthus annuus L.	Compositae
XIANG RI KUI JING SUI	Sunflower Stem Pith	Helianthus annuus L.	Compositae
XIANG RI KUI YE	Sunflower Leaf	Helianthus annuus L.	Compositae
XIANG RI KUI ZI	Sunflower Seed	Helianthus annuus L.	Compositae
XIANG ROU	Elephant Meat	Elephas maximus L.	Elephantidae
XIANG RU	Haichow Elsholtzia	Elsholtzia splendens Nakai ex F. Maekawa	Labiatae
XIANG SI TENG	Coralhead Plant	Abrus precatorium L.	Leguminosae
XIANG SI ZI	Coralhead Plant Seed	Abrus precatorium L.	Leguminosae
XIANG XUN	Champignon	Lentinus edodes (Berk.) Sing.	Tricholomataceae
XIANG YE	Roce Pelargonium	Pelargonium graveolens Lsymbol 162 \f "Symbol" \s 8′}Herit	Geraniaceae
XIANG YUAN	Medicinal Citron	Citrus medica L.	Rutaceae
	Wilson Citron	Citrus wilsonii Tanaka	Rutaceae
XIANG YUAN YE	Medicinal Citron Leaf	Citrus medica L.	Rutaceae
XIANG ZHANG	Yellow Cinnamon	Cinnamomum parthenoxylon (Jack) Nees [= Cinnamomum porrectum (Roxb.) Kosterm.]	Lauraceae
XIANG ZHANG YE	Yellow Cinnamon Leaf	Cinnamomum parthenoxylon (Jack) Nees [= Cinnamomum porrectum (Roxb.) Kosterm.]	Lauraceae
XIAO BAI BU	Officinal Asparagus	Asparagus officinalis L.	Liliaceae
XIAO BO	Amur Barerry	Berberis amurensis Rupr.	Berberidaceae
	Japanese Barerry	Berberis thunbergii DC.	Berberidaceae
	Poiret Barerry	Berberis poiretii Schneid.	Berberidaceae
XIAO CAO WU	Delavay Larkspur	Delphinium delavayi Franch.	Ranunculaceae
	Yunnan Larkspur	Delphinium yunnanense Franch.	Ranunculaceae

Index of Traditional Chinese Medicines by Chinese Name

TCM Name	Name in English	Origin Latin Name	Family
XIAO CHAO CAI	Pigeon Vetch	Vicia hirsuta (L.) S. F. Gray	Leguminosae
XIAO FEI YANG CAO	Thymifolious Euporbia	Euphorbia thymifolia L.	Euphorbiaceae
XIAO GEN SUAN (XIE BAI)	Longstamen Onion	Allium macrostemon Bge.	Liliaceae
XIAO HUA DUN YE SHU YU	Smallflower Yam Rhizome	Dioscorea parviflora C. T. Ting sp. Nov.	Dioscoreaceae
XIAO HUA SUAN TENG ZI	Smallflower Embelia	Embelia parviflora Wall. ex DC.	Myrsinaceae
XIAO JIAN CAO	Bulbiferous Stonecrop	Sedum bulbiferum Mak.	Crassulaceae
XIAO JIE JIN CAO	Selago-like Climbing Fern	Huperzia selago (L.) Bernh. ex Schrank et Mart. [= Lycopodium selago L.]	huperziaceae
XIAO LA BA	Verticillate Cladonia	Cladonia verticillata Hoffm.	Cladoniaceae
XIAO LIAN QIAO	Erect St. John'swort	Hypericum erectum Thunb.	Guttiferae
XIAO MAI	Wheat	Triticum aestivum L.	Gramineae
XIAO SHE ZI WAN	Smallligulatecorolla Aster	Aster albescens (DC.) Hand. -Mazz.	Compositae
XIAO TANG SONG CAO	Low Meadowrue	Thalictrum minus L.	Ranunculaceae
XIAO TOU DUI XIN JU	Littlehead Sneezeweed	Helenium microcephalum DC.	
XIAO XUE REN SHEN	Woolly Lespedeza	Lespedeza tomentosa (Thunb.) Sieb.	Leguminosae
XIAO YE HEI CHAI HU	Smallleaf Black Thorowax	Bupleurum smithii Wolff var. parvifolium Shan et Y. Li	Umbelliferae
XIAO YE HUA	Bridalwreath Spiraea	Spiraea prunifolia Sieb. et Zucc.	Rosaceae
XIAO YE JIU LI XIANG	Littleleaf Common Jasminorange	Murraya paniculata (L.) Jack var. exotica (L.) Huang	Rutaceae
XIAO YE MAI MA TENG	Smallleaf Jointfir	Gnetum parvifolium (Warb.) C.Y. Cheng	Gnetaceae
XIAO YE PI PA	Savoury Rhododendron	Rhododendron anthopogonoides Maxim.	Ericaceae
XIE BAI (XIAO GEN SUAN)	Longstamen Onion	Allium macrostemon Bge.	Liliaceae
XIE CAO	Common Valeriana	Valeriana officinalis L.	Valerianaceae
XIE KE	Mitten Crab Chelae	Eriocheir sinensis H. Milne-Edwards	Grapsidae
XIN JIANG GAO BEN (of GAO BEN)	Vaginate Hemlockparsley	Conioselinum vaginatum (Spr.) Thell.	Umbelliferae
XIN JIANG YI ZHI HAO	Sinkiang onetwig wormwood	Artemisia rupestris L.	Compositae
XIN YE CHI BO	Heartleaf Tubergourd	Thladiantha cordifolia (BL.) Cogn.	Cucurbhitaceae
XIN YE YIN YANG HUO (of YIN YANG HUO)	Shorthorned Epimedium	Epimedium brevicornum Maxim.	Berberidaceae
XIN YI	Lily Magnolia	Magnolia liliflora Desr.	Magnoliaceae
XING AN BAI ZHI (of DU HUO)	Dahurian Angelica	Angelica dahurica (Fisch. ex Hoffm.) Benth. et Hook. f. ex Franch. et Sav.	Umbelliferae
XING AN SHENG MA (of SHENG MA)	Dahurian Bugbane	Cimicifuga dahurica (Turcz.) Maxim.	Ranunculaceae
XING CAI	Shield Floatingheart	Nymphoides peltatum (Gmel.) O. Ktze.	Gentianaceae
XING REN	Ansu Apricot Seed	Prunus armeniaca L. var. ansu Maxim.	Rosaceae
	Apricot Seed	Prunus armeniaca L.	Rosaceae

Index of Traditional Chinese Medicines by Chinese Name

TCM Name	Name in English	Origin Latin Name	Family
XING ZI	Ansu Apricot	Prunus armeniaca L. var. ansu Maxim.	Rosaceae
	Apricot	Prunus armeniaca L.	Rosaceae
XIONG DAN	Bear Gall	Selenarctos thibetanus G. Cuvier;	Ursidae
		Ursus arctos L.	Ursidae
XIONG ZHANG	Bear's Paw	Selenarctos thibetanus G. Cuvier;	Ursidae
		Ursus arctos L.	Ursidae
XIU MAO JI SHENG	Rustyhair Taxillus	Taxillus levinei Merr.	Loranthaceae
XIU MAO YE TONG	Anomalus Mallotu	Mallotus anomalus	Euphorbiaceae
XIU XIAN JU YE	Japanese Spiraea Leaf	Spiraea japonica L. f.	Rosaceae
XU CHANG QING	Paniculate Swallowwort	Cynanchum paniculatum (bge.) Kitag.	Asclepiadaceae
XU DUAN	Japanese Teasel	Dipsacus japonicus Miq.	Dipsacaceae
XU DUAN	see CHUAN XU DUAN		
XU SUI ZI JING ZHONG BAI ZHI	Caper Euphorbia Latex	Euphorbia lathyris L.	Euphorbiaceae
XUAN CAO GEN	Orange Daylily	Hemerocallis fulva L.	Liliaceae
	Small Yellow Daylily	Hemerocallis minor Mill.	Liliaceae
	Yellow Daylily	Hemerocallis flava L.	Liliaceae
XUAN FU HUA	British Inula Flower	Inula britannica L.	Compositae
	Chinese Inula Flower	Inula britannica L. var. chinensis (Rupr.) Reg.	Compositae
	Linearleaf Inula Flower	Inula linariaefolia Turcz.	Compositae
XUE CHA	Vermiculate Thamnolia Thallus	Thamnolia vermicularis (Ach.) Asahina	Thamnoliaceae
XUE LIAN	Snow Lotus	Saussurea involucrata Kar. et Kir.	Compositae
XUE SHAN LIN	Japanese Pachysandra	Pachysandra terminalis Sieb. et Zucc.	Buxaceae
XUE SHANG YI ZHI HAO	Shortstalk Monkshood	Aconitum brachypodum Diels	Ranunculaceae
XUE YU	Human Hair	Homo sapiens L.	
XUN DAO NIU	Heterostemonous Biebersteinia	Biebersteinia heterostemon Maxim.	Geraniaceae
YA DAN ZI	Java Brucea	Brucea javanica (L.) Merr.	Simaroubaceae
YA ER QIN	Japanese Cryptotaenia	Cryptoaenia japonica Hassk.	Umbelliferae
YA JIAO AI	Ghostplant Wormwood	Artemisia lactiflora Wall. ex DC.	Compositae
YA MA	Common Flax	Linum usitatissimum L.	Linaceae
YA MA ZI	Common Flax Seed	Linum usitatissimum L.	Linaceae
YA PIAN	Opium	Papaver sommiferum L.	Papaveraceae
YA ZHI CAO	Common Dayflower Herb	Commelina communis L.	Commelinaceae
YAN BAI CAI	Purple Bergenia	Bergenin purpurascens (Hook. f. et Thoms.) Engl.	Saxifragaceae
	Thickleaf Bergenia	Bergenin crassifolia (L.) Fritsch	Saxifragaceae
	Thickleaf Boea	Boea crassifolia Hemsl.	Gesneriaceae
YAN CAO	Common Tobacco	Nicotiana tabacum L.	Solanaceae
YAN FU YE	Chinese Sumac Leaf	Rhus chinensis Mill.	Anacardiaceae
YAN FU ZI	Chinese Sumac Fruit	Rhus chinensis Mill.	Anacardiaceae
YAN GUO CAO	East-Asia Low Meadowrue	Thalictrum thunbergii DC.	Ranunculaceae
YAN HU SUO	Yanhusuo	Corydalis yanhusuo W. T. Wang [= Corydalis turtschaninovii Bess. f. yanhusuo Y. H. Chou et C. C. Hsu]	Papaveraceae
YAN JIAO CAO	White Chinaure Herb	Boenninghausenia albiflora (Hook.) Meissn.	Rutaceae
YAN JIN CAI	Tibet Berneuxine	Berneuxia thibetica Decne.	Diapensiaceae
YAN LAI HONG	Three-coloured Amaranth	Amaranthus tricolor L.	Amaranthaceae

Index of Traditional Chinese Medicines by Chinese Name

Index of Traditional Chinese Medicines by Chinese Name

TCM Name	Name in English	Origin Latin Name	Family
YE LI ZHI YE	Callery Pear Branch and Leaf	Pyrus calleryana Decne.	Rosaceae
YE MING SHA	Bat Dung	Vespertilio superans Thomas	Vespertilionidae
	Chinese Stauntonvine	Stauntonia chinensis DC.	Lardizabalaceae
YE MU GUA	Chinese Stauntonvine	Stauntonia hexaphylla Decne.	Lardizabalaceae
YE QI SHU YE	Woods Lcaquertree Leaf	Rhus sylvestris Sieb. et Zucc.	Anacardiaceae
YE SHENG MA	Kamchatka Bugbane	Cimicifuga simplex Wormsk.	Ranunculaceae
YE WU TONG	Japanese Mallotus	Mallotus japonicus Muell.-Arg.	Euphorbiaceae
YE XIA ZHU	Common Leafflower	Phyllanthus urinaria L.	Euphorbiaceae
YE XIANG MAO	Goering Lemongrass	Cymbopogon goeringii (Steud.) A. Camus	Gramineae
YE YAN YE	Mullein Nightbrier Leaf	Solanum verbascifolium L.	Solanaceae
YE YING SU	Chinese Poppy	Papaver nudicaule L.	Papaveraceae
YE YU	Taro	Colocasia antiquorum Schott et Endl.	Araceae
YE ZHI MA	Barbate Deadnettle	Lamium barbatum Sieb. et Zucc.	Labiatae
YE ZHU DAN	Wild Boar Gall	Sus scrofa L.	Suidae
YE ZI PI	Coconut Root-bark	Cocos nucifera L.	Palmae
YE ZI RANG	Coconut Albumen	Cocos nucifera L.	Palmae
YE ZI YOU	Coconut Oil	Cocos nucifera L.	Palmae
YI BEI MU (of CHUAN BEI MU)	Siberian Fritillary	Fritillaria pallidiflora Schrenk	Liliaceae
YI DIAN HONG	Sowthistle Tasselflower	Emilia sonchifolia (L.) DC.	Compositae
YI HE GUO	Smoothfruit Ventiago	Ventilago leiocarpa Benth.	Rhamnaceae
YI MU CAO	Wormwood-like Motherwort Herb	Leonurus heterophyllus Sweet	Labiatae
YI NIAN PENG	Annual Fleabane	Erigeron annuus (L.) Pers.	Compositae
YI YE BAI JIANG	Diversifolious Patrinia	Patrinia heterophylla Bge.	Valerianaceae
YI YE LIANG WANG CHA	David Falsepanax	Nothopanax davidii (Franch.) Harms	Arliaceae
YI YE QIU	Suffrutescent Securinega	Securinega suffruticosa (Pall.) Rehd.	Euphorbiaceae
YI YI GEN	Jobstears Root	Coix lachrymajobi L.	Gramineae
YI YI REN	Jobstears	Coix lachrymajobi L.	Gramineae
YI ZHI HAO	Alpine Yallow	Achillea alpina L.	Compositae
YI ZHI HUANG HUA	Common Goldenrod	Solidago virgaurea L. var. leiocarpa (Benth.) A. Gray [= Solidago decurrens Lour.]	Compositae
YI ZHI XIANG	Bastard Speedwell	Veronica spuria L.	Scrophulariaceae
YIN BIAN LONG SHE LAN	Silveredge Agave	Agave angustifolia var. marginata Hort.	Agavaceae
YIN BU HUAN	Barbate Cyclea	Cyclea barbata (Wall.) Miers	Menispermaceae
YIN CHAI HU	Lanceolate Starwort	Stellaria dichotoma L. var. lanceolata Bge.	Caryophyllaceae
YIN CHEN HAO	Capillary Wormwood	Artemisia capillaris Thunb.	Compositae
	Virgate Wormwood	Artemisia scoparia Wldst. et Kitaibel	Compositae
YIN DU JIU LI XIANG	Indian Common Jasminorange	Murraya koenigii Spreng	Rutaceae
YIN DU SHE GU	Indian Balanophora	Balanophora indica (Arn.) Griff. [= Langodorffia indica Arn.]	Balanophoraceae
YIN XIANG PI	Burmann Cinnamon Bark	Cinnamomum burmannii (Nees) Bl.	Lauraceae
YIN XIANG YE	Burmann Cinnamon Leaf	Cinnamomum burmannii (Nees) Bl.	Lauraceae
YIN XING CAO	Chinese Siphonostegia	Siphonostegin chinensis Benth.	Scroophulariaceae
YIN YANG HUO	Largeflower Epimedium	Epimedium grandiflorum Morr.	Berberidaceae

Index of Traditional Chinese Medicines by Chinese Name

TCM Name	Name in English	Origin Latin Name	Family
YIN YANG HUO GEN	Largeflower Epimedium Root	Epimedium grandiflorum Morr.	Berberidaceae
	Sagittate Epimedium Root	Epimedium sagittatum (Sieb. et Zucc.) Maxim.	Berberidaceae
	Shorthorned Epimedium Root	Epimedium brevicornum Maxim.	Berberidaceae
YIN YU	Reeves Skimmia	Skimmia reevesiana Fortune	Rutaceae
YING BU BO	Avicenna's Pricklyash	Zanthoxylum avicennae (Lam.) DC.	Rutaceae
YING SHAN HONG	Korean Rhododendron	Rhododendron mucronulatum Turcz.	Ericaceae
YING SHUI HUANG LIAN	Shortstalk Slimtop Meadowrue	Thalictrum simplex L. var. brevipes Hara	Ranunculaceae
YING SU	Opium Poppy	Papaver somniferum L.	Papaveraceae
YING SU KE	Opium Poppy Pericarp	Papaver somniferum L.	Papaveraceae
YING TAO	Falsesour Cherry	Prunus pseudocerasus Lindl.	Rosaceae
YING ZHUA	Sixpetal Tailgrape	Artabotrys hexapetalus (L. f.) Bhandari [= Annona hexapetalus L. f.]	Annonaceae
YONG NING DU HUO (of DU HUO)	Yungning Cowparsnip	Heracleum yungningense Hand.-Mass	Umbelliferae
YOU	Pummelo	Citrus grandis (L.) Osbeck	Rutaceae
YOU CHA GEN PI	Oiltea Camellia Root-bark	Camellia oleifera Abel	Theaceae
YOU GAN GEN	Emblic Leafflower Root	Phyllanthus emblica L.	Euphorbiaceae
YOU GAN LAN (QI DUN GUO)	Common Olive	Olea europaea L.	Oleaceae
YOU GAN MU PI	Emblic Leafflower Bark	Phyllanthus emblica L.	Euphorbiaceae
YOU GAN YE	Emblic Leafflower Leaf	Phyllanthus emblica L.	Euphorbiaceae
YOU HE	Pummelo Seed	Citrus grandis (L.) Osbeck	Rutaceae
YU BAI FU	Giant Typhonium	Typhoniun giganteum Engl.	Araceae
YU DAI GEN	Tithymalus-like Pedilanthus	Pedilanthus tithymaloides (L.) Poit.	Euphorbiaceae
YU ER	Incamate Gloeostereum	Gloeostereum incamatum S. Ito et Imai	Meruliaceae
YU ER QI	Tschonosk Trillium	Trillum tschonoskii Maxim.	Liliaceae
	Whiteflower Trillium	Trillum camtschaticum Pall.	Liliaceae
YU JIN	Common Turmeric	Curcuma longa L.	Zingiberaceae
YU JIN XIANG	Common Tulip	Tulipa gesneriana L.	Liliaceae
YU JIN XIANG GEN	Common Tulip Root	Tulipa gesneriana L.	Liliaceae
YU LAN (of XIN YI)	Yulan Magnolia	Magnolia denudata Desr.	Magnoliaceae
YU LI REN	Chinese Dwarf Cherry Seed	Prunus humilis Bge.	Rosaceae
	Dwarf Flowering Cherry Seed	Prunus japonica Thunb.	Rosaceae
	Longpedicel Chinese Buscherry Seed	Prunus japonica Thunb. var. nakaii (Lévl.) Rehd.	Rosaceae
YU MI XU	Maize Style	Zea mays L.	Gramineae
YU SHAN HU GEN	Jerusalemcherry Root	Solanum pseudocapsicum L.	Solanaceae
YU SHU SHU	Maize	Zea mays L.	Gramineae
YU TENG	Trifoliate Jewelvine	Derris trifoliata Lour.	Leguminosae
YU XIANG CAO	Apple Mint Herb	Mentha rotundifolia (L.) Huds.	Labiatae
YU XING CAO	Heartleaf Houttuynia Herb	Houttuynia cordata Thunb.	Saururaceae
YU YE SAN QI	Bipinnatifid Ginseng	Panax japonicus var. bipinnatifidus (Seem.) Wu et Feng [= Panax bipinnatifidus (Seem.) Li]	Arliaceae

Index of Traditional Chinese Medicines by Chinese Name

TCM Name	Name in English	Origin Latin Name	Family
ZE XIE	Oriental Waterplantain	Alisma orientale (Sam.) Juzepcz. [= Alisma plantagoaquatica L. var. orientale Samuels]	Alismataceae
ZHAI YE BAN FENG HE	Lanceleaf Wingseedtree	Pterospermum lanceaefolium Roxb	Sterculiaceae
ZHAN LONG JIAN (LUN YE PO PO NA)	Siberian Veronicastrum	Veronicastrum sibirica (L.) Pennell	Scroophulariaceae
ZHAN MAO CUI QUE HUA	Hair Larkspur	Delphinium kamaonense var. glabrescens W. T. Wang	Ranunculaceae
ZHANG GU GAN CAO (of GAN CAO)	Inflated Licorice	Glycyrrhiza inflata Batal.	Leguminosae
ZHANG LANG	Cockroach	Blatta orientalis L.	Blattidae
ZHANG LIU TOU	Canereed Spiralflagg	Costus speciosus (Koen.) Smith.	Zingiberaceae
ZHANG MU (ZHANG SHU)	Camphortree	Cinnamomum camphora (L.) Presl	Lauraceae
ZHANG SHU (ZHANG MU)	Camphortree	Cinnamomum camphora (L.) Presl	Lauraceae
ZHANG SHU YE	Camphortree Leaf	Cinnamomum camphora (L.) Presl	Lauraceae
ZHANG YA CAI	False Chinese Swertia	Swertia pseudochinensis Hara	Gentianaceae
ZHANG YE BAN XIA	Pedate Pinallia	Pinellia pedatisecta Schott	Araceae
ZHANG YE HU JIAO	Camphortreeleaf Pepper	Piper polysyphorum C. DC	Piperaceae
ZHANG YU	Common Atlantic Octopus	Octopus vulgaris Lamarck	Octopodidae
ZHAO SHAN BAI	Manchurian Rhododendron	Rhododendron micranthum Turcz.	Ericaceae
ZHE BEI MU	Thunberg Fritillary	Fritillaria verticillata Willd. var. thunbergii Bak. [= Fritillaria thunbergii Miq.]	Liliaceae
ZHE GU CAI	Leprieur Caloglossa Frond	Caloglossa leprieurii (Mont.) J. Ag.	Delesseriaceae
ZHEN CAI	Pungent Litse	Litsea pungens Hemsl. [= Lindera umbellata Thunb.]	Lauraceae
ZHEN MO	Mellea Armillaria Sporophore	Armillaria mellea (Vahl ex Fr.) Quél.	Tricholomataceae
ZHEN ZHU CAI (ZHEN ZHU YE)	Clethra Loosestrife	Lyaimachia Clethroides Duby	Primulaceae
ZHEN ZHU MEI	Tree Falsespiraea	Sorbaria arborea Schneid.	Rosaceae
	Ural Falsespiraea	Sorbaria sorbifolia (L.) A. Br.	Rosaceae
ZHEN ZHU YE (ZHEN ZHU CAI)	Clethra Loosestrife	Lyaimachia Clethroides Duby	Primulaceae
ZHI	Common Pheasant	Phasianus colchicus Gmelin	Phasianidae
ZHI GEN PI	Trifoliate-orange Root-bark	Poncirus trifoliata (L.) Raf.	Rutaceae
ZHI JIA HUA YE	Henna Leaf	Lawsonia inermis L.	Lythraceae
ZHI JU GEN	Japanese Raisin Tree Root	Hovenia dulcis Thunb.	Rhamnaceae
ZHI JU ZI	Japanese Raisin Tree Seed	Hovenia dulcis Thunb.	Rhamnaceae
ZHI KE	Bitter Orange (almost ripe fruit)	Citrus aurantium L.	Rutaceae
	Trifoliate Orange (almost ripe fruit)	Poncirus trifoliata (L.) Raf.	Rutaceae
	Wilson Citron (almost ripe fruit)	Citrus wilsonii Tanaka	Rutaceae
ZHI MU	Common Anemarrhena	Anemarrhena asphodeloides Bge.	Lilyaceae
ZHI SHI	Bitter Orange	Citrus aurantium L.	Rutaceae
	Trifoliate Orange	Poncirus trifoliata (L.) Raf.	Rutaceae
ZHI SHI	Wilson Citron Fruit	Citrus wilsonii Tanaka	Rutaceae

Index of Traditional Chinese Medicines by Chinese Name

TCM Name	Name in English	Origin Latin Name	Family
ZHI XIE MU PI	Droughtdysentery Holarrhena Bark	Holarrhena antidysenterica Wall.	Apocynaceae
ZHI ZHU BAO DAN	Common Aspidistra	Aspidistra elatior Bl.	Liliaceae
ZHI ZHU XIANG	Broadleaf Common Valeriana	Valeriana officinalis L. var. latifolia Miq.	Valerianaceae
ZHI ZHU XIANG	Jatamans Valeriana	Valeriana jatamansii Jones	Valerianaceae
ZHI ZI	Cape Jasmine Fruit	Gardenia jasminoides Ellis	Rubiaceae
ZHI ZI YE	Cape Jasmine Leaf	Gardenia jasminoides Ellis	Rubiaceae
ZHONG CHI MAO DANG GUI (of DU HUO)	Doubleteeth Pubescent Angelica	Angelica pubescens Maxim. f. biserrata Shan et Yuan	Umbelliferae
ZHONG HUA JIU LI XIANG	Chinese Common Jasminorange	Murraya exotica	Rutaceae
ZHONG JIAN WU WEI ZI	Intermediate Magnoliavine	Schisandra propinqua (Wall.) Baill. var. intermedia A. C. Smith	Schisandraceae
ZHU BAI	Nagai Podocarpus	Podocarpus nagi Zoll. et Mor.	Podocarpaceae
ZHU DAN	Pig Gall	Sus scrofa domestica Brisson	Suidae
ZHU JIE SAN QI	Japanese Ginseng	Panax pseudoginseng Wall. var. japonicus (Mey.) Hoo et Tseng	Araliaccac
ZHU LING	Popyporus Agaric	Polyporus umbellatus (Pers.) Fries	Polyporaceae
ZHU SHA LIAN	Kaempfer Dutchmanspipe	Aristolochia kaempferi Willd.	Aristolochiaceae
ZHU YA JIAN JU ZI JIN	see ZHU YA ZI JIN		
ZHU YA ZI JIN	Bulbiliferous Corydalis	Corydalis sheareri var. bulbillifera Hand. -Mazz.	Papaveraceae
ZHU YE JIAO	Bambooleaf Pricklyash	Zanthoxylum planispinum Sieb. et Zucc.	Rutaceae
ZHU YE JIAO GEN	Bambooleaf Pricklyash Root	Zanthoxylum planispinum Sieb. et Zucc.	Rutaceae
ZHU ZONG CAO	David's Maidenhair Fern	Adiantum davidii Franch.	Adiantaceae
	Maidenhair Fern	Adiantum capillusveneris L.	Adiantaceae
ZI BAI PI	Ovate Catalpa Bast	Catalpa ovata G. Don	Bignoniaceae
ZI BEI TIAN KUI CAO	Nudicaulous Grounsel Herb	Senecio nudicaulis Buch.-Ham.	Compositae
ZI CAI	Laver	Porphyra tenera Kjellm.	Bangiaceae
ZI CAO	Paniculate Onosma	Onosma paniculatum Bur. et Franch.	Boraginaceae
	Redroot Gromwell	Lithospermum erythrhizon Sieb. et Zucc.	Boraginaceae
	Sinkiang-Tibet Arnebia	Arnebia euchroma (Royle) Johnst.	Boraginaceae
ZI CAO RONG	Lac	Laccifer lacca Kerr.	Lacciferidae
ZI HE CHE	Human Placenta	Homo sapiens L.	
ZI HONG ZHANG YA CAI	Scarlet Swertia	Swertia punicea Hemsl.	Gentianaceae
ZI HUA BA BAO	see ZI HUA JING TIAN		
ZI HUA E BEI BEI MU	Purpleflower Fritillary	Fritillaria ebeiensis var. pvrpvrea G. D. Yu et P. Li	Liliaceae
ZI HUA JING TIAN	Purpleflower Stonecrop	Hylotelephium mingjinianum (S. H. Fu) H. Ohba	Crassulaceae
ZI HUA YU DENG CAO (LIE BAO ZI JING)	Incised Corydalis	Corydalis incusa (Thunb.) Pers.	Papaveraceae
ZI JIN LIAN	Willmott Ceratostigma	Ceratostigma willmottianum Stapf	Plumbaginaceae
ZI JIN NIU	Japanese Ardisia	Ardisia japonica (Hornst.) Bl.	Myrsinaceae

Index of Traditional Chinese Medicines by Chinese Name

Index of Traditional Chinese Medicines by English Name

Index of Traditional Chinese Medicines by English Name

English Name	TCM Name	Origin Latin Name
Abelmusk	SHE XIANG	*Moschus moschiferus* L.; *Moschus berezovskii* Flerov.; *Moschus sifanicus* Przewalski
Acuminate Epimedium	CU MAO YIN YANG HUO	*Epimedium acuminatum* Franch.
Acutangular Scopolia	SAN FEN SAN	*Scopolia acutangula* C. Y. Wu *et* C. Chen [= *Anisodus acutangulus* C. Y. Wu *et* C. Chen]
Acute Common Perilla Leaf	ZI SU YE	*Perilla frutescens* (L.) Britt. var. *acuta* (Thunb.) Kudo
Acute Common Perilla Seed	ZI SU ZI	*Perilla frutescens* (L.) Britt. var. *acuta* (Thunb.) Kudo
Acute Common Perilla Stem	ZI SU GEN	*Perilla frutescens* (L.) Britt. var. *acuta* (Thunb.) Kudo
Acute Sida	HUANG HUA REN	*Sida acuta* Burm. f.
Acutelobed Hornpoppy	JIAN LIE HAI YING SU	*Glaucium oxylobum* Boiss. *et* Bushse
Acutifoliate Podocarpium Herb	SHAN MA HUANG	*Desmodium racemosum* (Thunb.) DC. [=*Podocarpium podocarpum* var. *oxyphyllum* (DC.) Yang *et* Huang]
Adder's Tongue	PING ER XIAO CAO	*Ophioglossum vulgatum* L.
Adhesive Rehmannia Dried Root	GAN DI HUANG	*Rehmannia glutinosa* (Gaertn.) Libosch *ex* Mey.
African Myrsine	DA HONG PAO	*Myrsine africana* L.
Ailanthus-like Pricklyash Bark	CHU YE HUA JIAO PI	*Zanthoxylum ailanthoides* Sieb. *et* Zucc.
Ailanthus-like Pricklyash	CHU YE HUA JIAO (SHI ZHU YU)	*Zanthoxylum ailanthoides* Sieb. *et* Zucc.
Air-plant Herb	LUO DI SHENG GEN	*Bryophyllum pinnatum* (L. f.) Oken
Airpotato Yam	HUANG YAO ZI	*Dioscorea bulbifera* L
Aizoon Stonecrop Root	JING TIAN SAN QI GEN	*Sedum aizoon* L.
Aleppo Gall (Galla Halepensis)	MO SHI ZI	*Cynips gallae-tinctoriae* Olivier
Alfalfa Root	MU XU GEN	*Medicago sativa* L.
Alfalfa	MU XU	*Medicago sativa* L.
Alligator Alternanthera	KONG XIN XIAN	*Alternanthera philoxeroides* (Mart.) Griseb.
Alpine Gentian	BAI HUA LONG DAN	*Gentiana algida* Pall.
Alpine Yallow	YI ZHI HAO	*Achillea alpina* L.
Alpine Thermopsis	GAO SHAN HUANG HUA	*Thermopsis alpina* Ledeb.
Altai Heteropappus	A ER TAI ZI WAN	*Heteropappus altaicus* (Willd.) Novopokr.
Amanita Fungus	E GAO XUN	*Amanita strobilifomis* (Paul.) Quél.
Amanita	BAO PI JUN	*Amanita panthorina*
American Agave	FAN MA	*Agave americana* L.
American Ginseng	XI YANG SHEN	*Panax quinquefolium* L.
American Maidenhair Fern	TIE SI QI	*Adiantum pedatum* L.
American Pokeweed	MEI SHANG LU	*Phytolacca americana* L.
Ammbergris	LONG XIAN XIANG	*Physeter catodon* L.
Ampelopsis	SHE PU TAO	*Ampelopsis brevipedunculata* (Maxim.) Trautv.
Amphibious Knotweed	LIANG QI LIAO	*Polygonum amphibium* L.
Amur Adonis	FU SHOU CAO	*Adonis amurensis* Reg. *et* Radde
Amur Barerry	XIAO BO	*Berberis amurensis* Rupr.
Amur Corktree	HUANG BAI	*Phellodendron amurene* Rupr.
Amur Jackinthepulpit	TIAN NAN XING	*Arisaema amurense* Maxim.
Amur Lilac	BAO MA ZI	*Syringa amurensis* Rupr.
Amygdalate Apricot Seed	BA DAN XING REN	*Prunum amygdalus* Batsch
Ancients Euphorbia	HUO YANG LE	*Euphorbia antiquorum* L.

Index of Traditional Chinese Medicines by English Name

Index of Traditional Chinese Medicines by English Name

Index of Traditional Chinese Medicines by English Name

Index of Traditional Chinese Medicines by English Name

English Name	TCM Name	Origin Latin Name
Boreal Wild Chrysanthemum Flower	YE JU HUA	*Chrysanthemum boreale* Mak.
Boreal Wild Chrysanthemum	BEI YE JU	*Chrysanthemum boreale* Mak.
Borneol	BING PIAN	*Dryobalanops aromatica* Gaertn. f.
Bottle Gourd	HU LU	Lagenaria siceraria (Molina) Standl. var. *depressa* Ser.
Bottle-brush	WEN JING	*Equisetum arvense* L.
Bouquet Larkspur	CUI QUE HUA	*Delphinium grandiflorum* L.
Bower Actinidia	MI HOU LI	*Actinidia arguta* (Sieb. *et* Zucc.) Planch.
Boxleaf Atalantia Leaf	DONG FENG JU YE	*Atalantia buxifolia* (Poir.) Oliv.
Boxleaf Atalantia Root	DONG FENG JU GEN	*Atalantia buxifolia* (Poir.) Oliv.
Boxleaf Syzygium	CHI NAN	*Syzygium buxifolium* Hook. *et* Arn.
Brainea	GUAN ZHONG	*Brainea insignis* (Hook.) J. Sm.
Bretschneider Pear Leaf	LI YE	*Pyrus bretschneideri* Rehd.
Bridalwreath Spiraea	XIAO YE HUA	*Spiraea prunifolia* Sieb. *et* Zucc.
Brithsh Inula Herb	JIN FO CAO	*Inula britannica* L.
British Inula Flower	XUAN FU HUA	*Inula britannica* L.
Broadbean Leaf	CAN DOU YE	*Vicia faba* L.
Broadbean Pericarp	CAN DOU JIA KE	*Vicia faba* L.
Broadbean Spermoderm	CAN DOU KE	*Vicia faba* L.
Broadbean Stem	CAN DOU JING	*Vicia faba* L.
Broadbean	CAN DOU	*Vicia faba* L.
Broadleaf Cattail Pollen	PU HUANG	*Typha latifolia* L.
Broadleaf Common Valeriana	ZHI ZHU XIANG	*Valeriana officinalis* L. var. *latifolia* Miq.
Broadleaf Giantfennel Resin	A WEI	*Ferula conocaula* Eug.
Broadleaf Globethistle	HUA ZHOU LOU LU	*Echinops latifolus* Tausch
Broadleaf Holly	KU DING CHA	*Ilex latafolia* Thunb.
Broadleaf Vetch	SHAN YE WAN DOU	*Vicia amoena* Fisch.
Broomcorn Millet	SHU MI	*Panicum miliaceum* L
Buddha's Lamp	SHAN GAN CAO	*Mussaenda pubescens* Ait. f.
Buffalo Horn	SHUI NIU JIAO	*Bubalus bubalis* L.
Bulbiferous Stonecrop	XIAO JIAN CAO	*Sedum bulbiferum* Mak.
Bulbiliferous Corydalis	ZHU YA ZI JIN	*Corydalis sheareri* var. *bulbillifera* Hand. -Mazz.
Bullocksheart Custardapple	NIU XIN FAN LI ZHI	*Annona reticulata* L.
Bumalda Bladdernut	SHENG GU YOU	*Staphylea bumalda* DC.
Bunga Ash Bark	QIN PI	*Fraxinus bungeana* DC.
Bunge Giantfennel	SHA QIAN HU	*Ferula borealis* Kuan
Bunge Hackberry	BANG BANG MU	*Celtis bungeana* Bl.
Bunge Pricklyash Root	HUA JIAO GEN	*Zanthoxylum bungeanum* Maxim.
Bunge Pricklyash	HUA JIAO	*Zanthoxylum bungeanum* Maxim.
Bunge Swllowwort	BAI SHOU WU	*Cynanchum bungei* Decne.
Burmacoast Padauk	ZI TAN	*Pterocarpus indicus* Willd.
Burmann Cinnamon Bark	YIN XIANG PI	*Cinnamomum burmannii* (Nees) Bl.
Burmann Cinnamon Leaf	YIN XIANG YE	*Cinnamomum burmannii* (Nees) Bl.
Burrowed Click Beetle	KOU TOU CHONG	*Pleonomus canaliculatus* Faldermann
Bush Redpepper	LA JIAO	*Capsicum frutescens* L.
Cabbage	GAN LAN	*Brassica oleracea* L. var. *capiata* L.
Cablin Potchouli	GUANG HUO XIANG	*Pogostemon cablin* (Blanco) Benth.
Cairo Morningglory	WU ZHAO LONG	*Ipomoea cairica* (L.) Sweet
California Burclover Root	MU XU GEN	*Medicago hispida* Gaertn.
California Burclover	MU XU	*Medicago hispida* Gaertn.
Callery Pear Branch and Leaf	YE LI ZHI YE	*Pyrus calleryana* Decne.
Calycin Swertia	BAO E ZHANG YA CAI	*Swertia calycina* Franch.
Calyx-shaped Daphniphyllum Fruit	NIU ER FENG ZI	*Daphniphyllum calycinum* Benth.
Calyx-shaped Daphniphyllum Leaf	NIU ER FENG ZHI YE	*Daphniphyllum calycinum* Benth.

Index of Traditional Chinese Medicines by English Name

English Name	TCM Name	Origin Latin Name
Camphortree Leaf	ZHANG SHU YE	*Cinnamomum camphora* (L.) Presl
Camphortree	ZHANG MU (ZHANG SHU)	*Cinnamomum camphora* (L.) Presl
Camphortreeleaf Pepper	ZHANG YE HU JIAO	*Piper polysyphorum* C. DC
Campus-belu Aspidosperma	BAI JIAN MU	*Aspidosperma campus-belus* A. P. Duarte.
Canereed Spiralflagg	ZHANG LIU TOU	*Costus speciosus* (Koen.) Smith.
Canton Abrus Herb	JI GU CAO	*Abrus fruticulosus* Wall. *ex* Wight *et* Arn. [= *Abrus cantoniensis* Hance]
Canton Buttercup Herb	ZI KOU CAO	*Ranunculus cantoniensis* DC.
Cape Ganoderma	BAO GAI LING ZHI	*Ganoderma capense* (Lloyd) Teng
Cape Jasmine Fruit	ZHI ZI	*Gardenia jasminoides* Ellis
Cape Jasmine Leaf	ZHI ZI YE	*Gardenia jasminoides* Ellis
Cape of Good Hope Aloe Dried Juice	HAO WANG JIAO LU HUI	*Aloe ferox* Mill.
Caper Euphorbia Latex	XU SUI ZI JING ZHONG BAI ZHI	*Euphorbia lathyris* L.
Caper Euphorbia Seed	QIAN JIN ZI	*Euphorbia lathyris* L.
Capillary Wormwood	YIN CHEN HAO	*Artemisia capillaris* Thunb.
Capitate Cyathula	CHUAN NIU XI	*Cyathula capitata* (Wall.) Moq.
Capitateflower Velvetbean	LI DOU	*Stizolobium capitatum* (Sweet) O. Ktze.
Carp Gall	LI YU DAN	*Cyprinus carpio* L.
Carp Skin	LI YU PI	*Cyprinus carpio* L.
Carp	LI YU	*Cyprinus carpio* L.
Carrot Seed	HU LUO BO ZI	*Daucus carota* L. var. *sativa* DC.
Carrot	HU LUO BO	*Daucus carota* L. var. *sativa* DC.
Cassiabarktree Twig	GUI ZHI	*Cinnamomum cassia* Presl
Cassiabarktree	ROU GUI	*Cinnamomum cassia* Presl
Castorbean Leaf	BI MA YE	*Ricinus communis* L.
Castorbean Oil	BI MA YOU	*Ricinus communis* L.
Castorbean Root	BI MA GEN	*Ricinus communis* L.
Castorbean Seed	BI MA ZI	*Ricinus communis* L.
Catchweed Bedstraw	BA XIAN CAO	*Galium aparine* L.
Catnip	JIA JING JIE	*Nepeta cataria* L.
Caudate Milkwort	SHUI HUANG YANG MU	*Polygala caudata* Rehd. *et* Wils.
Caudate Sweetleaf Leaf	SHAN FAN YE	*Symplocos caudata* Wall.
Celery Wormwood	QING HAO	*Artemisia apiacea* Hance
Centipede	WU GONG	*Scolopendra subspinipes mutians* L. Koch
Cera Chinensis Wax	CHONG BAI LA	*Ericerus pela* (Chavannes)
Cernuous Clubmoss Herb	PU DI WU GONG	*Lycopodium cernnum* L.
Ceylon Helminthostachys	RU DI WU GONG	*Helminthostachys zeylanica* (L.) Hook.
Ceylon Persimmon Sawdust	WU MU XIE	*Diospyros ebenum* Koen.
Chachi Citrus Pericarp	GAN PI	*Citrus chachiensis* Hort.
Chachi Citrus	GAN	*Citrus chachiensis* Hort.
Chaffanjon Ampelopsis	YU YE SHE PU TAO	*Ampelopsis chaffanjonii* (Lévl.) Rehd.
Champac Michelia	HUANG MIAN GUI	*Michelia champaca* L
Champignon	XIANG XUN	*Lentinus edodes* (Berk.) Sing.
Champion Wood Fern	MAO GUAN ZHONG	*Dryopteris championii* (Benth.) C. Chr. *ex* Ching
Chaulmoogratree Seed	DA FENG ZI	*Hydrocarpus anthelmintica* Pierr. *ex* Less.
Chaxiong Ligusticum	CHA XIONG	*Ligusticum sinense* Oliv. cv. *chaxiong*
Cheliensis Goniothalamus	JING HONG GE NA XIANG	*Goniothalamus cheliensis*

Index of Traditional Chinese Medicines by English Name

English Name	TCM Name	Origin Latin Name
Cherokee Rose	JIN YING ZI	*Rosa laevigata* Michx.
Chicken Brain	JI NAO	*Gallus gallus domesticus* Brisson
Chicken	JI ROU	*Gallus gallus domesticus* Brisson
Chicken's Gizzard Endothelium	JI NEI JIN	*Gallus gallus domesticus* Brisson
Chinaberry-tree Bark	KU LIAN PI	*Melia azedarach* L.
Chinaberry-tree Flower	LIAN HUA	*Melia azedarach* L.
Chinaroot Greenbrier	BA QIA	*Smilax china* L.
Chinese Aloe Dried Juice	BAN WEN LU HUI	*Aloe vera* L. var. *chinensis* (Haw.) Berger
Chinese Angelica	DANG GUI	*Angelica sinensis* (Oliv.) Diels
Chinese Arborvitae Branch	BAI ZHI JIE (CE BAI ZHI JIE)	*Thuja orientalis* (L.) Endl. [= *Platycladus orientalis* (L.) Franco]
Chinese Arborvitae Leaf	CE BAI YE	*Thuja orientalis* (L.) Endl. [= *Platycladus orientalis* (L.) Franco]
Chinese Ash Bark	QIN PI	*Fraxinus chinensis* Roxb.
Chinese Astilbe Root	LUO XIN FU GEN	*Astilbe chinensis* (Maxim.) Franch. *et* Sav.
Chinese Astilbe	LUO XIN FU	*Astilbe chinensis* (Maxim.) Franch. *et* Sav.
Chinese Atractylodes	CANG ZHU	*Atractylodes chinensis* Koidz.
Chinese Aucuba	TIAN JIAO BAN	*Aucuba chinensis* Benth.
Chinese Azalea Flower	NAO YANG HUA	*Rhododendron molle* (Bl.) G. Don
Chinese Box Juvenile Leaf	HUANG YANG MU YE	*Buxus microphylla* Sieb. *et* Zucc. var. *sinica* Rehd. *et* Wils.
Chinese Buckeye Seed	SUO LUO ZI	*Aesculus chinensis* Bge.
Chinese Cedar	LIU SHAN	*Cryptomeria fortunei* Hooibrenk
Chinese Clematis	WEI LING XIAN	*Clematis chinensis* Osbeck
Chinese Clinopodium	FENG LUN CAI	*Clinopodium chinense* (Benth.) O. Ktze.
Chinese Common Jasminorange	ZHONG HUA JIU LI XIANG	*Murraya exotica*
Chinese Coriaria Leaf	MA SANG YE	*Coriaria sinica* Maxim.
Chinese Coriaria	MA SANG	*Coriaria sinica* Maxim. [= *Coriaria nepalensis* Wall.]
Chinese Corktree	HUANG BAI	*Phellodendron chinense* Schneid.
Chinese Cricket	XI SHUAI	*Gryllulus chinensis* Weber
Chinese Crinum Root	LUO QUN DAI GEN	*Crinum asiaticum* L. var. *sinicum* Bak.
Chinese Crossostephium Root	FU RONG JU GEN	*Crossostephium chinense* (L.) Mak. *ex* Cham. *et* Schltr.
Chinese Dandelion	JIAN DI PU GONG YING	*Taraxacum sinicum* Kitag.
Chinese Desmos	JIA YING ZHUA	*Desmos cochinchinensis* Lour. [= *Desmos chinensis* Lour.]
Chinese Diploclisia	QING FENG TENG	*Diploclisia chinensis* Merr.
Chinese Dodder Seed	TU SI ZI	*Cuscuta chinensis* Lam.
Chinese Dregea	KU SHENG	*Dregea sinensis* Hemsl.
Chinese Dwarf Cherry Seed	YU LI REN	*Prunus humilis* Bge.
Chinese Eaglewood	BAI MU XIANG	*Aquilaria sinensis* (Lour.) Gilg
Chinese Elm Bark	LANG YU PI	*Ulmus paruifolia* Jacq.
Chinese Ephedra	MA HUANG	*Ephedra sinica* Stapf
Chinese Fevervine Fruit	JI SHI TENG GUO	*Paederia scandens* (Lour.) Merr.
Chinese Fevervine	JI SHI TENG	*Paederia scandens* (Lour.) Merr.
Chinese Forgetmenot	GOU SHI HUA	*Cynoglossum amabile* Stapf *et* Drumm.
Chinese Galangal	LIAN JIANG	*Alpinia chinensis* Rosc.
Chinese Gambirplant	HUA GOU TENG	*Uncaria sinensis* (Oliv.) Havil.
Chinese Goldthread	HUANG LIAN	*Coptis chinensis* Franch.

Index of Traditional Chinese Medicines by English Name

Index of Traditional Chinese Medicines by English Name

Index of Traditional Chinese Medicines by English Name

English Name	TCM Name	Origin Latin Name
Cockroach	ZHANG LANG	*Blatta orientalis* L.
Coconut Albumen	YE ZI RANG	*Cocos nucifera* L.
Coconut Oil	YE ZI YOU	*Cocos nucifera* L.
Coconut Root-bark	YE ZI PI	*Cocos nucifera* L.
Coffee Senna Seed	WANG JIANG NAN ZI	*Cassia occidentalis* L.
Coffee Senna	WANG JIANG NAN	*Cassia occidentalis* L.
Collett Yam	CHA RUI SHU YU	*Dioscorea collettii* Hook. f.
Collybia Albuminosa Sporophore	JI ZONG	*Collybia albuminosa* (Berk.) Petch
Colophony	SONG XIANG	*Pinus massoniana* Lamb.
Colored Mistletoe	HU JI SHENG	*Viscum coloratum* (Kom.) Nakai
Combined Spicebush	WU YAO	*Lindera strychnifolia* (Sieb. *et* Zucc.) Villar [= *Lindera aggregata* (Sims) Kosterm.]
Common Alstonia	XIANG PI MU	*Alstonia scholaris* (L.) R. Br.
Common Andrographis	CHUAN XIN LIAN	*Andrographis paniculata* (Burm.f.) Nees
Common Anemarrhena	ZHI MU	*Anemarrhena asphodeloides* Bge.
Common Anisodus	SAI LANG DANG	*Anisodus luridus* Link *et* Otto
Common Aspidistra	ZHI ZHU BAO DAN	*Aspidistra elatior* Bl.
Common Atlantic Octopus	ZHANG YU	*Octopus vulgaris* Lamarck
Common Aucklandia (Costustoot)	MU XIANG	*Saussurea lappa* Clarke [= *Aucklandia lappa* Decne]
Common Banana	XIANG JIAO	*Musa paradisiaca* L. var. *sapientum* O. Ktze. [= *Musa sapientum* L.]
Common Baphicacanthus Leaf	DA QING YE	*Baphicacanthus cusia* (Nees) Bremek
Common Baphicacanthus Root	BAN LAN GEN	*Baphicacanthus cusia* (Nees) Brem.
Common Bombax Flower	MU MIAN HUA	*Gossampinus malabarica* (DC.) Merr.
Common Broadlily	LEI GONG QI	*Clintonia alpina* (Royle) Kunth
Common Buckwheat Stem	QIAO MAI JIE	*Fagopyrum esculentum* Moench
Common Buckwheat	QIAO MAI	*Fagopyrum esculentum* Moench
Common Burreed	SAN LENG	*Sparganium stoloniferum* Buch.-Ham.
Common Butterbush	FENG XIANG SHU YE (a)	*Cephalanthus occidentalis* L.
Common Camptotheac	XI SHU	*Camptotheca acuminata* Decne.
Common Caper	LAO SHU GUA	*Capparis spinosa* L.
Common Carpesium Fruit	HE SHI (TIAN MING JING)	*Carpesium abrotanoides* L.
Common Carpesium	TIAN MING JING	*Carpesium abrotanoides* L.
Common Cashew Fruit	DU XIAN ZI	*Anacardium occidentale* L.
Common Cerberustree	NIU XIN QIE ZI	*Cerbera manghas* L.
Common Chicory	JU QU	*Cichorium intybus* L.
Common Cissampelos	XI SHENG TENG	*Cissampelos pareira* L.
Common Cnidium	SHE CHUANG ZI	*Cnidium monnieri* (L.) Cusson
Common Coltsfoot	KUAN DONG HUA	*Tussilago farfara* L.
Common Crapemyrtle Flower	ZI WEI HUA	*Lagerstroemia indica* L.
Common Crapemyrtle Leaf	ZI WEI YE	*Lagerstroemia indica* L.
Common Crapemyrtle Root	ZI WEI GEN	*Lagerstroemia indica* L.
Common Cruculigo	XIAN MAO	*Curculigo orchioides* Gaertn.
Common Cyanotis	LU SHUI CAO (II)	*Cyanotis vaga* (Lour.) Roem. *et* Schult.
Common Dayflower Herb	YA ZHI CAO	*Commelina communis* L.
Common Devilpepper Stem and Leaf	LUO FU MU JING YE	*Rauwolfia verticillata* (Lour.) Baill.
Common Devilpepper	LUO FU MU	*Rauwolfia verticillata* (Lour.) Baill.
Common Ducksmeat	FU PING	*Spirodela polyrrhiza* Schleid.
Common Duckwood	FU PING	*Lemna mino*r L.

Index of Traditional Chinese Medicines by English Name

English Name	TCM Name	Origin Latin Name
Common Dysosma	GUI JIU	*Dysosma versipellis* (Hance) M. Cheng
Common Elsholtzia	BAN BIAN SU	*Elsholtzia ciliata* (Yhunb.) Hyland
Common Evolvulus	TU DING GUI	*Evolvulus alsinoides* L.
Common Fenugreek	HU LU BA	*Trigonella foenum-graecum* L.
Common Flax Seed	YA MA ZI	*Linum usitatissimum* L.
Common Flax	YA MA	*Linum usitatissimum* L.
Common Floweringquince	MU GUA	*Chaenomeles lagenaria* (Loisel.) Koidz.
Common Floweringquince	QIU MU GUA	*Chaenomeles speciosa* (Sweet) Nakai
Common Four-o'clock Leaf	ZI MO LI YE	*Mirabilis jalapa* L.
Common Four-o'clock Root	ZI MO LI GEN	*Mirabilis jalapa* L.
Common Ginger Dried Rhizome	GAN JIANG	*Zingiber officinale* Rosc.
Common Goldenrod	YI ZHI HUANG HUA	*Solidago virgaurea* L. var. *leiocarpa* (Benth.) A. Gray [= *Solidago decurrens* Lour.]
Common Heron's Bill Herb	LAO GUAN CAO	*Erodium stephanianum* Willd.
Common Hogfennel	QIAN HU	*Peucedanum decursivum* (Miq.) Maxim.
Common Houndstongue	YAO YONG DAO TI HU	*Cynoglossum officinale* L.
Common Indianmulberry	YANG JIAO TENG	*Morinda umbellata* L.
Common Japanese Clubmoss	SHEN JIN CAO	*Lycopodium clavatum* L.
Common Jasminorange	JIU LI XIANG	*Murraya paniculata* (L.) Jacks.
Common Jujube (Chinese Date)	DA ZAO	*Ziziphus jujuba* Mill.
Chinese Date (Common Jujube)	DA ZAO	*Ziziphus jujuba* Mill.
Common Jujube Seed	SUAN ZAO REN	*Ziziphus jujuba* Mill. var. *spinosa* (Bunge) Hu *ex* H. F. Chow [= *Zyziphs jujuba* Miller]
Common Knotgrass	BIAN XU	*Polygonum aviculare* L.
Common Lamiophlomis	DU YI WEI	*Lamiophlomis rotata* (Benth.) Kudo [= *Phlomis rotata* Benth.]
Common Lantana	WU SE MEI	*Lantana camara* L.
Common Leafflower	YE XIA ZHU	*Phyllanthus urinaria* L.
Common Lophatherum Root	DAN ZHU YE GEN (SUI GU ZI)	*Lophatherum gracile* Brongn.
Common Lophatherum	DAN ZHU YE	*Lophatherum gracile* Brongn.
Common Marsharigold	MA TI YE	*Caltha palustris* L.
Common Mayapple	DUN YE GUI JIU	*Podophyllum peltatum* L.
Common Monkshood	CHUAN WU TOU	*Aconitum carmichaeli* Debx.
Common Nandina Fruit	NAN TIAN ZHU ZI	*Nandina domestica* Thunb.
Common Nandina Root	NAN TIAN ZHU GEN	*Nandina domestica* Thunb.
Common Nandina Stem	NAN TIAN ZHU GENG	*Nandina domestica* Thunb.
Common Nasturtium	HAN LIAN HUA	*Tropaeolum majus* L.
Common Nutmeg	ROU DOU KOU	*Myristica fragrans* Houtt.
Common Olive	QI DUN GUO (YOU GAN LAN)	*Olea europaea* L.
Common onion	YANG CONG	*Allium cepa* L.
Common Origanum	TU XIANG RU	*Origanum vulgare* L.
Common Pearleverlasting	DA YE BAI TOU WENG	*Anaphalis margaritacea* (L.) Benth. *et* Hook. f.
Common Peganum Herb	LUO TUO PENG	*Peganum harmala* L.
Common Peganum Seed	LUO TUO PENG ZI	*Peganum harmala* L.
Common Peony (wild)	SHAO YAO	*Paeonia lactiflora* Pall.
Common peony	BAI SHAO YAO	*Paeonia lactiflora* Pall.
Common Perilla Fruit	BAI SU ZI	*Perilla frutescens* (L.) Britt.
Common Pheasant	ZHI	*Phasianus colchicus* Gmelin
Common Physochlaina	PAO NANG CAO	*Physochlaina physaloides* (L.) G. Don

Index of Traditional Chinese Medicines by English Name

English Name	TCM Name	Origin Latin Name
Common Pistache	HUANG LIAN YA	*Pistacia chinensis* Bge.
Common Quince	WEN PO	*Cydonia oblonga* Mill.
Common Ragweed	TUN CAO	*Ambrosia artemisiifolia* L.
Common Reed Rhizome	LU GEN	*Phragmites communis* Trin.
Common Rue Herb	CHOU CAO	*Ruta graveolens* L.
Common Sage Herb	LI ZHI CAO	*Salvia plebeia* R. Br.
Common Sassafras	CHA SHU	*Sassafras tzumu* Hemsl.
Common Scouring Rush	MU ZEI	*Equisetum hiemale* L.
Common Selfheal	XIA KU CAO	*Prunella vulgaris* L.
Common Sinopodophyllm	TAO ER QI	*Podophyllum emodi* Wall. var. *chinense* Sprague
Common Smoketree Branch and Leaf	HUANG LU ZHI YE	*Cotinus coggygria* Scop.
Common Smoketree	HUANG LU	*Cotinus coggygria* Scop.
Common Spiderflower Seed	BAI HUA CAI ZI	*Cleome gynandra* L.
Common Squill	MIAN ZAO ER	*Scilla sinensis* (Lour.) Merr.
Common St. John'swort	GUAN YE LIAN QIAO	*Hypericum perforatum* L.
Common St. Paulswort	XI XIAN	*Siegesbeckia orientalis* L.
Common Stelmatocrypton	SHENG TENG	*Stelmatocrypton khasianum* (Benth.) H. Baill.
Common Threewingnut	LEI GONG TENG	*Tripterygium wilfordii* Hook. f.
Common Tobacco	YAN CAO	*Nicotiana tabacum* L.
Common Tulip Root	YU JIN XIANG GEN	*Tulipa gesneriana* L.
Common Tulip	YU JIN XIANG	*Tulipa gesneriana* L.
Common Turmeric	JIANG HUANG	*Curcuma longa* L.
Common Turmeric	YU JIN	*Curcuma longa* L.
Common Valeriana	XIE CAO	*Valeriana officinalis* L.
Common Vetch	DA CHAO CAI	*Vicia sativa* L.
Common Vladimiria	MU XIANG	*Vladimiria souliei* (Franch.) Ling
Common Waterhyacinth	SHUI HU LU	*Eichhornia crassipes* Solms
Common Watershield	CHUN	*Brasenia schreberi* J. F. Gmel.
Common Wedgelet Fern	DA YE JIN HUA CAO	*Stenoloma chusanum* (L.) Ching
Common Yam	SHAN YAO	*Dioscorea opposita* Thunb.
Common Yarrow Herb	YANG SHI CAO	*Achillea millefolium* L.
Complanate Clubmoss	GUO JIANG LONG	*Lycopodium complanatum* L.
Concentrated Beef Extract	XIA TIAN GAO	*Bos taurus domesticus* Gmelin
Conic Gymnadenia	SHOU ZHANG SHEN	*Gymnadenia conopsea* R. Br.
Conical Redpepper	CHAO TIAN JIAO	*Capsicum annuum* L. var. *conoides* (Mill.) Irish
Contorted Tanglehead	DI JIN	*Heteropogon contortus* (L.) Beauv.
Coprinus Sporophore	GUI GAI	*Coprinus atramentarius* (Bull.) Fr.
Coralhead Plant Seed	XIANG SI ZI	*Abrus precatorium* L.
Coralhead Plant	XIANG SI TENG	*Abrus precatorium* L.
Cordateleaf Sida	HUANG HUA ZI	*Sida cordifolia* L.
Coriander Seed	HU SUI ZI	*Coriandrum sativum* L.
Corn Poppy Fruit	LI CHUN HUA GUO SHI	*Papaver rhoeas* L.
Corn Poppy	LI CHUN HUA	*Papaver rhoeas* L.
Corniculate Spurgentian	HUA MAO	*Halenia corniculata* (L.) Cornaz.
Coromandel Lannea	HOU PI SHU	*Lannea grandis* (Dennst.) Engl.
Coronarious Gingerlily	TU QIANG HUO	*Hedychium Coronarium* Koen.
Corrugate Chinese Dregea	GUAN JIN TENG	*Dregea sinensis* Hemsl. var. *corrugata* (Schneid) Tsiang *et* P. T. Li
Corymbose Hedyotis	SHUI XIAN CAO	*Oldenlandia corymbosa* L. [= *Hedyotis corymbosa* (L.) Lam.]
Cottonrose Hibiscus Flower	MU FU RONG HUA	*Hibiscus mutabilis* L.
Cow Milk	NIU RU	*Bos taurus domesticus* Gmelin; *Bubalus bubalis* Linnaeus

Index of Traditional Chinese Medicines by English Name

English Name	TCM Name	Origin Latin Name
Cow-bezoar (Ox-gallstone)	NIU HUANG	*Bos taurus domesticus* Gmelin; *Bubalus bubalis* Linnaeus
Ox-gallstone (Cow-bezoar)	NIU HUANG	*Bos taurus domesticus* Gmelin; *Bubalus bubalis* Linnaeus
Cowberry Fruit Leaf	YUE JU YE	*Vaccinium vitis-idaea* L.
Cowherb	WANG BU LIU XING	*Vaccaria segetalis* (Neck.) Garcke
Crassnerve Gymnadenia	SHOU ZHANG SHEN	*Gymnadenia crassinervis* Finet
Creeping Rockfoil	HU ER CAO	*Saxifraga stolonifera* (L.) Meerb.
Creeping Rostellularia	JUE CHUANG	*Rostellularia procumbens* (L.) Nees
Creeping Skyflower Leaf	JIA LIAN QIAO YE	*Duranta repena* L.
Crescent-shaped Euphorbia Herb	MAO YAN CAO	*Euphorbia lunulata* Bge.
Crispateleaf Ardisia Leaf	BAI LIANG JIN YE	*Ardisia crispa* (Thunb.) A. DC.
Crispateleaf Ardisia	BAI LIANG JIN	*Ardisia crispa* (Thunb.) A. DC.
Crisped Common Perilla Leaf	ZI SU YE	*Perilla frutescens* (L.) Britt. var. *crispa* (Thunb.) Hand. -Mazz.
Crisped Common Perilla Seed	ZI SU ZI	*Perilla frutescens* (L.) Britt. var. *crispa* (Thunb.) Hand. -Mazz.
Crisped Common Perilla Stem	ZI SU GEN	*Perilla frutescens* (L.) Britt. var. *crispa* (Thunb.) Hand. -Mazz.
Crisped Dock	NIU ER DA HUANG	*Rumex crispus* L.
Crownofhorns Euphorbia	TIE HAI TANG	*Euphorbia milii* Ch. des Moulins
Crucian Carp	JIN YU	*Carassium auratus* (L.)
Cubeba Piper	BI CHENG QIE	*Piper cubeba* L.
Cucumber	HUANG GUA	*Cuccumis sativus* L.
Cudweed	SHU QU CAO	*Gnaphalium affine* D. Don
Cultivate Sisalan Agave East-1	DONG YI HAO JIAN MA	*Agave east-one*
Cuneate Lespedeza	YE GUAN MEN	*Lespedeza cuneata* (Dum.Cours.) G. Don
Curly Bristlethistle	FEI LIAN	*Carduun crispus* L.
Curvebeak Monkshood	WAN ZHUO WU TOU	*Aconitum campylorrhynchum* Hand-Mazz
Cushaw Seed	NAN GUA ZI	*Cucurbita moschata* (Duch.) Poiret
Cushaw	NAN GUA	*Cucurbita moschata* (Duch.) Poiret
Cuspidate Mnium Herb	SHUI MU CAO	*Mnium cuspidatum* Hedw.
Custardapple	FAN LI ZHI	*Annona squamosa* L.
Cutechu	HAI ER CHA	*Acacia catechu* (L.) Willd
Daghestan Sweetclover Herb	PI HAN CAO	*Melilotus suaveolens* Ledeb.
Dahuria Gentian	QIN JIAO	*Gentiana dahurica* Fisch.
Dahurian Angelica	BAI ZHI	*Angelica dahurica* (Fisch. *ex* Hoffm.) Benth. *et* Hook. f. *ex* Franch. *et* Sav.
Dahurian Angelica	XING AN BAI ZHI	*Angelica dahurica* (Fisch. *ex* Hoffm.) Benth. *et* Hook. f. *ex* Franch. *et* Sav.
Dahurian Bugbane	XING AN SHENG MA	*Cimicifuga dahurica* (Turcz.) Maxim.
Dahurian Patrinia	HUANG HUA BAI JIANG	*Patrinia scabiosaefolia* Fisch.
Dahurian Rhododendron	MAN SHAN HONG	*Rhododendron dauricum* L.
Danshen	DAN SHEN	*Salvia miltiorrhiza* Bge.
Dateplum Persimmon	JUN QIAN ZI	*Diaspyros lotus* L.
David Epimedium	CHUAN DIAN YIN YANG HUO	*Epimedium davidii* Franch.
David Falsepanax	YI YE LIANG WANG CHA	*Nothopanax davidii* (Franch.) Harms
David Peach Bast	TAO JING BAI PI	*Prunus davidiana* (Carr.) Franch.
David Peach Flower	TAO HUA	*Prunus davidiana* (Carr.) Franch.
David Peach Juvenile Branch	TAO ZHI	*Prunus davidiana* (Carr.) Franch.
David Peach Leaf	TAO YE	*Prunus davidiana* (Carr.) Franch.
David Peach Resin	TAO JIAO	*Prunus davidiana* (Carr.) Franch.
David Peach Root	TAO GEN	*Prunus davidiana* (Carr.) Franch.
David's Maidenhair Fern	ZHU ZONG CAO	*Adiantum davidii* Franch.

Index of Traditional Chinese Medicines by English Name

Index of Traditional Chinese Medicines by English Name

Index of Traditional Chinese Medicines by English Name

Index of Traditional Chinese Medicines by English Name

Index of Traditional Chinese Medicines by English Name

English Name	TCM Name	Origin Latin Name
Glabrous Sarcandra	JIU JIE CHA	*Sarcandra glabra* (Thunb.) Nakai
Glabrousleaf Chinese Corktree	HUANG BAI	*Phellodendron chinense* Schneid. var. *glabriusculum* Schneid.
Glabrousleaf Erycibe	GUANG YE DING GONG TENG	*Erycibe schmidtii* Craib
Glabrousleaf Uvaria	GUANG YE ZI YU PAN	*Uvaria boniana* Finet *et* Gagnep.
Glandularstalk St. Paulswort	XIAN GENG XI XIAN	*Siegesbeckia orientalis* L. var. *pubescens* Mak.
Glaucousback Honeysuckle	JIN YIN HUA	*Lonicera hypoglauca* Miq.
Glaucousback Threewingnut	KUN MING SHAN HAI TANG	*Tripterygium hypoglaucum* (Lévl.) Hutch
Globeamaranth	QIAN RI HONG	*Gomphrena globosa* L.
Globefish	HE TUN	*Fugu ocellatus* (Osbeck)
Globose Condorvine	QIU HUA NIU NAI CAI	*Marsdenia globifera* Tsiang
Globular Pepper	DUAN JU	*Piper mullesua* D. Don.
Glossy Privet Fruit	NU ZHEN ZI	*Ligustrum lucidum* Ait.
Glutinose Bluebeard	NIAN YE YOU	*Caryopteris glutinosa* Rehd.
Gmelin Sealavender Herb	BU XUE CAO	*Limonium gmelinii* (Willd.) O. Ktze.
Goat Hide	YANG PI	*Capra hircus* L.; *Ovis aries* L.
Goat Milk	YANG RU	*Capra hircus* L.; *Ovis aries* L.
Goat Pancreas	YANG YI	*Capra hircus* L.; *Ovis aries* L.
Goering Lemongrass	YE XIANG MAO	*Cymbopogon goeringii* (Steud.) A. Camus
Golden Buckwheat Root	TIAN QIAO MAI GEN	*Fagopyrum cymosum* Meisr.
Golden Lycoris	DA YI ZHI JIAN	*Lycoris aurea* Herb.
Goldenflower Dendrobium	SHU HUA SHI HU	*Dendrobium chrysanthum* Wall.
Goldenshower Senna Fruit	PO LUO MEN ZAO JIA	*Cassia fistula* L.
Goldhair Hedyotis	JIN MAO ER CAO	*Hedyotis chrysotricha* (Polib.) Merr. [= *Oldenlandia chrysotricha* (Polib.) Chun]
Goldsaxifrage Herb	JIN QIAN KU YE CAO	*Chrysosplenium grayanum* Maxim.
Goose Fat	BAI E GAO	*Anser domestica* Geese
Goose Tail-meat	E CUI	*Anser domestica* Geese
Graceful Jessamine	GOU WEN	*Gelsemium elegans* Benth
Gram Chickpea	HUI HUI DOU	*Cicer arietinum* L.
Grandularflower Rabdosia	XIAN HUA XIANG CHA CAI	*Isodon adenanthus* (Diels.) Kudo
Grassleaf Sweetflag Leaf	SHI CHANG PU YE	Acorus gramineus Soland.
Grassleaf Sweetflag	SHI CHANG PU	*Acorus gramineus* Soland.
Great Burdock Fruit	NIU BANG ZI	*Arctium lappa* L.
Great Burdock Root	NIU BANG GEN	*Arctium lappa* L.
Great Willowherb (Firewood)	HONG KUAI ZI	*Chamaenerion angustifolium* (L.) Scop. [= *Epilobium angustifolium* L.]
Firewood (Great Willowherb)	HONG KUAI ZI	*Chamaenerion angustifolium* (L.) Scop. [= *Epilobium angustifolium* L.]
Greater Celandine	BAI QU CAI	*Chelidonium majus* L.
Grecian Laurel	YUE GUI ZI	*Laurus nobilis* L.
Green Alectoria Filament	JIN SI DAI	*Alectoria vivens* Tayl.
Greenish Lily	BAI HE	*Lilium brownii* F. E. Brown var. *colchesteri* Wils.
Greyblue Pericampylus	XI YUAN TENG	*Pericampylus glaucus* (Lam.) Merr.
Grosvenor Siraitia	LUO HAN GUO	*Siraitia grosvenorii* (Swingle) C. Jeffrey *ex* Lu *et* Z. Y. Zhang [= *Momordica grosvenorii* Swingle]
Guanabana	CI GUO FAN LI ZHI	*Annona muricata* L.
Guava Bark	FAN SHI LIU PI	*Psidium guajava* L.

Index of Traditional Chinese Medicines by English Name

English Name	TCM Name	Origin Latin Name
Guava Immature Fruit	FAN SHI LIU GAN	*Psidium guajava* L.
Guava Leaf	FAN SHI LIU YE	*Psidium guajava* L.
Gynura	SAN QI CAO	*Gynura segetum* (Lour.) Merr. [= *Cacalia procumbens* Lour.]
Gypsophila	HUANG JIE GU DAN	*Gypsophila acutifolia* Fisch.
Gypsum Fibrosum	SHI GAO	Calcium sulphate, $CaSO_4$symbol 215 \f "Symbol" \s 8·}H_2O.
Haichow Elsholtzia	XIANG RU	*Elsholtzia splendens* Nakai *ex* F. Maekawa
Hainan Devilpepper	HAI NAN LUO FU MU	*Rauvolfia verticillata* (Lour) Baill. var. *hainanensis* Tsiang
Hainan Goniothalamus	HAI NAN GE NA XIANG	*Goniothalamus howii* Merr.
Hainan Sarcococca	HAI NAN YE SHAN HUA	*Sarcococca vagans* Stapf
Hainan Tinospora	HAI NAN QING NIU DAN	*Tinospora hainanesis* H. S. Lo *et* Z. X. Li
Hair Larkspur	ZHAN MAO CUI QUE HUA	*Delphinium kamaonense* var. *glabrescens* W.T. Wang
Hairstalk St. Paulswort	MAO GENG XI XIAN	*Siegesbeckia orientalis* L. var. *glabrescens* Mak. [= *Siegesbeckia glabrescens* Mak.]
Hairstyle Poisonnut	MAO ZHU MA QIAN	*Strychnos nitida* G. Don
Hairy Antler	LU RONG	*Cervus nippon* Temminck; *Cervus elaphus* L.
Hairy Chestnut Bast	LI SHU PI	*Castanea mollissima* Bl.
Hairy Clivereshrub	DA HONG PAO	*Campylotropis hirtella* (Franch.) Schindl.
Hairy Datura Flower	YANG JIN HUA	*Datura inoxia* Mill.
Hairy Datura Leaf	MAN TUO LUO YE	*Datura inoxia* Mill.
Hairy Datura Root	MAN TUO LUO GEN	*Datura inoxia* Mill.
Hairy Datura Seed	MAN TUO LUO ZI	*Datura inoxia* Mill.
Hairy Rhynchotechum	MAO XIAN ZHU JU TAI	*Rhynchotechum vestitum* Hook. f. *et* Thoms.
Hairy Willowweed	SHUI JIE GU DAN	*Epilobium hirsutum* L.
Hairy Wormwood	MAO LIAN HAO	*Artemisia vestita* Wall.
Hairyleaf Aralia	TOU XU SONG MU	*Aralia dasyphylla* Miq.
Hairystalk Tinospora	JIN GUO LAN	*Tinospora capillipes* Gagn.
Hairyvein Agrimonia Root	LONG YA CAO GEN (XIAN HE CAO GEN)	*Agrimonia pilosa* Ledeb. var. *japonica* (Miq.) Nakai
Hairyvein Argimonia Rhizome	XIAN HE CAO GEN YA	*Argimonia pilosa* Ledeb. var. *japonica* (Miq.) Nakai
Hairyvein Argimonia	XIAN HE CAO	*Argimonia pilosa* Ledeb. var. *japonica* (Miq.) Nakai
Hance Pepper	SHAN JU	*Piper hancei* Maxim.
Hancock Swallowwort	HUA BEI BAI QIAN	*Cynanchum hancockianum* (Maxim) Al. Iljinski
Hard Bluegrass	LONG XU CAO (II)	*Poa sphondylodes* Trin.
Hard Clam Shell	WEN GE	*Meretrix meretrix* L.
Harrlequin Glorybower Leaf	CHOU WU TONG	*Clerodendron trichotomum* Thunb.
Harrlequin Glorybower Root	CHOU WU TONG GEN	*Clerodendron trichotomum* Thunb.
Hawaiian Elephantfoot	ROU MAO DI DAN CAO	*Elephantopus mollis* H. B. K.
Heartleaf Houttuynia Herb	YU XING CAO	*Houttuynia cordata* Thunb.
Heartleaf Tubergourd	XIN YE CIII BO	*Thladiantha cordifolia* (BL.) Cogn.
Hedge Sageretia	QUE MEI TENG	*Sageretia theezans* Brongn. [= *Sageretia thea* (Osbeck) Johnst.]
Hedgehog Brain	WEI NAO	*Erinaceus europaeus* L.; *Hemiechinus dauuricus* Sundevall
Hedgehog Heart and Liver	WEI XIN GAN	*Erinaceus europaeus* L.; *Hemiechinus dauuricus* Sundevall

Index of Traditional Chinese Medicines by English Name

Index of Traditional Chinese Medicines by English Name

Index of Traditional Chinese Medicines by English Name

English Name	TCM Name	Origin Latin Name
Indigo-coloured Woad Leaf	DA QING YE	*Isatis indigotica* Fort.
Indigoplant Leaf	DA QING YE	*Polygonum tinctorium* Ait
Indigoplant	LIAO LAN	*Polygonum tinctorium* Ait.
Indigowoad Root	BAN LAN GEN	*Isatis indigotica* Fort.
Inflated Licorice	ZHANG GU GAN CAO	*Glycyrrhiza inflata* Batal.
Inflatedfruit Senna	JIANG MANG	*Cassia sophera* L.
Inflexed Rabdosia	NEI ZHE XIANG CHA CAI	*Rabdosia inflexa* (Thunb.) Hara
Intermediate Ephedra	MA HUANG	*Ephedra intermeddia* Schrenk *et* Mey.
Intermediate Magnoliavine	ZHONG JIAN WU WEI ZI	*Schisandra propinqua* (Wall.) Baill. var. *intermedia* A. C. Smith
Involucrate Balanophora	TONG QIAO SHE GU	*Balanophora involucrata* Hook. f.
Involute Spikemoss	YAN ZHOU JUAN BAI	*Selaginella involvens* (Sw.) Spring
Ivy Glorybind	MIAN GEN TENG	*Calystegia hederacea* Wall.
Japanese Alder	CHI YANG	*Alnus japonica* Sieb. *et* Zucc.
Japanese Ampelopsis	BAI LIAN	*Ampelopsis japonica* (Thunb.) Mak.
Japanese Apricot	WU MEI	*Prunus mume* (Sieb.) Sieb. *et* Zucc.
Japanese Aralia	CI LAO YA	*Aralia elata* (Miq.) Seem.
Japanese Aralia	SONG MU BAI PI	*Aralia chinensis* L.
Japanese Ardisia Root	ZI JIN NIU GEN	*Ardisia japonica* (Hornst.) Bl.
Japanese Ardisia	ZI JIN NIU	*Ardisia japonica* (Hornst.) Bl.
Japanese Avens Root	SHUI YANG MEI (I) GEN	*Geum japonicum* Thunb.
Japanese Avens	SHUI YANG MEI (I)	*Geum japonicum* Thunb.
Japanese balanophora	GE XUN	*Balanophora japonica* Mak.
Japanese Barerry	XIAO BO	*Berberis thunbergii* DC.
Japanese Buckeye Seed	SUO LUO ZI	*Aesculus Turbinata* BL.
Japanese Butterbur	FENG DOU CAI	*Petasites japoniaus* (Sieb. *et* Zucc.) F. Schmidt
Japanese Buttercup	MAO GEN	*Ranunculus japonicus* Thunb.
Japanese Cayratia	WU LIAN MEI	*Cayratia japonica* (Thunb.) Gagn.
Japanese Chain Fern	GUAN ZHONG	*Woodwardia japonica* (L. f.) Sm.
Japanese Cinnamon	GUI PI	*Cinnamomum japonicum* Sieb.
Japanese Conehead	HONG ZE LAN	*Strobilanthes japonicus* (Thunb.) Miq.
Japanese Creeper	DI JIN	*Parthenocissus tricuspidata* (Sieb. *et* Zucc.) Planch.
Japanese Croomia	JIN GANG DA	*Croomia japonica* Miq.
Japanese Cryptotaenia	YA ER QIN	*Cryptoaenia japonica* Hassk.
Japanese Dock	YANG TI	*Rumex japonicus* Houtt.
Japanese Dodder Seed	DA TU SI ZI	*Cuscuta japonica* Choisy
Japanese Eel	MAN LI YU	*Anguilla japonica* Temminck *et* Schlegel
Japanese Eupatorium	CHENG GAN CAO	*Eupatorium japonicum* Thunb.
Japanese Eurya	LING MU	*Eurya Japonica* Thunb.
Japanese Farfugium Herb	LIAN PENG CAO	*Farfugium japonicum* (L.) Kitam.
Japanese Felt Fern Frond	SHI WEI	*Pyrrosia lingua* (Thunb.) Farw.
Japanese Fleeceflower (Giant Knotweed)	HU ZHANG	*Polygonum cuspidatum* Sieb. *et* Zucc.
Giant Knotweed (Japanese Fleeceflower)	HU ZHANG	*Polygonum cuspidatum* Sieb. *et* Zucc.
Japanese Galangal	TU SHA REN	*Alpinia japonica* Miq
Japanese Ginseng	ZHU JIE SAN QI	*Panax pseudoginseng* Wall. var. *japonicus* (Mey.) Hoo *et* Tseng
Japanese Honeysuckle	JIN YIN HUA	*Lonicera japonica* Thunb.
Japanese Hop Herb	LU CAO	*Humulus scandens* (Lour.) Merr.
Japanese Hylomecon	HE QING HUA	*Hylomecon japonica* (Thunb.) Prantl *et* Kündig
Japanese Inula Herb	JIN FO CAO	*Inula japonica* Thunb.

Index of Traditional Chinese Medicines by English Name

English Name	TCM Name	Origin Latin Name
Largehead Atractylodes	BAI ZHU	*Atractylodes macrocephala* Koidz. [= *Atractylis macrocephala* (Koidz.) Hand.-Mazz.]
Largeleaf Chinese Ash Bark	QIN PI	*Fraxinus rhynchophylla* Hance
Largeleaf Gamirplant	DA YE GOU TENG	*Uncaria macrophylla* Wall.
Largeleaf Gentian	QIN JIAO	*Gentiana macrophylla* Pall.
Largeleaf Hydrangea	BA XIAN HUA	*Hydrangea macrophylla* (Thunb.) Ser.
Largeleaf JapaneseGinseng	QIN LING ZHU ZI SHEN	*Panax japonicus* var. *major* (Burk.) Wu *et* Feng
Largeleaf Rabdosia	DA YE XIANG CHA CAI	*Rabdosia macrophylla* (Migo) C. Wu *et* H. Li
Largeleaf Spicebush Root-bark	DIAO ZHANG GEN PI	*Lindera umbellate* Thunb.
Largeseed Hemsleya	LUO GUO DI	*Hemsleya macrosperma* C. Y. Wu
Largeserrate Mosla	JI NING	*Mosla grosseserrata* Maxim.
Lateripening Bartsia Herb	CHI YE CAO	*Odontites serotina* Reich.
Laurelleaf Snailseed	HENG ZHOU WU YAO	*Cocculus laurifolius* DC.
Lavandulaleaf Chrysanthemum Flower	YE JU HUA	*Chrysanthemum lavandulaefolium* (Fisch.) Mak.
Lavandulaleaf Chrysanthemum	YAN XIANG JU	*Chrysanthemum lavandulaefolium* (Fisch.) Mak.
Lavandulaleaf Dendranthema	GAN JU	*Dendranthema lavandulifolium* (Fisch.) Ling *et* Shih
Laver	ZI CAI	*Porphyra tenera* Kjellm.
Laxleaf Sweetroot	XIANG GEN QIN	*Osmorhiza aristata* (Thunb.) Mak. *et* Yabe var. *laxa* (Royle) Constance *et* Shan
Leafy Euphorbia	JI CHANG LANG DU	*Euphorbia esula* L.
Leatherleaf Mahonia Fruit	SHI DA GONG LAO ZI	*Mahonia bealei* (Fort.) Carr.
Leatherleaf Mahonia Leaf	SHI DA GONG LAO YE	*Mahonia bealei* (Fort.) Carr.
Leatherleaf Mahonia	SHI DA GONG LAO MU	*Mahonia bealei* (Fort.) Carr.
Leatherleaf Millettia Root	KUN MING JI XUE TENG GEN	*Millettia reticulata* Benth.
Ledger Cinchona	JIN JI LE	*Cinchona ledgeriana* Moens.
Leiocarpus Goniothalamus	JIN PING GE NA XIANG	*Goniothalamus leiocarpus*
Lemon eucalyptus Leaf	NING MENG AN YE	*Eucalyptus citriodora* Hook f.
Lemon Leaf	NING MENG YE	*Citrus limon* Burm.
Lemon Root	NING MENG GEN	*Citrus limon* Burm.
Lemon	NING MENG	*Citrus limon* Burm.
Lemongrass	XIANG MAO	*Cymbopogon citratus* (DC.) Stapf
Lemonlike Citrus Leaf	NING MENG YE	*Citrus limonia* Osbeck
Lemonlike Citrus Root	NING MENG GEN	*Citrus limonia* Osbeck
Lemonlike Citrus	NING MENG	*Citrus limonia* Osbeck
Leprieur Caloglossa Frond	ZHE GU CAI	*Caloglossa leprieurii* (Mont.) J. Ag.
Lesser Galangal	GAO LIANG JIANG	*Alpinia officinarum* Hance
Lettuce Ulva Frond	SHI CHUN	*Ulva lactuca* L.
Levant Cotton Oil	MIAN ZI YOU	*Gossypium herbaceum* L.
Levant Cotton Root	MIAN HUA GEN	*Gossypium herbaceum* L.
Levant Cotton	MIAN HUA	*Gossypium herbaceum* L.
Licorice	GUANG GUO GAN CAO	*Glycyrrhiza glabra* L.
Lightyellow Sophora Seed	KU SHEN SHI	*Sophora flavescens* Ait.
Lightyellow Sophora	KU SHEN	*Sophora flavescens* Ait.
Likiang Hogfennel	LI JIANG QIAN HU	*Peucedanum govanianum* (Wall) Benth *ex* C. B. Clarke var. *bicolo* Wolff
Lilac Daphne Root	YUAN HUA GEN	*Daphne genkwa* Sieb. *et* Zucc.
Lilac Daphne	YUAN HUA	*Daphne genkwa* Sieb. *et* Zucc.
Lilac Pink	QU MAI	*Dianthus superbus* L.

English Name	TCM Name	Origin Latin Name
Lily Magnolia Bark	MU LAN PI	*Magnolia liliflora* Desr.
Lily Magnolia Flower	MU LAN HUA	*Magnolia liliflora* Desr.
Lily Magnolia	XIN YI	*Magnolia liliflora* Desr.
Lily	BAI HE	*Lilium brownii* F.E. Brown var. *viridulum* Baker
Lilyofthevalley	LING LAN	*Convallaria keiskei* Miq. [= *Convallaria majalis* L.]
Limpricht Begonia	JI YE QIU HAI TANG	*Begonia limprichtii* Irmsch.
Lindley Eupatorium	CHENG GAN SHENG MA	*Eupatorium lindleyanum* DC.
Linearleaf Gentian	LONG DAN	*Gentiana manshurica* Kitagawa
Linearleaf Inula Flower	XUAN FU HUA	*Inula linariaefolia* Turcz.
Linearleaf Inula Herb	JIN FO CAO	*Inula linariaefolia* Turcz.
Linearleaf Thistle	KU AO	*Cirsium chinense* Gardn. *et* Champ.
Little Groundcherry	TIAN PAO ZI	*Physalis minima* L.
Littleflower Plumbagella Herb	JI WA CAO	*Plumbagella micrantha* (Ledeb.) Spach
Littlehead Sneezeweed	XIAO TOU DUI XIN JU	*Helenium microcephalum* DC.
Littleleaf Common Jasminorange	XIAO YE JIU LI XIANG	*Murraya paniculata* (L.) Jack var. *exotica* (L.) Huang
Littleleaf Lemmaphyyllum Herb	LUO YAN CAO	*Lemmaphyllum microphyllum* Presl
Lobed Kudzuvine Leaf	GE YE	*Pueraria lobata* (Willd.) Ohwi
Lobed Kudzuvine Root	GE GEN	*Pueraria lobata* (Willd.) Ohwi
Lobedfruit Tacca	LIE GUO SHU	*Tacca plantaginea* (Hance) Drenth.
Lobedleaf Pharbitis Seed	QIAN NIU ZI	*Pharbitis nil* (L.) Choisy
Lobster	HAI XIA	*Panulirus ornatus* (Fabricius)
Loddiges Dendrobium	MEI HUA SHI HU	*Dendrobium loddigesii* Rolfe.
Long Pepper Root	BI BA GEN	*Piper longum* L.
Long Pepper	BI BA	*Piper longum* L.
Long Usnea Filament	SONG LUO	*Usnea longissima* Ach.
Longan Leaf	LONG YAN YE	*Euphoria longan* (Lour.) Steud.
Longbract Cattail Pollen	PU HUANG	*Typha angustata* Bory *et* Chaub.
Longbract Cattail	CHANG BAO XIANG PU	*Typha angustata* Bory *et* Chaub.
Longeared Epigynum	SI MAO TENG	*Epigynum auritum* (Schneid.) Tsiang *et* P. T. Li
Longleaf Rabdosia	CHANG YE XIANG CHA CAI	*Rabdosia stracheyi* (Benth. *ex* Hook. f.) Hara
Longpedicel Chinese Buscherry Seed	YU LI REN	*Prunus japonica* Thunb. var. *nakaii* (Lévl.) Rehd.
Longpeduncle Kadsura	CHANG GENG NAN WU WEI ZI	*Kadsura longepedunculata* Finet *et* Gagnép.
Longroot Onion	GE CONG	*Allium victorialis* L.
longstalk Gynostemma	CHANG GENG JIAO GU LAN	*Gynostemma longipes* C. Y. Wu
Longstamen Onion	XIE BAI	*Allium macrostemon* Bge.
Longtube Ground Ivy	JIN QIAN CAO	*Glechoma longituba* (Nakai) Kurp.
Longtube Rabdosia	CHANG GUAN XIANG CHA CAI	*Rabdosia longituba* (Miquel) Hara.
Lopseed Herb	LAO PO ZI ZHEN XIAN	*Phryma leptostachya* L.
Loquat Leaf	PI PA YE	*Eriobotrya japonica* (Thunb.) Lindl.
Loquat Seed	PI PA HE	*Eriobotrya japonica* (Thunb.) Lindl.
Lovely Hemsleya	LUO GUO DI	*Hemsleya amabilis* Diels
Low Lily	BAI HE	*Lilium pumilum* DC.
Low Meadowrue	XIAO TANG SONG CAO	*Thalictrum minus* L.
Low Uvaria	AI ZI YU PAN	*Uvaria Chamae* P. Beauv.
Lucid Ganoderma	CHI ZHI	*Ganoderma lucidum* (Leyss. *ex* Fr.) Karst.
Lunate Peltate Sundew	MAO GAO CAI	*Drosera peltata* Smith var. *lunata* (Buch.-Ham.) C. B. Clarke

Index of Traditional Chinese Medicines by English Name

English Name	TCM Name	Origin Latin Name
Lunathyrium Fern	GUAN ZHONG	*Lunathyrium acrostichoides* (Sw.) Ching
Lychee Seed	LI ZHI HE	*Litchi chinensis* Sonn.
Lychee	LI ZHI	*Litchi chinensis* Sonn.
Macropodous Solomonseal	HUANG JING	*Polygonatum macropodium* Turcz.
Madagascar Periwinkle	CHANG CHUN HUA	*Catharanthus roseus* (L.) G. Don.
Maidenhair Fern	ZHU ZONG CAO	*Adiantum capillusveneris* L.
Maire Alstonia	YANG JIAO MIAN	*Alstonia mairei* Lévl.
Maire Yew	MEI LI HONG DOU SHAN	*Taxus mairei* (Lemée *et* Lévl.) S. Y. Hu
Maize Style	YU MI XU	*Zea mays* L.
Maize	YU SHU SHU	*Zea mays* L.
Malabanut	DA BO GU	*Adhatoda vasica* Nees
Malay Blumea Herb	HONG TOU CAO	*Blumea lacera* (Burm. f.) DC.
Malaytea Scurfpea	BU GU ZHI	*Psoralea corylifolia* L.
Male Fern Rhizome	GUAN ZHONG	*Dryopteris crassirhizoma* Nakai
Manaplant Alhagi Sweet Secretion	CI MI (LUO TUO CI)	*Alhagi pseudalhagi* Desv.
Manchurian Dutchmanspipe	GUAN MU TONG	*Aristolochia manshuriensis* Kom.
Manchurian Rhododendron	ZHAO SHAN BAI	*Rhododendron micranthum* Turcz.
Manchurian Wildginger	XI XIN	*Asarum heterotropoides* F. Schm. var. *mandshuricum* (Maxim.) Kitag.
Mango Bark	MANG GUO SHU PI	*Mongifera indica* L.
Mango Leaf	MANG GUO YE	*Mongifera indica* L.
Mango Seed	MANG GUO HE	*Mongifera indica* L.
Mango	MANG GUO	*Mongifera indica* L.
Manyflower Garcinia	SHAN ZHU ZI	*Garcinia multiflora* Champ.
Manyflower Glorybower Leaf	DA QING YE	*Clerodendron cyrtophyllum* Turcz.
Manyflower Solomonseal	HUANG JING	*Polygonatum cyrtonema* Hua
Manyflower Tylophora	WA ER TENG	*Tylophora floribunda* Miq.
Manyhead Clinopodium	DENG LONG CAO	*Clinopodium polycephalum* (Vant.) C. Y. Wu *et* Hsuan
Manyleaf Meadowrue	MA WEI LIAN	*Thalictrum foliolosum* DC.
Manyleaf Paris	ZAO XIU	*Paris polyphlla* Smith
Manynerve Embelia	MA GUI HUA	*Embelia oblongifolia* Hemsl.
Manyprickle Acanthopanax Leaf	CI WU JIA YE	*Acanthopanax senticosus* (Rupr. *et* Maxim.) Harms
Manyprickle Acanthopanax Root-bark	CI WU JIA PI	*Acanthopanax senticosus* (Rupr. *et* Maxim.) Harms
Manyprickle Acanthopanax Root	CI WU JIA (WU JIA GEN)	*Acanthopanax senticosus* (Rupr. *et* Maxim.) Harms
Manyspike Knotweed	DUO SUI LIAO	*Polygonum polystachyum* Wall. *ex* Meisn
Manyspike Podocarpus	DUO SUI LUO HAN SONG SHI	*Podocarpus polystachyus* R. Br.
Manyspike Tanoak Leaf	DUO SUI SHI KE YE	*Lithocarpus polystachyus* Rehd.
Marchantia Polymorpha Lichen	DI SUO LUO	*Marchantia polymorpha* L.
Marginate American Agave	JIN BIAN LONG SHE LAN	*Agave americana* L. var. *marginata* Hort.
Marsh Horsetail Herb	GU JIE CAO	*Equisetum palustre* L.
Marshy Betony	GUANG YE SHUI SU	*Stachys palustris* L.
Mary Arthromeris	FENG WEI PA SHAN HU	*Arthromeris mairei* (Brause) Ching [= *Polypodium mairei* Brause]
Matteuccia Fern	GUAN ZHONG	*Matteuccia struthiopteris* (L.) Todaro
Maywood	MU JU	*Matricaria chamomilla* L. [= *Matricaria recutita* L.]
Meadow Cranesbill Herb	CAO YUAN LAO GUAN CAO	*Geranium pratense* L.
Medicinal Citron Leaf	XIANG YUAN YE	*Citrus medica* L.

Index of Traditional Chinese Medicines by English Name

Index of Traditional Chinese Medicines by English Name

Index of Traditional Chinese Medicines by English Name

Index of Traditional Chinese Medicines by English Name

Index of Traditional Chinese Medicines by English Name

English Name	TCM Name	Origin Latin Name
Phoenix Tree Seed	WU TONG ZI	*Firmiana simplex* (L.) W. F. Wight
Picrorhiza	HU HUANG LIAN	*Picrorrhiza kurrooa* Royle *ex* Benth.
Pig Gall	ZHU DAN	*Sus scrofa domestica* Brisson
Pigeon Vetch	XIAO CHAO CAI	*Vicia hirsuta* (L.) S. F. Gray
Pilose Asiabell	DANG SHEN	*Codonopsis pilosula* (Franch.) Nannf.
Pilose Gerbera	MAO DA DING CAO	*Gerbera piloselloides* Cass.
Pilular Adina	SHUI TUAN HUA	*Adina pilulifera* (Lam.) Franch. *ex* Drake
Pine Mushroom	SONG XUN	*Armillaria matsutake* Ito *et* Imai
Pineleaf Groundsel	SONG YE QIAN LI GUANG	*Senecio abrotanifolius* L.
Pink Plumepoppy	BO LUO HUI	*Macleaya cordata* (Willd.) R. Br.
Pink Reineckea Herb	JI XIANG CAO	*Reineckea carnea* (Andr.) Kunth
Plum Flower	BAI MEI HUA	*Prunus mume* (Sieb.) Sieb. *et* Zucc.
Poiret Barerry	XIAO BO	*Berberis poiretii* Schneid.
Poisonous Buttercup	SHI LONG RUI	*Ranunculus sceleratus* L.
Polymorphic Angelica	GUAI QIN	*Angelica polymorpha* Maxim.
Pomegranate Peel	SHI LIU PI	*Punica granatum* L.
Pomegranate Root	SHI LIU GEN	*Punica granatum* L.
Pomegranate	SUAN SHI LIU	*Punica granatum* L.
Pond Frog Gall	QING WA DAN	*Rana nigromaculata* Hallowell; *Rana plancyi* Lataste
Pond Frog	QING WA	*Rana nigromaculata* Hallowell; *Rana plancyi* Lataste
Poongaoil Pongamia	SHUI LIU DOU	*Pongamia pinnata* (L.) Merr.
Popyporus Agaric	ZHU LING	*Polyporus umbellatus* (Pers.) Fries
Potanin Larkspur	HEI SHUI CUI QUE	*Delphinium potaninii* W. T. Wang
Potmarigold Calendula	JIN ZHAN JU	*Calendula officinalis* L.
Prawn	HAI XIA	*Penaeus orientalis* Kishinouye
Prepared Common Monkshood Daughter Root	FU ZI	*Aconitum carmichaeli* Debx.
Prettyleaf Winchia	PEN JIA SHU	*Winchia calophylla* A. DC.
Pricklyfruit Licorice	CI GUO GAN CAO	*Glycyrrhiza pallidiflora* Maxim.
Prince's-feather Herb	HONG CAO	*Polygonum orientale* L.
Prinos-like salacia	SUO LA MU	*Salacia prinoides* DC.
Propolis	FENG JIAO	*Apis mellifera ligustica* Spin.
Przewalsk Fritillary	GAN SU BEI MU	*Fritillaria przewalskii* Maxim. *ex* Batal.
Pseudostapfia Monkshood	NI YU LONG WU TOU	*Aconitum pseudosta pfianum* W. T. Wang
Pubescent Angelica	MAO DANG GUI	*Angelica pubescens* Maxim.
Pukee Monkshood	PU GE WU TOU	*Aconitum pukeese* W. T. Wang
Pummelo Seed	YOU HE	*Citrus grandis* (L.) Osbeck
Pummelo	YOU	*Citrus grandis* (L.) Osbeck
Puncturevine Caltrap Root	JI LI GEN	*Tribulus terrestris* L.
Puncturevine Caltrap	CI JI LI	*Tribulus terrestris* L.
Pungent Litse	ZHEN CAI	*Litsea pungens* Hemsl. [= *Lindera umbellutu* Thunb.]
Purging Croton	BA DOU	*Croton tiglium* L.
Purple Bergenia	YAN BAI CAI	*Bergenin purpurascens* (Hook. f. *et* Thoms.) Engl.
Purple Puff-ball	MA BO	*Calvatia linacina* (Mont. *et* Berk.) Lloye
Purple Tephrosia Root	HUI YE GEN	*Tephrosia purpurea* (L.) Pers.
Purpleflower Crotalaria	YE BAI HE	*Crotalaria sessiliflora* L.
Purpleflower Fritillary	ZI HUA E BEI BEI MU	*Fritillaria ebeiensis* var. *pvrpvrea* G. D. Yu *et* P. Li

Index of Traditional Chinese Medicines by English Name

English Name	TCM Name	Origin Latin Name
Purpleflower Holly	DONG QING (SI JI QING)	*Ilex chinensis* Sims [= *Ilex purpurea*]
Purpleflower Stonecrop	ZI HUA JING TIAN	*Hylotelephium mingjinianum* (S. H. Fu) H. Ohba
Purplehair Rabdosia	ZI MAO XIANG CHA CAI	*Isodon enanderianus*
Purplestem Angelica	ZI JING DU HUO	*Angelica porphyrocaulis* Nakai *et* Kitag.
Purslane	MA CHI XIAN	*Portulaca oleracea* L.
Racemose Corydalis	HUANG JIN	*Corydalis racemosa* (Thunb.) Pers.
Racemose Cyclea	LUN HUAN TENG	*Cyclea racemosa* Oliv.
Rangooncreeper Leaf	SHI JUN ZI YE	*Quisqualis indica* L.
Rangooncreeper	SHI JUN ZI	*Quisqualis indica* L.
Red Clover	HONG CHE ZHOU CAO	*Trifolium pratense* L.
Red Fruit Leaf	SHAN ZHA YE	*Crataegus pinnatifida* Bge. var. *major* N. E. Br.
Red Fruit	SHAN ZHA	*Crataegus pinnatifida* Bge. var. *major* N. E. Br.
Red Knoxia	HONG YA DA JI	*Knoxia valerianoides* Thorel *ex* Pitard
Red Lady-bug	HONG NIANG ZI	*Huechys sanguinea* De Geer.
Red Nanmu Bark	HONG NAN PI	*Machilus thunbergii* Sieb. *et* Zucc.
Red Thorowax	HONG CHAI HU	*Bupleurum scorzonerifolium* Willd.
Red Vinespinach	LUO KUI HUA	*Basella rubra* L.
Red-knees	SHUI LIAO	*Polygonum hydropiper* L.
Redbark Cinchona	JIN JI LE	*Cinchona succirubra* Pav.
Redcalyx Glotybower	GUI DENG LONG	*Clerodendron fortunatum* L.
Reddish Jackinthepulpit	TIAN NAN XING	*Arisaema consanguineum* Schott
Redflower Magnoliavine	HONG HUA WU WEI ZI	*Schisandra rubriflora* Rhed *et* Wils
Redfruit Devilpepper	HONG GUO LUO FU MU	*Rauvolfia verticillata* (Lour.) Baill. f. *rubrocarpa* H. T. Chang.
Redroot Gromwell	ZI CAO	*Lithospermum erythrhizon* Sieb. *et* Zucc.
Reeves Skimmia	YIN YU	*Skimmia reevesiana* Fortune
Regel Threewingnut	HEI MAN	*Tripterygium regelii* Sprague *et* Takeda.
Reïndeer Moss	SHI RUI	*Cladonia rangiferina* Web.
Remote Lemongrass	YUN XIANG CAO	*Cymbopogon distans* (Nees) A. Camus
Rhinoceros Horn	XI JIAO	*Rhinoceros unicornis* L.; *Rhinoceros sondaicus* Desmarest; *Rhinoceros sumatrensis* (Fischer)
Rice Frog Gall	XIA MA DAN	*Rana limnocharis* Boie
Rice Spermoderm	MI PI KANG	*Oryza sativa* L.
Rice Straw	DAO CAO	*Oryza sativa* L.
Rice	JING MI	*Oryza sativa* L.
Rigescent Gentian	LONG DAN	*Gentiana rigescens* Franch.
Robust Leontice	HONG MAO QI	*Leontice robustum* (Maxim.) Diels
Roce Pelargonium	XIANG YE	*Pelargonium graveolens* Lsymbol 162 \f "Symbol" \s 8′}Herit
Rocket Consolida	FEI YAN CAO	*Consolida ajacis* (L.) Schur
Roof Iris	YUAN WEI	*Iris tectorum* Maxim.
Rorippa	HAN CAI	*Rorippa montana* (Wall.) Small
Rosemary	MI DIE XIANG	*Rosmarinus officinalis* L.
Rosemyrtle	TAO JIN NIANG	*Rhodomyrtus tomentosa* (Ait.) Hassk.
Rosthorn Snakegourd Root	GUA LOU GEN (TIAN HUA FEN)	*Trichosanthes rosthornii* Harms
Rosthorn Snakegourd	GUA LOU	*Trichosanthes rosthornii* Harms

Index of Traditional Chinese Medicines by English Name

English Name	TCM Name	Origin Latin Name
Rosthorn Yam Rhizome	CHAI HUANG JIANG	*Dioscorea nipponica* Makino subsp *rosthornii* (Prain *et* Burk) Ting
Rostratefruit Gynostemma	HUI GUO JIAO GU LAN	*Gynostemma yixingense* C. Y. Wu *et* SSK Chen
Rough Gentian	LONG DAN	*Gentiana scabra* Bunge
Roughleaf Bedstraw	BA XIAN CAO	*Galium asperifolium* Wall.
Roughleaf Raspberry	CU YE XUAN GOU ZI	*Rubus alceaefolius* Poir
Round Cardamom	BAI DOU KOU	*Amomun kravanh* Pierre *ex* Gagnep. [= *Amomum cardamomum* L.]
Roundfruit Licorice	YUAN GUO GAN CAO	*Glycyrrhiza squamulosa* Franch.
Roundleaf Pharbitis Seed	QIAN NIU ZI	*Pharbitis purpurea* (L.) Voigt
Roundpod Jute Leaf	HUANG MA YE	*Corchorus capsularis* L.
Roundpod Jute Seed	HUANG MA ZI	*Corchorus capsularis* L.
Roundwingfruit Cyclocarya	QING QIAN LIU	*Cyclocarya paliurus* (Batal.) Iljinskaja
Roxburgh Rose	CI LI	*Rosa roxburghii* Tratt.
Roxburgh Wormwood	HUI BAO HAO	*Artemisia roxbugiana* Bess.
Royal Jelly	FENG RU	*Apis cerana* Fabricius
Royal Paulownia Fruit	PAO TONG GUO	*Paulownia tomentosa* (Thunb.) Steud.
Royal Paulownia	PAO TONG (TONG MU)	*Paulownia tomentosa* (Thunb.) Steud.
Royle Euphorbia Latex	BA WANG BIAN	*Euphorbia royleana* Boiss.
Rufous Turtle Dove	BAN JIU	*Streptopelia orientalis* (Latham)
Rugose Rose	MEI GUI HUA	*Rosa rugosa* Thunb.
Russian Boschniakia	CAO CONG RONG	*Boschniakia rossica* Fedtsch. *et* Flerov
Russianolive Bark	SHA ZAO SHU PI	*Elaeagnus angustifolia* L.
Russianolive	SHA ZAO	*Elaeagnus angustifolia* L.
Rust-coloured Crotalaria	XIANG LING CAO	*Crotalaria ferruginea* Grah.
Rustyhair Taxillus	XIU MAO JI SHENG	*Taxillus levinei* Merr.
Safflower	HONG HUA	*Carthamus tinctrius* L.
Saffron Crocus Stigma	ZANG HONG HUA	*Crocus sativus* L.
Sagittate Epimedium Root	YIN YANG HUO GEN	*Epimedium sagittatum* (Sieb. *et* Zucc.) Maxim.
Sagittate Epimedium	JIAN YE YIN YANG HUO	*Epimedium sagittatum* (Sieb. *et* Zucc.) Maxim.
Sago Frond	FENG WEI JIAO YE (SU TIE YE)	*Cycas revoluta* Thunb.
Sago Seed	SU TIE SHU GUO (TIE SHU GUO)	*Cycas revoluta* Thunb.
Saline Cistanche	ROU CONG RONG	*Cistanche salsa* (C. A. Mey.) G. Beck
Saline Swainsonia	NIAO PAO CAO	*Swainsonia salsula* Taub.
Sanchi	SAN QI	*Panax pseudoginseng* Wall. var. *notoginseng* (Burk.) Hoo *et* Tseng [=*Panax notoginseng* (Burk.) F.H. Chen]
Sand Pear Leaf	LI YE	*Pyrus pyrifolia* (Burm. F.) Nakai
Sandal Beadtree Seed	HAI HONG DOU	*Adenanthera pavonina* L.
Sandalwood	TAN XIANG	*Santalum album* L.
Sappan Caesalpinia	SU MU	*Caesalpinia sappan* L.
Sargentgloryvine	DA XUE TENG	*Sargentodoxa cuneata* (Oeiv.) Rehd. *et* Wils.
Savin	CHOU BAI	*Sabina vulgaris* Antoine
Savoury Rhododendron	XIAO YE PI PA	*Rhododendron anthopogonoides* Maxim.
Scabrous Cowparsnip	BAI ZHI	*Heracleum scabridum* Franch.

Index of Traditional Chinese Medicines by English Name

Index of Traditional Chinese Medicines by English Name

English Name	TCM Name	Origin Latin Name
Sixpetal Tailgrape	YING ZHUA	*Artabotrys hexapetalus* (L. f.) Bhandari [= *Annona hexapetalus* L. f.]
Skin-carp	CHONG CHUN YU	*Hemibarbus labeo* (Pallas)
Skunk Bugbane	SHENG MA	*Cimicifuga foetida* L.
Skyblue Broomrape	LIE DANG	*Orobanche coerulescens* Steph.
Slender Dutchmanspipe Root	QING MU XIAN (MA DOU LING GEN)	*Aristolochia debilis* Sieb. *et* Zucc.
Slender Dutchmanspipe	MA DOU LING	*Aristolochia debilis* Sieb. *et* Zucc.
Slenderleaf Ligusticum	HUO GAO BEN	*Ligusticum tenuissimum* (Nakai) Kitag.
Slenderstyle Acanthopanax Leaf	WU JIA YE	*Acanthopanax gracilistylus* W. W. Smith
Slenderstyle Acanthopanax Root-bark	WU JIA PI	*Acanthopanax gracilistylus* W. W. Smith
Slimyhair Sida	HUANG HUA ZI	*Sida mysorensis* Wight *et* Arn.
Small Bugbane	SAN MIAN DAO	*Cimicifuga acerina* (Sieb. *et* Zucc.) Tanaka
Small Centipeda Herb	E BU SHI CAO	*Centipeda minima* (L.) A. Br. *et* Aschers
Small Yellow Daylily	XUAN CAO GEN	*Hemerocallis minor* Mill.
Smallflower Embelia	XIAO HUA SUAN TENG ZI	*Embelia parviflora* Wall. *ex* DC.
Smallflower Hemsleya	XI HUA XUE DAN	*Hemsleya graciliflora* (Harms) cogn. [= *Alsomitra graciliflora* Harms]
Smallflower Yam Rhizome	XIAO HUA DUN YE SHU YU	*Dioscorea parviflora* C. T. Ting sp. Nov.
Smallleaf Black Thorowax	XIAO YE HEI CHAI HU	*Bupleurum smithii* Wolff var. *parvifolium* Shan *et* Y. Li
Smallleaf Jointfir	XIAO YE MAI MA TENG	*Gnetum parvifolium* (Warb.) C.Y. Cheng
Smallligulatecorolla Aster	XIAO SHE ZI WAN	*Aster albescens* (DC.) Hand. -Mazz.
Smoothfruit Ventiago	YI HE GUO	*Ventilago leiocarpa* Benth.
Smoothstalk Madder	DAYE QIAN CAO	*Rubia schumannina* Pritz
Snake Sansevieria	HU WEI LAN	*Sansevieria trifasciata* Prain
Snake Slough	SHE TUI	*Elaphe taeniurus* Cope; *Elaphe carinata*; *Zaocys dhumnades*; *Dinodon rufozonatum*
Snow Azalea	BAI HUA YING SHAN HONG	*Rhododendron mucronatum* G. Don
Snow Lotus	XUE LIAN	*Saussurea involucrata* Kar. *et* Kir.
Snowbellleaf Tickclover	GUANG JIN QIAN CAO	*Desmodium styracifolium* (Osbeck) Merr.
Soda-apple Nightshade	YE DIAN QIE	*Solanum surattense* Burm. f.
Soft-hair Cowparsnip	RUAN MAO DU HUO	*Heracleum lanatum* Michx.
Sorghum	GAO LIANG	*Sorghum vulgare* Pers
Sorrel Rhubarb	DA HUANG	*Rheum palmatum* L.
South Dodder	NAN FANG TU SI ZI	*Cuscuta australis* R. Br.
South-western Honeysuckle	XI NAN REN DONG	*Lonicera bournei* Hemsl.
Southern Crapemyrtle	JU NA HUA	*Lagerstroemia subcostata* Koehne
Southwest pyrrosia frond	SHI WEI	*Pyrrosia gralla* (Gies.) Ching
Sowthistle Tasselflower	YI DIAN HONG	*Emilia sonchifolia* (L.) DC.
Soy Sauce	JIANG	Legume crop.
Soybean Oil	DOU YOU	*Glycine max* (L.) Merr.
Spicate Clerodendranthus	MAO XU CAO	*Clerodendranthus spicatus* (Thunb.) C. Y. Wu
Spiced Juice of Mature Winter-vegetable	CHEN DONG CAI LU ZHI	*Brassica chinensis* L.

Index of Traditional Chinese Medicines by English Name

Index of Traditional Chinese Medicines by English Name

Index of Traditional Chinese Medicines by English Name

Index of Traditional Chinese Medicines by English Name

English Name	TCM Name	Origin Latin Name
Tropic Ageratum	SHENG HONG JI	*Ageratum conyzoides* L.
Tropical American Hymenocallis Leaf	SHUI GUI JIAO YE	*Hymenocallis americana* Roem.
True Indigo	MU LAN	*Indigofera tinctoria* L.
True Lacquertree Seed	QI ZI	*Rhus verniciflua* Stokes
Tschonosk Trillium	YU ER QI	*Trillum tschonoskii* Maxim.
Tube Fleeceflower Stem	YE JIAO TENG	*Polygonum multiflorum* Thunb.
Tubeflower Dutchmanspipe	GUAN HUA MA DOU LING	*Aristolochia tubiflora* Dunn
Tuber Fleeceflower	HE SHOU WU	*Polygonum multiflorum* Thunb.
Tuber Onion	JIU CAI	*Allium tuberosum* Rottler
Tuber Stemona	BAI BU	*Stemona tuberosa* Lour.
Tuberculate Speranskia	TOU GU CAO	*Speranskia tuberculata* (Bge.) Baill.
Tuberousroot Jerusalemsage	KUAI JING CAO SU	*Phlomis tuberosa* L.
Tungoiltree Seed Oil	TONG YOU	*Aleurites fordii* Hemsl.
Twoanther Mosla	DA YE XIANG RU	*Mosla dianthera* (Ham.) Maxim.
Twodenntate Germander	ER CHI XIANG KE	*Teucrium bidentatum* Hemsl.
Twoflower Jerusalemcherry	YE HAI JIAO	*Solanum capsicastrum* Link
Twolobed Officinal Mangolia	HOU PO	*Magnolia biloba* (Rehd. *et* Wils.) Cheng
Twotooth Achyranthes	NIU XI	*Achyranthes bidentata* Bl.
Twotooth Achyranthes	TU NIU XI	*Achyranthes bidentata* Bl.
Udo	TU DANG GUI (I)	*Aralia cordata* Thunb.
Unarmed Glorybower	SHUI HU MAN	*Clerodendron inerme* (L.) Gaertn.
Undaria	KUN BU	*Undaria pinnatifida* (Harv.) Sur.
Unibract Fritillary	AN ZI BEI MU	*Fritillaria unibracteata* Hsiao *et* K. C. Hsiao
Uniclor Divid Lily	CHUAN BAI HE	*Lilium davidii* Duch. var. *uniclor* Cotton
Uniflower Swisscentaury	QI ZHOU LOU LU	*Rhaponticum uniflorum* (L.) DC.
Ural Falsespiraea	ZHEN ZHU MEI	*Sorbaria sorbifolia* (L.) A. Br.
Ural Licorice	GAN CAO	*Glycyrrhiza uralensis* Fisch.
Ural Licorice	WU LA ER GAN CAO	*Glycyrrhiza uralensis* Fisch.
Ussuri Falsehellebore	WU SU LI LI LU	*Veratrum nigrum* L. var. *ussuriense* Nakai
Ussuri Fritillary	PING BEI MU	*Fritillaria ussuriensis* Maxim.
Ussurian Pear Leaf	LI YE	*Pyrus ussuriensis* Maxim.
Vaginate Hemlockparsley	XIN JIANG GAO BEN	*Conioselinum vaginatum* (Spr.) Thell.
Vanillagrass	MAO XIANG HUA	*Hierochloe odorata* (L.) Beauv.
Veined Rabdosia	XIAN MAI XIANG CHA CAI	*Rabdosia nervosa* (Hemsl.) C. Y. Wu. *et* H. W. Li
Veitch Peony	CHUAN CHI SHAO	*Paeonia veitchii* Lynch
Vermiculate Thamnolia Thallus	XUE CHA	*Thamnolia vermicularis* (Ach.) Asahina
Versicolorous Dutchmanspipe	BIAN SE MA DOU LING	*Aristolochia versicolar* S. M. Hwang
Verticillate Acanthopanax Leaf	LUN SAN WU JIA YE	*Acanthopanax verticillatus* Hoo
Verticillate Acanthopanax Root-bark	LUN SAN WU JIA PI	*Acanthopanax verticillatus* Hoo
Verticillate Cladonia	XIAO LA BA	*Cladonia verticillata* Hoffm.
Vesper Iris	BAI HUA SHE GAN	*Iris dichotoma* Pall.
Vetchleaf Sophora Leaf	BAI CI HUA YE	*Sophora viciifolia* Hance
Vetchleaf Sophora Seed	BAI CI HUA ZI	*Sophora viciifolia* Hance
Vetchleaf Sophora	BAI CI HUA	*Sophora viciifolia* Hance
Villous Amomum	SHA REN	*Amomum villosum* Lour.
Vinegar.	CU	symbol 45 \f "Symbol" \s 8-
Virgate Wormwood	YIN CHEN HAO	*Artemisia scoparia* Wldst. *et* Kitaibel
Virginia Pepperweed Seed	TING LI ZI	*Lepidium virginicum* L.
Walking Maidenhair	BIAN YE TIE XIAN JUE	*Adiantum caudatum* L.

Index of Traditional Chinese Medicines by English Name

English Name	TCM Name	Origin Latin Name
Wamai Erycibe	WA MAI DING GONG TENG	*Erycibe elliptilimba* Merr. *et* Chun
Wanshan Epimedium	WAN SHAN YIN YANG HUO	*Epimedium wanshanense* S. Z. He *et* Guo.
Water Nightshade	SHUI QIE	*Solanum torvum* Sw.
Watermelon Seed	XI GUA ZI REN	*Citrullus vulgaris* Schrad.
Watermelon	XI GUA	*Citrullus vulgaris* Schrad.
Wayaka Yambean Seed	DI GUA ZI	*Pachyrhizus erosus* (L.) Urban
Weeping Forsythia	LIAN QIAO	*Forsythia suspensa* (Thunb.) Vahl
Wheat	XIAO MAI	*Triticum aestivum* L.
White Chinaure Herb	YAN JIAO CAO	*Boenninghausenia albiflora* (Hook.) Meissn.
White Clover Herb	SAN XIAO CAO	*Trifolium repens* L.
White Dendrobium	TIE PI SHI HU	*Dendrobium candidum* Wall. *ex* Lindl.
White Flax	BAI YA MA	*Linum album* Kotschy *ex* Boiss
White Mulberry Bast	SANG BAI PI	*Morus alba* L.
White Mulberry Branch	SANG ZHI	*Morus alba* L.
White Mulberry	SANG YE	*Morus alba* L.
White Mustard Seed	BAI JIE ZI	*Sinapis alba* L. [= *Brassica alba* (L.) Boiss.]
White Sweetclover Root	CHOU MU XU GEN	*Melilotus suaveolens* Ledeb.
Whiteflower Danshen	BAI HUA DAN SHEN	*Salvia miltiorrhiza* f. *alba* C. Y. Wu
Whiteflower Embelia	XIAN SUAN QIANG	*Embelia ribes* Burm. f.
Whiteflower Hogfennel	BAI HUA QIAN HU	*Peucedanum praeruptorum* Dunn
Whiteflower Leadword	BAI HUA DAN	*Plumbago zeylanica* L.
Whiteflower Mucuna	JI XUE TENG	*Mucuna birdwoodiana* Tutcher
Whiteflower Patrinia	BAI HUA BAI JIANG	*Patrinia villosa* Juss.
Whiteflower Trillium	YU ER QI	*Trillum camtschaticum* Pall.
Whitethroat Monkshood	BAI HOU WU TOU	*Aconitum leucostomum* Worosch.
Whorlleaf Litse	DIE DA LAO	*Litsea verticillata* Hance
Wild Boar Gall	YE ZHU DAN	*Sus scrofa* L.
Wild Carrot	HE SHI FENG	*Daucus carota* L.
Wild Honeysuckle	JIN YIN HUA	*Lonicera confusa* DC.
Wild Mint	BO HE	*Mentha haplocalyx* Briq.
Wild Spikenard	SHE BAI ZI	*Hyptis suaveolens* Poit
Wild Thermopsis	YE JUE MING	*Thermopsis lupinoides* (L.) Link.
Wildcelery	HAN QIN	*Apium graveolens* L. var. *dulce* DC.
Wilford Cranesbill Herb	LAO GUAN CAO	*Geranium wilfordii* Maxim.
Willmott Ceratostigma	ZI JIN LIAN	*Ceratostigma willmottianum* Stapf
Willowleaf Achyranthes	TU NIU XI	*Achyranthes longgifolia* Mak.
Willowleaf Swallowwort	LIU YE BAI QIAN	*Cynanchum stauntoni* (Decne.) Schltr. *ex* Lévl.
Wilson Buckeye Seed	SUO LUO ZI	*Aesculus wilsonee* Rehd.
Wilson Citron (almost ripe fruit)	ZHI KE	*Citrus wilsonii* Tanaka
Wilson Citron Fruit	ZHI SHI	*Citrus wilsonii* Tanaka
Wilson Citron	XIANG YUAN	*Citrus wilsonii* Tanaka
Wine	JIU	symbol 45 \f "Symbol" \s 8-
Winged Euonymus	GUI JIAN YU	*Euonymus alatus* (Thunb.) Sieb.
Winged Yam	MAO SHU	*Dioscorea alata L.*
Winged Yam	SHAN YAO	*Dioscorea alata* L.
Winked Marshweed	SHUI HUI XIANG	*Limnophila rugosa* (Roth) Merr.
Winter Daphne Flower	RUI XIANG HUA	*Daphne odora* Thunb.
Winter Daphne Root	RUI XIANG GEN	*Daphne odora* Thunb.
Winterberry Euonymus	SI MIAN MU	*Euonymus bungeanus* Maxim.
Wintergreen Barberry	TU HUANG LIAN	*Berberis Julianae* Schneid.
Wintersweet Immayure Flower	LA MEI HUA	*Chimonanthus praecox* (L.) Link
Woodland Beakchervil	E SHEN	Anthriscus sylvestris (L.) Hoffm.

Index of Traditional Chinese Medicines by English Name

Index of Traditional Chinese Medicines by English Name

English Name	TCM Name	Origin Latin Name
Yunnan Pholidota	YUN NAN SHI XIAN TAO	*Pholidota yunnanensis* Rolfe
Yunnan Pleurospermum	YUN NAN QIANG HUO	*Pleurospermum rivulorum* (Diels)
Yunnan Seseli	SONG YE FANG FENG	*Seseli yunnanense* Franch.
Yunnan Skullcap	DIAN HUANG QIN	*Scutellaria amoena* C. H. Wright
Yunnan Wintergreen	TOU GU XIANG	*Gaulthcria yunnanensis* (Franch.) Rehd.
Yunnan Yew	YUN NAN HONG DOU SHAN	*Taxus yunnanensis* Cheng *et* L. K. Fu
Yunnanwest Monkshood	DIAN XI WU TOU	*Aconitum bulleyanum* Diels
Zedoary Turmeric	PENG E SHU	*Curcuma zedoaria* (Berg.) Rosc.

Index of Origin of Traditional Chinese Medicines

Index of Origin of Traditional Chinese Medicines

Index of Origin of Traditional Chinese Medicines

Origin Latin Name	Family	English Name	TCM Name
Aconitum carmichaeli Debx.	*Ranunculaceae*	Prepared Common Monkshood Daughter Root	FU ZI
Aconitum chrysotrichum W. T. Wang	*Ranunculaceae*	Yellowhail Monkshood	HUANG MAO WU TOU
Aconitum gymnandrum Maxim	*Ranunculaceae*	Nakedstamen Monkshood	LU RUI WU TOU
Aconitum kusnezoffii Rchb.	*Ranunculaceae*	Kusnezoff Monkshood	BEI WU TOU (of CAO WU TOU)
Aconitum leucostomum Worosch.	*Ranunculaceae*	Whitethroat Monkshood	BAI HOU WU TOU
Aconitum pseudosta pfianum W. T. Wang	*Ranunculaceae*	Pseudostapfia Monkshood	NI YU LONG WU TOU
Aconitum pukeese W. T. Wang	*Ranunculaceae*	Pukee Monkshood	PU GE WU TOU
Aconitum sungpanense Hand. -Mazz.	*Ranunculaceae*	Sungpan Monkshood	SONG PAN WU TOU
Acorus calamus L.	*Araceae*	Drug Sweetflag	BAI CHANG
Acorus gramineus Soland.	*Araceae*	Grassleaf Sweetflag	SHI CHANG PU
Acorus gramineus Soland.	*Araceae*	Grassleaf Sweetflag Leaf	SHI CHANG PU YE
Acronychia pedunculata (L.) Miq.	*Rutaceae*	Pedunculate Acronychia	SHA TANG MU
Actinidia arguta (Sieb. *et* Zucc.) Planch.	*Actinidiaceae*	Bower Actinidia	MI HOU LI
Actinidia chinensis Planch.	*Actinidiaceae*	Yangtao Actinidia	MI HOU TAO
Actinidia polygama (Sieb. *et* Zucc.) Maxim.	*Actinidiaceae*	Silvervine Actinidia	MU TIAN LIAO
Adenanthera pavonina L.	*Leguminosae*	Sandal Beadtree Seed	HAI HONG DOU
Adenophora trachelioides Maxim.	*Campanulaceae*	Apricotleaf Ladybell	JI NI
Adhatoda vasica Nees	*Acanthaceae*	Malabanut	DA BO GU
Adiantum capillusveneris L.	*Adiantaceae*	Maidenhair Fern	ZHU ZONG CAO
Adiantum caudatum L.	*Adiantaceae*	Walking Maidenhair	BIAN YE TIE XIAN JUE
Adiantum davidii Franch.	*Adiantaceae*	David's Maidenhair Fern	ZHU ZONG CAO
Adiantum pedatum L.	*Adiantaceae*	American Maidenhair Fern	TIE SI QI
Adina pilulifera (Lam.) Franch. *ex* Drake	*Rubiaceae*	Pilular Adina	SHUI TUAN HUA
Adina rubella (Sieb. *et* Zucc.) Hance	*Rubiaceae*	Thinleaf Adina	SHUI YANG MEI (II)
Adonis amurensis Reg. *et* Radde	*Ranunculaceae*	Amur Adonis	FU SHOU CAO
Aeginetia indica L.	*Orobanchaceae*	Indian Aeginetia	YE GU
Aesculus chinensis Bge.	*Hippocastanaceae*	Chinese Buckeye Seed	SUO LUO ZI
Aesculus Turbinata BL.	*Hippocastanaceae*	Japanese Buckeye Seed	SUO LUO ZI
Aesculus wilsonee Rehd.	*Hippocastanaceae*	Wilson Buckeye Seed	SUO LUO ZI
Agaricus campestris L. *ex* Fr.	*Agaricaceae*	Mushroom	MO GU
Agastache rugosa (Fisch. *et* Mey.) O. Ktze.	*Labiatae*	Wrinkled Gianthyssop	HUO XIANG
Agave americana L.	*Agavaceae*	American Agave	FAN MA
Agave americana L. var. *marginata* Hort.	*Agavaceae*	Marginate American Agave	JIN BIAN LONG SHE LAN
Agave americana L. var. *variegata* Nichols	*Agavaceae*	Spineless Agave	WU CI FAN MA

Index of Origin of Traditional Chinese Medicines

Origin Latin Name	Family	English Name	TCM Name
Agave angustifolia Haw	*Agavaceae*	Narrowleaf Agave	DUAN YE LONG SHE LAN
Agave angustifolia var. *marginata* Hort.	*Agavaceae*	Silveredge Agave	YIN BIAN LONG SHE LAN
Agave cantala Roxb.	*Agavaceae*	Shortleaf Agave	XIA YE LONG SHE LAN
Agave east-one	*Agavaceae*	Cultivate Sisalan Agave East-1	DONG YI HAO JIAN MA
Agave sisalana Perr. *ex* Engelm.	*Agavaceae*	Sisal Hemp-plant (Sisal Agave)	JIAN MA
Ageratum conyzoides L.	*Compositae*	Tropic Ageratum	SHENG HONG JI
Aglaia odorata Lour.	*Meliaceae*	Chu-lan Tree	MI ZI LAN
Agrimonia pilosa Ledeb. var. *japonica* (Miq.) Nakai	*Rosaceae*	Hairyvein Agrimonia Root	LONG YA CAO GEN (XIAN HE CAO GEN)
Ailanthus altissima (Mill.) Swingle	*Simaroubaceae*	Tree of Heaven Ailanthus Bast	CHU BAI PI
Ajuga decumbens Thunb.	*Labiatae*	Decumbent Bugle Herb	BAI MAO XIA KU CAO
Ajuga forrestii Diels	*Labiatae*	Forrest Bugle	LI ZHI HAO
Akebia quinata (Thunb.) Decne.	*Lardizabalaceae*	Fiveleaf Akebia	MU TONG
Akebia quinata (Thunb.) Decne.	*Lardizabalaceae*	Fiveleaf Akebia Root	MU TONG GEN
Akebia quinata (Thunb.) Decne.	*Lardizabalaceae*	Fiveleaf Akebia Seed	YU ZHI ZI
Akebia trifoliata (Thunb.) Koidz.	*Lardizabalaceae*	Threeleaf Akebia	SAN YE MU TONG (of MU TONG)
Akebia trifoliata (Thunb.) Koidz.	*Lardizabalaceae*	Threeleaf Akebia Root	MU TONG GEN
Akebia trifoliata (Thunb.) Koidz.	*Lardizabalaceae*	Threeleaf Akebia Seed	YU ZHI ZI
Akebia trifoliata (Thunb.) Koidz. var. *australis* (Diels) Rehd.	*Lardizabalaceae*	Austral Akebia	BAI MU TONG (of MU TONG)
Akebia trifoliata (Thunb.) Koidz. var. *australis* (Diels) Rehd.	*Lardizabalaceae*	Austral Akebia Root	MU TONG GEN
Akebia trifoliata (Thunb.) Koidz. var. *australis* (Diels) Rehd.	*Lardizabalaceae*	Austral Akebia Seed	YU ZHI ZI
Albizzia julibrissin Durazz.	*Leguminosae*	Silktree Albizia Bark	HE HUAN PI
Alectoria vivens Tayl.	*Usneaceae*	Green Alectoria Filament	JIN SI DAI
Aleurites fordii Hemsl.	*Euphorbiaceae*	Tungoiltree Seed Oil	TONG YOU
Aleurites moluccana (L.) Willd.	*Labiatae*	Belgaum Walnut Seed	SHI LI ZI
Aleuritopteris argentea (Gmel.) Fée	*Sinopteridaceae*	Silvery Aleuritopteris	TONG JING CAO
Alhagi pseudalhagi Desv.	*Leguminosae*	Manaplant Alhagi Sweet Secretion	CI MI (LUO TUO CI)
Alisma orientale (Sam.) Juzepcz.	*Alismataceae*	Oriental Waterplantain	ZE XIE
Alisma plantagoaquatica L. var. *orientale* Samuels	*Alismataceae*	Oricntal Waterplantain	ZE XIE
Allium ascalonicum L.	*Liliaceae*	Shallot	HU CONG
Allium cepa L.	*Liliaceae*	Common onion	YANG CONG
Allium fistulosum L.	*Liliaceae*	Fistular Onion	CONG BAI
Allium macrostemon Bge.	*Liliaceae*	Longstamen Onion	XIE BAI
Allium sativum L.	*Liliaceae*	Garlic	DA SUAN
Allium schoenoprasum L.	*Liliaceae*	Chive	XI XIANG CONG
Allium tuberosum Rottler	*Liliaceae*	Tuber Onion	JIU CAI

Index of Origin of Traditional Chinese Medicines

Origin Latin Name	Family	English Name	TCM Name
Allium victorialis L.	*Liliaceae*	Longroot Onion	GE CONG
Allolobophora caliginosa trapezoides (Ant. Duges)	*Lumbricidae*	Earthworm	QIU YIN
Alnus japonica Sieb. *et* Zucc.	*Betulaceae*	Japanese Alder	CHI YANG
Aloe ferox Mill.	*Liliaceae*	Cape of Good Hope Aloe Dried Juice	HAO WANG JIAO LU HUI (of LU HUI)
Aloe vera L.	*Liliaceae*	Kulaso Aloe Dried Juice	KU LA SUO LU HUI (of LU HUI)
Aloe vera L. var. *chinensis* (Haw.) Berger	*Liliaceae*	Chinese Aloe Dried Juice	BAN WEN LU HUI (of LU HUI)
Alpinia chinensis Rosc.	*Zingiberaceae*	Chinese Galangal	LIAN JIANG
Alpinia galanga (L.) Swartz.	*Zingiberaceae*	Galanga Galangal	DA LIANG JIANG
Alpinia japonica Miq.	*Zingiberaceae*	Japanese Galangal	TU SHA REN
Alpinia katsumadai Hayata	*Zingiberaceae*	Katsumada Galangal	CAO DOU KOU
Alpinia officinarum Hance	*Zingiberaceae*	Lesser Galangal	GAO LIANG JIANG
Alpinia speciosa K. Schum.	*Zingiberaceae*	Beautiful Galangal	DA CAO KOU
Alsomitra graciliflora Harms	*Cucurbhitaceae*	Smallflower Hemsleya	XI HUA XUE DAN
Alstomia yunnanensis Diels	*Apocynaceae*	Yunnan Alstonia	DIAN JI GU CHANG SHAN
Alstonia mairei Lévl.	*Apocynaceae*	Maire Alstonia	YANG JIAO MIAN
Alstonia scholaris (L.) R. Br.	*Apocynaceae*	Common Alstonia	XIANG PI MU
Alternanthera philoxeroides (Mart.) Griseb.	*Amaranthaceae*	Alligator Alternanthera	KONG XIN XIAN
Althaea rosea (L.) Cav.	*Malvaceae*	Hollyhock Flower	SHU KUI HUA
Amanita panthorina	*Amanitaceae*	Amanita	BAO PI JUN
Amanita strobilifomis (Paul.) Quél.	*Amanitaceae*	Amanita Fungus	E GAO XUN
Amaranthus tricolor L.	*Amaranthaceae*	Three-coloured Amaranth	YAN LAI HONG
Ambrosia artemisiifolia L.	*Compositae*	Common Ragweed	TUN CAO
Amomum cardamomum L.	*Zingiberaceae*	Round Cardamom	BAI DOU KOU
Amomum villosum Lour.	*Trapaceae*	Villous Amomum	SHA REN
Amomun kravanh Pierre *ex* Gagnep.	*Zingiberaceae*	Round Cardamom	BAI DOU KOU
Ampelopsis brevipedunculata (Maxim.) Trautv.	*Vitaceae*	Ampelopsis	SHE PU TAO
Ampelopsis cantoniesis (H. *et* A.) Pl. var. *grossedentata* Hand. -Mazz.	*Vitaceae*	Bigdentate Ampelopsis	XIAN CHI SHE PU TAO
Ampelopsis chaffanjonii (Lévl.) Rehd.	*Vitaceae*	Chaffanjon Ampelopsis	YU YE SHE PU TAO
Ampelopsis grossedentata (Hand. -Mazz.) W.T. Wang	*Vitaceae*	Bigdentate Ampelopsis	XIAN CHI SHE PU TAO
Ampelopsis japonica (Thunb.) Mak.	*Vitaceae*	Japanese Ampelopsis	BAI LIAN
Anacardium occidentale L.	*Anacardiaceae*	Common Cashew Fruit	DU XIAN ZI
Anaphalis margaritacea (L.) Benth. *et* Hook. f.	*Compositae*	Common Pearleverlasting	DA YE BAI TOU WENG
Andrographis paniculata (Burm.f.) Nees	*Acanthaceae*	Common Andrographis	CHUAN XIN LIAN
Anemarrhena asphodeloides Bge.	*Lilyaceae*	Common Anemarrhena	ZHI MU
Anemone hupehensis Lem.	*Ranunculaceae*	Hupeh Anemone	DA PO WAN WAN HUA
Anethum graveolens L.	*Umbelliferae*	Dill Fruit	SHI LUO ZI
Angelica anomala Lallem.	*Umbelliferae*	Eumenol Angelica	BAI ZHI
Angelica dahurica (Fisch. *ex* Hoffm.) Benth. *et* Hook. f. *ex* Franch. *et* Sav.	*Umbelliferae*	Dahurian Angelica	BAI ZHI

Index of Origin of Traditional Chinese Medicines

Index of Origin of Traditional Chinese Medicines

Origin Latin Name	Family	English Name	TCM Name
Ardisia crispa (Thunb.) A. DC.	*Myrsinaceae*	Crispateleaf Ardisia Leaf	BAI LIANG JIN YE
Ardisia japonica (Hornst.) Bl.	*Myrsinaceae*	Japanese Ardisia	ZI JIN NIU
Ardisia japonica (Hornst.) Bl.	*Myrsinaceae*	Japanese Ardisia Root	ZI JIN NIU GEN
Ardisia pusilla A. DC.	*Myrsinaceae*	Tiny Ardisia	CHUAN CHAN JIU JIE LONG
Areca catechu L.	*Palmae*	Betenutpalm	BING LANG
Argimonia pilosa Ledeb. var. *japonica* (Miq.) Nakai	*Rosaceae*	Hairyvein Argimonia	XIAN HE CAO
Argimonia pilosa Ledeb. var. *japonica* (Miq.) Nakai	*Rosaceae*	Hairyvein Argimonia Rhizome	XIAN HE CAO GEN YA
Arisaema amurense Maxim.	*Araceae*	Amur Jackinthepulpit	TIAN NAN XING
Arisaema consanguineum Schott	*Araceae*	Reddish Jackinthepulpit	TIAN NAN XING
Arisaema heterophyllum Bl.	*Araceae*	Diversileaf Jackinthepulpit	TIAN NAN XING
Aristolochia contorta Bge.	*Aristolochiaceae*	Northern Dutchmanspipe	BEI MA DOU LING (of MA DOU LING)
Aristolochia contorta Bge.	*Aristolochiaceae*	Northern Dutchmanspipe Root	QING MU XIAN (MA DOU LING GEN)
Aristolochia debilis Sieb. *et* Zucc.	*Aristolochiaceae*	Slender Dutchmanspipe	MA DOU LING
Aristolochia debilis Sieb. *et* Zucc.	*Aristolochiaceae*	Slender Dutchmanspipe Root	QING MU XIAN (MA DOU LING GEN)
Aristolochia fangchi Wu	*Aristolochiaceae*	Fangchi	GUANG FANG JI (of FANG JI)
Aristolochia heterophylla Hemsl.	*Aristolochiaceae*	Yellowmouth Dutchmanspipe	HAN FANG JI (of FANG JI)
Aristolochia kaempferi Willd.	*Aristolochiaceae*	Kaempfer Dutchmanspipe	ZHU SHA LIAN
Aristolochia manshuriensis Kom.	*Aristolochiaceae*	Manchurian Dutchmanspipe	GUAN MU TONG
Aristolochia mollissima Hance	*Aristolochiaceae*	Wooly Dutchmanspipe	MIAN MAO MA DOU LING
Aristolochia moupinensis Franch.	*Aristolochiaceae*	Moupin Dutchmanspipe	HUAI TONG
Aristolochia tubiflora Dunn	*Aristolochiaceae*	Tubeflower Dutchmanspipe	GUAN HUA MA DOU LING
Aristolochia versicolar S. M. Hwang	*Aristolochiaceae*	Versicolorous Dutchmanspipe	BIAN SE MA DOU LING
Armillaria matsutake Ito *et* Imai	*Tricholomataceae*	Pine Mushroom	SONG XUN
Armillaria mellea (Vahl *ex* Fr.) Quél.	*Tricholomataceae*	Mellea Armillaria Sporophore	ZHEN MO
Armillariella tabescens (Scop. *ex* Fr.) Sing.	*Tricholomataceae*	Armillariella Tabescens	LIANG JUN
Arnebia euchroma (Royle) Johnst.	*Boraginaceae*	Sinkiang-Tibet Arnebia	ZI CAO
Artabotrys hexapetalus (L. f.) Bhandari	*Annonaceae*	Sixpetal Tailgrape	YING ZHUA
Artemisia annua L.	*Compositae*	Sweet Wormwood	QING HAO
Artemisia annua L.	*Compositae*	Sweet Wormwood	HUANG HUA HAO
Artemisia apiacea Hance	*Compositae*	Celery Wormwood	QING HAO
Artemisia argyl Lévl. *et* Vant	*Compositae*	Argy Wormwood Leaf	AI YE

Index of Origin of Traditional Chinese Medicines

Origin Latin Name	Family	English Name	TCM Name
Artemisia capillaris Thunb.	*Compositae*	Capillary Wormwood	YIN CHEN HAO
Artemisia cina (Berg. *ex* Poljak) Poljak	*Compositae*	Chinese Seriphidium	SHAN DAO NIAN HAO (HUI HAO)
Artemisia finita Kitag.	*Compositae*	Northeast Seriphidium	DONG BEI HUI HAO
Artemisia japonica Thumb.	*Compositae*	Japanese Wormwood	MU HAO
Artemisia lactiflora Wall. *ex* DC.	*Compositae*	Ghostplant Wormwood	YA JIAO AI
Artemisia roxbugiana Bess.	*Compositae*	Roxburgh Wormwood	HUI BAO HAO
Artemisia rupestris L.	*Compositae*	Sinkiang onetwig wormwood	XIN JIANG YI ZHI HAO
Artemisia scoparia Wldst. *et* Kitaibel	*Compositae*	Virgate Wormwood	YIN CHEN HAO
Artemisia sieversiana Ehrh. *ex* Willd.	*Compositae*	Sievers Wormwood	BAI HAO
Artemisia vestita Wall.	*Compositae*	Hairy Wormwood	MAO LIAN HAO
Arthraxon hispidus (Thunb.) Mak.	*Gramineae*	Hispid Arthraxon Herb	JIN CAO
Arthromeris mairei (Brause) Ching	*Polypodiaceae*	Mary Arthromeris	FENG WEI PA SHAN HU
Artocarpus heterophyllus Lam.	*Moraceae*	Diversileaf Artocarpus	BO LUO MI
Arundo donax L.	*Gramineae*	Giantreed Rhizome	LU ZHU GEN
Asarum forbesii Maxim.	*Aristolochiaceae*	Forbes Wildginger	DU HENG
Asarum heterotropoides F. Schm. var. *mandshuricum* (Maxim.) Kitag.	*Aristolochiaceae*	Manchurian Wildginger	XI XIN
Asarum maximum Hemsl.	*Aristolochiaceae*	Largeflower Wildginger	HUA LIAN XI XIN
Asarum sieboldii Miq.	*Aristolochiaceae*	Siebold Wildginger	XI XIN
Asclepias curassavica L.	*Asclepiadaceae*	Bloodflower Milkweed	LIAN SHENG GUI ZI HUA
Asparagus cochinchinensis (Lour.) Merr.	*Liliaceae*	Cochinchinese Asparagus	TIAN MEN DONG
Asparagus filicinus Buch. -Ham. *ex* D. Don	*Liliaceae*	Fernlike Asparagus	TU BAI BU
Asparagus officinalis L.	*Liliaceae*	Officinal Asparagus	XIAO BAI BU
Asparagus plumosus Bak.	*Liliaceae*	Setose Asparagus	WEN ZHU
Asparagus setaceus (Kunth) Jessop	*Liliaceae*	Setose Asparagus	WEN ZHU
Aspidistra elatior Bl.	*Liliaceae*	Common Aspidistra	ZHI ZHU BAO DAN
Aspidosperma campus-belus A. P. Duarte.		Campus-belu Aspidosperma	BAI JIAN MU
Aspongopus chinensis Dallas	*Pentatomidae*	Aspongopus	JIU XIANG CHONG
Aster albescens (DC.) Hand. -Mazz.	*Compositae*	Smallligulatecorolla Aster	XIAO SHE ZI WAN
Aster tataricus L. f.	*Compositae*	Tatarion Aster	ZI WAN
Astilbe chinensis (Maxim.) Franch. *et* Sav.	*Saxifragaceae*	Chinese Astilbe	LUO XIN FU
Astilbe chinensis (Maxim.) Franch. *et* Sav.	*Saxifragaceae*	Chinese Astilbe Root	LUO XIN FU GEN
Astragalus complanatus R. Br.	*Leguminosae*	Flatstem Milkvetch	BIAN JING HUANG QI
Astragalus membranaceus (Fisch.) Bge.	*Leguminosae*	Membranous Milkvetch	HUANG QI
Astragalus mongholicus Bge.	*Leguminosae*	Mongolian Milkvetch	MENG GU HUANG QI (of HUANG QI)

Index of Origin of Traditional Chinese Medicines

Origin Latin Name	Family	English Name	TCM Name
Astragalus sinicus L.	*Leguminosae*	Chinese Milkvetch	HONG HUA CAI (ZI YUN YING)
Astragalus sinicus L.	*Leguminosae*	Chinese Milkvetch Seed	ZI YUN YING ZI
Atalantia buxifolia (Poir.) Oliv.	*Rutaceae*	Boxleaf Atalantia Leaf	DONG FENG JU YE
Atalantia buxifolia (Poir.) Oliv.	*Rutaceae*	Boxleaf Atalantia Root	DONG FENG JU GEN
Atractylis macrocephala (Koidz.) Hand. -Mazz.	*Compositae*	Largehead Atractylodes	BAI ZHU
Atractylodes chinensis Koidz.	*Compositae*	Chinese Atractylodes	CANG ZHU
Atractylodes lancea (Thunb.) DC.	*Compositae*	Swordlike Atractylodes	CANG ZHU
Atractylodes macrocephala Koidz.	*Compositae*	Largehead Atractylodes	BAI ZHU
Aucklandia lappa Decne	*Compositae*	Common Aucklandia (Costustoot)	MU XIANG
Aucuba chinensis Benth.	*Cornaceae*	Chinese Aucuba	TIAN JIAO BAN
Auricularia aurivula (L. *ex* Hook.) Underw.	*Auriculariaceae*	Jew's Ear	MU ER
Baeckea frutescens L.	*Myrtaceae*	Shrubby Baeckea	GANG SONG
Baileya multiratiata Harv. *et* Gray.		Bailai's Chrysanthemum	BAI LAI SHI JU
Balanophora indica (Arn.) Griff.	*Balanophoraceae*	Indian Balanophora	YIN DU SHE GU
Balanophora involucrata Hook. f.	*Balanophoraceae*	Involucrate Balanophora	TONG QIAO SHE GU
Balanophora japonica Mak.	*Balanophoraceae*	Japanese balanophora	GE XUN
Balsamodendron ehrenbergianum Berg.	*Burseraceae*	Ehrenberg Myrrh	MO YAO
Baphicacanthus cusia (Nees) Brem.	*Cruciferae*	Common Baphicacanthus Root	BAN LAN GEN
Baphicacanthus cusia (Nees) Bremek	*Acanthaceae*	Common Baphicacanthus Leaf	DA QING YE
Basella rubra L.	*Basellaceae*	Red Vinespinach	LUO KUI HUA
Bauhinia hupehara Craib	*Leguminosae*	Hupeh Bauhinia	HU BEI YANG TI JIA
Beaumontia grandiflora Wall.	*Apocynaceae*	Easter Heraldtrumpet	PAO DAN GUO
Begonia limprichtii Irmsch.	*Begoniaceae*	Limpricht Begonia	JI YE QIU HAI TANG
Belamcanda chinensis (L.) DC.	*Iridaceae*	Blackberrylily	SHE GAN
Benincasa hispida (Thunb.) Cogn.	*Cucurbitaceae*	Chinese Waxgourd Seed	DONG GUA ZI
Berberis amurensis Rupr.	*Berberidaceae*	Amur Barerry	XIAO BO
Berberis Julianae Schneid.	*Berberidaceae*	Wintergreen Barberry	TU HUANG LIAN
Berberis poiretii Schneid.	*Berberidaceae*	Poiret Barerry	XIAO BO
Berberis thunbergii DC.	*Berberidaceae*	Japanese Barerry	XIAO BO
Berberis tschonoskiana Regel	*Berberidaceae*	Yellow Barberry	HUANG XIAO BO
Bergenin crassifolia (L.) Fritsch	*Saxifragaceae*	Thickleaf Bergenia	YAN BAI CAI
Bergenin purpurascens (Hook. f. *et* Thoms.) Engl.	*Saxifragaceae*	Purple Bergenia	YAN BAI CAI
Berneuxia thibetica Decne.	*Diapensiaceae*	Tibet Berneuxine	YAN JIN CAI
Betula luminifera H. Winkl.	*Betulaceae*	Shiningleaf Birch Bark	LIANG YE HUA PI
Betula platyphylla Suk.	*Betulaceae*	Asia White Birch Bark	BAI HUA PI (of HUA MU PI)

Index of Origin of Traditional Chinese Medicines

Origin Latin Name	Family	English Name	TCM Name
Betula platyphylla Suk. var. *japonica* (Sieb.) Hara	*Betulaceae*	Japanese White Birch Bark	HONG HUA PI (of HUA MU PI)
Biebersteinia heterostemon Maxim.	*Geraniaceae*	Heterostemonous Biebersteinia	XUN DAO NIU
Bischofia javanica Bl.	*Euphorbiaceae*	javan Bishopwood	QIU FENG MU
Blatta orientalis L.	*Blattidae*	Cockroach	ZHANG LANG
Blechnum orientale L.	*Blechnaceae*	Oriental Blechnum Frond	GUAN ZHONG
Blumea balsamifera DC.	*Compositae*	Balsamiferous Blumea	AI NA XIANG
Blumea lacera (Burm. f.) DC.	*Compositae*	Malay Blumea Herb	HONG TOU CAO
Boea crassifolia Hemsl.	*Gesneriaceae*	Thickleaf Boea	YAN BAI CAI
Boenninghausenia albiflora (Hook.) Meissn.	*Rutaceae*	White Chinaure Herb	YAN JIAO CAO
Bombyx mori L.	*Bombycidae*	Silk Cocoon	CAN JIAN
Bombyx mori L.	*Bombycidae*	Silkworm Egg	YUAN CAN ZI
Bombyx mori L.	*Bombycidae*	Silkworm Feculae	YUAN CAN SHA
Bombyx mori L.	*Bombycidae*	Silkworm King	YUAN CAN E
Bombyx mori L.	*Ombycidae*	Silkworm Larva	BAI JIANG CAN
Bos taurus domesticus Gmelin	*Bovidae*	Concentrated Beef Extract	XIA TIAN GAO
Bos taurus domesticus Gmelin	*Bovidae*	Cow Milk	NIU RU
Bos taurus domesticus Gmelin	*Bovidae*	Cow-bezoar (Ox-gallstone)	NIU HUANG
Bos taurus domesticus Gmelin	*Bovidae*	Ox Blood	NIU XUE
Bos taurus domesticus Gmelin	*Bovidae*	Ox Brain	NIU NAO
Bos taurus domesticus Gmelin	*Bovidae*	Ox Gall	NIU DAN
Bos taurus domesticus Gmelin	*Bovidae*	Ox Kindey	NIU SHEN
Bos taurus domesticus Gmelin	*Bovidae*	Ox Liver	NIU GAN
Bos taurus domesticus Gmelin	*Bovidae*	Ox Lung	NIU FEI
Bos taurus domesticus Gmelin	*Bovidae*	Ox Teeth	NIU CHI
Bos taurus domesticus Gmelin	*Bovidae*	Ox Thyroid	NIU YE
Bos taurus domesticus Gmelin	*Bovidae*	Oxhide Gelatin	HUANG MING JIAO
Boschniakia rossica Fedtsch. *et* Flerov	*Orobanchaceae*	Russian Boschniakia	CAO CONG RONG
Boswellia carterii Birdw.	*Anacardiaceae*	Olibanum	RU XIANG
Brainea insignis (Hook.) J. Sm.	*Blechnaceae*	Brainea	GUAN ZHONG
Brasenia schreberi J. F. Gmel.	*Nymphaeaceae*	Common Watershield	CHUN
Brassica alba (L.) Boiss.	*Cruciferae*	White Mustard Seed	BAI JIE ZI
Brassica campestris L.	*Cruciferae*	Bird Rape	YUN TAI ZI
Brassica campestris L. var. *oleifera* DC.	*Cruciferae*	Bird Rape	YUN TAI ZI
Brassica chinensis L.	*Cruciferae*	Spiced Juice of Mature Winter-vegetable	CHEN DONG CAI LU ZHI
Brassica juncea (L.) Czern. *et* Coss.	*Cruciferae*	India Mustart Seed	JIE ZI
Brassica oleracea L. var. *capiata* L.	*Cruciferae*	Cabbage	GAN LAN
Brucea javanica (L.) Merr.	*Simaroubaceae*	Java Brucea	YA DAN ZI
Bryophyllum pinnatum (L. f.) Oken	*Crassulaceae*	Air-plant Herb	LUO DI SHENG GEN
Bubalus bubalis Linnaeus	*Bovidae*	Buffalo Horn	SHUI NIU JIAO
Bubalus bubalis Linnaeus	*Bovidae*	Cow Milk	NIU RU
Bubalus bubalis Linnaeus	*Bovidae*	Cow-bezoar (Ox-gallstone)	NIU HUANG
Bubalus bubalis Linnaeus	*Bovidae*	Ox Blood	NIU XUE
Bubalus bubalis Linnaeus	*Bovidae*	Ox Brain	NIU NAO
Bubalus bubalis Linnaeus	*Bovidae*	Ox Gall	NIU DAN

Index of Origin of Traditional Chinese Medicines

Origin Latin Name	Family	English Name	TCM Name
Bubalus bubalis Linnaeus	*Bovidae*	Ox Kindey	NIU SHEN
Bubalus bubalis Linnaeus	*Bovidae*	Ox Liver	NIU GAN
Bubalus bubalis Linnaeus	*Bovidae*	Ox Lung	NIU FEI
Bubalus bubalis Linnaeus	*Bovidae*	Ox Teeth	NIU CHI
Bubalus bubalis Linnaeus	*Bovidae*	Ox Thyroid	NIU YE
Buddleia officinalis Maxim.	*Loganiaceae*	Pale Butterflybush	MI MENG HUA
Bufo bufo gargarizans Cantor	*Bufonidae*	Toad	CHAN CHU (GAN CHAN CHU)
Bufo bufo gargarizans Cantor	*Bufonidae*	Toad Gall	CHAN CHU DAN
Bufo bufo gargarizans Cantor	*Bufonidae*	Toad Skin	CHAN PI
Bufo bufo gargarizans Cantor	*Bufonidae*	Toad Skin Secretion Cake	CHAN SU
Bufo melanostictus Schneider	*Bufonidae*	Toad	CHAN CHU (GAN CHAN CHU)
Bufo melanostictus Schneider	*Bufonidae*	Toad Gall	CHAN CHU DAN
Bufo melanostictus Schneider	*Bufonidae*	Toad Skin	CHAN PI
Bufo melanostictus Schneider	*Bufonidae*	Toad Skin Secretion Cake	CHAN SU
Bupleurum chinense DC.	*Umbelliferae*	Chinese Thorowax	BEI CHAI HU (of CHAI HU)
Bupleurum longiradiatum Turcz.	*Umbelliferae*	Bigleaf Thorowax	DA YE CHAI HU (of CHAI HU)
Bupleurum scorzonerifolium Willd.	*Umbelliferae*	Red Thorowax	HONG CHAI HU (of CHAI HU)
Bupleurum smithii Wolff	*Umbelliferae*	Black Thorowax	HEI CHAI HU
Bupleurum smithii Wolff var. *parvifolium* Shan *et* Y. Li	*Umbelliferae*	Smallleaf Black Thorowax	XIAO YE HEI CHAI HU
Buthus martensi Karsch	*Buthidae*	Scorpion	QUAN XIE
Buxus microphylla Sieb. *et* Zucc. var. *sinica* Rehd. *et* Wils.	*Buxaceae*	Chinese Box Juvenile Leaf	HUANG YANG MU YE
Cacalia procumbens Lour.	*Compositae*	Gynura	SAN QI CAO
Caesalpinia sappan L.	*Leguminosae*	Sappan Caesalpinia	SU MU
Calcium sulphate, $CaSO_4$symbol 215 \f "Symbol" \s 8·}H_2O.		Gypsum Fibrosum	SHI GAO
Calendula officinalis L.	*Compositae*	Potmarigold Calendula	JIN ZHAN JU
Callicarpa arborea Roxb.	*Verbenaceae*	Tree Beautyberry	QIAO MU ZI ZHU
Callicarpa macrophylla Vahl.	*Verbenaceae*	Bigleaf Beautyberry	DA YE ZI ZHU
Caloglossa leprieurii (Mont.) J. Ag.	*Delesseriaceae*	Leprieur Caloglossa Frond	ZHE GU CAI
Caltha palustris L.	*Ranunculaceae*	Common Marsharigold	MA TI YE
Caltha scaposa Hook. f. *et* Thoms	*Ranunculaceae*	Scapose Marsharigold	MA TI YE
Calvatia gigantea (Batsch *ex* Pers.) Lloye	*Lycoperdaceae*	Large Puff-ball	MA BO
Calvatia linacina (Mont. *et* Berk.) Lloye	*Lycoperdaceae*	Purple Puff-ball	MA BO
Calystegia hederacea Wall.	*Convolvulaceae*	Ivy Glorybind	MIAN GEN TENG
Camellia oleifera Abel	*Theaceae*	Oiltea Camellia	CHA ZI XIN
Camellia oleifera Abel	*Theaceae*	Oiltea Camellia Root-bark	YOU CHA GEN PI
Camellia sinensis O. Ktze.	*Theaceae*	Tea	CHA YE
Camellia sinensis O. Ktze.	*Theaceae*	Tea Root	CHA SHU GEN
Camellia sinensis O. Ktze.	*Theaceae*	Tea Seed	CHA ZI
Camellia sinensis var. *assamica* (Masters) Kitamura	*Theaceae*	Assam Tea	PU ER CHA

Origin Latin Name	Family	English Name	TCM Name
Camptotheca acuminata Decne.	*Nyssaceae*	Common Camptotheac	XI SHU
Campylotropis hirtella (Franch.) Schindl.	*Leguminosae*	Hairy Clivereshrub	DA HONG PAO
Canarium album (Lour.) Raeusch.	*Burseraceae*	Olive	GAN LAN
Canavalia gladiata (Jacq.) DC.	*Leguminosae*	Sword Jackbean	DAO DOU
Canis familiaris L.	*Canidae*	Dog Heart	GOU XIN
Canis familiaris L.	*Canidae*	Dog Meat	GOU ROU
Cannabis sativa L.	*Moraceae*	Hemp Fimble	MA HUA
Cannabis sativa L.	*Moraceae*	Hemp Fimble Leaf	MA YE
Cannabis sativa L.	*Moraceae*	Hemp Fimble Seed	HUO MA REN
Capparis spinosa L.	*Capparidaceae*	Common Caper	LAO SHU GUA
Capra hircus L.	*Bovidae*	Goat Hide	YANG PI
Capra hircus L.	*Bovidae*	Goat Milk	YANG RU
Capra hircus L.	*Bovidae*	Goat Pancreas	YANG YI
Capsella bursapastoris (L.) Medic.	*Cruciferae*	Shepherdspurse	JI CAI
Capsella bursapastoris (L.) Medic.	*Cruciferae*	Shepherdspurse Seed	JI CAI ZI
Capsicum annuum L. var. *conoides* (Mill.) Irish	*Solanaceae*	Conical Redpepper	CHAO TIAN JIAO
Capsicum annuum L. var. *fasciculatum* (Sturt.) Irish	*Solanaceae*	Clustered Redpepper	CU SHENG JIAO
Capsicum frutescens L.	*Solanaceae*	Bush Redpepper	LA JIAO
Caragana jubata (Pall.) Poir.	*Leguminosae*	Shagspine Peashrub	GUI JIAN JIN JI ER
Caragana sinica (Buc'hoz) Rehd.	*Leguminosae*	Chinese Peashrub Root	JIN QUE GEN
Carassium auratus (L.)	*Cyprinidae*	Crucian Carp	JIN YU
Cardiospermum halicacabum L.	*Sapindaceae*	Balloonvine Heartseed	JIA KU GUA
Carduun crispus L.	*Compositae*	Curly Bristlethistle	FEI LIAN
Carica papaya L.	*Caricaceae*	Papaya Fruit	FAN MU GUA
Carica papaya L.	*Caricaceae*	Papaya Leaf	FAN MU GUA YE
Carpesium abrotanoides L.	*Compositae*	Common Carpesium	TIAN MING JING
Carpesium abrotanoides L.	*Compositae*	Common Carpesium Fruit	HE SHI (TIAN MING JING)
Carthamus tinctrius L.	*Compositae*	Safflower	HONG HUA
Caryopteris glutinosa Rehd.	*Verbenaceae*	Glutinose Bluebeard	NIAN YE YOU
Cassia acutifolia Del.	*Leguminosae*	Sharpleaf Senna Leaf	FAN XIE YE
Cassia angustifolia Vahl	*Leguminosae*	Narrowleaf Senna Leaf	FAN XIE YE
Cassia fistula L.	*Leguminosae*	Goldenshower Senna Fruit	PO LUO MEN ZAO JIA
Cassia mimosoides L.	*Leguminosae*	Sensitiveplant-like Senna	SHAN BIAN DOU ZI
Cassia nodosa L.	*Leguminosae*	Jointwood Senna	SHEN HUANG DOU
Cassia occidentalis L.	*Leguminosae*	Coffee Senna	WANG JIANG NAN
Cassia occidentalis L.	*Leguminosae*	Coffee Senna Seed	WANG JIANG NAN ZI
Cassia sophera L.	*Leguminosae*	Inflatedfruit Senna	JIANG MANG
Cassia tora L.	*Leguminosae*	Sickle Senna Seed	JUE MING ZI
Cassytha filiformis L.	*Lauraceae*	Filiform Cassytha	WU YE TENG
Castanea mollissima Bl.	*Fagaceae*	Hairy Chestnut Bast	LI SHU PI
Catalpa ovata G. Don	*Bignoniaceae*	Ovate Catalpa	ZI MU
Catalpa ovata G. Don	*Bignoniaceae*	Ovate Catalpa Bast	ZI BAI PI
Catalpa ovata G. Don	*Bignoniaceae*	Ovate Catalpa Fruit	ZI SHI
Catalpa ovata G. Don	*Bignoniaceae*	Ovate Catalpa Leaf	ZI YE

Index of Origin of Traditional Chinese Medicines

Origin Latin Name	Family	English Name	TCM Name
Catharanthus roseus (L.) G. Don.	*Apocynaceae*	Madagascar Periwinkle	CHANG CHUN HUA
Cayratia japonica (Thunb.) Gagn.	*Vitaceae*	Japanese Cayratia	WU LIAN MEI
Celastrus angulata Maxim.	*Celastraceae*	Angled Bittersweet	DIAO GAN MA
Celastrus flagellaris Rupt.	*Celastraceae*	Hookedspine Bittersweet	CI NAN SHE TENG
Celastrus hypoleucus (Oliv.) Warb.	*Celastraceae*	Pale Bittersweet	MIAN TENG
Celastrus orbiculatus Thunb.	*Celastraceae*	Oriental Bittersweet Leaf	NAN SHE TENG YE
Celastrus orbiculatus Thunb.	*Celastraceae*	Oriental Bittersweet Root	NAN SHE TENG GEN
Celtis bungeana Bl.	*Ulmaceae*	Bunge Hackberry	BANG BANG MU
Centella asiatica (L.) Urban	*Umbelliferae*	Asiatic Pennywort Herb	JI XUE CAO
Centipeda minima (L.) A. Br. *et* Aschers	*Compositae*	Small Centipeda Herb	E BU SHI CAO
Cephalanthus occidentalis L.	*Rubiaceae*	Common Butterbush	FENG XIANG SHU YE (a)
Cephalotaxus fortunei Hook. f.	*Cephalotaxaceae*	Fortune Plumyew Brench and Leaf	SAN JIAN SHAN
Cephalotaxus fortunei Hook. f.	*Cephalotaxaceae*	Fortune Plumyew Seed	TU XIANG FEI (SAN JIAN SHAN ZI)
Cephalotaxus sinesis (Rehd. *et* Wils.) Li	*Cephalotaxaceae*	Chinese Plumyew Brench and Leaf	SAN JIAN SHAN
Cephalotaxus sinesis (Rehd. *et* Wils.) Li	*Cephalotaxaceae*	Chinese Plumyew Seed	TU XIANG FEI (SAN JIAN SHAN ZI)
Ceratostigma willmottianum Stapf	*Plumbaginaceae*	Willmott Ceratostigma	ZI JIN LIAN
Cerbera manghas L.	*Apocynaceae*	Common Cerberustree	NIU XIN QIE ZI
Cervus elaphus L.	*Cervidae*	Hairy Antler	LU RONG
Cervus nippon Temminck	*Cervidae*	Hairy Antler	LU RONG
Chaenomeles lagenaria (Loisel.) Koidz.	*Rosaceae*	Common Floweringquince	MU GUA
Chaenomeles speciosa (Sweet) Nakai	*Rosaceae*	Common Floweringquince	QIU MU GUA
Chamaenerion angustifolium (L.) Scop.	*Onagraceae*	Great Willowherb (Firewood)	HONG KUAI ZI
Chelidonium majus L.	*Paraveraceae*	Greater Celandine	BAI QU CAI
Chenopodium album L.	*Chenopodiaceae*	Lambsquarters Juvenile	LI
Chenopodium ambrosioides L.	*Chenopodiaceae*	Mexican Tea	TU JING JIE
Chimonanthus praecox (L.) Link	*Calycanthaceae*	Wintersweet Immayure Flower	LA MEI HUA
Chrysanthemum boreale Mak.	*Compositae*	Boreal Wild Chrysanthemum	BEI YE JU (of YE JU)
Chrysanthemum boreale Mak.	*Compositae*	Boreal Wild Chrysanthemum Flower	YE JU HUA
Chrysanthemum indicum L.	*Compositae*	Indian Wild Chrysanthemum	YE JU
Chrysanthemum indicum L.	*Compositae*	Indian Wild Chrysanthemum Flower	YE JU HUA
Chrysanthemum lavandulaefolium (Fisch.) Mak.	*Compositae*	Lavandulaleaf Chrysanthemum	YAN XIANG JU (of YE JU)

Origin Latin Name	Family	English Name	TCM Name
Chrysanthemum lavandulaefolium (Fisch.) Mak.	*Compositae*	Lavandulaleaf Chrysanthemum Flower	YE JU HUA
Chrysanthemum morifolium Ramat.	*Compositae*	Florists Chrysanthemum Flower	JU HUA
Chrysosplenium grayanum Maxim.	*Saxifragaceae*	Goldsaxifrage Herb	JIN QIAN KU YE CAO
Cicer arietinum L.	*Leguminosae*	Gram Chickpea	HUI HUI DOU
Cichorium intybus L.	*Compositae*	Common Chicory	JU QU
Cicuta virosa L.	*Umbelliferae*	European Waterhemlock Root	DU QIN GEN
Cimicifuga acerina (Sieb. *et* Zucc.) Tanaka	*Ranunculaceae*	Small Bugbane	SAN MIAN DAO
Cimicifuga dahurica (Turcz.) Maxim.	*Ranunculaceae*	Dahurian Bugbane	XING AN SHENG MA (of SHENG MA)
Cimicifuga foetida L.	*Ranunculaceae*	Skunk Bugbane	SHENG MA
Cimicifuga simplex Wormsk.	*Ranunculaceae*	Kamchatka Bugbane	YE SHENG MA
Cinchona ledgeriana Moens.	*Rubiaceae*	Ledger Cinchona	JIN JI LE
Cinchona succirubra Pav.	*Rubiaceae*	Redbark Cinchona	JIN JI LE
Cinnamomum bodinieri Lévl.	*Lauraceae*	Bodinier Cinnamon	HOU ZHANG
Cinnamomum burmannii (Nees) Bl.	*Lauraceae*	Burmann Cinnamon Bark	YIN XIANG PI
Cinnamomum burmannii (Nees) Bl.	*Lauraceae*	Burmann Cinnamon Leaf	YIN XIANG YE
Cinnamomum camphora (L.) Presl	*Lauraceae*	Camphortree Leaf	ZHANG SHU YE
Cinnamomum camphora (L.) Presl	*Lauraceae*	Camphortree	ZHANG MU (ZHANG SHU)
Cinnamomum cassia Presl	*Lauraceae*	Cassiabarktree	ROU GUI
Cinnamomum cassia Presl	*Lauraceae*	Cassiabarktree Twig	GUI ZHI
Cinnamomum japonicum Sieb.	*Lauraceae*	Japanese Cinnamon	GUI PI
Cinnamomum parthenoxylon (Jack) Nees	*Lauraceae*	Yellow Cinnamon	XIANG ZHANG
Cinnamomum parthenoxylon (Jack) Nees	*Lauraceae*	Yellow Cinnamon Leaf	XIANG ZHANG YE
Cinnamomum porrectum (Roxb.) Kosterm.	*Lauraceae*	Yellow Cinnamon	XIANG ZHANG
Cinnamomum porrectum (Roxb.) Kosterm.	*Lauraceae*	Yellow Cinnamon Leaf	XIANG ZHANG YE
Cinnamomum tamala (Ham.) Nees *et* Eberm.	*Lauraceae*	Tibet Cinnamon Bark	SAN TIAO JIN
Cirsium chinense Gardn. *et* Champ.	*Compositae*	Linearleaf Thistle	KU AO
Cirsium japonicum DC.	*Conpositae*	Japanese Thistle	DA JI (b)
Cissampelos pareira L.	*Menispermaceae*	Common Cissampelos	XI SHENG TENG
Cistanche deserticola Y. C. Ma	*Orobanchaceae*	Desertliving Cistanche	ROU CONG RONG
Cistanche salsa (C. A. Mey.) G. Beck	*Orobanchaceae*	Saline Cistanche	ROU CONG RONG
Citrullus vulgaris Schrad.	*Cucurbitaceae*	Watermelon	XI GUA
Citrullus vulgaris Schrad.	*Cucurbitaceae*	Watermelon Seed	XI GUA ZI REN
Citrus aurantium L.	*Rutaceae*	Bitter Orange	ZHI SHI
Citrus aurantium L.	*Rutaceae*	Bitter Orange (almost ripe fruit)	ZHI KE
Citrus aurantium L. var. *amara* Engl.	*Rutaceae*	Bitter Citrus	DAI DAI HUA
Citrus chachiensis Hort.	*Rutaceae*	Chachi Citrus	GAN
Citrus chachiensis Hort.	*Rutaceae*	Chachi Citrus Pericarp	GAN PI

Origin Latin Name	Family	English Name	TCM Name
Citrus grandis (L.) Osbeck	*Rutaceae*	Pummelo	YOU
Citrus grandis (L.) Osbeck	*Rutaceae*	Pummelo Seed	YOU HE
Citrus junos Tanaka	*Rutaceae*	Fragrant Citrus	CHEN ZI
Citrus junos Tanaka	*Rutaceae*	Fragrant Citrus Seed	CHEN ZI HE
Citrus junos Tanaka	*Rutaceae*	Pericarp	CHEN ZI PI
Citrus limon Burm.	*Rutaceae*	Lemon	NING MENG
Citrus limon Burm.	*Rutaceae*	Lemon Leaf	NING MENG YE
Citrus limon Burm.	*Rutaceae*	Lemon Root	NING MENG GEN
Citrus limonia Osbeck	*Rutaceae*	Lemonlike Citrus	NING MENG
Citrus limonia Osbeck	*Rutaceae*	Lemonlike Citrus Leaf	NING MENG YE
Citrus limonia Osbeck	*Rutaceae*	Lemonlike Citrus Root	NING MENG GEN
Citrus medica L.	*Rutaceae*	Medicinal Citron	XIANG YUAN
Citrus medica L.	*Rutaceae*	Medicinal Citron Leaf	XIANG YUAN YE
Citrus medica L. var. *sarcodactylis* (Noot.) Swingle	*Rutaceae*	Fleshfingered Citron	FO SHOU (FO SHOU GAN)
Citrus reticulata Blanco	*Rutaceae*	Tangerine Pericarp	JU PI (CHEN PI)
Citrus reticulata Blanco	*Rutaceae*	Tangerine Seed	JU HE
Citrus sinensis (L.) Osbeck	*Rutaceae*	Sweet Orange	TIAN CHEN
Citrus suavissima Hort. *ex* Tanaka	*Rutaceae*	Sugary Citrus	GAN
Citrus suavissima Hort. *ex* Tanaka	*Rutaceae*	Sugary Citrus Pericarp	GAN PI
Citrus wilsonii Tanaka	*Rutaceae*	Wilson Citron	XIANG YUAN
Citrus wilsonii Tanaka	*Rutaceae*	Wilson Citron (almost ripe fruit)	ZHI KE
Citrus wilsonii Tanaka	*Rutaceae*	Wilson Citron Fruit	ZHI SHI
Cladonia alpestris (L.) Rabht.	*Cladoniaceae*	Stellate Cladonia Fruticose Thallus	TAI BAI HUA
Cladonia fallax Abbayes	*Cladoniaceae*	Cladonia fallax Lichen	JIN SHUA BA
Cladonia rangiferina Web.	*Cladoniaceae*	Reindeer Moss	SHI RUI
Cladonia stellaris (Opiz.) Pouzar *et* Vezda	*Cladoniaceae*	Stellate Cladonia Fruticose Thallus	TAI BAI HUA
Cladonia verticillata Hoffm.	*Cladoniaceae*	Verticillate Cladonia	XIAO LA BA
Clausena dentata (Willd.) Roem.	*Rutaceae*	Dunn Wampee	YE HUANG PI
Clausena excavata Burm. f.	*Rutaceae*	Hollowed Wampee	SHAN HUANG PI
Clausena lansium (Lour) Skeels	*Rutaceae*	Chinese Wampee Leaf	HUANG PI YE
Claviceps purpurea (Fr.) Turasne	*Clavicipitaceae*	Ergot	MAI JIAO
Clematis chinensis Osbeck	*Ranunculaceae*	Chinese Clematis	WEI LING XIAN
Clematis maximowicziana Franch. *et* Sav.	*Ranunculaceae*	Threeflower Clematis	BAI HUA TENG
Clematis terniflora DC.	*Ranunculaceae*	Threeflower Clematis	BAI HUA TENG
Cleome gynandra L.	*Capparidaceae*	Common Spiderflower Seed	BAI HUA CAI ZI
Clerodendranthus spicatus (Thunb.) C. Y. Wu	*Labiatae*	Spicate Clerodendranthus	MAO XU CAO
Clerodendron cyrtophyllum Turcz.	*Verbenaceae*	Manyflower Glorybower Leaf	DA QING YE
Clerodendron fortunatum L.	*Verbenaceae*	Redcalyx Glotybower	GUI DENG LONG
Clerodendron fragrans Vent.	*Verbenaceae*	Fragrant Glorybower	CHOU MO LI
Clerodendron indicum (L.) O. Ktze.	*Verbenaceae*	Indian Glorybower	CHANG GUAN JIA MO LI

Index of Origin of Traditional Chinese Medicines

Origin Latin Name	Family	English Name	TCM Name
Clerodendron inerme (L.) Gaertn.	*Verbenaceae*	Unarmed Glorybower	SHUI HU MAN
Clerodendron serratum (L.) Spr.	*Verbenaceae*	Serrate Glorybower	SAN TAI HONG HUA
Clerodendron trichotomum Thunb.	*Verbenaceae*	Harrlequin Glorybower Leaf	CHOU WU TONG
Clerodendron trichotomum Thunb.	*Verbenaceae*	Harrlequin Glorybower Root	CHOU WU TONG GEN
Clinopodium chinense (Benth.) O. Ktze.	*Labiatae*	Chinese Clinopodium	FENG LUN CAI
Clinopodium polycephalum (Vant.) C. Y. Wu *et* Hsuan	*Labiatae*	Manyhead Clinopodium	DENG LONG CAO
Clintonia alpina (Royle) Kunth	*Liliaceae*	Common Broadlily	LEI GONG QI
Cnidium monnieri (L.) Cusson	*Umbelliferae*	Common Cnidium	SHE CHUANG ZI
Cocculus laurifolius DC.	*Menispermaceae*	Laurelleaf Snailseed	HENG ZHOU WU YAO
Cocculus trilobus (Thunb.) DC.	*Menispermaceae*	Japanese Snailseed	MU FANG JI (of FANG JI)
Cocculus trilobus (Thunb.) DC.	*Menispermaceae*	Japanese Snailseed Stem	QING TAN XIANG
Cocos nucifera L.	*Palmae*	Coconut Albumen	YE ZI RANG
Cocos nucifera L.	*Palmae*	Coconut Oil	YE ZI YOU
Cocos nucifera L.	*Palmae*	Coconut Root-bark	YE ZI PI
Codium fragile (Sur.) Har.	*Codiaceae*	Fragile Codium Frond	SHUI SONG
Codonopsis Modesta Nannf.	*Campanulaceae*	Moderate Asiabell	DANG SHEN
Codonopsis pilosula (Franch.) Nannf.	*Campanulaceae*	Pilose Asiabell	DANG SHEN
Codonopsis pilosula Nannf. var. *modesta* (Nannf.) L.T. Shen	*Campanulaceae*	Moderate Asiabell	DANG SHEN
Codonopsis tangshen Oliv.	*Campanulaceae*	Szechwon Tangshen	DANG SHEN
Coix lachrymajobi L.	*Gramineae*	Jobstears	YI YI REN
Coix lachrymajobi L.	*Gramineae*	Jobstears Root	YI YI GEN
Collybia albuminosa (Berk.) Petch	*Tricholomataceae*	Collybia Albuminosa Sporophore	JI ZONG
Colocasia antiquorum Schott *et* Endl.	*Araceae*	Taro	YE YU
Commelina communis L.	*Commelinaceae*	Common Dayflower Herb	YA ZHI CAO
Commiphora myrrha Engl.	*Burseraceae*	Myrrh	MO YAO
Conioselinum vaginatum (Spr.) Thell.	*Umbelliferae*	Vaginate Hemlockparsley	XIN JIANG GAO BEN (of GAO BEN)
Consolida ajacis (L.) Schur	*Ranunculaceae*	Rocket Consolida	FEI YAN CAO
Convallaria keiskei Miq.	*Liliceae*	Lilyofthevalley	LING LAN
Convallaria majalis L.	*Liliceae*	Lilyofthevalley	LING LAN
Convolvulus arvensis L.	*Convolvulaceae*	Field Bindweed	TIAN XUAN HUA
Conyza blinii Lévl.	*Conpositae*	Blin Conyza	JIN LONG DAN CAO
Coprinus atramentarius (Bull.) Fr.	*Agaricaceae*	Coprinus Sporophore	GUI GAI
Coptis chinensis Franch.	*Ranunculaceae*	Chinese Goldthread	HUANG LIAN
Coptis deltoidea C. Y. Cheng *et* Hsiao	*Ranunculaceae*	Deltoid Goldthread	HUANG LIAN
Coptis omeiensis (Chen) C. Y. Cheng	*Ranunculaceae*	Omei Mountain Goldthread	HUANG LIAN
Coptis teeta Wall.	*Ranunculaceae*	Yunnan Goldthread	HUANG LIAN
Coptis teetoides C. Y. Cheng	*Ranunculaceae*	Yunnan Goldthread	HUANG LIAN
Corchorus capsularis L.	*Tiliaceae*	Roundpod Jute Leaf	HUANG MA YE
Corchorus capsularis L.	*Tiliaceae*	Roundpod Jute Seed	HUANG MA ZI

Index of Origin of Traditional Chinese Medicines

Origin Latin Name	Family	English Name	TCM Name
Cordyceps sinensis (Berk.) Sacc.	*Clavicipitaceae*	Aweto (Chinese Caterpillar Fungus)	DONG CHONG XIA CAO
Cordyline strcta Endl.	*Agavaceae*	Strictleaf Dracaena Leaf	JIAN YE TIE SHU YE
Coreopsis lanceolata L.	*Compositae*	Lance Coreopsis	XIAN YE JIN JI JU
Coriandrum sativum L.	*Umbelliferae*	Coriander Seed	HU SUI ZI
Coriaria nepalensis Wall.	*Coriariaceae*	Chinese Coriaria	MA SANG
Coriaria sinica Maxim.	*Coriariaceae*	Chinese Coriaria	MA SANG
Coriaria sinica Maxim.	*Coriariaceae*	Chinese Coriaria Leaf	MA SANG YE
Cornus capitata Wall.	*Cornaceae*	Evergreen Dogwood	JI SU ZI
Cornus Officinalis Sieb. *et* Zucc.	*Cornaceae*	Asiatic Cornelian Cherry (Common Macrocarpium)	SHAN ZHU YU
Corydalis decumbens (Thunb.) Pers.	*Papaveraceae*	Decumbent Corydalis	XIA TIAN WU
Corydalis incusa (Thunb.) Pers.	*Papaveraceae*	Incised Corydalis	ZI HUA YU DENG CAO (LIE BAO ZI JING)
Corydalis pallida (Thunb.) Pers.	*Papaveraceae*	Yellowflower Corydalis	JU HUA HUANG LIAN
Corydalis racemosa (Thunb.) Pers.	*Papaveraceae*	Racemose Corydalis	HUANG JIN
Corydalis sheareri var. *bulbillifera* Hand. -Mazz.	*Papaveraceae*	Bulbiliferous Corydalis	ZHU YA ZI JIN
Corydalis turtschaninovii Bess. f. *yanhusuo* Y. H. Chou *et* C. C. Hsu	*Papaveraceae*	Yanhusuo	YAN HU SUO
Corydalis yanhusuo W. T. Wang	*Papaveraceae*	Yanhusuo	YAN HU SUO
Costus speciosus (Koen.) Smith.	*Zingiberaceae*	Canereed Spiralflagg	ZHANG LIU TOU
Cotinus coggygria Scop.	*Anacardiaceae*	Common Smoketree	HUANG LU
Cotinus coggygria Scop.	*Anacardiaceae*	Common Smoketree Branch and Leaf	HUANG LU ZHI YE
Crataegus cuneata Sieb. *et* Zucc.	*Rosaceae*	Nippon Hawthorn	SHAN ZHA
Crataegus cuneata Sieb. *et* Zucc.	*Rosaceae*	Nippon Hawthorn Leaf	SHAN ZHA YE
Crataegus pinnatifida Bge.	*Rosaceae*	Chinese Hawthorn	SHAN ZHA
Crataegus pinnatifida Bge.	*Rosaceae*	Chinese Hawthorn Leaf	SHAN ZHA YE
Crataegus pinnatifida Bge. var. *major* N. E. Br.	*Rosaceae*	Red Fruit	SHAN ZHA
Crataegus pinnatifida Bge. var. *major* N. E. Br.	*Rosaceae*	Red Fruit Leaf	SHAN ZHA YE
Crinum asiaticum L. var. *sinicum* Bak.	*Amaryllidaceae*	Chinese Crinum Root	LUO QUN DAI GEN
Crocus sativus L.	*Iridaceae*	Saffron Crocus Stigma	ZANG HONG HUA
Croomia japonica Miq.	*Stemonaceae*	Japanese Croomia	JIN GANG DA
Crossostephium chinense (L.) Mak. *ex* Cham. *et* Schltr.	*Compositae*	Chinese Crossostephium Root	FU RONG JU GEN
Crotalaria albida Heyne	*Leguminosae*	Diluteyellow Crotalaria	HUANG HUA DI DING
Crotalaria assamica Benth.	*Leguminosae*	Assam Crotalaria	ZI XIAO RONG
Crotalaria ferruginea Grah.	*Leguminosae*	Rust-coloured Crotalaria	XIANG LING CAO
Crotalaria sessiliflora L.	*Leguminosae*	Purpleflower Crotalaria	YE BAI HE
Crotalaria spectabilis Roth.	*Leguminosae*	Beautiful Crotalaria	MEI LI ZHU SHI DOU

Index of Origin of Traditional Chinese Medicines

Origin Latin Name	Family	English Name	TCM Name
Crotalaria tetragona Andr.	*Verbenaceae*	Tetragonal Crotalaria	HUA JIN DAN
Crotalaria tetragona Roxb.	*Verbenaceae*	Tetragonal Crotalaria	HUA JIN DAN
Croton caudatus Geisel. var. *tomentosus* Hook.	*Euphorbiaceae*	Tomentose Caudate Croton	MAO YE BA DOU
Croton tiglium L.	*Euphorbiaceae*	Purging Croton	BA DOU
Cryptoaenia japonica Hassk.	*Umbelliferae*	Japanese Cryptotaenia	YA ER QIN
Cryptomeria fortunei Hooibrenk	*Taxodiaceae*	Chinese Cedar	LIU SHAN
Cuccumis sativus L.	*Cucurbitaceae*	Cucumber	HUANG GUA
Cucubalus baccifer L.	*Caryophyllaceae*	Berry-bearing Campion	BAI NIU XI
Cucumis melo L.	*Cucurbitaceae*	Muskmelon Fruit Pedicel	GUA DI
Cucurbita moschata (Duch.) Poiret	*Cucurbitaceae*	Cushaw	NAN GUA
Cucurbita moschata (Duch.) Poiret	*Cucurbitaceae*	Cushaw Seed	NAN GUA ZI
Cucurbita pepo L. var. *akoda* Mak.	*Cucurbitaceae*	Peachliking Pumpkin	TAO NAN GUA
Cupressus funebris Endl.	*Cupressaceae*	Chinese Weeping Cypress Leaf	BAI SHU YE
Curculigo orchioides Gaertn.	*Hypoxidaceae*	Common Cruculigo	XIAN MAO
Curcuma aromatica Salisb.	*Zingiberaceae*	Aromatic Turmeric	JIANG HUANG (of YU JIN)
Curcuma longa L.	*Zingiberaceae*	Common Turmeric	YU JIN
Curcuma longa L.	*Zingiberaceae*	Common Turmeric	JIANG HUANG
Curcuma zedoaria (Berg.) Rosc.	*Zingiberaceae*	Zedoary Turmeric	PENG E SHU (of YU JIN)
Cuscuta australis R. Br.	*Convolvulaceae*	South Dodder	NAN FANG TU SI ZI (of TU SI ZI)
Cuscuta chinensis Lam.	*Convolvulaceae*	Chinese Dodder Seed	TU SI ZI
Cuscuta japonica Choisy	*Convolvulaceae*	Japanese Dodder Seed	DA TU SI ZI (of TU SI ZI)
Cyanotis vaga (Lour.) Roem. *et* Schult.	*Commelinaceae*	Common Cyanotis	LU SHUI CAO (II)
Cyathula capitata (Wall.) Moq.	*Amaranthaceae*	Capitate Cyathula	CHUAN NIU XI
Cyathula officinalis Kuan	*Amaranthaceae*	Mediinal Cyathula	CHUAN NIU XI
Cycas revoluta Thunb.	*Cycadaceae*	Sago Frond	FENG WEI JIAO YE (SU TIE YE)
Cycas revoluta Thunb.	*Cycadaceae*	Sago Seed	TIE SHU GUO (SU TIE SHU GUO)
Cyclea barbata (Wall.) Miers	*Menispermaceae*	Barbate Cyclea	YIN BU HUAN
Cyclea racemosa Oliv.	*Menispermaceae*	Racemose Cyclea	LUN HUAN TENG
Cyclea sutchuenensis Gagnep.	*Menispermaceae*	Szechwan Cyclea	SI CHUAN LUN HUAN TENG
Cyclocarya paliurus (Batal.) Iljinskaja	*Juglandaceae*	Roundwingfruit Cyclocarya	QING QIAN LIU
Cydonia oblonga Mill.	*Rosaceae*	Common Quince	WEN PO
Cymbopogon citratus (DC.) Stapf	*Gramineae*	Lemongrass	XIANG MAO
Cymbopogon distans (Nees) A. Camus	*Gramineae*	Remote Lemongrass	YUN XIANG CAO
Cymbopogon goeringii (Steud.) A. Camus	*Gramineae*	Goering Lemongrass	YE XIANG MAO
Cynanchum auriculatum Royle *ex* Wight	*Asclepiadaceae*	Auriculate Swallowwort	ER YE NIU PI XIAO
Cynanchum bungei Decne.	*Asclepiadaceae*	Bunge Swllowwort	BAI SHOU WU
Cynanchum chinense R. Br.	*Asclepiadaceae*	Chinese Swallowwort	E RONG TENG
Cynanchum hancockianum (Maxim) Al. Iljinski	*Asclepiadaceae*	Hancock Swallowwort	HUA BEI BAI QIAN

Origin Latin Name	Family	English Name	TCM Name
Cynanchum paniculatum (bge.) Kitag.	*Asclepiadaceae*	Paniculate Swallowwort	XU CHANG QING
Cynanchum stauntoni (Decne.) Schltr. *ex* Lévl.	*Asclepiadaceae*	Willowleaf Swallowwort	LIU YE BAI QIAN
Cynanchum thesioides (Freyn) K. Schum.	*Asclepiadaceae*	Bastardtoadflaxlike Swallowwort	DI SHAO GUA
Cynips gallae-tinctoriae Olivier		Aleppo Gall (Galla Halepensis)	MO SHI ZI
Cynoglossum amabile Stapf *et* Drumm.	*Boraginaceae*	Chinese Forgetmenot	GOU SHI HUA
Cynoglossum officinale L.	*Boraginaceae*	Common Houndstongue	YAO YONG DAO TI HU
Cyperus rotundus L.	*Cyperaceae*	Nutgrass Galingale	XIANG FU
Cyprinus carpio L.	*Cyprinidae*	Carp	LI YU
Cyprinus carpio L.	*Cyprinidae*	Carp Gall	LI YU DAN
Cyprinus carpio L.	*Cyprinidae*	Carp Skin	LI YU PI
Cyrtomium fortunei J. Sm.	*Dryopteridaceae*	Fortune's Holly Fern	HUN JI TOU
Dactylicapnos torulosa (Hook. f. *et* Thoms.) Hutch.	*Fumariaceae*	Torulosous Dactylicapnos	DA TENG LING ER CAO
Dalbergia odorifera T. Chen	*Leguminosae*	Odorate Rosewood	JIANG ZHEN XIANG
Dammacanthus indicus Gaertn. f.	*Rubiaceae*	Indian Damnacanthus	HU CI
Damnacanthus officinarum Huang	*Rubiaceae*	Medicinal Damnacanthus	EN SHI BA JI
Damnacanthus subspinosus Hand. -Mazz.	*Rubiaceae*	Shortspine Damnacanthus	DUAN CI HU CI
Daphne genkwa Sieb. *et* Zucc.	*Thymelaeaceae*	Lilac Daphne	YUAN HUA
Daphne genkwa Sieb. *et* Zucc.	*Thymelaeaceae*	Lilac Daphne Root	YUAN HUA GEN
Daphne odora Thunb.	*Thymelaeaceae*	Winter Daphne Flower	RUI XIANG HUA
Daphne odora Thunb.	*Thymelaeaceae*	Winter Daphne Root	RUI XIANG GEN
Daphniphyllum calycinum Benth.	*Daphniphyllaceae*	Calyx-shaped Daphniphyllum Fruit	NIU ER FENG ZI
Daphniphyllum calycinum Benth.	*Daphniphyllaceae*	Calyx-shaped Daphniphyllum Leaf	NIU ER FENG ZHI YE
Datura inoxia Mill.	*Solanaceae*	Hairy Datura Flower	YANG JIN HUA
Datura inoxia Mill.	*Solanaceae*	Hairy Datura Leaf	MAN TUO LUO YE
Datura inoxia Mill.	*Solanaceae*	Hairy Datura Root	MAN TUO LUO GEN
Datura inoxia Mill.	*Solanaceae*	Hairy Datura Seed	MAN TUO LUO ZI
Datura metel L.	*Solanaceae*	Hindu Datura Flower	YANG JIN HUA
Datura metel L.	*Solanaceae*	Hindu Datura Leaf	MAN TUO LUO YE
Datura metel L.	*Solanaceae*	Hindu Datura Root	MAN TUO LUO GEN
Datura metel L.	*Solanaceae*	Hindu Datura Seed	MAN TUO LUO ZI
Daucus carota L.	*Umbelliferae*	Wild Carrot	HE SHI FENG
Daucus carota L. var. *sativa* DC.	*Umbelliferae*	Carrot	HU LUO BO
Daucus carota L. var. *sativa* DC.	*Umbelliferae*	Carrot Seed	HU LUO BO ZI
Delphinium delavayi Franch.	*Ranunculaceae*	Delavay Larkspur	XIAO CAO WU
Delphinium grandiflorum L.	*Ranunculaceae*	Bouquet Larkspur	CUI QUE HUA
Delphinium kamaonense var. *glabrescens* W. T. Wang	*Ranunculaceae*	Hair Larkspur	ZHAN MAO CUI QUE HUA
Delphinium potaninii W. T. Wang	*Ranunculaceae*	Potanin Larkspur	HEI SHUI CUI QUE
Delphinium yunnanense Franch.	*Ranunculaceae*	Yunnan Larkspur	XIAO CAO WU
Delphinus delphis L.	*Delphinidae*	Dolphin	HAI TUN YU
Dendranthema lavandulifolium (Fisch.) Ling *et* Shih	*Compositae*	Lavandulaleaf Dendranthema	GAN JU

Origin Latin Name	Family	English Name	TCM Name
Dendrobenthamia capitata (Wall.) Hutch	*Cornaceae*	Evergreen Dogwood	JI SU ZI
Dendrobium candidum Wall. *ex* Lindl.	*Orchidaceae*	White Dendrobium	TIE PI SHI HU(of the SHI HU)
Dendrobium chrysanthum Wall.	*Orchidaceae*	Goldenflower Dendrobium	SHU HUA SHI HU (of SHI HU)
Dendrobium chrysotoxum Lindl.	*Orchidaceae*	Yellowbow Dendrobium	GU CHUI SHI HU
Dendrobium fimbriatum Hook. var. *oculatum* Hook.	*Orchidaceae*	Eyeshaped Dendrobium	LIU SU SHI HU (of SHI HU)
Dendrobium loddigesii Rolfe.	*Orchidaceae*	Loddiges Dendrobium	MEI HUA SHI HU (of SHI HU)
Dendrobium nobile Lindl.	*Orchidaceae*	Noble Dendrobium	SHI HU
Derris trifoliata Lour.	*Leguminosae*	Trifoliate Jewelvine	YU TENG
Desmodium gangeticum (L.) DC.	*Leguminosae*	Hookedhairypod Tickclover	HONG MU JI CAO
Desmodium pulchellum (L.) Benth.	*Leguminosae*	Beautiful Phyllodium	PAI QIAN CAO
Desmodium pulchellum (L.) Benth.	*Leguminosae*	Beautiful Phyllodium Root	PAI QIAN CAO GEN
Desmodium racemosum (Thunb.) DC.	*Leguminosae*	Acutifoliate Podocarpium Herb	SHAN MA HUANG
Desmodium styracifolium (Osbeck) Merr.	*Leguminosae*	Snowbellleaf Tickclover	GUANG JIN QIAN CAO
Desmos chinensis Lour.	*Annonaceae*	Chinese Desmos	JIA YING ZHUA
Desmos cochinchinensis Lour.	*Annonaceae*	Chinese Desmos	JIA YING ZHAO
Dianthus chinensis L.	*Caryophyllaceae*	Chinese Pink	QU MAI
Dianthus superbus L.	*Caryophyllaceae*	Lilac Pink	QU MAI
Diaspyros lotus L.	*Ebenaceae*	Dateplum Persimmon	JUN QIAN ZI
Dicentra spectabilis (L.) Lem.	*Papaveraceae*	Showy Bleedingheart	HE BAO MU DAN GEN
Dichroa febrifuga Lour.	*Saxifragaceae*	Antifebrile Dichroa	CHANG SHAN
Dictamnus dasycarpus Turcz.	*Rutaceae*	Densefruit Pittany Root-bark	BAI XIAN PI
Digenea simplex (Wulf.) C. Ag.	*Rhodomelaceae*	Simple Digenea Frond	HAI REN CAO
Dinodon rufozonatum	*Colubredae*	Snake Slough	SHE TUI
Dioscorea alata L.	*Dioscoreaceae*	Winged Yam	SHAN YAO
Dioscorea alata L.	*Dioscoreaceae*	Winged Yam	MAO SHU
Dioscorea althaeoira Kunth sp. Nov.	*Dioscoreaceae*	Hollyhock-like Yam Rhizome	SHU KUI YE
Dioscorea bulbifera L	*Dioscoreaceae*	Airpotato Yam	HUANG YAO ZI
Dioscorea collettii Hook. f.	*Dioscoriaceae*	Collett Yam	CHA RUI SHU YU (of BEI XIE)
Dioscorea futschauensis R. Kunth	*Dioscoreaceae*	Foochow Yam Rhizome	FU ZHOU SHU YU (of BEI XIE)
Dioscorea gracillima Miq.	*Dioscoriaceae*	Thinnest Yam	XIAN XI SHU YU (of BEI XIE)
Dioscorea hispida Dennst.	*Dioscoreaceae*	Hispid Yam	BAI SHU LANG
Dioscorea hypoglauca Palib.	*Dioscoriaceae*	Hypoglaucous Collett Yam	FEN BEI SHU YU (of BEI XIE)
Dioscorea nipponica Mak.	*Dioscoreaceae*	Nippon Yam	CHUAN SHAN LONG (CHUAN LONG SHU YU)
Dioscorea nipponica Makino subsp *rosthornii* (Prain *et* Burk) Ting	*Dioscoreaceae*	Rosthorn Yam Rhizome	CHAI HUANG JIANG
Dioscorea opposita Thunb.	*Dioscoreaceae*	Common Yam	SHAN YAO

Index of Origin of Traditional Chinese Medicines

Origin Latin Name	Family	English Name	TCM Name
Dioscorea panthaica Prain *et* Burkill	*Dioscoreaceae*	Yellow Yam Rhizome	HUANG SHAN YAO
Dioscorea parviflora C. T. Ting sp. Nov.	*Dioscoreaceae*	Smallflower Yam Rhizome	XIAO HUA DUN YE SHU YU
Dioscorea septemloba Thunb	*Dioscoreaceae*	Sevenlobed Yam Rhizome	MIAN BI XIE
Dioscorea tokoro Mak.	*Dioscoriaceae*	Mountain Yam	SHAN BEI XIE (of BEI XIE)
Dioscorea zingiberensis C. H. Wright	*Dioscoreaceae*	Peltate Yam Rhizome	DUN YE SHU YU
Diospyros ebenum Koen.	*Ebenaceae*	Ceylon Persimmon Sawdust	WU MU XIE
Diospyros kaki L. f.	*Ebenaceae*	Immature Persimmon Fruit Juice	SHI QI
Diospyros kaki L. f.	*Ebenaceae*	Persimmon	SHI ZI
Diospyros kaki L. f.	*Ebenaceae*	Persimmon Leaf	SHI YE
Diospyros kaki L. f.	*Ebenaceae*	Persimmon Persistent Calyx	SHI DI
Diospyros kaki L. f.	*Ebenaceae*	Persimmon Root	SHI GEN
Diphylleia sinensis Li	*Berberidaceae*	Chinese Umbrellaleaf	WO ER QI
Diploclisia chinensis Merr.	*Menispermaceae*	Chinese Diploclisia	QING FENG TENG
Dipsacus asperoides C. Y. Cheng *et* T. M. Ai	*Dipsacaceae*	Himalayan Teasel	CHUAN XU DUAN (of XU DUAN)
Dipsacus japonicus Miq.	*Dipsacaceae*	Japanese Teasel	XU DUAN
Dodonaea viscosa (L.) Jacq.	*Sapindaceae*	Clammy Hopseedbush Leaf	CHE SANG ZI YE
Doellingeria scaber (Thunb.) Nees	*Compositae*	Scabrous Doellingeria	DONG FENG CAI
Dolichos lablab L.	*Leguminosae*	Hyacinth Dolichos Seed	BIAN DOU
Dracaena cochinchinensis (Lour.) S. C. Chen	*Liliaceae*	Swordleaf Dracaena	JIAN YE LONG XUE SHU (GUANG XI XUE JIE)
Dregea sinensis Hemsl.	*Asclepiadaceae*	Chinese Dregea	KU SHENG
Dregea sinensis Hemsl. var. *corrugata* (Schneid) Tsiang *et* P. T. Li	*Asclepiadaceae*	Corrugate Chinese Dregea	GUAN JIN TENG
Drosera peltata Smith var. *lunata* (Buch.-Ham.) C. B. Clarke	*Droseraceae*	Lunate Peltate Sundew	MAO GAO CAI
Drynaria baronii (Christ) Diels	*Polypodiaceae*	Baron's Drynaria Rhizome	GU SUI BU
Drynaria fortunei (Kunze) J. Sm.	*Polypodiaceae*	Fortune's Drynaria Rhizome	GU SUI BU
Dryobalanops aromatica Gaertn. f.	*Dipterocarpaceae*	Borneol	BING PIAN
Dryopteris championii (Benth.) C. Chr. *ex* Ching	*Dryopteridaceae*	Champion Wood Fern	MAO GUAN ZHONG
Dryopteris crassirhizoma Nakai	*Dryopteridaceae*	Male Fern Rhizome	GUAN ZHONG
Duchesnea indica (Andr.) Focke	*Rosaceae*	Indian Mockstrawberry	SHE MEI
Duranta repena L.	*Verbenaceae*	Creeping Skyflower Leaf	JIA LIAN QIAO YE
Dysosma pleiantha (Hance) Woods.	*Berberidaceae*	Sixangular Dysosma	BA JIAO LIAN
Dysosma versipellis (Hance) M. Cheng	*Berberidaceae*	Common Dysosma	GUI JIU
Dysoxylum hongkongense (Tufch.) Merr.	*Meliaceae*	Hongkong Pencilwood	XIANG GANG JIAN MU

Origin Latin Name	Family	English Name	TCM Name
Echinops latifolus Tausch	*Compositae*	Broadleaf Globethistle	HUA ZHOU LOU LU (of LOU LU)
Ecklonia kurome Okam.	*Alariaceae*	Tangle Thallus	KUN BU
Eclipta alba (L.) Hassk	*Compositae*	Yerbadetajo	MO HAN LIAN
Eclipta prostrata L.	*Compositae*	Yerbadetajo	MO HAN LIAN
Eichhornia crassipes Solms	*Pontederiaceae*	Common Waterhyacinth	SHUI HU LU
Elaeagnus angustifolia L.	*Elaeagnaceae*	Russianolive	SHA ZAO
Elaeagnus angustifolia L.	*Elaeagnaceae*	Russianolive Bark	SHA ZAO SHU PI
Elaphe carinata	*Colubredae*	Snake Slough	SHE TUI
Elaphe taeniurus Cope	*Colubredae*	Snake Slough	SHE TUI
Elephantopus mollis H. B. K.	*Compositae*	Hawaiian Elephantfoot	ROU MAO DI DAN CAO
Elephantopus scaber L.	*Compositae*	Scabrous Elephantfoot	KU DI DAN
Elephas maximus L.	*Elephantidae*	Elephant Bone	XIANG GU
Elephas maximus L.	*Elephantidae*	Elephant Gall	XIANG DAN
Elephas maximus L.	*Elephantidae*	Elephant Meat	XIANG ROU
Elsholtzia ciliata (Yhunb.) Hyland	*Labiatae*	Common Elsholtzia	BAN BIAN SU
Elsholtzia splendens Nakai *ex* F. Maekawa	*Labiatae*	Haichow Elsholtzia	XIANG RU
Embelia oblongifolia Hemsl.	*Myrsinaceae*	Manynerve Embelia	MA GUI HUA
Embelia parviflora Wall. *ex* DC.	*Myrsinaceae*	Smallflower Embelia	XIAO HUA SUAN TENG ZI
Embelia ribes Burm. f.	*Myrsinaceae*	Whiteflower Embelia	XIAN SUAN QIANG
Emilia sonchifolia (L.) DC.	*Compositae*	Sowthistle Tasselflower	YI DIAN HONG
Entada phaseoloides (L.) Merr.	*Leguminosae*	Climbing Entada Seed	KE TENG ZI
Ephedra equisetina Bge.	*Ephedraceae*	Mongolian Ephedra	MA HUANG
Ephedra intermeddia Schrenk *et* Mey.	*Ephedraceae*	Intermediate Ephedra	MA HUANG
Ephedra sinica Stapf	*Ephedraceae*	Chinese Ephedra	MA HUANG
Epicauta gorhami Mars.	*Meloidae*	Bean Blister Beetle	GE SHANG TING CHANG
Epigynum auritum (Schneid.) Tsiang *et* P. T. Li	*Apocynaceae*	Longeared Epigynum	SI MAO TENG
Epilobium angustifolium L.	*Onagraceae*	Great Willowherb (Firewood)	HONG KUAI ZI
Epilobium hirsutum L.	*Onagraceae*	Hairy Willowweed	SHUI JIE GU DAN
Epimedium acuminatum Franch.	*Berberidaceae*	Acuminate Epimedium	CU MAO YIN YANG HUO (of YIN YANG HUO)
Epimedium brevicornum Maxim.	*Berberidaceae*	Shorthorned Epimedium	XIN YE YIN YANG HUO (of YIN YANG HUO)
Epimedium brevicornum Maxim.	*Berberidaceae*	Shorthorned Epimedium Root	YIN YANG HUO GEN
Epimedium davidii Franch.	*Berberidaceae*	David Epimedium	CHUAN DIAN YIN YANG HUO
Epimedium fargesii Franch.	*Berberidaceae*	Fargesi Epimedium	CHUAN E YIN YANG HUO
Epimedium grandiflorum Morr.	*Berberidaceae*	Largeflower Epimedium	YIN YANG HUO
Epimedium grandiflorum Morr.	*Berberidaceae*	Largeflower Epimedium Root	YIN YANG HUO GEN

Index of Origin of Traditional Chinese Medicines

Origin Latin Name	Family	English Name	TCM Name
Epimedium koreanum Nakai	*Berberidaceae*	Korean Epimedium	CHAO XIAN YIN YANG HUO
Epimedium sagittatum (Sieb. *et* Zucc.) Maxim.	*Berberidaceae*	Sagittate Epimedium	JIAN YE YIN YANG HUO (of YIN YANG HUO)
Epimedium sagittatum (Sieb. *et* Zucc.) Maxim.	*Berberidaceae*	Sagittate Epimedium Root	YIN YANG HUO GEN
Epimedium wanshanense S. Z. He *et* Guo.	*Berberidaceae*	Wanshan Epimedium	WAN SHAN YIN YANG HUO
Epimedium wushanense T. S. Ying	*Berberidaceae*	Wushan Epimedium	WU SHAN YIN YANG HUO
Equisetum arvense L.	*Equisetaceae*	Bottle-brush	WEN JING
Equisetum hiemale L.	*Equisetaceae*	Common Scouring Rush	MU ZEI
Equisetum palustre L.	*Equisetaceae*	Marsh Horsetail Herb	GU JIE CAO
Ericerus pela (Chavannes)	*Coccidae*	Cera Chinensis Wax	CHONG BAI LA
Erigeron annuus (L.) Pers.	*Compositae*	Annual Fleabane	YI NIAN PENG
Erigeron breviscapus (Vant.) Hand. - Mazz.	*Compositae*	Shortscape Fleabane	DENG ZHAN XI XIN
Erigeron canadensis L.	*Compositae*	Horseweed Fleabane	QI ZHOU YI ZHI HAO
Erigeron multiradiatus (Wall.) Benth.	*Compositae*	Multiradiate Fleabane	DUO SHE FEI PENG
Erinaceus europaeus L.	*Erinaceidae*	Hedgehog Brain	WEI NAO
Erinaceus europaeus L.	*Erinaceidae*	Hedgehog Heart and Liver	WEI XIN GAN
Erinaceus europaeus L.	*Erinaceidae*	Hedgehog Hide	CI WEI PI (WEI PI)
Eriobotrya japonica (Thunb.) Lindl.	*Rosaceae*	Loquat Leaf	PI PA YE
Eriobotrya japonica (Thunb.) Lindl.	*Rosaceae*	Loquat Seed	PI PA HE
Eriocheir sinensis H. Milne-Edwards	*Grapsidae*	Mitten Crab Chelae	XIE KE
Erodium stephanianum Willd.	*Geraniaceae*	Common Heron's Bill Herb	LAO GUAN CAO
Erycibe elliptilimba Merr. *et* Chun	*Convolvulaceae*	Wamai Erycibe	WA MAI DING GONG TENG
Erycibe schmidtii Craib	*Convolvulaceae*	Glabrousleaf Erycibe	GUANG YE DING GONG TENG
Erysimum cheranthoides L.	*Cruciferae*	Wormseed Mustard	GUI ZHU TANG JIE
Erysimum diffusum Ehrh.	*Cruciferae*	Diffuse Erysimum	TANG JIE
Erythrina arborescens Roxb.	*Leguminosae*	Himalayan Coralbean	QIAO MU CI TONG
Erythrina variegata L. var. *orentalis* (L.) Merr.	*Leguminosae*	Oriental variegated Coralbean Bark	HAI TONG PI
Eucalyptus citriodora Hook f.	*Myrtaceae*	Lemon eucalyptus Leaf	NING MENG AN YE
Eucalyptus gloulus Labill.	*Myrtaceae*	Eucalyptus Leaf	AN YE
Eucalyptus robusta Smith	*Myrtaceae*	Swamp Mahogany	DAS YE AN YE
Eucalyptus tereticornis Smith	*Myrtaceae*	Forest Gray Gum Leaf	XI YE AN YE
Eucheuma muricatum (Gmel.) Web. V. Bos.	*Solieriaceae*	Muriculate Eucheuma Frond	QI LIN CAI
Eucommia ulmoides Oliv.	*Eucommiaceae*	Eucommia	DU ZHONG
Euonymus alatus (Thunb.) Sieb.	*Celastraceae*	Winged Euonymus	GUI JIAN YU
Euonymus bungeanus Maxim.	*Celastraceae*	Winterberry Euonymus	SI MIAN MU
Euonymus fortunei (Turcz.) Hand. - Mazz.	*Celastraceae*	Forture Euonymus	FU FANG TENG

Index of Origin of Traditional Chinese Medicines

Origin Latin Name	Family	English Name	TCM Name
Euonymus grandiflorus Wall.	*Celastraceae*	Largeflower Euonymus	YE DU ZHONG
Euonymus japonicus Thunb.	*Celastraceae*	Evergreen Euonymus	DIAO JING CAO
Euonymus mupinensis Loes. *et* Rehd.	*Celastraceae*	Paohsing Euonymus	BAO XING WEI MAO
Eupatorium adoratum L.	*Compositae*	Fragrant Eupatorium Herb	FEI JI CAO
Eupatorium fortunei Turcz.	*Compositae*	Fortune Eupatorium	PEI LAN
Eupatorium japonicum Thunb.	*Compositae*	Japanese Eupatorium	CHENG GAN CAO
Eupatorium lindleyanum DC.	*Compositae*	Lindley Eupatorium	CHENG GAN SHENG MA
Euphorbia antiquorum L.	*Euphorbiaceae*	Ancients Euphorbia	HUO YANG LE
Euphorbia ebracteolata Hayata	*Euphorbiaceae*	Ebracteolate Euphorbia	YUE XIAN DA JI (of LANG DU)
Euphorbia esula L.	*Euphorbiaceae*	Leafy Euphorbia	JI CHANG LANG DU
Euphorbia esula L. var. *cyparissoides* Boiss.	*Euphorbiaceae*	Narrowleaf Euphorbia	XI YE DA JI
Euphorbia fischeriana Steud.	*Euphorbiaceae*	Fischer Euphorbia	LANG DU DA JI (of LANG DU)
Euphorbia helioscopia L.	*Euphorbiaceae*	Sun Euphorbia	ZE QI
Euphorbia hirta L.	*Euphorbiaceae*	Garden Euphorbia Herb	DA FEI YANG CAO
Euphorbia humifusa Willd.	*Euphorbiaceae*	Humifuse Euphorbia	DI JIN CAO
Euphorbia kansui Liou	*Euphorbiaceae*	Kansui Euphoria	GAN SUI
Euphorbia lathyris L.	*Euphorbiaceae*	Caper Euphorbia Latex	XU SUI ZI JING ZHONG BAI ZHI
Euphorbia lathyris L.	*Euphorbiaceae*	Caper Euphorbia Seed	QIAN JIN ZI
Euphorbia lunulata Bge.	*Euphorbiaceae*	Crescent-shaped Euphorbia Herb	MAO YAN CAO
Euphorbia milii Ch. des Moulins	*Euphorbiaceae*	Crownofhorns Euphorbia	TIE HAI TANG
Euphorbia nematocypha Hand. -Mazz.	*Euphorbiaceae*	Large Euphorbia Root	DA LANG DU
Euphorbia pekinensis Rupr.	*Euphorbiaceae*	Peking Euphorbia	DA JI (a)
Euphorbia royleana Boiss.	*Euphorbiaceae*	Royle Euphorbia Latex	BA WANG BIAN
Euphorbia thymifolia L.	*Euphorbiaceae*	Thymifolious Euporbia	XIAO FEI YANG CAO
Euphoria longan (Lour.) Steud.	*Sapindaceae*	Longan Leaf	LONG YAN YE
Eurya Japonica Thunb.	*Theaceae*	Japanese Eurya	LING MU
Evodia lepta (Spr.) Merr.	*Rutaceae*	Thin Evodia	SAN CHA KU
Evodia rutaecarpa (Juss.) Benth.	*Rutaceae*	Medicinal Evodia	WU ZHU YU
Evolvulus alsinoides L.	*Convolvulaceae*	Common Evolvulus	TU DING GUI
Fagopyrum cymosum Meisr.	*Polygonaceae*	Golden Buckwheat Root	TIAN QIAO MAI GEN
Fagopyrum esculentum Moench	*Polygonaceae*	Common Buckwheat	QIAO MAI
Fagopyrum esculentum Moench	*Polygonaceae*	Common Buckwheat Stem	QIAO MAI JIE
Farfugium japonicum (L.) Kitam.	*Compositae*	Japanese Farfugium Herb	LIAN PENG CAO
Ferula asafoetida L.	*Umbelliferae*	Asafetida Giantfennel Resin	A WEI
Ferula borealis Kuan	*Umbelliferae*	Bunge Giantfennel	SHA QIAN HU
Ferula caspica Marsh.-Bieb.	*Umbelliferae*	Sinkiang Giantfennel Resin	A WEI

Index of Origin of Traditional Chinese Medicines

Origin Latin Name	Family	English Name	TCM Name
Ferula conocaula Eug.	*Umbelliferae*	Broadleaf Giantfennel Resin	A WEI
Ficus carica L.	*Moraceae*	Fig	WU HUA GUO
Ficus carica L.	*Moraceae*	Fig Leaf	WU HUA GUO YE
Ficus carica L.	*Moraceae*	Fig Root	WU HUA GUO GEN
Ficus pumila L.	*Moraceae*	Climbing Fig	BI LI
Fimbristylis dichotoma (L.) Vahl	*Cyperaceae*	Dichotomous Fimbristylis	PIAO FU CAO
Firmiana simplex (L.) W. F. Wight	*Sterculiaceae*	Phoenix Tree Bast	WU TONG BAI PI
Firmiana simplex (L.) W. F. Wight	*Sterculiaceae*	Phoenix Tree Leaf	WU TONG YE
Firmiana simplex (L.) W. F. Wight	*Sterculiaceae*	Phoenix Tree Seed	WU TONG ZI
Flemingia philippinensis (Merr. *et* Rolfe) Li	*Leguminosae*	Philippine Flemingia	MAN XING QIAN JIN BA
Foeniculum vulgare Mill.	*Umbelliferae*	Fennel Fruit	HUI XIANG
Foeniculum vulgare Mill.	*Umbelliferae*	Fennel Root	HUI XIANG GEN
Foeniculum vulgare Mill.	*Umbelliferae*	Fennel Stem and Leaf	HUI XIANG JING YE
Fomes officinalis (Vill. *et* Fr.) Ames	*Polyporaceae*	Fomes Officinalis Sporophore	A LI HONG
Formica fusca L.	*Formicidae*	Silky Ant	HEI MA YI
Forsythia suspensa (Thunb.) Vahl	*Oleaceae*	Weeping Forsythia	LIAN QIAO
Fortunella crassifolia Swingle	*Rutaceae*	Meiwa Kumquat	JIN JU
Fortunella crassifolia Swingle	*Rutaceae*	Meiwa Kumquat Leaf	JIN JU YE
Fortunella margarita (Lour.) Swingle	*Rutaceae*	Oval Kumquat	JIN JU
Fortunella margarita (Lour.) Swingle	*Rutaceae*	Oval Kumquat Leaf	JIN JU YE
Fraxinus bungeana DC.	*Oleaceae*	Bunga Ash Bark	QIN PI
Fraxinus chinensis Roxb.	*Oleaceae*	Chinese Ash Bark	QIN PI
Fraxinus paxiana Lingelsh	*Oleaceae*	Pax Ash Bark	QIN PI
Fraxinus rhynchophylla Hance	*Oleaceae*	Largeleaf Chinese Ash Bark	QIN PI
Fritillaria anhuiensis S. C. Chen *et* S. F. Yin	*Liliaceae*	Anhwei Fritillary	AN HUI BEI MU
Fritillaria cirrhosa D. Don	*Liliaceae*	Tendrilleaf	JUAN YE BEI MU (of CHUAN BEI MU)
Fritillaria cirrhosa D. Don var. *ecirrhosa* Franch.	*Liliaceae*	Blackflower Fritillary	WU HUA BEI MU (of CHUAN BEI MU)
Fritillaria delavayi Franch.	*Liliaceae*	Delavay Fritillary	LENG SHA BEI MU (of CHUAN BEI MU)
Fritillaria ebeiensis var. *pvrpvrea* G. D. Yu *et* P. Li	*Liliaceae*	Purpleflower Fritillary	ZI HUA E BEI BEI MU
Fritillaria hupehensis Hsiao *et* K. C. Hsiao	*Liliaceae*	Hupeh Fritillary	HU BEI BEI MU
Fritillaria ningguoensis S. C. Chen *et* S. F. Yin	*Liliaceae*	Ningguo Fritillary	NING GUO BEI MU
Fritillaria pallidiflora Schrenk	*Liliaceae*	Siberian Fritillary	YI BEI MU (of CHUAN BEI MU)
Fritillaria przewalskii Maxim. *ex* Batal.	*Liliaceae*	Przewalsk Fritillary	GAN SU BEI MU (of CHUAN BEI MU)
Fritillaria siechuanica	*Liliaceae*	Huaxi Fritillary	HUA XI BEI MU
Fritillaria taipaiensis P. Y. Li var. *ningxiaensis* Y.K. Yang et.J.K.Wu	*Liliaceae*	Ningxia Fritillary	NING XIA BEI MU
Fritillaria thunbergii Miq.	*Liliaceae*	Thunberg Fritillary	ZHE BEI MU

Index of Origin of Traditional Chinese Medicines

Origin Latin Name	Family	English Name	TCM Name
Fritillaria unibracteata Hsiao *et* K. C. Hsiao	*Liliaceae*	Unibract Fritillary	AN ZI BEI MU (of CHUAN BEI MU)
Fritillaria ussuriensis Maxim.	*Liliaceae*	Ussuri Fritillary	PING BEI MU (of CHUAN BEI MU)
Fritillaria verticillata Willd. var. *thunbergii* Bak.	*Liliaceae*	Thunberg Fritillary	ZHE BEI MU
Fugu ocellatus (Osbeck)	*Tetraodontidae*	Globefish	HE TUN
Galeola faberi Rolfe	*Orchidaceae*	Faber Galeola	SHAN HU LAN
Galium aparine L.	*Rubiaceae*	Catchweed Bedstraw	BA XIAN CAO
Galium asperifolium Wall.	*Rubiaceae*	Roughleaf Bedstraw	BA XIAN CAO
Galium verum L.	*Rubiaceae*	Yellow Bedstraw	PENG ZI CAI
Gallus gallus domesticus Brisson	*Phasianidae*	Chicken	JI ROU
Gallus gallus domesticus Brisson	*Phasianidae*	Chicken Brain	JI NAO
Gallus gallus domesticus Brisson	*Phasianidae*	Chicken's Gizzard Endothelium	JI NEI JIN
Gallus gallus domesticus Brisson	*Phasianidae*	Hen's Egg Yolk	JI ZI HUANG
Gallus gallus domesticus Brisson	*Phasianidae*	Hen's Egg-albumen	JI ZI BAI
Ganoderma capense (Lloyd) Teng	*Polyproraceae*	Cape Ganoderma	BAO GAI LING ZHI
Ganoderma japonicum (Fr.) Lloyd	*Polyporaceae*	Japonese Ganoderma	ZI ZHI (of LING ZHI CAO)
Ganoderma lucidum (Leyss. *ex* Fr.) Karst.	*Polyporaceae*	Lucid Ganoderma	CHI ZHI (of LING ZHI CAO)
Garcinia morella Desv.	*Guttiferae*	Gamboge Tree Resin	TENG HUANG
Garcinia multiflora Champ.	*Guttiferae*	Manyflower Garcinia	SHAN ZHU ZI
Gardenia jasminoides Ellis	*Rubiaceae*	Cape Jasmine Fruit	ZHI ZI
Gardenia jasminoides Ellis	*Rubiaceae*	Cape Jasmine Leaf	ZHI ZI YE
Gardenia jasminoides Ellis var. *grandiflora* Nakai	*Rubiaceae*	Bigflower Cape Jasmine	SHUI ZHI
Gardenia jasminoides Ellis var. *grandiflora* Nakai	*Rubiaceae*	Bigflower Cape Jasmine Leaf	SHUI ZHI YE
Gastrodia elata Blume	*Orchidaceae*	Tall Gastrodia	TIAN MA
Gaulthcria yunnanensis (Franch.) Rehd.	*Ericaceae*	Yunnan Wintergreen	TOU GU XIANG
Gelsemium elegans Benth	*Loganiaceae*	Graceful Jessamine	GOU WEN
Gentiana algida Pall.	*Gentianaceae*	Alpine Gentian	BAI HUA LONG DAN
Gentiana crassicaulis Duthie *ex* Burkill	*Gentianaceae*	Thickstemen Gentian	QIN JIAO
Gentiana dahurica Fisch.	*Gentianaceae*	Dahuria Gentian	QIN JIAO
Gentiana macrophylla Pall.	*Gentianaceae*	Largeleaf Gentian	QIN JIAO
Gentiana manshurica Kitagawa	*Gentianaceae*	Linearleaf Gentian	LONG DAN
Gentiana rigescens Franch.	*Gentianaceae*	Rigescent Gentian	LONG DAN
Gentiana scabra Bunge	*Gentianaceae*	Rough Gentian	LONG DAN
Gentiana straminea Maxim.	*Gentianaceae*	Straw-coloured Gentian	QIN JIAO
Gentiana tibetica King	*Gentianaceae*	Tibet Gentian	QIN JIAO
Gentiana triflora Pall.	*Gentianaceae*	Threeflower Gentian	LONG DAN
Geranium pratense L.	*Geraniaceae*	Meadow Cranesbill Herb	CAO YUAN LAO GUAN CAO
Geranium sibiricum L.	*Geraniaceae*	Siberian Cranesbill	SHU ZHANG LAO GUAN CAO
Geranium wilfordii Maxim.	*Geraniaceae*	Wilford Cranesbill Herb	LAO GUAN CAO
Gerbera anandria (L.) Sch.-Bip.	*Compositae*	Gerbera	DA DING CAO
Gerbera piloselloides Cass.	*Compositae*	Pilose Gerbera	MAO DA DING CAO

Index of Origin of Traditional Chinese Medicines

Origin Latin Name	Family	English Name	TCM Name
Gryllulus chinensis Weber	*Gryllidae*	Chinese Cricket	XI SHUAI
Gymnadenia conopsea R. Br.	*Orchidaceae*	Conic Gymnadenia	SHOU ZHANG SHEN
Gymnadenia crassinervis Finet	*Orchidaceae*	Crassnerve Gymnadenia	SHOU ZHANG SHEN
Gynostemma compressum X. X. Chen *et* D. R. Liang	*Cucurbitaceae*	Flatfruit Gynostemma	BIAN GUO JIAO GU LAN
Gynostemma longipes C. Y. Wu	*Cucurbhitaceae*	longstalk Gynostemma	CHANG GENG JIAO GU LAN
Gynostemma pentaphylla (Thunb.) Makino	*Cucurbitaceae*	Fiveleaf Gynostemma	QI YE DAN (JIAO GU LAN)
Gynostemma yixingense C. Y. Wu *et* SSK Chen	*Cucurbhitaceae*	Rostratefruit Gynostemma	HUI GUO JIAO GU LAN
Gynura segetum (Lour.) Merr.	*Compositae*	Gynura	SAN QI CAO
Gypsophila acutifolia Fisch.	*Caryophyllaceae*	Gypsophila	HUANG JIE GU DAN
Halenia corniculata (L.) Cornaz.	*Gentianaceae*	Corniculate Spurgentian	HUA MAO
Hedera ncpalensis K. Koch var. *sinensis* (Tobl.) Rehd.	*Araliaceae*	Chinese Ivy	CHANG CHUN TENG
Hedychium Coronarium Koen.	*Zingiberaceae*	Coronarious Gingerlily	TU QIANG HUO
Hedychium forrestii Diels.	*Zingiberaceae*	Forrest Gingerlily	YUAN BAN JIANG HUA
Hedychium spicatum Ham	*Zingiberaceae*	Spiked Gingerlily	TU LIANG JIANG
Hedyotis chrysotricha (Polib.) Merr.	*Rubiaceae*	Goldhair Hedyotis	JIN MAO ER CAO
Hedyotis corymbosa (L.) Lam.	*Rubiaceae*	Corymbose Hedyotis	SHUI XIAN CAO
Hedyotis diffusa Willd.	*Rubiaceae*	Spreading Hedyitis	BAI HUA SHE SHE CAO
Helenium microcephalum DC.		Littlehead Sneezeweed	XIAO TOU DUI XIN JU
Helianthus annuus L.	*Compositae*	Sunflower	XIANG RI KUI HUA
Helianthus annuus L.	*Compositae*	Sunflower Leaf	XIANG RI KUI YE
Helianthus annuus L.	*Compositae*	Sunflower Seed	XIANG RI KUI ZI
Helianthus annuus L.	*Compositae*	Sunflower Stem Pith	XIANG RI KUI JING SUI
Helicteres angustifolia L.	*Sterculiaceae*	Narrowleaf Screwtree	SHAN ZHI MA
Helicteres isora L.	*Sterculiaceae*	Tortedfruit Screwtree	HUO SUO MA
Heliotropium indicum L.	*Boraginaceae*	Indian Heliotrope	DA WEI YAO
Helleborus thibetanus Franch.	*Ranunculaceae*	Tibetan Hellebore	TIE KUAI ZI (II)
Helminthostachys zeylanica (L.) Hook.	*Helminyhostachyaceae*	Ceylon Helminthostachys	RU DI WU GONG
Hemerocallis flava L.	*Liliaceae*	Yellow Daylily	XUAN CAO GEN
Hemerocallis fulva L.	*Liliaceae*	Orange Daylily	XUAN CAO GEN
Hemerocallis minor Mill.	*Liliaceae*	Small Yellow Daylily	XUAN CAO GEN
Hemibarbus labeo (Pallas)	*Cyprinidae*	Skin-carp	CHONG CHUN YU
Hemiechinus dauuricus Sundevall	*Erinaceidae*	Hedgehog Brain	WEI NAO
Hemiechinus dauuricus Sundevall	*Erinaceidae*	Hedgehog Heart and Liver	WEI XIN GAN
Hemiechinus dauuricus Sundevall	*Erinaceidae*	Hedgehog Hide	CI WEI PI (WEI PI)
Hemsleya amabilis Diels	*Cucurbitaceae*	Lovely Hemsleya	LUO GUO DI
Hemsleya graciliflora (Harms) cogn.	*Cucurbhitaceae*	Smallflower Hemsleya	XI HUA XUE DAN

Index of Origin of Traditional Chinese Medicines

Origin Latin Name	Family	English Name	TCM Name
Hemsleya henryi Cogn.	*Cucurbitaceae*	Henry Hemsleya Root	SAI JIN GANG
Hemsleya macrosperma C. Y. Wu	*Cucurbitaceae*	Largeseed Hemsleya	LUO GUO DI
Hemsleya pengxianensis W. J. Chang	*Cucurbitaceae*	Pengxian Hemsleya	PENG XIAN XUE DAN
Heracleum hemsleyanum Diels	*Umbelliferae*	Hemsley Cowparsnip	HIU WEI DU HUO (of DU HUO)
Heracleum lanatum Michx.	*Umbelliferae*	Soft-hair Cowparsnip	RUAN MAO DU HUO (of DU HUO)
Heracleum moellendorffii Hance var. *Paucivitatum* Shan *et* Wang.	*Umbelliferae*	Paucivitat Cowparsnip	ZOU MA QIN
Heracleum scabridum Franch.	*Umbelliferae*	Scabrous Cowparsnip	BAI ZHI
Heracleum yungningense Hand.-Mass	*Umbelliferae*	Yungning Cowparsnip	YONG NING DU HUO (of DU HUO)
Hericium erinaceus (Bull. *ex* Fr.) Pers.	*Hydnaceae*	Bearded Tooth Carpophore	HOU TOU JUN
Heteropappus altaicus (Willd.) Novopokr.	*Compositae*	Altai Heteropappus	A ER TAI ZI WAN
Heteropogon contortus (L.) Beauv.	*Gramineae*	Contorted Tanglehead	DI JIN
Hibiscus mutabilis L.	*Malvaceae*	Cottonrose Hibiscus Flower	MU FU RONG HUA
Hibiscus rosasinensis L.	*Malvaceae*	Chinese Hibiscus Flower	FU SANG HUA
Hibiscus rosasinensis L.	*Malvaceae*	Chinese Hibiscus Leaf	FU SANG YE
Hibiscus syriacus L.	*Malvaceae*	Shrubalthea Bark	MU JIN PI (CHUAN JIN PI)
Hibiscus syriacus L.	*Malvaceae*	Shrubalthea Flower	MU JIN HUA
Hibiscus syriacus L.	*Malvaceae*	Shrubalthea Fruit	MU JIN ZI
Hierochloe odorata (L.) Beauv.	*Gramineae*	Vanillagrass	MAO XIANG HUA
Hippophae rhamnoides L.	*Elaeagnaceae*	Seabuckthorn Fruit	CU LIU GUO (SHA JI)
Holarrhena antidysenterica Wall.	*Apocynaceae*	Droughtdysentery Holarrhena Bark	ZHI XIE MU PI
Homo sapiens L.		Human Hair	XUE YU
Homo sapiens L.		Human Placenta	ZI HE CHE
Homo sapiens L.		Human Urine	REN NIAO
Homo sapiens L.		Human Urine Sediment	REN ZHONG BAI
Hordeum vulgare L.	*Gramineae*	Barley Germinating Fruit	MAI YA
Hosta sieboldiana Engl.	*Liliaceae*	Shortclustered Plantainlily	DA YU BIAO HUA
Houttuynia cordata Thunb.	*Saururaceae*	Heartleaf Houttuynia Herb	YU XING CAO
Hovenia dulcis Thunb.	*Rhamnaceae*	Japanese Raisin Tree Root	ZHI JU GEN
Hovenia dulcis Thunb.	*Rhamnaceae*	Japanese Raisin Tree Seed	ZHI JU ZI
Huechys sanguinea De Geer.	*Cicadidae*	Red Lady-bug	HONG NIANG ZI
Humulus lupulus L.	*Moraceae*	European Hop Female-flower	PI JIU HUA
Humulus scandens (Lour.) Merr.	*Moraceae*	Japanese Hop Herb	LU CAO
Huperzia selago (L.) Bernh. *ex* Schrank *et* Mart.	*huperziaceae*	Selago-like Climbing Fern	XIAO JIE JIN CAO
Huperzia serrata (Thunb.) Trev.	*Huperziaceae*	Serrate Clubmoss	QIAN CENG TA

Index of Origin of Traditional Chinese Medicines

Origin Latin Name	Family	English Name	TCM Name
Hydnum erinaceus Bull. *ex* Fr.	*Hydnaceae*	Bearded Tooth Carpophore	HOU TOU JUN
Hydrangea macrophylla (Thunb.) Ser.	*Saxifragaceae*	Largeleaf Hydrangea	BA XIAN HUA
Hydrangea paniculata Sieb.	*Saxifragaceae*	Paniculate Hydrangea	FEN TUAN HUA
Hydrangea paniculata Sieb. var. *grandiflora* Sieb.	*Saxifragaceae*	Largeflower Paniculate Hydrangea	FEN TUAN HUA
Hydrocarpus anthelmintica Pierr. *ex* Less.	*Flacourticeae*	Chaulmoogratree Seed	DA FENG ZI
Hylomecon japonica (Thunb.) Prantl *et* Kündig	*Papaveraceae*	Japanese Hylomecon	HE QING HUA
Hylotelephium mingjinianum (S. H. Fu) H. Ohba	*Crassulaceae*	Purpleflower Stonecrop	ZI HUA JING TIAN
Hymenocallis americana Roem.	*Amaryllidaceae*	Tropical American Hymenocallis Leaf	SHUI GUI JIAO YE
Hymenodictyon excelsum (Roxb.) Wall.	*Rubiaceae*	Tall Hymenodictyon	TU LIAN QIAO
Hyoscyamus niger L.	*Solanaceae*	Black Henbane Root	LANG DANG GEN
Hyoscyamus niger L.	*Solanaceae*	Black Henbane Seed	TIAN XIAN ZI (LANG DANG ZI)
Hypecoum leptocarpum Hook. f. *et* Thoms.	*Papaveraceae*	Thinfruit Hypecoum	XI GUO JIAO HUI XIANG
Hypericum chinense L.	*Guttiferae*	Chinese St. John'swort Fruit	JIN SI TAO GUO SHI
Hypericum erectum Thunb.	*Guttiferae*	Erect St. John'swort	XIAO LIAN QIAO
Hypericum perforatum L.	*Guttiferae*	Common St. John'swort	GUAN YE LIAN QIAO
Hypodematium sinense Iwatsuki	*Hypodematiaceae*	Shandong Hypodematium	SHAN DONG ZHONG ZU JUE
Hyptis suaveolens Poit	*Labiatae*	Wild Spikenard	SHE BAI ZI
Ilex chinensis Sims	*Aquifoliaceae*	Purpleflower Holly	SI JI QING (DONG QING)
Ilex cornuta Lindl.	*Aquifoliaceae*	Chinese Holly	KU DING CHA
Ilex cornuta Lindl.	*Aquifoliaceae*	Chinese Holly Bark	GOU GU SHU PI
Ilex cornuta Lindl.	*Aquifoliaceae*	Chinese Holly Leaf	GOU GU YE
Ilex latafolia Thunb.	*Aquifoliaceae*	Broadleaf Holly	KU DING CHA
Ilex purpurea	*Aquifoliaceae*	Purpleflower Holly	SI JI QING (DONG QING)
Ilex rotunda Thunb.	*Aquifoliaceae*	Ovateleaf Holly	JIU BI YING
Illicium difengpi K. I. B. *et* K. I. M.	*Illiciaceae*	Difengpi Anisetree	DI FENG PI
Illicium henryi Diels	*Illiciaceae*	Henry Anisetree	HONG HUI XIANG
Illicium minwanense B. N. Chang *et* S. D. Zhang	*Illiciaceae*	Minwan Anisetree	MIN WAN BA JIAO
Illicium simonsii Maxim.	*Illiciaceae*	Yunnan Anisetree	YUN NAN BA JIAO
Illicium verum Hook. f.	*Magnoliaceae*	Star Anise	BA JIAO HUI XIANG
Impatiens balsamina L.	*Balsaminaceae*	Garden Balsam	TOU GU CAO
Impatiens balsamina L.	*Balsaminaceae*	Garden Balsam Seed	JI XING ZI
Impatiens balsamina L.	*Balsaminaceae*	Garden Balsum Flower	FENG XIAN HUA
Impatiens balsamina L.	*Balsaminaceae*	Garden Balsum Root	FENG XIAN GEN
Impatiens siculifer Hook. *F.*	*Balsaminaceae*	Incurvedspur Snapweed	HUANG JIN FENG
Imperata cylindrica (L.) P. Beauv. var. *major* (Nees) C. E. Hubb.	*Gramineae*	Lalang Grass Leaf	MAO CAO YE

Index of Origin of Traditional Chinese Medicines

Origin Latin Name	Family	English Name	TCM Name
Imperata cylindrica (L.) P. Beauv. var. *major* (Nees) C. E. Hubb.	*Gramineae*	Lalang Grass Rhizome	BAI MAO GEN
Incarvillea arguta Royle	*Bignoniaceae*	Sharptooth Incarvillea	MA TONG HUA
Indigofera tinctoria L.	*Leguminosae*	True Indigo	MU LAN
Inula britannica L.	*Compositae*	Brithsh Inula Herb	JIN FO CAO
Inula britannica L.	*Compositae*	British Inula Flower	XUAN FU HUA
Inula britannica L. var. *chinensis* (Rupr.) Reg.	*Compositae*	Chinese Inula Flower	XUAN FU HUA
Inula helenium L.	*Compositae*	Elecampane Inula	TU MU XIANG
Inula helianthus-aguatica C. Y. Wu *ex* Ling	*Compositae*	Aquatic-sunflower Inula	SHUI CHAO YANG
Inula japonica Thunb.	*Compositae*	Japanese Inula Herb	JIN FO CAO
Inula linaraeifolia Turcz.	*Compositae*	Linearleaf Inula Herb	JIN FO CAO
Inula linariaefolia Turcz.	*Compositae*	Linearleaf Inula Flower	XUAN FU HUA
Iphigenia indica Kunth *et* Benth	*Liliaceae*	Indian Iphigenia	CAO BEI MU
Ipomoea cairica (L.) Sweet	*Convolvulaceae*	Cairo Morningglory	WU ZHAO LONG
Iris dichotoma Pall.	*Iridaceae*	Vesper Iris	BAI HUA SHE GAN
Iris japonica Thunb.	*Iridaceae*	Fringed Iris	HU DIE HUA
Iris sanguinea Donn	*Iridaceae*	Bloodred Iris	DOU CHI CAO
Iris sanguinea Hornem.	*Iridaceae*	Bloodred Iris	DOU CHI CAO
Iris tectorum Maxim.	*Iridaceae*	Roof Iris	YUAN WEI
Isatis indigotica Fort.	*Cruciferae*	Indigo-coloured Woad Leaf	DA QING YE
Isatis indigotica Fort.	*Cruciferae*	Indigowoad Root	BAN LAN GEN
Isatis tinctoria L.	*Cruciferae*	Dyers Woad Leaf	DA QING YE
Isatis tinctoria L.	*Cruciferae*	Dyers Woad Root	BAN LAN GEN
Isodon adenanthus (Diels.) Kudo	*Labiatae*	Grandularflower Rabdosia	XIAN HUA XIANG CHA CAI
Isodon enanderianus	*Labiatae*	Purplehair Rabdosia	ZI MAO XIANG CHA CAI
Isodon oresbia (Smith) Hara	*Labiatae*	Montane Rasbdosia	SHAN DI XIANG CHA CAI
Isodon pharicus (Prain) Murata	*Labiatae*	Szechwan-Tibet Rabdosia	CHUAN ZANG XIANG CHA CAI
Isodon ternifolius (D. Don) Kudo	*Labiatae*	Ternateleaf Rabdosia	CHONG YA YAO
Jasminum sambac (L.) Ait.	*Oleaceae*	Arabian Jasmine	MO LI HUA
Juglans regia L.	*Juglandaceae*	English Walnut Exocarp	HU TAO QING PI
Juglans regia L.	*Juglandaceae*	English Walnut Leaf	HU TAO YE
Juglans regia L.	*Juglandaceae*	English Walnut Seed	HU TAO REN
Juniperus rigida Sieb. *et* Zucc.	*Cupressaceae*	Stiffleaf Juniper Fruit	DU SONG SHI
Juniperus taiwaniana Hayata	*Cupressaceae*	Taiwan Juniper	SHAN CI BAI
Kadsura longepedunculata Finet *et* Gagnep.	*Schisandraceae*	Longpeduncle Kadsura	CHANG GENG NAN WU WEI ZI
Kaempferia galanga L.	*Zingiberaceae*	Galanga Resurrectionlily	SHAN NAI
Kalopanax septemlobus (Thunb.) Koidz.	*Araliaceae*	Septemlobate Kalopanax Bark	CI QIU SHU PI
Kerria japonica (L.) DC.	*Rosaceae*	Japanese Kerria Flower	DI TANG HUA
Knoxia valerianoides Thorel *ex* Pitard	*Rubiaceae*	Red Knoxia	HONG YA DA JI (of DA JI (a))

Index of Origin of Traditional Chinese Medicines

Origin Latin Name	Family	English Name	TCM Name
Koelreuteria paniculata Laxm.	*Sapindaceae*	Paniculate Goldraintree	LUAN HUA
Laccifer lacca Kerr.	*Lacciferidae*	Lac	ZI CAO RONG
Lactuca indica L.	*Compositae*	Indian Lettuce	SHAN WO JU
Lactuca sativa L.	*Compositae*	Garden Lettuce	WO JU
Lagenaria siceraria (Molina) Standl. var. *depressa* Ser.	*Cucurbitaceae*	Bottle Gourd	HU LU
Lagerstroemia indica L.	*Lythraceae*	Common Crapemyrtle Flower	ZI WEI HUA
Lagerstroemia indica L.	*Lythraceae*	Common Crapemyrtle Leaf	ZI WEI YE
Lagerstroemia indica L.	*Lythraceae*	Common Crapemyrtle Root	ZI WEI GEN
Lagerstroemia subcostata Koehne	*Lythraceae*	Southern Crapemyrtle	JU NA HUA
Laminaria japonica Aresch.	*Laminariaceae*	Kelp Thallus	KUN BU
Lamiophlomis rotata (Benth.) Kudo	*Labiatae*	Common Lamiophlomis	DU YI WEI
Lamium amplexicaule L.	*Labiatae*	Henbit Deadnettle Herb	BAO GAI CAO
Lamium barbatum Sieb. *et* Zucc.	*Labiatae*	Barbate Deadnettle	YE ZHI MA
Langodorffia indica Arn.	*Balanophoraceae*	Indian Balanophora	YIN DU SHE GU
Lannea grandis (Dennst.) Engl.	*Anacardiaceae*	Coromandel Lannea	HOU PI SHU
Lantana camara L.	*Verbenaceae*	Common Lantana	WU SE MEI
Lappula echinata Gilib.	*Boraginaceae*	European Stickseed	DONG BEI HE SHI
Laurus nobilis L.	*Lauraceae*	Grecian Laurel	YUE GUI ZI
Lawsonia inermis L.	*Lythraceae*	Henna Leaf	ZHI JIA HUA YE
Legume crop.	*Leguminosae*	Soy Sauce	JIANG
Leibnitzia anandria (L.) Nakai	*Compositae*	Gerbera	DA DING CAO
Lemmaphyllum microphyllum Presl	*Polypodiaceae*	Littleleaf Lemmaphyyllum Herb	LUO YAN CAO
*Lemna mino*r L.	*Lemnaceae*	Common Duckwood	FU PING
Lentinus edodes (Berk.) Sing.	*Tricholomataceae*	Champignon	XIANG XUN
Leontice robustum (Maxim.) Diels	*Berberidaceae*	Robust Leontice	HONG MAO QI
Leonurus heterophyllus Sweet	*Labiatae*	Wormwood-like Motherwort Herb	YI MU CAO
Lepidium apetalum Willd.	*Cruciferae*	Pepperweed Seed	TING LI ZI
Lepidium sophia (L.) Schur	*Cruciferae*	Flixweed Tansymustard Seed	TING LI ZI
Lepidium virginicum L.	*Cruciferae*	Virginia Pepperweed Seed	TING LI ZI
Lepisorus thunbergianus (Kaulf.) Ching	*Polypodiaceae*	Thunberg's Lepisorus	WA WEI
Lespedeza bicolor Turcz.	*Leguminosae*	Shrub Lespedeza	HU ZHI ZI
Lespedeza cuneata (Dum.Cours.) G. Don	*Leguminosae*	Cuneate Lespedeza	YE GUAN MEN
Lespedeza tomentosa (Thunb.) Sieb.	*Leguminosae*	Woolly Lespedeza	XIAO XUE REN SHEN
Ligularia dentata (A. Gray.) Hara	*Compositae*	Toothleaf Goldenray	HU LU QI
Ligularia fischeri (Ledeb.) Turcz.	*Compositae*	kindeyleaf Goldenray	HU LU QI
Ligusticum chuanxiong Hort.	*Umbelliferae*	Szechuan Lovage	CHUAN XIONG
Ligusticum jeholense Nakai *et* Kitag.	*Umbelliferae*	Jehol Ligusticum	LIAO GAO BEN (of GAO BEN)
Ligusticum sinense Oliv.	*Umbelliferae*	Chinese Ligusticum	GAO BEN
Ligusticum sinense Oliv. cv. *chaxiong*	*Umbelliferae*	Chaxiong Ligusticum	CHA XIONG

Index of Origin of Traditional Chinese Medicines

Origin Latin Name	Family	English Name	TCM Name
Ligusticum tenuissimum (Nakai) Kitag.	*Umbelliferae*	Slenderleaf Ligusticum	HUO GAO BEN (of GAO BEN)
Ligusticum wallichii Franch.	*Umbelliferae*	Chuanxiong (Wallich Ligusticum)	CHUAN XIONG
Ligustrum lucidum Ait.	*Oleaceae*	Glossy Privet Fruit	NU ZHEN ZI
Lilium brownii F. E. Brown var. *colchesteri* Wils.	*Liliaceae*	Greenish Lily	BAI HE
Lilium brownii F.E. Brown var. *viridulum* Baker	*Liliaceae*	Lily	BAI HE
Lilium davidii Duch. var. *uniclor* Cotton	*Liliaceae*	Uniclor Divid Lily	CHUAN BAI HE
Lilium longiflorum Thunb.	*Liliaceae*	Lanceleaf Lily	BAI HE
Lilium pumilum DC.	*Liliaceae*	Low Lily	BAI HE
Limnophila rugosa (Roth) Merr.	*Scrophulariaceae*	Winked Marshweed	SHUI HUI XIANG
Limonium gmelinii (Willd.) O. Ktze.	*Plumbaginaceae*	Gmelin Sealavender Herb	BU XUE CAO
Linaria vulgaris Mill.	*Scrophulariaceae*	Yellow Toadflax	LIU CHUAN YU
Lindera aggregata (Sims) Kosterm.	*Lauraceae*	Combined Spicebush	WU YAO
Lindera obtusiloba Bl.	*Lauraceae*	Japanese Spicebush	SAN ZUAN FENG
Lindera strychnifolia (Sieb. *et* Zucc.) Villar	*Lauraceae*	Combined Spicebush	WU YAO
Lindera umbellata Thunb.	*Lauraceae*	Pungent Litse	ZHEN CAI
Lindera umbellate Thunb.	*Lauraceae*	Largeleaf Spicebush Root-bark	DIAO ZHANG GEN PI
Linum album Kotschy *ex* Boiss	*Linaceae*	White Flax	BAI YA MA
Linum usitatissimum L.	*Linaceae*	Common Flax	YA MA
Linum usitatissimum L.	*Linaceae*	Common Flax Seed	YA MA ZI
Liparis nervosa (Thunb.) Lindl.	*Orchidaceae*	Nervate Twayblade	JIAN XUE QING
Lippia nodiflora (L.) L. C. Rich.	*Verbenaceae*	Knotteflower Phyla Herb	PENG LAI CAO
Liquidambar formosana Hance	*Hamamelidaceae*	Beautiful Sweetgum	FENG XIANG SHU
Liquidambar orientalis Mill.	*Hamamelidaceae*	Oriental Sweetgum Resin	SU HE XIANG
Liquidambar taiwaniana Hance	*Hamamelidaceae*	Beautiful Sweetgum Leaf	FENG XIANG SHU YE (b)
Liriope spicata (Thunb.) Lour. var. *prolifera* Y. T. Ma	*Liliaceae*	Hubei Liriope	HU BEI SHAN MAI DONG
Litchi chinensis Sonn.	*Sapindaceae*	Lychee	LI ZHI
Litchi chinensis Sonn.	*Sapindaceae*	Lychee Seed	LI ZHI HE
Lithocarpus polystachyus Rehd.	*Fagaceae*	Manyspike Tanoak Leaf	DUO SUI SHI KE YE
Lithospermum erythrhizon Sieb. *et* Zucc.	*Boraginaceae*	Redroot Gromwell	ZI CAO
Litsea cubeba (Lour.) Pers.	*Lauraceae*	Mountain Spicy Tree	BI CHENG QIE
Litsea pungens Hemsl.	*Lauraceae*	Pungent Litse	ZHEN CAI
Litsea verticillata Hance	*Lauraceae*	Whorlleaf Litse	DIE DA LAO
Lobelia chinensis Lour.	*Campanulaceae*	Chinese Lobelia	BAN BIAN LIAN
Lobelia radicans Thunb.	*Campanulaceae*	Chinese Lobelia	BAN BIAN LIAN
Lonicera bournei Hemsl.	*Caprifoliaceae*	South-western Honeysuckle	XI NAN REN DONG
Lonicera confusa DC.	*Captifoliaceae*	Wild Honeysuckle	JIN YIN HUA
Lonicera fulvotomentosa Hsu *et* S. C. Cheng	*Caprifoliaceae*	Yellowhair Honeysuckle	HUANG HE MAO REN DONG
Lonicera hypoglauca Miq.	*Captifoliaceae*	Glaucousback Honeysuckle	JIN YIN HUA
Lonicera japonica Thunb.	*Captifoliaceae*	Japanese Honeysuckle	JIN YIN HUA

Index of Origin of Traditional Chinese Medicines

Origin Latin Name	Family	English Name	TCM Name
Lonicera macranthoides Hand. -Mazz.	*Caprifoliaceae*	Largeflower-like Honeysuckle	DA HUA REN DONG
Lophatherum gracile Brongn.	*Gramineae*	Common Lophatherum	DAN ZHU YE
Lophatherum gracile Brongn.	*Gramineae*	Common Lophatherum Root	SUI GU ZI (DAN ZHU YE GEN)
Loranthus parasiticus (L.) Merr.	*Loranthaceae*	Parasite Scurrula	SANG JI SHENG
Loranthus yadoriki Sieb.	*Loranthaceae*	Yadirik Scurrula	MAO YE SANG JI SHENG (of SANG JI SHENG)
Loropetalum chinense (R. Br.) Oliv.	*Hamamelidaceae*	Chinese Loropetalum	JI HUA YE
Lotus corniculatus L.	*Leguminosae*	Birdsfoot Trefoil	DI YANG QUE
Luffa acutangula Roxb	*Cucurbitaceae*	Singkwa Towelgourd	SI GUA
Luffa acutangula Roxb	*Cucurbitaceae*	Singkwa Towelgourd Seed	SI GUA ZI
Luffa acutangula Roxb	*Cucurbitaceae*	Singkwa Towelgourd Stem	SI GUA TENG
Luffa cylindrica (L.) Roem.	*Cucurbitaceae*	Suakwa Vegetablesponge	SI GUA
Luffa cylindrica (L.) Roem.	*Cucurbitaceae*	Suakwa Vegetalesponge Seed	SI GUA ZI
Luffa cylindrica (L.) Roem.	*Cucurbitaceae*	Suakwa Vegetalesponge Stem	SI GUA TENG
Lunathyrium acrostichoides (Sw.) Ching	*Athyriaceae*	Lunathyrium Fern	GUAN ZHONG
Lyaimachia Clethroides Duby	*Primulaceae*	Clethra Loosestrife	ZHEN ZHU CAI (ZHEN ZHU YE)
Lycium barbarum L.	*Solanaceae*	Barbary Wolfberry Fruit	GOU QI ZI
Lycium barbarum L.	*Solanaceae*	Barbary Wolfberry Leaf	GOU QI YE
Lycium barbarum L.	*Solanaceae*	Barbary Wolfberry Root-bark	DI GU PI (GOU QI GEN PI)
Lycium chinense Mill.	*Solanaceae*	Chinese Wolfberry Root-bark	DI GU PI (GOU QI GEN PI)
Lycium chinense Mill.	*Solanaceae*	Chinese Wolfberry Fruit	GOU QI ZI
Lycium chinense Mill.	*Solanaceae*	Chinese Wolfberry Leaf	GOU QI YE
Lycopersicon esculentum Mill.	*Solanaceae*	Tomato	FAN QIE
Lycopodium cernnum L.	*Lycopodiaceae*	Cernuous Clubmoss Herb	PU DI WU GONG
Lycopodium clavatum L.	*Lycopodiaceae*	Common Japanese Clubmoss	SHEN JIN CAO
Lycopodium complanatum L.	*Lycopodiaceae*	Complanate Clubmoss	GUO JIANG LONG
Lycopodium selago L.	*huperziaceae*	Selago-like Climbing Fern	XIAO JIE JIN CAO
Lycopodium serrayum Thunb.	*Huperziaceae*	Serrate Clubmoss	QIAN CENG TA
Lycopus lucidus Turcz.	*Labiatae*	Shiny Bugleweed Root	DI SUN (ZE LAN GEN)
Lycopus lucidus Turcz.	*Labiatae*	Shiny Bugleweed Stem and Leaf	ZE LAN
Lycoris aurea Herb.	*Amaryllidaceae*	Golden Lycoris	DA YI ZHI JIAN
Lycoris radiata (L'Her.) Herb.	*Amaryllidaceae*	Shorttube Lycoris	SHI SUAN

Index of Origin of Traditional Chinese Medicines

Origin Latin Name	Family	English Name	TCM Name
Lyonia ovalifolia (Wall.) Drude	*Ericaceae*	Tibet Lyonia	LI MU
Lysimachia christinae Hance	*Primulaceae*	Christina Loosestrife Herb	DA JIN QIAN CAO
Lysimachia paridiformis Franch.	*Primalaceme*	Parisshape Loosestrife	CHONG LOU PAI CAO
Lysionotus paucylora Maxim.	*Gesneriaceae*	Fewflower Lysionotus	SHI DIAO LAN
Lythrum salicaria L.	*Lythraceae*	Spiked Loosestrife	QIAN QU CAI
Lytta caraganae Pallas	*Meloidae*	Mung Bean Blister Beetle	QING NIANG ZI
Machilus thunbergii Sieb. *et* Zucc.	*Lauraceae*	Red Nanmu Bark	HONG NAN PI
Macleaya cordata (Willd.) R. Br.	*Papaveraceae*	Pink Plumepoppy	BO LUO HUI
Macrocarpium officinalis (Sieb. *et* Zucc.) Nakai	*Cornaceae*	Asiatic Cornelian Cherry (Common Macrocarpium)	SHAN ZHU YU
Maesa japonica (Thunb.) Moritzi	*Myrsinaceae*	Japanese Maesa	DU JING SHAN
Magnolia biloba (Rehd. *et* Wils.) Cheng	*Magnoliaceae*	Twolobed Officinal Mangolia	HOU PO
Magnolia biondii Pamp.	*Magnoliaceae*	Biond Magnolia	WANG CHUN MU LAN (of XIN YI)
Magnolia coco (Lour.) DC.	*Magnoliaceae*	Chinese Magnolia Flower	YE HE HUA
Magnolia denudata Desr.	*Magnoliaceae*	Yulan Magnolia	YU LAN (of XIN YI)
Magnolia fargesii Cheng	*Magnoliaceae*	Biond Magnolia	WANG CHUN MU LAN (of XIN YI)
Magnolia liliflora Desr.	*Magnoliaceae*	Lily Magnolia	XIN YI
Magnolia liliflora Desr.	*Magnoliaceae*	Lily Magnolia Bark	MU LAN PI
Magnolia liliflora Desr.	*Magnoliaceae*	Lily Magnolia Flower	MU LAN HUA
Magnolia officinalis Rehd. *et* Wils.	*Magnoliaceae*	Officinal Mangolia	HOU PO
Magnolia rostrata W. W. Smith	*Magnoliaceae*	Bigleaf Magnolia	DA YE MU LAN (DA YE HOU PU)
Mahonia bealei (Fort.) Carr.	*Berberidaceae*	Leatherleaf Mahonia	SHI DA GONG LAO MU
Mahonia bealei (Fort.) Carr.	*Berberidaceae*	Leatherleaf Mahonia Fruit	SHI DA GONG LAO ZI
Mahonia bealei (Fort.) Carr.	*Berberidaceae*	Leatherleaf Mahonia Leaf	SHI DA GONG LAO YE
Mahonia fortunei (Lindl.) Fedde	*Berberidaceae*	Chinese Mahonia	SHI DA GONG LAO MU
Mahonia fortunei (Lindl.) Fedde	*Berberidaceae*	Chinese Mahonia Fruit	SHI DA GONG LAO ZI
Mahonia fortunei (Lindl.) Fedde	*Berberidaceae*	Chinese Mahonia Leaf	SHI DA GONG LAO YE
Mahonia japonica (Thunb.) DC.	*Berberidaceae*	Japanese Mahonia	SHI DA GONG LAO MU
Mahonia japonica (Thunb.) DC.	*Berberidaceae*	Japanese Mahonia Fruit	SHI DA GONG LAO ZI
Mahonia japonica (Thunb.) DC.	*Berberidaceae*	Japanese Mahonia Leaf	SHI DA GONG LAO YE
Mallotus anomalus	*Euphorbiaceae*	Anomalus Mallotu	XIU MAO YE TONG
Mallotus japonicus Muell.-Arg.	*Euphorbiaceae*	Japanese Mallotus	YE WU TONG
Mallotus philippinensis (Lam.) Muell.-Arg.	*Euphorbiaceae*	Kamalatree Pericarpial Glandular Hairs	LU SONG QIU MAO

Index of Origin of Traditional Chinese Medicines

Origin Latin Name	Family	English Name	TCM Name
Malus asiatica Nakai	*Rosaceae*	Chinese Pearleaf Crabapple	LIN QIN
Mangifera persiciformis C.Y. Wu *et* T. L. Ming	*Anacardiaceae*	Peachform Mango	BIAN TAO
Manis pentadactyla Linnaeus	*Manidae*	Pangolin	CHUAN SHAN JIA
Marchantia polymorpha L.	*Marchantiaceae*	Marchantia Polymorpha Lichen	DI SUO LUO
Marsdenia globifera Tsiang	*Asclepiadaceae*	Globose Condorvine	QIU HUA NIU NAI CAI
Marsdenia koi Tsiang	*Asclepiadaceae*	Ko Condorvine	DA YE NIU NAI CAI
Marsdenia oreophila Smith	*Asclepiadaceae*	Beakstyle Condorvine	HUI ZHU NIU NAI CAI
Matricaria chamomilla L.	*Compositae*	Maywood	MU JU
Matricaria recutita L.	*Compositae*	Maywood	MU JU
Matteuccia struthiopteris (L.) Todaro	*Onocleaceae*	Matteuccia Fern	GUAN ZHONG
Maytenus hookeri Loes.	*Celastraceae*	Yunnan Mayten	YUN NAN MEI DENG MU
Medicago hispida Gaertn.	*Leguminosae*	California Burclover	MU XU
Medicago hispida Gaertn.	*Leguminosae*	California Burclover Root	MU XU GEN
Medicago sativa L.	*Leguminosae*	Alfalfa	MU XU
Medicago sativa L.	*Leguminosae*	Alfalfa Root	MU XU GEN
Melia azedarach L.	*Meliaceae*	Chinaberry-tree Bark	KU LIAN PI
Melia azedarach L.	*Meliaceae*	Chinaberry-tree Flower	LIAN HUA
Melia toosendan Sieb. *et* Zucc.	*Meliaceae*	Szechwan Chinaberry Bark	KU LIAN PI
Melia toosendan Sieb. *et* Zucc.	*Meliaceae*	Szechwan Chinaberry Flower	LIAN HUA
Melia toosendan Sieb. *et* Zucc.	*Meliaceae*	Szechwan Chinaberry Fruit	CHUAN LIAN ZI (KU LIAN)
Melilotus suaveolens Ledeb.	*Leguminosae*	Daghestan Sweetclover Herb	PI HAN CAO
Melilotus suaveolens Ledeb.	*Leguminosae*	White Sweetclover Root	CHOU MU XU GEN
Melodinus hemsleyanus Diels	*Apocynaceae*	Hemsley Melodinus	CHUAN SHAN CHENG
Menispermum dauricum DC.	*Menispermaceae*	Asiatic Moonseed	BIAN FU GE
Menispermum dauricum DC.	*Menispermaceae*	Asiatic Moonseed Root	BIAN FU GE GEN
Mentha haplocalyx Briq.	*Labiatae*	Wild Mint	BO HE
Mentha rotundifolia (L.) Huds.	*Labiatae*	Apple Mint Herb	YU XIANG CAO
Menyanthes trifoliata L.	*Gentianaceae*	Bogbean	SHUI CAI
Menyanthes trifoliata L.	*Gentianaceae*	Bogbean Gen	SHUI CAI GEN
Meretrix meretrix L.	*Veneridae*	Hard Clam Shell	WEN GE
Metaplexis japonica (Thunb.) Mak.	*Asclepiadaceae*	Japanese Metaplexis	LUO MO
Metaplexis japonica (Thunb.) Mak.	*Asclepiadaceae*	Japanese Metaplexis Seed	LUO MO ZI
Michelia alba DC.	*Magnoliaceae*	Bailan Flower	BAI LAN HUA
Michelia champaca L	*Magnoliaceae*	Champac Michelia	HUANG MIAN GUI
Michelia yunnanensis Fr. *ex* Fin. *et* Gagn	*Magnoliaceae*	Yunnan Micheli	YUN NAN HAN XIAO
Millettia dielsiana Harms *ex* Diels	*Leguminosae*	Diels Millettia	JI XUE TENG
Millettia nitida Benth.	*Leguminosae*	Shiningleaf Millettia	JI XUE TENG
Millettia pachycarpa Benth.	*Leguminosae*	Thickfruit Millettia	KU TAN ZI
Millettia reticulata Benth.	*Leguminosae*	Leatherleaf Millettia Root	KUN MING JI XUE TENG GEN

Origin Latin Name	Family	English Name	TCM Name
Millingtonia hortensis L. f.	*Bignoniaceae*	Garden Millingtonia	ZI MEI SHU
Mimosa pudica L.	*Leguminosae*	Sensitiveplant Herb	HAN XIU CAO
Mirabilis jalapa L.	*Nyctaginaceae*	Common Four-o'clock Leaf	ZI MO LI YE
Mirabilis jalapa L.	*Nyctaginaceae*	Common Four-o'clock Root	ZI MO LI GEN
Miscanthus sinensis Anderss.	*Gramineae*	Chinese Silvergrass	MANG JING
Mnium cuspidatum Hedw.	*Mniaceae*	Cuspidate Mnium Herb	SHUI MU CAO
Momordica charantia L.	*Cucurbitaceae*	Balsampear	KU GUA
Momordica charantia L.	*Cucurbitaceae*	Balsampear Seed	KU GUA ZI
Momordica cochinchinensis (Lour.) Spr.	*Cucurbitaceae*	Cochinhina Momordica Root	MU BIE GEN
Momordica cochinchinensis (Lour.) Spr.	*Cucurbitaceae*	Cochinhina Momordica Seed	MU BIE ZI
Momordica dioica	*Cucurbhitaceae*	Mountain Balsampear	SHAN KU GUA
Momordica grosvenorii Swingle	*Cucurbitaceae*	Grosvenor Siraitia	LUO HAN GUO
Mongifera indica L.	*Anacardiaceae*	Mango	MANG GUO
Mongifera indica L.	*Anacardiaceae*	Mango Bark	MANG GUO SHU PI
Mongifera indica L.	*Anacardiaceae*	Mango Leaf	MANG GUO YE
Mongifera indica L.	*Anacardiaceae*	Mango Seed	MANG GUO HE
Monotropa uniflora L.	*Pyrolaceae*	Indianpipe	SHUI JINGLAN
Morinda officinalis How	*Rubiaceae*	Medicinal Indianmulberry	BA JI TIAN
Morinda umbellata L.	*Rubiaceae*	Common Indianmulberry	YANG JIAO TENG
Morus alba L.	*Moraceae*	White Mulberry	SANG YE
Morus alba L.	*Moraceae*	White Mulberry Bast	SANG BAI PI
Morus alba L.	*Moraceae*	White Mulberry Branch	SANG ZHI
Moschus berezovskii Flerov.	*Cervidae*	Abelmusk	SHE XIANG
Moschus moschiferus L.	*Cervidae*	Abelmusk	SHE XIANG
Moschus sifanicus Przewalski	*Cervidae*	Abelmusk	SHE XIANG
Mosla dianthera (Ham.) Maxim.	*Labiatae*	Twoanther Mosla	DA YE XIANG RU
Mosla grosseserrata Maxim.	*Labiatae*	Largeserrate Mosla	JI NING
Mosla scabra (Thunb.) C. Y. Wu *et* H. W. Li	*Labiatae*	Scabrous Mosla	SHI JI NING
Mucuna birdwoodiana Tutcher	*Leguminosae*	Whiteflower Mucuna	JI XUE TENG
Murica rubra (Lour.) Sieb. *et* Zucc.	*Myricaceae*	Chinese Waxmyrtle	YANG MEI
Murica rubra (Lour.) Sieb. *et* Zucc.	*Myricaceae*	Chinese Waxmyrtle Bark	YANG MEI SHU PI
Murraya crenulata	*Rutaceae*	Taiwan Common Jasminorange	TAI WAN JIU LI XIANG
Murraya euchrestifolia Hayata	*Rutaceae*	Euchretaleaf Common Jasminorange	DOU YE JIU LI XIANG
Murraya exotica	*Rutaceae*	Chinese Common Jasminorange	ZHONG HUA JIU LI XIANG
Murraya koenigii Spreng	*Rutaceae*	Indian Common Jasminorange	YIN DU JIU LI XIANG
Murraya microphylla	*Rutaceae*	Juvenileleaf Common Jasminorange	NEN YE JIU LI XIANG (2807-JIU LI XIANG)
Murraya paniculata (L.) Jack var. *exotica* (L.) Huang	*Rutaceae*	Littleleaf Common Jasminorange	XIAO YE JIU LI XIANG

Index of Origin of Traditional Chinese Medicines

Origin Latin Name	Family	English Name	TCM Name
Murraya paniculata (L.) Jacks.	*Rutaceae*	Common Jasminorange	JIU LI XIANG
Murraya siamensis	*Rutaceae*	Siamense Common Jasminorange	YUAN DONG JIU LI XIANG (2808-JIU LI XIANG)
Musa paradisiaca L. var. *sapientum* O. Ktze.	*Musaceae*	Common Banana	XIANG JIAO
Musa sapientum L.	*Musaceae*	Common Banana	XIANG JIAO
Mussaenda pubescens Ait. f.	*Rubiaceae*	Buddha's Lamp	SHAN GAN CAO
Mylabris cichorii Linnaeus	*Meloidae*	Blister Beetle	BAN MAO
Mylabris phalerata Pall.	*Meloidae*	Blister Beetle	BAN MAO
Myristica fragrans Houtt.	*Myristicaceae*	Common Nutmeg	ROU DOU KOU
Myroxylon pereirae (Royle) Klotzsch	*Leguminosae*	Peru Balmtree Resin	BI LU XIANG JIAO
Myrsine africana L.	*Leguminosae*	African Myrsine	DA HONG PAO
Nandina domestica Thunb.	*Berberidaceae*	Common Nandina Fruit	NAN TIAN ZHU ZI
Nandina domestica Thunb.	*Berberidaceae*	Common Nandina Root	NAN TIAN ZHU GEN
Nandina domestica Thunb.	*Berberidaceae*	Common Nandina Stem	NAN TIAN ZHU GENG
Narcissus tazeyya L. var. *chinensis* Roem.	*Amaryllidaceae*	Chinese Narcissus Bulb	SHUI XIAN GEN
Narcissus tazeyya L. var. *chinensis* Roem.	*Amaryllidaceae*	Chinese Narcissus Flower	SHUI XIAN HUA
Nardostachys chinensis Batal.	*Valerianaceae*	Chinese nardostachys	GAN SONG
Nauclea officinalis Pierre *ex* Pitard	*Rubiaceae*	Medicinal Fatheadtree	DAN MU
Nelumbo nucifera Gaertn.	*Nymphaeaceae*	Hindu Lotus Large Rhizome	OU
Nelumbo nucifera Gaertn.	*Nymphaeaceae*	Hindu Lotus Leaf	HE YE
Nelumbo nucifera Gaertn.	*Nymphaeaceae*	Hindu Lotus Leaf-base	HE YE DI
Nelumbo nucifera Gaertn.	*Nymphaeaceae*	Hindu Lotus Petiole	HE GENG
Nelumbo nucifera Gaertn.	*Nymphaeaceae*	Hindu Lotus Plumule	LIAN ZI XIN
Nelumbo nucifera Gaertn.	*Nymphaeaceae*	Hindu Lotus Seed	LIAN ZI
Nelumbo nucifera Gaertn.	*Nymphaeaceae*	Hindu Lotus Spermoderm	LIAN YI
Neocheiropteris palmatopedata (Bak.) Christ	*Polypodiaceae*	Palmatipartiteleaf Neocheiropteris	SHAN JUE
Nepeta cataria L.	*Labiatae*	Catnip	JIA JING JIE
Nerium indicum Mill.	*Apocynaceae*	Sweetscented Oleander	JIA ZHU TAO
Nicandra physaloides (L.) Gaerth.	*Solanaceae*	Peru Herb	JIA SUAN JIANG
Nicotiana tabacum L.	*Solanaceae*	Common Tobacco	YAN CAO
Nitraria Sibirica Pall.	*Zygophyllaceae*	Siberian Nitraria	KA MI
Notholirion hyacinthinum (Wils.) Stapf	*Liliaceae*	Hyacinth Falselily	JIA BAI HE
Nothopanax davidii (Franch.) Harms	*Arliaceae*	David Falsepanax	YI YE LIANG WANG CHA
Notopterygium forbesii Boiss.	*Umbelliferae*	Forbes Notopterygium	KUAN YE QIANG HUO (of QIANG HUO)
Notopterygium franchetii Boiss.	*Umbelliferae*	Szechwan Notopterygium	CHUAN QIANG HUO (of QIANG HUO)

Index of Origin of Traditional Chinese Medicines

Origin Latin Name	Family	English Name	TCM Name
Notopterygium incisum Ting *ex* H. T. Chang	*Umbelliferae*	Incised Notopterygium	QIANG HUO
Nymphoides peltatum (Gmel.) O. Ktze.	*Gentianaceae*	Shield Floatingheart	XING CAI
Nyssa sinensis Oliv.	*Nyssaceae*	Chinese Tupelo	ZI SHU
Ocimum basilicum L.	*Labiatae*	Basil Fruit	LUO LE ZI
Ocimum basilicum L.	*Labiatae*	Basil Herb	LUO LE
Octopus vulgaris Lamarck	*Octopodidae*	Common Atlantic Octopus	ZHANG YU
Odontites serotina Reich.	*Scrophulariaceae*	Lateripening Bartsia Herb	CHI YE CAO
Oenanthe javanica (Bl.) DC.	*Umbelliferae*	Javan Waterdropwort	SHUI QIN
Oenanthe javanica (Bl.) DC.	*Umbelliferae*	Javan Waterdropwort Flower	QIN HUA
Oldenlandia chrysotricha (Polib.) Chun	*Rubiaceae*	Goldhair Hedyotis	JIN MAO ER CAO
Oldenlandia corymbosa L.	*Rubiaceae*	Corymbose Hedyotis	SHUI XIAN CAO
Oldenlandia diffusa (Willd.) Roxb.	*Rubiaceae*	Spreading Hedyitis	BAI HUA SHE SHE CAO
Olea europaea L.	*Oleaceae*	Common Olive	YOU GAN LAN (QI DUN GUO)
Onopordum acanthium L.	*Compositae*	Scotch Cottonthistle	DA CHI JI
Onosma paniculatum Bur. *et* Franch.	*Boraginaceae*	Paniculate Onosma	ZI CAO
Ophiocephalus argus Cantor	*Ophiocephalidae*	Serpent-head (Black Fish)	WU LI
Ophioglossum vulgatum L.	*Ophioglossaceae*	Adder's Tongue	PING ER XIAO CAO
Ophiopogon japonicus (Thunb.) Ker-Gawl.	*Liliaceae*	Dwarf Lilyturf	MAI MEN DONG
Ophiorrhiza japonica Bl.	*Rubiaceae*	Japanese Ophiorrhiza	SHE GEN CAO
Oplopanax elatus Nakai	*Arliaceae*	Tall Oplopanax	CI REN SHEN (DONG BEI CI REN SHEN)
Origanum vulgare L.	*Labiatae*	Common Origanum	TU XIANG RU
Orixa japonica Thunb.	*Rutaceae*	Japanese Orixa	CHOU SHAN YANG
Ormosia hosiei Hemsl. *et* Wils.	*Leguminosae*	Hosie Ormosia Seed	HONG DOU
Orobanche coerulescens Steph.	*Orobanchaceae*	Skyblue Broomrape	LIE DANG
Orobanche pycnostachya Hance	*Orobanchaceae*	Yellowflower Broomrape	LIE DANG
Oroxylum indicum (L.) Vent.	*Bignoniaceae*	Indian Trumpetflower	MU HU DIE
Oroxylum indicum (L.) Vent.	*Bignoniaceae*	Indian Trumpetflower Bark	MU HU DIE SHU PI
Orthodon chinensis (Maxim.) Kudo	*Labiatae*	Chinese Orthodon	SHI XIANG ROU
Oryza sativa L.	*Gramineae*	Rice	JING MI
Oryza sativa L.	*Gramineae*	Rice Spermoderm	MI PI KANG
Oryza sativa L.	*Gramineae*	Rice Straw	DAO CAO
Oryza sativa L. (The pathogen is *Ustilaginoidea virens* (Cke.) Tak.)	*Gramineae*	Fungus-infected Rice Spike	JING GU NU
Osmanthus fragrans Lour.	*Oleaceae*	Sweet Osmanthus Flower	GUI HUA
Osmorhiza aristata (Thunb.) Mak. *et* Yabe var. *laxa* (Royle) Constance *et* Shan	*Umbelliferae*	Laxleaf Sweetroot	XIANG GEN QIN

Index of Origin of Traditional Chinese Medicines

Origin Latin Name	Family	English Name	TCM Name
Osmunda japonica Thunb.	*Osmundaceae*	Japanese Osmunda Fern	GUAN ZHONG
Ostrea gigas Thunberg	*Osteridae*	Oyster Meat	MU LI ROU
Ostrea rivularis Gould	*Osteridae*	Oyster Meat	MU LI ROU
Ostrea talienwhanensis Crosse	*Osteridae*	Oyster Meat	MU LI ROU
Ovis aries L.	*Bovidae*	Goat Hide	YANG PI
Ovis aries L.	*Bovidae*	Goat Milk	YANG RU
Ovis aries L.	*Bovidae*	Goat Pancreas	YANG YI
Oxytropis oxyphylla DC.	*Leguminosae*	Mountain Crazyweed	PAO PAO CAO
Pachyrhizus erosus (L.) Urban	*Leguminosae*	Wayaka Yambean Seed	DI GUA ZI
Pachysandra terminalis Sieb. *et* Zucc.	*Buxaceae*	Japanese Pachysandra	XUE SHAN LIN
Paederia scandens (Lour.) Merr.	*Rubiaceae*	Chinese Fevervine	JI SHI TENG
Paederia scandens (Lour.) Merr.	*Rubiaceae*	Chinese Fevervine Fruit	JI SHI TENG GUO
Paeonia lactiflora Pall.	*Ranunculaceae*	Common peony	BAI SHAO YAO
Paeonia lactiflora Pall.	*Ranunculaceae*	Common Peony (wild)	SHAO YAO (of CHI SHAO YAO)
Paeonia obovata Maxim.	*Ranunculaceae*	Obovate Peony	CAO SHAO YAO (of CHI SHAO YAO)
Paeonia suffruticosa Andr.	*Ranunculaceae*	Subshrubby Peony Bark	MU DAN PI
Paeonia veitchii Lynch	*Ranunculaceae*	Veitch Peony	CHUAN CHI SHAO (of CHI SHAO YAO)
Panax bipinnatifidus (Seem.) Li	*Arliaceae*	Bipinnatifid Ginseng	YU YE SAN QI
Panax ginseng C. A. Mey.	*Araliaceae*	Ginseng	REN SHEN
Panax ginseng C. A. Mey.	*Araliaceae*	Ginseng Buds	REN SHEN HUA LEI
Panax japonicus var. *bipinnatifidus* (Seem.) Wu *et* Feng	*Arliaceae*	Bipinnatifid Ginseng	YU YE SAN QI
Panax japonicus var. *major* (Burk.) Wu *et* Feng	*Arliaceae*	Largeleaf JapaneseGinseng	QIN LING ZHU ZI SHEN
Panax notoginseng (Burk.) F. H. Chen	*Araliaceae*	Sanchi	SAN QI
Panax pseudoginseng Wall. var. *japonicus* (Mey.) Hoo *et* Tseng	*Araliaceae*	Japanese Ginseng	ZHU JIE SAN QI
Panax pseudoginseng Wall. var. *notoginseng* (Burk.) Hoo *et* Tseng	*Araliaceae*	Sanchi	SAN QI
Panax quinquefolium L.	*Araliaceae*	American Ginseng	XI YANG SHEN
Pandanus tectorius Soland.	*Pandanaceae*	Thatch Screwpine Flower	LU DOU LE HUA
Panicum miliaceum L	*Gramineae*	Broomcorn Millet	SHU MI
Panthera tigris L.	*Felidae*	Tiger Fat	HU GAO
Panulirus ornatus (Fabricius)	*Palinuridae*	Lobster	HAI XIA
Papaver nudicaule L.	*Papaveraceae*	Chinese Poppy	YE YING SU
Papaver rhoeas L.	*Papaveraceae*	Corn Poppy	LI CHUN HUA
Papaver rhoeas L.	*Papaveraceae*	Corn Poppy Fruit	LI CHUN HUA GUO SHI
Papaver sommiferum L.	*Papaveraceae*	Opium	YA PIAN
Papaver somniferum L.	*Papaveraceae*	Opium Poppy	YING SU
Papaver somniferum L.	*Papaveraceae*	Opium Poppy Pericarp	YING SU KE
Paris polyphlla Smith	*Liliaceae*	Manyleaf Paris	ZAO XIU
Paris tetraphylla A. Gray	*Liliaceae*	Tetraphyllous Paris	WANG SUN
Parmelia saxatilis Ach.	*Parmeliaceae*	Parmelia Lichen	SHI HUA

Index of Origin of Traditional Chinese Medicines

Origin Latin Name	Family	English Name	TCM Name
Parthenocissus tricuspidata (Sieb. *et* Zucc.) Planch.	*Vitaceae*	Japanese Creeper	DI JIN
Passiflora caerulea L.	*Passifloraceae*	Passionflower	XI FAN LIAN
Patrinia heterophylla Bge.	*Valerianaceae*	Diversifolious Patrinia	YI YE BAI JIANG
Patrinia scabiosaefolia Fisch.	*Valerianaceae*	Dahurian Patrinia	HUANG HUA BAI JIANG (of BAI JIANG)
Patrinia villosa Juss.	*Valerianaceae*	Whiteflower Patrinia	BAI HUA BAI JIANG (of BAI JIANG)
Paulownia fortunei (Seem.) Hemsl.	*Scrophulariaceae*	Fortune Paulownia	TONG MU (PAO TONG)
Paulownia fortunei (Seem.) Hemsl.	*Scrophulariaceae*	Fortune Paulownia Fruit	PAO TONG GUO
Paulownia tomentosa (Thunb.) Steud.	*Scrophulariaceae*	Royal Paulownia	TONG MU (PAO TONG)
Paulownia tomentosa (Thunb.) Steud.	*Scrophulariaceae*	Royal Paulownia Fruit	PAO TONG GUO
Pedicularis muscicola Maxim.	*Scrophulariaceae*	Muscicolous Woodbetony	XIAN SHENG MA XIAN HAO
Pedilanthus tithymaloides (L.) Poit.	*Euphorbiaceae*	Tithymalus-like Pedilanthus	YU DAI GEN
Peganum harmala L.	*Zygophyllaceae*	Common Peganum Herb	LUO TUO PENG
Peganum harmala L.	*Zygophyllaceae*	Common Peganum Seed	LUO TUO PENG ZI
Pelargonium graveolens Lsymbol 162 \f "Symbol" \s 8′}Herit	*Geraniaceae*	Roce Pelargonium	XIANG YE
Pelargonium hortorum Bailey	*Geraniaceae*	Fish Pelargonium	SHI LA HONG
Penaeus orientalis Kishinouye	*Penaeidae*	Prawn	HAI XIA
Pericampylus glaucus (Lam.) Merr.	*Menispermaceae*	Greyblue Pericampylus	XI YUAN TENG
Perilla frutescens (L.) Britt.	*Labiatae*	Common Perilla Fruit	BAI SU ZI
Perilla frutescens (L.) Britt. var. *acuta* (Thunb.) Kudo	*Labiatae*	Acute Common Perilla Leaf	ZI SU YE
Perilla frutescens (L.) Britt. var. *acuta* (Thunb.) Kudo	*Labiatae*	Acute Common Perilla Seed	ZI SU ZI
Perilla frutescens (L.) Britt. var. *acuta* (Thunb.) Kudo	*Labiatae*	Acute Common Perilla Stem	ZI SU GEN
Perilla frutescens (L.) Britt. var. *crispa* (Thunb.) Hand. -Mazz.	*Labiatae*	Crisped Common Perilla Leaf	ZI SU YE
Perilla frutescens (L.) Britt. var. *crispa* (Thunb.) Hand. -Mazz.	*Labiatae*	Crisped Common Perilla Seed	ZI SU ZI
Perilla frutescens (L.) Britt. var. *crispa* (Thunb.) Hand. -Mazz.	*Labiatae*	Crisped Common Perilla Stem	ZI SU GEN
Periploca sepium Bge.	*Asclepiadaceae*	Chinese Silkvine Root-bark	XIANG JIA PI
Petasites japoniaus (Sieb. *et* Zucc.) F. Schmidt	*Compositae*	Japanese Butterbur	FENG DOU CAI
Peucedanum decursivum (Miq.) Maxim.	*Umbelliferae*	Common Hogfennel	QIAN HU
Peucedanum govanianum (Wall) Benth *ex* C. B. Clarke var. *bicolo* Wolff	*Umbellifera*	Likiang Hogfennel	LI JIANG QIAN HU
Peucedanum longshengense Shan *et* Sheh	*Umbelliferae*	Nanling Hogfennel	NAN LING QIAN HU

Index of Origin of Traditional Chinese Medicines

Origin Latin Name	Family	English Name	TCM Name
Peucedanum praeruptorum Dunn	*Umbelliferae*	Whiteflower Hogfennel	BAI HUA QIAN HU (of QIAN HU)
Peucedanum rubuicaule Shan *et* Shch	*Umbelliferae*	Yun Hogfennel	YUN QIAN HU
Pharbitis nil (L.) Choisy	*Convolvulaceae*	Lobedleaf Pharbitis Seed	QIAN NIU ZI
Pharbitis purpurea (L.) Voigt	*Convolvulaceae*	Roundleaf Pharbitis Seed	QIAN NIU ZI
Phaseolus vulgaris L.	*Leguminosae*	Kidney Bean Seed	BAI FAN DOU
Phasianus colchicus Gmelin	*Phasianidae*	Common Pheasant	ZHI
Phellinus igniarius (L. *ex* Fr.) Quél.	*Polyproraceae*	Phellinus Igniarius	SANG HUANG
Phellodendron amurene Rupr.	*Rutaceae*	Amur Corktree	HUANG BAI
Phellodendron chinense Schneid.	*Rutaceae*	Chinese Corktree	HUANG BAI
Phellodendron chinense Schneid. var. *glabriusculum* Schneid.	*Rutaceae*	Glabrousleaf Chinese Corktree	HUANG BAI
Pheretima aspergillum (E. Perrier)	*Megascolecidae*	Earthworm	QIU YIN
Philydrum lanuginosum Banks	*Phylydraceae*	Woolly Philydrum	TIAN CONG
Phlegmariurus fordii (Baker) Ching	*Huperziaceae*	Fordi Phlegmariurus	HUA NAN MA WEI SHAN
Phlomis mongolica Turcz.	*Labiatae*	Mongolian Jjerusalemsage	MENG GU CAO SU
Phlomis rotata Benth.	*Labiatae*	Common Lamiophlomis	DU YI WEI
Phlomis tuberosa L.	*Labiatae*	Tuberousroot Jerusalemsage	KUAI JING CAO SU
Phoebe nanmu (Oliv.) Gamble	*Lauraceae*	Nanmu Lignum	NAN MU
Phoenix dactylifera L.	*Palmae*	Phoenix Date	WU LOU ZI
Pholidota yunnanensis Rolfe	*Orchidaceae*	Yunnan Pholidota	YUN NAN SHI XIAN TAO
Photinia serrulata Lindl.	*Rosaceae*	Chinese Photinia Leaf	SHI NAN YE
Phragmites communis Trin.	*Gramineae*	Common Reed Rhizome	LU GEN
Phryma leptostachya L.	*Phrymataceae*	Lopseed Herb	LAO PO ZI ZHEN XIAN
Phyllanthus emblica L.	*Euphorbiaceae*	Emblic Leafflower	AN MO LE
Phyllanthus emblica L.	*Euphorbiaceae*	Emblic Leafflower Bark	YOU GAN MU PI
Phyllanthus emblica L.	*Euphorbiaceae*	Emblic Leafflower Leaf	YOU GAN YE
Phyllanthus emblica L.	*Euphorbiaceae*	Emblic Leafflower Root	YOU GAN GEN
Phyllanthus urinaria L.	*Euphorbiaceae*	Common Leafflower	YE XIA ZHU
Physalis alkekengi L. var. *franchetii* (Mast.) Mak.	*Solanaceae*	Franchet Groundcherry	SUAN JIANG
Physalis alkekengi L. var. *franchetii* (Mast.) Mak.	*Solanaceae*	Franchet Groundcherry Root	SUAN JIANG GEN
Physalis minima L.	*Solanaceae*	Little Groundcherry	TIAN PAO ZI
Physalis peruviana L.	*Solanaceae*	Peruvian Groundcherry Herb	DENG LONG CAO
Physalis pubescens L.	*Solanaceae*	Downy Groundcherry	KU ZHI
Physeter catodon L.	*Physeteridae*	Ammbergris	LONG XIAN XIANG
Physochlaina physaloides (L.) G. Don	*Solanaceae*	Common Physochlaina	PAO NANG CAO
Phytolacca acinosa Roxb.	*Phytolaccaceae*	Indian Pokeweed	SHANG LU
Phytolacca americana L.	*Phytolaccaceae*	American Pokeweed	MEI SHANG LU
Phytolacca esculenta Van Houtte	*Phytolaccaceae*	Indian Pokeweed	SHANG LU

Origin Latin Name	Family	English Name	TCM Name
Picrasma quassioides (D.Don) Benn.	*Simaroubaceae*	Indian Quassiawood	KU SHU PI
Picrorrhiza kurrooa Royle *ex* Benth.	*Scrophulariaceae*	Picrorhiza	HU HUANG LIAN
Picrorrhiza scrophulariaeflora Pennell	*Scrophulariaceae*	Figwortflower Picrorhiza	HU HUANG LIAN
Pimpinella thellungiana Wolff	*Umbelliferae*	Thellung Pimpinella	YANG HONG SHAN
Pinellia pedatisecta Schott	*Araceae*	Pedate Pinallia	ZHANG YE BAN XIA
Pinellia ternata (Thunb.) Breit.	*Araceae*	Ternate Pinellia	BAN XIA
Pinus koraiensis Sieb. *et* Zucc.	*Pinaceae*	Korean Pine Seed	HAI SONG ZI
Pinus massoniana Lamb.	*Pinaceae*	Colophony	SONG XIANG
Piper betle L.	*Piperaceae*	Betel Pepper Leaf	JU JIANG YE
Piper cubeba L.	*Lauraceae*	Cubeba Piper	BI CHENG QIE
Piper futo-kadsura Sieb.	*Piperaceae*	Kadsura Pepper Stem	HAI FENG TENG
Piper hancei Maxim.	*Piperaceae*	Hance Pepper	SHAN JU
Piper kadsura (Choisy) Ohwi	*Piperaceae*	Kadsura Pepper Stem	HAI FENG TENG
Piper longum L.	*Piperaceae*	Long Pepper	BI BA
Piper longum L.	*Piperaceae*	Long Pepper Root	BI BA GEN
Piper mullesua D. Don.	*Piperaceae*	Globular Pepper	DUAN JU
Piper nigrum L.	*Piperaceae*	Black Pepper	HU JIAO
Piper polysyphorum C. DC	*Piperaceae*	Camphortreeleaf Pepper	ZHANG YE HU JIAO
Pistacia chinensis Bge.	*Anacardiaceae*	Common Pistache	HUANG LIAN YA
Pisum sativum L.	*Leguminosae*	Garden Pea	WAN DOU
Plantago asiatica L.	*Plantaginaceae*	Asiatic Plantain	CHE QIAN
Plantago depressa Willd.	*Plantaginaceae*	Depressed Plantain	CHE QIAN
Platycarya strobilacea Sieb. *et* Zucc.	*Juglandaceae*	Dyetree Leaf	HUA XIANG SHU YE
Platycladus orientalis (L.) Franco	*Cupressaceae*	Chinese Arborvitae Branch	BAI ZHI JIE (CE BAI ZHI JIE)
Platycladus orientalis (L.) Franco	*Cupressaceae*	Chinese Arborvitae Leaf	CE BAI YE
Platycodon grandiflorum (Jacq.) A. DC.	*Campanulaceae*	Balloonflower	JIE GENG
Pleonomus canaliculatus Faldermann	*Elateridae*	Burrowed Click Beetle	KOU TOU CHONG
Pleurospermum rivulorum (Diels)	*Umbelliferae*	Yunnan Pleurospermum	YUN NAN QIANG HUO
Plumbagella micrantha (Ledeb.) Spach	*Plumbaginaceae*	Littleflower Plumbagella Herb	JI WA CAO
Plumbago indica L.	*Plumbaginaceae*	Indian Leadword	ZI XUE HUA
Plumbago zeylanica L.	*Plumbaginaceae*	Whiteflower Leadword	BAI HUA DAN
Poa sphondylodes Trin.	*Labiatae*	Hard Bluegrass	
Podocarpium podocarpum var. *oxyphyllum* (DC.) Yang *et* Huang	*Leguminosae*	Acutifoliate Podocarpium Herb	SHAN MA HUANG
Podocarpus gracilior Pilg.	*Podocarpaceae*	Musengerra Podocarpus	XI LUO HAN SONG
Podocarpus imbricatus Bl.	*Podocarpaceae*	Imbricate Podocarpus	JI MAO SONG
Podocarpus macrophyllus (Thunb.) D. Don	*Podocarpaceae*	Kusamaki Broadleaved Podocarpus Leaf	LUO HAN SONG YE
Podocarpus macrophyllus (Thunb.) D. Don	*Podocarpaceae*	Kusamaki Broadleaved Podocarpus Seed	LUO HAN SONG SHI

Index of Origin of Traditional Chinese Medicines

Origin Latin Name	Family	English Name	TCM Name
Podocarpus macrophyllus (Thunb.) D. Don var. *maki* (Sieb.) Endl.	*Podocarpaceae*	Chinese Podocarpus Leaf	LUO HAN SONG YE
Podocarpus macrophyllus (Thunb.) D. Don var. *maki* (Sieb.) Endl.	*Podocarpaceae*	Chinese Podocarpus Seed	LUO HAN SONG SHI
Podocarpus nagi Zoll. *et* Mor.	*Podocarpaceae*	Nagai Podocarpus	ZHU BAI
Podocarpus polystachyus R. Br.	*Podocarpaceae*	Manyspike Podocarpus	DUO SUI LUO HAN SONG SHI
Podophyllum emodi Wall. var. *chinense* Sprague	*Berberidaceae*	Common Sinopodophyllm	TAO ER QI
Podophyllum peltatum L.	*Berberidaceae*	Common Mayapple	DUN YE GUI JIU
Pogostemon cablin (Blanco) Benth.	*Labiatae*	Cablin Potchouli	GUANG HUO XIANG (of HUO XIANG)
Polygala arillata Buch.symbol 45 \f "Symbol" \s 8-Ham.	*Polygalaceae*	Yellowflower Milkwort	HUANG HUA YUAN ZHI
Polygala caudata Rehd. *et* Wils.	*Polygalaceae*	Caudate Milkwort	SHUI HUANG YANG MU
Polygala chinensis L.	*Polygalaceae*	Chinese Milkwort Herb	DA JIN NIU CAO
Polygala tenuifolia Willd.	*Polygalaceae*	Thinleaf Milkwort	YUAN ZHI
Polygonatum cirrhifolium (Wall.) Royle	*Liliaceae*	Tendrilleaf Solomonseal	HUANG JING
Polygonatum cyrtonema Hua	*Liliaceae*	Manyflower Solomonseal	HUANG JING
Polygonatum kingianum Coll. *et* Hemsl.	*Liliaceae*	King Solomonseal	HUANG JING
Polygonatum macropodium Turcz.	*Liliaceae*	Macropodous Solomonseal	HUANG JING
Polygonatum odoratum (Mill.) Druce	*Liliaceae*	Fragrant Solomonseal	YU ZHU
Polygonatum sibiricum Redoute	*Liliaceae*	Siberian Solomonseal	HUANG JING
Polygonum amphibium L.	*Polygonaceae*	Amphibious Knotweed	LIANG QI LIAO
Polygonum aviculare L.	*Polygonaceae*	Common Knotgrass	BIAN XU
Polygonum bistorta L.	*Polygonaceae*	Bistort	QUAN SHEN
Polygonum chinense L.	*Polygonaceae*	Chinese Knotweed Herb	HUO TAN MU CAO
Polygonum ciliinerve (Nakai) Ohwi	*Polygonaceae*	Ciliatenerve Knotweed Root	HONG YAO ZI
Polygonum cuspidatum Sieb. *et* Zucc.	*Poligonaceae*	Japanese Fleeceflower (Giant Knotweed)	HU ZHANG
Polygonum hydropiper L.	*Polygonaceae*	Red-knees	SHUI LIAO
Polygonum multiflorum Thunb.	*Polygonaceae*	Tube Fleeceflower Stem	YE JIAO TENG
Polygonum multiflorum Thunb.	*Polygonaceae*	Tuber Fleeceflower	HE SHOU WU
Polygonum orientale L.	*Polygonaceae*	Prince's-feather Herb	HONG CAO
Polygonum perfoliatum L.	*Polygonaceae*	Perfoliate Knotweed Root	GANG BAN GUI GEN
Polygonum polystachyum Wall. *ex* Meisn	*Polygonaceae*	Manyspike Knotweed	DUO SUI LIAO
Polygonum suffultum Maxim.	*Leguminosae*	Ovateleaf Knotweed	HONG SAN QI
Polygonum thunbergii Sieb. *et* Zucc.	*Polygonaceae*	Thunberg Knotweed	SHUI MA TIAO
Polygonum tinctorium Ait	*Polygonaceae*	Indigoplant Leaf	DA QING YE
Polygonum tinctorium Ait.	*Polygonaceae*	Indigoplant	LIAO LAN

Index of Origin of Traditional Chinese Medicines

Origin Latin Name	Family	English Name	TCM Name
Polypodium mairei Brause	*Polypodiaceae*	Mary Arthromeris	FENG WEI PA SHAN HU
Polypodium niponicum Mett.	*Polypodiaceae*	Japanese Polypody	SHUI LONG GU
Polyporus umbellatus (Pers.) Fries	*Polyporaceae*	Popyporus Agaric	ZHU LING
Poncirus trifoliata (L.) Raf.	*Rutaceae*	Trifoliate Orange	ZHI SHI
Poncirus trifoliata (L.) Raf.	*Rutaceae*	Trifoliate Orange (almost ripe fruit)	ZHI KE
Poncirus trifoliata (L.) Raf.	*Rutaceae*	Trifoliate-orange	GOU JU
Poncirus trifoliata (L.) Raf.	*Rutaceae*	Trifoliate-orange Leaf	GOU JU YE
Poncirus trifoliata (L.) Raf.	*Rutaceae*	Trifoliate-orange Root-bark	ZHI GEN PI
Poncirus trifoliata (L.) Raf.	*Rutaceae*	Trifoliate-orange Seed	GOU JU HE
Pongamia pinnata (L.) Merr.	*Leguminosae*	Poongaoil Pongamia	SHUI LIU DOU
Populus tomentosa Carr.	*Salicaceae*	Chinese White Poplar	MAO BAI YANG
Poria cocos (Schw.) Wolf	*Polyporaceae*	Indian Bread	FU LING
Porphyra tenera Kjellm.	*Bangiaceae*	Laver	ZI CAI
Portulaca grandiflora Hook.	*Labiatae*	Largeflower Purslane	BAN ZHI LIAN
Portulaca oleracea L.	*Portulacaceae*	Purslane	MA CHI XIAN
Potamogeton perfoliatus L.	*Potamogetonaceae*	Thorowort Pondweed	SUAN SHUI CAO
Potentilla reptons L.var. *sericophylla* Franch.	*Rosaceae*	Sericeous Cinquefoil	JIN JIN BANG
Prunella vulgaris L.	*Labiatae*	Common Selfheal	XIA KU CAO
Prunum amygdalus Batsch	*Rosaceae*	Amygdalate Apricot Seed	BA DAN XING REN
Prunus armeniaca L.	*Rosaceae*	Apricot	XING ZI
Prunus armeniaca L.	*Rosaceae*	Apricot Seed	XING REN
Prunus armeniaca L. var. *ansu* Maxim.	*Rosaceae*	Ansu Apricot	XING ZI
Prunus armeniaca L. var. *ansu* Maxim.	*Rosaceae*	Ansu Apricot Seed	XING REN
Prunus davidiana (Carr.) Franch.	*Rosaceae*	David Peach Bast	TAO JING BAI PI
Prunus davidiana (Carr.) Franch.	*Rosaceae*	David Peach Flower	TAO HUA
Prunus davidiana (Carr.) Franch.	*Rosaceae*	David Peach Juvenile Branch	TAO ZHI
Prunus davidiana (Carr.) Franch.	*Rosaceae*	David Peach Leaf	TAO YE
Prunus davidiana (Carr.) Franch.	*Rosaceae*	David Peach Resin	TAO JIAO
Prunus davidiana (Carr.) Franch.	*Rosaceae*	David Peach Root	TAO GEN
Prunus humilis Bge.	*Rosaceae*	Chinese Dwarf Cherry Seed	YU LI REN
Prunus japonica Thunb.	*Rosaceae*	Dwarf Flowering Cherry Seed	YU LI REN
Prunus japonica Thunb. var. *nakaii* (Lévl.) Rehd.	*Rosaceae*	Longpedicel Chinese Buscherry Seed	YU LI REN
Prunus mume (Sieb.) Sieb. *et* Zucc.	*Rosaceae*	Japanese Apricot	WU MEI
Prunus mume (Sieb.) Sieb. *et* Zucc.	*Rosaceae*	Mumeplant (Japanese Apricot)	MEI HE REN
Prunus mume (Sieb.) Sieb. *et* Zucc.	*Rosaceae*	Plum Flower	BAI MEI HUA
Prunus persica (L.) Batsch.	*Rosaceae*	Peach	TAO REN
Prunus persica (L.) Batsch.	*Rosaceae*	Peach Bast	TAO JING BAI PI
Prunus persica (L.) Batsch.	*Rosaceae*	Peach Juvenile Branch	TAO ZHI
Prunus persica (L.) Batsch.	*Rosaceae*	Peach Flower	TAO HUA
Prunus persica (L.) Batsch.	*Rosaceae*	Peach Leaf	TAO YE

Origin Latin Name	Family	English Name	TCM Name
Prunus persica (L.) Batsch.	*Rosaceae*	Peach Resin	TAO JIAO
Prunus persica (L.) Batsch.	*Rosaceae*	Peach Root	TAO GEN
Prunus pseudocerasus Lindl.	*Rosaceae*	Falsesour Cherry	YING TAO
Prunus salicina Lindl.	*Rosaceae*	Japanese Plum	LI ZI
Prunus salicina Lindl.	*Rosaceae*	Japanese Plum Kernel	LI HE REN
Prunus tomentosa Thunb.	*Rosaceae*	Downy Cherry	SHAN YING TAO
Pseudostellaria heterophylla (Miq.) Pax *ex* Pax *et* Hoffm.	*Caryophyllaceae*	Heterophylla Falsestarwort	TAI ZI SHEN
Psidium guajava L.	*Myrtaceae*	Guava Bark	FAN SHI LIU PI
Psidium guajava L.	*Myrtaceae*	Guava Immature Fruit	FAN SHI LIU GAN
Psidium guajava L.	*Myrtaceae*	Guava Leaf	FAN SHI LIU YE
Psilotum nudum (L.) Griseb.	*Psilotaceae*	Nude Fern	SHI SHUA BA
Psoralea corylifolia L.	*Papilionaceae*	Malaytea Scurfpea	BU GU ZHI
Pteridium aquilinum (L.) Kuhn var. *latiusculum* (Desv.) Underw	*Pteridaceae*	Eastern Bracken Fern	JUE
Pterocarpus indicus Willd.	*Leguminosae*	Burmacoast Padauk	ZI TAN
Pterocarya stenoptera DC.	*Juglandaceae*	Chinese Wingnut	MA LIU YE
Pteromys volans L.	*Petauristidae*	Trogopterus Dung	WU LING ZHI
Pterospermum lanceaefolium Roxb	*Sterculiaceae*	Lanceleaf Wingseedtree	ZHAI YE BAN FENG HE
Pueraria lobata (Willd.) Ohwi	*Leguminosae*	Lobed Kudzuvine Leaf	GE YE
Pueraria lobata (Willd.) Ohwi	*Leguminosae*	Lobed Kudzuvine Root	GE GEN
Pueraria mirifica	*Leguminosae*	Mirifica Kudzuvine	GUO YE GE
Pueraria thomsonii Benth.	*Leguminosae*	Thomson Kudzuvine Root	GE GEN
Pulsatilla chinensis (Bge.) Reg.	*Ranunculaceae*	Chinese pulsatilla	BAI TOU WENG
Punica granatum L.	*Punicaceae*	Pomegranate	SUAN SHI LIU
Punica granatum L.	*Punicaceae*	Pomegranate Peel	SHI LIU PI
Punica granatum L.	*Punicaceae*	Pomegranate Root	SHI LIU GEN
Pygeum topengii Merr.	*Rosaceae*	Topeng Pygeum	TUN XING GUO
Pyrola japonica Klenze *ex* Alef.	*Pyrolaceae*	Japanese Pyrola Herb	LU SHOU CAO
Pyrola rotundifolia L.	*Pyrolaceae*	European Pyrola Herb	LU XIAN CAO
Pyrola rotundifolia L. subsp. *chinensis* H. Andres	*Pyrolaceae*	Chinese Pyrola Herb	LU XIAN CAO
Pyrrosia davidii (Gies.) Ching	*Polypodiaceae*	Peking pyrrosia frond	SHI WEI
Pyrrosia drakeana (Franch.) Ching	*Polypodiaceae*	Felthair pyrrosia frond	SHI WEI
Pyrrosia gralla (Gies.) Ching	*Polypodiaceae*	Southwest pyrrosia frond	SHI WEI
Pyrrosia lingua (Thunb.) Farw.	*Polypodiaceae*	Japanese Felt Fern Frond	SHI WEI
Pyrrosia petiolosa (Christ) Ching	*Polypodiaceae*	Petioled pyrrosia frond	SHI WEI
Pyrrosia sheareri (Bak.) Ching	*Polypodiaceae*	Shearer's Pyrrosia Frond	SHI WEI
Pyrus betulaefolia Bge.	*Rosaceae*	Birchleaf Pear	TANG LI
Pyrus bretschneideri Rehd.	*Rosaceae*	Bretschneider Pear Leaf	LI YE
Pyrus calleryana Decne.	*Rosaceae*	Callery Pear Branch and Leaf	YE LI ZHI YE
Pyrus pashia Buch.-Ham. *ex* D. Don	*Rosaceae*	Pashi Pear Fruit	CHUAN LI GUO

Origin Latin Name	Family	English Name	TCM Name
Pyrus pyrifolia (Burm. F.) Nakai	*Rosaceae*	Sand Pear Leaf	LI YE
Pyrus ussuriensis Maxim.	*Rosaceae*	Ussurian Pear Leaf	LI YE
Python molurus bivittatus Schlegel	*Boidae*	Indian Python	MANG SHE
Quercus mongolica Fisch.	*Fagaceae*	Mongolian Oak	MENG GU LI
Quisqualis indica L.	*Combretaceae*	Rangooncreeper	SHI JUN ZI
Quisqualis indica L.	*Combretaceae*	Rangooncreeper Leaf	SHI JUN ZI YE
Rabdosia coetsoides C. Y. Wu	*Labiatae*	Falselittleconical Rabdosia	JIA XI ZHUI XIANG CHA CAI
Rabdosia inflexa (Thunb.) Hara	*Labiatae*	Inflexed Rabdosia	NEI ZHE XIANG CHA CAI
Rabdosia japonica (Burm. f.) Hara.	*Labiatae*	Japanese Rabdosia	MAO YE XIANG CHA CAI
Rabdosia longituba (Miquel) Hara.	*Labiatae*	Longtube Rabdosia	CHANG GUAN XIANG CHA CAI
Rabdosia macrophylla (Migo) C. Wu *et* H. Li	*Labiatae*	Largeleaf Rabdosia	DA YE XIANG CHA CAI
Rabdosia nervosa (Hemsl.) C. Y. Wu. *et* H. W. Li	*Labiatae*	Veined Rabdosia	XIAN MAI XIANG CHA CAI
Rabdosia rubescens (Hemsl.) Hara	*Labiatae*	Blushred Rabdosia	DONG LING CAO
Rabdosia serra (Maxim.) Hara	*Labiatae*	Serrate Rabdosia	XI HUANG CAO
Rabdosia stracheyi (Benth. *ex* Hook. f.) Hara	*Labiatae*	Longleaf Rabdosia	CHANG YE XIANG CHA CAI
Rana amurensis Boulenger	*Ranidae*	Dried Chinese (or Amur) Woodfrog	HA SHI MA
Rana limnocharis Boie	*Ranidae*	Rice Frog Gall	XIA MA DAN
Rana nigromaculata Hallowell	*Ranidae*	Pond Frog	QING WA
Rana nigromaculata Hallowell	*Ranidae*	Pond Frog Gall	QING WA DAN
Rana plancyi Lataste	*Ranidae*	Pond Frog	QING WA
Rana plancyi Lataste	*Ranidae*	Pond Frog Gall	QING WA DAN
Rana temporaria chensinensis David	*Ranidae*	Dried Chinese (or Amur) Woodfrog	HA SHI MA
Ranunculus cantoniensis DC.	*Ranunculaceae*	Canton Buttercup Herb	ZI KOU CAO
Ranunculus japonicus Thunb.	*Ranunculaceae*	Japanese Buttercup	MAO GEN
Ranunculus sceleratus L.	*Ranunculaceae*	Poisonous Buttercup	SHI LONG RUI
Raphanus sativus L.	*Cruciferae*	Garden Radish	LAI FU
Raphanus sativus L.	*Cruciferae*	Garden Radish Seed	LAI FU ZI
Rauvolfia verticillata (Lour) Baill. var. *hainanensis* Tsiang	*Apocynaceae*	Hainan Devilpepper	HAI NAN LUO FU MU
Rauvolfia verticillata (Lour.) Baill. f. *rubrocarpa* H. T. Chang.	*Apocynaceae*	Redfruit Devilpepper	HONG GUO LUO FU MU
Rauwolfia verticillata (Lour.) Baill.	*Apocynaceae*	Common Devilpepper	LUO FU MU
Rauwolfia verticillata (Lour.) Baill.	*Apocynaceae*	Common Devilpepper Stem and Leaf	LUO FU MU JING YE
Rehmannia glutinosa (Gaertn.) Libosch *ex* Mey.	*Scrophulariaceae*	Adhesive Rehmannia Dried Root	GAN DI HUANG
Rehmannia glutinosa Libosch. f. *hueichingensis* (Chao *et* Schih) Hsiao	*Scrophulariaceae*	Hueiching Rehmannia	HUAI QING DI HUANG (of GAN DI HUANG)
Reineckea carnea (Andr.) Kunth	*Liliaceae*	Pink Reineckea Herb	JI XIANG CAO
Rhamnus crenata Sieb. *et* Zucc.	*Rhamnaceae*	Oriental Buckthorn Root	LI LA GEN
Rhamnus davurica Pall.	*Rhamnaceae*	Davurian Buckthorn	SHU LI
Rhamnus leptophylla Schneid.	*Rhamnaceae*	Thinleaf Buckthorn Root	JIANG LI MU GEN

Origin Latin Name	Family	English Name	TCM Name
Rhaponticum uniflorum (L.) DC.	*Compositae*	Uniflower Swisscentaury	QI ZHOU LOU LU (of LOU LU)
Rheum officinale Baill.	*Polygonaceae*	Medicinal Rhubarb	DA HUANG
Rheum palmatum L.	*Polygonaceae*	Sorrel Rhubarb	DA HUANG
Rheum tanguticum Maxim. *ex* Balf.	*Polygonaceae*	Tangut Rhubarb	DA HUANG
Rheum wittrochii Lundstr	*Polygonaceae*	Tianshan Rhubarb	TIAN SHAN DA HUANG
Rhinoceros sondaicus Desmarest	*Rhinocerotidae*	Rhinoceros Horn	XI JIAO
Rhinoceros sumatrensis (Fischer)	*Rhinocerotidae*	Rhinoceros Horn	XI JIAO
Rhinoceros unicornis L.	*Rhinocerotidae*	Rhinoceros Horn	XI JIAO
Rhodiola crenulata (Hook. f. *et* Thoms.) S. H. Fu	*Crassulaceae*	Bigflower Rhodiola	DA HUA HONG JING TIAN
Rhodiola kirilowii (Reg.) Reg.	*Crassulaceae*	Kirilow Rhodiola	XIA YE HONG JING TIAN
Rhododendron anthopogonoides Maxim.	*Ericaceae*	Savoury Rhododendron	XIAO YE PI PA
Rhododendron dauricum L.	*Ericaceae*	Dahurian Rhododendron	MAN SHAN HONG
Rhododendron micranthum Turcz.	*Ericaceae*	Manchurian Rhododendron	ZHAO SHAN BAI
Rhododendron molle (Bl.) G. Don	*Ericaceae*	Chinese Azalea Flower	NAO YANG HUA
Rhododendron mucronatum G. Don	*Ericaceae*	Snow Azalea	BAI HUA YING SHAN HONG
Rhododendron mucronulatum Turcz.	*Ericaceae*	Korean Rhododendron	YING SHAN HONG
Rhododendron simsii Planch.	*Ericaceae*	Indian Azalea	DU JUAN HUA
Rhododendron simsii Planch.	*Ericaceae*	Indian Azalea Leaf	DU JUAN HUA YE
Rhodomyrtus tomentosa (Ait.) Hassk.	*Myrtaceae*	Downy Rosemyrtle Leaf	SHAN REN YE
Rhodomyrtus tomentosa (Ait.) Hassk.	*Myrtaceae*	Rosemyrtle	TAO JIN NIANG
Rhus chinensis Mill.	*Anacardiaceae*	Chinese Sumac Fruit	YAN FU ZI
Rhus chinensis Mill.	*Anacardiaceae*	Chinese Sumac Leaf	YAN FU YE
Rhus succedanea L.	*Anacardiaceae*	Field Lacquertree	LIN BEI ZI
Rhus sylvestris Sieb. *et* Zucc.	*Anacardiaceae*	Woods Lcaquertree Leaf	YE QI SHU YE
Rhus taishanensis S. B. Liang sp. nov	*Anacardiaceae*	Taishan Sumac	TAI SHAN YAN FU MU
Rhus verniciflua Stokes	*Anacardiaceae*	Lacquer	SHENG QI
Rhus verniciflua Stokes	*Anacardiaceae*	True Lacquertree Seed	QI ZI
Rhynchotechum vestitum Hook. f. *et* Thoms.	*Gesneriaceae*	Hairy Rhynchotechum	MAO XIAN ZHU JU TAI
Ricinus communis L.	*Euphorbiaceae*	Castorbean Leaf	BI MA YE
Ricinus communis L.	*Euphorbiaceae*	Castorbean Oil	BI MA YOU
Ricinus communis L.	*Euphorbiaceae*	Castorbean Root	BI MA GEN
Ricinus communis L.	*Euphorbiaceae*	Castorbean Seed	BI MA ZI
Robinia pseudoacacia L.	*Leguminosae*	Black Locust Flower	CI HUAI HUA
Rodgersia aesculifolia Batal.	*Saxifragaceae*	Fingerleaf Rodgersflower	MU HE
Rohdea japonica Roth.	*Compositae*	Aztec Marigold Leaf	WAN SHOU JU YE
Rohdea japonica Roth.	*Liliaceae*	Omoto Nipponlily Root	WAN NIAN QING GEN
Rorippa montana (Wall.) Small	*Cruciferae*	Rorippa	HAN CAI
Rosa laevigata Michx.	*Rosaceae*	Cherokee Rose	JIN YING ZI
Rosa multiflora Thunb.	*Rosaceae*	Japanese Rose Root	QIANG WEI GEN
Rosa roxburghii Tratt.	*Rosaceae*	Roxburgh Rose	CI LI
Rosa rugosa Thunb.	*Rosaceae*	Rugose Rose	MEI GUI HUA

Origin Latin Name	Family	English Name	TCM Name
Rosmarinus officinalis L.	*Labiatae*	Rosemary	MI DIE XIANG
Rostellularia procumbens (L.) Nees	*Acanthaceae*	Creeping Rostellularia	JUE CHUANG
Rubia cordifolia L.	*Rubiaceae*	India Madder Root	QIAN CAO GEN
Rubia schumannina Pritz	*Rubiaceae*	Smoothstalk Madder	DAYE QIAN CAO
Rubus alceaefolius Poir	*Rosaceae*	Roughleaf Raspberry	CU YE XUAN GOU ZI
Rubus hirsutus Thunb.	*Rosaceae*	Hirsute Respberry	CI BO
Rubus parviforlius L.	*Rosaceae*	Japanese Raspberry	MAO MEI
Rumex acetosa L.	*Polygonaceae*	Garden Sorrel	SUAN MO
Rumex acetosa L.	*Polygonaceae*	Garden Sorrel Leaf	SUAN MO YE
Rumex crispus L.	*Polygonaceae*	Crisped Dock	NIU ER DA HUANG
Rumex dentatus L.	*Polygonaceae*	Toothedfruit Dock	NIU SHE CAO
Rumex japonicus Houtt.	*Polygonaceae*	Japanese Dock	YANG TI
Rumex nepalensis Spr.	*Polygonaceae*	Nepal Dock	YANG TI
Rumex patientia L.	*Polygonaceae*	Patience Dock	NIU XI XI
Russula rosacea (Bull) Grray	*Russulaceae*	Bitter Russula	KU HONG GU
Ruta graveolens L.	*Rutaceae*	Common Rue Herb	CHOU CAO
Sabia japonica Maxim.	*Sabiaceae*	Japanese Sabia	QING FENG TENG
Sabia swinhoei Hemsl. *ex* Forb. *et* Hemsl.	*Sabiaceae*	Sharpleaf Sabia	JIAN YE QING FENG TENG
Sabina vulgaris Antoine	*Cupressaceae*	Savin	CHOU BAI
Saccharum sinensis Roxb.	*Gramineae*	Sweetcane Culm	GAN ZHE
Sageretia thea (Osbeck) Johnst.	*Rhamnaceae*	Hedge Sageretia	QUE MEI TENG
Sageretia theezans Brongn.	*Rhamnaceae*	Hedge Sageretia	QUE MEI TENG
Sagittaria sagittifolia L.	*Alismataceae*	Oldworld Arrowhead Corm	CI GU
Salacia prinoides DC.	*Hippocrateaceae*	Prinos-like salacia	SUO LA MU
Saliosphaera fenzlii Reich.	*Lycoperdaceae*	Bark-less Puff-ball	MA BO
Salix babylonica L.	*Salicaceae*	Babylon Weeping Willow Branch	LIU ZHI
Salix babylonica L.	*Salicaceae*	Babylon Weeping Willow Root-bast	LIU BAI PI
Salix purpurea L.	*Salicaceae*	Bitter Willow Bast	SHUI YANG MU BAI PI
Salix purpurea L.	*Salicaceae*	Bitter Willow Branch and Leaf	SHUI YANG ZHI YE
Salvia miltiorrhiza Bge.	*Labiatae*	Danshen	DAN SHEN
Salvia miltiorrhiza f. *alba* C. Y. Wu	*Labiatae*	Whiteflower Danshen	BAI HUA DAN SHEN
Salvia plebeia R. Br.	*Labiatae*	Common Sage Herb	LI ZHI CAO
Salvia prionitis Hance	*Labiatae*	Hispid Sage	HONG GEN CAO
Salvia trijuga Diels	*Labiatae*	Threeleaf Sage	SAN YE SHU WEI CAO
Sanguisorba officinalis L.	*Rosaceae*	Garden Burnet	DI YU
Sansevieria trifasciata Prain	*Agavaceae*	Snake Sansevieria	HU WEI LAN
Santalum album L.	*Santalaceae*	Sandalwood	TAN XIANG
Sapindus mukorossi Gaertn.	*Sapindaceae*	Chinese Soapberry Fruit	WU HUAN ZI PI
Sapindus mukorossi Gaertn.	*Sapindaceae*	Chinese Soapberry Leaf	WU HUAN ZI YE
Sapium discolor (Champ.) Muell.-Arg.	*Euphorbiaceae*	Mountain Tallowtree Leaf	SHAN WU JIU YE
Sapium discolor (Champ.) Muell.-Arg.	*Euphorbiaceae*	Mountain Tallowtree Root	SHAN WU JIU GEN
Sapium sebiferum (L.) Roxb.	*Euphorbiaceae*	Chinese Tallowtree Bark	WU JIU MU GEN PI

Index of Origin of Traditional Chinese Medicines

Origin Latin Name	Family	English Name	TCM Name
Sapium sebiferum (L.) Roxb.	*Euphorbiaceae*	Chinese Tallowtree Leaf	WU JIU YE
Saposhnikovia divaricata (Turcz.) Schischk.	*Umbelliferae*	Divaricate Saposhnikovia	FANG FENG
Sarcandra glabra (Thunb.) Nakai	*Chloranthaceae*	Glabrous Sarcandra	JIU JIE CHA
Sarcococca vagans Stapf	*Buxaceae*	Hainan Sarcococca	HAI NAN YE SHAN HUA
Sargassum fusiforme (Harv.) Setch.	*Sargassaceae*	Fusiform Sargasum	HAI ZAO
Sargassum pallidum (Turn.) C. Ag.	*Sargassaceae*	Palli Sargasum	HAI ZAO
Sargentodoxa cuneata (Oeiv.) Rehd. *et* Wils.	*Sargentodoxaceae*	Sargentgloryvine	DA XUE TENG
Sassafras tzumu Hemsl.	*Lauraceae*	Common Sassafras	CHA SHU
Saururus chinensis (Lour.) Baill.	*Saururaceae*	Chinese Lizardtail	SAN BAI CAO
Saussurea involucrata Kar. *et* Kir.	*Compositae*	Snow Lotus	XUE LIAN
Saussurea lappa Clarke	*Compositae*	Common Aucklandia (Costustoot)	MU XIANG
Saxifraga stolonifera (L.) Meerb.	*Saxifragaceae*	Creeping Rockfoil	HU ER CAO
Scabiosa comosa Fisch.	*Dipsacaceae*	Narrowleaf Scabious	MENG GU SHAN LUO BO
Schisandra chinensis (Turcz.) Baill.	*Schisandraceae*	Chinese Magnoliavine	WU WEI ZI
Schisandra propinqua (Wall.) Baill. var. *intermedia* A. C. Smith	*Schisandraceae*	Intermediate Magnoliavine	ZHONG JIAN WU WEI ZI
Schisandra rubriflora Rhed *et* Wils	*Schisandraceae*	Redflower Magnoliavine	HONG HUA WU WEI ZI
Schizonepeta tenuifolia (Benth.) Briq.	*Labiatae*	Fineleaf Schizonepeta	JING JIE
Scilla sinensis (Lour.) Merr.	*Liliaceae*	Common Squill	MIAN ZAO ER
Scolopendra subspinipes mutians L. Koch	*Scolopendridae*	Centipede	WU GONG
Scoparia dulcis L.	*Scrophulariaceae*	Sweet Broomwort	YE GAN CAO
Scopolia acutangula C. Y. Wu *et* C. Chen	*Solanaceae*	Acutangular Scopolia	SAN FEN SAN
Scopolia japonica Maxim.	*Solanaceae*	Japanese Scopolia	DONG LANG DANG
Scutellaria amoena C. H. Wright	*Labiatae*	Yunnan Skullcap	DIAN HUANG QIN
Scutellaria baicalensis Georgi	*Labiatae*	Baikal Skullcap	HUANG QIN
Scutellaria indica L.	*Labiatae*	Indian Skullcap	HAN XIN CAO
Securinega suffruticosa (Pall.) Rehd.	*Euphorbiaceae*	Suffrutescent Securinega	YI YE QIU
Sedum aizoon L.	*Crassulaceae*	Aizoon Stonecrop Root	JING TIAN SAN QI GEN
Sedum bulbiferum Mak.	*Crassulaceae*	Bulbiferous Stonecrop	XIAO JIAN CAO
Sedum kamtschaticum Fisch.	*Crassulaceae*	Orange Stonecrop	FEI CAI
Sedum sarmentosum Bge.	*Crassulaceae*	Stringy Stonecrop	SHI ZHI JIA
Selaginella doederleinii Hieron.	*Selaginellaceae*	Doederlein's Spikemoss Herb	DA YE CAI
Selaginella involvens (Sw.) Spring	*Selaginellaceae*	Involute Spikemoss	YAN ZHOU JUAN BAI
Selaginella tamariscina (Beauv.) Spring	*Selaginellaceae*	Tamariskoid Spikemoss	JUAN BAI
Selenarctos thibetanus G. Cuvier	*Ursidae*	Bear Gall	XIONG DAN
Selenarctos thibetanus G. Cuvier	*Ursidae*	Bear's Paw	XIONG ZHANG
Senecio abrotanifolius L.	*Compositae*	Pineleaf Groundsel	SONG YE QIAN LI GUANG

Index of Origin of Traditional Chinese Medicines

Origin Latin Name	Family	English Name	TCM Name
Senecio chrysanthemoides DC.	*Compositae*	Chrusanthemum-like Groundsel Herb	TU SAN QI
Senecio integerrimus Nutt.	*Compositae*	Entire Groundsel	QUAN YUAN QIAN LI GUANG
Senecio integrifolius (L.) Clairvill var. *fauriei* (Lévl. *et* Vant.) Kitam.	*Compositae*	Kirilow Groundsel Herb	GOU SHE CAO
Senecio nemorensis L	*Compositae*	Shady Groundsel	HUANG WAN
Senecio nudicaulis Buch.-Ham.	*Compositae*	Nudicaulous Grounsel Herb	ZI BEI TIAN KUI CAO
Senecio orgzetorum Diels	*Compositae*	Field Grounsel Herb	DA BAI DING CAO
Senecio scandens Buch.-Ham.	*Compositae*	Climbing Groundsel	QIAN LI GUANG
Seriphidium cinum (Berg. *ex* Poljak) Poljak	*Compositae*	Chinese Seriphidium	SHAN DAO NIAN HAO (HUI HAO)
Seriphidium finitum (Kitag.) Ling *et* Y. R. Ling	*Compositae*	Northeast Seriphidium	DONG BEI HUI HAO
Sesamum indicum DC.	*Pedaliaceae*	Oriental Sesame	BAI ZHI MA (HU MA ZI)
Sesamum indicum DC.	*Pedaliaceae*	Oriental sesame	HEI ZHI MA
Sesamum indicum DC.	*Pedaliaceae*	Oriental Sesame Leaf	HU MA YE
Seseli yunnanense Franch.	*Umbelliferae*	Yunnan Seseli	SONG YE FANG FENG (of FANG FENG)
Setaria italica (L.) Beauv.	*Gramineae*	Foxtail Millet	SU MI
Sida acuta Burm. f.	*Malvaceae*	Acute Sida	HUANG HUA REN
Sida cordifolia L.	*Malvaceae*	Cordateleaf Sida	HUANG HUA ZI
Sida mysorensis Wight *et* Arn.	*Malvaceae*	Slimyhair Sida	HUANG HUA ZI
Siegesbeckia glabrescens Mak.	*Compositae*	Hairstalk St. Paulswort	MAO GENG XI XIAN (of XI XIAN)
Siegesbeckia orientalis L.	*Compositae*	Common St. Paulswort	XI XIAN
Siegesbeckia orientalis L. var. *glabrescens* Mak.	*Compositae*	Hairstalk St. Paulswort	MAO GENG XI XIAN (of XI XIAN)
Siegesbeckia orientalis L. var. *pubescens* Mak.	*Compositae*	Glandularstalk St. Paulswort	XIAN GENG XI XIAN (of XI XIAN)
Sinapis alba L.	*Cruciferae*	White Mustard Seed	BAI JIE ZI
Sinocalamus oldhami (Munro) Mcclure	*Gramineae*	Oldham Bamboo Shoot	LU SUN PIAN
Sinomenium acutum (Thunb.) Rehd. *et* Wils.	*Menispermaceae*	Orientvine	QING FENG TENG
Siphonostegin chinensis Benth.	*Scroophulariaceae*	Chinese Siphonostegia	YIN XING CAO
Siraitia grosvenorii (Swingle) C. Jeffrey *ex* Lu *et* Z. Y. Zhang	*Cucurbitaceae*	Grosvenor Siraitia	LUO HAN GUO
Skimmia reevesiana Fortune	*Rutaceae*	Reeves Skimmia	YIN YU
Smilax china L.	*Liliaceae*	Chinaroot Greenbrier	BA QIA
Smilax glabra Roxb.	*Liliaceae*	Glabrous Greenbrier	TU FU LING
Smilax sieboldi Miq.	*Liliaceae*	Siebold Greenbrier	NIAN YU XU
Sobina chinensis (L.) Antoine	*Cupressaceae*	Chinese Juniper Leaf	GUI YE
Solanum capsicastrum Link	*Solanaceae*	Twoflower Jerusalemcherry	YE HAI JIAO
Solanum dulcamara L.	*Solanaceae*	Bitter Nightshade	BAI MAO TENG
Solanum dulcamara L.	*Solanaceae*	Bitter Nightshade	KU QIE
Solanum indicum L.	*Solanaceae*	Indian Nightshade	TIAN QIE ZI
Solanum khasianum C. B. Clarke	*Solanaceae*	Khasi Nightshade Fruit	CI TIAN QIE
Solanum lyratum Thunb.	*Solanaceae*	Bittersweet	BAI MAO TENG

Index of Origin of Traditional Chinese Medicines

Index of Origin of Traditional Chinese Medicines

Origin Latin Name	Family	English Name	TCM Name
Stauntonia chinensis DC.	*Lardizabalaceae*	Chinese Stauntonvine	YE MU GUA
Stauntonia hexaphylla Decne.	*Lardizabalaceae*	Chinese Stauntonvine	YE MU GUA
Stellaria dichotoma L. var. *lanceolata* Bge.	*Caryophyllaceae*	Lanceolate Starwort	YIN CHAI HU
Stellera chamaejasme L.	*Thymelaeaceae*	Chinese Stellera	RUI XIANG LANG DU (of LANG DU)
Stelmatocrypton khasianum (Benth.) H. Baill.	*Asclepiadaceae*	Common Stelmatocrypton	SHENG TENG
Stemona japonica (Bl.) Miq.	*Stemonaceae*	Japanese Stemona	BAI BU
Stemona sessilifolia (Miq.) Franch. *et* Sav.	*Stemonaceae*	Sessile Stemona	BAI BU
Stemona tuberosa Lour.	*Stemonaceae*	Tuber Stemona	BAI BU
Stenoloma chusanum (L.) Ching	*Lindsaeaceae*	Common Wedgelet Fern	DA YE JIN HUA CAO
Stephania cepharantha Hayata	*Menispermaceae*	Oriental Stephania	BAI YAO ZI
Stephania delavayi Diels	*Menispermaceae*	Delavay Stephania	DI BU RONG
Stephania hernandifolia (Willd.)Walp.	*Menispermaceae*	Hernandialeaf Stephania	RU LAN
Stephania japonica (Thunb.) Miers	*Menispermaceae*	Japanese Staphania	QIAN JIN TENG
Stephania sinica Diels	*Menispermaceae*	Chinese Stephania	JIN BU HUAN
Stephania tetrandra S. Moore	*Menispermaceae*	Fourstamen Stephania	FEN FANG JI (of FANG JI)
Stichopus japonicus Selenka	*Stichopodidae*	Sea-cucunber Intestines	HAI SHEN CHANG
Stizolobium capitatum (Sweet) O. Ktze.	*Leguminosae*	Capitateflower Velvetbean	LI DOU
Streptopelia orientalis (Latham)	*Columbidae*	Rufous Turtle Dove	BAN JIU
Strobilanthes japonicus (Thunb.) Miq.	*Acanthaceae*	Japanese Conehead	HONG ZE LAN
Strophanthus divaricatus (Lour.) Hook. *et* Arn.	*Apocynaceae*	Divaricate Strophanthus	YANG JIAO AO ZI
Strychnos ignatii Berg.	*Loganiaceae*	Ignat Poisonnut Seed	LU SONG GUO
Strychnos nitida G. Don	*Loganiaceae*	Hairstyle Poisonnut	MAO ZHU MA QIAN
Strychnos nux-vomica L.	*Loganiaceae*	Nut-vomitive Poisonnut	MA QIAN ZI
Styrax benzoin Dryand.	*Styracaceae*	Benzoin	AN XI XIANG
Styrax tonkinensis (Pier.) Craib *ex* Hart.	*Styracaceae*	Tonkin Snowbell	AN XI XIANG
Sus scrofa domestica Brisson	*Suidae*	Pig Gall	ZHU DAN
Sus scrofa L.	*Suidae*	Wild Boar Gall	YE ZHU DAN
Swainsonia salsula Taub.	*Leguminosae*	Saline Swainsonia	NIAO PAO CAO
Swertia angustifolia Buch.-Ham. *ex* D. Don	*Gentianaceae*	Narrowleaf Swertia	XIA YE ZHANG YA CAI
Swertia calycina Franch.	*Gentianaceae*	Calycin Swertia	BAO E ZHANG YA CAI
Swertia macrosperma C. B. Clarke	*Gentianaceae*	Bigseed Swertia	DA ZI ZHANG YA CAI
Swertia pseudochinensis Hara	*Gentianaceae*	False Chinese Swertia	ZHANG YA CAI
Swertia punicea Hemsl.	*Gentianaceae*	Scarlet Swertia	ZI HONG ZHANG YA CAI
Symplocos caudata Wall.	*Symplocaceae*	Caudate Sweetleaf Leaf	SHAN FAN YE
Syringa amurensis Rupr.	*Oleaceae*	Amur Lilac	BAO MA ZI
Syzygium aromaticum (L.) Merr. *et* Perry	*Myrtaceae*	Clove	DING XIANG

Index of Origin of Traditional Chinese Medicines

Origin Latin Name	Family	English Name	TCM Name
Syzygium brachyantherum Merr. *et* Perry	*Myrtaceae*	Duhat Bark	YE DONG QING PI
Syzygium brachyantherum Merr. *et* Perry	*Myrtaceae*	Duhat Fruit	YE DONG QING QUO
Syzygium buxifolium Hook. *et* Arn.	*Myrtaceae*	Boxleaf Syzygium	CHI NAN
Syzygium cumini (L.) Skeels	*Myrtaceae*	Shortanther Syzygium Bark	YE DONG QING PI
Syzygium cumini (L.) Skeels	*Myrtaceae*	Shortanther Syzygium Fruit	YE DONG QING QUO
Tacca plantaginea (Hance) Drenth.	*Taccaceae*	Lobedfruit Tacca	LIE GUO SHU
Tagetes erecta L.	*Compositae*	Aztec Marigold	WAN SHOU JU
Tagetes patula L.	*Compositae*	French Marigold Herb	KONG QUE CAO
Tamarindus indica L.	*Leguminosae*	Tamarind Fruit	SUAN JIAO
Tamarix chinensis Lour.	*Tamaricaceae*	Chinese Tamarisk	CHENG LIU
Taraxacum mongolicum Hand. -Mazz.	*Compositae*	Mongolian Dandelion	PU GONG YING
Taraxacum sinicum Kitag.	*Compositae*	Chinese Dandelion	JIAN DI PU GONG YING (of PU GONG YING)
Taxillus levinei Merr.	*Loranthaceae*	Rustyhair Taxillus	XIU MAO JI SHENG
Taxus cuspidata Sieb. *et* Zucc.	*Taxaceae*	Japanese Yew	ZI SHAN
Taxus mairei (Lemée *et* Lévl.) S. Y. Hu	*Taxaceae*	Maire Yew	MEI LI HONG DOU SHAN
Taxus yunnanensis Cheng *et* L. K. Fu	*Taxaceae*	Yunnan Yew	YUN NAN HONG DOU SHAN
Tephroseris kirilowii (Turcz. *ex* DC.) Holub	*Compositae*	Kirilow Groundsel Herb	GOU SHE CAO
Tephrosia purpurea (L.) Pers.	*Leguminosae*	Purple Tephrosia Root	HUI YE GEN
Terminalia chebula Retz.	*Combretaceae*	Medicine Terminalia Fruit	HE ZI
Terminalia chebula Retz.	*Combretaceae*	Medicine Terminalia Leaf	HE ZI YE
Tetracera asiatica (Lour.) Hoogl.	*Dilleniaceae*	Asian Tetracera	XI YE TENG
Teucrium bidentatum Hemsl.	*Labiatae*	Twodenntate Germander	ER CHI XIANG KE
Teucrium quadrifarium Buch-Ham	*Labiatae*	Fourfile Germander	TIE ZHOU CAO
Thalictrum baicalense Turcz.	*Ranunculaceae*	Baikal Meadowrue	MA WEI LIAN
Thalictrum foliolosum DC.	*Ranunculaceae*	Manyleaf Meadowrue	MA WEI LIAN
Thalictrum honanenae W.T. Wang *et* S. H. Wang	*Ranunculaceae*	Honan Meadowrue	HE NAN TANG SONG CAO
Thalictrum Incidum L.	*Ranunculaceae*	Narrowleaf Meadowrue	XIA YE TANG SONG CAO
Thalictrum minus L.	*Ranunculaceae*	Low Meadowrue	XIAO TANG SONG CAO
Thalictrum simplex L. var. *brevipes* Hara	*Ranunculaceae*	Shortstalk Slimtop Meadowrue	YING SHUI HUANG LIAN
Thalictrum thunbergii DC.	*Ranunculaceae*	East-Asia Low Meadowrue	YAN GUO CAO
Thamnolia vermicularis (Ach.) Asahina	*Thamnoliaceae*	Vermiculate Thamnolia Thallus	XUE CHA
Thermopsis alpina Ledeb.	*Leguminosae*	Alpine Thermopsis	GAO SHAN HUANG HUA
Thermopsis lanceolata R. Br.	*Leguminosae*	Lanceleaf Thermopsis	MU MA DOU

Index of Origin of Traditional Chinese Medicines

Origin Latin Name	Family	English Name	TCM Name
Thermopsis lupinoides (L.) Link.	*Leguminosae*	Wild Thermopsis	YE JUE MING
Thevetia peruviana (Pers.) K. Schum.	*Apocynaceae*	Yellow Oleander	HUANG HUA JIA ZHU TAO
Thladiantha cordifolia (BL.) Cogn.	*Cucurbhitaceae*	Heartleaf Tubergourd	XIN YE CHI BO
Thlaspi arvense L.	*Cruciferae*	Boor's Mustardd	XI MING
Thlaspi arvense L.	*Cruciferae*	Boor's Mustardd Seed	XI MING ZI
Thuja orientalis (L.) Endl.	*Cupressaceae*	Chinese Arborvitae Branch	BAI ZHI JIE (CE BAI ZHI JIE)
Thuja orientalis (L.) Endl.	*Cupressaceae*	Chinese Arborvitae Leaf	CE BAI YE
Thymus vulgaris L.	*Labiatae*	Thyme	SHE XIANG CAO
Tilia miqueliana Maxim.	*Tiliaceae*	Miquel Linden	PU TI SHU HUA
Tinospora capillipes Gagn.	*Menispermaceae*	Hairystalk Tinospora	JIN GUO LAN
Tinospora hainanesis H. S. Lo *et* Z. X. Li	*Menispermaceae*	Hainan Tinospora	HAI NAN QING NIU DAN
Tinospora sagittata Gagn.	*Menispermaceae*	Arrowshaped Tinospora	JIN GUO LAN
Toddalia asiatica (L.) Lam.	*Rutaceae*	AsiaticToddalia	FEI LONG ZHANG XUE
Toona sinensis (A. Juss.) Roem.	*Meliaceae*	Chinese Toona Root-bast	CHUN BAI PI
Toxicodendron succedaneum (L.) O. Kuntze	*Anacardiaceae*	Field Lacquertree	LIN BEI ZI
Trachelospermum jasminoides (Lindl.) Lem.	*Apocynaceae*	Chinese Starjasmine	LUO SHI TENG
Trapa bispinosa Roxb	*Trapaceae*	Singharanut	LING
Trema dielsiana Hard. -Mazz.	*Ulmaceae*	Diels Trema	SHAN YOU MA
Tribulus terrestris L.	*Zygophyllaceae*	Puncturevine Caltrap	CI JI LI
Tribulus terrestris L.	*Zygophyllaceae*	Puncturevine Caltrap Root	JI LI GEN
Trichosanthes cucumeroides (Ser.) Maxim.	*Cucurbitaceae*	Japanese Snakegourd	WANG GUA
Trichosanthes cucumeroides (Ser.) Maxim.	*Cucurbitaceae*	Japanese Snakegourd Seed	WANG GUA ZI
Trichosanthes hupehensis C.Y.Cheng *et* Yueh.	*Cucurbitaceae*	Hupeh Snakegourd	HU BEI GUA LOU
Trichosanthes kirilowii Maxim.	*Cucurbitaceae*	Mongolian Snakegourd	GUA LOU
Trichosanthes kirilowii Maxim.	*Cucurbitaceae*	Mongolian Snakegourd Root	TIAN HUA FEN (GUA LOU GEN)
Trichosanthes rosthornii Harms	*Cucurbhitaceae*	Oneflower Snakegourd	SHUANG BIAN GUA LOU
Trichosanthes rosthornii Harms	*Cucurbitaceae*	Rosthorn Snakegourd	GUA LOU
Trichosanthes rosthornii Harms	*Cucurbitaceae*	Rosthorn Snakegourd Root	TIAN HUA FEN (GUA LOU GEN)
Trichosanthes Uniflora Hao	*Cucurbhitaceae*	Oneflower Snakegourd	SHUANG BIAN GUA LOU
Trifolium pratense L.	*Leguminosae*	Red Clover	HONG CHE ZHOU CAO
Trifolium repens L.	*Leguminosae*	White Clover Herb	SAN XIAO CAO
Triglochin maritimum L.	*Juncaginaceae*	Shore Podgrass	HAI JIU CAI
Trigonella foenum-graecum L.	*Leguminosae*	Common Fenugreek	HU LU BA
Trillum camtschaticum Pall.	*Liliaceae*	Whiteflower Trillium	YU ER QI
Trillum tschonoskii Maxim.	*Liliaceae*	Tschonosk Trillium	YU ER QI

Index of Origin of Traditional Chinese Medicines

Origin Latin Name	Family	English Name	TCM Name
Vaccinium bracteatum Thunb.	*Ericaceae*	Oriental Blueberry Leaf	NAN ZHU YE
Vaccinium vitis-idaea L.	*Ericaceae*	Cowberry Fruit Leaf	YUE JU YE
Valeriana jatamansii Jones	*Valerianaceae*	Jatamans Valeriana	ZHI ZHU XIANG
Valeriana officinalis L.	*Valerianaceae*	Common Valeriana	XIE CAO
Valeriana officinalis L. var. *latifolia* Miq.	*Valerianaceae*	Broadleaf Common Valeriana	ZHI ZHU XIANG
Vallisneria spiralis L.	*Hydrocharitaceae*	Eelgrass Herb	KU CAO (I)
Ventilago leiocarpa Benth.	*Rhamnaceae*	Smoothfruit Ventiago	YI HE GUO
Veratrilla baillonii Franch	*Gantianaceae*	Baillon Veratrilla	HUANG QIN JIAO
Veratrum nigrum L.	*Liliaceae*	Black Falsehellebore	LI LU
Veratrum nigrum L. var. *ussuriense* Nakai	*Liliaceae*	Ussuri Falsehellebore	WU SU LI LI LU
Verbascum thapsus L.	*Scrophulariaceae*	Flannel Mullein	MAO RUI HUA
Verbena officinalis L.	*Verbenaceae*	European Verbena Herb	MA BIAN CAO
Veronica linariifolia Pall. *ex* Link. subsp. *dilatata* (Nakai *et* Kitagawa) Hong	*Scroophulariaceae*	Dilatata Speedwell	SHUI MAN QING
Veronica spuria L.	*Scrophulariaceae*	Bastard Speedwell	YI ZHI XIANG
Veronicastrum sibirica (L.) Pennell	*Scroophulariaceae*	Siberian Veronicastrum	ZHAN LONG JIAN (LUN YE PO PO NA)
Vespertilio superans Thomas	*Vespertilionidae*	Bat Dung	YE MING SHA
Vicia amoena Fisch.	*Leguminosae*	Broadleaf Vetch	SHAN YE WAN DOU
Vicia faba L.	*Leguminosae*	Broadbean	CAN DOU
Vicia faba L.	*Leguminosae*	Broadbean Leaf	CAN DOU YE
Vicia faba L.	*Leguminosae*	Broadbean Pericarp	CAN DOU JIA KE
Vicia faba L.	*Leguminosae*	Broadbean Spermoderm	CAN DOU KE
Vicia faba L.	*Leguminosae*	Broadbean Stem	CAN DOU JING
Vicia hirsuta (L.) S. F. Gray	*Leguminosae*	Pigeon Vetch	XIAO CHAO CAI
Vicia sativa L.	*Leguminosae*	Common Vetch	DA CHAO CAI
Viola tricolor L.	*Violaceae*	Garden Pansy	SAN SE JIN
Viscum articulatum Burm. f.	*Loranthaceae*	Flatshoot Mistletoe	FENG XIANG JI SHENG
Viscum coloratum (Kom.) Nakai	*Loranthaceae*	Colored Mistletoe	HU JI SHENG (of SANG JI SHENG)
Vitex negundo L.	*Verbenaceae*	Negundo Chastetree Leaf	HUANG JING YE
Vitex rotundifolia L.	*Verbenaceae*	Simpleleaf Shrub Chastetree	MAN JING ZI
Vitex rotundifolia L.	*Verbenaceae*	Simpleleaf Shrub Chastetree Leaf	MAN JING ZI YE
Vitex trifolia L.	*Verbenaceae*	Threeleaf Chastetree	MAN JING ZI
Vitex trifolia L.	*Verbenaceae*	Threeleaf Chastetree Leaf	MAN JING ZI YE
Vitis vinifera L.	*Vitaceae*	European Grape	PU TAO
Vitis vinifera L.	*Vitaceae*	European Grape Stem and Leaf	PU TAO TENG YE
Viverra zibetha L.	*Viverridae*	Civet	LING MAO XIANG
Vladimiria denticulata Ling	*Compositae*	Denticulate Vladimiria	MU XIANG
Vladimiria souliei (Franch.) Ling	*Compositae*	Common Vladimiria	MU XIANG
Waltheria americana L.	*Sterculiaceae*	Florida Waltheria	HE TA CAO

Index of Origin of Traditional Chinese Medicines

Origin Latin Name	Family	English Name	TCM Name
Wikstroemia indica (L.) C. A. Mey.	*Thymelaeaceae*	Indian Stringbush Root	LIAO GE WANG GEN
Winchia calophylla A. DC.	*Apocynaceae*	Prettyleaf Winchia	PEN JIA SHU
Wisteria sinensis Sweet	*Leguminosae*	Chinese Wisteria	ZI TENG
Wisteria sinensis Sweet	*Leguminosae*	Chinese Wisteria Seed	ZI TENG ZI
Woodwardia japonica (L. f.) Sm.	*Blechnaceae*	Japanese Chain Fern	GUAN ZHONG
Woodwardia orientalis Sm.	*Blechnaceae*	Oriental Chain Fern	DONG FANG GOU JI
Xanthium sibiricus Patr. *ex* Widd.	*Compositae*	Siberian Cocklebur	CANG ER
Zanthoxylum ailanthoides Sieb. *et* Zucc.	*Rutaceae*	Ailanthus-like Pricklyash	SHI ZHU YU (CHU YE HUA JIAO)
Zanthoxylum ailanthoides Sieb. *et* Zucc.	*Rutaceae*	Ailanthus-like Pricklyash Bark	CHU YE HUA JIAO PI
Zanthoxylum avicennae (Lam.) DC.	*Rutaceae*	Avicenna's Pricklyash	YING BU BO
Zanthoxylum bungeanum Maxim.	*Rutaceae*	Bunge Pricklyash	HUA JIAO
Zanthoxylum bungeanum Maxim.	*Rutaceae*	Bunge Pricklyash Root	HUA JIAO GEN
Zanthoxylum nitidum (Roxb.) DC.	*Rutaceae*	Shinyleaf Pricklyash	RU DI JIN NIU
Zanthoxylum planispinum Sieb. *et* Zucc.	*Rutaceae*	Bambooleaf Pricklyash	ZHU YE JIAO
Zanthoxylum planispinum Sieb. *et* Zucc.	*Rutaceae*	Bambooleaf Pricklyash Root	ZHU YE JIAO GEN
Zanthoxylum podocarpum Hemsl.	*Rutaceae*	Stalkedfruit Pricklyash	BING GUO HUA JIAO
Zanthoxylum schinifolium Sieb. *et* Zucc.	*Rutaceae*	Peppertree Pricklyash	QING HUA JIAO (of HUA JIAO)
Zanthoxylum schinifolium Sieb. *et* Zucc.	*Rutaceae*	Peppertree Pricklyash Root	HUA JIAO GEN
Zanthoxylum simulans Hance	*Rutaceae*	Flatspine Pricklyash Leaf	YE HUA JIAO YE
Zaocys dhumnades	*Colubredae*	Snake Slough	SHE TUI
Zea mays L.	*Gramineae*	Maize	YU SHU SHU
Zea mays L.	*Gramineae*	Maize Style	YU MI XU
Zephyranthes candida Herb.	*Amaryllidaceae*	Autumn Zephyrlily Herb	GAN FENG CAO
Zingiber officinale Rosc.	*Zingiberaceae*	Common Ginger Dried Rhizome	GAN JIANG
Zingiber officinale Rosc.	*Zingiberaceae*	Fresh Common Ginger	SHENG JIANG
Ziziphus jujuba Mill.	*Rhamnaceae*	Common Jujube (Chinese Date)	DA ZAO
Ziziphus jujuba Mill. var. *inermis* (Bge.) Rehd.	*Rhamnaceae*	Spineless Common Jujube	DA ZAO
Ziziphus jujuba Mill. var. *spinosa* (Bunge) Hu *ex* H. F. Chow	*Rhamnaceae*	Common Jujube Seed	SUAN ZAO REN
Ziziphus mauritiana Lam.	*Rhamnaceae*	Indian Jujube	MIAN ZAO
Ziziphus spinosus Hu	*Rhamnaceae*	Spine Data	SUAN ZAO
Zostera marina L.	*Potamogetonaceae*	Ellgrass	HAI DAI (DA YE ZAO)
Zyziphs jujuba Miller	*Rhamnaceae*	Common Jujube Seed	SUAN ZAO REN

Index of Chemicals in Traditional Chinese Medicines

Index of Chemicals in Traditional Chinese Medicines

References

References

Abbreviation:
ABY = Acta Botanica Yunnanica
APS = Acta Pharmaceutica Sinica
ASNUS = Acta Scientiarum Naturalium Universitatis Sunyatseni
CCMM = China Journal of Chinese Materia Medica
CTHD = Chinese Traditional and Herbal Drugs

1. Editing Group of the Handbook of Bio-activity Components from Medicinal Plants, Handbook of Bio-activity Components from Medicinal Plants, The People's Medical Publishing House, Beijing, 1986, in Chinese.
2. Jian Yin and Ligong Guo, Modern Study of Chinese Drugs and Clinical Applications (1), Xueyuan Press, 1993, in Chinese.
3. Jian Yin (chief editor), Modern Study of Chinese Drugs and Clinical Applications (3), Ancient Book Press of Chinese Medicine, 1997, in Chinese.
4. Yubin Ji (chief editor), Pharmacological Action and Application of Available Composition of Traditional Chinese Medicine, Heilongjiang Science and technology Press, Heilongjiang, 1995, in Chinese.
5. Yubin Ji and Guangmei Zhang (chief editors), Pharmacological Action and Application of Available Antitumor Composition of Traditional Chinese Medicine, Heilongjiang Science and technology Press, Heilongjiang, 1998, in Chinese.
6. Edited by Jiangsu New Medical College, Chinese Medicine Dictionary, Shanghai Science and technology Press, Shanghai, 1979.
7. Chinese Materia Medica Editing Committee of the National Chinese Medicine and Pharmacology Bureau, Chinese Materia Medica, Shanghai Science and Technology Press, Shanghai, 1998.
8. Qi Chen (chief editor), The Methodology of Studying the Pharmacology of Chinese Drugs, The People's Medical Publishing House, Beijing, 1993, in Chinese.
9. Crude Drug Company of China, A Complete Collection of Chinese Drug Sources in China, Science press, Beijing, 1994, in Chinese.
10. Yanyong Chen, Tiecheng Liu, Chapter 25, Raw Material Plants of Steroids Drugs, in Modern Studies of Chinese Herbal Medicine, edited by Institute of Materia Medica, Chinese Academy of Medical Sciences, Vol. 2, 226-254, 1996.
11. Jingxi Xie, Wanzhi Song, Naigong Wang, Chapter 28, JIU LI XIANG, in Modern Studies of Chinese Herbal Medicine, edited by Institute of Materia Medica, Chinese Academy of Medical Sciences, Vol. 2, 333-61, 1996.
12. Junshan Yang, Zhaoyi Zhu and Naigong Wang , Chapter 30, KU MU, in Modern Studies of Chinese Herbal Medicine, edited by Institute of Materia Medica, Chinese Academy of Medical Sciences, Vol. 2, 452-71, 1996.
13. Junshan Yang, Chapter 48, CHEN XIANG, in Modern Studies of Chinese Herbal Medicine, edited by Institute of Materia Medica, Chinese Academy of Medical Sciences, Vol. 3, 1-21, 1997.
14. Junshan Yang and Yuheng Chen, Chapter 39, HU MAN TENG, in Modern Studies of Chinese Herbal Medicine, edited by Institute of Materia Medica, Chinese Academy of Medical Sciences, Vol. 3, 123-147, 1997.
15. Guojun Xu et al., Chinese Materia Medica, 1154-6, Chinese Medicinal Science and Technology Press, 1996.
16. Weiliang Song and Dihua Chen, Chapter 1, FU ZI, in Modern Studies of Chinese Herbal Medicine, edited. by Institute of Materia Medica, Chinese Academy of Medical Sciences, Vol. 1, 21-47, 1995.
17. Guojun Xu et al., Chinese Materia Medica, 947-8, Chinese Medicinal Science and Technology Press, 1996.

References

18. Hongju Fang, et al., Chapter 17, DANG GUI, in Modern Studies of Chinese Herbal Medicine, edited by Institute of Materia Medica, Chinese Academy of Medical Sciences, Vol. 2, 1-51, 1996.
19. Junshan Yang, et al., Chapter 18, HAN QIN, in Modern Studies of Chinese Herbal Medicine, edited. by Institute of Materia Medica, Chinese Academy of Medical Sciences, Vol. 2, 52-70, 1996.
20. Liang Huang, et al., Chapter 21, in Modern Studies of Chinese Herbal Medicine, edited. by Institute of Materia Medica, Chinese Academy of Medical Sciences, Vol. 2, 128-152, 1996.
21. Jichun Zhou and Liang Huang, APS, 1985, **20**(1), 45-51.
22. Yonglong Liu and Yili Bai, APS, 1985, **20**(1), 53-8.
23. Cuiying Hou and Hong Xue, APS, 1985, **20**(2), 112-7.
24. Chenglai Liu and Yanyong Chen, APS, 1985, **20**(2), 143-5.
25. Yonghua Shu, Yuying Zhao and Ruyi Zhang, APS, 1985, **20**(3), 193-7.
26. Mao lin, Dequan Yu, Xin Liu, Fengyong Fu, Qitai Zheng, Cunheng He, Guanghong Bao and Changfu Xu, APS, 1985, **20**(3), 198-202.
27. Wen Lin, Rentong Chen and Zhi Xue, APS, 1985, **20**(4), 283-7.
28. Junxian Wei, Liangan Wang, Hua Du and Rui Li, APS, 1985, **20**(4), 288-93.
29. Renling Jin, Peiyuan Cheng and Guangyi Xu, APS, 1985, **20**(5), 366-71.
30. Jizhou Wu and Quanlong Pu, APS, 1985, **20**(5), 372-6.
31. Haiyin He and Luoqing Ling, APS, 1985, **20**(6), 433-5.
32. Xianjun Meng, Yaozu Chen, Ruilin Nie and Jun Zhou, APS, 1985, **20**(6), 446-9
33. Yongmin Liu and Dequan Yu, APS, 1985, **20**(7), 514-8.
34. Houwei Luo, Baojin Wu, Meiyu Wu, Zhonggen Yong and Yi Jin, APS, 1985, **20**(7), 542-4.
35. Xuefen Wang, Jiayuan Chen and Wenjie Lu, APS, 1985, **20**(8), 615-8.
36. Chengjun Xu, Xianyi Zeng and Dequan Yu, APS, 1985, **20**(9), 652-7.
37. Bizhu Chen and Qicheng Fang, APS, 1985, **20**(9), 658–61.
38. Deyun Kong, Xingjie Liu, Maikun Teng and Zihe Rao, APS, 1985, **20**(10), 747-51.
39. Hongjie Wang and Yanyong Chen, APS, 1985, **20**(11), 832-41.
40. Weiguo Liu and Mingshi Wang, APS, 1985, **20**(11), 842-51.
41. Mao Lin, Xin Liu, Deqan Yu, Shiqi Dou, Youji Zhang and Qingmei Li, APS, 1985, **20**(12), 902-5.
42. Weiming Chen, Ying Yan, Yongji Wang and Xiaotian LIang, APS, 1985, **20**(12), 906-12.
43. Fang Sun and Dequan Yu, APS, 1985, **20**(12), 913-7.
44. Tingmo Hu and Shouxun Zhao, APS, 1986, **21**(1), 29-34.
45. Peiyuan Cheng, Meijuan Xu, Yongle Lin, Jincheng Shi and Guangyi Xu, APS, 1986, **21**(2), 109-13.
46. Mao Lin, BaoqiYang and Dequan Yu, APS, 1986, **21**(2), 114-8.
47. Wenhao Xu and Zhi Xue, APS, 1986, **21**(3), 177-82.
48. Xiuchun Wang, Yuehu Pei, Xian Li and Tingru Zhu, APS, 1986, **21**(3), 183-6.
49. Weiming Chen, Ying Yan and Xuemei Ma, APS, 1986, **21**(3), 187-90.
50. Jin YU Huiying Lang and Peigen Xiao, APS, 1986, **21**(3), 191-7.
51. Ju Zhang and Linxing He, APS, 1986, **21**(4), 273-8.
52. Shanhao Jiang, Suhua Guo, Bingnan Zhou, Shengxin Wang, Fusheng Yi and Lanju Ji, APS, 1986, **21**(4), 279-84.
53. Guowei Li, Qichao Pan, Xiaoping Yang and Baiping Ying, APS, 1986, **21**(4), 303-5.
54. Guiqiu Han, Shuming Li and Changling Li, APS, 1986, **21**(5), 361-5.
55. Shishan Jia, Yongrong Liu, Chaomei Ma APS, 1986, **21**(6), 441-6.
56. Xiaoyong Fu, Wenzao Liang and Guoshi Tu, APS, 1986, **21**(6), 447-53.
57. Ruyi Zhang, Jianhua Zhang and Maotian Wang, APS, 1986, **21**(7), 510-5.

58. Junshan Yang and Yuwu Chen, APS, 1986, **21**(7), 516-20.
59. Jizhou Wu, Yongyao Wang and Dakui Ling, APS, 1986, **21**(7), 546-50.
60. Weijiang Zhang, Deji Pan, Luoxiu Zhang and Yide Shao, APS, 1986, **21**(8), 592-8.
61. Soujin Wu, Deyu Li, Li Zhang, Xiaodong Du and Yukun Zhang, APS, 1986, **21**(8), 599-604.
62. Huikang Wang, Zhang dai Lin, Kan He and Shuwen Wan, APS, 1986, **21**(9), 680-2.
63. Dekang Qin, APS, 1986, **21**(9), 683-5.
64. Fengchang Lou, Linsheng Ding, Meiyu Wu and Lingling Li, APS, 1986, **21**(9), 702-5.
65. Qinghua Li and Zonghao Wu, APS, 1986, **21**(10), 767-71.
66. Chengjun Xu, Xiaofang Sun, Junshan Yang, Dequan Yu, Qingmei Li , Youji Zhang and Shiqi Dou, APS, 1986, **21**(10), 772-5.
67. Yuqi Gu and Gongyu Han, APS, 1986, **21**(10), 792-5.
68. Yang Lu, Tianrong Yao and Zenai Chen, APS, 1986, **21**(11), 829-35.
69. Yingqin Li, Ranru Lu and Luxue Wei, APS, 1986, **21**(11), 836-51.
70. Weizao Liang, Dakui Ling, Songjiu Tian and Guoshi Tu, APS, 1986, **21**(12), 906-11.
71. Jiasheng Guo, Suxian Wang, Xian Li and Tinglu Zhu, APS, 1987, **22**(1), 28-32.
72. Minghe Yang, Yanhuai Cao, Weixun Li, Yongqing Yang, Yanyong Chen and Liang Huang, APS, 1987, **22**(1), 33-40.
73. Lu Zeng , Ruyi Zhang and Xu Wang, APS, 1987, **22**(2), 114-20.
74. Guangyi Liang, APS, 1987, **22**(2), 121-5.
75. Shuming Li, Guiqiu Han, B.H. Arison and M. N. Chang, APS, 1987, **22**(3), 196-202.
76. Guangyi Li, Yulan Wang, Wanzhi Song and Qingyi Ji, APS, 1987, **22**(4), 269-71.
77. Lihong Gu, Suxian Wang, Xian Li and Tingru Zhu, APS, 1987, **22**(4), 272-7.
78. Fuxiao Deng, Jianhong Cao, Zhiling Xa, Sui Lin, Dayuan Zhu and Shanhao Jiang, APS, 1987, **22**(5), 377-9.
79. Jingxian Pan, LAMY K, ARISON B, SMITH J and Guiqiu Han, APS, 1987, **22**(5), 380-4.
80. Lifeng Xu, Suxian Wang, Tingru Zhu and Dequan Yu, APS, 1987, **22**(6), 433-7.
81. Jifu Zhao, Yunzhen Guo and Xianshu Meng, APS, 1987, **22**(7), 507-11.
82. Yonghua Shu, Ruyi Zhang, Yuying Zhao, Junwei Zhang and Weidong Tong, APS, 1987, **22**(7), 512-4.
83. Yongxin Zhu, Kedong Yan and Guoshi Tu, APS, 1987, **22**(9), 679-84.
84. Yingjie Chen, Suixu Xu, Qifeng Ma, Yuping Pei, Hua Xie and Xinsheng Yao, APS, 1987, **22**(9), 685-9.
85. Mokun Yang, Yaoshu Tang, Liangmu Cai, Jingyi Xie, Fujin Shen, Xiuyun Lin and Qitai Zheng, APS, 1987, **22**(9), 711-5.
86. Dingxian Han, Jianwei Han, Ming Jiao, Zichuan Yu, Wwnjie Tan and Suixu Xu, APS, 1987, **22**(10), 746-9.
87. Suixu Xu, Yngjie Chen, Zhongjun Cai and Xinsheng Yao, APS, 1987, **22**(10), 750-5.
88. Dongming Yang, Shiwen Su, Xian Li and Tingru Zhu, APS, 1987, **22**(10), 756-60.
89. Mao Lin, BaoqiYang and Dequan Yu, APS, 1987, **22**(11), 833-6.
90. Dequan Yu and Fengzhi Xie, APS, 1987, **22**(11), 837-40.
91. Guoming Gu, APS, 1987, **22**(12), 886-8.
92. Hairui Liang, Wenmei Yan, Jiashi Li and Chuishu Yang, APS, 1988, **23**(1), 34-7.
93. Wenhao Xu and Zhi Xue, APS, 1988, **23**(1), 61-3.
94. Aiqing Wang, Shengchu Feng, Xiang He and Rensheng Xu rheumatic arthritis, APS, 1988, **23**(1), 64-6.
95. Binmeng Chu and Jun Li, APS, 1988, **23**(2), 115-21.
96. Guangshun Xu, Xiyuan Chen and Dequan Yu, APS, 1988, **23**(2), 122-5.
97. Baiping Ying, Jiu Han, Guowei Li and Yi Zhong, APS, 1988, **23**(2), 126-9.
98. Longze Lin, Jinsheng Zhang, Jihui Shen, Tong Zhou and Wenyi Zhang, APS, 1988, **23**(2), 186-8.
99. Miaohua Chen and Fengshan Liu, APS, 1988, **23**(3), 218-20.

100. Jiashen Liu and Qianru Zhou, APS, 1988, **23**(3), 221-3.

101. Junshan Yang Dequan Yu and Xiaotian Liang, APS, 1988, **23**(4), 267-72.

102. Longze Lin, Xiaoming Wang, Xiulan Huang, Yong Huang and Baojin Yang, APS, 1988, **23**(4), 273-5.

103. Shusheng Gong, Chengdi Liu, Suolan Liu, Yingrong Du, Wui Kang and Xiuqin Dong, APS, 1988, **23**(4), 276-80.

104. Sheng Lai, Tongfang Zhao and Xiankai Wang, APS, 1988, **23**(5), 356-60.

105. Qinghua Li, Zonghao Wu, Lianlong Zhang and Li Shao, APS, 1988, **23**(6), 415-21.

106. Jin Chen, Guilan Geng, Guanghua Ye, Fengde Xi, Shufeng Chen, Cunheng He and Qitai Zheng, APS, 1988, **23**(6), 422-5.

107. Honggang Li and Guangyi Li, APS, 1988, **23**(6), 460-3.

108. Shanqin Yuan and Tongtai Wei, APS, 1988, **23**(7), 516-20.

109. Jun Li, Yanyi Han and Jiashen Liu, APS, 1988, **23**(7), 549-52.

110. Xuemei Ma and Yongqi Qin, APS, 1988, **23**(8), 588-92.

111. Deyun Kong, Siqi Luo, Huiting Li and Xinghan Lei, APS, 1988, **23**(8), 593-600.

112. Feng Li and Yonglong Liu, APS, 1988, **23**(9), 672-81.

113. Deyun Kong, Siqi Luo, Huiting Li and Xinghan Lei, APS, 1988, **23**(9), 707-10.

114. Feng Li and Yonglong Liu, APS, 1988, **23**(10), 739-48.

115. Yanqing Jiang and Chunxu Zuo, APS, 1988, **23**(10), 749-55.

116. HouweiLuo, Xiaojie Hu, Ning Wang and Jiang Ji, APS, 1988, **23**(11), 830-4.

117. Dongming Xu, Shuqing Wang, Enxi Huang, Maoli Xu, Yuxin Zhang and Xiaoguang Wen, APS, 1988, **23**(12), 902-5.

118. Mao Lin, Shouzhen Li, Xin Liu and Denquan Yu, APS, 1989, **24**(1), 32-36.

119. Lijuan Ren, Fengzhi Xie and Jinxi Xie, APS, 1989, **24**(1), 67-70.

120. Guomao Pang, Chunjiu Zhao, H. Hori and S. Inayama, APS,1989, **24**(1), 75-79.

121. Shixuan Liao,Gongyu Han, Yunru Zhang, Qitai Zheng and Chunheng He, APS, 1989, **24**(2), 110-113.

122. Zhenchun Miao, Zhensheng Yang and Rui Feng, APS, 1989, **24**(2), 114-117 .

123. Baoliang Cui, Yunru Lu and Luxue Wei, APS, 1989, **24**(3), 189-193.

124. Bihuang Hu and Yonglong Liu, APS, 1989, **24**(3) , 200-206.

125. Chongpu Zhang, Yonggang Zhang, Qitai Zheng and Cunheng He, APS, 1989, **24**(3), 225-228.

126. Qing Mao and Xiansheng Jia, APS, 1989, **24**(4), 269-274.

127. Fengchang Lou, Linsheng Ding and PG Wateriman, APS, 1989, **24**(4), 305-307.

128. Qi Jia, Bin Wang, Yonghua Shu, Ruyi Zhang, Congyuan Gao, Liang Qiao and Jihai Pang, APS, 1989, **24**(5), 348-351.

129. Yuehu Pei, Xian Li and Tingru Zhu, APS, 1989, **24**(6), 431-437.

130. Guiqiu Han, Lihua Wei, Changling Li, Liang Qiao, Yuzhen Jia and Qitai Zheng, APS, 1989, **24**(6), 438-443.

131. Huaibin Wang, Dequan Yu, Xiaotian Liang, N. Watanabe, M. Tamai and S Omura, APS, 1989, **24**(6), 444-451.

132. Xuefen Wang, Wenjie Lu, Qitai Zheng, Cunheng He, Jiayuan Chen, Rongfang Wei, Yihuan Wen and Yipeng Tao, APS, 1989, **24**(7), 522-524.

133. Qin Liu and Yonglong Liu, APS, 1989, **24**(7), 525-531.

134. Qirui Jin and Quanzhang Mu, APS, 1989, **24**(8), 587-592.

135. Daqi Wang, Juan Fan, Baoshu Feng, Shurong Li, Xibin Wang, Congren Yang and Jun Zhou, APS, 1989, **24**(8), 593-599.

136. Jizhou Wu, Xiping Pan, Minan Lou, Xiaosheng Wang and Dakui Ling, APS, 1989, **24**(8), 600-605.

137. Daqi Wang, Baoshu Feng, Xibin Wang, Congren Yang and Jun Zhou, APS, 1989, **24**(8), 633-635.

138. Dongming Xu, Shuqin Wang, Enxi Huang, Maoli Xu and Xiaoguang Wen, APS, 1989, **24**(9), 668-672.
139. Zhida Min, Hong Jiang and Jingyu Liang, APS, 1989, **24**(9), 673-677.
140. Junshan Yang, Yulan Wang and Yalun Su, APS, 1989, **24**(9), 678-683.
141. Lihong Gu, Xian Li, Siqing Yan and Tingru Zhu, APS, 1989, **24**(10), 744-748.
142. Wei Liu, Zhulu Wang and Huaqin Liang, APS, 1989, **24**(10), 749-754.
143. Xiangying Dong, Min Chen, Wei Jing, Daxian Huang, Shanmei Shen and Huiting Li, APS, 1989, **24**(11), 833-836.
144. Yuehu Pei, Xian Li and Tingru Zhu, APS, 1989, **24**(11), 837-840.
145. Changdai Wang, H. Takayanagi, Caifeng Mi, Boling Qiao, Jing Yang, Qitai, Zheng and Cunheng He, APS, 1989, **24**(12), 913-915.
146. Huizhong Xue, Jiu Zhang, Linxing He, Cunheng He, Qitai Zheng and Rui Feng, APS, 1989, **24**(12), 917-921.
147. Junshan Yang, Yalun Su, Yulan Wang, Xiaozhang Feng, Dequan Yu and Xiaotian Liang, APS, 1990, **25**(1), 24-8.
148. Wenji Sun, Dengke Zhang, Zhenfang Sa, Hengli Zhang and Xiaoli Zhang, APS, 1990, **25**(1), 29-34.
149. HuiMin Zhou and Yongji Liu, APS, 1990, **25**(2), 123-6.
150. Dongming Xu, Cunheng He, Shuqin Wang, Enxi Huang, Maoli Xu and Xiaoguang Wen, APS, 1990, **25**(2), 127-30.
151. Shanqin Yuan, Guoming Gu and Tongtai Wui, APS, 1990, **25**(3), 191-7.
152. Yuehu Pei, Xian Li, Tingru Zhu and Lijun Wu, APS, 1990, **25**(4), 267-70.
153. Bihuang Hu, Yonglong Liu, Tian Zhang and Wuanzhi Song, APS, 1990, **25**(4), 302-6.
154. Junshan Yang, Yalun Su, Yulan Wang, Xiaozhang Feng, Dequan Yu, Xiaotian Liang, Cunheng He, Qitai Zheng, Jingjing Yang and Jing Yang, APS, 1990, **25**(5), 353-6.
155. Yngjie Chen, Shaolin Zhang, Jixing Wang, Yongjun Lu, Suixu Xu, Xinshen Yao, CB. Cui, Y. Tezuka, T. Kikuchi, Y. Ogihara and T. Tadahiro, APS, 1990, **25**(5), 379-81.
156. Yanan Yu and Xian Li, APS, 1990, **25**(5), 382-6.
157. Lixin Ding and Weixin Chen, APS, 1990, **25**(6), 438-40.
158. Lisheng Ding and Weixin Chen, APS, 1990, **25**(6), 441-4.
159. Yi Ding and Chongren Yang, APS, 1990, **25**(7), 509-14.
160. Lu Zeng, Ruyi Zhang, Ping Wei, Dong Wang, Congyuan Gao and Zhicen Lou, APS, 1990, **25**(7), 515-21.
161. Fugang Qian, Guangyi Xu, Shangjian Du and Minhua Li, APS, 1990, **25**(7), 522-5.
162. Guolin Zhang, Weien Pan, Shulin Peng, Lei Chen and Weixin Chen, APS, 1990, **25**(8), 604-7.
163. Deyun Kong, Huiteng Li and Siqi Luo, APS, 1990, **25**(8), 608-11.
164. Jingguang Yu, Raoyun Chen, Zhixi Yao, Yunfeng Zhai, Shilin Yang and Junli Ma, APS, 1990, **25**(8), 612-6.
165. Qiduan Jin and Jinzhang Mu, APS, 1990, **25**(8), 617-6.
166. Jianghua Liu, Songsong Yang, Yuqin Fu, Changlu Yuan and Bo Liu, APS, 1990, **25**(9), 689-93.
167. Zhengquan He and Baoqing Wang, APS, 1990, **25**(9), 694-6.
168. Guangming Liu, Zenai Chen, Tianrong Yao and Weigong Ding, APS, 1990, **25**(9), 699-704.
169. Yanghua Yi and Xiang Huang, APS, 1990, **25**(10), 745-9.
170. Lu Zeng, Ruyi Zhang, Dong Wang, Jihai Pang, Zhiliang Zhang, Cingyuan Gao and Zhicen Lou, APS, 1990, **25**(10), 750-7.
171. Shishan Jia, Chaomei Ma and Jianmin Wang, APS, 1990, **25**(10), 758-62.
172. Dongming Xu, S. Arihara, N. Shoji, Xiuwei Yang, Enxi Huang and Chaosheng Li, APS, 1990, **25**(10), 795-7.
173. Chuguo Liu, Xinfu Pan, Changying Chen and Jisheng Chen, APS, 1990, **25**(11), 830-3.

174. Yafang Jiao, Suxian Wang, Lijun Wu, Xian Li and Tengru Zhu, APS, 1990, **25**(11), 834-9.
175. Maotian Wang, Yianzi Li, Tianzeng Zhao, Chunru Ji, Weisheng Feng and Tengzhai Liu, APS, 1990, **25**(11), 866-8.
176. Zhaojing Zhu, Zhichang Zhong, Zhaiyuan Luo and Zhuoyin Xiao, APS, 1990, **25**(12), 898-903.
177. Gaoxiong Rao, Handong Sun, Zhongwen Lin and Ruoying Hu, APS, 1991, **26**(1), 30-6.
178. Jinhai Yi, Zhichang Zhong, Zeyuan Luo and Zhuoyin Xiao, APS, 1991, **26**(1), 37-41.
179. Min Chen, Siqi Luo and Junhong Chen, APS, 1991, **26**(1), 42-8.
180. Yamin Chen, Yinghua Lu, Yanjun Chen, Cunsheng Ma and Dequan Yu, APS, 1991, **26**(2), 123-7.
181. Cailan Wang, Ruyi Zhang, Longsheng Han, Xigu Dong and Wenbin Liu, APS, 1991, **26**(2), 147-51.
182. Xuezhao Lu, Houwei Luo, Jiang Ji and Hao Cai, APS, 1991, **26**(3), 193-6.
183. Wenji Sun, Dengke Zhang, Zhenfang Sha, Hengli Zhang, Xiaoli Zhang, APS, 1991, **26**(3), 197-202.
184. Cuiying Ma, Kaixian Zhu, Dingming Yang, Junshan Yang and Dequan Yu, APS, 1991, **26**(3), 203-8.
185. Zhitian Li, Baojin Yang and Guangen Ma, APS, 1991, **26**(3), 209-213.
186. Jianxing Zhang, Guangen Ma, Aina Lao and Rensheng Xu, APS, 1991, **26**(3), 231-3.
187. Shishan Yu and Zhuoyin Xiao, APS, 1991, **26**(4), 261-6.
188. Raoyun Chen and Dequan Yu, APS, 1991, **26**(4), 267-73.
189. Manfei Li, Y. Hirata, Guojun Xu, M. Niwa and Houming Wu, APS, 1991, **26**(4), 307-10.
190. Dongming Zhang, Dequan Yu and Fengzhi Xie, APS, 1991, **26**(5), 341-4.
191. Ying Ma, Guiqiou Han, Changling Li and Jingrong Cheng, APS, 1991, **26**(5), 345-50.
192. Ruoyun Chen and Dequan Yu, APS, 1991, **26**(6), 430-6.
193. Jianbei Li, Mao Lin, Shouzhen Li and Wanzhi Song, APS, 1991, **26**(6), 437-41.
194. Dean Guo, Zhicen Lou, Congyuan Gao, Liang Jiao and Jiarou Peng, APS, 1991, **26**(6), 442-6.
195. Lining Cai, Ruyi Zhang, Zhiliang Zhang, Bin Wang, Liang Jiao, Liru Huang and Jingrong Cheng, APS, 1991, **26**(6), 447-50.
196. Guangshun Xu, Wen Zhao, Dan Wu, Dequan Yu, Cunheng He, Jingjing Yang and Fang Sun, APS, 1991, **26**(7), 505-9.
197. Liang Zhang, Zhinghang Zhang, Dengkui An and Chen Kong, APS, 1991, **26**(7), 515-8.
198. Hongxiang Lou, Xian Li and Tingru Zhu, APS, 1991, **26**(8), 584-92.
199. Dong Guo, Shu Li, Qun Chi, Wenji Sun, Zhenfang Sha and Xiaowen Zhao, APS, 1991, **26**(8), 619-21.
200. Jinlan Yuan, Yaowen Wan, Guixian Chen and Weipei Ding, APS, 1991, **26**(9), 667-71.
201. Yongwen Zhang and Zhi Xue, APS, 1991, **26**(9), 676-81.
202. Weiming Chen, Peiling Zhang, Bin Wu and Qitai Zheng, APS, 1991, **26**(10), 747-54.
203. Haisheng Chen, Huaqing Liang and Shixuan Liao, APS, 1991, **26**(10), 755-8.
204. Pengcheng Ma, Xieyu Lu, Jingjing Yang and Qitai Zheng, APS, 1991, **26**(10), 759-63.
205. Qinghua Li, Zonghao Wu, Lianlong Zhang Jiande Pan, APS, 1991, **26**(10), 794-7.
206. Jizhou Wu, Ming Tang Rui Wang, APS, 1991, **26**(11), 829-35.
207. Suolan Liu, Luxue Wei, Dong Wang and congyuan Gao, APS, 1991, **26**(11), 836-40.
208. Qirui Jin and Quanzhang Mu, APS, 1991, **26**(11), 841-5.
209. Jiu Zhang, Linxing He, Huizhong Xue, Rui Feng and Quanlong Pu, APS, 1991, **26**(11), 846-51.
210. Zhongmei Zhou and Puzhu Cong, APS, 1991, **26**(12), 906-10.
211. Yongwen Zhang and Zhi Xue, APS, 1991, **26**(12), 911-7.
212. Yude Wu, Fuquan Zhang, Mei Zhang, Qianshun Yan, Baoshan Huang and Zhongliang Chen, APS, 1991, **26**(12), 918-92.
213. Junxing Dong and Gongyu Han, APS, 1992, **27**(1), 26-32.

References

214. Ju Gao, Dechao Yao, Keli Cheng, Shuchun Wang, Kaibei Yu, Qitai Zheng and Junshan Yang, APS, 1992, **27**(1), 33-6.
215. Fengchang Lou, Meiyu Wu, Hongzhe Sun, Yuanzhu Chen and Benjie Xu, APS, 1992, **27**(1), 37-41.
216. Shishan Geng and Zhuoyin Xiao, APS, 1992, **27**(1), 42-7.
217. Huiyan Zhang, Wenmei Yan and Dechang Chen, APS, 1992, **27**(2), 113-6.
218. Shu Wang and Fengpeng Wang, APS, 1992, **27**(2), 117-20.
219. Yajuan Xu, Dongming Xu, Enxi Huang, Xiuying Wu, Xxiangqun Jin, Dongbin Ccui and Shiyue Liu, APS, 1992, **27**(2), 121-4.
220. Yaohua Luo and Ruilin Nie, APS, 1992, **27**(2), 125-9.
221. Xiaojiang Yang, Lizhen Xue, Nanjun Sun, Shuchun Wang and Qitai Zheng, APS, 1992, **27**(3), 185-90.
222. Dequan Yu, Fengzhi Xie, Wenyi He and Xiaotian Liang, APS, 1992, **27**(3), 191-6.
223. Jinhai Yi, Chichang Zhong, Zhaiyuan Luo and Zhuoyin Xiao, APS, 1992, **27**(3), 204-6.
224. Shenru xue, Jinqi Liu, Gang Wang, Jianqiu Shi, Jiangjin Wu and Shengzhi Hu, APS, 1992, **27**(3), 207-12.
225. Fengpeng Wang, Rong Zhang and Xinzhai Tang, APS, 1992, **27**(4), 273-8.
226. Huiming Hua, Suxian Wang, Lijun Wu, Xian Li Tingru Zhu, APS, 1992, **27**(4), 279-82.
227. Junping Xu and Rensheng Xu, APS, 1992, **27**(5), 353-7.
228. Yanjun Yang Huiyi Shu and Zhida Min, APS, 1992, **27**(5), 358-64.
229. Lisheng Ding, Fenge Wu and Yaozu Chen, APS, 1992, **27**(5), 394-6.
230. Bihuang Hu, Lidong Zhou and Yonglong Liu, APS, 1992, **27**(5), 397-400.
231. Shishan Jia, Chaomei Ma, Yinghe Li and Junhai Hao, APS, 1992, **27**(6), 441-4.
232. Dong Cao, Yalun Su and Junshan Yang, APS, 1992, **27**(6), 445-51.
233. Jianxing Zhang, Aina Lao, Heizhu Huang, Guangen Ma and Rensheng Xu, APS, 1992, **27**(6), 472-5.
234. Wendou Pan, Yujing Li, Langtian Mai, K. Ohtani, R. Kasai, and O. Tanaka, APS, 1992, **27**(7), 515-21.
235. Longtao Jiang, Suixu Xu, Xiaohua Gu, Li Ren, Yingjie Chen, Xinsheng Yao and Zhenchun Liao, APS, 1992, **27**(7), 528-32.
236. Huiqing Yuan and Chunxu Zuo, APS, 1992, **27**(8), 589-94.
237. Hongxiang Lou, Xian Li and Tingru Zhu, APS, 1992, **27**(8), 595-602.
238. Mingsheng Liu, Yingjie Chen, Yinghua Wang, Shirui Xing, Chuanxian An and K Yasukawa, APS, 1992, **27**(9), 667-9.
239. Weidong Zhang, Gongyu Han and Huaqing Liang, APS, 1992, **27**(9), 670-3.
240. Yongji You, Jingao Lin and Lianfang Ji, APS, 1992, **27**(9), 674-8.
241. Lihong Yang, Huozhong Zhang, Bing Zhang, Feng Chen, Zhaohui Lai, Lifeng Xu and Xiangqun Jin, APS, 1992, **27**(9), 679-83.
242. Suxian Wang, Huiming Hua, Lijun Wu, Xian Li and Tingru Zhu, APS, 1992, **27**(10), 743-7.
243. Lining Cai, Ruyi Zhang, Bin Wang, Liang Qiao Liru Huang and Zhiliang Zhang, APS, 1992, **27**(10), 748-51.
244. Hongxiang Lou, Xian Li and Tingru Zhu, APS, 1992, **27**(10), 752-7.
245. Lijuan Liu, XiouKun Wang and Haixue Kuang, APS, 1992, **27**(11), 837-40.
246. Dajian Yang, Zhichang Zhong and Zhaoming Xie, APS, 1992, **27**(11), 841-4.
247. Shiping Zhao and Zhi Xue, APS, 1992, **27**(11), 845-8.
248. Zilian Pu, Zhenchun Liao and Hui Zhao, APS, 1992, **27**(12), 908-11.
249. Yongwen Zhang and Zhi Xue, APS, 1992, **27**(12), 912-7.
250. Junpeng Peng, Yan Wu, T. Okuyama, T. Narui, APS, 1992, **27**(12), 918-22.
251. Shishan Jia, Dong Liu, Xiuping Zheng, Yong Zhang and Yongkang Li, APS, 1993, **28**(1), 28-31.

252. Liang Zhang, Zhengxing Zhang, Longsheng Sheng, Dengkui An, Yang Lu, Qitai Zheng and Shuchun Wang, APS, 1993, **28**(1), 32-34

253. Wendou Pan, Langtian Mai, Lujing Li, Lanxing Xu and Dequan Yu, APS, 1993, **28**(1), 35-39.

254. Wendou Pan, Yujin Li, Langtian Mai, KH. Ohtani, RT. Kasai, O. Tanaka and Dequan Yu, APS, 1993, **28**(1), 40-43.

255. Jingfang Mi, Rensheng Xu, Yiping Yang and Peiming Yang, APS, 1993, **28**(2), 105-109.

256. Chongpu Zhang, Xieyu Lu, Pengcheng Ma, Yun Cheng, Yonggang Zhang, Zheng Yan, Guofang Chen, Qitai Zheng, AP930 Chunheng He and Dequan Yu, APS, 1993, **28**(2),110-115.

257. AP930 Hong Liang and Ruyi Zhang, APS, 1993, **28**(2), 116-121 .

258. Xuefeng Wang, Wenjie Lu, Jiayuan Chen, Rongfang Wei, Jun Le, Yang Lu, Zhiyue Tian and Qitai Zheng, APS, 1993, **28**(2), 122-125.

259. Yajuan Xu, Dongming Xu, Dongbin Cui, Enxi Huang, Xiangqun Jin, Shiyue Liu and Mingming Yan, APS, 1993,**28**(3),192-195.

260. Junshan Yang, Yalun Su and Yulan Wang, APS, 1993, **28**(3), 197-201.

261. Wenhan Lin, Mengshen Cai, Baiping Ying and Rui Feng, APS, 1993, **28**(3), 202-206.

262. Xiangqun Jin, Dongming Xu, Yajuan Xu, Dongbin Cui, Yanwen Xiao, Zhiyue Tian, Yang Lu and Qitai Zheng, APS, 1993, **28**(3), 212-215 .

263. Qing Mao, Dong Cao and Xiansheng Jia, APS,1993, **28**(4), 273-281.

264. Xikui Chen, Ruyi Zhang, Zhiliang Zhang, Tianyi Jiang and Bin Wang, APS, 1993, **28**(5), 352-357.

265. Yongwen Zhang and Zhi Xue, APS, 1993, **28**(5), 358-363.

266. Shuli Ding and Zhaoyi Zhu. APS, 1993, **28**(5), 364-369.

267. Ying Ma, Guiqui Han and Yinye Wang, APS, 1993, **28**(5),370-373.

268. Lingyi Kong, Yuehu Pei, Xian Li, Tingru Zhu and Sanche Ao, APS, 1993, **28**(6), 432-435 .

269. Mao Lin and Shouzhen Li. APS, 1993, **28**(6), 437-441.

270. Zhaoming Li, Xianming Zhang, Yunli Zhou, Liying Huang and Guoda Tao, APS, 1993, **28**(7), 512-515.

271. Chenghao Hu, Erning Shang, Wenhan Lin and Mengsheng Çai, APS, 1993, **28**(7), 516-521 .

272. Pei Tan, Yonglong Liu and Cuiying Hou, APS, 1993, **28**(7), 522-525.

273. Junpeng Peng, Xuan Wang and Xinsheng Yao, APS, 1993, **28**(7), 526-531.

274. Sheng Lai, Tongfang Zhao, Xiankai Wang, Y. Shizuri and S. Yamamura, APS, 1993, **28**(7), 599-603.

275. Shishan Jia, Dong Liu, Hongqin Wang and Zhixin Suo, APS, 1993, **28**(8), 623-625.

276. Qinghua Zhang, Xiaojuan Wang, Zhenchun Miao and Rui Feng, APS, 1993, **28**(9), 673-678 .

277. Yuanyuan Zhu and Guangyi Li, APS, 1993, **28**(9), 679-683.

278. Xiaolin Yan, Shiying Liao, Huaqing Liang and Ping Zhou, APS, 1993, **28**(9), 684-689.

279. Chen Ma, Junshan Yang and Shurong Luo, APS, 1993, **28**(9), 690-694.

280. Yiming Li, Zhuolun Zhou and Yongfu Hong, APS, 1993, **28**(10), 766-771.

281. Lingyi Kong, Yuehu Pei, Xian Li, Suxian Wang, Boling Hou and tingru Zhu, APS, 1993, **28**(10), 772-774.

282. Congjun Li, Dihua Chen, Peigen Xiao, APS, 1993, **28**(10), 777-781.

283. Qingqiang Yao and Chunxu Zuo, APS, 1993, **28**(11), 829-835.

284. Long liang, Lingen Lu and Yuancong Cai, APS, 1993, **28**(11), 836-839.

285. Jingguang Yu, Puzhu Cong, Jitian Lin, Youju Zhang, Shaoliang Hong and Guangzhong Tu, APS, 1993, **28**(11), 840-843.

286. Mingkui Wang, Fenge Wu and Yaozu Chen, APS, 1993, **28**(11), 845-848.

287. Hongmei Liu, Zhong Jiang and Xiaozhang Feng, APS, 1993, **28**(11), 849-853.

288. Haiyan Wang and Junshan Yang, APS, 1993, **28**(12), 911-917.

289. Huaibin Wang, Guohua Yang, Shaofang, Wang, Guangyi Li, Weikun Xu, Lishan Meng ZhongYao Li, APS, 1994, **29**(1), 39-43.
290. Lingyi Kong, Xian Li, Yuhu Pei and Tinglu Zhu, APS, 1994, **29**(1), 49-54.
291. Xiaojie Tong, Weisuo Fang, Jinyun Zhou, Cunheng He, Weiming Chen and Qicheng Fang, APS, 1994, **29**(1), 55-60.
292. Lixin Zhou, Mao Lin, Jianbei Li and Shouzhen Li, APS, 1994, **29**(2), 107-10.
293. Kefang Mi, Zhongliang Chen and Jihui Shen, APS, 1994, **29**(2), 111-5.
294. Congjun Li, Dihua Chen and Peigen Xiao, APS, 1994, **29**(3),195–9.
295. Yujiang Ren, Haisheng Chen, Genjin Yang and Hao Zhu, APS, 1994, **29**(3), 204-6.
296. Weiming Chen, Peiling Zhang and Jinyun Zhou, APS, 1994, **29**(3), 207-14.
297. Lingyi Kong, Xian Li, Yuhu Pei, Rongmin Yu, Zhida Min and Tinglu Zhu, APS, 1994, **29**(4), 276-80.
298. Yue Zhang, Jinlan Yuan and Weipei Ding, APS, 1994, **29**(4), 281-4.
299. Shuangcheng Ma, Dechang Chen and Shujie Zhao, APS, 1994, **29**(4), 285-9.
300. Chang Rao, Jinyun Zhou, Weiming Chen, Yang Lv and Qitai Zheng, APS, 1994, **29**(5), 355-9.
301. Kun Zou, Yuying Zhao and Ruyi Zhang, APS, 1994, **29**(5), 393-6.
302. Kun Zou, Ruyi Zhang and Xianbin Yang, APS, 1994, **29**(5), 397-9.
303. Jingguang Yu, Xiuzhen Luo, Chunyu Liu, Lan Sun, Shaoliang Hong and Libin Ma, APS, 1994, **29**(6), 443-8.
304. Congjun Li, Yinghuo Li, Shunfeng Chen and Pegen Xiao, APS, 1994, **29**(6), 449-53.
305. Haijun Zhang, Yuan Liu and Ruyi Zhang, APS, 1994, **29**(6), 471-4.
306. Yayan Chen, Bin Wang, Congyuan Gao, Liang Qiao and Guiqiou Han, APS, 1994, **29**(7), 506-10.
307. Feng Wei, Zhicen Lou, Yimin Liu and Zhenchun Miao, APS, 1994, **29**(7), 511-8.
308. Guishan Tan and Chunxu Zuo, APS, 1994, **29**(7), 519-25.
309. Junpeng Peng, Xinsheng Yao, Y. Okada and T. Okuyama, APS, 1994, **29**(7), 526-31.
310. Sui Lin, N. Sakurai, Youlan Zheng and Yuanchao Li, APS, 1994, **29**(8), 599-602.
311. Min Chen, Weiwei Wu, Guoqiang Shen, Siqi Luo and Huiting Li, APS, 1994, **29**(8), 617-20.
312. Jiuhong Wu, Shixuan Liao, Huaqing Liang and Shilong Mao, APS, 1994, **29**(8), 621-3.
313. Ruyi Zhang, Xikui Chen, Xianbin Yang, Li Tan and Wenyi He, APS, 1994, **29**(9), 684-8.
314. Haiyan Pu and Fengpeng Wang, APS, 1994, **29**(9), 689-92.
315. Jialin Wang, Chunshu Yang, Lunan Yan, Bing Yao and Xianbin Yang, APS, 1994, **29**(9), 693-6.
316. Weiming Chen, Peiling Zhang, Jinyun Zhou, Xxin Liu and Qicheng Fang, APS, 1994, **29**(10), 751-7.
317. Jingfang Mi, Weimin Zhao, Yong Tao, Rensheng Xu, Guowei Qin and Meifen Huang, APS, 1994, **29**(10), 758-62.
318. Guoxiang Ma, Guojun Xu, Luoshan Xu, Zhengtao Wang and Chiche Ju, APS, 1994, **29**(10), 763-6.
319. Aiguo Wang, Yang Lu and Xiaozhang Feng, APS, 1994, **29**(12), 899-904.
320. Congjun Li, Yinghe Li and Peigen Xiao, APS, 1994, **29**(12), 937-6.
321. Jinfeng Hu Zhonglin Ye and Fengjia Shen, APS, 1995, **30**(1), 27-33.
322. Qing Zhao, Xiaojiang Hao, Yaozu Chen and Cheng Zou, APS, 1995, **30**(2), 119-22.
323. Jinhai Yi, Xianzhong Yan, Zhaiyuan Luo and Zhichang Zhong, APS, 1995, **30**(3), 206-10.
324. Xiaofeng Zhang, Bailin Hu and Binnan Zhou, APS, 1995, **30**(3), 211-4.
325. Yongqing Xiao, M. Taniguchi, Xiaohong Liu, Youfu Sun and M. Kozawa, et al. APS, 1995, **30**(4), 274-9.
326. Guangyi Liang, Kongyun Wu, Rensheng Xu, Deyuan Chen and Zhuying He, APS, 1995, **30**(5), 367-71.
327. Hesheng Luo, Yuying Zhao, Libin Ma, Yizhu Jin, Jiarou Peng and Ruyi Zhang, APS, 1995, **30**(6), 435-9.
328. Yanbin Yang, Xiangyu Pu, Xia Peng and Hong Yin, APS, 1995, **30**(6), 440-2.
329. Qi Chang, Dihua Chen, Jianyong Si, Liangang Shen and Zhaoyi Zhu, APS, 1995, **30**(7), 506-5.
330. Sui Lin, Yuanchao Li, N. Sakurai, Youlan Zheng and Fuxiao Deng , APS, 1995, **30**(7), 513-6.

331. Zhimao chao and Jingming Liu, APS, 1995, **30**(7), 517-20.
332. Guoping Peng, Fengchang Lou and Shouxun Zhao, APS, 1995, **30**(7), 521-5.
333. Ruoyun Chen and Dequan Yu, APS, 1995, **30**(7), 526-30.
334. Fengchang Lou, Guoping Peng, Ying Wang and Shouxun Zhao, APS, 1995, **30**(8), 588-93.
335. Qianqun Gu, S. Fushiya and S. Nozoe, APS, 1995, **30**(9), 685-8.
336. Yijun Yi, Zhengzhong Cao, Wenhong Yang, Wuqi Hong, Yuan Cao and Zongkang Leng, APS, 1995, **30**(9), 718-20.
337. Wenhan Lin, Yaoxin Wang, Mengshen Cai and Shanger Ning, APS, 1995, **30**(10), 752-6.
338. Rengeng Shu, Changrui Xu and Liannang Li, APS, 1995, **30**(10), 757-61.
339. Feng Wui, Zhicen Lou, Ming Gao and Zhenchun miao, APS, 1995, **30**(11), 831-7.
340. Caifeng Mi, Changdai Wang, Huili Shi and Fuxian Li, APS, 1995, **30**(12), 910-3.
341. Lifu Shi, Peng Wang, Haisheng Chen and Jianping Dong, APS, 1995, **30**(12), 935-8.
342. Wenkui Li, Jingqi Pan, Mujian Lu, Ruyi Zhang, Maochuan Liao and Peigen Xiao, APS, 1996, **31**(1), 29-32.
343. Jinlan Zhang, Dequan Yu and Zhihua Zhou, APS, 1996, **31**(6), 33-7.
344. Jianghua Liu, Suixu xu, Xinsheng Yao and Yuqiang Wu, APS, 1996, **31**(1), 63-7.
345. Shilong Mao, Shixuan Liao, Jiuhong Wu, Huaqing Liang, Haisheng Chen and Cankun Zhang, APS, 1996, **31**(1), 118-21.
346. Long Liang, Changyu Liu, Guangyu Li, Lingen Lu and Yuancong Cai, APS, 1996, **31**(2), 122-5.
347. Yuanqing Tang, Xiaozhang Feng and Liang Huang, APS, 1996, **31**(2), 151-5.
348. Yinan zheng, etc., APS, 1996, **31**(3), 191-5.
349. Mei Zhang and Yayan Chen, APS, 1996, **31**(3), 196-9.
350. Fangsheng Wang, Hui Cai, Junshan Yang, Yumei Zhang and Yingju Zhao, APS, 1996, **31**(3), 200-4.
351. Guoxiang Ma, Guojun Xu, Luoshan Xu, Zhengtao Wang and Chiche Ju, APS, 1996, **31**(3), 222-5.
352. Jinna Cai, Zhengtao Wang, Guojun Xu and Zhentao Che, APS, 1996, **31**(3), 267-70.
353. Baiping Ma, Junxing Dong, Bingji Wang and Xianzhong Yan, APS, 1996, **31**(4), 271-7.
354. Ping Huang, Min Yang, Maoxiang Lai, Xuezhong Zheng, Zhengmin Xi and Xiqin Zhong, APS, 1996, **31**(4), 278-81.
355. Yongping Qin, Xiping Pan, Ruoyun Chen and Dequan Yu, APS, 1996, **31**(5), 381-6.
356. Yuru Sun and Youfu Sun, APS, 1996, **31**(6), 437-40.
357. Wenkui Li, Jingqi Pan, Mujian Lu, Ruyi Zhang and Peigen Xiao, APS, 1996, **31**(6), 441-5.
358. Guoping Peng, Fengchang Lou, Ying Wang, Shouxun Zhao and Dongjun Chen, APS, 1996, **31**(6), 446-50.
359. Haifeng Tang, Yanghua Yi, Zhongzhuang Wang, Wenjun Hu and Yinqing Li, APS, 1996, **31**(7), 517-23.
360. Lingyi Kong and Zhida min, APS, 1996, **31**(7), 524-9.
361. Pengyue Sun, Yingjie Chen, Ye Wen, Yuping Pei, Zhenhua Liu, Xinsheng Yao, etc., APS, 1996, **31**(8), 602-6.
362. Junpeng Peng, Hao Chen, Yanqiu Qiao, Liren Ma, etc., APS, 1996, **31**(8), 607-12.
363. Xiaoling Shen, Yingjie Hu, Jie Xu, Haidong Chen and Yumao Shen, APS, 1996, **31**(8), 613-6.
364. Zzh*Acta Pharmaceutica Sinica*u Fang and Xianyi Zeng, APS, 1996, **31**(9), 680-3.
365. Haifeng Hao, Lijuan Ren and Yuwu Chen, APS, 1996, **31**(9), 689-94.
366. Yiqing Li, Yanghua Yi, Haifeng Tang and Kai Xiao, APS, 1996, **31**(2), 761-3.
367. Zhimin Wang, Hao Feng, Xiaotian Liang Sitong Yuan and Meijuan Xu, APS, 1996, **31**(10), 764-9.
368. AP960 Liang Ye and Junshan Yang, APS, 1996, **31**(11), 844-8.
369. Jiaoshe Li, Yuying Zhao, Bin Wang, Xiulan Li Libin Ma, APS, 1996, **31**(11), 849-54.
370. Guangshu Wang, Yanping Chen, Jingda Xu, T. Murayama and J. Shoji, APS, 1996, **31**(12), 940-4.
371. Beling Qiao, Changdai Wang, Caifeng Mi, Fuxian Li, Huili Shi and J Takashima, APS, 1997, **32**(1), 56-8.

372. Ying Gu, Zhongda Huang and Yonghe Liu, APS, 1997, **32**(1), 56-61.

373. Ping huang, Xuezhong Zheng, M Nishi and T Nakanishi, APS, 1997, **32**(1), 62-4.

374. Siping Chen, Luyi Zhang, Libin Ma and Guangzhong Tu, APS, 1997, **32**(2), 110-5.

375. Siping Chen and Ruyi Zhang, APS, 1997, **32**(2), 144-6.

376. Bin Wang, Kun Zou, Xianbin Yang, Wenyi He, Yuying Zhao and Ruyi Zhang, APS, 1997, **32**(3), 199-202.

377. Dean Guo, Zhenggao Zhang, Guoqing Ye and Zhicen Lou, APS, 1997, **32**(4), 282-5.

378. Xiping Pan and Dequan Yu, APS, 1997, **32**(4), 286-93.

379. Yumei Zhang, Xudong Xu, Bihuang Hu Qin Liu Cuiying Hou Yonglong Liu and Junshan Yang, APS, 1997, **32**(4), 301-4.

380. Wui Meng and wenzao JIn, APS, 1997, **32**(5), 352-6.

381. Jinhai Yi, Xiaoping Huang, Yan Chen, Zhaiyuan Luo and Chichang Zhong, APS, 1997, **32**(5), 357-60.

382. Shilong Mao, Shixuan Liao, Jiuhong Wu, Na Ling, Hua Chen, Huaqing Liang and Mingzhu Liu, APS, 1997, **32**(5), 360-4.

383. Weiming Chen, Peiling Zhang, Jinyun Zhou and Qicheng Fang, APS, 1997, **32**(5), 363-7.

384. Mingan Wang, Jun Liu and Fuheng Chen, APS, 1997, **32**(5), 368-72.

385. Jingguang Yu, Huaqing Gui, Xiuzhen luo, Lan Sun, Ping Zhu and Zhili Yu, APS, 1997, **32**(5), 431-7.

386. Lifu Shi, Yingying Cao, Haisheng Chen and Jianping Dong, APS, 1997, **32**(6), 442-6.

387. Fangsheng Wang, Hui Cai, Junshan Yang, Yumei Zhang , Junqiou Liu and Moju chao, APS, 1997, **32**(6), 447-50.

388. Yixing Shen, Lihui Quan, Ling Guan, Jianmin Chen, APS, 1997, **32**(6), 451-4.

389. Zhipeng You, Meijiang Liao, Yuhu Shi and Yaozu Chen, APS, 1997, **32**(6), 455-7.

390. Xulin Guo, Tiejun Wang and Baolin Bian, APS, 1997, **32**(7), 524-9.

391. Linsheng Ding, Qiaoli Liang and Yanfen Teng, APS, 1997, **32**(8), 600-2.

392. Mei Zhang, Yayan Chen Xiaohui Di and Mei Liu, APS, 1997, **32**(8), 633-4.

393. Guolin Li, Jiafeng Zeng and Dayuan Zhu, APS, 1997, **32**(9), 682-4.

394. Haifeng Tang, Yanghua Yi, Zhongzhuang Wang, Yongpei Jiang and Yinqing Li, APS, 1997, **32**(9), 685-90.

395. Ping Huang, Zhengmin Xi, Xuezhong Zheng, Maoxiang Lai and Xiqin Zhong, APS, 1997, **32**(9), 704-7.

396. Long Liang, Changyu Liu, Guangyu Li, Lingen Lu and Yuancong Cai, APS, 1997, **32**(10), 761-4.

397. Feng Wei and Wenmei Yan, APS, 1997, **32**(10), 765-8.

398. Yanghua Yi, Jingqin Gu, Kai Xiao, Zhongzhuang Wang and Houwen Lin, APS, 1997, **32**(10), 769-72.

399. Shishan Geng, Zhongmei Zou, Jie Zheng, Dequan Yu and Puzhu Cong, APS, 1997, **32**(11), 852-6.

400. Jiangnan Peng, Xiaozhang Feng, Guangyu Li and Xiaotian Liang, APS, 1997, **32**(6), 908-13.

401. Jingguang Yu, Dong Liu, Lizhen Xu and Shilin Yang, APS, 1997, **32**(6), 914-9.

402. Dekang Qin and Liping Yu, APS,1.998, **33**(1), 34-6.

403. Hong Liang, Yuying Zhao, Haiyun Qiu, Ji Huang and Ruyi Zhang, APS,1.998, **33**(1), 37-41.

404. Wenxiang Wang and Xingbao Ding, APS,1.998, **33**(2),128-31.

405. Zhimin Wang, Hao Feng, Qing Zhang, Fengshan Liu, Wenshan Jin, Min Mu, Qiuhua Fan, Man Kong and Wenyi He , APS,1.998, **33**(3), 207-11.

406. Xiping Pan, Yongping Qin, Ruoyun Chen and Dequan Yu, APS,1.998, **33**(4), 275-81.

407. Hong Liang, Yuying Chao,Yanjing Bai, Ruyi Zhang and Guangzhong Tu, APS, 1998, **33**(4), 282-5.

408. Youying Guo, Lianpo Lin and Jing Shen, APS,1.998, **33**(5), 350-4.

409. Yong Jiang, Naili Wang, Xingsheng Yang and Zhongjin Bei, APS,1.998, **33**(5),355-61.

410. Ruoyun Chen, Dequan Yu, Lin Ma, Feng Wu and Wanzhi Song, APS, 1998, **33**(6), 453-6.

411. Tongmei Li and Jingguang Yu, APS, 1998, **33**(8), 591-6.

412. Kexu Yan, Shaoliang Hong and Xiaozhang Feng, APS, 1998, **33**(8), 597-9.

413. Hong Wei, Fanjian Zeng, Minyi Lu and Renjiu Tang, APS, 1998, **33**(9), 688-92.

414. Wenjie Lu, Xuefen Wang, Jiayuan Chen, Yang Lu, Nan Wu, Wenjun Kang and Qitai Zheng, APS, 1998, **33**(10), 755-8.

415. Yinjun Zhang, Liangqiong Li, Peiquan Yang and Hao Zhang, APS, 1998, **33**(11), 836-86.

416. Yijun Yi, Zhengzhong Cao, Dalong Yang, Yuan Cao, Yongping Wu, and Shouxun Zhao, APS, 1998, **33**(11), 873-5.

417. Pengyue Sun, Ye Wen, Ying Xu, Yuping Pei, Yingjie Chen, Noriko Shimizu and Tadahiro Takeda, APS, 1998, **33**(12), 919-22.

418. Xiuyun Hou and Fakei Chen, APS, 1998, **33**(12), 923-6.

419. Zhaoming Li, Qing Mu, Handong Sun, Bin Xu and Weidong Tang, ABY, 1998, **20**(1), 102-4

420. Qing Mu, Chaoming Li, Handong Sun, Huilan Zheng and Guoda Tao, ABY, 1998, **20**(1), 123-5

421. Haihui Xie, Xiaoyi Wei and Biyu Wei, ABY, 1998, **20**(2), 238-40

422. Qifeng Zhang, Shide Luo and Huilan Wang, ABY, 1998, **20**(3), 362-8

423. Xikui Liu, Zhongrong Li, Minghua Qiu and Ruilin Nie, ABY, 1998, **20**(3), 369-73

424. Ke Zhang, Wei Ni, Changxiang Chen and Yidan Liu,ABY, 1998, **20**(3), 374-6

425. Zhongrong Li, Minghua Qiu, Xueping Xu, Jun Tian, Ruilin Nie, Zhihong Duan and Zemo Lei, ABY, 1998, **20**(3), 379-82

426. Xin Hong, Bingui Wang, Jun Zhou and Xiaojiang Hao, ABY, 1998, **20**(4), 464-8.

427. Kun Zhang, Yanhong Wang, Yaozu Chen, Handong Sun and Zhongwen Lin, ASNUS, 1998, **37**(2), 49-51.

428. Lisheng Ding, Peiqing Chen, Shulin Peng and Yuanzheng Huang, Natural Product R&D, 1998, **10**(1), 6-8.

429. Tingzhai Liu, Aijun Hou and Chunru Ji, Natural Product R&D, 1998, **10**(1), 14-18.

430. Renwen Zhang, Yongyue Lin and Yufang Qi, Natural Product R&D, 1998, **10**(1), 31-33.

431. Hong Cai and Mingkui Wang, Natural Product R&D, 1998, **10**(1), 48-50.

432. Dong Liu, Jingguang Yu, Lan Sun, Xiuzhen Luo, Shaorong Guo and Jitian Lin, Natural Product R&D, 1998, **10**(2), 1-6.

433. Yongli Zhong, Sujin Yan, Jingyu Su and Longmei Zeng, Natural Product R&D, 1998, **10**(2), 15-18.

434. Wenwu Li, Lisheng Ding and Bogang Li, Natural Product R&D, 1998, **10**(2), 19-20.

435. Jian Shen, Huyi Zhang, Bo Xu and Jingxian Pan, Natural Product R&D, 1998, **10**(2), 33-36.

436. WC981017 Jian Feng, West China Journal of Pharmaceutical Science, 1998, **13**(1), 17-18.

437. WC982095 Jiayuan Chen, Wenjie Lu, Xuefen Wang, Rongfang Wei and Qun Shi, West China Journal of Pharmaceutical Science, 1998, **13**(2), 95-96.

438. Weijie Zhao, Yongtian Guo, Yasuhiro Tezuka and Tohro Kikuchi, Chinese Journal of Medicinal Chemistry, 1998, **8**(1), 35-37.

439. Ting Xiang, Lijun Wu, Mei Dong, Xiaochuan Zhou, Qi Huang and Bochong Zhang, Chinese Journal of Medicinal Chemistry, 1998, **8**(1), 44-45.

440. Yun Ling,Yalin Zhang, Shaoqing Cai and Junhua Zheng, Chinese Journal of Medicinal Chemistry, 1998, **8**(1), 46-47.

441. Xiuyun Hou, Fakui Chen and Lijun Wu, Chinese Journal of Medicinal Chemistry, 1998, **8**(1), 49.

442. Pengyue Sun, Yng Xu, Ye Wen, Yuping Pei, Yingjie Chen, Noriko Shimizu and Tadahiro Takeda, Chinese Journal of Medicinal Chemistry, 1998, **8**(2),122-126.

443. Zhiyun Meng and Suixu Xu, Chinese Journal of Medicinal Chemistry, 1998, **8**(2), 135-136.

444. Xiqiang Li, Jinhui Wang, Suxian Wang and Xian Li, Chinese Journal of Medicinal Chemistry, 1998, **8**(3), 199-200

445. Jinhui Wang and Xian Li, Chinese Journal of Medicinal Chemistry, 1998, **8**(3), 201-202.

References

446. Feng Qiu, Zhongze Ma, Yuping Pei, Zhentao Che, Xusui Xu, Xinsheng Yao and Yingjie Chen, Chinese Journal of Medicinal Chemistry, 1998, **8**(3), 205-207.
447. Xiaojie Tong, Jinyun Zhou and Qicheng Fang, Chinese Pharmaceutical Journal, 1993, **28**(3), 133-135.
448. Haisheng Chen, Shixuan Liao and Zhijun Hong, Chinese Pharmaceutical Journal, 1993, **28**(3), 137-138.
449. Jinlan Yuan, Juying Wang and Weipei Ding, Chinese Pharmaceutical Journal, 1993, **28**(4), 213-214.
450. Jinping Liu, Guangxuan Wu and Yongmao Zhang, Chinese Pharmaceutical Journal, 1993, **28**(5), 277-279.
451. Xingyuan Ma, Guangshu Wang, Luli Wang Ping Sun, Chinese Pharmaceutical Journal, 1993, **28**(12), 718-720.
452. Xiuwei Yang, Zhongkai Yan, Zheming Gu, Guangchun Zhou, Masao Hattori and Tsuneo Namba, Chinese Pharmaceutical Journal, 1994, **29**(3), 141-143.
453. Jianhua Wang, Wenzhe Huang, Zenghui Zhang, Changgui Wang, Peiquan Yang and Rong Xiao, Chinese Pharmaceutical Journal, 1994, **29**(5), 268-270.
454. Heng Zhao, Baozhen Wang, Bingru Ma and Jinyan Sun, Chinese Pharmaceutical Journal, 1994, **29**(9), 523-524
455. Liping Zhang and Changqi Hu, Chinese Pharmaceutical Journal, 1994, **29**(10), 600-601.
456. Yongming Luo, Jinhai Zhang, Jiahu Pan, Songlin Yao, Honglin Huang, Ying Zhu and Qisheng Li, Chinese Pharmaceutical Journal, 1994, **29**(12), 714-715.
457. Guangshu Wang, Ping Sun, Chunjie Shao Jingda Xu, Chinese Pharmaceutical Journal, 1995, **30**(6), 333-336.
458. Wenkui Li, Peigen Xiao, Jingqi Pan, Mujian Lu and Ruyi Zhang, Chinese Pharmaceutical Journal, 1995, **30**(8), 455-457.
459. Zheng Cui, Dan Yuan, Zerong Jiang, Yushan Li, Jun Yin, Dequan Yu and Jinhe Li, Chinese Pharmaceutical Journal, 1995, **30**(9), 524-526.
460. Xiankai Wang, Tongfang Zhao and Sheng Lai, Chinese Pharmaceutical Journal, 1995, **30**(12), 716-719.
461. Xiankai Wang, Tongfang Zhao and Sheng Lai, Chinese Pharmaceutical Journal, 1996, **31**(2), 74-77
462. Haifeng Tang, Yanghua Yi, Zhongzhuang Wang, Wenjun Hu and Yiqing Li, Chinese Pharmaceutical Journal, 1996, **31**(4), 204-206.
463. Jiaping Chi, Bingwen xue Haisheng Chen, Chinese Pharmaceutical Journal, 1996, **31**(5), 264-266.
464. Juying Wang and Jinlan Yuan, Chinese Pharmaceutical Journal, 1996, **31**(5), 266-269.
465. Wenkui Li, Peigen Xiao, Jingqi Pan, Mujian Lu and Ruyi Zhang, Chinese Pharmaceutical Journal, 1996, **31**(6), 332-334.
466. Tianda Zhou and Xuexian Zhou, Chinese Pharmaceutical Journal, 1996, 31(8), 458-461.
467. Guangshu Wang, Qin Meng, et al., Chinese Pharmaceutical Journal, 1996, **31**(9), 522-524.
468. Cheng Guo, Gongyu Han and Zhongwu Su, Chinese Pharmaceutical Journal, 1997, **32**(1), 8-10.
469. Guangshu Wang, Yanping Chen, Jingda Xu, Xiangjie Yuan and Yaling Zhou, Chinese Pharmaceutical Journal, 1997, **32**(1), 11-13.
470. Haifeng Tang, Yanghua Yi, Zhongzhuang Wang, Yaxuan Fan and Yiqing Li, Chinese Pharmaceutical Journal, 1997, **32**(2), 78-80.
471. Mingyu Gui, Honggui Zhang, Yongri Jin, Guangxuan Wu and Wanru Peng, Chinese Pharmaceutical Journal, 1997, **32**(4), 204-206.
472. Haiming Lei, Rong Zhu and Luxue Wei, Chinese Pharmaceutical Journal, 1997, **32**(5), 271-273.
473. Jing Li, Hong Li and Jin Xu , Chinese Pharmaceutical Journal, 1997, **32**(7), 401-403.
474. Yinjuan Bai, Yu Li, Yanping Shi and Youhua Hu, Chinese Pharmaceutical Journal, 1997, **32**(8), 462-465.
475. Yun Ling, Yanyan Bao, Lili Zhu, Junhua Zheng, Shaoqing Cai and Yue Xiao, Chinese Pharmaceutical Journal, 1997, **32**(10), 584-586.
476. Hongzheng Fu, Zhicen Lou, Shaoqing Cai, Xujia Hu, and Zengwei Zhang, Chinese Pharmaceutical Journal, 1998, **33**(3), 140-142.

477. Wenjuan Qin, Rui Wang, Yuesheng Wen, Lan Yang and Libin Ma, CTHD, 1995, **26**(1), 3-6.
478. Xuemei Ma, Manfei Li, Qingrong Zhang, CTHD, 1995, **26**(2), 59-61.
479. Lizhen Xu, Huiying Li, Lei Tian, Chen Xie, Keming Li, Bin Li, Tianxiu Qian and Nanjun Sun, CTHD, 1995, **26**(2), 62-65.
480. Weidong Zhang, Kai Xiao, Genquan Yang , Haisheng Chen, CTHD, 1995, **26**(3), 125-6.
481. Kangli Miao, Jianzhong Zhang, Feiyin Wang and Yongjiao Qin, CTHD, 1995, **26**(4), 171-3.
482. Fenggang Chang and Jianmei Li, CTHD, 1995, **26**(6), 281-4.
483. Xiaoyi Wei, Biyu Wei and Ji Zhang, CTHD, 1995, **26**(7), 344-6.
484. Ping Chen, Jingyun Sun, Niangeng Xie and Yinyu Shi, CTHD, 1995, **26**(8), 397-9.
485. Qinli Wu, Yanqing Zhao and Zhulian Li, CTHD, 1995, **26**(9), 451-2.
486. Ziyan Li, Liang Li and Hongbin Zhang, CTHD, 1996, **27**(1), 3-4.
487. Ying Chen, Lisheng Ding, Mingkui Wang, et al., CTHD, 1996, **27**(1), 5-8.
488. Guifang Liu, Chuanling Zhao, et al., CTHD, 1996, **27**(2), 67-9.
489. Liping Zhang, Meihua Ju, Changqi Hu, CTHD, 1996, **27**(3), 134-6.
490. Xiaoling Shen, Yuemao Shen, et al., CTHD, 1996, **27**(5), 259-60.
491. Jicheng Li, Baomei Yuan, Jinling Su, et al., CTHD, 1996, **27**(6), 323-4.
492. Zhili Chen, Yongming Luo, Wenshu Xiong, CTHD, 1996, **27**(6), 325-7.
493. Ruijian Zhong, Youheng Gao, Changrui Xu and Liannian Li, CTHD, 1996, **27**(7), 387-9.
494. Tianbo Ma, Sizhen Liu, Chuanling Liu and Yuxia Liu, CTHD, 1996, **27**(8), 451-3.
495. Xuefen Wang, Wenjie Lu, Jiayuan Chen, Minyang Gong, Yuhong Li, Duo Lu, Yang Lu and Qitai Zheng, CTHD, 1996, **27**(9), 515-8.
496. Youheng Gao, Shenhua Wu, Ruijian Zhong and Guangyi Li, CTHD, 1996, **27**(10), 579-80.
497. Weidong Zhang, Luping Qin and Yonghong Wang, CTHD, 1996, **27**(11), 643-5.
498. Xiuwei Yang, Yumei Jiang, Junshan Li and Zhicen Lou, CTHD, 1996, **27**(12), 707-11.
499. Yiqing Li, Yanghua Yi, Haifeng Tang and Kai Xiao, CTHD, 1996, **27**(12), 712-4.
500. Youfo Sun, Yongqing Xiao and Xiaohong Liu, CCMM, 1994, **19**(2), 99-100.
501. Lutai Pan, et al., CCMM, 1994, **19**(2), 102-3.
502. Yansheng Zhou and Muyun Ni, CCMM, 1994, **19**(3), 162-3.
503. Youhua Hu and Yu Li, CCMM, 1994, **19**(3), 164-5.
504. Youheng Gao, Zhenxian Wan, et al., CCMM, 1994, **19**(5), 295-6.
505. Ling Guan, Lihui Quan, et al., CCMM, 1994, **19**(6), 355-6.
506. Youfu Sun, Yongqing Xiao and Xiaohong Liu, CCMM, 1994, **19**(6), 357-8.
507. Yongqing Xiao Youfu Sun, and Xiaohong Liu, CCMM, 1994, **19**(7), 421-2.
508. Hui Xu, Zhihua Zhou and Junshan Yang, CCMM, 1994, **19**(8), 485-6.
509. Xianrong Wang, Anquan Du and Hongping Wang, CCMM, 1994, **19**(8), 486-7.
510. Shengxiang Qiu, CCMM, 1994, **19**(8), 488-9.
511. Shilan Feng, Lan He, et al., CCMM, 1994, **19**(10), 611-2.
512. Jing Liao, Wenzao Liang and Guoshi Tu, CCMM, 1994, **19**(10), 612-3.
513. Jiaming Zhang, Fenge Wu and Yaozu Chen, CCMM, 1994, **19**(10), 613-4.
514. Xiaoping Dong, Chonghou Xiao, et al., CCMM, 1994, **19**(10), 614-5.
515. Li zhen Xu, Xiaojiang Yang and Bin Lin, CCMM, 1994, **19**(11), 675-6.
516. Jiangnan Peng, Chengyu Ma and Yongchao Ge, CCMM, 1994, **19**(11), 676-7.
517. Honggen Tan and Yingquan Liu, CCMM, 1994, **19**(11), 677-8.
518. Xin Fan, Yuanchong Du and Junxian Wei, CCMM, 1994, **19**(12), 734-6.
519. Enjuan Zhang, Qinshu Kang and Zhao Zhang; CCMM, 1993, **18**(1), 37-38.

520. Jinlan Yuan, Rengsheng Jiang, et al., CCMM, 1993, **18**(2), 100-1.
521. Guirong Qu, Suxian Wang, et al.; CCMM, 1993, **18**(2), 101-2.
522. Jianjun Gao, Dongliang Cheng and Xiaoping Liu, CCMM, 1993, **18**(2), 102-3.
523. Honggui Zhang, Guangxuan Wu and Yongmao Zhang, CCMM, 1993, **18**(2), 104-5.
524. Jiyan Wang, Xianggao Li and Yinan Zheng, CCMM, 1993, **18**(2), 105-7.
525. Qi Chang, Dihua Chen, et al., CCMM, 1993, **18**(3), 162-4.
526. Puhai Wang, Jun Xu and Meiyu Wu, CCMM, 1993, **18**(3), 164-5.
527. Haoru Zhao, Mingshi Wang, et al., CCMM, 1993, **18**(4), 226-8.
528. Jianxing Zhang, Aina Lao and Rensheng Xu, CCMM, 1993, **18**(6), 354-5.
529. Miaohua Chen, Fengshan Liu and Jianping Xu, CCMM, 1993, **18**(7), 424-6.
530. Yuqing Zhao, Songsong Yang, et al., CCMM, 1993, **18**(7), 428-9.
531. Wenshu Xiong and Jiagu Pan, CCMM, 1993, **18**(8), 486-8.
532. Luqi Huang and Santao Yao, CCMM, 1993, **18**(8), 491-2.
533. Wensheng Yu, Hong Li, et al., CCMM, 1993, **18**(9), 548-9.
534. Axing Yuan, CCMM, 1993, **18**(10), 609-11.
535. Yong Ju, Mei Du, et al., CCMM, 1993, **18**(10), 611-13.
536. Liya Wand, Huijie Wan, et al., CCMM, 1993, **18**(10), 613-4.
537. Yunning Yan and Schiff L. Paul, CCMM, 1993, **18**(10), 615-6
538. Baoyuan Jin and Jeonghill Park, CCMM, 1993, **18**(11), 675-7.
539. Hairui Liang, Wenmei Yan, et al., CCMM, 1993, **18**(11), 677-9.
540. Jianhong Cao and Yiping Qi, CCMM, 1993, **18**(11), 681-2.
541. Gaoxiong Rao, Yan Wu, and Wansheng Dai, CCMM, 1993, **18**(12), 736-7.
542. Xiuwei Yang and Zhongkai Yan, CCMM, 1993, **18**(12), 739-40.
543. Yuliang Ma and Guiqiu Han, CCMM, 1995, **20**(2), 102-4.
544. Shihai Gu, Lizhen Xu and Nanjun Sun, CCMM, 1995, **20**(2), 105-6.
545. Li Ji and Zhiling Xu, CCMM, 1995, **20**(2), 120-122.
546. Xiukun Wang, Jiashi Li and Luxue Wei, CCMM, 1995, **20**(3), 168-9.
547. Kuijun Zhao, Suolan Liu, et al., CCMM, 1995, **20**(3), 169-70.
548. Jiang Du and Junwen Xu, CCMM, 1995, **20**(4), 232-3.
549. Yongqing Xiao, Lixin Yang, et al., CCMM, 1995, **20**(5), 294-5.
550. Xiuling Si and Song Wei, et al., CCMM, 1995, **20**(5), 295-6.
551. Yongqing Xiao, Shulian Cui, et al., CCMM, 1995, **20**(7), 423-4.
552. Zhihong Xu, Xinjie Liu and Guangsheng Xu, CCMM, 1995, **20**(8), 484-6.
553. Shuyun Zhang, CCMM, 1995, **20**(8), 486-7.
554. Peiquan Yang, Yaqin Shi and Qin Pan, CCMM, 1995, **20**(9), 551-553.
555. Haiqing Hua, CCMM, 1995, **20**(9), 564-567
556. Guifang Liu, Yuqin Fu, et al., CCMM, 1995, **20**(12), 738-40.
557. Gaoxiong Rao, Wansheng Dai, et al., CCMM, 1995, **20**(12), 740-42.
558. Shulian Cui, Xiaohong Liu, et al., CCMM, 1995, **20**(12), 743-4.
559. Liangqiong Li, Meirong Li and Aijiang Zhu, CCMM, 1996, **21**(1), 34-35.
560. Chengzhong Zhang, Chong Li, et al., CCMM, 1996, **21**(1), 36-37.
561. Xiukun Wang, Jiashi Li and Luxue Wei, CCMM, 1996, **21**(3), 165-6.
562. Xianyi Zeng, Zhapu Fang, et al., CCMM, 1996, **21**(3), 167-8.
563. Zhangyu Chen and Yushu Chen, CCMM, 1996, **21**(4), 230-232.
564. Yuning Yan, Xiukun Wang, et al., CCMM, 1996, **21**(4), 232-3.

565. Baolin Guo, Jingguang Yu and Peigen Xiao, CCMM, 1996, **21**(5), 290-292.
566. Shu Wang and Tianzhi Wang, CCMM, 1996, **21**(5), 295-296.
567. Baolin Guo, Jingguang Yu and Peigen Xiao, CCMM, 1996, **21**(6), 353-355.
568. Guangyao Chen, Liansheng Shen and Peifen Jiang, CCMM, 1996, **21**(6), 355-357.
569. Zenai Chen, Yang Lu, et al., CCMM, 1996, **21**(7), 420-422.
570. Xuezhao Lu and Houwei Luo, CCMM, 1996, **21**(7), 424-425.
571. Gaoxiong Rao, Handong Sun and Qixing Liu, CCMM, 1996, **21**(8), 482-483
572. Lan He, Dongliang Cheng and Xuan Pan, CCMM, 1996, **21**(8), 483-4.
573. Weidong Zhang, Yonghong Wang and Luping Qin, CCMM, 1996, **21**(9), 550-1.
574. Wenkui Li, Baolin Guo and Peigen Xiao, CCMM, 1996, **21**(10), 614-6.
575. Fengming Xu, Huiping Hu and Zhaoquan Wang, CCMM, 1996, **21**(11), 678-9.
576. Zhiping Gu, Tongmei Li, et al., CCMM, 1997, **22**(1), 40-41.
577. Zhong Jiang and Guangyi Li, CCMM, 1997, **22**(2), 105.
578. Jingduan Chi, Lixin Xu, et al., CCMM, 1997, **22**(2), 106-7.
579. Jinguo Kang and Zhongjian Jia, CCMM, 1997, **22**(3), 167-8.
580. Shihai Gu, Dan Zhang, et al., CCMM, 1997, **22**(3), 169-170.
581. Junxian Wei, Qunying Zuo and Yan Zhu, CCMM, 1997, **22**(4), 228-30.
582. Song Wei, Hong Liang, et al., CCMM, 1997, **22**(5), 293-295.
583. Shengzhen Yin, Baoyuan Jin, et al., CCMM, 1997, **22**(5), 296-297.
584. Xiangri Li and Luxue Wei, CCMM, 1997, **22**(5), 298-299.
585. Wei Song, Jihua Liu and Rongluan Jin, CCMM, 1997, **22**(6), 359-360.
586. Rui Wang, Yuesheng Wen, et al., CCMM, 1997, **22**(7), 421-423.
587. Dongbin Cui, Shuqin Wang and Xiaokun Ding, CCMM, 1997, **22**(8), 485-6.
588. Dong Wang, Hui Sun, et al., CCMM, 1997, **22**(8), 486-7.
589. Gengsheng Li and Yayan Chen, CCMM, 1997, **22**(9), 548-550.
590. Yanjun Zhang, Haifeng Pan, et al., CCMM, 1997, **22**(9), 550-551.
591. Xudong Xu, Cuiying Hou, et al., CCMM, 1997, **22**(11), 679-80.
592. Xuezhao Lu, Wenhao Xu and Jiaxiang Shen, CCMM, 1997, **22**(11), 680-82.
593. Lanzhen Zhang, Jiashi Li, et al., CCMM, 1997, **22**(12), 740-3.
594. Lei Tian, Lizhen Xu and Shilin Yang, CCMM, 1997, **22**(12), 743-5.
595. Hao Huang, Shouxun Zhao, et al., CCMM, 1998, **23**(1), 37-38.
596. Peiyu Liang, Qi Zhou and Faxing Zhou, CCMM, 1998, **23**(1), 39-40.
597. Jingduan Chi and Lixin Xu, CCMM, 1998, **23**(1), 40-41.
598. Yinghau Wang and Shirui Xing, et al., CCMM, 1998, **23**(2), 96-8.
599. Xiansheng Jia, Jiaqi Wu and Qing Mao, CCMM, 1998, **23**(3), 162-4.
600. Faxing Zhou, Peiyu Liang, et al., CCMM, 1998, **23**(3), 164-5.
601. Haiyan Wang, Ruxian Chen and Hongzhang Xu, CCMM, 1998, **23**(3), 167-8.
602. Yun Ling, Yonglin Zhang, et al., CCMM, 1998, **23**(4), 232-3.
603. Jingduan Chi and Lixin Xu, CCMM, 1998, **23**(4), 233-4.
604. Liping Xu, Jiansheng Liu, et al., China Journal of Chinese Materia Medica, 1998, **23**(5), 293-5.
605. Axing Yuan, Xiaomei Huang and Jin Chen, CCMM, 1998, **23**(6), 359-360.
606. Lu Gan, Yuying Zhao, et al., CCMM, 1998, **23**(6), 361-2.
607. Ying Zhong, Chunxu Zuo, et al., CCMM, 1998, **23**(6), 363-4.
608. De Min, Liping Xu, et al., CCMM, 1998, **23**(7), 416-418.
609. De Min, Liping Xu, et al., CCMM, 1998, **23**(8), 486-488.

610. Xuemin Guo, Ling Zhang, et al., CCMM, 1998, **23**(9), 546-547.
611. Jiuzhi Yuan and Qishi Sun, CCMM, 1998, **23**(9), 548-549.
612. Liang Zhang, Zhihong Jiang, et al., CCMM, 1998, **23**(9), 549-550.
613. Yu Zhou, Fengrui Song and Shuying Liu, CCMM, 1998, **23**(9), 551-552.
614. Liping Xu, Jiansheng liu, et al., CCMM, 1998, **23**(9), 552-553.
615. Mingying Shang, Shaoqing Cai, et al., CCMM, 1998, **23**(10), 614-616.
616. Hong Wei, Dongxu Wen, et al., CCMM, 1998, **23**(10), 616-618.
617. Yujun Chen, Jin Xiang, et al., CCMM, 1998, **23**(10), 620-621.
618. Xiaoqiang Ma, Shanhao Jiang and Dayuan Zhu, CCMM, 1998, **23**(11), 679-680.
619. Ying Han, Chao Xia, et al., CCMM, 1998, **23**(11), 680-682.
620. Haiyan Du, Sitong Yuan, and Peifen Jiang, CCMM, 1998, **23**(11), 682-683.
621. Qiuan Wang, Jingyu Shu and Longmei Zeng, CCMM, 1998, **23**(11), 683-684.
622. Xudong Xu, Yumei Yang, et al., CCMM, 1998, **23**(12), 733-4.
623. Wenmei Yan, Ying Fu, et al., CCMM, 1998, **23**(12), 735-6.
624. Xiansheng Jia, Jiaqi Wu and Qing Mao, CCMM, 1998, **23**(12), 737-9.
625. Guande Zhang, CCMM, 1998, **14**(9), 53-56.
626. Gangli Wang, et al., CCMM, 1996, **21**(2), 67-9.
627. Haiqing Hua, CCMM, 1995, **20**(9), 564-7.
628. Xiulian Jin and Qingrong Zhang, CCMM, 1994, **19**(11), 695-7.
629. Muyun Ni and Baolin Bian, CCMM, 1989, **14**(7), 41-43.
630. Ji Li and Zhining Xi, CCMM, 1995, **20**(2), 120-124.
631. Lee BL, Koh D, Ong HY, Ong CN, J Chromatog. A, 1997, **763**(1-2), 221-6.
632. Guiru Han, et al., CCMM, 1990, **15**(2), 41-42.
633. Chaoming Li, et al., ABY, **20**(2), 244-246.
634. Qingya Bian, Cuiying Hou and Jianmin Chen, Natural Product R&D, 1998, **10**(1), 1-5.
635. Meizhen Xu and Zhiming Cheng, CCMM, 1997, **22**(10), 631-2.
636. Guiren Cheng, Jinglan Jin and Yongxin Wen, APS, 1987, **22**(3), 203-7.
637. Qiang Li, et al., CCMM, 1998, **23**(9), 570-3.
638. Xifeng Huang, CCMM, 1997, **22**(4), 247-9.
639. Shiping Zhao and Guixiang Fu, CTHD, 1997, **28**(3), 187-8.
640. Xiaohe Xiao, et al., CTHD, 1997, **28**(2), 114-9.
641. Zenglai Xu and Zhizun Ding, CTHD, 1998, **29**(2), 125-8.
642. Mingyan Chu, et al., CTHD, 1998, **29**(8), 564-6.
643. Ying Gao, Weiming Cheng and Guangyi Li, CCMM, 1993, **18**(7), 426-8.
644. Yanmei Li and Qingming Che, Acta Pharmaceutica Sinica, 1998, **33**(8), 626–8.
645. Lei Luo, Zuqiang Li, Yuanqing Zhang and Rong Huang, AP, 1998, **33**(11), 839-42.
646. Xingliang Chen, Xiuping Yang, Aijin Hou, Bei Jiang, Zhongwen Lin and Handong Sun, Acta Botanica Yunnanica, 1998, **20**(2), 241-3.
647. Qingya Bian, Cuiying Hou and Jianmin Chen, Natural Product R&D, 1998, **10**(1), 1-5.
648. Jiu Han, Wenhan Lin, Rensheng Xu, Wenlu Wang and Shanhuan Zhao, Acta Pharmaceutica Sinica, 1991, **26**(5), 426-9.
649. Chunshu Yang, Jialin Wang, Zhiliang Zhang and I. Kouno, Acta Pharmaceutica Sinica, 1991, **26**(2), 128-31.
650. Yanhong Wang, Yaozu Chen, Handong Sun and Zhongwen Lin, Acta Scientiarum Naturalium Universitatis Sunyatseni, 1998, **37**(1), 122-4.
651. Shiyue Feng, Zhisheng He and Yongmao Ye, CTHD, 1996, 27(3), 131-4.

652. AS981122 Yanhong Wang, Yaozu Chen, Handong Sun and Zhongwen Lin, ASNUS, 1998, **37**(1), 122-4.

653. AS982049 Kun Zhang, Yanhong Wang, Yaozu Chen, Handong Sun and Zhongwen Lin, Acta Scientiarum Naturalium Universitatis Sunyatseni, 1998, **37**(2), 49-51

654. Jing Huang, Maoli Tu and Jingyi Xie, APS, 1987, **22**(4), 264-8.

655. XIUCAI LI, CCMM, 1997, **22**(1), 53-56.

656. Yajuan Xu, Dongming Xu, Dongbin Cui, Jishan Gao, Enxi Huang, Shiyue Liu and Dequan Yu, APS, 1994, **29**(3), 200-3.

657. Taikang Huang (chief editor), A Handbook of the Composition and Pharmacology of Common Chinese Drugs, Medicinal Science and Technology Press of China, Beijing, 1994, in Chinese.

Additional Reading

1. Huiyuan Zhang, Zhiying Zhang, Zunsan Yue, Rongling Guo et al., China Resources Brief Flora of Chinese Medicine, Beijing, 1994.
2. Jiangsu New Medical College, Chinese Materia Medica, Shanghai, Shanghai Science and Technology Press, 1977.
3. Dictionary of Seed-plants Names Latin-Chinese-English, Beijing, 1983.
4. Nigel Wiseman, English-Chinese Chinese-English Dictionary of Chinese Medicine, Chang Sha, Hunan Science and Technology Press, 1996.
5. Yanwen Li , Yunhui Huang, Yuezhong Huang. Dictionary of Chinese Medicinal Herb Names in Chinese-Latin-English, Guangzhou , Guangdong Science and Technology Press, 1998.
6. Dictionary of Seed-Plants Names in Latin-Chinese-English , Beijing, 1983.
7. Yixiang Yuan, Jixue Ren, Long Huang, Guangzhen Gao, Chinese-English Dictionary of Traditional Chinese Medicine, Beijing, 1997.
8. Zhufan Xie, Zhicen Lou, Xiaokai Huang, Classified Dictionary of Traditional Chinese Medicine, New World Press, Beijing, 1994.
9. Chao Zhu (chief editor) et al., The Chinese-English Medical Dictionary, Beijing, 1987.
10. Jingfeng Qu, Shaohua Zhang, Rong Xie, The Chinese Materia Medica, Publishing House of Shanghai College of Traditional Chinese Medicine, Shanghai, 1990.
11. Guojun Xu, Hongxian He, Luoshan Xu, Rongluan Jin, Chinese Materia Medica, Chinese Medicinal Science and Technology Press, 1996.
12. Yikui Ling, Zhenghua Yan, et al., The Chinese Materia Medica, Shanghai, Shanghai Science and Technology Press, 1984.
13. Renan Ren, Ruihua Chen, et al., Determinative Chinese Materia Medica, Shanghai, Shanghai Science and Technology Press, 1984.
14. Jinghe Ding, Wanzhang Zeng, et al. Pharmaceutical Botany, Shanghai, Shanghai Science and Technology Press, 1985.
15. Junmo Wang, Mingying Jiang et al., Pharmacology of Traditional Chinese Drugs, Shanghai, Shanghai Science and Technology Press, 1985.
16. Zhenyu Song (chief editor), Tonghui Zhou, Qicheng Fang, Xinming Chao (Institute of Materia Medica, Chinese Academy of Medical Sciences), Modern Studies of Chinese Herbal Medicine, Vol. 1, 2, 3, Beijing, Union Press of Beijing Medical University and Peking Union Medical College, 1995, 1996, 1997.
17. Sixun Peng (chief editor), Pharmaceutical Chemistry, Beijing, 1988.
18. Rensheng Xu (chief editor), Natural Products Chemistry, Beijing, 1993.